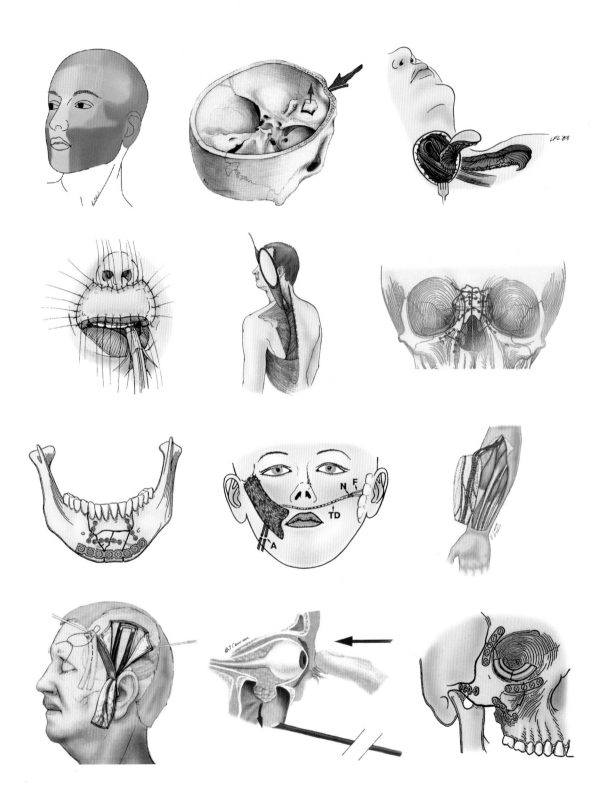

Plastic Surgery

Plastic Surgery

First Edition

Editor:
Joseph G. McCarthy, MD

Editors, Hand Surgery volumes:
James W. May, Jr., MD
J. William Littler, MD

Plastic Surgery

Second Edition

Editor
Stephen J. Mathes, MD
Professor of Surgery
Chief, Division of Plastic Surgery
University of California, San Francisco
School of Medicine
San Francisco, California

Editor, Hand Surgery Volumes
Vincent R. Hentz, MD
Professor of Surgery
Chief, Division of Plastic and Hand Surgery
Stanford University School of Medicine
Stanford, California

With illustrations by Kathy Hirsh and Scott Thorn Barrows, CMI, FAMI

Shireen L. Dunwoody, Editorial Coordinator

VOLUME *III*

THE HEAD AND NECK, PART 2

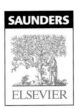

SAUNDERS
ELSEVIER

Volume I General Principles
Volume II The Head and Neck, Part 1
Volume III The Head and Neck, Part 2
Volume IV Pediatric Plastic Surgery
Volume V Tumors of the Head, Neck, and Skin
Volume VI Trunk and Lower Extremity
Volume VII The Hand and Upper Limb, Part 1
Volume VIII The Hand and Upper Limb, Part 2

SAUNDERS
ELSEVIER

1600 John F. Kennedy Blvd.
Ste 1800
Philadelphia, PA 19103-2899

PLASTIC SURGERY, 2nd ed.

Volume I 0-7216-8812-8/978-0-7216-8812-1
Volume II 0-7216-8813-6/978-0-7216-8813-8
Volume III 0-7216-8814-4/978-0-7216-8814-5
Volume IV 0-7216-8815-2/978-0-7216-8815-2
Volume V 0-7216-8816-0/978-0-7216-8816-9
Volume VI 0-7216-8817-9/978-0-7216-8817-6
Volume VII 0-7216-8818-7/978-0-7216-8818-3
Volume VIII 0-7216-8819-5/978-0-7216-8819-0
8-Volume Set 0-7216-8811-X/978-0-7216-8811-4

Notice

Knowledge and best practice in this field are constantly changing. As new research and experience broaden our knowledge, changes in practice, treatment and drug therapy may become necessary or appropriate. Readers are advised to check the most current information provided (i) on procedures featured or (ii) by the manufacturer of each product to be administered, to verify the recommended dose or formula, the method and duration of administration, and contraindications. It is the responsibility of the practitioner, relying on his or her own experience and knowledge of the patient, to make diagnoses, to determine dosages and the best treatment for each individual patient, and to take all appropriate safety precautions. To the fullest extent of the law, neither the Publisher nor the Editors assume any liability for any injury and/or damage to persons or property arising out of or related to any use of the material contained in this book.

The Publisher

Previous edition copyrighted 1990.

Library of Congress Cataloging-in-Publication Data
Mathes, Stephen J.
    Plastic surgery / Stephen J. Mathes ; editor Vincent R. Hentz.—2nd ed.
      p.   cm.
    ISBN 0–7216–8811–X
    1. Surgery, Plastic.   I. Hentz, Vincent R.   II. Title.
RD118.M388 2006
617.9′5—dc21

                                        2003041541

Acquisitions Editors: Sue Hodgson, Allan Ross, Joe Rusko, Judith Fletcher
Senior Developmental Editor: Ann Ruzycka Anderson
Publishing Services Manager: Tina Rebane
Senior Project Manager: Linda Van Pelt
Design Direction: Steven Stave
Cover Designer: Shireen Dunwoody

Printed in China

Last digit is the print number: 9   8   7   6   5   4   3   2   1

This text is dedicated to Mary H. McGrath, who is my inspiration and a source of joy in our daily life together, our adventures at home and away, and our shared enthusiasm and excitement as plastic surgeons.

✦ CONTRIBUTORS

HIROTAKA ASATO, MD, PhD
Associate Professor and Deputy Chair
Department of Plastic and Reconstructive Surgery
Graduate School of Medicine and Faculty of Medicine
University of Tokyo
Tokyo, Japan

AMARDIP S. BHULLER, MD
Physician in Residence
Department of Plastic Surgery
The Cleveland Clinic
Cleveland, Ohio

BURTON D. BRENT, MD
Adjunct Associate Clinical Professor of Surgery
Stanford University School of Medicine
Stanford, California
Staff Surgeon
El Camino Hospital
Mountain View, California

JOHN J. COLEMAN III, MD, FACS
James E. Bennett Professor of Surgery
Indiana University School of Medicine
Chief, Division of Plastic Surgery
Roudebush Veterans Affairs Medical Center
Indianapolis, Indiana

JOSEPH J. DISA, MD, FACS
Associate Professor of Surgery
Weill Medical College of Cornell University
Associate Attending Surgeon
Memorial Sloan-Kettering Cancer Center
New York, New York

MATTHIAS B. DONELAN, MD, FACS
Associate Clinical Professor of Surgery
Harvard Medical School
Chief of Plastic Surgery
Shriners Burns Hospital
Associate Visiting Surgeon
Massachusetts General Hospital
Boston, Massachusetts

CRAIG R. DUFRESNE, MD, FACS
Associate Professor of Plastic Surgery
Division of Plastic Surgery
Department of Surgery
Johns Hopkins University School of Medicine
Baltimore, Maryland
Staff Surgeon
Center for Craniofacial Development and Disorders
Washington, DC

LOREN H. ENGRAV, MD, FACS
Professor of Surgery
Division of Plastic Surgery
University of Washington School of Medicine
Plastic Surgeon
Harborview Medical Center
Seattle, Washington

GREGORY R. D. EVANS, MD, FACS
Professor of Surgery and the Center for Biomedical
  Engineering
University of California, Irvine, School of Medicine
Chief, Division of Plastic Surgery
University of California, Irvine, Medical Center
Orange, California

CHRISTOPHER R. FORREST, MD, MSc, FRCS(C)
Associate Professor of Surgery
Head, Division of Plastic Surgery
Department of Surgery
University of Toronto Faculty of Medicine
Medical Director
Centre for Craniofacial Care and Research
The Hospital for Sick Children
Toronto, Ontario, Canada

CHRISTOPHER B. GORDON, MD
Assistant Professor of Surgery
Division of Plastic Surgery
University of Cincinnati College of Medicine
Plastic Surgeon
Cincinnati Children's Hospital Medical Center
Cincinnati, Ohio

KIYONORI HARII, MD
Professor Emeritus
University of Tokyo
Professor and Chair
Department of Plastic and Reconstructive Surgery
Kyorin University School of Medicine
Tokyo, Japan

DAVID A. HIDALGO, MD
Clinical Professor of Surgery
Weill Medical College of Cornell University
Associate Attending Surgeon
Manhattan Eye, Ear and Throat Hospital
New York, New York

GAZI HUSSAIN, MBBS, FRCS(A)
Clinical Faculty
University of Sydney Faculty of Medicine
Plastic Surgeon
Plastic Surgery Unit
Concord Hospital
Sydney, New South Wales, Australia

CHEN LEE, MD, MSc, FRCS(C), FACS
Associate Professor and Chairman
Division of Plastic Surgery
McGill University School of Medicine
Attending Surgeon
McGill University Health Center
Montreal, Quebec, Canada

JOANNE J. LENERT, MD
Assistant Professor of Surgery
George Washington University School of Medicine
Plastic Surgeon
Medical Faculty Associates of George Washington
    University Medical Center
Washington, DC

MALCOLM ALAN LESAVOY, MD, FACS
Clinical Professor of Plastic and Reconstructive Surgery
David Geffen School of Medicine at the University of
    California, Los Angeles (UCLA)
Los Angeles, California
Former Chief, Division of Plastic Surgery
Harbor/UCLA Medical Center
Torrance, California
Director, Encino Outpatient Surgery Center
Encino, California

ERNEST K. MANDERS, MD, FACS
Professor of Surgery
Devision of Plastic and Reconstructive Surgery
Department of Surgery
University of Pittsburgh School of Medicine
Medical Director, Facial Nerve Center
Chief, Plastic and Reconstructive Surgery
Oakland Veterans Administration Medical Center
Pittsburgh, Pennsylvania

MAHESH H. MANKANI, MD, FACS
Assistant Professor
Division of Plastic and Reconstructive Surgery
Department of Surgery
University of California, San Francisco (UCSF), School of
    Medicine
Attending Surgeon
UCSF Medical Center
San Francisco General Hospital
San Francisco, California

RALPH T. MANKTELOW, MD, FRCS(C)
Professor of Surgery
University of Toronto Faculty of Medicine
Staff Surgeon
Division of Plastic Surgery
Toronto General Hospital
Toronto, Ontario, Canada

PAUL N. MANSON, MD, FACS
Professor of Surgery
Division of Plastic Surgery
Department of Surgery
Johns Hopkins University School of Medicine
Chief, Plastic Surgery
Johns Hopkins Hospital
Baltimore, Maryland

STEPHEN J. MATHES, MD, FACS
Professor of Surgery
University of California, San Francisco, School of
    Medicine
Professor of Growth and Development
University of California, San Francisco, School of
    Dentistry
Chief, Division of Plastic Surgery
Department of Surgery
University of California, San Francisco, Medical Center
San Francisco, California

DELORA L. MOUNT, MD, FACS
Assistant Professor of Surgery
Assistant Professor of Pediatrics
University of Wisconsin Medical School
Chief, Pediatric Plastic Surgery
University of Wisconsin Children's Hospital
Director, Craniofacial Anomalies Clinic
Madison, Wisconsin

REID V. MUELLER, MD
Associate Professor of Surgery
Oregon Health and Science University School of Medicine
Attending Surgeon
Oregon Health and Science University Hospitals and
    Clinics
Portland, Oregon

OMER OZERDEM, MD
Consultant in Plastic Surgery
Department of Plastic and Reconstructive Surgery
Baskent University Faculty of Medicine
Adana, Turkey

MARIA TERESA RIVAS-TORRES, MD
Plastic Surgeon
Coordinadora de Investigación
Hospital de Traumatología del Instituto Mexicano del
    Seguro Social
Mexico, Distrito Federal

STEPHEN A. SCHENDEL, MD, DDS, FACS
Professor of Surgery
Division of Plastic Surgery
Stanford University School of Medicine
Stanford, California
Director, Craniofacial Surgery Program
Lucile Packard Children's Hospital at Stanford
Stanford, California

ANDREW D. SMITH, MD
Private Practice
Irvine, California

AKIHIKO TAKUSHIMA, MD, PhD
Assistant Professor
Department of Plastic and Reconstructive Surgery
Kyorin University School of Medicine
Tokyo, Japan

ANDREW E. TURK, MD, FACS
Staff Plastic Surgeon
Department of Plastic and Reconstructive Surgery
The Cleveland Clinic, Florida
Naples, Florida

MARK D. WELLS, MD, FRCS(C), FACS
Plastic Surgeon
Grant Regional Trauma Center
Columbus, Ohio

S. ANTHONY WOLFE, MD, FACS
Director, Craniofacial Fellowship
Clinical Professor of Surgery–Voluntary
University of Miami School of Medicine
Chief, Plastic Surgery
Miami Children's Hospital
Chief, Plastic Surgery
Cedars Medical Center
Miami, Florida

MICHAEL J. YAREMCHUK, MD, FACS
Clinical Professor of Surgery
Harvard Medical School
Associate Visiting Surgeon
Massachusetts General Hospital
Boston, Massachusetts

RONALD M. ZUKER, MD, FRCS(C), FACS
Professor of Surgery
University of Toronto Faculty of Medicine
Staff Plastic Surgeon
The Hospital for Sick Children
Toronto, Ontario, Canada

✦ PREFACE

It is a great thing to start life with a small number of really good books which are your very own. *Through the Magic Door* (1908), Sir Arthur Conan Doyle

My meeting for lunch with Joseph McCarthy in Boston in 1998 during the annual meeting of the Society of Plastic Surgery was arranged to discuss the possibility of my becoming the editor of the new edition of *Plastic Surgery*. I was well aware of the responsibility of assuming this giant project. My admiration of the past editors, including Joseph McCarthy for the 1990 edition of *Plastic Surgery* and John Marquis Converse for the 1964 and 1977 editions of *Reconstructive Plastic Surgery*, was great since these texts in my estimation really defined our specialty of plastic surgery and provided the platform for future advances in treating congenital and acquired deformities. My memory of Converse's first edition started with my residency in plastic surgery on my first rotation at the private practice of William Schatten, John Hartley, and John Griffith in Atlanta, Georgia. There, in moments when I was not involved in patient care activities, I would enjoy reading the pages of clinical advice on all subjects related to plastic surgery in the five volumes of *Reconstructive Plastic Surgery*. Subsequently, in 1977, as a faculty member at Washington University, I was privileged to be able to purchase my own copy of the then six-volume edition of *Reconstructive Plastic Surgery*, again edited by Converse. This time, my reading of the exciting pages was less relaxed, since I was using the text as the reference in preparation for my plastic surgery board examinations.

By 1990, I was able to contribute a chapter to *Plastic Surgery*, edited by Joseph McCarthy, and I personally knew most of the contributors, having witnessed the evolution of many of the new advances and unique contributions contained within the then eight volumes. With this background, I was excited and honored to have been recommended as the next editor of this text, which has so well reflected the greatness of the specialty of plastic surgery. My meeting was punctuated by advice regarding the importance of the text and the selection of experts who would provide both guidance and stimulation to future readers on the many subjects important to physicians involved in plastic surgery. The complexity of orchestrating so many contributors in a timely fashion was also emphasized. I left this luncheon inspired to undertake this project, with the anticipation of capturing the best and most innovative surgeons as contributors to achieve an edition in keeping with the unique traditions of excellence of the past editions of *Plastic Surgery* and *Reconstructive Plastic Surgery*.

My first step was to find an academic hand surgeon to edit the two hand volumes. J. William Littler had served as the editor of the hand and upper extremity volume in Converse's two editions of *Reconstructive Plastic Surgery*. Littler was a master hand surgeon and one of the foremost innovators in hand surgery. McCarthy selected a unique combination of academic hand surgeons, James W. May and J. William Littler, to edit the two volumes dedicated to upper extremity and hand surgery in the 1990 edition of *Plastic Surgery*. With the many new techniques related to microvascular surgery, the space devoted to this important aspect of plastic surgery had been expanded into two volumes. Jim May, like Bill Littler, is a master hand surgeon, a gifted teacher, and an innovator in all aspects of plastic surgery and was able to include both his contributions and those of many other hand surgeons, who all took part in advancing this important discipline.

Fortunately, the decision regarding who should be the hand editor for this edition of *Plastic Surgery* was obvious. Vincent R. Hentz is a master hand surgeon and past president of the American Society of Surgery of the Hand. As an accomplished educator and chief of the division of plastic and hand surgery at Stanford, he is the ideal person to follow in the footsteps of Littler and May. In keeping with the many innovations and new techniques in upper extremity and hand surgery, this edition contains two volumes devoted to hand surgery. Of interest, we have shifted the editorial geography from the East Coast (New York City and Boston) to the West Coast (San Francisco and Palo Alto). Unfortunately, despite the improvement in weather characteristics of the western coastline of the United States, the commitment to continue the excellence of this text has kept the editors mostly indoors during the complex editing process necessary to complete these volumes.

The goal of this edition is to cover the scope of plastic surgery. The key was to select the best contributors to define the problems encountered in plastic surgery, to provide both the most current and the most successful solutions, and to deliver the challenge for future innovation in each area of plastic surgery. In this new edition, there are 219 chapters with 293 contributors. Each of the senior authors of the 219 chapters was carefully selected for his or her recognized expertise in the assigned subject of the chapter. Each author has personally contributed to the advancement in knowledge related to his or her area of expertise in our specialty.

The authors selected are inspirational leaders due to their many innovations toward improvement in the management of the plastic surgery patient. After the manuscripts were submitted, each chapter was carefully reviewed by the editors to ensure that all aspects of the authors' assigned topics were adequately covered and well illustrated so that the reader could readily incorporate the chapter content into the practice of plastic surgery.

In the eight volumes included in this edition, all subjects pertinent to the scope of plastic surgery are covered. Many new topics, 67 in all, have been developed or were enlarged from broader subjects and warranted a new individual chapter. Thirteen of these new chapter topics are included in Volume I: General Principles. The enlargement of the volume containing general principles reflects the continuing expansion of our specialty, the emphasis on experimental and clinical research, and the impact of research on the practice of plastic surgery. In the remaining volumes, devoted to specific clinical topics, two new types of chapter formats were added: 25 technique chapters and 7 secondary chapters. The technique chapters are added to complement the overview chapters and are designed to focus on particular techniques currently in use for a clinical problem. Likewise, the secondary chapters are again an extension of the overview chapters on particular subjects but focus on problems that persist despite the application of primary plastic surgery solutions. These secondary chapters are designed to demonstrate areas where operations may fail related to improper patient or technique selection or technique failures. They also discuss procedures to correct unsatisfactory outcomes following primary plastic surgery.

Volumes II through VII are divided into specific topographical areas of plastic surgery. Volume II: The Head and Neck (Part 1) is devoted to cosmetic procedures and contains six new topic chapters, seven new technique chapters, and three new secondary chapters. This volume now contains color illustrations, which will help the reader evaluate problems and results following cosmetic procedures. Many important subjects are expanded and introduced. For instance, there are now five chapters on the face lift, which provide the reader with the ability to compare techniques and focus on specific aspects of the procedure. Volume III: The Head and Neck (Part 2) is dedicated to reconstructive procedures and contains 10 new topics as well as the traditional subjects used in the previous edition. Volume IV: Pediatric Plastic Surgery contains five new topics and provides multispecialty approaches to children presenting with congenital facial anomalies. Volume V: Tumors of the Head, Neck, and Skin has seven new topics. Along with management principles of head and neck cancer, identification and treatment of melanoma and non-melanoma skin cancer have been added in new topic chapters. Volume VI: Trunk and Lower Extremity contains 34 added topics. For example, in the area of postmastectomy reconstruction, 12 new chapters have been added to provide specific diagnostic, management, and technical information on breast reconstruction issues. Similarly, four new chapter topics have been added on body contouring procedures. With emphasis on bariatric surgery and body contouring procedures, these chapters provide a complete array of information on techniques and outcomes. Volume VII: The Hand and Upper Limb (Part 1) contains introductory and general principles related to diagnosis and management of acquired disorders, both traumatic and nontraumatic. Volume VIII: The Hand and Upper Limb (Part 2) contains three parts: congenital anomalies, paralytic disorders, and rehabilitation. The two volumes on hand and upper extremity surgery contain an additional 22 chapters introducing new subjects to this edition of *Plastic Surgery*.

Education involves the process of observation as well as contact with teachers, mentors, colleagues, and students and the literature. Each component is essential to learning a specialty in medicine and maintaining competence in the specialty over the course of one's career. In plastic surgery, the abundance of master surgeons gives everyone the opportunity to observe excellence in technique, during residency and later through educational programs. Contact with teachers and colleagues must be maintained in order to keep abreast of the new innovations in medicine and to measure one's outcomes in the context of standard of care. Our professional society meetings and symposia, both locally and nationally, provide us with this opportunity. Contact with mentors and students is critical for innovation. The physician must seek out these sources of inspiration and stimulation to improve patient care. Collaboration with professionals is a unique opportunity to allow further growth in our specialty and is available in every medical environment. The literature allows the physician to see where we have been, where we are currently, and what the future holds. The physician can hold a piece of literature in the hand and review its message both in critical times, when patient management decisions must be made on a timely basis, and during leisure times, when a subject is studied and carefully measured against personal experience and knowledge acquired through professional contacts. It is hoped that this edition of *Plastic Surgery*, like its predecessors, can serve the purpose of literature in teaching. Its eight volumes contain more than 6800 pages of information carefully formulated by recognized experts in our specialty in plastic surgery. It is designed, as initially stated, to define the current knowledge of plastic surgery and to serve as a platform for future creativity to benefit the patient we see with congenital and acquired deformities.

Stephen J. Mathes, MD, 2005

✦ ACKNOWLEDGMENTS

So many talented and dedicated professionals are necessary to complete a text of this magnitude. It is impossible to really thank everyone adequately, since there are so many people behind the scenes who were silently working toward the completion of this project. However, I shall endeavor to acknowledge the people who provided scientific, technical, and emotional support to make this edition of *Plastic Surgery* possible.

My first contact with the publisher (Saunders, now Elsevier) started with my meeting with Allan Ross and Ann Ruzycka Anderson. Allan Ross, executive editor, was assigned to guide this text to publication. He is a dedicated publishing executive who was most supportive at the inception of this project. Ann Ruzycka Anderson, senior developmental editor, has been working in medical publishing for 20 years. This text was most fortunate to have Allan and Ann assigned as the guiding forces at the onset. Ann states that working on this text is "something exciting, worthwhile, and important" because she is helping to "produce the largest book in medical publishing history."

Because this book took 5 years to complete, there were changes in the personnel involved in the project. Joe Rusko, medical editor, assumed the responsibilities of guiding the development of the text, with Allan Ross taking on the role of consultant. Joe has great enthusiasm and provided great ideas for the format of this book and for associated advertising. During the past year, the project was turned over to the leadership of Sue Hodgson, currently the publishing director and general manager for Elsevier Ltd. With Sue living in London, the project took on a more international outlook, with Sue flying between London, Philadelphia, New York, and San Francisco to keep the project moving ahead to completion. Both Sue Hodgson and Allan Ross have a great deal of success in guiding complex publications to press. Sue has published highly successful books in dermatology, and now, it is hoped, she will be able to make the same claim for the field of plastic surgery. For sure, she can now lay claim to publishing the largest medical book in existence. Recently, Sue Hodgson summed up her role in the publishing industry as follows: "The opportunity to create new products to answer the market's educational needs and handling high-profile and demanding projects are what get me out of bed in the morning." All plastic surgeons who use this text are indebted to the perseverance and commitment of these publishing leaders: Allan Ross, Joe Rusko, and Sue Hodgson.

"The quality of a person's life is in direct proportion to their commitment to excellence, regardless of their chosen field of endeavor."
—Vince Lombardi

After the authors were selected for the 219 chapters, it was obvious that we needed someone special to serve as the editorial coordinator between the editors and the authors. Thanks to the advice of Allan Ross and Ann Ruzycka Anderson, Shireen Dunwoody was recommended for this position. Shireen is an accomplished computer programmer and musician and has served as a senior medical writer, media programmer/editor, and developmental editor since 1991. Among the high-profile medical texts on which she has worked are *Clinical Oncology* (Martin Abeloff et al., editors), *Surgery of the Liver and Biliary Tract* (Leslie Blumgart, editor), and *Fundamentals of Surgery* (John E. Niederhuber, editor). Shireen has worked closely with the editors and our assigned authors during every step of the process—obtaining the manuscripts (including a multitude of meetings and phone calls with authors), helping find artists when needed, confirming references, discovering historical information as related to the many subjects covered in *Plastic Surgery,* and coordinating all these data with the publishing staff in Philadelphia and New York. When asked to describe what this job was like, she described the process as follows: "At times, this project has been a struggle, but most of the time it has been a joy (kind of like raising eight children). On any given day, working on this project has given me a reason to (1) get up in the morning; (2) stay up all night; (3) despise the morning; (4) stay sober; (5) get drunk; (6) laugh; (7) cry; (8) live; (9) lie; (10) rejoice. Who could ask for anything more? It has certainly kept things interesting!" Shireen credits special members of the publishing staff for helping this immense project move ahead at a fairly steady pace. In Philadelphia, Linda Van Pelt, senior project manager, book production, and RoseMarie Klimowicz, freelance copyeditor, have been with this project since its inception. They have both dedicated vast amounts of blood, sweat, tears, and personal time. Ann Ruzycka Anderson has been dedicated to this project since the onset and has also worked closely with Shireen. Judy Fletcher, publishing director, provided the support needed for timely layouts and served as an advocate for this project even when layout or illustrations were changed to maintain the continuity and artistry of the chapters. Finally, Shireen acknowledges her two amazing assistants in Palm Springs, California, Donna Larson and Carla Parnell, who have helped her scan, copy, crop, sort, mail, and stay sane. Without the dedication and brilliance of Shireen Dunwoody in bringing out the best in the editors, publishers, authors, and artists, this text would not have the quality and completeness it now possesses.

My immediate family was always supportive of this project despite the time-consuming work associated with text preparation. I wish to acknowledge and thank my family for their exciting accomplishments, which are a source of pride and enjoyment: Mary, Norma, Paul, Leslie, Isabelle, Peter, David, Brian, Vasso, Zoe, Ned, Erin, Maggie, and Rick.

In any profession, the support and encouragement of one's colleagues are essential for productivity. I wish to thank the faculty in our division of plastic surgery for their specific contributions to the text and their active roles as outstanding teachers for our residents and students at the University of California in San Francisco. The faculty, both full time and clinical, include the following: Bernard Alpert, Jim Anthony, Ramin Behmand, Kyle Bickel, Greg Buncke, K. Ning Chang, Tancredi D'Amore, Keith Denkler, Issa Eschima, Robert Foster, Roger Friedenthal, Gilbert Gradinger, Ronald Gruber, William Hoffman, Clyde Ikeda, Gabriel Kind, Chen Lee, Pablo Leon, Mahesh Mankani, Robert Markeson, Mary McGrath, Sean Moloney, Douglas Ousterhout, John Owsley, Lorne Rosenfield, Vivian Ting, Bryant Toth, Philip Trabulsy, D. Miller Wise, and David Young.

During the time span in which this book was edited, a group of outstanding residents completed their plastic surgery residencies at UCSF. All these residents contributed to both the care of many of the patients included in the chapters written by our faculty and the development of concepts used in the chapters of this edition. Each resident listed has contributed to the advancement of our knowledge in plastic surgery: Delora Mount, Richard Grossman, Jeff Roth, Laura McMillan, Kenneth Bermudez, Marga Massey, Yngvar Hvistendahl, Duc Bui, Te Ning Chang, Hatem Abou-Sayed, Farzad Nahai, Hop Nguyen Le, Clara Lee, Scott Hansen, Jennifer Newman-Keagle, and Wesley Schooler. General surgery residents, research fellows, and students who participated in the project include Lee Alkureishi, Julie Lang, Edward Miranda, and Cristiane Ueno.

Without the dedication of our staff, the preparation of this text would not have been possible. Crystal Munoz served as our office manager during most of the preparation time. My patient coordinators, Marian Liebow and, later, Skye Ingham, are patient advocates and made the arrangements necessary to treat the patients discussed in our chapters. Our nurses, Janet Tanaka and, later, Ann Hutchinson, were essential to the overall care of patients presenting to our clinical practice. Our staff provides the support needed to allow the faculty to have the time necessary to participate in the creative activities expected in academic plastic surgery.

Plastic surgeons depend on visual assessment of problems; thus, illustrations are an essential part of our scientific literature. Numerous artists were involved in the chapters selected by the individual authors. However, two artists were available to all the contributors and provided outstanding art to accompany many of the chapters. Kathy Hirsh, located in Shanghai, China, and Scott Barrows, in Chicago, have worked diligently to provide accurate artistic interpretations of the surgical procedures recommended throughout this text.

"Mental toughness is many things. It is humility because it behooves all of us to remember that simplicity is the sign of greatness and meekness is the sign of true strength. Mental toughness is spartanism with qualities of sacrifice, self-denial, dedication. It is fearlessness, and it is love."

—Vince Lombardi

All the authors who contributed to these volumes exemplify mental toughness. To complete a chapter for a text is often considered an unappreciated task. However, thanks to the great reputation established by the prior editors of this comprehensive work, John M. Converse and Joseph G. McCarthy, and the previous editors of the hand volumes, William Littler and James May, the top plastic surgeons in their respective fields have given their time and efforts to maintain the excellence associated with past editions of this text. Thanks to these contributors, this book provides information at the forefront of innovation and current practice in the specialty of plastic surgery. The contributors and their families are thanked for their perseverance and sacrifice in the completion of these chapters and for their dedication to our specialty, plastic surgery.

SJM

✦ C O N T E N T S

✦ VOLUME I
General Principles

1 **Plastic Surgery: The Problem-Solving Specialty** 1
STEPHEN J. MATHES, MD, FACS

2 **Historical Perspectives** 27
WILLIAM D. MORAIN, MD

3 **Outcomes Research: The Path to Evidence-Based Decisions in Plastic Surgery** 35
E. DALE COLLINS, MD
CAROLYN L. KERRIGAN, MDCM, MSc

4 **Genetics** 51
DEEPAK NARAYAN, MS, MD, FRCS (ENG), FRCS (EDIN)

5 **Psychological Aspects of Plastic Surgery** 67
LAURIE STEVENS, MD
MARY H. MCGRATH, MD, MPH, FACS

6 **Ethics in Plastic Surgery** 93
THOMAS J. KRIZEK, MD, MA (HON)

7 **Liability Issues in Plastic Surgery: A Legal Perspective** . . . 127
ERLE E. PEACOCK, Jr., MD, JD

8 **Liability Issues in Plastic Surgery: An Insurance Perspective** 139
MARK GORNEY, MD, FACS

9 **Photography in Plastic Surgery** 151
WILLIAM Y. HOFFMAN, MD, FACS

10 **Anesthesia for Plastic Surgery** 167
PAUL F. WHITE, PhD, MD
JEAN P. WADDLE, MD

11 **Wound Healing: Repair Biology and Wound and Scar Treatment** 209
H. PETER LORENZ, MD, FACS
MICHAEL T. LONGAKER, MD, FACS

12 **Scar Revision** 235
NICHOLAS PARKHOUSE, DM, MCh, FRCS
TANIA C. S. CUBISON, FRCS
M. DALVI HUMZAH, MBBS, FRCS, MBA

13 **Transplantation in Plastic Surgery** 269
W. P. ANDREW LEE, MD, FACS
PETER E. M. BUTLER, MD, FRCS (ENGL), FRCSI, FRCS (PLAST)
DAVID W. MATHES, MD

14 **Skin Grafts** 293
CHRISTIAN E. PALETTA, MD, FACS
JEFFREY J. POKORNY, MD
PETER M. RUMBOLO, MD, FACS

15 **Vascular Territories** 317
G. IAN TAYLOR, MBBS, MD, FRACS, FRCS, FACS
ANDREW IVES, MBChB
SHYMAL DHAR, MD

16 **Flap Classification and Applications** 365
STEPHEN J. MATHES, MD, FACS
SCOTT L. HANSEN, MD

17 **Flap Physiology** 483
NICHOLAS B. VEDDER, MD, FACS

18 **Principles and Techniques of Microvascular Surgery** 507
FU-CHAN WEI, MD
SINIKKA SUOMINEN, MD, PhD

19 **Principles of Tissue Expansion** . . 539
LOUIS C. ARGENTA, MD, MBA, FACS
MALCOLM W. MARKS, MD, FACS

20 **Repair and Grafting of Dermis, Fat, and Fascia** 569
THOMAS R. STEVENSON, MD, FACS
THOMAS P. WHETZEL, MD, FACS

21 **Repair and Grafting of Tendon** 591
PHYLLIS CHANG, MD, FACS

22 **Repair, Regeneration, and Grafting of Skeletal Muscle** 605
    GEORGE H. RUDKIN, MD, FACS
    TIMOTHY A. MILLER, MD, FACS

23 **Repair, Grafting, and Engineering of Cartilage** 621
    MARK A. RANDOLPH, MAS
    MICHAEL J. YAREMCHUK, MD, FACS

24 **Repair and Grafting of Bone** . . . 639
    BABAK J. MEHRARA, MD
    JOSEPH G. MCCARTHY, MD, FACS

25 **Repair and Grafting of Peripheral Nerve** 719
    SALEH M. SHENAQ, MD, FACS
    JOHN Y. S. KIM, MD

26 **Alloplastic Materials** 745
    TANYA A. ATAGI, MD
    V. LEROY YOUNG, MD, FACS

27 **Prostheses in Plastic Surgery** 769
    ARIAN MOWLAVI, MD
    DIMITRIOS DANIKAS, MD
    MICHAEL W. NEUMEISTER, MD, FRCS(C), FACS
    ROBERT C. RUSSELL, MD, FRACS, FACS

28 **Exfoliative Disorders** 793
    ROBERT C. CARTOTTO, MD, FRCS(C)
    JOEL S. FISH, MD, MSc, FRCS(C)

29 **Burn and Electrical Injury** 811
    DAVID M. YOUNG, MD, FACS

30 **Radiation Injury** 835
    STEPHAN ARIYAN, MD, MBA

31 **Cold Injuries** 855
    ROSS I. S. ZBAR, MD, FACS
    JOHN W. CANADY, MD, MS, FACS, FAAP

32 **Pharmacologic and Mechanical Management of Wounds** 863
    CHRISTOPHER ATTINGER, MD, FACS
    ERWIN J. BULAN, MD
    PETER A. BLUME, DPM

33 **Problem Wounds and Principles of Closure** 901
    SCOTT L. HANSEN, MD
    STEPHEN J. MATHES, MD, FACS

34 **Principles of Endoscopic Surgery** 1031
    FELMONT F. EAVES III, MD, FACS

35 **Principles of Cancer Management** 1053
    STEPHAN ARIYAN, MD, MBA

36 **Prenatal Detection of Fetal Anomalies** 1067
    JUDITH R. CHIN, DDS, MS
    ARNOLD J. KAHN, MS, PhD

37 **Tissue Engineering** 1081
    JENNIFER J. MARLER, MD
    JOSEPH UPTON III, MD

38 **Fetal Surgery** 1117
    MARC H. HEDRICK, MD
    MICHAEL T. LONGAKER, MD, FACS

39 **Telemedicine** 1137
    SUBHAS C. GUPTA, MD, CM, PhD, FRCS(C), FACS

40 **Robotics in Plastic Surgery** . . . 1147
    JOSEPH ROSEN, MD
    ROBERT COHEN, MD
    ELIOT GRIGG, BA

✦ VOLUME II

The Head and Neck, Part 1

41 **Anthropometry and Cephalometric Facial Analysis** 1
    BRETT E. LEHOCKY, DDS, MD

42 **Analysis of the Aesthetic Surgery Patient** 31
    GILBERT P. GRADINGER, MD, FACS
    EUGENE H. COURTISS, MD

43 **Forehead Correction of Aging** . . . 47
    CHARLES R. DAY, MD, FACS ABPS (DIPL)
    FOAD NAHAI, MD, FACS

44 **Aesthetic Periorbital Surgery** 77
    ROBERT S. FLOWERS, MD, FACS
    JOHN M. NASSIF, MD, FACS

45 **Aesthetic Techniques in Periorbital Surgery** 127
    JAMES H. CARRAWAY, MD, FACS
    DENTON D. WEISS, MD, FACS

46 **Aging Face and Neck** 159
    JAMES M. STUZIN, MD, FACS
    THOMAS J. BAKER, MD

47 **Rejuvenation of the Upper
    Face and Midface: Current
    Techniques** 215
    BRENT MOELLEKEN, MD, FACS

48 **Face Lift (Midface): Current
    Techniques** 253
    JOHN Q. OWSLEY, MD, FACS

49 **Face Lift (Lower Face): Current
    Techniques** 275
    DEAN J. FARDO, MD
    JAMES E. ZINS, MD, FACS
    FOAD NAHAI, MD, FACS

50 **Face Lift (Neck): Current
    Techniques** 297
    JOHN Q. OWSLEY, MD, FACS

51 **Facial Resurfacing** 339
    JOHN T. ALEXANDER II, MD, FACS
    MITCHEL P. GOLDMAN, MD
    THOMAS L. ROBERTS III, MD, FACS

52 **Pharmacologic Skin
    Rejuvenation** 385
    NIA TEREZAKIS, MD, FACP, FAAD
    DEIRDRE O'BOYLE HOOPER, MD
    VENETIA N. PATOUT, MD

53 **Facial Skeletal Augmentation** . . . 405
    MICHAEL J. YAREMCHUK, MD, FACS

54 **Primary Rhinoplasty** 427
    ROD J. ROHRICH, MD, FACS
    ARSHAD R. MUZAFFAR, MD, FACS

55 **Open Rhinoplasty: Concepts
    and Techniques** 473
    RONALD P. GRUBER, MD, FACS
    SIMEON H. WALL, JR., MD
    DAVID KAUFMAN, MD

56 **Closed Rhinoplasty: Current
    Techniques, Theory, and
    Applications** 517
    MARK B. CONSTANTIAN, MD, FACS

57 **Aesthetic Reconstruction
    of the Nose** 573
    GARY C. BURGET, MD, FACS

58 **Aesthetic Orthognathic
    Surgery** 649
    HARVEY M. ROSEN, MD, DMD, FACS

59 **Hair Restoration** 687
    JACK FISHER, MD, FACS

60 **Secondary Rejuvenation
    of the Face** 715
    TIMOTHY J. MARTEN, MD, FACS

61 **Secondary Rhinoplasty** 765
    JOHN H. HARTLEY, JR., MD, FACS

62 **Secondary Aesthetic Periorbital
    Surgery** 801
    ROBERT S. FLOWERS, MD, FACS
    JOHN M. NASSIF, MD, FACS

63 **Secondary Blepharoplasty:
    Current Techniques** 823
    GLENN W. JELKS, MD, FACS
    ELIZABETH B. JELKS, MD
    ERNEST S. CHIU, MD

✦ VOLUME III

THE HEAD AND NECK, PART 2

64 **Facial Trauma: Soft Tissue
    Injuries** 1
    REID V. MUELLER, MD

65 **Acute Care and Reconstruction
    of Facial Burns** 45
    LOREN H. ENGRAV, MD, FACS
    MATTHIAS B. DONELAN, MD, FACS

66 **Facial Fractures** 77
    PAUL N. MANSON, MD, FACS

67 **Pediatric Facial Injuries** 381
    CRAIG R. DUFRESNE, MD, FACS
    PAUL N. MANSON, MD, FACS

68 **Endoscopic Facial Fracture
    Management: Techniques** 463
    CHEN LEE, MD, MSC, FRCS(C), FACS
    CHRISTOPHER R. FORREST, MD, MSC, FRCS(C)

69 **Endoscopic Mandible Fracture
    Management: Techniques** 511
    REID V. MUELLER, MD

70 **Temporomandibular Joint Dysfunction** 535
STEPHEN A. SCHENDEL, MD, DDS, FACS
ANDREW E. TURK, MD, FACS

71 **Acquired Cranial Bone Deformities** 547
MICHAEL J. YAREMCHUK, MD, FACS

72 **Acquired Facial Bone Deformities** 563
S. ANTHONY WOLFE, MD, FACS
MARIA TERESA RIVAS-TORRES, MD
OMER OZERDEM, MD

73 **Scalp Reconstruction** 607
MARK D. WELLS, MD, FRCS(C), FACS

74 **Reconstruction of the Auricle** . . . 633
BURTON D. BRENT, MD

75 **Forehead Reconstruction** 699
MAHESH H. MANKANI, MD, FACS
STEPHEN J. MATHES, MD, FACS

76 **Reconstruction of the Periorbital Adnexa** 733
S. ANTHONY WOLFE, MD, FACS
MARIA TERESA RIVAS-TORRES, MD
OMER OZERDEM, MD

77 **Subacute and Chronic Respiratory Obstruction** 763
CHRISTOPHER B. GORDON, MD
ERNEST K. MANDERS, MD, FACS

78 **Lower Third Face and Lip Reconstruction** 799
MALCOLM ALAN LESAVOY, MD, FACS
ANDREW D. SMITH, MD

79 **Midface Reconstruction** 859
KIYONORI HARII, MD
HIROTAKA ASATO, MD, PhD
AKIHIKO TAKUSHIMA, MD, PhD

80 **Facial Paralysis** 883
RONALD M. ZUKER, MD, FRCS(C), FACS
RALPH T. MANKTELOW, MD, FRCS(C)
GAZI HUSSAIN, MBBS, FRCS(A)

81 **Oral Cavity Reconstruction** 917
JOANNE J. LENERT, MD
GREGORY R. D. EVANS, MD, FACS

82 **Mandible Reconstruction** 957
DAVID A. HIDALGO, MD
JOSEPH J. DISA, MD, FACS

83 **Hypopharyngeal and Esophageal Reconstruction** 993
JOHN J. COLEMAN III, MD, FACS
AMARDIP S. BHULLER, MD

84 **Neck Reconstruction** 1025
DELORA L. MOUNT, MD, FACS
STEPHEN J. MATHES, MD, FACS

✦ VOLUME IV
Pediatric Plastic Surgery

85 **Embryology of the Craniofacial Complex** 1
JILL A. HELMS, DDS, PhD
RANDALL P. NACAMULI, MD, FACS
ALI SALIM, MD
YUN-YING SHI, BS

86 **Embryology, Classifications, and Descriptions of Craniofacial Clefts** 15
JAMES P. BRADLEY, MD
DENNIS J. HURWITZ, MD, FACS
MICHAEL H. CARSTENS, MD, FACS

87 **Classification, Varieties, and Pathologic Anatomy of Primary Labial Clefts** 45
PETER D. WITT, MD
JAN RAPLEY, MD

88 **Classification and Anatomy of Cleft Palate** 55
ANIL P. PUNJABI, DDS, MD
ROBERT A. HARDESTY, MD, FACS

89 **Anatomy and Classification of Alveolar and Palatal Clefts** 69
DAVID M. KAHN, MD
STEPHEN A. SCHENDEL, MD, DDS, FACS

90 **Craniofacial Syndromes** 91
CRAIG A. VANDER KOLK, MD, FACS
JOHN M. MENEZES, MD

91 **Craniofacial Microsomia** 113
JOSEPH G. McCARTHY, MD, FACS
RICHARD A. HOPPER, MD, FACS
BARRY H. GRAYSON, DDS

92 Nonsyndromic
   Craniosynostosis 135
   JEFFREY L. MARSH, MD, FACS
   JUDITH M. GURLEY, MD
   ALEX A. KANE, MD, FACS

93 Unilateral Cheiloplasty 165
   M. SAMUEL NOORDHOFF, MD
   PHILIP KUO-TING CHEN, MD

94 Bilateral Cleft Lip Repair 217
   COURT BALDWIN CUTTING, MD

95 Cleft Palate Repair 249
   WILLIAM Y. HOFFMAN, MD, FACS
   DELORA L. MOUNT, MD, FACS

96 Orthodontics in Cleft Lip and
   Palate Management 271
   ALVARO A. FIGUEROA, DDS, MS
   JOHN W. POLLEY, MD

97 Velopharyngeal Dysfunction . . . 311
   GERALD M. SLOAN, MD, FACS
   DAVID J. ZAJAC, PhD, CCC-SLP

98 Secondary Deformities of the
   Cleft Lip, Nose, and Palate 339
   SAMUEL STAL, MD, FACS
   LARRY H. HOLLIER, Jr., MD, FACS

99 Reconstruction: Orbital
   Hypertelorism 365
   JOSEPH G. MCCARTHY, MD, FACS

100 Reconstruction: Facial Clefts . . 381
    DAVID J. DAVID, MD, FRCS

101 Reconstruction:
    Craniosynostosis 465
    JOSEPH G. MCCARTHY, MD, FACS
    LARRY H. HOLLIER, Jr., MD, FACS

102 Reconstruction: Craniofacial
    Syndromes 495
    SCOTT P. BARTLETT, MD, FACS
    JOSEPH E. LOSEE, MD, FACS, FAAP
    STEPHEN B. BAKER, DDS, MD

103 Reconstruction: Craniofacial
    Microsomia 521
    JOSEPH G. MCCARTHY, MD, FACS
    BARRY H. GRAYSON, DDS

104 Hemifacial Atrophy 555
    JOHN W. SIEBERT, MD
    HOOMAN SOLTANIAN, MD
    ALEXES HAZEN, MD

✦ VOLUME V

Tumors of the Head, Neck, and Skin

105 Pediatric Tumors 1
    JULIANA E. HANSEN, MD, FACS
    RICHARD CHAFFOO, MD, FACS

106 Vascular Anomalies 19
    JENNIFER J. MARLER, MD
    JOHN B. MULLIKEN, MD, FACS

107 Salivary Gland Tumors 69
    STEPHAN ARIYAN, MD, MBA
    DEEPAK NARAYAN, MS, MD, FRCS (ENG),
      FRCS (EDIN)
    CHARLOTTE E. ARIYAN, MD, PhD

108 Tumors of the Craniofacial
    Skeleton 91
    IAN T. JACKSON, MD, DSc (HON), FRCS,
      FACS, FRACS (HON)

109 Tumors of the Lips, Oral Cavity,
    and Oropharynx 159
    DAVID L. LARSON, MD, FACS

110 Tumors of the Mandible 189
    GREGORY L. BORAH, MD, DMD, FACS
    SHAHID R. AZIZ, MD, DMD

111 Carcinoma of the Upper
    Aerodigestive Tract 217
    STEVEN A. GOLDMAN, MD
    EDWARD A. LUCE, MD, FACS

112 Benign Tumors of the Skin 251
    PABLO LEÓN, MD

113 Malignant Tumors of the
    Skin 273
    RONALD M. BARTON, MD, FACS

114 Malignant Melanoma 305
    STEPHAN ARIYAN, MD, MBA

115 Local Flaps for Facial
    Coverage 345
    IAN T. JACKSON, MD, DSc (HON), FRCS,
      FACS, FRACS (HON)

116 Management of Nonmelanoma
    Skin Cancer 391
    KEITH DENKLER, MD
    WILLIAM F. KIVETT, MD, FACS

117 Management of Regional
Metastatic Disease of the
Head and Neck: Diagnosis
and Treatment 465
STEPHAN ARIYAN, MD, MBA

✦ VOLUME VI

Trunk and Lower Extremity

118 Breast Augmentation 1
G. PATRICK MAXWELL, MD, FACS
R. WINFIELD HARTLEY, Jr., MD

119 Breast Augmentation
Techniques 35
MALCOLM ALAN LESAVOY, MD, FACS

120 Mastopexy 47
JAMES C. GROTTING, MD, FACS
ANN P. MARX, MD
STEPHEN M. CHEN, MD

121 Abdominoplasty 87
LUIS O. VÁSCONEZ, MD, FACS
JORGE I. DE LA TORRE, MD, FACS

122 Abdominoplasty Techniques . . . 119
TE NING CHANG, MD, PhD
RICARDO BAROUDI, MD

123 Body Contouring:
Comprehensive Liposuction . . . 193
GERALD H. PITMAN, MD, PC, FACS
SHARON Y. GIESE, MD, FACS

124 Body Contouring:
Large-Volume Liposuction 241
JEFFREY M. KENKEL, MD, FACS
ROD J. ROHRICH, MD, FACS

125 Body Contouring: Trunk and
Thigh Lifts 257
TED E. LOCKWOOD, MD, FACS

126 Liposuction of the Trunk and
Lower Extremities 273
MARY K. GINGRASS, MD, FACS
LAUREN GREENBERG, MD

127 Body Contouring: Upper
Extremity 291
PETER A. VOGT, MD, FRCS(C), FACS

128 Secondary Breast
Augmentation 315
V. LEROY YOUNG, MD, FACS
MARLA E. WATSON, MA
TANYA A. ATAGI, MD

129 Secondary Abdominoplasty . . . 361
KLAUS J. WALGENBACH, MD, FACS
KENNETH C. SHESTAK, MD, FACS

130 Secondary Liposuction 381
MARY K. GINGRASS, MD, FACS
JOHN M. HENSEL, Jr., MD

131 Aesthetic Genital Surgery 389
GARY J. ALTER, MD

132 Reconstruction of the Chest . . . 411
JAMES KNOETGEN III, MD
CRAIG H. JOHNSON, MD
PHILLIP G. ARNOLD, MD, FACS

133 Reconstruction of the Back . . . 441
JULIUS W. FEW, MD, FACS
FOAD NAHAI, MD, FACS

134 Congenital Anomalies of the
Chest Wall 457
STEPHEN J. MATHES, MD, FACS
ALAN E. SEYFER, MD, FACS
EDWARD P. MIRANDA, MD

135 Breast Reduction 539
GLYN E. JONES, MD, FACS

136 Vertical Reduction:
Techniques 585
KRISTIN BOEHM, MD, FACS
FOAD NAHAI, MD, FACS

137 Inferior Pedicle Reduction:
Techniques 601
STEPHEN J. MATHES, MD, FACS
WESLEY SCHOOLER, MD

138 Breast Cancer: Diagnosis,
Therapy, and Postmastectomy
Reconstruction 631
STEPHEN J. MATHES, MD, FACS
JULIE LANG, MD

139 Reconstruction of the
Nipple-Areola Complex 791
STEPHEN J. MATHES, MD, FACS
CRISTIANE M. UENO, MD

140 Immediate Postmastectomy
Reconstruction: Latissimus
Flap Techniques 819
SCOTT L. SPEAR, MD, FACS
AMER A. SABA, MD

141 Immediate Postmastectomy
Reconstruction: TRAM Flap
Transposition Techniques 835
SCOTT L. SPEAR, MD, FACS
JASON C. GANZ, MD

142 Postmastectomy
Reconstruction: Free TRAM
Flap Techniques 849
JAMES C. GROTTING, MD, FACS
MICHAEL S. BECKENSTEIN, MD, FACS
STEPHEN M. CHEN, MD

143 Postmastectomy
Reconstruction: Expander-
Implant Techniques 875
STEPHEN J. MATHES, MD, FACS
MARGA MASSEY, MD

144 Delayed Postmastectomy
Reconstruction: TRAM
Transposition Techniques 973
GLYN E. JONES, MD, FACS

145 Delayed Postmastectomy
Reconstruction: Free TRAM
Techniques 1001
STEPHEN S. KROLL, MD

146 Delayed Postmastectomy
Reconstruction: Latissimus
Flap Techniques 1023
SCOTT L. SPEAR, MD, FACS
CHRISTOPHER L. HESS, MD

147 Perforator Flaps for Breast
Reconstruction 1039
PETER C. NELIGAN, MB, BCh, FRCS(I),
   FRCS(C), FACS
STEVEN F. MORRIS, MD, MSc, FRCS(C)

148 Postmastectomy
Reconstruction: Alternative
Free Flaps 1053
L. FRANKLYN ELLIOTT II, MD, FACS
PATTI BERGEY, PA-C

149 Secondary Reconstructive
Surgery: Mastopexy and
Reduction 1067
DAVINDER J. SINGH, MD
R. BARRETT NOONE, MD, FACS

150 Secondary Breast
Reconstruction 1083
STEPHEN J. MATHES, MD, FACS
LEE W. T. ALKUREISHI, MBChB, Bsc (HONS)

151 Reconstruction of the
Abdominal Wall 1175
MOTOHIRO NOZAKI, MD
KENJI SASAKI, MD
TED T. HUANG, MD, FACS

152 Reconstruction of Male
Genital Defects: Congenital
and Acquired 1197
DAVID A. GILBERT, MD, FRCS(C), FACS
GERALD H. JORDAN, MD, FACS

153 Hypospadias 1259
DAVID J. COLEMAN, MS, FRCS (PLAST)
PAUL E. BANWELL, BSc, FRCS

154 Reconstruction of Female
Genital Defects:
Congenital 1281
MALCOLM ALAN LESAVOY, MD, FACS
EUGENE J. CARTER, MD

155 Reconstruction of Acquired
Vaginal Defects 1295
PETER G. CORDEIRO, MD, FACS
ANDREA L. PUSIC, MD, MHS, FRCS(C)

156 Surgery for Gender Identity
Disorder 1305
DAVID KAUFMAN, MD
JUDY VAN MAASDAM, MA
DONALD R. LAUB, Sr., MD, FACS

157 Pressure Sores 1317
ROBERT D. FOSTER, MD, FACS

158 Reconstructive Surgery:
Lower Extremity Coverage . . . 1355
DOUGLAS J. MACKENZIE, MD
ALAN E. SEYFER, MD, FACS

159 Reconstructive Surgery:
Skeletal Reconstruction 1383
EDWARD J. HARVEY, MD, MSc
L. SCOTT LEVIN, MD, FACS

160 Foot Reconstruction 1403
LAWRENCE B. COLEN, MD, FACS
THEODORE UROSKIE, JR., MD, FACS

161 Vascular Insufficiency of the
Lower Extremity: Lymphatic,
Venous, and Arterial 1455
ELISABETH K. BEAHM, MD, FACS
ROBERT L. WALTON, MD, FACS
ROBERT F. LOHMAN, MD, FACS

✦ VOLUME VII

The Hand and Upper Limb, Part 1

INTRODUCTION AND GENERAL PRINCIPLES 1

162 Plastic Surgery: Contributions to
Hand Surgery 3
JAMES CHANG, MD, FACS

163 Anatomy and Biomechanics
of the Hand 13
JAMES CHANG, MD, FACS
FRANCISCO VALERO-CUEVAS, PhD
VINCENT R. HENTZ, MD, FACS
ROBERT A. CHASE, MD, FACS

164 Examination of the Upper
Extremity 45
DONALD R. LAUB, JR., MD

165 Diagnostic Imaging of the
Hand and Wrist 55
MICHAEL W. NEUMEISTER, MD, FRCS(C), FACS
E. GENE DEUNE, MD
ARIAN MOWLAVI, MD

166 Anesthesia for Upper Extremity
Surgery 87
J. C. GERANCHER, MD
ROBERT S. WELLER, MD

167 General Principles 109
MICHAEL E. PANNUNZIO, MD
WILLIAM C. PEDERSON, MD, FACS

168 Arthroscopy of the Wrist 125
DANIEL J. NAGLE, MD, FACS

169 Principles of Internal Fixation
as Applied to the Hand
and Wrist 139
MICHAEL E. JABALEY, MD, FACS
ERIC E. WEGENER, MD, FACS

ACQUIRED DISORDERS— TRAUMATIC 151

170 Fingertip Reconstruction 153
PARHAM A. GANCHI, MD, PhD, FACS
W. P. ANDREW LEE, MD, FACS

171 Surgery of the Perionychium . . 171
NICOLE Z. SOMMER, MD
RICHARD E. BROWN, MD, FACS
ELVIN G. ZOOK, MD, FACS

172 Reconstructive Surgery of
Individual Digits
(Excluding Thumb) 207
ROGER K. KHOURI, MD, FACS
ALEJANDRO BADIA, MD, FACS

173 Thumb Reconstruction:
Microvascular Methods 253
NICHOLAS B. VEDDER, MD, FACS
BENJAMIN M. MASER, MD, FACS

174 Thumb Reconstruction:
Conventional Techniques 281
GUY FOUCHER, MD
ALLEN BISHOP, MD

175 Thumb Reconstruction:Pollicization
for Traumatic Loss 295
JOSEPH UPTON III, MD
J. WILLIAM LITTLER, MD

176 Reconstructive Surgery: Extensive
Injuries to the Upper Limb 317
WILLIAM C. PEDERSON, MD, FACS
MILAN STEVANOVIC, MD
CHARALAMPOS ZALAVRAS, MD, PhD
RANDY SHERMAN, MD, FACS

177 Flexor Tendon Injuries and
Reconstruction 351
DAVID G. WILLIAMSON, MD, FRCS(C)
ROBERT S. RICHARDS, MD, FRCS(C)

178 Extensor Tendon Injuries and
Reconstruction 401
WILLIAM B. NOLAN, MD

179 Fractures and Joint Injuries
Involving the Metacarpals
and Phalanges 423
R. Christie Wray, Jr., MD, FACS

180 Fractures and Dislocations
of the Wrist and Distal
Radioulnar Joint 453
Doron I. Ilan, MD
Timothy R. McAdams, MD

181 Peripheral Nerve Injuries:
Repair and Reconstruction 471
Jonathan M. Winograd, MD
Susan E. MacKinnon, MD, FACS

182 Adult Brachial Plexus
Injuries 515
David Chwei-Chin Chuang, MD

183 Obstetric Brachial Plexus
Palsy 539
Vincent R. Hentz, MD, FACS

184 Replantation and
Revascularization 565
Gregory M. Buncke, MD, FACS

   Appendix 583
   Shirley Chan, CHT

185 Acute Management of the
Burned Hand and Electrical
Injuries 587
David G. Greenhalgh, MD, FACS
Hugh L. Vu, MD, MPH

186 Upper Extremity Burn
Reconstruction 605
Robert L. McCauley, MD, FACS
Malachy E. Asuku, MD, FWACS

187 Cold and Chemical Injury
of the Upper Extremity 647
Timothy R. McAdams, MD

188 The Stiff Hand 659
David T. Netscher, MD, FACS
Paula Lee-Valkov, MD

ACQUIRED DISORDERS—
NONTRAUMATIC 673

189 Tenosynovitis and Cumulative
Trauma Syndrome 675
Anthony A. Smith, MD, FACS
Craig H. Johnson, MD
Stephan J. Finical, MD, FACS

190 Disorders of Musicians'
Hands 693
Ian Winspur, LLM, FRCS

191 Management of Osteoarthritis
of the Hand 707
Daniel Vincent Egloff, MD

192 Management of Dupuytren
Disease 729
Caroline Leclercq, MD

193 Infections of the Hand 759
David T. Netscher, MD, FACS
Paula Lee-Valkov, MD

194 Ischemic Conditions of the
Hand 791
Michael A. McClinton, MD
E. F. Shaw Wilgis, MD

195 Reflex Sympathetic Dystrophy/
Chronic Regional Pain
Syndrome 823
Wyndell H. Merritt, MD, FACS

196 Nerve Entrapment
Syndromes 875
A. Lee Dellon, MD, FACS

197 Painful Neuromas 929
A. Lee Dellon, MD, FACS

198 Benign and Malignant Soft
Tissue Tumors of the Upper
Limb 949
Earl J. Fleegler, MD

199 Benign and Malignant Bone
Tumors of the Hand 979
Catherine M. Curtin, MD
Kevin C. Chung, MD, FACS

200 **Lymphedema in the Upper Extremity** 995
CHARLES L. PUCKETT, MD, FACS
MATTHEW J. CONCANNON, MD, FACS
CARLOS L. FARIAS, MD

♦ VOLUME VIII

The Hand and Upper Limb, Part 2

THE HAND AND UPPER LIMB: CONGENITAL ANOMALIES 1

201 **Embryology of the Upper Limb** . . . 3
LOREN J. BORUD, MD
JOSEPH UPTON III, MD

202 **Classification of Upper Limb Congenital Differences and General Principles of Management** 25
JOSEPH UPTON III, MD

203 **Management of Transverse and Longitudinal Deficiencies (Failure of Formation)** 51
JOSEPH UPTON III, MD

204 **Management of Disorders of Separation—Syndactyly** 139
JOSEPH UPTON III, MD

205 **Constriction Ring Syndrome** . . . 185
JOSEPH UPTON III, MD

206 **Disorders of Duplication** 215
JOSEPH UPTON III, MD

207 **Failure of Differentiation and Overgrowth** 265
JOSEPH UPTON III, MD

208 **Hypoplastic or Absent Thumb** . . 323
JOSEPH UPTON III, MD

209 **Vascular Anomalies of the Upper Extremity** 369
JOSEPH UPTON III, MD
JENNIFER J. MARLER, MD

210 **Pediatric Upper Extremity Trauma** 417
EDWARD J. HARVEY, MD, MSc
L. SCOTT LEVIN, MD, FACS

211 **Hand Management for Patients with Epidermolysis Bullosa** 431
AMY L. LADD, MD
JOHN M. EGGLESTON III, MD

212 **Effect of Growth on Pediatric Hand Reconstruction** 439
ALAIN GILBERT, MD

PARALYTIC DISORDERS 451

213 **Tendon Transfers in the Upper Limb** 453
NEIL F. JONES, MD, FRCS
KAYVAN T. KHIABINI, MD, MSc, FRCS(C), FACS

214 **Free Functioning Muscle Transfers in the Upper Limb** . . . 489
RALPH T. MANKTELOW, MD, FRCS(C)
RONALD M. ZUKER, MD, FRCS(C), FACS

215 **Restoration of Upper Extremity Function in Tetraplegia** 507
VINCENT R. HENTZ, MD, FACS
TIMOTHY R. MCADAMS, MD

216 **Management of the Spastic Hand** 543
ANN VAN HEEST, MD
JAMES HOUSE, MD, MS

REHABILITATION 555

217 **Hand Therapy** 557
CAROLYN GORDEN, OHT, CHT
DONNA LASHGARI, OTR, CHT
PREM LALWANI, OTR, CHT

218 **Upper Limb Functional Prosthetics** 573
MAURICE LEBLANC, MSME, CP
GERALD STARK, BSME, CP, FAAOP

219 **Upper Limb Aesthetic and Functional Prosthetics** 583
JEAN PILLET, MD
ANNIE DIDIER-JEAN PILLET, MD

Index i

Facial Trauma: Soft Tissue Injuries

Reid V. Mueller, MD

IDENTIFICATION OF THE PROBLEM

INCIDENCE AND ETIOLOGY

EVALUATION
   Anatomy
   Clinical Examination
   Diagnostic Studies
   Consultations and Multispecialty Approach to Care

TREATMENT
   Anesthesia
   Irrigation and Débridement
   Scalp and Forehead
   Eyebrows
   Eyelids
   Cheek
   Nose
   Ears
   Mouth

IDENTIFICATION OF THE PROBLEM

Soft tissue injuries are commonly encountered in the care of traumatized patients. Many of these injuries are simple superficial lacerations that require nothing more than a straightforward closure. Other seemingly uncomplicated wounds harbor injuries to the facial skeleton, teeth, motor and sensory nerves, parotid duct, eyes, or brain. The types of soft tissue injuries encountered include abrasions, tattoos, simple or "clean" lacerations, complex or contusion-type lacerations, bites, avulsions, and burns. Recognition of the full nature of the injury and a logical treatment plan determine whether there will be future aesthetic or functional deformities. All wounds will benefit from cleaning, irrigation, conservative débridement, and minimal tension closure. Some wounds will benefit from local or regional flaps for closure; a few wounds will need tissue expansion or free tissue transfer for complete restoration of function and appearance.

INCIDENCE AND ETIOLOGY

The etiology of facial soft tissue trauma varies considerably, depending on age, sex, and geographic location. Many facial soft tissue injuries are relatively minor and are treated by the emergency department without a referral to a specialist. There are few data about the cause of facial trauma that is subsequently referred to a specialist, but it is weighted toward more significant traumas such as road crashes and assaults. Facial soft tissue trauma tends to occur in certain areas of the head, depending on the causative mechanism. When all causes of facial trauma are taken into account, the distribution is concentrated in a T-shaped area that includes the forehead, nose, lips, and chin. The lateral brows and occiput also have localized frequency increases (Fig. 64-1).

When the cause of facial trauma is considered for all patients who present to emergency departments (Fig. 64-2), falls are by far the most common cause, accounting for 48% to 51% of the injuries.[1,2] The peak age is 2 to 3 years, when toddlers are beginning to walk and frequently fall into objects. There is a smaller peak during the 20s to 30s and then a steady rise after the age of 50 years. Alcohol consumption is a major factor for those between the ages of 30 and 50 years; concomitant medical conditions, such as epilepsy, are a causative factor for up to 8% of fall injuries. There is an 8% risk of associated craniofacial fracture; however, this figure rises to 77% in those older than 50 years.[1] The distribution of injuries is concentrated in the T-shaped area (see Fig. 64-1) of the forehead, nose, lips, and chin, followed by the occiput and anterior temporal areas.[1,3]

Approximately 16% of facial soft tissue trauma is the result of a non-fall impact with a structural element such as a door (72%), wall (15%), or window frame (15%). Other collisions with furnishings such as tables or radiators account for the remainder. These types of injuries peak in children younger than 5 years

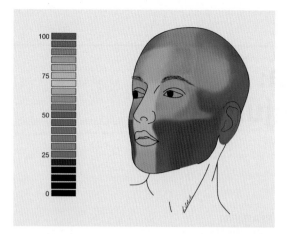

FIGURE 64-1. Segregation of 700 facial soft tissue injuries into the number of injuries for different facial areas indicated by color. Note the T distribution across the forehead, nose, lips, and chin. Also note the concentration of injuries at the lateral brow. (Data from Hussain K, Wijetunge DB, Grubnic S, et al: A comprehensive analysis of craniofacial trauma. J Trauma 1994;36:34.)

and are rarely associated with a fracture. The most common areas injured are the forehead, nose, and anterior temples.[1-3]

Assaults account for 16% to 32% of facial soft tissue injuries.[1-3] Assaults and brawling have a peak incidence in young men, as might be expected. The male predominance persists until after the age of 60 years. Alcohol consumption is a factor in two thirds of these patients. The assaults were most commonly caused by fists (56%), kicks (17%), and blunt instruments (15%). Injuries were more common on the left side of the head consistent with a statistical predominance of right-handed assailants. Up to 20% of assaults resulted in concomitant isolated nasal, zygoma, or mandible fractures. The locations of the lacerations

were primarily in T distribution over the forehead, nose, and lips and in anterior temporal areas.[1]

Road accidents cause 6% to 13% of facial trauma,[2,4] but up to 49% of those injuries are subsequently referred to a specialist.[3] In some European countries, bicycle injuries account for the majority of crash injuries[2]; in the United States, automobile crashes are responsible for 50% of the facial soft tissue injuries from road accidents, followed by bicycle (24%), motorcycle (7%), truck or van (5%), and pedestrian-vehicle collisions (4%).[5] The peak incidence is seen in young men at 15 to 24 years of age.[5] There is a male preponderance from the ages of 15 to 60 years. Impact with the steering wheel (51%) and windshield (27%) resulted in the majority of lacerations.[6,7] The most commonly lacerated areas are the forehead and nose. The overall incidence of facial fracture associated with soft tissue injury is 22% in patients involved in a road crash.[8] Bicyclists, motorcyclists,[9] and pedestrians are more likely to have an associated facial fracture.

Sporting injuries account for about 8% of facial soft tissue trauma and tend to occur more commonly in young men. Clashing of heads and kicks to the face are the most common causes; the forehead and nose are the most likely areas to be injured. Concomitant facial fracture resulted in 17% to 40% of sporting injuries to the head, with nose and mandible fractures being most common.[1,10-12]

Other causes account for the remainder of facial soft tissue traumas. These include occupational injuries, bites from humans or animals, and other miscellaneous causes. Occupation injury from falls or falling objects accounts for 5% of facial trauma and is primarily seen in young men.

In 2001, approximately 368,245 persons were treated for dog bite injuries (129.3 per 100,000 population). The risk of dog bite was highest for children aged 5 to 9 years and decreased with age. Approximately 42% of dog bites occurred in children younger than

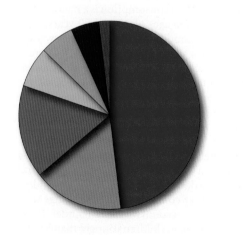

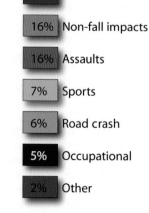

48% Falls

16% Non-fall impacts

16% Assaults

7% Sports

6% Road crash

5% Occupational

2% Other

FIGURE 64-2. Etiology of soft tissue injuries from facial trauma in 950 consecutive patients presenting to an urban university emergency department. (From Hussain K, Wijetunge DB, Grubnic S, et al: A comprehensive analysis of craniofacial trauma. J Trauma 1994;36:34.)

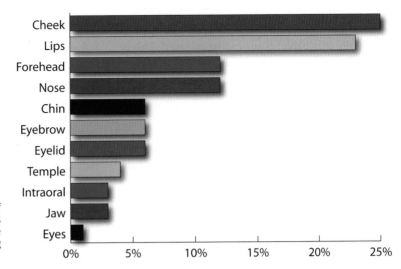

FIGURE 64-3. The distribution of hospital-treated facial lacerations from dog bites. (From Karlson TA: The incidence of facial injuries from dog bites. JAMA 1984;251:3265.)

14 years, and boys were at greater risk than girls. The frequency of facial injuries was highest in children younger than 4 years, in whom nearly 65% of dog bite injuries involve the face; in adults, the likelihood of a dog bite on the face is about 9%.[13] Most bite injuries are from dogs known to the person and occur near or in the home. One study of children younger than 4 years found that 47% were bitten by their own dog and 90% were bitten at home. Facial injuries from dog bites have a distribution different from that of other forms of common trauma and typically involve the cheek, lips, forehead, and nose (Fig. 64-3).[14]

EVALUATION

Anatomy

SKIN

Almost all soft tissue injuries of the head involve the skin in some manner. The skin of the head shows more variety than any other area of the body in terms of thickness, elasticity, mobility, and texture. Consider the profound differences between the thick, inelastic, hair-bearing skin of the scalp and the thin, elastic, mobile skin of the eyelids. Consider also the transitions from external skin of the face to the orbital, nasal, and oral linings. Significant differences in the structure of the facial skin in different areas require different methods for the repair and reconstruction.

All skin is composed of an epithelial outer layer supported by the underlying dermis. The underlying structure of the dermis gives skin its elasticity and structural integrity and thereby determines how the skin will respond to the stresses of injury and repair. The reticular layer of the dermis is composed of a dense mass of collagenous and elastic fibers that are generally oriented perpendicular to the underlying muscle fibers. The elastic fibers maintain the skin in a constant state of tension. In 1861, Langer deduced the patterns of these fibers by punching circular holes in the skin of cadavers and noting the orientation of the long axis of the resultant ellipses.[15-20] The patterns formed by these lines have come to be known as lines of least tension or the so-called Langer's lines. Langer's lines run parallel to the main fiber bundles in the reticular layer of the dermis and are thought to originate from the ultrastructural organization of the dermis.[21] Langer's lines should not be confused with the wrinkle lines of the face. Wrinkle lines are caused by mechanical forces from the underlying muscle fibers and as such are orientated perpendicular to the direction of contraction.

Langer's lines are not visible features of the skin but a map of the biomechanical properties of the skin for strain response to load. Langer's lines are perpendicular to the direction of greatest force on the skin. Wounds and surgical incisions that parallel these lines will therefore have less force across the wound and presumably better wound healing and less scar spreading. Langer's lines normally but not always parallel wrinkle lines, and thus wrinkle lines offer an inconspicuous and suitable location for many surgical incisions.

PERFUSION

Anyone who has suffered a cut lip or scalp as a child knows firsthand from the torrent of blood that the face is well perfused. The generous vascular network and robust perfusion of the face have implications for the surgeon.

The dense interconnected network of collateral vessels in the face means that injured and partially avulsed tissue with seemingly insufficient blood supply due to a narrow pedicle will in fact survive, whereas the same injury would result in tissue necrosis in other areas of the body. The implication is that more (and potentially invaluable) tissue can be salvaged. This is especially important for areas with little or no excess tissue or areas that are difficult to reconstruct later (e.g., the oral commissure). In repair of the face, conservative débridement is often preferable. If a segment of tissue appears only marginally viable but is indispensable from a reconstructive standpoint, it should be loosely approximated and re-examined in 24 to 48 hours. At that time, a line of demarcation will usually delineate what will survive and what will die. Nonviable tissue may then be débrided during a second-look procedure.

INNERVATION

The trigeminal nerve provides the majority of the sensory innervation in the face, with lesser contributions from the cervical plexus, facial, and glossopharyngeal nerves (Fig. 64-4). The sensory innervation of the scalp, top of the head, forehead, conjunctiva, eye, paranasal sinuses, oral cavity, and teeth is from the trigeminal. The trigeminal nerve has three main divisions (ophthalmic, maxillary, and mandibular), each of which has three subdivisions. The ophthalmic (CN V1) division further subdivides into the lacrimal, frontal (bifurcating into the supraorbital and supratrochlear), and nasociliary (dividing into the infratrochlear and external nasal) nerves. The maxillary (CN V2) division trifurcates to give rise to the zygomaticotemporal, zygomaticofacial, and infraorbital nerves. The mandibular (CN V3) division also has three subdivisions: mental, buccal, and auriculotemporal.

The cervical plexus confers sensation to the angle and border of the mandible as well as to the neck. This plexus gives rise to the great auricular, transverse cervical, and supraclavicular nerves. These three nerves all pass across the midpoint of the posterior border of the sternocleidomastoid at Erb point, providing a convenient location for local nerve block.

The facial nerve (CN VII) gives off sensory fibers that travel with the auricular branch of the vagus nerve (CN X) to provide sensation to the external auditory meatus and portions of the concha. This nerve, known as Arnold nerve, will continue to have sensation after a ring block of the ear because of its anatomic course.

The glossopharyngeal nerve (CN IX) also supplies sensation to a variable portion of the auditory canal, concha, and middle ear. This nerve is known as Jacobson nerve.

The motor innervation of the face is supplied from the facial and trigeminal nerves. The facial nerve exits

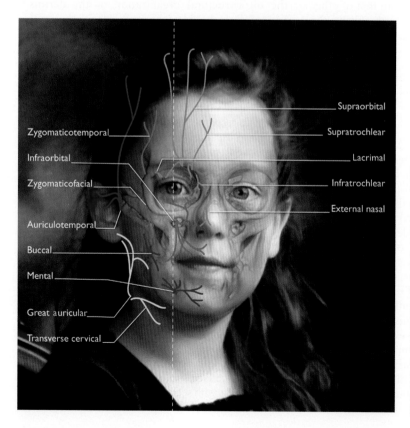

Zygomaticotemporal

Infraorbital

Zygomaticofacial

Auriculotemporal

Buccal

Mental

Great auricular

Transverse cervical

Supraorbital

Supratrochlear

Lacrimal

Infratrochlear

External nasal

FIGURE 64-4. The course of the sensory nerves to the face in relation to bone and external landmarks. The ophthalmic division (CN V1) depicted in blue gives rise to the supraorbital, supratrochlear, lacrimal, infratrochlear, and external nasal branches. The maxillary division (CN V2) in green divides into the zygomaticotemporal, infraorbital, and zygomaticofacial nerves. The mandibular division (CN V3) depicted in red gives rise to the auriculotemporal, buccal, and mental nerves. The cervical plexus shown in yellow gives rise to the great auricular, transverse cervical, and supraclavicular (not shown) nerves. Note the proximity of the supraorbital, infraorbital, and mental nerves as they exit the facial skeleton to the pupillary midline *(dashed white line)*.

the skull through the stylomastoid foramen and passes through the parenchyma of the parotid gland between the superficial and deep lobes. It splits into six major branches: temporal, zygomatic, buccal, mandibular, cervical, and auricular (Fig. 64-5). Within the parotid, the nerve splits into two main divisions, the temporofacial and the cervicofacial. The temporofacial further divides into temporal and zygomatic branches. The cervicofacial divides into the buccal, mandibular, and cervical branches. The auricular branch diverges from the main facial nerve trunk before the nerve enters the body of the parotid and innervates the superior auricular, posterior auricular, and occipitalis muscles. The facial nerve remains deep to the superficial musculoaponeurotic system along its entire course and innervates the deep surfaces of the muscles of facial animation except the levator anguli oris, mentalis, and buccinator muscles. The buccal and zygomatic branches usually have a number of communicating branches, whereas the frontal and mental branches do not. Therefore, injuries to the buccal and zygomatic branches are much less likely

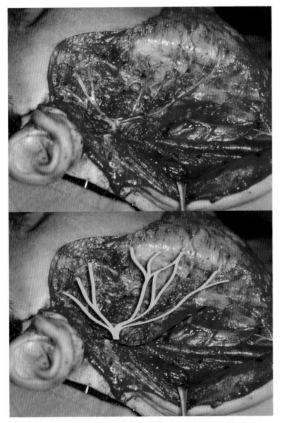

FIGURE 64-5. The superficial parotid has been removed to reveal the facial nerve branches. The lower photograph highlights the facial nerve in yellow and the border of the mandible with a dashed black line. Note the interconnections in the buccal branch.

to produce permanent paralysis compared with injuries to the frontal and mental branches. The facial nerve innervates all the muscles of facial expression as well as the posterior belly of the digastric and stapedius muscles.

The mandibular division of the trigeminal nerve (CN V3) is the motor nerve to the muscles of mastication (temporalis, masseter, medial pterygoid, and lateral pterygoid muscles) and several suprahyoid muscles (mylohyoid, posterior digastric, and geniohyoid muscles). The deep location of this nerve makes injury uncommon.

Clinical Examination

The external manifestations of craniofacial soft tissue injuries are more dramatic because of the alteration of appearance; however, one should not be distracted from a methodical examination to search for other injuries. Seemingly straightforward wounds often harbor injuries to the facial skeleton, teeth, motor and sensory nerves, parotid duct, eyes, or brain.

Evaluation of an injured patient always starts with establishment of an airway and ventilation, volume resuscitation, control of hemorrhage, and stabilization of other major injuries—the ABCs of an initial trauma assessment. Although the plastic surgeon is rarely "on the front lines" of trauma care, one cannot be complacent and assume that the emergency or trauma physician has completed a trauma assessment.

Once it is ascertained that there are no immediate life-threatening injuries, the examination begins. The assessment of facial injuries is guided by the nature of the mechanism of injury. A thermal burn will be approached differently from a dog bite avulsion injury. The history of the injury, if it is known, will often provide some clue as to what other injuries one might expect to find. A child who falls against a coffee table is unlikely to have any associated fractures, whereas a soccer player has a 17% chance of having an underlying fracture. Practitioners will have their own style of examination, but one should stick to a routine to decrease the likelihood of forgetting to check something. It is preferable to begin externally and proceed internally.

Initial observation, inspection, and palpation generally provide most of the information a practitioner will need. Ideally, the examination is performed with adequate anesthesia and sterile technique as well as with good lighting, irrigation, and suction.

Inspection of the skin will reveal abrasions, traumatic tattoos, simple or clean lacerations, complex or contusion-type lacerations, bites, avulsions, or burns. Systematic palpation of the skull, orbital rims, zygomatic arches, maxilla, and mandible may reveal asymmetry, bone step-off, crepitation, or other evidence of underlying facial fracture. Palpation within the wound is also useful. Sensation of the face is tested with a light touch, and motor activity of the facial nerve should be tested before the administration of local anesthetics.

Any injury near the eye should prompt a check of visual acuity and diplopia or evidence of globe injury, such as hyphema. The extraocular movements should be tested, and an examination is conducted for vertical dystopia and enophthalmos that might suggest orbital blowout fracture. The condition of the eyelids and integrity of the medial and lateral canthi should be tested. Any laceration near the medial third of the eye may harbor a canalicular injury. The canthi should have a snug and discernible endpoint when traction is applied. Rounding or laxity of the canthi suggests nasal-orbital-ethmoidal fracture. If there is any suggestion of globe injury, an immediate ophthalmology consultation is needed.

The contours of the nose are noted, and the nasal framework is palpated for fracture or crepitation. A speculum examination of the internal nose should be undertaken to look for mucosal lacerations, exposed cartilage or bone, or septal hematoma (a bluish boggy bulge of the septal mucosa).

Any laceration of the cheek that is near any facial nerve branch or along the course of the parotid duct will need to be investigated. If there is facial paralysis on the side of the injury, there is a high likelihood of facial nerve injury. Injury to the parotid duct can be evaluated by cannulation of the duct and irrigation with fluid (see later).

The oral cavity is inspected for loose or missing teeth. Any unaccounted for teeth may be loose in the wound, lost at the scene, or aspirated. A radiograph may be needed. The oral lining should be inspected for lacerations, and the occlusion should be checked. Palpation of the maxillary buttresses and mandible may reveal fractures. A sublingual hematoma suggests mandible fracture.

Diagnostic Studies

Any diagnostic studies are directed toward defining injuries to underlying structures. Most soft tissue injuries do not need any special diagnostic studies; however, concomitant facial fractures are common, and any suspicion should be followed up with a radiographic evaluation.

Consultations and Multispecialty Approach to Care

Any patient with an underlying orbital fracture or ocular injury should have an evaluation by an ophthalmologist. Dental injuries, such as fractured or missing teeth, should be evaluated by a dentist once the patient has recovered from the initial injury.

TREATMENT

The ultimate goal is to restore form and function with minimum morbidity. Function generally takes precedence over form; however, the face plays a fundamental role in emotional expression and social interaction, and therefore the separation of facial appearance from function is not possible. Different areas of the face require different approaches for treatment, but there are underlying principles that have broad application.

Anesthesia

Good anesthesia is necessary for the patient's comfort and cooperation, and it is often needed to complete a comprehensive evaluation. Most soft tissue injuries of the head and neck can be managed with simple infiltration or regional anesthesia blocks (Table 64-1). Patients who are uncooperative because of age, intoxication, or head injury may require general anesthesia. Patients with extensive injuries requiring more involved reconstruction or who would require potentially toxic doses of local anesthetics will likewise require general anesthesia.

Local anesthetics have a long history in the repair of facial injuries. Cocaine was first extracted from the leaves of the *Erythroxylon coca* bush in 1860, becoming the first local anesthetic.[22] In 1864, Sigmund Freud and Karl Koller used cocaine for anesthesia during an ophthalmologic procedure. Procaine, the first synthetic anesthetic, was developed in 1904; in 1943, lidocaine was synthesized, becoming the first amide anesthetic and ultimately the most commonly used prototypical short-acting anesthetic. Procaine and other ester-type anesthetics are metabolized by plasma pseudocholinesterase, and one of the byproducts of hydrolysis is *p*-aminobenzoic acid, which is a known allergen. Amide anesthetics, on the other hand, are metabolized by microsomal cytochrome P-450 3A4 in the liver and rarely cause allergic reactions. Further developments in anesthetics have given us many drugs from which to choose, but only a few are frequently needed or used. Lidocaine is the hallmark short-acting anesthetic; mepivacaine, bupivacaine, and ropivacaine are long acting. All of the anesthetics with the letter *i* in the prefix (e.g., lidocaine, ropivacaine) are amide anesthetics.

EPINEPHRINE

With the exception of cocaine, all of the local anesthetics cause some degree of vasodilatation. Epinephrine is commonly added to anesthetic solutions to counteract this effect to cause vasoconstriction, decrease bleeding, slow absorption, and increase duration of action. Most anesthetic solutions are available with epinephrine concentrations ranging from 1:100,000 to 1:200,000. When epinephrine is added to

TABLE 64-1 ◆ ANESTHETICS USED FOR LOCAL INFILTRATION AND LOCAL NERVE BLOCKS OF THE FACE

Anesthetic	Duration without Epinephrine (min)	Duration with Epinephrine (min)	Maximum Dose without Epinephrine (mg/kg)	Maximum Dose with Epinephrine (mg/kg)
Amides				
Lidocaine	30-120	60-400	4.5	7
Mepivacaine	30-120	30-120	4.0	7
Prilocaine	30-120	60-400	5.7	8.5
Bupivacaine	120-240	240-480	2.5	3.2
Ropivacaine	120-360		2.5	
Esters				
Cocaine	45		2.8	
Procaine	15-30	30-90	7.1	8.5
Tetracaine	120-240	240-480	1.5	2.5

the local anesthetic, 0.1 mL of 1:1000 epinephrine for each 10 mL of solution will give a final concentration of 1:100,000. Epinephrine can have systemic effects from as little as 2 mL of a 1:100,000 solution. Epinephrine should not be use in patients with pheochromocytoma, hyperthyroidism, severe hypertension, or severe peripheral vascular disease or in patients taking propranolol. There is the risk of tissue necrosis with higher concentrations of epinephrine. Every medical student has also learned that epinephrine should never be injected in the "finger, toes, penis, nose, or ears." This admonition is based on anecdotal reports or simple assumptions. There are few data to support the notion, and plastic surgeons routinely use epinephrine in the face, including the ears and nose, with rare complications. Unfortunately, from a medicolegal standpoint, it is probably best to avoid epinephrine in these areas unless clinical judgment determines the specific need for epinephrine.

SODIUM BICARBONATE BUFFERING

Local anesthetics are acidic and painful on injection. When the pH is buffered with sodium bicarbonate, the pain of injection is decreased. Lidocaine 1% solution can be buffered with 8.4% sodium bicarbonate (1 mEq/mL) in a 1:10 ratio (1 mL sodium bicarbonate in 10 mL of lidocaine). Different concentrations of lidocaine will take proportionately more or less buffer. Mepivacaine and bupivacaine may be buffered with 8.4% sodium bicarbonate solution in ratios of 1:10 and 1:150, respectively.[23] If too much buffer is added, the solution may precipitate and should be discarded. Once the solution is buffered, its shelf-life is significantly reduced; one third of a buffered lidocaine solution will degrade after 4 weeks at room temperature.

Refrigeration will extend the lifetime, but it is probably best to discard buffered solutions after several weeks.

LOCAL INFILTRATION

Local anesthetics should usually be injected into the deep dermis. More superficial infiltration will cause a peau d'orange appearance and unnecessary discomfort for the patient. Intradermal infiltration has the advantage of rapid onset of anesthesia and control of bleeding if epinephrine has been added. However, injection may distort some facial landmarks needed for alignment and accurate repair (such as the vermilion border of the lip), and therefore anatomic landmarks should be noted and marked before injection.

Lidocaine is the prototypical short-acting amide local anesthetic that is used for local infiltration and local nerve blocks. It is commonly prepared with epinephrine to decrease the rate of absorption, prolong the duration of action, and reduce the risk of systemic toxicity. The maximal safe dose for lidocaine is 4.5 mg/kg without epinephrine and 7 mg/kg with epinephrine. A 0.5% (5 mg/mL) lidocaine solution is generally used for local infiltration when larger volumes are needed; 1% (10 mg/mL) or 2% (20 mg/mL) solutions are used for nerve blocks.

Bupivacaine is a long-acting amide local anesthetic that is also used for local infiltration and nerve blocks. Maximum dosage limits must be individualized for each patient after evaluation of the size and physical status of the patient as well as the rate of systemic absorption from a particular injection site. The safe dosage for adults is 2.5 mg/kg without epinephrine and 3.2 mg/kg with epinephrine; more or less drug may be used, depending on the patient. Cardiac toxicity is the most dreaded systemic side effect. Because of the long duration of action, adverse cardiac effects may persist for hours. Inadvertent intravascular injection of long-acting local anesthetics has been associated with death. Bupivacaine or other long-acting anesthetics should not be injected intravascularly or used as part of a Bier block. Ropivacaine is a newer long-acting amide anesthetic that is a pure *S* enantiomer with some data to suggest reduced cardiac toxicity.

TOPICAL ANESTHETICS

Topical anesthetics are well established for the treatment of children with superficial facial wounds and to decrease the pain of injection. The most widely used topical agent is a 5% eutectic mixture of local anesthetics (EMLA) containing lidocaine and prilocaine.[23,24] EMLA has been shown to provide adequate anesthesia for split-thickness skin grafting[25] and minor surgical procedures such as excisional biopsy and electrosurgery.[26] Successful use of EMLA requires 60 to 90 minutes of application for adequate anesthesia. The most common mistake leading to failure is not allowing sufficient time for diffusion and anesthesia. Some areas, such as the face with a thinner stratum corneum, may have onset of anesthesia more quickly. Mucosal application (without a stratum corneum) may produce analgesia in 10 to 15 minutes. Because the prilocaine component may exacerbate methemoglobinemia, caution should be used in patients with methemoglobinemia or in patients younger than 12 months who are receiving medication known to exacerbate methemoglobinemia. The dosage recommendation[24] for patients weighing less than 10 kg is no more than 2 g on an area less than 100 cm². For patients weighing 10 to 20 kg, the maximum dose is 10 g on an area less than 100 cm². EMLA should not be used near the eyes.

FIELD BLOCKS FOR THE FACE

Field block of the face can provide anesthesia of a larger area with less discomfort and fewer needle sticks for the patient. A field block may provide better tolerance of the patient for multiple painful injections of anesthetic when local infiltration of an epinephrine-containing solution is needed. Field blocks are more challenging to perform and require time to take effect. Impatient surgeons often fail to wait a sufficient amount of time (at least 10 to 15 minutes) for most blocks to take effect.

Forehead, Anterior Scalp to Vertex, Upper Eyelids, Glabella (Supraorbital, Supratrochlear, Infratrochlear Nerves)

ANATOMY. The supraorbital nerve is located at the superior medial orbital rim about a fingerbreadth medial to the midpupillary line. The supratrochlear nerve lies about 1.5 cm farther medially near the medial

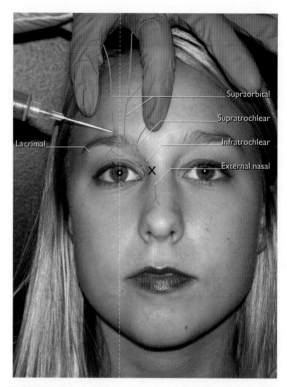

FIGURE 64-6. The majority of the forehead, medial upper eyelid, and glabella can be anesthetized with a block of the ophthalmic division of the trigeminal nerve (CN V1). Identify the supraorbital notch by palpation and enter the skin just lateral to that point near the pupillary midline. Aim for a point just medial to the medial canthus (marked by an *x*) and advance the needle about 2 cm. Inject 2 or 3 mL while withdrawing the needle.

margin of the eyebrow. The infratrochlear nerve is superior to the medial canthus.

METHOD. Identify the supraorbital foramen or notch along the superior orbital rim and enter just lateral to that point. Direct the needle medially and advance it to just medial of the medial canthus (about 2 cm). Inject 2 mL while withdrawing the needle (Fig. 64-6).

Lateral Nose, Upper Lip, Upper Teeth, Lower Eyelid, Most of Medial Cheek (Infraorbital Nerve)

ANATOMY. The infraorbital nerve exits the infraorbital foramen at a point that is medial to the midpupillary line and 6 to 10 mm below the inferior orbital rim.

METHOD. Identify the infraorbital foramen along the inferior orbital rim by palpation. An intraoral approach is better tolerated and less painful (Fig. 64-7). Place the long finger of the nondominant hand on the foramen and retract the upper lip with thumb and

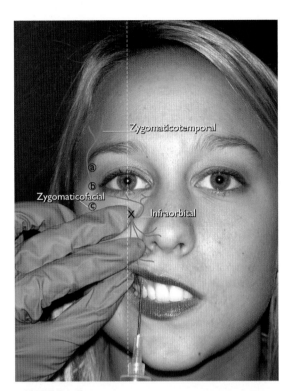

FIGURE 64-7. The lower eyelid, medial cheek, and lower nose can be anesthetized with an infraorbital nerve block. The infraorbital foramen may be palpable about 1 cm below the orbital rim just medial to the midpupillary line. The intraoral approach is less painful and anxiety provoking for most patients. Place the long finger of the nondominant hand on the orbital rim at the infraorbital foramen. Grasp and retract the upper lip. Insert the needle in the superior gingival buccal sulcus above the canine tooth root and direct the needle toward your long finger and the foramen while injecting 2 or 3 mL.

index finger. Insert the needle in the superior gingival buccal sulcus above the canine tooth root and direct the needle toward your long finger while injecting 2 mL. You may also inject percutaneously by identifying the infraorbital foramen about 1 cm below the orbital rim just medial to the midpupillary line. Enter perpendicular to the skin, advance the needle to the maxilla, and inject about 2 mL (Fig. 64-8).

Lower Lip and Chin (Mental Nerve)

ANATOMY. The mental nerve exits the mental foramen about 2 cm inferior to the alveolar ridge below the second premolar. The nerve can often be seen under the inferior gingival buccal mucosa when lower lip and cheek are retracted. It branches superiorly and medially to supply the lower lip and chin.

METHOD. The lower lip is retracted with the thumb and index finger of the nondominant hand, and the needle is inserted at the apex of the second premolar. The needle is advanced 5 to 8 mm, and 2 mL is injected

(Fig. 64-9). When the percutaneous approach is used, insert the needle at the midpoint of a line between the oral commissure and inferior mandibular border. Advance the needle to the mandible and inject 2 mL while slightly withdrawing the needle (Fig. 64-10).

Posterior Auricle, Angle of the Jaw, Anterior Neck (Cervical Plexus: Great Auricular, Transverse Cervical)

ANATOMY. Both the great auricular nerve and transverse cervical nerve emerge from the midpoint of the posterior border of the sternocleidomastoid muscle at Erb point. The great auricular nerve parallels the external jugular vein as it passes up toward the ear. The transverse cervical nerve is about 1 cm farther

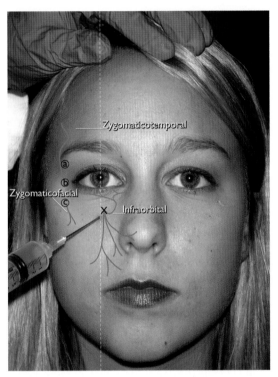

FIGURE 64-8. The lower eyelid, medial cheek, and lower nose can be anesthetized with an infraorbital nerve block. The infraorbital foramen may be palpable about 1 cm below the orbital rim just medial to the midpupillary line. Enter the skin directly over the palpable or anticipated location of the infraorbital foramen and advance to the maxilla. Inject about 2 mL of anesthetic. Anesthesia of the anterior temple area can be achieved with a block of the zygomaticotemporal nerve. Enter just posterior to the lateral orbital rim at a level above the lateral canthus *(a)* and advance toward the chin to a point level with the lateral canthus *(b)*. Inject 2 or 3 mL while withdrawing the needle. The zygomaticofacial nerve supplies the lateral malar prominence. To block this nerve, enter at a point one fingerbreadth inferior and lateral to the intersection of the inferior and lateral orbital rim. Advance the needle to the zygoma and inject 1 or 2 mL.

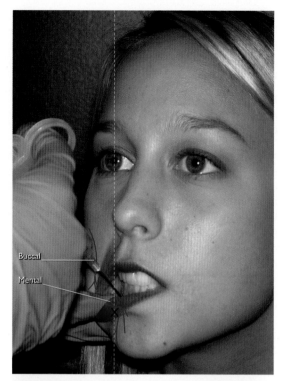

FIGURE 64-9. The lower lip and chin can be anesthetized with a block of the mental nerve (CN V3). Retract the lower lip with the thumb and index finger of the nondominant hand. Many times, the mental nerve is visible under the mandibular gingival buccal sulcus near the apex of the second premolar. Insert the needle at the apex of the second premolar and advance it 5 to 8 mm while injecting 2 mL.

inferiorly and passes parallel to the clavicle, then curves toward the chin. Both are in the superficial fascia of the sternocleidomastoid muscle.

METHOD. Locate Erb point by having the patient flex against resistance. Mark the posterior border of the sternocleidomastoid muscle and locate the midpoint between clavicle and mastoid. Insert the needle about 1 cm superior to Erb point and inject transversely across the surface of the muscle toward the anterior border. A second more vertically oriented injection may be needed to block the transverse cervical nerve.

Ear (Auriculotemporal Nerve, Great Auricular Nerve, Lesser Occipital Nerve, and Auditory Branch of the Vagus [Arnold] Nerve)

ANATOMY. The anterior half of the ear is supplied by the auriculotemporal nerve that branches from the mandibular division of the trigeminal nerve (CN V3). The posterior half of the ear is innervated by the great auricular and lesser occipital nerves that are both branches from the cervical plexus (C2, C3). The

auditory branch (Arnold nerve) of the vagus nerve (CN X) supplies a portion of the concha and external auditory canal.

METHOD. Insert a 1.5-inch needle at the junction of the earlobe and the head and advance it subcutaneously toward the tragus while infiltrating 2 or 3 mL of anesthetic (Fig. 64-11). Pull the needle back and redirect it posteriorly along the posterior auricular sulcus, again injecting 2 or 3 mL. Reinsert the needle at the superior junction of the ear and the head. Direct the needle along the preauricular sulcus toward the tragus and inject 2 or 3 mL. Pull the needle back and redirect it along the posterior auricular sulcus while injecting the anesthetic. It may be necessary to insert the needle a third time along the posterior sulcus to complete a ring block. Care should be taken to avoid the temporal artery when the needle is directed along the preauricular sulcus. If the artery is inadvertently

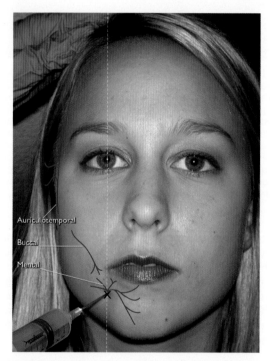

FIGURE 64-10. The lower lip and chin can be anesthetized with a block of the mental nerve (CN V3). The mental foramen is near the midpoint of a line between the oral commissure and the mandibular border. Enter the skin at this point and advance to the mandible. Inject 2 or 3 mL while slightly withdrawing the needle. The auriculotemporal nerve emerges deep and posterior to the temporomandibular joint and travels with the temporal vessels to supply the temporal scalp, lateral temple, and anterior auricle. Palpate the temporomandibular joint and base of the zygomatic arch. Enter the skin superior to the zygomatic arch just anterior to the auricle. Aspirate to ensure that you are not within the temporal vessels and inject 2 or 3 mL.

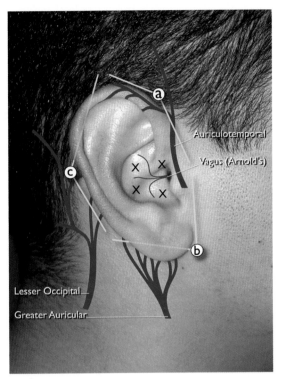

FIGURE 64-11. The majority of the external ear can be anesthetized with a ring block. Insert a 1.5-inch needle at the superior junction of the ear and the head at *a*. Direct the needle along the preauricular sulcus toward the tragus and inject 2 or 3 mL. Pull the needle back and redirect it along the posterior auricular sulcus while injecting. Reinsert the needle at the junction of the earlobe and head at *b* and advance it subcutaneously toward the tragus while infiltrating 2 or 3 mL of anesthetic. Pull the needle back and redirect it posteriorly along the posterior auricular sulcus, again injecting 2 or 3 mL. It may be necessary to insert the needle a third time, at *c*, along the posterior sulcus to complete a ring block. If anesthesia of the concha or external auditory canal is needed, local infiltration (marked with *x*'s) will be required to anesthetize the auditory branch of the vagus nerve (Arnold nerve).

soft tissue damage. The process starts by irrigation of the wound with a bulb syringe, or a 60-mL syringe with an 18-gauge angiocatheter attached, to forcibly irrigate the wound. More contaminated wounds will benefit from pulsed lavage systems.

After irrigation, hemostasis is secured to give the surgeon a better opportunity to inspect the wound. The use of epinephrine in the local anesthetic will cause some degree of vasoconstriction and assist in this regard. Electrocautery should be applied to specific vessels at the lowest setting conducive to coagulation. Wholesale indiscriminate application of electrocautery causes unnecessary tissue necrosis. Use electrocautery cautiously in areas where important nerves might be located to avoid iatrogenic injury. Remember that nerves are often in proximity to vessels.

Limited sharp débridement is used to remove clearly nonviable tissue. In areas where there is minimal tissue laxity or irreplaceable structures (e.g., tip of nose, oral commissure), débridement should be kept to a minimum and later scar revision undertaken if needed. Areas such as the cheek and lip have significant tissue mobility and will tolerate more aggressive débridement.

After the preliminary débridement and irrigation, a methodical search for foreign material is undertaken. Small fragments of automobile glass become embedded through surprisingly small external wounds. They are usually evident on radiographic examination or computed tomographic scan or by careful palpation. Patients thrown from vehicles will often have dirt, pebbles, or plant material embedded in their wounds. Patients who have blast injuries from firearms or fireworks will have paper, wadding, or bullet fragments present. One should not undertake a major dissection for the sake of retrieving a bullet fragment; however, one should make sure that other identifiable pieces of foreign matter are removed. Failure to do so will result in later infection.

punctured, apply pressure for 10 minutes to prevent formation of a hematoma.

If anesthesia of the concha or external auditory canal is needed, local infiltration will be required to anesthetize the auditory branch of the vagus nerve (Arnold nerve).

Irrigation and Débridement

Once good anesthesia has been obtained, the wound is cleaned of foreign matter and clearly nonviable tissue is removed. This is the process of converting an untidy wound to a tidy one. Clean lacerations from a sharp object will result in little collateral tissue damage or contamination, whereas a wound from an impact with the asphalt will have significant foreign material and

ABRASIONS

Abrasions result from tangential trauma that removes the epithelium and a portion of the dermis, leaving a partial-thickness injury that is painful. This type of injury is often the result of sliding across pavement or dirt and therefore embeds small particulate debris within the dermis. If dirt and debris are not promptly removed, the dermis and epithelium will grow over the particulates and establish a traumatic tattoo that is difficult to manage later. Topical anesthetic, if it is properly applied and given sufficient time for onset, can give good anesthesia for cleaning of simple abrasions. This can be accomplished with generous irrigation and cleaning with a surgical scrub brush (Fig. 64-12). If more involved débridement is needed, general anesthesia is advisable.

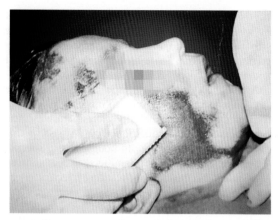

FIGURE 64-12. Facial abrasions should be cleaned of any dirt and debris with generous irrigation and gentle scrubbing with a surgical scrub brush.

TRAUMATIC TATTOO

There are two basic types of traumatic tattoo, those that result from blast injuries and those that result from abrasive injuries. In either instance, various particles of dirt, asphalt, sand, carbon, tar, explosives, or other particulate matter are embedded into the dermis.

Abrasive traumatic tattoos are more common. Typically, a person is ejected from a vehicle or thrown from a bicycle, and the face is subsequently ground into the pavement. This causes a simultaneous traumatic dermabrasion of the epidermis and superficial dermis and embedding of the pigment (dirt). If this is left untreated, the dermis and epidermis heal over the pigment, resulting in a permanent tattoo (Fig. 64-13).

Blast-type injuries seen in military casualties and civilian powder burns as well as in firework and bomb mishaps produce numerous particles of dust, dirt, metal, combustion products, unignited gunpowder, and other foreign materials that act like hundreds of small missiles, each penetrating the wound to various depths. The entry wounds collapse behind the particle, trapping them within the dermis.

Regardless of the mechanism of injury, prompt removal of the particulate matter results in a far better outcome than with later removal. Once the skin has healed, the opportunity to remove the particles with simple irrigation and scrubbing is lost. The initial treatment is vigorous scrubbing with a surgical scrub brush or gauze and copious irrigation.[27-31] Wounds treated within 24 hours show substantially better cosmetic outcome than do those treated later[29]; however, some improvement has been seen as late as 10 days.[32] Larger particles should be searched for and removed individually with fine forceps or needles, loupe magnification, and generous irrigation.[33] The tedious and time-consuming nature of these maneuvers may require serial procedures during several days for completion. However, meticulous débridement of

the acute injury is the best opportunity for optimal outcome.

The treatment of traumatic tattoo remains an unresolved problem in plastic surgery, and as such, there are multiple techniques, none of which is perfect. Some of the treatment options are surgical excision and microsurgical planing[34,35]; dermabrasion[36-39]; salabrasion[40]; application of various solvents, such as diethyl ether[30]; cryosurgery, electrosurgery, and treatment with carbon dioxide and argon lasers[27,28,30,41]; and treatment with Q-switched Nd:YAG laser,[42,43] erbium:YAG laser,[44] Q-switched alexandrite laser,[45,46] and Q-switched ruby laser.[47,48] The mechanism for laser removal is not entirely understood but is thought to involve the fragmentation of pigment particles, rupture of pigment-containing cells, and subsequent phagocytosis of the tattoo pigment.[49,50] Laser therapy for pigment tattoos will require slightly higher fluences than those used for removal of professional tattoos.[47]

A note of caution is in order for treatment of gunpowder traumatic tattoos. Several authors have noted ignition of retained gunpowder during laser tattoo removal,[43,51] resulting in spreading of the tattoo or formation of significant dermal pits. If initial laser treatment suggests the presence of unignited gunpowder

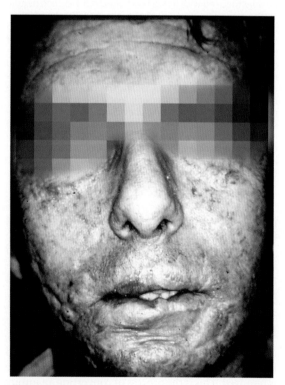

FIGURE 64-13. This man has an established traumatic tattoo. The best opportunity to prevent such an outcome is at the time of injury by meticulous débridement. Secondary treatment of traumatic tattoo is difficult and includes dermabrasion, excision, and laser treatments.

in the dermis, laser removal should be discontinued in favor of other treatments, such as dermabrasion or surgical microexcision of the larger particles.

LACERATIONS

Simple or clean lacerations are usually caused by cutting of the tissue by sharp objects. Lacerations from window and automobile glass or knife wounds are typical examples (Fig. 64-14). Simple lacerations may be repaired primarily after irrigation and minimal débridement, even if the patient's condition has delayed closure for several days. When immediate closure is not feasible, the wound should be irrigated and kept moist with a saline and gauze dressing. Before repair, foreign bodies such as window glass should be removed. Wounds of this type usually require little or no débridement. A few well-placed absorbable 4-0 or 5-0 sutures will help align the tissue and relieve tension on the skin closure. The temptation to place numerous dermal sutures

should be avoided because excess suture material in the wound will only serve to incite inflammation and impair healing. The skin should be closed with 5-0 or 6-0 nylon interrupted or running sutures; alternatively, 5-0 nylon or monofilament absorbable running subcuticular pull-out sutures can be placed. Any suture that traverses the epidermis should be removed from the face in 4 or 5 days. If sutures are left in place longer than this, epithelialization of the suture tracks will lead to permanent suture marks known as railroad tracks. Sutures of the scalp may be left in place for 7 to 10 days. Removal of pull-out sutures should usually follow the same guidelines; however, there is less risk of permanent suture marks.

COMPLEX OR CONTUSION-TYPE LACERATIONS

When soft tissue is compressed between a bone prominence and an object, it will burst or fracture,

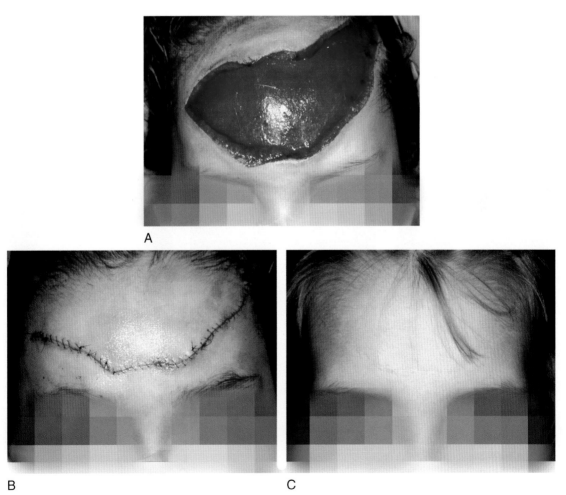

A

B

C

FIGURE 64-14. *A* and *B,* A clean forehead laceration sustained in a motor vehicle crash requires nothing more than irrigation and closure. *C,* Several months later, a good result can be expected.

resulting in a complex laceration pattern and significant contusion of the tissue. A typical example of these types of lacerations is the brow laceration, sustained when a toddler falls onto a coffee table or an occupant is ejected from a vehicle in a crash and strikes an object (Fig. 64-15). Many wounds on first impression suggest significant tissue loss. However, after irrigation, minimal débridement, and careful replacement of the tissue fragments piece by piece, it becomes apparent that most of the tissue is present. Contused and clearly nonviable tissue should be débrided. Tissue that is contused but has potential to survive should usually be returned to anatomic position. Elaborate repositioning of tissue with Z-plasties and the like should usually be reserved for secondary reconstructions after primary healing has finished. Limited undermining may be used to decrease tension and achieve closure; however, wide undermining in the face of widespread contusions and lacerations is rarely indicated. It is probably better to accept a modest area of secondary intention healing and plan for later scar revision rather than to risk tissue necrosis from overzealous undermining of already injured tissue.

AVULSIONS

Many wounds of the face suggest tissue loss on initial inspection, but closer examination reveals that the tissue has simply retracted or folded over itself. Avulsive injuries that remain attached by a pedicle will often survive, and the likelihood of survival depends on the size of the pedicle relative to the segment of tissue it must nourish. Human and animal bites account for many avulsions of the nose, lip, and ears. Fortunately, the remarkably good perfusion of the face allows survival of avulsed portions on surprisingly small pedicles. If there is any possibility that the avulsed tissue may survive, one should attempt to repair it. Venous congestion of the repaired portion should be treated with medicinal leeches until the congestion resolves. Reconstruction of a failed reattachment can always be undertaken later, but a discarded portion of tissue can never be replaced.

Many avulsed and amputated portions of soft tissue are amenable to replantation, provided the patient does not have underlying injuries or medical conditions that would preclude a lengthy operation. Examples of facial segments that have been successfully replanted include scalp, nose, lip, ear, and cheek. Vein grafts are often needed to complete the replantation, and venous congestion is a common complication that can be successfully managed with leeches or bleeding of the congested segment.

KELOIDS

Any scar has the potential to form a hypertrophic scar or keloid. Keloids may be distinguished from hypertrophic scars because they grow outside the bounds of the original injury; hypertrophic scar is simply thickened or spread. A keloid may form after seemingly

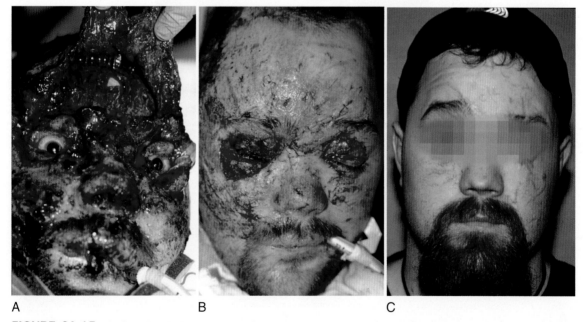

A   B   C

FIGURE 64-15. *A,* Complex facial laceration after a motor vehicle crash that gives the impression of significant tissue loss. *B,* Irrigation, minimal débridement, and careful repositioning of the tissue fragments—"solving the jigsaw puzzle"—reveal that most of the tissue is present and usable. *C,* Postoperative result.

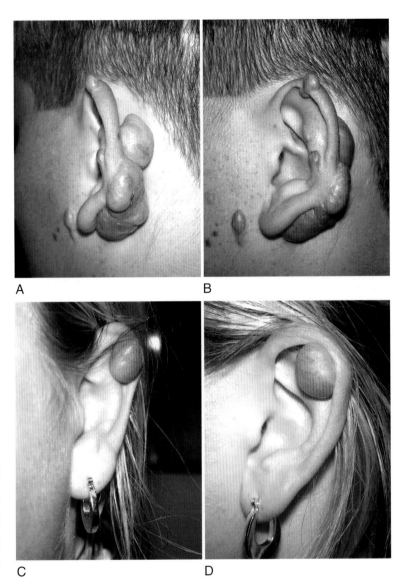

FIGURE 64-16. Keloids can form after soft tissue injury and are commonly seen on the ears and neck. *A* and *B* show several recurrent ear keloids from a motor vehicle crash. *C* and *D* show an isolated ear keloid after an ear piercing. Note that the lobule did not form a keloid. Both were treated with excision and postoperative low-dose irradiation.

minor trauma (an ear piercing) or after major injuries (Fig. 64-16). It is not uncommon for one wound to form a keloid while another wound 2 cm away does not. Keloids are more common on the ears and neck and less common on the rest of the face.

Scalp and Forehead

ETIOLOGY

Most scalp injuries are the result of blunt force sustained in road crashes, assaults, and falls. Motor vehicle crashes result in most of the avulsive injuries; complete avulsion of the scalp usually occurs in industrial or farm accidents when the hair becomes entangled around a rotating piece of machinery.

EVALUATION

Anatomy

The scalp is composed of five layers that can be remembered by the mnemonic SCALP (**S**kin, sub**C**utaneous, **A**poneurosis and muscle, **L**oose areolar tissue, and **P**ericranium). The outer three layers are fused together and glide over the loose areolar tissue and pericranium. The thickness of the skin of the scalp ranges from 3 to 8 mm, making it some of the thickest on the body.[52] The frontalis muscles anteriorly and occipitalis muscles posteriorly are connected over the majority of the scalp by the galea aponeurotica. The galea is a strong, relatively inelastic layer that is an important structure in repair of scalp wounds. It plays a role in protecting the skull and pericranium from superficial subcutaneous infections, provides a strength layer in suturing, and limits elastic deformation of the scalp that often makes closure more difficult.

The subgaleal fascia is a thin, loose areolar connective tissue that lies between the galea and the pericranium and allows scalp mobility. The emissary veins cross this space as they drain the scalp into the intracranial venous sinuses. This is a potential site of ingress for bacteria contained within a subgaleal abscess, leading to meningitis or septic venous sinus thrombosis,[53-56] although the incidence is low.

The tightly adherent pericranium is simply the periosteum of the skull. The pericranium derives its blood supply from the diploic circulation with numerous small perforating vessels through the outer table. It can often provide a sufficiently vascularized layer of tissue to accept a skin graft for a scalp wound when primary closure is not possible. The pericranium fuses with the deep temporal fascia above the superior temporal line.[57,58] The deep temporal fascia then divides at the superior orbital margin into the superficial leaflet, which attaches to the superficial superior margin of the zygomatic arch, and the deep leaflet, which attaches to the deep surface of the zygoma. Between these two leaflets is the temporal fat pad.[57]

The vascular supply of the scalp is rich and replete with an extensive collateral circulation. Five major paired vessels supply this network. The anterior scalp is supplied by the supraorbital and supratrochlear arteries that exit the orbit through a notch or foramen superior to the medial limbus or medial canthus, respectively. The lateral aspect of the skull is supplied by the superficial temporal artery (the terminal branch of the external carotid artery). The artery courses preauricularly and bifurcates near the top of the ear into the frontal branch and parietal branches. The posterior lateral scalp is supplied by the posterior auricular artery that branches off the superficial temporal artery just inferior to the ear and then passes posteriorly and superiorly across the mastoid process. The posterior scalp is supplied by the medial and lateral branches from the occipital artery. Both enter the scalp near the supranuchal line and pass superiorly. Inferior to this line, small perforators from the splenius and trapezius are the primary blood supply.

Venous drainage occurs through veins traveling with the named arteries as well as from parietal and mastoid emissary veins. These veins traverse the skull, thereby connecting the scalp veins to the cranial venous sinuses. The parietal emissary veins find passage just anterior to the lambda at the junction of the sagittal and lambdoid sutures.[59] There are scattered reports of meningitis or septic intracranial sinus thrombosis that resulted from extension of a scalp infection into the cranium; however, the actual incidence is probably low.[53-56]

The collateral circulation of the scalp is so robust that the majority of the scalp can be supported on a single vessel. It has been reported, however, that the reliability of midline crossover circulation declines after the sixth decade of life.[60]

The sensory innervation of the scalp comes from the auriculotemporal branch of the mandibular nerve; the zygomaticotemporal branch of the maxillary nerve; the supraorbital and supratrochlear branches of the trigeminal nerve; and the lesser, greater, and third occipital nerves.[57] The frontal branch of the facial nerve (CN VII) is the motor nerve to the frontalis muscle; the auricular branch innervates the occipitalis muscle.

Diagnostic Studies

Treatment is based on clinical examination findings. Radiographic images are obtained for diagnosis of associated closed head injury and skull, facial, or cervical spine injuries.

TREATMENT

Treatment Goals

The goal of treatment is to provide stable soft tissue coverage of the skull and a normal appearance. These goals are often achieved in a single procedure; but under certain circumstances, a staged approach is needed.

Nonsurgical Versus Surgical Management

Closed scalp injuries such as abrasions and contusions will heal without surgical intervention. Small scalp hematomas are common and do not need to be evacuated acutely. Large hematomas may benefit from evacuation after bleeding has stopped from tamponade and the patient is otherwise stabilized. Large hematomas left unevacuated have the potential to organize into a fibrotic or calcified mass. This is of minimal consequence in the hair-bearing scalp but may be a cosmetic deformity on the forehead.

Full-thickness scalp wounds with tissue loss may be treated with nonsurgical management as a bridge to later reconstruction. The bone must be kept moist at all times if there is to be any growth of granulation tissue over it. If the bone becomes desiccated, it will die. Once a bed of granulation tissue has formed, a skin graft may be applied, or it may be allowed to epithelialize from the margins of the wound.

Algorithm for Surgical Treatment

The treatment of other life-threatening injuries will take precedence over the scalp with the exception of bleeding. The adventitia of the scalp arteries is intimately attached to the surrounding dense connective tissue so that the cut ends of vessels do not collapse and tend to remain patent and bleeding. This coupled with the rich blood supply can make the scalp a source of significant and ongoing blood loss.[61] A pressure dressing or rapid mass closure will provide time for treatment of other more urgent injuries with deferred treatment of the scalp up to 24 hours later.

Infiltration with 0.5% lidocaine with 1:100,000 epinephrine into the wound margins will provide some degree of vasoconstriction and adequate anesthesia for the emergency department treatment of most lacerations. Patients with extensive wounds or those who are unable to cooperate should be managed with general anesthesia.

The wound is thoroughly irrigated, and hemostasis of major vessels is completed with electrocautery or suture ligature. All foreign material such as dirt, glass, rocks, hair, plant matter, grease, and small bone fragments should be removed. The wound is explored for any previously unrecognized skull fractures. There is seldom a need for radical débridement of the scalp because of the rich blood supply. Surprisingly large segments of scalp can survive on relatively small vascular pedicles, and therefore it is often preferable to preserve any scalp tissue that has even a remote probability of survival. Shaving of the scalp in nonemergent neurosurgery has not been shown to be of any benefit in reducing wound infections.[62-65] It is reasonable to shave sufficient hair for clear visualization of the injury. There is little or no benefit to shaving the scalp for simple clean lacerations.

Specific Surgical Repairs

In general, scalp closure involves closure of the galea and subcutaneous tissue to control bleeding and provide strength, followed by skin closure. Absorbable 3-0 sutures are used for the galea and subcutaneous tissue in either a running or an interrupted manner. The skin can be closed with staples or sutures. In children, a rapidly absorbable suture is often used to avoid the need for later removal.

Repair of the scalp will depend on the nature of the injury, the extent of tissue loss, and the condition of the underlying pericranium and bone. Simple cuts from sharp objects require nothing more than simple closure. Blows to the head from assaults, falls, and road crashes often crush the soft tissue against the skull, resulting in a jagged bursting of the tissue. In these injuries, the initial impression may be that of extensive tissue loss; but after careful inspection and systematic replacement of tissue (solving the jigsaw puzzle), it becomes apparent that little tissue is missing. The pieces should be reassembled, and any areas of dubious survival are watched carefully. They often will survive.

Defects of 2 cm or less in diameter can usually be closed with wide undermining of the scalp at the subgaleal level (Fig. 64-17). The scalp is notoriously inelastic and will often require scoring of the galea with multiple incisions perpendicular to the desired direction of stretch. This is best accomplished with electrocautery on low power or a scalpel. Care should be taken to cut through only the galea, leaving the subcutaneous tissue and vessels within unharmed.

Scalp defects too large for primary closure may be closed in several ways. If the underlying pericranium is intact, a skin graft may be placed immediately without waiting for granulation. If the pericranium is not intact, a pericranial flap may be elevated from the adjacent uninjured areas and placed over the defect and subsequently skin grafted.[66] These flaps should generally be designed to follow a major vascular pedicle and not cross the midline. This method is applicable to defects up to 7 cm in diameter.[66] Alternatively, the outer table of the skull can be removed with a burr to expose the diploë, which is dressed for 5 to 7 days to allow ingrowth of granulation tissue and subsequent skin grafting. Skin grafts of this type have poor mechanical durability because of the thin dermis and no underlying shear plane. This may be a problem in certain areas, such as the occiput, that have more significant mechanical demands.

Larger defects of the scalp will require scalp reconstruction with tissue expansion, local Juri or Orticochea flaps, or free tissue transfer. Total scalp avulsion is best treated with microsurgical replantation whenever possible (Fig. 64-18). Avulsion injuries are most commonly caused when long hair becomes entangled around a rotating piece of industrial or agricultural machinery. The scalp detaches at the subgaleal plane, with the skin tearing at the supraorbital, temporal, and auricular areas. Many authors have reported excellent results with scalp replantation, even when only one vein and artery were available for revascularization.[67-89] The scalp will tolerate up to 18 hours of cold ischemia. Because the injuries are usually avulsive in nature, the veins and arteries needed for replantation have sustained significant intimal stretch injury. Because of this, vein grafts are frequently needed to bridge the zone of injury. Blood loss can be significant, and blood transfusion is common. If possible, the venous anastomoses should be completed before anastomosis of the arteries to minimize unnecessary blood loss.[75] The scalp can survive on a single vessel, but other vessels should be repaired if possible.

Outcomes

Scalp wounds tend to heal well because of their robust blood supply. Complications are rare.

Eyebrows

EVALUATION

Anatomy

The eyebrows are agile structures that are an important cosmetic part of the face. The eyebrows serve as

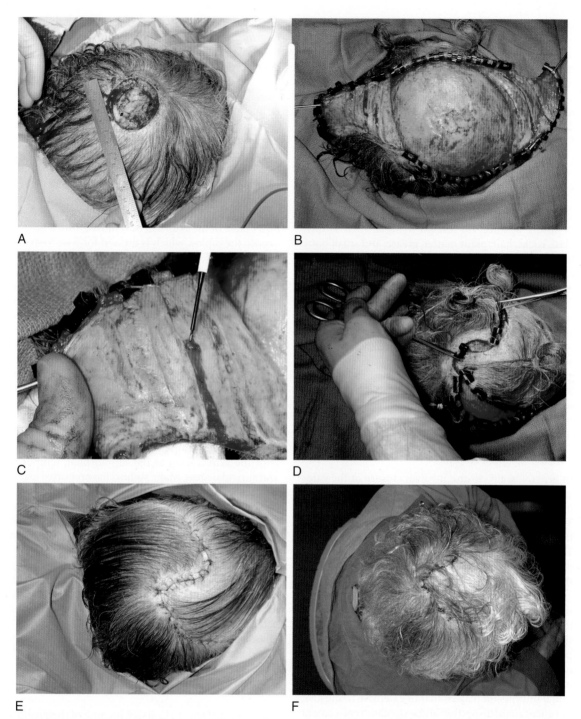

FIGURE 64-17. Scalp defects of more than 2 cm *(A)* will often require formation of scalp flaps *(B)* for closure. Scoring the galea with the electrocautery *(C)* or a scalpel will allow advancement of the flaps *(D)* and wound closure *(E)*. It is not necessary to shave any hair as a matter of routine in repair of scalp wounds unless visualization is impaired. The scalp tends to heal well *(F)*. Sutures are removed in about 14 days.

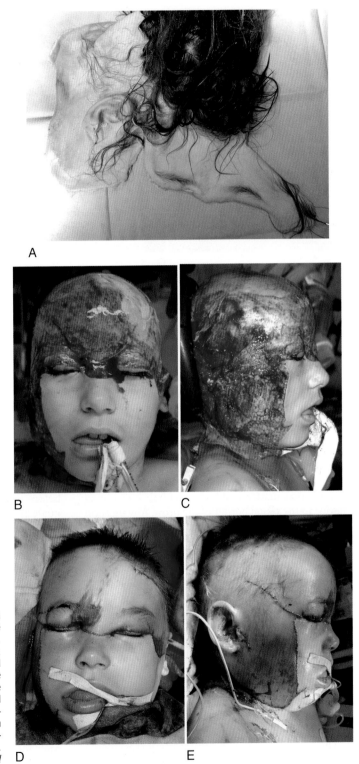

FIGURE 64-18. A 15-year-old girl with a total scalp avulsion after her hair became entangled in a machine. *A,* The avulsed scalp. *B* and *C,* The entire scalp, eyelids, right ear, face, and a portion of the neck were avulsed with the defect. Multiple vein grafts were needed for vascular anastomosis to the superficial temporal, supraorbital, and facial vessels. *D* and *E,* The patient is shown immediately after replantation with multiple vein grafts. The right side of the face was congested and required leech therapy for 6 days.

Continued

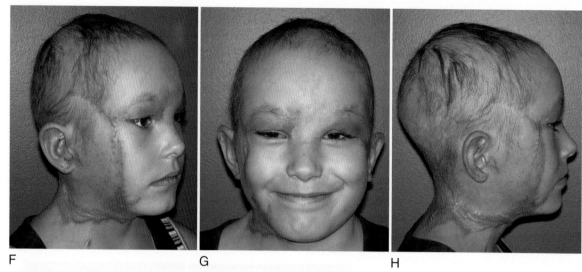

F   G   H

FIGURE 64-18, cont'd. *H,* The patient is shown 2 months after replantation of scalp, eyelids, right side of the face, and ear. An area on the posterior neck needed skin grafting.

nonverbal organs of communication and facial expression.[90-93] Several notable anatomic considerations are important in the treatment of soft tissue injuries in this area.

The most conspicuous aspect of the eyebrow is the pattern and direction of the associated hair follicles. The hair bulbs of the eyebrows extend deeply into the subcutaneous fat, placing them at risk if undermining is undertaken too superficially. The hairs grow from an inferior medial to superior lateral direction; therefore, an incision placed along the inferior aspect of the brow may inadvertently transect hair bulbs lying inferior to the visual border of the brow. Any incision in the brow should be beveled along an axis parallel to the hair shafts to avoid injury to the hair bulbs or shafts.

The temporal branch of the facial nerve innervates the frontalis muscle along its lateral margin at a point somewhat superior to the eyebrow. The nerve passes along a path from a point 0.5 cm inferior to the tragus to a point 1.5 cm superior to the outer extent of the eyebrow.[94] It travels in the deep portions of the superficial fascia in association with the anterior branches of the superficial temporal artery. The number of branches varies,[94] and there are few nerve crossovers.[57,95] When the area lateral to the eyebrow is undermined, the plane of dissection should be subcutaneous and thereby superficial to the nerve.

The supraorbital and supratrochlear nerves emerge from the supraorbital foramen or notch and medial aspect of the superior orbit, respectively. They pass superiorly deep to the frontalis and orbicularis oculi muscles to provide sensory innervation to the forehead and scalp. The supraorbital and supratrochlear vessels travel along with the nerves.

The lacrimal gland lies within the superior and lateral aspect of the orbit. With age, the gland becomes ptotic and subject to injury as it descends beyond the superior orbital margin.

Clinical Examination

Lacerations of the lateral brow area are common and place the temporal branch of the facial nerve at risk. The administration of local anesthetics will cause loss of temporal nerve function and mimic a nerve injury; therefore, temporal branch injury should be tested before the administration of anesthetics. After adequate anesthesia and irrigation, the underlying structures are inspected and palpated. In particular, the wound is inspected for possible frontal sinus fracture, orbital rim fractures, and foreign bodies.

TREATMENT

Treatment Goals

Reconstruction of the brow is difficult because the short, thick hair of the brows and the unique orientation of the hair shafts are nearly impossible to reproduce accurately. Therefore, every effort should be made to preserve and repair the existing brow tissue with as little distortion as possible.

Algorithm for Surgical Treatment

After the integrity of the frontal branch of the facial nerve has been tested, local infiltration with anesthetic will provide good anesthesia in most patients. Although generations of medical students have heard that the brow should never be shaved for fear that it will not grow back, there is no scientific evidence to support this belief.[96] It is rarely necessary to shave the brow, and it may make proper alignment of the eyebrow repair more difficult. If the brow prevents proper visualization, it may be lightly clipped.

After irrigation, the underlying structures are inspected and palpated. In particular, the wound is inspected for possible frontal sinus fracture, orbital rim fractures, and foreign bodies. Débridement of the wound should be conservative. Any tissue that has a potential to survive should be carefully sutured into position (Fig. 64-19). If clearly nonvital tissue must be removed, the incision should be made parallel to the hair shafts to minimize damage to the underlying hair follicles. The closure should not be excessively tight because constricting sutures may damage hair follicles and cause brow alopecia.

Most brow wounds are simple lacerations and as such may be closed by approximation of the underlying muscle layer with fine resorbable suture and of the skin with 5-0 or 6-0 nylon. Areas of full-thickness brow loss (up to 1 cm) with little or no injury to the

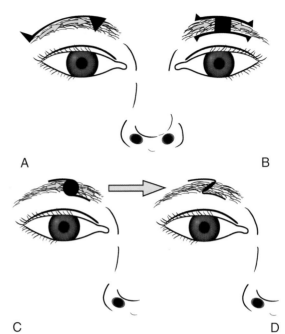

FIGURE 64-20. *A,* A Burow wedge triangle closure favors movement of the lateral brow medially. It affords easy alignment of the hair-bearing margin and a broad-based flap design. *B,* Two opposing rectangular flaps can be advanced with the aid of the Burow wedge triangle excisions. This flap also provides easy alignment of the brow margins but has a greater scar burden. The O to Z excision *(C)* and closure *(D)* result in some distortion of the eyebrow's hair orientation.

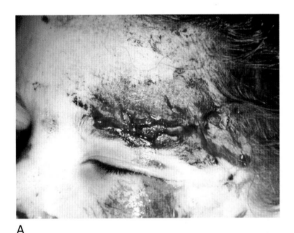

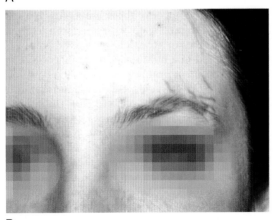

FIGURE 64-19. *A* and *B,* Initial débridement of eyebrow lacerations should be minimal. Even severely contused tissue will survive and usually lead to a result better than with any graft, flap, or hair transplantation.

surrounding area can be repaired primarily with a number of local advancement flaps including a Burow wedge advancement flap,[97] double advancement flap,[98] and O to Z repair (Fig. 64-20).[99] Primary closure of larger defects may distort the remainder of the brow excessively. The medial half of the brow is thicker and cosmetically more prominent, and therefore the illusion of symmetry is easier to preserve if the medial brow position is not disturbed. For this reason, it is generally better to advance the lateral brow medially to accommodate closure.[97] Small areas of tissue loss not amenable to primary closure should be allowed to heal by secondary intention. The resulting scar or deformity can be revised 6 to 12 months after the injury when the tissues have softened. Wound contracture and the passage of time may allow local flap reconstruction that was not initially possible. Larger defects may need to be reconstructed with a variety of scalp pedicle flaps[100-108] or individual hair follicle transplants.[109,110]

Specific Surgical Techniques

LOCAL FLAP. A variety of local brow advancement flaps have been described for brow reconstruction of smaller defects. The cosmetic focus of the brow is in its medial half where the hair growth is thickest. When possible, it is usually preferable to advance the lateral brow medially, rather than to advance the medial brow laterally, to close a defect. This is most important for defects of the medial brow. A Burow wedge advancement flap is suitable for these defects (Fig. 64-20A). On elevation of the flap to be advanced, it is important for the dissection to be of sufficient depth that the vulnerable hair follicles are not damaged. Defects of the lateral brow can be closed by advancing tissue from both directions with two advancement flaps (the so-called A to T closure) as long as there is no undue distortion of the medial brow.

The double advancement flap method that uses two rectangular flaps for closure affords capabilities similar to those of the Burow wedge rotation flap but requires four incisions (Fig. 64-20B). It is important for the margins of the hair-bearing skin to be accurately aligned in much the same way as the vermilion border is aligned for lip lacerations. Inaccurate repair will result in an unsightly step-off. Both the Burow wedge rotation flap and the double advancement flap closures make alignment of the hair-bearing margin relatively easy.

The O to Z closure that has also been advocated for repair of brow defects is not as easily applied (Fig. 64-20C and D). The movement of the flaps includes a vertical component and a larger degree of rotation. This means that the alignment of the hair-bearing margin is more difficult, and the orientation of the follicles is somewhat distorted.

LOCAL GRAFT. Full-thickness eyebrow grafting may be used for smaller defects of the brow when significant trauma of the surrounding tissue is not present (Fig. 64-21). It is best used for circular or elliptical defects. This technique is essentially a brow-sharing procedure that harvests a portion of the contralateral brow corresponding to the defect site. The graft is rotated 180 degrees and sutured into the defect. The donor site and the non–hair-bearing portion of the original defect are closed primarily. This technique has the advantage of simplicity and excellent hair quality match. The hair follicle is oriented properly in a medial to lateral direction; however, the orientation is not correct in an inferior to superior direction. It also has the disadvantage of producing an abnormality in the previously normal brow. Because this technique borrows from one brow to fix the other, the patient must have sufficiently thick brows.

Composite full-thickness grafts from the scalp have been used for brow reconstruction but rarely for the initial repair.[106,111] The grafts are usually taken full thickness from the occipital region because the hair grows in a circular pattern that more closely approximates a natural growth pattern when it is transposed

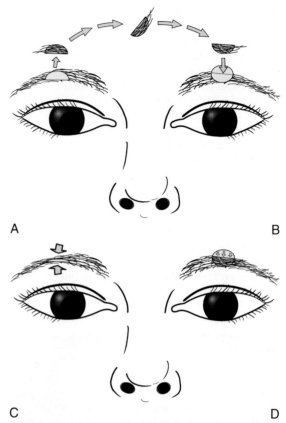

A   B

C   D

FIGURE 64-21. A and B, An eyebrow graft is harvested from the contralateral eyebrow and rotated 180 degrees before placement into the defect. C, The donor site is undermined and closed primarily. D, The brow defect extending above the hair-bearing skin is undermined and closed primarily. This results in some narrowing of both eyebrows, making this reconstruction better suited for patients with thicker eyebrows.

to the brow. A template of the missing brow is transferred to the occipital scalp, with care taken to orient the direction of hair growth to mimic the brow. The graft is excised in a full-thickness manner with scissors or knife. Electrocautery will burn the hair follicles and result in graft alopecia. The graft is carefully thinned of subcutaneous fat, leaving the follicles undisturbed. The graft is sutured into place with nonconstrictive sutures and covered with a light pressure dressing, both of which are removed in a week. Because the graft is full thickness, there is little graft retraction; thus, the graft will remain the same size.

Defects that include the eyebrow and a significant portion of non–hair-bearing skin can be reconstructed with a full-thickness graft that incorporates hair-bearing and non–hair-bearing scalp. Hair-bearing grafts have been harvested from the temporal hairline,[112] but the size of the graft for larger defects will result in visible scars that may not be acceptable. The postauricular region may allow a larger graft to be harvested from a more acceptable donor site.[111] A template is made from the defect that denotes hairless and hair-bearing areas of the defect. The template is transferred to the postauricular area, where the full-thickness graft is harvested at the junction of the subcutaneous tissue and galea. The graft is then placed in the recipient bed and sutured into position; a protective compression bandage is placed.

Many authors have described eyebrow reconstruction with pedicle grafts based on branches from the temporal artery.[100,101,104,106] Early descriptions used a frontal branch from the superficial temporal artery to support a flap from the frontal area. The disadvantage with this donor site is that it is a frequent site of hair loss in men, and the orientation of the hair follicles is not correct after flap transfer. The temporal and parietal areas are better donor sites and can be transferred by use of the temporal parietal artery.

Areas of brow alopecia can be camouflaged with hair transplantation.[109,110] Strips of hair-bearing scalp are harvested from the occipital area with a multibladed scalpel. The grafts are divided into single- and double-follicle grafts (Fig. 64-22). The two-hair grafts are inserted with a 1.3-mm round punch or large needle; the single grafts are inserted by small knife or needle punctures. The hairs are inserted obliquely to establish the normal angle and orientation of eyebrow hairs. That is to say that medially, the hairs are almost vertical, with a smooth progression to a more horizontal orientation laterally. The advantages of this technique are decreased hair density and more normal orientation of the hair compared with pedicle or free scalp grafts. The disadvantage is that the procedure is tedious and time-consuming, and the hairs must be regularly trimmed to proper length.

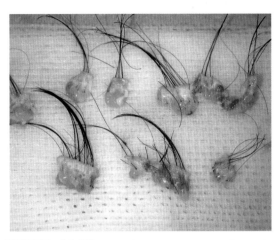

FIGURE 64-22. Hair follicles harvested from the occiput can be subdivided further into single and double follicles for transplantation into an eyebrow to camouflage an area of scar alopecia.

Eyelids

Treatment of eyelid injuries is important for preservation of the vital functions of the eyelids, namely, protection of the globe, prevention of drying, and appearance.

EVALUATION

Anatomy

The eyelids are composed of skin, areolar tissue, orbicularis oculi muscle, tarsus, septum orbitale, tarsal (meibomian) glands, and conjunctiva (Fig. 64-23). At the lid margin, the conjunctiva meets the skin at the gray line. Embedded within the margins of the lids are the hair follicles of the eyelashes. The tarsal plates are dense condensations of connective tissue that support and

FIGURE 64-23. Lower eyelid seen in cross section shows the lamellar nature of the eyelids. Repair of full-thickness eyelid lacerations should include repair of the conjunctiva, tarsal plate, and skin. The lash line or gray line should be used as an anatomic landmark to ensure proper alignment of the lid margin during repair.

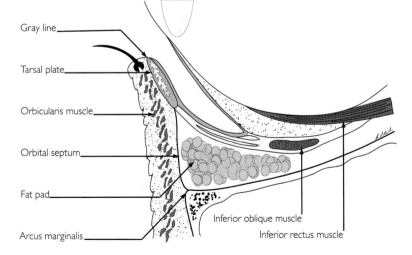

Gray line

Tarsal plate

Orbicularis muscle

Orbital septum

Fat pad

Arcus marginalis

Inferior oblique muscle

Inferior rectus muscle

give form to the eyelids and assist in keeping the conjunctiva in apposition to the globe.

The levator palpebrae muscle inserts into the skin of the upper lid and to the tarsal plate by Müller muscle. It is responsible for elevation of the upper lid and is innervated by the oculomotor nerve (CN III). The orbicularis oculi muscle surrounds the ocular aperture and is responsible for closing the eyelids; it is innervated by the facial nerve (CN VII). The pretarsal portion of the orbicularis oculi muscle is anchored medially and laterally to the medial and lateral canthus, respectively. The orbital septum is a thin fibrous sheet that extends from the tarsal plates to the circumference of the orbital rim. The orbital septum maintains the periorbital fat within the confines of the bony orbital cone.

The arterial supply of the eyelids is from the ophthalmic and facial arteries. The ophthalmic artery gives rise to the lacrimal and supraorbital arteries as it passes toward the medial orbital wall. The lacrimal artery traverses the lateral orbit to supply the lacrimal gland, pierce the orbital septum, and divide into the lateral palpebral branches of the lids. The supraorbital artery passes along the orbital roof before joining the supraorbital nerve to exit through the supraorbital foramen. The ophthalmic artery traverses the medial orbital wall, giving off the posterior ethmoidal and anterior ethmoidal arteries before dividing into the dorsal nasal, supratrochlear, and medial palpebral arteries. The medial and lateral palpebral arteries form tarsal arcades across the upper and lower lids about 2 to 4 mm from the lid's margins.[113]

The orbicularis oculi, procerus, and corrugator supercilii muscles are supplied by the zygomatic branches of the facial nerve (CN VII). The levator muscle opens the upper lid and is supplied by the oculomotor nerve (CN III). Sensory innervation of the upper lids is from the ophthalmic (CN V1) division of the trigeminal nerve by the lacrimal, supraorbital, supratrochlear, and infratrochlear nerves. The lower lid is supplied from the maxillary (CN V2) division of the trigeminal nerve by the zygomaticofacial and infraorbital nerves (see Fig. 64-4). The lacrimal gland is located in the upper outer margin of the orbit and produces tears that flow across the surface of the cornea toward the medial canthus, where they enter the superior and inferior puncta. The canaliculus passes about 2 mm perpendicular to the lid margin before heading medially toward the lacrimal sac and nasolacrimal apparatus, ultimately draining into the nose through the inferior meatus.

Clinical Examination

The eyelids are inspected for ptosis (suggesting levator apparatus injury) and rounding of the canthi (suggesting canthus injury or nasal-orbital-ethmoidal fracture). It may be helpful to tug on the lid with fingers

or forceps to check the integrity of the canthi. A firm endpoint should be felt. Epiphora may be a tip-off for canalicular injury. A search for concomitant globe or facial fractures should be undertaken.

Consultations and Multispecialty Approach to Care

Any injury to the eyelids should suggest a globe injury. If there is any doubt about ocular injury, an ophthalmology consultation is needed.

TREATMENT

Nonsurgical Versus Surgical Management

In general, nonsurgical treatment of eyelid injuries is not advisable because the natural contraction of secondary intention healing may distort the lid and result in lagophthalmos, ectropion, or distortion of the lid architecture (Fig. 64-24). However, some wounds are

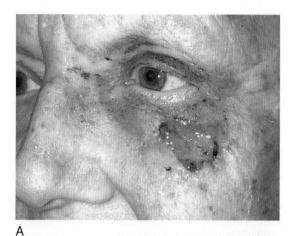

A

B

FIGURE 64-24. A superficial cheek avulsion injury *(A)* was allowed to heal by secondary intention *(B)*, resulting in a cicatricial ectropion. Any injury to the eyelids or on the upper cheek has the potential to distort the eyelid from the normal contractile forces of healing.

amenable to nonsurgical treatment[114-116]; wounds of the medial canthal area that do not involve the lid margin or lacrimal apparatus tend to do well, especially in the elderly, who have greater intrinsic laxity of the skin. Nonsurgical treatment should be reserved for those patients in whom primary closure is not possible because of tissue loss or when secondary intention healing is preferable to skin grafting or other reconstruction.

Specific Surgical Repairs

Simple lacerations of the eyelid that do not involve the lid margin or deeper structures may be minimally débrided and closed primarily. The eyelid is a layered structure; as such, full-thickness injuries should be repaired in layers. Repair of the conjunctiva, tarsal plate, and skin is usually sufficient. Small injuries to the conjunctiva do not require closure, but larger lacerations should be repaired with 5-0 gut suture. The tarsal plate should be repaired with a 5-0 absorbable suture, the skin with 6-0 nylon.

Lacerations that involve the lid margin require careful closure to avoid lid notching and misalignment. The technique involves placement of several "key" sutures of 6-0 nylon at the lid margin to align the gray line and lash line. These sutures are not initially tied but used as traction and alignment sutures. The conjunctiva and tarsal plate are repaired, and then the key sutures may be tied. The sutures are left long. Placement of subsequent skin sutures starts near the lid margin and works away. As each subsequent suture is placed and tied, the long ends of the suture nearer the lid margin are tied under the subsequent suture to prevent the loose ends from migrating toward the eye and irritating the cornea (Fig. 64-25). Avulsive injuries to the lids that involve only skin may be treated with full-thickness skin grafts from the postauricular region or contralateral upper eyelid. Lid-switch pennant flaps are also an option. Injuries that involve full-thickness loss of 25% of the lid may be débrided and closed primarily like any other full-thickness laceration. Loss of more that 25% of the lid will require more involved eyelid reconstruction covered in other chapters.

Any laceration to the medial third of the eyelids should suggest a canalicular injury (Fig. 64-26). The canaliculus is a white tubular structure that is more easily seen with 3× loupe magnification. If the proximal end of the canaliculus cannot be found, a lacrimal probe may be inserted into the punctum and passed distally out the cut end of the canaliculus. The canaliculus travels perpendicular to the lid margin for 2 mm and then turns medially to parallel the lid margin.

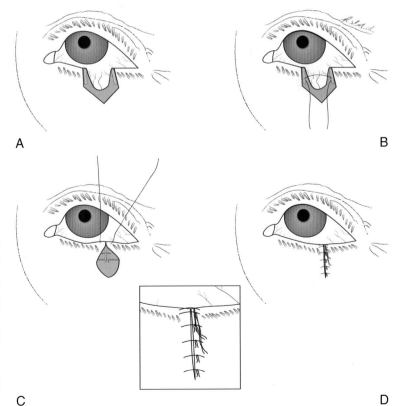

FIGURE 64-25. *A,* A full-thickness eyelid injury involves skin, tarsal plate, and conjunctiva. *B,* Repair starts with the conjunctiva and tarsal plate. *C,* A "key" suture is placed at the lash line to align the eyelid margin and prevent an unsightly step-off. The repair progresses from the lid margin outward (*D* and *inset*). The ends of each suture are left long, such that they are captured under the subsequent sutures. This prevents the loose suture ends from migrating up and irritating the eye.

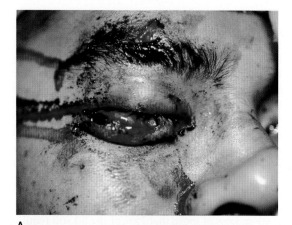

A

B

C

FIGURE 64-26. *A,* A lower lid laceration involving the medial third of the lid. *B,* A lacrimal probe is passed through the inferior punctum to identify the proximal end of the canaliculus. *C,* The canaliculus was repaired over a Silastic stent after the distal canalicular duct was located, and the lid was repaired in layers.

The distal end of the inferior canaliculus may be located by placing a pool of saline in the eye while instilling air into the other (intact) canaliculus. Bubbles will reveal the location of the distal canalicular stump. Once it is identified, the canaliculus is repaired over a small double-ended Silastic or polyethylene lacrimal stent with 8-0 absorbable sutures. The stent is left in place for 2 to 3 months.

Most patients with one intact canaliculus will not experience epiphora.[117,118] However, if repair can be accomplished at the time of injury without jeopardizing the intact canaliculus, most plastic surgeons would repair it. Good results are generally possible with repair over a stent.[119,120]

Cheek

EVALUATION

In repair of lacerations of the cheek, primary concern is for injury to the underlying structures, namely, facial nerve, facial muscles, parotid duct, and bone.

Anatomy

The blood supply of the cheek is derived primarily from the transverse facial and superficial temporal arteries. Generous collaterals and robust dermal plexus provide reliable perfusion after injury and reconstruction.

The facial nerve exits the stylomastoid foramen. It divides into five main branches within the substance of the parotid gland. The temporal and zygomatic branches run over the zygomatic arch; the buccal branch travels over the masseter along with the parotid duct. The mandibular branch usually loops below the inferior border of the mandible, but rarely more than 2 cm, and then rises above the mandibular border anterior to the facial artery and vein.[57,94,95,121-124] The zygomatic and buccal branches are at particular risk from cheek lacerations. The buccal branches usually have a number of interconnections, and therefore a laceration of a single buccal branch may not be clinically apparent.

The parotid gland is a single-lobed gland with superficial and deep portions determined by their relation to the facial nerve running between them. The superficial part of the gland is lateral to the facial nerve and extends anteriorly to the border of the masseter. The parotid duct exits the gland anteriorly and passes over the superficial portion of the masseter, penetrating the buccinator to enter the oral cavity opposite the upper second molar. The course of the parotid may be visualized on the external face by locating the middle third of a line drawn from the tragus to the middle of the upper lip (Fig. 64-27). The parotid duct travels adjacent to the buccal branches of the facial nerve. If buccal branch paralysis is noted in conjunction with a cheek laceration, parotid duct injury should be suspected.

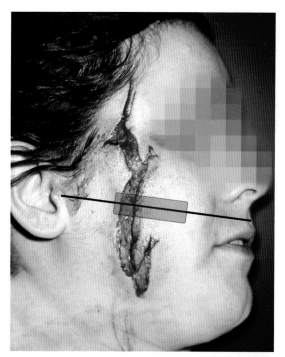

FIGURE 64-27. The middle third of a line between the tragus and the middle of the upper lip defines the course of the parotid duct. Evidence of injury to the zygomatic or buccal branch of the facial nerve or lacerations of the cheek near the area shaded in green should raise concern for parotid duct injury.

Clinical Examination

Clinical examination is directed toward identifying underlying injury to bone, facial nerve, or parotid duct. The function of facial nerve branches should be tested before administration of local anesthetics. Some patients will exhibit asymmetry in facial movement simply because of pain and edema not related to any underlying facial nerve injury.

Diagnostic Studies

If parotid duct injury is suspected, a 22-gauge catheter may be inserted into Stensen duct, and a small quantity of saline or methylene blue solution can be injected. This can be facilitated with a lacrimal probe, but care must be taken not to injure the duct with overzealous probing. If egress of the fluid from the wound is noted, the diagnosis of parotid duct injury has been made.

TREATMENT

Specific Surgical Repairs

REPAIR OF PAROTID GLAND OR DUCT. Laceration to the parotid gland without duct injury may result in a sialocele but will rarely cause any long-term problems. If a gland injury is suspected, the overlying soft tissue should be repaired and a drain left in place. If a sialocele develops, serial aspirations and a pressure dressing should be sufficient (Fig. 64-28).

FACIAL NERVE INJURY REPAIR. Facial nerve injuries should be primarily repaired. Surgical exploration and 3× magnification with good lighting and hemostasis will assist in locating the cut ends of the nerve. Wounds with contused, stellate lacerations will provide greater challenges to finding the nerve ends. A nerve stimulator can be used to locate the distal nerve segments within 48 hours of injury. After 48 hours, the distal nerve segments will no longer conduct an impulse to the involved facial musculature, rendering the simulator useless. If the proximal ends of the facial nerves cannot be located, the uninjured proximal nerve trunk can be located and followed distally to the cut end of the nerve. The nerves should be repaired primarily with 9-0 nylon. If primary repair is not possible, nerve grafts should be placed, or the proximal and distal nerve ends should be tagged with nonabsorbable suture for easy location during later repair.

Nose

The prominent position of the nose on the face places it at risk for frequent trauma. Many injuries result in nasal fractures without any soft tissue involvement. Nasal injuries are not life-threatening; however, failure to treat nasal injuries appropriately at the time of injury may result in distorted appearance or nasal obstruction due to loss of tissue, scarring, or misalignment of normal structures.

EVALUATION

Anatomy

The nose is a layered structure that in simplest terms can be thought of as an outer soft tissue envelope composed of skin, subcutaneous fat, and nasal muscles. A support structure to give the envelope shape is composed of cartilage and bone, and an endonasal mucosal lining filters particulates and exchanges heat and moisture.

The skin is thick and rich in dermal appendages, especially in the caudal half of the nose. The skin of the caudal nose is adherent to the lower lateral cartilage; in contrast, the skin over the bone and upper lateral cartilage is mobile. A rich vascular network of blood vessels runs just superficial to the musculoaponeurotic layer and is supplied by the lateral nasal, angular, alar, septal, external nasal, and superior labial arteries. The venous drainage is through the facial and ophthalmic veins.[125,126] Sensation to the external nose is provided by the supratrochlear nerve to the glabella, the infratrochlear nerve to the upper nasal sidewall, the infraorbital nerve to the ala and columella, and the external nasal branch of the anterior ethmoidal

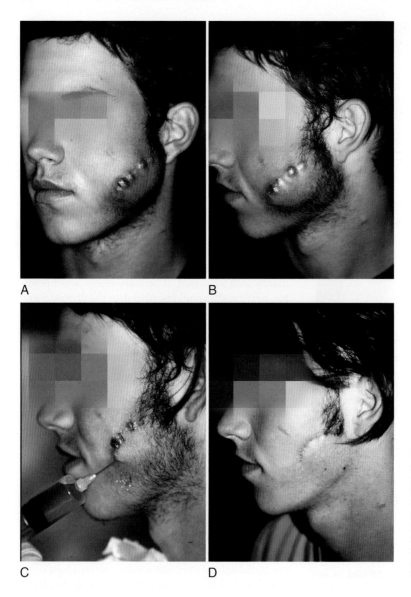

A   B

C   D

FIGURE 64-28. *A* and *B,* A laceration of the cheek may injure the substance of the parotid gland, resulting in an accumulation of saliva under the skin or a sialocele. If this is recognized at the time of injury, a drain may be left in place and a pressure dressing applied. *C* and *D,* When a sialocele presents after initial repair, serial aspirations and a pressure dressing will resolve the problem.

nerve to the caudal half of the dorsum and the tip. The nasal septum is supplied by the internal nasal branches of the anterior ethmoidal nerve anteriorly and the nasopalatine nerve inferiorly.[127]

The internal support structure of the nose is composed of bone and cartilaginous components. The bone component of the nose is made up of the nasal bone, the frontal process of the maxilla, and the nasal process of the frontal bone. Internally, the roof is formed by the cribriform plate of the ethmoid bone, frontal bone, and sphenoid bone. The cartilaginous framework is composed of paired lower lateral and upper lateral cartilages, quadrilateral cartilage of the septum, and several cartilaginous sesamoids.

The septum separates the left and right nasal passageways and provides support for the nasal dorsum. The structural component of the septum is composed of the septal cartilage, vomer bone, perpendicular plate of the ethmoid, maxillary crest, and premaxilla.

Internal nasal lining is covered by a mucous membrane of pseudostratified ciliated columnar epithelium except for the vestibule and nares, which are covered with stratified squamous epithelium, and the olfactory areas, which are covered with nonciliated pseudostratified columnar epithelium. Sensation of the lateral nasal lining is from the anterior ethmoidal nerve anteriorly, the posterolateral nasal branch from the pterygopalatine ganglion, the nasal branch of the anterior superior alveolar nerve to the anterior floor, and the internal nasal branch of the infraorbital nerve to the nares. The septum is also supplied by the anterior ethmoidal and internal nasal branches of the infraorbital nerves as well as by the nasopalatine nerves. The nasal lining is supplied by the anterior ethmoid, posterior ethmoid, and sphenopalatine arteries that supply both the medial and lateral lining. The septum is also supplied anteriorly by the superior labial and greater palatine arteries. The nasal septum is supplied by the internal nasal branches of the anterior ethmoidal nerve anteriorly and the nasopalatine nerve inferiorly.[127]

Clinical Examination

On examination of the nose, the three primary components (external covering, support structures, and lining) should be considered. The external soft tissue envelope can be quickly assessed after anesthesia and irrigation of lacerations or tissue loss. The support structures of the nose can be assessed by observation for asymmetry or deviation of the nasal dorsum. Fractures can usually be ascertained with palpation for bone step-off or crepitation. Significant nasal fractures are usually evident from clinical examination; radiographs rarely add significant information. If lacerations are present, they will provide a window to the underlying structures of the nose. After adequate anesthesia and irrigation, any open wounds are inspected for evidence of laceration or fractures of the upper lateral or lower lateral cartilages.

Examination of the internal nose requires a nasal speculum, good lighting, and suction if there is active bleeding. The mucosa is examined for any evidence of septal hematoma, mucosal laceration, or exposed or fractured septal cartilage. Septal hematomas will appear as a fusiform bluish boggy swelling of the septal mucosa. After adequate anesthesia and irrigation, the full nature of the injury to the support framework of the nose and lining can be appreciated.

Diagnostic Studies

Nasal fractures are common and should be suspected after blunt nasal trauma. Plain radiographs rarely add significant information to a thorough clinical examination in most isolated nasal injuries. If any other fractures of facial or paranasal structures are suspected, a facial computed tomographic scan should be acquired. The incidence of orbital injuries after major midfacial fractures has been reported to be as high as 59%.[128]

TREATMENT

Treatment Goals

The goal is to restore normal nasal appearance without subsequent nasal obstruction.

Anesthesia

Less complex nasal injuries can be managed with local anesthesia; major nasal injuries are best managed with general anesthesia. For injuries that involve the septum or nasal mucosa, topical application of 4% cocaine on cotton pledgets is used to provide anesthesia and vasoconstriction. The cotton pledgets are saturated with the cocaine solution and then squeezed out to remove excess cocaine. The placement of the pledgets should not be haphazard but should be specifically targeted. One pledget is placed into the nose anteriorly just under the dorsum where the anterior ethmoidal nerve enters the nose. A second pledget is placed just under the middle turbinate and posteriorly in the area of the nasopalatine nerve. A third pledget may be placed on the floor of the nose.

After the topical anesthesia has been placed, local infiltration with 0.5% lidocaine with 1:100,000 epinephrine is commenced. Some recommend mixing a fresh solution to augment the final epinephrine concentration to 1:50,000. In general, local infiltration into the wound is preferable to block anesthesia because of the vasoconstrictive effects of the epinephrine.

Nonsurgical Versus Surgical Management

Laceration of the nose should be repaired primarily when possible. Smaller avulsive injuries of the cephalic third of the nose may be allowed to heal by secondary intention because of the mobility and laxity of the overlying skin in this area. Avulsive injuries to the remainder of the nose, if they are allowed to heal by secondary intention, will cause distortion of the nasal architecture by contractile forces during healing.

Algorithm for Surgical Treatment

In general, the repair of nasal trauma begins with the nasal lining and proceeds from internal structures to external by repair of the lining, framework, and finally skin.

Specific Surgical Repairs and Techniques

ABRASIONS. Nasal abrasions tend to heal rapidly and well because of the rich vascular supply. The skin of the caudal half of the nose is rich in skin appendages that allow rapid epithelialization. Traumatic tattooing is not uncommon after nasal abrasions. Late treatment of an established traumatic tattoo is difficult. The best opportunity to avoid this difficult problem is at the time of the injury. Meticulous cleaning of the wound with pulsed lavage, loupe magnification to remove embedded particles, and conservative débridement are needed. On occasion, one is faced with the difficult decision to débride further, thereby forming a full-thickness wound, or to leave some embedded material within the dermis. In general, faced with such a decision, it is best to stop the débridement and proceed with excision and reconstruction later if needed for cosmesis.

SEPTAL HEMATOMA. A septal hematoma should be evacuated to prevent subsequent infection and septic necrosis of the septum or organization of the clot into a calcified, subperichondrial fibrotic mass. If a clot has yet to form within the hematoma, aspiration is possible with a large-bore needle. Evacuation that is more reliable can be achieved with a small septal incision in the mucosa of the hematoma. The blood and clot are evacuated with a small suction cannula, and a through-and-through running 4-0 chromic gut suture is placed across the septum to close the dead space and prevent reaccumulation of the blood.

LACERATION

Lining. The lining of the nose should be repaired with thin absorbable sutures such as 5-0 chromic gut sutures. Because of the confined working space, a needle with a small radius of curvature will facilitate placement of the sutures. The knots should be placed facing into the nasal cavity. Small areas of exposed septal cartilage associated with septal fractures or mucosal lacerations will not pose a significant problem as long as intact mucosa is present on the other side. If lining is missing from both sides, a mucosal flap should be used to cover at least one side.

Framework. Fractures of the septum should be reduced, and if the septum has become subluxed off the maxillary ridge, it should be reduced back toward the midline. Lacerations of the upper or lower lateral cartilages should be repaired anatomically if they are structurally significant. Usually 5-0 absorbable or clear nonabsorbable sutures should be used. Displaced bone fragments within the wound should be repositioned anatomically and wired or removed if they are not needed to maintain the structure or shape of the nose. One should make an effort not to detach bone from its soft tissue attachments to preserve its blood supply. If loss of important support structures has occurred, reconstruction of the nasal support must be undertaken within a few days. Delay will result in contraction and collapse of the soft tissues of the nose. Later reconstruction is almost impossible. Reconstruction of this type will usually involve bone or cartilage grafts. If there is doubt about the viability of lining or coverage over the area where grafted cartilage or bone will be placed, reconstruction should be delayed for a few days until the survival of the soft tissue coverage is no longer in doubt, or secondary soft tissue reconstruction can be accomplished.

Covering. After repair of the lining and framework, the skin of the nose can be repaired. Key sutures should be placed at the nasal rim to ensure proper alignment before the remainder of the closure with 6-0 nylon suture. The mobile skin of the cephalic nose is forgiving and can be undermined and mobilized to close small avulsive wounds. To prevent suture track scarring, the sutures should be removed in 4 days.

AVULSIVE INJURIES. Avulsive injuries are frequently the result of automobile crashes and animal or human bites. They usually involve only skin but may involve portions of the underlying cartilage. One is frequently faced with the decision to proceed with nasal reconstruction with a local flap or to cover temporarily with a skin graft. Smaller defects of the cephalic portion of the dorsum and sidewalls will heal by secondary intention without significant distortion of the anatomy. The skin of the caudal dorsum, tip, and ala is adherent and less mobile and will often defy primary closure. Secondary intention healing will result in contraction and distortion of the nasal anatomy, and treatment with a retroauricular skin graft is best (Fig. 64-29). Retroauricular full-thickness skin grafts have excellent color and texture match. The healed skin graft limits most wound contraction. If secondary reconstruction is needed, the skin graft can be excised and a local flap reconstruction can be performed later.

DEGLOVING. Degloving is an extension along a continuum from laceration to amputation. Degloving is typically seen in motor vehicle accidents and animal bites. The soft tissues of the nose may be attached by a small superiorly or laterally based flap.[129] The nasal tissue has a remarkable blood supply and may survive on surprisingly small pedicles. The repair follows the logical sequence of mucosa, bone and cartilaginous support structures, and then the degloved skin. If the skin flap is not viable, microvascular salvage can be attempted; however, the likelihood of finding undamaged vessels of adequate caliber is low. Some have advocated closure of the wounds followed by anticoagulation and cooling as well as multiple small stab wounds or leech therapy for venous drainage.[130]

AMPUTATED FRAGMENTS. Small amputated fragments can be reattached as a composite graft,[131,132] but some warn of the risk of poor outcome and infection after reattachment of bite amputations.[133,134] Davis and Shaheen[135] have reported up to 50% failure of composite grafts even under ideal conditions. They recommend that composite grafts be attempted only when the wound edges are cleanly cut, there is little risk of infection, the repair is not delayed, no part of the graft is more than 0.5 cm from viable cut edge of the wound, and all bleeding is controlled. Others have advocated hyperbaric oxygen therapy[132] or cooling[130] to improve tissue survival. Microsurgical replantation may be possible with larger amputated nasal segments[136] or with nose and lip composites.[137]

Outcomes

Late complications of nasal injury include nasal stenosis, septal deviation, loss of nasal support, and scar contractures.

Ears

Traumatic ear injuries may result from mechanical trauma by motor vehicle crashes, boxing, wrestling, sports, industrial accidents, ear piercing, and animal or human bites. Thermal burns to the ear are seen in

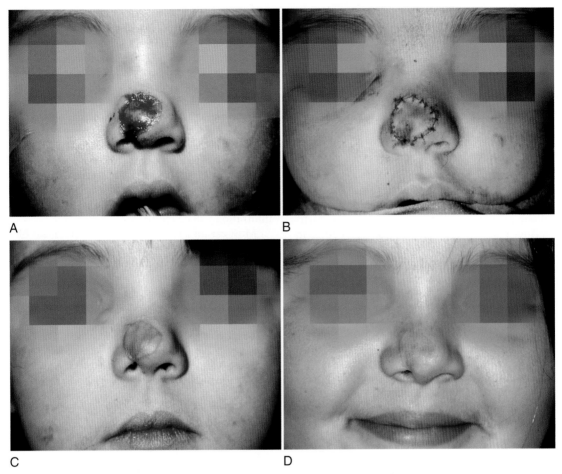

FIGURE 64-29. *A* and *B*, A full-thickness dog bite avulsion injury to the nose was treated with a full-thickness retroauricular skin graft. *C*, The patient is shown 6 weeks after grafting. *D*, Two years later, there is good contour and color match.

more than 90% of patients with other head and neck burns.[138] The ears are at particular risk because they are thin and exposed on two sides.

EVALUATION

Anatomy

STRUCTURE. The skin of the anterior ear is tightly adherent to the underlying auricular fibrocartilage that gives shape to the external ear. The posterior skin is somewhat thicker and more mobile. The anterior surface is rich in topography; the posterior surface is simple. The external ear has some function in assisting with sound gathering and localization.

BLOOD SUPPLY. The ear has a rich blood supply primarily from branches of the superficial temporal artery and the posterior auricular artery. The superficial temporal artery supplies the lateral surface of the auricle from upper, middle, and lower branches that are interconnected with branches of the posterior auricular artery. The posterior auricular artery sup-

plies the posterior surface, lobule, and retroauricular skin from three to five branches that pass toward the auricular rim. Cartilaginous fenestrations allow the posterior auricular branches to pass to the anterior surface of the ear, forming a dense interconnected network of vessels.[139] The occipital artery may contribute to the posterior ear and in 7% of the population will be the dominant supply to the posterior ear.[140] The venous drainage of the ear is by the posterior auricular veins into the external jugular vein and the superficial temporal and retromandibular veins that drain the anterior auricle.

NERVE SUPPLY. The great auricular nerve (cervical plexus C2, C3) ascends from Erb point at the midpoint of the posterior border of the sternocleidomastoid muscle and ascends toward the ear, often traveling next to and slightly posterior to the external jugular vein to supply sensation to the lower half of the anterior and posterior surfaces of the ear. The auriculotemporal branch from the mandibular branch (V3) of the trigeminal nerve (see Fig. 64-4) ascends with the superficial temporal vessels and gives several branches to supply the anterior superior portions of the auricle and external auditory canal. The lesser occipital nerve (cervical plexus C2, C3) supplies sensation to the posterior superior aspect of the ear. The concha and posterior auditory canal are supplied by the auricular branch of the vagus nerve (CN X) known as Arnold nerve. This nerve travels along the ear canal and is not anesthetized by a ring block of the ear.

Clinical Examination

A clinical examination is generally all that is required for diagnosis and treatment of ear trauma. The pinna should be examined to determine whether there has been any tissue loss or injury to the auricular cartilage. After blunt trauma or a surgical procedure, an auricular hematoma may develop; this is a collection of blood under the perichondrium that can take several hours to accumulate. It presents as a painful swelling that obliterates the normal contours of the anterior surface of the ear (Fig. 64-30).

TREATMENT

Treatment Goals

The goals of treatment are to restore cosmetic appearance of the ear, to maintain a superior auricular sulcus that can accommodate eyeglasses, and to minimize later complications from infection or fibrosis.

Algorithm for Surgical Treatment

ANESTHESIA

Ear Block. The four nerves supplying the majority of the external ear can be anesthetized by placing a ring of local anesthetic around the ear. Insert a 1.5-inch needle at the junction of the earlobe and the head and advance it subcutaneously toward the tragus while infiltrating 2 or 3 mL of anesthetic. Pull the needle back and redirect it posteriorly along the posterior auricular sulcus, again injecting 2 or 3 mL. Reinsert the needle at the superior junction of the ear and the head. Direct the needle along the preauricular sulcus toward the tragus and inject 2 or 3 mL. Pull the needle back and redirect it along the posterior auricular sulcus while injecting anesthetic to complete a ring block. Care should be taken to avoid the temporal artery along the preauricular sulcus. If it is inadvertently entered, apply pressure for 10 minutes. Remember that Arnold nerve supplies a portion of the concha and external auditory canal; if anesthesia is needed in this area, local infiltration will be required.

Most ear injuries will not require a total ear block and can be managed with local infiltration of anesthetic. Although there is a theoretical concern of tissue necrosis when epinephrine is used in any appendage (in medical school we learned "finger, toes, penis, nose, and ears"), there are no good data to support this. Most plastic surgeons routinely use 1:100,000 epinephrine in the local anesthetics for ear infiltration. The advantages are prolonged duration of anesthesia and less bleeding. Complications attributed to the anesthetic infiltration are extremely rare.

Specific Surgical Repairs

HEMATOMA. The most common complication of blunt trauma to the ear is the development of an auricular hematoma. Blunt trauma may cause a shearing force that separates the cartilage from the overlying soft tissue and perichondrium. Inevitably, there is bleeding into the space that further separates the cartilage and perichondrium. The clinical appearance is of a convex ear with loss of the normal contours (see Fig.

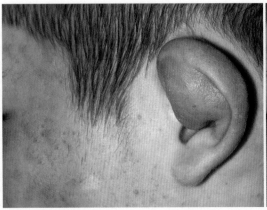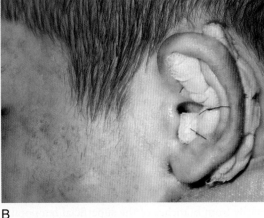

A   B

FIGURE 64-30. *A,* An auricular hematoma after a wrestling injury. The collection of blood must be drained to prevent organization and calcification of the hematoma. Untreated hematomas will result in "cauliflower ear." *B,* After evacuation, a through-and-through bolster should be molded and secured to the ear to prevent reaccumulation of the hematoma.

64-30). If it is left untreated, the blood will clot and eventually develop into a fibrotic mass that obliterates the normal ear topography. Over time (and with repeated injury), the fibrotic mass may develop into a calcified bumpy irregular mass, leading to what is known as a cauliflower ear. Ear cartilage depends on the adjacent soft tissue for blood supply, and therefore separation of the cartilage from the perichondrium places the cartilage at risk for necrosis and infection.

The treatment of ear hematoma is evacuation of the hematoma, control of the bleeding, and pressure to prevent an accumulation of blood and to encourage adherence of the soft tissues to the cartilage. Simple aspiration within a few hours of the injury may evacuate the blood, but without any other treatment, hematoma or seroma will reaccumulate.[141,142] Some have advocated use of a small liposuction cannula to more effectively evacuate the hematoma.[143] Aspiration with subsequent pressure dressing has been used effectively.[144,145] Most authors recommend a surgical approach for more reliable removal of adherent fibrinous material that may delay healing of the soft tissue to the cartilage.[141,145-155]

Surgical drainage can be accomplished with an incision placed parallel to the antihelix and just inside of it where the scar can be hidden. The skin and perichondrial flap are gently elevated, and a small suction cannula is used to evacuate the hematoma. If adherent fibrinous material remains, it should be removed with forceps. After the wound is irrigated, it is inspected for bleeding that may require cautery for control. There are many different methods of pressure dressing. Some mold saline-soaked cotton behind the ear and then mold more cotton into the anterior contours of the ear.[147] This is followed by a head wrap dressing. Others have used thermoplastic splints molded to the ear.[156] It is preferable to mold Xeroform (petrolatum jelly and bismuth tribromophenate impregnated) gauze into the ear contours and to secure the bolsters with several 3-0 nylon through-and-through mattress sutures (see Fig. 64-30B). A head wrap dressing is applied, and the sutures and bolsters are removed in 1 week.

LACERATIONS. Simple lacerations should be irrigated and minimally débrided. As in other areas of the face, the blood supply of the ear is robust and will support large portions of the ear on small pedicles. The cartilage depends on the perichondrium and soft tissue for its blood supply; as long as one surface of the cartilage is in contact with viable tissue, it should survive. Known landmarks such as the helical rim or antihelix should be reapproximated with a few key sutures. The remainder of the repair is accomplished with 5-0 or 6-0 nylon skin sutures. It is important that the closure be accurate with slight eversion of the wound edges, by use of vertical mattress sutures if

needed. Any inversion will persist after healing and result in unsightly grooves across the ear.[157] It is usually not necessary to place sutures in the cartilage, and most authors prefer to rely on the soft tissue repair alone.[147,154,158-162] There is some concern that suturing of the cartilage is detrimental,[163] leading to necrosis and increased risk of infection. If cartilage must be sutured, an absorbable 5-0 suture is best.[164]

There are no good data on the use of postoperative antibiotics after repair of ear lacerations. However, many authors recommend a period of prophylactic antibiotics to prevent suppurative chondritis, especially for larger injuries or those with degloved or poorly perfused cartilage.[165-171] There is no role for postoperative antibiotics after repair of simple lacerations of the ear.

THERMAL BURN. The most important consideration in the treatment of thermal burns of the ear is prevention of suppurative chondritis. A full-thickness burn of the ear invariably damages and exposes the underlying cartilage. Because the cartilage is avascular, a burn may result in loss of coverage and blood supply, setting the stage for loss or infection of the cartilage. The overall risk of complete loss of the ear in a series of 100 ear burns was 13%.[172]

The management of the burned ear is aimed at preventing a partial-thickness burn from becoming a full-thickness injury. Avoidance of pressure on the ear is of paramount importance in preventing compromise of an already injured ear.[173] This is best accomplished by use of a ring-shaped pad rather than a conventional pillow. The application of topical antibiotics, such as 0.5% silver nitrate solution on gauze and p-aminomethylbenzene sulfonamide (Sulfamylon) ointment, will reduce surface contamination. Regular cleaning and application of topical antibiotics are effective in allowing partial-thickness burns to heal.[138,173]

The management of a full-thickness burn depends on whether there is exposed cartilage and personal preference. In the absence of exposed cartilage, some authors recommend allowing the wound to form a dry eschar that becomes a protective biologic dressing for the cartilage.[174] They allow the eschar to separate spontaneously over time and apply skin grafts to the resultant granulation tissue at a later date. Others advocate early excision of the damaged skin with a dermabrader and immediate grafting. If cartilage becomes exposed, they excise it and approximate the adjacent soft tissue.[173]

When there is exposed cartilage, it must be covered with vascularized tissue. Either the framework is buried under a postauricular skin flap or a local flap of cervical skin and platysma muscle[175] or a temporoparietal fascial flap is placed with skin graft.[176,177]

SUPPURATIVE CHONDRITIS. Suppurative chondritis is most commonly seen in patients with ear burns, but it may develop after other ear trauma and even ear piercings.[178] It is most commonly seen 3 to 5 weeks after injury and is characterized by a dull progressive ear pain associated with edema and inflammation. An abscess will occasionally develop and drain with temporary relief of the symptoms. The most common organism implicated in suppurative chondritis is *Pseudomonas aeruginosa,* often in association with *Staphylococcus aureus* or *Proteus mirabilis.*[138]

Simple incision and drainage are insufficient treatment because the stiff cartilage cannot contract to obliterate the abscess cavity as soft tissue would. Some advocate a "bivalve" technique, in which the ear is incised along the helical rim and antibiotic-soaked gauze is inserted and changed daily.[138,179] This technique may be associated with an increased risk of subsequent deformity. Others have used irrigation of polymyxin B 0.25% solution through small polyethylene catheters every 3 hours for 5 days.[180] Others have had success by simply injecting culture-specific antibiotics directly into the ear for 7 to 10 days.[181] Iontophoresis has been successfully used to deliver antibiotics into the ear.[182,183] The technique relies on the migration of gentamicin or penicillin through an applied electrical field into the ear cartilage.

AUDITORY CANAL STENOSIS. When an injury involves the external auditory canal, scarring and contracture may result in stenosis or occlusion of the canal. Canal injuries should be stented to prevent stenosis.[154] If a portion of the canal skin is avulsed out of the bony canal, it may be repositioned and stented into place as a full-thickness skin graft.

AVULSIVE INJURIES. Avulsive injuries to the ear are most often the result of human and animal bites or motor vehicle crashes. Every attempt should be made to salvage an avulsed segment because an ear restored with meticulous repair will usually be superior to any that can be reconstructed de novo. If the avulsed segment dies, the subsequent deformity can be severe and require complex reconstruction. Ear avulsions may be classified into four general categories on the basis of pedicle size relative to the avulsed part and the availability of any amputated portions of the ear:

- partial amputation with a wide pedicle
- partial amputation with a narrow pedicle
- complete amputation with all or a portion of the amputated ear available
- complete amputation with no portion of the ear available

This classification provides a general framework for understanding the injuries and guiding treatment.[184]

Partial Amputation with a Wide Pedicle. If the pedicle is relatively large, it should provide adequate perfusion and venous drainage of the segment or fragment (Fig. 64-31). The prognosis is excellent after conservative débridement and meticulous repair. Because there is no way to quantitatively assess for the adequacy of venous drainage, the ear should be observed during the first 4 to 6 hours for any signs of venous congestion if there is any concern that drainage may not be adequate. If venous congestion develops, leech therapy should be instituted.

Partial Amputation with a Narrow Pedicle. When the amputated portion of the ear is attached by a small pedicle, one must consider the size of the pedicle relative to the amputated portion and make a judgment about whether the pedicle can provide adequate perfusion to sustain the amputated segment. An ear fragment that contains primarily soft tissue (e.g., the lobule) is more likely to survive than is a similarly sized fragment that contains more cartilage.[147,184,185] Surprisingly small pedicles can provide for good arterial inflow, but the risk of venous congestion is much higher. The avulsed portion must be observed during the first 4 to 6 hours for venous congestion; if it develops, leech therapy should be instituted. In 5 to 7 days or more, adequate venous drainage will re-establish itself. Ongoing blood loss during this time will require blood transfusion, typically 4 to 6 units. Prophylactic antibiotics to cover *Aeromonas hydrophila* (a commensal organism in the leech gut) should be given.

If the pedicle is narrow with inadequate or no perfusion, the avulsed portion should be treated like a complete amputation (see next section) or the perfusion should be augmented with local flaps.[162,176,177,186-191] Many varieties of local or regional flaps have been devised for ear salvage; all rely on apposition of the flap to dermabraded dermis or denuded cartilage. Some have advocated elevation of a mastoid skin flap and application of the flap to a dermabraded portion on the lateral[186] or medial[162] surface of the avulsed ear; others have dermabraded the avulsed part and placed it into a subcutaneous retroauricular pocket. In 2 to 4 weeks, the ear is removed from the pocket and allowed to spontaneously epithelialize.[154,163,190,192-194] These techniques are simple and provide a period of nutritive support until the wound heals and the ear becomes self-sustaining. They further preserve the delicate relationship between cartilage and dermis so important in maintaining the subtle folds and architecture that give an ear its shape.

Some authors have recommended similar techniques that remove the entire dermis and then cover denuded cartilage under retroauricular skin,[195] under a cervical flap,[196] or with a tunnel procedure.[197,198] Others have used a temporoparietal fascial flap to cover the denuded cartilage and then cover the temporoparietal fascial flap with a skin graft.[199] Another method involves removal of the posterior skin from the avulsed part and fenestration of the remaining cartilage in

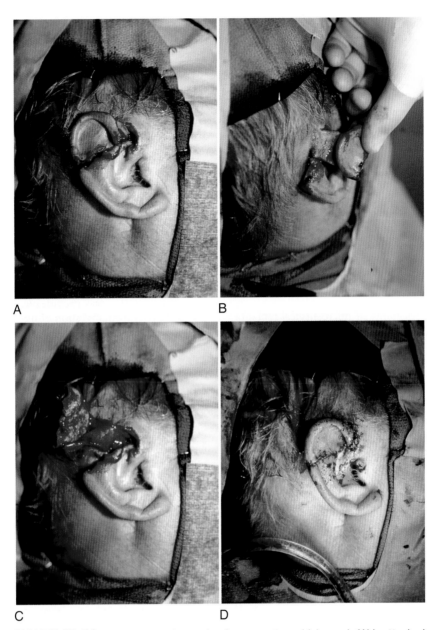

A   B

C   D

FIGURE 64-31. An upper ear laceration from a motor vehicle crash *(A)* is attached by a posterior skin bridge *(B* and *C)*. The upper auricle survived on this pedicle because of the generous blood supply of the ear. The helical rim was sutured first for alignment *(D)*, and the remainder of the skin was closed with 6-0 nylon.

several areas, then surfacing of the posterior part with a mastoid skin flap.[200] The idea behind the cartilage fenestrations is to allow vascular ingrowth from the posterior to the anterior surface to increase the likelihood of survival. One criticism of all of the methods that attempt to cover denuded cartilage is that the subtle architecture of the ears is often lost, resulting in a distorted, thick, formless disk.[184]

When the pedicle is small, one may choose to proceed as if the avulsed portion were a complete ampu-

tation (see following section). In this instance, do not divide the small pedicle for the sake of convenience; even a very small pedicle can provide some perfusion and, more important, some venous drainage over time.

Complete Amputation (Complete or Partial Segment Available). Amputated ear fragments are difficult to reconstruct; and the larger the defect, the more challenging and time-consuming the reconstruction. Reattachment of amputated facial fragments as composite grafts has a long history dating at least to 1551.[201] Contemporary reports describe occasional successes and many failures.[166,184,190,200-203] A good outcome after simple reattachment of a composite graft is more often the exception rather than the rule. The final outcome is often marred by scar, hyperpigmentation, partial loss, and deformity.[154] Spira and Hardy[174] stated that "if the amputated portion consists of anything more than the lobe or segment of helix, replacement is invariably doomed."

In an effort to salvage the cartilage, many authors have advocated burying it in a subcutaneous pocket in the abdomen[174,204-208] or under a postauricular flap.[195] Mladick[163,194,209,210] improved on these techniques by dermabrading the skin, rather than removing it, before placement in a subcutaneous pocket. This has the advantage of preserving the delicate relationship between the dermis and cartilage, which is important for maintaining the subtle architecture of the ear.

In 1966, the feasibility of microsurgical replantation of an amputated ear was demonstrated in rabbits by Buncke and Schulz,[211] and in 1976, the first ear replantation (as part of a scalp replantation) was reported.[70] Many reports of ear replantation followed, and it became clear that venous congestion was a common occurrence that accounted for the majority of failures.[212] Some authors have recommended prophylactic medicinal leech therapy because of the high incidence of venous congestion.[213]

Microsurgical replantation should be considered whenever it is feasible for patients who do not have concomitant trauma or medical conditions that would preclude a lengthy operation. The ear has fairly low metabolic demands and will tolerate prolonged periods of ischemia; successful replantation has been reported after 33 hours of cold ischemia time.[214] After sharp injuries, the branches from the superficial temporal artery or posterior auricular artery may be identifiable and repairable. In some patients, a leash of superficial temporal artery may be brought down to the ear. In a similar manner, veins may be repaired primarily or with vein grafts. Nerves may be repaired if they can be identified; surprisingly, however, a number of replanted ears without any nerve repair are reported to have had good sensation.[215] A protective dressing is placed that will allow clinical monitoring for arterial or venous compromise.

There is no consensus about whether anticoagulation is beneficial in ear replantation. Most authors would advocate intravenous dextran 40 at 20 to 30 mL/hr or aspirin for 5 to 7 days. Heparin is usually reserved for those patients who have had vascular problems intraoperatively. If venous congestion is encountered, leech therapy should be instituted until the congestion resolves. A review of the ear replantation literature reveals that the average operative time is 6 hours, with an average hospital stay of 11.4 days. The average number of blood transfusions is 5.94 units, and the most common complication is venous congestion.[216]

Complete Amputation (No Portion Available). When the amputated segment is unavailable, the ear should be reconstructed by the standard reconstructive methods appropriate for the particular defect.

Mouth

EVALUATION

Anatomy

The lips are the predominant feature of the lower third of the face; they are important for oral competence, articulation, expression of emotion, kissing, sucking, and playing of various musical instruments and as a symbol of beauty. In addition, the lips are important sensory organs that may provide pleasure and protect the oral cavity from ingestion of unacceptably hot or cold materials.

The external landmarks of the lips are the philtral columns and interposed philtral dimple extending from the columella down to the Cupid's bow at the central upper vermilion border. The central portion of the upper lip has a central tubercle. The upper and lower lips are joined at the commissure. The upper lip is set apart from the surrounding cheek by the nasolabial fold; the lower lip is divided from the chin by a curved mental crease. The nasolabial and mental creases are important to facial aesthetics and afford a location for camouflage of scar.

The lip is a laminar structure composed of inner mucosal lining and associated minor salivary glands, orbicularis oris muscle, and outer subcutaneous tissue and skin. Closure of lip lacerations should include repair of all of these structures.

The primary function of the lips is sphincteric. This function is accomplished by the action of the orbicularis oris muscle. Other facial muscles are important for facial expression and clearing the gingival sulci but are not important in maintaining oral competence. The primary motor nerves of the lips are the buccal and marginal mandibular branches of the facial nerve. The orbicularis oris muscle is innervated entirely by the buccal branch; the depressors of the lower lip are innervated by the marginal mandibular branch. The sensory innervation of the lips is by the infraorbital (V2) and mental (V3) branches of the trigeminal nerve.

The arterial supply to the lips is by the superior and inferior labial arteries branching from the external maxillary artery. The venous drainage of the lips is into the anterior facial vein. Lymphatic drainage is primarily through the submental and submandibular lymph nodes.[217]

Clinical Examination

The oral cavity should be carefully examined for dental, dentoalveolar, oral mucosal, tongue, and palate injuries.

TREATMENT

Treatment Goals

Repair of the lip must provide for oral competence, adequate mouth opening, sensation, complete skin cover, oral lining, and the appearance of vermilion.[218] The restoration of the mental and nasolabial crease lines, philtral columns, and precisely aligned vermilion border is an important cosmetic goal.

Nonsurgical Versus Surgical Management

Nonsurgical management is appropriate for smaller intraoral lacerations of the buccal mucosa, gingiva, or tongue. Nonsurgical management of electrical cord burns to the commissure is appropriate as well.

Specific Surgical Repairs

The majority of lip lacerations can be managed in the outpatient setting after infiltration of local anesthetic with epinephrine. If the laceration involves the white roll or vermilion border, it may be useful to mark this important landmark with a needle dipped in Bonnie blue or methylene blue before infiltration with larger amounts of local anesthetic because subsequent vasoconstriction may obscure the vermilion border.

A good rule of thumb is to work from the inside of the mouth outward. To this end, urgent dental or dentoalveolar injuries should be treated first so that repaired soft tissue does not limit access for treatment later. The wounds are gently irrigated to remove any loose particles and debris. In most patients, normal saline applied with a 30-mL syringe and an 18-gauge angiocatheter will be sufficient. If there is evidence of broken teeth and the fragments are not accounted for, a radiograph is obtained to make sure the tooth fragments are not embedded within the soft tissues. Dead or clearly nonviable tissue is débrided; once again, tissue of the face, and of the lips in particular, can survive on small pedicles that would be inadequate on any other part of the body. Fortunately, the lips have sufficient redundancy and elasticity that loss of up to 25% to 30% of the lip can be closed primarily. This also means that unlike in many other areas of the face, more aggressive débridement may be undertaken.

Tongue Repair. The tongue has a rich blood supply, and injuries to the tongue may cause significant blood loss. In addition, subsequent tongue swelling after larger injuries may cause oropharyngeal obstruction. Most tongue lacerations, such as those associated with falls and seizures, are small, linear, and superficial and do not require any treatment. Larger lacerations or those that gape open or continue to bleed should be repaired.

Repair of the tongue can be challenging for the patient and physician alike. Gaining the patient's confidence is important if cooperation is to be had. Topical 4% lidocaine on gauze can be applied to an area of the tongue for 5 minutes and will provide some anesthesia that will allow local infiltration of anesthetic or lingual nerve block. General anesthesia is frequently needed for repair of such lacerations in children. The laceration can be closed with an absorbable suture such as 4-0 or 5-0 chromic gut or polyglycolic acid.

Oral Mucosa Repair. The muscle and overlying mucosa can be approximated in a single layered closure. The subsequent edema of the tongue may be profound, and therefore the sutures should be loosely approximated to allow some edema.

Lip Repair. Lip lacerations can result in prominent cosmetic defects if they are not treated in a precise and proper manner. In particular, small misalignments of the white roll or vermilion border are conspicuous to even the casual observer.

Anesthesia of lip wounds is best accomplished with regional nerve blocks and minimal local infiltration. This will prevent distention and distortion of anatomic landmarks critical for accurate repair. An infraorbital nerve block is used for the upper lip, a mental nerve block for the lower.

When simple superficial lip lacerations involving the vermilion border are repaired, the first suture should be placed at the vermilion border for alignment. The remainder of the laceration is then closed with 6-0 nonabsorbable sutures. If the laceration extends onto the moist portion of the lip, 5-0 or 6-0 gut sutures are preferred because they are softer when moist and therefore less bothersome for the patient.

Full-thickness lip lacerations are repaired in three layers from the inside out. The oral mucosa is repaired first with absorbable suture, such as 5-0 chromic or plain gut. If the oral mucosa and gingiva have been avulsed from the alveolus, the soft tissue may be reattached by passing a suture from the soft tissue around the base of a neighboring tooth. In general, proceeding from buccal sulcus toward the lip makes the most sense. The muscle layer is approximated with 4-0 or 5-0 absorbable suture, such as polyglactin-polylactic acid. Failure to approximate the orbicularis oris muscle or later dehiscence will result in an unsightly depression of the scar. It is best to include some of the fibrous tissue surrounding the muscle for more strength in placement of these sutures. A key suture of 5-0 or 6-0 nylon is placed at the vermilion border, and then the remainder of the external sutures are placed.

Avulsive wounds of the lip will often survive on surprisingly small pedicles. It is usually advisable to approximate even marginally viable tissue because of the possibility of survival (Fig. 64-32).

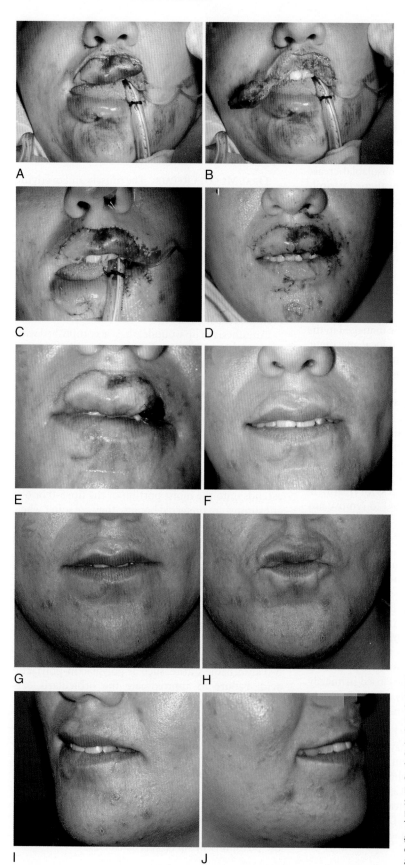

FIGURE 64-32. *A* and *B*, An upper lip avulsion after a motor vehicle crash is attached by a small lateral pedicle. *C*, After conservative débridement, the landmarks were approximated and the wound was closed. *D*, An area of poor perfusion was present, resulting in a small area of necrosis 4 days later. *E* and *F*, The necrotic area was allowed to heal by secondary intention and ultimately resulted in a healed wound. *G* to *J*, Three months after repair, there is good orbicularis oris function and oral competence as well as an acceptable cosmetic result.

CONCLUSION

As humans, we live in a complex social structure that depends not only on the words we use for communication but also on the emotive subtext of facial expression that imbues our words with greater meaning. Our faces are able to express a wide range of subtle emotions and silent messages. Because the face is so important for negotiating the complex social interactions that are part of our everyday lives, an important task is careful repair and restoration of function, one that must not be engaged in lightly. Historical and recent advances have enabled repair of most soft tissue injuries to the face, provided the nature of the injury is carefully considered and a thoughtful reconstructive plan is used.

REFERENCES

1. Hussain K, Wijetunge DB, Grubnic S, et al: A comprehensive analysis of craniofacial trauma. J Trauma 1994;36:34.
2. Key SJ, Thomas DW, Shepherd JP: The management of soft tissue facial wounds. Br J Oral Maxillofac Surg 1995;33:76.
3. Koonin AJ: Findings in 300 patients with facial lacerations. Plast Reconstr Surg 1973;52:525.
4. Hussain K: Management of soft tissue facial wounds. Br J Oral Maxillofac Surg 1995;33:265.
5. Karlson TA: The incidence of hospital-treated facial injuries from vehicles. J Trauma 1982;22:303.
6. Huelke DF, Moore JL, Ostrom M: Air bag injuries and occupant protection. J Trauma 1992;33:894.
7. Huelke DF, Compton CP: Facial injuries in automobile crashes. J Oral Maxillofac Surg 1983;41:241.
8. Nakhgevany KB, LiBassi M, Esposito B: Facial trauma in motor vehicle accidents: etiological factors. Am J Emerg Med 1994;12:160.
9. Gopalakrishna G, Peek-Asa C, Kraus JF: Epidemiologic features of facial injuries among motorcyclists. Ann Emerg Med 1998;32:425.
10. Frenguelli A, Ruscito P, Bicciolo G, et al: Head and neck trauma in sporting activities. Review of 208 cases. J Craniomaxillofac Surg 1991;19:178.
11. Hackl W, Hausberger K, Sailer R, et al: Prevalence of cervical spine injuries in patients with facial trauma. Oral Surg Oral Med Oral Pathol Oral Radiol Endod 2001;92:370.
12. McGregor JC: Soft tissue facial injuries in sport (excluding the eye). J R Coll Surg Edinb 1994;39:76.
13. Nonfatal dog bite-related injuries treated in hospital emergency departments—United States, 2001. MMWR Morb Mortal Wkly Rep 2003;52:605.
14. Karlson TA: The incidence of facial injuries from dog bites. JAMA 1984;251:3265.
15. Langer K: On the anatomy and physiology of the skin: conclusions by Professor K. Langer. Br J Plast Surg 1978;31:277.
16. Langer K: On the anatomy and physiology of the skin. IV. The swelling capabilities of skin by Professor K. Langer, presented at the meeting of 27th November 1861. Br J Plast Surg 1978;31:273.
17. Langer K: On the anatomy and physiology of the skin. III. The elasticity of the cutis by Professor K. Langer, presented at the meeting of 27th November 1861. Br J Plast Surg 1978;31:185.
18. Langer K: On the anatomy and physiology of the skin. II. Skin tension by Professor K. Langer, presented at the meeting of 27th November 1861. Br J Plast Surg 1978;31:93.
19. Langer K: On the anatomy and physiology of the skin. I. The cleavability of the cutis. [Translated from Langer K: Zur Anatomie und Physiologie der Haut. I. Über die Spaltbarkeit der Cutis. Sitzungsbericht der mathematisch-naturwissenschaftlichen Classe der Kaiserlichen Academie der Wissenschaften 1861;44:19.] Br J Plast Surg 1978;31:3.
20. Gibson T: Karl Langer (1819-1887) and his lines. Br J Plast Surg 1978;31:1.
21. Pierard GE, Lapiere CM: Microanatomy of the dermis in relation to relaxed skin tension lines and Langer's lines. Am J Dermatopathol 1987;9:219.
22. Wildsmith JA, Strichartz GR: Local anaesthetic drugs—an historical perspective. Br J Anaesth 1984;56:937.
23. Chen BK, Eichenfield LF: Pediatric anesthesia in dermatologic surgery: when hand-holding is not enough. Dermatol Surg 2001;27:1010.
24. Friedman PM, Mafong EA, Friedman ES, et al: Topical anesthetics update: EMLA and beyond. Dermatol Surg 2001;27:1019.
25. Ohlsen L, Englesson S, Evers H: An anaesthetic lidocaine/prilocaine cream (EMLA) for epicutaneous application tested for cutting split skin grafts. Scand J Plast Reconstr Surg 1985;19:201.
26. Gupta AK, Sibbald RG: Eutectic lidocaine/prilocaine 5% cream and patch may provide satisfactory analgesia for excisional biopsy or curettage with electrosurgery of cutaneous lesions. A randomized, controlled, parallel group study. J Am Acad Dermatol 1996;35(pt 1):419.
27. Agris J: Traumatic tattooing. J Trauma 1976;16:798.
28. Apfelberg DB, Manchester GH: Decorative and traumatic tattoo biophysics and removal. Clin Plast Surg 1987;14:243.
29. Bohler K, Muller E, Huber-Spitzy V, et al: Treatment of traumatic tattoos with various sterile brushes. J Am Acad Dermatol 1992;26(pt 1):749.
30. Parsons RW: The management of traumatic tattoos. Clin Plast Surg 1975;2:517.
31. Zook EG: Care of the traumatic tattoo. Med Times 1974;102:90.
32. Hohenleutner U, Landthaler M: Effective delayed brush treatment of an extensive traumatic tattoo. Plast Reconstr Surg 2000;105:1897.
33. Furnas DW, Somers G: Microsurgery in the prevention of traumatic tattoos. Plast Reconstr Surg 1976;58:631.
34. Kurokawa M, Isshiki N, Taira T et al: The use of microsurgical planing to treat traumatic tattoos. Plast Reconstr Surg 1994;94:1069.
35. Sun B, Guan W: Treating traumatic tattoo by micro-incision. Chin Med J (Engl) 2000;113:670.
36. Peris Z: Removal of traumatic and decorative tattoos by dermabrasion. Acta Dermatovenerol Croat 2002;10:15.
37. Notaro WA: Dermabrasion for the management of traumatic tattoos. J Dermatol Surg Oncol 1983;9:916.
38. Horowitz J, Nichter LS, Stark D: Dermabrasion of traumatic tattoos: simple, inexpensive, effective. Ann Plast Surg 1988;21:257.
39. Cronin ED, Haber JL: A new technique of dermabrasion for traumatic tattoos. Ann Plast Surg 1996;36:401.
40. Neely JL, Kovach RF: Traumatic tattoos treated by salabrasion. W V Med J 1986;82:5.
41. Dufresne RG Jr, Garrett AB, Bailin PL, et al: CO_2 laser treatment of traumatic tattoos. J Am Acad Dermatol 1989;20:137.
42. Suzuki H: Treatment of traumatic tattoos with the Q-switched neodymium:YAG laser. Arch Dermatol 1996;132:1226.
43. Fusade T, Toubel G, Grognard C, et al: Treatment of gunpowder traumatic tattoo by Q-switched Nd:YAG laser: an unusual adverse effect. Dermatol Surg 2000;26:1057.
44. Kunzi-Rapp K, Krahn GM, Wortmann S, et al: Early treatment of traumatic tattoo by erbium-YAG laser. Br J Dermatol 2001;144:219.

45. Alster TS: Successful elimination of traumatic tattoos by the Q-switched alexandrite (755-nm) laser. Ann Plast Surg 1995;34:542.

46. Chang SE, Choi JH, Moon KC, et al: Successful removal of traumatic tattoos in Asian skin with a Q-switched alexandrite laser. Dermatol Surg 1998;24:1308.

47. Ashinoff R, Geronemus RG: Rapid response of traumatic and medical tattoos to treatment with the Q-switched ruby laser. Plast Reconstr Surg 1993;91:841.

48. Achauer BM, Nelson JS, Vander Kam VM, et al: Treatment of traumatic tattoos by Q-switched ruby laser. Plast Reconstr Surg 1994;93:318.

49. Taylor CR, Gange RW, Dover JS, et al: Treatment of tattoos by Q-switched ruby laser. A dose-response study. Arch Dermatol 1990;126:893.

50. Taylor CR, Anderson RR, Gange RW, et al: Light and electron microscopic analysis of tattoos treated by Q-switched ruby laser. J Invest Dermatol 1991;97:131.

51. Taylor CR: Laser ignition of traumatically embedded firework debris. Lasers Surg Med 1998;22:157.

52. Dingman RO, Argenta LC: The surgical repair of traumatic defects of the scalp. Clin Plast Surg 1982;9:131.

53. Freedman RM, Baltimore R: Fatal *Streptococcus viridans* septicemia and meningitis: relationship to fetal scalp electrode monitoring. J Perinatol 1990;10:272.

54. Jonkhoff-Slok TW, Weyerman ME: Scalp electrode associated neonatal *Escherichia coli* meningitis—a case report. J Perinat Med 1991;19:217.

55. Chillag S, Chillag KL, Bhanot VK: Self-mutilation resulting in bacterial meningitis. W V Med J 1991;87:115.

56. Luo CB, Teng MM, Chen SS, et al: Pneumocephalus secondary to septic thrombosis of the superior sagittal sinus: report of a case. J Formos Med Assoc 2001;100:142.

57. Stuzin JM, Wagstrom L, Kawamoto HK, et al: Anatomy of the frontal branch of the facial nerve: the significance of the temporal fat pad. Plast Reconstr Surg 1989;83:265.

58. Tolhurst DE, Carstens MH, Greco RJ, et al: The surgical anatomy of the scalp. Plast Reconstr Surg 1991;87:603.

59. Welch TB, Boyne PJ: The management of traumatic scalp injuries: report of cases. J Oral Maxillofac Surg 1991;49:1007.

60. Corso P: Variations of the arterial, venous, and capillary circulation of the soft tissues of the head. Plast Reconstr Surg 1961;27:160.

61. Paff G: Anatomy of the Head and Neck. Philadelphia, WB Saunders, 1973.

62. Horgan MA, Piatt JH Jr: Shaving of the scalp may increase the rate of infection in CSF shunt surgery. Pediatr Neurosurg 1997;26:180.

63. Kumar K, Thomas J, Chan C: Cosmesis in neurosurgery: is the bald head necessary to avoid postoperative infection? Ann Acad Med Singapore 2002;31:150.

64. Siddique MS, Matai V, Sutcliffe JC: The preoperative skin shave in neurosurgery: is it justified? Br J Neurosurg 1998;12:131.

65. Ratanalert S, Saehaeng S, Sripairojkul B, et al: Nonshaved cranial neurosurgery. Surg Neurol 1999;51:458.

66. Terranova W: The use of periosteal flaps in scalp and forehead reconstruction. Ann Plast Surg 1990;25:450.

67. Nahai F, Hurteau J, Vasconez LO: Replantation of an entire scalp and ear by microvascular anastomoses of only 1 artery and 1 vein. Br J Plast Surg 1978;31:339.

68. Biemer E, Stock W, Wolfensberger C, et al: Successful replantation of a totally avulsed scalp. Br J Plast Surg 1979;32:19.

69. Frank IC: Avulsed scalp replantation. J Emerg Nurs 1979;5:8.

70. Miller GD, Anstee EJ, Snell JA: Successful replantation of an avulsed scalp by microvascular anastomoses. Plast Reconstr Surg 1976;58:133.

71. Buncke HJ, Rose EH, Brownstein MJ, et al: Successful replantation of two avulsed scalps by microvascular anastomoses. Plast Reconstr Surg 1978;61:666.

72. Van Beek AL, Zook EG: Scalp replantation by microsurgical revascularization: case report. Plast Reconstr Surg 1978;61:774.

73. Chater NL, Buncke H, Brownstein M: Revascularization of the scalp by microsurgical techniques after complete avulsion. Neurosurgery 1978;2:269.

74. Tantri DP, Cervino AL, Tabbal N: Replantation of the totally avulsed scalp. J Trauma 1980;20:350.

75. Gatti JE, LaRossa D: Scalp avulsions and review of successful replantation. Ann Plast Surg 1981;6:127.

76. Hentz VR, Palma CR, Elliott E, et al: Successful replantation of a totally avulsed scalp following prolonged ischemia. Ann Plast Surg 1981;7:145.

77. Stratoudakis AC, Savitsky LB: Microsurgical reimplantation of avulsed scalp. Ann Plast Surg 1981;7:312.

78. Alpert BS, Buncke HJ Jr, Mathes SJ: Surgical treatment of the totally avulsed scalp. Clin Plast Surg 1982;9:145.

79. Nahai F, Hester TR, Jurkiewicz MJ: Microsurgical replantation of the scalp. J Trauma 1985;25:897.

80. Khoo CT, Bailey BN: Microsurgical replantation of the avulsed scalp. Ann Acad Med Singapore 1983;12(suppl):370.

81. Sakai S, Soeda S, Ishii Y: Avulsion of the scalp: which one is the best artery for anastomosis? Ann Plast Surg 1990;24:350.

82. Juri J, Irigaray A, Zeaiter C: Reimplantation of scalp. Ann Plast Surg 1990;24:354.

83. Borenstein A, Yaffe B, Seidman DS, et al: Microsurgical replantation of two totally avulsed scalps. Isr J Med Sci 1990;26:442.

84. Eren S, Hess J, Larkin GC: Total scalp replantation based on one artery and one vein. Microsurgery 1993;14:266.

85. Zhou S, Chang TS, Guan WX, et al: Microsurgical replantation of the avulsed scalp: report of six cases. J Reconstr Microsurg 1993;9:121.

86. McCann J, O'Donoghue J, Kaf-al Ghazal S, et al: Microvascular replantation of a completely avulsed scalp. Microsurgery 1994;15:639.

87. Rivera ML, Gross JE: Scalp replantation after traumatic injury. AORN J 1995;62:175.

88. Chen IC, Wan HL: Microsurgical replantation of avulsed scalps. J Reconstr Microsurg 1996;12:105.

89. Cheng K, Zhou S, Jiang K, et al: Microsurgical replantation of the avulsed scalp: report of 20 cases. Plast Reconstr Surg 1996;97:1099.

90. Boucher JD, Ekman P: Facial areas and emotional information. J Commun 1975;25:21.

91. Prkachin KM, Mercer SR: Pain expression in patients with shoulder pathology: validity, properties and relationship to sickness impact. Pain 1989;39:257.

92. Sullivan LA, Kirkpatrick SW: Facial interpretation and component consistency. Genet Soc Gen Psychol Monogr 1996;122:389.

93. Kirkpatrick SW, Bell FE, Johnson C, et al: Interpretation of facial expressions of emotion: the influence of eyebrows. Genet Soc Gen Psychol Monogr 1996;122:405.

94. Pitanguy I, Ramos AS: The frontal branch of the facial nerve: the importance of its variations in face lifting. Plast Reconstr Surg 1966;38:352.

95. Gosain AK, Matloub HS: Surgical management of the facial nerve in craniofacial trauma and long-standing facial paralysis: cadaver study and clinical presentations. J Craniomaxillofac Trauma 1999;5:29.

96. Fezza JP, Klippenstein KA, Wesley RE: Cilia regrowth of shaven eyebrows. Arch Facial Plast Surg 1999;1:223.

97. Gormley DE: Use of Burow's wedge principle for repair of wounds in or near the eyebrow. J Am Acad Dermatol 1985;12(pt 1):344.

98. Albom MJ: Closure of excisional wounds with "H" flaps. J Dermatol Surg 1975;1:26.

99. Hammond RE: Uses of the O-to-Z-plasty repair in dermatologic surgery. J Dermatol Surg Oncol 1979;5:205.

100. Sutterfield TC, Bingham HC: Reconstruction of the eyebrow and eyelid following traumatic deformity. Case report. Mo Med 1971;68:259.

101. Mantero R, Rossi F: Reconstruction of hemi-eyebrow with a temporoparietal flap. Int Surg 1974;59:369.

102. Brent B: Reconstruction of ear, eyebrow, and sideburn in the burned patient. Plast Reconstr Surg 1975;55:312.

103. Sloan DF, Huang TT, Larson DL, et al: Reconstruction of eyelids and eyebrows in burned patients. Plast Reconstr Surg 1976;58:340.

104. McConnell CM, Neale HW: Eyebrow reconstruction in the burn patient. J Trauma 1977;17:362.

105. Pensler JM, Dillon B, Parry SW: Reconstruction of the eyebrow in the pediatric burn patient. Plast Reconstr Surg 1985;76:434.

106. Juri J: Eyebrow reconstruction. Plast Reconstr Surg 2001;107:1225.

107. Kim KS, Hwang JH, Kim DY, et al: Eyebrow island flap for reconstruction of a partial eyebrow defect. Ann Plast Surg 2002;48:315.

108. Goldman BE, Goldenberg DM: Nape of neck eyebrow reconstruction. Plast Reconstr Surg 2003;111:1217.

109. Van Droogenbroeck JB: Eyebrow transplantation. Int J Lepr Other Mycobact Dis 1971;39:629.

110. Goldman GD: Eyebrow transplantation. Dermatol Surg 2001;27:352.

111. Fritz TM, Burg G, Hafner J: Eyebrow reconstruction with free skin and hair-bearing composite graft. J Am Acad Dermatol 1999;41:1008.

112. Dzubow LM: Basal-cell carcinoma of the eyebrow region. J Dermatol Surg Oncol 1984;10:609.

113. Tyers A, Collin J: Colour Atlas of Ophthalmic Plastic Surgery. New York, Churchill Livingstone, 1995.

114. Zitelli JA: Wound healing by secondary intention. A cosmetic appraisal. J Am Acad Dermatol 1983;9:407.

115. Zitelli JA: Secondary intention healing: an alternative to surgical repair. Clin Dermatol 1984;2:92.

116. Goldwyn RM, Rueckert F: The value of healing by secondary intention for sizeable defects of the face. Arch Surg 1977;112:285.

117. Ortiz MA, Kraushar MF: Lacrimal drainage following repair of inferior canaliculus. Ann Ophthalmol 1975;7:739.

118. Canavan YM, Archer DB: Long-term review of injuries to the lacrimal drainage apparatus. Trans Ophthalmol Soc U K 1979;99:201.

119. Dortzbach RK, Angrist RA: Silicone intubation for lacerated lacrimal canaliculi. Ophthalmic Surg 1985;16:639.

120. Shafer D, Bennett J: Associated soft tissue injuries. Atlas Oral Maxillofac Surg Clin North Am 1994;2:47.

121. Dingman RO, Grabb WC: Surgical anatomy of the mandibular ramus of the facial nerve based on the dissection of 100 facial halves. Plast Reconstr Surg 1962;29:266.

122. Furnas DW: Landmarks for the trunk and the temporofacial division of the facial nerve. Br J Surg 1965;52:694.

123. Grabski WJ, Salasche SJ: Management of temporal nerve injuries. J Dermatol Surg Oncol 1985;11:145.

124. Davis RE, Telischi FF: Traumatic facial nerve injuries: review of diagnosis and treatment. J Craniomaxillofac Trauma 1995;1:30.

125. Ritter FN: The vasculature of the nose. Ann Otol Rhinol Laryngol 1970;79:468.

126. Toriumi DM, Mueller RA, Grosch T, et al: Vascular anatomy of the nose and the external rhinoplasty approach. Arch Otolaryngol Head Neck Surg 1996;122:24.

127. Oneal RM, Beil RJ Jr, Schlesinger J: Surgical anatomy of the nose. Clin Plast Surg 1996;23:195.

128. Holt GR, Holt JE: Incidence of eye injuries in facial fractures: an analysis of 727 cases. Otolaryngol Head Neck Surg 1983;91:276.

129. Hallock GG: Nasal degloving injuries. Ann Plast Surg 1984;12:537.

130. Fuleihan NS, Natout MA, Webster RC, et al: Successful replantation of amputated nose and auricle. Otolaryngol Head Neck Surg 1987;97:18.

131. Wynn SK: Immediate composite graft to loss of nasal ala from dog bite: case report. Plast Reconstr Surg 1972;50:188.

132. Rapley JH, Lawrence WT, Witt PD: Composite grafting and hyperbaric oxygen therapy in pediatric nasal tip reconstruction after avulsive dog-bite injury. Ann Plast Surg 2001;46:434.

133. Stucker FJ, Shaw GY, Boyd S, et al: Management of animal and human bites in the head and neck. Arch Otolaryngol Head Neck Surg 1990;116:789.

134. Stucker FJ, Hoasjoe DK: Soft tissue trauma over the nose. Facial Plast Surg 1992;8:233.

135. Davis P, Shaheen O: Soft tissue injuries of the face. In Rowe N, Williams J, eds: Maxillofacial Injuries. Edinburgh, Churchill Livingstone, 1985.

136. Hussain G, Thomson S, Zielinski V: Nasal amputation due to human bite: microsurgical replantation. Aust N Z J Surg 1997;67:382.

137. Mueller R: Microsurgical replantation of amputated upper lip and nose. Personal communication, 2003.

138. Dowling JA, Foley FD, Moncrief JA: Chondritis in the burned ear. Plast Reconstr Surg 1968;42:115.

139. Park C, Lineaweaver WC, Rumly TO, et al: Arterial supply of the anterior ear. Plast Reconstr Surg 1992;90:38.

140. Allison GR: Anatomy of the auricle. Clin Plast Surg 1990;17:209.

141. Butt WE: Auricular haematoma—treatment options. Aust N Z J Surg 1987;57:391.

142. Schuller DE, Dankle SD, Strauss RH: A technique to treat wrestlers' auricular hematoma without interrupting training or competition. Arch Otolaryngol Head Neck Surg 1989;115:202.

143. Krugman ME: Management of auricular hematomas with suction assisted lipectomy apparatus. Otolaryngol Head Neck Surg 1989;101:504.

144. Kelleher JC, Sullivan JG, Baibak GJ, et al: The wrestler's ear. Plast Reconstr Surg 1967;40:540.

145. Cochran JH Jr: "How I do it"—otology and neurotology. A specific issue and its solution. Treatment of acute auricular hematoma. Laryngoscope 1980;90(pt 1):1063.

146. Davis PK: An operation for haematoma auris. Br J Plast Surg 1971;24:277.

147. Elsahy NI: Acquired ear defects. Clin Plast Surg 2002;29:175.

148. Giffin CS: Wrestler's ear: pathophysiology and treatment. Ann Plast Surg 1992;28:131.

149. Lee D, Sperling N: Initial management of auricular trauma. Am Fam Physician 1996;53:2339.

150. Liston SL, Cortez EA, McNabney WK: External ear injuries. JACEP 1978;7:233.

151. O'Donnell BP, Eliezri YD: The surgical treatment of traumatic hematoma of the auricle. Dermatol Surg 1999;25:803.

152. Punjabi AP, Haug RH, Jordan RB: Management of injuries to the auricle. J Oral Maxillofac Surg 1997;55:732.

153. Starck WJ, Kaltman SI: Current concepts in the surgical management of traumatic auricular hematoma. J Oral Maxillofac Surg 1992;50:800.

154. Templer J, Renner GJ: Injuries of the external ear. Otolaryngol Clin North Am 1990;23:1003.

155. Zohar Y, Strauss M: A technique to treat wrestler's auricular hematoma. Arch Otolaryngol Head Neck Surg 1990;116:359.

156. Henderson JM, Salama AR, Blanchaert RH Jr: Management of auricular hematoma using a thermoplastic splint. Arch Otolaryngol Head Neck Surg 2000;126:888.

157. Grabb WC, Smith JW: Basic techniques of plastic surgery. In Grabb WC, Smith JW: Plastic Surgery. Boston, Little, Brown, 1973:3.

158. Lacher AB, Blitzer A: The traumatized auricle—care, salvage, and reconstruction. Otolaryngol Clin North Am 1982;15:225.

159. Turbiak TW: Ear trauma. Emerg Med Clin North Am 1987;5:243.

160. Kirsch JP, Amedee RG: Management of external ear trauma. J La State Med Soc 1991;143:13.

161. Holmes RE: Management of traumatic auricular injuries in children. Pediatr Ann 1999;28:391.

162. Powers M, Bertz J, Fonseca R: Management of soft tissue injuries. In Fonseca R, Walker R, eds: Oral and Maxillofacial Trauma, vol 1. Philadelphia, WB Saunders, 1991:616.

163. Mladick RA: Salvage of the ear in acute trauma. Clin Plast Surg 1978;5:427.

164. Humber P, Kaplan I, Horton C: Trauma to the ear: hematoma, laceration, amputation, atresia, and burns. In Stark R, ed: Plastic Surgery of the Head and Neck. New York, Churchill Livingstone, 1987.

165. Earley MJ, Bardsley AF: Human bites: a review. Br J Plast Surg 1984;37:458.

166. Bardsley AF, Mercer DM: The injured ear: a review of 50 cases. Br J Plast Surg 1983;36:466.

167. Brandt FA: Human bites of the ear. Plast Reconstr Surg 1969;43:130.

168. Stierman KL, Lloyd KM, De Luca-Pytell DM, et al: Treatment and outcome of human bites in the head and neck. Otolaryngol Head Neck Surg 2003;128:795.

169. Chidzonga MM: Human bites of the face. A review of 22 cases. S Afr Med J 1998;88:150.

170. Scheithauer MO, Rettinger G: Bite injuries in the head and neck area [in German]. HNO 1997;45:891.

171. Tomasetti BJ, Walker L, Gormley MB, et al: Human bites of the face. J Oral Surg 1979;37:565.

172. Goel TK, Law EJ, MacMillan BG: Management of the acutely burned ear. Burns Incl Therm Inj 1983;9:218.

173. Grant DA, Finley ML, Coers CR 3rd: Early management of the burned ear. Plast Reconstr Surg 1969;44:161.

174. Spira M, Hardy SB: Management of the injured ear. Am J Surg 1963;106:678.

175. McGrath MH, Ariyan S: Immediate reconstruction of full-thickness burn of an ear with an undelayed myocutaneous flap. Case report. Plast Reconstr Surg 1978;62:618.

176. Tegtmeier RE, Gooding RA: The use of a fascial flap in ear reconstruction. Plast Reconstr Surg 1977;60:406.

177. Cotlar SW: Reconstruction of the burned ear using a temporalis fascial flap. Plast Reconstr Surg 1983;71:45.

178. Margulis A, Bauer BS, Alizadeh K: Ear reconstruction after auricular chondritis secondary to ear piercing. Plast Reconstr Surg 2003;111:891.

179. Martin R, Yonkers AJ, Yarington CT Jr: Perichondritis of the ear. Laryngoscope 1976;86:664.

180. Wanamaker HH: Suppurative perichondritis of the auricle. Trans Am Acad Ophthalmol Otolaryngol 1972;76:1289.

181. Apfelberg DB, Waisbren BA, Masters FW, et al: Treatment of chondritis in the burned ear by the local instillation of antibiotics. Plast Reconstr Surg 1974;53:179.

182. Greminger RF, Elliott RA Jr, Rapperport A: Antibiotic iontophoresis for the management of burned ear chondritis. Plast Reconstr Surg 1980;66:356.

183. LaForest NT, Cofrancesco C: Antibiotic iontophoresis in the treatment of ear chondritis. Phys Ther 1978;58:32.

184. Elsahy NI: Ear replantation. Clin Plast Surg 2002;29:221.

185. Safak T, Kayikcioglu A: A traumatic ear amputation attached with a narrow pedicle. Ann Plast Surg 1998;40:106.

186. Elsahy NI: Ear replantation combined with local flaps. Ann Plast Surg 1986;17:102.

187. Ariyan S, Chicarilli ZN: Replantation of a totally amputated ear by means of a platysma musculocutaneous "sandwich" flap. Plast Reconstr Surg 1986;78:385.

188. Weston GW, Shearin JC, DeFranzo AJ: Avulsion injuries of the external ear. N C Med J 1985;46:51.

189. Turpin IM, Altman DI, Cruz HG, et al: Salvage of the severely injured ear. Ann Plast Surg 1988;21:170.

190. Pribaz JJ, Crespo LD, Orgill DP, et al: Ear replantation without microsurgery. Plast Reconstr Surg 1997;99:1868.

191. Chun JK, Sterry TP, Margoles SL, et al: Salvage of ear replantation using the temporoparietal fascia flap. Ann Plast Surg 2000;44:435.

192. Clayton JM, Friedland JA: Ear reattachment by the pocket principle. Ariz Med 1980;37:91.

193. Lehman JA Jr, Cervino AL: Replantation of the severed ear. J Trauma 1975;15:929.

194. Mladick RA: Replantation of severed ear parts [letter]. Plast Reconstr Surg 1976;57:374.

195. Sexton RP: Utilization of the amputated ear cartilage. Plast Reconstr Surg 1955;15:419.

196. Conroy WC: Salvage of an amputated ear. Plast Reconstr Surg 1972;49:564.

197. Converse JM: Reconstruction of the auricle. II. Plast Reconstr Surg 1958;22:230.

198. Converse JM: Reconstruction of the auricle. I. Plast Reconstr Surg 1958;22:150.

199. Jenkins AM, Finucan T: Primary nonmicrosurgical reconstruction following ear avulsion using the temporoparietal fascial island flap. Plast Reconstr Surg 1989;83:148.

200. Baudet J: Successful replantation of a large severed ear fragment. Plast Reconstr Surg 1973;51:82.

201. Grabb WC, Dingman RO: The fate of amputated tissues of the head and neck following replacement. Plast Reconstr Surg 1972;49:28.

202. Godwin Y, Allison K, Waters R: Reconstruction of a large defect of the ear using a composite graft following a human bite injury. Br J Plast Surg 1999;52:152.

203. Gifford GH Jr: Replantation of severed part of an ear. Plast Reconstr Surg 1972;49:202.

204. Tanzer RC: The reconstruction of acquired defects of the ear. Plast Reconstr Surg 1965;35:355.

205. Suraci A: Plastic reconstruction of acquired defects of the ear. Am J Surg 1944;66:196.

206. Spira M: Early care of deformities of the auricle resulting from mechanical trauma. In Tanzer R, Edgerton M, eds: Symposium on Reconstruction of the Auricle. St. Louis, CV Mosby, 1974:204.

207. Greeley P: Reconstruction of the external ear. Naval Bull 1944;62:1323.

208. Conway H, Neumann C: Reconstruction of the external ear. Ann Surg 1948;128:226.

209. Mladick RA, Carraway JH: Ear reattachment by the modified pocket principle. Case report. Plast Reconstr Surg 1973;51:584.

210. Mladick RA, Horton CE, Adamson JE, et al: The pocket principle: a new technique for the reattachment of a severed ear part. Plast Reconstr Surg 1971;48:219.

211. Buncke HJ Jr., Schulz WP: Total ear reimplantation in the rabbit utilising microminiature vascular anastomoses. Br J Plast Surg 1966;19:15.

212. Katsaros J, Tan E, Sheen R: Microvascular ear replantation. Br J Plast Surg 1988;41:496.

213. Sadove RC: Successful replantation of a totally amputated ear. Ann Plast Surg 1990;24:366.

214. Shelley OP, Villafane O, Watson SB: Successful partial ear replantation after prolonged ischaemia time. Br J Plast Surg 2000;53:76.
215. Nath RK, Kraemer BA, Azizzadeh A: Complete ear replantation without venous anastomosis. Microsurgery 1998;18:282.
216. Kind GM: Microvascular ear replantation. Clin Plast Surg 2002;29:233.
217. Zitsch RP 3rd: Carcinoma of the lip. Otolaryngol Clin North Am 1993;26:265.
218. Tobin GR, O'Daniel TG: Lip reconstruction with motor and sensory innervated composite flaps. Clin Plast Surg 1990; 17:623.

Acute Care and Reconstruction of Facial Burns

Loren H. Engrav, MD ✦ Matthias B. Donelan, MD

EXCISION AND GRAFTING OF ACUTE FACE AND NECK BURNS

GENERAL PRINCIPLES OF RECONSTRUCTION

COMMON RESULTS OF EXCISION AND GRAFTING
    Hypertrophic Scars
    Hypertrophic Graft Juncture Scars
    Missing Eyebrows
    Retraction of Upper Lid
    Ectropion of the Lower Lid
    Medial Canthal Webs
    Deformed Nasal Tip with Retracted or Missing Alar
      Margins
    Flat Upper Lip with No Philtrum, Philtral Ridges, or
      Cupid's Bow and Retracted Upper Lip

Deformed Lower Lip with Ectropion, Flat Chin, and
    Thick Lower Lip
Microstomia and Skin Graft Yoke from Cheek to Chin
    to Cheek
Mandibular Growth Retardation
Color Mismatch
Neck Contracture
Wrinkled Neck Graft
Neck Webs
Thin Skin Grafts
Three-dimensional Tissue Loss from Fourth-, Fifth-,
    and Sixth-Degree Burns
Poor Gestalt
Hypertrophic Donor Sites

ELECTRICAL BURNS OF THE ORAL COMMISSURES

Excision with grafting of nonfacial acute burns has become the standard of care. Several historical figures also favored excision of facial burns (Fig. 65-1). Nevertheless, there is still controversy about whether this technique should be applied to facial burns. There are now eight manuscripts in the literature supporting the method with published results.[1-8] On the contrary, six manuscripts argue against the procedure, but none presented illustrative or supportive results.[9-14] It is the opinion of the authors that the answer is yes, and the method is described. The technique eliminates late grafting of large, flat areas and the misery of two prolonged periods of pressure therapy, one after the acute care and the second after the grafting for reconstruction. However, the technique does not totally solve the problem of facial burns because it is routinely followed by a collection of deformities involving the eyes, nose, and mouth that require late reconstruction. These, too, are described.

Although early excision and grafting of facial burns may be the standard of care in certain centers, there are still many burn patients with facial burns that are allowed to heal spontaneously, often resulting in contraction and hypertrophic scarring. Patients frequently present to the plastic surgeon with recurring patterns of facial deformity, which require late reconstructive surgery. These deformities are discussed individually.

EXCISION AND GRAFTING OF ACUTE FACE AND NECK BURNS

The method of excision and grafting as previously described[2,15-17] continues to be our standard method with one slight modification, which is described later. Facial burns are débrided of loose blisters on admission. Burns that are clearly full thickness are scheduled for excision and grafting within the next 7 to 10 days. Indeterminate burns are treated with once- or twice-daily hydrotherapy, débridement, and topical antibacterials, usually silver sulfadiazine. The hydrotherapy and topical antimicrobials are continued until day 10. At that time, the face burns are evaluated to determine which areas will not be healed within

Portions of this chapter were previously published in Engrav LH, Donelan MB: Face burns: acute care and reconstruction. Operative Techniques Plast Reconstr Surg 1997;4:53-85; and Engrav LH: Secondary reconstruction of the burned face and neck. In Grotting JC: Reoperative Aesthetic and Reconstructive Surgery. St. Louis, Quality Medical Publishing, 1995, 657-676.

```
PROF. DR. Zora JANŽEKOVIČ
Vinarska 10 b

62 000  M A R I B O R              Maribor, 5 September 1981

Y U G O S L A V I A


     Mr. LOREN H. ENGRAV, M.D.
     University of Washington zdg
     Division of Plastic Surgery, ZA-16
     SEATLE, WASHINGTON  98 104


     Dear Prof. L.M. ENGRAV,

     Thank you very much for your letter and your interest on
early excisions in burns.

     We never ignore the burns of the face; on contrary we do
excise them in the first operation and cover them immidiately.
On full thickness defects we put thicker grafts with small
incisions in them. In size they must fit to the anatomical
areas (forehead, lips, chin etc.) and must be  fixed on the
edges and on some perforations holes in order to ensure 100
per cent take. The defects of deep dermal burns are grafted
with thin epidermal grafts.

     The first dressing is performed after 24 hours.




                         Sincerely
```

FIGURE 65-1. Letter from Zora Janžekovič, 1981.

3 weeks of the injury. Fortunately, most facial burns (90% to 95%) will be healed by 3 weeks with the treatment described. When this is not the case, plans are made for excision and grafting of the laggard areas.

The goal is to have the excision and grafting of the face completed by 21 days after injury. In patients with extensive total body surface area burns, this permits immediate treatment of the large body surfaces and the hands. Between days 10 and 14, one can then deal with the face. The technique for the excision and grafting is described later and has not changed since the 1986 publication except for one thing—the delay between allografting and autografting is 1 week instead of 2 days.

The operation is carried out with general anesthesia and the patient in the reverse Trendelenburg position. Ace bandages are used on the lower extremities to prevent venous stasis. The endotracheal tube is wired to the teeth and suspended from overhead hooks. Contact lenses are used to protect the corneas. The feeding tube is left in place without ties. Perioperative antibiotics are administered.

Those aesthetic units[2,17,18] (Fig. 65-2A and B) judged to be incapable of healing within 3 weeks of the injury are outlined with markers. Small unburned or healed areas must frequently be included in the excision to preserve the aesthetic unit. In some circumstances, a portion of an aesthetic unit will clearly not heal in 3 weeks, but the area is small enough to be reconstructed later by excision and closure or with tissue expanders. In this situation, excision and grafting either are not performed or are done with routine grafts; valuable thick grafts from special donor sites are not used. It is also common that some areas to be excised are shallower than others. One must excise deeply enough to prevent the bed from healing underneath the graft with resultant graft loss. This is accomplished by excising deeply enough to remove the hair follicles.

On some occasions, after the burn excision has begun, it becomes apparent that the burn is not as deep as originally thought. In this case, it is wise either to excise shallowly or to merely scrape off any loose debris and apply allograft or xenograft. Then, if the burn is healed in 3 weeks, all is done. If not, one can

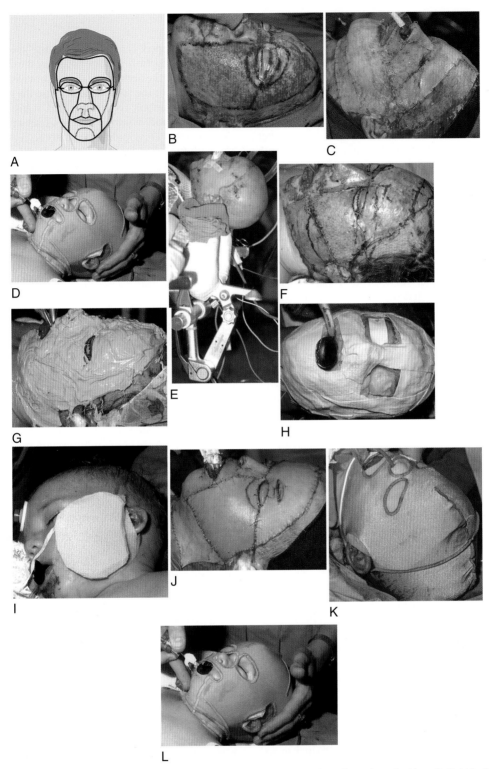

FIGURE 65-2. *A*, Aesthetic units. *B*, Aesthetic unit markings. *C*, Allograft at time of application. *D*, Bubble facemask. *E*, Mayfield headrest. *F*, Allograft at 1 week. *G*, Duplicast mold. *H*, Plaster reinforcement. *I*, Foam. *J*, Autograft placement. *K*, Bubble and elastomer. *L*, Bubble and foam.

return to the operating room and resume the planned procedure.

The eyelids are usually excised first. Three traction stitches are placed through the lids near the margin and used to stretch the lids. The Goulian dermatome with a 0.008-inch guard is used to excise the lids; multiple passes are made until normal, bleeding tissue is visualized. Portions of the orbicularis muscle must frequently be removed but rarely anything deeper. After the excision is complete, hemostasis is achieved with bipolar cautery and epinephrine (1 : 10,000)–soaked Telfa pads. The nature of the bleeding seen during the excision is key to determining if all the eschar has been removed, and the vasoconstriction caused by epinephrine that has leaked onto unexcised areas can interfere with this determination. For this reason, leakage of the epinephrine solution onto areas yet to be excised must be avoided.

The medial canthal regions are done next. This may be the most difficult area of the face to excise because the Goulian dermatome is too large to move nicely in and out of the region. The excision is usually done piecemeal with curved iris scissors or a No. 15 blade. Again, hemostasis is accomplished with bipolar cautery and epinephrine-soaked Telfa pads.

The next area to be excised is the nose, again with the Goulian dermatome and the 0.008-inch guard. The upper nose is well supported by bony and cartilaginous structures, so it is simply excised. Placing the tip of the little finger into the nares to provide support facilitates excision of the eschar over the nares. It is important that the excision over the nares and the tip of the nose be minimal and to stop at the first sign of normal tissue. This tissue is vital to the appearance of the grafted nose, so everything possible must be left. It is better to have to redo the nose for graft loss than to remove significant living tissue, which results in a flat nose. Hemostasis is achieved with bipolar cautery and epinephrine-soaked Telfa pads.

The upper lip is then excised. Although it is well supported by the teeth, it is loose, and therefore three traction stitches are used to apply tension. The Goulian dermatome with the 0.008-inch guard is used. The tissue of the philtral columns and the philtrum is crucial to the ultimate appearance; therefore, the excision of this region must also stop at the first sign of living tissue. Again, it is better to have to redo the lip for graft loss than to excise deeply to ensure graft survival. Hemostasis is achieved with bipolar cautery and epinephrine-soaked Telfa pads.

The Goulian dermatome with the 0.008-inch guard is next used for the lower lip and chin. Again, three traction stitches are used, and again there is a zone wherein the excision must be kept minimal—the mental prominence. A flat chin is unattractive, and therefore all tissue possible must be spared from the excision. When the excision is complete, hemostasis is achieved with bipolar cautery and epinephrine-soaked Telfa pads.

The T-shaped central area of the face is now excised, leaving the four large flat areas: the cheeks, the forehead, and the neck. Typically, it is not wise to excise all four areas at the same time because the blood loss can be substantial, requiring rapid transfusions to maintain blood volume. These areas are usually done serially. The Goulian dermatome is again used but with the 0.010-inch or 0.012-inch guard, and the excision continues to normal bleeding tissue with no remaining hair follicles. Each area is excised in an orderly fashion. When each area is completely excised, hemostasis is achieved with bipolar cautery and epinephrine-soaked Telfa pads. In doing the forehead, the area of the eyebrows is not excised. This is allowed to heal in the hope that some or all of the eyebrow will recover.

Ear burns are not excised because there is no instrument adequate to excise the three-dimensional structure of the ear. The historical method of spontaneous separation of eschar followed by split-thickness skin grafting works well in these small areas.

After excision is complete, each area is covered with allograft. Multiple teams can be used to speed the process. The allograft (Fig. 65-2C) is placed with all of the attention to detail that is used for autograft, that is, it must be snug and well secured with staples, sutures, and Steri-Strips. Staples are used for the large flat areas, whereas sutures are used for the eyelids, nose, and lips and wherever staples seem to be inadequate. Steri-Strips are used everywhere as added support. A bubble pressure garment facemask is applied to support the allograft and to promote hemostasis (Fig. 65-2D).

Approximately 1 week postoperatively, the patient is returned to the operating room for autografting. The head is supported with a Mayfield neurosurgical headrest applied in a nonstandard fashion (Fig. 65-2E). The allograft (Fig. 65-2F) is carefully inspected to determine whether it is adherent to the bed underneath. If the allograft is loose, it may mean that the excision was not deep enough, in which case the excision and allografting must be repeated. If the allograft is adherent, and if elastomer is later to be applied under pressure garments, which is usually the case, a Duplicast or Jeltrate negative impression (Fig. 65-2G) with plaster reinforcement (Fig. 65-2H) is made over the allograft by the burn occupational and physical therapists. While the procedure continues, the therapists make a plaster positive mold, then an elastomer negative mold to be worn under the compression garment. On occasion, a simple piece of foam is sufficient (Fig. 65-2I). The allograft is then removed, again examining for adherence and viability of the underlying bed. Hemostasis is achieved with epinephrine-soaked Telfa pads. While waiting for hemostasis, split-thickness skin is obtained. It is usually 0.018 to 0.021 inch in thickness in adults and 0.008 to 0.012 inch in children and obtained from the scalp if graft color must be matched with the color of healed or unburned areas. If the entire face is to be grafted, the scalp is insufficient, and the harvesting must be done elsewhere. The thicknesses mentioned are merely estimates and greatly influenced by the dermatome used and the technique of harvesting.

To harvest the scalp, a Mayfield neurosurgical headrest is useful (Fig. 65-2E). However, it is used in a nonstandard fashion. It is positioned such that the ends of the U-shaped piece project directly upward and are placed under the neck. To distribute the pressure and achieve more stability, several folded towels are placed between the U-shaped piece and the neck. This positioning permits access to nearly the entire scalp. One or more persons then check each screw and nut on the headrest to be sure it is tight.

The scalp is then shaved, and the pattern of scalp harvesting to be used is planned. One strip is usually obtained with a Padgett air dermatome from ear to ear over the top of the skull, one from top of skull to nape of neck over the occipital region, and two smaller residual pieces from each posterolateral area, resulting in four pieces of autograft. This is insufficient to do an entire face but is useful for partial face grafting. Each area is then infiltrated with large volumes of saline containing 1 : 500,000 epinephrine to make it flat or nearly so. To achieve this, more solution is injected around the perimeter of the site to be harvested than in the center. This is done just before harvesting because the fluid leaves the scalp rapidly. A powered dermatome is then used to harvest the skin. Usually, the first pass proceeds from ear to ear, the second from nape of neck to the first harvest. On occasion, two transverse passes can be obtained. Assistance is critical because the skull must be absolutely immobile. This requires one assistant on each side to press against the lateral skull, which leaves the entire area around the top of the skull available to the person running the dermatome. The assistants must be ready to change the direction of pressure. When the harvesting is occurring on the right side of the skull, there must be pressure on the left ear. When the harvesting passes over the top of the skull and moves to the left side of the skull, the pressure must change to the right ear. This pressure change should be rehearsed before harvesting. After harvesting, epinephrine-soaked Telfa pads and epinephrine-soaked gauze are immediately applied because the blood loss from scalp donors sites can be considerable. The other three pieces of scalp skin are then obtained in a similar fashion, if needed.

If the entire face is to be grafted, it is not possible to obtain sufficient skin from the scalp. Color match becomes moot, except that the entire face should be of the same color. In this situation, the graft may be obtained wherever adequate skin is available. However, it is generally unwise to obtain these thick grafts from the upper chest or neck in women because the donor sites tend to develop hypertrophic scarring. It is important that the donor site be planned shortly after admission, before all donor sites have been used to resurface other body parts.

Wherever on the body is chosen to harvest these large, thick face grafts, the Padgett manual dermatomes (small, medium, and wide) are clearly the instruments of choice; they yield pieces of skin of uniform thickness, large enough to cover the entire cheek with one piece. Use of the device is slow, so a common maneuver is to first harvest one large piece for a cheek and then to have the grafting team begin while further harvesting continues. In any event, a piece for each facial area is obtained. Common thicknesses are 0.016 inch for the eyelids and 0.018 to 0.021 inch for the remainder of the face in adults. In children, 0.008 to 0.012 inch is used. In some instances, full-thickness grafts are used for the eyelids, both upper and lower.[19]

Once obtained, the grafts are carefully stitched into place with 4-0 plain gut by several teams, making sure that each piece is snug (Fig. 65-2J). If all four lids are to be grafted, three traction stitches are placed in the margin of each lid, and each is grafted in a stretched-out position. The traction stitches in the lower lid are passed under the upper lid and brought out through the upper lid and tied over bolsters. This keeps the lower lids stretched, albeit under the upper lids. The traction stitches through the upper lid are later pulled down and anchored to the tissue of the cheek to keep the upper lids stretched out. There are no tricks to stitching the grafts in place on the nose, lips, chin, cheeks, and forehead except that it should be meticulous, snug, and applied in aesthetic units. On the neck, if only a portion of the neck is being grafted, or at the lateral aspect of the neck where skin graft meets posterior unburned skin, darts and half Z-plasties are indicated to prevent webs. These are simple half Z-plasties in which a skin flap from the adjacent normal skin is created and inset into an incision in the graft. A "dressing" is then applied that consists of fine mesh gauze, the elastomer mold (or foam if sufficient), and a pressure garment bubble (Fig. 65-2K and L). Bioclusive (Johnson & Johnson) is applied to the scalp, if it was harvested, and is held in place by the pressure garment bubble.

Postoperatively, these devices are removed twice daily. The grafts are inspected and any hematomas removed, through 1-cm incisions placed in the relaxed skin tension lines. If hematomas are large, we do not hesitate to return to the operating room and remove the hematoma with general anesthesia. Patients are given nothing by mouth for 3 days and are encouraged to refrain from talking.

Until the grafts are mature, usually for several months, the patient wears pressure garments. If the pressure garment does not fit the contours of the face well, the occupational and physical therapists fabricate inserts. Some patients object to the pressure garments but will wear transparent, rigid masks, also fabricated by the therapists. Silicone sheeting is also sometimes placed under the garments or masks in an effort to reduce hypertrophic scarring.[20] The garments, masks, inserts, and silicone sheeting may need to be removed for a sufficient time each day to prevent maceration.

Stents are occasionally necessary for the nostrils. These are usually ordered from Porex Corporation*; they come in several sizes and are worn 23 hours per day.

After circumoral grafting, splinting and exercises to minimize microstomia are necessary. The Therabite system† is used for mouth stretching. Two types of splints are used. One is held in place by a retainer to the teeth. The other is a pair of commissure splints held in place by a tension strap around the head.

Steroid injections are used only rarely. They are painful, must be repeated monthly for several months, are not applicable to large scars, and do not totally eliminate the scar. Nevertheless, there are circumstances in which they are indicated (e.g., small hypertrophic scars). The usual dose is 40 mg/mL triamcinolone, 40 to 80 mg monthly for 6 to 9 months.

Although synthetic and semisynthetic skin substitutes are used for many burn procedures, we have not used them for these facial operations. It seems unlikely that they will match the function and appearance of thick autograft. Similarly, xenograft is not used as the temporary biologic dressing between excision and grafting. One of the functions of the allograft is to test the bed remaining after excision, and xenograft will not do this.

GENERAL PRINCIPLES OF RECONSTRUCTION

Unless the surgeon and the patient are surrounded by a well-functioning support system, they probably should not embark on a complex reconstruction plan. Following a patient from an acute facial burn to completion of reconstruction successfully simply cannot be done without a team consisting of the patient, the surgeon, one or more nurses, and one or more therapists. It is far too complex for the surgeon to take on alone and far too stressful for the patient to take on alone. It is better to leave things unreconstructed than to consume valuable reconstructive tissues to no avail or to compound the problem with further scars.

There are times after reconstruction has begun when it is wise to stop. No reconstruction plan should keep a patient from usual activities for longer than a couple

of years. It is simply not in the best interest of the patient to make him or her a reconstruction addict. The team, including the patient, should make a plan that can be completed in that period. Most patients will come to agree with this philosophy. Some will not; these patients should be seen in the clinic at periodic intervals, but further surgery should not be planned. They should merely receive kind and understanding support until it is no longer needed. Unfortunately, some will continue for years to look for the surgeon who can erase the scars.

It is not possible to do everything for everybody. There are many difficulties in following a patient from the acute injury to the completion of reconstruction, a sequence of events that may take 2 to 3 years or longer. Some patients have deformities that are technically difficult, if not impossible, to correct. Some of the deformities to be described are simply not reconstructable. When this is the case, the authors will clearly indicate so, hoping that a reader might become interested and solve the problem. Other patients have no support systems and therefore cannot keep clinic appointments, manage splints and pressure garments, or participate in therapy programs. Others, for financial reasons, must return to work and cannot be bothered by time off work for operations and clinic visits. Therefore, the patient/surgeon/nurse/therapist team must be willing to admit that it is impossible to do everything for everybody. Some patients will need to be discharged before all surgically possible reconstructions are completed. The team must be willing to admit that some less than perfect results will have to be good enough. However, just because this is the case at one point in time does not mean that it will always be the case. Some patients, who for whatever reason could not deal with reconstruction immediately after the injury, may return years later ready to begin.

All members of the team must have patience. As with other wounds, grafts on the face require many months to mature. At 3 to 5 months, the grafts, even very thick split grafts, are usually stiff and erythematous. The patient's usual reaction is one of depression and despair. All members of the team simply must "keep the faith" and "stay the course." The patient and the team must be constantly reminded that by 12 to 18 months, the appearance of the grafts will improve markedly. In fact, at 12 to 18 months, these thick grafts are usually very much like normal skin. Without this mindset, the patient and the rest of the team will fall apart.

Most of the deformities after excision and grafting of deep facial burns will be found in the T-shaped area composed of the eyes, nose, lips, and mouth. With the thick grafts applied as described, in most instances the forehead and cheeks do not need reconstruction. In fact, they are quite like normal skin. But in the T-shaped area, things are different. Hypertrophic scarring and

---

*www.porex.com.
†Therabite Corporation, www.therabite.com.

wound contraction result in the deformities described later. Virtually all of the secondary reconstructions involve this area, and nearly all patients who have undergone excision and grafting of facial burns will need revision. This will remain the problem until there is a method of controlling contraction of wounds and grafts and hypertrophic scarring. This being the case, one might question the prudence of excision and grafting of facial burns. The answer is that most patients can tolerate relatively small procedures in the T-shaped area but cannot tolerate months of struggling with facial burns only to be told that they must now start all over with facial grafting of large areas, especially if the prime donor sites have already been used.

The general guidelines for reconstruction described by Feldman[21] and Achauer[22] are important and true.

1. A precise, comprehensive, prospective plan is important for the patient, family, nurses, therapists, physicians, insurance companies, and lawyers. None of the persons listed can accept an open-ended plan. Furthermore, donor sites must be rationed, complementary procedures done together, and conflicting procedures done separately. It is usually not possible for the surgeon or the patient to make such a plan in one 10-minute clinic visit. Several visits are usually necessary, and each may require 30 to 60 minutes.

2. The timing of the procedures must match all the constraints. In general, no reconstructions should be done in the first couple of months after discharge. The patients need time to resume other aspects of their lives, and usually at this time they are already overwhelmed by splints and pressure garments and exercises anyway. No reconstructive procedures should be done until the patient understands what will be done, the patient knows what will be required of him or her, and he or she is emotionally ready. If the patient does not understand that the pressure garment will be required 23 hours per day or is too depressed to wear it, the resurfacing will fail. Reconstruction of the extremities should generally precede reconstruction of the face. Facial reconstruction will usually not succeed if the patient cannot use the hands and feet. When it is time to reconstruct the face, functional needs should generally be addressed before cosmetic needs, although in dealing with the face and neck, the difference between the two is not so distinct. Last, it is usually wise to allow scars to mature before starting the reconstruction. Many scars will mature sufficiently enough that reconstruction is not necessary, and in fact the mature scar is as good as or better than the reconstruction would have been. However, in some situations, this last principle must be overlooked. If the nasal tip is totally destroyed, the appearance is too unattractive to wait months for the scars to mature.

3. Several general technical guidelines are aimed at restoring the contour and the surface of the face and correcting contractures. Identify and relieve intrinsic and extrinsic contractures. Resurface according to aesthetic units. Do not, if at all possible, resurface only portions of aesthetic units because this results in patches of differing color and texture. Use residual scar to build up areas where the burn or the excision destroyed the original tissue (e.g., the philtral ridges and the mental prominence). Maintain symmetry, for asymmetric reconstruction is intrinsically unattractive. If one cheek has been well resurfaced with a thick graft, do not use a flap if reconstruction is necessary for the other cheek. Match adjacent skin. If scalp skin was used to resurface a portion of the upper lip, do not use trunk skin to resurface the other portion. Orient scars parallel to the relaxed skin tension lines. Use epinephrine injections and bipolar coagulation to minimize bleeding and cautery damage. Use splints, pressure garments, and steroid injections just as for the original excision and grafting. Offer the patient aesthetic rhinoplasty and other facial cosmetic procedures if these would improve the facial appearance.

COMMON RESULTS OF EXCISION AND GRAFTING

Cole[15] has compiled and described our 20-plus year experience with more than 100 patients with this technique. Because there is no useful, numeric method to evaluate the results, we have included postoperative photographs of all patients found to have complete photographic sets including 1-year follow-up. Patients with essentially full-face burns are shown in Figure 65-3A (n = 25). Patients with partial face burns are shown in Figure 65-3B (n = 20). It is our opinion that the technique yields results that permit burn victims to function in the world with a shorter period of morbidity and fewer and smaller reconstructive procedures than in the classic method of spontaneous healing followed by reconstruction. On the other hand, it is not a panacea. The common problems and reconstructive methods for each are considered.

Hypertrophic Scars

After excision and grafting of face burns, hypertrophic scarring is uncommon, as can be seen in Figure 65-3. Therefore, revision of significant hypertrophic scars is usually not necessary. However, graft loss, although uncommon, is not totally prevented by the two-stage grafting and the deep excisions. It may result from hematoma, but a more common reason is shallow excision resulting in healing of the bed underneath the graft and sloughing of the graft. Such defects are usually small and are allowed to heal spontaneously, and this may result in two-dimensional areas of hypertrophic scarring.

Another cause of hypertrophic scarring is failure to excise and graft an area. As described before, the usual method is to excise and graft those areas that at 10 days are not healed or essentially healed. Sometimes the areas allowed to heal spontaneously become hypertrophic. In the male patient, these areas may incorporate whiskers and form a purulent hypertrophic scar.

Pressure garments and Silastic sheeting are used commonly to prevent and treat these lesions, but not all respond. The unsatisfactory area may be small, moderate, or large in dimension and located in a grafted area or an area that healed spontaneously.

Small scars within skin-grafted areas are excised and closed in the facial skin lines under general or local anesthesia. An ellipse is drawn around the scar in the facial skin lines and the scar excised, leaving all normal

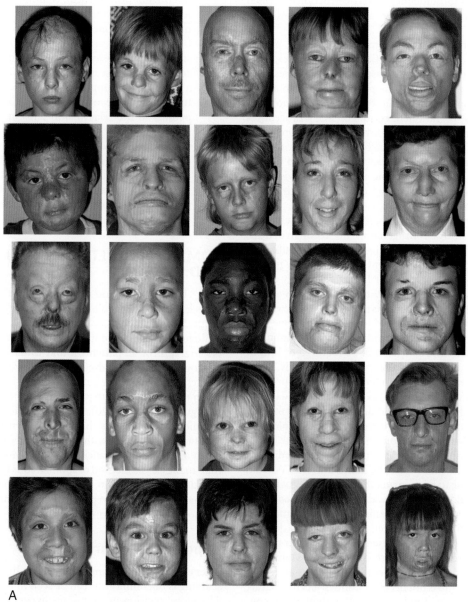

A

FIGURE 65-3. *A,* "Total" face results.

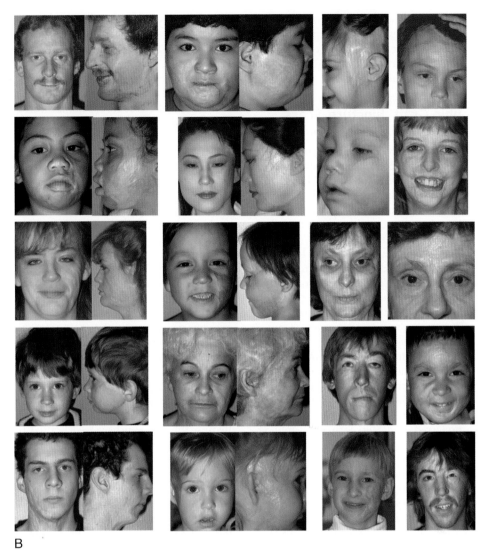

B

FIGURE 65-3, cont'd. *B,* "Partial" face results.

tissue in place. The surgeon must be careful not to excise too much. Grafted cheeks are already contracted, and after the "small" scar is removed, the defect may become quite large. The wound is then closed in layers in whatever fashion the surgeon prefers. Nonabsorbable sutures are generally indicated because these wounds can be tense. Steri-Strips are applied. Hypertrophic scarring after this procedure is uncommon, and the linear scar is usually much less unsightly than the previous two-dimensional scar.

Some hypertrophic scars in grafted areas are much too large to excise and close. Tissue expansion under the surrounding skin graft is not possible. In this case, the aesthetic unit must be re-excised and regrafted. The operative technique is identical to that used originally and described before.

On occasion, the scar within a grafted area cannot be included in an ellipse in the skin lines because of either size or shape but is still too small for complete re-excision and regrafting. In this case, serial excision as it lies seems the best alternative. Under general or local anesthesia, as much of the scar as possible is removed and the wound is closed in layers, again with use of nonabsorbable sutures and Steri-Strips. This may then be repeated in several months. This is of course a compromise, but patients are generally pleased with efforts to make these scars simply smaller.

If one is unfortunately faced with a hypertrophic scar in an area of the cheeks and forehead that was not grafted, reconstruction with skin grafts is inappropriate because it will result in a patched appearance. Rather, one must use other standard methods that are not unique to the deformities seen after excision and grafting. These include staged excision, skin expansion, and local or distant flap tissue. Fortunately, excision and grafting of deep facial burns as described diminishes the need for these procedures.

Hypertrophic Graft Juncture Scars

Hypertrophic scars are common at graft junctures, especially in the lower face and, in particular, at the nasolabial creases (Fig. 65-4). Careful edge-to-edge suturing of the grafts at the time of the initial grafting does not prevent this. When severe, and in conjunction with the yoke of graft made up of the two cheek grafts and the neck graft, a condition to be described later, these prevent full mouth opening.

If mild and small, the scars are ignored. If moderate in severity and small in dimensions, steroid injections may be used (40 mg/mL triamcinolone, 40 to 80 mg monthly for 6 to 9 months), but many patients object to the monthly clinic visits and the pain of the injections. Therefore, the use of steroids is not a common practice for these lesions.

If these are small enough, the procedure of choice is simple excision and closure under general or local anesthesia. Again, all normal tissue is left in the depths of the wound, and the wound is closed in layers in whatever fashion the surgeon prefers. Nonabsorbable sutures are preferred, and Steri-Strips are applied. Recurrence of scar as significant as that excised is unusual.

If the scar is too wide for simple excision and closure, serial excision is again an option with techniques similar to those already described. This is usually preferable to Z-plasty and other tissue-rearranging techniques at the juncture between graft and normal skin because the shape of the flap-plasty remains visible and is usually less acceptable than a small linear hypertrophic scar. Z-plasty or W-plasty is occasionally indicated.

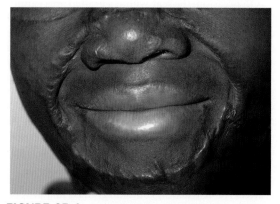

FIGURE 65-4. Hypertrophic juncture scars.

Missing Eyebrows

This deformity is common after deep facial burns (Fig. 65-5A). Two methods have been described for eyebrow reconstruction, strip scalp grafts and vascularized island pedicle flaps. Unfortunately, neither is truly useful after the forehead has been grafted. The residual bed after thermal injury and excision and grafting is usually thin and scarred, making strip grafts difficult to inset. On the other hand, tunneling the pedicle of the island pedicle flap under the forehead skin graft is also difficult. As a consequence, this deformity is often left unreconstructed and is clearly an unresolved aspect of facial burns. Some patients decide to merely pencil in the eyebrows. In fact, one author (L.E.) has reconstructed eyebrows in only two burn patients in 23 years, both with the method described here.

If reconstruction seems warranted, the strip scalp graft method described by Brent[23] is usually tried first. With local or general anesthesia, the position of the eyebrow is marked either to match a remaining eyebrow or, if there is no brow to match, by hand and by eye, trying not to place the eyebrow too high. Two separate incisions are made for the medial aspect of the eyebrow (Fig. 65-5B). Hemostasis is achieved with the bipolar cautery or simple pressure, with care taken to minimize thermal damage to the recipient bed. Because this area may have been grafted, there may be little subcutaneous tissue, and the edges of the graft may need to be undermined for a millimeter or two to achieve sufficient tissue to receive the graft. The grafts are then harvested from posterosuperior to the ears, choosing a location where the direction of the hairs will produce an upward and lateral direction in the reconstructed eyebrows (Fig. 65-5E). To achieve this, it may be necessary to harvest the graft from the contralateral side of the head. The grafts should be no more than 3 mm wide or the hairs in the middle of the graft will not survive, and the incisions should be made in slanted fashion to avoid cutting as many hair follicles as possible. The grafts are minimally defatted with care to avoid damage to hair follicles and then sutured in place, with minimal stitches passing through only the epidermis and the very uppermost dermis. Tie-over dressings are used, with the tie-over stitches not passing through the grafts. These are removed at 10 days. At a later time, the strip of hairless skin between the two medial grafts can be excised under local anesthesia, resulting in a thicker medial portion of the eyebrow (Fig. 65-5C). Further strip grafts can be added later to strengthen the medial brow (Fig. 65-5D).

The results of these procedures in burn patients are not truly remarkable (Fig. 65-5F), but they do reduce the amount of pencil work required.

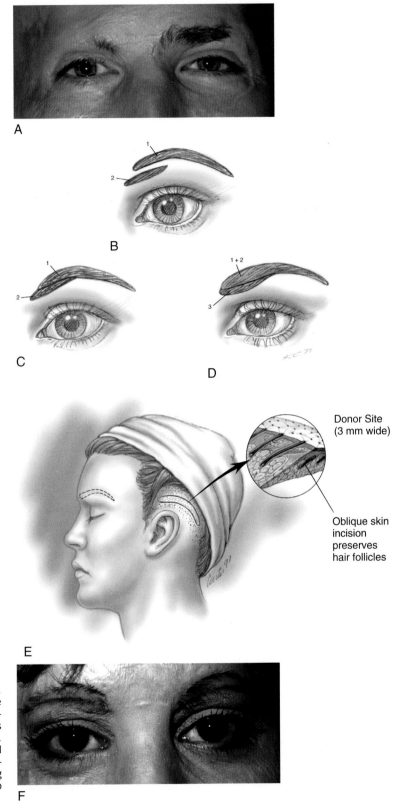

FIGURE 65-5. *A,* Missing eyebrow. *B,* Two strips of graft-scar are removed and grafted with full-thickness skin. *C,* Intervening hairless skin is removed and the defect closed. *D,* Further strip grafts can be added to strengthen the medial brow. *E,* Harvesting full-thickness hair-bearing scalp skin. *F,* Eyebrows after strip grafting.

Retraction of Upper Lid

The complex three-dimensional anatomy of the periorbital region requires abundant skin to appropriately drape its extensive surfaces. The propensity of skin grafts and scars to contract until opposed by equal forces causes flattening of periorbital contours and distortion of the normal relationships between eyelids and globe. When contractures are severe, they result in eversion of the eyelids and ectropion (Fig. 65-6A).

Satisfactory correction of both upper and lower eyelid deformities requires adherence to several basic principles. The goal of reconstruction should be step-by-step restoration of normal eyelid anatomy as much as possible. The thin specialized eyelid skin should be maintained or restored to its normal location. When upper lid contractures are extensive, an effective release will often result in an exceedingly large defect, which necessitates the use of split-thickness skin grafts. For smaller defects, full-thickness skin grafts may sometimes be appropriate. Full-thickness grafts work best when they make up the entire length of the supratarsal fold or are limited to the aesthetic units above the fold or in the pretarsal area. If the junction between a full-thickness graft and normal eyelid skin or a full-thickness graft and split-thickness graft crosses the supratarsal fold, the different thicknesses of the skin may cause unsightly distortions of this delicate anatomic feature. The shape of the palpebral fissure is of paramount importance. If complete release of extrinsic and intrinsic contractures is carried out, the upper lid will drape normally around the globe and normal relationships will be restored. The lower eyelids should cover the inferior corneoscleral limbus to avoid scleral show and the clinical appearance of ectropion.

Careful analysis of the eyelid deformity should be carried out to determine whether it is the result of an intrinsic or extrinsic contracture. If the contracture is extrinsic with preservation of normal eyelid skin, the extrinsic forces should be corrected. Carrying out a release and graft at the eyelid margin in such cases can create significant iatrogenic deformities and should be avoided (Fig. 65-6B to D).

When retraction of the upper eyelids is the result of intrinsic contracture of skin grafts and scars, release should be carried out at the ciliary margin. Typically, the deep concavity in the region of the medial canthus and nasal bridge has been obliterated and the upper eyelid skin crosses in a straight plane from the supraorbital ridge to the free border of the lid (Fig. 65-6E and F). Surgery is performed under general anesthesia. Releasing incisions are marked along the eyelid margin and are carried out well beyond the medial and lateral canthi (Fig. 65-6G). It is important to "fishtail" or "dart" the incisions medially and laterally so that the deep concavity of the medial canthal area

and the contour of the lateral canthal area can be appropriately resurfaced. This helps to minimize postoperative contracture. Local anesthesia is infiltrated in the incisions before preparation and draping for postoperative pain control and hemostasis. Two traction sutures are placed in the gray line of the eyelid at the junction between the medial and lateral thirds.

The release is carried out 1 to 2 mm from the ciliary margin and is carefully limited to the superficial fibrous scarring. When pretarsal eyelid skin is present, the release should be carried out at the margin of the eyelid skin and scar. Most often, there is partial or complete preservation of the orbicularis oculi. The muscle has been "bunched up" or "rolled up" by the contracting process rather than injured. The muscle must be carefully unfurled and the eyelid allowed to drape freely over the globe (Fig. 65-6H and I). Upper eyelid releases should always be carried out separately from lower eyelid releases so that overcorrection can be accomplished. Split-thickness skin grafts are most often used for resurfacing upper lids because of the extent of the resulting defect and the need for overcorrection. These are taken from the best available donor site in terms of color and texture match. Full-thickness skin grafts may sometimes be appropriate but have disadvantages. The relatively thick dermis from even the thinnest donor sites can inhibit formation of a normal delicate supratarsal fold. The limited size of full-thickness grafts may lead to undercorrection. The one exception is full-thickness skin grafts from the contralateral upper eyelid, but this donor site is rarely available and is appropriate only for the most minor upper lid contractures.

The split-thickness skin graft is harvested at a thickness of 0.016 inch. The graft should be laid in with significant redundancy, anticipating that this will be taken up by the tie-over stent (Fig 65-6J). The skin graft is sutured into place with interrupted 4-0 silk sutures. A Xeroform and cotton stent is applied. When the stent is tied down, there is a deliberate overcorrection of the eyelid position. No effort is made to preserve a visual field. Visual obstruction is usually minimal and transient and can be corrected with appropriate head positioning. Adequate skin must be provided in a transverse as well as in a vertical dimension. If the graft is not wide enough, there can be artificial indentations of the normal convex curvature of the lid from medial to lateral.

The stents are left in place for 10 days to 2 weeks, if possible. After the stent is removed, a pressure mask can be fashioned to compress the portion of the grafts in the area above the supratarsal fold and against the orbital rim. Any persisting raised margins of the graft can be corrected at a later date by either excision or Z-plasty revision. Recontraction of upper eyelid grafts is unusual if an adequate release has been carried out and the grafts heal without complication (Fig. 65-6K to N).

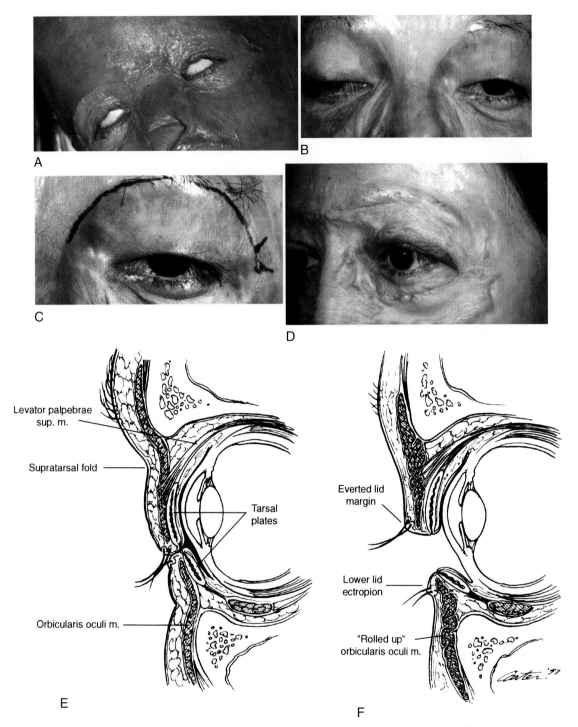

FIGURE 65-6. *A*, Retraction of the upper lid. *B*, Extrinsic contracture of upper lids. Right upper lid shows previous inadequate release with graft placed in the center of unburned upper lid skin. *C*, Proper location of releasing incision at outer edge of unburned lid skin. *D*, Postoperative result with lid skin restored to normal location and configuration. *E*, Normal eyelid anatomy. *F*, Eyelid anatomy after burn contracture. There is shortening and eversion of the lids with flattening of contours and bunching of the orbicularis oculi muscle.   *Continued*

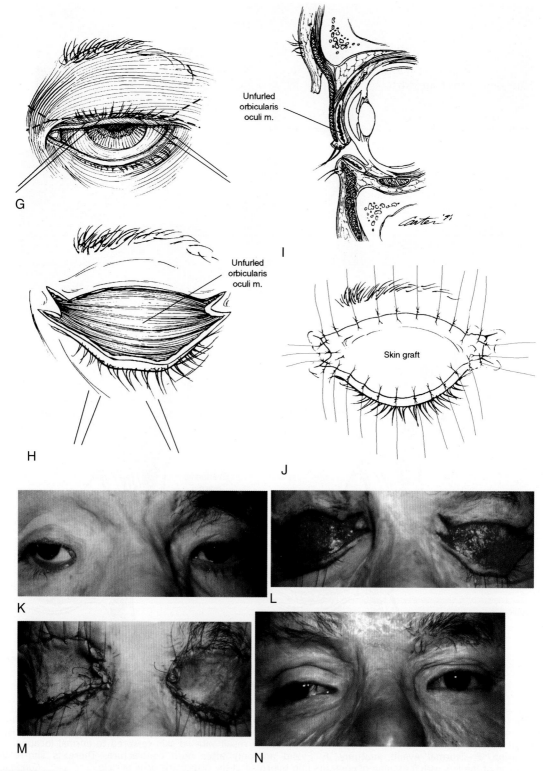

FIGURE 65-6, cont'd. *G,* Upper eyelid releasing incisions. *H* and *I,* After release, the orbicularis oculi has been restored to its thin, flat shape with the lid draping over the globe and the supratarsal fold restored. *J,* Skin graft sutured in place. *K,* Bilateral upper and lower lid contractures. *L,* Incisions marked for upper lid release adjacent to the ciliary margin. *M,* Intraoperative release with orbicularis oculi muscle unfurled and contracture overcorrected. *N,* Split-thickness skin grafts used to resurface the defect.

Ectropion of the Lower Lid

Lower eyelid ectropion (Fig. 65-7A) can be the result of either intrinsic or extrinsic contracture. The importance of accurate diagnosis cannot be overemphasized. Attempting to correct an extrinsic contracture by releasing and grafting through normal eyelid skin in the lower eyelids causes a significant iatrogenic deformity, which is difficult to correct.

The goal of lower eyelid reconstruction should be more than correction of frank ectropion. The normal shape of the palpebral fissure should be restored,

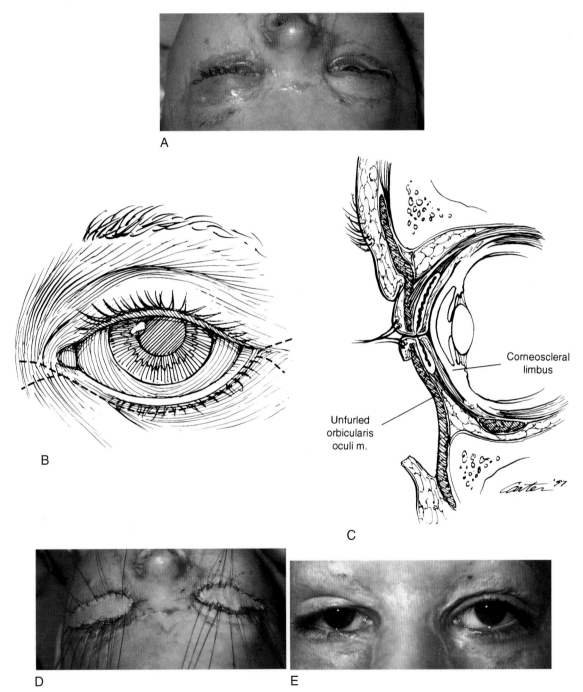

FIGURE 65-7. *A,* Eyelid ectropion. *B,* Lower eyelid releasing incision. *C,* Lower eyelid after complete release of superficial scarring. The orbicularis oculi muscle is flat and retains its integrity. *D,* Grafts inserted. *E,* Healed mature grafts.

and the lower eyelid should cover the inferior margin of the corneoscleral limbus in neutral gaze. Correction will be satisfactory only if this endpoint is reached.

Surgery is carried out under general anesthesia. Local anesthesia is infiltrated before preparation and draping to minimize bleeding. Traction sutures are placed in the lid margin at the medial and lateral thirds. The releasing incision is made 1 to 2 mm below the ciliary margin and carried beyond the medial and lateral canthi with darts (Fig 65-7B). These darts avoid straight-line scars and are important to minimize the "bowstringing" of grafts and scars across concave contours. Care should be taken to carry out the release in the superficial layer where the contracture has occurred. Incising through the fibers of the orbicularis oculi muscle must be avoided. The muscle has usually been rolled up by the superficial contracted scar to an even greater extent than occurs in the upper eyelid. If the releasing incision is carried through this muscle mass to the septum orbital and a skin graft placed, a permanent unsightly crevice is created. The muscle must carefully be teased apart under tension until it is restored to its normal flat contour (Fig. 65-7C). When all of the superficial tethering scar has been divided, the margin of the lower lid can easily be raised above the upper corneoscleral limbus.

Split-thickness or full-thickness skin grafts can be used for lower eyelid resurfacing. The decision should be based on the size of the defect, color and texture of surrounding tissues, and donor site availability. For severe contractures, most often the size of the defect requires thick, split-thickness skin grafts.

The graft is sutured into place with interrupted 4-0 silk sutures (Fig. 65-7D). Care should be taken to provide adequate skin in both a vertical and transverse dimension. A tie-over bolster dressing is then constructed from Xeroform and cotton. The stent is left in place for 10 days to 2 weeks. A pressure mask can be advantageous. This is constructed to put pressure along the inferior orbital rim to achieve the final result (Fig. 65-7E).

Medial Canthal Webs

In virtually all cases when the lids and nose must be grafted, canthal webs form (Fig. 65-8A). It seems impossible to fashion the grafts to avoid this result, nor does it seem possible to devise splinting devices to prevent the deformity. These webs come in all shapes and sizes, so no one method will suffice for all. In fact, it is classic plastic surgery in which the surgeon must analyze the defect and decide on a method of repair, which may be creative and spontaneous.

If the web is merely a ridge, a simple Z-plasty will suffice. This may be done under local or general anesthesia and closed in whatever manner the surgeon prefers. If the web is large, there is no alternative but to incise it, remove the scar tissue, and regraft the area. This again may be done under local or general anesthesia. After the web is removed, the area is resurfaced, usually with a small, postauricular, full-thickness skin graft covered with a tie-over dressing. This leaves a patch but is more attractive than a large canthal web.

When the web is of medium dimensions, it can be corrected with any of several flap-plasties, all done under local or general anesthesia. The VM-plasty[24-26] and the double opposing Z-plasty[27] are simple and work well for these mild to moderate deformities. Under local or general anesthesia, the VM-plasty (Fig. 65-8B) or double opposing Z-plasty (Fig. 65-8C to E) is marked with the limbs being 2 to 10 mm in length, depending on the shape of the web. The wound is then closed in whatever manner the surgeon prefers. For larger defects, the elongation method of Converse is used.[27] The location of the canthus is marked, and then an oblique incision is made through the skin graft that forms the outer layer of the web (Fig. 65-8F to I). With the second incision, this is converted into a flap that is raised off the lining. An oblique incision opposite the first is then made through the lining of the web. Each flap is then sutured over a raw edge, exposing the caruncle. The wound may be closed in any manner the surgeon prefers. Because these webs come in many shapes and sizes, the surgeon should be prepared to use any flap-plasty that seems indicated for the defect at hand. The three described have been useful, however (Fig. 65-8J to L).

Deformed Nasal Tip with Retracted or Missing Alar Margins

The contracting forces of thermal injury typically shorten the nose and cause alar flaring (Fig. 65-9A and B). With increasing severity of burn injury, there can be tissue loss of varying degrees. Mild to moderate alar flaring is best treated by releasing and grafting in the area of the alar groove. The releasing incision can be placed in the alar groove following its contour around the lobule. The bulky soft tissue that makes up the lobule is often compressed by overlying scar; with release, this can be rolled out to restore adequate contour. The resulting defect is resurfaced with either full-thickness or split-thickness grafts, depending on the adjacent tissues (Fig. 65-9C and D).

When there has been focal loss of tissue on the alar rim, notching can be addressed by carrying out a release in the area of the alar groove, lowering the alar rim an appropriate amount. The rim position can then be maintained by use of a composite graft from the ear containing cartilage. This can be used to support the rim in the best position.

When the nose has been significantly shortened, additional length must be obtained. This task is made easier if the nose will require resurfacing in the future. An inferiorly based turndown flap of dorsal skin graft and scar can be used to lengthen the nose. The rich blood supply makes such flaps reliable despite the scarred base. Deep tissues can be used to simulate the missing bulk of the alar lobules and tip. This technique can be repeated more than once, if necessary, to obtain sufficient nasal length and to position and shape the lobules and nasal tip satisfactorily. After the nose has been lengthened and the position of the lobule and tip is satisfactory, the entire nasal dorsum and columella can be resurfaced with a graft, eliminating irregularities in contour, color, and texture.

When extensive nasal damage has resulted from thermal injury, there is almost always extensive damage to the remainder of the face, resulting in extensive scarring and skin grafts. In this context, the use of distant flap tissue, such as a Tagliacozzi flap or radial forearm free flap, is rarely indicated for nasal reconstruction. The unburned tissues of the nasal reconstruction contrast sharply with the remainder of the face and do not provide a satisfactory aesthetic result. If flap tissue is required to allow reconstruction of a supporting framework of bone and cartilage, it must, of course, be used. After a satisfactory supporting framework has been restored, the cutaneous portion of the flap can be excised and replaced with a skin graft if this will provide a better color and texture match. Median forehead flap reconstruction in the context of burn injury is infrequently indicated in our experience.

There is a postburn nasal tip deformity that responds to reduction rhinoplasty and alar rim

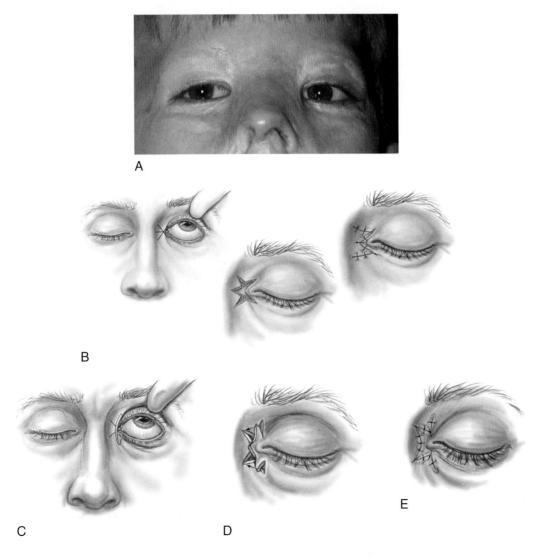

FIGURE 65-8. *A,* Canthal webs. *B,* VM-plasty. *C,* Skin markings of the double opposing Z-plasty. *D,* Incisions made and flaps moved. *E,* Flaps sutured into place.   *Continued*

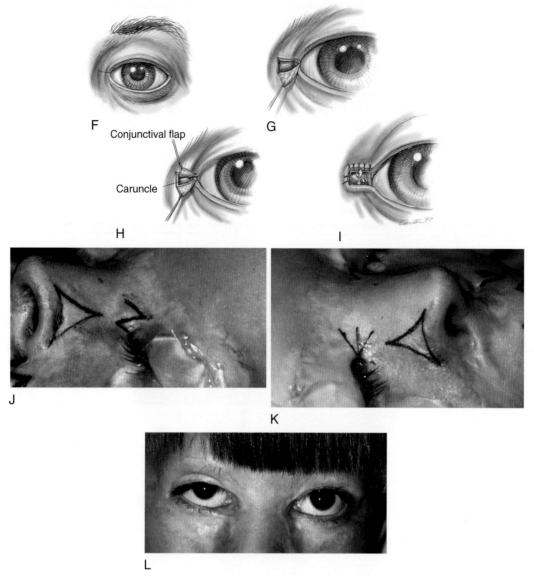

FIGURE 65-8, cont'd. *F,* Skin markings. *G,* Skin flap raised and markings of the conjunctival flap. *H,* Conjunctival flap raised. *I,* Flaps sutured into place. *J,* Z-plasty marking to the canthal web. *K,* VM-plasty markings on medial canthus. *L,* Medial canthal webs corrected.

advancement flaps. This defect includes moderate alar rim notching, exposed columella, and open nares (Fig. 65-9*E* and *F*). Under local or general anesthesia, the alar rim flaps are marked (Fig. 65-9*G* and *H*). These must be fashioned in accord with the defect. Figure 65-9*G* shows an alar rim flap to be advanced anteriorly into the incised alar rim. Figure 65-9*H* shows a modified bilobed flap; the anterior flap is advanced into the incision in the rim, and the posterior flap is used to fill the defect created by the first flap. In addition, the columella is shortened and, if necessary, the dorsum narrowed. This produces a small nose but with proper proportions (Fig. 65-9*I* and *J*).

Flat Upper Lip with No Philtrum, Philtral Ridges, or Cupid's Bow and Retracted Upper Lip

The contractile forces of burn trauma easily distort the subtle lines and contours that make up normal lip anatomy. The upper lip becomes shortened and loses its concave shape. Early excision and grafting can minimize or prevent the shortening of the lip and eversion of the vermilion, but the philtral hollow and philtral ridges are flattened and the Cupid's bow is obliterated (Fig. 65-10*A* and *B*). Successful reconstruction of the upper lip requires restoring appropriate length,

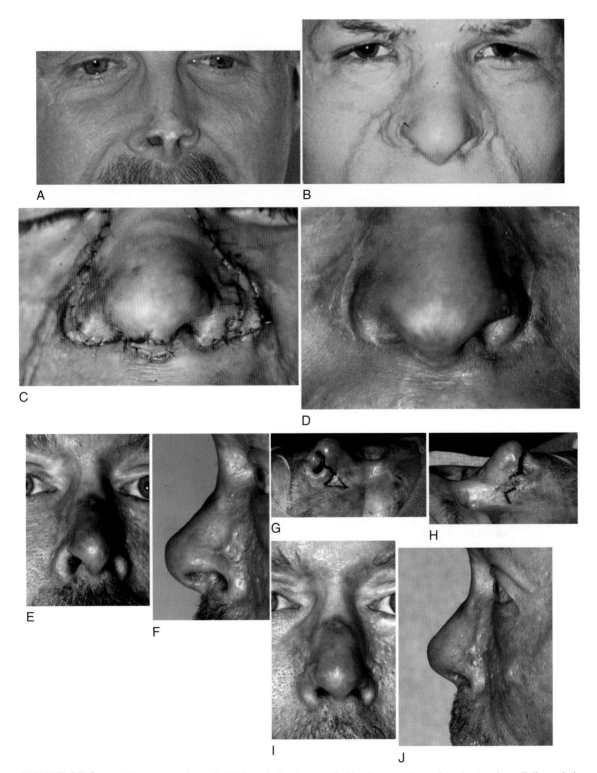

FIGURE 65-9. *A,* Missing alar rims. *B,* Widened alar bases. *C,* Alar bases released and moved medially and the defect grafted. *D,* The final result. *E,* Alar rims notched, columella visible, and nares open. *F,* Lateral view. *G,* Alar rim flap marked. *H,* Alar rim flap marked. *I,* Final result. *J,* Lateral view.

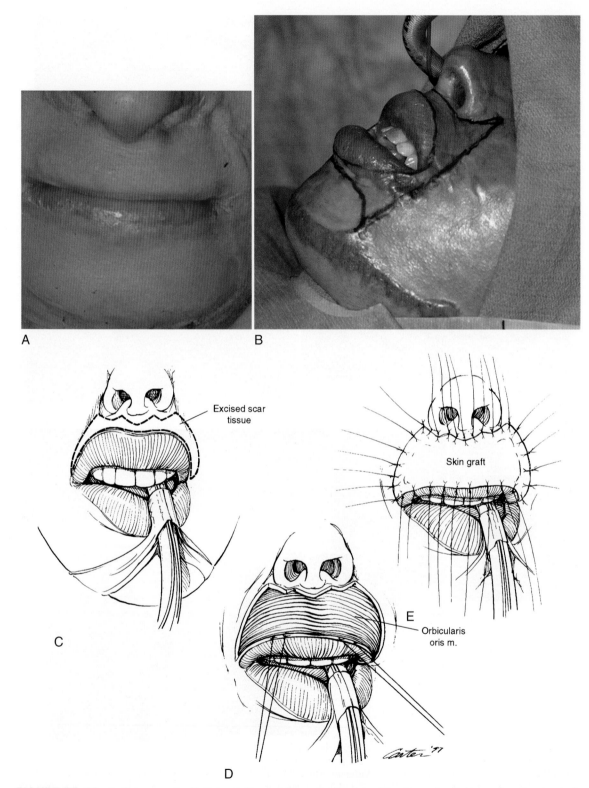

FIGURE 65-10. *A,* Flat upper lip. *B,* Retracted upper lip and ectropion of the lower lip. *C,* Upper lip releasing incision. Scar is excised when indicated. *D,* Release is carried beyond the oral commissures. The orbicularis oris muscle is unfurled, creating a concave upper lip. *E,* Skin graft sutured in place.

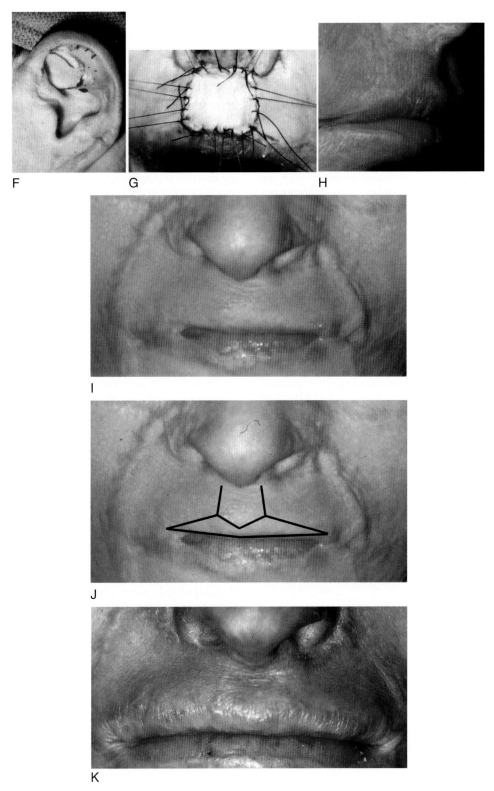

FIGURE 65-10, cont'd. *F,* Design for harvesting composite graft of cartilage and preauricular skin from the triangular fossa. *G,* Composite graft in place after lengthening of lip and release of transverse tension. *H,* Cartilage graft aids in positioning of upper lip as well as in creating philtral dimple. *I,* Flat upper lip with no Cupid's bow. *J,* Markings. *K,* Final result.

reconstructing a philtrum with a Cupid's bow, and ensuring that the width of the upper lip is slightly greater than the lower lip and that the upper lip precedes the lower lip in lateral view.

Surgery is carried out under general anesthesia with an orotracheal tube. A REA tube can be helpful. Skin graft or scar in the upper lip can be used to fashion local flaps for reconstruction of the columella and alar margins when this is necessary. A releasing incision is marked out as shown in Figure 65-10C. Unfavorable scars and skin grafts in the upper lip are excised according to the upper lip aesthetic unit. In many cases, the shortening of the upper lip and eversion of the mucosa result in little skin graft or scar between the base of the columella and the free border of the lip. In such cases, minimal or no scar excision is necessary. After the releasing incision has been made as shown and the contracted tissues teased apart, a defect in the shape of the upper lip aesthetic unit will be created and no scar excision will be required (Fig. 65-10D). Release is carried lateral to the oral commissure. The scarring is usually superficial to the orbicularis oris muscle. With patient, careful dissection in this plane, the lip can be restored to normal length. Dissection should be kept superficial to the substance of the orbicularis oris to avoid creating iatrogenic contour deformities. The bunched muscle will unfurl and resume its normal shape. The release should not be "overcorrected" in the vertical dimension. Contraction is moderate after release and satisfactory resurfacing, and the lip can easily be made too long.

The transverse release of the upper lip must be complete so that it can resume its bowed convex shape from commissure to commissure in the anterior-posterior dimension. Inadequate transverse release can result in tightening across the free border of the lip at the graft-vermilion junction. This prevents restoration of a normal pouting shape. Tightness at the vermilion-cutaneous junction also makes the lip convex in profile view, a hallmark of the postburn lip deformity.

The best reconstructive material for the upper lip, in our experience, has been full-thickness skin grafts (Fig. 65-10E). The graft must be of adequate dimensions, particularly transversely, so that a loose free border of the upper lip can be created. Flaps are usually a poor reconstructive option in this area and rarely allow normal facial animation and expression.

The best technique for reconstruction of the philtral dimple is that described by Schmid using the triangular fossa of the ear. This has been a key element in effective aesthetic restoration of upper lip contour. The Schmid[28] graft can be used either at the time of the initial release or as a secondary procedure. Either way can be successful. Better control of the lip length and contour can be obtained when a previously placed upper lip graft is divided in the middle and the Schmid graft placed as a secondary procedure. The composite graft is harvested and the resulting ear defect resurfaced with either a thick split- or full-thickness graft. An ideal donor site is the retroauricular skin, when available. The resulting composite graft measures approximately 2.2 cm in height by 1.2 cm in width. Each case will vary. The cartilage is taken somewhat smaller than the skin and can be thinned in the central portion. The stiffness of the cartilage helps in setting the length of the lip and preserving the concavity of the dimple. When the reconstruction is done as one procedure, the philtrum is first reconstructed with a composite graft to set the lip length. Full-thickness skin grafts are then harvested to resurface the lateral thirds of the lip. The grafts are sutured into place with interrupted 4-0 silk sutures. The composite philtral reconstruction is sutured to the medial borders of the graft. A Xeroform and cotton stent is applied. The stent is left in place for 2 weeks. Postoperative management consists of conformers and a mask (Fig. 65-10F to H).

A lesser procedure will occasionally suffice to rebuild the philtrum and Cupid's bow (Fig. 65-10I to K). Under local or general anesthesia, the proper position of the Cupid's bow is drawn, as is each philtral column and the vermilion-graft juncture. The philtral column markings are merely incised into the graft and sutured, so as to create a subtle scar. The surgeon then dissects under the middle of the graft in the location of the philtrum and removes scar and muscle until graft and mucosa can be sutured together to mimic the philtral dimple. The graft included in the Cupid's bow markings is then excised. All wounds are then closed in whatever manner the surgeon prefers. The subtle improvement can be seen in Figure 65-10K.

Deformed Lower Lip with Ectropion, Flat Chin, and Thick Lower Lip

Deformities of the lower lip–chin complex have a recurring pattern (Fig. 65-11A; see also Fig. 65-10A). The lower lip vermilion and mucosa are everted and inferiorly displaced; the lower teeth and gum may be visible in the absence of mentalis spasm. The lower lip appears wider than the upper lip in anterior view, the reverse of the normal relationship. The contractile forces of skin graft and scarring eliminate the normal concavity between the vermilion-cutaneous junction of the lip and the chin pad. The chin pad is compressed, creating a "pseudomicrogenia." Correction of this constellation of deformities requires attention to each component at the time of reconstruction.

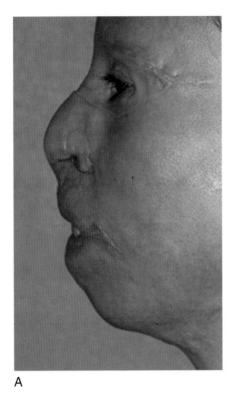

A

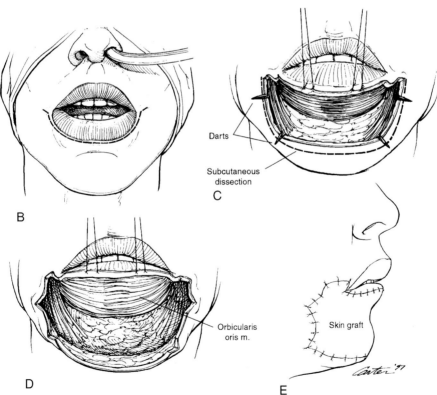

B

C

Darts

Subcutaneous
dissection

D

Orbicularis
oris m.

E

Skin graft

Carter '97

FIGURE 65-11. *A,* Thick lower lip and flat mental prominence. *B,* Lower lip releasing incision. Note extension lateral to oral commissures. *C,* Lateral darts expand the release. *D,* After complete release, the lower lip can be elevated above the upper incisors, and the defect has expanded to include the entire lower lip–chin aesthetic unit. *E,* The skin graft sutured in place with a concave lip-chin sulcus.   *Continued*

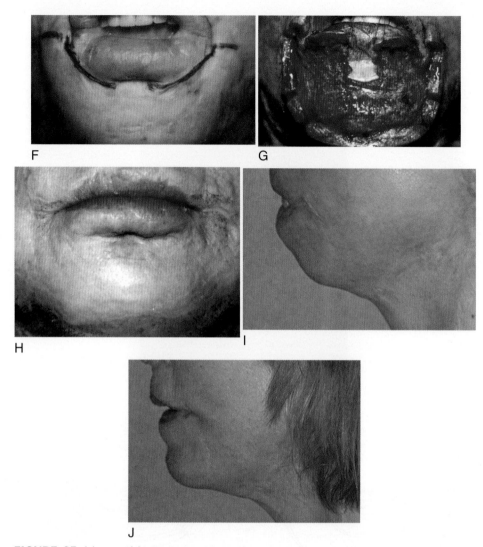

FIGURE 65-11, cont'd. *F,* Lower lip ectropion with eversion and inferior displacement and initial releasing incisions. *G,* Complete release of lip with lateral darts. *H,* Restoration of normal lip-chin anatomy with restoration of balance between upper and lower lips. *I,* Thick lower lip and flattened mental prominence. *J,* Final result after chin advancement. (Surgery performed by Dr. Mark Egbert.)

Surgery is performed under general anesthesia. Nasotracheal anesthesia is preferred because it eliminates any distortion of the lower lip and commissures. A releasing incision is outlined 1 to 2 mm into the cutaneous scar and extended an appropriate distance beyond the oral commissures bilaterally (Fig. 65-11*B*). Local anesthesia with epinephrine is injected for postoperative pain control and hemostasis. The releasing incision is made along the lip margin. The lip is then released, with care taken to preserve the integrity of the orbicularis oris muscle. This flat muscle is unfurled in the same fashion as the orbicularis oculi. It is again

essential to avoid dividing the muscle because this creates unsightly troughs and crevices in the contour of the lip-chin complex. At the lateral edges of the release, the incision is darted or fishtailed. This results in a W-plasty roughly along the infracommissural fold. The compressive scar over the chin pad may need to be excised to allow complete release. At the margin of the overall defect, multiple releasing incisions are made that allow the cheek and neck skin to retract around the prominence of the chin (Fig. 65-11*C*). Release of the lip and commissures must be complete. At the completion of the procedure, the lip should be able to be completely turned in. The free border of the lower lip should be well above the inferior border of the upper incisors at the completion of the release. The oral commissure must be completely mobile and inverted (Fig. 65-11D).

The lip-chin complex is then resurfaced, with the best possible skin for each individual case. This will often be full-thickness skin grafts (Fig. 65-11E). A flap may sometimes be appropriate if the remainder of the face is made up of flap tissue. Split-thickness skin grafts are often the best available material. All of these resurfacing modalities can be satisfactory.

When the deformity does not involve the entire lip-chin complex, a lesser release can be carried out. The lip-chin sulcus can be used as an aesthetic subunit, and the release of the lip can be limited to this area. The lateral extent of the release should be the same as previously described. The resurfacing then goes from infra-commissural fold to infracommissural fold with appropriate W-plasties in the area of the fold.

The importance of complete correction of the lower lip contracture cannot be overemphasized. Persistent inferior displacement resulting in chronic mentalis spasm is one of the most common of the postburn facial stigmata. Adequate release, allowing the lower lip to completely cover the lower teeth without tension, can dramatically improve facial appearance and improve lip function. Even if a release and graft somewhat violate the principles of aesthetic units, overall improvement in facial appearance will be obtained when the lower lip is restored to its natural position.

Regardless of whether skin grafts or flaps are used to resurface the chin, there is a tendency for compression to occur. Chin implants can help prevent compression and therefore maintain an adequate chin prominence. The grafts are sutured in with 4-0 silk sutures. A Xeroform and cotton stent is applied. The stent dressing is left in place for 2 weeks or longer. This is the best possible postoperative conformer, and there is nothing to be gained by earlier removal (Fig. 65-11F to H).

In spite of treatment as described, there may be a thick lower lip and a flattened mental prominence from thermal injury, surgical excision, or contraction (Fig. 65-11I). In this case, the lower lip should be debulked. This may be done by incising the vermilion-graft juncture, undermining the graft for a limited distance, and removing scar and orbicularis muscle. The groove between the lower lip and chin should also be sculpted. This may be done through a curved incision between the lip and chin. If the defect is severe, a silicone implant may be inserted through the submental approach in a supraperiosteal pocket. These implants are usually small. If the problem is compounded by skeletal deformities that existed before the injury, they too should be corrected because the burn residuals will make the

general appearance even worse. In the patient in Figure 65-11J, chin advancement was done.

Microstomia and Skin Graft Yoke from Cheek to Chin to Cheek

This occurs after grafting for two reasons. First, the unyielding skin grafts at the commissures prevent full mouth opening. Second, the yoke of skin graft created by the grafts of the cheeks and the neck also prevents full opening of the mouth (Fig. 65-12A). Patients who have healed without skin grafting may present with the same problem secondary to a continuous band of inelastic scar tissue extending from zygoma to zygoma (Fig. 65-12B).

The length of the mouth can be reconstructed as described by Converse.[29] Under local or general anesthesia, the position of the new angle of the mouth is determined by inspection, but it is generally placed at a line dropped from the medial margin of the limbus. A triangle of skin graft and underlying scar is removed at each commissure, and the mucosa is then wrapped out and used to close the defect (Fig. 65-12C to F). The method of closure is critical. The sutures should be robust (i.e., 3-0 plain gut or 3-0 permanent), and the bites should be large. These wounds tend to fall apart, and strong sutures with large tissue bites are necessary. This procedure works nicely to eliminate the appearance of a narrow mouth and does to some degree allow a greater degree of opening. Because it is better to err on the short side, the procedure may need to be repeated if the lengthening obtained by the first procedure is insufficient (Fig. 65-12G to I).

The second cause is much more difficult to correct. Describing the problem is simple. The grafts on the cheeks and the neck simply do not expand enough to allow full mouth opening. Correcting the problem requires more tissue, but adding grafts creates a patched appearance, and starting over with cheek and neck flaps is usually rejected by the patient. The surgeon and the patient usually agree to leave it alone. In some patients, breaking the contracture band by carrying out releasing incisions below the mandibular margin and extending across the submental triangle allows the addition of either full-thickness or split-thickness grafts in a relatively inconspicuous location. This serves the double purpose of improving oral opening as well as decreasing tension on facial features and improving jaw line definition.

Mandibular Growth Retardation

This problem occurs in young children after wearing of a pressure garment on the face for several months.[30,31] Fortunately, the problem resolves spontaneously after the garments are discontinued, but it is wise to discuss this with the parents. Because the problem does exist, if the potential for scarring is minimal, the pressure garments are omitted in these patients.

Color Mismatch

These are common and, to our knowledge, are neither preventable nor repairable (Fig. 65-13). Bleaching creams containing hydroquinone are minimally effective in treating hyperpigmented scars and grafts. Chemical peeling agents such as phenol and trichloroacetic acid have unpredictable results and can be harmful. For pigmented lesions, use of lasers, such as the yttrium-aluminum-garnet and alexandrite lasers, is traumatic and can result in further hyperpigmentation. The pulsed dye laser can be effective in decreasing chronic hyperemia in facial burn scars. The ability to control pigment changes would greatly enhance burn care.

Neck Contracture

The voluminous literature dealing with the problem of cervical contractures after burn injury attests to both the frequency and difficulty of this reconstructive

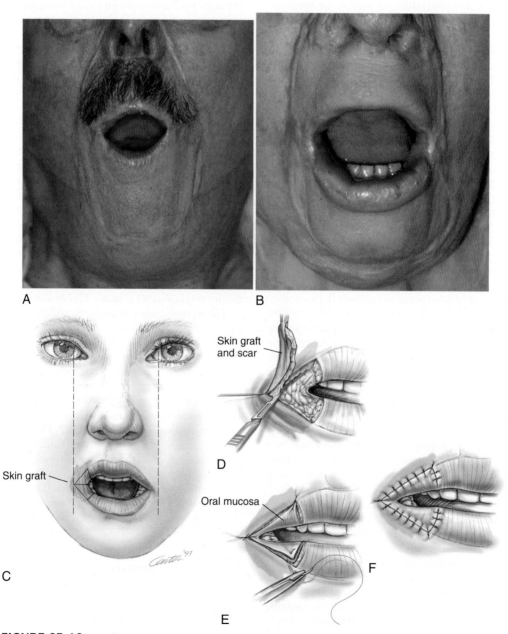

FIGURE 65-12. *A,* Microstomia. *B,* Cheek, neck, cheek yoke. *C,* The scarred commissure. *D,* Removing the scar. *E,* Oral mucosa advanced into the defect. *F,* Oral mucosa sutured in place.

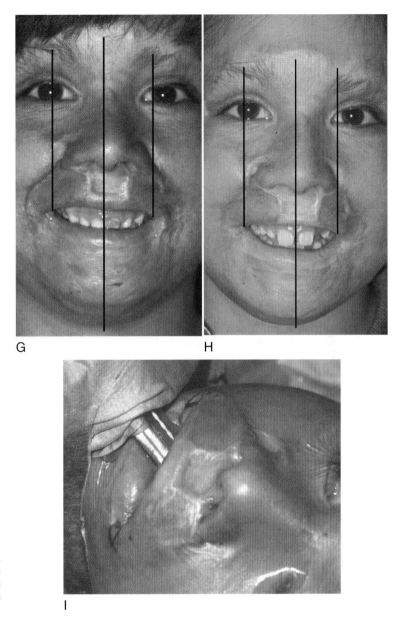

FIGURE 65-12, cont'd. *G,* Preoperative appearance. *H,* Postoperative appearance. Note right commissure has been moved laterally but left has not. *I,* Intraoperative markings.

challenge (Fig. 65-14A). Every deformity is different, and the tissue available for reconstruction varies greatly from patient to patient. Selecting the best reconstructive plan for each patient is a challenging exercise that requires familiarity with all of the reconstructive options.

Several basic goals must be accomplished for reconstruction to be successful. The neck contracture should be released to the point where all extrinsic forces causing distortion of facial features have been eliminated, if at all possible. Contracting forces in the neck tend to obliterate the jaw line and pull the neck skin forward into the same plane as the cheeks. Satisfactory correction must restore jaw line definition and separate the plane of the cheek from that of the neck. Restoration of a pleasing chin-neck angle is exceedingly important and may be facilitated by chin augmentation.

When the entire cervicopectoral region has been resurfaced with skin grafts, the neck reconstruction is usually best carried out with skin grafting (Fig. 65-14A to C). Intensive postoperative splinting with conformers and pressure garments is mandatory. More than one release and grafting procedure is frequently required. When the cervicopectoral region consists of grafted areas, healed second-degree burn, and uninjured skin, local flaps with or without skin grafts are

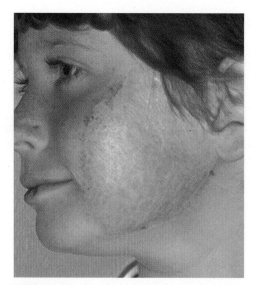

FIGURE 65-13. Color mismatch.

often most advantageous. Distant flaps with microvascular free tissue transfer have also been used effectively for cervical contractures. The best reconstructive option usually becomes manifest as each deformity is analyzed.

When local flaps are used for reconstruction, a number of principles are worth emphasizing. Tension is poorly tolerated in the vertical dimension. However, the neck usually tolerates transverse tension well. Vertical scars and contractures are often amenable to lengthening with Z-plasty variations. The Z-plasty flaps can be designed in such a way that the transverse tension resulting from flap transposition can be used to increase jaw line definition and help define the cervical-mental angle. Placement of releasing incisions in inconspicuous areas such as the submental triangle and beneath the mandibular margin can make skin grafts less noticeable and can actually help to define the jaw line. The overall goal should be the complete release of all extrinsic contracture forces that are deforming the mobile features of the face.

The technique selected for correction of neck contractures is not nearly as important as having a clear target in mind at the outset. If facial distortion is eliminated, a jaw line defined, and a pleasing chin-neck angle created, the outcome will be satisfactory from a functional and aesthetic standpoint. If the reconstruction focuses on color and texture of the neck skin and ignores the goals stated, the skin may look pleasing but the face and neck will be suboptimal.

Wrinkled Neck Graft

This unfortunate event is uncommon on the face but common on the neck after excision and grafting (Fig.

65-15). It is presumably a result of wound contraction that was not prevented by pressure garments and splints. The first step is to merely wait. Sometimes the wrinkling will disappear with time. If it does not, the only alternatives depend on whether an entire aesthetic unit or a partial unit is involved. If an entire aesthetic unit is involved, it must be re-excised and regrafted as described for the original burn. If a partial unit is involved, reconstruction with local flaps is indicated. This again requires the creativity of the plastic surgeon.

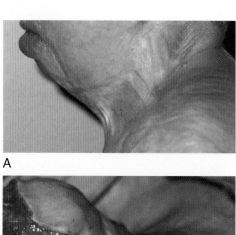

A

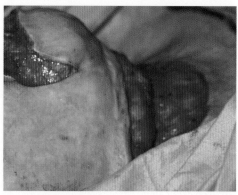

B

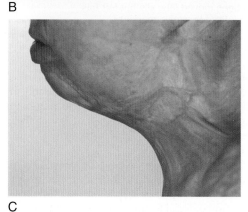

C

FIGURE 65-14. *A,* Contracted neck. *B,* Neck incised and widely opened. *C,* Final result.

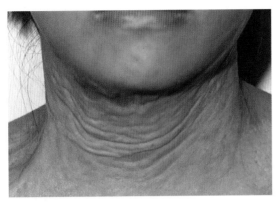

FIGURE 65-15. Wrinkled neck graft.

Neck Webs

These may occur at the lateral aspect of the neck where anterior grafts meet posterior unburned skin or at the edge of a graft that covered only a portion of the neck (Fig. 65-16A). They can be prevented by including darts or half Z-plasties with the original grafting. If the adjacent normal skin and grafts are acceptable to use as flaps (which is usually the case), this deformity is usually correctable with one or more Z- or VY-plasties done under local or general anesthesia (Fig. 65-16B to D). The flaps must be cut thickly because the vascularity of burned and grafted tissue is precarious but may be closed with the method of the surgeon's choice. A soft collar splint for 3 weeks is indicated.

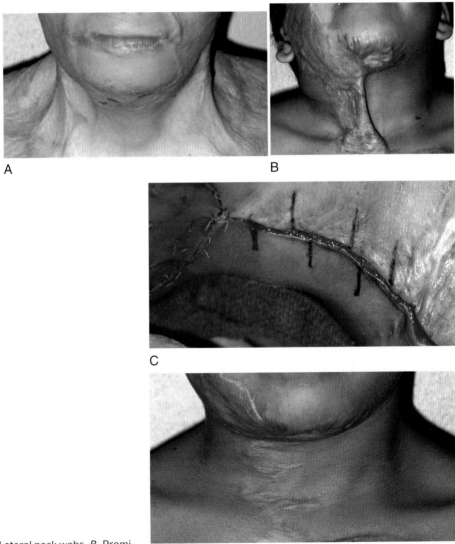

FIGURE 65-16. *A*, Lateral neck webs. *B*, Prominent neck web. *C*, Z-plasty outlined. *D*, Final result.

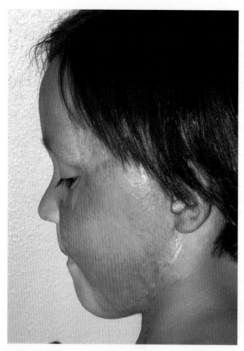

FIGURE 65-17. Thin, atrophic graft.

Thin Skin Grafts

Thin skin grafts should not be used for face grafting; they always appear atrophic and frequently become hyperpigmented (Fig. 65-17). There is no alternative but to remove them and resurface the area as described before.

Three-dimensional Tissue Loss from Fourth-, Fifth-, and Sixth-Degree Burns

If the three-dimensional structure of the face is missing, everything described here will be inadequate (Fig. 65-18). Methods must be used to rebuild the structure (e.g., the nose or the ear).

Poor Gestalt

Even if the described procedures go well, the overall gestalt after grafting of face burns is lacking

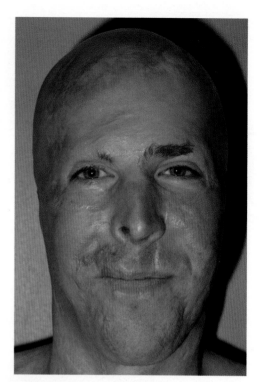

FIGURE 65-18. Three-dimensional tissue loss of the ears due to fourth- to sixth-degree burn.

(Fig. 65-19). This will not be solved by yet another technique, another suture material, another flap, another dermatome. It will be solved only by control of contraction and hypertrophic scarring. The authors hope that these come in their lifetimes.

Hypertrophic Donor Sites

As mentioned, the grafts used are thick. This is commonly followed by hypertrophic scarring of the donor sites (Fig. 65-20). It is for this reason that we rarely use the upper anterior chest as a donor site if there is any alternative. If hypertrophic scarring does occur, it can be excised and closed if small, excised and resurfaced with local flaps if medium, and excised and grafted if large.

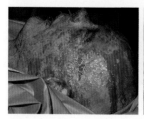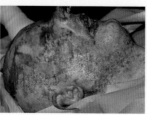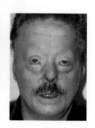

FIGURE 65-19. Poor gestalt.

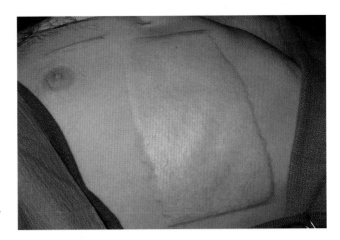

FIGURE 65-20. Hypertrophic scar in the donor site.

ELECTRICAL BURNS OF THE ORAL COMMISSURES

Electrical burns of the oral commissure are not a sequela of standard face burns but are logically included in this chapter. They include a broad spectrum of injuries ranging from relatively superficial ulceration of vermilion and mucosa to devastating full-thickness destruction of lips and cheek. The injury occurs in small children and is usually the result of placing extension cord outlets in the mouth.

Acute care should be nonoperative, allowing the wounds to heal by contraction and epithelialization. Splints should be tried to preserve the dimensions of the mouth, but they often fail because these children are so young. Parents must be counseled about the risk of bleeding from the labial artery. Early surgical intervention has been advocated but seems to offer no advantage and runs the risk of iatrogenic deformity. Late reconstruction with use of local flaps is well described in the literature.[32-34] When patients sustain injuries that result in extensive tissue loss, reconstruction with distant tissue from the ventral surface of the tongue can be advantageous.[35]

Acknowledgments

The authors are grateful to the countless burn team members who struggled with these problems for the past 20-plus years. The authors are also grateful to the burn survivors who struggled with these problems and who permitted their photographs to be used in this effort to improve burn outcomes.

REFERENCES

1. Bloem JJAM, Hermans RP: The deeper burn of the face and surrounding areas. Burns 1976;2:124.
2. Engrav LH, Heimbach DM, Walkinshaw MD, et al: Excision of burns of the face. Plast Reconstr Surg 1986;77:744.
3. Fraulin FO, Illmayer SJ, Tredget EE: Assessment of cosmetic and functional results of conservative versus surgical management of facial burns. J Burn Care Rehabil 1996;17:19.
4. Housinger TA, Hills J, Warden GD: Management of pediatric facial burns. J Burn Care Rehabil 1994;15:408.
5. Hunt JL, Purdue GF, Spicer T, et al: Face burn reconstruction—does early excision and autografting improve aesthetic appearance? Burns Incl Therm Inj 1987;13:39.
6. Jonsson CE, Dalsgaard CJ: Early excision and skin grafting of selected burns of the face and neck. Plast Reconstr Surg 1991;88:83.
7. Warden GD, Saffle JR, Schnebly A, et al: Excisional therapy of facial burns. J Burn Care Rehabil 1986;7:24.
8. Warpeha RL: Resurfacing the burned face. Clin Plast Surg 1981;8:255.
9. Bell JL: Treatment of acute thermal burns of the face. Am J Surg 1959;98:923.
10. Boswick JA Jr: Burns of the head and neck. Surg Clin North Am 1973;53:97.
11. Janžekovič Z: The dermal burn. In Dergranc M, ed: Present Clinical Aspects of Burns: A Symposium. Maribor, Yugoslavia, Mariborski Tisk, 1968:215.
12. MacMillan BG: Indications for early excision. Surg Clin North Am 1970;50:1337.
13. McIndoe AH: Total reconstruction of the burned face. The Bradshaw Lecture 1958. Br J Plast Surg 1983;36:410.
14. Neale HW, Billmire DA, Carey JP: Reconstruction following head and neck burns. Clin Plast Surg 1986;13:119.
15. Cole JK, Engrav LH, Heimbach DM, et al: Early excision and grafting of face and neck burns in patients over 20 years. Plast Reconstr Surg 2002;109:1266.
16. Engrav L, Donelan M: Face burns: acute care and reconstruction. Operative Techniques Plast Reconstr Surg 1997;4:53.
17. Engrav LH: Primary and secondary reconstruction of the burned face. In Grotting J, ed: Reoperative Aesthetic and Reconstructive Surgery. St. Louis, Quality Medical Publishing, 1995:657-676.
18. Gonzalez-Ulloa M: Restoration of the face covering by means of selected skin in regional aesthetic units. Br J Plast Surg 1956;9:212.
19. Lille S, Engrav L, Caps M, et al: Full-thickness grafting of acute eyelid burns results in less ectropion and fewer reconstructive procedures and should not be considered taboo. Plast Reconstr Surg 1999;104:637.
20. Perkins K, Davey RB, Wallis KA: Silicone gel: a new treatment for burn scars and contractures. Burns Incl Therm Inj 1983;9:201.
21. Feldman JJ: Facial burns. In McCarthy JG, ed: Plastic Surgery. Philadelphia, WB Saunders, 1990:2153.
22. Achauer BM: Reconstructing the burned face. Clin Plast Surg 1992;19:623.

23. Brent B: Reconstruction of ear, eyebrow, and sideburn in the burned patient. Plast Reconstr Surg 1975;55:312.

24. Alexander JW, MacMillan BG, Martel L: Correction of post-burn syndactyly: an analysis of children with introduction of the VM-plasty and postoperative pressure inserts. Plast Reconstr Surg 1982;70:345.

25. Lin SD: Correction of the epicanthal fold using the VM-plasty. Br J Plast Surg 2000;53:95.

26. Onishi K, Maruyama Y, Chang CC: Further application of VM-plasty. Ann Plast Surg 1987;18:480.

27. Converse JM, McCarthy JG, Dobrkovsky M, et al: Facial burns. In Converse JM, ed: Reconstructive Plastic Surgery. Philadelphia, WB Saunders, 1977:1628.

28. Schmid E: The use of auricular cartilage and composite grafts in reconstruction of the upper lip, with special reference to reconstruction of the philtrum. In Broadbent TR, ed: Transactions of the Third International Congress of Plastic Surgery. Amsterdam, Excerpta Medica, 1964:306.

29. Converse JM, Wood-Smith D: Techniques for the repair of defects of the lips and cheeks. In Converse JM, ed: Reconstructive Plastic Surgery. Philadelphia, WB Saunders, 1977:1574.

30. Fricke N, Omnell M, Dutcher K, et al: Skeletal and dental disturbances after facial burns and pressure garments. J Burn Care Rehabil 1996;17:338.

31. Fricke NB, Omnell ML, Dutcher KA, et al: Skeletal and dental disturbances in children after facial burns and pressure garments: a 4-year follow-up. J Burn Care Rehabil 1999;20:239.

32. Converse JM: Technique of elongation of the oral fissure and restoration of the angle of the mouth. In Kazanjian VH, Converse JM, eds: The Surgical Management of Facial Injuries. Baltimore, Williams & Wilkins, 1959:795.

33. Gillies H, Millard DR Jr: The Principles and Art of Plastic Surgery. Boston, Little, Brown, 1957.

34. Kazanjian VH, Roopenian A: The treatment of lip deformities resulting from electrical burns. Am J Surg 1954;88:884.

35. Donelan M: Reconstruction of electrical burns of the oral commissure with a ventral tongue flap. Plast Reconstr Surg 1995;95:1155.

Facial Fractures

Paul N. Manson, MD

GENERAL CONSIDERATIONS
    Mechanism of Injury
    Concomitant Injuries
    Timing of Intervention for Facial Fractures
    Diagnosis
GENERAL MANAGEMENT PRINCIPLES
    Surgical Access
    Fracture Reduction by Dental Fixation
    Fracture Stabilization
MANAGEMENT OF SPECIFIC FRACTURES OF THE
CRANIOFACIAL SKELETON
    Mandible
    Nasal Bone and Cartilage

Zygoma
Maxilla
Complex Maxillary (Panfacial) Fractures
Orbit
Nasoethmoidal-Orbital Fractures
Frontobasilar Region
GUNSHOT WOUNDS OF THE FACE
    Low Velocity
    Intermediate and High Velocity
POST-TRAUMATIC FACIAL PAIN
    Nerve Injuries
    Treatment

Few injuries are as challenging as those of the face. Surgeons who undertake treatment of facial injuries have a dual responsibility: repair of the aesthetic defect (restoration of the preinjury appearance) and restoration of function. A third goal is to minimize the period of disability.

A unique aspect of facial injury treatment is that the restoration of appearance alone may be the chief indication for treatment. In other patients, injuries might require surgery solely for restoration of function, but commonly, both goals are evident. Although there are few facial emergencies, the literature has underemphasized the advantages of prompt definitive reconstruction of facial injuries and the contribution of early operative intervention to superior aesthetic and functional results. Economic, sociologic, and psychological factors operating in a competitive society make it imperative that an aggressive, expedient, and well-planned surgical program be outlined, executed, and maintained to return the patient to an active and productive life as soon as possible while minimizing aesthetic and functional disabilities.

Greater emphasis has recently been placed on minimizing operative techniques and exposures, whereas the decade of the 1980s witnessed the widespread application of craniofacial principles of broad exposure and fixation at all buttresses for fracture injuries of all degrees of severity. The treatment of injuries is currently classified both by degree of severity and by anatomic area to permit the smallest exposure possible to achieve a good result with the least surgery for a particular injury.

Since the late 1970s, the application of craniofacial techniques of exposure has improved the ability to restore the preinjury facial appearance by providing access to any area of the facial skeleton.[1,2] These techniques had their adverse sequelae, however, particularly soft tissue damage and loss of soft tissue position. Current facial injury treatment protocols minimize the use of potentially morbid exposures (such as lower eyelid incisions). The techniques of extended open reduction[3,4] and immediate repair or replacement of bone and microvascular tissue transfer of bone or soft tissue have made extensive and challenging injuries manageable.[3,5-8] The principle of immediate skeletal stabilization in anatomic position[9,10] has been enhanced by the use of rigid fixation.[5] Soft tissue volume over this expanded skeleton has been maintained, particularly preventing soft tissue shrinkage and contracture. Complicated external devices and the mobility of interfragment wires have been eliminated by plate and screw fixation. These techniques improve both the functional and aesthetic results of facial fracture treatment.

GENERAL CONSIDERATIONS

Mechanism of Injury

The causes of facial injuries in the United States include motor vehicle accidents, assaults, altercations, bicycle and motorcycle accidents, home and industrial accidents, and athletic injuries. A review of 7296 patients with facial injuries during an 11-year period at the Maryland Institute of Emergency Medical Services Systems showed motor vehicle accidents to be the most common mechanism of injury.[11] Whereas the automobile is frequently responsible for some of the most devastating facial injuries, the increased use of seat belts and air bags, the implementation of strict drunk driving laws, and the enforcement of speed limits have reduced the incidence and severity of facial injuries.

Lee et al[12] in 2000 published a definitive article analyzing the records of 73,000 patients admitted from 1983 to 1994 with craniofacial injuries. The average age was 33 years, with 2:1 male predominance. The most common mechanism of injury was motor vehicle collision. Overall, mortality was 5.9%. Mortality increased to 17% with brain injury. Soft tissue injuries occurred generally along a T-shaped distribution involving the forehead, periorbital area, nose, lip, and chin. The midface was the region most susceptible to fracture.

Lim et al,[13] in 1993, studied the incidence of concomitant injuries in a population of 839 facial trauma patients. Approximately 11% sustained injuries outside the facial skeleton, 8% had injuries of the extremities, 5% had associated neurosurgical injuries, 4% had ocular injuries, and 1% had a spinal injury. In automobile accidents, injuries to the head, face, and cervical spine occur in more than 50% of all victims. Alcohol, drug abuse, and emotional problems are common contributing factors.

Concomitant Injuries

Facial injury victims often sustain multiple injuries to other organ systems. Too often, patients with dramatic facial injuries are prematurely and inappropriately assigned to a subspecialty service. It is important, therefore, that subspecialists first consider whether the patient has been adequately evaluated for the presence of multiple injuries. Definitive care of the maxillofacial injury should be rendered only after a thorough multisystem evaluation, which must include an examination of the airway,[14] profuse blood loss, and central nervous system (head and cervical spine) for injury.[13,15]

AIRWAY

One of the most important considerations in the clinical management of the patient with acute facial injury is evaluation and control of the airway. Early concerns focus on securing the airway; late concerns may include surgical access for repair during general anesthesia. Asphyxia is an ever-present threat in patients with injuries to the jaws, combined facial injuries, or laryngeal trauma. Traumatic asphyxia rarely occurs.[16] The mouth must be cleared of broken teeth, fractured dentures, foreign bodies, and clots that might cause obstruction. Similarly, the nasal passages must be patent and unobstructed. Traction on the mandible and tongue can pull these structures away from the pharynx and permit removal or retrieval of objects displaced into the pharynx. In fractures of the mandible that are unstable, the jaw may be displaced posteriorly, with the tongue falling against the posterior wall of the pharynx, obstructing respiration. In these patients, placement in a prone or sitting position with the head down or forward, if the patient can be turned or moved without aggravation of other injuries, may assist respiration. Anterior traction on the jaw or tongue may avert asphyxia in patients who cannot be turned so that the tongue is displaced forward by gravity. An oropharyngeal airway is a simple device placed to prevent displacement of the tongue and jaw and to open the pharyngeal airway. Respiratory obstruction is most likely to occur with combined fractures of the maxilla, mandible, and nose or in patients with profuse hemorrhage or with massive soft tissue swelling, especially in the tongue, pharynx, or floor of the mouth. Patients especially likely to have difficulty are those with stupor or coma resulting from head injury and those whose reflexes are not alert. Endotracheal intubation is the most expedient method to secure an airway in the majority of patients with an acutely compromised airway. In extremely urgent situations, when oral or nasal intubation is not feasible, cricothyroidotomy[17] or a coniotomy is the preferred treatment, incising transversely through the skin and cricothyroid ligament (conoid ligament) between the thyroid and cricoid cartilages. Cricothyroidotomy is an *emergency* surgical treatment of airway obstruction, as is percutaneous tracheostomy (Table 66-1).[14] After the cricothyroidotomy procedure, the cricothyroidotomy should be formally converted to a tracheostomy.[18,19] The conversion avoids the damage that occurs when a cricothyroidotomy is used for long-standing intubation.

When the facial fracture disrupts the dental occlusion, maxillomandibular fixation is required during the operative course of management. The method of securing an airway that does not interfere with the technical aspect of repair and ensures safe postoperative care must be planned. Nasotracheal anesthesia is usually satisfactory for the reduction and fixation of fractures of the maxilla and mandible. Nasotracheal anesthesia facilitates application of arch bars and study of the occlusion and clears the view for intraoral operative therapy.

Endotracheal anesthesia with oral intubation may be possible for maxillary or mandibular fractures that require intermaxillary fixation if the tube can be placed

TABLE 66-1 ✦ COMPLICATIONS OF PERCUTANEOUS TRACHEOSTOMY

Minor Complications	PCT (n = 31)	OT (n = 29)
Air leak	6	4
Bleeding	1	2
Local infection	1	3
Subcutaneous emphysema	1	1
Pneumothorax (no chest tube)	1	1
Pneumomediastinum	1	1
Post-tracheal hematoma	1	1
Total	12 (39%)	13 (41%)

Major Complications	PCT (n = 31)	OT (n = 29)
Aspiration	0	1
Bleeding (conversion to OT)	2	0
Local infection (antibiotics)	1	0
Pneumothorax (chest tube)	1	2
Airway loss during procedure	1	1
Delayed airway loss	2	0
Pneumonia	0	1
Total	7 (23%)	5 (17%)

PCT, percutaneous tracheostomy; OT, open tracheostomy.
From Graham JS, Mulloy RH, Sutherland FR, Rose S: Percutaneous versus open tracheostomy: a retrospective cohort outcome study. J Trauma 1996;41:245.

through a gap in the dentition or behind the last molar tooth. The requirement for placing the patient in intermaxillary fixation before fracture fixation may prevent the use of oral intubation in some patients. Oral intubation is satisfactory for fractures of the upper face when it is not necessary to establish intermaxillary fixation. Endotracheal anesthesia, with oral intubation, is the preferred route for fractures of the orbit, zygoma, and frontal bone.

Some clinicians have passed the tube through the floor of the mouth, making an incision for exit of the tube in the submental area. Reintubation of the patient on the floor is of course not possible; although the technique does eliminate the interference of an oral tube with establishing intermaxillary fixation, the tube is still in the oral cavity, sometimes impairing surgical vision.

Fractures of the maxilla and mandible necessitate maxillomandibular fixation during the course of surgical repair. A tracheotomy is indicated in patients with panfacial fractures, in whom the presence of an endotracheal tube would unnecessarily complicate the repair, or in those patients with significant head or chest injuries who are unlikely to manage their own airway within a 1-week period. Dunham et al[20] have an excellent article on guidelines for emergency tracheal intubation and tracheostomy. They relate in detail the threats to the airway versus mechanism of treatment. Tracheotomy facilitates placement of the patient in intermaxillary fixation and clears the oral and nasal areas of obstructing tubes. Patients in whom the floor of the mouth, tongue, and hypopharynx are to become increasingly edematous and those requiring maintenance of intramaxillary fixation who have inadequate ventilation because of swelling should be considered for tracheotomy. Tracheostomy, in these situations, makes pulmonary management easier. A tracheostomy provides a route by which a general anesthetic may be administered and one that does not interfere with a reduction of fractures in the facial area. A tracheostomy also minimizes the chance of inadvertent extubation in a swollen patient. Such an event precipitates chaotic attempts at reintubation and has resulted in death of patients even in level I trauma units. Anesthesia by transtracheal route permits unobstructed reduction and fixation of facial fractures, placement of intermaxillary fixation, intranasal packing, application of arch bars, and placement of internal fixation devices, without the need to worry about airway obstruction. With oral intubation and extubation, these conditions in the postoperative period can impair respiration and cause respiratory obstruction. The use of a tracheostomy, rather than prolonged nasotracheal or oral-tracheal intubation, is dictated by the experience of the surgeon, the team that is to provide postoperative monitoring, and the adequacy of alert nursing care in the intensive care unit.

PROFUSE BLOOD LOSS

Life-threatening hemorrhage is defined by the loss of more than 3 units of blood or a hematocrit below 29%.[21] Lacerations and crush injuries of the facial region may result in significant hemorrhage that may be life-threatening.[22] Life-threatening hemorrhage occurs in 1.2% to 5% of Le Fort fractures[21]; 70% is from the internal maxillary artery or branches. Rarely, skull base fractures present with exsanguinations through the nose. When bleeding is from a superficial facial site, control of blood loss can be achieved by local pressure, dressings, and the application of clamps, ligation, or packing. Approximation of large wound edges with a few sutures or temporary reduction of fractures manually (placement of the jaws in intermaxillary fixation) often diminishes hemorrhage. Final wound suturing may be accomplished when adequate exposure and time permit a precise repair. With an anterior nasal bleed, packing the nasal cavity with hemostatic material may be required (Fig. 66-1). As soon as the patient's general condition improves and

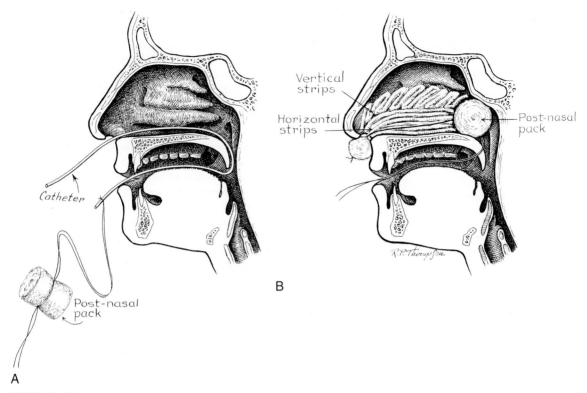

FIGURE 66-1. Technique of anterior-posterior nasal packing for the arrest of severe nasopharyngeal bleeding. *A,* The "posterior pack" is guided into the nasopharynx by a suture attached to a Foley catheter. Alternatively, a Foley catheter can have its balloon inflated in the posterior pharynx and brought to the posterior choanal nasal opening. *B,* With either a Foley catheter balloon or posterior nasal pack in place, the nasal cavity is packed with strips of antibiotic ointment-impregnated gauze. The entire cavity of the nose should be thoroughly packed, applying a light pressure. If the bleeding persists, the anterior pack should be removed and the recesses of the nasal cavity carefully repacked. In severe fractures, one should take care not to enter the anterior cranial fossa or the orbit through areas of disrupted bone.

the hemorrhage has ceased, these packs may be gradually removed during a 2- to 3-day period.

However, access to and control of closed hemorrhage from the nasopharyngeal region are difficult.[23-25] Bleeding often originates from the posteriorly located internal maxillary artery. Rapid and efficient anterior-posterior nasal packing may be achieved by placing two 30- to 50-mL balloon Foley catheters, one in each nostril. The catheter should be placed into the pharynx and then pulled to occlude the posterior nasopharyngeal opening on each side. This maneuver provides a posterior obturator against which several packs of antibiotic-impregnated petrolatum gauze are packed into the recesses of each nasal cavity. Care must be taken to avoid entering the orbit or anterior cranial fossa in patients with severe comminuted fractures. The packing provides compression, which can be supplemented by tying or securing the ends of the Foley catheters over the columella. Necrosis of the columella and palate must be avoided by intermittently relaxing this pressure. Necrosis of the soft palate has also

been reported after excess intracranial pressure. A period of several hours of pressure is usually sufficient to stop the bleeding. The columella, palate, or intranasal pressure can be relaxed after an hour. The packing is removed after 24 to 48 hours. If a cerebrospinal fluid (CSF) leak is present, most surgeons prefer that the packing be removed as early as possible to permit free nasal drainage. It is thought that obstruction of the nasal cavity increases the possibility for an infection to ascend into the meningeal area, although proof of this mechanism remains to be established.[26] Blindness has occurred after nasal packing.[27]

Frequently, closed midface fractures bleed because of displacement. Manual reduction of fractures, including placement of patients in temporary intermaxillary fixation, will frequently decrease traction on veins and arteries in the walls and sinuses and allow cessation of bleeding (Fig. 66-2). External compression dressings have been the practice in the past, but it is doubtful whether they have any strongly positive effect in con-

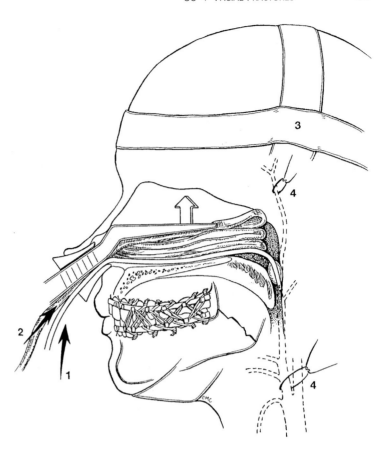

FIGURE 66-2. If nasal packing does not suffice to control bleeding, one may employ a Barton bandage, but these are of limited usefulness. Placement of the patient in intermaxillary fixation, however, is extraordinarily effective in Le Fort fracture bleeding. Selective angiography with embolization is the procedure of choice in persistent bleeding. Application of external pressure and ligation of the superficial temporal and external carotid arteries are performed if selective embolization by angiography has failed. Selective arterial embolization requires angiographic definition of the bleeding point. (From Manson P: Complications in facial injuries. In Maull KI, Wiles CE 3rd, Wiles CE, et al, eds: Complications in Trauma and Critical Care. Philadelphia, WB Saunders, 1996.)

trolling bleeding. They are known as Barton bandages and circle the head, applying pressure.

Embolization under radiographic control is reserved for those few patients who continue to hemorrhage despite these measures.[21,26,28] On the average, 7 liters of blood and crystalloid are infused before angiography. Complications include stroke, tongue necrosis, and facial nerve palsy. If a patient continues to bleed, the anterior-posterior nasal packing should be removed and then replaced. If this is not successful, selective arterial embolization may be able to stop the bleeding. An angiogram indicates the source, which may be embolized. Massive uncontrolled hemorrhage secondary to closed craniofacial trauma occasionally occurs; it may be due to fractures through the anterior cranial fossa (Fig. 66-3) that transect the carotid artery or large veins, such as the dural venous sinuses. Coagulation factor abnormalities should be searched for, and one must be ready to administer multiple transfusions and blood products. Obviously, control of lacerations of the internal carotid artery at the skull base or within the intracranial cavity is difficult. These injuries may be defined by selective arteriography at the time of attempted embolization, but death from hemorrhage is frequent.

Selective arterial ligation is reserved for those few patients who continue to hemorrhage despite all of these measures. In patients with severe hemorrhage, the bilateral external carotid and superficial temporal arteries are ligated, which decreases flow through the midportion of the face (see Fig. 66-2).

HEAD INJURY

Cerebral injury includes that due to mechanical damage to neurons and that resulting from secondary ischemia, edema, and hematoma.[29] Ischemia is aggravated by mass lesions, brain swelling, and hypothermia; hypoxia and hypoperfusion are poor prognostic signs.[30] Increased intracranial pressure leads in a progressive cycle to intracranial hypertension, increased intracranial pressure, and progressive ischemia. Patients with head injuries should be evaluated by a clinical examination that classifies the severity of injury according to the Glasgow Coma Scale (Table 66-2). This scale relates the patient's level of consciousness, eye opening response, and ability to speak and move extremities to a prognostic grade. There is evidence that motor score alone is a good predictor of survival,[31] and the pupil size and pupil

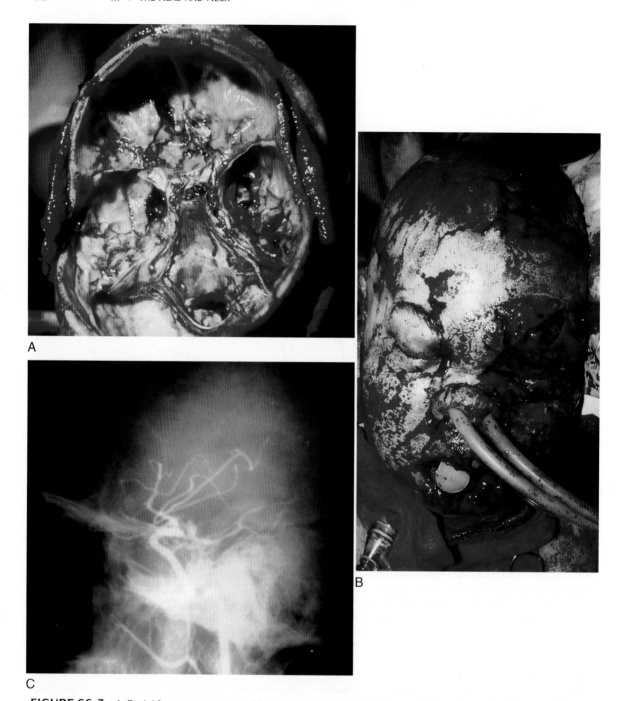

FIGURE 66-3. *A,* Facial fractures may extend into the anterior and middle cranial fossa, lacerating the carotid artery and dural venous sinuses. *B,* Severe hemorrhage may result in exsanguination. An autopsy view shows skull base fractures in a patient who expired after experiencing massive bleeding. *C,* Arteriogram demonstrates bleeding from pharynx in a patient with a Le Fort fracture. The arteriogram also demonstrates blood leaking from the carotid as it goes through a skull base fracture.

TABLE 66-2 ♦ GLASGOW COMA SCALE

Best Verbal Response

None	1
Incomprehensible sound	2
Inappropriate words	3
Confused	4
Oriented	5

Eyes Open

None	1
To pain	2
To speech	3
Spontaneously	4

Best Motor Response

None	1
Abnormal extension	2
Abnormal flexion	3
Withdraws from pain	4
Localizes pain	5
Obeys	6

reactivity are predictors as good as a more extensive scale.[32] Patients with a Glasgow Coma Scale score of 3 and fixed dilated pupils have no reasonable chance of survival.[33-37]

A computed tomographic (CT) scan of the face, brain, and skull should be taken in *every* facial injury and for *anyone* with an abnormal Glasgow Coma Scale score. The CT scan should identify mass lesions, cerebral contusion, shift of the midline, extradural or intradural hematoma, skull fractures, and intracranial air. Patients with head injuries have a less favorable prognosis with increasing age, decreasing Glasgow Coma Scale score, decreasing systemic blood pressure, abnormal posturing, and prolonged intracranial hypertension. Additional factors correlating with better prognosis include spontaneous and reflex eye movements and pupil reactivity to light. Accompanying spinal injuries, pulmonary injuries, and shock worsen the prognosis of head injuries. In general, children have a more favorable prognosis than do adults for head injuries. Even minor head injuries, however, often establish permanent symptoms and deserve CT evaluation.

The presence of coma alone should never contraindicate the operative treatment of a maxillofacial injury.[33,38,39] Neurosurgical studies have shown that patients in coma that has lasted more than 1 week have a hopeful prognosis in terms of returning to a functional role in society. In one study, one fourth of patients in coma whose duration exceeded 1 week died, and one fourth were disabled; however, half were returned to useful work.[38]

Although the presence of coma should never be used as an excuse to defer the treatment of a facial injury, even minor head injuries produce behavioral sequelae that affect socialization, relationships with loved ones, and ability to work. For these reasons, head-injured patients who survive greatly benefit from improved aesthetic and functional results, which can be obtained by early, proper treatment. Safe anesthesia is achieved with intracranial pressure monitoring, when it is indicated.[40]

Despite the progress that has occurred in the treatment of major head injuries, one should not assume that minor head injuries do not have permanent sequelae. In patients in whom the duration of coma was less than 20 minutes (minor head injuries), 80% demonstrated some late symptoms such as headaches, memory difficulty, and problems within interpersonal relationships or behavior alterations.[41] Decreased attention span, poor concentration, and judgment problems directly reflect the degree of organic brain damage. When patients frequently complain of problems in work, school, and home, they could benefit from intervention by a head injury rehabilitation center program and from early psychological guidance.[38]

CERVICAL SPINE INJURIES

Injuries to the cervical spine often accompany those of the head and face.[42,43] A significant cervical cord injury exists in 1 of 300 accident victims and in 1 of 14 occupants who are ejected from their cars.[43] All patients (especially those who are unconscious) should be considered to have a spinal injury until it has been excluded. Spinal cord injury without radiographic abnormality exists.[44] Diagnostic failures occur in one third of patients evaluated with plain film,[45] especially those with neurologic damage (Glasgow Coma Scale score < 12).[46] Patients who are unable to move their extremities on command or sternal pressure, those who have penetrating trauma to the neck, and those who complain of pain in the neck or who describe disturbances in sensation or motor function must be assumed to have a cervical cord injury.[43] The association of facial injuries and cervical injuries has been suggested in several large studies in which 10% of those with a facial fracture had a cervical spine injury and 18% of those with a cervical spine injury had a maxillofacial injury.[29,47] Blunt injury to the cervical artery occurs with upper (C1-3) dislocation-subluxation.[48] Studies also document an association between fractures of the mandible and those of the upper cervical spine and the association of upper facial injuries with cervical hyperextension injuries at all levels.[29,47]

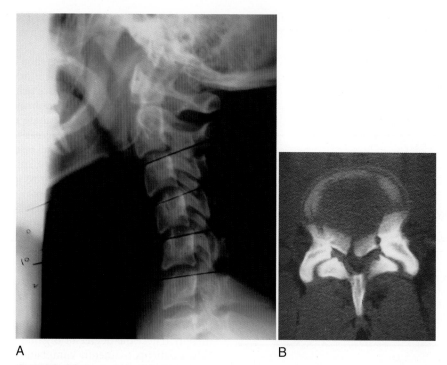

A   B

FIGURE 66-4. *A,* Mandible fractures are associated with fractures at the upper and lower cervical spine, which are the most difficult to visualize (plain film). *B,* Frontal fractures imply the delivery of large forces to the cervical spine, which cause subluxation (CT scan).

Careful reviews of cervical injuries indicate that the most commonly missed lesions are those at the upper or at the lower ends of the cervical spine, such as C1-2 and C6-7.[42-45,49-51] Whiplash can be documented on single-photon emission computed tomography.[52] These areas are notoriously more difficult to visualize on radiographs, and the failure to adequately demonstrate these areas allows fractures to be missed. In general, CT scans are more accurate than plain radiographs, and CT scans frequently require less neck movement. Both cerebral and cervical spine injuries may occur secondary to whiplash without head contact or skull or facial fracture. The diagnostic principle to be emphasized is that if one is unable to visualize the whole cervical spine radiographically to confirm that the patient is asymptomatic by examination, the patient must be treated as if he or she had a cervical fracture by neck immobilization and limiting the movement of the head[52] (Fig. 66-4).

Cervical cord injuries are initially overlooked in 10%, and approximately 50% of these injuries are mismanaged.[53] Harris[53] recommends the following: vigilance (think of diagnosis); protect the spine; perform neurologic examination; use consultants; supplement a normal conventional radiographic examination by CT scan or magnetic resonance imaging, and always when the findings on a neurologic examination are abnormal.

Anterior cervical cord compression produces a syndrome of motor paralysis and loss of pain and temperature sense below the level of the lesion with preservation of dorsal column sensation (pain, touch, and vibration). Posterior cord compression affects dorsal column sensation. Acute central cord compression results in greater motor impairment of the upper limbs than of the lower and is usually due to central hemorrhage and bruising. Many cervical cord injuries are incomplete and thus may be aggravated by improper diagnosis and treatment. There is evidence that the cycle of ischemia and vasoconstriction, mentioned in the cycle of vasospastic cerebral injury progression, may also occur and aggravate cervical cord or spinal cord lesions. Some think that "spinal cord dose steroids" protect against this cycle of ischemia.[54,55]

Hendey et al[44] studied the characteristics of spinal cord injuries without radiographic abnormality in

35,000 patients. They reported that 2.4% of patients had cervical spine injury and 0.08% had spinal cord injury without radiographic abnormality. Magnetic resonance imaging findings included central disk herniation, spinal stenosis, cord edema, contusion, and central cord syndrome.

Timing of Intervention for Facial Fractures

Once life-threatening injuries have been stabilized and managed, the patient's principal concerns frequently involve residual facial deformity. The timing of facial injury treatment is important in optimum outcomes.[37] Bone and soft tissue injuries in the facial area should be managed as soon as is consistent with the patient's general condition and with the particular characteristics of ancillary injuries. It is the author's impression that early, skillful facial injury management decreases permanent facial disfigurement and limits serious functional disturbances.[9,56] However, one should carefully evaluate each patient in terms of ability to tolerate early operative intervention and possess as much knowledge of the multi-injured patient, and the ancillary injuries, as of the face.[57-59]

Classically, facial soft tissue and bone injuries are rarely acute surgical emergencies as far as closure of wounds or immediate reduction of fractures is concerned. However, both the ease of obtaining a good result and the quality of the result are better with immediate fracture management.[9] Less soft tissue stripping is required, and bones are often easily replaced into their anatomic position. There are few patients, however, whose injuries cannot be definitively managed within a short time if an aggressive plan for facial rehabilitation is considered preeminent. Exceptions to acute treatment include patients who have ongoing or significant blood loss (such as pelvic fractures),[57] those whose intracranial pressure exceeds normal limits, those with coagulation problems,[9] and those with pulmonary ventilation pressures that are abnormal or increasing. These patients *do not* tolerate operative intervention of any length. In the admitting area, however, their lacerations are closed, the patient is placed in intermaxillary fixation, and grossly displaced fractures are returned to their approximate position. Many patients with brain injuries or multiple system trauma, however, do not have criteria preventing operative management, and they may receive facial injury management at the time that other injuries are being stabilized.[8]

Diagnosis

The management of facial fractures depends on an initial physical examination and an accurate radiologic evaluation accomplished with CT scanning. These scans should visualize both soft tissue and bone. It is generally no longer feasible or economically justifiable to obtain plain radiographs in facial injury diagnostics with certain exceptions, such as the Panorex mandible examination or dental films.

CLINICAL EXAMINATION OF THE FACE

A careful history and a thorough clinical examination form the basis for the diagnosis of almost all facial injuries. Facial injuries are more difficult to diagnose in children and in the elderly.[60] Thorough examination of the face is indicated even if the patient has only minor superficial wounds or abrasions. Abrasions, contusions, and lacerations may be the most apparent symptom of an underlying fracture or abnormality that will surface later as a problem. A facial laceration may be the only sign of a penetrating injury that has entered the eye, nose, ear, or cranial cavity. Face lacerations may often be repaired during the treatment of injuries in other parts of the body without the need for an additional operative session. The treatment of facial lacerations should therefore not be deferred. Superficial lacerations or abrasions may leave disfiguring scars despite their apparently inconsequential appearance if they are not adequately managed. Careful cleaning of all wounds, meticulous débridement, and, when necessary, layered closure minimize conspicuous permanent deformity.

Bone injuries are suggested by soft tissue symptoms such as contusions, abrasions, ecchymosis, edema, and distortion of the facial proportions or position of facial fractures. These symptoms should prompt a clinical examination and radiographic evaluation to confirm or to exclude fractures. Subconjunctival hemorrhage with ecchymosis and edema in the region of the orbit and a palpebral hematoma suggest a fracture of the zygoma or orbit. Bilateral hematomas suggest a Le Fort, nasal-ethmoid, or anterior cranial fossa fracture. Ecchymotic, contused intraoral tissue, loose teeth, and malocclusion suggest the possibility of lower jaw fracture (Fig. 66-5).

An orderly examination of all facial structures should be accomplished, progressing from either superior to inferior or inferior to superior in a systematic fashion. A meticulous examination in search of dysfunction of the periorbital, masticatory, and neurosensory systems of the face will often reveal the anatomy of the underlying fracture pattern to the facial skeleton.

Symptoms and signs produced by facial injuries include pain or localized tenderness, crepitation from areas of underlying bone fracture, hypesthesia or anesthesia in the distribution of a specific sensory nerve, paralysis in the distribution of a specific motor nerve, malocclusion, visual acuity disturbance, double vision, facial asymmetry, facial deformity, obstructed

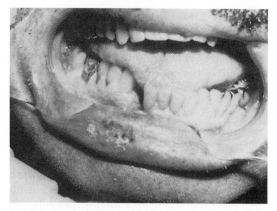

FIGURE 66-5. An intraoral examination demonstrates a fracture, a gingival laceration, and a gap in the dentition. These alveolar and gingival lacerations sometimes extend along the floor or roof of the mouth for a considerable distance. Floor of the mouth lacerations should be explored, irrigated, and drained dependently through the neck to prevent deep space neck infection.

respiration, lacerations, bleeding, and contusions. The clinical examination should begin with the evaluation for symmetry and deformity and with inspection of the face, comparing one side with the other. Palpation of all bone surfaces follows in an orderly manner. The superior orbital rim (Fig. 66-6A), the inferior orbital rim (Fig. 66-6B), the nose, the brows, the zygomatic arches (Fig. 66-7), the malar eminence, and the border of the mandible should be evaluated.

Periorbital Region

A thorough palpation of all areas of the facial bones should be performed, systematically, checking for tenderness, crepitus, or contour defects (see Fig. 66-6). Unequal globe levels (dystopia of the globe), enophthalmos, proptosis, or double vision indicates zygomatic, orbital, or maxillary fractures. In all severe injuries in the periorbital area, consultation with an ophthalmologist may be desirable to fully evaluate the internal portions of the eye to detect retinal detachment or a subtle globe rupture.[61] If an ophthalmologist is not available, visual acuity as well as extraocular muscle and pupillary function should be ascertained *before* any surgical treatment is undertaken. Intraocular pressure should be measured. The minimum visual system examination includes an assessment of vision and the adequacy of extraocular motion, an evaluation for double vision, an ophthalmoscopic examination, and a measurement of intraocular pressure.[62]

Visual acuity in each eye should be assessed by a Snellen visual acuity chart or a Rosenbaum pocket vision card (Fig. 66-8). Alternatively, printed material may be shown to the patient and the response noted. In uncooperative patients, the response to light stimuli, such as photophobia, pupillary constriction, aversion of the head, or lid closure, indicates probable light perception. Any decrease or loss of visual function should be documented *preoperatively,* and the patient should be asked about any history of visual loss. In patients with amblyopia, it is common for one eye to have 20/200 or 20/400 vision, and therefore patients should be counseled as if they had one eye. Operating on a

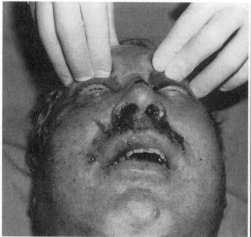
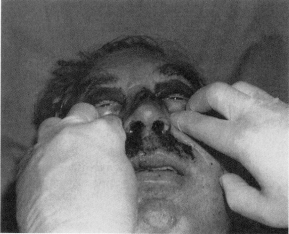

A   B

FIGURE 66-6. Palpation of the superior and inferior orbital rims. *A,* The superior orbital rims are palpated with the pads of the fingertips. *B,* Palpation of the inferior orbital rims. One should feel for discontinuity and level discrepancies in the bone of the rim and evaluate both the anterior and vertical position of the inferior orbital rims, comparing the prominence of the malar eminence of the two sides of the face.

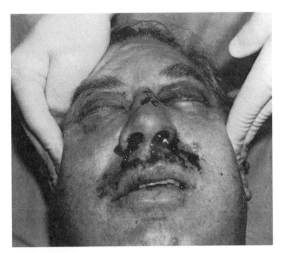

FIGURE 66-7. The zygomatic arches are palpated.

and measurements of globe pressure should be performed.[62] The presence of hyphema, corneal abrasion or visual disturbance (field defect), visual loss, double vision, decreased vision, or absent vision should be noted and appropriate consultation requested.

Masticatory Dysfunction

A thorough inspection of the intraoral area should be made to detect lacerations, loose teeth, or abnormalities of the dentition. Palpation of the dental arches follows the inspection, noting mobility of dental-alveolar arch segments. The maxillary and mandibular dental arches are carefully visualized and palpated to detect an irregularity of the bone, loose teeth, intraoral lacerations, bruising, hematoma, swelling, movement, tenderness, or crepitus. An evaluation of sensory and motor nerve function in the facial area is performed.

single good eye risks total blindness if a problem occurs. Litigation after surgical treatment is not uncommon,[63] and visual loss may be inappropriately ascribed to a surgical procedure in the absence of a proper preoperative documentation of the visual acuity.

An assessment of pupillary reactivity is of critical importance because the direct pupillary response to light is thought by many to be the most reliable sign of the extent of optic nerve injury. Pupillary inequality should be assessed and a focused neurologic examination performed. The absence of pupillary reactivity is an indication of serious visual compromise. Radiographic studies, history of accompanying head trauma, and ophthalmoscopic findings are all considerably less valuable than the status of the pupillary light reflex. After an ipsilateral optic nerve injury, the pupil on the side of the injured nerve is equal in size to the opposite pupil but less reactive to direct light stimulation. The pupil on the side of the optic nerve lesion, however, usually reacts consensually. This indicates an afferent lesion in the pupillary light reflex pathway, specifically a conduction defect involving the optic nerve on the side of the less reactive pupil. The difference in pupillary reactions, with the light first in one and then in the other eye, may be enhanced by swinging a flashlight back and forth from one eye to the other. When the light is moved from the intact eye to the abnormal eye, a paradoxical dilation of the pupil in the abnormal eye is seen (the Marcus Gunn pupillary phenomenon) (Figs. 66-9 and 66-10).[64]

Extraocular movements (cranial nerves III, IV, and VI) and the muscles of facial expression (cranial nerve VII) are examined in the conscious, cooperative patient. Pupillary size and symmetry, speed of pupillary reaction, globe turgor, globe excursion, eyelid excursion, double vision, and visual acuity and visual loss are noted.[62,65] An ophthalmoscopic examination

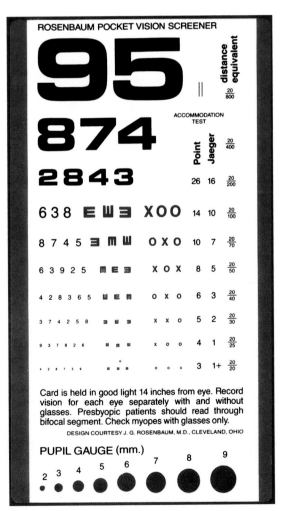

FIGURE 66-8. The Rosenbaum pocket visual examination card. (© J. G. Rosenbaum, MD, Cleveland, Ohio.)

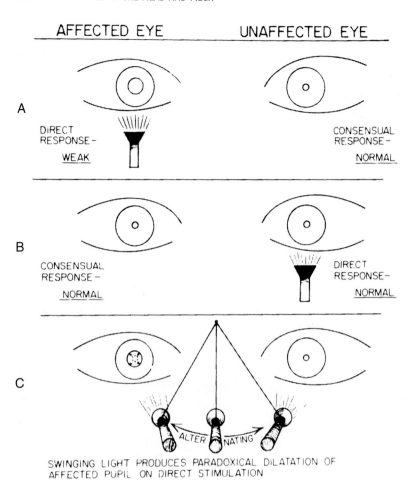

AFFECTED EYE   UNAFFECTED EYE

A

DIRECT
RESPONSE –
WEAK

CONSENSUAL
RESPONSE –
NORMAL

B

CONSENSUAL
RESPONSE –
NORMAL

DIRECT
RESPONSE –
NORMAL

C

ALTER—NATING

SWINGING LIGHT PRODUCES PARADOXICAL DILATATION OF
AFFECTED PUPIL ON DIRECT STIMULATION

FIGURE 66-9. The Marcus Gunn test for pupillary response. *A,* The test should be conducted in a dark room with the patient's eyes fixed on a distant object. *B,* Shining a light in the affected eye produces minimal or no constriction of that pupil. Shining a light in the unaffected eye produces normal constriction of the pupils of both eyes (consensual response). *C,* When the light is moved from the unaffected eye to the affected eye, a paradoxical dilation rather than a constriction of the affected pupil designates a positive test result. (From Jabalay ME, Lerman M, Sanders HJ: Ocular injuries in orbital fractures: a review of 119 cases. Plast Reconstr Surg 1975;56:410.)

Fractures of the facial bones may be diagnosed on the basis of malocclusion of the teeth (see Fig. 66-5) or an open bite deformity due to fracture displacement involving the upper or the lower jaw. A fracture of the mandibular condyle (Fig. 66-11), for instance, may produce pain, deviation with motion to the side of the injury, and inability to occlude the upper and the lower jaw properly. Pain with movement of the jaw (trismus) may be caused by a fracture of the zygoma or upper or lower jaw.

The excursion and deviation of the jaws with motion, the presence of pain on opening of the jaw, the relationship of the teeth, the ability of the patient to bring the teeth into occlusion, the symmetry of the dental arches, and the intercuspal dental relationship are important clues to the diagnosis of fractures involving the dentition. One finger in the ear canal and another over the condylar head can detect condylar movement (Fig. 66-11), or crepitus, either by the patient's movement or when the jaw is pulled forward. A gingival laceration, a fractured or missing tooth, or a split alveolus (Fig. 66-12; see also Fig. 66-5) should imply the possibility of more significant maxillary or

mandibular injuries, which must be confirmed by further examinations for mobility (Fig. 66-12) and appropriate CT radiographs. Fractures of the mandible may be detected by pulling forward on the jaw (see Fig. 66-11) or by applying "up-and-down" manual pressure on the anterior portion of the mandible, having supported the angle, or lateral pressure on the dentition. Instability, crepitus, and pain may be noted when this maneuver is performed. Edema and hemorrhage may mask the perception of facial asymmetry. Bleeding from lacerations of vessels accompanying facial fractures may disguise a CSF leak. Bleeding or fluid draining from the ear canal may indicate a laceration in the ear canal, a condylar dislocation, or a middle cranial fossa fracture with a CSF leak. Bleeding from the nose may indicate nasal or septal injuries; Le Fort, nasoethmoidal, or orbital fractures; or fractures of the anterior cranial fossa. Mobility of the middle third of the facial skeleton indicates a fracture of the Le Fort type (Fig. 66-13). Anterior or middle basilar skull fractures or cribriform plate fractures should be suspected when CSF rhinorrhea or clear drainage from the ears is present. Central nervous system injury is implied by

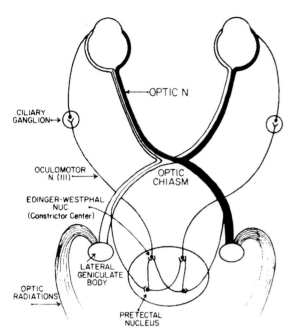

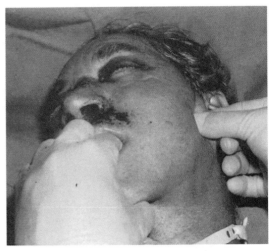

FIGURE 66-11. Condylar examination. The mandible is grasped with one hand, and the condyle area is bimanually palpated with one finger in the ear canal and one finger over the head of the condyle. Abnormal movement, or crepitation, indicates a condylar fracture. In the absence of a condylar fracture, a noncrepitant movement of the condylar head should occur synchronously with the anterior mandible. Disruption of the ligaments of the condyle will permit dislocations of the condylar head out of the fossa in the absence of fracture.

FIGURE 66-10. The normal pupillary reflex pathway and the relationship to the Marcus Gunn pupil. In the normal eye, light striking the retina produces an impulse in the optic nerve that travels to the pretectal nucleus, both Edinger-Westphal nuclei via cranial nerve III to the ciliary ganglion, and the pupillary constrictor muscles. In lesions involving the retina or the optic nerve anterior to the chiasm, a light in the unaffected eye produces consensual constriction of the pupil of the affected eye, but a light in the affected eye produces a paradoxical dilation of the affected pupil. (From Jabalay ME, Lerman M, Sanders HJ: Ocular injuries in orbital fractures: a review of 119 cases. Plast Reconstr Surg 1975;56:410.)

to occur at connections, over bone prominences, and in the midlines (brows, nose, lips).[12,66,67] The sensory branches of the trigeminal (fifth cranial) nerve in the region of the skin are small, and approximation is usually impractical and unnecessary. Partial recovery of sensation usually occurs within several months to a year. Larger branches of the nerve, such as the infraorbital, supraorbital mental, or inferior alveolar nerve, are amenable to primary repair.[68]

paralysis of one or more of the cranial nerves, impaired consciousness, unconsciousness, depressed sensorium, unequal size of the pupils, paralysis of one or more of the extremities, abnormal neurologic reflexes, convulsions, delirium, or irrational behavior.

Neurosensory Dysfunction

Hypesthesia or anesthesia in the distribution of the supraorbital, infraorbital, and mental nerves should suggest a fracture occurring somewhere along the bony path of these sensory nerves (cranial nerve V). Cutaneous branches of these nerves might have been interrupted by a facial laceration as well. Contusion of trigeminal nerve branches also results from fractures producing impairment of sensation. Whereas some loss is permanent, partial recovery is the rule. The nerve branches travel through foramina, which form weak points in the bone, and therefore the nerves are often crushed between bone fragments. For example, the infraorbital nerve is often crushed in its exit from the infraorbital canal in zygomatic or maxillary fractures. Lacerations from auto accidents or blunt injuries tend

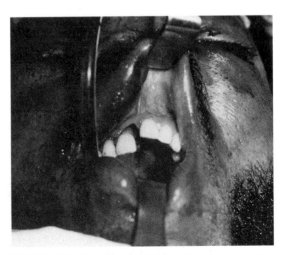

FIGURE 66-12. A split palate (sagittal fracture of the maxilla) is often accompanied by a laceration in the upper buccal sulcus adjacent to the frenulum.

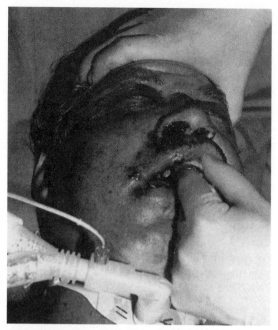

FIGURE 66-13. With the head securely grasped, the midface is assessed for movement by grasping the dentition. Loose teeth, dentures, or bridgework should not be confused with mobility of the maxilla. Le Fort fractures demonstrate, as a rule, less mobility if they exist as large fragments, and especially if they are a "single fragment," than do lower Le Fort fractures. More comminuted Le Fort fractures demonstrate extreme mobility ("loose" maxillary fractures).

RADIOGRAPHIC DIAGNOSIS

A thorough clinical examination can provide much of the information necessary for emergency diagnosis and treatment. Bedside radiographs (and even plain films in this situation) provide useful information. However, the definitive radiographic evaluation is the craniofacial CT scan with axial and coronal sections and bone and soft tissue windows.[69-71]

A definitive radiographic CT evaluation[72] is indispensable in the evaluation of a patient with head and face injuries. However, the CT examination does not, under any circumstances, replace the clinical examination, which is the most sensitive indication of the character and functional implications of the facial injury. A complete radiographic evaluation of the cranial and facial bone structures, however, should be obtained when any clinical symptoms are present. A craniofacial CT scan, with axial and coronal views and bone and soft tissue windows, provides the definitive radiologic evaluation. Even though the clinical evaluation may demonstrate obvious fractures and suggest a standard type of management, a thorough radiographic examination must be completed before any significant treatment is undertaken. For instance, it

may be obvious that the patient has a fracture of the parasymphysis region of the mandible, with malocclusion. These fractures are commonly accompanied by subcondylar fractures, and the documentation of the subcondylar fracture may require radiographic evaluation. Even if the plan of treatment involves closed treatment of the subcondylar fracture, the displacement of the fragments, degree of gap, and amount of shortening should be known to the surgeon to explain the choice of treatments to the patient.[73] The significant incidence of litigation arising from injuries makes it of prime importance to have a thorough documentation of all bone injuries, even if treatment is not required.[72] Three-dimensional CT scans may help evaluate proportionality and asymmetry, especially in secondary corrections (Fig. 66-14).[74,75]

Plain Facial Films

Plain facial films are of limited usefulness unless CT examinations cannot be obtained. The facial bone series is the most valuable and includes the most often employed views of the face—the Caldwell, submental vertex, Waters, Towne, and lateral skull films.[76,77] Anteroposterior and lateral oblique views of the mandible are also obtained, as is the Panorex mandible examination. The specialized view of the mandible, such as the panoramic radiograph, and the occlusal or apical views of the teeth, bite-wing and root films, may disclose detailed dental anatomy. Special radiographs, such as cephalometric examinations (see Chapters 41 and 58), to evaluate proportional changes in the face and to compare the existing sizes to skeletal norms may be helpful. Soft tissue views may be included with profile views to assess soft tissue proportions. The middle and upper facial structures are most accurately evaluated with a detailed CT examination. The evaluation of the frontal bone, sinuses, orbit, and midface may require both axial and coronal CT sections for the most accurate examinations.[72,73]

Radiographic Positions

WATERS POSITION. The posterior-anterior projection is employed for an oblique anterior view of the upper facial bones; the orbits, malar bones, and zygomatic arches are well shown. This view is helpful in the diagnosis of fractures of the maxilla, maxillary sinuses, orbital floor, infraorbital rim, zygomatic bone, and zygomatic arches. To a lesser extent, the view documents the nasal bones, nasal processes of the maxilla, and supraorbital rim (Fig. 66-15).

CALDWELL POSITION. The posterior-anterior projection is primarily used to demonstrate the frontal sinuses, frontal bone, anterior ethmoidal cells, and zygomaticofrontal suture. The orbital margin, the lateral walls of the maxillary sinuses, the petrous ridges, and

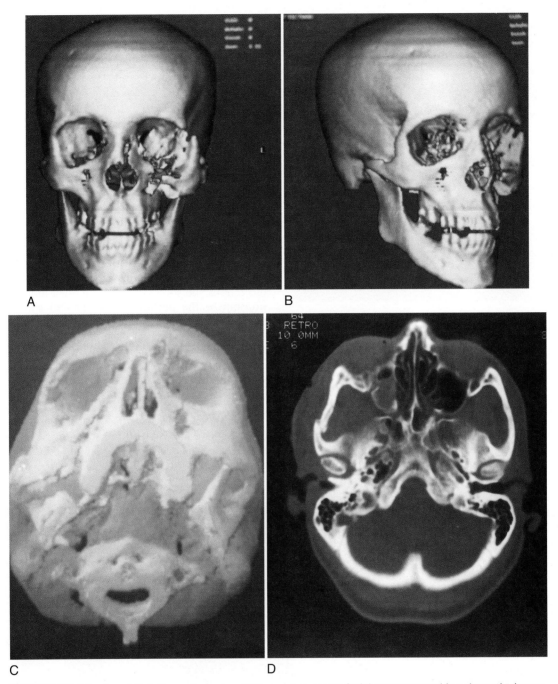

FIGURE 66-14. *A* and *B*, A three-dimensional CT scan documents facial symmetry and is a dramatic demonstration of the skeletal deformity. *C*, Another three-dimensional CT scan documents the fixation of a zygoma in malreduction. *D*, Another type of isolated zygomatic arch fracture.   *Continued*

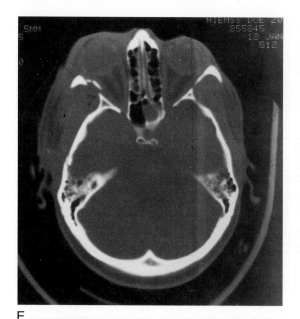

E

FIGURE 66-14, cont'd. *E,* Fracture of the greater wing of the sphenoid accompanies a zygomatic fracture with lateral arch displacement.

the mandibular rami are also demonstrated in this projection (Fig. 66-16).

FRONTAL OCCIPITAL PROJECTION. This view is used when injuries prevent examination of the facial bones with the patient in a more prone or seated position. This projection gives a satisfactory view of the orbits and the lesser and greater wings of the sphenoid, frontal bone, frontal and ethmoid sinuses, nasal septum, floor of the nose, hard palate, mandible, and upper and lower dental arches (Fig. 66-17).

REVERSE WATERS POSITION. The middle occipital position is also used to demonstrate the facial bones when the patient cannot be placed in the prone position. This projection is used to demonstrate fractures of the orbits, maxillary sinuses, zygomatic bone, and zygomatic arches. The increased distance of patient to film magnifies the upper facial structures, but otherwise, the film is similar to that obtained with the Waters position (Fig. 66-18).

OPTIC FORAMEN-OBLIQUE ORBITAL POSITION. This view is best demonstrated by stereoscopic projections and shows the optic foramen in its relationship to the posterior ethmoid and sphenoid sinuses. It also demonstrates the lateral wall of the frontal sinus, the vertical plate of the frontal bone, and the roof and lateral wall of the deep portion of the orbit. Under a bright spotlight, the lateral wall of the opposite orbit may be clearly defined (Fig. 66-19).

SEMIAXIAL (SUPEROINFERIOR) CLOSED PROJECTION (TITTERINGTON POSITION). The zygomatic arches, facial bones, and orbits may be viewed in this projection (Fig. 66-20).

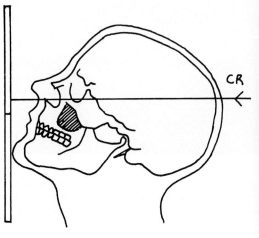

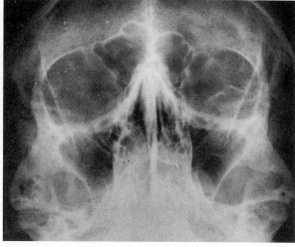

A   B

FIGURE 66-15. Waters position. Posterior-anterior view for visualization of the maxillary sinuses, maxilla, orbits, and zygomatic arches. This projection may also be helpful in demonstrating fractures of the nasal bones and nasal processes of the maxilla. In this view, the petrous ridges are projected just below the floors of the maxillary sinuses. *A,* Position of the patient in relation to the film and the central ray. *B,* Waters view showing fractures of the middle third of the face. (From Kazanjian VH, Converse J: Surgical Treatment of Facial Injuries, 3rd ed. Baltimore, Williams & Wilkins, 1974.)

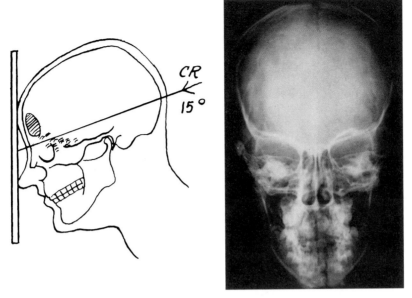

FIGURE 66-16. Caldwell position. Posterior-anterior view of the skull. This position is used to study fractures of the frontal bone, orbital margins, zygomaticofrontal sutures, and lateral walls of the maxillary sinuses. The paranasal sinuses are shown in this projection. The petrous ridges are shown at a level between the lower and the middle thirds of the orbits. (From Kazanjian VH, Converse J: Surgical Treatment of Facial Injuries, 3rd ed. Baltimore, Williams & Wilkins, 1974.)

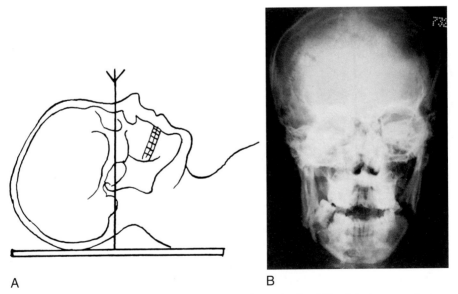

A   B

FIGURE 66-17. Frontal occipital anterior-posterior projection. When injuries prevent prone or seated posterior-anterior positioning of the patient, this position, or the reverse Waters projection, may be used. A, The examination is made with the patient in the dorsal recumbent position. B, Fractures of the lateral mandibular areas are demonstrated with the frontal occipital anterior-posterior projection. (From Kazanjian VH, Converse J: Surgical Treatment of Facial Injuries, 3rd ed. Baltimore, Williams & Wilkins, 1974.)

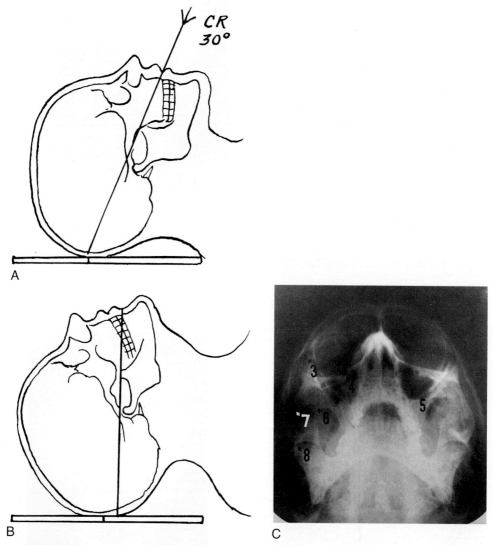

FIGURE 66-18. The reverse Waters position. *A* and *B,* The mento-occipital position, or the reverse Waters projection, is a view of the facial bone similar to the Waters view, except for the greater magnification of the facial bones because of the increased distance between the face and the film. *C,* Fractures of the orbits, maxillary sinuses, zygomatic bones, and zygomatic arches are identified. (From Kazanjian VH, Converse J: Surgical Treatment of Facial Injuries, 3rd ed. Baltimore, Williams & Wilkins, 1974.)

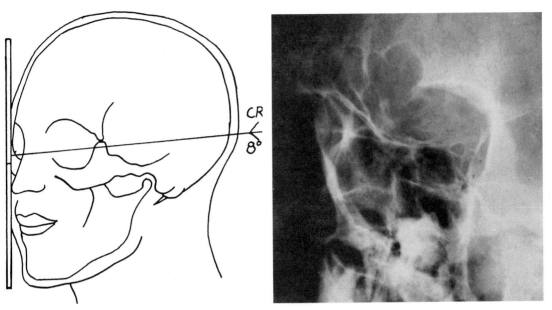

FIGURE 66-19. Optic foramen-oblique orbital position. The oblique posterior-anterior view of the facial bones shows the optic foramen in the lower inferior quadrant of the orbit in relation to the posterior ethmoid and sphenoid sinuses. (From Kazanjian VH, Converse J: Surgical Treatment of Facial Injuries, 3rd ed. Baltimore, Williams & Wilkins, 1974.)

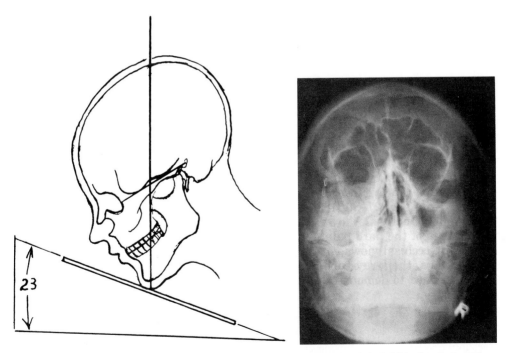

FIGURE 66-20. The semiaxial (Titterington) position. The projection is helpful in the study of fractures of the zygomatic arches, lateral walls of the maxilla, orbital floors, and orbital margins. The maxillary, ethmoid, and frontal sinuses and the inferior border of the mandible are clearly shown in this projection. (From Kazanjian VH, Converse J: Surgical Treatment of Facial Injuries, 3rd ed. Baltimore, Williams & Wilkins, 1974.)

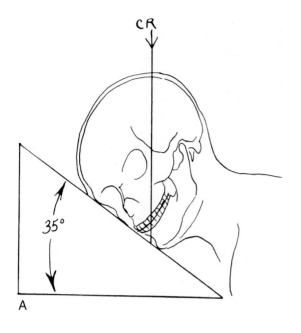

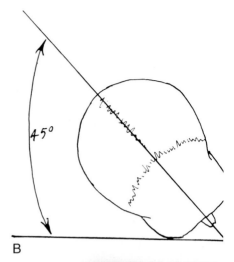

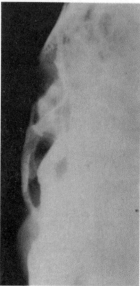

FIGURE 66-21. *A* and *B*, The lateral anterior projection is an excellent view of the zygomatic arch projected free of superimposed structures. Fractures of the lateral wall of the maxillary sinus may also be studied in this view. *C*, Fractures of the zygomatic arch are demonstrated by the lateral anterior projection. (From Kazanjian VH, Converse J: Surgical Treatment of Facial Injuries, 3rd ed. Baltimore, Williams & Wilkins, 1974.)

LATERAL ANTERIOR PROJECTION (FUCHS POSITION). An oblique view of the zygomatic arch, projected free of superimposed structures, is provided by this projection. The lateral wall of the maxillary sinus is also well shown in this view (Fig. 66-21).

LATERAL AND PROFILE VIEW OF THE FACE. Stereoscopic projections may be made with this view because of the complexity of the superimposed shadows of the face. This projection demonstrates the lateral profile of the facial bones and soft tissues of the face. The study is important in the evaluation of maxillary-

mandibular relationships and fractures of the vertical plate of the frontal bone (Fig. 66-22).

NASAL BONES, LATERAL VIEWS. A detailed view of the nasal bone on the side nearest the film and of the soft tissue structures of the nose is possible with this projection. Both sides must be examined radiographically. One view, with this projection, may be made with intensifying screens to show the frontal sinuses. Fractures of the nasal bones, the anterior nasal spine, and the frontal process of the maxilla are demonstrated in this view (Fig. 66-23*A*).

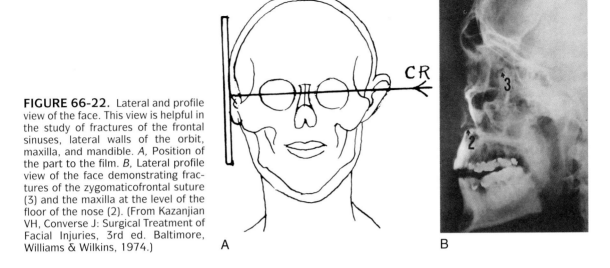

FIGURE 66-22. Lateral and profile view of the face. This view is helpful in the study of fractures of the frontal sinuses, lateral walls of the orbit, maxilla, and mandible. *A,* Position of the part to the film. *B,* Lateral profile view of the face demonstrating fractures of the zygomaticofrontal suture (3) and the maxilla at the level of the floor of the nose (2). (From Kazanjian VH, Converse J: Surgical Treatment of Facial Injuries, 3rd ed. Baltimore, Williams & Wilkins, 1974.)

A   B

NASAL BONES, AXIAL PROJECTION. The axial superoinferior view of the nasal bones is used to demonstrate medial or lateral displacement of the bone fragments that are not shown on lateral views. The thin nasal bones do not have sufficient body to cast a shadow through the superimposed frontal bone or the anterior maxillary structures. This view demonstrates only those portions of the nasal bones that project beyond the line anterior to the glabella and upper incisor teeth. The view is not helpful in children or adults who have short nasal bones, a concave face, or protruding maxillary teeth (Fig. 66-23*B*).

SUPEROINFERIOR OCCLUSAL VIEWS OF THE HARD PALATE. Fractures of the hard palate may be demonstrated by occlusal views with superoinferior projections. The x-ray tube is focused in position to demonstrate the angle of interest.

Superoinferior Central Occlusal View. This view demonstrates the palatine process of the maxilla and the horizontal plates of the palatine bones in the entire dental arch (Fig. 66-24).

Superoinferior Anterior Occlusal View. This view of the anterior part of the hard palate, the alveolar process, and the upper incisor teeth gives more bone detail than the central occlusal view because the obliquely focused central ray does not penetrate any superimposed structures (Fig. 66-25).

Oblique Superoinferior Posterior Occlusal View. This projection provides an oblique, occlusal view of the posterior part of the hard palate (unilateral), the alveolar processes, and all the teeth of the upper quadrant of the maxilla. Fractures of the teeth, or alveolar process, may also be demonstrated (Fig. 66-26).

SUBMENTOVERTEX AND VERTICOSUBMENTAL POSITIONS FOR BASE OF SKULL. This view provides an axial projection of the mandible, coronoid and condyloid processes of the mandible, mandibular rami, zygomatic arches, base of the skull and its foramina, petrous pyramid, sphenoid sinus, posterior ethmoid sinus, maxillary sinus, and bony septum (Fig. 66-27).

OCCLUSAL INFEROSUPERIOR VIEWS OF THE MANDIBLE. Medial or lateral bone displacement and anterior mandibular fractures are shown by occlusal inferosuperior views of the mandible. This view affords bone detail of the entire lower dental arch, mandibular body, symphysis, lower alveolar process, and teeth.

Occlusal Inferosuperior Projection. The occlusal inferosuperior projection view demonstrates medial (or lateral) displacement of fragments and fractures of the anterior portion of the mandible (Fig. 66-28).

Oblique Inferosuperior Projection. An oblique occlusal view of the anterior mandibular area shows the symphysis, alveolar process, and incisor teeth. The bone detail is excellent, and a fracture of the symphysis region, alveolar process, or teeth can clearly be demonstrated (Fig. 66-29).

OBLIQUE SUPEROINFERIOR SUBMENTAL PROJECTION OF THE MANDIBULAR SYMPHYSIS. This projection provides an oblique anteroposterior projection of the mandibular symphysis (Fig. 66-30).

OBLIQUE LATERAL VIEWS OF THE MANDIBLE. Oblique lateral views of the mandible are used to demonstrate fractures of the mandibular ramus, body of the mandible, and symphysis region.

Body of the Mandible. This projection provides a lateral view of the mandible, posterior to the cuspid

Text continued on p. 103

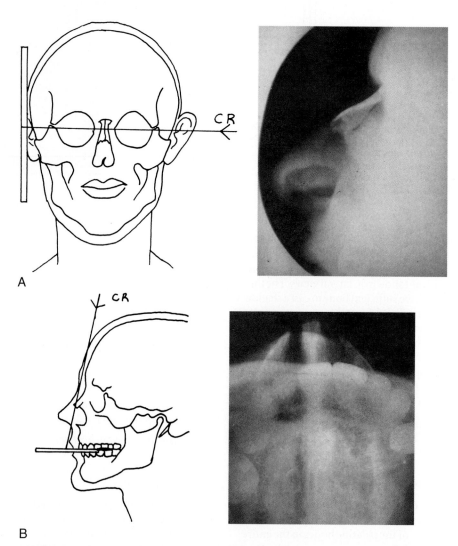

A

B

FIGURE 66-23. *A,* Nasal bones, lateral view. This projection provides a detailed view of the nasal bones nearest the side of the film. Views from both sides are helpful in the study of fractures of the nasal bones, anterior nasal spine, and nasal processes of the maxilla. *B,* The axial view of the nasal bones may reveal fractures with medial or lateral displacement that are not demonstrated on lateral views. Only those portions of the nasal bones that project anteriorly to the line between the glabella and the upper incisor teeth can be demonstrated in this projection. This view is not helpful in the examination of children or adults who have relatively smaller or depressed nasal bones, which do not project satisfactorily through the upper teeth or forehead. (From Kazanjian VH, Converse J: Surgical Treatment of Facial Injuries, 3rd ed. Baltimore, Williams & Wilkins, 1974.)

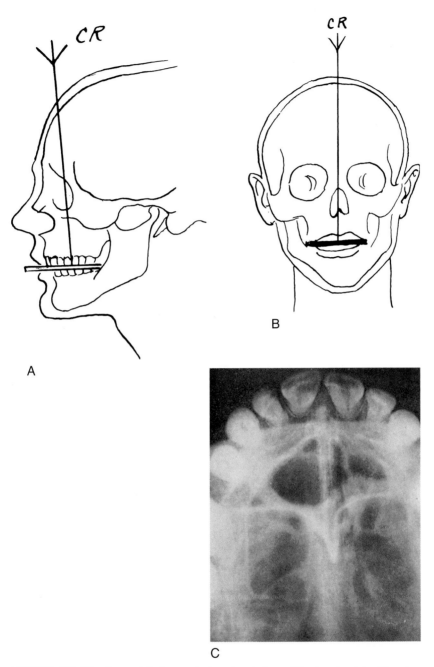

FIGURE 66-24. Superoinferior central occlusal view of the hard palate. The view helps demonstrate fractures of the alveolar process, or hard palate. Cysts and bone malformations or defects of the upper dental arch may be shown by this view. *A* and *B* demonstrate the path of the central ray. *C*, A radiographic example showing a fracture immediately off the midline of the hard palate. (From Kazanjian VH, Converse J: Surgical Treatment of Facial Injuries, 3rd ed. Baltimore, Williams & Wilkins, 1974.)

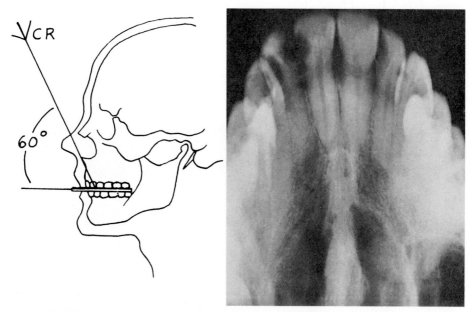

FIGURE 66-25. Superoinferior anterior occlusal view of the hard palate. This view gives details of the maxillary anterior teeth, the alveolar processes, and the anterior portion of the hard palate. The incisive canal is well demonstrated in this view. (From Kazanjian VH, Converse J: Surgical Treatment of Facial Injuries, 3rd ed. Baltimore, Williams & Wilkins, 1974.)

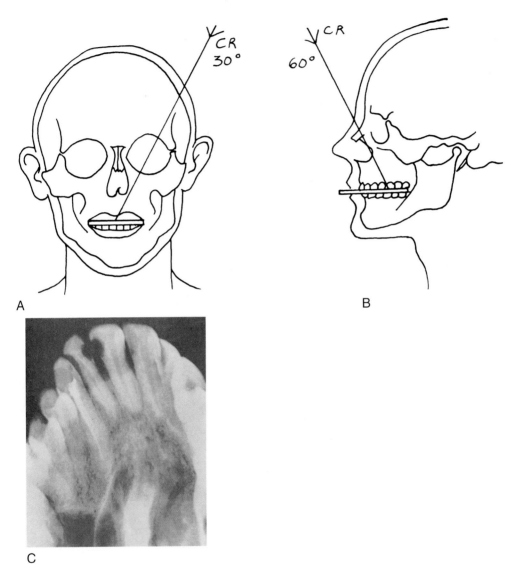

A

B

C

FIGURE 66-26. The oblique superoinferior posterior occlusal view of the hard palate. This projection gives an oblique occlusal view of the posterior part of the hard palate on one side. *A* and *B,* The path of the central ray. *C,* The alveolar process of the teeth and upper quadrant of the maxilla are demonstrated in detail. Fractures of the alveolar process or teeth may be demonstrated by this view. (From Kazanjian VH, Converse J: Surgical Treatment of Facial Injuries, 3rd ed. Baltimore, Williams & Wilkins, 1974.)

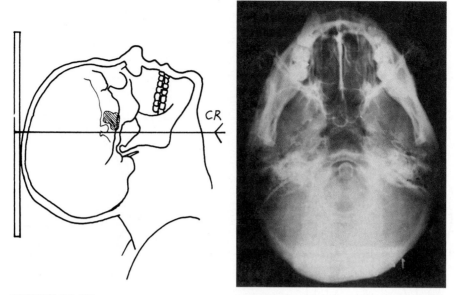

FIGURE 66-27. Submental vertex and verticosubmental positions for base of skull. The submentovertex projection of the base of the skull gives an axial projection of the mandible, including the coronoid and condyloid processes and the ramus of the mandible. The zygomatic arches, the base of the skull and its foramina, the petrous pyramids, the sphenoid sinus, the posterior ethmoid sinus, the maxillary sinus, and the nasal septum are seen in this view. (From Kazanjian VH, Converse J: Surgical Treatment of Facial Injuries, 3rd ed. Baltimore, Williams & Wilkins, 1974.)

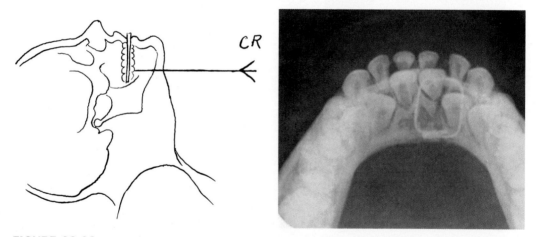

FIGURE 66-28. Inferosuperior occlusal projection of the mandible. The symphysis area is well demonstrated. A fracture has been wired in the parasymphysis area. The dentition in this child, with the unerupted teeth, is clearly visualized. A small gap is noted on the lingual surface of the mandibular cortex. (From Kazanjian VH, Converse J: Surgical Treatment of Facial Injuries, 3rd ed. Baltimore, Williams & Wilkins, 1974.)

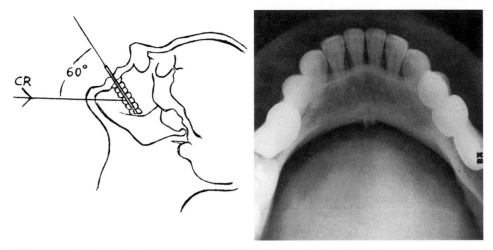

FIGURE 66-29. Oblique inferosuperior position. This projection shows the mental symphysis, the incisor and canine teeth, and the alveolar process with excellent bone detail. (From Kazanjian VH, Converse J: Surgical Treatment of Facial Injuries, 3rd ed. Baltimore, Williams & Wilkins, 1974.)

tooth, and includes a portion of the ramus of the mandible (Fig. 66-31).

Ramus of the Mandible. Posteriorly directed, oblique, lateral views show fractures of the ramus, mandibular condyle, coronoid and condyloid processes, and posterior body of the mandible (Fig. 66-32).

Symphysis of the Mandible. An anteriorly directed, oblique, lateral projection of the symphysis of the mandible demonstrates fractures of the mandibular symphysis, mental foramen region, and body of the mandible (Fig. 66-33).

Posteroanterior View of the Mandible. Medial and lateral displacement of the fractured segments of the mandible may be demonstrated by this view. It demonstrates the symphysis, body, and rami of the mandible, coronoid and condyloid processes, and temporomandibular joints (Fig. 66-34).

Temporomandibular Joints

Oblique Anteroposterior View. Oblique, anteroposterior, frontal occipital view of the temporomandibular joints provides an oblique, posterior view of the condyloid processes of the mandible, mandibular fossa, temporal bones, petrous bones, internal auditory canals, occipital bone, posterocranial fossa, and

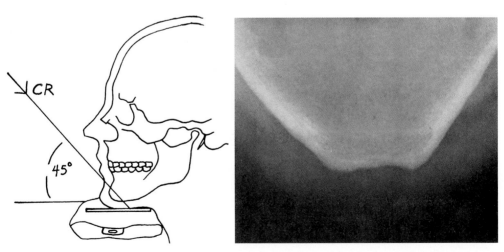

FIGURE 66-30. Oblique superoinferior submental projection of the mental symphysis. (From Kazanjian VH, Converse J: Surgical Treatment of Facial Injuries, 3rd ed. Baltimore, Williams & Wilkins, 1974.)

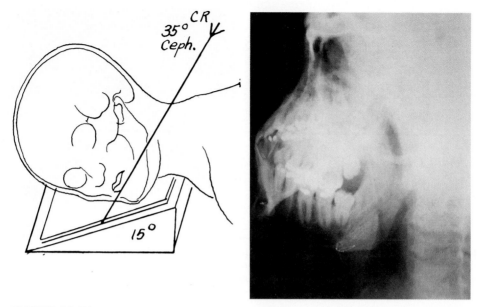

FIGURE 66-31. The body of the mandible: oblique lateral views of mandible. These positions are used to demonstrate fractures of the mandibular ramus, body of the mandible, and symphysis regions. The angle and most of the mandibular ramus are demonstrated in this projection. (From Kazanjian VH, Converse J: Surgical Treatment of Facial Injuries, 3rd ed. Baltimore, Williams & Wilkins, 1974.)

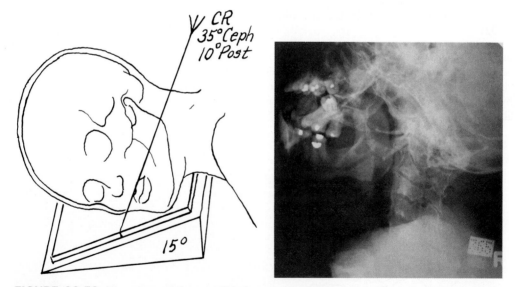

FIGURE 66-32. The ramus of the mandible in a posteriorly directed oblique lateral view. (From Kazanjian VH, Converse J: Surgical Treatment of Facial Injuries, 3rd ed. Baltimore, Williams & Wilkins, 1974.)

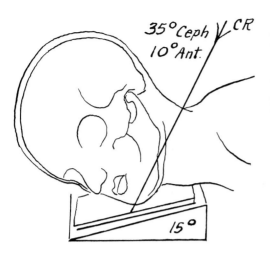
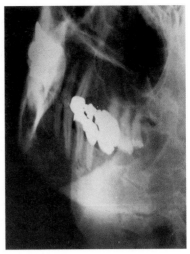

FIGURE 66-33. The symphysis of the mandible is shown by an anteriorly directed oblique lateral view. The regions of the mental foramen and the body of the mandible are also shown in detail. (From Kazanjian VH, Converse J: Surgical Treatment of Facial Injuries, 3rd ed. Baltimore, Williams & Wilkins, 1974.)

foramen magnum. Fractures in the region of the temporomandibular joints, with displacement medially or laterally, can be detected in these views (Fig. 66-35).

Oblique Lateral Views. The views are taken by the lateral, transcranial projection and demonstrate the temporomandibular joints in opened and closed mouth positions. The closed mouth view demonstrates the temporomandibular joint, the relation of the mandibular condyle to the condylar fossa, and the width of the joint cartilage. The open mouth view demonstrates the excursion of the head of the condyle downward and forward in relation to the glenoid fossa and tubercle. This projection is useful in demonstrating fractures and dislocations of the mandibular condyle and the condylar process. The external auditory meatus and the mastoid process are also shown (Fig. 66-36).

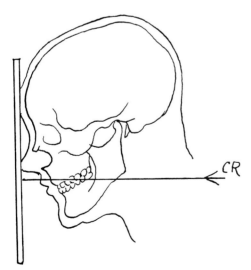
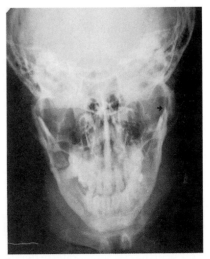

FIGURE 66-34. Posteroanterior view of the mandible. This view demonstrates the symphysis, the body and the rami of the mandible including the coronoid and condyloid processes, and the articular surfaces of the temporomandibular joints. Angle and bilateral subcondylar fractures are demonstrated in the radiographs. (From Kazanjian VH, Converse J: Surgical Treatment of Facial Injuries, 3rd ed. Baltimore, Williams & Wilkins, 1974.)

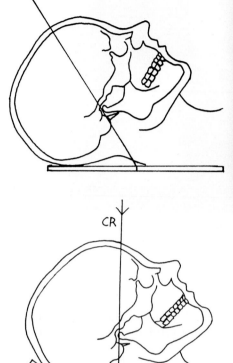

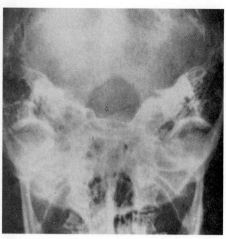

FIGURE 66-35. Oblique, anteroposterior, frontal occipital view of the temporomandibular joints. The view is helpful in the study of fractures of the condyle and the mandible and in demonstrating medial or lateral displacement. (From Kazanjian VH, Converse J: Surgical Treatment of Facial Injuries, 3rd ed. Baltimore, Williams & Wilkins, 1974.)

Mayer View. The temporomandibular joint, external auditory canal, mastoid process, and petrous pyramid are shown in the unilateral, superoinferior view (Fig. 66-37). Medial or lateral displacement of the bone fragments of the mandibular condyle can be shown by this projection. Fracture-dislocation of the bony portion of the external auditory canal may also be demonstrated by this technique.

Panoramic Films. Panoramic films are helpful in defining location and displacement of mandibular fractures. A study by Chayra et al[78] reported that it is the most accurate plain view, from which approximately 92% of mandibular fractures were diagnosed. A diagnostic accuracy rate of 92% for the panoramic radiograph and 67% for the traditional mandibular series was reported. CT scans have accuracy rates better than or similar to those of panoramic films.[79,80] The sites in which mandibular fractures are most commonly underdiagnosed on the panoramic view are the condylar, angle, and symphyseal regions, especially if there

is some blurring by the patient's movement or hardware. In the traditional mandibular series, fractures were missed in every site except the ramus (Figs. 66-38 and 66-39).

Computed Tomographic Scans

CT evaluation of every area of the face can be accomplished, depending on the patient's cooperation and ability to flex the cervical spine. Bone and soft tissue windows, axial or coronal views[75] (Figs. 66-40 and 66-41), and specialized views, such as the longitudinal orbital projection (Fig. 66-42), can be obtained. The bone windows allow definition of bone fractures, whereas the soft tissue views allow definition of the various kinds of soft tissue injury to the area of the fracture. Artifacts in CT scans have been extensively described.[81-84]

Three-dimensional CT scans[73-75] (see Fig. 66-14*A* and *B*) may be obtained to compare symmetry and volume of the two sides of the bones of the face.

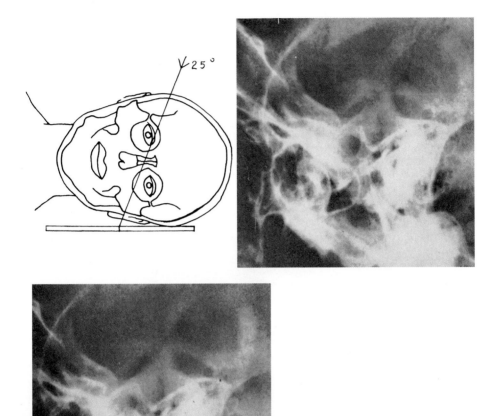

FIGURE 66-36. Lateral transcranial projections of the temporomandibular joints, taken in the open and closed positions, are useful in demonstrating motion of the mandibular condyle in relation to the glenoid fossa. The view may show fractures of the condylar process. (From Kazanjian VH, Converse J: Surgical Treatment of Facial Injuries, 3rd ed. Baltimore, Williams & Wilkins, 1974.)

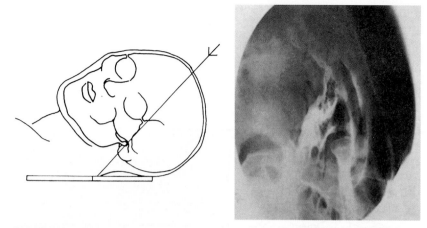

FIGURE 66-37. The Mayer view gives a unilateral superoinferior view of the temporomandibular joint, external auditory canal, and mastoid and petrous processes. The view is helpful in the demonstration of fractures and malformations of the temporomandibular joint and in the study of bony atresia of the external auditory canal. (From Kazanjian VH, Converse J: Surgical Treatment of Facial Injuries, 3rd ed. Baltimore, Williams & Wilkins, 1974.)

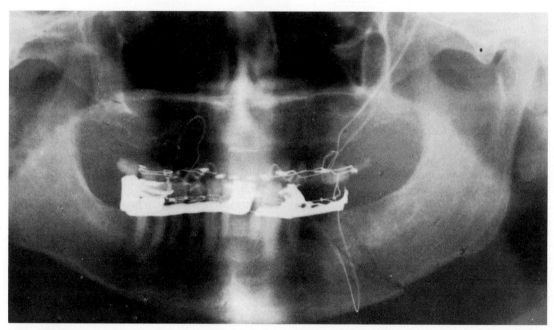

FIGURE 66-38. Panoramic postreduction radiograph showing a comminuted fracture of the mandibular body, in a partially edentulous patient, treated by circumferential wiring of the partial denture. This has been stabilized with a skeletal wire attached to the arch bars. This treatment is cumbersome and often does not align the fracture or provide much postoperative stability. It is uncomfortable for the patient, and it is difficult to maintain nutrition and oral hygiene.

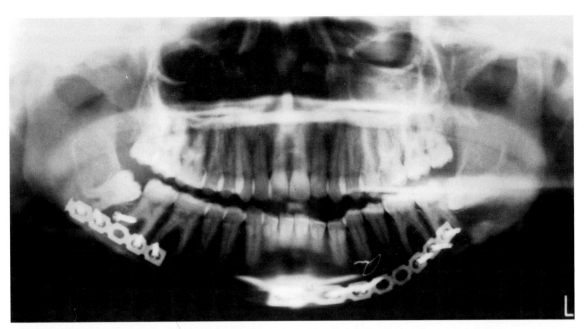

FIGURE 66-39. Panorex of a mandible fracture, treated with internal fixation.

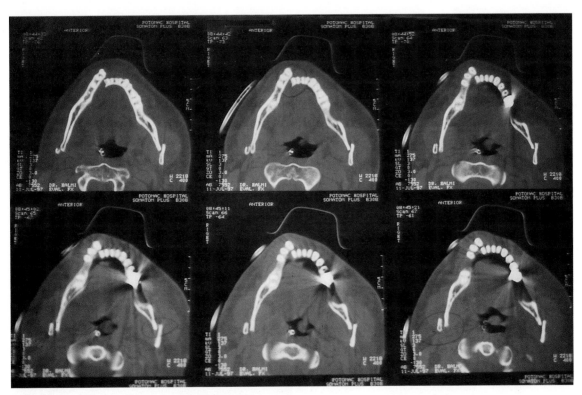

FIGURE 66-40. CT scan of a complex mandible fracture.

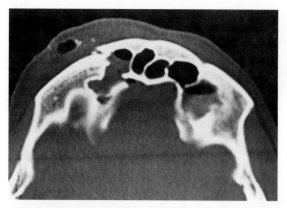

FIGURE 66-41. CT scan of a complex frontal bone-frontal sinus fracture.

Specialized views, such as those of the orbital apex, allow a special magnified visualization. Fractures with little or no bone displacement are missed in CT scans or in those films that show only soft tissue views or thicker cuts. Specialized CT examination of facial fractures is discussed with each region.

GENERAL MANAGEMENT PRINCIPLES

Regardless of the complexity of the fracture pattern, the technical aspects of repair are most expediently achieved by a succinct organized anatomic approach. Accurate anatomic imaging permits rational planning of access incisions, sequences of fracture reduction, and stabilization. Severe bone comminution or loss

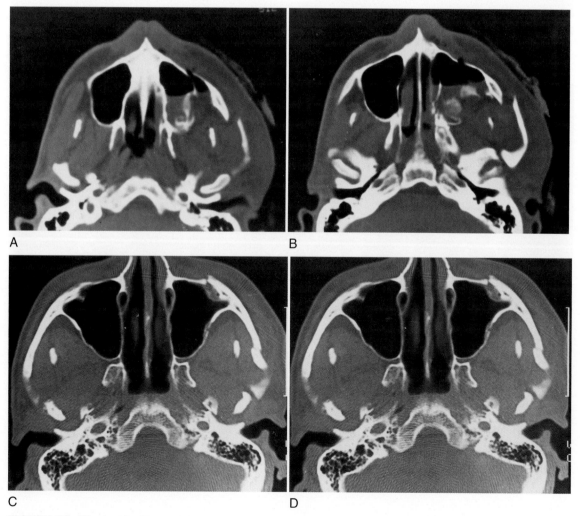

FIGURE 66-42. *A* to *D*, CT scans of a complex orbital-zygomatic fracture. "Cuts" are inferior to superior.

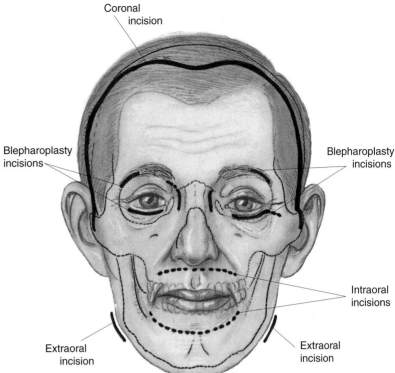

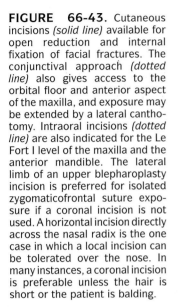

FIGURE 66-43. Cutaneous incisions *(solid line)* available for open reduction and internal fixation of facial fractures. The conjunctival approach *(dotted line)* also gives access to the orbital floor and anterior aspect of the maxilla, and exposure may be extended by a lateral canthotomy. Intraoral incisions *(dotted line)* are also indicated for the Le Fort I level of the maxilla and the anterior mandible. The lateral limb of an upper blepharoplasty incision is preferred for isolated zygomaticofrontal suture exposure if a coronal incision is not used. A horizontal incision directly across the nasal radix is the one case in which a local incision can be tolerated over the nose. In many instances, a coronal incision is preferable unless the hair is short or the patient is balding.

may necessitate primary replacement. In this section, techniques commonly applied to multiple regions of the facial skeleton are discussed.

Surgical Access

Fracture exposure must be sufficiently extensive so as not to compromise the repair yet to respect the aesthetic soft tissue envelope (Fig. 66-43). When possible, facial lacerations may be employed in the repair. Almost all regions of the facial skeleton can be accessed from the incisions described in the following sections.

CORONAL INCISION

A coronal incision generally provides the most appropriate superior exposure of the nasoethmoidal-orbital and the frontal bone area. In young patients and in those who have no suitable lacerations, the incision provides unexcelled exposure of the entire frontal, temporal, zygomatic, and orbital regions. The incision is begun with a straight or zigzag ("stealth") incision to the periosteum from ear to ear. Supraperiorbital dissection is performed to the midforehead unless intracranial surgery is required, and then a subperiosteal dissection is performed. Subperiosteal dissection is begun at the midforehead. The supraorbital nerves[85-87] are freed from the groove (two thirds) or canal (one third) in the upper medial orbital rim, and

dissection laterally on the deep temporalis fascia is used to approach the zygomatic arch. The supraorbital passage is single (supraorbital foramen) in 80% and double (frontal and supraorbital) in 20%.[86] The distance is 2.5 mm from the midline to the supraorbital foramen and 20 mm to the frontal. The foramina are separated by 5 mm.[87] The coronal incision allows exposure of the entire zygomatic arch, nasal root, frontal sinus, and superior and lateral orbital rims. The frontal branch of the facial nerve lies close to the periosteum of the zygomatic arch and must be dissected with care to prevent injury.

MODIFIED BLEPHAROPLASTY INCISIONS

Upper

By use of a shortened upper blepharoplasty incision in direct proximity to a fracture site, injuries to the lateral and superior orbital rim can be accessed.

Lower

The inferior orbital rim, orbital walls, upper maxilla, and nasofrontal process can be accessed by a lower eyelid incision. A number of incisions have been employed to approach the facial skeleton through the lower eyelid. The "one-stroke" cutaneous incision to the orbital rim has the disadvantage of causing a unified line of cicatricial tissue, which can result in a retracted, scarred lower eyelid with vertical shortening.[61] The

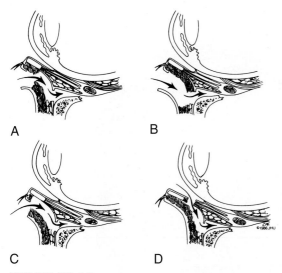

A   B

C   D

FIGURE 66-44. Types of lower lid incisions for zygomatic and orbital reduction. *A,* The Converse subtarsal muscle-splitting incision. A skin flap is dissected to the lower level of the tarsus and then a composite skin-muscle flap developed to the level of the orbital rim. *B,* A skin-only flap. This incision is hazardous and should *not* be used. It results in a high incidence of ectropion, and loss of skin is possible when the eyelid has been contused because of interruption of the cutaneous circulation. *C,* A composite skin-muscle flap is the preferred subciliary incision. The Converse incision is the second choice. *D,* A transconjunctival incision with lateral canthotomy provides excellent exposure. This is a higher transconjunctival incision made below the tarsal plate that divides the lower lid retractors. It is also possible to make this incision in the conjunctival fornix, dissecting through the orbital fat to approach the orbital rim. This variation results in less lower lid retraction, but the inferior oblique must be avoided in dissection through anterior intraorbital fat; the globe and inferior oblique are displaced backward with a malleable retractor.

incision in the lower portion of the eyelid is also frequently beyond finely textured eyelid skin and is surprisingly noticeable with the formation of a permanent scar even if the tissue is not contracted. Incisions into the lower eyelid are also more prone to edema. Incisions into the lower eyelid do have the least incidence of lower eyelid ectropion of any lid incision.[88-90]

The subciliary skin-muscle flap incision (Fig. 66-44) near the upper margin of the lower lid leaves the least conspicuous scar in most patients.[91-93] This incision, however, has the highest incidence of lid retraction (scleral show and ectropion). The incision should begin 2 to 3 mm below the lash line and extend only 8 to 10 mm lateral to the lateral canthus. It should not be taken beyond this dimension laterally as the incision begins to invade cheek skin rather than eyelid skin, and the scar becomes more noticeable. Incisions through lower lid skinfolds (midlid or midtarsal incisions) require less vertical dissection, and the scar is

usually inconspicuous (Fig. 66-45). Visualization is not quite as good as with subciliary incisions. The incidence of ectropion or scleral show in midlid incisions is considerably reduced.

The Converse subciliary incision[94] (see Fig. 66-44) is made by initially transecting the skin just beneath the eyelashes, then dissecting superficial to the orbicularis muscle until one is 2 to 3 mm below the tarsal plate. The dissection at this point incises the orbicularis muscle and then involves raising a combined "skin and muscle" flap to the inferior orbital rim. The septum orbitale is followed below the tarsus until the rim of the orbit is reached. An incision is then made on the anterior aspect of the orbital rim to avoid damage to the septum, which inserts on the superior margin of the inferior orbital rim except for the lateral portion of the inferior orbital rim, where the recess of Eisler is present.

Incisions in the inferior orbital rim periosteum should always be in the periosteum *below* the insertion of the septum orbitale to minimize scarring of the septum, which produces vertical shortening of the lid.[64] The periosteal edges of the incision can be marked with a fine silk suture cut short on each side to identify the edges for closure.

Incisions in a midlid crease (midtarsal incision) (see Fig. 66-45) may be dissected initially with a few millimeters of skin dissection and then deepened through the orbicularis. The dissection plane is then identical to that used for the subciliary skin-muscle flap incision.

The skin-flap-alone incision should *not* be used as it is a random skin flap. In the presence of severe contusion, elevation of a skin-only flap may result in infarction of the skin. Skin flap incisions are also unusually complicated by vertical lid shortening, which produces scleral show and ectropion.

The conjunctival approach (Fig. 66-46) is another incision initially advocated by Tessier[95] in 1973 for correction of craniofacial anomalies and by Converse et al[96] in 1973 for post-traumatic deformities. The conjunctival approach may be performed by making an incision below the tarsus through the lower eyelid retractors, which theoretically allows a preseptal dissection plane to be established. The orbital fat does not prolapse in this approach. A retroseptal dissection plane can be established as well, which allows prolapse of fat. A conjunctival fornix incision may also be employed (Fig. 66-46), which avoids the lower lid retractors; fat prolapses in this approach. Any conjunctival incision may be combined with a lateral canthotomy, which provides exposure nearly equal to that of the subciliary incision. Medial orbital rim visualization is more difficult with a conjunctival versus a subciliary incision. The conjunctival incision avoids an external scar, except when it is extended in the skin lateral to the lateral canthus. It can be complicated,

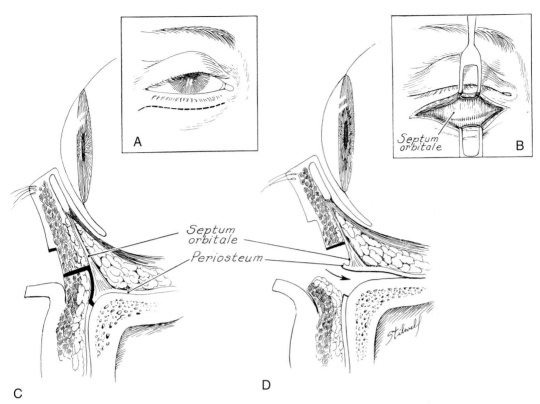

FIGURE 66-45. Converse technique of exposure of the orbital floor through a midtarsal incision. *A,* Outline of the lower eyelid incision. *B,* The septum orbitale is exposed. The skin and muscle incisions are "stepped" to avoid a notch. The septum orbitale is used as a guide for dissection underneath the orbicularis muscle. *C,* Sagittal section showing the skin incision through the orbicularis oculi muscle and the path of dissection from the septum orbitale to the orbital rim. *D,* The periosteum of the orbit (periorbita) is raised from the orbital floor. The periosteal incision should be on the anterior face of the rim, and the cut periosteal edges should be marked with sutures to facilitate closure at the end of the reconstruction. (From Converse JM, Cole JG, Smith B: Late treatment of blow-out fracture of the floor of the orbit. Plast Reconstr Surg 1961;28:183.)

however, to repair the lateral canthus, which is prone to deformities.

The conjunctival incision is preferred by many surgeons because of its inconspicuous scarring and lower incidence of ectropion. In the absence of a lateral canthotomy, excessive retraction may tear the lid either in its midportion or adjacent to the lacrimal system. The conjunctival incision is usually accompanied by less lid shortening than in a subciliary approach. In any approach that interferes with the lower eyelid retractors, some lagophthalmos may be noted in the lower lid. Increased scleral show, ectropion, and entropion may be complications of any lid approach. Often, scleral show and ectropion are temporary conditions that resolve after resolution of the initial mild cicatricial contracture that follows surgery. The contraindications to conjunctival and cutaneous incisions are outlined by Soparkar and Patrinely[97] (Table 66-3).

The infratarsal transconjunctival incision permits the surgeon to avoid perforation of the septum orbitale

with the consequent extrusion of orbital fat.[98,99] The dissection may be performed by making an incision in the conjunctiva in the lower eyelid retractors just beneath the lower lid tarsal plate, then dissecting anterior to the orbital septum in the same plane that one would use for a skin-muscle flap. Alternatively, one may make an incision in the conjunctival fornix (Fig. 66-47), which goes directly through the lower eyelid retractors and the intraorbital fat to approach the orbital rim.

Conceptually, the fornix transconjunctival incision has less chance of lower eyelid retraction (secondary to scar tissue) with a lower fornix conjunctival incision than with a subtarsal conjunctival incision. In making conjunctival incisions, the globe should be pushed backward to retract the inferior oblique from the path of the surgical incision. Lower eyelid conjunctival incisions may be confined to the lower eyelid, or additional exposure may be provided by making a lateral canthotomy and dividing the skin

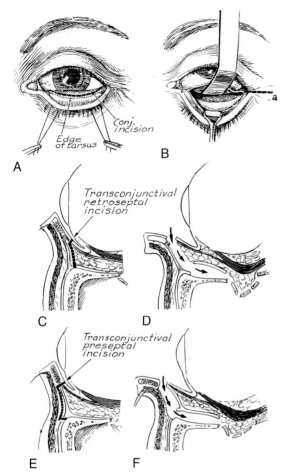

FIGURE 66-46. Transconjunctival approach. *A,* Conjunctival incision below the lower border of the tarsus. The lower lid retractors are transected, and a dissection plane is established either in front of or behind the orbital septum. *B,* Subperiosteal dissection of the orbital floor is performed. The dotted line at *a* represents the lateral canthal extension required for additional exposure. The extension should not measure more than 1 cm laterally to avoid going outside the skin of the eyelid. (Eyelid skin produces a fine scar, but cheek skin does not.) The lower limb of the lateral canthus is severed from the remainder of the canthal attachment, which requires reconstruction at the time of eyelid closure. *C,* Retroseptal approach. *D,* Sagittal view of the retroseptal approach to the fracture. *E,* Preseptal approach. *F,* Sagittal view of the preseptal approach to the fracture.

lateral to the canthus. This addition provides exposure almost equal to that of the subciliary skin-muscle flap incision, which exceeds that of any other lid incision. In general, a corneal protector is placed over the eye to protect the globe and cornea from instruments, retractors, or rotating drills. Ocular lubricant is flammable and should not be used where cautery is to be employed.

The conjunctival incision avoids an external scar, except in the skin lateral to the lateral canthus. This

lateral extension of the incision, if it is used, should not be extended more than 8 to 10 mm, or one will dissect out of eyelid skin. As cheek skin is entered, a more prominent scar is produced. The conjunctival incision is inconspicuous; however, it can still be accompanied by septal shortening, but less than that experienced in the subciliary skin-muscle flap approaches.[100-102] Conjunctival incisions may be accompanied by entropion or ectropion.[103,104] With any lower eyelid approach, some lagophthalmos may be noted in the lower lid in upward gaze. Further, the lid may not depress inferiorly (because of the transection of lower lid retractors) in inferior gaze. Increased scleral show may be noted secondary to contracture of the orbital septum and fibrosis. In general, these are temporary conditions that resolve after resolution of the mild scar contraction (2 to 6 months).

Contraindications to conjunctival incisions are noted when the orbital rim has been reached by following the septum orbitale anteriorly; on reaching the orbital rim, an incision through the periosteum is made several millimeters below the insertion of the orbital septum into the periosteum on the anterior face of the orbital rim. The incision should therefore be squarely on the anterior aspect of the rim of the orbit beneath the insertion of the orbital septum. Laterally, the recess of Eisler (which drapes over the anterior aspect of the lower orbital rim) should be avoided by making the incision a few millimeters lower on the anterior rim. Subperiosteal dissection is then begun by first clearing the anterior face of the orbital rim, then extending the dissection posteriorly over the posterior edge of the orbital rim, following the complex curvature of the internal orbit first downward and inward and then backward and upward over the contours of the orbital floor.

INTRAORAL BUCCAL SULCUS INCISION
Upper

The intraoral approach is one of the most important approaches for exposure of the maxilla and body of the zygoma. A gingivobuccal incision is made 1 cm above the attached gingiva and then deepened through the buccinator straight to the anterior maxillary wall until the mucoperiosteum is identified. The periosteum is incised and reflected superiorly as a mucoperiosteal flap, exposing the entire anterior wall and lateral buttress of the maxilla and all of the anterior and lateral portions of the zygomaticomaxillary buttress. The dissection may be extended medially to the piriform aperture as required. The dissection then progresses superiorly, and the malar eminence is exposed. One should visualize the anterior edge of the masseter muscle inserting on the lower aspect of the malar prominence. The infraorbital foramen is reached after

TABLE 66-3 ✦ CONTRAINDICATIONS TO SUBCILIARY TRANSCUTANEOUS AND TRANSCONJUNCTIVAL INCISIONS

Relative Contraindications to the Subciliary Transcutaneous Approach

"Scarophobic" patient: The larger the skin incision, the greater the chance of visible scar formation or localized lymphedema. Even the normal, mild amount of scarring from a subciliary approach may be unacceptable to certain patients.

Cutaneous inflammatory disorders (acute or chronic): Inflammation increases the risk of visible scar formation. Inflammation may be due to infection, as in cellulitis; acute trauma, as in deep abrasion or severe sunburn; chronic disease, as in psoriasis (Koebner reaction); or collagen vascular diseases with cutaneous manifestations.

History of keloid formation: Eyelid keloids are extremely rare, even among individuals with a clear history of keloid formation elsewhere; yet cutaneous incisions in such individuals, when other options exist, might best be avoided.

Frank lower eyelid retraction or ectropion that will not be addressed: Transcutaneous approaches seem to have a higher incidence of postoperative lower eyelid retraction and ectropion. If such conditions already exist, risking further exacerbation may be inadvisable.

Orbicularis dysfunction

Significant anterior lamella shortage that will not be addressed

Relative malar hypoplasia or exophthalmos that will not be addressed

Lower eyelid laxity or need for lateral canthal suspension: If a transconjunctival approach with canthotomy is performed, this problem can be surgically addressed at the time of orbital fracture repair.

Child or mentally handicapped patient: Cutaneous approaches are more apparent, with skin sutures and possible eschar formation. Additionally, transconjunctival incisions supported by lateral canthal suspension are stronger and less available for manipulation and patient-induced wound dehiscence.

Patients with prior transcutaneous incision undergoing reoperation: Operating through established scar tissue will make surgery more difficult and increase the chance for further postoperative scarring and possible eyelid retraction.

Relative Contraindications to the Transconjunctival Approach

Ipsilateral monocular status: This approach places the patient's only eye more directly into the surgical field and increases the risk of inadvertent damage (e.g., dropped instrument).

Ipsilateral enucleated eye: Conjunctival incisions following prior enucleation may set up severe conjunctival scarring and socket contraction, making it impossible for the patient to wear the ocular prosthesis. This is not true for anophthalmic sockets following less commonly performed ocular evisceration procedures.

Severe dry eye syndrome: Conjunctival incisions and scarring may further decrease tear production by damaging remaining tear-producing glands.

Ipsilateral conjunctival infection: Conjunctivitis (bacterial or viral) is a setup for conjunctival scarring, and bacterial contamination of implants or hardware could prove disastrous.

Ipsilateral nasolacrimal duct obstruction with infection: High bacterial colony counts increase the risk of implant or hardware contamination.

History of conjunctival inflammatory disorder: Diseases that cause inflammation or scarring of the conjunctiva, such as ocular cicatricial pemphigoid, are relative contraindications to further conjunctival trauma.

Severe conjunctival scarring that will not be addressed: If fornix shortening already exists, small amounts of further scarring may lead to entropion or lower eyelid retraction.

Existing transverse skin laceration: If nearby transverse cutaneous scar already exists and would benefit from excision, a transcutaneous approach may be more appropriate.

Prior scleral buckle procedure with porous sponge: Some forms of retinal detachment are treated with ocular encircling elements and porous, silicone sponges. If exposed and contaminated during surgery, these implants may become infected, with serious consequences.

Surgeon's inexperience with canthoplasty or periocular and eyelid surgery: Transconjunctival approaches are generally considered to be more technically difficult than transcutaneous ones due to the frequent need for cantholysis. Also, these approaches theoretically offer greater risk to the nasolacrimal outflow system (canaliculus and nasolacrimal sac), the extraocular muscles, the tear-producing glands, and the globe itself.

From Soparkar CN, Patrinely J: Palpebral surgical approach for orbital fracture repair. Semin Plast Surg 2002;16:273.

detachment of the levator anguli oris muscle. The infraorbital foramen is seen just above this muscle, and the contents of the infraorbital canal should be protected by careful dissection. An elevator may also be placed intraorally underneath the arch, if desired, and medial arch fractures reduced.

Lower

Alantar et al[105] have studied the lower labial branches of the mental nerve and suggested that incisions should be made in a U-shaped fashion, with the two sides of the U parallel to the lower labial branches of the mental nerve (Fig. 66-48). It is essential to reclose the

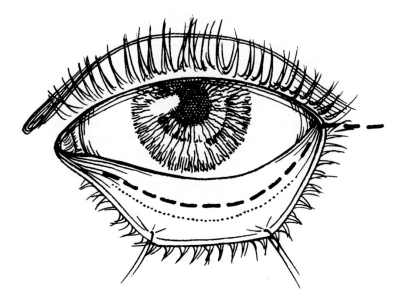

FIGURE 66-47. A conjunctival incision may also be made in the conjunctival fornix, with avoidance of the lower lid retractors and transection of the fat behind the septum. The inferior oblique should be avoided by pushing the globe backward with a soft retractor, keeping dissection anterior to the inferior oblique origin at the rim. The dotted line represents the lower edge of the tarsal plate. (© Johns Hopkins University.)

mentalis muscle anteriorly, or lip ptosis and lip ectropion will occur. In the edentulous mandible with reduced bone height, the inferior alveolar nerve and artery may be located in the soft tissue on top of the remaining bone. An incision slightly off the crest of the body of the mandible to the buccal side provides protection for these structures in the intraoral reduction of edentulous mandible fractures. The fracture site is exposed widely with subperiosteal dissection on the buccal aspect, and superior (Figs. 66-49 and 66-50) or superior and inferior border rigid fixation devices are applied, depending on the height of the mandible.

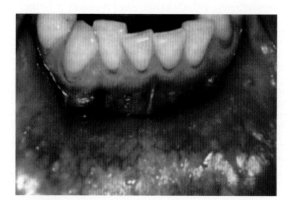

FIGURE 66-48. Incision design for intraoral buccal subcutaneous approach. The incision is made in a slightly U-shaped manner, with the two sides of the U parallel to the lower labial branches of the mental nerve. (From Alantar A, Roche Y, Maman L, Carpentier P: The lower labial branches of the mental nerve: anatomic variations and surgical relevance. J Oral Maxillofac Surg 2000; 58:415.)

Keeping the mucosal incisions slightly out of the most inferior extent of the buccal sulcus ("the gutter") keeps the suture line out of the pool of secretions that occurs more inferiorly and provides a cuff of muscle for closure. After intraoral incisions, some contracture of the vestibule is always noticed. A two-layer closure involving individual muscle and mucosa layers is always the most effective. In general, sutures that absorb slowly or that need to be removed are preferred for a stable intraoral closure. The use of rapidly absorbing sutures, like chromic catgut, predisposes to early wound breakdown when the wound has not achieved sufficient tissue strength to prevent a dehiscence.

EXTRAORAL AND PREAURICULAR INCISIONS

Extraoral approaches may use the Risdon, submandibular, or retromandibular incision for subcondylar fractures or the preauricular or retroauricular incision for higher condylar fractures. With practice, the intraoral approach is much more rapid than the extraoral approach for open reduction, and the visualization is often enhanced, especially for the horizontal mandible anteriorly. Most important, the intraoral approach avoids an external scar. However, comminuted body and angle fractures are best treated with an extraoral approach and reconstruction plate (Figs. 66-51 and 66-52). The incision should correspond to a relaxed line of skin tension 1 cm below the inferior border of the mandible. The skin creases in the neck serve as guides to the location of incisions. The incision should be only long enough to provide adequate exposure of the fracture site for the length of the plate to be used.

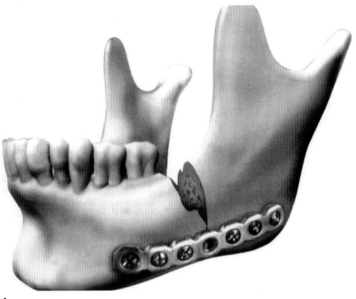

A

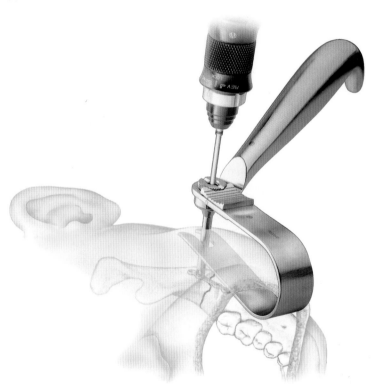

B

FIGURE 66-49. *A,* Treatment of an angle fracture with a lower border reconstruction plate. *B,* Use of a percutaneous trocar for placement of screws in the angle region. (Illustrations courtesy of Synthes Maxillofacial, Paoli, Pa.)

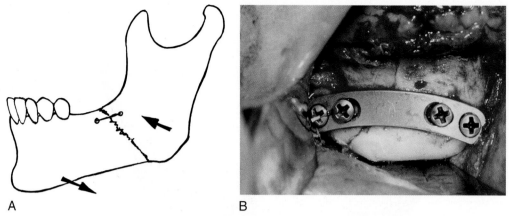

A   B

FIGURE 66-50. *A,* Fixation of a fracture with a wire near the upper border of the bone placed through an intraoral approach. Symphyseal and angle fractures are particularly amenable to intraoral exposure. *B,* Compression plating intraorally of a symphysis fracture.

In some instances, the combination of a dislocated condylar head with fracture of the neck requires both a preauricular incision and a retromandibular incision (upper and lower condylar approaches). However, this dual approach may require a specific exposure for protection of the facial nerve. A transparotid incision has also been described for subcondylar exposure with dissection in the direction of facial nerve fibers to expose the bone through the parotid gland. This incision carries the risk of a parotid glandular fistula as well as facial nerve injury but has the advantage of being directly over the fracture site. In patients with medial dislocation of the condylar head, a preauricular approach is necessary.

Fracture Reduction by Dental Fixation

Fractures of the craniofacial skeleton frequently involve the jaws. Fractures of the jaws invariably produce alterations in the relationship of the upper and lower teeth, or malocclusion. In the edentulous patient, the relationships alter the occlusal bond between the dentures. Knowledge of the dentition is thus an absolute prerequisite for the proper treatment of jaw fractures.

DENTITION

The deciduous teeth begin to erupt at 5 to 6 months of age (see Chapter 67). The lower central incisors are generally first to be noted. By the age of 20 to 24 months, the child has a total of 20 teeth, 10 in the upper and 10 in the lower dental arch. The teeth consist of the incisors, the cuspid teeth, and the deciduous molars. This complement of teeth is known as the deciduous, or temporary, dentition. At the age of 6 years, in addi-

tion to the temporary dentition, the first permanent or 6-year molars erupt behind the second deciduous molars. At the age of 6 years, the maxillary and mandibular central incisor teeth are replaced by the permanent incisors. At the age of 9 years, the permanent lateral incisors have erupted. At the age of 10 to 11 years, the deciduous molar teeth are replaced by the permanent premolar teeth. At the age of 12 to 13 years, the second permanent molar teeth come into position; the deciduous canine teeth are lost and replaced by the permanent canine teeth. At the age of 14 years, all the deciduous teeth usually have been exfoliated and replaced by the permanent teeth. The first and second permanent molars, in all quadrants, are present. The third molars may be missing, partially erupted, impacted, or totally unerupted in some but erupt in most persons after the age of 16 years. When all of the permanent teeth have erupted, the adult has 32 permanent teeth, 8 in each quadrant. The teeth are numbered as follows: the maxillary dental arch, right to left, 1 to 16; the mandibular dental arch, left to right, 17 to 32 (Fig. 66-53). The deciduous teeth are numbered 1 to 8 in the maxillary arch, right to left, and 9 to 16 in the mandibular arch, left to right.

The occlusal relationships between the first molar and cuspid teeth are indicated in Figure 66-54. The Angle[106] classification of malocclusion describes the skeletal relationship between the teeth of the maxilla and the mandible (Fig. 66-54).

Missing teeth in the partially dentulous patient can produce changes in dental relationships. Teeth that have not developed can also produce changes in the usual dental relationships. The first step in identifying abnormal occlusal patterns is to count the teeth, identifying those that are missing and those that are present. Frequently, this will explain an occlusal deviation. The

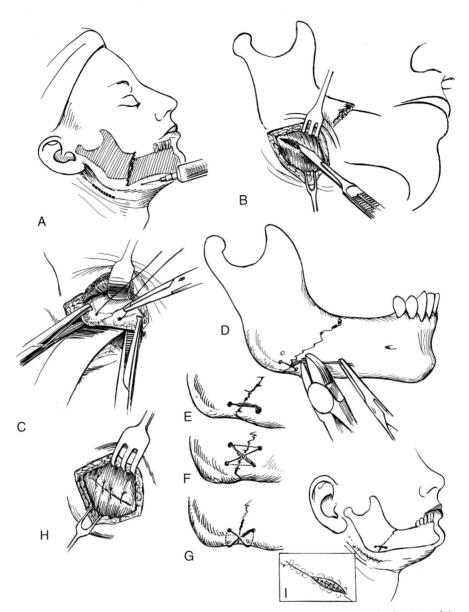

FIGURE 66-51. Open reduction and interosseous wire or plate fixation for fracture of the angle of the mandible. *A,* The incision is made 1 cm or more below the lower border of the mandible (and preferably in the hyoid crease) or in a retromandibular (illustrated) location. The soft tissue is lifted, and dissection is carried beneath the platysma fascia to expose the angle of the mandible. The marginal mandibular branch of the facial nerve beneath the muscle must be identified and protected. The attachment of the masseter must be incised over the inferior mandibular border and the incision carried entirely through the muscle to the bone of the inferior border. *B,* Dissection, avoiding the marginal branch of the mandibular nerve, has been performed to the angle. The attachments of the masseter muscle at the inferior border are divided and elevated. *C,* Small drill holes are passed through the bone, one on each side of the fracture site. The drill holes should be perpendicular to the fracture plane as much as possible to ensure a good reduction. *D,* No. 24 stainless steel wires used for wire fixation. *E,* The cut ends of the wire, after twisting over one of the drill holes, are tucked to prevent prominence underneath the skin. *F* and *G,* Two methods of using crossed (figure-of-eight or double-wire) technique to minimize fracture displacement. There is a tendency for dislocation of the fragments to occur if only a single wire is used. Alternatively, two sets of separate wires may be placed to prevent or to limit the dislocation. *H,* The wound is closed in layers. A dependent or suction drain should be used unless the wound is open intraorally. *I,* A continuous subcuticular suture is an excellent means of skin approximation.

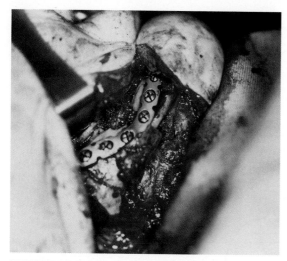

FIGURE 66-52. Comminuted body and angle fractures are best treated with an extraoral incision and reconstruction plate.

use of dental impressions and formation of study models provide a leisurely ability to accurately study dental relationships and wear patterns, which suggest how the teeth came together. The relationship between the central incisors of the mandible and maxilla (the midline relationship to the jaws) and the relationships of the cuspid and first molar teeth on each side serve as the principal guides to the establishment of proper occlusion. These three points should be examined, noted, recorded, and used intraoperatively to align the occlusion and postoperatively to tell whether any deviation has occurred. By study of models, the preexisting occlusion can often easily be recognized by the wear facets. Wear facets indicate where the teeth have habitually come together. A patient who had a class III occlusal relationship (skeletal malocclusion) before injury would be impossible to treat by attempting to force the teeth into a neutral occlusal relationship. A class I (neutral) occlusion is one in which the mesial buccal cusp of the upper first molar occludes with the mesial buccal groove of the mandibular first molar. The protruding or jetting type of jaw is known as class III malocclusion (mesial occlusion), and the retrusive or undeveloped jaw is termed class II malocclusion (distoclusion or mesial occlusion). In addition, there are abnormalities of occlusal relationship in a lateral direction, which are referred to as crossbite or laterognathism. Open bite or absence of occlusal contact in any area should be noted. An open bite may occur laterally, anteriorly, or anterolaterally and may be unilateral or bilateral (Figs. 66-55 and 66-56). In the injured patient in whom teeth or segments of bone are missing, it may be difficult to determine what the normal occlusal relationship should be. Usually, the

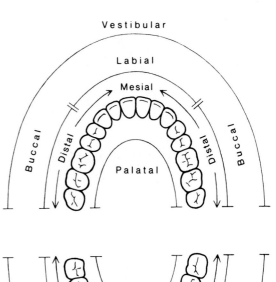

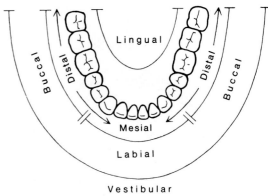

A

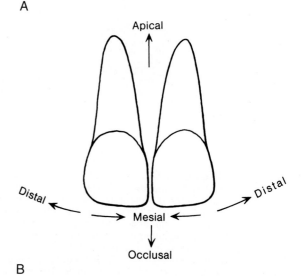

B

FIGURE 66-53. *A* and *B,* Dental terminology describing maxillary and mandibular relationships. (From Texhammar R, Schmoker R: Stable Internal Fixation in Maxillofacial Bone Surgery—A Manual for Operating Room Personnel. New York, Springer-Verlag, 1984:12.)

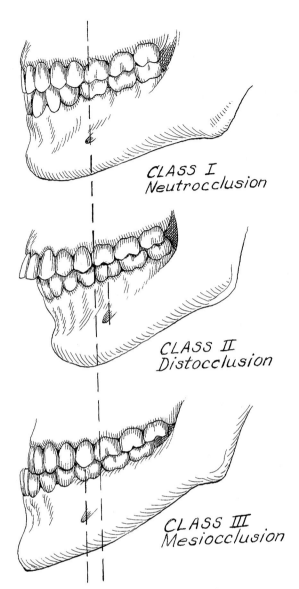

FIGURE 66-54. The classification of occlusion has three categories and is based on the relation of the mesial buccal cusp of the maxillary first molar to the mesial buccal cusp of the mandibular first molar. The position of the cuspid teeth should also be noted, as should the midline of the central incisor teeth. Subdivisions of the three main classes of occlusion and malocclusion are identified by differences in the mesial or lateral positioning of the teeth in the dental arches.

injured patients, when cooperation is not possible, study models become more important (Fig. 66-57). Information may also be obtained from the patient's family, from old photographs that demonstrate the dentition, or from dentists or orthodontists who may have treated the patient previously or perhaps have taken radiographs or have models. In older patients, wear facets on the teeth give clues to preexisting relationships. A patient in neutroclusion, for instance, often shows more wear surfaces on the outer (labial) edges of the lower anterior teeth and on the under (lingual) surfaces of the maxillary anterior teeth. The wear facets show that the teeth previously occluded in a normal relationship. The patient with a severely retruded jaw usually has no wear facets on the incisal edges of the lower anterior teeth. The patient who has a protruding lower jaw may have worn surfaces on the outer anterior edge of the maxillary teeth. If the patient has premolar and molar teeth in both segments of the upper jaw, these teeth usually fit into the contours of the opposing teeth on the lower jaw. Dental consultation may be helpful when the apparent occlusion does not fit a precise, preexisting pattern. It is impor-

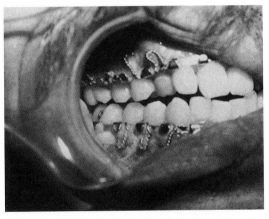

FIGURE 66-55. Lateral open bite and edge incisor occlusion developing following initial reduction and release of intermaxillary fixation in a complicated panfacial fracture. The cause of malocclusion may be displacement of the maxilla (usually posterior and inferior displacement of the nonreduced posterior maxilla), mandibular ramus shortening (as in a displaced, overlapped subcondylar fracture), or both. In this patient, the maxilla has drifted posteriorly and inferiorly in its posterior section, and there is a premature contact in the incisor dentition. The open bite was subsequently closed and the occlusal alignment obtained with light anterior intermaxillary elastic traction for a brief period to move the maxilla forward. The open bite was closed with strong anterior elastic traction. The anterior arch bars may have to be supported with skeletal wires to sustain such traction, and one must be careful not to extrude the anterior teeth by strong traction. Incisor tooth length should be precisely measured and repeatedly checked to notice any tooth extrusion by elastic tension.

patient is helpful in advising the physician about the preexisting occlusal pattern and can comment on whether the teeth are coming together properly. The patient's perception is one of the most sensitive indicators of proper alignment after jaw fracture treatment. Slight differences in the way the teeth fit together are usually perceived by the patient with ease. In head-

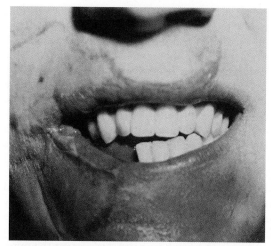

FIGURE 66-56. Malocclusion due to lingual rotation of fragments in a right parasymphyseal fracture. The lingual rotation of the left fragment causes an anterior open bite and lingual version of the left side of the mandible.

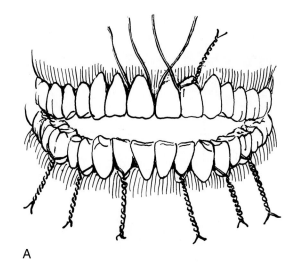

A

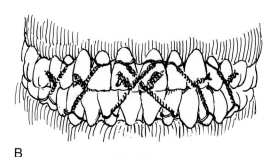

B

FIGURE 66-58. The Gilmer method of intermaxillary fixation of the teeth, which have been brought into occlusion by intermaxillary wiring. *A,* Application of wires to the maxillary and mandibular dentition. *B,* Intermaxillary fixation has been established.

tant to restore the occlusion in fractures of the jaws to the preexisting dental relationships. Alternatively (and less desirably), the occlusion should be brought into a range where it can easily be corrected with orthodontic manipulation. It is necessary that the teeth be brought into the best possible occlusal relationship so that adequate chewing surface and joint function occur after the reduction, fixation, and consolidation of jaw fractures.

WIRING TECHNIQUES

Gilmer Method

The simplest way to establish intermaxillary fixation is by the Gilmer method, first described by Gilmer[107] in 1887 (Fig. 66-58). In that year, he recognized the

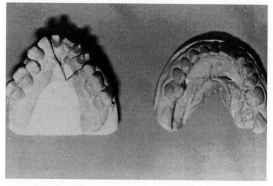

FIGURE 66-57. Models for the construction of crowns or bridgework are often useful in defining previous dental relationships.

importance of the teeth with regard to the fixation of fractures and described this technique in the American literature. The technique is simple and effective but has the disadvantage that the mouth cannot be opened for inspection of the fracture site without removal of the wire fixation. The method consists of passing wire ligatures around the necks of the available teeth and twisting them in a clockwise direction until the wire is tightened around each tooth. After an adequate number of wires have been placed on the upper and lower teeth, the teeth are brought into occlusion and the wires are twisted, one upper to one lower wire. Stainless steel 24-gauge and 26-gauge wires are usually employed. With the Gilmer method, the wires are twisted with a vertical direction to prevent slipping in an anterior-posterior direction (Fig. 66-58).

Eyelet Method

The eyelet method[108] (Fig. 66-59) of intermaxillary fixation has the advantage that the jaws may be opened for inspection by removal of only the intermaxillary

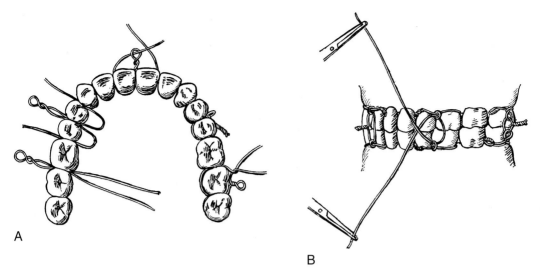

FIGURE 66-59. The eyelet method of intermaxillary fixation (popularized by Ivy). *A*, Establishment of wires. *B*, Intermaxillary fixation is established by No. 24 wires cut in thirds and passed around the loops.

ligatures. This method consists of twisting a 20-cm length of 24-gauge or 26-gauge wire around an instrument to establish a loop. Both ends of the wire are passed through the interproximal space from the outer surface. One end of the wire is passed around the anterior tooth, the other around the posterior tooth. One end of the wire may be passed through the loop. The eyelet should project in the upper jaw above and in the lower jaw below the horizontal twists to prevent the ends from impinging on each other. After the establishment of sufficient number of eyelets, the teeth are brought into occlusion, and ligatures are passed in "loop" fashion between one upper and one lower eyelet. The interjaw wires are twisted tightly to provide intermaxillary fixation. If it is necessary to open the mouth for inspection, the ligature loop wires may be cut and then replaced without much difficulty. A heavy No. 24 wire is used to form the eyelets in most patients. If heavy wire is used to form the eyelets, they may be turned to form hook-like projections to which intermaxillary orthodontic rubber bands are attached to provide occlusion between the jaws.

Arch Bar Method

In most patients, prefabricated arch bars, which are commercially available, should be used to establish intermaxillary fixation. These represent the usual method of establishing intermaxillary fixation (Figs. 66-60 and 66-61). They are ligated to the external surface of the dental arch by passing 24- or 26-gauge steel wires around the arch bar and around the necks of the available teeth. The wires are twisted tightly to individual teeth to hold the arch bars in the form of an arch, completely around the dental arch. All teeth,

including the second molars, should be ligated, with the possible exception of the incisor teeth. The incisor teeth have conical roots and may be extruded by aggressive wire tightening to the arch bar. If segments of teeth are missing or if anterior support of the arch bar is required to balance the forces generated by elastic traction anteriorly, the arch bar may be stabilized by additional wires passed and connected to the skeleton (skeletal wires). Acrylic interdental splints between the incisor occlusal surfaces and an acrylated segment of arch bar (acrylic is applied and allowed to dry over the arch bar) are two other ways that incisor teeth can be stabilized. If traction is to be exerted in the anterior section of the mandible or maxilla, this traction may result in loosening of the incisor teeth unless the arch bar is stabilized to the jaw by skeletal wires. Arch bar stability may be obtained by suspension of a wire from a screw at the piriform margin to the maxillary arch bar. Suspension wires may be passed through drill holes at the piriform margin or around screws (Fig. 66-62). Access to the piriform aperture is provided by a small gingival buccal sulcus incision. This technique is particularly applicable in children, in whom the structure of the teeth tends to render arch bars less stable. The mandibular arch bar may also be stabilized by wires passed to a screw at the lower mandibular border or by the technique of circummandibular wiring (Fig. 66-62). It is helpful to have a special instrument set for arch bar application, which can be used and sterilized separately. The arch bars are applied before the rest of the operation is begun. It cannot be overemphasized that the stability and the alignment of a fracture reduction depend, to a great extent, on the alignment of the teeth

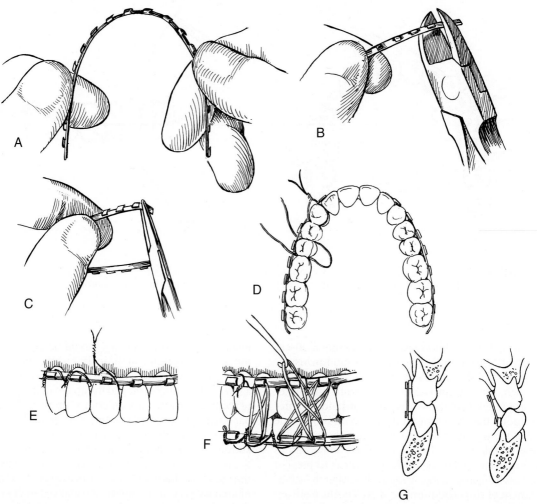

FIGURE 66-60. In almost all patients, there is no substitute for the flexibility and control obtained by the use of a full Erich arch bar applied to the upper or lower teeth. Either intermaxillary elastics (rubber bands) or wires can be used to establish intermaxillary fixation. *A,* Selection of an appropriate length and contouring of the Erich arch bar. *B,* Trimming the bar to length as established by measurements on the patient. *C,* The posterior edges of the bar should be bent to conform to the contour of the posterior maxillary arch and dentition to prevent soft tissue injury. *D* and *E,* Wires are passed above and below the arch bar and tightened so as not to obstruct the lug. It is important to make sure that these wires have been tightly applied by checking whether any vertical movement of the arch bar is possible at the site of the wire loop. The bar may be grasped with a clamp and movement attempted. *F,* Intermaxillary fixation may be established by either wires or elastics. Elastics apply a constant force and, if light, permit some movement of the jaws. They do exert a constant force on the dentition, which may not be desirable. Wires are stable, permit no movement, and do not constantly apply undesirable forces to the dentition as elastics do. *G,* Elastic forces tend to displace (rotate) the dentition.

achieved by this initial application of arch bars. Further, the stability of the fracture reduction depends on an arch bar securely applied to the dentition. Wires should be stretched, tightened, and guided down with periosteal elevators to the proper location on the tooth and stabilized as they are tightened. No "slack" should be permitted. Wires should be tightened until "secondary spiraling" is seen in the twisted wire. In most instances, 26-gauge wires do not take much secondary manipulation without breaking, and the use of

24-gauge wires is recommended in most patients, especially young adult men.

Wires should be seated away from the arch bar lugs, twisted with the use of a periosteal elevator, and tucked appropriately so they will not pierce the patient's lips or mucosa. Wires or elastic bands (Fig. 66-63) anterior to the cuspid teeth should be used with caution for intermaxillary fixation, unless specific precautions have been taken to prevent incisor extrusion from anterior traction, such as skeletal wire placement to the

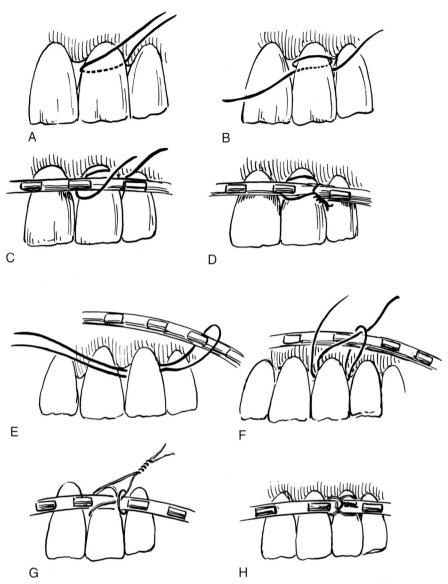

FIGURE 66-61. The single root and conical shape of the maxillary anterior teeth may require special wiring techniques to keep the wire and arch bar from slipping. The method of Rowe and Killey[373] is another way of providing fixation of the arch bar in the maxillary incisor and cuspid area. *A,* Passage of the wire. *B,* An extra loop is passed. *C,* The wire is passed above and below the arch bar. *D,* The wire is tightened and tucked in to prevent soft tissue injury. *E* and *F,* A double wire may be passed around each tooth and circles the arch bar. *G,* One wire end is placed through the loop, and the other goes behind the arch bar to be twisted over the top. *H,* Completed fixation with the wire end tucked to prevent soft tissue injury.

arch bars or the use of an occlusal wafer (a wafer between the incisal edges of the teeth). Because the incisor teeth do not contact (oppose) one another as in the lateral dentition, one can extrude them from their sockets with strong anterior traction. The use of an occlusal wafer or skeletal wire allows an "occlusal contact" to be generated between the incisor teeth, and

this opposes the forces of extrusion. Rubber orthodontic bands (Fig. 66-63) can be used to occlude the two dental arches by applying these bands between the arch bars. The rubber bands exert constant traction, which will occlude the teeth in their proper relationship. The elastic fatigues over time, and the rubber bands must be periodically replaced. Rubber bands

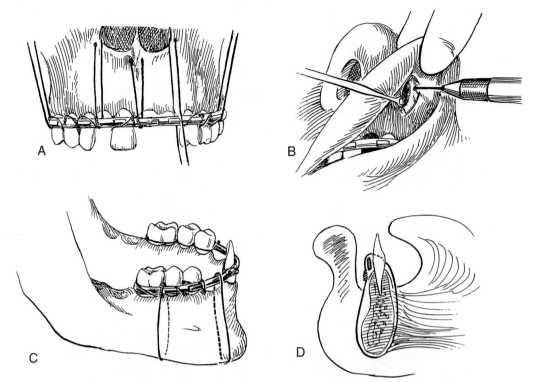

FIGURE 66-62. Supplementary fixation of arch bars is necessary in partially edentulous jaws. Teeth may be missing because of previous extraction or injury and may be insufficient in numbers to secure the arch bar adequately. *A,* Support in the maxillary anterior region may be obtained by passing additional wires through small drill holes at the piriform aperture or by use of a screw in this area, passing the wire around the screw. Additional wires may be placed through the piriform aperture at the nasal spine, around the zygomatic arches, or to drill holes placed in the inferior orbital rims. *B,* The approach to the piriform margin is through a small vertical incision in the labial vestibule of the upper lip. *C* and *D,* Circumferential wires may be used to give stability to the lower arch bars when an insufficient number of teeth are available for attachment of the bar. The bar may also be strengthened by the application of a small amount of acrylic, after the initial wiring, to increase its rigidity.

are useful if one is trying to overcome muscle forces or to move a dental segment into another occlusal relationship. If not, the teeth are better held in occlusion with wires. Rubber bands may be applied, for example, in a class III or a class II relationship to provide traction anteriorly or posteriorly on the jaws to change or guide the occlusion.

Dental relationships should be used to describe movements of the teeth and interdental relations (see Fig. 66-53*A* and *B*). A malocclusion can sometimes be corrected by the simple use of orthodontic rubber bands. Once the proper occlusal relationship of the teeth has been obtained, the rubber bands are replaced with wires. In some patients who have concomitant fractures of the condyle, it is desirable to allow the patient to begin motion and yet reapply rubber band traction at night to re-establish occlusal relationships and provide some rest and lengthening of the vertical segment of the mandible, for instance, in a condylar

head fracture that is being treated with a closed reduction. This technique allows mobilization of the temporomandibular joint and yet continues to re-establish periodic occlusal relationships with interval elastic traction. Patients can learn to apply and change the elastics themselves. Patients are often sensitive to minor changes in occlusal relationships and can report new abnormalities. Mobilization additionally improves dental hygiene and prevents joint stiffness. The use of rubber bands is advantageous because they are more easily removed than wires, and patients can apply them with minimal instruction. Wires are frequently less bulky than rubber bands, are easier to clean with a toothbrush or forced water (e.g., WaterPik) appliance, but have sharp ends that have to be protected. At the end of a course of fracture treatment, if there is mobility at the fracture site, fixation may easily be re-established for a short period by reconnecting the intermaxillary fixation.

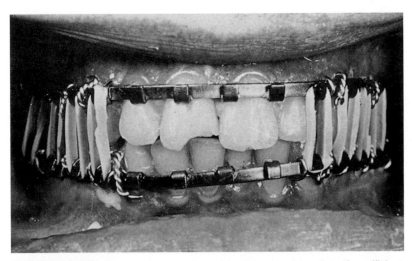

FIGURE 66-63. Intermaxillary fixation with rubber band traction. If a sufficient number of posterior teeth are present to give stability to the arch bars, the anterior teeth (distal to the cuspid) are not ligated. Heavy traction on the anterior teeth may loosen the teeth from the alveolar bone because of their single conical root structure. This method provides a quick, easy, and effective means of intermaxillary fixation and exerts constant slight traction. The author prefers wire for most patients because no constant traction is necessary. If traction is to be placed in the incisor dentition, the use of an occlusal wafer or the supplementary stabilization of the arch bar with skeletal wires is required. Anterior traction is necessary in the closed treatment of condylar fractures, where one is trying to prevent an open bite. Anterior elastic forces applied to arch bars close the open bite most effectively.

Orthodontic Bands

One of the nicest ways to provide intermaxillary fixation is by orthodontic bands and brackets (Fig. 66-64). This is a precise and accurate method of holding occlusion, but the technique is not as strong as arch bars and can be used only where no force is to be exerted on the fracture segments and in cooperative patients. The appliances require special expertise to construct and apply. They are more expensive to use in fracture treatment and usually require an orthodontist as a member of the fracture team.

Adaptations of the use of wire ligatures are many. A fracture in which there is a stable complement of teeth on each side can be secured with a single wire circling the teeth across the line of the fracture or with several wires twisted around adjacent teeth and linked together by twisting. Seldom, however, do these techniques align fractures properly or provide enough stability. Further, any problems that occur require intermaxillary fixation by the use of a full arch bar.

Acrylic Splints

Acrylic splints are useful in the maintenance of intermaxillary fixation and in establishing the continuity of the maxillary and mandibular dental arches. In particular, segments of missing teeth can be compensated with a suitably designed maxillary or mandibular splint. These splints are wired to the maxillary or mandibular teeth. Alternatively, a fracture can be reduced and stabilized by the application of a palatal or a lingual splint for certain fractures (Fig. 66-65). Intermaxillary fixation is then sometimes not necessary. Appliances of this type are effective but require detailed dental knowledge and skeletal models for splint construction. Their use was formerly routine in complicated fractures of the jaws with wire interfragment fixation, and they were particularly important before plate and screw fixation. The splints were fabricated by specially educated physicians with dental training, dental personnel, or a dental laboratory; some prosthodontic laboratories are able to fabricate acrylic splints for those less familiar with the intricacies of fabrication. Acrylic splints provide precise dental alignment during healing and are specifically useful in complicated fractures, such as those mandible fractures with combined alveolar fractures. Splints prevent alveolar segment fracture rotation and telescoping of the fragments, and they may also be designed to provide an occlusal "stop" to compensate for missing sections of teeth. An acrylic splint is occasionally placed to facilitate dental occlusal alignment before plate and screw fixation of a fracture is employed, and then it is removed after fixation.

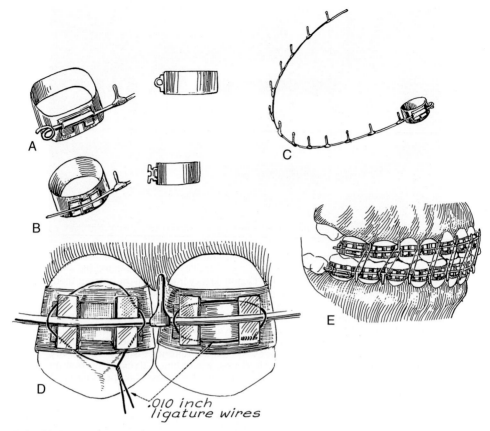

FIGURE 66-64. Orthodontic appliances may be used to provide fixation. These consist of a combination of bands and glued appliances for fixation. *A,* Edgewise appliance consists of molar bands with rectangular sheaths (internal dimensions, 0.022 × 0.028 inch) through which an edgewise arch bar is inserted at each end. *B,* Remaining teeth in each dental arch carry bands with twin brackets (slot dimensions, 0.022 × 0.028 inch) to permit insertion of an edgewise wire (0.021 × 0.025 inch) and secure it in position with ligature wires (0.010 inch). *C,* Arch wire with spurs soldered to the gingival side as it appears before final insertion for planned surgery. *D,* Arch wiring and position are maintained with wire ligatures placed around the brackets. *E,* Appliance as it appears at the time of surgery with intermaxillary wires (0.028 inch) placed between the arches to fix one jaw to the other. (From Kazanjian VH, Converse J: Surgical Treatment of Facial Injuries, 3rd ed. Baltimore, Williams & Wilkins, 1974.)

Monomaxillary Versus Bimaxillary Fixation

When several teeth are present on each side of a fracture, the use of a suitable splint and prefabricated arch bar augmented by acrylic stabilization may entirely obviate the need for postoperative intermaxillary fixation to the considerable increase of a patient's comfort and nutrition (Fig. 66-65E). These techniques require specialized dental knowledge, and today open reduction with plate and screw fixation is equally effective in preventing postoperative motion.

INTERMAXILLARY FIXATION SCREW TECHNIQUE

Intermaxillary fixation screws have been introduced as "labor-saving" devices.[109] Intermaxillary fixation screws provide a rapid method of immobilization of the teeth, given good dentition and uncomplicated fracture type (Fig. 66-66). The number and position of the intermaxillary fixation screws to be inserted are based on the fracture type, the location of the fracture, and the surgeon's preference. Screws must be positioned superior to the maxillary tooth roots and inferior to the mandibular tooth roots.

Their disadvantages are the minimal and focused points of force application to maintain good intermaxillary fixation. The focused points of force application may result in malocclusion by leaving the posterior dentition in an open bite.

Fracture Stabilization

Control and maintenance of fracture reduction require a thorough understanding of the biomechanical forces

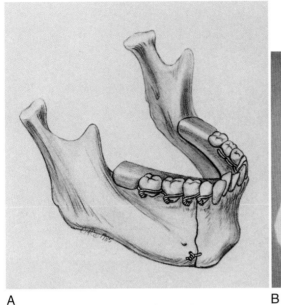

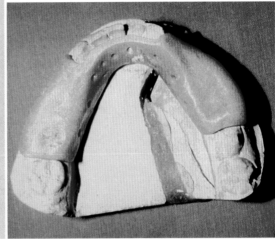

A

B

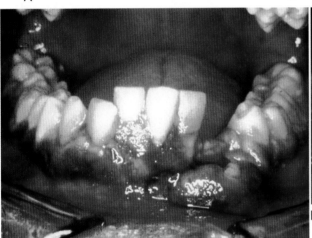

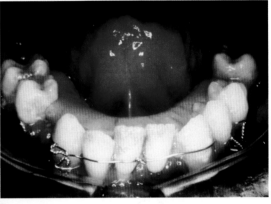

C

D

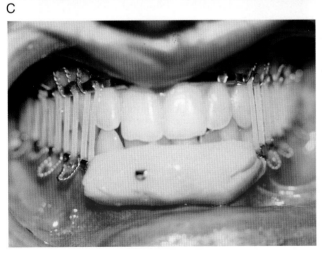

E

FIGURE 66-65. *A,* The application of a lingual splint supports an open reduction of a parasymphyseal fracture with a wire. The use of the splint prevents lingual deviation of the fracture and provides control of the width of the mandible in the angle region. The action of the splint prevents lingual rotation of the upper border of the mandible at the dentition. It is most often used together with arch bars but is more cumbersome than plate and screw fixation, which would prevent the same rotation because of its three-dimensional stability. The arch bars were omitted in the illustration for clarity of splint position. *B,* A lingual splint in place. Splint has occlusal stop for missing dentition. *C,* Alveolar fractures involving incisor teeth. *D,* Lingual splint supports treatment of alveolar fracture. *E,* Acrylic on arch bar may also provide additional stabilization for alveolar fractures.

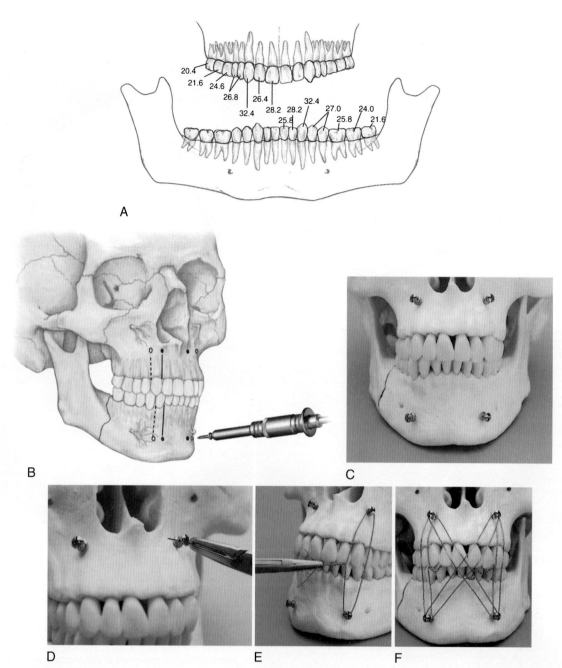

A

B

C

D

E

F

FIGURE 66-66. The use of intermaxillary fixation screws for intermaxillary fixation. These devices do not provide the stability or flexibility obtained from arch bars and full intermaxillary fixation. Numbers of patients have been thought to be in good occlusion with this technique when actually they were in an open bite, were malreduced, and required osteotomy or fracture revision. *A,* Estimates of the average lengths of the teeth including a 10% magnification associated with the radiograph. *B,* Pay attention to the canine root (the longest) and the mental nerve. Screws should be inserted 5 mm inferior or superior and medial or lateral to the canine root, which may be visualized on the bone surface. •, medial to canine roots; ○, lateral to canine roots. *C and D,* Four screws should be inserted. No. 24 wire is passed through the cross holes or alternatively wrapped around the screw heads. *E,* The wires are tightened. *F,* Crossed wires may also be used to buttress the screw support obtained. (*A* modified from Wheeler RC: Dental Anatomy, Physiology and Occlusion. Philadelphia, WB Saunders, 1974. *B* to *F* courtesy of Synthes Maxillofacial, Paoli, Pa.)

acting on the site of injury. Specific techniques of stabilization are discussed for each site. However diverse and seemingly different the techniques, they all are similar in the basic biomechanics of fracture stabilization. This section deals with the principles and similarities of various techniques of fracture stabilization.

Stabilization of displaced facial fractures can be enhanced with a variety of techniques. External techniques include maxillomandibular fixation and external fixators. These techniques generally allow some degree of fracture mobility and are considered nonrigid and inaccurate but benefit from ease of application and reduced morbidity from a reduced surgical dissection. Internal methods of fixation include interosseous wire, K-wire, plate and screw, and lag screw techniques. These techniques have the potential to yield highly accurate and stable fixation of the three-dimensional facial skeleton form. One-stage accurate reconstruction of the highly vascular facial skeleton is now routinely achieved by judicious and meticulous application of these techniques.

DEFINITIONS: FUNCTIONAL STABILITY, RIGIDITY, LOAD SHARING, LOAD BEARING

Rigid fixation is defined as internal fixation that is stable enough to prevent micromotion of the bone fragments under normal function. Rigidity of the bone fragments is not necessary for healing of a fracture to occur under functional loading. Ellis[110] applies the term *functionally stable fixation* to those forms of internal fixation recognized as not being "rigid." Load-bearing fixation devices are of sufficient strength and rigidity that the devices can bear the entire loads during functional activities without impaction of the bone ends. Load-sharing fixation is a form of internal fixation that is of insufficient stability to bear all the functional loads applied across the fracture. It relies on the impaction of the bone on each side of the fracture to bear the majority of the functional load.

BONE PLATES AND SCREWS, COMPRESSION PLATES, LOCKING PLATES, LAG SCREWS

Currently, the most advanced methods of fracture stabilization involve the surgical implantation of an appliance to impart stability to a fracture. Bone plates and screws achieve fracture stabilization by design of the implant to absorb part or all of the functional load acting at the fracture interface. Therefore, screw anchorage of the plate to the bone by friction permits force transmission from the bone to the plate. There are a plethora of commercial systems widely available. They all bear similarity in that they are designed so that the plate composition, size, thickness, and security of screw anchorage allow custom application to meet the varied loads expected at each anatomic site of the face. Originally, screws were not self-tapping and required an initial tapping procedure to cut screw threads into the bone. Nontapped screws are the system with the least trauma to the bone, as self-tapping screws further damage the bone by virtue of the cutting flute. Self-tapping screws are now universally used.

The dynamic compression plate is designed with elliptical beveled holes in such a way that the screw head will glide in the plate to its center on engagement. The result produced from tightening the initial screws of the plate is movement of the bone such that the ends of the bone are compressed together. Compression of the bone ends conceptually speeds fracture healing (primary bone healing) and also places more of the functional load needed for fracture stabilization on the bone instead of on the hardware. In the absence of compression and bone contact, the hardware bears the entire functional load of the fracture. Compression was developed for extremity fracture treatment. Its application in the facial skeleton can change the fracture reduction sufficiently to result in a malunion, and it must be used judiciously in the craniofacial skeleton. The disadvantage of compression plates in the facial skeleton is the undesirable movement of well-reduced fractures. Small movements that minimally affect the bone alignment are capable of producing malocclusion or causing the interface of bone at the fracture site to necrose from excess pressure of the compression (Figs. 66-67 to 66-69). The author's usual practice is to use noncompressive fixation (Fig. 66-70). In plates with compression holes (Figs. 66-71 and 66-72), as the screw is tightened, the screw-bone unit is moved toward the fracture site, impacting against the bone on the opposite side of the fracture (Fig. 66-73; see also Fig. 66-72). Only a single hole on each side of the fracture should be drilled in the "compression mode." The compression screw, if it is used, must always be inserted first. In compression plates, if the drill is placed to the outside of the slot for the screw, a "compression" hole is formed, whereas if the hole is drilled toward the inside of the hole, the sliding plane of the hole is not used by the screw and the screw is considered a "neutral screw." The compression mode is activated only by drilling the hole at the outer margin of the drill hole in the plate. If the inner margin of the drill hole is used, the screw is placed in a neutral position and no compression force is delivered across the fracture site.

Drilling at the outer margin of the hole allows the screw to slip down an inclined plane toward the fracture as screw tightening occurs, and the screw and bone move as a unit toward the fracture site to achieve compression at the fracture site as the screw is tightened. This motion occurs because of the inclined plane in the screw holes of the plate (the so-called spherical

Text continued on p. 138

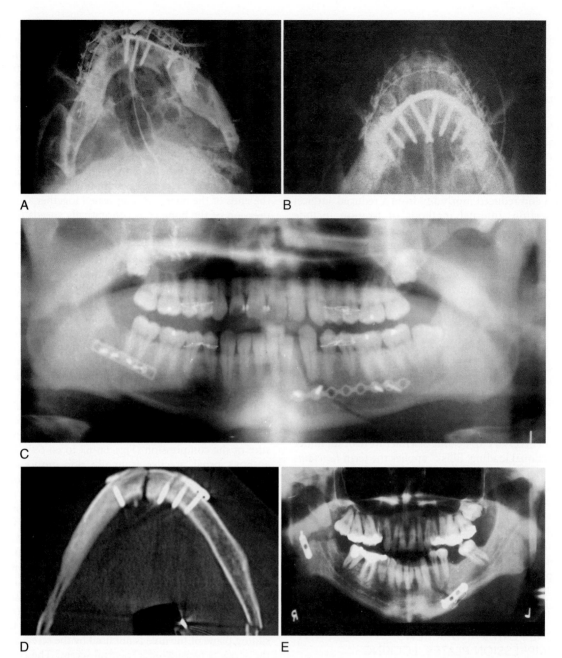

FIGURE 66-67. *A,* Malalignment of a distal body fracture is seen from a submental vertex view. This view, or a CT scan, is helpful in assessing alignment of the lingual cortex of the mandible after open reduction. Malalignment is likely to occur in intraoral open reductions, in which full visualization of the basal part of the mandible is difficult to obtain. *B,* Another fracture demonstrating correct alignment. Note the combination of plate, interosseous wiring, and intermaxillary fixation. The plate has sufficient holes and a length sufficient to prevent the mandibular angles from rotating outward. *C,* Panorex demonstrating poor alignment of a mandibular fracture after reduction. Small plates were used with screws in the fracture sites. The comminuted bone at the angle was unstable, as was the bone in the parasymphysis. *D,* Computed tomographic (CT) image of a symphysis in malalignment. A nontreated angle fracture is also malaligned. *E,* Small plates with too few screws result in nonunion and malocclusion.

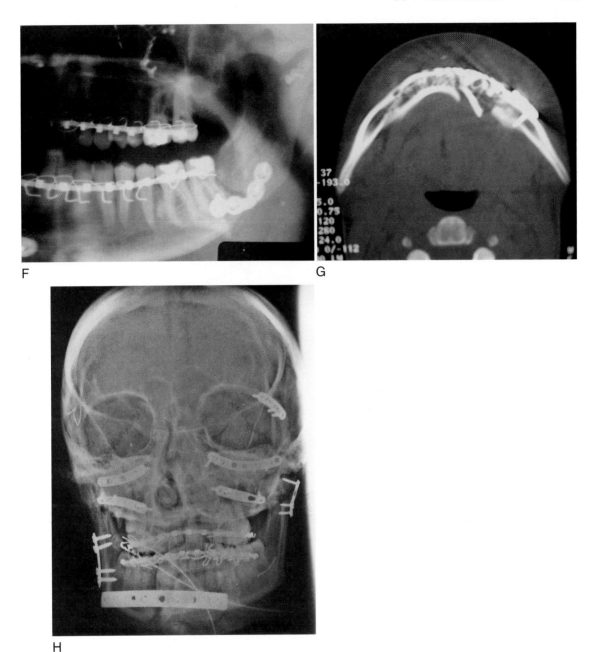

F

G

H

FIGURE 66-67, cont'd. *F,* Insufficient plate length results in instability. *G,* Comminution and use of a small plate result in widening of the mandible. *H,* Malocclusion and wide face result from a poor reduction.

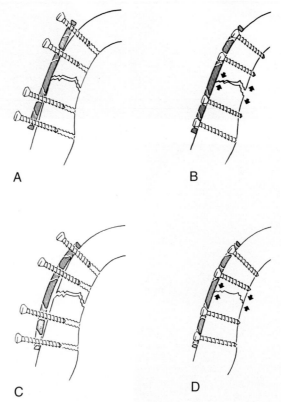

FIGURE 66-68. *A,* Incorrect internal fixation due to the use of a poorly adapted dynamic compression plate in the form of an insufficiently bent plate. *B,* After tightening of the screws, there is complete adaptation of the plate against the surface of the bone. This results in distraction of the fracture edges at the lingual cortex. Compression forces are acting only on the closest surface of the fractured area to the plate. *C,* Correct application of a dynamic compression plate, taking the curve or shape of the jaw into consideration. The plate is slightly overbent (2 mm) above the surface of the mandible. *D,* After tightening of the screws, the overbent plate produces compression of the entire fractured area and fracture alignment. (From Spiessl B: New Concepts in Maxillofacial Bone Surgery. New York, Springer-Verlag, 1976.)

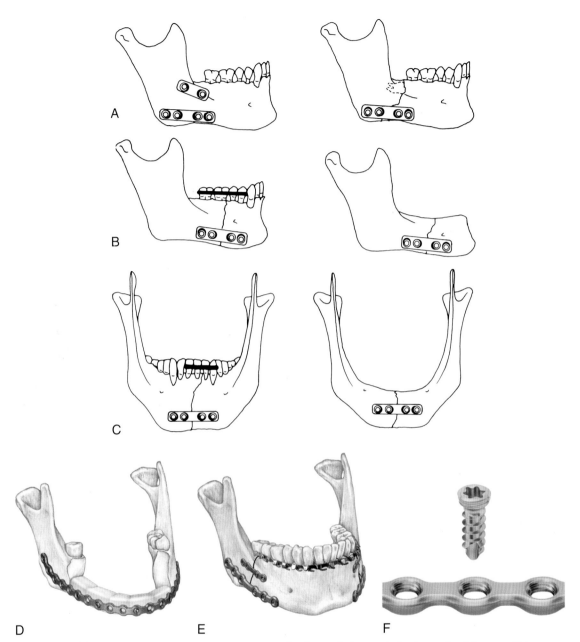

FIGURE 66-69. Indications for various different plate fixation techniques. *A,* At the angle of the mandible, a compression tension band plate and stabilization plate are used superiorly and inferiorly, respectively. *B,* In the area of the lateral dentulous mandible, a compression plate at the inferior border with an arch bar may be used. The arch bar functions as a tension band for the dentulous jaw. In an edentulous jaw or edentulous segment (and probably preferentially), a superior border plate should be placed in addition to the inferior border plate, even with an arch bar in place. *C,* In the area of the anterior teeth, a compression plate with an arch bar functioning as a tension band is satisfactory. However, in practice, it is almost always better to use an upper border unicortical plate and a lower border stabilization plate. Three holes should be used for each side of the fracture and an additional (fourth) hole added if a bone gap or comminuted fracture is present. *D* to *F,* Locking plate technology. (*A* to *C* from Spiessl B: New Concepts in Maxillofacial Bone Surgery. New York, Springer Verlag, 1976. *D* to *F* courtesy of Synthes Maxillofacial, Paoli, Pa.)

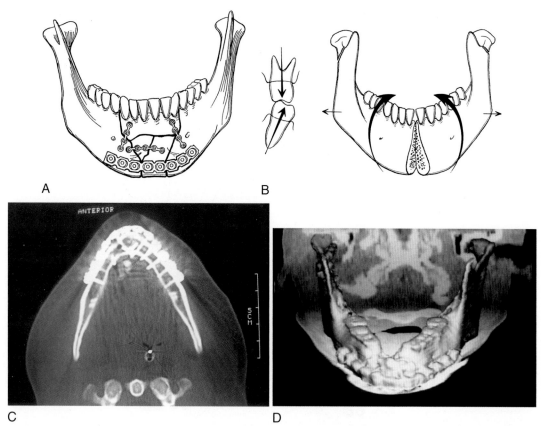

FIGURE 66-70. *A,* Smaller bone fragments should be coapted to the larger bone fragments first with small plates, then the larger bone segments may be stabilized with a reconstruction plate. *B,* Comminuted symphysis and subcondylar fractures tend to splay, rotating lingually in the lateral mandibular segments and thereby increasing the width of the mandible at the angle and subcondylar areas. *C,* A comminuted fracture of the symphysis is stabilized with a long (10- to 12-hole) plate. The length of this plate prevents lingual version (rotation) of the lateral mandibular segments and maintains the width of the mandible at the angle and subcondylar areas. The suprahyoid muscles were attached to a small bone fragment that was incorporated in the reduction. *D,* Three-dimensional CT scan (cut planes) of the reduction in *C.*

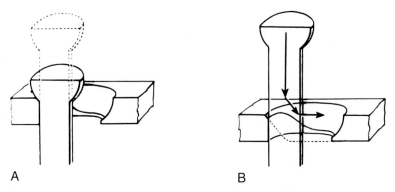

FIGURE 66-71. The spherical gliding principle in a dynamic compression plate. *A,* A spherically shaped screw head is caused to move down an inclined plane in a hole in a dynamic compression plate. When the spherical screw head is turned, it glides in the section of the inclined plane because of pressure of the screw against the plate. The bone segment, grasped by the screws, is thus moved horizontally (spherical gliding principle) toward the fracture gap. By the horizontal movement, a locking action between the screw and plate is avoided. The bone is compressed across the fracture site by this application of force. *B,* The path taken by the screw in the vertical and horizontal direction as it is tightened. (From Spiessl B: New Concepts in Maxillofacial Bone Surgery. New York, Springer-Verlag, 1976.)

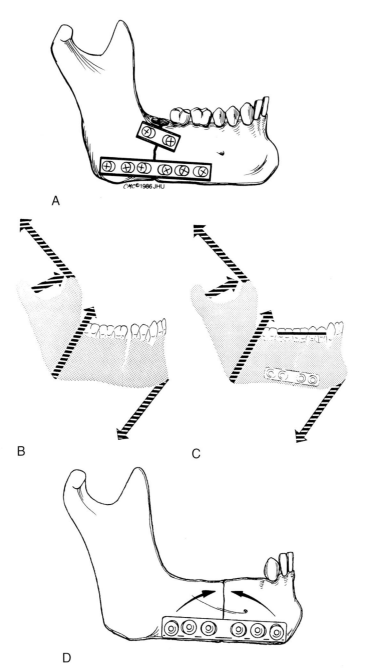

FIGURE 66-72. *A,* A body fracture is treated by the application of a dynamic compression plate at the inferior border. A small dynamic compression plate, which is placed unicortically at the upper border, acts as a tension band in this edentulous region. *B* and *C,* Muscle forces on a body fracture. The action of a tension band and a dynamic compression plate will resist these muscle forces. In *B,* the muscle forces are indicated by arrows, and they tend to open the fracture at the superior border. It is difficult for a single plate at the inferior border to entirely resist this action. In *C,* the fracture is closed and securely reduced by the tension band at the upper border (arch bar), and these forces would be further neutralized by use of a unicortical upper border plate. The dynamic compression plate at the inferior border provides considerable stability. *D,* Treatment of an edentulous body fracture with a long compression plate alone. (*B* and *C* from Spiessl B: New Concepts in Maxillofacial Bone Surgery. New York, Springer-Verlag, 1976.)

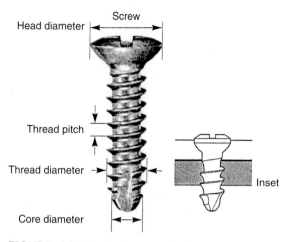

FIGURE 66-73. Basic screw design comparing the thread (major) and core diameters as well as the pitch (distance between the threads). A cutting "flute" is seen in the inferior end of the screw. The inset shows the relation of pitch and thickness of bone. At least two threads should engage in cortical bone to provide sufficient holding capacity. (From Assael LA: Craniofacial fractures. In Prein J, ed: Manual of Internal Fixation in the Craniofacial Skeleton: Techniques as Recommended by the AO/ASIF Group. New York, Springer-Verlag, 1997:120.)

gliding principle; see Fig. 66-71). As the screw is tightened, the screw-bone unit moves in a horizontal direction with vertical tightening of the screw. It is important that at least two screws be used for each main fragment to prevent rotation of the fragments. Only *one* screw on each side of the plate can be used in the compression mode, and *all* of the rest of the screws must be in the *neutral* position.

The most recent modification to plate design is the inclusion of plate threads that permit the screw head to lock into the plate to essentially form a single-piece implant. Locking plate and screw systems function as "internal-external fixators," achieving stability by locking the screw to the plate.[111,112] The potential advantage of these fixation devices is that precise adaptation of the plate to the underlying bone is not necessary. As the screws are tightened, they "lock" to the plate, thus stabilizing the segments without the need to compress the bone to the plate. This makes it impossible for the screw insertion to alter the reduction. This theoretically makes it less important to have good plate bending; other plates must be perfectly adapted to the contour of the bone. This hardware should be less susceptible to inflammatory complications from loosening as it is known that loose hardware propagates an inflammatory response and promotes infection.

A lag screw generally refers to a principle in fracture stabilization and not a special device. This technique achieves stability at a fracture interface by compressing the bone ends together. The technique uses an overdrilled hole in the first cortex of a fractured bone, with the drill hole diameter exceeding the major diameter of the screw. The second segment of the screw path is drilled to the minor diameter of the screw. Only the screw head will engage bone in the first section of the path, and therefore, as the screw is tightened into the second section of the fracture, the screw head impacts the cortex toward the fracture site as it is tightened. In general, two lag screws are recommended for each fracture to be stable, for if one becomes loose, the fracture would be unstable by virtue of the rotation (Fig. 66-74A). With only one screw, the fracture could still rotate around the single screw. A sleeve or drill guide is used to protect soft tissue (Fig. 66-74B). In screw placement, the angle between the bone and the direction of the screw should bisect a 90-degree angle from the bone in a plane parallel to the bone.

PRIMARY BONE GRAFTS

Primary bone grafting is routinely used to restore the integrity of orbital walls, midfacial buttresses, and nose and frontal bone areas. Bonanno and Converse,[113] in 1975, reported the use of primary bone grafting in the management of severely comminuted maxillary fractures. They thought that bone grafting maintained the projection of the fractured maxilla and the contour of the nose and established bone continuity in areas of severe comminution of the craniofacial skeleton. Thin onlay bone grafts (iliac, calvaria, or ribs) (Fig. 66-75) restored the contour and provided coverage of the bone gap. Gruss[114-118] and Manson[5,56,119,120] described these treatments in the acute management of midfacial fractures and popularized their use.

Areas in which primary bone grafting is applicable include the nasal skeleton; the frontal bone; the roof, floor, and medial and lateral walls of the orbit; the orbital rims; and the Le Fort I level. Primary bone grafting is usually not indicated in the mandible as there is a significant incidence of infection. Experience in the other areas of the face has shown that bone grafts are partially successful even though one surface of the bone graft may be lying totally exposed to a sinus cavity (such as bone grafts at the Le Fort I level over the maxillary sinus or in the orbital floor). The success of bone grafting depends on dependent drainage and surrounding well-vascularized soft tissue to provide adequate cover of most of the bone graft. It is obvious that when the soft tissue lining or cover has been destroyed, it must be restored before primary bone grafting can be successfully performed. The aesthetic results of primary bone grafting exceed those obtained with secondary bone grafting in most patients.

In severely comminuted midfacial fractures, after reduction and plate and screw fixation, bone grafting can be employed to increase stability if mobility is

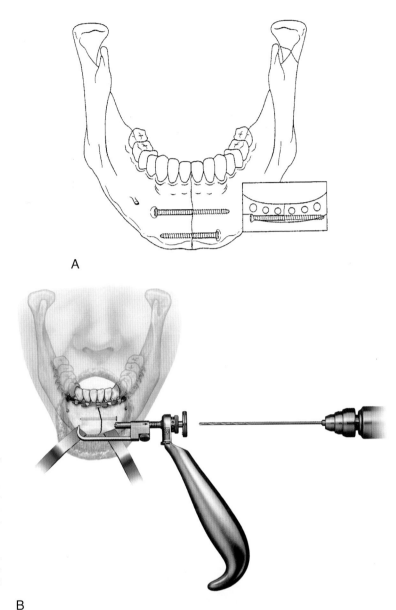

FIGURE 66-74. *A,* Placement of two horizontal lag screws to reduce and stabilize a parasymphysis fracture. *B,* Use of a percutaneous trocar for placement of screws in the angle region. (*A* from Assael LA: Mandibular fractures. In Prein J, ed: Manual of Internal Fixation in the Craniofacial Skeleton: Techniques as Recommended by the AO/ASIF Group. New York, Springer-Verlag, 1997:62. *B* courtesy of Synthes Maxillofacial, Paoli, Pa.)

present. The use of inlay bone grafts as buttresses can increase stability. These supporting bone grafts increase the adequacy of stabilization. Bone grafts provide buttress material to maintain the facial height and projection. They also fill structural voids, and additional bone graft may aid the healing potential and augment the strength of bone consolidation at the Le Fort I level, avoiding weeks of intermaxillary fixation. Restoration of the strength of critical maxillary buttresses may prevent secondary recession of the maxilla.

Bone grafting of the nasoethmoidal-orbital area restores the medial orbital walls and the orbital floors to prevent enophthalmos (Fig. 66-76). In conjunction with bone grafting of the nasal dorsum, the correction of traumatic telecanthus is improved. The indications for primary bone grafting are to replace critical structural support, such as missing portions of the buttresses, and to provide contour. Despite extensive soft tissue injury, bone grafting is a successful technique, provided the wounds can be surgically cleaned by débridement and irrigation. Proper soft tissue coverage of most of the bone graft should be ensured. Contraindications include infected or severely contaminated soft tissue wounds that cannot be properly cleaned, marginally viable soft tissue, and avulsive or

Text continued on p. 144

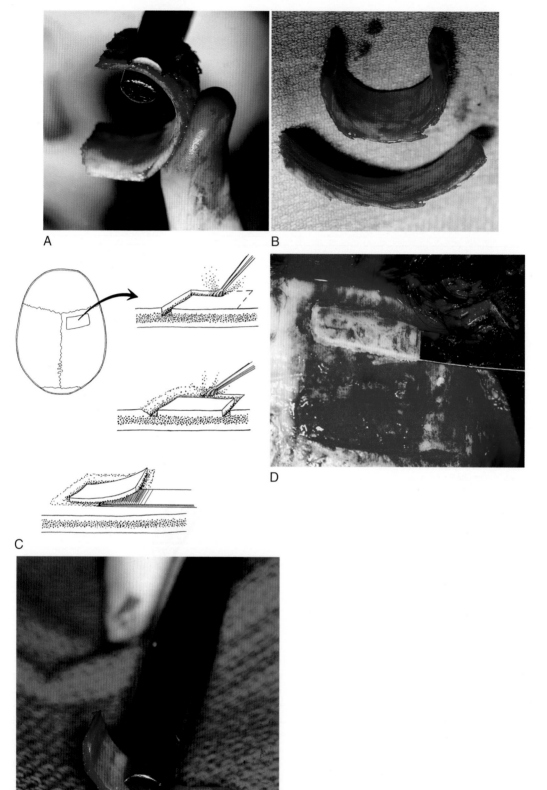

FIGURE 66-75. *A,* Rib grafts may be bent with a Tessier forceps. *B,* Curve of a rib graft for the anterior or posterior orbit. *C,* "Trough" cut for calvarial bone harvest and technique. *D,* Harvesting of strip calvarial grafts. *E,* Bending of brittle calvarial grafts must be performed carefully.

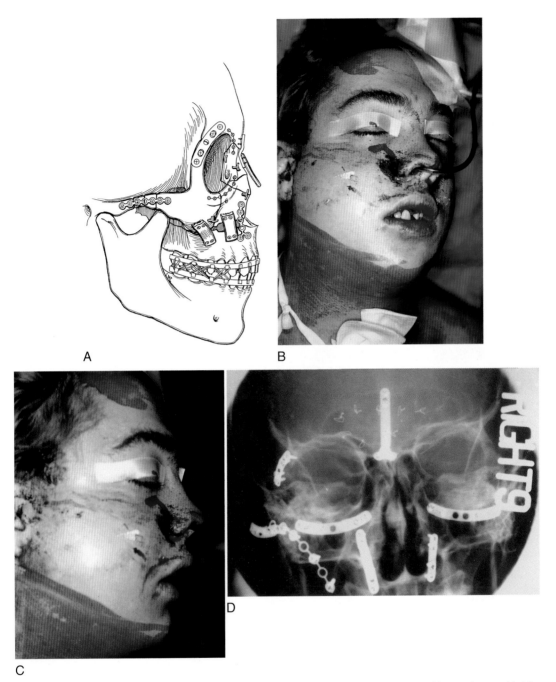

A

B

C

D

FIGURE 66-76. *A,* Fixation of central midface to the outer facial frame and the frontal bar to the nasal bridge with the 1.3 system. Fixation at the nasal bridge area with one 2.0 plate is another option. The vertical buttresses are stabilized with the 2.0 system or a bone graft. Intermaxillary fixation is maintained during fracture treatment and may be released postoperatively by employing the principles elaborated in the section on mandible fractures. *B* and *C,* Preoperative appearance of comminuted facial fractures involving the maxilla, nasoethmoid, and mandibular areas. *D,* Radiograph of fracture treatment. The high right condyle fracture was treated closed and the left, open. Limited intermaxillary fixation for 2 weeks was followed by nighttime elastic traction.

Continued

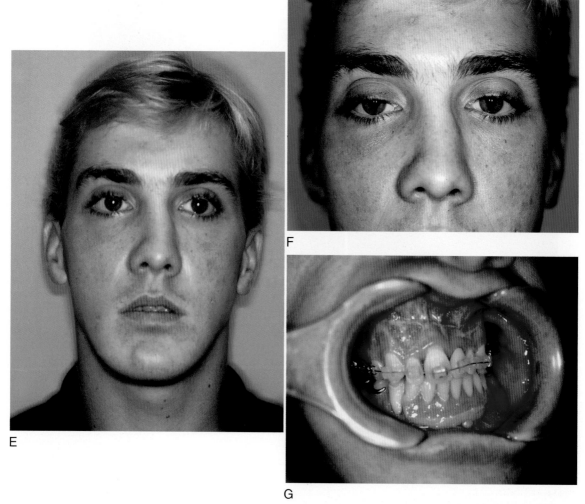

FIGURE 66-76, cont'd. *E,* Postoperative result of patient, frontal. *F,* Postoperative result, orbital. *G,* Occlusion.

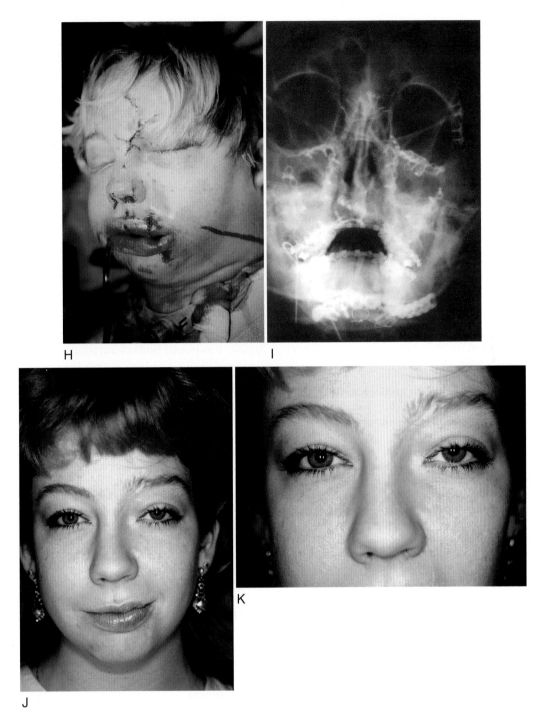

FIGURE 66-76, cont'd. *H,* Frontal, midface, and nasoethmoidal-orbital fractures. *I,* Another patient. *J* and *K,* Postoperative results. (*B* and *E* from Manson PN, Clark N, Robertson B, et al: Subunit principles in midface fracture treatment: the importance of sagittal buttresses, soft-tissue reductions, and sequencing treatment of segmental fractures. Plast Reconstr Surg 1999;103:1287.)

shotgun wounds where critical areas of lining or soft tissue cover are missing.

Bone grafts may be anchored either by plates or with lag (or "tandem") screws (Fig. 66-76). In the tandem screw technique, the first bone cortex is not overdrilled. Bone grafts may be secured to a buttress plate by using one of the plate holes at the desired location.

Rib

Rib grafts may be used whole or may be split for reconstruction of the calvaria, nose, internal orbit, and buttresses. Split ribs are prone to more resorption than calvaria, but they are easy to contour to curved shapes without fracture. They are perhaps the easiest material to contour to internal orbital shapes. The marrow may be curetted out of a split rib to make a very thin nasal onlay graft to provide a smooth contour.

Split rib grafts may be harvested in situ, leaving the posterior section intact to reduce postoperative pain, or they may be split with a Tessier osteotome on the instrument table. In harvesting of a rib, an incision is made down to the rib and through the periosteum. The periosteum is reflected with an Alexander periosteal elevator, and the periosteum is carefully reflected from the superior and inferior edges of the rib. The neurovascular bundle runs adjacent to the inferior edge of the rib, and the rib has a shallow groove on the posterior aspect of its inferior surface. Careful dissection is necessary to try to avoid injury to the neurovascular bundle. Moderate pain is common in the donor site for 6 weeks, and occasional chronic pain can be encountered that generally responds to nerve blocks. One may also apply alcohol blocks of this nerve by using 0.2 mL of absolute alcohol at three locations along the bundle.

For large bone requirements, multiple ribs are harvested, and the chest is stabilized by harvesting every other rib. On completion of the rib harvest, an inspection to exclude pleural tear should be conducted with direct-vision water seal. If it is torn, the pleura may be reclosed, or the chest cavity is placed on water seal

drainage with the chest tube in the superior aspect of the pneumothorax. An upright chest film is mandatory to exclude pneumothorax after rib harvest. Small pneumothoraces (>10%) may be treated with serial observation and chest radiograph.

Iliac

The iliac bone may be harvested for cortical bone for onlay or for its rich cancellous bone. The incision should be over the crest near the anterior superior iliac spine and placed in the relaxed lines of skin tension. The incision is deepened through the periosteum. Care should be taken to avoid the ilioinguinal, iliohypogastric and lateral femoral cutaneous nerves, which can be damaged if the dissection strays.[121-123]

The cortical lip of the crest may be included in the bone harvest, or it may be osteotomized and replaced to preserve contour. Alternatively, the inner lip of the crest only may be taken for a unicortical graft. If the whole thickness of the crest is obtained, a bicortical graft is possible with considerable thickness. If it is desired, only cancellous bone can be harvested for a use, such as frontal sinus obliteration.

Calvarial

Tessier popularized the calvarial bone graft as a donor site for adults.[124] Pensler and McCarthy[125] have specified the thickness of the calvaria in various regions (Table 66-4). Calvarial bone may be harvested full thickness and split on the instrument table with a portion replaced to the donor site, or a cranioplasty may be performed in the donor area. The most popular technique is harvest of split-thickness calvarial bone with osteotomy of the diploic layer, or a partial thickness of one cortex (after Kawamoto[126]) can be obtained with the periosteum attached for continuity.

For the split-thickness technique, a groove around the area of harvest is burred into the cortical bone to the level of the diploë. The peripheral margin of the groove is further beveled so that an osteotome may be placed in the diploic layer and used to section the

TABLE 66-4 ✦ COMPARISON OF RIGHT AND LEFT SIDES*

Variable	Number	Mean	SD	Median	Minimum	Maximum
Right side 1	200	6.80	1.04	6.80	3.50	10.00
Right side 2	200	7.03	1.06	7.01	3.50	10.25
Right side 3	200	7.45	1.03	7.38	4.25	11.25
Right side 4	200	7.72	1.07	7.60	4.00	12.00
Left side 1	200	6.86	0.99	6.89	3.75	10.25
Left side 2	200	7.03	1.05	7.00	3.75	10.25
Left side 3	200	7.46	1.09	7.49	3.00	11.50
Left side 4	200	7.72	1.11	7.55	4.00	12.00

* Measurements taken in 200 cadavers. Values given in millimeters. SD, Standard deviation.
From Pensler J, McCarthy JG: The calvarial donor site: an anatomic study in cadavers. Plast Reconstr Surg 1985;75:648.

external table from the skull. The area of the harvest can be divided by grooves to narrow the area of harvest and facilitate the proper level of cleavage being obtained. The "feel" and the sound of the tapping of the Tessier osteotome change when the osteotome tip is in cortical versus cancellous bone. The donor site can be left as a depression, or a cranioplasty can be performed with methyl methacrylate anchored to screws in the remaining internal table to achieve a smooth contour.

Calvarial bone has the greatest persistence of any bone donor material. It is avascular, brittle, and difficult to shape to curved defects. Its use in the elderly has been defined.[127]

Calvarial shavings may be harvested with a neurotome for uses such as frontal sinus obliteration.[128,129] Calvarial shavings may have less bone-forming potential than iliac cancellous bone.

COMPLICATIONS OF CALVARIAL BONE GRAFTS. Kline and Wolfe[130] reported findings on complications associated with harvesting of cranial bone grafts. They reported 13,000 bone grafts with 0.02% neurologic complications. Half of the complications were permanent and half were temporary. They recommended the technique of in situ bone graft harvesting, in which a pericranial flap is first raised from the area of the proposed graft and a 3- to 4-mm-wide graft is designed, usually in several pieces. They stress the importance of burring into the cortex on at least one side of the graft so that the proper angle of incidence may be established to allow the osteotome to cleave the skull in the diploic space. A curved osteotome is used to avoid damage to the inner table. The osteotome is carefully introduced into the diploic space and used to separate the inner and outer cortices. Considerable patience and many reapplications of the osteotome are sometimes necessary to safely achieve the desired split. Although the size of each individual graft is limited, as much bone as is needed can be obtained by sequential removal of adjacent strips. When a large piece is required, a neurosurgical approach with splitting after harvesting is performed. The harvested graft is split, and the inner or outer cortex can be used to reconstruct the donor site. The depression in the donor area can be left as is or grafted with alloplastic material (e.g., Norian), or a cranioplasty may be performed. The issue of strength of the remaining donor site bone requires some consideration and perhaps cranioplasty for protection. About half of the replaced bone would be expected to survive, which might make the donor area equal to one fourth of its original strength.

The prompt recognition and appropriate management of complications are essential. Inadvertent exposure of the dura during in situ harvesting is not considered a complication, but all areas of exposed dura should be covered with bone graft. Dural lacerations are dealt with by first extending the craniotomy beyond the limits of the tear.[131] A careful search is then made for underlying injury of the cerebral cortex. If injury is found, immediate neurosurgical consultation is indicated. If no injury is found, any bleeding from the dural edges is precisely controlled with bipolar cautery. Meticulous dural repair is then carried out with the addition of a pericranial patch if necessary. The repaired dura should be covered with bone graft. Bleeding from bone edges should be controlled with the judicious use of bone wax. Hemorrhage from dural or epidural vessels should be controlled with precise bipolar cautery and Gelfoam application. The commentary on this article by Paul Tessier describes his entire experience with cranial bone grafting and is essential reading for anyone harvesting calvarial bone grafts.

MANAGEMENT OF SPECIFIC FRACTURES OF THE CRANIOFACIAL SKELETON

Mandible

Any external force can fracture the mandible. Fractures may occur in the course of a difficult tooth extraction or during treatments such as electroshock therapy. They also may occur from weakness at areas of dental infection or in areas where metastatic tumors lodge in the mandible. The most common causes are automobile accidents, falls, fistfights, missile injuries, and sporting accidents. Fischer et al[132] looked at mandible fractures that were caused by motor vehicle collisions and found associated injuries in 99%. Facial and head lacerations and facial fractures were the leading associated injuries, occurring in more than half of the patients who had a mandible fracture. Closed head injury is the major life-threatening associated injury and cause of mortality.[133,134] Life-threatening injuries occurred in 64.8% of patients in this study. The mortality rate was 8.1%. These data suggest that a mandible fracture from a motor vehicle collision should never be viewed as an isolated injury but rather as part of a spectrum of significant and sometimes life-threatening injuries that require trauma evaluation at the time of presentation.

Direct trauma indicates that a force at the site of the fracture has resulted in discontinuity of the bone. A blow to the opposite side of the jaw or at a distance from the fracture site may produce a fracture in the contralateral portion of the mandible in a weak area. This type of injury is seen in fractures of the condyle or subcondylar area, which frequently follow a blow on the chin on the contralateral side. A blow on the symphysis may result in a fracture of both mandibular condyles and no fracture of the symphysis. A fracture of the left body, the result of a direct blow, may be accompanied by a contralateral fracture of the right subcondylar area or angle. Less commonly, a fracture of the right parasymphysis area may be accompanied by a left angle fracture. In practice, more mandibular fractures are bilateral than unilateral, especially after the forces experienced in automobile accidents. There is a saying that "like a LifeSaver," the mandible cannot be broken in only one spot."

ANATOMY

The prominence, position, and anatomic configuration of the mandible are such that it is one of the most frequently injured facial bones, like the nose and zygoma.[11] After automobile accidents, the mandible is the most commonly encountered fracture at many major trauma centers. The mandible is a movable, predominantly U-shaped bone consisting of horizontal and vertical segments. The horizontal segment consists of the body on each side and the symphysis area centrally. The vertical segments consist of the angles and the rami, which articulate with the skull through the condyles and temporomandibular joints. The mandible is attached to other facial bones by a complex system of muscles and ligaments. The mandible articulates with the maxilla through the occlusion of the teeth.

The mandible is a strong bone but has several areas of weakness that are prone to fracture. The body of the mandible is composed principally of dense cortical bone with a small substantial spongiosa through which blood vessels, lymphatic vessels, and nerves pass. The mandible is thin at the angles where the body joins with the ramus and can be further weakened by the presence of an unerupted third molar in this area or by a previous dental extraction.[135] The mandible is also weak at the neck of the condyle, at the root of the cuspid tooth (which has the longest root), and at the mental foramen, through which the mental nerve and vessels extend into the soft tissue of the lateral aspect of the lower lip. Foramina and deeply rooted teeth weaken areas of bone. Fractures often traverse the mandible adjacent to the mental foramen. The weak areas for fractures of the dentulous mandible are the subcondylar area, the angle and distal body areas, and the mental foramen.[136-138]

With a loss of teeth from the mandible, atrophic changes occur in the alveolar bone and alter the structural characteristics of the mandible. Fractures then often occur in the partially dentulous mandible through the edentulous areas (proximal body) rather than through the areas better supported by adequate tooth and alveolar bone structures.[137,138]

Mandibular movements are determined by the action of reciprocally placed muscles attached to the bone. When fractures occur, displacement of the segments is influenced by the pull of the muscles attaching to the segments. The direction of the fracture line may oppose forces exerted by these muscles.

Muscle function is an important variable influencing the degree and direction of displacement of fractured mandibular segments. Overcoming the forces of displacement is also important in reduction and fixation of mandibular fragments.[139,140]

The posterior group of muscles are commonly referred to as the muscles of mastication. The muscles are short, thick, and capable of exerting extremely strong forces on the mandible. The muscles of mastication are the temporalis, the masseter, and the medial (internal) and lateral (external) pterygoid muscles. The overall activity of this group is to move the mandible in a general upward, forward, and medial direction (Fig. 66-77).

The masseter muscle is a thick, short, powerful, heavy muscle attached to the inferior portion of the zygomatic eminence and the zygomatic arch. It arises from tendinous fibers on the inferior two thirds of the lower border of the zygomatic bone and from the medial surfaces of the zygomatic arch; it inserts onto the lateral surface of the ramus and densely onto the bone along the inferior border of the mandible at the region of the angle. The masseter muscle is an elevator of the jaw and functions to pull the mandible upward and forward.

The temporalis muscle arises from the limits of the temporal fossa. It is a broad, fan-shaped muscle whose fibers converge to descend under the zygomatic arch and insert on the coronoid process, the lateral and medial surfaces of the coronoid, and the anterior surface of the ramus as far down as the occlusal plane of the third molar tooth. The anterior fibers are elevators and the posterior fibers are retractors of the mandible.

The medial pterygoid muscle originates in the pterygoid fossa, mainly from the medial surface of the lateral pterygoid process, and from the pyramidal process of the palatine bone and maxillary tuberosity. It inserts on the medial surface of the ramus and angle of the mandible. The fibers of the medial pterygoid muscle pass in a downward, posterior, and lateral direction to the angle of the mandible. The function of the medial pterygoid muscle is upward, medial, and forward traction on the mandible.

The lateral pterygoid muscle has two heads of origin. The upper head arises from the infratemporal crest, the infratemporal surface of the greater wing of the sphenoid bone, and a small area of the squamous part of the temporal bone. The lower head arises from the lateral surface of the lateral pterygoid plate. The upper head inserts into the capsule of the temporomandibular joint and into the articular disk of the temporomandibular joint (Fig. 66-78). The lower head inserts onto the anterior surface of the neck of the condyle. The innermost or upper portion pulls the mandible upward, medially, and forward; the external portion

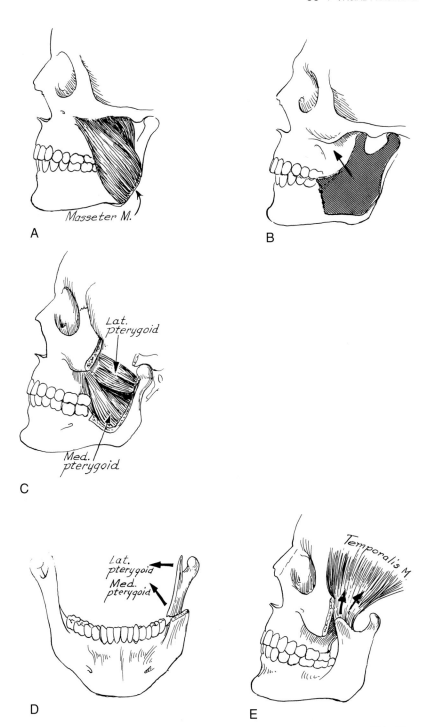

FIGURE 66-77. The posterior group of muscles attached to the mandible. The overall force from the activity of this group of muscles results in movement of the mandible upward, forward, medially, or laterally. *A,* The masseter muscle. *B,* Upward displacement in a fractured mandible produced by the pull of the masseter muscle on the edentulous proximal fragment. *C,* The medial and lateral pterygoid muscles. *D,* Directional pull of the medial and lateral pterygoid muscles. *E,* The temporalis muscle and the direction of pull. (From Kazanjian VH, Converse J: Surgical Treatment of Facial Injuries, 3rd ed. Baltimore, Williams & Wilkins, 1974.)

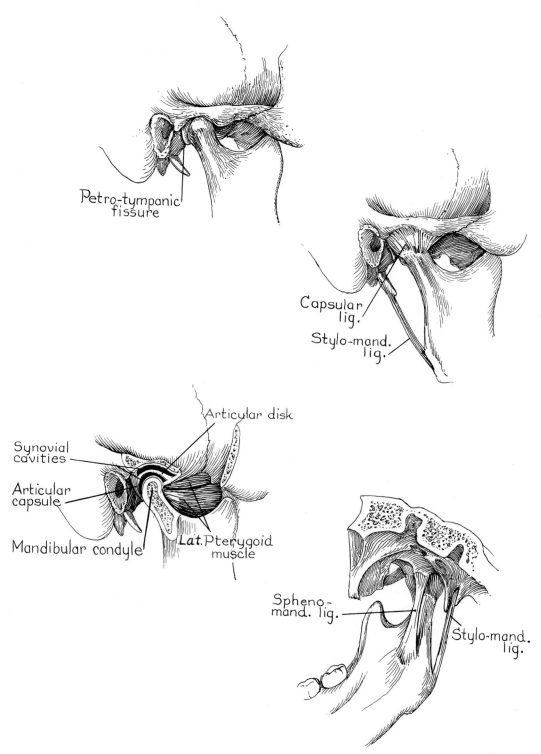

FIGURE 66-78. The temporomandibular joint and its associated ligaments. (From Kazanjian VH, Converse J: Surgical Treatment of Facial Injuries, 3rd ed. Baltimore, Williams & Wilkins, 1974.)

pulls the condyle downward, medially, and forward. Simultaneous contraction of the muscle segments on one side pulls the mandible to the opposite side. Simultaneous contraction of both lateral pterygoid muscles protrudes the mandible.

The anterior or depressor group of mandibular muscles are considered the opening muscles of the mandible (Fig. 66-79). With the hyoid bone fixed, they depress the mandible. When the mandible is fractured, they displace the fracture segments downward, posteriorly, and medially. This group is made up of the geniohyoid, genioglossus, mylohyoid, and digastric muscles. The geniohyoid muscle arises on the inferior medial spine of the mandible and passes downward

and posteriorly to insert on the body of the hyoid bone. Its function is to elevate the hyoid and to depress the mandible. The genioglossus muscle, the main muscle of the tongue, is attached to the genial tubercles on the inferior surface of the anterior mandible. Its fibers pass primarily into the substance of the tongue and into the upper surface of the hyoid bone. Its function is to protrude the tongue, elevate the hyoid, and depress the mandible. The mylohyoid muscle is a fan-shaped muscle that acts as a diaphragm for support of the floor of the mouth. It arises from the mylohyoid line on the inner surface of the body of the mandible. Its fibers pass medially to insert into a median raphe and posteriorly to insert onto the hyoid bone. Its function

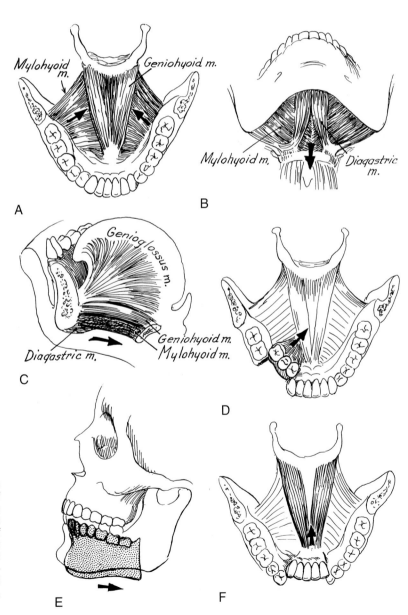

FIGURE 66-79. *A* to *F,* The anterior or depressor group of muscles of mastication, the suprahyoid muscles. The arrows indicate the direction and pull of the displacement of the fragments in fractures of the mandible. (From Kazanjian VH, Converse J: Surgical Treatment of Facial Injuries, 3rd ed. Baltimore, Williams & Wilkins, 1974.)

is to elevate the hyoid bone and to depress the mandible. Its fibers pull medially, posteriorly, and downward. The digastric muscle arises from the digastric fossa at the inferior medial portion of the mandible bilaterally and extends posteriorly to pass beneath the fiber sling attached near the lesser cornus of the hyoid bone. Its tendon is continuous with that of the posterior portion, which originates from the digastric fossa on the temporal bone. The function of this muscle is to elevate the hyoid and to depress the anterior portion of the mandible.

The lingual nerve was found to be in an "unsafe" position in relation to some angle fracture procedures. Behnia et al[141] have diagrammed the location and pathways of the nerve (Fig. 66-80 and Table 66-5).

CLASSIFICATION

Mandibular fractures are classified according to the location, the condition of the teeth, the direction of the fracture and its favorability for treatment, the presence of a compound injury through the skin or through the mucosa, and the characterization of the anatomic area and fracture pattern (Fig. 66-81). Dingman and Natvig[142] classified mandibular fractures by anatomic location (Fig. 66-81B). Alternatively, the fracture pattern and presence of an open wound may be further used in classification.

The direction and extent of displacement of the fragments depend on the site of the fracture, the direction of the fracture, the direction of pull of the muscles attached to the mandible, the direction and intensity of displacement forces, the presence of overlying muscle, and the presence or absence of teeth in the fragments. In fractures of the mandible, the segments may be displaced in the direction of the strongest muscle action.

Fry et al[143] pointed out that fractures may be "favorable" or "unfavorable" for displacement according to their direction and bevel. The muscle forces on some fracture fragments are opposed by the direction and bevel of the fracture line. Thus, in some fractures, the muscle force would pull the fragments into a position favorable for healing, whereas in other fractures, the muscle pull is unfavorable and separation of the frac-

ture fragments occurs by action of the muscle forces (Fig. 66-82). Mandibular fractures that are directed downward and forward are classified as *horizontally favorable* because the posterior group of muscles and the anterior group of muscles pull in antagonistic directions, favoring stability at the site of the fracture. Fractures running from above, downward, and posteriorly are classified as *horizontally unfavorable*. The bevel of the fracture may also influence a displacement medially. If a fracture runs from posteriorly forward and medially, displacement would take place in a medial direction because of the medial pull of the elevator muscles of mastication *(vertically unfavorable)*. The fracture that passes from the lateral surface of the mandible posteriorly and medially is a favorable fracture because the muscle pull tends to prevent displacement. It is called a *vertically favorable* fracture (Fig. 66-82).

DIAGNOSIS

Clinical Examination

Fractures occurring along the course of the inferior alveolar nerve may produce numbness in the distribution of the nerve, which represents the ipsilateral lower lip (mental nerve), and numbness of the ipsilateral teeth. There is usually exquisite tenderness over the site of the fracture. Excessive saliva is often produced as a result of local irritation (drooling). Small lacerations of the gingiva and mucosa or gaps between the mucosa and the gingiva attached to the teeth indicate the possibility of a fracture with displacement. These gaps make the fracture compound into the mouth. Loose or missing teeth may indicate the site of a fracture. A gap may be the result of slight fracture or dental displacement and permit contamination and the initial development of an infection. The jaw may deviate to one side, or there may be an abnormal contour to the jaw line. An open bite deformity, for example, may be present, a finding that indicates that the patient cannot bring the teeth into proper occlusion in the anterior or lateral portion of the dentition. The mandible may be shifted to one side or the other (crossbite) or, in bilateral fractures, may be dislocated posteriorly, giving a bizarre retruded appearance to the

TABLE 66-5 ✦ VERTICAL AND HORIZONTAL DISTANCES OF THE LINGUAL NERVE FROM THE LINGUAL CREST AND THE LINGUAL PLATE OF THE MANDIBLE

	Mean Distance (mm)	Minimum Distance (mm)	Maximum Distance (mm)	Standard Deviation (mm)
Horizontal	2.06	0.00	3.20	±1.10
Vertical	3.01	1.70	4.00	±0.42

From Behnia H, Kheradvar A, Shahrokhi M: An anatomic study of the lingual nerve in the third molar region. J Oral Maxillofac Surg 2000;58:649.

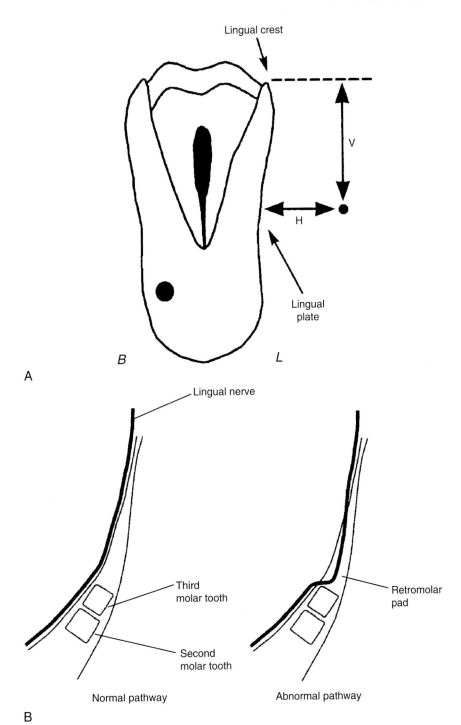

FIGURE 66-80. *A,* Coronal sections through the third molar region showing methods of measurement. V, vertical distance from lingual crest; H, horizontal distance from the lingual plate; B, buccal; L, lingual. *B,* Irregular pathway of the lingual nerve alongside the mandibular molar teeth in comparison with normal pathway (occlusal view). (From Behnia H, Kheradvar A, Shahrokhi M: An anatomical study of the lingual nerve in the third molar region. J Oral Maxillofac Surg 2000;58:649.)

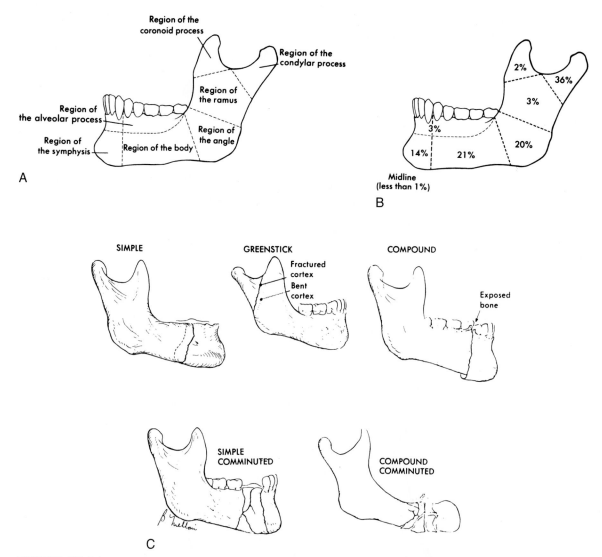

FIGURE 66-81. *A,* The regions of the mandible. *B,* The percentage of fractures occurring within each region. *C,* Types of mandibular fractures. (*A* and *B* from Dingman RO, Natvig P: Surgery of Facial Fractures. Philadelphia, WB Saunders, 1964. *C* from Kruger GO: Textbook of Oral Maxillofacial Surgery, 6th ed. St. Louis, CV Mosby, 1984.)

whole lower facial area. After a day or two, debris often accumulates in an intraoral laceration with food, blood clots, and devitalized tissue undergoing bacterial putrefaction, giving rise to an offensive breath (fetor oris).

Bimanual manipulation of the mandible is useful to determine the degree of instability and mobility at the site of the fracture. One hand should stabilize the ramus while the other manipulates the symphysis or the body area. The fracture will be demonstrated by abnormal movement. The mandible may be pulled forward with one hand while the other hand is placed with one finger in the ear canal and one finger over the condylar process (see Fig. 66-11). Abnormal mobil-

ity or crepitus indicates a fracture in the condylar-sub-condylar area or ligament laxity, indicating a temporomandibular joint injury. The most reliable finding in fractures of the mandible, in dentulous patients, is malocclusion. Often, the most minute dislocation caused by the fracture is obvious to the patient, as the teeth do not mesh or come together in the proper occlusal relationship.

Upper displacement of the posterior segment is prevented by occlusal contact of the lower teeth against the upper teeth. The elevator muscles of the mandible pull the posterior segment forward. The anterior group of muscles depresses the anterior segments of the mandible, separating the teeth anterior to the fracture

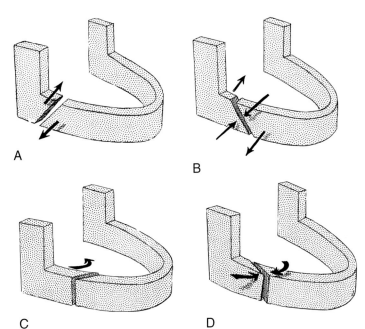

FIGURE 66-82. In *A* and *C,* the direction and bevel of the fracture line did not resist displacement due to muscle action. The arrows indicate the direction of muscle pull. In *B* and *D,* the bevel and direction of the fracture line resist displacement and oppose muscle action. The direction of the muscle pull in fractures beveled in this direction would tend to impact the fractured bone ends. (After Fry WK, Shepherd PR, McLeod AC, Parfitt GJ: The Dental Treatment of Maxillofacial Injuries. Oxford, Blackwell Scientific, 1942.)

from the upper teeth. A single tooth in the posterior fragment may be extremely important and should be retained; the tooth acts as an occlusal stop and provides some stability for fracture alignment (Fig. 66-83).[144,145]

Damage of the anterior teeth occurs more often than damage of the posterior teeth because of their forward position and single conical root structure. Teeth may be completely avulsed from the bone or may fracture at the gingival line, with the roots remaining in the bone, or segments of the alveolar bone may be fractured, with the teeth remaining firmly attached or dislocated. The fracture line may traverse the tooth at any level. The fracture line may parallel the border of the

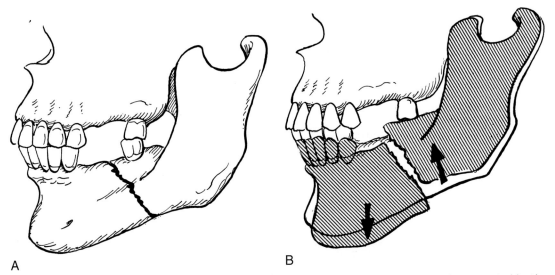

FIGURE 66-83. *A,* Upward displacement of the posterior segment of the mandible can be prevented by the presence of a tooth on the posterior fragment occluding against a maxillary tooth. *B,* When these teeth are not present, displacement of the posterior fragment occurs because of the absence of the occluding teeth. A dental splint with an occlusal stop segment substituting for the distance of the missing occluding teeth would prevent this displacement; however, an open reduction with plate and screw fixation is preferred.

tooth, or if a fracture of the crown or edges of the tooth occurs, the dental pulp may be exposed.

Radiographic Examination

Radiographic examination is imperative for confirmation. One study has indicated that in up to 10% of patients, the clinical examination is responsible for the diagnosis of a fracture that cannot be fully supported by radiographs obtained at the time of the injury. Thus, the patient should be treated for a fracture if there is sufficient clinical indication. A careful radiologic examination should be performed in all suspected fractures with particular attention to the condyle and subcondylar area (see Figs. 66-28 to 66-38). Plain films are less useful at present because of the superiority of CT scans taken in the axial and coronal planes (see Figs. 66-40 to 66-42). The panoramic radiograph (Panorex) (see Figs. 66-38 and 66-39) is still helpful but may be difficult to obtain in patients with multiple trauma who cannot be transported to a dental unit. It may also blur fractures in the midline. Specialized examinations, such as occlusal films, palatal films, and apical views of the teeth, are helpful in detecting alveolar fractures and in analyzing the degree of tooth injury (see Figs. 66-28 to 66-30).

TREATMENT

The primary consideration in the management of fractures of the mandible is to restore the function and efficiency of the jaws and the occlusion of the dentition. Conceptually, mandibular fracture treatment requires establishment of occlusion (intermaxillary fixation) and then upper or lower border fracture fixation of the bone (usually rigid fixation). Either intermaxillary fixation or (rarely) both intermaxillary fixation and rigid fixation may not be necessary, depending on the characteristics and completeness of the fracture. However, most commonly, both will be required. Usually, the simplest treatment that will obtain and satisfy these requirements is chosen. The methods of fixation may vary with the age and the general health of the patient, the training of the surgeon, the facilities and circumstances available for treatment, and the conditions under which the patient is to be treated. A satisfactory end result may be accomplished by the use of any one of a number of methods. No method is without its specific requirements and approaches and, of course, advantages, disadvantages, cost, and particular complications.

Laskin[146] has reported variations and current trends in the treatment of maxillofacial injuries in the United States. He found that there is a wide variation in treatment of fractures, with arch bars and maxillomandibular fixation alone being a popular treatment for simple mandible fractures. Lower border wiring and closed treatment of Le Fort I fractures are also

common. He found that rigid internal fixation is accompanied by maxillomandibular fixation postoperatively in more than 50% of patients for 1 to 2 weeks, in 30% for several days, and in 10% for several hours. Only 10% of practitioners used no maxillomandibular fixation postoperatively. There is a wide variation in methods and types of treatment for open reduction, with rigid fixation slowly gaining popularity. Laskin documented increasing use of rigid fixation in the treatment of mandible fractures, largely conservative condylar fracture treatment, and persistent use of splints and arch bars. Schmidt et al,[147] in 2000, documented that closed reduction with maxillomandibular fixation is considerably less expensive, considering all factors in a financial analysis, than rigid internal fixation for the treatment of mandibular fractures.

Intravenous administration of antibiotics at the time of the surgery is recommended.[148-151] Antibiotics are especially helpful in patients undergoing delayed treatment, patients having long operations, patients with severely contused soft tissue when the fracture treatment is delayed and the tissues are heavily contaminated, and patients with multiple intraoral lacerations. Administration of antibiotics is also indicated in patients who are medically compromised, who are diabetic, who have poor nutritional status, or who have systemic illness or local conditions of poor dental hygiene or periodontal or dental infections.

Abubaker and Rollert[152] published a study in 2001 in which they were not able to discern a benefit of postoperative oral antibiotics in uncomplicated fractures of the mandible. They conducted a prospective randomized double-blind study. Their criteria for infection included purulent drainage from the fracture site, increased facial swelling beyond postoperative day 7, fistula formation at the surgical site or fracture with evidence of drainage, and fever associated with local evidence of infection (swelling, erythema, and tenderness). Fractures whose treatment is delayed have an increased risk of potential infection. In these patients, without use of prophylactic antibiotics, wound infection ranges from 22% to 50%. Many studies have indicated that the risk of infection should be as low as 10% with the use of prophylactic antibiotics. In mandible fractures treated by experienced practitioners, the incidence of infection should be as low as 5% or 7%. In other studies, it has been difficult to prove that prophylactic antibiotics in otolaryngologic surgery or elective oral and maxillofacial surgery are of value. Chole and Yee[151] concluded that antibiotic prophylaxis is of value only in certain procedures. However, they noted that the majority of the studies they surveyed were retrospective and the criteria used for diagnosis of an infection were subjective. They reduced the incidence of infection from 42% to 8.9% in compound mandibular fractures by antibiotic use in facial fractures. Angle fractures have the most significant risk for infection, and body fractures are second in frequency. Zallen[150] recommended preoperative, intraoperative, and postoperative antibiotics for 5 days. The antibiotic agent should be appropriate against aerobic and anaerobic oral flora. Antibiotics, however, are *never* a replacement for proper surgical technique, including débridement of devitalized tissue, removal of any soft tissue in the fracture, stabilization (immobility) of the fracture, and proper closure of the soft tissue over the repaired fracture with the liberal use of a dependent drain.

Reimplantation of avulsed teeth may be successful if it is prompt; it is reportedly more appropriate in children. Presumably, the open structure of the root apex in children allows a more successful re-establishment of blood supply. Reimplantation is most successful if the tooth is reimplanted within $1/2$ to 1 hour and if the tooth is firmly supported after reimplantation by splinting. In adults, the pulp is occasionally removed and the canal filled and treated before the tooth is reimplanted. Such teeth "ankylose" to the alveolar bone. If the crown of the tooth has been fractured with exposure of the dental pulp, it may be advisable to protect the pulp in some way at the time of establishing intermaxillary fixation. If this is not done, infection and severe pain may be troublesome. If segments of the alveolus contain teeth that have been fractured and have adequate blood supply by virtue of the soft tissue attachments, attempts should be made to replace the segments along with their contained teeth and to hold them securely into position with interdental wires, a splint, orthodontic bands, or small plates and screws. The arch bar and dental ligatures assist positioning of the dental segment. Most of these tooth-bearing segments survive and produce a satisfactory masticatory surface. One presumes that some teeth in

this segment will ultimately need root canal therapy, and care should be taken not to unnecessarily strip surrounding soft tissues, which further devascularizes the segment.

Even completely avulsed bone may be replaced if it is stabilized and covered with mucosa. Injury to the teeth without avulsion or fracture may result in devitalization from hemorrhage into the dental pulp. The teeth become insensitive and discolored as a result of infiltration of the blood pigments into the tooth structure. If infection occurs, the teeth must be treated, the infection drained, and the tooth extracted. Some teeth (even though discolored and nonvital) remain asymptomatic and useful teeth. As mentioned, teeth in the line of fracture should be retained if they offer any degree of stability of the bone fragments and if they have solid attachments. It is important that loose teeth with extensive periodontal disease be considered for removal and that steps are taken to prevent infection, such as administration of antibiotics. Antibiotic therapy protects against infection; some studies have demonstrated a twofold advantage if antibiotics are employed when teeth are involved in the fracture, but others have not. If teeth are loose or interfere with reduction, they should be removed. In general, third molars in a fracture line are removed if an open reduction is required and the tooth is blocking reduction of the fracture. If the fracture would otherwise be amenable to closed reduction, the tooth may be left, employing antibiotic therapy until healing has occurred, and the third molar can then be removed (Fig. 66-84). The removal of a third molar tooth from a fracture of the angle, which would otherwise be treated with a closed reduction, often precipitates a need for an open reduction, and the increased soft tissue stripping and trauma often increase the chance of infection.

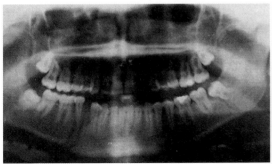
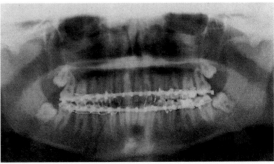

A   B

FIGURE 66-84. *A,* The fracture of the right body and left angle of the mandible. *B,* The fracture was treated by closed reduction and immobilization. The third molar in the left angle fracture, partially erupted, was extracted after healing. Extraction of the molar at the time of closed reduction would surely have precipitated the need for an open reduction. Although this fracture was treated with a closed reduction, the success depends on periosteal continuity, and in retrospect, the fracture was probably better treated by open reduction with more certainty of success.

After the mandibular fracture is healed and the patient has opened the mouth sufficiently, the teeth should be given the necessary cleaning and attention by the patient's dentist. Apical views of the teeth and sensory stimulation studies detect apical disease or devitalization. Such teeth must be carefully observed for periapical abscesses, and they may require root canal treatment. A typical Jaw Fracture Protocol, such as that of John Doyle, DDS, at the University of Wisconsin, is helpful for coordinating care in the postoperative period (Table 66-6).

Closed Reduction and Intermaxillary Fixation

If intermaxillary fixation alone is to be used for treatment, that period of fixation should constitute 4 to 6

weeks,[144,153-155] with the emphasis on 6 weeks. During 4 to 6 weeks of intermaxillary fixation, the average patient loses 15 to 20 pounds.[136] Weight loss may be minimized by appropriate dietary counseling, including the use of nutritional and vitamin supplements, which are important to ensure proper nutrition. Books have been published that emphasize cooking techniques, the use of liquid diets, and dietary supplements.[156] This technique is most efficacious in dentate compliant patients with minimally displaced fractures.

Open Reduction and Internal Fixation

Indications for osteosynthesis include patients who desire to minimize intermaxillary fixation, medically compromised patients, uncooperative patients,

TABLE 66-6 ✦ JAW FRACTURE PROTOCOL, JOHN DOYLE, DDS

Diagnosis	*Treatment of Condylar Fractures*

Mandibular condyle fracture
Mandibular subcondylar fracture
Mandibular body fracture
	Closed reduction and immobilization
	  Immobilized until bone union—up to 6 weeks
	  Risk of fibroankylosis with increased length of
	    immobilization
	Immobilization without reduction and active range of
	  motion
	  Brief period of immobilization (1-3 weeks)
	  Obtain bone union of condyle in new relationship to
	    glenoid fossa
	  Post-fixation function and therapy produce
	    neuromuscular adaptation to restore activity of
	    joint, teeth, and muscles
	Active range of motion/active therapy as single modality
	  Elimination of immobilization phase, initiating active
	    therapy immediately
	  Indications:
	    When risk of immobilization is high (i.e.,
	      intracapsular fracture)
	    Fracture in child
	    Patient with epilepsy
	    Uncooperative patient
	Open reduction and immobilization
	  Means of restoring preinjury position of fractured
	    segments in a precise way
	  Indications:
	    See Kaplan AS, Assael LA: Temporomandibular
	      Disorders: Diagnosis and Treatment.
	      Philadelphia, WB Saunders, 1991:232.
	    May be delayed—decision to perform open
	      reduction should be made in 3 weeks; success
	      rates decrease after this time

Patient-Related Problems	
Hypomobility Possible scarring Decreased functional tolerance Post-condylar fracture syndrome Soft tissue and muscle spasm Decreased joint mobility	
Acute Clinical Findings	

Tenderness over site of injury exacerbated by
  movement and palpation
Swelling
Crepitation
Interfragmentary mobility
Muscle spasm
Mandible may be deviated to side of injury at rest
Ipsilateral occlusal prematurity when maximum
  intercuspation is attempted
Decreased lateral excursion to contralateral side
Post–condylar fracture syndrome: Late functional
  occlusal findings vary, depending on type of
  injury and therapeutic intervention employed
  Adaptations to restore function after injury
  Deviation of mandible to side of injury
  Short ramus on side of injury
  Decreased translation of injured condyle
  Canting of occlusal plane and other dental
    adaptations
  Loss of condylar guidance with lateral excursion away
    from side of injury
  Functional occlusal abnormalities
  Muscle adaptation, atrophy, and shortening
  Internal derangement of injured temporomandibular
    joint
  Growth and developmental abnormalities
	Condylar Fracture in Growing Child

	Usually follows fall on chin Rarely discovered Late findings of ankylosis or growth disturbance Condylar fractures have greatest propensity to produce growth disturbance Unilateral fracture—no immobilization with active therapy Bilateral fracture—brief immobilization with guiding elastics

TABLE 66-6 ◆ JAW FRACTURE PROTOCOL, JOHN DOYLE, DDS—cont'd

THERAPEUTIC INTERVENTION

Time Frame	Intervention	Goals
1-3 weeks; see in clinic with dentist or physician	In fixation Liquid diet Icing	Stabilization and joint protection Treatment of inflammation and pain
3-4 weeks; see in clinic with dentist or physician	Removal of elastics Evaluation of opening pattern Home exercise program: controlled rotation with manual and visual cues to increase symmetry; use of guiding elastics if necessary	Active range of motion to prevent ankylosis Symmetric opening pattern
4-5 weeks	Removal of arch bars	Symmetric vertical opening

1-2 times per week as determined by therapist	Evaluation: opening pattern, range of motion, joint mobility, soft tissue and scars
	Treatment
	  Diet: mechanical soft
	  Active range of motion (vertical opening)
	  Soft tissue stretching and mobilization
	  Moist heat/icing
	  Scar massage
	  Joint mobilization: long axis distraction, gentle within pain tolerance
		Increase active range of motion in all planes
		Increase soft tissue mobility

6-8 weeks	Begin joint mobilization and all grades within pain tolerance—all planes Begin lateral and protrusive movements Home exercise program to include passive stretching of temporomandibular joint, soft tissue mobilization and stretching Ice/heat and scar massage Begin to progress diet to semisoft foods Address parafunctional habits: education in joint protection, normal resting position of tongue and jaw, and self-cueing to decrease parafunctional habits	Increase joint mobility Increase active range of motion in all planes Increase tolerance of functional activities
8-10 weeks 1 time per week	Evaluation for discharge	Range of motion within functional limits of jaw: 35 mm vertical opening and 5 mm lateral excursion bilateral Patient demonstrates symmetric opening pattern Patient demonstrates increased tolerance of normal function and diet

fractures in the edentulous maxilla and mandible, panfacial fractures, comminuted fractures, complicated fractures, open fractures, dislocated fractures, and the multiply fractured mandible, especially where condylar and subcondylar fractures occur with other mandible fractures.

With practice, the intraoral approach is much more rapid than the extraoral approach (see Fig. 66-48) for open reduction, and the visualization is often enhanced, especially for the horizontal mandible anteriorly. Most important, the intraoral approach avoids an external scar. The biggest disadvantage of the intraoral approach is that only the labial cortex of the mandible is visualized, and it is possible to have a significant gap in the lingual cortex. Care must be taken in this approach to achieve an exact reduction, and positioning wires may be helpful. The CT examination is important in planning the approach to detect the exact internal anatomy of the fracture (the length of the mandibular segment involved by the fracture) (Fig. 66-85). Superior border plates have a biomechanical advantage over inferior border plates in the horizontal mandible. Superior border fixation alone is often sufficient for noncomminuted angle or body fractures, but the preference in the horizontal arch of the mandible is for both superior and inferior border fixation. Comminuted angle fractures are best managed by an extraoral approach with an upper

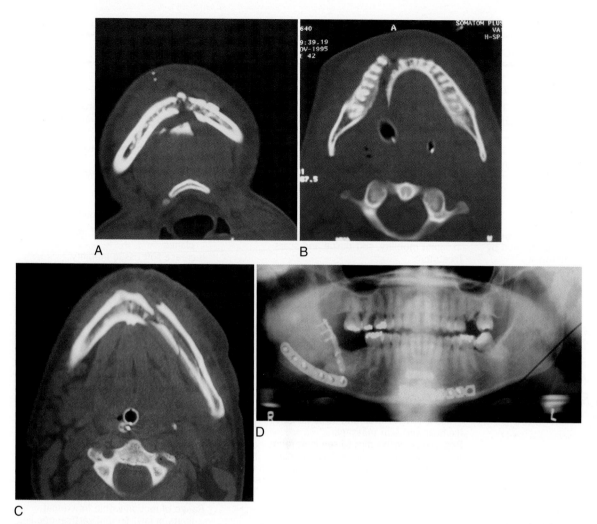

A

B

C

D

FIGURE 66-85. *A,* A CT scan detects the exact length of the mandible involved in the fracture. "Good screws" are those placed beyond the fractured area in good (noninvolved) bone. *B* and *C,* A comminuted mandible fracture is seen in this CT radiograph. The nature and length of the comminuted segment would be difficult to perceive in a Panorex or plain film, but it is clearly visible in the axial CT scan. *D,* Panorex of bone defect, angle fracture, and parasymphysis fracture.

border unicortical plate and lower border reconstruction plate (Fig. 66-86; see also Fig. 66-51).

In general, fractures of the symphysis-parasymphysis area are best exposed with an intraoral degloving technique (see Fig. 66-48) versus an external incision. Broader exposure is possible with the intraoral technique. Periosteal attachments should be retained where possible as the periosteal blood supply is often the only remaining circulation (the medullary blood supply is generally injured by the fracture).[157] Adequate exposure, especially for plate and screw fixation, frequently demands wider soft tissue mobilization (Figs. 66-87 to 66-90). Experience has shown that "free" bone fragments will generally survive if stabilization is sufficient and if they are covered by well-vascularized soft tissue. Secure intraoral closure is important, and either nonabsorbable or slowly absorbable sutures are preferred. The use of both interrupted and running lock sutures simultaneously forms a "watertight" seal in the intraoral closure. The periosteum, therefore, is not thought to be so important a blood supply that preservation is preferable to improper fracture reduction or an inadequate fracture stabilization. It is always more important to reduce and stabilize the fracture properly than to preserve periosteal attachments. A mentalis muscle stump on the bone should always be preserved, and the muscle must be reconnected at the time of soft tissue closure. In general, closure of muscle and mucosa in intraoral incisions is always preferred to closure of mucosa alone.

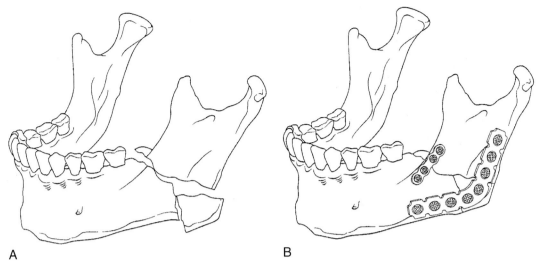

A   B

FIGURE 66-86. *A,* Angle fracture with basal comminution exceeding 25% of the height of the mandible is treated with a lateral upper border tension band plate and a lower border reconstruction plate. *B,* Open reduction with superior border miniplate and inferior border 2.4 reconstruction plate. (From Assael LA: Mandibular fractures. In Prein J, ed: Manual of Internal Fixation in the Craniofacial Skeleton: Techniques as Recommended by the AO/ASIF Group. New York, Springer-Verlag, 1997:78.)

The lingual surface of the fracture is better visualized with an extraoral approach to open reduction. Protection of the marginal mandibular branch of the facial nerve is necessary in exposing the inferior border of the mandible when cutaneous incisions are used.[158] This nerve is located up to 1 to 2 cm below the inferior edge of the mandible posterior to the facial artery. Anterior to the facial artery, the nerve should be above the inferior aspect of the mandible.

Rigid mandibular repair requires a mastery of nonsurgical fracture treatment involving manual repositioning of the fracture segments and the restoration of proper occlusal relationships by the establishment of intermaxillary fixation and the proper use of arch bars, upper border fixation, splints, or provisional wires. Both the teeth (upper border) and the lower border of the mandible need to be reduced in mandibular open reductions. The teeth are generally reduced with arch bars and intermaxillary fixation. The lower border wire and arch bar placement is completed. Upper and lower border plate and screw fixation can then be completed, with a small miniplate[159] (see Fig. 66-87) superiorly and a larger stabilization plate (see Figs. 66-89 and 66-90) inferiorly or a plate size dependent on the strength of fixation desired. The use of the locking plate minimizes the requirement for precise plate bending. Comminuted fractures (Fig. 66-91) require larger fixation plates and are conceptually treated as fractures with bone loss, where the plate itself must bear the entire load of fixation. Visual basal bone repositioning at the inferior border is essential to confirm three-dimensional restoration of the mandibular arch.

Stabilization can then follow with plate and screw application. Care is taken to maintain an inferior position of the plate so that damage to the apices of the tooth roots and inferior alveolar canal structures is avoided. For rigid internal fixation, it is necessary to have two tight secure screws in each major bone frag-

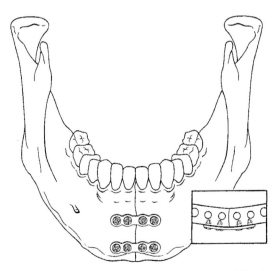

FIGURE 66-87. Open reduction and internal fixation with upper and lower border miniplates. (From Assael LA: Mandibular fractures. In Prein J, ed: Manual of Internal Fixation in the Craniofacial Skeleton: Techniques as Recommended by the AO/ASIF Group. New York, Springer-Verlag, 1997:61.)

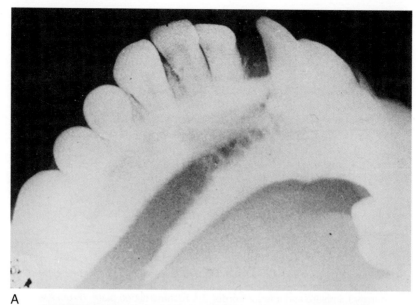

A

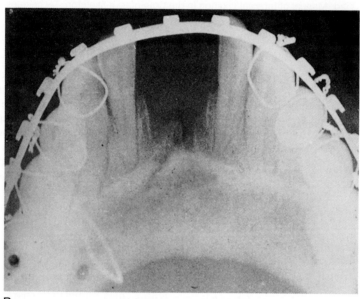

B

FIGURE 66-88. Oblique fracture through the symphyseal region. *A,* Displacement from the pull of the mylohyoid muscle. This type of fracture does not respond well to intermaxillary fixation alone, and plating is indicated. A complete exposure of the inferior border of the mandible is necessary to permit accurate alignment of this "lingually split" fragment. *B,* Symphyseal fracture fixation by interosseous wiring supplemented by arch bar intermaxillary fixation.

ment. In general, a large plate is initially "overbent" so that it stands 2 to 3 mm off the fracture site. This over-bending technique achieves an even compression throughout the width of the fracture site (see Figs. 66-68 and 66-72). The overbent plate flattens itself against the outer border of the mandible and tends to reduce the lingual cortex properly. After the fixation is secure,

maxillomandibular fixation should be released to confirm restoration of the dental occlusion.

For the horizontal portion of the mandible, the best fixation principles employ a tension band plate placed along the upper mandibular border; this should usually be a small unicortical 2.0-mm plate from the mandibular system. Some consider that the arch bar

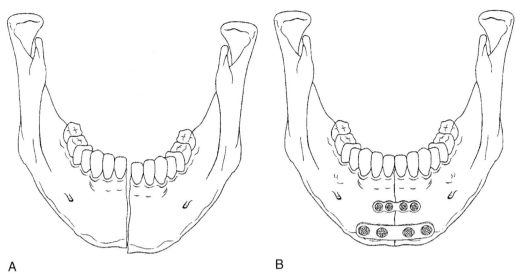

A   B

FIGURE 66-89. *A,* Transverse fracture of the symphysis with dislocation. *B,* Use of a four-hole miniplate superiorly and a dynamic compression plate inferiorly. (From Assael LA: Mandibular fractures. In Prein J, ed: Manual of Internal Fixation in the Craniofacial Skeleton: Techniques as Recommended by the AO/ASIF Group. New York, Springer-Verlag, 1997:63.)

can substitute for this plate, but it is better to have both an arch bar and the upper plate to neutralize displacement forces. It is the author's strong recommendation that tension band (upper border) plates be used; both the superior and inferior borders of the mandible

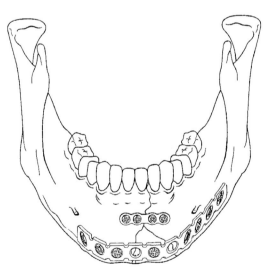

FIGURE 66-90. Reduction of a symphysis fracture with a basal triangle exceeding 25% of the height of the anterior mandible with a miniplate superiorly and a 10-hole reconstruction (noncompression) plate at the inferior border. The basal fragment makes compression treatment unfeasible as movement (and malocclusion) will occur with compression. (From Assael LA: Mandibular fractures. In Prein J, ed: Manual of Internal Fixation in the Craniofacial Skeleton: Techniques as Recommended by the AO/ASIF Group. New York, Springer-Verlag, 1997:65.)

are then kept in approximation by rigid fixation at each surface. The upper border tension band plate effectively balances the muscle forces, which tend to open the fracture at the superior border and rotate the distal mandibular fragment inferiorly (see Figs. 66-68 and 66-72).

Technical Considerations

Ellis[110] has clarified the issues regarding selection of internal fixation devices for mandibular fractures. To begin with, fixation devices must counter bite forces. In the mandible, rigid fixation is defined as internal fixation that is stable enough to prevent micromotion of the bone fragments under normal bite loads. Large, difficult-to-contour load-bearing implants were traditionally endorsed by the Association for the Study of Internal Fixation,[160] Luhr,[161] and others.[162,163] However, patients who have sustained mandible fractures do not generate normal bite forces for months after the injury. These difficult-to-perform traditional techniques are overengineered and are best reserved for the complicated mandible fracture. Champy[164,165] has shown that smaller implants in uncomplicated fractures can be strategically placed to reliably achieve implant load sharing at the fracture interface. Absolute rigidity of the bone fragments is not necessary for healing of the fracture to occur under functional loading. Functionally stable fixation is technically easier to perform and can reliably achieve fracture repair with a low risk of complications.

Common mistakes observed in treatment with rigid internal fixation devices include poor reduction of the fracture with interposition of soft tissue between the

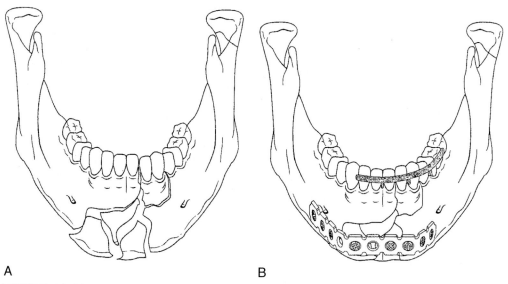

FIGURE 66-91. *A,* Comminuted fracture of the parasymphysis area. *B,* Treatment with a superior border arch bar and a large reconstruction plate (noncompression plate) inferiorly. (From Assael LA: Mandibular fractures. In Prein J, ed: Manual of Internal Fixation in the Craniofacial Skeleton: Techniques as Recommended by the AO/ASIF Group. New York, Springer-Verlag, 1997:66.)

fracture surfaces; poor alignment of fracture segments; poor plate bending; insufficient screw placement beyond the fractured (microfractured) bone areas; inadequate plate length; soft tissue damage by rotating instruments; poor or loose application of intermaxillary fixation; insufficient strength of plate; and inadequate plate strength, length, or placement for load bearing by the fracture.[166-168]

Soft tissue must be removed when it is interposed between the bone surfaces as proper alignment cannot be achieved nor healing anticipated without bone-to-bone contact. In delayed treatment of malaligned fractures, extra callus must be removed to permit fracture reduction in occlusion. Interposed soft tissue will impair or prevent bone healing, and soft tissue that is "pinched," crushed, or devitalized acts as a focus for infection. The fracture segments must sometimes be significantly displaced to remove all soft tissue from the fracture site; distraction may abnormally stretch or tear the inferior alveolar nerve. Excessive stretching of the inferior alveolar nerve in treating the fracture should be avoided. A soft tissue "cuff" can be left around the mental foramen to prevent traction injury to the mental nerve in the anterior mandible. Displacement of angle or body fracture fragments moderately can injure the inferior alveolar nerve within its canal.

Poor positioning of the screwdriver, screws, or reduction instruments or inadequate exposure may tear, pinch, or avulse the mental nerve. Rotating instruments may damage nerves or tooth roots or the inferior alveolar canal in its mandibular nerve channel.[169] Screw holes must be placed in such a way that the holes bypass these structures. One should stay 5 mm away from the mental foramen as the nerve bends inferiorly just before its exit. If it is necessary to place a screw adjacent to a tooth root or adjacent to the inferior alveolar canal, a carefully drilled monocortical hole should be considered. A drill sleeve provides adequate soft tissue protection. *Constant* cooling of the bone by irrigation must be achieved to prevent *any* heating of the bone. Heating of the bone causes bone necrosis and early screw loosening. Any bone that heats beyond 40°C is going to necrose, making screw failure a certainty (Fig. 66-92). A drill guide not only protects soft tissue but also reduces "whipping" of the drill, which causes a wider hole to be drilled in the bone, leading to poor purchase of the screw threads.

In fractures treated late or secondarily, where a fracture gap has been present and callus has attempted to bridge the gap, the callus should be removed from the bone ends by a curet or rongeur. The bone ends are reshaped toward their original configuration; otherwise, an anatomic reduction cannot be achieved. Sometimes, both extraoral and intraoral approaches are necessary in difficult fractures (Fig. 66-93). Wear facets on the teeth (Fig. 66-94) provide a guide to reestablishment of the proper occlusal pattern. In fractures treated late, the bone architecture after removal of callus generated by poor bone healing from the fracture ends may be such that a bone gap exists and

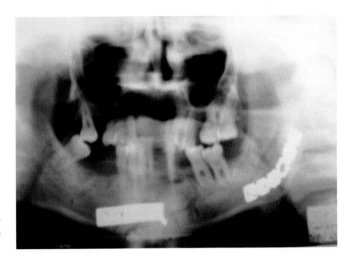

FIGURE 66-92. Malalignment after treatment with lag screws in a parasymphysis fracture.

cancellous bone grafting, preferably immediate but perhaps delayed, is necessary.

Although young men with head injuries (who are uncooperative) generally require the longest, strongest plates and extra screws, the functional forces in elderly patients and in edentulous and atrophic mandibles are frequently underestimated. In these situations, the plate must be load bearing and have enough screw holes to absorb the considerable forces sustained without the load-sharing effect of bone contact and bone compression. In thin edentulous fractures, the teeth do not serve to prevent fracture displacement and "upper border stabilization" is not possible,

making a long sturdy reconstruction plate the plate of choice. In fractures with comminution, partial bone loss, or a bone defect, where the plate must bear the entire fracture load without sharing the load through bone impaction, a reconstruction plate with at least four holes to each side of the fracture defect in good bone must be used. Small fixation plates will be inadequate in all these circumstances. Even strong plates that span bone defects will eventually fatigue and fracture if bone continuity is not eventually restored.

Most commercial plating systems are strong enough to bear the weight without bone impaction. In non-compression techniques, the bone is not used as a

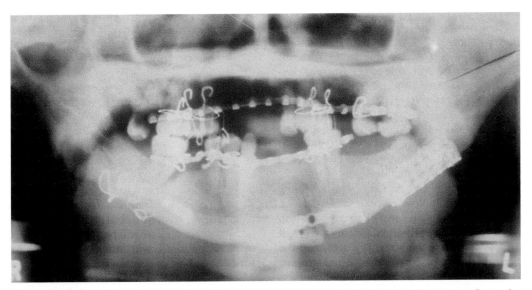

FIGURE 66-93. Microfractures render the center segment unstable for fixation. "Good screws" must be placed in bone well beyond the fracture area.

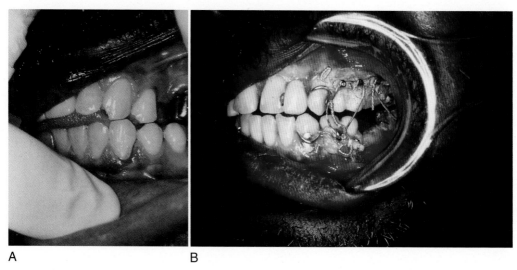

FIGURE 66-94. *A,* Wear facets (flattened areas of occlusal contact) help determine the proper interdigitation of the teeth. *B,* Loose, poorly applied intermaxillary fixation facilitates malreduction.

component of the stabilization forces as in compression techniques. In compression techniques, the bone actually bears a major portion of the load of the forces of fixation. Compression techniques are suitable *only* for non-bone gap, noncomminuted fractures (Fig. 66-95). When more than 25% of the bone height of the mandible is rendered unstable by comminution, the fracture must be considered a "bone gap" fracture and treated with a *noncompression* reconstruction plate with four screws per major segment whose fixation is in good bone beyond the fracture area.[170,171] The plate must bear the entire load of the fracture.

Many fractures are oblique, and it is easy to place a screw from a buccal exposure that parallels or lies in a fracture gap on the lingual side. Failure to achieve bicortical purchase may not be realized during the operative procedure, and early screw loosening and fixation failure are possible. Placement of a third or fourth screw in good bone beyond each side of the fracture conceptually is not necessary, but practically, if the first two screws loosen or are poorly placed, the extra screws add "insurance." Therefore, the use of at least three screws placed outside the fracture area, as defined by the CT scan, is recommended for secure fixation. If one screw becomes loose, there are still two good screws in good bone maintaining stability.

Repeated insertion and removal of self-tapping screws, drilling of multiple screw holes close together, and whipping of the drill bit make screw fixation weak or unobtainable. Self-tapping screws will cut new threads each time the screw is seated, and the process is especially problematic in weak and atrophic bone. Overtightening of screws strips the threads, as does drilling into an area of bone microfracture or drilling with a drill bit that is dull (heats excessively),

whips, or is too large for the minor diameter of the screws.

Plate bending errors are increased with use of stronger plates[172] (see Fig. 66-68). This is why many prefer small plates or the locking system. Small plates are malleable and adaptable and can easily bend to the fracture contour. With stronger plates, gaps on the lingual side of the fracture after fixation can be avoided by slight initial overbending (3 mm) of the plate off the fracture surface. If the plate is not overbent properly, it exerts torsional forces in tightening that may change the occlusion and produce dental interference. Intraoperative observation of the occlusion before and after fracture treatment is necessary. After fracture stabilization, the patient is taken out of intermaxillary fixation; the occlusion is confirmed as correct after the fracture reduction has been completed with the condyle seated in the fossa by finger pressure applied to the inferior surface of the angle as the jaws are closed in occlusion. If the occlusion is not adequate, the rigid fixation devices have to be removed and reapplied. The condyle may be seated in the fossa by finger pressure applied simultaneously over the condylar head laterally and on the inferior border of the mandible at the angle. The occlusion may be checked by releasing the intermaxillary fixation, pressing up on the angle to see that the condyle is seated, and lightly closing the mouth to see that the occlusion is acceptable and complete throughout the whole dental arch. Repeated applications of fixation plates will perforate the cortex of the mandible excessively with multiple screw holes, making further purchase of fixation screws difficult.

SYMPHYSIS AND PARASYMPHYSIS FRACTURES. Surgical exposure is generally achieved by a lower buccal

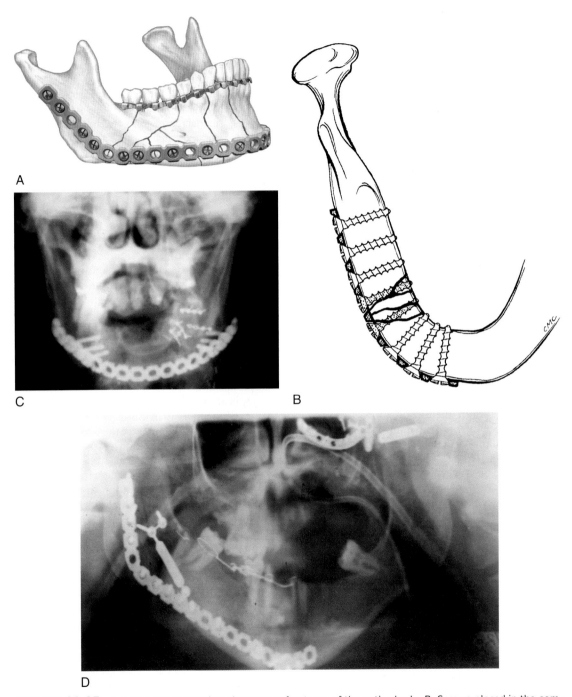

FIGURE 66-95. *A*, Large reconstruction plate spans fractures of the entire body. *B*, Screws placed in the comminuted bone segment are considered unstable. At least three or four screws must be placed in good bone (bicortically stable) to each side of the entire comminuted bone segment. *C*, Comminuted mandible fracture with the use of small screws to unite comminuted fragments of the left body. A reconstruction plate spans the anterior defect. *D*, Bone defect fracture spanned by reconstruction plate. (*A* courtesy of Synthes Maxillofacial, Paoli, Pa.)

sulcus incision. The mental nerve must be protected. Mental nerve branches may be seen submucosally in the tissue of the lip.[105,173] The mentalis muscle bundles must also have a cuff left on the bone and should be specifically reapproximated to prevent lip ectropion.

Torsional forces tend to rotate the mandible segments inward (lingually) after central mandibular fractures, and this displacement is aggravated by the application of elastics and overly tight intermaxillary fixation. In this displacement, the tooth-bearing mandible rotates inward and the inferior aspects of the angles rotate outward, increasing facial width. Reduction maneuvers, described by Ellis,[174] require pushing on the angles until the labial cortex begins to gap to ensure that the lingual cortex is in approximation. Gapping of the labial border means that the lingual border of the fracture is in approximation as the labial border cannot gap without approximation of the lingual border. This maneuver allows the operator to achieve a good reduction of both the labial and lingual surfaces of the fracture without actually observing the inferior border at the lingual surface.

Even nondisplaced symphysis fractures are better treated with internal fixation, so that the torsional forces remain neutralized for the entire period of bone healing. Champy[164,165] recommended both upper and lower border plates in the symphysis-parasymphysis area to help neutralize the torsional forces and keep the lower border in approximation. Stability can be achieved by traditional plates and screws or with a lag screw technique. Two lag screws are recommended for each fracture to be stable to guard against rotation. In general, these screw lengths require 35 to 45 mm anteriorly (Fig. 66-96; see also Fig. 66-74).[175]

BODY FRACTURES. Body fractures are anatomically located from the cuspid through the first molar. They require upper and lower border plating and represent fractures prone to displacement because of muscle forces applied to the fractures. An intraoral incision is preferred, but a trocar may be required (see Figs. 66-48 and 66-49) for screw placement. The upper border unicortical tension band plate is applied, following which the lower border is fixated. Compression techniques in the lower border work well for noncomminuted fractures and may use small or larger plates in noncomminuted fractures. The use of a lag screw either alone in a fracture or in a plate in one of the center holes will rigidly fix a fracture in the body that is oblique and "unfavorable."

ANGLE FRACTURES. Patients with third molars have an increased risk of an angle fracture. This risk still exists for a period of 2 months postoperatively after extraction.[135,176] Long-term studies show that even remote third molar extraction results in a slightly increased risk of fractures of the angle.

In angle fracture treatment, the use of extraction techniques to remove an impacted third molar in a fracture must be carefully considered.[135] In some circumstances, when the third molar is partially erupted and inflamed, it should be removed at the time of fracture treatment.[177] Otherwise, it makes little sense to do osteotomies to remove a fully impacted third molar, as further damage to the bone and mucosa in the area of the fracture may actually cause bone necrosis, further expose the fracture to the intraoral environment, and contribute to bone instability and infection. Bone support of the fracture fragments may be lost after extraction, and a linear fracture may be converted to a comminuted, less stable fracture by third molar removal.[178] The fracture site is often less vascularized after third molar removal by virtue of periosteal stripping. Fully impacted third molars can be electively removed when angle fracture healing is completed, unless the operative treatment of the fracture exposes the tooth or tooth removal is necessary to achieve alignment of the fracture.[144,168,179]

What constitutes adequate fixation of the angle is debated. Conceptually, an upper border plate alone can be used for noncomminuted fractures, as in the mandibular angle fracture. In the author's experience, the application of an upper border at the angle plate frequently forms a gap in the lower border of the fracture, but the gap may not alter the occlusion or jeopardize bone healing (nonunion). If the gap is small, it rarely poses a problem, but it is most effectively reduced by the application of a second plate at the lower border. The upper border is the location in the horizontal mandible that most effectively resists the pull of the suprahyoid musculature, which tends to open the mandible along the superior border.

Choi and Suh[180] have specified a method for plating angle fractures without having the patient in intermaxillary fixation. The technique involves the use of a reduction forceps for pressing the fracture together initially for the upper border mylohyoid ridge plate; the reduction forceps is removed, and then a contralateral mouth prop is used to open the occlusion on the contralateral side, which compresses the inferior aspect of the opposite angle fracture.

Haug et al[181] performed an extensive biomechanical evaluation of mandibular angle fracture plating.[111,139,182,183] Comparing miniplates (one or two) and large plates (including monocortical tension band systems and bicortical stabilization plates) subjected to loads, Haug found that all systems met or currently exceeded postoperative functional requirements for stability in incisal edge loading. All systems, however, failed to meet stability requirements for contralateral molar loading, which indicates that all plating systems may have problems generated by immediate indiscriminate molar use.

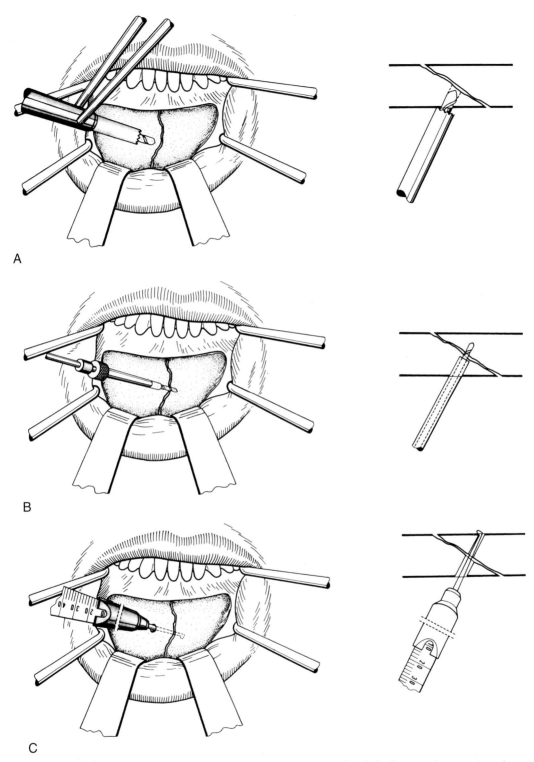

FIGURE 66-96. The lag screw concept involves drilling a "gliding" hole in the outer bone cortex whose diameter is the same diameter as the screw threads. The inner cortex is drilled to the minor or core diameter of the screw. The screw therefore does not engage the outer cortex but engages only the inner cortex, pulling the inner cortex toward the outer cortex as the screw is tightened. *A,* A gliding hole is drilled in the outer fragment. The gliding hole is the same diameter as the threads of the screw. *B,* A guide is placed through the gliding hole, and the smaller drill bit, the size of the core diameter of the screw, is used to drill a hole across the fracture into the other fragment. *C,* The screw length is determined by a depth gauge.

Continued

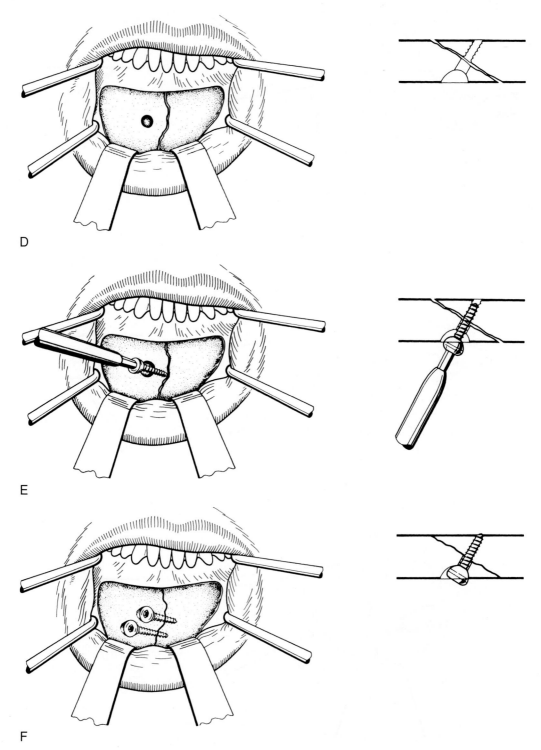

D

E

F

FIGURE 66-96, cont'd. *D,* The prepared gliding hole, thread holes, and "bed" for the screw head are seen. The bed has been shaved by a shaping bit. Care should be taken not to drill this bed too deeply, or the entire thickness of the cortical bone on the outer surface of the mandible will be penetrated. *E,* Placement of the first lag screw. *F,* Final fixation of the fracture by two lag screws as demonstrated. They engage the inner cortex and pull across the fracture to compress the outer cortex to the inner cortex. This technique may be used alone, or it may be performed through a hole in a plate by angling one of the screws as a lag screw and leaving it long enough to go through both bone fragments obliquely. (From Niederdellmann H: Rigid internal fixation by means of lag screws. In Kruger E, Schilli W, eds: Oral and Maxillofacial Traumatology, vol I. Chicago, Quintessence Publishing, 1982:376.)

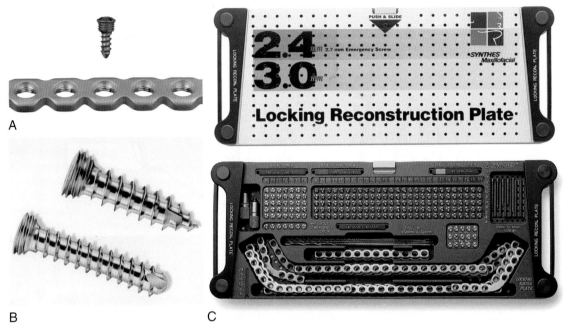

FIGURE 66-97. *A,* Use of a locking plate to unite the bone to the screws. *B,* Design of a locking screw. *C,* The locking system. (Courtesy of Synthes Maxillofacial, Paoli, Pa.)

Ellis,[184-189] in the most extensive clinical comparisons of various types of plating systems in mandibular angle fractures, found that an upper border miniplate was as successful as any other miniplate or compression plate combination in the treatment of noncomminuted angle fractures. He thought that periosteal stripping devitalized bone and that larger compression plates contributed to bone loss by compression of devitalized bone edges. It must be noted that Ellis is a strong believer in immediate full function. A reconstruction plate provided the best result for comminuted fractures.

Theoretically, a lag screw may be driven from the proximal body somewhat sagittally through the angle to stabilize a transverse fracture of the angle. This technique, advocated by Niederdellmann et al,[190,191] is not commonly practiced because it is difficult to execute and it is easy to achieve inadequate fixation. Poor purchase of the bone in the proximal mandibular segment makes this technique problematic.

In complicated or comminuted angle or body fractures, an extraoral approach is preferred as it maximizes the ability to achieve a precise reduction and stable fixation. Comminuted fractures may be difficult to reduce and stabilize with an intraoral approach alone. Comminuted angle or body fractures should be treated extraorally with reconstruction locking plates whose length is set by bone defect criteria to bear the entire load of fixation (Fig. 66-97).

CORONOID FRACTURES. The coronoid process of the mandible is sheathed by its overlying musculature and by the zygomatic arch.[192] The temporalis muscle has broad attachments surrounding the ramus and extending along the anterior surface of the ramus and the coronoid areas. With the mouth closed, the coronoid process is under the zygomatic arch so that it is protected from injury. Fractures of the coronoid may involve only the tip of the coronoid process, may involve the whole process, or may extend along the surface of the ramus of the mandible to comminute the whole anterior portion of the ramus and separate it from the rest of the mandible (Fig. 66-98). Coronoid fractures may either be isolated or occur with a complex, complicated fracture of the angle portion of the mandible (combined angle, ramus, and condyle). Coronoid fractures frequently show little dislocation because of the broad, dense sheath of insertions of the temporalis muscle and its fascia. In many patients, treatment is unnecessary because little displacement has been produced. Intermaxillary fixation may be used as a temporary splinting maneuver for pain for 2 weeks. If displacement is observed, open reduction through an intraoral, a retromandibular, or a Risdon approach is recommended. Some fractures of the coronoid are accompanied by other fractures of that region, such as the zygoma or the zygomatic arch. The classification of Natvig et al[192] describes coronoid fractures as intramuscular and submuscular, with submuscular types

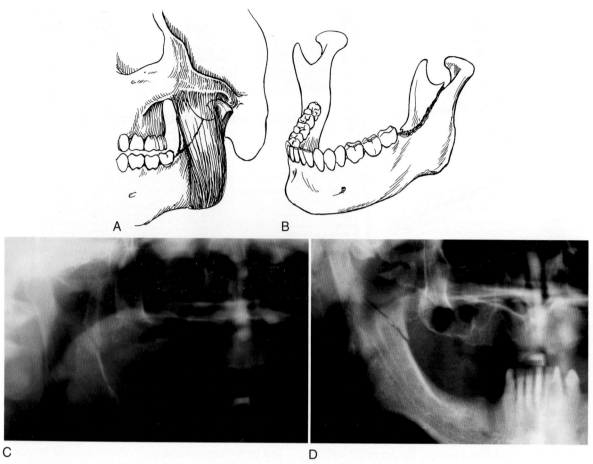

FIGURE 66-98. In ramus fractures, the heavy musculature and the periosteum surrounding the ramus of the mandible provide protection and tend to prevent displacement of fractured segments. *A,* The heavy musculature. *B,* Fractures of the coronoid process are uncommon, and displacement (because they are ensheathed within the temporalis muscle) is usually minimal. *C,* High coronoid fracture. *D,* Submarginal coronoid fracture.

being the marginal submuscular and the submarginal submuscular. If the entire region (including the angles, coronoid, and subcondylar region) is fractured, the whole area benefits from reduction and plate and screw fixation.

CONDYLAR AND SUBCONDYLAR FRACTURES. When anatomically classifying condylar and subcondylar fractures, one must consider dislocation, angulation between the fragments, fracture override (which translates to ramus vertical length shortening), fracture angulation, and bone gaps between the fragments (Fig. 66-99). In children, growth considerations[193] not present in adults establish a capacity for both regenerative and restitutional remodeling that is not present in later years.[194,195] Adults are capable of only partial restitutional remodeling.

High condylar (intracapsular) fractures (head and upper neck) are generally treated with closed reduc-

tion with a limited (2-week) period of postoperative intermaxillary fixation, followed by early "controlled" mobilization with elastics for re-establishment of occlusion in a rest position day and night, at night alone, or intermittently as required.[196] Most neck and low subcondylar fractures with good alignment, reasonable contact of the bone ends, and preservation of ramus vertical height without condylar head dislocation may be treated by intermaxillary fixation for 4 to 6 weeks, with weekly or biweekly observation of the occlusion for at least an additional 4 weeks after release of fixation if fracture alignment is initially reasonable. Some shortening of the ramus height of the mandible is almost inevitable with a closed approach to condylar or subcondylar fracture treatment, which may lead to a premature contact in the ipsilateral molar occlusion with function. Angulation between the fractured fragments in excess of 30 degrees and fracture gap between the bone ends exceeding 4 or 5 mm, lateral

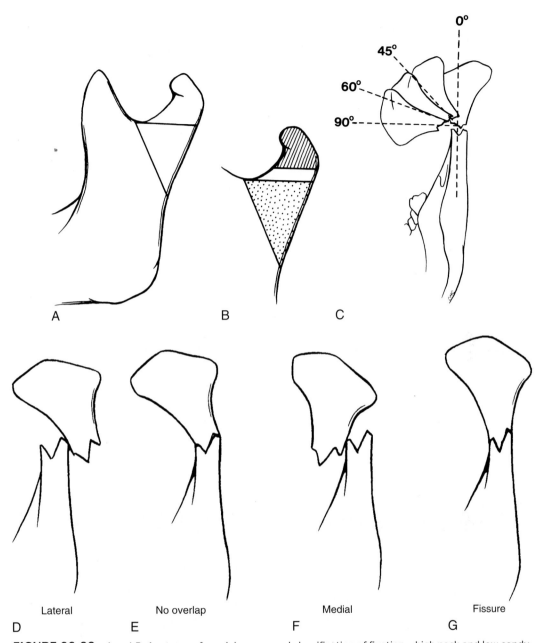

FIGURE 66-99. *A* and *B,* Anatomy of condylar area and classification of fixation—high neck and low condylar regions. *C,* Angulation and condylar fractures. *D* to *G,* Classification of condylar fractures.

Continued

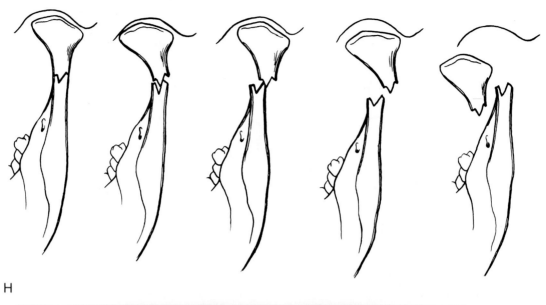

H

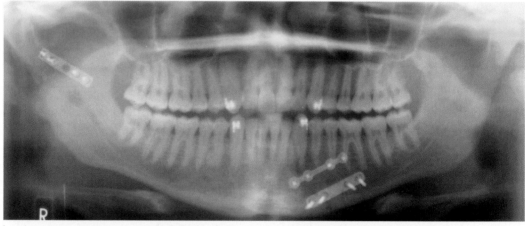

I

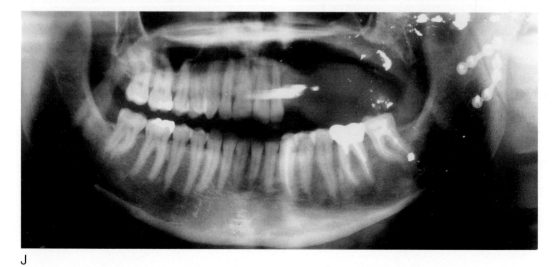

J

FIGURE 66-99, cont'd. *H,* Gap in fracture alignment. *I,* Open reduction of condyle with one plate (right condyle). *J,* Open reduction of condyle with two plates (left condyle).

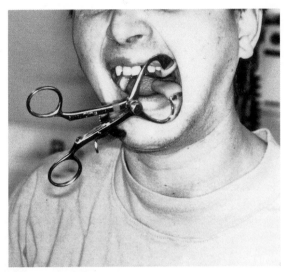

K

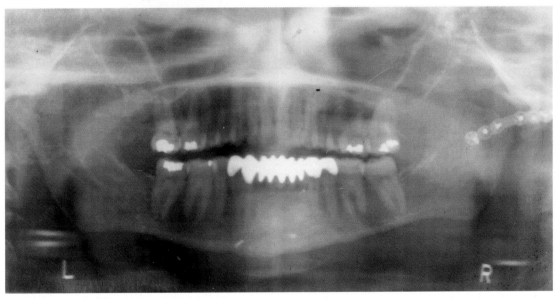

L

FIGURE 66-99, cont'd. *K,* Mouth gap for increasing motion. *L,* Malreduction of condyle by open reduction and internal fixation with nonunion.   *Continued*

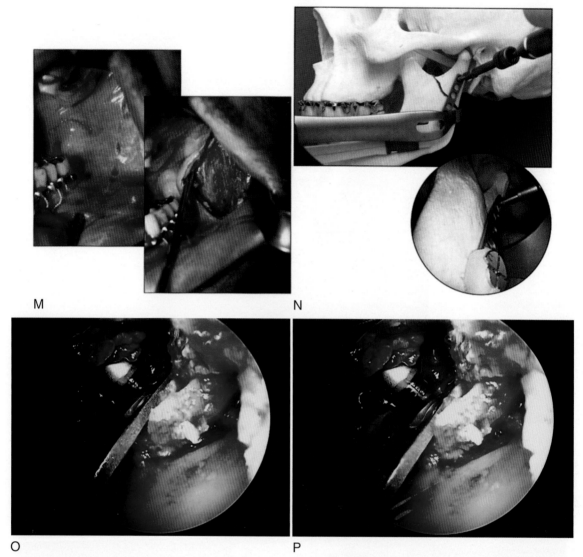

M   N

O   P

FIGURE 66-99, cont'd. *M* to *P,* Endoscopic reduction of a condylar fracture. (*M* courtesy of Reid Mueller, MD. *N* courtesy of Synthes Maxillofacial, Paoli, Pa.)

override, and lack of contact of the fractured fragments should be considerations justifying open reduction (Fig. 66-99).[197-200] Loss of ramus height is heralded by a premature contact in the molar dentition on the fractured side, which first produces a subtle open bite in the contralateral occlusion, a lack of the "cuspid contact" that is present in normal occlusion in most individuals.

Open reduction of subcondylar fractures is preferred for any low, dislocated fracture; the low condylar fracture that occurs with a multiply fractured mandible; or a low fracture that occurs simultaneously with maxillary or Le Fort fractures, where the maxilla requires support from the intact mandible for Le Fort I level maxillary stability.[201,202] Open treatment of a dislocated condylar head fracture brings with it the possibility of necrosis of the condylar head due to stripping of its blood supply and the possibility of damage to the upper trunk or temporal branch of the facial nerve if a preauricular incision is used or the mandibular branch (cranial nerve VII) if a lower (retromandibular or Risdon) incision is used for subcondylar fractures.[203] A scar, hypertrophic in 10% of patients, is often a sequela to external approaches.[203] Open reduction of condylar fractures can be approached either intraorally or extraorally.

Intraoral[204,205] approaches may make use of specialized fixation and operative field televised viewing.

Intraoral endoscopic special instruments are assisted by percutaneous instrument use (Fig. 66-99*M* and *N*). Short percutaneous incisions for trocar placement are required to place screws and drill holes in the endoscopic technique.

Extraoral approaches may use the Risdon, submandibular, or retromandibular incision for subcondylar fractures or the preauricular or retroauricular incision for higher condylar fractures[203,206] (Fig. 66-100). Sometimes, the combination of a dislocated condylar head with fracture of the neck requires both a preauricular incision and a retromandibular incision (upper and lower condylar approaches). This simultaneous approach gives a panoramic view but may require a specific exposure for protection of the facial nerve. A transparotid incision has also been described for subcondylar exposure with dissection in the direction of facial nerve fibers to expose the bone through the parotid gland. This incision carries the risk of a parotid glandular fistula as well as facial nerve injury but has the advantage of being directly over the fracture site. In patients with medial dislocation of the condylar head, a preauricular approach is necessary.

The most common form of condylar head dislocation is medial and anterior with the condylar head fractured at the neck. The pull of the medial pterygoid muscle retracts the condyle toward the area of the pterygoid plates. The capsular ligaments are torn, and the disk may be dislocated. The condyle occasionally can be dislocated without fracture.

Dislocations of the condylar head lateral to the joint, posteriorly into the ear canal, or superiorly into the intracranial fossa[207] have been recorded. A variety of exposures and techniques for the dislocated condylar head into the middle cranial fossa are listed in the excellent paper by Kroetsch,[207] which summarizes the literature. Reconstruction consists of retrieval of the fragment, closure of any dural fistula, and closure of the bone perforation with a graft to complete the repair. Condylar dislocations treated more than a few days after injury often require stripping of the condylar head from its blood supply to replace the head into the fossa. Partial resorption after replacement is universal and complete resorption more frequent than expected. Some authors[208] have used costochondral grafts in this situation rather than retrieval of the damaged condylar head. Lateral or posterior dislocations are absolute indications for open reduction as joint function is often blocked.

In general, low subcondylar fractures benefit from two sets of plates and screws,[178] one toward the anterior border and one toward the posterior border[209] (see Fig. 66-99). The dynamic compression plates used in this area should equal or exceed the mandibular strength.[181] A variety of fixation devices have been used for subcondylar fixation, including plates, K-wires, and lag screws. Stability and bite forces seem to be improved

after open reduction, but condylar resorption may be prominent.[210,211] Inferior alveolar and lingual nerve injuries occur occasionally as complications of ramus and angle fracture treatment.[212]

Sugiura et al[213] compared osteosynthesis of the condylar process with lag screws, miniplates, and K-wires. K-wires demand a 4-week period of immobilization in intermaxillary fixation. Acceptable position immediately and postoperatively was found in 90% of patients, and a shortening of the ramus more than 5 mm was observed significantly more frequently in the miniplate group than in the lag screw group. The authors noted that instability makes for greater loads, which yield a malposition. Adequate stability is difficult to obtain with a single miniplate and depends really on bone impaction, such as may be achieved with the lag screw. Most authors reduce the incidence of problems by having a short period of maxillomandibular fixation postoperatively. Interestingly, the use of two plates resulted in more bone deviation than with one plate. The authors suggest that the stripping of the bone necessary for plate and screw application results in poorer bone healing conditions, possibly because of multiple drill holes or microfractures.

Ellis et al[203,214-216] have concluded that bite forces after closed and open treatment of mandibular condylar fractures are about 60% of normal at 6 weeks. Yang et al[217] have summarized their functional results after treatment of 61 patients with unilateral condylar process fractures; 36 patients had open reduction, and groups were separated into condylar and subcondylar fractures. Condylar fractures treated closed had more mobility, whereas those treated open had less chin deviation on opening and less pain.

In a questionnaire, 57% of surgeons preferred open reduction.[218] Previous studies have suffered because of lack of or random selection of patients, no qualification of clinical variables, confusion of fracture levels, different treatment protocols, and different methods of results evaluation. Clinical variables include age, degree of displacement, fracture level, unilateral or bilateral fracture, and associated fractures. In general, mobility is the same when closed reduction and open reduction are compared.[217,219,220]

Takenoshita[221,222] reported 39 mm of opening for the open group and 50 mm for the closed group. Postoperative pain, muscle stripping, and scarring might contribute to hypomobility in the open group. Chin deviation is twice as common in the closed group (40% versus 22%) as it is in the open group.[223,224] The incidence of transient frontal branch palsy in the open group is 8%.[196,217] All patients recovered nerve function by 2 months. Conceptually, the endoscopic approach would decrease the incidence of facial nerve injury.[204]

Ellis[206] has thoroughly analyzed a large series of condylar fractures and concluded that those treated

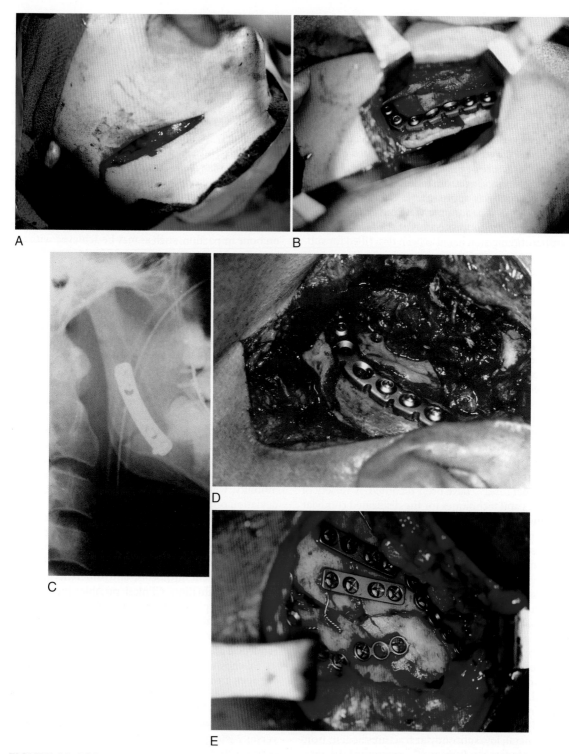

A

B

C

D

E

FIGURE 66-100. *A,* Risdon incision. *B,* Open reduction of a complex fracture of the coronoid, condyle, and ramus through a neck incision (retromandibular); clinical approach and plate. *C,* Radiograph of another reconstruction. *D,* Malreduction of angle fracture by compression plate. *E,* Less stable reduction of angle fracture with multiple small plates.

closed had shorter posterior facial height, more tilting of the occlusal plane, more malocclusion, and less excursion toward the fractured side than those treated open. He found a 17.2% incidence of hypertrophic scarring and a similar incidence of transient nerve injury.[203] Worsaae and Thorn[225,226] found malocclusion, mandibular asymmetry, mastication dysfunction, and pain to be significantly more common in patients treated closed (39% complications) versus open (4% complications). Takenoshita et al[221,222] and Konstantinovic and Dimitrijevic,[196] in separate nonrandomized series, found similar results in groups treated both closed and open. However, the patients with the worst defects were treated open, implying that open treatment may yield the best results in the more difficult fractures.

Silvennoinen et al[227] classified the factors leading to problems after nonsurgical treatment of condylar fractures and reviewed the literature. They focused on angulation of the fracture and reduction in ramus height. Most of the problem fractures were in the subcondylar region, had a ramus height reduction of 5 to 10 mm, and had an angulation of more than 23 degrees in the anterior-posterior plane. Most of these fractures had no contact between fracture fragments and demonstrated override at the fracture level, with medial override being slightly less problematic than lateral override. Haug et al,[209,228] in analyzing the long-term outcomes of open versus closed treatment of mandibular subcondylar fractures, determined that no statistically significant differences existed between open reduction, internal fixation and closed reduction and maxillomandibular fixation for age, maximum inner incisal opening, lateral excursion, protrusive movement, deviation on opening, or occlusal position. The open reduction group was associated with perceptible scars and the closed reduction group with chronic pain.

Haug[228] thought that when fewer than three functional teeth per quadrant exist, maxillomandibular fixation is compromised. He thought that open reduction and internal fixation permitted earlier function, enhanced nutrition, and contributed to a protected airway. Many times, in an edentulous patient, he noted that a patient's denture was old, ill-fitting, broken, or lost. Although a splint may be fabricated, it requires a dental impression, curing a plaster model, fabrication of the splint, and then surgical application with circumferential wiring or screw or pin fixation. Modification of an intact denture for fixation often ruins the denture. The more atrophic the ridge, the more difficult it is to achieve stability with closed reduction. He also thought that open reduction with internal fixation is contraindicated for the management of condylar head fractures, whether single fragment, comminuted, or medial pole at or above the ligamentous attachment.

A high risk of avascular necrosis is associated with open reduction of a dislocated condylar head fracture.[210,211] These patients should be managed by a brief (2-week) period of maxillomandibular fixation with training elastics if occlusal prematurity is associated with a loss in vertical dimension. Haug[229] thought that the condylar neck fracture in the thin constricted region inferior to the condylar head is a relative contraindication to open reduction and internal fixation. In condylar neck fractures, a predictable amount of bone is not always available to permit the placement of two screws per segment. Thus, the precepts of rigid immobilization fall short of what is obtainable to prevent an increased risk of nonunion or infection. The possibility of loosening of hardware exists. Zide,[230-232] in a discussion following the article, has two indications for condylar fracture treatment, dislocation of the condylar head and loss of ramus height with instability of reduction. He mentions that Haug[228] might have a third critical indication for open reduction and internal fixation, and that is to lessen pain. Zide pointed out that about 70% of closed reduction patients have a good result and 30% do not; he tried to determine the "black and white" feature that characterizes the 30% with less than good results, but these patients cannot be characterized. He comments that with 20 years of "anecdotal certainty," his open reduction, internal fixation patients have been easier to manage postoperatively, have routinely had better symmetry, and have shown better occlusal results than his closed reduction patients, in spite of the more difficult surgery, the facial scar, and the occasional but "always temporary" facial nerve palsy.

One of the best summaries of the literature regarding the closed versus open reduction controversy on mandibular condylar fractures appeared in November of 2003.[201] The literature was summarized and emphasized the importance of classification in deciding which condylar fractures needed an operation. The considerations involved alignment of the fractured ends, shortening of the ramus, and level of the fracture. The "shortening" refers to angulation with override and "displacement" movement away from each other of the fractured ends, which can be either medial or lateral. Displacement of the condylar head out of the glenoid fossa, medial tilt of the condylar fragment more than 14 degrees, and shortening of the ramus by more than 5% were listed by Haug as indications for open reduction. Bilateral fractures with an open bite, gross fracture end malalignment, fracture-dislocation, partly or completely healed fractures with arthralgia, abnormal function, and malocclusion were also listed.

Condylar head fractures that are intracapsular, whether single fragment, medial pole, or comminuted, should be managed according to the preceding criteria or with closed reduction: a brief 1- or 2-week period of intermaxillary fixation and early free or guided

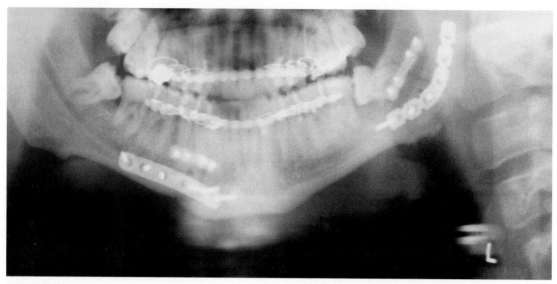

FIGURE 66-101. Locking plate for angle fracture. (Courtesy of Synthes Maxillofacial, Paoli, Pa.)

(elastic) motion with frequent observation of the occlusion. The patient may even apply elastics at night, placing the mandible in full normal occlusion.

Zide[230-232] emphasizes that condylar segment displacement and ramus height instability are really the only orthopedic indications for the open reduction and internal fixation of mandibular condylar fractures. Thus, displaced and unstable low condylar neck or subcondylar fractures are the ones for which open reduction is generally indicated.

Assael[201] emphasized that symptoms similar and often attributed to condylar fractures occur frequently in a normal, nonfractured population. He emphasized that most condylar fractures could be treated closed according to the classification system agreed on by Brandt and Haug.[233] He emphasized that each component decision in contemporary meaningful condylar fracture treatment must be considered individually and assessed individually.

COMMINUTED FRACTURES. These fractures require a long plate over the comminuted segments with at least three screws placed in good bone beyond the CT-established length of the fracture. The comminuted bone pieces are initially attached to the large fragments with small plates and screws. An arch bar and tension band plate with neutral screws are applied to the upper border. The larger plate is applied to the lower border, spanning the fracture site. In comminution extending to the upper border, longer spanning reconstruction plates must be used (Fig. 66-101; see also Fig. 66-97), and the locking plate variety is recommended.

EDENTULOUS MANDIBLE. Fractures in the edentulous mandible are seen less commonly than fractures in the dentulous or partially dentulous mandible.[153,234-237] They represent less than 5% of the mandibular fractures in most series.[238] The fractures commonly occur through portions of the bone where atrophy is the most advanced or where the bone is thin and weak.[136,153] Therefore, the body is a common site for fracture compared with the angle and subcondylar region in dentulous patients.[137,138,238,239] Many mandible fractures are bilateral or multiple, and displacement of a bilateral edentulous body fracture is often severe and a challenging condition to treat. There are tremendous forces on the edentulous fracture site. The fractures in the horizontal mandible may be closed or open to the oral cavity. Closed fractures demonstrating minimal displacement may be treated with a soft diet and avoidance of dentures; however, in these patients, observation is critical to be sure that healing occurs within several weeks without further displacement. In practice, most fractures are better treated with open reduction with a load-bearing plate (Fig. 66-102).

The edentulous mandible is characterized by the loss of the alveolar ridge and the teeth.[239] The atrophy of the bone has been related to arteriosclerotic changes in the inferior alveolar artery and external carotid circulation, and progressive loss of bone is seen first in the mandibular alveolus with loss of the teeth and bone until the mandible becomes pencil thin.[240] The bone atrophy may be minimal if there is sufficient height (>20 mm) of the mandibular body to ensure good bone healing. In patients with moderate atrophy, the height of the mandibular body ranges from 10 to 20 mm, and healing is usually satisfactory but not as certain as when the height is more than 20 mm.[241]

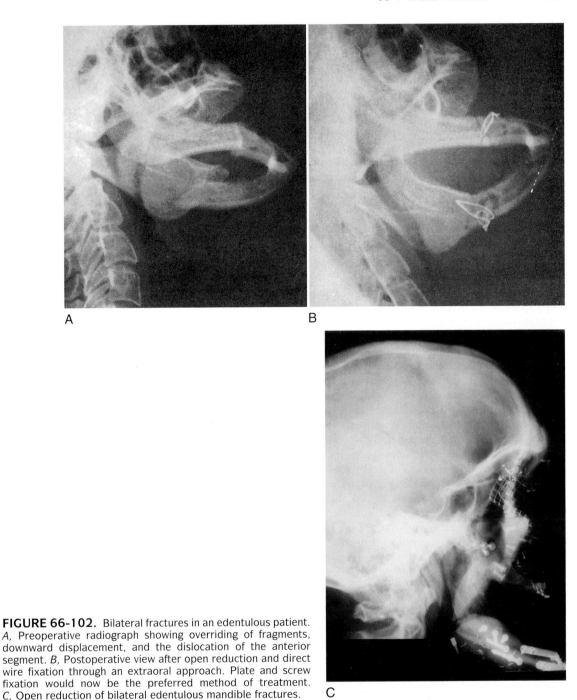

FIGURE 66-102. Bilateral fractures in an edentulous patient. *A,* Preoperative radiograph showing overriding of fragments, downward displacement, and the dislocation of the anterior segment. *B,* Postoperative view after open reduction and direct wire fixation through an extraoral approach. Plate and screw fixation would now be the preferred method of treatment. *C,* Open reduction of bilateral edentulous mandible fractures.

Intraoral appliances (dentures or splints) were previously useful largely in simple fractures that had a substantial alveolar ridge in which displacement was minimal (Fig. 66-102). Often, a wire would be placed between the bone ends, and patients would be stabilized in their own dentures, which were circumferentially wired to the upper or lower jaws. This method was cumbersome and did not permit any oral hygiene to be accomplished. The splints were often left in place for a 6- to 8-week period until consolidation of the fracture fragments had occurred. When dentures were not present or not usable, impressions of the alveolar ridges were taken and models were prepared and sectioned, and suitable splints or "bite blocks" were constructed. Splints were not helpful when the height of the mandible was less than 15 mm, as there was no "alveolar ridge" present that could be stabilized by the flanges of the splint or denture. Baudens[242] was the first to use circumferential wiring techniques for the reduction of mandibular fractures. He described the use of a wire inserted around the mandible in the molar area. Robert,[243] in 1852, used a single circumferential wire to reduce a mandibular fracture, twisting the wire close to the bone and approximating the segments in an oblique fracture. The circumferential wiring technique may be used alone or in combination with a splint or denture.

Plate and screw fixation is now the preferred method of treatment of all displaced edentulous fractures; the selection of the plate is keyed to how much bone buttressing the height of bone provides (<15 mm of bone height provides poor bone buttressing). Many individuals underestimate the size of a plate that is necessary to stabilize the edentulous body fracture in the atrophic mandible. Small plates with few screws often fail in patients with atrophic mandibles as there is insufficient bone to provide buttressing support for the fracture treatment, and the plate must bear the entire load of the fracture. Large reconstruction locking plates with four screws per side are recommended.[111] In patients in whom the mandibular height is less than 10 mm, the atrophy is described as severe, and one can assume that the patient has a disease of "poor bone healing." Complications that follow fracture of the edentulous mandible directly parallel the extent of mandibular atrophy. Obwegeser and Sailer,[244] in 1973, documented that 20% of the complications in mandible fractures that were edentulous were seen in the 10- to 20-mm mandibular height group, and 80% of the complications (consisting mostly of poor or unsatisfactory bone union) were experienced in patients demonstrating a mandibular height of less than 10 mm. Virtually no complications are seen in those fractures that exceed 20 mm in height.

This experience caused some authors to recommend primary bone grafting for the severely atrophic edentulous mandible (10 mm or less in height) that requires an open reduction.[245] The addition around the fracture area of cancellous bone graft should be considered, especially if there is no intraoral communication with the fracture site. However, some of the fractures of the severely atrophic edentulous mandible may be treated without fixation (soft diet alone) if there is minimal instability and no displacement. In this treatment technique, the patient's dentures should be taken away until healing has occurred, so that they do not overly traumatize the fracture site. Many patients with edentulous mandibles have other health problems, are not well nourished, and are often elderly. Therefore, this group of patients is likely to have a result that includes poor wound and bone healing, and such factors must be considered in treatment selection.

The location of the inferior alveolar nerve and canal should be noted in screw or drill hole (wire) placement. In the severely atrophic mandible, the nerve is in the soft tissue directly over the surface of the superior border of the mandible because of bone atrophy. It must be avoided in intraoral open reduction techniques.

The use of plating through either an intraoral or extraoral approach is simple and direct and provides tremendous mechanical advantage. Plates placed near the upper border of a body fracture provide a fulcrum against which the muscle forces tending to displace the anterior mandible inferiorly are most effectively neutralized, but in mandibles less than 20 mm in height, an upper border plate may not be possible. The posterior fragment of the mandible is displaced upward by the posterior (elevator) mandibular muscles. The anterior fragment of the mandible is displaced downward by the pull of the anterior (suprahyoid) mandibular muscles. Some plates placed in the inferior portion of the mandible for fractures of the mandibular body do not as effectively oppose the tendency of the superior border to "gap." This unfavorable situation results in a tendency for the fracture fragments to separate at the superior border, and the forces are best neutralized by a superior border plate. A long reconstruction plate technique in fractures in which bone height is less than 20 mm is recommended. In edentulous mandible fractures that are less than 20 mm in height, the two-plate technique is not possible because of technical considerations, and a long reconstruction plate is preferred.

In extraoral open reductions, cancellous bone graft may be packed around the fracture site to assist healing in fractures in which the bone height is less than 15 mm. The rate of infection is higher in intraoral open reductions with bone graft compared with extraoral procedures.

EXTERNAL PIN FIXATION. An external pin fixation device has been used for long bone fractures since the 19th century and was described by Lambotte[246] for facial injuries in 1913. Roger Anderson[247] popularized its use in fractures of the facial bones in 1936. Currently, this technique is rarely used in facial injury treatment because of the reliability, technical superiority, rigidity, and improved nursing and comfort of the patient available with internal fixation. The most popular device used in the 1980s was the Joe Hall Morris biphasic fixation appliance, which was described by Morris[248] in 1949. This is a stable, easily used device that employs an acrylic connector between Vitallium bone pins. The pins are set in hand-drilled holes to minimize bone resorption. External fixation was most popular in the period from 1936 to 1945.

Indications for external fixation include the multiply fractured mandible (to provide additional stability), fractures in the edentulous mandible, infected fractures or fractures with nonunion, and mandibular fractures with bone or bone and soft tissue defects. Light mobilization of the jaws may be accomplished with an external fixation device in place. The devices are less stable than internal fixation with large plates. Little can be added to Morris' excellent original description of the technique,[248] which involves the initial use of a primary connector that is a mechanical set of metal arms to hold the screws (which have first been inserted into the bone fragments) in a certain relationship. A good illustrated description also exists in the Walter Lorenz catalogue. The primary connector is a metal "rig" that is used to position the bone fragments and their screws until the secondary phase, employing an acrylic connector bar, can be completed. The connector bar is mixed from acrylic components, then placed onto the threaded portions of the screws and allowed to harden (see Fig. 66-65). The primary connector (initial reduction device) is then removed. The external fixation device can be worn for a considerable time (patients have worn them for up to 6 months) and permits motion, making possible oral hygiene, diet, speech, and absence of intermaxillary fixation. The disadvantages of the device include the lack of total rigidity, possible facial nerve or parotid damage from the placement of pins, cutaneous scarring in the pin sites, and possibility of less accurate occlusal relationships because of some differences in the reduction stability. Currently, locking plates are preferred where feasible.[112]

EARLY COMPLICATIONS

Hemorrhage

The early complications seen in the treatment of mandibular fractures include hemorrhage into soft tissues that requires drainage if it is localized. Extensive bone and soft tissue injury may accompany fractures. Some symphysis and parasymphyseal fractures, for instance, are accompanied by a tear in the soft tissues longitudinally in the floor of the mouth, which may extend as far as the pharynx. This tear opens the deep spaces of the neck to blood and saliva and potentially permits infection of the deep spaces of the neck, which may track from the neck into the thorax.[173,249] If such a tear is present, the tissue in the floor of the mouth should (after irrigation and débridement) be closed in layers with a drain in the dependent portion of the wound led externally, and antibiotic coverage is employed.

Carotid Injury

Severe mandibular dislocations may damage the carotid artery, resulting in aneurysm formation or thrombosis with stroke. The condyle is frequently driven into the auricular canal, because it is adjacent to it, lacerating the canal and resulting in bleeding.[250]

Facial Nerve Injury

Fractured fragments of the ramus of the mandible may contuse or lacerate the facial nerve, causing palsy or paralysis.[158,250]

Infection

It has been proved that achieving adequate stability of bone fragments in the fracture area reduces the possibility of infection. These considerations are even more important than the potential adverse consequences of periosteal stripping, which decreases blood supply. In infected fractures, the necrotic (nonbleeding) bone can be débrided and a longer, stronger plate applied, and function may be permitted while the infection is clearing. The infected area may then be bone grafted as early as the soft tissue integrity and absence of infection permit. The soft tissue must be free of purulence, cellulitis must be eliminated, and dead space and intraoral contamination must be controlled. Although some individuals have primarily bone grafted such fractures acutely despite the presence of infection and made claims of success in this challenging situation, it is the author's recommendation that mandibular bone grafting be completed secondarily when intraoral mucosal integrity is certain and the soft tissue infection *has* been clinically cleared. "Take" of a bone graft is optimized only by optimal soft tissue conditions. Nonvascularized bone grafting (when intraoral communication with the graft site exists) is hazardous and not recommended. Antibiotics are useful in acute fracture treatment, but fracture stability, a surgically clean wound, and the integrity of mucosal closure are much more important than antibiotics, and antibiotic use is of lesser importance than achieving good fixation and good soft tissue closure. Nerves must be protected in fracture reduction.

In the face of an infection, appropriate exploration, drainage and removal of any purulent collections, and assessment of the security of fixation should be accomplished.[251,252] Any dead tissue or dead bone should be débrided. Extraoral drainage is recommended and is mandatory if the process is extensive and penetrates into the deep tissue of the neck. Any procrastination in instituting drainage of an abscess leads to the spread of infection into the bone or into the soft tissue of the neck. Devitalized fragments of bone and soft tissue must be removed.[166] It is often not necessary to remove internal fixation devices such as plates and screws. They should be checked to make sure that they are still secure and replaced if they are loose with a longer, stronger stable reconstruction plate with its screws out of the area of infection.[253] In the face of severe or persistent infection, such as osteomyelitis, it may rarely be necessary to remove the plates and screws and convert to an external fixation device. This maneuver allows control of the fracture site and bone position by use of areas of the mandible remote from the site of infection. Only rarely must bone and all internal fixation hardware be removed to clear the infection.[254]

Avascular Necrosis, Osteitis, and Osteomyelitis

The mandible has both a periosteal and a medullary blood supply. When the bone is fractured, the medullary blood supply is disturbed.[157] Stripping of the periosteum in fracture reduction will sacrifice the mandible of its secondary or cortical blood supply. The inferior alveolar artery and vein provide the medullary blood supply. Devascularized bone has the potential to experience avascular necrosis. This complication may be minimized by early replacement of well-vascularized soft tissue and limiting the motion and displacement of the bone and soft tissue. The author is a firm believer in an initial period of soft tissue rest maintained by intermaxillary fixation, which reduces the incidence of infection. This period of soft tissue rest cannot be achieved when the mandible is moving. In the presence of abscess formation, "osteitis" (infection in bone without blood supply) may progress to osteomyelitis (invasive infection) in adjacent bone with blood supply.

True osteomyelitis in the mandible is a relatively uncommon complication in the management of facial fractures and may progress through the entire mandible.[157] Localized (osteitis) infections occur with considerable frequency, but the condition rarely progresses to true osteomyelitis. The use of antibiotics and prompt drainage in an area of suppuration prevent invasive colonization of bone in most circumstances. If osteomyelitis has occurred, it is usually demonstrable radiographically as increased fluffiness and varying opacity of the bone. All sequestra of devitalized bone and any internal fixation devices in the osteomyelitis area should be removed. Control of soft tissue spread of infection is indicated with soft tissue rest, antibiotics, and removal of devitalized soft tissue. Appropriate drainage is important. The bone should be stabilized with external fixation.

LATE COMPLICATIONS

The delayed complications of mandibular fractures include delayed union, nonunion, malalignment, tooth or bone loss, coronoid or temporomandibular joint ankylosis, loss of the gingival buccal sulcus, scar tissue contracture, and malocclusion.

Temporomandibular Joint Ankylosis

Ankylosis of the temporomandibular joint may follow injury to the articular structures, including bone in the temporomandibular joint and the fibrous meniscus.[255,256] Temporomandibular joint ankylosis produces stiffness, pain, and limitation of mandibular motion. The loss of motion may be difficult to differentiate from ankylosis involving the coronoid process of the mandible.[257] The restrictive ankylosis may consist of either fibrous tissue or bone. Ankylosis of the temporomandibular joint involving bone most commonly follows intracapsular fractures involving the articular surface of the condylar head. After severe fractures, there may be aseptic necrosis with loss of the articular surface and destruction of cartilage with replacement by fibrous scar tissue. The bone proliferation and scarring that occur may produce fibrous or osseous ankylosis of the condyle to any of the surrounding structures, such as the glenoid fossa or zygomatic arch. Fibro-osseous ankylosis may occur in the ligaments surrounding the bone, such as the joint capsule and temporomandibular meniscus. Often, bony ankylosis is more common on the medial aspect of the condyle. On occasion, infection is a complicating factor in patients with ankylosis, probably occurring through communication with the ear canal. In these patients, partially vascularized or nonvascularized fragments of bone that are colonized must be removed, and a condylectomy is required. The patient must then go for a time without any joint while absence of infection is confirmed. After complete healing and confirmed absence of infection, the joint may be reconstructed with costochondral grafting or with a temporomandibular joint prosthesis.[208,258] Although CT scans taken in axial and coronal planes and Panorex examinations are helpful in determining the cause of the problem (the CT scans must have bone and soft tissue windows and axial and coronal orientation), it is sometimes difficult to differentiate coronoid from temporomandibular joint stiffness. Sometimes, operations must proceed with the ability to deal with either problem if the initial approach does not satisfy the required range of motion.

Replacement of the condylar head is most physiologic with a costal chondral graft[208,258] or by an alloplastic temporomandibular joint replacement, which may involve structures for both the condyle and the glenoid fossa. A sagittal split osteotomy may be used if the range of motion is satisfactory and malocclusion is the problem.[259]

Nonunion

In most instances, healing of the site of a mandibular fracture is accomplished within a 4- to 8-week period. Remodeling and bone healing continue histologically for 26 weeks.[260] Several studies, such as those of Amaratunga,[144,153,155] have shown that healing in many mandibular fractures is sufficient to permit early guarded motion 3 weeks after wire fixation (4 to 6 weeks is routine). The use of plate and screw fixation techniques has conceptually allowed immediate guarded motion, but most clinicians, including the author, believe in a period of rest. The controversy about immediate motion involves the potential for bone instability (such as with the use of small plates in parasymphysis fractures) and principally the detrimental effect of motion on soft tissue rest. In the author's experience, rest of 1 week is recommended, especially when there is significant soft tissue injury. Younger patients do not require as much time for healing as older patients do. Some patients with deficient bone structure, such as the atrophic edentulous mandible (<10 mm in height), may actually require bone grafts in the area of the fracture to promote healing. Healing in membranous bones is affected by the degree and type of fracture, the blood supply to the bone, the age and general nutritional condition of the patient, the presence of other conditions such as atrophy of the alveolar process, and the dental health and condition of the teeth.[261] Most investigators think that significant motion at the fracture site aggravates bone healing, but some orthopedic surgeons believe that micromotion stimulates bone healing.[262] In some fractures, interposition of soft tissue (such as muscle and fascia between the fracture bone ends) will delay or prevent healing. Anything that keeps the bone edges apart or sets them in motion begins the stage for nonunion. The largest gap that can be expected to heal is 3 mm.[263] When the mandibular body area splits in the sagittal plane, for instance, it is easy for soft tissue to be interposed between the long edges of this fracture.[264] Unless one completes a full inspection of the fracture site on all sides or a CT scan is obtained, it is easy to miss a "sagittal extension" of a mandibular body fracture from a parasymphysis or anterior body fracture and therefore fail to position the buccal and lingual cortices in proper approximation (Fig. 66-103). This fracture extension is often not appreciated on a plain film or Panorex examination.[78,265]

Poor position and reduction of fracture fragments with gaps in alignment predispose to delayed union or nonunion.[266] One of the most common predisposing factors is improper immobilization with motion at the fracture site.[267] In fractures that are comminuted, portions of bone are devascularized and may become sequestered if they are exposed to the intraoral environment. Lack of watertight intraoral closure bathes the fracture ends in bacteria, contributing to nonunion and bone infection. Debilitated or poorly nourished patients can be expected to heal more slowly and to have an increased chance for development of nonunion. If one examines series of patients with nonunion of fractures, the body of the mandible is the site most often affected.

The healing of mandibular fractures is best assessed by clinical examination. Radiographic examinations

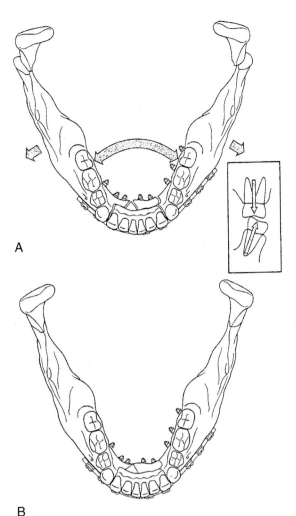

A

B

FIGURE 66-103. As the proper width of the mandible is achieved, fractures in the anterior symphysis-parasymphysis area tend to "gap" on their labial surface. *A,* If insufficient correction of mandibular width is achieved, the fractures appear to be in reduction on the buccal surface anteriorly, but there is actually excessive width at the angles, allowing the lateral mandibular segments to rotate lingually, tipping the direction toward the tongue and causing a lingual open bite by bringing the lingual palatal cusps out of alignment. *B,* Correct fixation of the symphysis fracture by means of a long, correctly bent reconstructive plate. (From Assael LA: Craniofacial fractures. In Prein J: Manual of Internal Fixation in the Craniofacial Skeleton: Techniques as Recommended by the AO/ASIF Group. New York, Springer-Verlag, 1997:102.)

may show persistent radiolucency at the fracture site, even in the presence of solid bone union. In membranous bones of the facial region, it is not necessary to demonstrate the radiopacity of a fracture site as a criterion of bone union. Craft[268] studied the mineralization patterns of membranous bones and found that bone healing was present, but the mineralization was not of the character to demonstrate radiopacity.

In many instances, "nonunion" is really a "delayed union" and responds to a short period of increased immobilization. Any nonunion or delayed union should prompt a thorough assessment of the fracture site, both clinically and radiographically. The degree of motion in three planes (transverse, vertical, and anteroposterior) should be assessed. In most instances, some motion is observed in one or two planes, but not in all three. These findings indicate the potential for union, and either a brief period of immobilization (such as intermaxillary fixation) or re-exploration of the fracture with bone gap plating (four solid fixation screws in good bone on each side of the fracture) should be employed. A thorough radiologic examination of the fracture site should be performed to detect abscessed teeth, the presence of tooth fragments in the fracture site (e.g., root tips), periapical infection in fractured teeth, or other factors that might predispose to poor bone healing. Rounding or sclerosis at the fractured ends with radiolucency suggests nonunion. In patients with more advanced defects, dense eburnated bone is noted covering the ends of the fracture segments. These patients require resection of the nonunion to good bone, bone gap-type plate stabilization (reconstruction plate), and possible bone grafting.

Nonunion may occur under plate and screw fixation by resorption of comminuted bone and not be detectable until the plate and screw fixation is removed. Therefore, if one is removing large plates for palpability or cold sensitivity, the patient should be warned that if the area of bone healing is not complete, additional fracture fixation will be required, that is, revision of the fracture with débridement of the products of nonunion, with plate and screw bone gap fixation of the nonunion and bone grafting. In this situation, cancellous bone is compacted and placed into the area between the resected bone ends, or cortical-cancellous bone graft may be cut to fit the defect, interposed, and stabilized, and the defect site is then surrounded with compressed cancellous bone.

In most instances, management of nonunited fractures is surgical. The bone ends must be exposed, preferably through an extraoral approach, and an attempt made to avoid intraoral communication. The eburnated bone and edges of the bone at the fracture site should be removed with bone burrs or rongeurs back to normal bleeding bone. Any evidence of infection should prompt eradication of the infection and delay in grafting. There are those who have described the immediate treatment of infected fractures with simultaneous bone grafting.[259] It is still wise to totally eliminate soft tissue infection before any definitive bone grafting is performed. One may span the defect in the bone with bone gap plate and screw fixation, using the principles of bone defect fracture treatment or external (Joe Hall Morris) fixation.[248] When the conditions are surgically appropriate, bone continuity should be reconstructed with a bone graft. This can be a combination of cortical bone cut to fit the defect with packed cancellous bone around it, or it may consist entirely of packed cancellous bone. These bone grafts are generally taken from the anterior or posterior iliac crest.[269] Wolfe and Kawamoto[270] described the approach in detail. The use of an external fixation device or reconstruction plate fixation eliminates the motion permitted with interosseous wires and the need for intermaxillary fixation. It is the author's preference to immobilize the mandible for a brief period, such as a week, to allow soft tissue consolidation and soft tissue rest. In many patients with nonunion, there is insufficient bone present to bridge the gap between the bone ends without forming a defect or a weak area in the dental arch, which will ultimately fracture. Bone grafts are always preferable to questionable bone contact. One may assume that bone is weak in this area, otherwise consolidation would have been obtained previously. Consideration must be given to the adequacy of soft tissue and to the integrity of the intraoral lining, which determines the soft tissue blood supply for healing. Integrity of intraoral lining is important to prevent infection.

Mathog[263,271] has written two good papers on nonunion of the mandible. The significance is that one was before and one after rigid fixation. Nonunion of the mandible, based on a series of 1432 fractures, had an incidence of 2.8%. Patients likely to sustain nonunions were men who had fractures as the result of an altercation; factors associated with nonunion were body fracture location, multiple fractures (especially delayed treatment), teeth in the fracture line, alcohol and drug abuse, and early removal by the patient of fixation devices. He found osteomyelitis to be a common complication; one fourth of the patients were believed to be stabilized insufficiently, and 1 of 25, or 4% of the nonunion group, had a poor initial reduction. Secondary treatment included external fixation with or without bone grafting in half and plate fixation with or without bone grafting in half. Only one of the patients was able to be treated with maxillomandibular fixation alone. More than half of the patients were thought to have associated osteomyelitis. Under those conditions listed for mandibular fractures, 80% of the patients are men with an altercation history in 77%, history of drug or alcohol abuse in 72%, premature removal of maxillomandibular fixation in 20%, and delay in initial treatment of more than 5 days in 32%.

Maloney,[267,272] in an editorial on Mathog's paper, thinks that the primary pathophysiologic process is the lack of early immobilization in compound fractures. He thinks that simple fractures or compound fractures of the mandible treated within 72 hours of the initiating trauma will heal uneventfully whether they are treated by closed or open reduction in a patient who is compliant with postoperative instructions. Maloney's group firmly believes that delay in treatment of a compound fracture is the central factor placing the patient at increased risk for development of a bone infection or nonunion. This delay is usually intertwined with the social history of the patient.[273] They believe that treatment of a compound fracture, when it is delayed more than 72 hours, is hazardous for development of chronic bone infection if an open reduction is immediately performed, including the possibility of a chronic suppurative osteomyelitis. Osteomyelitis is initially an acute infection of the medullary bone; its progression is characterized by a gradual impairment of blood supply to the bone that may be followed by infection and nonunion.

Maloney et al[267,272] think that the primary initial management in delayed treatment of a compound fracture is to first resolve the intramedullary infection before performing an open reduction. The patient is placed in maxillomandibular fixation and given intravenous antibiotics for a period approximately equal to the period of the delay. In their protocol, a 5-day-old compound fracture is first treated with maxillomandibular fixation and 5 days of intravenous antibiotic administration before an open reduction is performed. The underlying principle of their approach is to maximize the perfusion of blood as well as antibiotics at the fracture site. In their protocol dealing with compound fractures of the mandible that are more than 72 hours old, they have successfully minimized the likelihood of the occurrence of chronic suppurative osteomyelitis and nonunion.

Malunion

Malunion of mandibular fractures results from inadequate fixation or inadequate reduction. The bone therefore heals in an abnormal position. In most patients, malunion results from inadequate fixation or inadequate initial alignment. Many times, this begins with inadequate application of arch bars. One of the most critical alignment maneuvers at the time of fracture repair is the placement of the patient in adequate intermaxillary fixation. Intermaxillary fixation should be tight, but not excessively tight, as the fragments may rotate lingually or palatally with excessive wire tightening. Temporary positioning plates and screws or wires can be used to adjust the position of the mandibular fragments before the application of definitive plate and screw fixation. Rotation of the mandible in a lingual direction at the alveolus or at the tooth margin is a common occurrence in comminuted fractures and in the parasymphyseal and bilateral subcondylar fracture, especially if the subcondylar fractures are treated closed (Fig. 66-104). Previously, the use of a lingual splint placed against the lingual surface of the teeth acted to prevent lingual rotational displacement. Visualization of the surfaces of the fracture may provide evidence of proper alignment so the plate and screw fixation can securely appose the bone fragments. Telescoping of bone segments in the ramus of the mandible may result from strong muscle forces of mastication. Shortening of the ramus occurs in condyle and subcondylar fractures and gives rise to a premature contact in the molar dentition and an open bite anteriorly and contralaterally. The first sign of this open bite is the lack of a cuspid contact. Patients with mandibular fractures must be examined at least weekly with regard to their ability to bring themselves into proper occlusion. Malunion is first observed generally in the anterior dentition, with lack of cuspid contact. At this point, if the patient is replaced in intermaxillary fixation, the malunion may sometimes be overcome by elastic traction with rubber bands applied between the mandible and maxilla. Elastic traction is effective only in early incomplete unions. When there is sufficient bone union, rubber band traction will only extract teeth rather than move the fracture site. It is emphasized that rubber band traction should never be applied anterior to the cuspid teeth without skeletal wires or an occlusal splint, which provides protection for the more delicate incisor teeth against extrusion.

The treatment of established malunion consists of a planned osteotomy, either at the site of the malunion or at another area (Fig. 66-105).[259] A condylar fracture malunion with shortening of the ramus height may be best approached by a sagittal split osteotomy secondarily if joint motion is good (>35 mm) (Fig. 66-106). This avoids the potential for mandibular ankylosis from re-entering the area of the condylar fracture about the temporomandibular joint.[256] If there is temporomandibular ankylosis and a malunion at the temporomandibular area, the preferred treatment is temporomandibular joint replacement, such as with a costal chondral graft.[258] When mandibular nonunion occurs in the body or parasymphysis area, the preferred treatment consists of an osteotomy at the site of the malunion with rigid fixation and bone grafting. Osteotomies should be designed to be oblique or "stepped" to permit realignment of bone edges and yet provide some bone contact across the osteotomized area. Bone grafting should be considered in all of these secondary patients. In all patients, only brief periods of intermaxillary fixation should be employed after the procedure to prevent further stiffness.

Malocclusion

Malocclusion is most commonly the result of insufficient or inaccurate alignment in initial reduction, which is especially common when intermaxillary fixation is poorly applied or loose. Improper intermaxillary fixation may hold a fracture in nonre-

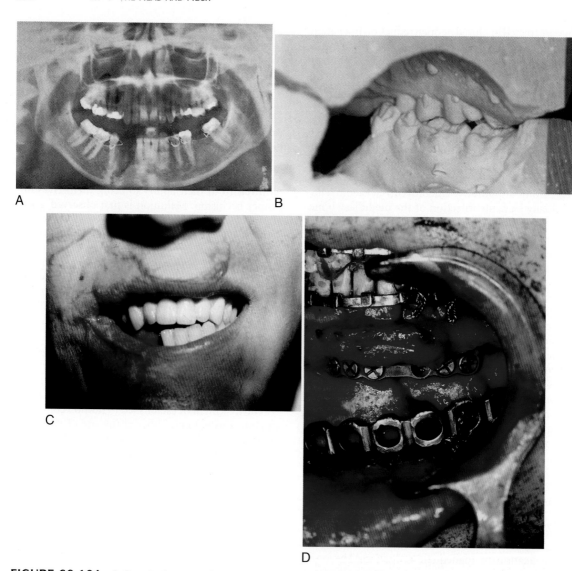

FIGURE 66-104. *A,* Developing nonunion in a parasymphyseal fracture. Bone loss and lack of contact across the fracture site are evident. Rounding and eburnation of the bone ends are apparent. *B,* A lingual splint to minimize lingual rotation of the lateral segments of the mandible. This model shows lingual rotation. *C,* Lingual rotation of fragments. *D,* The treatment involves a thorough removal of all artificial material including any abortive products of fracture healing. A resection of all the infected and nonunion portions of the fracture edges, débridement, and stabilization with a rigid internal fixation device are completed. Such fractures may be secondarily or primarily bone grafted, depending on the presence of infection and intraoral continuation.

duction. Other causes include inadequate final reduction, inadequate contouring with a plate that induces a malocclusion, and failure of fixation (such as with small plates with an insufficient number of screws, which become loose and permit dislocation). Although subtle malocclusions may be corrected by grinding the occlusal facets of the teeth, any significant malocclusion requires refracture or osteotomy. The use of small plates with minimal screws, although conceptually and technically attractive, produces malocclusion when they become unstable, which is possible when such

plates are used in fractures where there are microfractures or comminution, where the bone cannot bear the load required in fracture reduction, or in the multiply fractured mandible where a large plate is necessary to form the correct shape of the mandible.

Increased Facial Width and Rotation of the Mandible

Broadening of the distance between the mandibular angles is produced by rotation of the lateral mandibular segments lingually at the occlusal surface of the

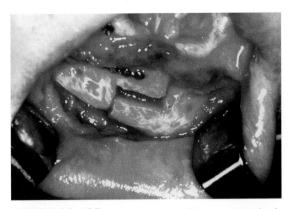

FIGURE 66-105. An osteotomy of the parasymphysis in a stepped fashion allows good bone contact plus flexibility for dealing with the movements necessary to correct the malocclusion. Such osteotomies permit more bone contact than would be provided by a straight osteotomy, where a bone graft might be required.

teeth. The lateral mandibular segments rotate externally at the lower border and angle. The distance between the mandibular angles increases as the mandible and lower face widen. This rotation (aggravated by tight intermaxillary fixation and the presence of subcondylar fractures) (see Fig. 66-103) produces a malocclusion of the buccal cusps (open bite between the buccal and palatal cusps) and a characteristic broadening and rounding of the face, which is aesthetically and functionally unacceptable. The lingual and palatal "open bite" is best observed in a dental model obtained after reduction, looking internally at the posterior dentition (the perspective is as if one were standing on the tongue viewing the inner surface of the teeth). It may also be noticed on opening the mouth by observing the lingually oblique inclination of the lateral mandibular dentition. This complication cannot be treated by orthodontia and requires refracture.[8] The use of a long, strong reconstruction plate to keep the mandibular angles rotated properly and the width (or distance between the angles) narrow is required. In symphysis and parasymphysis fractures, the body and angle segments of the mandible must be held upright by the anteriorly placed plate. Remotely, some surgeons used a lingual splint or a threaded K-wire driven through the angles to prevent this complication, but the use of a 10- to 12-hole reconstruction plate anteriorly provides the most secure and straightforward fixation. Overtightening of intermaxillary fixation wires, because they exert forces at the labial and buccal aspects of the dentition, has the tendency to result in lingual diversion of the lateral mandibular segments.

Implant Failure

Implant failures include plate fracture and screw head fracture. Most of the failures occur in defect fractures or when too *light* fixation is used. Hirai et al,[274] in 2001, found that the formation of new bone was observed around titanium bone screws in all patients. Some black particles were observed in the bone and soft tissues around titanium bone screws, and multinuclear giant cells resembling macrophages were observed near these particles. This was thought to represent "metalosis."

The feasibility of biodegradable plates[275-278] for internal fixation in the mandible in the horizontal portion, such as the angle, has not been well studied clinically. Some studies have been based on computer modeling alone.

Screw removal[183,279,280] occurs in 5% to 10% of patients, but fortunately teeth transfixed by osteosynthesis screws generally do not have problems.[229] Bone adjacent to titanium screws has been noted to have fretting corrosion.[274]

Borah and Ashmead[169] studied 387 patients during a 5-year period at a level I trauma center and documented the long-term outcome of teeth that have been transfixed by osseous fixation screws. There were 191 mandibular fractures and 281 midfacial fractures. They documented 565 plates and 2300 screws employed in the treatment. Eleven teeth were observed to be transfixed by a screw. Mandibular third molars were most common and mandibular first molars, maxillary cuspid, and mandibular cuspid next most common, in that order. All transfixed teeth mesial to a mandibular fracture site tested nonvital, as did other adjacent mesial teeth, and 100% of the erupted teeth in the proximal segment tested vital. Teeth impinged by screws did not become abscessed, nor did they require extraction more frequently than "normal" adjacent teeth. Borah concluded that impingement of tooth roots by fixation screws during osteosynthesis does not appear to adversely affect the survival of affected teeth. He also postulated that the integrity of tooth sensory innervation is primarily determined by fracture location. Unerupted teeth that were transfixed did not become infected and did not appear to require extraction more than adjacent teeth did. He concluded that although avoidance of tooth root structures during osteosynthesis with plates and screws is generally advisable, tooth root impingement by screws appears to have minimal adverse consequences.

Nasal Bone and Cartilage

The external nose is a triangular pyramid composed of cartilaginous and osseous structures that support the skin, musculature, mucosa, nerves, and vascular structures. The upper third of the nose is supported by bone that connects to the maxilla and frontal bone; the lower two thirds gains its support from a complicated interrelationship of the upper and lower lateral cartilages and the nasal septum (Fig. 66-107).

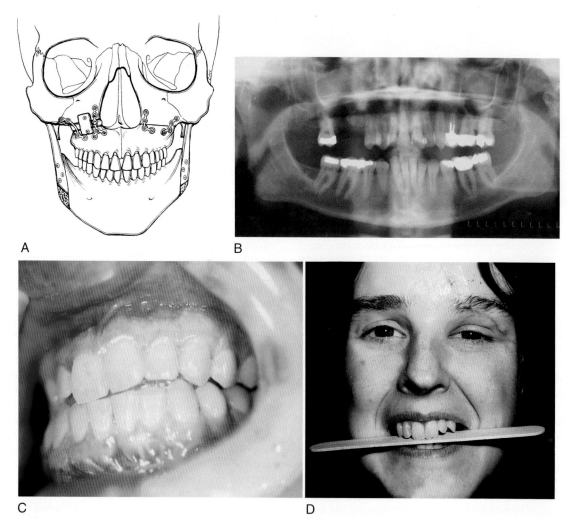

A

B

C

D

FIGURE 66-106. *A*, Sagittal split osteotomies have the potential of lengthening the ramus and reorienting the horizontal segment of the mandible and maxilla (features of malreduced condylar fractures) without re-entering the joint area. If range of motion of the joint is good, this sagittal split approach is favored. If joint range of motion is poor (<25 mm), condylar replacement should be considered. *B*, Malunion and dislocation of a condyle fracture. *C*, Occlusion reveals subtle left anterior open bite (lack of cuspid contact). No revisional surgery was performed. *D*, Lack of a level occlusal plane of the closed treatment of Le Fort and subcondylar fractures. (*A* from Manson P: Reoperative facial fracture repair. In Grotting J, ed: Reoperative Aesthetic and Reconstructive Plastic Surgery. St. Louis, Quality Medical Publishing, 1995:677.)

ANATOMY

The skin in the upper portion of the nose is freely movable and thin; in the lower portion, the skin is thick and has prominent sebaceous glands. It is densely adherent, flexible, and difficult to move, and the loss of even a small portion of nasal tip skin results in distortion. In the distal nose, the attachment of the skin to the underlying cartilaginous structures is more intimate. The entire nose skin has an excellent blood supply that permits extensive dissection with safety in the submuscular plane. The generous blood supply of the nose results in early rapid healing of both the soft tissues and the bone.

The supporting framework of the nose is made up of semirigid cartilaginous structures that are attached to the solid and inflexible bone structure of the nose (Fig. 66-107). The cartilaginous tissues include the lateral nasal cartilages, the alar cartilages, and the septal cartilage. There are several sesamoid cartilages in the lateral portions of the alae and in the base of the nasal cartilage. The cartilaginous structures support the overlying subcutaneous tissue, skin, mucosa, and lining of the nose. The cartilages are intimately attached to the bone structures, which consist of the frontal process of the maxilla, the nasal spine of the frontal bone, the paired nasal bones, and the bones of the septum, which are the vomer and the perpendicular plate of the

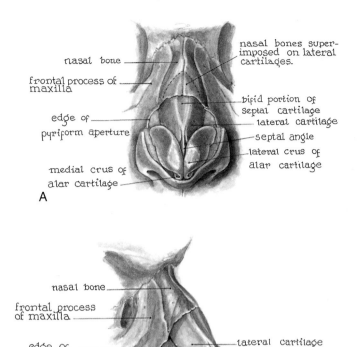

FIGURE 66-107. Anatomy of the nasal framework. *A,* Anterior view. *B,* Lateral view. (From Converse JM: Cartilaginous structures of the nose. Ann Otol Rhinol Laryngol 1955;64:220.)

ethmoid. The paired nasal bones articulate in the midline with each other, and each is supported laterally by the frontal processes of the maxilla and superiorly by the "nasal spine" of the frontal bone. The lower third of the nasal bones is thin and broad. In the proximal portion, the nasal bones are thicker and narrow in their articulation with the frontal bone. The thin portion of the nasal bones is fragile and easily fractured, whereas the thicker portions are more difficult to injure. The nasal bones seldom fracture in the upper portions, but fractures commonly occur in the lower half. In the upper portions, the bones are also firmly supported by an intimate articulation with the frontal bone and the frontal process of the maxilla and by a thickened perpendicular plate of the ethmoid.

TYPES AND LOCATIONS OF FRACTURES

Fractures in adults vary with the site of the impact and with the direction and intensity of force. Direct frontal blows over the nasal dorsum result in fracture of the thin lower half of the nose or, if more severe, may cause separation at the nasofrontal suture. The margins of the piriform aperture are thin and also may be easily fractured. Piriform aperture fractures may be associated with fractures of the nasal bones and may

extend through the frontal process of the maxilla (Fig. 66-108).

Lateral forces[281] account for the majority of nasal fractures and produce a wide variation of fractures and deformities, depending on the age of the patient and intensity and direction of force. Younger patients tend to have fracture-dislocations of larger segments, whereas older patients with more dense, brittle bone often exhibit comminution. Kazanjian and Converse[94] and Murray et al[282] confirmed that most nasal fractures occur in thin portions of the nasal bone. In the Kazanjian and Converse series, 80% of a series of 190 nasal fractures occurred at the junction of the thick and thin portions of the nasal bones.

An anteroposterior blow results in decreased stability; the septum "telescopes," losing height, and the nasal bridge drops. Violent blows result in multiple fractures of the nasal bones and frontal processes of the maxilla, lacrimal bone, septal cartilages, and ethmoidal areas, the nasoethmoidal-orbital fracture.[283,284] These bones are driven into the nose, and displaced fractures occur with damage to the bony portion of the nasolacrimal apparatus, the perpendicular plate of the ethmoid, the ethmoid sinuses, the cribriform plate, and the orbital plate of the frontal bone. Displacement in these severe comminuted fractures

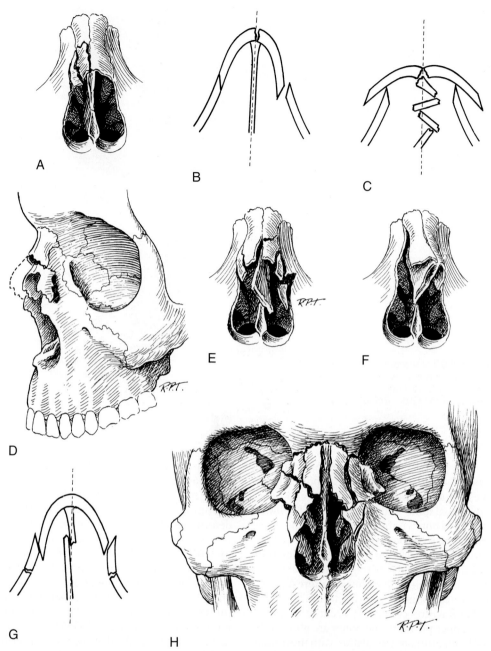

FIGURE 66-108. Various types of fractures of the nasal bones. *A* and *B,* Depressed fracture of one nasal bone. *C,* "Open book" type of fracture as seen in children. *D,* Fracture of the nasal bones at the junction of the thick upper and thin lower portions. *E,* Comminuted fractures of the distal nasal bone. *F* and *G,* Fracture-dislocation of the nasal bones. *H,* Comminuted fracture of the nasal bones involving the frontal processes of the maxilla. The canthal ligament-bearing bone has been fractured, causing a true nasoethmoidal-orbital fracture. On the left side, the central fragment (bone to which the canthal ligament is attached) is intact. On the right side, the canthal ligament-bearing bone fragment is split horizontally. Note the fractures of the piriform aperture. (From Kazanjian VH, Converse J: Surgical Treatment of Facial Injuries, 3rd ed. Baltimore, Williams & Wilkins, 1974.).

(nasoethmoid) results in broadening and widening of the interorbital space with a posterior displacement of the nasal bones and lateral displacement of the medial canthal ligaments, producing post-traumatic telecanthus (Fig. 66-109; see also Fig. 66-108).[285] These fractures are true nasoethmoidal-orbital fractures, which occur in a variety of combinations with associated fractures of adjacent bones, such as the frontal bones, zygoma, and maxilla, or fractures of the Le Fort variety.[286] Fractured bone segments in more severe nasal injuries may be driven into the nasolacrimal system at various levels, resulting in obstruction. Permanent epiphora may occur. Telescoped and comminuted nasal fractures involving the nasoethmoidal and frontal area are commonly seen after severe "frontal impact" injuries. Frequently, the entire central middle third of the face has struck an object, such as an instrument panel or some other projecting object inside an automobile. These fractures are not isolated nasal injuries but represent the end stage of the frontal impact or central midfacial fracture, that is, the nasoethmoidal-orbital injury.

Fractures and dislocations of the septal cartilages and septal bone may occur independently of or concomitantly with fractures of the distal nasal bone framework. Most commonly, the two injuries occur together, but frontal impact nasal fractures carry the worst prognosis regarding preservation of nasal height.[287,288] Because of the intimate association of the bones of the nose with the nasal cartilages and bony nasal septum, it is unusual to observe fractures of either structure without damage to the other.[289] In particular, the caudal or cartilaginous portion of the septum is almost always injured in nasal fractures.[290,291] The caudal portion of the septum has a degree of flexibility and bends to absorb moderate impact.[288] The first stage of nasal septal injury is fracturing and bending of the septum; the next stage involves overlap between fragments, which reduces nasal height. In midlevel severity injuries, the septum fractures, often initially with a C-shaped or double transverse component in which the septum is fractured and dislocated out of the vomerine groove.[292] Displacement of the fractured segment occurs with partial obstruction of the nasal airway. The cartilage may be fractured in any plane, but the most frequent location of the fracture is that described with horizontal and vertical components separating the anterior and posterior portions of the septum. As the cartilage heals, it can exhibit progressive deviation with warping forces due to the stresses exerted by the perichondrium. Ten Koppel[293] has classified the depth of cartilage injury necessary to produce distortion. In general, the injury must extend more than halfway through the thickness of the septum to produce distortion by release of elastic forces. Cartilage is thought to possess an inherent springiness; internal stresses are released when tearing of the perichondrium on one side of the cartilage occurs. If the perichondrium and cartilage are torn, the septum tends to deviate away from the torn area toward the intact perichondrial side. Severe fractures of the septum are additionally associated with telescoping displacement, resulting in a collapse with a Z-shaped overlapping and displacement of the septum[294,295] (see Fig. 66-108). The septum is shortened, giving rise to a retruded appearance in profile of the cartilage and also the columellar portion of the nose (Fig. 66-110). Slight loss of the dorsal nasal height can give rise to a nasal hump, at the junction of the septum with the nasal bones. The loss of septal projection distally produces a retrusion and slumping in the dorsum below the bone that looks like a nasal hump, whereas the bone remains in better position. Superior angulation of the caudal portion of the septum is frequent and can be indicative of a septal fracture with loss of columellar support. It is confirmed by palpation of the caudal septum with absence of resistance beneath the columella. A dual component loss of septal support occurs in both the dorsum and the columella.

CLASSIFICATION

Nasal fractures can be divided into lateral impact and frontal impact varieties (see Fig. 66-109) after Stranc and Robertson.[281] Frequently, components of each type of displacement may be seen in the same injury.

Lateral Impact

In plane I (see Fig. 66-109) lateral impact nasal fractures, a unilateral displacement of one nasal bone into the nasal cavity occurs. In plane II lateral impact injuries, moderate medial (internal) displacement of the ipsilateral nasal bone is accompanied by some outward displacement of the contralateral nasal bone. Plane III lateral impact injuries involve the frontal process of the maxilla at the piriform aperture on one side and are in fact heminasoethmoidal-orbital fractures.

Frontal Impact

Plane I frontal impact injuries involve the distal ends of the nasal bones and are usually bilateral but worse on one side. Plane II frontal impact nasal fractures displace at least the lower half of both the nasal bones and are accompanied by some telescoping of the septum. There is almost always a reduction in nasal height, with the bone decrease usually less than the height decrease of the cartilaginous septum. This deformity presents clinically as a dorsal nasal hump. This can be managed primarily or secondarily by a reduction rhinoplasty, which reduces the height of the existing bony nasal dorsum to match the height of the

Text continued on p. 196

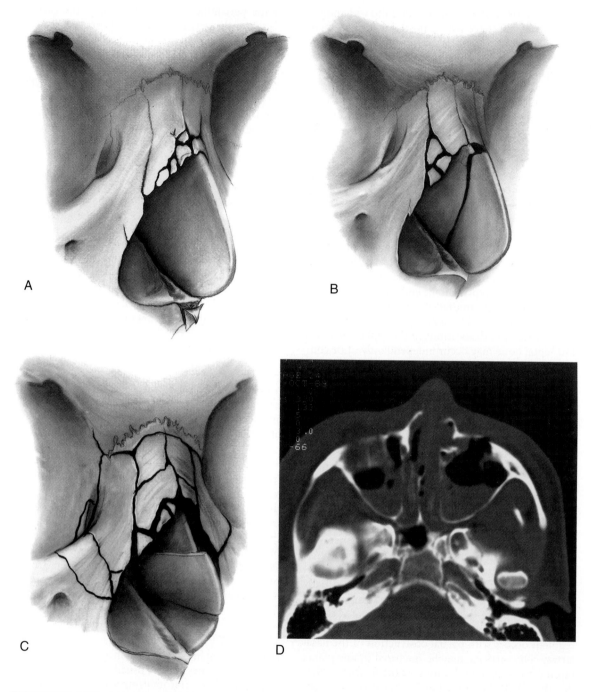

FIGURE 66-109. Stranc classification of displacement after nasal fractures. Frontal impact nasal fractures are classified by degrees of displacement, as are lateral fractures. *A,* Plane I frontal impact nasal fracture. Only the distal ends of the nasal bones and the septum are injured. *B,* Plane II frontal impact nasal fracture. The injury is more extensive, involving the entire distal portion of the nasal bones and the frontal process of the maxilla at the piriform aperture. The septum is comminuted and begins to lose height. *C,* Plane III frontal impact nasal fractures involve one or both frontal processes of the maxilla, and the fracture extends to the frontal bone. These fractures are in reality nasoethmoidal-orbital fractures because they involve the lower two thirds of the medial orbital rim (central fragment of the nasoethmoidal-orbital fracture) as well as the bones of the nose. *D,* CT scan of plane I frontal impact nasal fracture.

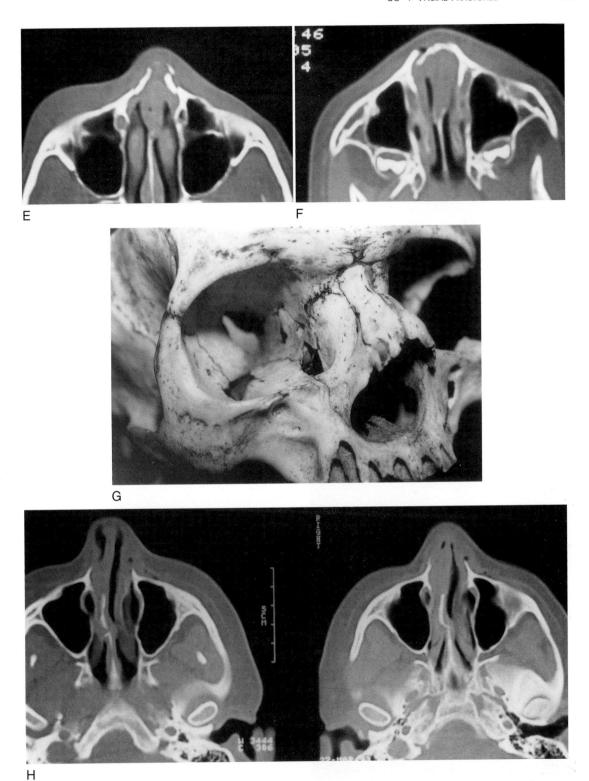

FIGURE 66-109, cont'd. *E,* CT scan of plane II frontal impact nasal fracture. *F,* Depressed frontal impact nasal fracture, plane II. *G,* Skull with heminasoethmoidal-orbital fracture. *H,* CT scan of plane I laterally deviated nasal fracture.

Continued

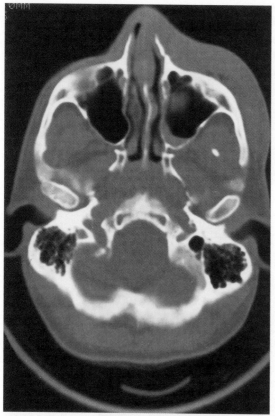

I

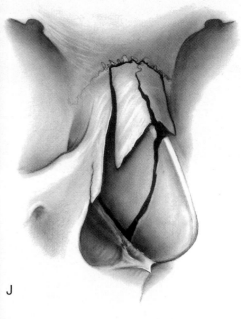

J

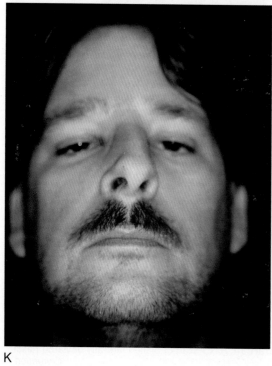

K

FIGURE 66-109, cont'd. *I,* CT scan of plane I laterally deviated nasal fracture. *J,* Plane II laterally deviated nasal fracture. *K,* Laterally deviated nasal fracture, plane II.

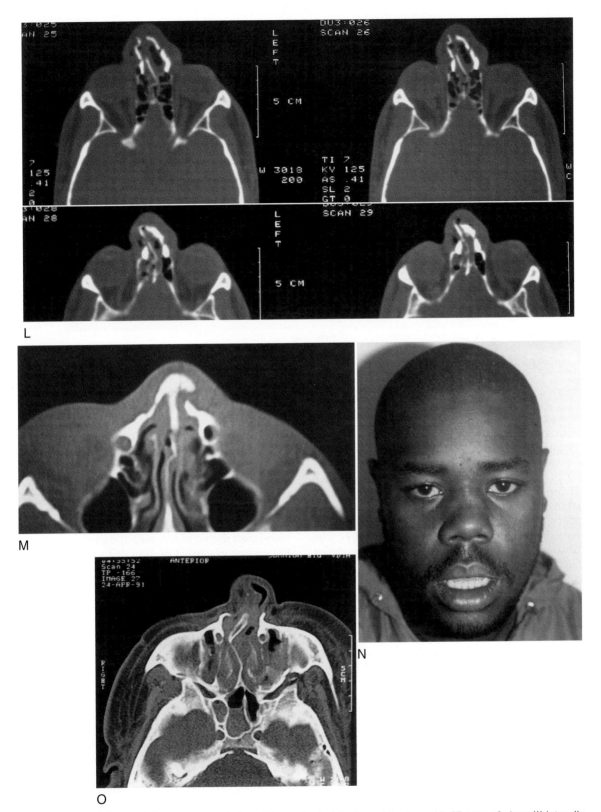

FIGURE 66-109, cont'd. *L,* CT scan of plane II laterally deviated nasal fracture. *M,* CT scan of plane III laterally deviated nasal fracture (heminasoethmoidal-orbital fracture). *N* and *O,* Patient with plane II frontal and lateral impact nasal fracture. (*A* to *C, G, J,* and *L* © Johns Hopkins University.)

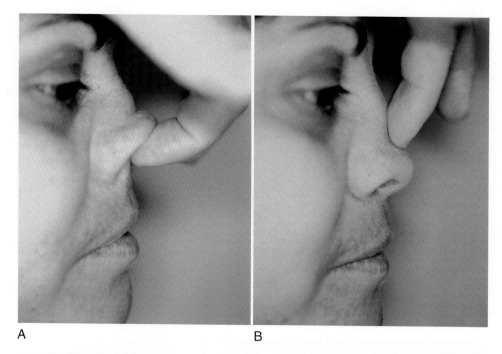

A   B

FIGURE 66-110. Palpation of the columella *(A)* and dorsum *(B)* detects superior rotation of the septum and lack of dorsal support. There is an absence of columellar support and dorsal septal support.

cartilaginous septum. Conversely, one may (by open reduction with onlay cartilage grafting over the depressed [telescoped] portion of the dorsal septum) match the height of the existing bony dorsum. Plane III frontal impact injuries are true nasoethmoidal-orbital fractures. In some patients, a severe plane II injury may mimic a plane III injury, suggesting a nasoethmoidal-orbital injury (see Fig. 66-109). The bimanual nasal examination (Fig. 66-111) to detect canthal bone-bearing (central fragment) mobility will exclude a true nasoethmoidal-orbital fracture. Palpation of the nose will also indicate the degree of existing structural support. When structural support of the dorsal nose is weak, one can depress the skin against the collapsed septum or to the superiorly rotated septum or columella. The loss of septal and columella support in the distal nose is obvious by the flattened, depressed, foreshortened nose.

DIAGNOSIS

Clinical Examination

On physical examination, there is mobility and crepitus on palpation of the nose, with tenderness over the areas of the fracture. A hematoma over the nose and extending into the periorbital area is present, which can be differentiated from the hematoma of an orbital fracture in that it is not confined to the area delineated by the insertion of the orbital septum (spectacle

hematoma). On intranasal examination, there is deviation of the septum with swelling and laceration of the mucosa and perhaps hematoma. Periorbital and nasal edema, ecchymosis, and dislocation may mask displacement of the bones or cartilages. The intranasal findings are more accurately evaluated if the mucosa is vasoconstricted by oxymetazoline (Afrin). Any blood clots should be removed and any hematoma of the septum evacuated or aspirated to prevent cartilaginous deformity and possibly septal or mucosal necrosis from the expanding pressure of a resolving hematoma. Drainage of the septal hematoma also minimizes the possibility of infection and minimizes the possibility of pressure necrosis. A straight or L-shaped mucosal incision is used after injection of 0.5% lidocaine and 1:200,000 epinephrine. "Quilting sutures" of 4-0 plain gut are used to prevent the reaccumulation of hematoma.

Radiographic Examination

Plain radiographs will define the nasal bone fracture (Fig. 66-112). However, CT scans provide a definitive view of the dislocation of both the bones and the cartilages of the septum. Cartilage dislocation also must be diagnosed by physical examination. Radiographic examination serves to guide treatment and to provide a legal documentation of the injury. Many individuals think that radiographs or CT scans are not absolutely necessary in nasal fracture treatment, but they do serve

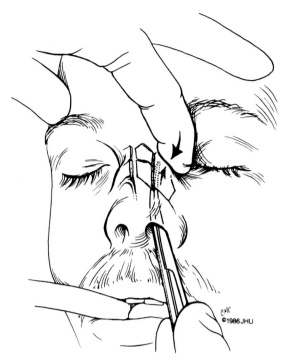

FIGURE 66-111. A bimanual examination detects central fragment instability of the nasoethmoid fracture by moving the central fragment between an external palpating finger and a clamp placed intranasally with its tip underneath the canthal ligament. (From Paskert J, Manson PN: Bimanual examination for detection of medial canthal ligament instability. Plast Reconstr Surg 1989;83:165.)

to confirm the absence of injury to adjacent bones, such as the maxilla and orbit, and to diagnose the exact pattern and displacement of the nasal and septal fracture, which may be somewhat obscured by swelling. Standard plain radiographs do not clearly reveal the exact displacement and pattern of nasal fractures. Following the suggestion of Gillies and Millard,[296] radiographs that increase the backward tilt of the occipitomental view from 15 to 30 degrees to 45 degrees provided better illustration of fractures not apparent in the usual occipitomental projection. Soft tissue techniques and profile views demonstrate fractures of the thin anterior edge of the nasal bones and the nasal spine. In practice, however, CT scans accurately demonstrate all nasal fractures and their displacement as well as exclude injury to adjacent structures, such as the frontal sinus, orbit, and nasoethmoidal-orbital area (Fig. 66-113).

TREATMENT

Nasal Fractures

Most fractures of the nasal bones are initially reduced by closed reduction techniques. In more severe frontal impacts, in which loss of nasal height and length occurs,

particularly in plane II or nasoethmoidal-orbital fractures, the use of open reduction and primary bone or cartilage grafting is beneficial to restore the support of the nose to its original volume, filling the original soft tissue envelope to prevent soft tissue contracture.[297-299] Verwoerd[300] summarized the indications for closed and open reduction in 1992, which are here modified by Metzinger et al.[288] Closed reduction is indicated in (1) unilateral depressed nasal pyramid fractures with a stable dorsum, (2) bilateral fractures with dislocation without significant loss of septal height, and (3) disruption of an upper lateral cartilage from the septal aperture. Open reduction is indicated in (1) bilateral fractures with or without lateral dislocation of the nasal dorsum and significant septal injury (potential for loss of septal height); (2) bilateral fractures with buttress dislocation (e.g., hemilateral greenstick nasoethmoidal-orbital or nasofrontal dysfunction), with or without major septal pathologic changes; and (3) fractures or dislocation of the cartilaginous pyramid with or without upper lateral dislocation, with or without injury to the bony nasal dorsum. Conceptually, the contusion and hematoma of the skin may increase the risk of skin necrosis in the open rhinoplasty approach.

It is helpful to perform a closed reduction before edema prevents accurate palpation and visual inspection to confirm the reduction (Fig. 66-114). Most simple nasal fractures may be managed on an outpatient basis.

OPEN REDUCTION. Where extensive fractures exist or open lacerations provide appropriate exposure, open reduction may be accomplished with definitive reduction and cartilage or bone grafting, when appropriate. In severe injury of the nose, that is, the plane II nasal injury, an open reduction with bone or cartilage grafting to restore nasal height may be required. Semiclosed reductions[301] may be performed with limited incisions by use of small K-wires to stabilize the nasal bones. Internal splinting[302] may be required. Some nasal fractures are sufficiently dislocated that they can only be stabilized with an open rhinoplasty reduction.[303,304] In practice, closed reduction of most nasal fractures is often deferred until the edema has partially subsided and the accuracy of the reduction may be confirmed by visual inspection and palpation. Treatment may be postponed for 5 to 7 days when required. After 2 weeks, it becomes more difficult to reduce a nasal fracture, as partial healing in malalignment has occurred, and for those fractures resulting in a reduced volume, soft tissue contracture has occurred.

A fiberoptic headlight is an essential instrument for intranasal illumination. Intranasal specula of various lengths should be provided for adequate intranasal investigation. Depressed or dislocated nasal fractures are first reduced by an upward and outward force, gen-

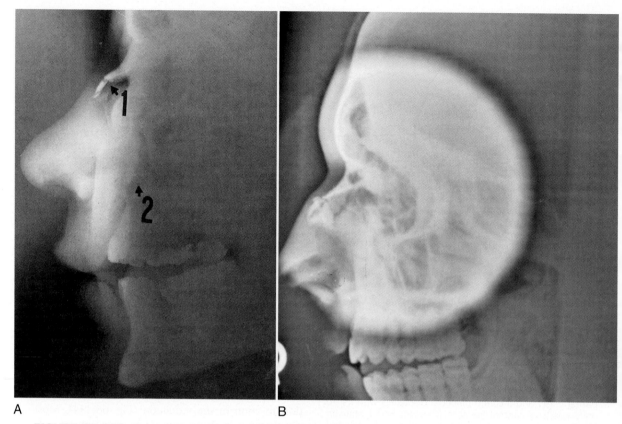

A   B

FIGURE 66-112. *A,* Lateral low-density, soft tissue radiographs are the best plain films to demonstrate the small bones of the nasal dorsum. Fractures of the nasal bones (1) are seen along with a fracture of the anterior nasal spine (2). *B,* Magnified view of the nasal bones in a comminuted nasal fracture.

erated by an instrument placed in the nose underneath the ipsilateral nasal bone. There are forceps designed for intranasal and extranasal reduction of facial fractures, such as the Asch (Fig. 66-114*B*) and Walsham (Fig. 66-115). The use of a compression forceps, such as the Walsham, can damage the skin, and sufficient control is available with the use of the back of a No. 3 scalpel handle (*without* the blade), which is the preferred method of reduction. An Asch forceps (Fig. 66-114*B*) is the required instrument for a septal fracture reduction.

The nasal bone or septal fracture must first be completed and then the bone replaced into its proper location. This is true for both the septum and the nasal bones, each as a separate maneuver. The nasal bones are manipulated upward and outward with an instrument in one hand as the other hand is used either to apply external pressure or to palpate the proper displacement and reduction of the nasal bone fragments with the pads of the fingertips. In practice, it is preferable to dislocate both nasal bones outward to each side (see Fig. 66-114), completing any fractures, and then to remold the bones inwardly with digital pressure. The septum is then grasped

with an Asch forceps, placed first in a high and then in a low position to complete the septal fractures and replace the septum into the midline. Reduction of the bony nasal pyramid often facilitates the reduction of the septum, or vice versa, in patients with complex fractures. If the nasal bones are comminuted or loose and sink posteriorly after reduction, it is preferable to support them internally with packing placed underneath the nasal bone fragments to prevent

---

FIGURE 66-113. CT scan of a severe fracture of the nasal bones. *A,* The nasal bones are comminuted. The orbit and sinus are also seen. *B,* CT scan of a laterally dislocated deviated nasal fracture. *C,* CT scan of a plane II (moderately posteriorly impacted) nasal fracture. *D,* Buttresses of the nose. *E* and *F,* Buttress disruption with plane II laterally deviated nasal fractures. *G,* Buttress disruption with plane III laterally deviated nasal fractures. *H,* Buttress deviation with plane I posteriorly dislocated fractures. *I,* Buttress deviation with plane II posteriorly dislocated fractures. *J* and *K,* Buttress deviation with plane III posteriorly dislocated fractures. (© Johns Hopkins University.)

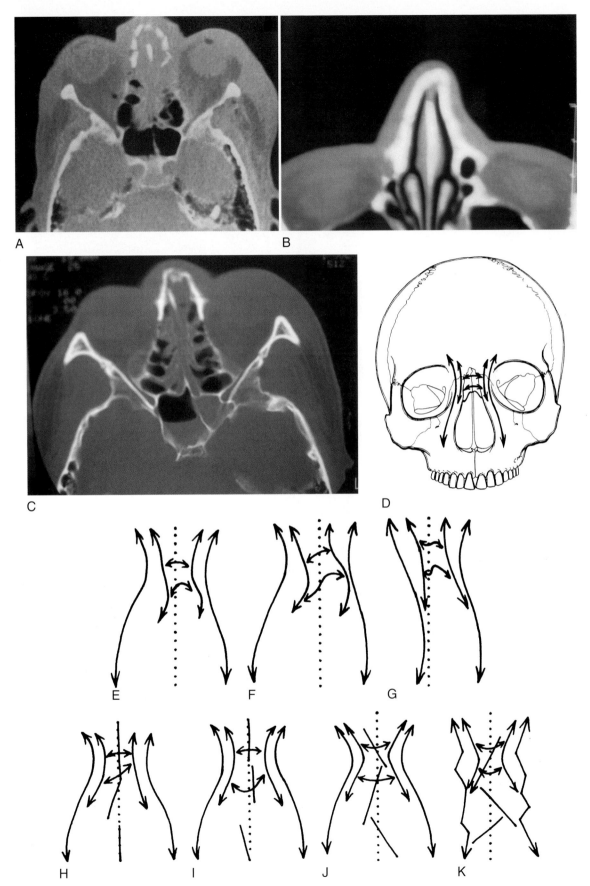

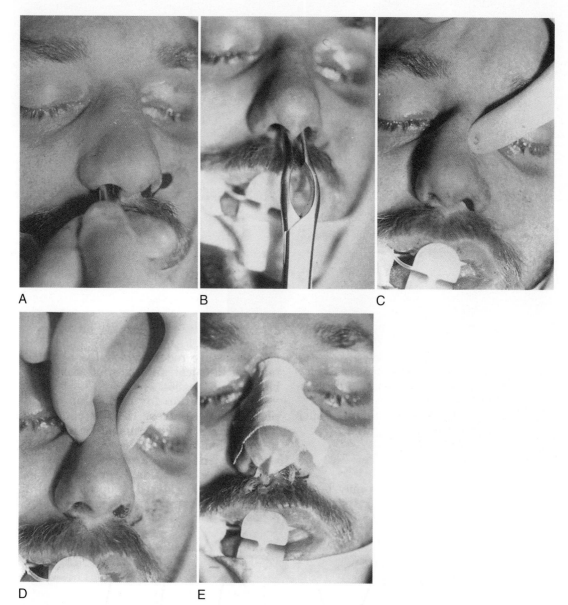

A   B   C

D   E

FIGURE 66-114. Reduction of a nasal fracture. *A,* After vasoconstriction of the nasal mucous membrane with oxymetazoline-soaked cotton applicators, the nasal bones are "outfractured" with the handle of a No. 3 scalpel *without* the blade. *B,* The septum is then straightened with an Asch forceps. Both the nasal bones and the septum should be able to be freely dislocated in each direction *(C)* if the fractures have been completed. If the incomplete fractures have been completed properly, the nasal bones may then be molded back into the midline and remain in reduction *(D).* Care must be taken to avoid placing the reduction instruments into the intracranial space through a fracture or congenital defect in the cribriform plate. The cribriform plate (vertical level) may be detected with a cotton-tipped applicator by light palpation and its position noted and avoided with reduction maneuvers. *E,* Steri-Strips and adhesive tape are applied to the nose, and a metal splint is applied over the tape. The tape keeps the edges of the metal splint from damaging the skin. A light packing material is placed inside the nose (such as Adaptic or Xeroform gauze) to minimize clot and hematoma in the distal portion of the nose. The author dislikes "adhesive-backed" splints as they place undesirable traction on nasal skin.

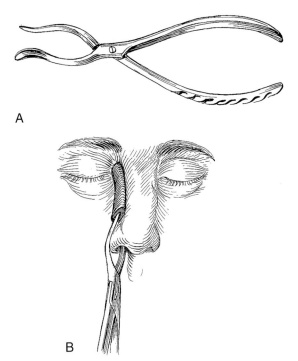

FIGURE 66-115. *A,* The Walsham forceps. *B,* Reduction of the fractured nasal bone by application of rubber tubing over the blade of a Walsham forceps. The skin may be injured by crushing, and the author prefers either the handle of a scalpel used intranasally or a small (2-mm) osteotome to complete any incomplete fractures.

the distal nasal bones from slumping posteriorly. Burm and Oh[301] have described K-wires for this purpose. This packing may be saturated with antibiotic ointment to minimize odor and infection. An external nasal splint then provides some protection and molding for the nose. Some nasal fractures may remain in position without the need for nasal packing or splints.

After the nasal bone and cartilaginous structures have been reduced and manipulated in position, intranasal packing is used to keep the septum in position, or one may use a Doyle nasal splint.* Each splint should be trimmed appropriately for smaller noses. The splint provides a section for breathing and a flat side for positioning the nasal bones and septum. Quilting sutures (4-0 plain gut on a short, straight needle) also assist approximation of the septal mucosa to the cartilage. In depressed fractures involving the distal portion of the nasal bones, a small amount of intranasal packing may be used for support of the depressed fragment to prevent displacement into the nasal cavity. It is much more comfortable for a patient to have soft

silicone (Doyle) splints than nasal packing. In addition, they do not produce as much discomfort on removal. The ability to breathe through the openings in the splint does permit an equalization of pressure in the nasopharynx during the act of swallowing and prevents the discomfort of negative pressure in the middle ear. The external splints may be of metal, plaster, or dental compound. The Brown cloth-backed nasal splint, which is a fiber-backed metal splint without adhesives (see Fig. 66-114*E*), named after Barrett Brown, is the preferred external splint. The cloth layer of the splint is moistened with collodion and placed over a two-layer dressing of Steri-Strips and one layer of $^1/_2$-inch regular adhesive tape. Collodion is applied with a cotton applicator to the cloth on the back of the splint. Both intranasal and external splints are removed, generally, in a week. A 1 × 4-inch strip of Xeroform gauze is placed anterior to the Doyle splint in each nostril and removed the day after the reduction. The gauze prevents the collection of blood in the anterior portion of the nose, which, if it is clotted and adherent, sticks to the sutures, obliterates the airway, and is difficult to clean or remove.

PERCUTANEOUS COMPRESSION. Closed techniques for severe plane II frontal impact nasal fractures include placement of Doyle nasal splints internally and use of percutaneous compression bolsters, which are used in moderately depressed plane II frontal impact nasal fractures in which there is loss of septal height and a tendency to slumping of the nasal dorsum and lateral splaying of the nasal bone fragments with loss of nasal height and increased width of the nose. In these injuries, there is often telescoping, overlap, and depression of the nasal bone and cartilages, especially in the cartilaginous portion. The cartilaginous injury and displacement are not visible on radiographic examination. There is a tendency for the nasal bones to sink posteriorly, pulled by gravity, scar tissue, and the forces of spherical contracture. The structures are displaced laterally, and a wide flat nose occurs.

Adequate control of the width of the nose in displaced nasal bone and cartilage fractures in significant plane II frontal impact fractures is facilitated by the application of a Xeroform gauze compression bolster wrapped over a nasal bone-sized half-thickness of orthopedic felt, compressed by a 2.0-mm Supramid plastic plate applied external to the Xeroform-wrapped orthopedic felt padding. Percutaneous wires are placed inferior to the base of the nose just distal to the bones of the nose and just above the piriform aperture and through fractures of the nasal bones or across the nasal fossa. The wires are led through the septum and passed across the nose with a straight No. 18 spinal needle, or a curved (Mayo) needle is used to "walk" the wire through the sites of the nasal bone fractures (Fig. 66-116).

*Xomed, Jacksonville, Florida.

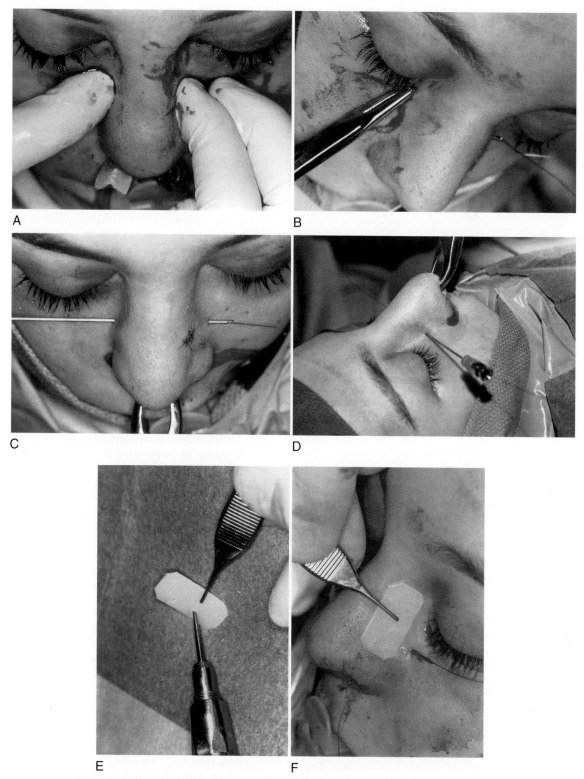

FIGURE 66-116. *A,* Treatment of a severe plane II nasal fracture with soft compression plates. *B,* The wires are "walked" through sites of nasal fracture on a large needle. *C* and *D,* Distal septal wire is passed below the piriform aperture with a spinal needle; light pressure is applied to the skin for molding of nasal bones, controlling the width and height of the nose, and for reapproximation of the skin to the bone, preventing hematoma, fibrosis, and thickening. *E,* Compression plate is 2.0 mm Supramid. *F,* Plate is sized to the nose.

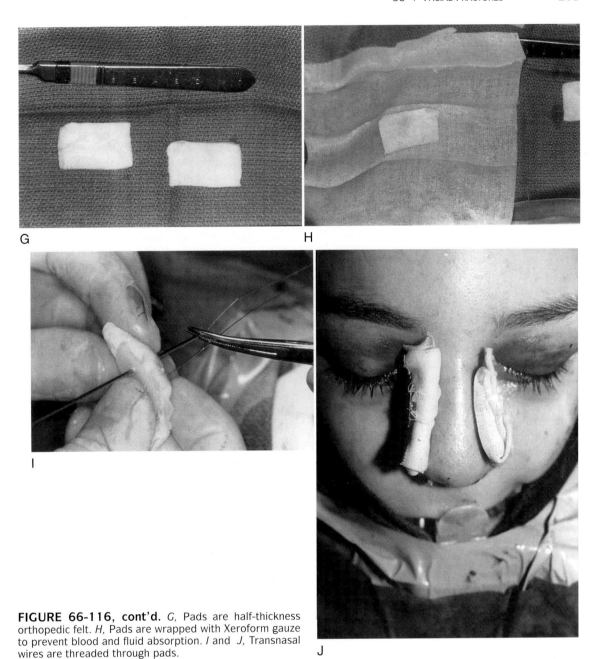

FIGURE 66-116, cont'd. *G,* Pads are half-thickness orthopedic felt. *H,* Pads are wrapped with Xeroform gauze to prevent blood and fluid absorption. *I* and *J,* Transnasal wires are threaded through pads.

The distal wire is placed just inferior to the nasal bone margin at the junction with the maxilla at the piriform aperture and across the septum. The nasal structures are elevated at the time of transfixion by placing an Asch forceps underneath the nasal bones and lifting upward.

These "compression plates" prevent hematoma from occurring between the skin of the nose and the nasal bones, or cartilages, and they serve to narrow the nose and improve the height of the nasal dorsum by medial compression. These maneuvers cannot be accomplished as accurately with closed reduction or standard nasal splints because the bones slip "out from under" the splint.

Plane III (or nasoethmoidal-orbital) fractures *always* require open reduction and cannot be treated by transnasal wiring or compression plates alone. Similarly, plane II nasal fractures may have an open reduction through lacerations or an open rhinoplasty approach. More extensive fractures in which height is lost require a complete open reduction, interfragment wiring, or plate and screw fixation. External plates can serve only to narrow the nose, to preserve nasal height, and to prevent hematoma from thickening the skin. These bolsters and plates remain in place for about 1 to 2 weeks, and one must clean thoroughly underneath them on a *daily* basis with antiseptics to prevent infection at the site where the wire goes through the nose. Ulceration occurs quickly, facilitated by the moist environment, with *Pseudomonas* causing skin necrosis. Any ulceration should be allowed to heal spontaneously by contraction. Troublesome nasal bleeding may be controlled by packing or Merocel splints.

COMPOUND NASAL FRACTURES AND ACUTE OPEN REDUCTION. Compound nasal fractures permit an accurate open reduction of the nasal bones or cartilages. It may be performed through the laceration, but if a laceration does not exist, an open rhinoplasty, conventional closed rhinoplasty, or transverse incision in the radix could be considered. The external wound is used for an open reduction, and the nasal fracture fragments are accurately reduced with fine No. 30 or No. 32 wires or small 1.0-mm plate and screw fixation. The cartilage structures may be reunited to the bony dorsum with clear nylon sutures or with fine wires. Careful repair of the nasal lining and the muscle and subcutaneous layers of the nose in layers permits accurate, level skin closure. One is often impressed by the dramatically superior result that can be obtained from such open reduction techniques, in contrast to that obtained by closed reductions (Fig. 66-117). Immediate bone or cartilage grafting may be considered for restoration of dorsal contour or columellar support where nasal height and length are lost.

Fractures and Dislocations of the Septum

The nasal septum should be straightened and repositioned as soon after the injury as possible. When fractures of the nasal bones and septum occur simultaneously, it is important at the time of reduction that the bone fragments can be freely deviated in all directions to ensure completion of the fracture. In terms of the nasal bones, they should be able to be deviated freely in both lateral directions to indicate satisfactory completion of any greenstick fractures. Incomplete fractures will cause the nasal bones to slowly "spring" back toward their original deviated position. When the reduction is incomplete, there is early recurrence of displacement. This is true for both the nasal bones and the septum. When the nasal bones are reduced, the intimate relationship of the nasal bones with the upper and lower lateral cartilages tends to reduce the upper septal cartilage as well. Displacement of the cartilaginous septum out of the vomerine groove will not be reduced with nasal bone reduction alone. The correction of the position of the bony and cartilaginous septum must be completed with an Asch forceps, and the septal fragments must be maintained

in position with an intranasal splint. In some patients, the septum should be reunited with the anterior nasal spine with a direct wire or suturing technique. This is commonly required in nasoethmoidal-orbital fractures. Cartilage, by virtue of the elastic forces in the perichondrium, is subject to deforming forces that even further displace the cartilage after injury.

When nasal fractures are treated more than a week after the injury, and especially after 2 weeks, it may not be possible to obtain the desired result with a single operation (Fig. 66-118). Osteotomies may be necessary.[305] Partial healing may make the reduction of the displaced or overlapped fragments difficult and less stable, and these patients often require a subsequent rhinoplasty. Although some individuals have performed open reductions routinely in nasal fractures, this amounts to resecting telescoped portions of the septum and additional osteotomies, and such procedures are generally best performed secondarily when the initial swelling has disappeared and bone healing is complete. A more predictable result is usually obtained with secondary elective (late) rhinoplasty. The exception is a unilateral greenstick nasoethmoid fracture.

Acute open reductions of the septum are usually performed by removal of overlapped cartilage, and therefore they inevitably result in a loss of nasal height. It is possible to establish a septal perforation by too much dissection or to excessively reduce nasal height by removal of too much cartilage. All patients with nasal fractures should be warned that a late rhinoplasty may be indicated for correction of residual or recurrent deviation of the nose, irregular nasal height, or nasal airway obstruction. They should be warned about the natural characteristic of healing cartilage to warp, resulting in displacement.

EARLY COMPLICATIONS

Complications of nasal fractures are common and include bruising and ecchymosis with subsequent pigmentation of the skin and eyelids, nasal bleeding (either early or late), and hematoma of the nasal septum with the possibility of infection and perforation. Hematomas develop between the septal mucoperichondrium and the cartilage in fractures or dislocations of the septum as a result of bleeding (Fig. 66-119). The mucoperichondrium of the nose is profusely supplied with blood vessels, and bleeding is common. Indeed, if bleeding from the nose does not occur, the diagnosis of a nasal or septal fracture should be in question. Hematomas of the septum are often bilateral because fractures within the cartilaginous septum permit the passage of blood from one side to the other. Undrained septal hematomas lead to septal perforation or fibrosis, and the organization of the hematoma results in a thick section of cartilage material. If excess

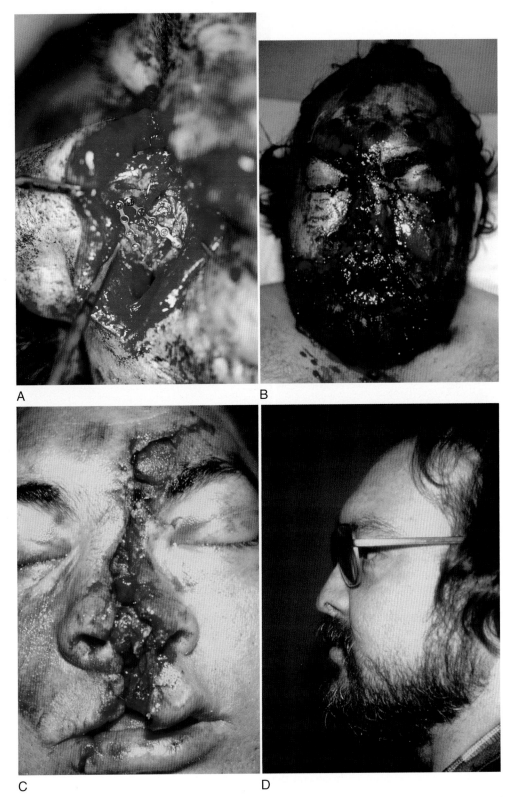

FIGURE 66-117. *A,* Open reduction with fine wires or microfixation plates should be accomplished if there are suitable nasal skin lacerations. *B,* Another patient with a heavily contaminated open nasal, nasoethmoid, Le Fort, and palatal fracture. *C,* The cleaned hemifacial laceration. *D,* Result after open reduction.

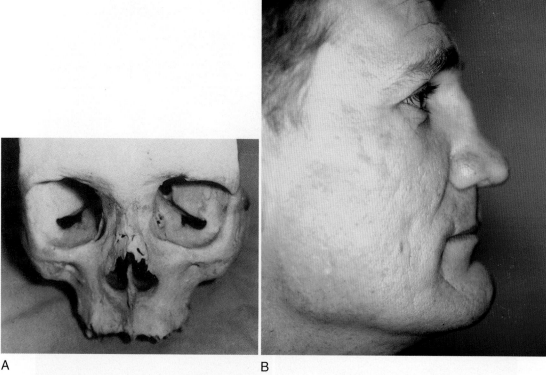

A   B

FIGURE 66-118. *A,* A healed fracture of the distal portions of both nasal bones is seen in a skull. *B,* Loss of height (saddle nose) after plane II fractures.

pressure occurs, the septum can undergo necrosis and result in perforation of the septum with symptoms of whistling, dryness, or crusting. Permanent thickening of the septum may obstruct the nasal airway. The condition is similar to the subperichondrial thickening of the auricle, commonly referred to as a cauliflower ear, that is observed after healing in undrained hematomas of the auricle. Loss of the septum is usually associated with collapse of the cartilaginous dorsum of the nose. In septal hematomas, both surgical and antibiotic therapy should be routine. Growth may be impaired in children.[306,307]

A septal hematoma is treated by incising the mucoperichondrium over the hematoma. Suction and irrigation facilitate thorough evacuation of the hematoma. The mucosa should be reapproximated to the cartilage of the nasal septum with quilting sutures (4-0 plain gut on a short [1-cm] straight needle) to prevent reaccumulation of hematoma. The incision is loosely closed to permit some drainage. In general, the hematoma should not be incised on both sides, which may facilitate a septal perforation. Drainage should not be accompanied by resection of the septal cartilage, or a septal perforation may occur.

Swelling after nasal fractures is temporary and usually disappears within 21 days. Bleeding from the nose is usually of short duration and usually ceases by 2 or 3 days. Some patients may experience rebleeding at 7 to 10 days after the initial injury. Nasal bleeding usually ceases spontaneously and may be controlled with light intranasal packing or the use of Merocel splints. In rare instances, vasoconstriction, anteroposterior nasal packing, or intranasal coagulation after identification of the bleeding point may be required.

Infection is treated by antibiotics, warm compresses, and appropriate hygiene of the skin and mucosa. Soft tissue emphysema of the face and neck may occur after displacement of air into soft tissues but rarely results in infection. Some individuals consider any nasal fracture an indication for antibiotic treatment. Patients who experience emphysema should be warned not to partially obstruct the nose as it is "blown" or air and nasal secretions will be driven into soft tissues.

LATE COMPLICATIONS

Untreated hematomas of the nasal septum may become organized, resulting in subperichondrial

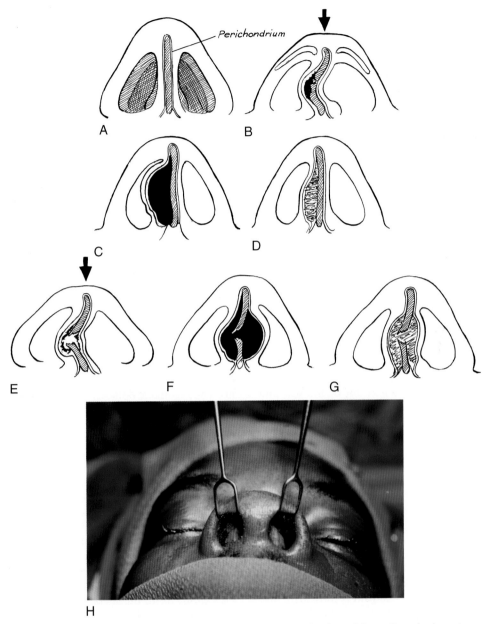

FIGURE 66-119. Hematoma of the septum. *A* and *B*, Mechanism of formation of a hematoma as a result of excessive bleeding of the mucous membrane without septal fracture. *C*, A hematoma is present. *D*, Thickening of the septum resulting from fibrosis when the hematoma is not evacuated. Pressure necrosis of the septum may occur with formation of an abscess and nasal septal perforation. *E* to *G*, Fracture of the nasal septal cartilage with hematoma and thickening of the septum with fibrosis. The hematoma may be drained by making a small incision at the proximal edge of the hematoma and aspirating it with suction. The nasal mucous membrane should be vasoconstricted to minimize rebleeding. The mucoperichondrium may be reapproximated to the septum and the dead space reduced by the use of quilting sutures, which reinforce the adhesion of the nasal mucous membrane to the septal cartilage. Splints and lubricated packing material also assist the process. *H*, Septal hematoma. (*A* to *G* from Kazanjian VH, Converse J: Surgical Treatment of Facial Injuries, 3rd ed. Baltimore, Williams & Wilkins, 1974.)

fibrosis and thickening with partial nasal airway obstruction. The septum may become as thick as 1 cm in areas and may require sculpturing or resection. In patients who have sustained repeated trauma, the cartilages of the septum may be largely replaced with calcified or chondrified material. Submucous resection of thickened portions of the nasal septum may be required; in many patients, turbinate outfracture, anterior turbinate cautery, or partial resection of enlarged turbinates may be advisable.

Synechiae may form between the septum and the turbinates in areas where soft tissue lacerations occur and the tissues are in contact.[308] These may be treated by division with placement of a splint or a nonadherent petrolatum-impregnated gauze material between the cut surfaces for a period of 5 days. During this time, partial epithelialization begins.

Obstruction of the nasal vestibule may result from malunited fractures of the piriform margin, especially if they are displaced medially. It also occurs from telescoping and overlap of the nasal septum or lateral dislocation of the nasal septum into the airway. Soft tissue contracture and loss of vestibular lining produce narrowing, which is difficult to correct without grafting material. Osteotomy of the bone fragments can correct displaced fractures; however, contracture due to loss of soft tissue may require excision of the scar and replacement with mucosal or composite grafts within the nasal vestibule or flap reconstruction.

Residual osteitis or infection of the bone or cartilage is occasionally seen in the compound fractures of the nose or fractures associated with infected hematomas, when exposed septal cartilage or bone fragments are left to be sequestered intranasally. These conditions are usually treated by repeated conservative débridement until the infected fragments are removed or sequestered. Débridement and antibiotic therapy constitute the preferred regimen of treatment. Secondary grafting may be performed where needed after an absence of infection and inflammation has persisted for 6 months. Chronic pain is infrequent and usually affects the external nasal branches.[309]

Malunion of nasal fractures is common after closed reductions. The exact anatomic position of the bone fragments can be difficult to detect by palpation alone, and closed splinting may not prevent subsequent deviation due to the release of "interlocked stresses" after fracture of the cartilage.[310,311] Any external or internal deformity of significance may require secondary reconstructive rhinoplasty, which may consist of repositioning the bone fragments alone, or it may involve cartilage or grafting techniques, such as dorsal grafts or the use of spreader grafts between the upper lateral cartilage and the septum to widen the internal nasal valve area to improve nasal airway obstruction.

The management of a nasoethmoidal-orbital fracture as a nasal fracture (mistaken diagnosis) is surprisingly frequent and may produce a severe deformity consisting of telecanthus and nasal airway obstruction, loss of nasal height, and upward tilting of the caudal nose. The skin and mucosa shrink to fit the reduced skeletal volume. Secondary corrections must involve soft tissue expansion by repeated grafting. It is preferable that severe fractures be detected and corrections completely managed at the initial treatment. A plan for operative intervention consisting of definitive open reduction techniques can be instituted only if the diagnosis and severity of injury are correctly identified.

Zygoma

ANATOMY AND SURGICAL PATHOLOGY

The zygomatic bone is a major buttress of the midfacial skeleton. It forms the malar eminence, giving prominence to the cheek, and forms the lateral and inferior portions of the orbit (Fig. 66-120). The zygomatic bone is commonly called the malar bone and has a quadrilateral shape with several processes that extend to reach the frontal bone, the maxilla, the temporal bone (zygomatic arch), and the orbital processes. The zygoma meets the maxilla medially at the inferior orbital rim and inferiorly at the maxillary alveolus. The zygomatic bone articulates with the external angular process of the frontal bone superiorly and with the greater wing of the sphenoid in the lateral orbit. In the inferior orbit, it articulates with the maxilla. The outer surface of the zygoma is convex and forms the malar eminence. On the inner surface, beyond the orbital rim, it is concave and then convex and participates in the formation of the temporal fossa. The bone has its broadest and strongest attachment with the frontal bone and with the maxilla. Thinner and weaker attachments occur with the sphenoid and through the zygomatic arch. The zygoma forms the greater portion of the lateral and inferior orbit, including the anterior half of the lateral wall of the orbit. In most skulls, the zygoma forms the lateral and superior wall of the maxillary sinus. The zygoma may thus be partially pneumatized with air cells connecting to the maxillary sinus. The bone furnishes attachments for the masseter, temporalis, zygomaticus major and minor, and zygomatic head of the quadratus labii superioris muscles. The zygomaticotemporal and zygomaticofacial nerves[312] pass through small foramina in the lateral orbit and malar eminence, respectively, to innervate the soft tissues over the region of the zygomaticofrontal junction and malar eminence.

Although the zygoma is a sturdy bone, it is frequently injured because of its prominent location. Moderately severe blows are absorbed by the bone and its buttresses and transferred to its buttressing attachments. Severe blows, such as from a fall or a fist, may cause separation of the zygoma at its articulating surfaces, and high-

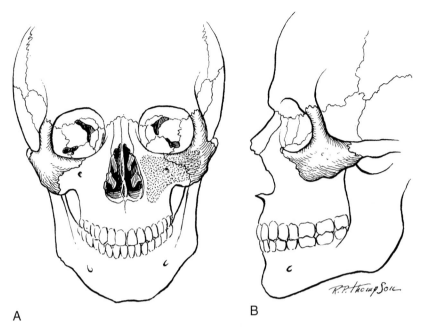

FIGURE 66-120. The zygoma and its articulating bones. *A,* The zygoma articulates with the frontal, sphenoid, and temporal bones and the maxilla. The dotted area shows the portion of the zygoma and maxilla occupied by the maxillary sinus. *B,* Lateral view of the zygoma. (From Kazanjian VH, Converse J: Surgical Treatment of Facial Injuries, 3rd ed. Baltimore, Williams & Wilkins, 1974.)

energy injuries may cause shattering of the body of the zygoma, often through weak areas such as the zygomaticofacial foramen.[312] As the zygoma is disrupted, it is usually displaced in a downward, medial, and posterior direction. The direction of displacement, however, varies with the direction of the injuring force and with the pull of the muscles, such as that of the masseter. The zygoma may be shattered, resulting in extensive comminution not only of the body of the zygoma but also of the zygoma's articulating attachments. As comminution increases, the buttressing attachments shatter into smaller pieces such that comminution through the zygomatic arch, the inferior orbital rim, and the zygomaticomaxillary buttress is seen.

The zygoma is the principal buttressing bone between the maxilla and the cranium. Fractures usually involve the inferior orbital rim and result in hematoma or extravasation of blood into tissue, which is limited by the orbital septum in terms of diffusion. A periorbital hematoma and subconjunctival hematoma are the most accurate physical signs of an orbital fracture, which can include a fracture of the zygoma (Fig. 66-121). Numbness of the infraorbital nerve is a common symptom as well. The infraorbital nerve runs in a groove in the posterior portion of the orbit and enters a canal in the antral third of the orbit behind the infraorbital rim.[313] It may be crushed in a fracture as the fracture occurs first in the rim in the

weak area of bone penetrated by the infraorbital foramen. Direct force to the lateral face may result in isolated fractures of the temporal extension of the zygoma and the zygomatic process of the temporal bone, which make up the zygomatic arch. The zygomatic arch may be fractured in the absence of a fracture of the remainder of the zygoma and its articulations (Fig. 66-122).

Medial displacement of an isolated arch fracture is usually observed, and if its displacement is sufficient, the arch itself may impinge against the temporalis muscle and coronoid process of the mandible. Fractures in the posterior portion of the zygomatic arch may enter the glenoid fossa and produce stiffness or a change in occlusion because of the swelling in the joint or muscles. Restriction of mandibular motion may be caused by displacement of the zygomatic arch medially or by posterior displacement of the body of the zygoma against the coronoid process (Fig. 66-123). Hematoma in and around the zygomatic arch and infratemporal fossa and contusion of the muscles of mastication may also interfere with mandibular motion. Swelling and bruising in these areas temporarily impair motion of the mandible and sometimes prohibit full intercuspation with regard to the occlusion. Difficulty in opening or inability to open the mouth because of interference with the forward and downward movement of the coronoid process may occur from either soft tissue swelling or bone obstruc-

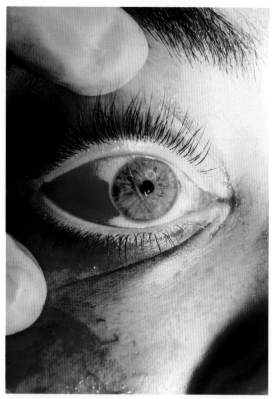

FIGURE 66-121. The combination of a palpebral and subconjunctival hematoma is suggestive of a fracture somewhere within the orbit. There is frequently a zygomatic or orbital floor fracture present when these signs are confirmed.

tion. Accurate CT examinations will disclose the nature of the impingement. In high-energy injuries or gunshot wounds, fragments of bone can be driven through the temporal muscle and make contact with the coronoid process and precipitate the formation of

a fibrous or bony ankylosis, necessitating excision of the bone of the coronoid process and any scar tissue as a secondary procedure. Zygomatico-coronoid ankylosis is particularly common after gunshot wounds.

Fracture-dislocation of the zygoma with sufficient displacement to impinge on the coronoid process requires considerable backward dislocation of the malar eminence (Fig. 66-123). About half of fracture-dislocations of the zygoma result in separation at the zygomaticofrontal suture, which is palpable through the skin over the upper and lateral margins of the orbit. Level discrepancies or step deformities at the infraorbital margin can usually be palpated in the presence of inferior and medial orbital rim displacement. The lateral and superior walls of the maxillary sinuses are involved in fractures of the zygoma, and the tear of the maxillary sinus lining results in the accumulation of blood within the sinus with unilateral epistaxis. The lateral canthal attachment is directed toward the Whitnall tubercle, located approximately 10 mm below the zygomaticofrontal suture. The ligament extends toward a shallow eminence on the internal aspect of the frontal process of the zygoma. When the zygoma is displaced inferiorly, the lateral attachment of the eyelids is also displaced inferiorly, giving rise to the visible deformity of an antimongoloid slant of the palpebral fissure (Fig. 66-124). The globe follows the inferior displacement of the zygoma with a lower (inferior) position after fracture-dislocation. Displacement of the orbital floor allows displacement of the rim. Dysfunction of the extraocular muscles may be noted as a result of the disruption of the floor and lateral portion of the orbit. The mechanism of diplopia is usually muscle contusion. Displacement of the globe and orbital contents may also result from downward displacement of the suspensory ligament of Lockwood, which forms an inferior "sling" for the globe and orbital contents. Lockwood ligament attaches to the lateral wall of the orbit adjacent to Whitnall tubercle (Fig.

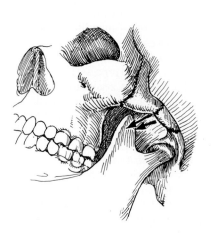

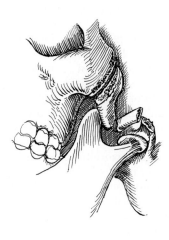

FIGURE 66-122. Fracture of the zygomatic arch with medial displacement against the coronoid process of the mandible. This may limit mandibular motion or produce an anterior open bite by blocking full occlusion of the mandible.

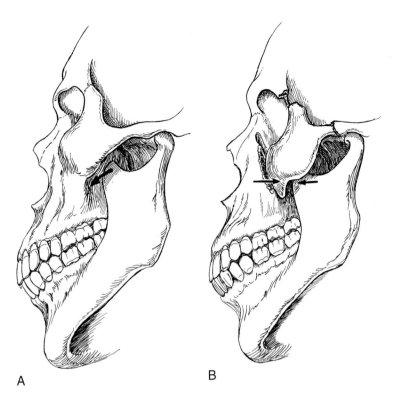

FIGURE 66-123. The intimate anatomic relationship between the zygoma and the coronoid process. *A,* As the mandible moves forward, the coronoid process must have room between the posterior aspect of the body of the zygoma and itself to permit opening movements of the mandible. *B,* If the fractured body of the zygoma is displaced backward sufficiently to impinge on the coronoid process, opening movements of the mandible are impaired. A slight open bite may be produced as a result of this impingement.   *A*   *B*

66-124). Fragmentation of the bony orbital floor may disrupt the continuity of the suspensory ligaments of the globe and orbit, and orbital fat may be extruded from the intramuscular cone and herniate into the maxillary sinus, where it may become incarcerated or attached to sinus lining or bone segments by the devel-

opment of adhesions. Double vision is usually transient in uncomplicated fractures of the zygoma, which always involve the orbital floor. Diplopia may persist when the fracture is more extensive, especially if a fracture extends to comminute the inferior orbital floor. This diplopia may be based on muscle contusion, incar-

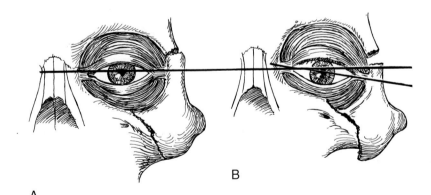

A   *B*

FIGURE 66-124. When the frontal process of the zygoma is depressed inferiorly, the lateral canthal mechanism and the canthus of the eye follow. *A,* Normal position of the lateral canthus in a fracture without displacement. The palpebral fissure slants slightly upward from the medial to the lateral canthus by several millimeters. *B,* Downward displacement of the globe and lateral canthus results from a frontozygomatic separation with inferior displacement of the zygoma. The globe and periorbita are permitted to sink into an enlarged orbital cavity, and the lateral canthus with the attachment of the eyelids and orbicularis are dragged inferiorly as a result of the displacement, producing an antimongoloid slant to the palpebral fissure.

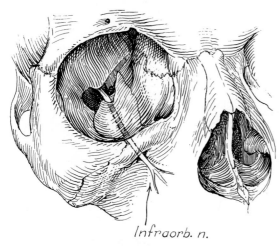

Infraorb. n.

FIGURE 66-125. The infraorbital nerve has an intimate relationship with the floor of the orbit and is almost always damaged in a fracture-dislocation of the zygoma or of the orbital floor. The resultant hypesthesia may involve the lower lid, lateral wall of the nose, upper lip, and ipsilateral medial cheek. Branches of the infraorbital nerve travel in the anterior wall of the maxilla to reach the anterior maxillary teeth. Portions or all of these nerve branches may be involved. In the anterior portion of the orbit at the rim, the infraorbital nerve is in a canal. In the midportion of the orbit, it begins to lie only in a groove, and a communication is present from the infraorbital neurovascular bundle to the inferior rectus muscle. The nerve enters the orbit posteriorly through the posterior portion of the inferior orbital fissure. (From Converse JM, Smith B: Enophthalmos and diplopia in fractures of the orbital floor. Br J Plast Surg 1957;9:65.)

ceration of perimuscular soft tissue, actual muscle incarceration, or simply drooping of the muscle sling. The orbital portion of the fracture communicates with fractures of the inferior rim of the orbit. Frequently, one or two small fragments of the maxilla at the inferior orbital rim are fractured adjacent to its junction with the zygoma, and they are called butterfly fragments. These rim fractures result in considerable instability of the rim with inferior and posterior displacement. The orbital septum attaches to the orbital rim and is also displaced downward and backward, resulting in a downward pull on the lower eyelid. The lower eyelid then has a tendency to eversion, resulting in further anatomic derangement produced by the fracture.

The infraorbital nerve (Fig. 66-125) travels obliquely from lateral to medial across the floor of the orbit.[313,314] In the posterior portion of the orbit, the nerve is in a groove; in the anterior portion of the orbit, it is located in a canal. Adjacent to the orbital rim, the canal turns downward and exits approximately 10 mm below the upper edge of the inferior orbital rim. The foramen is aligned parallel with the medial margin of the cornea when the eye is in straightforward gaze. The infraorbital nerve is often compressed by fractures because the canal and groove represent a weak portion of the bone. Laceration of the nerve in the canal, when it is crushed by impaction of bone fragments, may result in permanent anesthesia. The nerve is frequently contused, and although temporary symptoms of infraorbital nerve hypesthesia are present initially, they usually partially resolve. After zygomatic fractures, sensory disturbances of a more minimal nature have been detected in up to 40% of patients.[315-317] Persistent total anesthesia after fracture may represent an indication for exploration and decompression of the infraorbital nerve with neurolysis to free it from scar tissue, although the efficacy of the procedure has not been confirmed in large series. The infraorbital nerve enters the orbit from the pterygoid space through the posterior orbit, crossing the posterior aspect of the inferior orbital fissure. Anterior to the nerve in the fissure are located veins and lymphatics and the orbitalis muscle.

CLASSIFICATION

Knight and North[318] proposed a classification in 1961 of fractures of the zygoma based on the direction of anatomic displacement and pattern formed by the fracture. This classification, which was used for predicting the success of a closed reduction, is presented for acquaintance with classical knowledge about postreduction stability. The Knight and North[318] classification, clarified by Yanagisawa,[319] identified fractures with complete dislocation of the zygomaticofrontal suture and comminuted fractures with external rotation as unstable (Table 66-7).

Currently, surgical practice is to explore the zygoma and the articular processes involved in complete frac-

TABLE 66-7 ✦ KNIGHT AND NORTH CLASSIFICATION

Group I	No significant displacement; fractures visible on radiograph, but fragments remain in line: 6%
Group II	Arch fractures, which involve inward buckling of the arch with no orbital or anterior involvement (10%)
Group III	Unrotated body fractures; downward and inward displacement, but no rotation: 33%
Group IV	Medially rotated body fractures; downward, inward, and backward displacement with medial rotation: 11%
Group V	Laterally rotated body fractures; downward, backward, and medial displacement with lateral rotation of the zygoma: 22%
Group VI	All cases in which additional fracture lines cross the main fragment: 18%

From Knight JS, North JF: The classification of malar fractures: an analysis of displacement as a guide to treatment. Br J Plast Surg 1961;13:315.

tures in an effort to achieve direct anatomic alignment and to provide fixation. In current practice, closed reductions are employed only in isolated zygomatic arch fractures. Limited reductions are popular today, such as the use of the gingival buccal sulcus approach alone.[320-322] Such an approach is indicated in greenstick fractures that are at the zygomaticofrontal suture, in fractures with a minimal or linear orbital floor component that would be reduced by the zygomatic reduction, and in fractures that are displaced principally at the zygomaticomaxillary buttress at the maxillary alveolus. These limited reductions reduce considerably the number of the incisions and thus the morbidity of open reduction, accounting for rapid and efficient procedures with reduced scarring and eyelid morbidity.

DIAGNOSIS

A history of the injury can provide an indication of the direction and magnitude of force. In penetrating wounds, the soft tissue must be searched for the presence of foreign material driven underneath the skin by the force of the injury. The history of the injury is often helpful in arriving at a diagnosis, but the main findings are identified on clinical examination and should be supported and confirmed by CT radiographs.

Clinical Examination

Fractures of the zygoma frequently result from altercations, such as a fist's striking the malar eminence, as the right hand strikes the left cheek. Falls against a hard object also are a frequent source of injury. Zygomatic fractures may also be the result of shattering forces, such as those produced by automobile accidents or gunshot wounds.

Fractures of the zygoma, with the exclusion of fractures of the arch, are invariably accompanied by periorbital ecchymosis, edema, and subconjunctival hematoma. The combination of a periorbital ecchymosis and subconjunctival hematoma suggests a fracture within the orbit but does not specifically identify the location. The characteristic feature about the ecchymosis in the periorbital skin is that it is confined to the distribution of the lids by the insertion of the orbital septum on the bone; therefore, a spectacle hematoma is produced, with a clear demarcation. Edema is present and may extensively involve the conjunctiva. Numbness of the ipsilateral cheek, nose, upper lip, and anterior teeth is an almost invariable accompaniment of orbital floor or zygomatic fractures. One may see ecchymosis intraorally over the fractured zygomaticomaxillary buttress. The amount of swelling in the face and cheek is variable. With direct blows to the cheek, the physical findings are sometimes obscured by swelling of the eyelids and soft tissues. Inspection of the globe may be difficult in patients with extensive hematoma. The lateral canthal ligament[323] may be displaced downward, producing an antimongoloid slant to the palpebral fissure and inferior displacement of the lateral canthus. Retraction of the lower eyelid may be observed because of the same mechanism. If the orbital floor is lowered with the zygoma, the ocular globe may follow the downward displacement, producing (on resolution of the swelling) a deeply sunken upper lid. The eye may sink backward into the orbit as well as downward, producing enophthalmos and orbital dystopia.[324-326]

Unilateral retraction of the lower lid may be observed because of the depression of the zygoma, to which the lid is attached by the orbital septum. Unilateral epistaxis occurs on the involved side, indicating a fracture in the maxillary sinus. The patient may demonstrate a malocclusion or difficulty in moving the lower jaw because of swelling about the coronoid process of the mandible or because of the direct interference with coronoid excursion. This interference may be produced by either medial dislocation of the zygomatic arch or posterior displacement of the malar eminence. The patient may complain on movement of the mouth and may demonstrate only a short distance of mandibular movement. The patient may volunteer that the teeth do not fit together properly. Sometimes, a minimal "lateral open bite" is present because of swelling and edema, which interfere with the ability to bring the teeth into full occlusion.

Hypesthesia or anesthesia may involve the branches of the infraorbital nerve to the ipsilateral skin of the medial face (i.e., the upper lip, eyelid, medial cheek, and lateral nose) or the branch of the nerve that comes off within the infraorbital canal and travels in the anterior wall of the maxillary sinus to the upper anterior teeth. Depending on the extent of involvement of both branches, variable patterns of numbness are present. Double vision or decreased visual acuity accompanies some fractures in which there has been cornea damage, hyphema, retinal damage, optic nerve injury, or direct contusion or involvement of an extraocular muscle or one of the cranial nerves,[327-329] such as the abducens nerve (cranial nerve VI) to the lateral rectus muscle.

Palpation of the zygoma may be helpful in documenting the degree of displacement. The patient should be examined seated, from a frontal perspective and then from a superior view approach. The inferior orbital rim on both sides is palpated, as is the lateral orbit and orbital roof. The zygomaticomaxillary suture as well as the external angular process of the frontal bone should be palpated. The malar arch should be palpated and compared. Viewed from above, a finger resting on the malar eminence can compare malar prominence. A finger may be placed on the infraorbital rim with a fingernail parallel to the horizontal portion of the rim on both sides. In this way, the fingertips may be used to establish the vertical level of the zygoma on both sides and the anterior projection. Step or level discrepancies palpated in the inferior orbital rim suggest inferior and posterior displacement of the zygoma. Frequently, comminution is present in the zygomaticomaxillary buttress and the infraorbital rim, with extension of the rim fracture medial to the infraorbital foramen. This butterfly rim fragment must be carefully aligned before reduction of the main portion of the zygoma. This small fracture fragment extends almost to the area of the lacrimal duct. In general, the periosteal attachment just inside the rim providing the origin of the inferior oblique muscle has to be dissected to visualize this medial fracture completely.

Hematoma may be visible in the mouth, and intraoral palpation may demonstrate irregularity or narrowing of the space between the malar eminence and the maxilla. The groove normally present between the undersurface of the zygoma and first portion of the zygomatic arch and the maxilla may be narrow or absent if the zygoma is displaced downward, medially, and posteriorly.

Malar fractures that are medially displaced may narrow the volume of the orbit, producing exophthalmos. This is the so-called blow-in fracture described by Antonyshyn and Gruss[330] and Stanley.[331,332]

Radiographic Examination

Confirmation of a zygomatic fracture may be documented by plain films, but such fractures are always better imaged on a CT scan. Therefore, the value of plain films in the presence of a CT scan is minimal. The findings after a zygomatic fracture include the possibility of disjunction at the zygomaticofrontal and zygomaticotemporal suture lines. Always, there is fluid in the maxillary sinus. The presence of bilateral maxillary sinus fluid should suggest the possibility of a bilateral maxillary or a Le Fort fracture, and the maxilla must be examined for mobility and the occlusion confirmed as preinjury.

The Waters view is the single best plain film to demonstrate depression and malalignment of the zygoma at its buttresses, depression of the orbital floor, and fractures through the inferior orbital rim, zygomaticofrontal suture, and zygomaticomaxillary buttress. The second most helpful plain film is the Caldwell view, which demonstrates the zygomaticofrontal suture. Any fracture with displacement at the zygomaticofrontal suture requires open reduction in this area. The zygomatic arches as well as the forward projection of the zygoma may be documented in the submentovertex view or by the Titterington position, the semiaxial superoinferior projection.

A CT scan should be done in axial and coronal planes and with both bone and soft tissue windows

(Fig. 66-126).[333] It provides an unexcelled documentation of the displacement of the zygoma at each of its articulations. In particular, the degree of involvement of the orbital floor and the status of the soft tissue contents of the orbit, such as the extraocular muscles, can be documented in coronal views. Views obtained in the axial and the coronal planes show the degree of comminution and the displacement of the medial and inferior walls of the orbit as well as the zygoma. Although three-dimensional examinations[74,75] are interesting, they do not provide the detail of thin-slice axial and coronal views, and these views are required for intraorbit evaluation (see Fig. 66-14). The three-dimensional CT examination is most helpful in comparing the normal versus the abnormal rim and malar eminence (see Fig. 66-14). Because of averaging techniques, visualization and documentation of small fractures or thin bones such as the internal orbital walls may be eliminated from three-dimensional calculations.

CT scans may be done in the longitudinal orbital projection, which shows the orbit in an oblique anterior-posterior axis demonstrating the orbital floor viewed laterally. There is a great deal of value in obtaining a postoperative CT scan. Specifically, these scans are one of the best learning techniques for evaluating the accuracy of open reduction procedures. Recent techniques of intraoperative evaluation by imaging, either fluoroscopy or intraoperative CT scanning, have emphasized that these techniques are also of potential value,[334] although they are more cumbersome. In the final analysis, the intraoperative or postoperative radiographs serve to document the reduction examination and to suggest what improvements might allow precise anatomic reduction and fixation of the fracture. In most patients, more exposures are required for confirmation of reduction than for achieving fixation stability. Nevertheless, an exposure required for the purposes of reduction should then be generally used for fixation.

TREATMENT

In the analysis of zygoma fractures, one should examine each area of fractured articulation, evaluating first the presence of fracture and then the degree of comminution and displacement. The direction and amount of displacement and the degree of comminution determine the plan for operative management of fractures of the zygoma. Cranial fixation appliances, direct fixation with percutaneous pins such as K-wires, and finally direct fixation of interosseous wires led to improved results in the period from 1960 to 1980.[335,336] In comminuted fractures, interfragment wiring techniques were supplemented by immediate bone grafting to strengthen buttress areas. In the mid-1980s, plate and screw fixation techniques became

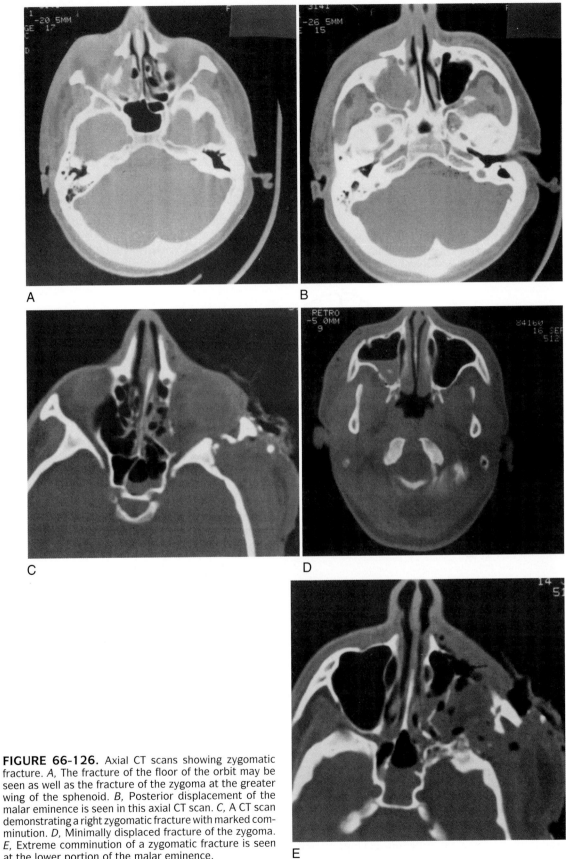

FIGURE 66-126. Axial CT scans showing zygomatic fracture. *A,* The fracture of the floor of the orbit may be seen as well as the fracture of the zygoma at the greater wing of the sphenoid. *B,* Posterior displacement of the malar eminence is seen in this axial CT scan. *C,* A CT scan demonstrating a right zygomatic fracture with marked comminution. *D,* Minimally displaced fracture of the zygoma. *E,* Extreme comminution of a zygomatic fracture is seen at the lower portion of the malar eminence.

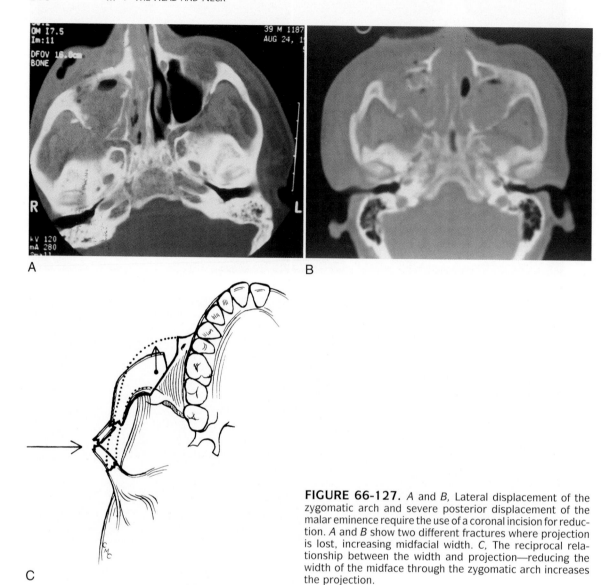

FIGURE 66-127. *A* and *B,* Lateral displacement of the zygomatic arch and severe posterior displacement of the malar eminence require the use of a coronal incision for reduction. *A* and *B* show two different fractures where projection is lost, increasing midfacial width. *C,* The reciprocal relationship between the width and projection—reducing the width of the midface through the zygomatic arch increases the projection.

popular, replacing interfragment wires and decreasing the need for bone grafts.

Buttress Articulations and Their Alignment

For the zygoma, six points of alignment with adjacent bone may potentially be confirmed with craniofacial exposure techniques: the zygomaticofrontal suture, the infraorbital rim, the zygomaticomaxillary buttress, the greater wing of the sphenoid in the lateral portion of the orbit, the orbital floor, and through the zygomatic arch. The orbital floor may require reconstruction with bone or artificial materials such as titanium[337] or MEDPOR.[338,339] The inferior orbital fissure is a particular area where undercorrection of volume of the orbit is frequent, as are the inferomedial buttress and the medial orbital wall.

Anterior Approach

The majority of zygoma fractures require an anterior approach for treatment (partial or complete), but some may require a simultaneous anterior and posterior approach (Fig. 66-127; see also Fig. 66-126).

The anterior approach may be partial or complete and potentially involves up to three incisions: (1) an incision to approach the zygomaticofrontal suture; (2) an incision to approach the inferior orbital rim; and (3) an incision to approach the zygomaticomaxillary buttress, anterior face of the maxilla, and malar prominence. Sometimes, (1) and (2) may be accomplished with the same incision, such as a subciliary incision with canthal detachment. Many surgeons do not like to detach the canthus because of the need to replace it on the frontal process.

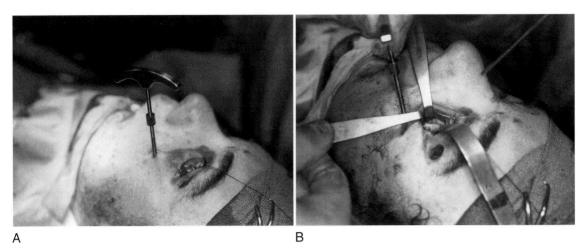

A   B

FIGURE 66-128. *A,* A Carroll-Girard screw may be placed through a small incision in the malar eminence into the body of the zygoma and the position of the zygomatic bone manipulated. *B,* The screw is placed in position to align the rim.

Most zygoma fractures are medially and posteriorly dislocated. Frequently, displacement is minimal and requires no treatment. In about 50% to 75% of fractures, an anterior or even a gingival sulcus alone approach can be used.

Approximately half of these simple fractures requiring reduction are large segments and are able to be managed with an inferior or gingivobuccal sulcus approach alone. In this approach, the gingivobuccal sulcus is opened, and the anterior face of the maxilla and zygoma are degloved. The infraorbital rim and infraorbital nerve are visualized from an inferior direction. Palpation with a finger on the rim avoids entry of elevators into the orbit as the maxilla and zygoma are dissected. The infraorbital nerve is protected by the technique of dissection—it is immediately seen after detachment of the levator anguli oris muscle. The zygoma may often be reduced by placing the tip of an elevator in the lateral aspect of the maxillary sinus directly underneath the solid bone of the malar eminence (not up into the orbit) and levering the body of the zygoma first outward and then forward. Alternatively, a Carroll-Girard screw* can be placed in the solid bone of the malar eminence through a percutaneous incision and the position of the zygomatic bone manipulated (Fig. 66-128). Another reduction approach involves placing a "hook" elevator beneath the anterior zygomatic arch and malar eminence and raising both the arch and the body of the zygoma. In gingival buccal sulcus alone approaches, after the reduction maneuver has been completed, zygomatic stability depends on a relatively intact, greensticked, zygomaticofrontal suture. The floor of the orbit can

be inspected for adequacy of support and alignment either with an intraoperative CT scan or with an endoscope through the maxillary sinus. It is also possible to tell from a preoperative CT scan the degree of comminution of the orbital floor. Fractures that have comminution of the orbital floor are not suitable for an approach that does not involve an inferior lid incision for orbital floor exploration.

In the endoscopic confirmation of orbital integrity, ballottement of the soft tissue by finger pressure on the eye allows the integrity of floor support to be determined by an endoscope placed in the maxillary sinus, visualizing the area of movement and the degree of soft tissue prolapse. If there is significant motion over an area that exceeds a nickel in size, the orbital floor should be explored and grafted or repaired through the sinus. This may be accomplished with an alloplastic wafer of material, such as barrier MEDPOR,[340-342] or by replacement of the orbital floor fracture fragments themselves, uniting them with rigid fixation.

FRACTURES WITH ZYGOMATICOFRONTAL SUTURE DIASTASIS. If the zygomaticofrontal suture demonstrates diastasis (complete fracture permitting dislocation), an exposure of this suture needs to be accomplished for stabilization. This could be accomplished through the lateral portion of an upper blepharoplasty incision (<1 cm) that is made directly over the zygomaticofrontal suture 8 to 10 mm above the lateral canthus (Fig. 66-129). By palpation of the frontal process of the zygoma between the thumb and index finger, the frontal process can be marked precisely in *eyelid* skin. The incision should be short and not progress laterally out of eyelid skin, as it will then scar and be noticeable. Alternatively, the zygomaticofrontal suture may be approached through a brow laceration

*Walter Lorenz, Jacksonville, Florida.

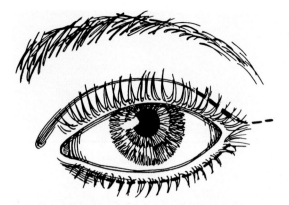

FIGURE 66-129. Lateral blepharoplasty incision for zygomatic fracture reduction.

or by superior dissection from a subciliary or conjunctival lower lid incision by canthal detachment.

The inferior portion of the orbit may be approached through a midtarsal, lower orbital rim, subciliary, or conjunctival incision (either below the tarsus or in the conjunctival fornix). Conceptually, the conjunctival fornix incision produces the least cutaneous scarring, but the exposure may be restricted by fat prolapse. The therapy for a zygoma fracture has recently become quite specific and directed only at areas that require open reduction for confirmation of alignment or for fixation.

Although a brow incision has been advocated for the exposure of the zygomaticofrontal suture, it is *not* an acceptable approach because of the unpredictability of scarring in this area. Incisions within brow hair should never be considered because the hairless intrabrow scar is never able to be improved. In addition, it is slightly superior to the area being explored. Incisions in brow skin outside the hair also leave a prominent scar.

Coronal Incisions (Posterior Approach)

Fractures with extreme posterior displacement of the malar eminence and those with lateral displacement of the zygomatic arch benefit from the addition of a coronal incision to the anterior approach incisions. The coronal incision allows exposure of the entire zygomatic arch and roof of the glenoid fossa for precise arch reconstruction. It also exposes the zygomaticofrontal junction and the lateral wall of the orbit. Any sagittally oriented split of the glenoid fossa should be reduced first, following which reduction and fixation of the remainder of the zygomatic arch may be accomplished, confirming alignment in the lateral wall of the orbit, which confirms proper medial position of the arch. When the orbital process of the zygoma comes in line with the broad surface of the greater wing of the sphenoid, the arch is of the proper length (which

guarantees the proper projection of the malar eminence) and is properly medially positioned.

Dingman Approach

After disappointing results of closed fixation techniques, Dingman and Alling[343] suggested that any significant fracture-dislocation of the zygoma should be treated by exposure of the fractured areas, including open reduction and direct wire fixation. Open reduction has proved to be the standard treatment, resulting in a high degree of satisfaction.

In this approach, an incision (or laceration) is used in the lateral brow approximately 1.5 cm in length. Another incision is made in the lower eyelid in a midtarsal, subciliary, or conjunctival location. Dissection exposes the zygomaticofrontal and zygomaticomaxillary suture lines. A moderately heavy periosteal elevator is passed through the upper incision behind the malar eminence and into the temporal fossa. The elevator is used to control the position of the zygoma and to reduce it by upward, forward, and outward forces. Depending on the displacement of the fracture segments, the bone is elevated into position. After the reduction of the zygoma, the orbital floor can be explored and any herniation of orbital contents reduced. The defect in the orbital floor is corrected by means of autogenous or alloplastic material.

Dingman and Natvig[142] recommended that drill holes be placed through the bone, 5 mm to each side of the fracture. Interosseous wires are then used to secure the position by means of interfragment wiring. The zygomatic arch fracture may be either a component of an isolated arch injury or a significant zygoma fracture, and both types usually may be reduced through any one of the approaches described by passing the elevator beneath the arch. This semiclosed technique is effective only for medially displaced arch fractures. The heavy fascial and muscle attachments to the arch hold it in relative position after closed reduction unless displacement or comminution has been extreme. Patients in whom laterally displaced zygomatic arch fractures are present frequently require a coronal incision and direct arch reduction and fixation to provide reduction stability. The periosteum is extremely disrupted in an arch fracture.

Subsequently, a more complete exposure of the fracture sites, including the zygomaticomaxillary buttress, has been recommended.[9,10,118] These exposures provide the ability to clearly visualize the anatomic accuracy of the skeletal reduction. In zygomatic fractures accompanied by the Le Fort fractures, considerable lateral displacement of the zygoma is often observed with comminution of the arch. Extreme anteroposterior depression of the zygoma can also be observed. In these types of fractures, exposure and anatomic reduction of the arch through a coronal incision help restore proper anterior projection of the malar eminence and alignment in the lateral orbit between the greater wing of the sphenoid and the orbital process of the zygoma.

Intraoral Approach

The intraoral approach is one of the most important approaches for reduction of zygomatic fractures. A Kelly clamp or elevator may be placed through the anterior wall of the fractured maxillary sinus (a Caldwell-Luc exposure) with the tip placed directly under the malar eminence. Gentle pressure is used to elevate the body of the zygoma anteriorly and laterally. An elevator may also be placed intraorally underneath the arch, if desired, and medial arch fractures reduced. Impacted or partially healed fractures may be dislodged by elevator pressure or preferably by passing an elevator or osteotome through the line of the fracture, completing the fracture. This is particularly necessary when greenstick (or incomplete) fractures are treated late, which requires an osteotomy to complete the incomplete fracture, which is usually at the zygomaticofrontal suture. The zygomaticomaxillary buttress may be reconstructed by either temporary positioning of the bone pieces with interfragment wires or provisional reduction with plates and a single screw in each fragment. A bone graft may be placed into any existing gap in the zygomaticomaxillary buttress, over the anterior wall of the maxillary sinus, or it may be placed in a bone gap and lag screwed to existing plates in the surrounding buttress suture or maxillary sinus wall.

Fixation with a 1.5- or 2-mm system at the Le Fort I level is recommended[344]; 1.0 or 1.3 systems are recommended for the maxillary sinus wall. An L-shaped plate is generally used at the zygomaticomaxillary buttress, and its solid fixation depends on at least two stable screws beyond the areas of fracture in intact bone on each side. Tooth roots inferiorly should be avoided. The butterfly buttress bone pieces may be screwed to the plate already in alignment.

The intraoral approach alone is not an effective method when the zygomatic arch is laterally displaced or when there is disjunction at the zygomaticofrontal suture. These conditions require simultaneous extensive exposures of the zygomaticofrontal suture, inferior orbital rim, zygomaticomaxillary buttress, lateral orbit, and zygomatic arch. An attempt should be made to avoid penetrating tooth roots in screw placement. In practice, screws that penetrate teeth have not had the frequency of adverse sequelae initially predicted.[169]

Endoscopically Assisted Repair

The endoscope may be used to assist the repair of zygomatic fractures by defining the orbital floor defect or by visualizing the zygomatic arch reduction.[345,346]

For reduction of the zygomatic arch, a 4- to 6-cm incision is made preauricularly and extended into the temporal hair. The arch is dissected, with the endoscope communicating with an intraoral buccal sulcus incision and approach to the anterior face of the zygoma.

The arch fragments may be dissected and removed and reassembled on a "back table," united by plate and screw fixation and replaced into the defect, and the reassembled structure fixated at its margins. Another approach involves leaving the segments of the arch in situ. They may be positioned and fixed to a reduction plate with the assistance of simultaneous percutaneous and endoscopic manipulation. Branches of the facial nerve[347] must be avoided with this technique; they are just superficial to the condensation of the deep temporal fascia, which splits to enclose the arch. Both techniques avoid the use of a coronal incision. Little long-term outcome analysis is available to justify the superiority of endoscopic over traditional approaches.

Maxillary Sinus Approach (With or Without Endoscopic Assistance)

The maxillary sinus approach to comminuted fractures now includes endoscopic visualization of the orbital floor and the sinus ostia. Some clinicians are beginning to approach the orbital floor through this mechanism, replacing and stabilizing the orbital floor either with small plates and screws or by insertion of a piece of alloplastic material. In general, the sinus should have any blood or devitalized bone fragments removed and discarded if they are not to be used for replacement of the anterior wall of the maxilla or floor of the orbit. In all patients, one should be able to irrigate into the nose through the sinus, confirming the integrity of the maxillary sinus ostium. In the past, it was common to pack the maxillary sinus blindly to reduce the orbital floor or zygoma. This was a dangerous maneuver, as it involved insertion of packing without visualization of the floor, and blindness has resulted from excessive pressure of packing material. The techniques of endoscopic evaluation through the maxillary sinus allow precise visualization of the fracture areas to be treated.

Fixation Required to Achieve Stability

Several individuals have examined the issues of zygomatic stability after open reduction and specifically how much, where, what kind, and how many sites of fixation are necessary to achieve stability.

Rinehart and Marsh[348] studied cadaver heads with use of one, two, or three miniplate and assessed stability of noncomminuted zygoma fractures submitted to static and oscillating loads to simulate the effect of the masticatory apparatus on postoperative displacement. Neither single-miniplate nor triple-wire fixation was enough to stabilize the zygoma against simulated masseter forces; however, three miniplates were sufficient to stabilize the zygomaticofrontal, zygomaticomaxillary, and infraorbital rim areas.

Dal Santo et al[349] thought that Rinehart and Marsh overestimated the postoperative forces that could be generated by the masseter muscle and suggested that stability with fewer than three plates would be possible. Conclusions were based on actual human measurements of bite forces after zygomatic fracture treatment.

Davidson et al[350] studied combinations of wires and plates at the anterior fixation sites and determined that three-point fixation was the best (either plates or wires) at preventing displacement. Miniplates were recommended as at least one strong buttress as well as two- and three-point fixation. Plate bending and bone splitting at the screw or drill holes was the mechanism of the failure.

Kasrai et al[351] studied the miniplate versus the bioresorbable systems. Titanium provided 39% of the strength of the nonfractured area, and bioresorbable systems provided 13% of the intact breaking strength. Deformation or bending of miniplates was the primary mode of failure.

Gosain et al[352] in parietal calvarial bone demonstrated that in both compression and distraction, titanium miniplates were considerably stronger than the bioresorbable systems.

Manson et al[353] performed experiments with stainless steel systems and found that bone fractures were the primary mode of failure. This study implied that the titanium and resorbable systems are considerably less strong than the bone itself, but the stainless steel system compared favorably with the bone strength.

Rohrich and Watumull[354] and Rohrich et al[321] found plate fixation to be superior to wire fixation after a thorough study. They also found that fixed deformities were quite challenging to correct.

O'Hara et al[355] demonstrated that two- and three-point fixation with miniplates was superior to other methods of fixation.

Rohner et al[356] studied combinations of plate fixation and concluded that the addition of fixation within the lateral wall of the orbit was one of the most stable constructs. They demonstrated that titanium systems had one third and bioresorbable systems less than 10% of the strength of the intact zygomatic complex. Plate bending was the cause of the failure of the titanium system, whereas plate and screw breakage was the cause of the failure in the resorbable system.

Therefore, there seems to be justification for using three plates, one each at the zygomaticofrontal suture, the infraorbital rim, and the zygomaticomaxillary buttress (Fig. 66-130). The upper two plates could be of the 1.3-mm system, and the lower plate of the 1.5- or 2.0-mm system. Whereas single-plate fixation and single-lag screw fixation have been recommended, there seems to be little justification for use of the other

incisions for fixation because they are required for alignment.

K-WIRE OR PIN FIXATION. Brown et al[357] devised a technique using one or more stainless steel pins, Kirschner wires, or Steinmann pins for fixation. The zygoma was first reduced with a closed reduction and then held in place while a hand-driven or electric drill was used to drive a stainless steel K-wire through the zygoma in a transverse or oblique direction into the adjacent bones of the maxilla and palate or contralateral maxilla and zygoma. Care must be taken to avoid penetrating the contralateral orbit. The pins were then cut at skin level, or just beyond skin level, or covered with a rubber protector. They were left in for a period of 4 weeks, during which time the fracture fragments consolidated. Although effective results have been reported in the hands of experienced surgeons, this technique, although rapid, does not confirm satisfactory fracture alignment by open reduction. It has been replaced by direct open reduction and plate and screw fixation. K-wire fixation is a rapid and inexpensive technique that may still have some use in areas where medical care is severely limited by financial considerations. The technique also has some use in patients with bone loss in which plate and screw fixation may be more difficult to use, where some stability can be maintained by the use of a threaded K-wire. Complications include external scars, malunion, nonunion, displacement, and facial deformity.

OPEN REDUCTION, PLATE AND SCREW FIXATION, INTERFRAGMENT WIRING (MANSON APPROACH). The "Manson approach" technique is the most effective in obtaining accurate reduction and positive fixation. Absolute anatomic accuracy may be achieved by direct visualization of the fracture sites to be stabilized. In general, the zygomaticomaxillary buttress and inferior orbital rim are always exposed, and this is true in discontinuity at the zygomaticofrontal suture. In addition, some individuals[358] prefer direct fracture fixation in the lateral wall of the orbit, over the junction of the greater wing of the sphenoid and orbital process of the zygoma. Finally, fractures demonstrating lateral displacement through the arch generally require an arch exposure (coronal incision). In this technique, the body of the zygoma and the processes identified for open reduction are exposed with appropriate incisions.

After anatomic alignment of the various buttresses is achieved, interfragment wiring is performed at the zygomaticofrontal suture, at the infraorbital rim, and possibly in the zygomatic arch or zygomaticomaxillary buttress. This wiring provides several axes for temporary positioning of the zygoma (Fig. 66-130G). Next, these areas are serially stabilized with plate and screw fixation, with removal of the wires after fixation has been completed; 1.3-mm plates are placed at the zygomaticofrontal suture or under the inferior orbital rim. Many individuals place the inferior orbital rim plate at a distance inferior to the rim, so it does not generate eyelid fibrosis and retraction from titanium metal reactions near the orbital septum. After orbital rim continuity is restored, the integrity of the floor of the orbit may be restored by either bone grafts or alloplastic material. Because the zygoma conceptually requires three or four incisions for visualization of all of its buttress alignments, and one can look through only one incision at a time, the use of temporary interfragment wire positioning for several of these fracture sites allows temporary control of displacement of the zygoma fracture while one is looking through the other fracture exposures. The technique allows more control of the displacement before permanent fixation.

In zygomatic fractures demonstrating only medial types of displacement, management with anterior approaches alone is satisfactory. A coronal incision is not required. The medially displaced zygomatic arch may be managed by a supplemental Gillies-type approach used to perform a closed reduction of the arch segment. Open anterior approaches permit the reduction of the anterior portion of the zygoma. For the arch, an elevator is placed through the temporal fascia (Fig. 66-131), and the arch is reduced. Palpation is used to determine the proper alignment. A towel clamp may also be placed about the arch, and the arch is pulled into position. After exposure of the principal zygomatic fragments, drill holes are placed through

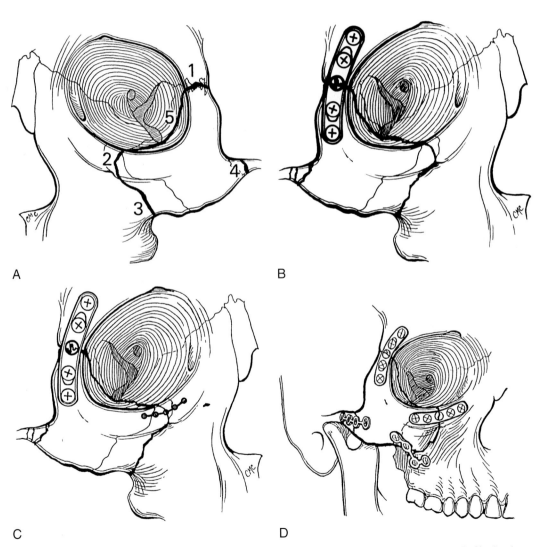

FIGURE 66-130. Plate and screw fixation of a zygomatic fracture. *A,* Areas of alignment. *B,* Single plate. *C,* Two plates. *D,* Complete anterior fixation.   *Continued*

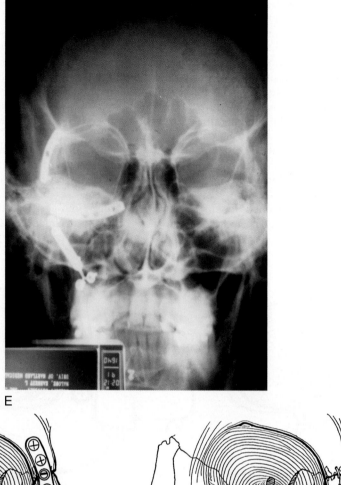

E

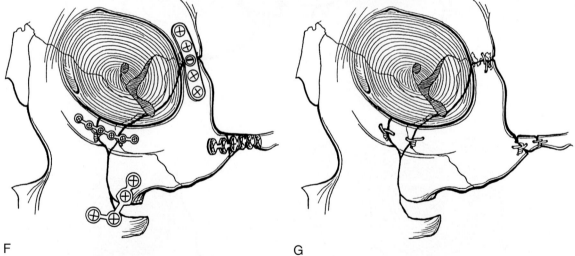

F   G

FIGURE 66-130, cont'd. *E,* Radiograph. *F,* Complete anterior and posterior fixation. *G,* Setup for preliminary positioning wires.

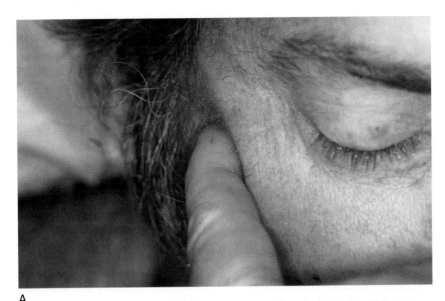

A

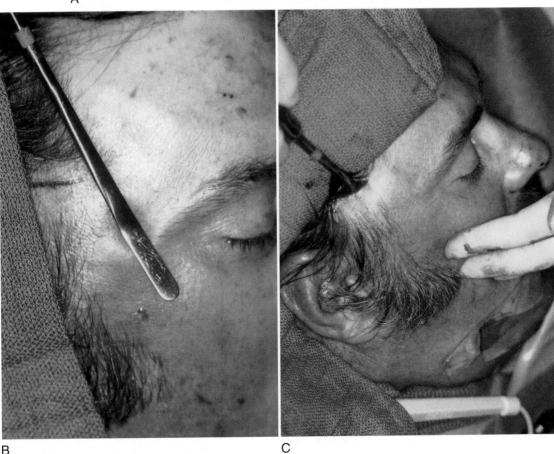

B   C

FIGURE 66-131. *A,* Palpation of a depressed zygomatic arch. *B,* Incision marked and checking position of eleva-tor. *C,* Elevator placed beneath deep temporal fascia superficial to muscle to reach depressed segment of arch, which is elevated in a smooth maneuver.

the margins of the bone adjacent to fracture sites and at a distance of 4 to 5 mm from the fracture ends, and temporary No. 26 or No. 28 positioning wires are placed. Small plates and screws can then be used to span the fracture sites and provide positive fixation once the rest of the buttress alignment has been confirmed. Two screws per fragment in solid bone provide good immobilization. Often, a five-hole plate is selected for the zygomaticofrontal suture, with the central hole placed over the zygomaticofrontal fracture site. Screws placed in comminuted bone do not provide secure fixation. In providing plate and screw fixation for a comminuted fracture of the orbital rim, the fragments may be removed and pieced together on a back table with a plate applied, and then the center fragments are reinserted into the defect. This technique is usually more difficult than in situ reduction and fixation. Alternatively, the defect can be spanned by a plate and then the intervening fragments individually lag screwed to the plate after plate and screw fixation to the more stable, large peripheral bone fragments.

"High-Energy" Zygoma Fractures

Violent injury to the zygoma results in shattering of the bone into multiple fragments. The approaches described before are satisfactory for simple, noncomminuted, minimally displaced fractures. The method of management of more complicated types of fractures must include a thorough visualization of the body, the frontal and maxillary processes of the zygoma (Fig. 66-132), and the zygomatic arch.[359,360] The zygomaticomaxillary buttress is restored by direct intraoral rigid fixation with plate and screw fixation after initial wire placement at the zygomaticofrontal suture, the infraorbital rim, and perhaps the zygomatic arch for temporary positioning. A wire placed at the zygomaticofrontal suture provisionally positions this buttress (Figs. 66-133 and 66-134). A subciliary incision may provide exposure of the inferior rim, the lateral wall, and potentially the frontal process of the zygoma by canthal detachment. Wires in the infraorbital rim complete a provisional reduction. The wires then may be replaced by plate and screw fixation, adjusting the position of the zygoma before rigid fixation placement because wires allow minimal adjustments to be achieved to improve reduction. The entire lower and lateral zygoma may be exposed with a subciliary incision, dissecting the lateral canthal ligament off the Whitnall tubercle. The lateral aspect of the incision may therefore be retracted upward to expose the zygomaticofrontal suture.[361] The lateral wall of the orbit is best inspected through a coronal incision (Fig. 66-134), stripping the canthal ligament for exposure, but exposure may be provided with a subciliary or conjunctival incision. The lateral wall visualization may be used to confirm alignment of the orbital process of the zygoma with the greater wing of the sphenoid. There are some who think that plating of the lateral wall of the orbit intraorbitally is a desired point of fixation.[362] The orbital floor and inferior orbital rim are approached by any of the lower lid approaches: conjunctival, subciliary, midtarsal, or orbital rim. Care must be taken to place lower lid cutaneous incisions in eyelid skin, or the scar will be noticeable as it enters cheek skin.

Compound Comminuted Zygoma Fractures

Fractures of the zygoma may be compounded intraorally or extraorally when the force is severe enough to cause soft tissue wounds. These wounds may or may not extend to the bone. A thorough inspection of the wound must be made to rule out the presence of foreign material, grass, debris, road dirt, and blood clots. Wood fragments are especially hazardous because they are colonized, driven in the soft tissue, and not easily perceived at the time of wound inspection. The fractured pieces of the zygoma are reconstituted by plate and screw fixation (see Fig. 66-132). Careful cleaning, débridement, and closure of soft tissue in layers over the comminuted repaired fracture generally results in satisfactory cutaneous healing, but all the layers of the soft tissue need to be repaired and the soft tissue then fixed to bone at appropriate locations. In these patients, the laceration may provide a preferred approach for a fracture reduction. Care must be taken, however, not to extend lacerations, increasing cutaneous scarring and possibly producing lymphedema by transection of lymphatics or injury to sensory or motor nerve branches, such as those of the trigeminal and facial nerves. Antibiotics are usually indicated at the discretion of the surgeon, and tetanus prophylaxis is indicated in open injuries.

In isolated zygomatic arch fractures that demonstrate the tendency to recurrent medial displacement, the arch segments may be supported after reduction by placement of packing underneath the medial surface of the arch, removing it after 1 or 2 weeks.[363] Some individuals use a protective splint, externally, to prevent redisplacement of the arch. If the reduction is performed carefully and precisely (serial back-and-forth motions of the arch should be attempted), the heavy periosteum of the arch is then still relatively intact, the segments of the fractures are wedged, and the arch fracture will be stable without external support.

Delayed Treatment of Zygoma Fractures

The best results are obtained when patients with zygomatic fractures are treated relatively early. Consolidation begins to occur in the fracture site within 1 week, and it is reasonably well organized in 3 weeks, at which time it may be difficult to mobilize and reposition the bone by reduction maneuvers alone.

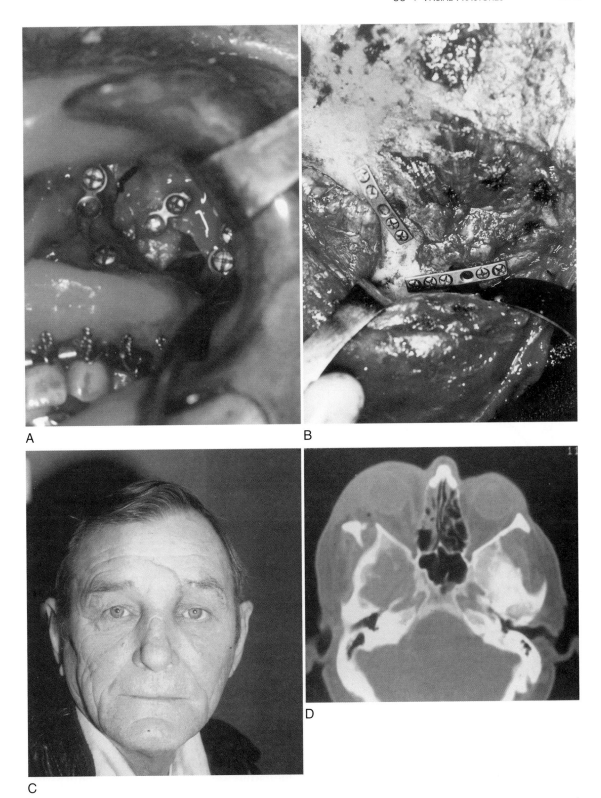

FIGURE 66-132. *A,* Plate and screw fixation of the zygomaticomaxillary buttress. *B,* Use of a coronal incision for exposure and fixation of the zygoma. *C,* Appearance of the patient in *D* after healing. *D,* Preoperative displacement.

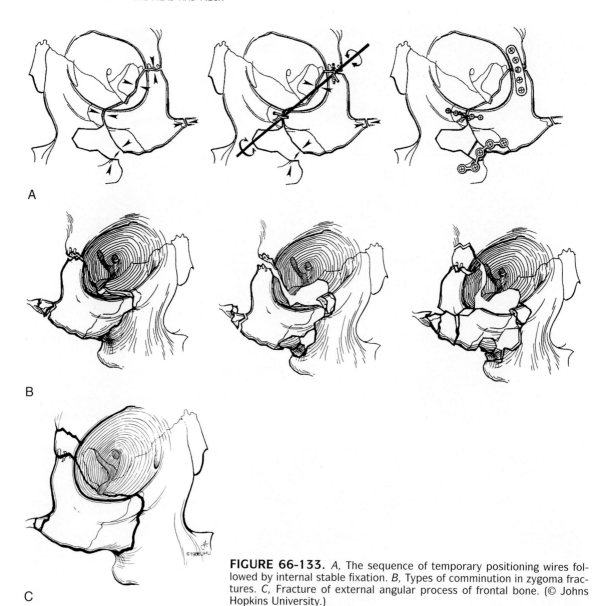

A

B

C

FIGURE 66-133. *A,* The sequence of temporary positioning wires followed by internal stable fixation. *B,* Types of comminution in zygoma fractures. *C,* Fracture of external angular process of frontal bone. (© Johns Hopkins University.)

Repositioning after 2 weeks frequently requires an osteotome-facilitated reduction. An osteotome is placed in the fracture sites to free the fracture for reduction; this maneuver can be accomplished through the usual exposures. The malunited bone is mobilized by osteotomies through the old fracture lines and through the area of fibrous or bony ankylosis. After the bone has been mobilized, an inspection of each fracture site should be conducted to remove any area of fibrous ankylosis or any proliferative bone that was not present originally because it will produce malalignment.[73] Plate and screw fixation then unites the fractures (see Fig. 66-134). In fractures treated late, the masseter muscle may need to be divided or mobilized from the inferior surface of the malar eminence and arch to allow the bone to be repositioned superiorly. The masseter muscle contracts in length in the malreduced fracture, and it may not be able to be extended to length after several weeks have elapsed.

Fractures treated in a delayed stage are more safely treated with osteotomy than by trying to remobilize the fracture with blunt force. Mobilization of partially healed fractures may result in new fracture lines extending deep within the orbit, occasionally precipitating blindness. These forcible reduction techniques carry the risk of radiating fractures extending into the apex of the orbit, with cranial nerve injury.

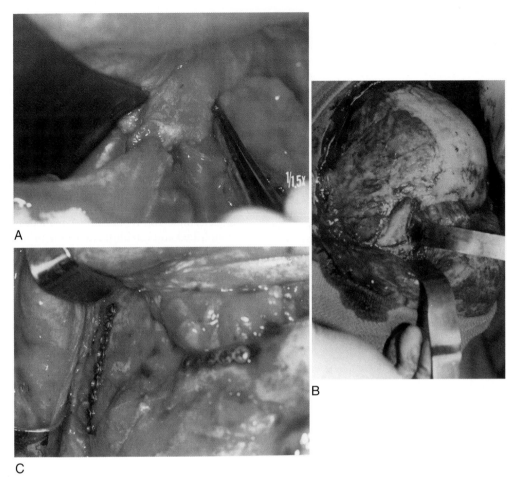

FIGURE 66-134. *A* and *B,* Inspection of the lateral orbital wall through a coronal incision. Alignment in the lateral orbit between the orbital process of the zygoma and the greater wing of the sphenoid confirms proper medial position of the zygomatic arch. *C,* The reduced zygomatic arch should be as straight as possible.

EARLY COMPLICATIONS

Fractures of the zygoma are occasionally accompanied by complications. Bleeding into the maxillary sinus is usually of short duration. It may be necessary to irrigate blood clots from the antrum and to remove any devitalized bone fragments, which become sequestered if they are left. Rarely, the ostia of the maxillary sinus will be occluded by the fractures and require endoscopic sinus surgery. In those patients with pre-existing sinus disease, acute exacerbation may be a complicating factor. Proper sinus drainage into the nose must be confirmed by free irrigation of saline into the nose at the time of Caldwell-Luc exposure. Otherwise, a persistent oral-antral fistula may result in the sublabial area.[364] Malfunction of the extraocular muscles is a result of damage from fracture forces (contusion) or less frequently interference by segments of bone, orbital floor injury, or fat or muscle entrap-

ment. Several instances of blindness have occurred after malar fracture reduction.[365,366]

LATE COMPLICATIONS

Late complications of zygomatic fractures include nonunion, malunion, double vision, persistent infraorbital nerve anesthesia or hypesthesia, and chronic maxillary sinusitis.[367] Scarring may result from laceration or malpositioned incisions (Fig. 66-135). In general, ectropion and scleral show are mild and resolve spontaneously. About 10% of patients having subciliary incisions of the lower eyelid develop a temporary ectropion. Gross downward dislocation of the zygoma results in diplopia and orbital dystopia (Fig. 66-136). Usually, an excess of 5 mm of inferior globe dystopia is required to produce diplopia. Treatment involves zygomatic mobilization by osteotomy, with bone grafting to augment the malar eminence when malar

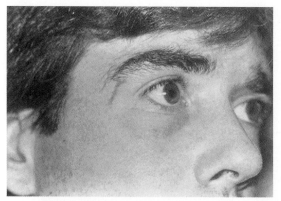

FIGURE 66-135. Malposition of incision used for zygomatic fracture reduction in the brow. Both the brow and subciliary incisions are improperly placed. The brow incision should have been at the upper lateral aspect of the brow and never within the brow, and the subciliary incision should follow the lower lid cilia and not extend more than 1 cm lateral to the lateral canthus. These incisions will be noticeable because they are in cheek skin and not in eyelid skin. Eyelid skin is forgiving in terms of scar formation, but cheek skin is not. The author never uses brow incisions unless a laceration is present but prefers an upper blepharoplasty approach.

projection is deficient.[367,368] The position of the eye must be restored with intraorbital bone grafts or artificial material such as MEDPOR.[339] Infection is not common and usually responds to sinus drainage or lacrimal drainage. Preexisting maxillary sinusitis or

obstruction predisposes to infection, and the maxillary sinus should be cleared by endoscopic surgery before an elective osteotomy is performed. Sinus or lacrimal infection is possible.

Late complications result mainly from malposition.[367] In these patients, correction is obtained either by osteotomy or by osteotomy and bone grafting. When an osteotomy is performed, the zygoma should be directly aligned and plate and screw fixation used. The buttresses may have to be modified in length by resection or bone grafting. Onlay bone and cartilage grafts are usually necessary to supplement the result, overcoming the loss of bone that occurs in displaced fractures. A three-dimensional CT scan and plain films help determine the repositioning maneuvers to be accomplished and establish size of the orbital cavity to be achieved.

Orbital Complications

Orbital complications consist of diplopia, visual loss, globe injury, enophthalmos or exophthalmos, and lid position abnormalities. (Orbital blowout fractures and ocular complications resulting from zygoma fractures are discussed in the section on the orbit.) Infection is not common but usually involves a lacrimal system or maxillary sinus blockage. Therapy is directed toward the cause of the problem.

Malposition of the arch or body of the zygoma may interfere with mandibular motion of the coronoid process and require osteotomy.[92,369] In these patients,

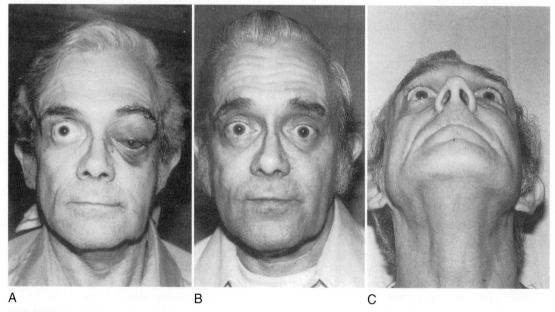

A   B   C

FIGURE 66-136. Fracture-dislocation of the zygoma with severe comminution of the orbit allowing marked inferior globe displacement. *A,* The canthal ligament system is markedly depressed inferiorly and the globe is enophthalmic. *B,* Frontal view after reduction. *C,* Result obtained after reduction and bone grafting, inferior perspective.

the zygomatic reduction has usually been performed in a "closed" fashion, and perhaps with excessive vigor in an attempt to mobilize a partially consolidated fracture. Impacted fractures of the zygomatic arch that abut the coronoid process may result in fibro-osseous ankylosis, with limited motion of the mandible. The gunshot wound is especially prone to this problem. If the zygomatic arch cannot be adequately repositioned, resection of the coronoid process through an intraoral route usually frees the mandible from the fibrous ankylosis and permits normal function. It is important that the patient vigorously exercise to preserve and to improve the range of motion obtained, which may take 6 months.

Numbness

Persistent anesthesia or hypesthesia in the distribution of the infraorbital nerve usually lasts only a short time.[250,370] If total anesthesia exists for more than 6 months, it is likely that the nerve is severely damaged or perhaps transected. If the nerve is impinged by bone fragments, especially in a medially and posteriorly impacted zygoma fracture, reduction or decompression of the infraorbital canal and neurolysis are indicated. Bone spurs or constricting portions of the canal should be removed so that the nerve has an adequate opportunity for regeneration and relief of pressure. The nerve must be explored throughout the floor of the orbit so that it is free from any compression by bone fragments, scar tissue, or callus. Permanent anesthesia is annoying, especially immediately after the injury. Patients generally become somewhat accustomed to any neurologic deficit, and some spontaneous reinnervation may occur from adjacent facial regions as well as regrowth of axons through the infraorbital nerve. Some vague sensation is usually then present.

Oral-Antral Fistula

An oral-antral fistula requires débridement of bone or mucosa, confirmation of maxillary sinus drainage into the nose, and closure with a marginally based flap for mucosal reconstruction and a transposition mucosal flap for cover. A two-layer closure is required. A bone graft may be placed between the layers of soft tissue. A marginally based flap may be used for intraoral mucosal covering closure over a buccal fat pad[364,371] mobilized and sewn into the defect before the mucosa is sutured over it. On occasion, a free tissue transfer or a more distant flap is required for difficult persistent fistulas.

Plate Complications

Complications of internal fixation include screw loosening or extrusion, plate exposure requiring removal, and tooth root penetration by screws.[169] Prominence of plates over the zygomatic arch is directly due to associated fat and soft tissue atrophy (temporalis) and to malreduction of the zygomatic arch laterally. Probably 10% of plates placed at the Le Fort I level need to be removed for exposure, nonhealing wound, or cold sensitivity.[279,372]

Maxilla

Maxillary fractures are encountered far less commonly than are fractures of the mandible, zygoma, or nose. The ratio of mandible fractures to maxillary fractures is 4:1.[373] In centralized trauma units, there is a higher incidence of maxillary fractures in relation to mandibular fractures.[59]

ANATOMY AND SURGICAL PATHOLOGY

The maxilla forms a large part of the bone structure of the middle third of the facial skeleton. The maxilla itself is attached to the cranium through the zygomatic bones and medially by its nasofrontal buttress (medial orbital rim) in the nasoethmoidal area. There is a strong vertical and horizontal system of buttresses (or thick sections of bone) that architecturally and structurally arrange the maxilla into a mass capable of resisting considerable force.[5] Sagittal buttresses, which are relatively weak, are also present.[10] Many think that the maxilla is stronger in compression vertically than it is horizontally (in terms of being able to resist horizontal fracture forces).[69,374] The midfacial and orbital areas form an important protection to the brain and intracranial structures. Violent forces and injuries of the midface are dissipated and energy is absorbed without transmitting fractures or energy to the brain and skull base.[375] The pattern of fractures in the orbit almost always protects the globe from rupturing because of the alternating thin and thick structure of the bones of the midfacial skeleton (Fig. 66-137).

The maxilla is formed from two irregular pyramidal component parts. It contributes to the formation of the midportion of the face and forms part of the orbit, nose, and palate. It is hollowed on its anterior aspect, providing space for the maxillary sinuses (Fig. 66-138). The maxilla thus forms a large portion of the orbit, the nasal fossa, and the oral cavity and a major portion of the palate, the nasal cavity, and the piriform aperture. The frontal processes of the maxilla provide anchorage for the medial canthal ligaments and support for the nasal bones and nasal cartilages. Anteriorly, these include the nasal bones and frontal processes of the maxilla, which attach to the cranium and cranial base at the glabella medially, and the zygoma and its articulations laterally. The zygoma articulates with both the frontal cranium and the greater wing of the sphenoid and also through the arch to the temporal bone. The maxilla contributes to stability only by its intimate association with the other bones of the midface and the base of the cranium.

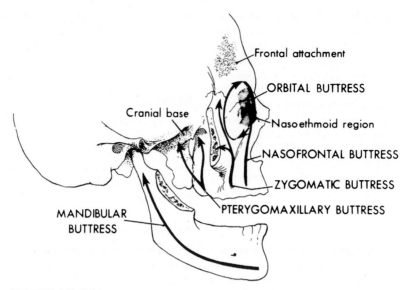

FIGURE 66-137. The vertical buttresses of the midfacial skeleton. Anteriorly, the nasofrontal buttress skirts the piriform aperture inferiorly and composes the bone of the medial orbital rim superiorly to reach the frontal bone at its internal angular process. Laterally, the zygomaticomaxillary buttress extends from the zygomatic process of the frontal bone through the lateral aspect of the zygoma to reach the maxillary alveolus. A component of the zygomaticomaxillary buttress extends laterally through the zygomatic arch to reach the temporal bone. Posteriorly, the pterygomaxillary buttress is seen. It extends from the posterior portion of the maxilla and the pterygoid fossa to reach the cranial base structures. The mandibular buttress forms a strong structural support for the lower midface in fracture treatment. This support for maxillary fracture reduction must conceptually be achieved by placement of both jaws in intermaxillary fixation. The other "transverse" maxillary buttresses include the palate, the inferior orbital rims, and the superior orbital rims. The superior orbital rims and lower sections of the frontal sinus are also known in the supraorbital regions as the frontal bar and are technically frontal bone and not part of the maxilla. (From Manson PN, Hoopes JE, Su CT: Structural pillars of the facial skeleton: an approach to the management of Le Fort fractures. Plast Reconstr Surg 1980;66:54.)

Posteriorly, the maxilla is attached to the cranium by strong buttresses to the skull base in the pterygoid region. The maxilla consists of a body and four processes—frontal, zygomatic, palatine, and alveolar. The body of the bone contains the large maxillary sinuses. In childhood, the sinuses are small; but in adults, sinus structures become large and penetrate most of the central structure of the midface, nose, and periorbital area medially and superiorly. Only a thin orbital floor and thin anterior and posterior medial wall of the maxilla remain.[376] The growth of the sinuses occurs in combination with the development of the permanent dentition. Tooth buds, present in the infant's and young child's maxilla, descend and are absent in adult structures, which results in further weakening of the bone of the midface. The surrounding bone is thus thinned to eggshell thickness with alternating areas of stronger bone, which are the buttresses of the midfacial skeleton.[10]

The alveolar process of the maxilla is strong and thick and provides excellent support to the teeth. The bone provides good support also for the horizontal processes of the maxilla through the palate and, by virtue of the strong horizontal buttresses, protects the upper portion of the maxilla. As the teeth are lost, the alveolar process thins, weakens, and resorbs.[377] The entire maxilla may thus become weaker, and recession may occur. The entire alveolar portion of the bone may recede to the extent that the nasal spine is evident, and the bone of the alveolar ridge may recede to the level of the floor of the nose and maxillary sinuses. Resorption of the anterior surfaces of the maxilla may occur simultaneously.

The nerves, passing through the maxilla, pass through the anterior wall of the bone as branches from the infraorbital nerve to the anterior teeth. Additional nerves exit the infraorbital canal to supply the soft tissue of the upper lip and lateral aspect of the nose (Fig. 66-138). The mucosa overlying the bony palate and the mucosa of the soft palate are innervated by palatine branches of the second division of the trigeminal nerve. These branches pass through the palatine

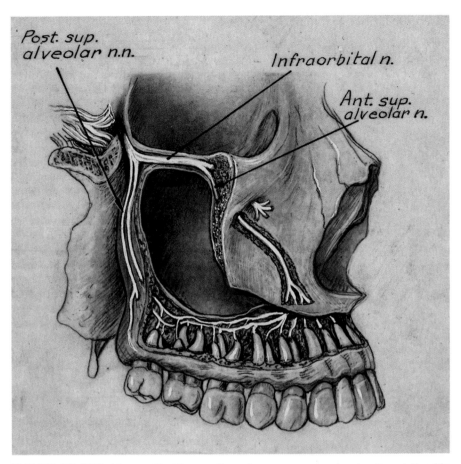

FIGURE 66-138. The maxilla. The maxillary sinuses are open, showing the relationship with the floor of the orbit. Note also the interface between the pterygoid plates and the tuberosity of the maxilla. The sensory nerves traveling in the walls of the maxillary sinus are outlined. The anterior superior dental alveolar nerve travels in the anterior wall of the maxilla to reach the anterior maxillary teeth. Branches of the posterior superior dental alveolar nerves travel in the lateral walls of the maxilla to reach the middle and posterior maxillary teeth. (From Kazanjian VH, Converse J: Surgical Treatment of Facial Injuries, 3rd ed. Baltimore, Williams & Wilkins, 1974.)

canal between the maxilla and the palatine bones in the posterior portion of the palate. The nasopalatine nerves traverse each side of the vomer and pass from the nasal cavity through a small incisive foramen to provide the innervation of the mucoperiosteum of the anterior third of the hard palate.

The maxilla is designed to absorb forces of mastication and to provide a strong vertical buttress for the occluding teeth of the mandible.[378] By virtue of the buttress system, the load is distributed over the entire craniofacial skeleton.[376,379] The forces are distributed through the arch of the palate near the articulation of the maxilla against the frontomaxillary, zygomaticomaxillary, and ethmoidal maxillary sutures. The palatine bone and pterygoid plates of the sphenoid give additional stability posteriorly to the maxilla. These structures extend to the strong buttresses of the sphenoid bone in the skull base. The vomer, the perpendicular plate of the ethmoid, and the zygoma distribute the load to the temporal and frontal bones and to the anterior cranial fossa. The upper half of the nasal cavity, situated below the anterior cranial fossa between the orbits, is designated the interorbital space.

Fractures of the maxilla are usually the result of a direct impact. They vary from simple incomplete fractures of a portion of the alveolar process of the maxilla to comminuted fractures of the entire midface area. Their pattern and distribution depend on the magnitude and the direction of force (from a frontal, lateral, or inferior impact).[380]

Muscle contraction plays a less important role in displacement of maxillary compared with mandibular fractures. The muscles attaching to the maxilla include the muscles of facial expression anteriorly and the pterygoid muscles posteriorly. The muscles of facial expression have weaker forces but have some influence on the displacement of the fractured maxillary segments; segmental fractures are displaced posteriorly by the pterygoid muscles. A so-called sagittal fracture of the maxilla[119] (a fracture that splits the palate in the anterior-posterior direction) can be pulled laterally by these facial muscle attachments.[381] The pull of the pterygoid muscles posteriorly exerts downward and backward displacement forces in higher maxillary fractures. When maxillary fractures are associated with fractures of the zygoma, the action of the masseter muscle may be a factor in displacement through its strong attachments to the body of the zygoma,[10] pulling fragments posteriorly and medially.

CLASSIFICATION

Le Fort Classification

The heavier portions of the maxilla give strength to the bone; the thinner areas represent weakened sections through which fracture lines are likely to occur. The fracture lines travel adjacent to the thicker portions of the bone. Le Fort[382] completed experiments that determined the areas of structural weakness of the maxilla, which he designated "lines of weakness." Between the lines of weakness were "areas of strength." This classification led to the Le Fort classification of maxillary fractures, which identifies the patterns of midfacial fractures. The usual Le Fort fracture consists of combinations and permutations of these patterns so that straightforward pure bilateral Le Fort I, Le Fort II, or Le Fort III fractures are less common than combination patterns.[383] The level of fracture on one side is different from that on the other, and the fracture is usually more comminuted on the side of the injury (Table 66-8).[5] Thus, it is common to see a Le Fort III superior level fracture on one side with a Le Fort II superior level fracture on the other side, with the shape of the segment carrying the dentition of a Le Fort I or II fracture.

TRANSVERSE (GUÉRIN) FRACTURES OR LE FORT I LEVEL FRACTURES. Fractures that traverse the maxilla horizontally above the level of the apices of the maxillary teeth section the entire alveolar process of the maxilla, vault of the palate, and inferior ends of the pterygoid processes in a single block from the upper craniofacial skeleton. This type of injury is known as the transverse Le Fort I or Guérin fracture (Fig. 66-139).[382] This horizontal fracture extends transversely across the base of the maxillary sinuses and is almost always bilateral. The fracture level varies from just beneath the zygoma to just above the floor of the maxillary sinus and the inferior margin of the piriform aperture. Le Fort I level fractures may almost reach the inferior orbital rims and sometimes produce a pattern similar to that seen in a low Le Fort II fracture or a high Le Fort I osteotomy.

TABLE 66-8 ✦ CLASSIFICATION OF LE FORT FRACTURES

The highest level and components of the fracture on each side
   Le Fort I: Maxillary alveolus
            Split palate
            Alveolar tuberosity fracture
   Le Fort II: Pyramidal fracture
   Le Fort III: Craniofacial disjunction
   Le Fort IV: Frontal bone

Pattern of fragment that includes the maxillary dentition ("occlusal fragment")

Associated fractures
   Mandible
   Nasoethmoido-orbital
   Frontal sinus

From Manson PN: Some thoughts on the classification and treatment of Le Fort fractures. Ann Plast Surg 1986;17:356.

PYRAMIDAL FRACTURES OR LE FORT II LEVEL FRACTURES. Blows to the central maxilla, especially those involving a frontal impact, frequently result in fractures with a pyramid-shaped central maxillary segment. This is a Le Fort II central maxillary segment; the fracture begins above the level of the apices of the maxillary teeth laterally and posteriorly in the zygomaticomaxillary buttress and extends through the pterygoid plates in the same fashion as the Le Fort I fracture. Fracture lines travel medially and superiorly to pass through the medial portion of the inferior orbital rim and extend across the nose to separate a pyramid-shaped central maxillary segment from the superior cranial and midfacial structures. The fracture line centrally may traverse the nose high or low to separate superior cranial from midfacial structures (Fig. 66-139). This fracture, because of its general shape and configuration, has become known as the pyramidal fracture of the maxilla or the Le Fort II fracture. The degree of variability of the fracture in terms of the level at which it crosses the nose is extreme. It may extend through the nasal cartilages on one side (low) or through the distal nasal bone on the other side or may separate the nasal bones from the glabella at the junction of the nasal bones and frontal bone (high). With high-energy central midface impacts, the frontal sinus may be fractured and even comminuted because it is adjacent to the upper part of a high Le Fort II segment. Damage to the ethmoidal areas is routine in pyramidal fractures; these are weak areas through which fracture lines traverse the medial orbit. The lacrimal system may be involved if fracture lines traverse the lacrimal fossa. With increasing force of fracture, fractures include the combination of Le Fort I and II fractures with or without a split palate.[119,384]

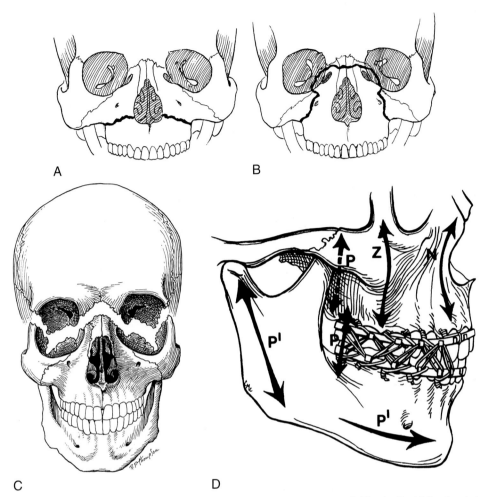

FIGURE 66-139. The Le Fort classification of midfacial fractures. *A,* The Le Fort I (horizontal or transverse) fracture of the maxilla, also known as Guérin fracture. *B,* The Le Fort II (or pyramidal) fracture of the maxilla. In this fracture, the central maxilla is separated from the zygomatic areas. The fracture line may cross the nose through its cartilages or through the middle nasal bone area, or it may separate the nasal bones from the frontal bone through the junction of the nose and frontal sinus. *C,* The Le Fort III fracture (or craniofacial disjunction). In this fracture, the entire facial bone mass is separated from the frontal bone by fracture lines traversing the zygoma, nasoethmoid, and nasofrontal bone junctions. *D,* Buttresses of the midface. N, nasofrontal buttress; Z, zygomatic buttress; p, pterygomaxillary buttress; p', posterior height and anteroposterior projection must be maintained in complicated fractures. This is especially true in Le Fort fractures accompanied by bilateral subcondylar fractures. (*A* to *C* from Kazanjian VH, Converse J: Surgical Treatment of Facial Injuries, 3rd ed. Baltimore, Williams & Wilkins, 1974.)

CRANIOFACIAL DISJUNCTION OR LE FORT III FRACTURES. Craniofacial disjunction may occur when the fracture extends through the zygomaticofrontal suture and the nasal frontal suture and across the floor of the orbits to effectively separate all midfacial structures from the cranium (Fig. 66-139). In these fractures, the maxilla is usually separated from the zygoma, but occasionally (5% of Le Fort III fractures) the entire midface may be a large single fragment, which is often only slightly displaced and immobile.[373] These fractures are usually minimally displaced and present only with "black eyes" and with subtle occlusal problems. The Le Fort III segment may or may not be separated through the nasal structures. In these fractures, the entire midfacial skeleton is incompletely detached from the base of the skull and suspended by the soft tissues and greenstick fracture.[385]

Vertical or Sagittal Fractures

Less common fractures of the maxilla may occur in a sagittal direction and section the maxilla in a sagittal, anterior-posterior plane (Fig. 66-140).[119] A common fracture splits the maxillary alveolus longitudinally near

Text continued on p. 238

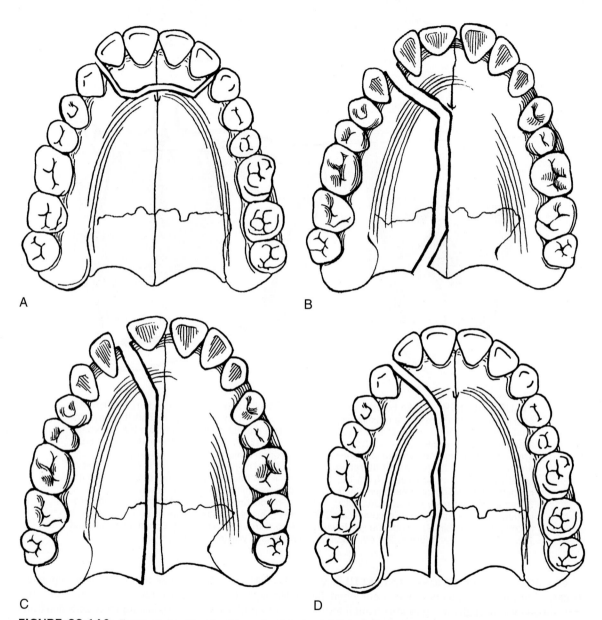

FIGURE 66-140. Types of maxillary fractures. *A*, Anterior (alveolar). *B*, Sagittal (center). *C*, Parasagittal (right). *D*, Para-alveolar.

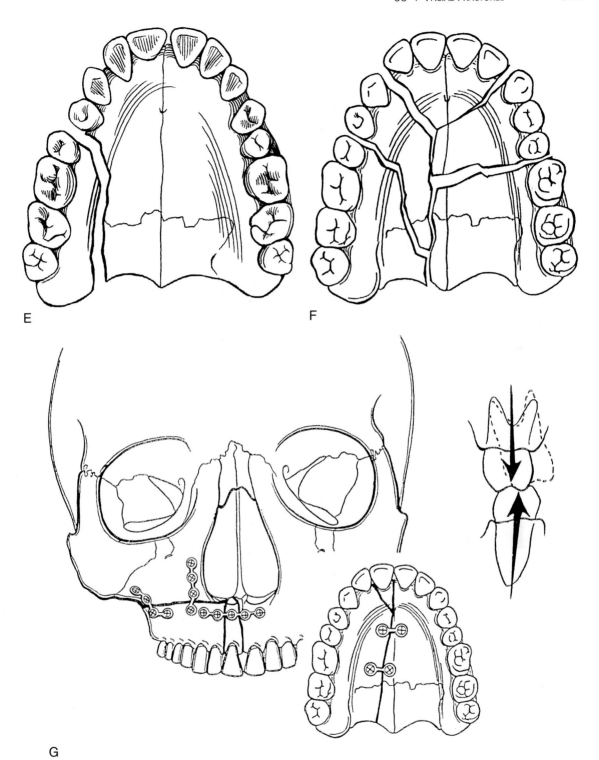

E

F

G

FIGURE 66-140, cont'd. *E,* Posterolateral (tuberosity) (left). *F,* Complicated. *G,* Scheme for reconstruction.

Continued

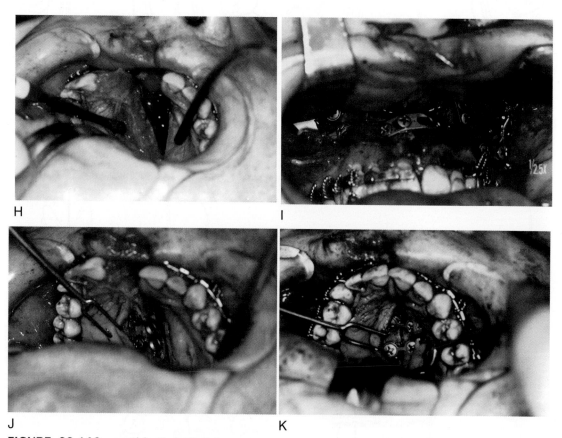

FIGURE 66-140, cont'd. *H,* Sagittal fracture—clearing enough periosteum to plate fracture. *I,* Piriform aperture reduction in a patient. Le Fort I reduction has also been completed. *J,* Palatal vault plate applied to side. *K,* Palatal vault plate reduced with double plates of 2.0-mm system.

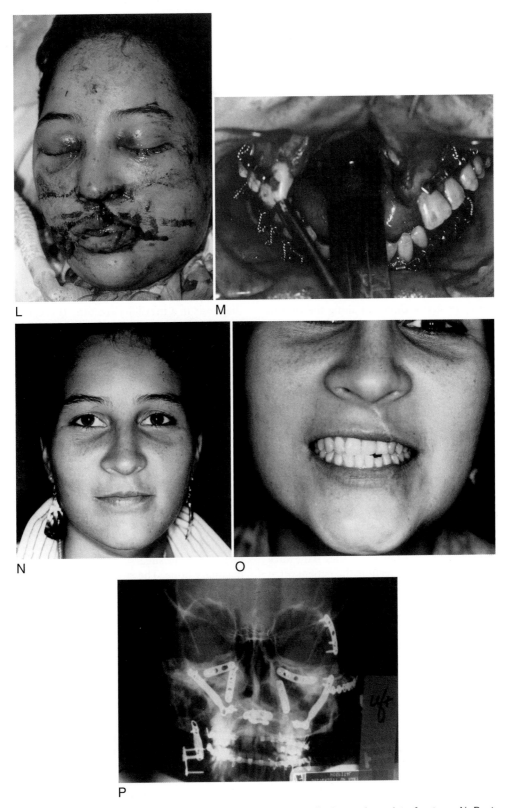

FIGURE 66-140, cont'd. *L,* Injury appearance. *M,* Note lip laceration, plate fracture. *N,* Post-operative appearance. *O,* Occlusion. *P,* Radiograph.

the junction of the maxilla with the vomer.[386] The fracture exits anteriorly to traverse between the cuspid teeth. These fractures usually involve the palate alone and Le Fort I level but occasionally extend to the Le Fort II level; 50% of sagittal fractures are usually associated with other fractures of the maxilla.[387] When present, they increase the comminution of the Le Fort fracture and make the treatment of the Le Fort fracture considerably more difficult because of the instability in the alveolar segments. The potential does exist for transverse (facial and dental arch) width problems as well as vertical and anterior or posterior displacement.[388] Displacement depends on the direction and degree of fracture and muscle forces involved.[384] Some fractures can have sufficient periosteal integrity that they may be stable even though a fracture line may be demonstrated on CT scans or plain radiographs of the palate. These fractures are usually not accompanied by the characteristic laceration in the upper buccal mucosa, lip laceration, or the laceration that travels in an anterior-posterior direction along the roof of the palate.

DIAGNOSIS

The most common cause of fractures of the maxilla is a frontal or lateral impact. The victim of the accident is thrown forward, striking the middle third of the face against an object such as an instrument panel, dashboard, or steering wheel of an automobile. If the force is sustained on the lower maxilla in the region of the upper lip, an alveolar or transverse fracture of the maxilla is likely to occur. If the force is more violent and sustained at a higher level, comminuted fractures of the maxilla may be expected. If the force is largely from a frontal impact, the fragment carrying the maxillary dentition is frequently a Le Fort II fracture. The combination of the Le Fort I and Le Fort II fractures is frequent in higher energy impact injuries. If the force is sustained from a lateral direction, the patient often has a Le Fort III level fracture on one side and a Le Fort II level fracture on the other side. The shape of the fracture fragment of the maxilla that carries the maxillary dentition in these patients may be a Le Fort I or a Le Fort II fragment, which describes the shape of the most inferior broken segment.

Although the most dramatic forces are directed from an anterior or lateral direction, there may be upward forces on the maxilla caused by impaction of the mandible against the maxilla. It is also possible to fracture the maxilla by upward force on the mandible alone, and this has been shown both clinically and experimentally.[389,390]

Displacement after maxillary fractures generally occurs in a posterior and inferior direction. The patient has an elongated, retruded appearance in the middle third of the facial skeleton. Overall elongation of the midfacial structures occurs. The maxillary occlusal fragment tilts downward, causing a premature occlusal

contact in the molar occlusion. An anterior open bite is present, often more prominent on one side than on the other, and the maxillary dentition is frequently rotated. The pterygoid musculature aids the posterior and downward forces of maxillary displacement. Partial fracture of the maxilla or alveolar processes with displacement of the segments into the sinus or region of the palate may occur from laterally directed impacts. Impacted (immobile) fractures of the maxilla are less frequent, but in some patients, the entire maxilla is driven upward and backward into the interorbital space or pharyngeal region and may be so securely impacted that no movement of the maxilla can be elicited on clinical examination.[385] Le Fort fractures of all types usually have *bilateral maxillary sinus fluid and malocclusion.*, and upper Le Fort (II and III) fractures have bilateral periorbital ecchymosis.

Clinical Examination

Mobility of the maxillary dentition is the hallmark of diagnosis in a maxillary fracture. It is exceeded only by malocclusion in diagnostic sensitivity. Certain fractures of the maxilla are incomplete (greenstick) and thus display little or no maxillary mobility. Characteristically, a single-fragment pure Le Fort III level fracture without comminution is revealed only by the presence of bilateral periorbital ecchymosis and a minor malocclusion consisting of a fraction of a cusp of malocclusion. Maxillary mobility usually cannot be detected in this rarer type of fracture. Rowe[373] thought that these fractures occurred about 5% of the time. Maxillary sinus fluid, present bilaterally on CT scans, is the most reliable CT finding. Actual fracture lines may be difficult to demonstrate on CT examination because of a lack of displacement.[385]

Epistaxis, bilateral ecchymosis (periorbital, subconjunctival, scleral), facial edema, and subcutaneous hematoma are suggestive of fractures involving the maxillary bone. The swelling is usually moderate to severe, indicating the severity of the fracture. Malocclusion with an anterior open bite and rotation of the maxilla suggests a fracture of the maxilla. The maxillary segment is frequently displaced downward and posteriorly, resulting in a class III malocclusion and premature occlusion in the posterior dentition with an anterior open bite. On internal examination, there may be tearing of the soft tissues in the labial vestibule of the lip or the palate, a finding that indicates the possibility of an alveolar or palate fracture. A sagittal fracture of the maxilla may be suspected in these patients and is confirmed by lateral digital pressure on the maxillary (palatal aspect) dentition, demonstrating lateral movement of the lateral maxillary dentition. Any movement or instability indicates a fracture of the teeth, palate, or alveolus. Hematomas may be present in the buccal or palatal mucosa. The face, after several days, may have an elongated, retruded appearance, the so-called donkey-like facies suggestive of a craniofacial disjunction. An increase in midfacial length is seen.

Bilateral palpation may reveal step deformities of the zygomaticomaxillary suture, indicating fractures of the inferior orbital rims. These findings suggest a pyramidal fracture of the maxilla or confirm the zygomatic component of a more complicated injury, such as a Le Fort III fracture. If the maxilla medially is higher than the zygoma, a zygomatic fracture is suggested, whereas if the maxilla medially is lower than the zygoma, a pyramidal fracture is suggested. Intraoral palpation may reveal fractures of the anterior portion of the maxilla or fractured segments of the alveolar bone. Fractures of the junction of the maxilla and zygoma may be detected by digital palpation along the inferior rim of the orbit. Movement of the nasal bones by palpation suggests that a nasal fracture is associated with a maxillary fracture. Nasal fractures are a routine component of Le Fort II and III fractures.

The bone should be palpated with the tips of the fingers both externally through the skin and internally intraorally. Movement of the alveolar process of the maxilla by grasping the anterior portion of the maxilla between the thumb and index finger demonstrates mobility of the maxilla. Zygomatic mobility may also be demonstrated. The manipulation test for maxillary mobility is not entirely diagnostic because impacted or greenstick fractures may exhibit no movement but still possess bone displacement. Nonmobile (impacted or incomplete) fractures are easily overlooked unless a specific and careful examination of the occlusion is performed. The occlusal discrepancy in high Le Fort III, incomplete, or single-segment fractures may be minor (i.e., within half- to one cusp displacement) (Fig. 66-141). No movement of the maxilla can be confirmed. Curiously, patients may be unable to discern this degree of occlusal discrepancy as abnormal shortly after the injury. Manipulation of the maxilla may confirm movement in the entire middle third of the face, including the bridge of the nose. This movement is appreciated by holding the head securely with one hand and moving the maxilla with the other hand. Crepitation may be heard when the maxilla is manipulated in loose fractures.

CSF may leak from the anterior or middle cranial fossa in high Le Fort fractures and is then apparent in the nose or ear canal.[391] A fluid leak signifies a dural fistula extending from the intracranial subarachnoid space through the skull and into the nose or ear.[392] The drainage is frequently obscured by bloody secretions in the immediate postinjury period.[393] Fractures of the anterior or middle cranial fossa frequently accompany severe midfacial (Le Fort II or III) injuries, and a CSF leak or pneumocephalus should be diligently sought on physical examination and by review of appropriate CT scans to detect simultaneous cranial base injuries.

If the mandible is intact, malocclusion of the teeth is highly suggestive of a maxillary fracture (Fig. 66-141). It is possible, however, that the malocclusion relates to a preinjury condition. A thorough study of the patient's dentition with reference to previous dental records and pictures is helpful. Impressions may be taken, models poured, and wear facets of the teeth studied to determine the preinjury occlusal pattern. It is possible to have a high craniofacial disjunction and still have reasonable occlusion of the teeth (high Le Fort III level fracture, single fragment). If the maxilla is rotated and markedly displaced backward and downward, there is a complete disruption of occlusal relationships with failure of all but a single posterior tooth to make contact with the mandibular dentition.

Radiographic Examination

The diagnosis of a fracture of the maxilla should be suspected clinically and then confirmed radiographically. Maxillary fractures may be difficult to demonstrate on routine plain radiographs but are easily demonstrated in craniofacial CT scans, with the exception that fracture lines in minimally displaced fractures are more difficult to see in CT scans.[69,70] CT scans are required for diagnosis of the maxillary fracture, especially those within the orbit. Plain films used for maxillary fracture diagnosis are now superfluous but include the Waters, Caldwell, and submental vertex views as well as those of the lateral skull. Bilateral maxillary sinus opacity should always suggest the possibility of a maxillary fracture. Separation at the inferior orbital rims, zygomaticofrontal sutures, nasal frontal area, and Le Fort I levels may be noted as fractures through the lateral portion of the maxillary sinus and pterygoid plate region. Fractures of the pterygoid plates are diagnosed by CT scan, as are fractures of the palate.

Fractures of the maxilla are best documented by careful axial and coronal CT scans. These scans should be taken from the palate through the anterior cranial fossa and may be oriented both in axial and coronal planes. Bone and soft tissue windows are helpful in the evaluation of the orbital portion of the fracture and in the evaluation of the brain. Bilateral maxillary sinus fluid should always be suspected of representing a maxillary fracture until it is proved otherwise. Incomplete maxillary fractures are nondisplaced, but bilateral fluid in the maxillary sinuses may still be visualized. This sign should suggest a bilateral Le Fort maxillary fracture.

TREATMENT

Treatment of maxillary fractures is initially oriented toward the establishment of an airway, control of hemorrhage, closure of soft tissue lacerations, and placement of the patient in intermaxillary fixation. The last maneuver manually reduces the fracture, reduces movement and bleeding, and is the single most important treatment of a maxillary fracture.[10] Intermaxillary fixation may be accomplished despite the general

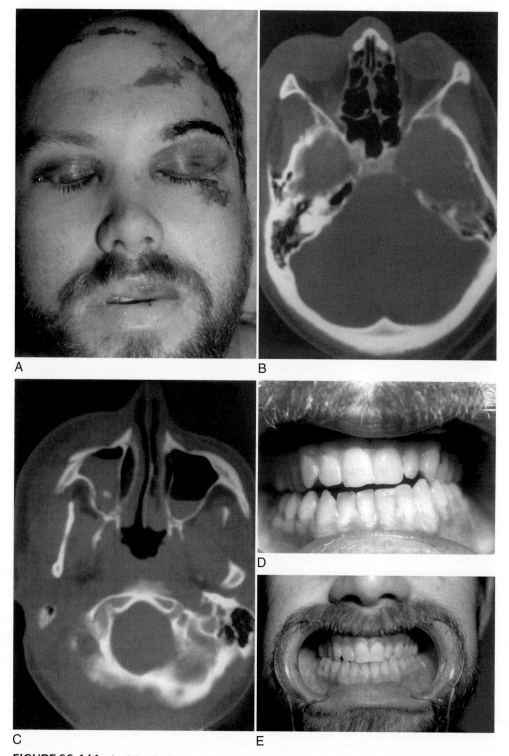

FIGURE 66-141. A minimally displaced (the displacement of the fracture is only half a cusp) impacted or incomplete fracture of the maxilla will present with a subtle malocclusion but usually with bilateral bleeding from the nose and bilateral maxillary sinus air-fluid levels from fractures in the maxillary sinuses. A displaced zygoma fracture is also frequently present with periorbital and subconjunctival hematoma unilaterally. *A,* Clinical photograph. *B* and *C,* CT radiograph. *D,* Occlusion preoperatively. *E,* Occlusion postoperatively.

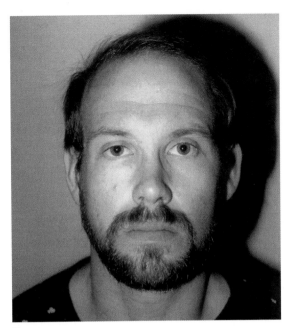

F

FIGURE 66-141, cont'd. *F,* Post-treatment appearance. (From Romano JJ, Manson PN, Mirvis WE, et al: Le Fort fractures without mobility. Plast Reconstr Surg 1990;85:355.)

condition of the patient. An arch bar tray should be taken to the admitting area or intensive care unit, and local anesthesia is used for application.

In significantly displaced fractures, considerable displacement of the maxilla can occur, blocking the airway. Hemorrhage, swelling, and secretions may render breathing difficult. The upper airway is occasionally blocked by structures forced into the pharyngeal region, such as loose teeth, pieces of broken bone, broken dentures, blood clot, or other foreign material. These obstructing materials must be removed, and if an adequate airway cannot be established, endotracheal intubation or tracheostomy should be performed.

Some fractures require anterior exposures alone (less complicated); others require exposure of the entire anterior and posterior craniofacial skeleton (Fig. 66-142). There are two steps in soft tissue closure and repositioning: (1) closure of the skin, periosteum, muscle, and fascia where incisions have been made (this step prevents soft tissue diastasis) and (2) refixation of the periosteum or fascia to the skeleton (see Fig. 66-43). The areas for periosteal closure are the zygomaticofrontal suture, infraorbital rim, deep temporal fascia, and muscle layers of the maxillary and mandibular incisions. The areas for periosteal reattachment are the malar eminence at the infraorbital rim, the temporal fascia over the zygomatic arch, the medial and lateral canthi, and the gingival (buccinator and mentalis) and zygomatic musculature over the malar eminence.

The preferred reconstructive approach proposes graded requirements for exposure, depending on the number of areas of buttress alignment required for reduction and fixation of each fractured bone. Each critical area may then have an initial and a final fixation.[5] In each subunit of the face, the important dimension to be considered first is facial width. In less severe fractures, correction of facial width is not challenging; an anterior approach alone is sufficient (see Fig. 66-43). Control of facial width in more severe injuries requires more complete dissection and alignment of each fracture component with all the peripheral and cranial base landmarks. Reconstructions that emphasize control of facial width are in fact the scheme that reciprocally restores facial projection.

The timing of soft tissue reduction is critical. The soft tissue, after complete degloving, drops inferiorly, developing thickness and an internal pattern of scarring (Fig. 66-143). Even if the bone is moved secondarily after initial healing to another location, the soft tissue retains its internal deformity and thickness because of internal fibrosis and memory. Thus, repositioning of the bone and replacement of the soft tissue must be accomplished *before* the soft tissue has developed significant memory (internal scarring) in the pattern of an abnormal bone configuration if a truly natural result is to be achieved.

In reconstruction of a nasoethmoid fracture, if the canthal ligament is partially stripped from the bone, telecanthus results because of the soft tissue displacement when the bone reduction may actually be satisfactory. Excessive width of the soft tissue may also result from soft tissue thickening secondary to scarring from internal hemorrhage and may mimic the telecanthus observed from bone malposition in the nasoethmoid area. A common mechanism of error is identification and suture of the canthal ligament inside the coronal incision rather than externally at the eyelid commissure. Fixation of the ligament at the internal aspect of the coronal incision grasps only the medial edge of the tendon, which may add 5 mm per side to the intercanthal distance.

Palatal fractures that are not corrected for width, especially if they accompany fractures of the anterior mandible, tend to result in a wide maxillary arch. Intermaxillary fixation and elastic traction result in "off axis" forces, which tend to tip the inferior aspect of the lateral maxillary dentition toward the palate. The most common deformity seen with parasymphysis or parasymphysis-subcondylar mandibular fracture combinations is increased width of the lower face at the mandibular angles (Fig. 66-143). These deformities are not prevented by the use of small plates in the anterior mandible, but only a long strong plate in the ante-

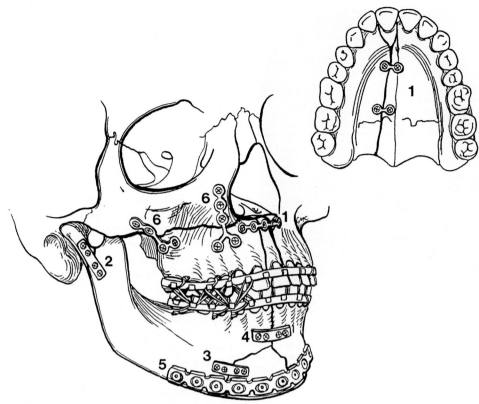

FIGURE 66-142. Reconstruction sequence in the lower facial unit. The reduction sequence is as follows: 1, split palate; 2, ± intermaxillary fixation and vertical segment of the mandible; 3, minor segment reduction in horizontal mandible; 4, horizontal mandible upper border tension band plate; 5, major segment horizontal mandible reduction; and 6, Le Fort I buttress reduction. (From Manson PN, Clark N, Robertson B, et al: Subunit principles in midface fracture treatment: the importance of sagittal buttresses, soft-tissue reductions, and sequencing treatment of segmental fractures. Plast Reconstr Surg 1999;103:1287.)

rior mandible can maintain the preferred width and prevent flaring of the mandible at the angles and prevent lingual rotation of the lateral mandibular dentition (Fig. 66-143).

The most common positional deformities seen in the frontal region that lead to midfacial subunit malposition are posterior and inferior positioning of the superior orbital rims and flattened frontal contour (Fig. 66-143). Lack of periosteal closure over the zygomaticofrontal suture produces the appearance of temporal wasting because of the gap in the temporal aponeurosis and skeletonization of the frontal process of the zygoma (Fig. 66-144). Incisions for arch exposure made higher in the posterior layer of the deep temporal fascia with dissection through the syssarcosis of fat to reach the zygomatic arch produce fat atrophy by direct fat damage (interference with its middle temporal blood supply). Incisions in the deep temporal fascia just immediately above the arch minimize damage to the fat. Arch reductions have been known to be displaced postoperatively, and stronger

plates are recommended, such as the Zydaption plate,* which is designed for strength and thinness.

The midface, because of its thin bone, should be considered a dependent structure.[5] Most of its injuries are comminuted and occur with fractures of the frontal bone or mandible more frequently than isolated midface fractures do. The bone structure of the midface is thin and not particularly conducive to stability. The use of malleable plates and small screws in thin midfacial bone (which is often affected by microfractures and has a lack of guides to correct anterior positioning) must be viewed as a relative positioning device rather than rigid fixation. The maxilla has weak sagittal buttresses. Further, with rare exception, the posterior or pterygoid buttresses of the maxilla are not addressed in current facial fracture reduction schemes. Incomplete maxillary reductions are prone to instability. Therefore, some period of postoperative

---

*Synthes Maxillofacial, Paoli, Pa.

intermaxillary fixation and frequent observation of the occlusion are both indicated to detect displacement or malocclusion.

There is considerable theoretical support, therefore, for the concept that the midface should be addressed in two sections, divided at the Le Fort I level, and then reassembled in anatomic subunits, relating each segment to anatomic areas with strong sagittal buttresses, which are correctly positioned. It is more predictable to stabilize the occlusion in comminuted

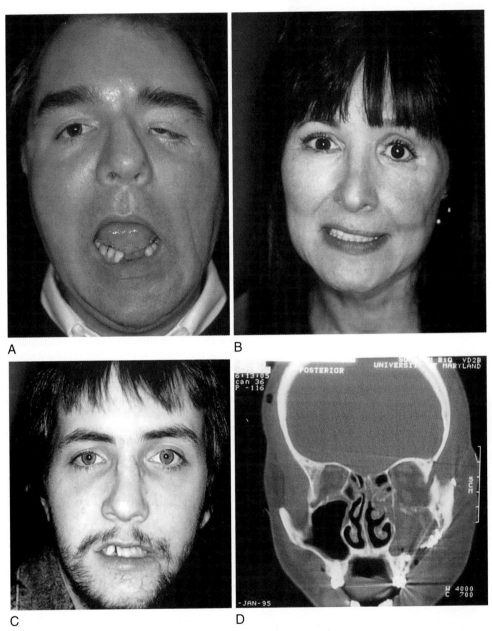

FIGURE 66-143. *A,* Soft tissue and bone deformity with enophthalmos, lateral canthal dystopia, ectropion, and soft tissue slippage in the midface. The lateral mandibular dentition is rotated lingually. *B,* Enophthalmos, skeletonization of the orbital rim, scleral show, and retraction ("balling up") of midface soft tissue; slippage of the thick tissue off the malar eminence is caused by lack of soft tissue closure and lack of stabilization and fixation of the soft tissue onto the bone. *C,* Right enophthalmos and soft tissue slippage off the malar eminence because of postoperative displacement of a zygoma fracture after plate and screw fixation. The lower incisors are seen because of failure to close the mentalis muscle in the gingival buccal sulcus incision, producing lower lip ectropion and incisor show. *D,* Orbital enlargement after disruption of fixation. *Continued*

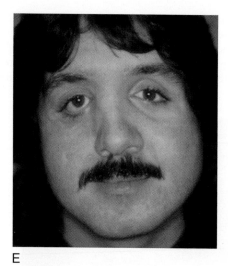

E

FIGURE 66-143, cont'd. *E,* Disruption of fixation in zygomatic arch.

fractures by relating the maxilla to the mandible than by relating the inferior maxilla to the superior maxilla. The most common bony facial deformities after midface fracture treatment relate to lack of projection, enophthalmos, malocclusion, and increased facial width (see Fig. 66-143). Such deformities are seen especially in the central midface, which lacks sagittal

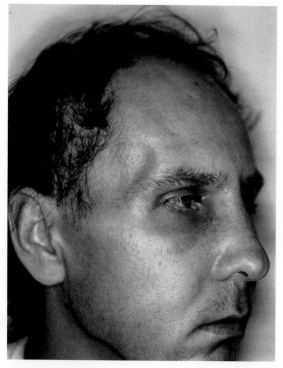

FIGURE 66-144. "Skeletonization" of the frontal process of the zygoma from failure to close the temporal fascia to the orbital periosteum over the frontal process.

buttresses—thus the difficulty of restoration and projection. The most common soft tissue deformities are descent, diastasis, fat atrophy, ectropion, thickening, and rigidity.

Patients with large-segment fractures may be adequately stabilized by plate and screw fixation to permit early release of intermaxillary fixation. Patients with comminuted midface or panfacial fractures are best served by varying periods of postoperative intermaxillary fixation. Patients with accompanying palatal fractures routinely benefit from more prolonged intermaxillary fixation in terms of preservation of occlusal alignment. The split palate should be repaired first before the buttresses are plated. Whenever intermaxillary fixation is released, the occlusion must be observed carefully and frequently. Some authors have implied that intermaxillary fixation is not necessary postoperatively for midface fractures. This depends entirely on the amount of stability obtained, the nature of the fractures and their comminution, and the muscle forces placed on the fractures. Intermaxillary fixation has more importance than has been emphasized in the recent literature. It is an unexcelled positioning and stabilizing device for the lower midface segment, both acutely at the initial reduction and postoperatively as required.

The usual midface fracture is not isolated; also it is usually comminuted. Midfacial bone is thin and often involved with microfractures; titanium fixation devices are thin, malleable, and not necessarily able to hold these thin bones stable when there are strong muscle and soft tissue forces, when the fractures are impacted and not fully mobilized, or when incomplete fractures are present and not completed. Titanium plates are not sufficient in themselves to control displacement of the Le Fort I fragment in comminuted facial fracture treatment.

The use of craniofacial exposure techniques has produced increased accuracy and refinement of bone positioning. When the soft tissue is degloved from the facial skeleton, malposition and thinning of soft tissue over the skeleton can be expected unless specific maneuvers are used for reconstruction and replacement. Soft tissue repairs must be designed so that layered closures reapproximate the muscles and the periosteum, re-forming the inner layer of the soft tissue envelope. The periosteum, which is inflexible and therefore of correct length, may then be reattached to the craniofacial skeleton at appropriate locations, preventing soft tissue descent.

Recognizing the importance of realigning both bone and soft tissue, craniofacial surgeons are able to improve their results in facial fracture treatment. The midface must be treated as a dependent structure because of its thin bone and comminuted fracture patterns. The buttresses of the midface are weak; the frontal bone and the mandible are therefore the best sagittal buttresses of the midface in comminuted fracture treatment. The technique of postoperative CT scanning, although adding considerable cost, increases operator precision by identifying common treatment errors.

Importance of Intermaxillary Fixation

The simplest treatment of a maxillary fracture, and the one that is surprisingly the most effective and almost always can be accomplished, involves placing the patient in occlusion in intermaxillary fixation.[10,394] Arch bars should be ligated to the upper and lower dentition, and then the arch bars are linked with either elastic or wire intermaxillary fixation. Intermaxillary fixation should be accomplished as soon after a maxillary injury as possible. Much of the deformity of a midfacial fracture may be eliminated by the simple act of placing the patient in intermaxillary fixation. This maneuver also reduces the distraction of the fragments, frequently facilitates cessation of hemorrhage, and places the maxilla at rest, which is an important treatment when dural fistulas exist. If the mandible is intact, this maneuver immediately limits the downward and posterior displacement of the lower portion of the midface and keys a major portion of the lower midface into proper anterior-posterior reduction. The elongated, retruded midface is effectively avoided because of the tendency of the mandibular musculature to assume a balanced or "rest" position, close to centric rest.

Alveolar Fractures

Simple fractures of the portions of the maxilla involving the alveolar process and the teeth can usually be digitally repositioned and held in reduction while an arch bar is applied to these teeth. The arch bar may be acrylated for stability, or an open reduction may use unicortical plates and screws to unite the alveolar fragment to the remainder of the maxilla. Previously, an occlusal splint was placed across the palate to provide alignment and additional stability for loose teeth or support for an alveolar fracture. An acrylated arch bar would also provide dental stability. Orthodontic appliances may also effectively manage an alveolar fracture. The position of the teeth may be maintained by ligating the teeth in the fractured segment to adjacent teeth with the use of an arch bar and interdental wiring technique. Acrylation of the arch bar results in additional support, once reduction is achieved. The fabrication of a splint or the acrylation of an arch bar may be simply accomplished with quick-curing acrylic resin molded to a lubricated model of the teeth and alveolus. The acrylic material may be cooled as it cures. If the fragments cannot be adequately reduced manually, or if there is consistent premature contact between the teeth of the maxilla and the mandible, the teeth of the fractured segment are placed in jeopardy by this premature contact. A more definitive reduction of the fractured segment should be considered that allows the segment to be seated in proper position. An incomplete fracture or intervening soft tissue is usually the problem. Fixation of the alveolar segment should be maintained for at least 4 to 12 weeks or until clinical immobility has been achieved.[119] The teeth involved in the fractured alveolar segment may be subject to damage of the neurovascular structures within the pulp and are often insensitive; appropriate endodontic evaluation should be obtained when feasible. For alveolar fractures, the model of the dentition may have to be segmented and repositioned and the fracture segment placed in a better position, cementing it and then making the splint.[395]

Le Fort Fractures

Le Fort,[382] a French orthopedic surgeon, described his findings on the pattern of maxillary fractures based on cadaver experiments performed around 1900. Milton Adams described in 1942[335] and in 1956[336] internal fixation with suspension and open reduction of the upper parts of these midface fractures by use of wires (Fig. 66-145). In Le Fort fractures, Adams advocated open reduction and internal fixation of the orbital rims in midfacial fractures by a combination of closed reduction of the lower midface, placement of intermaxillary fixation devices, and placement of suspension wires leading to a point above the fracture on each side (Fig. 66-145). These suspension wires were meant to compress or impact the maxillary segments, achieving a reduction. His principles were welcome because the external fixation devices were avoided in many patients. The limitation of the Adams technique related to the incomplete exposure and fixation of all fractured fragments and the use of compression with suspension wires as a means of facial fracture stabilization.

However, the midface would often be shorter and wider after Adams fixation. Although Adams' technique served to simplify and improve the results of treatment and was satisfactory for simple, noncomminuted fractures, the technique failed to provide an opportunity to open or reduce the complete fracture patterns and restore all the comminuted segments of the fractures occurring between the maxillary alveolus and the orbit to their proper position. The technique also relied only on the bone fragments present, no matter what their condition. No early bone grafting was performed.

Advances in the last 20 years have revolutionized the treatment of Le Fort fractures, primarily with regard to the aesthetic (as opposed to functional) criteria.[9,115,120,396-400] The advances are predicated on a better definition of the soft tissue and bone injury from CT scans and the use of extended open reduction techniques first involving exposures with fixation by wires, bone grafts, and internal fixation with plate and screw techniques. The use of bone grafts primarily to replace or to augment unusable bone structure was pioneered by Gruss[114] and rapidly spread throughout North America for the treatment of all facial injuries. These two techniques, rigid fixation of the facial skeleton and

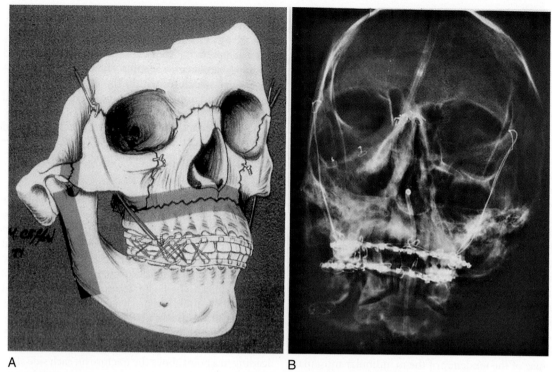

A   B

FIGURE 66-145. Fixation in Le Fort fractures originally described by Milton Adams and used up to the 1980s. *A,* Orbital rim fractures treated by open reduction at the zygomaticofrontal sutures and inferior orbital rim areas. The patient was placed in intermaxillary fixation. Wires were passed from the arch bars to a point above the most superior level of the Le Fort fracture on each side, which were called suspension wires. The suspension wires were expected to contribute to stability by compression of the midfacial skeleton. Their action, however, was frequently to reduce the vertical height of the midface and retrude the midface, especially in comminuted fractures involving the middle levels of the midfacial skeleton or when fractures of the subcondylar areas of the mandible accompanied loose midface fractures. The goals in midface fracture treatment are now to allow complete "expansion" of the midfacial skeleton, achieving the original dimensions of the facial bones, and to stabilize these dimensions with bone grafts and plate and screw fixation. *B,* Radiograph of Adams fracture treatment and suspension wires.

primary bone grafting, allowed the preinjury bone architecture to be established before soft tissue contracture had occurred over a malpositioned bony skeleton. These techniques greatly improved the aesthetic results of treatment and have reduced the residual deformity by establishing a more accurate restoration of the preinjury craniofacial architecture.

Initially, wire interfragment fixation was used for bone alignment and reduction. These techniques did not produce rigid bone stabilization, as interfragment wires provide only a one-dimensional force of apposition.[5] Three-dimensional stabilization of facial fracture fragments is achieved only by multiple wire points of fixation per fragment or preferably the use of a plate and screw technique that prevents rotation of facial fracture fragments. Stability is provided by the placement of two screws (two points of fixation) per bone fragment (one point would still permit rotation).

The use of the Adams technique[335,336] (Fig. 66-145) in comminuted fractures results in excessive midfa-

cial compression and overlap, especially in crushed facial fractures. Midfacial height may be maintained only by a proper anatomic reconstruction of the vertical height of the maxillary buttresses. In the past, attempts were made to establish restoration of midfacial height and projection with a head frame in addition to open reduction and interfragment wire techniques in complicated fractures. The midface was set and stabilized to an exact relationship with the cranial base.

The bone reconstruction may now be more simply and securely performed by an anatomic surgical reconstruction of the horizontal and vertical structural pillars of the midface.

GOALS OF LE FORT FRACTURE TREATMENT. The goals of the treatment of Le Fort fractures are to reestablish midfacial height and projection,[383] to provide proper occlusion, and to restore the integrity of the nose and orbit. The structural supports between the areas of the buttress and maxillary alveolus must also be restored to provide for the proper soft tissue contour. Fracture patterns exist as comminuted but standard discrete fracture segments corresponding in their boundaries to the lines of weakness at the various levels of the Le Fort fracture. The present Le Fort classification system is actually a simplification of the fracture pattern described in his experiments and represents the application of the techniques of open reduction to Le Fort's description. The Le Fort classification may be practically used to describe the most superior level of the fracture on each side because the fractures usually are bilaterally asymmetric. When Adams[335,336] suspension wires were employed, the highest level of the fracture was the point beyond which the suspension had to be carried to achieve a stable reduction by compression[10] (Fig. 66-146). Now, the use of rigid fixation allows the stable point on each side to be the keystone to reduction of the lower midfacial fractures.[120,386]

Ferraro and Berggren[401] were the first to document the reduced facial height that accompanies the usual Le Fort fracture treatment. Thus, in the treated Le Fort injury, the most common disturbance is reduced midfacial height and projection rather than the facial elongation and retrusion seen in the untreated Le Fort fracture. It becomes important, therefore, to restore the facial height and projection by anatomic reconstruction of the buttresses of the maxilla. Anteriorly, the nasomaxillary and zygomaticomaxillary buttresses are reconstructed after alignment, providing bone grafts and rigid fixation for stability. The fracture is usually worse (more extensive and comminuted) on one side. The more intact side is often the best key to the facial height. Correction of the posterior facial height does not involve accurate reconstruction of the pterygoid buttresses but is achieved by intermaxillary fixation of the maxilla to an intact or anatomically reconstructed mandible. Therefore, the posterior (ramus) height of the mandible must be correct for a proper reconstruction of posterior maxillary midface height to be accomplished. Because the posterior maxilla is reduced by placing the maxilla in occlusion with the mandible, it becomes important to have the mandible anatomically reconstructed as a buttress for restoration of midfacial height and projection. Ramus and subcondylar fractures are stabilized by open reduction and rigid fixation. The importance of diagnosing the sagittally split palate fracture is emphasized by the increase in lower midfacial width and malocclusion that complicates the Le Fort I segment in these injuries.[119,381]

Fractures of the Edentulous Maxilla

Fractures of the edentulous maxilla[245,377,402] are seen less frequently and are usually associated with other extensive fractures of the bones of the middle third of the face. The absence of teeth through which the fracturing forces are usually transmitted can provide a measure of protection for the edentulous elderly patient. In addition, older patients are not usually exposed to the traumatic hazards of the lifestyle of the younger age groups, which reduces the incidence of maxillary fractures in the edentulous patient. Dentures provide some protection from fracture by absorbing traumatic forces, which are partially dissipated by the breaking of the denture. If the displacement of an edentulous Le Fort fracture is minimal, causing little facial deformity, it is reasonable to expect a discrepancy in the maxillary-mandibular relationships to be corrected by means of adjustment or construction of a new denture. Treatment is therefore nonoperative. Fractures selected for this type of treatment may be expected to heal within 3 to 8 weeks on a soft diet. The denture is not worn until healing has occurred. As soon as the edema and hematomas have disappeared and healing has been confirmed, the patient may have a new denture constructed.

If there is mobility or significant displacement such that it results in deformity of the middle third of the face or if there is significant displacement that precludes correction with a new denture, efforts should be made to reduce and to immobilize the midface fracture segments (Fig. 66-147). In some instances, the Le Fort I level segments are so comminuted that accurate reduction is difficult. For the operation, the use of a denture or a splint designed to key the position of the lower midface segments to the mandible is recommended, just as intermaxillary fixation provides this relationship in dentulous patients (Fig. 66-147).

A full open reduction is performed, anatomically uniting the areas of the facial buttresses. Plate and screw fixation is helpful, decreasing the time required for fixation. In many patients, bone grafts at the Le Fort I level and over the retruded piriform aperture and over the maxillary sinus may be required. In patients in whom the dentures are used as splints, one may screw them temporarily to the alveolus of the maxilla, palate, or mandible, which provides a straightforward and rapid initial fixation of the denture. Intermaxillary fixation is usually released at the completion of reduction. In many instances, good bone inferiorly will be found only at the maxillary alveolus, and the screws may have to extend to this level. They will therefore interfere with wearing of a new denture and must be removed before new denture construction.

EARLY COMPLICATIONS

Hemorrhage

The early complications associated with fractures of the maxilla include extensive hemorrhage. Hemorrhage may be managed by carefully identifying and ligating vessels in cutaneous lacerations and by tamponade in closed midface injuries with anterior-posterior nasopharyngeal packing, manual reduction of the

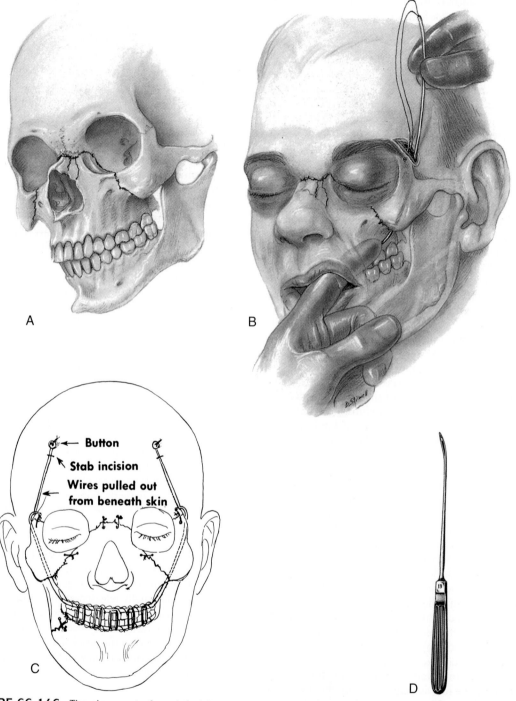

A

B

C

Button

Stab incision

Wires pulled out
from beneath skin

D

FIGURE 66-146. The placement of craniofacial suspension wires is occasionally used with present-day treatment to stabilize arch bars or to prevent the jaws from opening in uncooperative patients. *A,* A pyramidal (Le Fort II) fracture is seen. *B,* Suspension wires are passed through a spinal needle or with a wire passer that has a perforated pointed tip that is inserted through the brow incision, traverses the area medial to the zygomatic arch and posterior to the body of the zygoma, and enters the oral cavity opposite the maxillary first molar. *C,* The area of direction of the interosseous fixation and the direction of the wires used for craniofacial suspension. The suspension wires are removed after healing has taken place by cutting the wires in the mouth and pulling them out by traction on the "pull-out" wires in the forehead area. *D,* Wire passers are used in passing these wires. These techniques are currently infrequently used for arch bar stabilization and almost never for fracture reduction. They are sometimes used in uncooperative (head-injured) patients to prevent the mouth from opening.

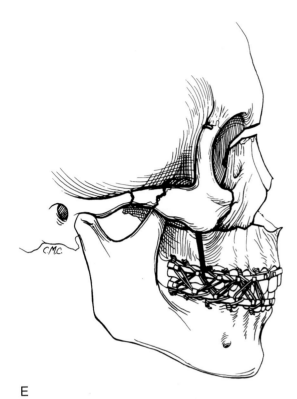

E

FIGURE 66-146, cont'd. *E,* Overlap of fragments, producing a reduced midface height, was inevitable with Adams suspension alone. (*E* from Manson PN: Some thoughts on the classification and treatment of Le Fort fractures. Ann Plast Surg 1986;17:356.)

displaced maxilla, reduction in intermaxillary fixation, angiographic embolization and external carotid and superficial temporal artery ligation, and other appropriate techniques.

Airway

The maxilla forms a significant part of the boundary of the nasogastric cavities. In almost all patients with extensive fractures, the airway is partially compromised by posterior displacement of the fracture fragments and by edema and swelling of the soft tissues in the nose, mouth, and throat. In some patients, a nasopharyngeal airway may assist in establishing a pathway for ventilation. In other patients, intubation or tracheostomy may be indicated to provide a secure airway.

Infection

Maxillary fracture wounds are less complicated by infection than are mandibular fractures.[403] Although they are contaminated at the time of the injury by entry into adjacent sinuses and by fractures of the teeth and open wounds, fractures passing through the sinuses do not usually result in infection unless there has been preexisting nasal or sinus disease or persistent obstruction of the sinus orifice by displaced bone fractures or blood clot. Appropriate methods of managing local infection are instituted if infection occurs; these include evaluation for the source of the infection, removal of any devitalized bone fragments or

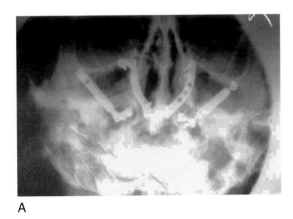

A

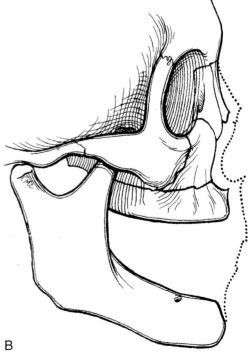

B

FIGURE 66-147. An edentulous Le Fort II-III level fracture. *A,* Radiograph. *B,* Artist's diagram of edentulous fracture displacement. If maxillary and mandibular arches are not aligned, the alignment of the upper jaw may appear to be correct but actually is too posterior.

Continued

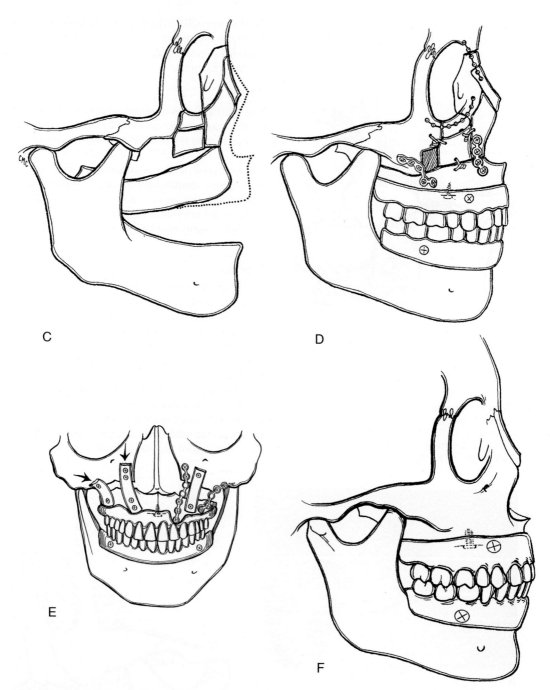

C

D

E

F

FIGURE 66-147, cont'd. *C* to *E,* Illustration of edentulous fracture treatment. *F,* Screw fixation of dentition.

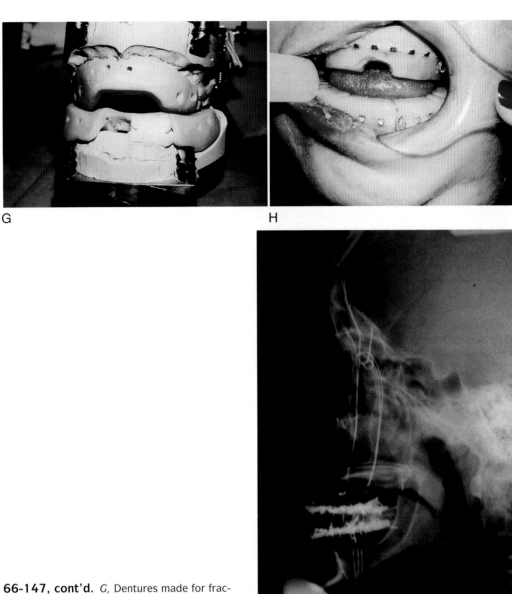

G

H

I

FIGURE 66-147, cont'd. *G,* Dentures made for fracture alignment. *H,* Dentures in place with arch bars incorporated. *I,* Radiograph of reduction with dentures. (From Crawley WA, Azman P, Clark N, et al: The edentulous Le Fort fracture. J Craniofac Surg 1997;8:298.)

devitalized soft tissue from the sinus cavities, provision for sinus drainage, extraction of loose or devitalized teeth, removal of foreign material, and administration of antibiotics as appropriate, confirmed by culture and sensitivity testing. If the maxillary sinuses are obstructed, a nasal-antral window or preferably endoscopic drainage of the maxillary sinus by enlarging its orifice may be required.

Lacrimal Obstruction

Obstruction of the lacrimal system produces dacryocystitis[404] and may require external drainage. Infections may spread into orbital soft tissues, requiring decompression of the orbit. Orbital cellulitis is a potentially serious complication resulting in blindness from excess intraorbital pressure.[405]

Cerebrospinal Fluid Rhinorrhea

High Le Fort (II and III) level fractures may be associated with fractures of the cribriform area, which produce CSF rhinorrhea or pneumocephalus. Antibiotic therapy may be used in these fractures at the discretion of the attending surgeon. Although antibiotic prophylaxis in CSF rhinorrhea has been widely employed, it is difficult to prove that antibiotics have substantially reduced the incidence of meningitis accompanying CSF rhinorrhea when they are administered during a prolonged period. Blowing of the nose and placement of obstructing nasal packing should be avoided. Nasal packing tends to cause CSF drainage to pool, forming a stagnant environment that allows bacterial proliferation. Blowing of the nose with the fingers over the nostrils, producing partial obstruction of the nasal orifices, forces nasal secretions into soft tissue, the sinuses, or the intracranial CSF in the presence of a leak. In general, prophylactic antibiotics are employed around the time of fracture reduction or for a brief (48-hour) period. The prolonged administration of antibiotics in CSF rhinorrhea merely selects an organism to colonize the meninges as one that will be resistant to the particular antibiotic used for long-term prophylaxis.

Blindness

Blindness is a rare complication of fractures of the orbit and may complicate fractures of the Le Fort II and III level. It is rare for the optic nerve to be severed by bone fragments. The most common cause is swelling of the nerve within the tight portion of the optic canal or interference with the capillary blood supply of the optic nerve by swelling and edema. Blindness is dealt with in the section on the orbit.

LATE COMPLICATIONS

Late complications of fractures of the maxilla include those referable to the orbit and zygoma because these areas form a portion of the upper Le Fort (II and III) fractures. Specific complications referable to the maxilla include nonunion, malunion, plate exposure, lacrimal system obstruction, infraorbital and lip hypesthesia or anesthesia, and devitalization of teeth. There may be changes in facial appearance due to differences in midfacial height and projection and differences in the transverse width of the face or dental arch. Complications referable to the nasal portion of the injury include reduced nasal airway from restriction of passage diameter, septal deviation, cartilage warping and altered appearance, and aesthetic deformities of the nose. If the maxillary alveolus is impacted upward, the size of the nasal cavity is reduced and the superior edge of the palate is often visible above the level of the nasal floor.

Nonunion of fractures of the maxilla is rare,[406,407] but delayed union is frequent because of the thin characteristics of the bone of the maxillary sinuses. Slower union is common, especially in comminuted fractures, because of the thin bone; this slower union frequently results in subtle drift to malocclusion, especially if it is not detectable by maxillary mobility. If the arch bars or intermaxillary fixation is removed too soon, the maxilla may slowly drift into malocclusion and malalignment despite being "clinically immobile." The patients most prone to this complication usually have

considerable comminution of the thin bones forming the structural supports of the maxilla at the Le Fort I level, and destruction of this bone or poor fixation results in collapse and retrusion. The only real nonunions have followed closed reductions of extremely comminuted fractures and are thus very uncommon.

The maxilla is normally healed within 6 to 8 weeks after the fracture. Patients with comminuted fractures must be watched for an additional period on a weekly basis to ensure that no occlusal displacement is occurring (Fig. 66-148). Patients who still demonstrate mobility of the maxilla after 8 weeks usually heal within an additional 4 weeks. Careful postoperative observation of the occlusion when the intermaxillary fixation is released is required and is too frequently omitted. Patients are generally seen once or twice a week to confirm that no change is occurring in occlusion after intermaxillary fixation is released. The arch bars should stay in place so that elastic traction can easily be reinstituted by elastics. The first sign of occlusal deviation is usually an anterior open bite, first detected by lack of a cuspid contact (Fig. 66-148). After 4 weeks of confirmed stability in function where no occlusal deviation or open bite has occurred, the arch bars are removed. The patients may eat a *soft* diet when the intermaxillary fixation is released and progress to a regular diet.

The timing of release of the intermaxillary fixation depends on the degree of comminution of the fracture, the presence of associated fractures, such as fractures of the mandible (especially the subcondylar area), and the degree of stability obtained by rigid fixation. Rigid fixation in maxillary fractures is not really "rigid" because of the thin bone and the somewhat malleable nature of smaller titanium plates, which makes all reductions potentially unstable. Therefore, patients with their intermaxillary fixation released must be carefully watched in terms of their occlusion. In general,

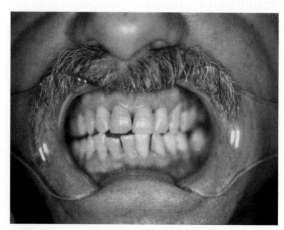

FIGURE 66-148. Lack of contact between the maxillary and mandibular cuspid teeth is usually the first indication of an open bite deformity.

the first occlusal deformity to be noted is the lack of a cuspid contact and the development of a slight open bite anteriorly or an edge incisal relationship. Normally, the maxilla will be displaced slightly inferiorly in the posterior dentition, resulting in an open bite anteriorly. If the surgeon notices a slight difference in the occlusion on close observation, the fracture has not completely healed even though the maxilla may consistently be immobile on a manual test for clinical mobility. These patients should be placed in intermaxillary fixation with light elastic (class III) traction to guide the maxilla back into the proper relationship and to continue to achieve maximal intercuspation of the teeth. Diet should be reduced in consistency (light or soft diet). The retention of arch bars for several weeks after the initial release of intermaxillary fixation is a helpful adjunct because it is a simple matter just to reapply some elastics. If the arch bars are removed too early and the patient does not return, a malocclusion may not be noticed until the maxilla has healed in the wrong position, necessitating refracture by osteotomy.

Nonunion and Bone Grafting

True nonunion of the maxilla is rare and usually follows failure to provide even the most elementary type of intermaxillary fixation or open reduction. If nonunion occurs, the treatment consists of exposure of the fracture site, resection of the fibrous tissue in the fracture site, reduction of the displaced segments, removal of any proliferative bone edges, placement of bone grafts in all the existing gaps, and stabilization plate and screw fixation.[268,408,409]

Healing almost always follows this approach. It is essential to bone graft significant (>3 to 5 mm) defects[410,411] in the buttress system and to bone graft between buttresses over the anterior wall of the maxillary sinus or to replace this bone if it is destroyed, as it ultimately strengthens the repair and also prevents prolapse of soft tissue into the sinus.[268,409]

Malunion or Partial Healing

Impacted fractures or those seen several weeks after injuries that have partially healed may be impossible to reduce without an osteotomy and full open reduction.[412] The reduction may be difficult even though one does perform an open reduction. In some patients, intermaxillary fixation with elastic traction can be employed, which is then used to accomplish displacement of the fractured fragments.[407] In other patients, however, the maxilla will need to be mobilized either by direct osteotomies (which are preferred) or through the use of Rowe disimpaction forceps (which is not recommended) (Fig. 66-149). Experience gained in craniofacial surgery has shown that open reduction and osteotomies may be employed safely and efficiently.[405] The result is always superior to that obtained by forcible closed methods. After osteotomy

and rigid fixation, the patient is more comfortable and more stable and is permitted more dietary options, and oral hygiene is greatly improved.

In malunited completely or partially consolidated fractures of the maxilla, the direct approach, transcutaneous and intraoral as appropriate for the Le Fort fracture level, is indicated. The Le Fort I malunited fracture is approached through a gingival buccal sulcus incision. The areas of fracture are exposed and the segments mobilized. A Le Fort I osteotomy is completed, and the maxillary alveolus is mobilized with finger pressure. The technique is similar to performing a Le Fort I osteotomy. Mobilization of Le Fort II and III malpositioned fractures with Rowe forceps applied at the Le Fort I level may establish undesirable new fracture lines in the orbit that may extend to the orbital apex. Osteotomies are a safer method of repositioning fractures.[412]

The lower maxillary segment may then be repositioned in the correct occlusal relationship with the mandibular teeth and maintained in intermaxillary fixation while plate and screw fixation at the Le Fort I level is completed. In some maxillary malunited fractures, the posterior maxilla has increased in length and the anterior maxilla is about the same or shortened. These fractures require resection of bone at the posterior aspect of the maxillary sinus and pterygoid plate area to be able to be returned to the proper midface vertical height. Study of the patient's preinjury photographs, old models from orthodontia, and recent models is helpful, as is evaluation of previous midfacial height and projection in photographs. Bone grafts may be necessary in some of these fractures because of the lack of good bone or bone gaps in the buttress areas. The bone grafts may be taken from the calvarial, iliac, or rib donor sites and are bent to correspond to the contour of the maxilla and attached with plate and screw fixation. Bone grafts may supplement (but do not replace) plates for rigid fixation.

Fractures at the Le Fort II and III levels are approached through the appropriate cutaneous and intraoral incisions. The use of coronal or lower lid exposures bilaterally provides complete exposure of the upper midfacial skeleton. Malunited portions of the facial skeleton are osteotomized, disimpacted, and repositioned according to the principles established in craniofacial surgery. In most instances, the bone gaps that occur require the use of bone grafts. Plate and screw fixation assists the control of fracture fragments. In some instances, initial placement of interfragment wires provides temporary positioning of the fracture segments before the application of rigid fixation.

Plates may become exposed early or late after repair, especially at the Le Fort I level.[178] The screws may become loose and migrate.[169] Plates may, if extended to the alveolus in edentulous fractures, require removal to permit wearing of a denture without discomfort.

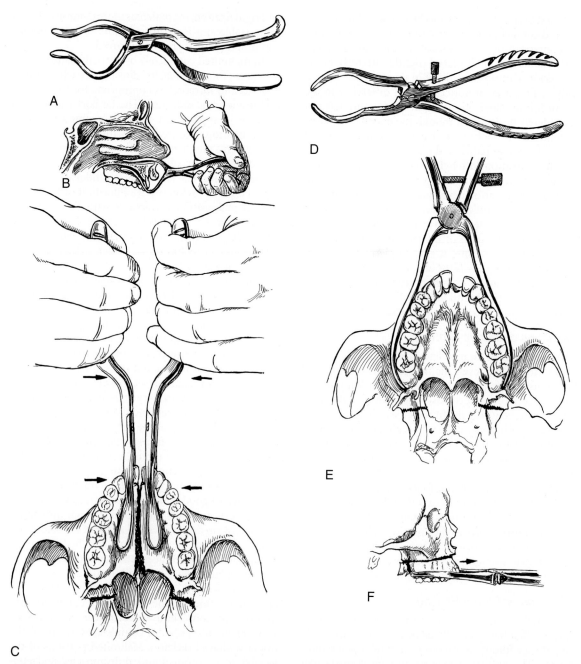

FIGURE 66-149. *A,* Rowe disimpaction forceps. *B,* Forceps in position. *C,* Two forceps may be applied to exert greater force and approximate the edges of a paramedian (sagittal) fracture of the maxilla. *D,* Hayton-Williams forceps for "maxillary disimpaction." *E,* Position of the forceps, which embrace the maxillary tuberosities. The screw that penetrates the branches of the forceps permits regulation of the pressure exerted against the bone. The forceps are not necessary in open reduction techniques, which are preferred. *F,* The use of the forceps in low maxillary fractures.

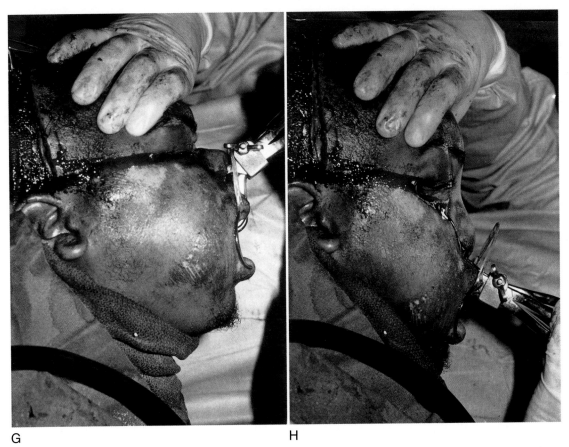

G

H

FIGURE 66-149, cont'd. *G* and *H,* Rowe disimpaction forceps used for completion of a fracture. (*A* to *F* from Kazanjian VH, Converse J: Surgical Treatment of Facial Injuries, 3rd ed. Baltimore, Williams & Wilkins, 1974.)

Nasolacrimal Duct Injury

The nasolacrimal duct may be transected or obstructed by the fractures extending across the middle third of the facial skeleton between the Le Fort I and Le Fort III levels.[413,414] The obstruction is frequently due to fracture displacement in the bones composing the nasal lacrimal duct or bone proliferation after fracture near the nasal lacrimal canal that obstructs the duct in its bony path. The duct may also be transected in the canal. The canalicular portion of the lacrimal system may be obstructed in lacerations that transect the system or in displacement of the medial canthus. When the canalicular lacrimal system is intact and the patient's lacrimal system is obstructed by a bony block of the nasal lacrimal duct, a dacryocystorhinostomy is indicated.[415] In Le Fort II or III fractures associated with nasoethmoidal-orbital fractures, the nasal lacrimal sac and canaliculi may be injured by displacement of bone fragments around the upper portion of the nasolacrimal duct at the orbital rim level. Anatomic repositioning of the fracture fragments of the medial portion of the maxilla and nasoethmoidal-orbital area provides the best protection against obstruction, but if it occurs,

external drainage and a formal secondary dacryocystorhinostomy may be necessary.[61]

Extraocular Muscle Injury

The extraocular muscles may be injured by contusion or surgical dissection in Le Fort fractures. Disturbances of the oculorotatory mechanism of the eye are more frequent in maxillary fractures with significant orbital, nasoethmoidal-orbital, and zygomatico-orbital components. The eye may not be at the proper level after treatment of fractures of the orbit. This represents the sequela of displacement of the orbital rim and orbital walls in most patients. Enlargement of the orbit is discussed more fully in the section on nasoethmoidal-orbital fractures and enophthalmos.

Complex Maxillary (Panfacial) Fractures

In panfacial fractures, fractures of various areas of the face occur in combination.[115,120,400,416] For the sake of simplicity, the individual patterns of treatment described in the previous sections can be combined so that the anatomic integrity of all the bones of the face can be restored. These multiply fractured facial skeletons are common after motor vehicle injuries. The multiply injured patient is a significant challenge since the advent of high-speed transportation, producing multiple injuries in various organ systems. The reader is referred to the initial segments of this chapter, which describe evaluation of the patient, selection and timing of emergency and definitive treatments, and selection of incisions.

No matter how severely the patient is injured, cutaneous wounds can be cleaned and closed, devitalized tissue removed, and the patient placed in intermaxillary fixation. This is the *minimum* urgent treatment of a significant maxillary or mandibular injury and may always be accomplished, despite the condition of the patient. In complex injuries of the jaws, impressions can be taken for the construction of study models, which may be used to determine patterns of preinjury occlusion by analysis of the wear pattern. The patient may also have old orthodontic models and dental radiographs or records that may be of value. Old pictures also provide clues to the prominence and shape of the nose; the prominence of the eyes; the length, projection, and width of the various portions of the face; and the relationship of the lips to the teeth. These data provide additional clues to facial height, and most pictures provide some idea of occlusal relationships.

Although much attention has been paid to the shattered bones themselves in panfacial fractures, the soft tissue overlying the bones is contused and suffused with blood. In these massively contused injuries, the soft tissue quickly fills with scar tissue, which assumes the shape of the underlying malreduced or malaligned bone fragments. The soft tissue develops an internal thickening and rigidity that becomes difficult to restructure to its original shape as it heals. Thus, in major injuries, and despite multiple system involvement, it becomes important to achieve an early anatomic alignment of the bony facial skeleton. The skeleton forms a framework over which the injured soft tissue drapes and restructures. Only early accurate treatment of the bone can restore the preinjury appearance of the soft tissue and thus of the patient.

DEFINITION OF THE PANFACIAL INJURY

Conceptually, panfacial fractures involve all three areas of the face: frontal bone, midface, and mandible.[120] In practice, when two of these three areas are involved, the term *panfacial fracture* has been applied to these more extensive injuries (Fig. 66-150).

TIMING OF TREATMENT

There are several contraindications to the immediate definitive management of panfacial fractures. These include uncontrolled intracranial pressure (>20 mm

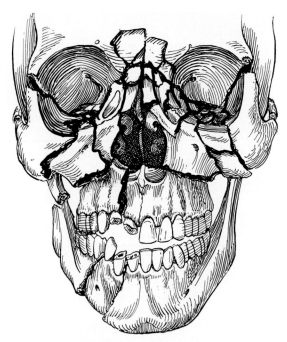

FIGURE 66-150. Panfacial fractures. The drawing shows multiple fractures involving all the facial bones.

Hg), acute hemorrhage with depleted clotting factors (such as occurs with massive pelvic fractures or intra-abdominal hemorrhage), development of a coagulopathy (such as occurs in severe central nervous system injuries), and acute respiratory distress syndrome (decreasing PO_2). In almost all other instances, the patient may be adequately monitored and the facial fractures treated despite the presence of coma, mechanical ventilation, or other injuries such as mild coma without intracranial hypertension. Sometimes, the face can be managed simultaneously with extremity fractures when surgeons are willing to cooperate with regard to equipment placement. Intraoperative monitoring of all injuries allows safe anesthesia. In patients with coma, the use of a CT scan and an intracranial pressure monitor can provide an exact monitor of the state of the head injury by a continuous indication of intracranial pressure. In general, the patient with multiple system injury should first be resuscitated; then, after physiologic stabilization, the diagnostic evaluation of injuries is undertaken in a sequence, and an appropriate plan for treatment is determined. The maxillofacial surgeon should work closely with other specialty colleagues, such as ophthalmologists and neurosurgeons, in providing an early plan for maxillofacial injury treatment.

TREATMENT

There are certain overriding considerations in the management of panfacial fractures that call for early operative intervention. The optimal time for the easiest treatment of these injuries is within hours of the accident, before the development of massive edema and soft tissue rigidity that follows these injuries. This early treatment is possible only when other systems either are not injured or are evaluated to exclude significant problems, managed, and stabilized. Fractures in specific anatomic areas of the facial skeleton may be evaluated for their severity, and a treatment plan for each area is determined according to severity. Most facial injuries can be accurately diagnosed on physical examination and are confirmed on CT scan.

A one-stage restoration of the architecture of the craniofacial skeleton is currently the preferred method of treatment for severely comminuted, multiply fractured facial bones.[120,398] Open reduction of all fracture sites is performed with plate and screw fixation, supplementing bone defects with bone grafts. Although local incisions may be useful in select patients, regional incisions, such as the coronal, lower eyelid, upper and lower gingival buccal sulcus, and retromandibular incisions, provide the preferred exposure. In some patients, these preferred exposures may not be possible because of lacerations. Wide exposure is the key to anatomic reduction of the facial skeleton.

In recent years, plate and screw fixation techniques have been used to provide maximum rigidity. In some areas, such as the zygoma, temporary placement of positioning wires in certain fractures allows provisional control of the position of the fracture while other areas are being aligned. In the zygoma, for instance, one may, for a complicated zygomatic injury, require gingival buccal sulcus, lower eyelid, and coronal incisions. Because one cannot look through these three incisions simultaneously, positioning wires stabilize the reductions in the other two exposed areas while the third area is being reduced. Then, plate and screw fixation can be applied, replacing the wires sequentially as final position and stability are achieved.

The use of a coronal incision, bilateral lower eyelid incisions (see Fig. 66-43), and a maxillary degloving (intraoral gingival buccal sulcus) incision provides exposure for the treatment of the entire middle and upper face. The frontal bone, frontal sinus, supraorbital areas, upper orbits, and zygomatic arches are effectively visualized, repositioned, and stabilized through the coronal incision. The nasoethmoidal area, frontal process of the zygoma, and lateral and medial orbits are likewise preferentially exposed through a coronal incision. The inferior portion of the orbit and remainder of the zygoma are exposed with a lower lid incision—subciliary, midtarsal, or conjunctival. The lower portion of the maxilla is exposed through the maxillary degloving incision. The bone fragments are repositioned, and buttress reconstruction is completed. Significant bone gaps of more than 3 to 5 mm should be treated by insertion of bone grafts to reconstruct

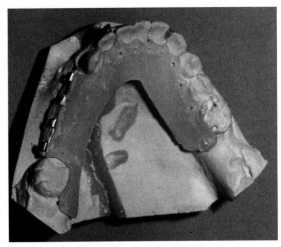

FIGURE 66-151. Dental splint with an occlusal stop preserves the relationship of the jaws and alveolar ridges when significant numbers of teeth are missing.

the structural buttresses of the facial skeleton.[410] Plate and screw fixation may also be used.

When a number of teeth or a section of the dental alveolar process is lost, a dental splint[395] with an occlusal stop (which replaces the height of the teeth) might be necessary to provide support for the intermaxillary fixation and to support the lips and cheeks during the period of healing (Fig. 66-151). This is especially helpful if the lips and cheeks have been subjected to full-thickness lacerations or extensive contusions. This approach requires the application of a number of principles of combined bone and soft tissue management.

Although the procedure may begin at any location, priorities such as neurosurgical intervention may dictate that the procedure begin in one anatomic area. If there are no such urgent neurosurgical or ophthalmologic priorities, the procedure may begin in a sequence determined by the surgeon. Various sequences have been suggested, such as top to bottom, bottom to top, outside to inside, or inside to outside. In reality, it does not make any difference what the order is as long as the order makes sense and the order leads to a reproducible, anatomically accurate bone reconstruction.

PREFERRED ORDER OF RECONSTRUCTION

1. Arch bars are applied to the mandible and maxilla, and the mandible and maxilla are placed in intermaxillary fixation.
2. If the palate is split, or if mandibular fractures occur in the horizontal portion of the mandible, these fractures should be initially aligned before the arch bar is applied. A split palate, for instance, can be anatomically repositioned and plated, and then the maxillary arch bar will act

as a tension band; the single Le Fort I fragment thus obtained can then be placed in occlusion with the mandible. The mandible and the dental arches must be provisionally realigned before a proper arch bar length can be determined for the mandible. The combination of intermaxillary fixation and basal bone reduction in mandibular fractures is managed in sequence, adjusting the occlusion to a best fit.

3. In alveolar fractures, palatal fractures, or mandible fractures, impressions are taken and stone models constructed to aid in the determination of the desired occlusion. A splint can be provided for comminuted palatal fractures or for replacement of missing segments of dentition if an occlusal stop is necessary. This requires model surgery; the fractured fragments in the model are sectioned and reconfigured to the proper arch form.

4. Intraoral incisions are used to approach the angle of the mandible, body of the mandible, symphysis, and parasymphysis portions of the mandible.

5. For comminuted fractures of the body or angle, an extraoral incision in the area of fracture is preferred. The fractured fragments are keyed into proper position, and interfragment wires may be used for temporary positioning before plate and screw fixation and intermaxillary fixation are applied. In condylar fractures, the condyle is usually restabilized by plate and screw fixation through an open approach before the basal bone of the mandible is united.

6. The anteriorly reconstructed maxillary arch should serve as a guide for the assembly and realignment of the mandible. The anatomically reconstructed maxilla in palate fractures provides the best guide for mandibular width, dental inclination, and occlusal position. The fragments of the Le Fort I area of the maxilla are exposed with a maxillary gingival buccal sulcus degloving incision, and reduction and fixation are accomplished. When the maxillary alveolus and palate are severely comminuted, they must be anatomically positioned and stabilized with rigid fixation. A splint may provide an occlusal stop or stability in patients with missing or highly comminuted sections of the dental arch or palate. Open reduction of any other fractures involving the mandible may then be performed. In large-segment sagittal fractures of the maxilla, an open reduction at the piriform aperture and in the fracture in the palatal vault assists stabilization of the bone fragments. The open reduction in the roof of the mouth (palate) may be accomplished through a laceration that exists over this frac-

ture or through a longitudinal or "palatal flap"[417] exposure. This roof of the mouth plate controls the width of the maxilla.

The mandibular reduction is now keyed to the maxillary dental relationship. After placement of the mandibular fractures into their proper position, rigid fixation of the mandible is accomplished, and the patient's occlusion is again checked. Sometimes, a dental splint can be helpful. Alignment of the basal portion of the mandible is achieved through the exposures described, and interfragment wiring may temporarily position these fragments before internal fixation. An external fixation appliance may be used to stabilize mandibular continuity through an area of missing bone, especially where there is also soft tissue missing. Preferably, internal fixation with a large stable plate such as the 2.4-mm locking plate acts as an internal "external fixator." This bone gap may also be spanned by a reconstruction plate and stabilized until a definitive reconstruction of the missing bone and soft tissue is accomplished. The sequence usually begins with temporary reduction of the horizontal portion of the mandible followed by open reduction of the ramus of the mandible exposed with a Risdon, retromandibular, or preauricular incision. If the entire ramus is comminuted, the combination of a preauricular incision and a retromandibular incision allows exposure of the entire ramus through two incisions that expose and protect the facial nerve between them. Open reduction of the basal portion of the mandible is then accomplished. In this instance, it is essential that the patient be in intermaxillary fixation in proper occlusion when definitive stabilization of the mandible or maxilla is performed. After the mandible and maxilla are initially stabilized, the intermaxillary fixation is released and the occlusion checked with the condyle carefully seated in the fossa by finger pressure. Reduction of the lower face by reconstruction of the lower maxillary-mandibular unit is now completed.

7. The coronal incision is then used to accomplish exposure of the frontal bone, frontal sinus, nasoethmoidal, and zygomaticofrontal fractures including the zygomatic arches. In the upper midface, it is the author's practice to reduce the nasoethmoidal areas first so that the zygoma can be repositioned to the medial maxilla. The medial to lateral position of the zygoma is best determined by inspecting alignment in the lateral orbit of the orbital process of the zygoma with the greater wing of the sphenoid. Zygomatic fracture reduction is often

slightly lateral unless these keys to position are appreciated. The zygomatic arches should be anatomically reduced and plated to maintain the straight character of the arch (Fig. 66-152). The medial to lateral position of the arch is best determined by observing alignment within the orbit of the orbital process of the zygoma and the greater wing of the sphenoid.

8. The orbital floor should be reconstructed anatomically. Small "ledges" of bone are usually present in the orbital floor 35 to 38 mm behind the rim. These serve as a guide to the angle of the bone graft to be used in orbital floor reconstruction. The orbital rim may be restored by realignment of all fragments and then use of interfragment wires to establish initial position. A 1.3-mm straight plate and screw fixation system is used to stabilize the individual orbital rim fragments. In the comminuted inferior orbital rim, the multiple rim segments tend to sag downward and backward. Therefore, rigid fixation must follow this reduction technique; the surgeon must hold these rim segments upward and forward as the fixation is applied.

The rim should be flat, not curved inferiorly or allowed to slip posteriorly. The basic principle of panfacial fracture reduction is to provide secure interosseous fixation throughout the entire area of bone fracture.

9. The nasoethmoid areas (frontal processes of the maxilla or central fragments of the nasoethmoid fracture) are reduced and linked with a transnasal reduction wire. The nasoethmoid area is united by junctional rigid fixation to the frontal bone and inferior orbital rim. When the mandible is severely comminuted, the maxillary arch should be used as a guide for establishment of proper dental arch form of the mandible.

10. The medial and lateral orbit is preferably bone grafted through a coronal approach. Bilateral lower lid incisions expose the inferior portion of the zygomas, the superior portion of the maxilla, and the orbital floor. The orbital rim fragments are aligned with interfragment wires and prepared for plate and screw fixation. Appropriate bone graft reconstruction of the orbital floors is accomplished. In severe floor

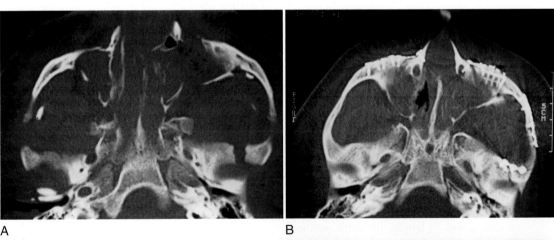

A   B

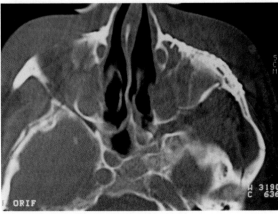

FIGURE 66-152. *A,* The zygomatic arch is laterally displaced and cleaved off the skull base. *B,* Reconstruction must begin by replacing this posterior "glenoid fossa segment" of the arch (the roof of the condylar fossa) onto the skull. *C,* Failure to restore the posterior arch by secure fixation results in disruption of the reduction. (*A* and *B* from Manson P: Reoperative facial fracture repair. In Grotting J, ed: Reoperative Aesthetic and Reconstructive Plastic Surgery. St. Louis, Quality Medical Publishing, 1995:677.)

C

injuries, the bone grafts may need to be supported with small plates or titanium mesh[418,419] employed for orbital reconstruction. Some authors prefer that orbital reconstruction be accomplished with titanium orbital floor plates alone when the critical inferomedial orbital buttress is missing.[419,420]

11. Before fixation of the Le Fort I level, it is essential to complete reconstruction of the mandibular ramus if fractures of the mandible in the ramus have produced a disturbance in the anterior projection of the mandible or loss of ramus height. Any fractures in the vertical portion of the mandible must have an open reduction with plate and screw fixation technique. The Le Fort I segment is positioned appropriately through precise intermaxillary fixation. It is also essential to be sure that the condyles are seated properly in the glenoid fossae at the time of intermaxillary fixation. In patients in whom the condylar head is not fractured but is dislocated partially out of the fossa, an open reduction may be needed to position the condyle squarely within the condylar fossa. Drilling through the roof of the glenoid fossa from a superior approach allows a wire to be loosely passed through the condylar head to keep it in position.

    After completion of the reduction of the nasoethmoidal and zygomatic areas (the upper midface), attention is then turned to uniting the upper face and the lower face at the Le Fort I level. The Le Fort I level is then linked to the upper portion of the midface by plate and screw fixation at the medial (nasomaxillary) and lateral (zygomaticomaxillary) buttresses on each side of the maxilla. Usually one or more buttresses can be anatomically repositioned to provide an index of the height at the Le Fort I level. If no Le Fort I level buttresses permit exact reconstruction to length, lip-tooth position should be used as the guide for length of buttress reconstruction.

12. The soft tissue of the face needs to be replaced on the facial skeleton, and the soft tissue layers need to be closed (Fig. 66-153). Closure must include the periosteum over the zygomaticofrontal suture, linking the orbital periosteum to the temporalis fascia; the periosteal incision over the zygomatic arch; the muscle layer of the gingival buccal sulcus incisions; and the periosteum over the inferior orbital rim. Routinely, the periosteal layers in the lower lid incision should be marked at the time of making the periosteal incision so that they can easily and accurately be identified during closure. The muscle layer (the mentalis) must be specifically

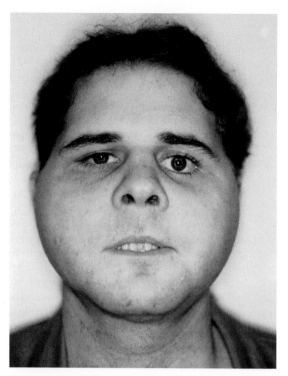

FIGURE 66-153. Lack of restoration of the preinjury appearance, even if the underlying bone is finally replaced into its proper anatomic position, is the result of scarring within soft tissue. Examples of soft tissue rigidity accompanying malreduced fractures include the conditions of enophthalmos, medial canthal ligament malposition, short palpebral fissure, rounded canthus, and inferiorly displaced malar soft tissue pad. The lower lip has a disrupted mentalis attachment. Secondary management of any of these conditions is more challenging and less effective than is primary reconstruction. A unique opportunity thus exists in immediate fracture management to maintain expansion shape and position of the soft tissue envelope and to determine the geometry of soft tissue fibrosis by providing an anatomically aligned facial skeleton as support. Excellent restoration of appearance results from primary soft tissue positioning.

closed or ectropion of the lower lip will follow because of dehiscence of the mentalis muscle insertion. Closure of the soft tissue of the face in these incisions is an important technique that prevents inferior displacement of the soft tissue after anatomic reconstruction of the facial skeleton. The thorough soft tissue degloving provides broad exposure of the bone; however, the soft tissue may slip inferiorly if it is not closed in layers and reattached to the facial skeleton. Before closure, the soft tissue is reattached to the facial skeleton at the inferior orbital rim and at the medial and lateral canthi; the soft tissue of the anterior cheek is reattached to the temporalis and malar eminence; and the deep temporal fascial incisions are closed.

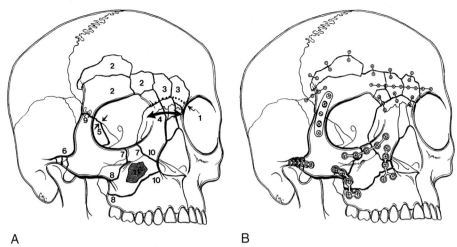

FIGURE 66-154. *A,* Reconstruction sequence in the upper facial unit. The reduction sequence is as follows: 1, anterior cranial base reconstruction (orbital roof and frontal sinus obliteration or cranialization); 2, frontal bone reassembly (back table); 3, frontal sinus fracture segment assembly or bone graft replacement of anterior wall; 4, nasoethmoid reduction after transnasal reduction of the medial orbital rims; 5, lateral orbital reduction; 6, zygomatic arch reduction; 7, inferior orbital rim reduction; 8, zygomaticomaxillary buttress reduction; 9, zygomaticofrontal suture reduction; 10, medial Le Fort I maxillary buttress reduction; and 11, anterior maxillary sinus wall bone grafting. Facial injury treatment may be organized by the need for anterior (type I, anterior facial frame) and posterior (type II, posterior facial frame) exposures *(dotted area)* based on the fracture location, the pattern of displacement, and the comminution in the individual fracture areas. *B,* Completed reconstruction of the upper facial units. (From Manson PN, Clark N, Robertson B, et al: Subunit principles in midface fracture treatment: the importance of sagittal buttresses, soft-tissue reductions, and sequencing treatment of segmental fractures. Plast Reconstr Surg 1999;103:1287.)

In patients with fractures of the frontal sinus, frontal bone, or anterior cranial fossa, a combined neurosurgical and plastic surgery approach must be used. A bifrontal craniotomy with removal of a frontal bone flap exposes the anterior cranial fossa, orbital roof, and base of the frontal and any supraorbital ethmoid sinuses. This approach may require a cranial bone flap to repair a dural laceration or to débride devitalized frontal lobe; the dural laceration usually extends toward the sphenoid sinus along the skull base. In patients with brain contusions, or if there is an epidural hematoma, and in patients in whom the brain has been penetrated by bone fragments, there may be destruction of the dura over a portion of the frontal lobe. A portion of the frontal lobe may require débridement because of severe contusion. Necrotic brain tissue should be removed and the dura sutured or reinforced with a dural patch graft of temporalis fascia, fascia lata, or pericranium. CSF fistula is controlled by suture of the dura with a reinforcing graft of fascia. The dura of the floor of the anterior cranial fossa is thin, and supplementing the strength with a graft is frequently indicated. The frontal bone fragments are cleaned and repositioned, and any defects in the orbital roof are reconstructed by primary bone

grafting. The frontal bar (or supraorbital rims) must be rigidly reconstructed, including the anterior wall of the frontal sinus. It is essential to remove fragments of sinus mucosa by light abrasive burring of the inner surfaces of the bone of the frontal sinus walls to remove microscopic invaginations of the mucosa that follow the veins (foramina of Breschet).[421] The frontal sinus mucosa should be thoroughly stripped down into the nasal frontal duct. The duct is plugged with a form-fitted bone graft, which is pressed into the duct area to form a seal. The frontal sinus cavities should be obliterated by bone graft and the intrasinus septum removed; cancellous iliac graft is preferred for obliteration. Fragments of the anterior sinus wall are restored by interfragment wiring by the "chainlink fence" technique[422] or preferably plate and screw fixation (Fig. 66-154).

COMPLICATIONS

Complications of panfacial fractures include complications referable to the bone and the soft tissue. Fixation in comminuted fractures may be troubled by disruption; screws can be placed in microfractures in apparently stable bone and may pull out, and deviation can occur (Fig. 66-155).

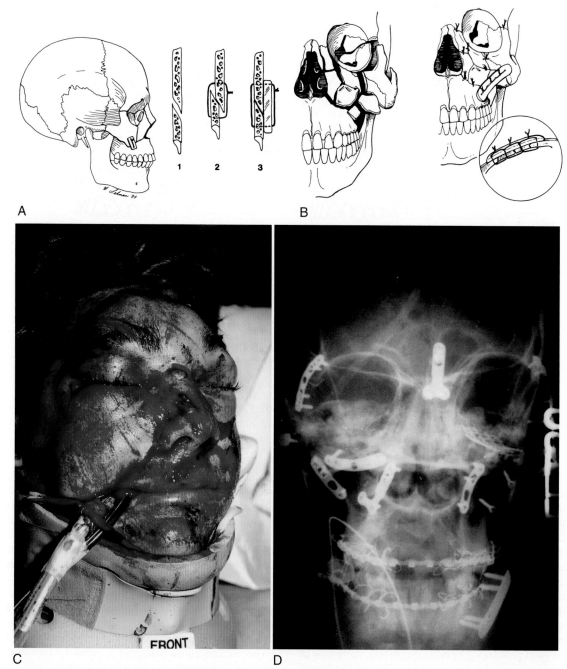

FIGURE 66-155. *A,* Buttress stabilization. Unstable oblique fracture of the anterior maxillary buttress is stabilized by the incorporation of a small bone graft at the site. *B,* Incorporation of a carefully contoured and measured bone graft into the site of comminuted or segmental fracture of the anterior buttress produces buttress reinforcement and stabilization. The height of the buttress is re-established by the open reduction. For both *A* and *B,* stabilization is now accomplished by a miniplate. *C,* Complex frontal Le Fort, mandible, and nasoethmoid fractures in a boy struck by a car while on a bicycle, with an occipital epidural hematoma and ruptured spleen. After these were managed, his facial fractures were repaired with rigid fixation and bone grafts. *D,* Radiograph of bone fixed to an orbital floor plate is seen.

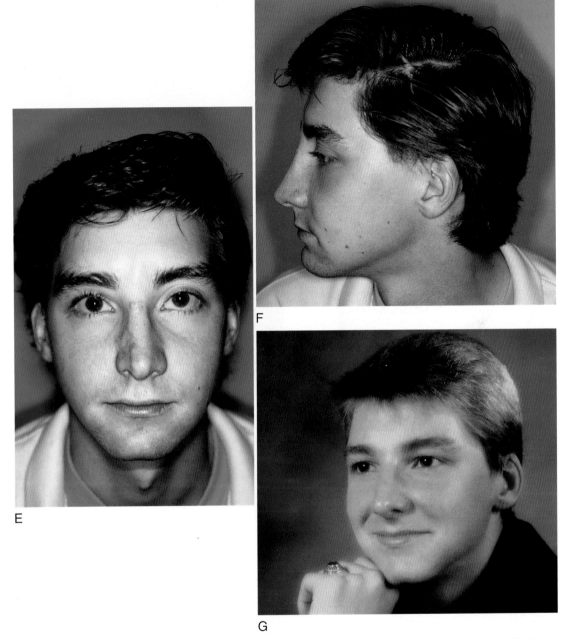

FIGURE 66-155, cont'd. *E* and *F*, Postoperative result. *G*, Preinjury picture. (*A* and *B* from Gruss JS, Mackinnon SE: Complex maxillary fractures: the role of buttress reconstruction and immediate bone grafts. Plast Reconstr Surg 1986;78:9.)

Failure to stabilize the mandible may displace the maxilla. The plates in maxillary fractures are placed in thin bone at the Le Fort I level and may not be able to stabilize the fracture (Fig. 66-156).

When the condylar area is fractured, it may, because of the magnitude of large muscle forces on the mandible, effectively shorten and retrude the lower face (Fig. 66-157). Condylar fractures may also cause strong traction forces on the lower maxilla, especially at the Le Fort I level where the bone is thin. It may be difficult to keep the mandible stable when a dislocated condylar fracture is present and allows too much mobility. If the mandible is placed into occlusion (forced to move anteriorly, pulling the condyle forward in the fossa to meet an impacted maxilla) (Fig. 66-157C), on release of intermaxillary fixation, the patient will drop

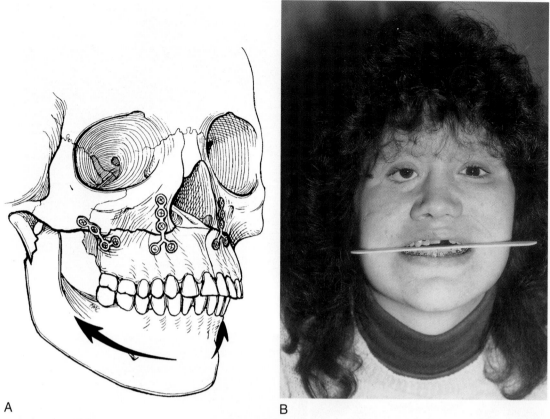

A   B

FIGURE 66-156. *A,* Fixation in the thin bone of the Le Fort I level may not be sufficient to stabilize a condylar fracture treated closed. *B,* The occlusal plane has shifted to an oblique position because of shortening of the ramus due to malposition of a condylar fracture. (From Manson P: Reoperative facial fracture repair. In Grotting J, ed. Reoperative Aesthetic and Reconstructive Plastic Surgery. St. Louis, Quality Medical Publishing, 1995:677.)

into an open bite (Fig. 66-157*D*) because the condyle will return to the fossa.

Current facial fracture reductions emphasize complete degloving of all bones by incising fascial layers and detaching soft tissue. It has only recently been appreciated that there are potential deformities caused by complete exposures and tissue stripping. Many times, a less complete exposure of a particular bone may suffice and may potentially prevent some soft tissue deformity. In facial injuries treated early, the injury itself has performed a portion of the dissection; soft tissue contracture and stiffness are absent, the bone is mobile, and a bone reduction can be performed with less dissection without scarred soft tissue opposing the reduction.

It is important to repair the soft tissue in layers and to replace the soft tissue onto the bone when it has been completely mobilized to accomplish bone repair. Soft tissue replacement requires layered closure and reattachment of this closed soft tissue to the facial skeleton so that the tissue is realigned and then repositioned

onto an anatomically assembled craniofacial skeleton at the proper position (see Fig. 66-142).

Orbit

Orbital fractures may occur as isolated fractures of the internal orbit or may involve both the internal orbit and the orbital rim.[423-425] Commonly, they are associated with other facial fractures, such as zygoma, nasoethmoidal-orbital, and Le Fort fractures. Patients presenting with orbital injuries, periorbital ecchymosis, or lacerations around the eye should have a thorough ophthalmologic examination to exclude the possibility of globe injury,[62] injury to extraocular muscles or the levator tendon, retinal detachment, or global rupture.[64,426-429] A history of the accident and a history of visual integrity including preexisting visual disturbances, visual correction, previous operations or treatment, and visual acuity should be obtained. Specific details of the accident, how it happened, and any visual disturbance that may have occurred, such

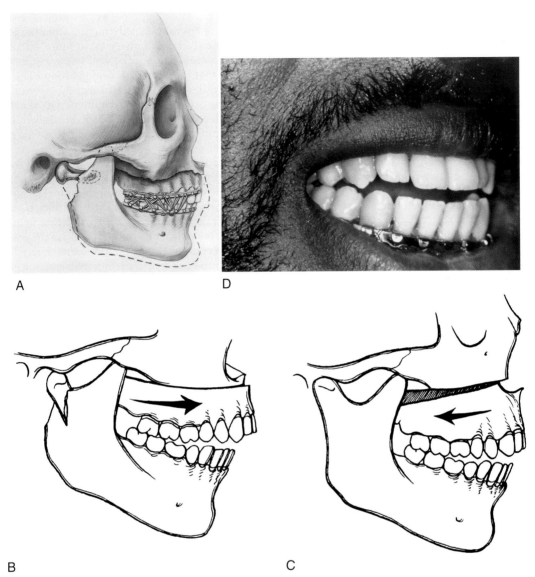

A   D

B   C

FIGURE 66-157. *A,* The whole lower face may be displaced despite fixation at the Le Fort I level because of strong muscle forces of the mandible exerted by a dislocated condylar fracture. *B,* If a dislocated condylar fracture occurs with a loose Le Fort I fracture, open reduction of the mandible and maxilla is necessary to properly align the fractures. *C,* The condyle of the mandible may be dislocated from the fossa if the mandible is forced into occlusion with an impacted Le Fort fracture that has not been mobilized and reduced. *D,* Malocclusion after release of intermaxillary fixation when the mandible has been tracked forward to meet a displaced but impacted maxilla. (*A* from Manson PN: Midface fractures: advantages of immediate open reduction and bone grafting. Plast Reconstr Surg 1985;76:1. *C* from Manson P: Reoperative facial fracture repair. In Grotting J, ed: Reoperative Aesthetic and Reconstructive Plastic Surgery. St. Louis, Quality Medical Publishing, 1995:677. *D* from Manson P: Complications of facial injuries. In Goldwyn R, Cohen MN: The Unfavorable Result in Plastic Surgery. New York, Lippincott Williams & Wilkins, 2001:489.)

as blurring, loss of vision, or double vision, should be recorded. Previous visual loss or a history of a visual disturbance ("lazy eye" or amblyopia, when the vision in one eye often may be relatively poor) should be noted. A visual acuity examination is required in any cooperative patient undergoing periorbital surgery. Bleeding from the nose and a period of uncon-

sciousness or confusion are important clues to the diagnosis of ancillary injuries, as is malocclusion. Any prior medical evaluation or surgical treatment involving the eye is important, including the use of contacts or glasses. Diminished vision is a frequent preexisting condition, and patients are often unaware of diminished vision because of the bilateral compensating nature of vision. Patients are likely to blame the surgeon for a preexisting visual defect if the preoperative visual acuity is not documented. The ophthalmologic examination must be performed routinely in patients with orbital injuries, and findings should be confirmed by the plastic surgeon even if an ophthalmologist has examined the patient. Identification of ocular problems, such as corneal abrasion or hyphema, should be confirmed. If the patient is unconscious, an ocular physical examination must be performed despite the absence of a clear history or voluntary confirmation of visual acuity. In conscious patients, cooperation facilitates an accurate examination.

The treatment of orbital fractures should not be delayed more than absolutely necessary. As soon as the injury has occurred, the process of an inflammatory reaction begins and ultimately results in fibrosis of any contused or entrapped orbital tissue. Circulation in the entrapped tissue could be impaired by the entrapment, and in true muscle entrapment, urgent surgical release of the entrapped muscle conceptually leads to better function.[430-436] It also seems reasonable to assume that orbital contents replaced early into their proper position will have scarring occur in an anatomically correct position, which may facilitate function and appearance.

ANATOMY

The orbits are paired bone structures forming cavities for the globes, separated in the midline by the interorbital space, which contains the ethmoid and frontal sinuses.[92,369,437] Above, the orbit is delimited by the floor of the anterior cranial fossa. The anterior cranial fossa partition is formed by the roof of the orbit, the roof of each ethmoid sinus, the floor of the frontal sinus, and the cribriform plate medially. The orbits are situated immediately below the floor of the anterior cranial fossa, and a portion of the floor of the anterior cranial fossa is formed by the roof of the orbit.

Orbital contents are protected by strong bone structures, which include the nasal bones, the nasal spine of the frontal bone, the frontal processes of the maxilla medially, the supraorbital rims of the frontal bones superiorly, the frontal process of the zygoma and zygomatic process of the frontal bone laterally, and inferiorly the thick inferior orbital rim formed by the zygoma laterally and the maxilla medially. The skeletal components of the orbital cavity are the frontal bone, the lesser and greater wings of the sphenoid, the zygoma, the maxilla, the lacrimal bone, a small portion of the palatine bone, and the ethmoid bones.

The bony orbit is described as a roughly conical or pyramid-shaped structure. Both of these comparisons are actually somewhat inaccurate. The widest diameter of the orbit is just behind the orbital rim approximately 1 to 1.5 cm within the orbital cavity. From this point posteriorly, the orbit begins to narrow dramat-

ically in its middle and posterior thirds. The orbital rim is an elliptically shaped structure, whereas the orbit immediately behind the rim is more circular in configuration. The medial wall has a quadrangular rather than a triangular configuration. The optic foramen lies on a medial and slightly superior plane in the apex of the orbit. In children, the orbital floor is situated at a lower level in relation to the orbital rim because of the incomplete development of the maxillary sinuses.

Functionally, and particularly in terms of fracture treatment, the orbits may be conceptualized in thirds progressing from anterior to posterior (Fig. 66-158). Anteriorly, the orbital rims consist of thick bone. The middle third of the orbit consists of relatively thin bone, and the bone structure thickens again in the posterior portion of the orbit (Fig. 66-159; see also Fig. 66-158). The orbital bone structure is thus analogous to a "shock-absorbing" device in which the middle portion of the orbit frequently breaks first, followed by the anterior portion of the rim. This combination of fractures actually protects the important nervous and vascular structures in the posterior third of the orbit from severe displacement. In effect, the globe is able to fracture the thin portions of the orbit, protecting the globe from rupture. If the orbit were composed of thick bone in its middle section, the globe would rupture with almost every orbital impact.

The floor of the orbit is a frequent site of fracture.[438-440] It has no sharp line of demarcation with the medial wall but proceeds into the medial wall by tilting upward in its medial aspect at a 45-degree angle. Stated another way, the lower portion of the medial orbital wall has a progressively lateral inclination. The floor is separated from the lateral wall by the inferior orbital (sphenomaxillary) fissure. The floor of the orbit (the roof of the maxillary sinus) is composed mainly of the orbital plate of the maxilla, a paper-thin structure medial to the infraorbital groove, and partly of the zygomatic bone interior to the inferior orbital fissure and the orbital process of the palatine bone. The inferior orbital groove and canal traverse the floor of the orbit from medial to lateral. The nerve canal begins anteriorly about the middle of the inferior orbital fissure, and the nerve lies in a groove in the posterior and middle portion of the orbit. Anteriorly, the nerve lies in a canal that turns downward to pass through the thick inferior orbital rim parallel to the medial limbus of the cornea in straightforward gaze. The canal angles downward, opening on the anterior surface of the maxilla as the infraorbital foramen. A branch of the nerve passes in the anterior wall of the maxilla to the anterior superior maxillary dentition.

The orbital floor bulges upward immediately behind the globe, which contributes to forward globe support. The anterior portion of the floor (the first 1.5 cm) is concave, and the remainder of the orbital floor is

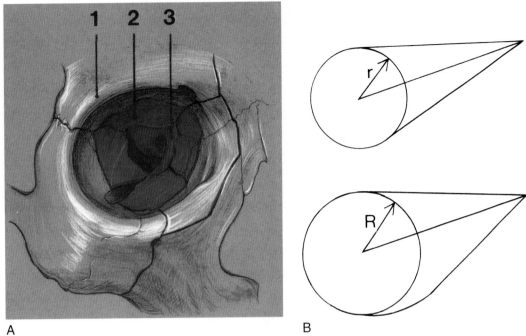

A   B

FIGURE 66-158. *A,* The segments of the anterior orbit (1) (three portions of the anterior rim), the four sections of the middle orbit (2), and the single section of the posterior orbit (3) are seen. The rim (the anterior third of the orbit) has supraorbital, zygomatic, and nasoethmoidal sections; the middle third of the orbit has medial wall, floor, lateral wall, and roof areas. *B,* Orbital enlargement (below) may occur with increase in the size of the rim or internal orbit. The most effective way to increase the size of the orbit is to expand the rim versus displacement of the orbital walls because the radius is squared in volume calculations ($\pi r^2 h$).

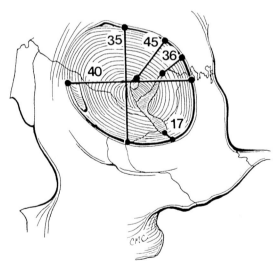

FIGURE 66-159. Orbital dimensions (in millimeters) from the rim to internal landmarks of the internal orbit. (From Manson PN, Iliff N: Surgical anatomy of the orbit. In Marsh J, ed: Current Therapy in Plastic and Reconstructive Surgery. Philadelphia, BC Decker, 1989:117.)

convex. In "blowout" fractures, the force is transmitted by the incompressible orbital contents to the thin walls of the orbit. Fractures may occur from this soft tissue pressure alone, or on bending of the rim, the orbital floor may flex first, breaking at an area remote from the point of contact of an object with the orbital rim. The theory of Pfeiffer[441] is that the globe is displaced posteriorly by a force, fracturing the ethmoid and orbital floor area, and then recoils into its usual position.[442]

Fractures first occur at thin areas in the floor and medial orbital wall; these are the convex portion of the orbital floor medial to the infraorbital nerve and the medial (ethmoidal) orbit. The posterior portion of the orbit (the inclined plane of the orbital floor) presents an especially thin area of bone. This "weak area" represents some of the thinnest bone of the orbit. It extends directly into the thin bone of the medial ethmoid and the lamina papyracea, which is a thin paper-like "plate" of bone that is easily fractured. Fractures in the lamina papyracea of the ethmoid often compress the bone symmetrically rather than displace small pieces individually (Fig. 66-160). Surgeons must be aware that this symmetric ethmoid displacement is a characteristic mechanism of orbital enlargement.

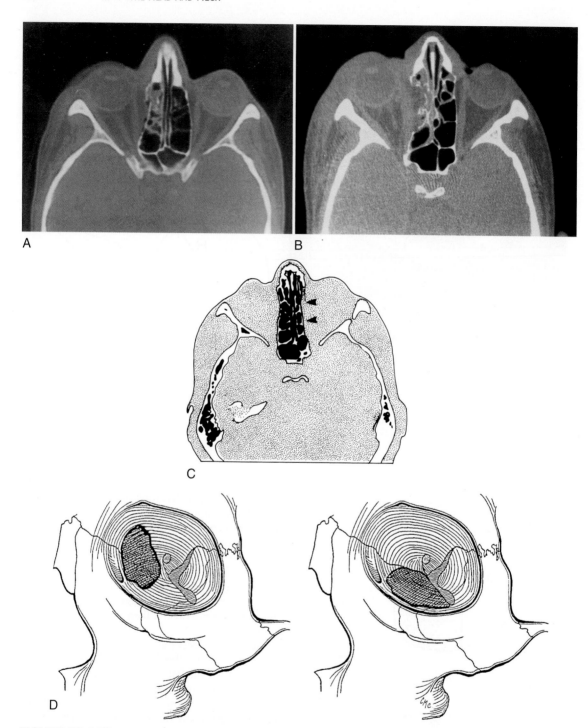

FIGURE 66-160. *A,* Unilateral compression of the medial ethmoidal cells (lamina papyracea, the usual medial orbital blowout fracture). *B,* Medial blowout fracture with swelling of the medial rectus muscle. *C,* Illustration of symmetric compression of medial wall (ethmoid) cells. *D,* Orbital floor and medial orbital wall defects.

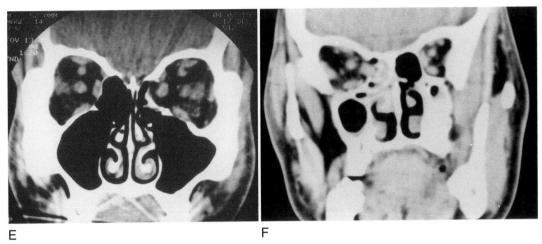

E   F

FIGURE 66-160, cont'd. *E,* Coronal view of medial orbital fracture, soft tissue window. *F,* Soft tissue coronal view of medial rectus muscle prolapsed into a medial orbital wall fracture.

Because the displacement is gradual, it is a more elusive injury than disordered comminution of the medial orbital wall in terms of recognizing the need to correct orbital enlargement. The "compressed ethmoid" must be recognized as displaced to be used as a criterion of fracture treatment (Fig. 66-160).

The inferior oblique muscle arises from the maxillary portion of the orbital floor immediately behind the rim and lateral to the lacrimal groove. The inferior rectus muscle is situated immediately above the infraorbital canal and the undersurface of the orbital contents. Both can easily be visualized in CT scans (Fig. 66-161). It is not surprising, therefore, that these two muscles are often involved in fractures of the medial wall and floor and the rim of the orbit. The absence of elasticity in the incarcerated inferior rectus muscle would restrict motion in the field of action of its antagonist, the superior rectus. Because the two inferior muscles are intimately connected at the point where the inferior oblique crosses beneath the inferior rectus, disturbance of function of the inferior oblique muscle may also be due to this mechanism in blowout fractures. When the fracture is lateral to the infraorbital groove or canal, the inferior rectus and inferior oblique muscles may not be involved. These variations in the site of the blowout fracture explain variations in the symptoms and clinical signs of the fractures.

The medial wall of the orbit is reinforced anteriorly by the frontal process of the maxilla. This wall is relatively fragile and is formed by the combination of the frontal bone, the lacrimal bone, the lamina papyracea, and the ethmoid bone and part of the lesser wing of the sphenoid around the optic foramen. The lamina papyracea is the largest component of the medial orbital wall and accounts for the structural weakness of the area. The lamina is actually reinforced by the transverse septa crossing and segmenting the ethmoid sinuses. The lesser wing of the sphenoid and the optic foramen are posterior to the lamina papyracea.

The optic foramen is close to the posterior portion of the ethmoid sinus and not at the true apex of the orbit. Consequently, in severe fractures involving the medial wall in its posterior portion, fracture lines may extend through the optic canal.

The groove for the lacrimal sac is a broad, vertical fossa lying partly on the anterior aspect of the lacrimal bone and partly on the posterior frontal process of the maxilla; the anterior and posterior margins of the lacrimal groove form the respective anterior and posterior lacrimal crests. The groove is continuous with the nasolacrimal duct at the junction of the floor and medial wall of the orbit, which passes down under the inferior turbinate to a meatus that empties into the nose. Between the roof and the medial wall of the orbit are the anterior and posterior ethmoid foramina, which are canals communicating with the medial portion of the anterior cranial fossa, the ethmoid sinus, and the nose that transmit anterior and posterior ethmoidal vessels and nerves.

The lateral wall of the orbit is relatively stout in its anterior portion. It is formed by the orbital process of the zygoma and the greater wing of the sphenoid. The rim is formed by the frontal process of the zygomatic bone, and the lateral wall by the greater and lesser wings of the sphenoid lateral to the optic foramen. The superior orbital fissure is a cleft that runs outward, forward, and upward from the apex of the orbit, between the roof and lateral wall. This fissure, which separates the greater and lesser wings of the sphenoid, gives passage to three motor nerves to the extraocular muscles of the orbit (cranial nerves III, IV, and VI). The ophthalmic division of the trigeminal nerve (cranial nerve V) also enters the orbit through this fissure. The fissure leads into the middle cranial fossa.

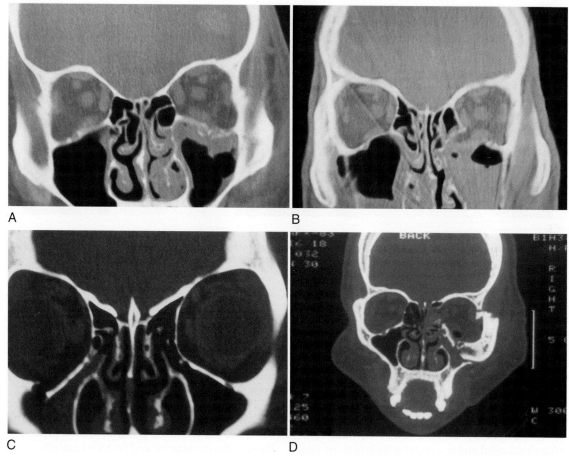

FIGURE 66-161. *A,* Small blowout fracture of the orbital floor with incarceration of a small amount of fat lateral to the inferior rectus muscle. *B,* A larger blowout fracture of the medial orbital floor incarcerating the inferior rectus and inferior oblique muscles by trapping of adjacent fat. *C,* Single-hinged fracture of orbital floor. *D,* Fracture of three sections of the internal orbit (medial floor, lateral wall, and zygoma). A dramatic expansion of orbital volume is produced.

The lateral wall of the orbit is situated in an anterior, lateral, and posterior medial plane. It is related to the temporal fossa. Posteriorly, a small part of the wall lies between the orbit and middle cranial fossa and the temporal lobe of the brain. Between the floor and lateral wall of the orbit is the inferior orbital fissure, which communicates with the infratemporal fossa. The inferior orbital fissure has divisions of the maxillary portion of the trigeminal nerve and veins communicating with the infratemporal fossa.

The roof of the orbit is composed mainly of the orbital plate of the frontal bone, but posteriorly, it receives a minor contribution from the lesser wing of the sphenoid. The fossa lodging the lacrimal gland is a depression situated on the anterior and lateral aspect of the inner orbit, which is sheltered by the zygomatic process of the frontal bone. The anterior medial portions of the roof can be invaded by supraorbital extension of the ethmoid or frontal sinuses or frontoethmoidal air cells. The roof separates the orbit from the anterior cranial fossa and from the middle cranial fossa on its posterior aspect.

The roof often consists of thin brittle bone; it is especially thin in its medial portion. The supratrochlear and supraorbital nerves and more medially the trochlea (or pulley of the superior oblique muscle) are located in the superior rim of the orbit. The tendon of the superior oblique muscle functions as a cartilaginous pulley or trochlea, which is fixed by ligamentous fibers immediately behind the superior medial angle of the orbital rim. Fractures involving the superior medial portion of the rim may result in compression of the supraorbital nerve within its foramen and the development of anesthesia in the area of distribution of this sensory nerve, which is the forehead and anterior portion of the scalp. Double vision or diplopia may also result from injury to the superior oblique muscle, thus affecting the balance of the extraocular movement.

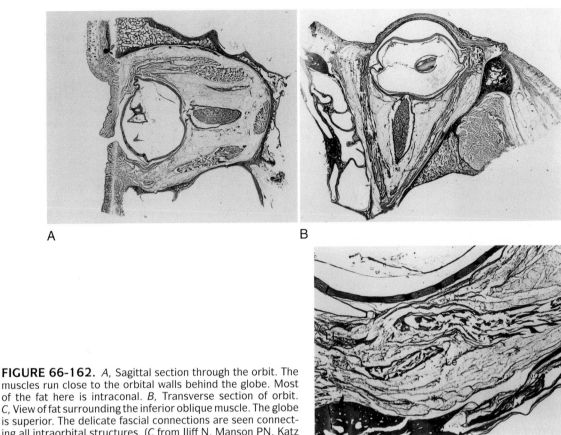

A   B

C

FIGURE 66-162. *A,* Sagittal section through the orbit. The muscles run close to the orbital walls behind the globe. Most of the fat here is intraconal. *B,* Transverse section of orbit. *C,* View of fat surrounding the inferior oblique muscle. The globe is superior. The delicate fascial connections are seen connecting all intraorbital structures. (*C* from Iliff N, Manson PN, Katz J, et al: Mechanisms of extraocular muscle injury in orbital fractures. Plast Reconstr Surg 1999;103:787.)

Orbital Fat and the Ocular Globe

The ocular globe is surrounded by a cushion of orbital fat within the orbital cavity. The extraocular muscles and their ligaments contain an intraconal fat compartment, which is separated by means of thin fascial connections from the extraconal fat. The ocular globe is in the anterior half of the orbital cavity. The posterior half of the orbital cavity is filled with fat, muscles, vessels, and nerves that supply the ocular globe and the extraocular muscles and provide sensation to the tissues around the orbit (Fig. 66-162*A* and *B*). The orbital cavity may thus be conceptualized in two halves from anterior to posterior. They are separated by the Tenon capsule (Figs. 66-162*C* and 66-163), a fascial structure that subdivides the orbital cavity into an anterior (or precapsular) segment and a posterior (or retrocapsular) segment.

Koornneef[443] has demonstrated that fine ligaments extend throughout the extraocular fat as thin, discrete but supple communications that diffusely divide the fat into small compartments and provide diffuse ligament interconnections that attach from the bony orbital walls and the periosteum to the extraocular muscle fascia and to the Tenon capsule. Thus, the fine

ligament structures of the orbit provide a diffuse network of support and organization for the orbital soft tissue contents and conceptually limit displacement and maintain the shape of the soft tissue. These ligament structures decrease in density as one progresses from anterior to posterior (Fig. 66-164). The orbital fat may be divided into anterior and posterior portions. The anterior extraocular fat is largely extraconal, which means that it exists outside the muscle cone and external to the ocular globe. Posteriorly, the muscle cone is an approximate rather than an exact anatomic structure, as there are only fine fascial connections separating the extraconal and the intraconal fat compartments. Intraconal fat constitutes three fourths of the fat in the posterior orbit and may be displaced outside the muscle cone by trauma, contributing to a loss of globe support from a loss of soft tissue volume. Loss of intraconal fat is one mechanism of enophthalmos. The cushion of fat above the levator muscle is extraconal, as is the fat underneath the globe on the anterior portion of the orbital floor. The extraconal fat does not contribute to globe support but does contribute to lid prominence. In the anterior portion of the orbit, the extraocular muscles,

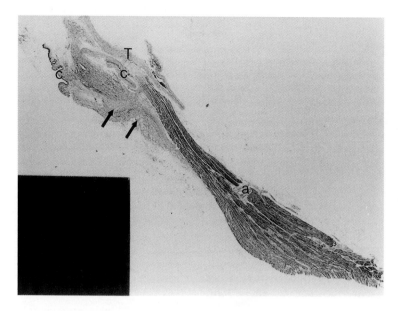

FIGURE 66-163. Tenon capsule (T) and the inferior rectus muscle (a) are seen; c is the lower eyelid retractors, and the arrows indicate the anterior fascia of the muscle insertion. (From Iliff N, Manson PN, Katz J, et al: Mechanisms of extraocular muscle injury in orbital fractures. Plast Reconstr Surg 1999;103:787.)

with the exception of the superior and inferior obliques, are separated from the bony wall of the orbit and periosteum by a layer of extraconal fat. In the posterior orbit, the extraocular muscles run adjacent to the orbital walls, rendering them susceptible to injury from either bone fracture or surgical dissection.

Septum Orbitale

The orbital contents are maintained in position by the bony walls of the orbit and anteriorly the septum orbitale, a fascial structure inserting on the inner aspect of the orbital rims. The septum orbitale attaches to and blends with the levator aponeurosis in the upper eyelid for a distance of a few millimeters above the upper border of the tarsus. In the lower eyelid, the septum orbitale is attached to the lower border of the tarsus. The septum orbitale attaches to the margin of the orbital rim; in the lateral lower orbit, it attaches on the

anterior surface of the inferior orbital rim, contributing to a small recess called the recess of Eisler.

Periorbita

The periosteum lining of the periphery of the orbit is also known as the periorbita. The periorbita is continuous with the dura at those sites where the orbit communicates with the intracranial cavity. Those are the optic foramen, the superior orbital fissure, and the anterior and posterior ethmoid canals. The extraocular muscles have a longitudinal blood supply, which can be contused after fracture (Fig. 66-165).

Optic Foramen and Optic Canal

The optic foramen is situated at the junction of the lateral and medial walls of the orbit in its far posterior portion (Fig. 66-165). The foramen is not on a horizontal plane with the orbital floor but is located above

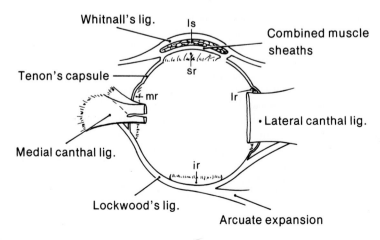

FIGURE 66-164. View of the ligament sling for the globe, which attaches to the sclera. (From Manson PN, Clifford CM, Su CT, et al: Mechanisms of global support and posttraumatic enophthalmos: I. The anatomy of the ligament sling and its relation to intramuscular cone orbital fat. Plast Reconstr Surg 1986;77:193.)

TABLE 66-9 ✦ OPTIC CANAL MEASUREMENTS

	Average (mm)	Range (mm)
Optic canal length	9.22	5.5-11.5
Horizontal canal width		
Proximal	7.18	5.0-9.5
Distal	4.87	4.0-6.0
Roof thickness	2.09	1.0-3.0
Medial canal wall thickness	.021	0.1-0.31
Optic ring thickness	.57	.04-0.74
Anterior to posterior		
ethmoidal foramen	12.25	8.0-19.0
Posterior ethmoidal		
foramen to optic ring	6.78	5.0-11.0

From Maniscalco JE, Habal MB: Microanatomy of the optic canal. J Neurosurg 1973;48:402.

the horizontal plane. The foramen is 40 to 45 mm behind the inferior orbital rim. Inferior orbital dissection should be performed with precise knowledge of this position and location. The position of instruments in floor dissection may easily be checked by putting a Freer elevator into the maxillary sinus and feeling the back of the sinus. This intrasinus location is 5 to 10 mm in front of and 10 mm below the optic foramen.

The optic canal is 4 to 10 mm in length and is a passage through which the optic nerve and ophthalmic artery pass from an intracranial to an intraorbital position. The canal is framed medially by the body of the sphenoid and laterally by the lesser wing of the sphenoid. It is thus in close approximation to the sphenoid sinus and the posterior ethmoidal air cells. The bony optic canal forms a straight tight bony sheet about the optic nerve and is most dense anteriorly. Posteriorly, its thickness decreases. Because of the close approximation of the bone to the nerve, fracture with swelling predisposes to vascular compression of the nerve within the canal (Table 66-9).

DIAGNOSIS

Clinical Examination

The examination of the eye should detect edema, corneal abrasion, laceration, contusion, or hematoma. A subconjunctival and periorbital hematoma confined to the distribution of the orbital septum is evidence of a facial fracture involving the orbit until it is proved otherwise. The extraocular movements should be checked as far as possible, noting double vision or restricted globe movement. In cooperative patients, visual acuity can be assessed at both near and far distances. A gross visual field examination is performed by having the patient stare at a fixed point and noting peripheral vision for an object, such as a cotton-tipped applicator, passed into the field of gaze. Globe pressure may be assessed by tonometry and should be less than 15 mm Hg. The results of a fundus examination should be recorded. Diminished vision may be assessed by recording the patient's ability to read newsprint or an ophthalmic examination card, such as the Rosenbaum pocket card (see Fig. 66-8). Diminished vision or no light perception indicates optic nerve damage or globe rupture. Light perception without usable vision indicates optic nerve damage, retinal detachment, hyphema, vitreous hemorrhage, or anterior or posterior chamber injuries of significance. Many internal globe injuries require expert ophthalmologic consultation. The globe should be inspected for globe lacerations, which may be hidden by swollen lids.

When eyelid lacerations occur adjacent to the medial canthus[444] or in nasoethmoidal-orbital fractures having canthal ligament avulsion, the integrity of the lacrimal system must be assessed.[323] The lacrimal punctum may be dilated with a pediatric punctum dilator, and a small irrigating cannula, such as a 24-mL Angiocath sleeve, may be used to irrigate the lacrimal drainage system. It may be helpful to occlude the opposite punctum with finger pressure. Drainage of fluid into the nose indicates continuity of the lacrimal system. The appearance of fluid in a laceration indicates the possibility of a divided lacrimal system, which must be repaired under loupe magnification. The lacrimal system repair should be stented with fine silicone (0.25 mm) tubing made for this purpose.[413-415]

Fractures of the orbit frequently occur in association with zygomaticomaxillary, nasoethmoidal-orbital, and high Le Fort (II and III) fractures. In these injuries, fracture lines traverse the orbital floor, medial and lateral orbit, and orbital rim. These fractures may cause simple linear fractures of the orbital floor, or there may be comminution of the floor with thin portions of the floor falling into the maxillary sinus. When orbital fractures are accompanied by displacement of large sections of the orbit, such as the zygoma, discontinuity occurs in the area of the lateral orbital wall adjacent to the greater wing of the sphenoid and inferior orbital fissure. These defects allow herniation of orbital contents (where the periosteum is torn) into the maxillary sinus and temporal fossa. The most frequent orbital wall displacement observed involves the lower medial orbital wall and a portion of the floor medial to the infraorbital groove and canal. These thin sections of bone are easily displaced inferiorly and posteriorly, allowing displacement of orbital soft tissue. In injuries that displace the inferior orbital rim posteriorly, there is generally comminution of the thin portion of the orbital floor. In fractures of the zygoma, downward displacement results in the separation of the lateral and inferior portions of the floor with a lowering of the orbital floor and an outward rotation of the lateral orbit. In some fractures, such as

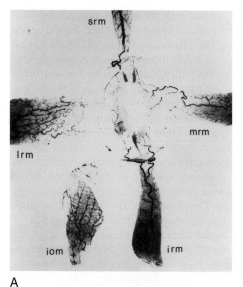

A

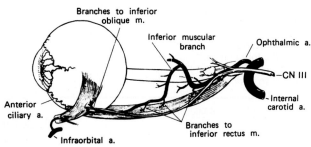

B

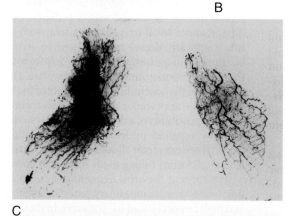

C

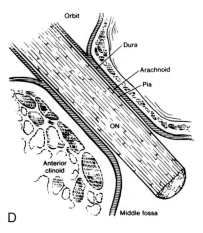

D

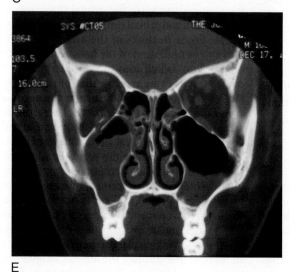

E

FIGURE 66-165. *A,* An angiographic view of the extraocular muscles, demonstrating their longitudinal circulation. *B,* Diagram of orbital anatomy of the inferior orbit. *C,* After an experimental orbital fracture, contusion of the inferior rectus muscle and loss of the continuity of the longitudinal circulation through the muscle are seen. *D,* Schematic drawing of the optic canal and optic nerve sheaths. The dura is tightly adherent to bone within the optic canal. Within the orbit, the dura splits, forming the outer sheath of the optic nerve and the periorbita. *E,* Blow-in fracture in a radiograph. (*A* to *C* from Iliff N, Manson PN, Katz J, et al: Mechanisms of extraocular muscle injury in orbital fractures. Plast Reconstr Surg 1999;103:787. *D* from Miller NR, ed: Walsh & Hoyt's Clinical Neuro-ophthalmology, 4th ed. Philadelphia, Lippincott Williams & Williams, 1982.)

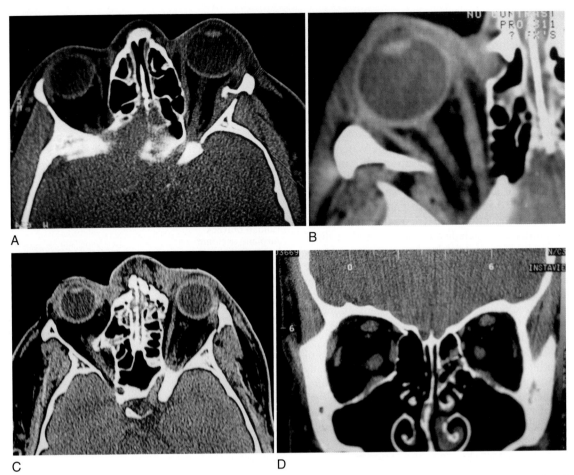

FIGURE 66-166. *A,* A blow-in fracture has been produced by medial dislocation of the zygoma, compressing the orbital volume. A bone fragment of the lateral orbit has been displaced into the lateral rectus muscle. The patient had diplopia looking laterally. *B,* Medially impacted zygoma fracture impaling the lateral rectus muscle. *C,* Nasoethmoidal fracture with impaction into the medial rectus muscle. *D,* True incarceration (rare) of the medial rectus muscle.

medially displaced zygoma fractures, the volume of the orbit is actually constricted (blow-in fracture),[445-447] and the patients present with exophthalmos (Fig. 66-166). This is also true with supraorbital fractures that are inferiorly and posteriorly displaced. They push the eye downward and forward. If the lids do not cover and protect the globe in patients with marked anterior ocular displacement, immediate reduction of the fracture should be considered.

Many orbital fractures are complicated by double vision. The usual cause of double vision is contusion of an extraocular muscle.[448,449] Frequently, incarceration of perimuscular orbital soft tissue causes limitation of extraocular muscle excursion by virtue of its tethering through the fine ligament system described by Koornneef.[443,450]

Radiographic Examination

Radiographic evaluation of any orbital fracture is essential. Plain films are able to diagnose larger frac-

tures but in practice have been completely replaced by a CT scan done in the axial and coronal planes with both bone and soft tissue windows. In the author's experience, actual coronal cuts are more useful than CT reconstructions. Reconstructions[451] are now achieving the technical sophistication to be more useful in patients who cannot, because of a head or neck injury, submit to a true coronal examination. Both bone and soft tissue windows are useful to define the anatomy and for complete examination of the orbital walls and soft tissue contents and the relation of the muscle to the fracture. A careful radiographic examination reveals a variety of findings; it defines the anatomic area of the fractures, their comminution and displacement, and the involvement of soft tissue structures and their relationship to the fracture. Because of the supraimposition of thick and thin bones, the radiographic picture on plain films is difficult to interpret. They are included here for completeness. Plain films should never be cited as evidence that a blowout fracture does not exist. Rather, the clinical examination provides the most important evidence of a blowout fracture. Almost all significant inferior orbital fractures involve the periorbita or manifest with a periorbital and subconjunctival hematoma and anesthesia of the infraorbital nerve. The absence of these signs should make the diagnosis questionable.

Plain films may suggest the presence of a fracture in the internal portion of the orbit by means of a variety of positions: the Caldwell position, the Waters position, the frontal occipital position, the anteriorposterior projection, the reverse Waters position, and the oblique orbital-optic foramen view (see section on radiographic diagnosis). The diagnosis of a blowout fracture is frequently missed if the radiographic examination does not include a CT scan. On plain films, fracture lines may be mistaken for superimposed bony septa or suture lines or may be hidden by disease processes in the underlying maxillary sinus. The thin orbital floor, partially transparent on radiographs, may be obscured against the background of other bones of the skull. CT scans disclose the exact presence of a blowout fracture and its location.

With adequate examination, blowout fractures of the orbit can be radiologically confirmed in virtually 100% of patients. The type of blowout fracture varies. A punched-out orbital fracture produces a "hanging" area of soft tissue, as the orbital fat has been extruded into the maxillary sinus. Single-hinged or double-hinged fractures may involve one or two bone fragments hanging into the sinus on a periorbital "hinge" (see Fig. 66-161). Medial wall fractures include those with a symmetric compression of the ethmoid air cells (see Fig. 66-160) or more punched-out defects. The presence of maxillary sinus fluid should suggest that a fracture might be present. In patients with massive floor destruction, the globe may drop away from the eyelid, which is an acute problem arguing for urgent repair as the displaced globe may dry out if air exists underneath the eyelids. In the absence of positive clinical signs suggesting the need for early surgical intervention, on the basis of volume correction or double vision, surgery should be postponed while the patient's orbital symptoms are kept under direct observation. Lisman[452] and Millman[453] suggest that contusion diplopia resolves faster if steroids are given in the peri-injury period. Mild diplopia, with an initially equivocal finding on forced duction examination, often resolves after a short (7- to 14-day) period of observation.[454]

BLOWOUT FRACTURES OF THE ORBITAL FLOOR

Mechanism of Production

A blowout fracture is caused by the application of a traumatic force to the rim or soft tissues of the orbit. Blowout fractures are generally assumed to be accom-

TABLE 66-10 ✦ ETIOLOGIC FEATURES IN 100 BLOWOUT FRACTURES

Automobile	49
Human fist	18
Human elbow	4
Wooden plank	1
Ball	5
Snowball	2
Ski pole	2
Edge of table	1
Blunt object	1
Shoe kick	2
Steel bar	1
Machinery	2
Boxing glove	1
Mop handle	1
Human buttock	1
Airplane accident	1
Water ski accident	1
Ice bank	1
Fall on face	4
Iatrogenic (surgical)	1
Military casualty (shell fragment)	1

From Converse JM, Smith B, Obear MF, Wood-Smith D: Orbital blowout fractures: a ten year survey. Plast Reconstr Surg 1967;39;20. Copyright 1967, The Williams & Wilkins Company, Baltimore.

panied by a sudden increase in intraorbital pressure (Tables 66-10 to 66-13). The concept of the blowout fracture was advanced by Lang,[455] in 1889, following the descriptions of Gessier, von Becker, Helsingfors, and Tweedy.[456] Lagrange[457] and Le Fort[382] had thought that orbital fractures were produced by force transmitted from the orbital rim to the orbital floor. Raymond Pfeiffer,[441] studying 140 orbital fractures, said, "It is evident that the force of the blow received by the eyeball was transmitted by it to the walls of the orbit with fracture of more delicate portions." Linhart,[458] in 1943, in the *Journal of the American Medical Association,* stated, "Contusion over the orbital area with resultant driving of the eyeball into the orbit and recession of the orbital fat to one side may alone result in fracture by direct contact of the eyeball and orbital wall. The common points of fracture are in the lacrimal and ethmoidal bones. The lamina papyracea of the ethmoid bone, a smooth, very thin quadrilateral plate which encloses the ethmoid cells and forms a large part of the medial wall of the orbit, is the most logical point of fracture." The term *orbital blowout fracture* was introduced in a study in 1957 by Smith and Regan,[440] who defined the term as a fracture of the orbital floor caused by sudden increase in intraorbital or hydraulic pressure. They had performed an experiment to simulate a clinical scenario in which a blow to the eyeball caused a fracture of the orbital floor, whereas blows to the rim on the contralateral side caused no fracture. Fujino and Sato,[459] some 20 years later, produced impacts on the eyeball alone and on

TABLE 66-11 ✦ CLASSIFICATION OF ORBITAL FRACTURES

Orbital Blowout Fractures

Pure blowout fractures: fractures through the thin areas of the orbital floor, medial and lateral wall. The orbital rim is intact.

Impure blowout fractures: fractures associated with fracture of the adjacent facial bones. The thick orbital rim is fractured, and its backward displacement causes a comminution of the orbital floor; the posterior displacement of the orbital rim permits the traumatizing force to be applied against the orbital contents, which produces a superimposed blowout fracture.

Orbital Fractures Without Blowout Fracture

Linear fractures, in upper maxillary and zygomatic fractures. These fractures are often uncomplicated from the standpoint of the orbit.

Comminuted fracture of the orbital floor with prolapse of the orbital contents into the maxillary sinus is often associated with fracture of the midfacial bones.

Fracture of the zygoma with frontozygomatic separation and downward displacement of the zygomatic portion of the orbital floor and of the lateral attachment of the suspensory ligament of Lockwood.

From Converse JM, Smith B, Obear MF, Wood-Smith D: Orbital blowout fractures: a ten year survey. Plast Reconstr Surg 1967;39:20. Copyright 1967, The Williams & Wilkins Company, Baltimore.

TABLE 66-12 ✦ DIPLOPIA AND ENOPHTHALMOS IN ORBITAL FRACTURES

With diplopia, with enophthalmos	This condition results from incarceration of the orbital contents into the area of the fracture and from tearing of the periorbita and escape of the orbital fat.
With diplopia, without enophthalmos	This condition may occur with fixation of the orbital contents in a linear fracture. There is no escape of orbital fat, no enlargement of the orbit, and no enophthalmos.
Without diplopia, with enophthalmos	There is no fixation of the inferior orbital contents into the area of the fracture. The periorbita is torn and an opening has occurred that allows escape of orbital fat, or the orbital cavity is sufficiently enlarged to result in enophthalmos.
Without diplopia, without enophthalmos	This condition occurs when the fracture does not cause fixation of the orbital contents or disturb the anatomy of the periorbita or orbital cavity.

the infraorbital margin alone and performed a third study in which both the eyeball and infraorbital margin were struck simultaneously. Striking of the eyeball independently produced an isolated floor fracture, but this fracture required more force for its production than if the infraorbital margin was struck either independently or in conjunction with the eyeball (Fig. 66-167). Their studies did propose an explanation for tissue entrapment in these fractures in that the recoil (recovery) time from impact was more than twice as long for soft tissue as for bone, thus promoting the incarceration of muscle, fat, and connective tissue as the bone more quickly returned to its original position, trapping the slower rebounding soft tissue. They confirmed the results of their two-dimensional test with three-dimensional and computer-generated mathematical simulations, but little detail was given about these experiments. In 1988, Takizawa et al[460] performed two-dimensional computer simulations analyzing orbital blowout fractures. Using the technique of the finite element method, they analyzed structural deformations and stress distributions on the floor and roof. The study was based on Smith and Regan's proposal that increases in orbital pressure alone caused orbital blowout fractures with no reference to the "buckling force" transferred to the middle orbital segment from the rim impact as theorized by Fujino and Sato. Their computer simulations emphasize the role that the contour of the bony orbital floor plays in vulnerability to these fractures.

TABLE 66-13 ✦ ANALYSIS OF COMPLICATIONS IN ORBITAL FRACTURES PERSISTENT AFTER FLOOR REPAIR (50 PATIENTS)*

	Preoperative	Postoperative	
		3 Months	1 Year
Extraocular muscle imbalance	43	30	20
Enophthalmos	27	15	11
Ptosis	12	3	2
Medial canthal deformity	12	12	9
Lacrimal obstruction	3	3	0
Vertical shortening of lower lid	4	4	2
Visual impairment	5	5	5
Trichiasis–symblepharon	2	1	0

*These complications were observed in patients referred to the author after unsuccessful treatment.

From Converse JM, Smith B, Obear MF, Wood-Smith D: Orbital blowout fractures: a ten year survey. Plast Reconstr Surg 1967;39:20. Copyright 1967, The Williams & Wilkins Company, Baltimore.

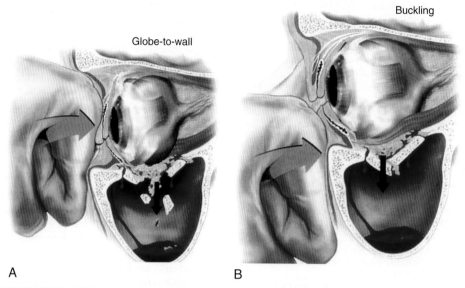

Globe-to-wall   Buckling

A   B

FIGURE 66-167. *A,* Mechanism of blowout fracture from displacement of the globe itself into the orbital walls. The globe is displaced posteriorly, striking the orbital walls and forcing them outward, causing a "punched out" fracture the size of the globe. *B,* "Force transmission" fracture of orbital floor. (*A* and *B* © Montage Media Corp.)

Erling et al,[442] in 1999, elaborated on the theory of Pfeiffer,[441] which predicted that the globe itself might have been impacted into the orbital walls, producing a "globe-sized" internal orbital defect. They proved in a series of blowout fractures that the size of the defect was often equal to the globe and that the fracture occurred at the point where the orbit became too narrow to accommodate a globe being displaced posteriorly.

In 1985, McCord[461] performed an experiment to determine orbital volume increases through the formation of wall defects as a model of treatment for exophthalmos. Using dried skulls, he inflated balloons in the orbit and developed pressure volume and compliance curves and related them to the floor, medial and lateral orbital wall, and roof defects. The results showed a 21% volume increase when combined floor and medial orbital wall were removed and a 3% increase with lateral wall removal; 9% was added to the orbit volume after the roof was removed.

Parsons and Mathog[462] used human skulls and disassembled sections of the orbit to note the volume increase. They noted a 7.5% difference between the right and left orbits and a 22% difference in orbital volume between subjects. They filled the orbits with Silastic material after their simulated surgery and used water displacement to determine the volume difference. Floor defects resulted in twice the volume increase as did medial wall defects. A 5-mm displacement resulted in a volume change of 10%, and a 2.8% volume change resulted in a globe position change of 1 mm. Medial wall displacement of 1 mm caused

1 mm of globe displacement, whereas a 1-mm displacement of the inferior wall caused a 1.5-mm change in globe position. Fries[463] found that 0.5 mL of volume change resulted in 1 mm of globe positional change. Stabile and Trekel,[464] in exophthalmos correction, found that the most profound volume increases were produced by a loss of the inferomedial orbital wall.

Pearl,[465] in a primate model, found that only volume changes posterior to the axis of the globe produce significant globe positional change. He also described intramuscular cone fat loss as a cause of a portion of the globe displacement.

Roncevic and Stajcic[466] treated 72 patients with enophthalmos with early and late treatment for pure and impure orbital injuries. Residual enophthalmos was three times as common (41% versus 18%) in late- as in early-treated patients, and diplopia was also much more common (32% versus 5%) in late-treated patients. Six percent of early-treated patients with diplopia had residual diplopia, whereas 45% of late-treated patients with diplopia had residual diplopia. Hawes and Dortzbach[467] found that more than 15 fracture volume units were necessary to cause enophthalmos. Fracture volume units were calculated by multiplying length, width, and displacement of the fracture. In their series, early corrections had better results (7% residual enophthalmos) than did late corrections (50% residual enophthalmos). Those fractures exceeding 15 volume units tended to have residual enophthalmos. With regard to motility, 88% of patients treated early and 40% of patients treated late had good outcomes.

Dolynchuk et al[468] demonstrated that patients with an orbital volume difference after injury of less than 4% had no enophthalmos. Enophthalmos proportional to the wall displacement was present in those patients with volume differences greater than 5% based on a 23-mL orbital soft tissue volume.

Stahlnecker and Whitaker[469] found that 3.3 mL of change in a 25-mL orbital soft tissue volume was the average difference in orbital volume increase in patients with enophthalmos. Postoperatively, enophthalmos was corrected in 75% of their patients with an average 3.1-mL bone graft volume (perhaps those with fat atrophy were the other 25%).

Raskin et al[470] studied 30 patients with orbital floor blowout fractures. They found that volume differences of greater than 13% correlated with 2 mm or more of enophthalmos in 92% of their patients. Only one patient with less than a 13% volume expansion demonstrated enophthalmos. Any patient presenting with enophthalmos had extensive simultaneous floor and medial wall fractures. No distinct correlations between the degree of enophthalmos and motility problems were found; 75% of anteroinferior wall fractures had motility restriction on presentation, and 90% of posterior fractures had this limitation. Each centimeter of orbital volume increase produced a 0.47-mm change in globe position or enophthalmos.

Yab et al[471] studied patients with CT scans and determined that most of the patients with enophthalmos had stabilized their eye position within 10 days. "Late enophthalmos" was not seen. Enophthalmos of 1 to 2 mm was produced by volume defects of less than 2 mL. They found, for medial wall fractures alone, that enophthalmos increased to 4 mL and then plateaued. When the inferior wall enlargement was less than 2 mL, enophthalmos was proportional to medial wall displacement. When the inferior wall displacement was greater than 2 mL (what they are describing here is the loss of the buttress between the medial orbital wall and the orbital floor), enophthalmos of 3 to 4 mm was produced irrespective of the amount of medial wall involvement. In their experiments, the proportionality between medial wall involvement and enophthalmos was good, but the proportionality between floor involvement did not have as precise a relationship between volume increase and enophthalmos. It is likely that in humans, the restricting action of the ligament sling results in a plateau in enophthalmos at around 4 mm. Rim disruption and soft tissue displacement are required for greater globe displacement to be produced.

Pearl[472,473] experimentally established fractures in fresh cadavers with a screwdriver after transconjunctival exposure of the chosen wall. The fractures were made in the medial and lateral walls and in the floor both anterior and posterior to the axis of the globe. Evaluation after each fracture revealed all medial and lateral wall fractures and half of the posterior floor

fractures resulted in enophthalmos. No enophthalmos was produced in any isolated anterior floor fracture or in half of the posterior fractures. Other experiments in Pearl's study determined the effect of the three regions of orbital fat: superficial, anterior, and deep posterior. He related these distinct fat compartments to globe positional changes through cadaver dissection, CT imaging, and magnetic resonance imaging. Finally, he produced medial wall and anterior floor fractures in chimpanzees to determine the incidence of early and late enophthalmos. Enophthalmos proportional to the defect occurred in medial wall fractures, but no enophthalmos (early or late) occurred in the anterior floor fractures. Pearl, in studying exophthalmos, found 1 mL of volume increase to produce 1.5 mm of exophthalmos correction.

In 1990, Schubert[474] presented a volumetric study that determined bone graft requirements for orbital reconstruction and enophthalmos. Dried skeletal orbits were lined with plastic and aluminum foil, and a floating sphere the size of the globe was placed inside the orbital aperture upright. The volume of water was recorded for each 2-mm increase in globe height until normal globe protrusion was reached. The study suggested the volume needed to return the globe to a normal position for each fracture pattern; 1 mL for each millimeter of enophthalmos was the baseline relationship achieved.

Matsuo et al[269] suggested that the determination of volume necessary for reconstruction of individual patients could be assessed from models. A plastic cast was made of the patient's face, and wax was added in increments to the enophthalmic eye on the cast until normal protrusion was reached. The amount of wax corresponded to the amount of bone graft necessary for reconstruction. Others have used CT imaging and models for orbital implant reconstruction.

Studies using three-dimensional CT scans[468,470,475-477] have been performed to analyze orbital volume in normal versus post-traumatic orbits experiencing enophthalmos. In all studies, the CT imaging enabled specific volume determinations to be completed for different categories of orbital tissue (bone, total soft tissue, fat, globe, and muscle). Each study showed that the bony orbital volume generally increased after trauma, whereas there was generally little volume change in the soft tissue orbital components. These results support the principal mechanism of enophthalmos as increased bony orbital volume (>5%). Decreased soft tissue volume from fat atrophy was seen in approximately 10% of patients, and slight volume increases in soft tissues were commonly seen, presumably because of scar tissue deposition in contused tissues.

Manson et al[477] performed an extensive study of orbital fracture patterns and displacements and then constructed an experimental model for orbital volume calculation. The initial volume of the orbit containing the globe was 26 cm calculated from the scans. An isolated floor displacement of 7 mm resulted in a volume increase of 12%. Total volume increase was linear, with 4% increments from 0 to 3, 3 to 5, and 5 to 7 mm. The 7-mm lateral wall displacement increased initial orbital volume 16%. In this instance, the amount of volume increase tripled with the increment from 3 to 7 mm. The 7-mm isolated medial wall displacement increased initial volume a total of 20% from 0 to 3, 3 to 5, and 5 to 7 mm. The percentage increase was not as steep as that of lateral wall displacement. The lateral wall area included the orbital process of the zygoma and the anterior lip of the greater wing of the sphenoid. The 7-mm roof out, rim out configuration, although clinically the least common fracture pattern, increased orbital volume 38%, which is more than any single wall and rim configuration. The volume difference for isolated floor fractures increased 30% between 5 and 7 mm from 2.2 to 3.2 mL, but the volume difference more than doubled when its associated rim, the zygoma, was displaced along with it.

The percentage increase in volume from 5 to 7 mm is not much changed in medial wall and medial wall with associated floor displacements; 7-mm medial wall displacement increased volume 38% more than the 5-mm displacement of the medial wall, showing the importance of medial wall displacement. The most pronounced enophthalmos occurred with a 7-mm zygoma, floor, and medial wall displacement and a 7-mm roof and supraorbital rim displacement.

Jin et al[478] studied nine patients with isolated medial blowout fractures by CT volume calculation associated with 2 mm of enophthalmos. They found 1.9 cm^2 to be the volume of displaced tissue, which correlated with 0.9 mm of enophthalmos.

Waterhouse et al[479] have produced one of the most elegant studies. This study was the first to compare the two mechanisms of force transmission and hydraulic force under identical experimental conditions, to quantify the striking force, to use unfixed intact human cadaver orbits, and to quantify restoration of intraocular pressure. They found that a buckling force produced a linear or a small fracture pattern in the anterior or middle portion of the orbital floor. The medial wall remained intact. None of the fractures resulted in herniation of soft tissue, and the fractures produced were remarkably consistent in size, anatomic location, and character. In contrast, the hydraulic study, in which blows were delivered to the globe, produced a simultaneous orbital floor and medial wall fracture; and in one third of the globes studied, the fracture extended into the orbital roof. The fractures demonstrated herniation of orbital contents. The study demonstrated that fractures are consistently produced by both mechanisms under the same experimental conditions.

Kersten[434] reported a fracture occurring in a patient with an intraocular lens and concluded that the absence of destruction of the lens excluded the possi-

bility of a striking force to the globe. Fujino[480] also applied lacquer to the skull, which showed strain lines after impacts. Impacts to the infraorbital rim revealed a concentration of lines in the orbital floor and infraorbital canal. This offered further evidence of force transmission as a mechanism of the orbital floor fracture after rim impacts. Phalen[481] repeated Fujino's studies[480,482,483] using human cadaver specimens in 1990. Impacts were delivered to the infraorbital rim of skulls, and it was demonstrated that blowout fractures could be produced without impacts to the globe.

Jones and Evans[484] studied 33 orbits and published their results in 1967. Fractures were consistently produced in the orbital floor and in the medial wall of 10 orbits. They noted that the globe was closer to the medial wall and floor than it was to the other walls and proposed that the globe established the fracture by being driven back along the axis of the orbit, striking the orbital walls when the size of the globe prevented further posterior displacement. They found the most frequent areas of fracture. Fracture of the floor alone occurred in two thirds of the globes. Fracture of the medial wall alone occurred in one sixth, and fracture of the floor and medial wall together occurred in 10%. The most common site of a blowout fracture was in the floor medial to the infraorbital nerve in the posterior portion of the orbit. They also investigated the thickness of the orbital floor and found that the anterior, middle, and posterior portions of the ethmoid were as thin as the posterior portion of the orbital floor. Variations occurred in the thickness of the orbital floor, with some areas being five times as thick as others. Measurements ranged from 0.23 to 1.25 mm in thickness. They measured the average length of the infraorbital groove and the infraorbital canal and found the total length of the groove and canal to be 2.8 cm, the length of the groove 1.5 cm, and the length of the canal 1.3 cm. They found that the orbital walls were closer to the geometric orbital axis between 2.0 and 2.5 cm anterior to the apical point of the orbit. They also noted that the vertical projection of the geometric orbital axis (along which the globe was driven by force) passed directly over the most common site of a blowout fracture 2.0 to 2.5 cm anterior to the apical point of the orbit.

Greene et al[485] studied the forces necessary to cause fracture in an experimental model involving live primates in 1990. At forces above 2.08 newtons, blowout fractures were consistently produced. Globe rupture was frequently observed and was attributed to the absence of the ethmoid sinuses and the strong maxillary buttresses in monkeys.

Considering the volume displacements, the "buttresses of the orbit" must be analyzed and, if missing, must be reconstructed by some technique to permit stable bone grafts or wall reconstructions. Loss of the inferior medial buttress and the inferolateral wall buttresses must be reconstituted to permit stable inferior, medial, and lateral wall position. When multiple walls of the orbit are fractured simultaneously, the roof and floor must be reconstructed with rigid fixation (two of the four orbital walls must be stable). The medial and lateral wall reconstructions may be "rested" between the "stable" floor and roof (Fig. 66-168).

Fan et al,[486] in 2003, studied the change in orbital volume and correlated that with the clinical enophthalmos produced in orbital blowout fractures. They analyzed orbital volume measurement from axial CT scans, correlated this with Hertel exophthalmometer measurements, and found that 1 mL of orbital volume caused 0.89 mm of enophthalmos.

Burm et al,[487] in 1999, evaluated the frequency of medial blowout fractures and emphasized that these might be produced by blows to the nose alone in the manner of force transmission to the infraorbital rim producing orbital floor blowout fractures. The paper also characterized the internal orbit inferomedial buttress. They noted that actual diplopia was four times more frequent than observation of restricted muscle gaze. They also described "hinged, double-hinged, and punched-out fracture types" and "hooking, catching, hanging, and herniation" to indicate how the relative origin, insertion, and path of extraocular muscles are changed (Figs. 66-169 to 66-171) (see also Chapter 67).

IMPURE BLOWOUT FRACTURES

The orbital floor may fracture alone, and the fracture may then be termed *pure*. However, if there is rim involvement, the fracture may be defined as *impure*. In a typical high-energy injury, the thick orbital rim may be fractured and displaced backward, resulting in an eggshell comminution of the thin or "middle portion" of the orbit. Because of the continuing momentum and the pressure against the soft tissue orbital contents, a portion of the contents is extruded through fracture sites that may incarcerate or prolapse orbital soft tissues. In two studies, automobile accidents were listed as the most common cause of orbital floor fractures, followed by physical assault, sports-related injuries, and falls.[488,489] In one study, the ratio of impure to pure orbital floor fractures was 3:1. In both studies, there was a higher percentage of male than female patients (90% of 250 patients[488] and quoted as >2:1 ratio of 199 patients[489]) because men engage in a wider range of behaviors resulting in orbital floor fractures. Serious ocular injury occurred in 19.6% of patients and 17.1% prospectively, with globe rupture quoted as the most prevalent (40.5% of serious injuries studied).

ORBITAL EXPANSION AND CONTRACTION

The volume occupied by the soft tissue contents (the eye and adnexa) may expand or contract secondary to the direction of orbital fracture displacement. *Blow-in fracture*[446,447,490] (see Fig. 66-166) has been used to describe the orbital volume contraction that occurs secondary to some types of bone displacement. Blow-in fractures may occur with either zygomatic or supra-orbital fractures. Dingman[142] and other authors have occasionally observed pure blow-in fractures of the orbital floor. A typical fracture causing orbital contraction is an orbital roof fracture in which the displacement of the roof is downward and backward, resulting in downward and forward displacement of the globe. The term *blowout* generally applies to destruction of the floor and medial wall of the orbit and signifies the potential for displacement of orbital contents into the sinus cavities (see Fig. 66-168). In the typical blowout fracture, displacement of the globe is posterior, medial, and inferior. This occurs because of the prolapse of orbital soft tissues into the maxillary and ethmoid sinuses. Fractures of the orbital floor and the lateral portion of the orbit accompany zygomatic fractures (see Fig. 66-166) and may vary from linear fractures to displacement of actual sections of the orbital walls.

SURGICAL PATHOLOGY

Diplopia

Extraocular muscle imbalance and subjective diplopia are usually the result of muscle contusion, but they can be the result of incarceration of either the muscle or the soft tissue adjacent to the muscles or be due to nerve damage to the third, fourth, and sixth cranial nerves.[491-493] Deviation of the visual axes can account for diplopia. It is also thought that positioning of the globe 1 cm beyond its usual position can account for diplopia.[6,271,494] The major issue for surgeons is to differentiate those fractures in which diplopia is caused by muscle contusion, which are expected to maximally heal spontaneously, from those in which entrapment of the soft tissue or muscle is actually caused by the bone fracture. Both mechanisms may produce a vertical muscle imbalance with diplopia on looking superiorly or inferiorly. For instance, when the inferior rectus muscle is tethered, inferior diplopia is much more incapacitating than superior diplopia for most patients. The soft tissue structures involved in inferior rectus diplopia include the muscle itself,[495] possibly the inferior oblique muscle (especially at its origin[496]), the suspensory ligaments of the globe, the periorbita, the fascial expansions, and fat, which tethers the muscle by virtue of its fine musculofascial ligament connections.[497-499] Also, an altered path or sagging of the muscle may contribute to double vision.[500,501] Most authors think that displacement of the globe must exceed 5 mm and probably 10 mm for diplopia to be reasonably attributed to globe displacement. The eye is able to accommodate a range of superior and inferior displacement without diplopia

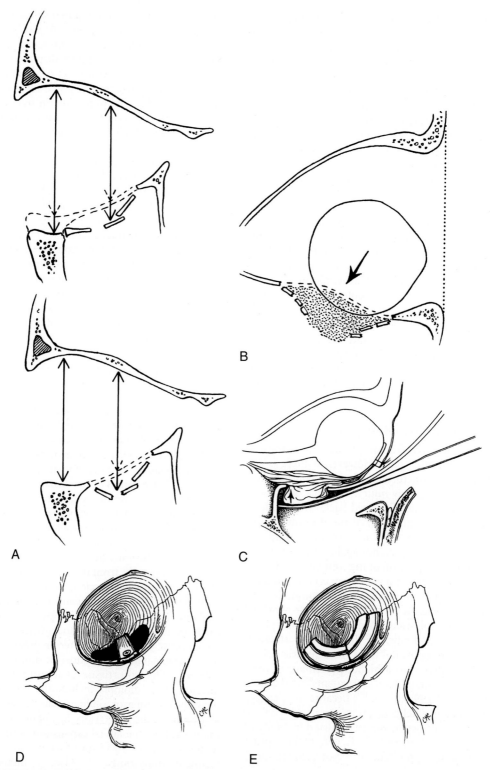

FIGURE 66-168. *A,* Orbital floor blowout fracture with displacement of orbital contents into the maxillary sinus cavity. *B,* The extraorbital volume and globe displacement accompanying the fracture. *C,* Locating the "ledge" (the posterior margin of the fracture) by placing a Freer elevator in the back of the maxillary antrum. Troublesome visualization is produced by prolapse of fat over the posterior edge of the fracture. *D* and *E,* Technique of orbital reconstruction by stacking bone grafts on a strut.

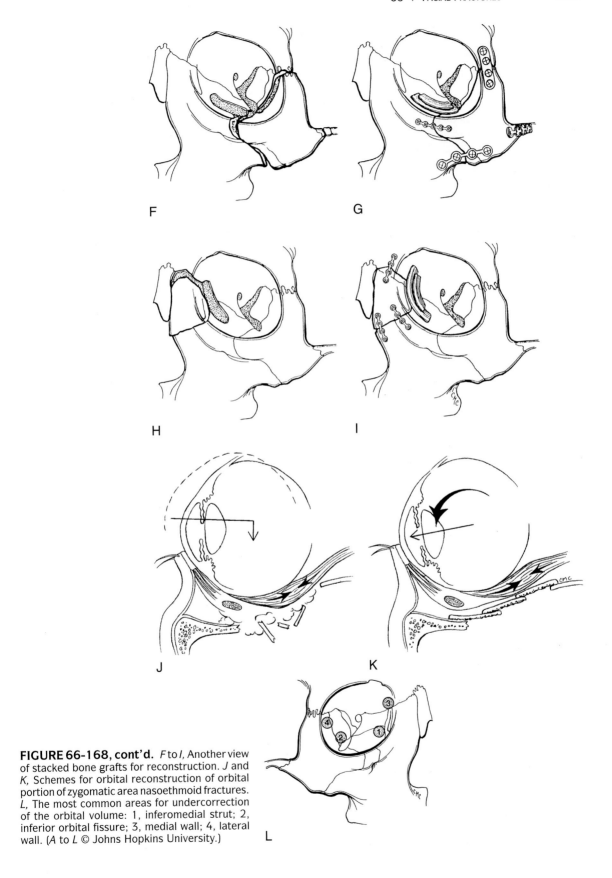

FIGURE 66-168, cont'd. *F* to *I*, Another view of stacked bone grafts for reconstruction. *J* and *K*, Schemes for orbital reconstruction of orbital portion of zygomatic area nasoethmoid fractures. *L*, The most common areas for undercorrection of the orbital volume: 1, inferomedial strut; 2, inferior orbital fissure; 3, medial wall; 4, lateral wall. (*A* to *L* © Johns Hopkins University.)

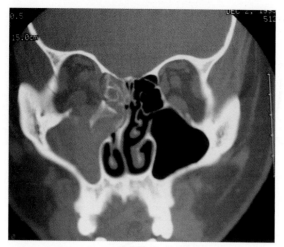

FIGURE 66-169. A patient with diplopia on the basis of displacement of the inferior oblique muscle.

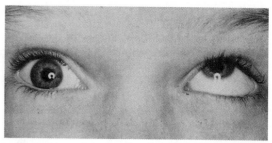

FIGURE 66-171. Blowout fracture in a child produced by a snowball. Note the nearly complete immobility of the ocular globe and the enophthalmos. Such severe loss of motion implies actual muscle incarceration, an injury that is more frequent in children than in adults. This fracture deserves *immediate* operation with release of the incarcerated extraocular muscle system. It is often accompanied by pain on attempted rotation of the globe and sometimes nausea and vomiting. These symptoms are unusual in orbital floor fractures without true muscle incarceration.

in most patients. Indeed, significant globe displacement occurring slowly is often asymptomatic. Significant loss of the orbital floor accounts for downward and posterior displacement of the ocular globe. In these large orbital fractures, there is frequently no actual entrapment unless the action of the muscle is severely limited by a fibrous adhesion. Compartment syndromes producing a Volkmann contracture[502,503] are also a possibility, although Iliff et al[504] have shown that it would be difficult to produce a true compartment syndrome.

Injury of the cranial nerves supplying the inferior oblique and the inferior rectus muscles must also be

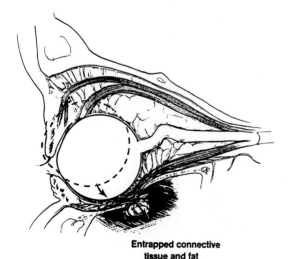

Entrapped connective tissue and fat

FIGURE 66-170. Incarceration of perimuscular fat adjacent to an extraocular muscle may tether the muscle by virtue of the interconnections of the fine ligament system. If the fat necroses, more mobility of the muscle may be obtained. The globe may be held inferiorly.

considered a cause of double vision. The inferior oblique and inferior rectus muscles are innervated by the inferior division of cranial nerve III. The branch to the inferior rectus muscle passes along its upper surface to pierce the muscle at the junction of the posterior and middle thirds of the muscle. The branch to the inferior oblique muscle runs along the lateral edge of the inferior rectus muscle and can clearly be seen in orbital dissections, entering the ocular surface of the inferior oblique muscle. In the anterior third of the orbit, the nerve is therefore exposed to injury by the contusion in blowout fractures. The relatively short course of the nerve to the inferior rectus muscle with its superior location renders it less vulnerable to injury. Visual field examination will help determine whether muscle function is disturbed. Saccadic velocities,[505] which measure the acceleration velocity of muscle movement, also assess the speed of acceleration of the extraocular muscle movement by monitoring globe speed and motion and can sometimes distinguish muscle contusion from actual muscle entrapment. Lesions of more proximal cranial nerves, such as cranial nerve IV or VI, may cause diplopia from intracranial mechanisms.[293,492]

Injury to cranial nerves III, IV, and VI or direct injury to the extraocular muscles may occur secondary to laceration by bone fragments, disruption of muscle attachments, contusion, and hemorrhage.[65] Alternatively, it has been postulated that a change in muscle balance can be caused by a change in orbital shape. Muscle imbalance occurs when ptosis of the globe is associated with enophthalmos. Secondary deviations are caused by overaction of the "yoke" or conjugate muscles of the opposite eye.[497,498] A factor to be remembered is that no extraocular muscle acts alone to produce ocular movements. Ocular rotation is the sum of the action, counteraction, and relaxation in concert of the 12 extraocular muscles (6 per globe). The subject of the physiology of the ocular rotatory muscles is so complex that in all universities, eye muscle specialists exist. Visual field examinations record the dominant actions of each of the extraocular muscles.

The cause of muscle imbalance may include paralytic problems, tropias (constant imbalance), or phorias (latent imbalance) occurring only with disruption of fusion. Phorias occur after temporary immobilization of the injured eye and are usually horizontal in nature.

Enophthalmos

Enophthalmos,[271,368,463,506-509] the second major complication of a blowout fracture, has a number of causes. The major cause, enlargement of the bony orbit with herniation of the orbital soft tissue structures into an enlarged cavity, is well documented.[468-470,474,476,477] This enlargement allows soft tissue structural displacement with a remodeling of the shape of the soft tissue into a sphere. Another postulated mechanism of enophthalmos is the retention of the ocular globe in a backward position when structures are entrapped in a fracture site. A popular postulated theory was fat atrophy, but the computerized volume studies show that fat atrophy is significant in only 10% of orbital fractures. A lowered fat volume has been shown to occur in some orbital injuries, but the several studies mentioned indicate that this is not the major mechanism in the production of enophthalmos. Other mechanisms of enophthalmos production include the neurogenic theories, in which fat atrophy secondary to sympathetic nerve disruption has been postulated; however, this has not been proved to be a major mechanism.[510] It has been shown by Manson et al[498] that part of the support of the globe is produced by the quantity and position of the intramuscular (or intraconal) fat. In the anterior portion of the orbit, fat is located in an extraconal as well as in an intraconal position. In the posterior portion of the orbit, very little of the fat is extraconal. The intraconal fat, after fracture, may be dislocated ("extruded") to an extraconal location; thus, its absence in the intraconal compartment provides a lack of globe support and contributes to enophthalmos.

When enophthalmos is conspicuous, and particularly when the orbital contents are downwardly displaced, a ptosis of the upper eyelid occurs with a deepening and hollow appearance of the supratarsal fold. A shortening of the horizontal dimension of the palpable fissure often accompanies the enophthalmos. This mechanism of lid ptosis was discussed by Pearl and Vistnes.[511] Ptosis of the lid is especially common when nasoethmoidal-orbital fractures are associated with significant fractures of the deep orbit.

Lower animals possess an "orbitalis muscle" that spans the area corresponding to a greatly enlarged infe-rior orbital fissure. In some animals, this muscle occupies a major portion of the lateral and inferior portion of the orbit. It is the orbitalis muscle with its sympathetic innervation that causes the animal to protrude its eyeball when frightened. The muscle contracts and the globe is moved forward for the purpose of focusing and improving the visual field. In humans, this muscle is vestigial, and most anatomists discount its importance. It has sometimes been claimed that this muscle is a factor in the enophthalmos of Horner syndrome, caused by paralysis of cranial nerve III. Most authors think that the suggestion of the appearance of enophthalmos in this condition is actually due to ptosis and perhaps fat atrophy produced by the sympathetic denervation.[510] It is possible that atrophic changes that occur in traumatized orbital fat may be partly responsible for the positional change of the globe. Some rarer factors that have been thought responsible for the development of post-traumatic enophthalmos include dislocation of the trochlea and dislocation of the trochlea and superior oblique muscle. Scar contracture of the postbulbar soft tissue, producing a fibrosis that pulls the globe backward, accompanied by rupture of the orbital ligaments and fascial bands, has also been postulated as a mechanism of enophthalmos. This phenomenon occurs routinely when scar tissue pulls the orbital soft tissue into an enlarged bony cavity.[498]

Koornneef[443,450] postulated that downward traction on the globe by entrapped orbital contents contributes to the production of globe positional change (Fig. 66-172). Actually, as time passes, the soft tissue of the orbit "contracts" and pulls the soft tissue backward to contact the bone fragments by the mechanism of scar contracture. In orbital dissection, on release of this adherence, there is an immediate improvement in globe position, but the globe position would relapse if no graft were placed between the bone wall and desired soft tissue position to prevent recurrence of the contracture. The bone graft volume required must correspond at least to the volume difference between the position of the displaced bone fragments and the released soft tissue, plus additional graft to guide the globe into its proper position.

The enlargement of the orbital cavity, from the depression of the floor, is the frequent factor in the production of enophthalmos. However, there may be no entrapment of the orbital structures and no diplopia in severe enophthalmos because of the lack of incarceration of ocular muscles or the fat adjacent to the muscles, which is tethered to the muscles by the fine ligament system.[450,512] Enophthalmos frequently accompanies major injuries involving the orbit, such as the zygomatic or upper Le Fort (II and III) fractures. In these injuries, fractures occur through the lateral wall and floor and medial walls of the orbit.

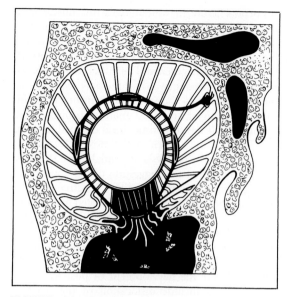

FIGURE 66-172. After fracture, the fine ligament system may be entrapped within the fracture site, tethering the extraocular muscle motion. (From Koornneef L: Current concepts on the management of blowout fractures. Ann Plast Surg 1982;9:185.)

EXAMINATION AND DIAGNOSIS

In the typical blowout fracture, the patient may not spontaneously comment about double vision. Double vision must be elicited both in the primary position and looking straight ahead, or in upward, downward, medial, or lateral gaze (Fig. 66-172). The patient may not recognize double vision early if the eye is temporarily closed by edema of the eyelids or if a dressing has closed the eyelids. Initially, after fracture, swelling appears, and it may be difficult to determine globe displacement or to detect enophthalmos. As the swelling disappears, enophthalmos becomes more noticeable. Those patients with acute enophthalmos need orbital volume correction by surgical repositioning or reconstruction of the displaced orbital walls, particularly the floor. The backward and downward displacement of the globe and the deep supratarsal sulcus may be initially absent but appear as the swelling resolves (Fig. 66-173). The patient should be examined for the possibility of ocular globe injury, eyelid damage, scleral lacerations, corneal damage, hyphema, and hematoma in the anterior or posterior chamber. The action of the levator muscle and integrity of the levator aponeurosis should also be confirmed.

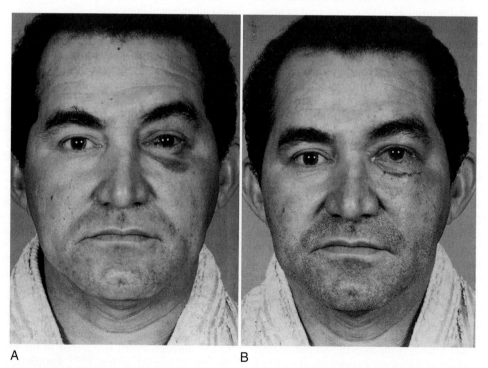

A   B

FIGURE 66-173. Blowout fracture of the left orbit. *A,* Forward gaze. Note the enophthalmos. *B,* Forward gaze after release of the herniated structures and restoration of the continuity of the orbital floor. Note the lower eyelid incision along the rim. This incision causes the least ectropion but produces the most visible scarring. The enophthalmos has been corrected. The left orbit is structurally situated in a higher preinjury position than the right. A preinjury picture is required to identify the goals of reconstruction.

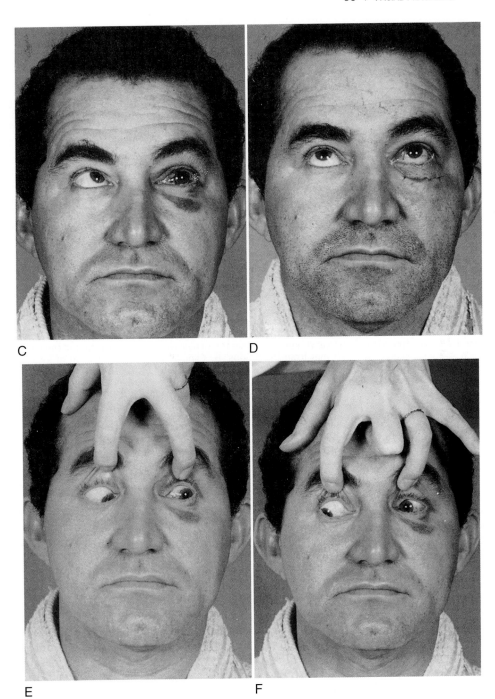

C   D

E   F

FIGURE 66-173, cont'd. *C,* Restriction in upper and lateral gaze before the operation. *D,* Upward gaze after surgery, demonstrating the release of the entrapment of the orbital muscle and ligament structures. *E,* The restriction in the dominant lateral gaze of the left ocular globe before the operation. *F,* The restriction of downward and inward gaze before surgery. The patient was one of the first to be treated for a blowout fracture. Diplopia in the downward gaze or reading position is more disabling than diplopia in "up gaze" for most patients. (From Converse JM, Smith B: Blow-out fracture of the floor of the orbit. Trans Am Acad Ophthal Otolaryngol 1960;64:676.)

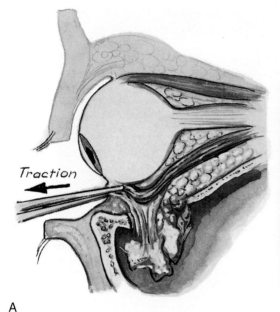

A

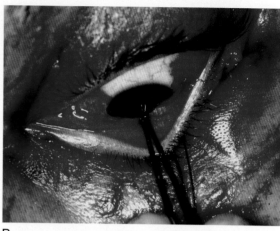

B

FIGURE 66-174. The forced duction test. *A,* Forceps grasp the ocular globe at the insertion of the inferior rectus muscle, which is approximately 7 to 10 mm from the limbus. *B,* Clinical photograph. A drop of local anesthetic instilled into the conjunctival sac precedes the procedure.

Globe rupture or injury or retinal detachment may accompany blunt injury to the periorbital structures.

Forced Duction Test

Limitation of forced rotation of the eyeball is the forced duction test or the eyeball traction test (Fig. 66-174). This test provides a means of differentiating entrapment of the ligaments of the inferior rectus muscle from weakness, paralysis, and sometimes contusion. Presumably, lack of muscle function will not cause any resistance to motion when the globe is grasped and rotated. Incarceration of the inferior rectus muscle fascial system, however, produces limitation to forced rotation of the globe, which is considered to be a pathognomonic sign of muscle or fine ligament incarceration in a fracture. Practically, fibrosis may produce limitation of motion, as may muscle contusion. Fibrosis should be absent in early examinations, but severe edema and hemorrhage in the muscle may also produce limitation of movement.

For performance of the test, a few drops of local anesthetic solution, such as proparacaine, are instilled into the conjunctival sac. Sufficient anesthesia is provided by the drops to permit grasping of the insertion of the inferior rectus muscle onto the eyeball, which is at a point 7 to 10 mm from the limbus. The globe should be gently rotated upward and downward and medially and laterally, confirming any resistance to motion. Extraocular motion should normally be free and unencumbered. The degree to which a muscle con-

tusion contributes to limited extraocular motion must be estimated.

CLASSIFICATION

Globe ruptures occasionally accompany blunt ocular injury (Fig. 66-175).[513] Pieramici[513] has summarized the basis of the classification system, which depends on type of injury, mechanism of injury, grade of injury (visual acuity), pupillary response (presence or absence of a relative afferent pupillary defect), and zone of injury (location of eye wall opening). In general, blunt injuries have a poorer prognosis than sharp injuries, and posterior injuries have worse prognoses than anterior injuries. The author has not seen significant ocular function occur after midface fractures and globe rupture from automobile accidents, but good visual function after zygoma fracture and globe rupture from a fall has occurred after globe repair. Patients with glaucoma must be carefully managed to exclude abnormal elevations of the intraocular pressure. In assessment of ocular movement, an object is held approximately 2 feet from the patient's eye and the patient is asked to look at the object. The object is then rotated into each field of gaze, and if the affected eye is not able to rotate to the normal range, restriction of extraocular motion is documented. The function of the muscles may be restricted by entrapment, contusion, scarring, hematoma, or fibrosis (Fig. 66-176). Release of entrapment allows fuller motion of the extraocular muscles. In children's fractures with

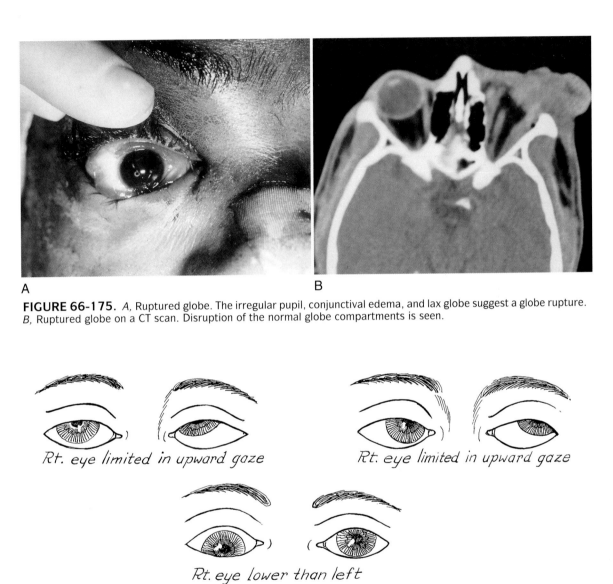

FIGURE 66-175. *A,* Ruptured globe. The irregular pupil, conjunctival edema, and lax globe suggest a globe rupture. *B,* Ruptured globe on a CT scan. Disruption of the normal globe compartments is seen.

Rt. eye limited in upward gaze

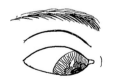

Rt. eye limited in upward gaze

Rt. eye lower than left

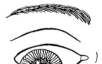

Rt.eye limited in downward gaze

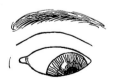

Very little restriction

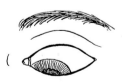

FIGURE 66-176. The limitation of oculorotatory movements after a blowout fracture of the right orbit.

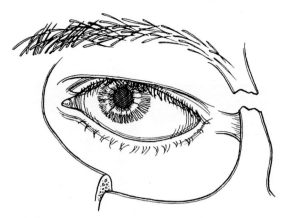

FIGURE 66-177. The lateral canthus and both lids are draped inferiorly by a displaced zygoma fracture. (© Johns Hopkins University.)

the bone in hinged fractures, plating it into position from within the maxillary sinus with endoscopic techniques.

A combined subconjunctival and periorbital hematoma is one of the most common symptoms in orbital fractures. An exception to this is the "white-eyed blowout" (Fig. 66-178).[435]

In fractures involving the orbital floor, the canal and groove for the infraorbital nerve are often the site of the fracture. This type of fracture produces an anesthesia or hypesthesia in the infraorbital nerve distribution.[515] Numbness of the ipsilateral upper lip and cheek are produced by contusion of the branches that innervate the cutaneous portion of the medial aspect of the face, nose, and upper lip. Numbness of the anterior superior maxillary teeth may be produced by involvement of the branches that travel in the anterior wall of the maxilla. Either the teeth or the soft tissue may be affected individually or collectively.

muscle incarceration and in some adults, the author has observed nearly complete fixation of the globe, which is an urgent indication for emergency release of the muscle and extraocular muscle system.[6]

In fractures in which the infraorbital rim is comminuted, one can observe that the lower lid is vertically shortened with a tendency toward eversion. The inferior orbital rim is displaced downward and backward and carries with it the insertion of the septum orbitale, which accounts for the vertical shortening and malposition of the lower eyelid (Fig. 66-177).

Burm[487,514] has categorized the types of blowout fractures as trap-door, single hinge, double hinge, and punched out. This has implication for the type of orbital reconstruction to be used. Some have actually replaced

TREATMENT

The primary objectives of treatment are achieved by the release of the soft tissue contents from their displaced position or adherent structures (Table 66-14). The accurate definition and extent of the bone fracture must then be determined. This involves an exploration of the intact bone and a definition of the location by surgical dissection of the intact bone around the orbital defect. Identification of intact bone landmarks permits a plan for reconstruction of the bony wall of the orbit in its anatomic position. In the face of a fracture requiring surgical intervention, the timing of surgery should be as early as practical. Early restoration prevents soft tissue scarring in nonanatomic positions and presumably relates to better function.

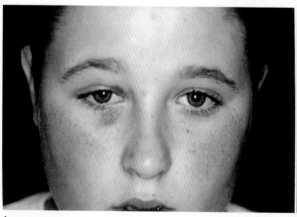
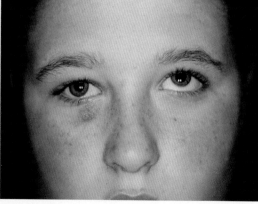

A   B

FIGURE 66-178. *A,* White-eyed blowout fracture. No subconjunctival hematoma is present. *B,* Attempting to look upward.

TABLE 66-14 ✦ ORBITAL BLOWOUT FRACTURE TREATMENT GOALS

Disengage entrapped midface ligamental structures and restore ocular rotatory function.
Replace orbital contents into the usual confines of the normal bony orbital cavity, including restoration of orbital volume and shape.
Restore orbital cavity walls, which in effect replaces the tissues into their proper position and dictates the shape into which the soft tissue can scar.

Indications

The indications for surgical treatment include a change in globe position (either enophthalmos or exophthalmos) and double vision with CT evidence of incarcerated soft tissue or an abnormal finding on forced duction examination—confirming incarceration of the extraocular muscles or the extraocular fine ligament system. Anesthesia or hypesthesia of the infraorbital nerve in the author's experience is an indication for surgical intervention only when blowout fractures are accompanied by orbital rim fractures that are medially impacted and therefore compress the canal of the infraorbital nerve. Some believe that progressive numbness is an indication.[515] Double vision caused by extraocular muscle incarceration must be differentiated from that caused by hematoma, edema, and neurogenic factors, which do not respond to operative release of the muscle system (Table 66-15).

Timing

In isolated blowout fractures, it is not necessary to operate immediately unless true muscle incarceration

TABLE 66-15 ✦ INDICATIONS FOR SURGICAL TREATMENT OF A BLOWOUT FRACTURE

Double vision caused by incarceration of muscle or the fine ligament system, documented by forced duction examination and CT scan
Radiographic evidence of extensive fracture, such that enophthalmos would be produced
Enophthalmos or exophthalmos or significant globe positional change produced by an orbital volume change
Visual acuity deficit, increasing and not responsive to medical-dose steroids, implying that optic canal decompression is indicated
Rarely, orbital fractures of a "blow-in" character may be produced. On occasion, these involve the medial or the lateral walls of the orbit (see Fig. 66-166) and severely constrict orbital volume, causing increased intraorbital pressure.

or severe restriction of vision is present. In the presence of significant edema, retinal detachment, or other significant globe injuries, such as hyphema, it is advisable to wait a number of days. Forcing an edematous soft tissue mass into a much smaller volume can be problematic and harmful. It is also advisable to wait when clinical signs indicating the necessity for surgery are equivocal. The symptoms may subside in a few days and indicate that surgery is not required.

Major significant orbital fractures are, however, best treated by early surgical intervention, and the author firmly believes that the earlier significant orbital volume or muscle derangement can be corrected, the better the aesthetic and functional result. The clinician is thus responsible for making a clear decision about operative intervention in the evaluation of the extent of injury and determining the necessity for surgical correction. In children, delay of operation is not desirable because bone regeneration is rapid and osteotomy will be required, and freeing of incarcerated orbital soft tissue contents then becomes less effective. Scarring of the periorbita in an abnormal position may persist after release of incarcerated orbital contents and therefore negate the results of surgical intervention. Late motility problems from significant incarceration persist if treatment is postponed for 2 to 3 weeks despite the late release of orbital contents. Undue delay therefore is *not* advocated; judicious consideration of all aspects of operative versus nonoperative treatment is required. In a large series of facial fractures studied by Hakelius and Ponten,[516] 22% of the patients with midfacial fractures had double vision. In comparing a series of patients treated within 2 weeks after the accident with another series in which treatment was delayed, Hakelius and Ponten[516] found that 16% of the patients in the first group reported the presence of diplopia only when they were tired (93% were completely free of diplopia). In the second group, 24% still had unchanged diplopia. As a result of this study, an early active surgical approach is recommended for significant fractures. Fractures requiring surgery can be assessed and defined by accurate CT scan examinations. It is the author's impression that disruptions in the orbital floor exceeding an area of 2 cm^2 set the stage for globe positional change; thus, fractures that exceed this dimension can be considered for surgical treatment. It is also significant that in a series of 50 patients referred with blowout fractures and other complications after unsuccessful and delayed treatment (mean time between trauma and surgery, 4 weeks), 43 patients showed extraocular muscle imbalance.[517,518] Emery et al[519] also reported the clinical findings in 159 patients with orbital floor fractures. They noted late double vision in 60% of patients with untreated blowout fractures when double vision was present initially. It was still present 15 days after the injury. However, the cause of the diplopia can vary according to the mechanisms described previously.

The author has occasionally observed that the forced duction test will free an entrapment; these patients do not require further treatment. Today, it is difficult to agree with the advice of Putterman et al,[520] who advocated the initial nonsurgical management of almost all isolated blowout fractures of the orbital floor, but their observations were made before the advent of the CT scan. These authors reported 25% residual diplopia in a retrospective study and 27% residual diplopia in a prospective study. Enophthalmos occurred in 65% of the patients in a retrospective study and in 36% of those involved in a prospective study. With the advent of CT scans, patients who are likely to have persistent diplopia or significant enophthalmos may be predicted with reasonable certainty. Thus, each patient should be considered individually, and the decision for or against exploratory surgery should be made on the basis of the criteria outlined before. Double vision in a functional field of gaze with positive evidence of muscle incarceration or fat trapping on CT scans should be treated surgically.[56,499] It is usually more difficult to correct enophthalmos as a secondary than as a primary procedure, and certainly muscle damage more frequently accompanies secondary corrections for enophthalmos when scar tissue and contracture are present. The extraocular muscles travel close to the orbital walls in the posterior half of the orbit and are vulnerable to surgical injury. Bringing a globe forward secondarily may also stretch a shortened muscle or produce diplopia on the basis of rotating the globe into the field of action of the shortened muscle as the globe is brought forward.

Techniques

A number of methods have been advocated for the treatment of blowout fractures. The surgical approaches have involved the eyelid, the canine fossa through the maxillary sinus, and, recently, endoscopic procedures. The eyelid or conjunctival approach to the orbital floor is preferred because it allows direct visualization and disengagement of any entrapped or prolapsed orbital tissue. It also permits anatomic replacement of the orbital floor fractures.

ENDOSCOPIC APPROACHES. Endoscopic approaches through the maxillary sinus have permitted direct visualization of the orbital floor and manipulation of the soft tissue and floor repair with this approach, which avoids an eyelid incision (Fig. 66-179).[521-525] Any approach that does not provide the operating surgeon with a precise view of the orbital contents to ensure their protection should not be used. Previously, blowout fractures were approached through the maxillary sinus "blind," and the eye position was changed by packing without the endoscopic evaluation of entrapped soft tissue. The maxillary sinus approach is useful as a means of removing dislocated bone fragments from the sinus cavity, which will become sequestered. It is important in the management of comminuted fractures of the maxilla and other bones of the midfacial area in that any bone fragments can be removed and the sinus irrigated, confirming free entry of sinus fluid into the nose (absence of sinus obstruction). Previously, some authors recommended that maxillary sinus packing be inserted to provide support for comminuted orbital floor fragments; however, with current orbital floor reconstruction materials, this approach appears to have no indications. Packing of the maxillary sinus without direct observation of the floor has been associated with blindness. Suppuration has also been observed after gauze packing of the maxillary sinus. McCoy et al[407] reported instances in which packing of the maxillary sinus caused fragments of the bone to damage the optic nerve, leading to blindness. In one study, the maxillary sinus approach was documented to be inadequate in one fourth of patients, and an eyelid approach was required to release incarcerated orbital contents from the surrounding impacted bone fragments. The efficacy of the endoscopic approaches to the orbital floor may be limited by the same issues. Some authors use a combined endoscopic and conjunctival approach to orbital repair.[526] Some authors drain the maxillary sinus into the mouth or the eyelid to the skin after orbital explorations. Some authors have restored the integrity of the orbit by repositioning the trap-door, single-hinged, or double-hinged fractures and reconstructing the integrity of the orbit floor with small plate unicortical fixation performed endoscopically through the sinus. Others have repositioned the displaced floor bone, angling it slightly so that it "catches" on adjacent bone. Artificial materials have also been used either alone, placed endoscopically, or over the replaced orbital floor (titanium mesh) to stabilize the reconstruction.

There are several approaches to fractures of the orbital floor through the endoscope[527] (Fig. 66-179). In single- or double-hinged or punched-out fractures, the bone fragments may be replaced and stabilized with a plate or mesh applied through the maxillary sinus. A Caldwell-Luc window is formed in the anterior wall with a perforating drill and replaced after the floor repair. The prolapsed orbital contents are gently teased into the orbit, and the bone is replaced. Alternatively, a MEDPOR sheet may be cut to size and stabilized with fixation. Another option is to size the MEDPOR slightly larger in one direction and "wedge" it over the edges of the intact orbital floor so that it is supported by the edges of the bone. Combined lower eyelid (conjunctival) and endoscopic approaches have been described that reportedly improve visualization by use of multiple approaches.

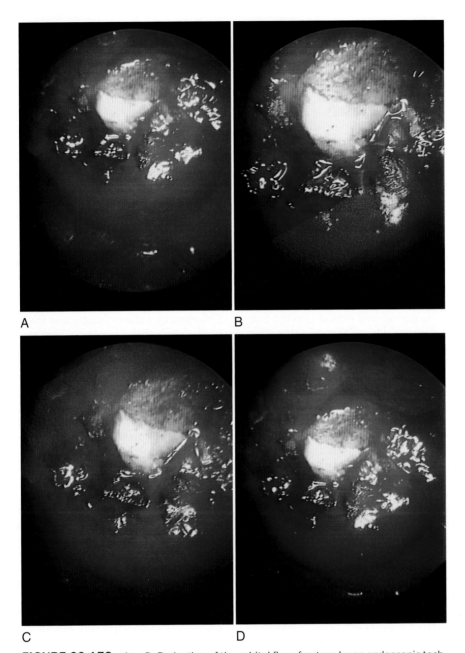

A

B

C

D

FIGURE 66-179. *A to D,* Reduction of the orbital floor fracture by an endoscopic technique through the maxillary sinus. (Courtesy of Navin Singh, MD.)

Endoscopic approaches to the medial orbital wall occur through the nose, conjunctiva, or upper eyelid. The eyelid and conjunctival approaches are "facilitated" by the endoscope in that visualization is magnified.

In the eyelid or conjunctival approach, an incision is made in the medial upper eyelid in the area of an upper blepharoplasty, or the medial extension of a transconjunctival incision is used.[528] Dissection proceeds subperiosteally along the medial orbital wall until the defect is identified. The ethmoidal vessels require

diversion and coagulation. After identification of the defect, MEDPOR may be placed in layers to achieve reconstruction of the inwardly bulging contour of the medial orbital wall.

The intranasal approach requires resection of the ethmoid sinus so a sheet of polyethylene can be placed in an upside-down U between the septum and the medial orbital wall, effectively wedging the medial orbital wall in place. The polyethylene sheet requires removal intranasally in 4 to 6 weeks.

Replacement of the fractured bone with a bone graft is the preferred technique of orbital floor reconstruction. Many orbital fractures, however, are managed by introduction of a plastic sheet, preferably of a thickness and strength to provide support for orbital contents. The efficacy of thin plastic sheets, which do not provide firm support, is questioned.

There are contraindications to the subciliary transcutaneous and transconjunctival incisions (see Table 66-3).[97]

SUBPERIOSTEAL DISSECTION AND SOFT TISSUE CLOSURE.

It is recommended that the edges of the periosteal incision be marked with 5-0 silk sutures left with 1-cm tags so that these structures can be accurately reapproximated at the time of soft tissue closure. It is surprising how difficult it is to put these structures together in the correct alignment after the operation is completed unless marking sutures are used. The subperiosteal dissection should begin in areas where the bone is normal and extend into the fractured area first from one side and then from the other. This allows easier identification and protection of important structures. The levator labii superioris muscle is above the infraorbital nerve, and the levator anguli oris muscle inserts below the infraorbital nerve. Therefore, in approaching the infraorbital nerve from either above or below, one must first detach the muscle insertions. The author thinks that first dissecting the medial maxillary buttress and then laterally along the lateral maxillary buttress allows the nerve to "appear between dissections." If any orbital contents are incarcerated in the floor, the defect can easily be made larger to allow visualization and gentle retraction of orbital contents without retraction damage. The zygomaticofacial nerve exits directly from the lateral malar eminence and should be protected in acute fracture treatment. In lateral fracture treatment, the nerve often has to be divided to mobilize the osteotomy. Division of this nerve leaves a small spot of numbness over the malar eminence and may give rise to chronic pain. Tugging on soft tissue incarcerated in the orbital floor with strong traction movements may damage delicate orbital structures. In some instances, it may be preferable to enlarge the opening or make an additional opening into the maxillary sinus beyond the fracture with a small chisel or rongeur to assist the recovery of orbital soft tissue with less traction, in effect making the fracture defect larger to allow easy retrieval of soft tissue from the maxillary sinus.

The infraorbital nerve runs in a canal in the anterior third of the orbit and in a groove in the posterior two thirds of the orbit. It enters the inferior orbital fissure at its midpoint. Therefore, it is frequently involved in fractures as it forms a weak point in the floor where fractures preferentially occur. The location of the infraorbital nerve should be respected in orbital floor dissection. There is a small communicating branch from the infraorbital artery to the inferior rectus muscle about 20 mm back in the orbit, which often has to be divided to achieve posterior orbit dissection. Loupe magnification aids visualization. In the posterior half of the orbit, the inferior rectus muscle travels close to the orbital floor, and it can easily be injured in dissection. One must be careful always to dissect subperiosteally and not penetrate the orbital contents to avoid blunt injury to orbital muscles and fat. Blunt, rough dissection and strong retraction easily damage muscle or nervous tissue and fascial connections within the orbit and may produce postoperative double vision. The author prefers to place a small retractor over the lid; an assistant gently holds the lower lid inferiorly *without any* traction. Orbital retractors should merely be lightly positioned, and if the incisions and dissection are sufficient, one can see perfectly. A Freer periosteal elevator is held in one hand and a small suction tube (7 or 8 French) in the other. This maneuver allows the operator to visualize the area of dissection with a headlight; light retraction on the lid with a right-angled and a malleable retractor placed between the orbital contents and the dissection area is a good technique. Therefore, two persons, a surgeon and an assistant, are required for orbital explorative surgery. A headlight and loupe magnification are essential. Various sizes of malleable retractors should be used to provide retraction of the orbital soft tissue contents, putting no pressure on the ocular globe. These retractors can be gently placed and readjusted in the proper location and held in location with light finger pressure by an assistant. Exposure of the lower medial, lateral, and floor portions of the orbit is provided by a properly performed eyelid incision. Some individuals suture a segment of a split Penrose drain over the lid margin to avoid retractor or cautery burns and drill injuries. It is easy to traumatize the lid margins with cautery or rotating instruments or to damage or tear the lid with strong retraction. The lower lid may occasionally tear adjacent to the lacrimal punctum from excessive traction, especially when a short conjunctival incision is used for a large fracture.

When the inferior orbital rim is fractured (impure blowout fracture), the fragments of the rim are realigned and temporary positioning is maintained by the placement of interosseous wires. After the interosseous wires have been linked, a small plate, such as a 1.3-mm titanium plate, can be placed across the fractured segments. Comminuted orbital rim fragments frequently must be supported in position anteriorly and superiorly because the fracture fragments tend to sag inferiorly and posteriorly. This positioning maneuver is necessary to restore cheek prominence and to prevent any vertical shortening of the rim attachment for the lower eyelid. If the rim is positioned too inferiorly, the orbital septum is of fixed length, and the lid will be positioned inferiorly because it will adhere to the rim. The tendency for a comminuted fracture of the orbital rim to be fixed in an inferior and posteriorly displaced position should be scrupulously avoided by meticulous attention to the reduction maneuver.

The inferior rectus muscle, the orbital fat, and any orbital soft tissue structures should be carefully dissected free from the areas of the blowout fracture. Any intact pieces of orbital floor that had been dislocated into the maxillary sinus should be removed, as otherwise they will become sequestered and cause cellulitis. The maxillary sinus should be irrigated, and confirmation of patency into the nose should be confirmed by observation of the irrigating fluid in the ipsilateral nostril. Intact orbital floor must be located around all the edges of the displaced blowout fracture. The floor must be explored sufficiently far back into the orbit that the posterior edge of the intact orbital floor beyond the defect can be identified. Many individuals call this the *ledge*. In major blowout fractures, a small ledge is located near the back of the maxillary sinus 35 to 38 mm behind the orbital rim. Identification of the intact ledge may be verified on CT scan (best shown in a longitudinal projection in the plane of the optic nerve). The ocular globe and its surrounding structures are freed from the fracture site. Proper rotation of the ocular globe after freeing of this orbital soft tissue may be confirmed by an intraoperative forced duction test.

RESTORATION OF CONTINUITY OF THE ORBITAL FLOOR. Restoration of the continuity of the orbital floor is required in all orbital floor fractures, except in small fractures in which the entrapped structures may be freed readily and the forced duction test shows that the free rotation of the eyeball has been re-established and there is no tendency to herniation of soft tissue into the fracture defect. In practice, the author reconstructs any orbital floor fracture that demonstrates a bone defect or a malpositioned, comminuted, or weakened orbital floor. The practice of putting Gelfilm, a thin, malleable membrane, or other extremely malleable, weak material as the sole support for an orbital floor reconstruction is inadequate. Gelfilm works only to prevent adhesions and does not provide support for positioning for the soft tissue of the orbit. MEDPOR barrier implant 0.8 mm may be used for small orbital defects, but 1.5 mm MEDPOR barrier implant must be used for larger defects.

BONE GRAFTS. Split calvarial, iliac, or split rib bone grafts provide the next ideal physiologic substitute material for reconstruction of the internal orbital fractures (see Fig. 66-75).[128,129] The smooth surface may be placed toward the muscles and the grafts thinned so that they may be appropriately contoured. It is sometimes difficult, in extensive orbital floor fractures, to contour iliac or calvarial bone grafts as easily as a split

rib can be molded to conform to the curvature of the orbit, especially in the posterior orbit. Calvarial bone grafts are firm and often crack when they are bent into the curves required by orbital reconstruction. The technique of taking a thinner, partial-thickness anterior table calvarial graft, with the periosteum attached (rather than a full thickness of the anterior table), provides small "shaved" grafts that are malleable and useful for thinner orbital reconstructions. One is impressed with the ease of the dissection and the lack of significant adhesions in secondarily dissecting an orbit that has been reconstructed with bone. Titanium and MEDPOR generate dense adhesions, and many think that these have adverse effects on the contracture of orbital septum and adhesion of the extraocular muscles to the graft.

It is not necessary to have the sinus lining present; there is often a wide area of communication between the orbit and maxillary sinus. Rather, the bone graft becomes a scaffold for the reconstitution of a new sinus lining. Increased bone graft resorption must be expected in this situation, but infections are not common. As the bone graft becomes vascularized, it is better able to resist bacterial invasion. It is not known whether bone grafts resist bacterial colonization better than inorganic implants do, but that is the presumption. The author prefers bone graft reconstruction in all major fractures in which the orbital walls are significantly disrupted for acute treatment. Bone grafts may be tailored to fit the precise contour of the orbital floor accurately and may be bent with a Tessier bone bending forceps (Fig. 66-180). Bone grafts should be anchored with either a screw or a plate to stable orbital floor or to the orbital rim. This provides positional stability.

Other bone or cartilage graft donor sites have been described for the orbit, such as the cortex of the mandible, anterior wall of the maxillary sinus, perpendicular plate of the ethmoid, septal or ear cartilage, or costal cartilage. These provide lesser quantities of material and are thinner, difficult to shape, and suitable only for smaller defects. In addition, some cartilage is too thin, small, or brittle to be of much use. Costal cartilage has been employed and constitutes a satisfactory but seldom-used transplant material because it is more difficult to carve and shape, it may warp, and its width is limited. Dingman and Grabb[529] described the use of irradiated cartilage allografts, and some authors have used irradiated or banked bone for orbital reconstruction, but given the availability of adequate bone donor sites in most patients, there seems to be little justification for not using autogenous bone because of its improved vascularity. Bone grafts are presumed to survive at the 50% to 80% level. The author has witnessed the entire disappearance of some calvarial bone grafts in the orbit in the absence of infection during a 1-year period postoperatively.

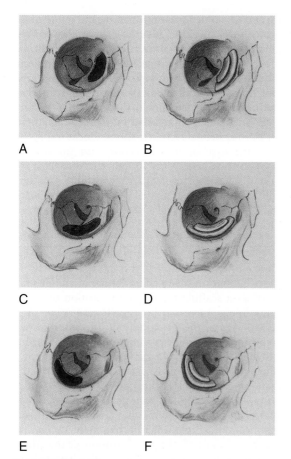

A   B

C   D

E   F

FIGURE 66-180. *A,* A medial blowout fracture involving about half of the medial orbital wall. *B,* The blowout fracture has been treated by bone grafts. *C,* Fracture involving the floor of the orbit. *D,* The fracture has been treated by several bone grafts placed over the defect. *E,* Fracture of the lateral portion of the orbit (the thin portion of the greater wing of the sphenoid and the inferior orbital fissure area). This is a fracture that often occurs in the "multiply fractured" comminuted orbit. *F,* The fracture has been treated by two bone grafts. (From Manson PN, French JA: Fractures of the midface. In Georgiade NG, Riefkohl R, Georgiade GS, Barwick WI, eds: Essentials of Plastic, Maxillofacial and Reconstructive Surgery. Baltimore, Williams & Wilkins, 1987.)

ALLOPLASTIC IMPLANTS. Alloplastic implants offer the advantage of obtaining the material necessary for the reconstruction of the orbital floor without the need for a second operation for bone graft harvest. Inorganic implants are certainly satisfactory for defects of a limited size and orbital fractures, and some authors use titanium mesh alone for large defects where stabilization of a bone graft becomes impractical. One may even obtain successful results in large defects where wide areas of communication with the maxillary and ethmoid sinuses occur. In some patients, limited bone regeneration has also been observed adjacent to the implant as well as the expected regeneration of the

sinus lining. In other patients, absence of complete sinus lining regeneration leads to episodes of recurrent cellulitis. Endoscopy of the sinus in these patients demonstrates exposed mesh or implants, which then require removal and late secondary orbital bone grafting for new structural support of the orbit.

Alloplastic implant materials employed in the orbital region have included Silastic materials, solid sponges, tantalum, stainless steel, Vitallium, titanium, polymethyl methacrylate, polyvinyl sponge, polyurethane, polyethylene, Teflon, hydroxyapatite, Gelfoam, Gelfilm, and Supramid. The author's preference is for an inorganic smooth implant material, such as polyethylene, with a smooth surface on one side (MEDPOR barrier implant or Supramid) to be placed adjacent to the orbital soft tissues (extraocular muscles). The opposite textured surface of the MEDPOR barrier implant is thought to be penetrated to 200 μm by vascularized host tissue and thus aids in resisting infection.

The author's experience with artificial materials confirms that most patients with reconstruction of limited fractures do very well. In particular, porous MEDPOR receives some soft tissue ingrowth into the pores, and almost no patients require removal. The incidence of late infection is certainly less than 1%, and displacement should not occur if the material has been properly anchored. MEDPOR is available in several thicknesses (0.4, 0.8, 1.5 mm) and an 8-mm block. Implants with special anchoring fixators are also available.* The 0.8-mm material does not have enough strength to support the periorbita in a larger defect (more than one buttressed section), and the 1.5-mm material is required. This material may be curved with finger pressure or a Tessier bone bending forceps to conform the material to fit a particular curve of the orbital defect. Light heating will increase pliability. Materials such as MEDPOR, polyethylene, and Silastic also come in blocks that can be carved to fit a specific defect or shape. The use of thin sheets of MEDPOR (<0.8 mm) does not usually provide enough soft tissue support for a fracture larger than 2.5 cm. MEDPOR barrier is preferred to place a smooth surface (non-adherent) next to the musculature.

The purpose of the orbital floor replacement, whether a bone graft or an inorganic implant, is to re-establish the size and the shape of the orbital cavity. Less importantly, it begins to seal off the orbit from the maxillary sinus. This replaces the orbital soft tissue contents and allows scar tissue to form in an anatomic position. The author prefers to place the smooth side of bone graft materials or implants (such as the smooth side of a MEDPOR barrier implant) toward the orbital contents to decrease potential muscle adherence. Titanium implants will soon be available with small poly-

---

*Porex, Fairburn, Georgia.

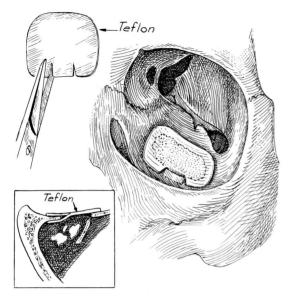

FIGURE 66-181. Technique to prevent forward displacement of a plastic implant. A tongue of implant material may be slipped under the anterior border of the bone defect, blocking the forward migration of the implant. It is the author's preference to use small screws to anchor implants.

ethylene coating for the same purpose, to resist adhesions. Any material used for floor reconstruction should preferably be anchored or otherwise fixed so that displacement is unlikely, and screw fixation is preferred (Fig. 66-181). Otherwise, migration or extrusion of the material may occur, as the material may press on the skin of the eyelid and slowly erode the eyelid.

The orbital implant must conform to the proper contour of the floor and not provide a place where the dead space causes fluid accumulation. Some implants are perforated so that they cannot retain fluid. At the time of implant placement, the maxillary sinus should be irrigated to make sure that sinus drainage freely occurs into the nose. If free communication with the nose cannot be demonstrated, a nasal-antral window or endoscopic opening into the maxillary sinus should be undertaken through the ostium. Any blood or devitalized bone fragments that have dropped into the sinus should be removed. The sinus may be temporarily drained through a Caldwell-Luc incision with a Penrose drain, but one does not want to establish this site as a chronic fistula. Infection (cellulitis of the orbit and cheek) usually accompanies improper surgical cleaning of the maxillary sinus, blocked drainage of the sinus into the nose, or dead pieces of orbital floor bone that have fallen into the sinus and become sequestered. A blocked maxillary sinus ostium will cause the sinus to drain through the Caldwell-Luc opening as an oral-antral fistula.

Oral-antral fistula must be closed (*after* establishment of proper antral drainage into the nose) with a two-layer closure (marginally based flaps and covering rotation flap). A bone graft may be interfaced between the two flaps. Alternatively, the oral-antral fistula may have the opening obturated with the buccal fat pad[364,371] mobilized to enter the opening and sutured to occlude the fistula. The buccal fat pad is then covered with a local rotation flap of intraoral mucosa.

The failure to reconstruct the proper size and shape of the bony orbital cavity is the most frequent cause of enophthalmos. The medial orbital wall and the floor must be reconstructed in their proper shape and location. Small fragments of bone may be present, all connected, but displaced with different contour and unstable against the forces of orbital contracture. They frequently hang "hammock-like" into the sinus, effectively enlarging the orbit. Pressing on these with an elevator convinces the surgeon that their attachments are too weak to provide structural support to the soft tissue contents of the orbit, and they should therefore be replaced with a stronger bone graft that is inserted over the existing comminuted fragments and perched on the ledges of intact bone that surround the orbital defect. The orbital floor graft must angle upward from anterior to posterior and upward toward the medial wall.

Orbital reconstruction for two or more adjacent missing walls is most easily accomplished with material that can reconstruct, in a stable fashion, the buttress supports of the orbit; metal meshes, bone graft stabilized by plates, or specialized plates designed for the orbit make this difficult task straightforward (Figs. 66-182 to 66-185). The orbital floor plate has multiple arms, most of which must be trimmed, as only one or two will be necessary for secure placement. The floor plate (see Fig. 66-182) is "universal," meaning it can be used for right or left. It is also too long and too wide for the usual defect. These plates require significant trimming because they are meant for either orbit or for any reconstructive problem (see Fig. 66-185). The orbital plate must first be contoured to the orbital shape, then unnecessary wings must be trimmed.

Larry Sargent (Chattanooga, Tennessee) has designed an orbital mesh (see Fig. 66-184) that is easily contoured to the orbit and "off the shelf."[418] It is a flat sheet, literally an "unfolded" orbital shape. This plate may easily be cut to the desired size, bent to contour shape, and attached within the orbit. Porex has designed MEDPOR implants stabilized by a titanium plate inserted within the plastic implant for conforming stability.

LINEAR ORBITAL FLOOR FRACTURES

The signs and symptoms of a linear fracture of the orbital floor (without blowout) are similar to those

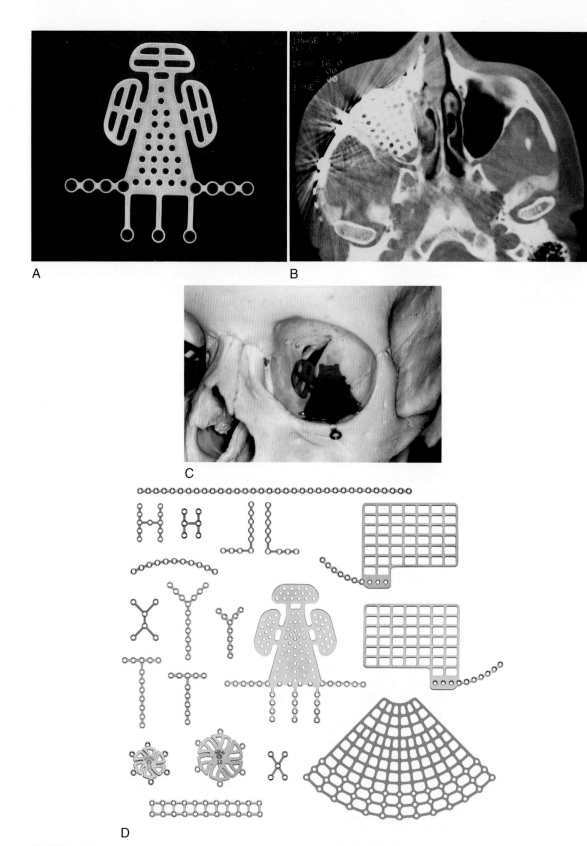

FIGURE 66-182. *A,* Orbital floor plate designed by Manson. *B,* Radiograph of orbital floor reconstruction. *C,* Plate trimmed for a specific floor defect. *D,* Materials for orbital and cranial reconstruction (fine plates, mesh burr hole covers). (*A* and *C* courtesy of Synthes Maxillofacial, Paoli, Pa.) Note: No royalties are received by the author for any products.

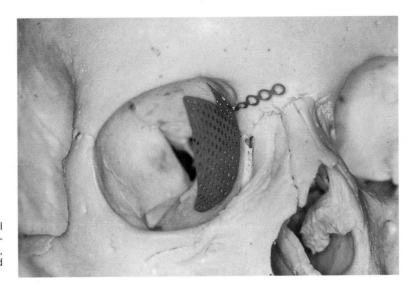

FIGURE 66-183. Medial orbital plate designed by Manson. (Courtesy of Synthes Maxillofacial, Paoli, Pa.) Note: No royalties are received by the author for any products.

of a blowout fracture. There is usually less concern about enophthalmos in these fractures unless an accompanying dislocation of the zygoma is present, which depresses a large segment of the floor. It has been demonstrated that simple contusion of orbital soft tissue and hematoma without fracture can produce the same symptoms as an orbital blowout fracture,[530] that is, double vision and impaired oculorotatory movements; these "nonfractures" frequently have numbness in the infraorbital nerve distribution and a disturbance of oculorotatory movements. These fractures do not need surgical exploration and may easily be differentiated on CT scan from fractures with incarcerated soft tissue. It is therefore imperative that accurate CT scans with both axial and coronal sections with bone and soft tissue windows demonstrate the exact nature of the fracture and the soft tissue involvement in the fracture site. In contusions without

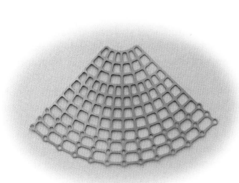

A

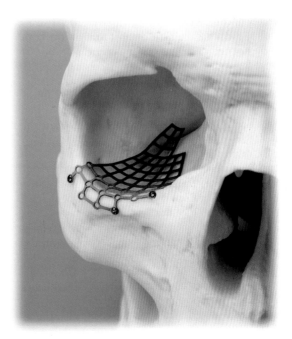

B

FIGURE 66-184. *A,* Orbital mesh "fan" plate designed by Larry Sargent. *B,* Orbital bone plate in orbit for reconstruction. (Courtesy of Synthes Maxillofacial, Paoli, Pa.) Note: No royalties are received by the designer for any products.

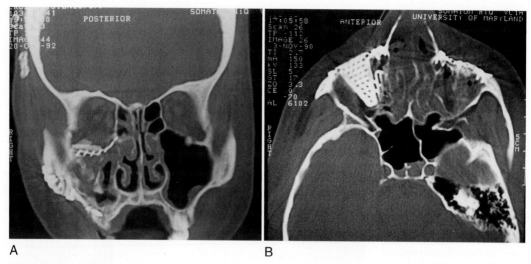

FIGURE 66-185. *A,* Inferior orbital bone graft stabilized by a plate. *B,* Trimmed orbital floor plate in orbit. Plate is "universal" (for right or left orbit) but must be trimmed before insertion to correspond to a size only just larger than the defect.

fracture, findings on the forced duction test should be normal in early stages unless the muscle has a hematoma, which tightens the muscle. If there is hematoma, edema, or fibrosis in extraocular muscles, the forced duction test findings may be abnormal. The CT scan will differentiate patients who do not have soft tissue entrapment or muscle entrapment. Frequently, transient diplopia accompanies hematoma, edema, and muscle contusion; usually, the diplopia partially or completely resolves with time. If CT scans do not show a characteristic discontinuity of the floor and do not demonstrate prolapse or incarceration of orbital soft tissue, no operation is necessary. Approximately one third of zygomatic fractures are undisplaced or minimally displaced, resulting in a linear fracture (anterior-posterior fracture) of the orbital floor. Careful examination is required to estimate the benefit that might be provided by surgery for the minimally displaced zygoma or orbital floor fracture. Linear fractures of the orbital floor occurring in zygomatic or maxillary fractures frequently do not require an orbital exploration. In these large-segment fractures, repositioning of the zygoma often repositions the floor of the orbit, and no formal orbital exploration is required. When one is uncertain about the integrity of the orbital floor, an exploration or an endoscopic examination of the floor through the maxillary sinus may be performed. If a defect larger than 2 cm is seen, exploration and replacement or endoscopic repair is indicated. In fractures in which the bone is displaced, the risk of enlargement of the orbital cavity and enophthalmos should be an important consideration governing treatment.

The treatment of an orbital fracture must be performed in conjunction with the reduction and fixation of fractures of the orbital rim and other bones of the midfacial area. The only technique that can adequately restore the continuity of displaced or fragmented bones is based on the full exploration of the usual sites of fracture, including the medial, inferior, and lateral orbit. Anatomic alignment of the bony skeleton, which includes the internal orbit, must reconstitute the bone defects. This is best done by direct exposure of the fractured area and bone graft reconstruction of the missing portions of the orbit in conjunction with reduction of the rim fractures. It is easy to underestimate the extent of an orbital fracture if only axial CT scans are obtained with soft tissue windows alone.

COMMINUTED FRACTURES

In patients with exceptionally severe crush injuries, such as high-speed automobile accidents, the orbital injury is uniformly associated with other fractures of the frontal and midfacial skeleton and the nasoethmoid area. In these situations, the orbital rim and the internal walls of the orbit may be completely comminuted. Thin fragments of bone in small pieces, whether they are attached to fragments of periosteum or not, may not be useful for the reconstruction. The orbital contents will sink into the maxillary and ethmoid sinuses, producing a severe enophthalmos. The soft tissue, which normally has a pyramid- or cone-shaped configuration, remodels into a spherical shape with a loss of supporting bone in the medial, inferior, and lateral orbit. For the soft tissue to undergo remodeling, the ligaments holding the orbital soft tissue structures in approximation and the fine ligaments connecting the extraocular muscles with the periosteum and extending through the intramuscular cone fat are disrupted by the force of the injury. Ligament disruption allows the soft tissue to remodel to whatever shape the underlying bone fragments provide in terms of shape and volume. After remodeling has occurred, the soft tissue scarring is "fixed" and opposes late anatomic soft tissue repositioning despite late bone reconstruction in the proper location. It is thus emphasized that early treatment of significant orbital fractures obtains superior aesthetic results because soft tissue scarring is initially absent at the time of treatment, then occurs in an anatomic position dictated by the bone graft reconstruction.

Small fragments of bone displaced into the sinuses may be removed or, if they are attached to lining, left in position and a new bone graft placed above them. Some are useful for replacement, particularly for endoscopic reconstruction. Completely loose fragments in the bottom of the maxillary sinus must be removed because they provide a nidus for infection.

The bone fragments of the orbital rims must always be salvaged and retrieved to reconstruct the orbital rims. The lateral wall of the orbit must be stabilized by interosseous fixation of the rim before the internal orbital walls can be bone grafted. Some surgeons use the lateral orbital wall as a point of fixation. The orbital floor may or may not be intact laterally adjacent to the edges of the inferior orbital fissure. The orbital floor is usually intact posteriorly 35 to 38 mm posterior to the orbital rim. This ledge forms a guide for reconstruction of the orbital floor and may be located by "walking" a Freer elevator up the back wall of the maxillary sinus, then running the Freer elevator upward until the posterior wall meets the floor; here, one feels the intact "lip" of bone or the intact ledge of the orbital floor. The orbital fat may be gently lifted off the ledge, and the ledge is thereby exposed. The inferior rectus muscle itself is often prolapsed over the ledge, and careful, precise dissection is required with no force exerted on the retractor. Medially, the normal orbital floor curves upward at approximately a 45-degree angle to meet the medial orbital wall. Because a bone graft placed in this area may be displaced in the absence of structurally sound fixation, the author has used metal mesh for severe two-wall medial and floor orbital fractures. Otherwise, in two-wall orbital fractures with loss of the inferomedial buttress, one must think of a way to re-establish the inferomedial orbital strut, such as a plate attached to a bone graft or a bone graft angled and stabilized,[531] to reconstruct this area. The same considerations apply to loss of the thicker bone or inferolateral strut, which composes the edges of the inferior orbital fissure.

MEDIAL ORBITAL WALL FRACTURES

Medial orbital wall fractures occur in conjunction with orbital floor fractures and nasoethmoidal-orbital frac-tures and as an isolated orbital fracture. Medial orbital wall fractures have a substantial propensity for producing enophthalmos but only a very small chance of tethering the medial rectus muscle. Frequently, one can see a medial wall fracture with medial rectus swelling, or one sees a medial wall fracture with diffuse symmetric enlargement of the medial orbital wall (see Fig. 66-160). There is usually no incarceration, but swelling of the muscle indicates contusion. Most double vision in medial orbital wall fractures is in fact due to medial rectus contusion and not to medial rectus, musculofibrous ligament system, or fat incarceration. Medial orbital wall fractures accompany nasoethmoid fractures as a routine component of the fracture. Rarely (<1%), the medial rectus may actually be entrapped in the fracture. Actual inferior rectus entrapment is seen in about 10% of orbital floor fractures. The clinical signs associated with medial orbital wall blowout fractures include progressively increasing enophthalmos, narrowing of the palpebral fissure, subcutaneous emphysema, horizontal diplopia with restriction of adduction or abduction, intraorbital emphysema, and medial position of the globe. Subcutaneous and intraorbital emphysema is a common sign of a medial wall fracture and is not usually present in isolated orbital floor fractures. Blood usually drips from the nose through the ipsilateral nostril.

It has been demonstrated that medial orbital wall fractures are associated with orbital floor fractures in an incidence varying from 5% to 70%. This relationship is explained by the structural relationships between the orbital floor and the medial orbital wall described earlier in this chapter. In the author's experience as well as that of Prasad,[532] true entrapment of the medial rectus muscle is rare. All medial wall fractures frequently demonstrate a moderate amount of orbital emphysema. The need for open reduction and volume correction of the orbit, which is restored by bone grafting, is determined by the amount of orbital enlargement. The cellular structure of the ethmoid bone offers some resistance to compression beyond the strength provided by the thickness of the bone because of the vertical struts that reinforce the medial orbital wall. Such structural reinforcement is not found in the maxillary sinus beneath the orbital floor. Floor fractures may stop at the inferomedial strut of the orbit (see Fig. 66-161) or extend up higher in the medial orbital wall. More extensive fractures extend posteriorly back to the posterior ethmoid foramen (the foramen for the posterior ethmoidal vessels), which is the ledge that one has to dissect to medially to reach normal bone beyond the fracture. This medial ledge area is directly in line with the optic nerve and directly in front of it. The optic nerve and the optic canal are about 5 mm behind the posterior ethmoid foramen. Although the ledge may be anywhere in the medial orbital wall, frequently, the posterior ethmoid is the ledge for the fracture.

The diagnosis of medial wall fractures is confirmed after an axial and coronal CT scan with bone and soft tissue windows is obtained. Air within the orbit (orbital emphysema) is suggestive of a medial orbital wall fracture. Often, one sees clouding of the ethmoid and perhaps the sphenoid sinuses. Both axial and coronal views and soft tissue and bone windows are necessary.

Treatment of medial orbital wall fractures depends on the anatomic location of the displaced wall and the geographic extent of the fracture. A substantial increase in orbital volume may occur, especially with loss of the inferomedial orbital buttress. Displacement of the medial orbital wall is one of the most effective ways to increase orbital volume. The lower half of the medial orbital wall can be exposed from a floor approach, but the upper half requires a local approach (horizontal limb alone of the open-sky incision), an appropriate laceration, or a coronal, medial upper lid, or extended conjunctival incision (medially around the caruncle). The coronal incision, although a dramatic approach for this fracture, provides the best visualization for the reduction. In treating medial orbital wall fractures, one simply augments the medial wall volume with bone or artificial material, adding layers on top of the displaced bone until the proper orbital volume reduction has been obtained. In circumstances when the inferomedial strut is lost, this first must be replaced from a floor approach. The medial wing of an orbital floor plate is meant to provide a strut for medial wall reconstruction. A medial wall plate may be used (see Fig. 66-183), but it has no strut for inferior support. It is solely supported by its upper fixation. The bone or artificial material is then placed between the displaced medial orbital wall and the periorbita and is supported by an inferomedial strut (Fig. 66-186). Therefore, the concept is that the inferior wall of the orbit (the floor) must be stable and rigid enough

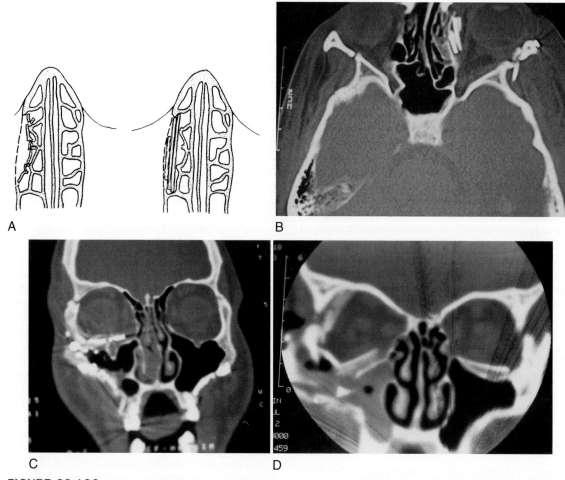

FIGURE 66-186. *A*, Bone grafting of a medial orbital defect. *B*, Radiograph of grafted medial orbit. *C*, MEDPOR in a medial orbital fracture stabilized with a plate. *D*, Right orbit bone graft reconstruction and left orbit plate reconstruction.

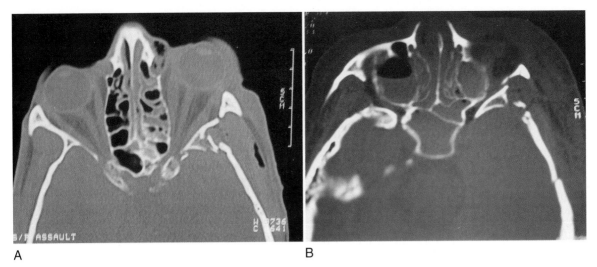

A   B

FIGURE 66-187. *A,* A sphenotemporal buttress fracture occurring with a fracture of the lateral orbital wall. Visual acuity may be compromised. The fracture extends into the optic canal. *B,* A sphenotemporal buttress fracture showing compression of inferior and superior orbital fissures.

to support the medial orbital reconstruction. The contour of the medial orbital wall, which has a slight bulge inward behind the globe, must be respected and reconstructed by a properly shaped bone.

LATERAL ORBITAL WALL FRACTURES

The lateral orbital wall consists of the strong, resistant anterior frontozygomatic rim, which is frequently exposed to trauma. The wall becomes thinner behind the rim and consists of the thin, orbital portion of the zygoma that joins the greater wing of the sphenoid at its orbital process. Severe fractures of the lateral wall of the orbit occur in conjunction with high-energy trauma to the zygomatic area (Fig. 66-187) and the zygomaticofrontal junction, with downward displacement of the zygoma and portions of the orbital floor. In severe fractures, the greater wing of the sphenoid and the orbital process of the zygoma are both comminuted, permitting a large volume increase in this area. In simpler fractures, there is a linear fracture between the orbital process of the zygoma and the greater wing of the sphenoid that extends through the inferior orbital fissure to communicate with the orbital floor fractures. In significant zygoma fractures, the canthus and lid are displaced and dislocated, because they are both attached to the downwardly displaced zygoma by virtue of the lateral canthus and the orbital septum at the Whitnall tubercle 10 mm below the zygomaticofrontal sutures. In rare instances, there may be an isolated fracture of the lateral orbital wall (Fig. 66-188).

Complex fractures require direct approaches to expose all fracture sites, similar to those employed in the multiply fractured midfacial skeleton. Direct interosseous fixation of the fragments and primary bone grafting to restore the integrity of the thin walls of the orbit (including the floor, the medial and lateral orbital wall, and the inferior orbital fissure areas) are required. The sequence generally involves interfragment wiring of the zygomaticofrontal suture, the inferior orbital rim fragments, and possibly the zygomatic arch. One may then begin to stabilize zygomatic position with rigid fixation. If the arch is severely fractured, a strong plate, such as the Zydaption plate, should be used. In severe fractures, the ocular globe may suffer varying degrees of injury from simple contusion to

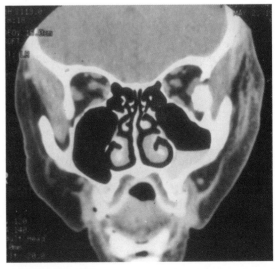

FIGURE 66-188. Rare isolated fracture of the lateral orbital wall.

globe rupture with loss of vision. It is imperative that a thorough visual examination to detect visual loss, retinal detachment, and hyphema be concluded *before* operative intervention is undertaken.

LATERAL ORBITAL WALL AND FLOOR FRACTURES

Fractures of the lateral orbital wall and floor routinely accompany every zygoma fracture except for isolated zygomatic arch fractures (see Fig. 66-161). When the fracture is simple, reduction of the major buttresses of the zygoma reduces the fracture as the displacement is corrected by open reduction of the rim. In more severe fractures, in which the greater wing of the sphenoid and orbital process of the zygoma are also comminuted, bone grafts must be placed for stability. Conceptually and practically, proper alignment of the zygomatic arch (medial to lateral arch position) in comminuted fractures should result in alignment in the lateral wall of the orbit.[5,115,356,418] The relationship (when arch length is restored) between the greater wing of the sphenoid and the orbital process of the zygoma should be a straight line. Soft tissue herniation through a gap in the lateral wall of the orbit results in loss of soft tissue contents into the temporal fossa.

Some authors have described a direct approach to these fractures, taking the temporalis muscle out of its temporal location,[533] plating that area of the zygomaticosphenoid junction through the coronal incision, and replacing the temporal muscle. A second solution, application of a plate while the globe is displaced medially, works within the orbit.[186,362] When the temporalis muscle is to be taken out of its fossa and retracted, closure is facilitated by making an anterior to posterior (horizontal) incision directly in the muscle 1 cm inferior to the temporal crest in the periphery of the temporalis. A cuff of muscle and fascial tissue is left at the superior periphery of the muscle so that replacement of the muscle to its normal location can easily be performed with sutures. Otherwise, the muscle must be reattached to screws placed in the anterior table of the skull. The muscle is stabilized by suturing it to these fixation struts. A blowout or "blow in" fracture of the lateral wall occasionally occurs in the absence of a rim fracture. Treatment depends on displacement and symptoms; the same determinants apply to consideration for operation as apply to the orbital floor fractures. Operations are then determined by the potential for enophthalmos or the possible interference of the fractures with extraocular motion. Volume consideration relates to 2 cm^2 and 3 to 5 mm of displacement.

ORBITAL ROOF FRACTURES

Lagrange,[457] in his classic monograph, showed that the thin medial portion of the orbital roof may be fractured and displaced in its posterior portion in the region of the superior orbital fissure and optic foramen. Isolated roof fractures may be accompanied by serious ocular complications, such as optic nerve contusion and visual injury loss or damage to nerves that travel through the superior orbital fissure. Dodick,[534] in a series of 22 patients with blowout fractures, obtained radiologic evidence of fractures of the orbital roof in two patients. Fractures of the orbital roof may occur as isolated fractures and also by the mechanism of blunt force delivered to the midfrontal bone, with reciprocal displacement and fracture occurring in an area remote from the force application in a weak area (such as the orbital roof).[535,536] The medial portion of the orbital roof is thinner than the lateral portion and thus more susceptible to fracture. Fractures of the orbital roof also occur in conjunction with frontal bone and nasoethmoidal fractures.[537] If the superior rim of the orbit is fractured, the trochlea of the superior oblique muscle is concomitantly damaged. Some double vision in the field of action of the superior oblique may occur.[538] Almost always, double vision from this mechanism is temporary unless the muscles have been inadvertently injured by surgical dissection. Pulsating exophthalmos may occur.[438]

Fractures of the orbital roof may involve only its thin portion; therefore, displacement is usually limited. Displacement may be superior or inferior.[536-539] These fractures may also involve the superior orbital rim.[540-543] In the presence of medial rim fractures, roof fractures occur either medially in the region of the frontal sinus or laterally in the supraorbital area. Lateral orbital rim fractures may be small, involving only the rim, or large, usually occurring in conjunction with more extensive fractures of the frontal bone and temporal area and producing the so-called lateral frontal-temporal-orbital fracture. The craniofacial or coronal approach is required in these patients for proper neurosurgical exposure, repair of dural lacerations, and débridement of any damaged frontal or temporal lobe of the brain. The dura is frequently torn or penetrated by comminuted bone fragments where displacement exceeds 3 to 5 mm. Bone fragments may be removed, cleaned, and placed on a back table in antiseptic-soaked medium until the brain exposure and repair are complete. After the anterior cranial fossa and frontal region are exposed and the brain and dural repairs completed, the orbital roof defect should be repaired by a thin bone graft placed *external* (within the cranial cavity and not the orbit) to the intact rim of bone in the orbital roof. Bone grafts placed within the orbit (under the edges of the intact roof) take up additional orbital space necessary for the globe and may produce a downward and forward position of the globe. The displacement of the supraorbital rim and orbital roof is generally downward and posterior, producing an anterior and inferior displacement of the globe and orbital soft tissue (Fig. 66-189). Ptosis of the eyelid is present, depending on the degree of displacement, and the contusion of the extraocular muscles first includes the levator. If structures in the superior orbital fissure are damaged, there may be paralysis of cranial nerves III, IV, and VI, and anesthesia may be present in the supraorbital branches of the ophthalmic division of the trigeminal nerve (cranial nerve V). When the fractures involve cranial nerves III, IV, and VI and the ophthalmic division of the trigeminal nerve (cranial nerve V), a superior orbital fissure syndrome is present.[325,544,545] If the nerve injury also involves the optic nerve as well as the superior orbital fissure structures, an orbital apex syndrome is present, which implies involvement of both posterior orbital foramina by fracture. Orbital roof fractures are best reduced intracranially with a bone graft placed external to the orbital cavity and secured to the frontal bar with plate and screw fixation (Fig. 66-190).

Nasoethmoidal-Orbital Fractures

The central feature characterizing nasoethmoidal-orbital fractures is the displacement of the section of the medial orbital rim carrying the attachment of the medial canthal ligament (Fig. 66-191). Fractures that separate the frontal process of the maxilla and its canthal-bearing tendon allow canthal displacement. Therefore, the simplest fracture that could be called a nasoethmoidal-orbital fracture is isolated to the medial orbital rim. Mobility of this fragment may be

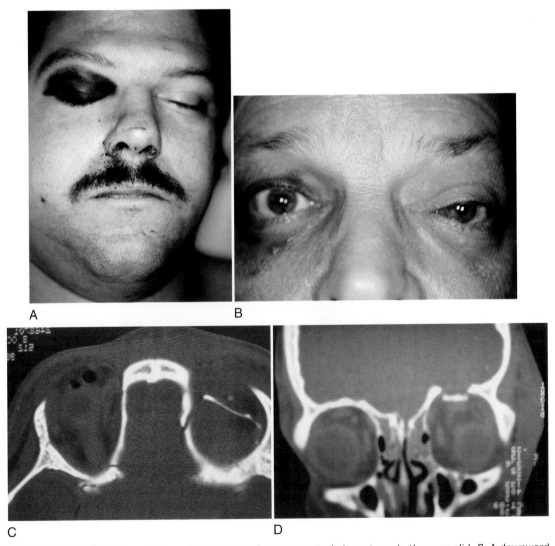

A   B

C   D

FIGURE 66-189. *A,* An orbital roof fracture produces a spectacle hematoma in the upper lid. *B,* A downward and forward position of the globe is caused by an inferiorly displaced orbital roof fracture. *C* and *D,* A pure blow-in fracture of the orbital roof.   *Continued*

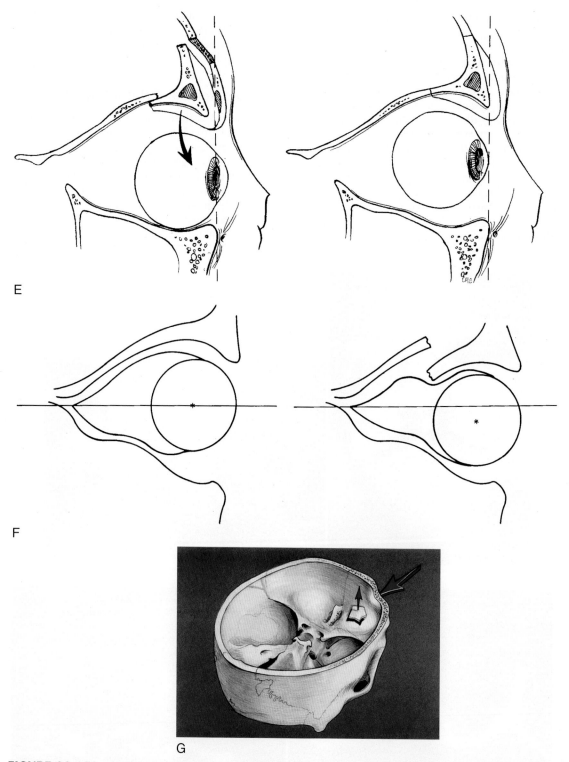

E

F

G

FIGURE 66-189, cont'd. *E,* Artist's diagram of globe displacement produced by an anterior roof fracture *(left)* versus normal placement *(right). F,* Displaced orbital roof fracture *(right)* versus normal *(left). G,* Mechanism of orbital roof fracture from frontal bone impact.

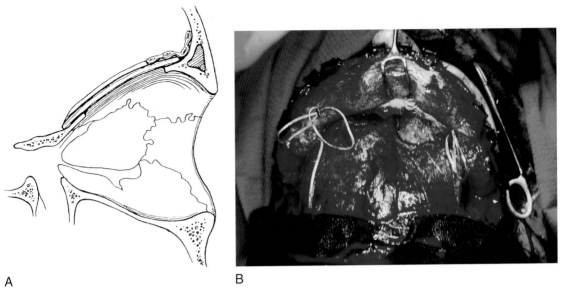

A   B

FIGURE 66-190. *A,* Intracranial bone graft reconstruction of the orbital roof. *B,* Stabilization of an intracranial bone reconstruction of the orbital roof by plate fixation to the frontal bar. The roof bone graft must be external to the orbit so that it does not constrict orbital volume.

assessed by direct digital palpation over the canthal ligament.

The central midfacial skeleton is the nasoethmoidal-orbital area. It may be fractured as an isolated medial orbital rim section (Fig. 66-192) by a direct blow, or fractures in the nasoethmoidal-orbital area may be associated with fractures of the maxilla, nasal bones, zygomas, and orbits. The bones of the middle third of the face are in a close anatomic relationship to the floor of the anterior cranial fossa and

the frontal lobes of the brain through the frontal and ethmoid sinuses and the cribriform plate.[546,547] The certainty of orbital floor and medial orbital wall fractures in nasoethmoidal-orbital injuries has been established.[548-551] The fractures of the medial and inferior orbital rims may be several large pieces, or the medial and inferomedial orbital rim may be comminuted into small fragments. Fractures of the frontal bone and anterior cranial fossa may accompany nasoethmoidal-orbital injuries. Any basal skull frac-

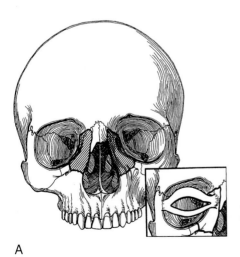

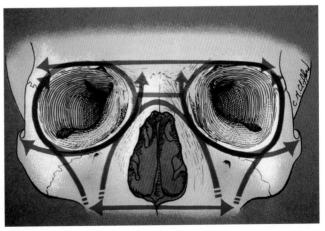

A   B

FIGURE 66-191. *A,* Illustration of the central fragment of the nasoethmoid fracture. *B,* The buttresses of the nasoethmoid area. (From Markowitz B, Manson PN, Sargent L, et al: Management of the medial canthal ligament in nasoethmoid orbital fractures: the importance of the central fragment in diagnosis and treatment. Plast Reconstr Surg 1991;87:843.)

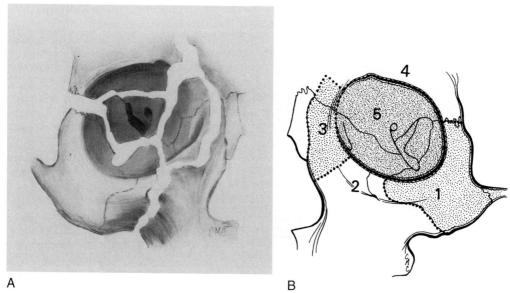

A   B

FIGURE 66-192. *A,* The orbital rim may be divided into thirds for the purpose of classifying fractures of the orbit. The superior portion is the supraorbital section, which contains a portion of the frontal sinus medially. The inferior and lateral portions of the orbit are the zygoma. The nasoethmoidal area is represented by the lower two thirds of the medial orbital rim. *B,* Parts of the rim: 1, zygoma; 2, medial maxilla; 3, medial orbital rim in nasoethmoidal-orbital area; 4, superior orbital rim (supraorbital area); and 5, internal orbit.

ture raises the possibility of pneumocephalus and CSF rhinorrhea from dural fistulas. Depressed skull fractures should signal the need for neurosurgical evaluation and operative treatment.

The signs of frontal lobe brain injury are often less obvious than those from injuries to other areas of the brain, such as the motor cortex. These more subtle signs include confusion, loss of consciousness, and inappropriate behavior. Radiographic signs of frontal lobe injury may be noted on CT scans and include brain contusion, epidural hematoma, pneumocephalus, subdural hematoma, and depressed skull fracture. The association of skull, brain, and facial injuries and cervical fractures has been reported.[58] Head injury may be complicated by other conditions, such as pulmonary edema and a disturbance in coagulation factors. A complete evaluation of these patients is therefore mandatory before any operative treatment is undertaken.

ANATOMY

The nasoethmoidal-orbital area forms the central third of the upper midfacial skeleton (Fig. 66-193).[550,551] The thin areas of the medial orbital walls transilluminate readily and contrast with the heavier abutments formed by the nasal process of the frontal bone, the frontal process of the maxilla, and the thick upper portions of the nasal bones. Posteriorly, the frontal process of the maxilla, the thinner lacrimal bone, and the

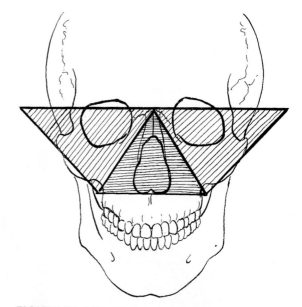

FIGURE 66-193. The bones forming the skeletal frame of the nose are situated in the upper and central portion of the midfacial skeleton. The diagram illustrates the concept by which the middle third of the face is divided into three triangles, essentially a nasal-maxillary triangle and two lateral orbital-zygomatic triangles. These three sections represent the upper half of the midfacial skeleton. The lower half is the Le Fort I level or alveolar processes and teeth of the maxilla.

delicate lamina papyracea are vulnerable to trauma. The anterior and posterior ethmoidal foramina are situated along the upper border of the lamina papyracea and the frontal ethmoidal suture where the orbital plate of the frontal bone and lamina papyracea of the ethmoid are joined. The anterior ethmoidal foramen transmits the nasociliary nerve and the anterior ethmoidal vessels. The posterior ethmoidal foramen gives passage to the posterior ethmoidal nerves and vessels. These vessels frequently rupture in significant nasoethmoidal-orbital fractures. Otherwise, in exposure of the medial orbital wall, the nerves and vessels must be divided, and they serve as landmarks to the depth of dissection. Bone fragments may penetrate the soft tissue of the orbit, and the vessels may be lacerated. Frequently, a symmetric medial compression of the ethmoidal labyrinth of sinuses is produced by fractures, with the ocular globe being driven against the medial orbital wall.[442] The rupture of these vessels in nasoethmoidal-orbital fractures is one of the causes of significant orbital hematoma. Usually, comminution of the bone fragments lacerates the periosteum, and the intraorbital pressure is thereby relieved, preventing a significant retrobulbar hematoma or an orbital compartment syndrome. It is unusual for a retrobulbar hematoma, despite its invariable presence in these injuries, to cause a significant intraorbital pressure increase or to require decompression in itself because the fractures decompress the intraorbital pressure. The most medial posterior portion of the medial orbital wall is formed by the body of the sphenoid, immediately in front of the optic foramen. In severe skeletal disruption of this area, the fracture lines involve the optic foramen and superior orbital fissure. These fractures may produce shearing of nerve fibers or a disturbance of circulation to the optic nerve or a pressure injury to the nerve, which might result in blindness. It is less common for the bones in the posterior third of the orbit to undergo significant displacement, but they are involved by linear fractures, and there is scant excess room for any nerve swelling or hematoma.

The term *interorbital space* designates an area between the orbits and below the floor of the anterior cranial fossa. The interorbital space contains two ethmoidal labyrinths, one on each side. The interorbital space is roughly pear shaped in transverse section, being wider in the middle than in the posterior portion. It is limited above by the cribriform plate in the midline and by the roof of each ethmoidal mass on the sides, and it is divided into two approximately equal halves by the nasal septum. The interorbital space is limited below at the level of the horizontal line through the lower border of the ethmoidal labyrinths. The lateral wall is the medial wall of the orbit. Anteriorly, the interorbital space is limited by the frontal process of the maxilla and by the nasal process and spine of the frontal bone. The nasal process of the frontal bone is also called the internal angular process.

The interorbital space contains many cellular ethmoid sinus bone structures, each lined by mucosa. These include the ethmoidal cells, the superior and middle turbinates, and a median thicker plate of septal bone, the perpendicular plate of the ethmoid, which forms the posterior superior portion of the nasal septal framework.

The size, shape, and septation of the frontal sinus vary greatly. It may occupy most of the frontal bone or only a small portion of the lower central portion. The two sides are usually strikingly asymmetric. Developing in teenage years to reach their full size, the frontal sinuses may be the size of an ethmoid cell or may be quite large, pneumatizing the entire frontal bone and roof of the orbits. The frontal sinus is always larger on one side than on the other. On occasion, one or both frontal sinuses may be absent. The frontal sinus contains highly variable partial and complete septa.

The sinus has the shape of a pyramid with inferior, anterior, and posterior walls. The inferior wall, or floor of the frontal sinus, corresponds to the roof of the orbit and is the thinnest portion of the frontal sinus. The anterior wall is thickest and is composed of compact and some cancellous bone; the amount of cancellous bone is variable. The posterior wall is thinner than the anterior wall and is composed almost entirely of compact bone, which separates the sinus from the frontal lobe. A median partition is usually present, and frequently each side of the sinus is divided by one to several subsinus partitions. The nasofrontal ducts descend from the posterior inferior portion of the sinus through the ethmoidal labyrinth to exit into the nose somewhat posteriorly at the level of the middle turbinate. Frequently, fractures isolated to the nasoethmoidal-orbital area do not block the nasofrontal duct because of its posterior location.

The ethmoid bone occupies the lateral portion of the interorbital space. Below the interorbital space, the lower half of the nasal cavity is flanked by the maxillary sinuses. Each lateral mass of the ethmoid is connected medially to the cribriform plate; the roof of each ethmoidal mass is inclined upward from the cribriform plate and projects in its lateral portion approximately 0.25 cm above it. The level of the cribriform plate is variable and must be individually identified on coronal cut CT scans to guide surgical treatment.

The ethmoid areas are pyramidal or cuboidal and are 3.5 to 5 cm long and 1.5 to 2.5 cm wide. They are cellular in structure and contain 8 to 10 cells with thin lamellar walls. They are usually divided into anterior and posterior sections. These cells drain into the middle meatus of the nose. The frontal sinus drains through the ethmoid either as a distinct nasofrontal duct or by emptying into the anterior ethmoidal cells and thereby into the middle meatus. There is thus an intimate anatomic relationship between the frontal and ethmoid sinuses, both anatomically and in view of the nasofrontal duct. A large ethmoidal cell, the frontoethmoidal, may be seen in the frontal bone between the frontal sinus and the roof of the orbit. This extension of the "supraorbital ethmoidal cells" may be dramatic, pneumatizing the medial orbital roof. Such extended ethmoidal cells are a frequently neglected problem in fractures involving the frontal bone, frontal sinus, and anterior cranial fossa. Proper management of ethmoidal injuries should apply the same treatment to the ethmoidal cells involved in the supraorbital area that is given to fractures of the frontal sinus, which includes ensuring drainage into the nose and débridement (collapse and bone grafting) of nonfunctional "crushed" areas.

SURGICAL PATHOLOGY

The bones that form the skeletal framework of the nose are projected backward between the orbits when they are subjected to strong traumatic forces. The term *naso-orbital* was employed to designate this type of fracture and was suggested by Converse and Smith[547] in 1963. The bones involved are situated in the upper central portion of the middle third of the face anterior to the anatomic crossroads between the cranial, orbital, and nasal cavities (Fig. 66-193). A typical cause of a nasoethmoidal-orbital fracture is a blunt impact applied over the upper portion of the bridge of the nose by projection of the face against a blunt object, such as a steering wheel or dashboard. The occupant of an automobile, for instance, is thrown forward, striking the nasofrontal area. A crushing injury with comminuted fractures is thus produced in the upper central midface. Bursting of the soft tissues, due to the severity of the impact and penetrating lacerations of the soft tissues resulting from projection of objects, may transform the closed fractures into an open, compound, comminuted injury. If the impact force suffered by the strong nose and anterior frontal sinus is sufficient to cause backward displacement of these structures, no further resistance is offered by the delicate "matchbox-like" structures of the interorbital space; indeed, these structures "collapse and splinter like a pile of matchboxes struck by a hammer."[547] The orbital roof, the interorbital space, and the perpendicular plate of the ethmoid are frequently involved in these fractures, and the anterior cranial fossa may be fractured or penetrated when fractures occur either adjacent to or through the cribriform plate area. In the medial upper orbit, these structures also involve the roofs of the ethmoid sinuses and the lateral walls of the ethmoid sinuses.

Some of the neurologic complications resulting from nasoethmoidal-orbital fractures are laceration of the dura covering the frontal lobes, laceration of the tubular sheaths enveloping the olfactory nerves and contusion or severance of the nerves as they perforate the cribriform plate, penetration of the brain by sharp-edged ethmoidal or frontal cell walls, and blunt contusion of brain tissue.

An additional point of interest in the skeletal structure of this area is the continuity of the thin lamina papyracea of the medial orbital wall with the thin portion of the medial floor of the orbit. A "bulge" of the maxillary sinus distinctly narrows the orbital volume in this area. Splintering of the lamina papyracea facilitates an enlarged blowout fracture in this area. Fractures of the medial portion of the inferior orbital rim and orbital floor are invariably present in nasoethmoidal-orbital fractures, as are fractures of the upper piriform aperture. Lacerations of the soft tissue may sever the levator palpebrae superioris or penetrate through the medial canthal ligament and lacrimal system. Less commonly, the medial canthal tendon may be avulsed from bone with its contained lacrimal system (canaliculi and upper portion of the lacrimal sac), divided, or partially avulsed from bone fragments. Fractures of the adjacent facial bones, particularly the midfacial skeleton, are frequently seen in combination with nasoethmoidal-orbital fractures. In many patients, the frontal bone and other bones of the orbit are involved.

Studies confirm that the nasal area is the weakest portion of the facial skeleton; fractures occur in this area with an impact load of 35 to 80 g. In Swearingen's study,[390] 45 impacts were made on cadaver heads to determine the fracture points of various portions of the facial skeleton (Fig. 66-194). With the exception of the neck of the condyle, the zygomatic arch area is the next weakest area, being able to sustain impact forces of greater than 50 g. The upper portion of the middle third of the face, which includes both the nasal and orbital areas, is also structurally susceptible to fracture. In contrast, the lower portion of the maxilla sustains impact forces up to 150 g, and the major portion of the body of the frontal bone, with the exception of the central portion, which is weakened by the frontal sinus cavities, sustains impact forces of up to 200 g. Although padding of the rigid dashboard decreases the severity of injuries sustained, the padded dashboard edges in many automobiles have a contour suitable for the production of the "pushback" type of nasal fractures between the orbits. Such fractures may occur even though the passenger is wearing a lap and shoulder belt. They occur less frequently when passengers are protected by the shoulder harness type of belt. These frontal-ethmoidal fractures are most effectively prevented by the combination of an air bag and a complete shoulder harness and seat belt. The passenger without a seat belt is often projected through the windshield and suffers various types of soft tissue lacerations, which occur concomitantly with facial

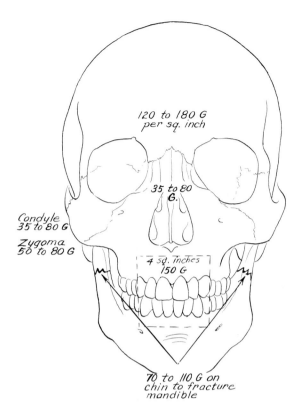

FIGURE 66-194. Forces causing facial fractures after impact on a padded deformable surface. This diagram illustrates a comparison of forces that cause fracture in the various areas of the face. (After Swearingen JJ: Tolerances of the human face to crash impact. Report from the Office of Aviation Medicine, Federal Aviation Agency, July 1965.)

fractures.[378,389] These include penetrating lacerations of the nasal and orbital areas.

The forces described by Swearingen[390] are the minimal forces necessary for fracture. In practice, the actual force delivered to the area in many of these injuries exceeds the minimal forces for fracture by a multiple almost exceeding comprehension. Therefore, the forces are sufficient to comminute many bones of the middle third of the facial skeleton.

In all but the first stage of nasoethmoidal-orbital fractures, the patient has a characteristic appearance. The bony bridge of the nose is depressed and widened, and the angle between the lip and the columella may be opened into an obtuse relationship. The eyes may appear far apart, as in orbital hypertelorism.[552,553] This phenomenon may simply be due to traumatic telecanthus,[286] or in the presence of bilateral zygomatic fractures,[554] there may be a true hyperteloric appearance. Traumatic telecanthus implies an increase in the distance between the medial canthi. This may or may not be present acutely in many nasoethmoidal-orbital fractures, as it is masked by swelling and may be noted

with further bone displacement that occurs as time passes. Swelling usually masks the exact degree of bone displacement or may itself simulate a fracture. Nasoethmoidal-orbital fractures may be unilateral (36%) or bilateral (64%).[286] The unilateral type is common in upper Le Fort II or III injuries or in fractures involving the frontal area, which are predominantly unilateral, progressing into the nasoethmoidal region. The final type of common unilateral nasoethmoidal fracture involves the zygoma and the medial inferior orbit. Traumatic orbital hypertelorism[554] (as opposed to telecanthus) is a deformity characterized by an increase in the distance between the orbits *and* the ocular globe; it occurs rarely in massive disruption of the midfacial skeleton and frontal bone.[551,554]

Converse and Smith[551] postulated that traumatic telecanthus is produced by two types or varieties of backward and lateral displacement of the bone structures. In the first type, the frontal process of the maxilla and the nasal bones penetrate the interorbital space, comminuting the ethmoidal cells and outfracturing the medial walls of the orbit. The medial canthal tendon attachments are displaced with the bone, and the medial canthi are displaced laterally. As they settle laterally, the inner commissures of the eyelids may be deformed, assuming a rounded shape and a lateral position with shortening of the palpebral fissures. It is rare for the medial canthus to be avulsed from a significantly sized bone fragment in the absence of lacerations near the medial canthal area.

In the second and more common type of fracture, the nasal bones and the frontal process of the maxilla are splayed outward and projected backward into the medial portion of the orbital cavity along the lateral surface of the medial orbital wall. Again, the medial canthal tendon usually is not severed from bone, nor is the lacrimal or canalicular system transected in the absence of cutaneous lacerations. Traumatic telecanthus may be contributed to by an increase in the thickness of the medial orbital wall from the overlapping bone fragments.

CLASSIFICATION

In the first stage of nasoethmoidal-orbital fractures, the bone bearing the medial canthal attachment is greensticked at the internal angular process of the frontal bone and displaced posteriorly and medially at the inferior orbital rim and piriform aperture.[286,555,556] The medial canthus is thus actually displaced posteriorly, medially, and slightly inferiorly, in effect "bowstringing" the medial canthus.[555] This phenomenon represents the first stage of the nasoethmoidal-orbital fracture and is an incomplete fracture at the internal angular process of the frontal bone.

In patients with nasoethmoidal-orbital fractures, one must identify and classify what is happening to the bone of the medial orbital rim, which bears the medial canthal attachment, as it has a direct relationship to the treatment techniques of the various fractures. Displacement of this medial canthal bone fragment is the sine qua non of the nasoethmoidal injury, and the correct definition and management of this fragment, the central fragment (see Fig. 66-191), determine the outcome of the fracture.

In many nasoethmoidal fractures, the medial orbital rim and walls are thin bone and thus diffusely splintered. Small bone pieces are not useful in reconstruction and must conceptually be replaced by bone grafts. In patients treated late, many of these small bone fragments have literally disappeared secondary to bone resorption.

The patterns of nasoethmoidal-orbital injuries consist of four types: a localized central midface injury; a unilateral injury extended superiorly in the frontal bone or inferiorly into the inferior orbital rim and zygoma; a high Le Fort II or III fracture with a nasoethmoidal-orbital component; and a panfacial fracture, which may or may not involve the frontal bone. Superior and inferior groups of incisions are necessary for visualization of the peripheral buttresses of a nasoethmoidal-orbital fracture. A laceration may occasionally substitute for one of the exposures. Lacerations should not be extended, as the scar is generally worse than what would have occurred if an elective incision were used. The inferior incisions consist of a lower lid incision, which is frequently a midtarsal incision, conjunctival or subciliary incision, and a gingival buccal sulcus incision to expose the lower aspect of the piriform aperture and the Le Fort I level. The lower eyelid incision exposes the infraorbital rim and the upper portion of the piriform aperture. The superior incision is generally a coronal incision, but two local incisions may be used in localized fractures to substitute a smaller approach for the coronal incision. These two localized incisions are a vertical midline incision over the root of the nose (not extended into the distal nose) and the horizontal limb alone of the Converse open-sky approach. Either one of these local two incisions may be used for exposure of the upper portion of a nasoethmoid fracture. They are inadequate for exposure of the frontal sinus and the frontal bone.

In nasoethmoid fractures displaced only inferiorly (type I), the superior incisions are unnecessary. Thus, a type I fracture may be treated with inferior exposures alone. The internal orbit must be brought to proper size by the addition of bone grafts or alloplastic material inferiorly and medially.

The author prefers to divide nasoethmoidal-orbital fractures into four types.

TYPE I. Type I is an incomplete fracture, mostly unilateral but occasionally bilateral, that is displaced only inferiorly at the infraorbital rim and piriform margin. Inferior-alone approaches are necessary.

TYPE II. Type II nasoethmoidal-orbital fractures section the entire nasoethmoidal area as a unit. These are perhaps not true nasoethmoidal-orbital fractures because telecanthus cannot occur. The central fragment is usually rotated and posteriorly displaced, and considerable canthal distortion occurs. Conceptually, these are treated with the same superior and inferior approaches as for a complete nasoethmoidal-orbital fracture, but neither type I nor type II requires canthal repositioning because the canthus is not unstable and remains attached to a large bone fragment.

TYPE III. Type III nasoethmoidal-orbital fractures are comminuted nasoethmoidal fractures with the fractures remaining outside the canthal ligament insertion. The central fragment may be dealt with as a sizable bone fragment and united to the canthal ligament-bearing fragment of the other side with a transnasal wire reduction. The remainder of the pieces of the nasoethmoidal-orbital skeleton are assembled with interfragment wiring and then united by junctional plate and screw fixation to the frontal bone, the infraorbital rim, and the Le Fort I level of the maxilla.

TYPE IV. Type IV nasoethmoidal-orbital fractures either have avulsion of the canthal ligament (uncommon) or extend underneath the canthal ligament insertion. The fracture fragments are small enough that a reduction would require detachment of the canthus for the bone reduction to be accomplished. Therefore, canthal ligament reattachment is required, a separate step accomplished with a separate set of transnasal wires for each canthus. In general, the bone reduction of the intercanthal distance should be 5 to 7 mm per side less than the soft tissue distance. Bone grafts are frequently required for the dorsal nose to add height and smoothness of contour. A cartilage graft may be needed for the columella to stabilize this area to prevent nasal shortening. The nasal septum is frequently perforated and should be repaired. If dislocated, the septum may be reattached to the anterior nasal spine with a wire reduction.

DIAGNOSIS

Clinical Examination

The appearance of patients who suffer nasoethmoidal-orbital fractures is typical. A significant frontal impact nasal fracture is generally present, with the nose flattened and appearing to have been pushed between the eyes. There is a loss of dorsal nasal prominence, and an obtuse angle is noted between the lip and columella. Finger pressure on the nose (Fig. 66-195) may document inadequate distal septal or proximal bone support, especially distally. Finger palpation of the columella or septum assesses the degree of superior rota-

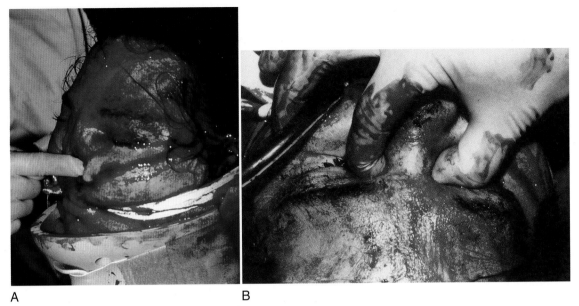

FIGURE 66-195. *A,* Finger pressure on the nasal dorsum and columella documents the lack of skeletal support in nasoethmoid fractures. *B,* If the fingertips are pressed over the medial orbital rim (not the nasal bones), a click or movement confirms a mobile nasoethmoidal-orbital fracture.

tion of the septum. The medial canthal areas are swollen and distorted with palpebral and subconjunctival hematomas. The lacrimal caruncles and plicae semilunaris may be covered by the edematous and displaced structures. Ecchymosis and subconjunctival hemorrhage are the usual findings. Directly over the medial canthal ligaments, crepitus or movement may be palpated with external pressure deeply over the canthal ligament. A bimanual examination[556] of the medial orbital rim is helpful if the diagnosis is uncertain. The bimanual examination is performed by placement of a palpating finger deeply over the canthal ligament and a clamp inside the nose with its tip directly under the finger. The frontal process of the maxilla may then, if it is fractured, be moved between the index finger and the clamp, indicating instability (see Fig. 66-111) and confirming both the diagnosis and the need for an open reduction. If the clamp is placed under the nasal bones (and not the medial orbital rim–medial canthal ligament attachment), it erroneously identifies a nasal fracture as canthal instability.

Intranasal examination generally shows swollen, bulging mucosa with fractures of the septum. Septal fractures may be severe, and indeed septal perforations are common in these injuries. Fracture of the septum is suggested by its displacement, swollen mucous membranes, and septal hematoma. Septal hematomas should be specifically searched for and drained to avoid a septal perforation from mucosal necrosis. Nasoethmoidal-orbital fractures are often accompanied by the signs of bilateral orbital blowout fractures or fractures of the frontal bone, maxilla, and zygoma. Edema and hematoma often mask the extent of the skeletal disruption in these areas, particularly if the patient is not seen during the first hours after the accident.

The patient may be unconscious or may have had a loss of consciousness of a long or short duration. This symptom is suggestive of significant brain injury. If the patient is irritable, restless, or even thrashing about, a frontal brain injury should be suspected. As in other fractures of the orbit, extensive edema of the periorbital structures and the lids may cause mechanical limitation of eyelid motion or extraocular movement. There may be little confirmatory evidence of skeletal deformity because of the hematoma or swelling. In some patients, the deformity is evident when the frontal bone has been crushed inward and the nasal structures have been projected into the interorbital space. The bones may be loose, and crepitation may be felt when they are mobilized. The entire upper jaw may be movable, and the motion may be felt in the bones of the interorbital space. A portion of the forehead or nasal skin may be avulsed in compound fractures, exposing the bone or revealing the sites of the fracture. Nasal lining may be torn and devascularized by the injury, prejudicing the survival of existing bone.

Clear fluid escaping from the nose is strongly suggestive of CSF rhinorrhea.[391] In acute injuries, this is often masked by bloody drainage. CSF rhinorrhea should be expected in any nasoethmoidal-orbital injury because of the direct path of extension of the fracture to the cribriform plate area through the thicker portion of the perpendicular plate of the ethmoid. Patients with CSF rhinorrhea always show an initial escape of blood from the fracture sites. During several days, the fluid becomes brownish and finally clear. The CSF may be distinguished from blood by the "double ring" sign. A small amount of nasal drainage is placed on a paper towel; the blood remains toward the center, whereas the CSF migrates laterally, forming an inner red and outer clear ring, the double ring sign.

BIMANUAL EXAMINATION. A bimanual examination[556] (see Fig. 66-111) may be performed for confirmation with a clamp inside the nose with its tip underneath the canthal ligament and an index finger pad palpating externally over the canthal ligament insertion. Digital manipulation allows the central fragment to move between the palpating index finger and the intranasal clamp. Any mobility indicates the need for an open reduction.

When the degree of comminution of the fracture is sufficient, the medial canthal ligament and its attached frontal process of the maxilla move laterally, producing telecanthus, or an increased distance between the medial commissures of the palpebral fissures. Initially, perception of modest increases in the intercanthal distance may be obscured by swelling. As time passes, the palpebral fissure shortens, the internal commissure of the eyelids becomes rounded, and enophthalmos, due to an enlarged orbit, occurs, with the globe sinking downward, medially, and posteriorly.

Radiographic Examination

CT examination is essential to document the injury. Plain radiographs often mask the fractures, and critical detail is obscured and always incomplete. Careful interpretation of CT scans shows diagnostic or implied signs of a nasoethmoidal fracture.[557] Four fractures must be present: the frontal process of the maxilla, the nose, the medial and inferior orbital rims, and the medial orbital wall and orbital floor. The fractures may extend into adjacent structures, but in their simplest form, the fractures surround the entire lower two thirds of the medial orbital rim and therefore isolate the nasoethmoidal-orbital fracture segment as a potentially "free" segment. Fractures of the anterior cranial fossa may be difficult to detect in the ordinary axial CT section, especially if displacement is minimal. Air in the subdural or extradural space or rarely in a ventricle is a sign of communication of the intracranial area with the nasal cavity or sinuses. A direct pathway for infection is therefore established, and it is an indication for consideration of neurosurgical intervention to close the fistula definitively or at least for prophylactic administration of perioperative antibiotics. Fractures of the frontal sinus frequently accompany

nasoethmoidal fractures, and depression of the anterior or posterior walls of the frontal sinus, or an air-fluid level implying nasofrontal duct obstruction, may be observed.[558,559] Displacement of either the anterior wall alone or the anterior and posterior walls of the sinus may be observed. The patency of the nasofrontal duct must be evaluated as a separate consideration.

Fragmentation and a "buckled" appearance of the cribriform plate are suggestive of penetration of bone fragments toward the base of the brain. This finding is an indication for neurosurgical intervention. One may also see brain tissue in the nose, which is an indication for neurosurgical intervention.

A CT scan taken in both the axial and coronal planes defines the extent of the fracture unilaterally and bilaterally[77,560,561] and documents any associated fractures, such as zygomatic, frontal, cranial vault or base, or high Le Fort (II or III). In the author's series, 36% of the nasoethmoidal fractures were unilateral.[286] These are usually associated with zygomatic or supraorbital fractures and may involve circumferential fractures around one orbit. On occasion, an isolated "point blow" may fracture only the frontal processes of the maxilla on one side. A high Le Fort II or III fracture often contains a unilateral nasoethmoidal-orbital component (Fig. 66-196).[562]

Bilateral fractures of the nasoethmoidal-orbital region are isolated to the central midface area or may be extended to other areas.[563] The bilateral injury may accompany a Le Fort II or III maxillary fracture or a frontal bone fracture, such as occurs with a craniofacial injury.[564] The bilateral "extended" nasoethmoidal-orbital fracture is often a part of a craniofacial injury consisting of a "Le Fort IV" fracture level on one side (frontal bone involvement) and a Le Fort III fracture (zygoma) level on the other (less involved) side. In its

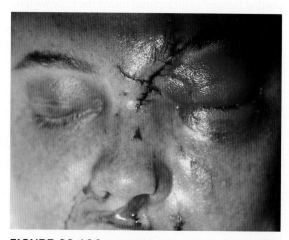

FIGURE 66-196. A high Le Fort fracture containing a nasoethmoid fracture. A CSF leak is present. The nose is flattened. Bilateral spectacle hematomas are present.

simplest form, the nasoethmoidal-orbital fracture must involve at least one medial orbital rim. The base of the frontal sinus and the nasofrontal ducts are in proximity but are frequently unimpaired in many nasoethmoidal fractures.[559,565] With extension of fractures into the frontal cranial area, the anterior and posterior walls of the frontal sinus become more involved in the fracture.

To have the simplest nasoethmoidal fracture, the fracture lines must separate the lower two thirds of the medial orbital rim from the adjacent bones (type I) (Fig. 66-197). The entire bilateral nasoethmoidal-orbital area may be detached as a single fragment (type II). This produces a bone segment to which the canthal ligaments remain attached but that can be displaced, depending on periosteal continuity, usually posteriorly and inferiorly. In this type of fracture, telecanthus cannot occur. In type II fractures, the bilateral nasoethmoid area is comminuted worse on one side, but the canthal ligament-bearing bone fragments are "free" and can be displaced (Fig. 66-198). In type III fractures, reduction can be performed without detachment of the canthal ligament from the central fragment, which is the canthal ligament-bearing bone fragment (Fig. 66-199). In type IV fractures, the canthal ligament-bearing bone fragment is comminuted or the ligament has been avulsed from the central fragment such that actual canthal reattachment is required in the bone reduction.[566,567] In some patients, fracture lines may be observed on CT radiographs; however, there is sufficient periosteal continuity to prevent displacement of the fractured segment. No surgery is required for undisplaced fractures, and stability may be confirmed by a stable bimanual examination (see Fig. 66-111).[556] As in zygomatic fractures that demonstrate greensticking at the zygomaticofrontal suture, a nasoethmoidal-orbital fracture may reveal greensticking at the junction of the frontal process of the maxilla with the internal angular process of the frontal bone (type I; see Fig. 66-197). Characteristically, the first fracture displacement occurs through the piriform aperture and the medial orbital rim and at the inferior orbital rim. The frontal process of the maxilla is fractured in a hinge-type manner at its junction with the frontal bone and is displaced last. When this junction is completely fractured, the frontal process of the maxilla is free to be displaced laterally, and telecanthus occurs.

The diagnosis of a nasoethmoidal-orbital fracture on radiographs requires at a minimum four fractures that isolate the frontal process of the maxilla from adjacent bones. These include (1) fractures of the nose, (2) fractures of the junction of the frontal process of the maxilla with the frontal bone, (3) fractures of the medial orbit (ethmoidal area), and (4) fractures of the inferior orbital rim extending to involve the piriform aperture and orbital floor. These fracture lines, therefore, define the central fragment of bone bearing the medial canthal ligament as free, and depending on periosteal integrity, the medial orbital rim could be displaced.

TREATMENT

Brain trauma should always be suspected in these injuries and excluded. Brain is occasionally observed in the nose, despite fractures not being clearly visible or dramatic on radiographic examination. This finding signifies a discontinuity in the integrity of the anterior cranial base, which requires neurosurgical repair. Neurosurgical intervention is required in patients who have depressed or open frontal skull or cranial base fractures. The isolated nasoethmoidal-orbital fracture may demonstrate fractures adjacent to the cribriform plate, and a CSF leak may persist for several days. A CSF leak must be assumed in *any* patient with a nasoethmoidal-orbital fracture. It has been the author's experience that in the absence of frontal bone or frontal sinus involvement, anterior cranial fossa fractures are usually short, linear, and minimally displaced and do not require a separate neurosurgical procedure to close the dural fistula. Few patients with these simple, linear basilar skull fractures accompanying isolated nasoethmoidal fractures require neurosurgical intervention. The need for such intervention depends on the presence of depressed fractures involving the frontal bone, orbital roofs, or frontal sinus. Pneumocephalus implies a communication from the nasal cavity or sinuses to the intradural space, and these patients should receive careful evaluation for possible neurosurgical exploration. Careful neurologic examination must assess the level of consciousness, motor response, eye movements, and response to questions. Any patient with a possibility of brain injury requiring observation may receive immediate surgical treatment by monitoring of the intracranial pressure. In practice, any patient receiving general anesthesia who does not have an examination and a history that exclude the possibility of brain injury should be carefully monitored. It is not necessary to delay surgical treatment to intermittently clarify the neurosurgical status of the patient when monitoring of this type is performed. This type of monitoring allows the earliest facial injury repair to be achieved with safety.

The technique of treatment in nasoethmoidal-orbital fractures consists of a thorough exposure of the naso-orbital region by means of three incisions: a coronal incision (or an appropriate laceration or local incision), a lower eyelid incision, and a gingival buccal sulcus incision. In some patients, a laceration may be present over the forehead or nose, which provides sufficient access for a localized fracture to be treated. Nasal and forehead lacerations are common, but often they are not quite long enough to provide sufficient exposure (Fig. 66-200). Judgment must be exercised

Text continued on p. 320

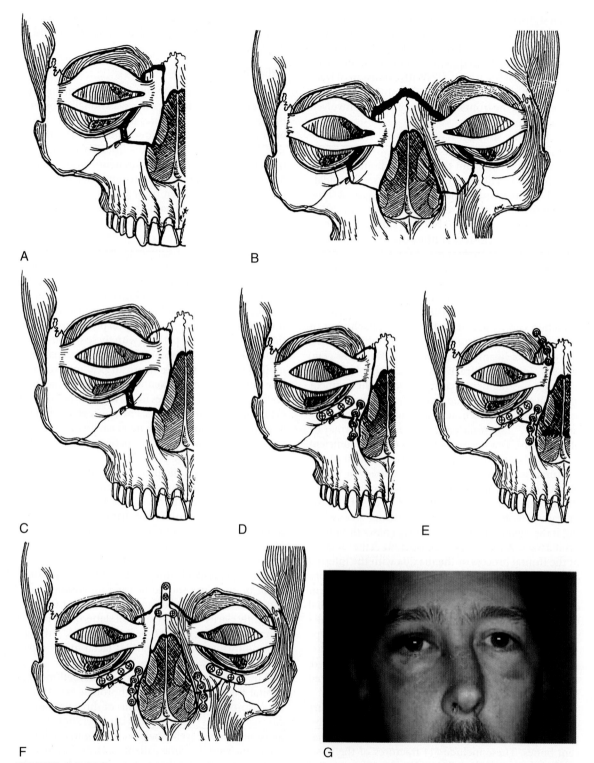

A

B

C

D

E

F

G

FIGURE 66-197. A single-fragment nasoethmoidal-orbital fracture. *A,* Unilateral. *B,* Bilateral. *C,* Greenstick fracture at the nasofrontal suture displaced only inferiorly. *D,* Repair of greenstick fracture with inferior- and orbital-only approaches. *E,* Complete dislocation repair with all approaches. *F,* Bilateral single-segment naso-orbital fracture. *G,* Injury photograph.

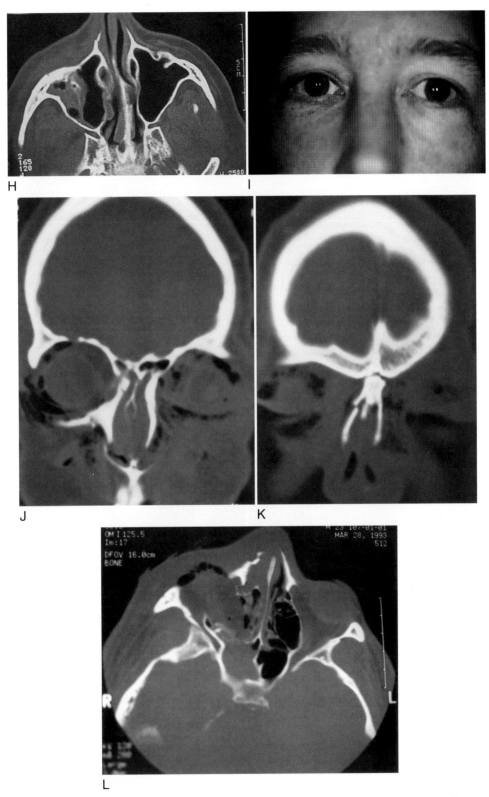

FIGURE 66-197, cont'd. *H,* Radiograph. *I,* Results after open reduction. *J,* Radiograph of a complete unilateral fracture. *K,* Radiograph of a complete nasoethmoidal-orbital fracture, nasal component. *L,* Unilateral complete nasoethmoidal-orbital fracture. (From Markowitz B, Manson PN, Sargent L, et al: Management of the medial canthal ligament in nasoethmoid orbital fractures: the importance of the central fragment in diagnosis and treatment. Plast Reconstr Surg 1991;87:843.)

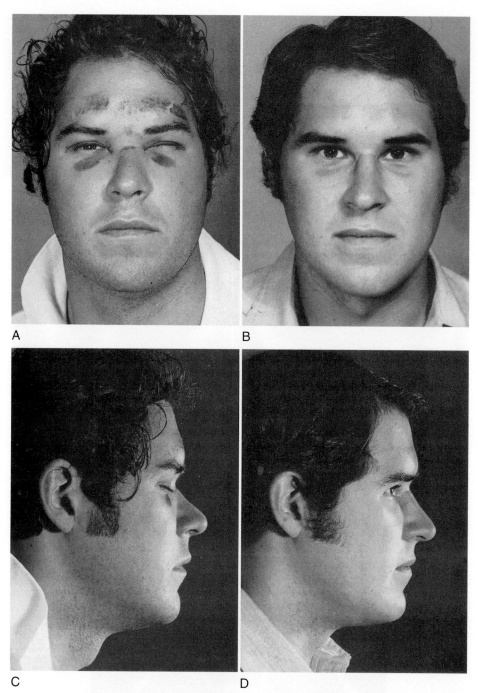

FIGURE 66-198. Primary bone grafting after treatment of a nasoethmoidal-orbital fracture and comminuted blowout fracture of the orbital floor. *A* and *C,* The appearance of the patient 9 days after trauma. The left eye is enophthalmic and the nasal bridge is collapsed. There is reasonable preservation of the distal height of the nose. The patient, an automobile racing driver, was involved in a crash. The helmet descended over the face, and the rim of the helmet struck the dorsum of his nose. This caused a fracture with backward recession of the bones of the nasal framework into the interorbital space, with splaying apart of the medial orbital walls, telecanthus *(A),* depression of the root of the nose *(C),* and bilateral orbital blowout fractures. *B* and *D,* The appearance 4 months postoperatively. A trap-door flap was raised at the laceration sites, and the comminuted fragments were reassembled and stabilized. The orbital fractures were treated by release of entrapped orbital contents and placement of Supramid implants. A primary bone graft was used for the nose.

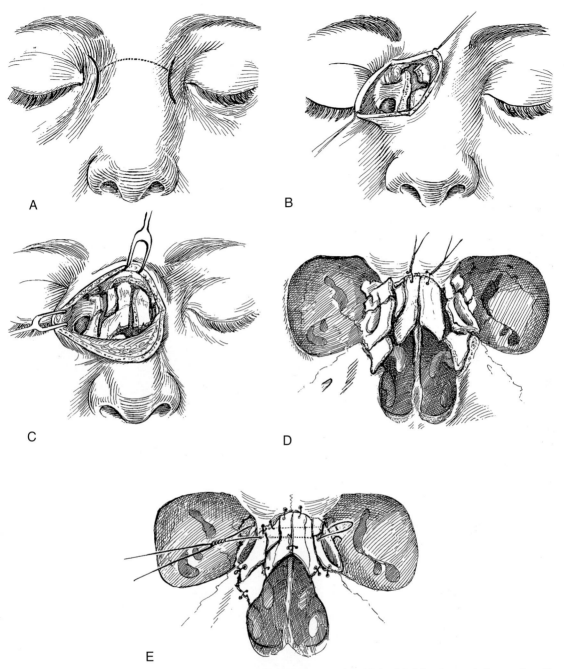

FIGURE 66-199. Open-sky technique in the treatment of nasoethmoidal-orbital fractures. *A*, In practice, the lateral superior and inferior oblique extensions of the open-sky incisions in the eyelids are seldom necessary. One may do the operation adequately with *only* the horizontal incision over the root of the nose. The lateral extensions into the eyelids frequently result in hypertrophic scarring and "web" contractures in the medial orbits. *B*, Exposure obtained through the external incision. *C*, Comminuted bone fragments, the lacrimal sac, and the medial canthal tendon are examined. *D*, Interosseous wiring of the main fragments of the orbital rims and nasal bones establishes an initial linkage of bone fragments, one to the other. *E*, Before the smaller fragments have been joined by loose interosseous wiring, a through-and-through transnasal wire is passed from one medial canthal ligament-bearing bone fragment to the other and back to maintain the anatomic position of the medial orbital walls. This is the most important step in nasoethmoidal fracture reduction. (After Converse JM, Hogan VM: Open-sky approach for reduction of naso-orbital fractures. A case report. Plast Reconstr Surg 1970;46:396).

in the extension of these lacerations, as the scar deformity from extension is sometimes worse than making a separate coronal incision. The ipsilateral inferior orbital rim and floor must be exposed in unilateral nasoethmoidal-orbital fractures, and the bilateral lower orbital rims must be exposed in bilateral nasoethmoidal-orbital fractures. The unilateral or bilateral gingival buccal sulcus incision is required to visualize the lower aspects of the fracture.

There is no place for closed treatment in dislocated nasoethmoidal-orbital fractures by external splints alone or intranasal manipulation alone. The surgical

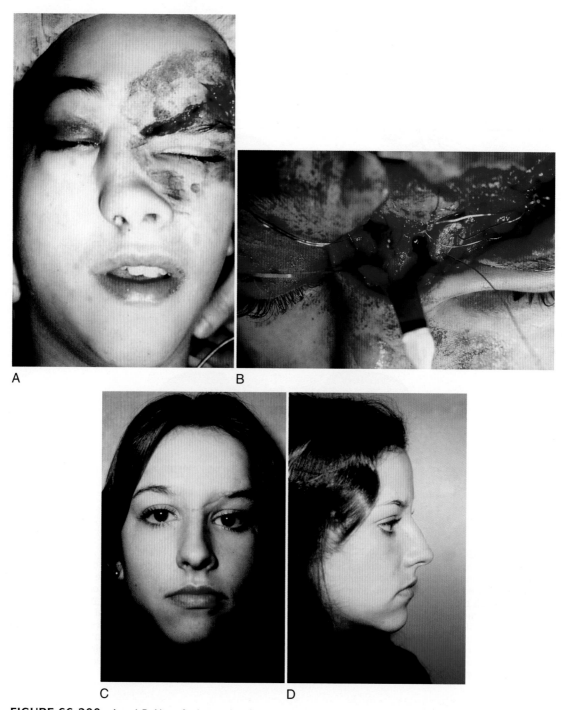

A   B

C   D

FIGURE 66-200. *A* and *B,* Use of a laceration for exposure. *C* and *D,* Postoperative result.

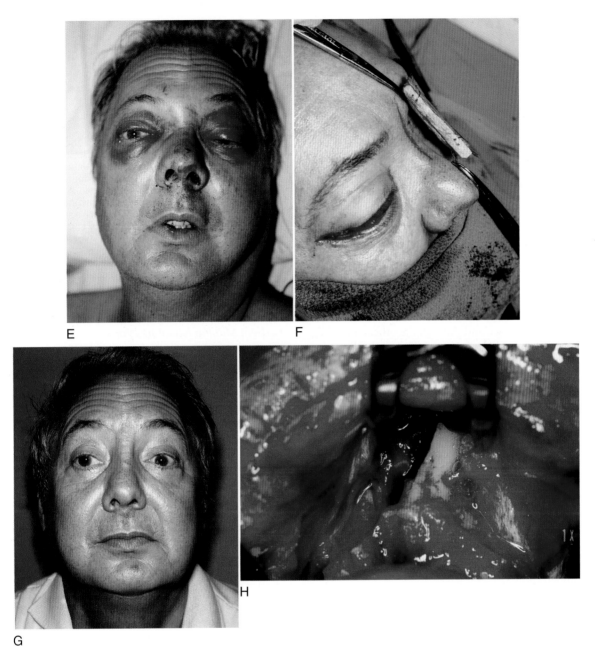

FIGURE 66-200, cont'd. *E* and *F,* Use of a vertical incision for exposure. *G,* Postoperative result. *H,* View through a coronal incision—the nasal bones will be removed for exposure.

treatment of nasoethmoidal-orbital fractures consists of a thorough exposure of all dislocated fracture sites and, in significant fractures, a transnasal wire reduction of the medial orbital rims and cross-linking of all bone fragments to adjacent bone with interosseous wiring. The periphery of the fractures may then be stabilized to adjacent areas with junctional rigid fixation. The most essential feature of a nasoethmoidal reduction is the transnasal reduction of the medial

orbital rims by a wire placed posterior and superior to the canthal ligament insertion. This wire may be placed by lifting the bone bearing the canthal ligament (the central fragment) out of its position in the interorbital space, up toward the operator so that it can be turned and drilled. The drill holes should be posterior and superior to the lacrimal fossa. Full-length No. 26 wires can be passed through one medial canthal ligament-bearing bone fragment across the

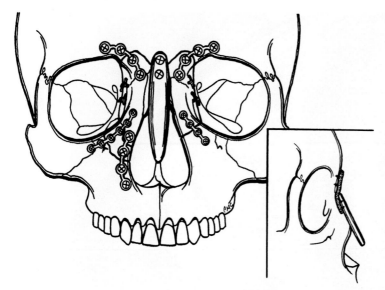

FIGURE 66-201. The author's favorite technique is to attach a plate by short screws to the underside of the proximal portion of the bone graft to stabilize it to the frontal bone. A dorsal nasal bone graft may be used to increase nasal height or simply produce a smooth nasal dorsal contour. In this case, a thin rib graft works well, its marrow hollowed out to produce a shell of the bone graft, which provides only thin, smooth covering over the reassembled fracture fragments.

interorbital space and through the other canthal ligament-bearing bone fragment. The canthal ligament-bearing bone fragments are then replaced into their proper position, and the wires are tightened while a forceps holds the fragments in position. Interfragment wires then link the central fragment to adjacent bones. Nasal bone fragments are placed in their proper position, and the interfragment wires are tightened to approximate the bone fragments, including the intranasal wires (see Figs. 66-198 and 66-199).

The transnasal wires are tightened to reduce the central fragments, with care being taken to hold these fragments in their proper position *before* the wires are tightened. Forcing the reduction of the fracture by tightening the wires without an initial reduction of the bone of the central fragment may cause the wires to split through the thin bone fragments, which generally have imperceptible microfractures.

Primary bone grafting is essential to restore the orbital and nasal bone continuity and contour. When the cartilaginous septum is destroyed and does not provide support, this area should be strengthened by a bone graft attached to the proximal portion of the nasal bones (Fig. 66-201). In some patients, a cartilage graft may be placed in the columella for columella support as well, or a columellar bone graft may be connected to the dorsal nasal bone graft to improve projection. In severe "telescoped" nasoethmoidal-orbital fractures, the cartilaginous support of the columella is destroyed. Bone grafting is essential to restore the size and the shape of the orbital cavity. The fractures usually begin in the medial portion of the orbital roof and extend to at least the infraorbital nerve in the orbital floor on each side. A properly curved bone graft can be used to replace missing floor segments or to strengthen comminuted fragments.

Vertical Midline Nasal Incision

Because scars on the nose may be of variable quality, local incisions are conceptually avoided. The vertical midline nasal incision is a local incision occasionally used to expose the nasoethmoidal-orbital region[286,548] (see Fig. 66-200). Elderly or bald patients with limited fractures often obtain a superior result from this incision compared with the more visible scar in these individuals from the standard coronal incision. Healing generally occurs as a fine line scar. Separate canthal incisions are not required. This vertical incision is most appropriate in patients who have glabellar rhytids, and it is a satisfactory exposure only for treatment of fractures *localized* to the nasoethmoidal-orbital area. The incision should *not* extend beyond the finely textured skin on the proximal portion of the nose. The skin of the distal two thirds of the nose responds poorly to elective incisions.

Coronal Incision

For exposure of the medial orbital rims, all periosteal attachments of the orbital soft tissue must be freed from the roof of the orbit and the entire frontal processes of the zygoma and maxilla, except for the medial canthal ligament attachment, by subperiosteal dissection. The zygomaticofrontal suture and the tissue in the lateral portions of the roof of the orbits must be dissected to allow the soft tissue to "drop out" of the orbital roof, which allows clear visualization of the nasoethmoidal-orbital area medially. The supraorbital neurovascular bundles must be released from the canal or groove, and careful dissection releases the trochlea medial to the nerve. Dissecting the tissue away from the roof of the orbits allows exposure of the entire nose and the nasal, medial orbital rim, and wall areas.

The nasal bones are dorsally dissected fully to the cartilaginous septum, and the dissection is continued inferiorly down the lateral nasal bone to communicate with the piriform aperture dissection, which was performed through the gingival buccal sulcus incisions. The medial orbital rim with its attached canthal ligament-bearing segment is then dislocated anteriorly and laterally, and brought clearly into view next to the nasal bones, where its superficial position facilitates drilling and wire passing of the central fragment. Nasal bone fragments can be temporarily dislocated or removed to permit better exposure of the medial orbital rim segments. Removal of the nasal bones is especially helpful in passing a transnasal wire from the posterior and superior aspect of one central fragment (medial orbital rim canthal ligament-bearing bone fragment) to the other. After the placement of two transnasal wires, one should pass one extra wire for soft tissue reapproximation to bone. The medial orbital rims are linked to adjacent nasal and frontal bone fragments by interfragment wiring. This is an essential step "linking" these fragments to the nasal bones, frontal bone, and maxilla; the entire medial orbital structures then begin to develop some structural integrity. Junctional plate and screw fixation is employed after the initial interfragment wiring (Fig. 66-202) is tightened.

The transnasal reduction wires must be passed posterior and superior to the lacrimal fossa to provide the proper direction of force to establish the preinjury bone position of the central fragments. The transnasal reduction is not a "transnasal canthopexy," as it usually does not involve the canthal ligament. It is a reduction *only* of the central bone fragment of the nasoethmoidal-orbital fracture.

Canthal Reattachment

If the canthal ligament requires reattachment (the canthal tendon is rarely stripped from bone), the canthal tendon may be grasped by one or two passes of 2-0 nonabsorbable suture adjacent to the medial commissure of the eyelids.[568-570] The canthal tendon requires approximately 4 to 6 weeks to solidly reattach.[566] This area is accessed through a separate 3-mm external incision on the canthus oriented vertically or horizontally. Probes may be placed through the lacrimal system to avoid needle penetration of the lacrimal ducts. The lacrimal system may be intubated with disposable Quickert tubes where required. The 2-0 nonabsorbable suture is then passed into the internal aspect of the coronal incision by dissecting above the medial canthal ligament medially, and the suture is connected to a separate set of No. 28 transnasal wires, one set for each canthal ligament, separate from those required for the bone reduction of the central fragment. The transnasal canthal ligament wires are tightened only as the last step of the reduction, after medial

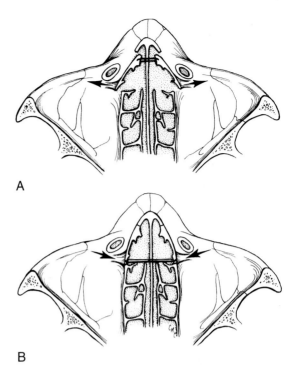

A

B

FIGURE 66-202. *A* and *B,* Transnasal wire in front of the canthal ligament will allow splaying of the posterior aspects of the fracture. Only a posterior transnasal wire will prevent rotation of the medial orbital rim. (From Markowitz B, Manson P, Sargent L, et al: Management of the medial canthal ligament in nasoethmoid orbital fractures: the importance of the central fragment in diagnosis and treatment. Plast Reconstr Surg 1991;87:843.)

orbital and nasal bone grafting and just before closure of the incision. Each set of canthal wires is tightened gently, after a manual reduction of the canthus to the bone with forceps is performed, to reduce stress on the canthal sutures. The canthal reduction wire pairs are then each separately twisted over a screw in the frontal bone. Although some have advocated unilateral plates, Mitek anchors, or special (Callahan) screws for canthal reattachment, the bone is often too fragile to accept these techniques. The author's experience is that the result, even if the bone is satisfactory, is invariably slightly laterally displaced.

The medial canthal tendon is a somewhat triangular band attached to the lacrimal fossa and frontal process of the maxilla stretching over the anterior lacrimal crest and the posterior nasal bone.[568,571] It has a distinct lower free border; superiorly, it becomes continuous with the periosteum over the internal angular process of the frontal bone, providing a roof for the lacrimal sac. The posterior portion of the medial canthal ligament continues as the cover for the lacrimal sac posteriorly; posteriorly, it is continuous with the lacrimal fascia inserting to the posterior lacrimal crest. The commissure of the eyelids is only several millimeters from the bone of the lacrimal fossa and the canthal apex. Branches of the canthal tendon divide to extend through the upper and lower lids to attach to the medial margins of the tarsal plates. There is a complicated relationship of various parts of the orbicularis muscle, the lacrimal sac, the divisions of the canthal tendon, and the attachments to bone. Both Anderson[568] and Zide and McCarthy[572] stress the importance of a vertical component of the medial canthal tendon. Surgeons have for some time appreciated that the direction of the posterior and superior limbs of the medial canthal tendon is important in procedures that reposition the canthal apparatus. The posterior limb of the medial canthal tendon exerts a force that keeps the eyelids tangent to the globe. Thus, redirecting the canthal tendon posteriorly maintains the position of the rest of the medial canthus after either accidental or surgical avulsion of the tendon. Anderson,[568] Zide and Jelks,[571] and Zide and McCarthy[572] thought that the strong posterior and superior branches that travel along the orbital rim to the frontonasal suture act to maintain vertical canthal position. The posterior branch is weak and has little structural integrity, which is why the tendon must be accessed and sutured in the anterior limb and then the fixation directed toward the posterior limb attachment.

After disinsertion of the canthal apparatus, one must establish, by canthal reattachment, a single summary vector of force that resuspends the entire canthal complex and provides the optimal architecture in proper vertical position. Converse[550,551,573] empirically determined that the optimal position for surgical repositioning is posterior and superior to its normal insertion. Most anatomic texts overemphasize the anterior limb of the medial canthal tendon and its attachment onto the frontal process of the maxilla and anterior lacrimal crest, thus distorting the true three-dimensional nature of the entire canthal apparatus and the need to reconstruct the posterior limb, which is the most delicate. The author's preferred surgical technique for reattachment involves placement of a suture through or around the canthal ligament; this approach is best accomplished by a 3-mm horizontal or vertical incision immediately adjacent to the medial commissure of the eyelids. The lacrimal system may be avoided by the insertion of fine probes. A braided suture is passed at least twice in the canthal tendon and then passed over the tendon superiorly through to the inside of the coronal exposure, medial to the orbital nasal soft tissue where a complete subperiosteal dissection has been performed. In most patients, it is necessary to mobilize most of the soft tissue contents of the orbit merely to allow an unstressed repositioning of the canthal ligament to be accomplished. Cutaneous incisions, such as Z-plasties, W-plasties, and other repositioning flaps, are usually not necessary for all primary and most secondary canthal procedures when proper mobilization of all the orbital soft tissue has been performed. In secondary procedures,[124,574] thinning of the scarred soft tissue is commonly required to achieve the canthal mobility and the required soft tissue thinness. The nasolacrimal duct may be dissected from its canal to achieve length for superior canthal positioning; rarely, the duct needs to be transected to be able to move the canthus superiorly. In this instance, a simultaneous dacryocystorhinostomy should be performed.[3,415]

In patients requiring late repair, excision of the periosteum and scar tissue from within the soft tissue must be completed to facilitate mobilization of the canthus. Often, resection of the periosteum may be required to release soft tissue stiffness, to thin the soft tissue, and to position the canthal ligament properly. Indeed, the thickness of the soft tissue adjacent to the medial portion of the nose and orbit may have to be thinned to simulate normal skin thickness. Skeletonization of the skin by excision of excess scar tissue dramatically increases the mobility of the dissected canthus. In some post-traumatic patients, the thickness of the skin in this area is impressive and represents a proliferation of scar tissue after hemorrhage and edema. This excess thickness must be resected and the skin contoured to its normal dimensions. This maneuver also usually frees the scar tissue, which allows more soft tissue flexibility. A braided suture in the canthus is attached to a separate pair of transnasal wires (reserved for this use alone), again positioned posterior and superior to the edge of the lacrimal fossa. The wires may be pulled tight to check the canthal alignment position and then released and finally tightened at the close of the procedure just before closure of the coronal incision.

COMPLICATIONS OF ORBITAL AND NASOETHMOIDAL-ORBITAL FRACTURES

The early diagnosis and adequate treatment of nasoethmoidal-orbital fractures achieve optimal aesthetic results with the least number of late complications. Depending on the quality of initial treatment and the results of healing, further reconstructive surgery may be required in some patients. Late complications, such as frontal sinus obstruction, occur in less than 5% of isolated nasoethmoidal-orbital fractures.[575,576] Deformities and functional impairment are late complications that can be minimized by early diagnosis and proper open reduction. A nasoethmoidal-orbital fracture may be obscured by the swelling of other facial injuries and may escape detection. An unconscious patient cannot volunteer information about double vision or cooperate for examinations. The diagnosis of a nasoethmoidal-orbital fracture should be suspected and confirmed by a bimanual examination[556] in questionable injuries. After several weeks, nasal deformity and enophthalmos are more evident. At this time, fibrous cicatrization is established, and the reconstruction of the nose and orbital cavity and restoration of symmetric ocular function and proper soft tissue position must be undertaken in the presence of scarred skin and soft tissue structures. Soft tissue, when it is injured, assumes the configuration of the underlying unreduced bone fragments as scar tissue forms in the geometric pattern of the unreduced bones. The soft tissue tends to develop a "memory" of the abnormal position and to return to this position despite late reconstruction of the bone in a more acceptable anatomic position because of its internal network of scar tissue, which was produced after the injury.[2]

Empty, deep orbital space should be minimized between bone grafts or implants and adjacent soft tissue margins by adding more graft materials.[577] Orbital suppuration is usually precipitated by infection of the obstructed lacrimal system or infection in an obstructed maxillary or ethmoid sinus. Antibiotic therapy is routinely employed in all patients at the time of operation, and the maxillary sinus is débrided of any bone fragments and irrigated to make sure that it communicates freely with the nose (duct functions). CT scans and orbital landmarks are useful in the evaluation of the bony orbital reconstruction.[578]

Implant or Bone Graft Complications

In the typical blowout fracture caused by blunt trauma, care must be taken to restore proper eye position. Excesses of vertical height of the implant may cause the globe to be elevated in proportion to the eyelid or cause proptosis. These problems should be noted and corrected on the operating table. In the early postoperative period, proptosis but no elevation of the globe is expected. As the swelling subsides, the globe should assume a more anatomic anterior-posterior position. If the globe remains displaced by an implant, the implant must be repositioned or removed and replaced by one that is either thinner or of a different shape so that the globe can rest in its proper position. Improperly designed implants can place excessive pressure on the globe, extraocular muscles, or lacrimal system or less commonly posteriorly on the optic nerve.[579,580]

Migration of an implant anteriorly may occur with extrusion if the implant is not secured to the orbital floor or to a plate that attaches to the rim. Spontaneous late proptosis can be caused by hemorrhage from long-standing low-grade infection around orbital implants or obstruction of the lacrimal system.[581] The author recommends curving bone grafts and implants to the desired contours of the orbit in the location where they are to be placed. Rib or calvarial grafts are easy to structure to the exact curvature of the desired orbital segment requiring replacement. The grafts are well tolerated by the patient and sufficiently strong to support the orbital contents, yet malleable enough to bend properly. More brittle types of bone, such as the calvaria and iliac crest, are more difficult to contour to the posterior dimensions of the orbit. Rib grafts have the highest percentage of resorption, and calvarial grafts are the most resistant to resorption.

Whereas autogenous bone is well tolerated by the patient and is the most physiologic substitute, it is not immune to resorption or infection, and it requires the use of a donor site with its attendant morbidities. Teflon, Silastic, Supramid, polyethylene, and metal titanium implants have been widely employed for orbital reconstruction and provide suitable inorganic implant materials. MEDPOR, a porous polyethylene, can be contoured, and it assumes the desired orbital curvature, much like a rib graft. The MEDPOR barrier implant has one smooth and one textured surface, limiting adherence of extraocular muscles. Any of these materials may be bent, shaped, shaved, carved, and fitted to the orbital defect without preliminary preparation or much delay. They are entirely satisfactory for most simple isolated orbital fractures. Metal implants are required in complex comminuted fractures where most of the orbital "buttress" supports have been lost and where it would be difficult to secure the position of several internal orbital bone grafts simultaneously (see Fig. 66-181).

Retrobulbar Hematoma

In severe trauma, retrobulbar hematoma may displace the ocular globe. Retrobulbar hematoma is signaled by globe proptosis, congestion, and prolapse of the edematous conjunctiva. Diagnosis is confirmed by a CT scan imaged with soft tissue windows. Globe displacement may be superior or inferior. It is usually not possible to drain retrobulbar hematomas because they are diffuse. If large in volume, they may not permit primary restoration of the bony volume of the orbit, and one may have to complete the internal portion of the orbital reconstruction several weeks later when the hemorrhage, swelling, and congestion have subsided. The orbital rim, however, may frequently be stabilized initially.

Diplopia

Despite early treatment of orbital fractures, ocular muscle imbalance, diplopia, and enophthalmos may occur.[327,329,448,449] Some adequately treated orbital fractures do not recover complete extraocular motion. If the patient has no double vision in any functional field of gaze, no treatment is required. Double vision present at the extremes of gaze is usually not a functionally limiting problem, and most patients do not generally require surgery. Double vision is most limiting when it occurs centrally or inferiorly in the downward gaze (reading or walking) position. Patients cannot read when this type of incapacitating double vision is present. Extraocular muscle surgery is often required if it persists, so early release of any muscle entrapment should be pursued.

Complicated blowout fractures are often accompanied by multiple fractures of the facial bones and injuries of the soft tissues. Many of these fractures may be complicated, and patients may have residual impairment of ocular movement and functionally disabling diplopia. These patients generally come to secondary extraocular muscle surgery when spontaneous improvement has ceased, which usually takes about 6 months. Enophthalmos should always be corrected before the eye muscles are adjusted with muscle surgery. Ptosis of the upper eyelid, downward displacement of the orbital contents, medial canthal deformities, shortening of the horizontal dimension of the palpebral fissure, reduction of the vertical dimension of the lower eyelid, saddle nose deformities, widening or foreshortening of the nose, and nasal airway obstruction all may require secondary reconstruction. Depression or lowering of the supraorbital rim may also be present.

In complicated orbital fractures, it is not unusual to have two or three secondary procedures done 6 to 12 months after the injury to adjust eye position and eyelid position and to remove prominent hardware. Diplopia occurring after repair may be due to muscle tear, surgical injury, impairment of muscle movement by the implant, enophthalmos, Volkmann contracture, motility issues, interference with scarring of the ligament system, head injury, cranial nerve paralysis (IV, VI), paresis, and enophthalmos.[582] Diplopia has been produced by muscle damage from orbital penetration by intranasal manipulation. Steroids are thought to improve diplopia.[453,583]

Ocular (Globe) Injuries and Visual Loss

The incidence of ocular injuries after orbital fractures has been reported to vary between 14% and 30%.[584] The incidence depends on the scrutiny of the examination and the recognition of minor injuries, such as corneal abrasion. Ocular globe injury may vary in severity from a corneal abrasion to loss of vision to globe rupture, retinal detachment, vitreous hemorrhage, or fracture involving the optic canal. Blindness or loss of an eye is remarkably infrequent despite the severity of some of the injuries sustained because of the "shock absorber" type of construction of the orbit; the thin bone gives way, allowing the globe to be pushed backward. In effect, the fracturing and blowout nature of the bone deformity and the nature of the bone collapse allow the globe to escape without rupture by dropping back into the orbit, where the thin bone is fracture-dislocated.

The importance of the ophthalmologic examination in all fractures of the orbit has already been discussed. Vitreous hemorrhage, dislocated limbus, rupture of the sclera, traumatic cataract, choroid rupture, retinal detachment, anterior or posterior chamber hemorrhage, rupture of the iris sphincter, and glaucoma are only some of the complications that follow blunt or penetrating injury of the globe, resulting in diminution or loss of vision. Globe injury[513] must be suspected in any patient who has contusion of the periorbital area. When lacerations exist, they must be probed and gently explored to exclude penetration of the globe by a sharp, thin object. Many complications may be avoided or minimized (or at least the condition not aggravated) if early diagnosis, treatment, and protection are instituted.

Verification of visual acuity is the *essential* step in the course of a preoperative or postoperative ophthalmologic examination. In the event of coma or uncooperative behavior on the part of the patient, the assessment of pupillary reaction to light must be accomplished. An ominous prognostic sign is the Marcus Gunn pupillary phenomenon.[64] A light is moved rapidly from one eye to the other, alternating the light position by swinging it back and forth (see Figs. 66-9 and 66-10). In the presence of a conduction defect of the optic nerve, the pupil on the involved side appears to dilate as the light is brought from the uninvolved to the involved eye, whereas it should constrict in the presence of an intact visual system. When a visual acuity deficit is documented, the surgeon must establish whether preinjury visual acuity was impaired or different. Diminished or monocular vision is common in patients who have amblyopia by history.

Ocular globe injury may vary in severity from a corneal abrasion to anterior or posterior chamber hematoma to retinal detachment. In the presence of hyphema, most ophthalmologists wish to wait a number of days before orbital fracture reduction with globe manipulation is undertaken so that the chance of rebleeding with orbital fracture reduction is reduced. Vitreous hematoma demands a specific protocol for management, which minimizes the possibility of rebleeding. A globe with a detached retina must be handled carefully, as must a ruptured globe that has been repaired, and these conditions delay bony orbital reconstruction. Although the prognosis of a ruptured globe in the face of major orbital fractures is poor, it is not appropriate to diminish the chance of recovery by vigorous fracture reduction unless hope for vision is lost. Many times, however, the orbital rim can be repaired without putting too much pressure on the globe, deferring the reduction of the internal orbit. The posterior third of the orbit is frequently involved by linear fractures, which often show little displacement. Such fractures may compromise (by virtue of their involvement of an orbital apex structure, such as the superior orbital fissure or optic canal) the circulation to the intracanalicular portion of the optic nerve as it travels through the optic canal. Blindness or loss of the eye is remarkably infrequent in view of the severity of some of the injuries sustained, a finding that attests to the great capacity of the structure of the orbital bones to absorb force without serious ocular injury. The eye socket is also constructed to collapse in its anterior rim and middle thirds so that the posterior third is protected from displacement.

The need for preliminary ophthalmologic examination is often dramatically illustrated by patients who demonstrate decreased vision, although no operation was performed. Miller[585] described such a patient with a midfacial fracture whose vision in the left eye was 20/70 a few hours after the injury and dropped to no light perception by the fifth day. No surgery had been performed. If surgery had taken place before the fifth day, the resulting blindness would probably have been attributed to the operation. Further deterioration of vision is common in facial injuries that cause diminished visual acuity. Several days after the initial event, one may find that visual acuity has dropped substantially.

Converse, in his landmark papers[517,518,551,573,586] describing the surgery of orbital repair, did not describe a single patient with blindness resulting from the repair of these fractures. The author has had several patients who have lost vision after operative intervention for Le Fort, nasoethmoidal, or frontal-orbital fractures.[365] One patient was prescribed systemic heparin on the second postoperative day for a subclavian vein thrombosis and bled into the orbit, becoming blind. One patient who had a straightforward Le Fort II fracture without the need for much orbital dissection was blind after the operation. Decompression of the orbit and optic nerve was performed, but no visual improvement occurred. Another patient had a severe frontal-orbital fracture and had neurosurgical exploration of the anterior cranial base and orbital roof reconstruction. Blindness in that eye was noted postoperatively. None of the patients had visual acuity return after decompression.

Nicholson and Guzak[587] described six patients in whom vision was lost in a series of 72 patients who underwent orbital fracture repair by means of silicone implants inserted by various surgeons in the same hospital. This is an extreme (8%) incidence of visual loss occurring at a reputable hospital, and it is largely unexplained because most competent experienced specialists have not encountered a single visual loss after orbital fracture repair.[588]

A summary of the literature has demonstrated that the incidence of blindness or visual damage after small

orbital blowout fracture repair should be much less than 0.1%.[588,589] Girotto et al,[365] in the most comprehensive description of blindness after orbital fracture repair, estimated that the incidence of blindness after facial fracture repair is about 2%. These findings were confirmed by MacKinnon et al,[590] who reported that 13% of patients with midface fractures had a documented ophthalmologic deficit on admission. They described the eye problems and defined blindness as a visual acuity of 60/60 or worse, a visual field of 10 degrees or less in the affected eye, or a destroyed globe. MacKinnon et al[590] noted that the incidence of eye injuries in other papers (depending on the definition of the problem) ranges from 4% to 91%. This extreme range of incidence is due to the methods of data collection and reporting and to the definition of what causes an eye injury. MacKinnon et al[590] found the incidence of blindness or severe visual impairment to be 0.8%, with motor vehicle fractures the most common cause. Even relatively insignificant fractures can be associated with loss of vision. Anderson[591] described blunt injury to the forehead resulting in blindness and proved in experiments that deformation of the posterior orbital roof was produced by frontal bone contusion without fracture, which caused optic nerve injury. In the study by MacKinnon et al,[590] the lateral wall was the most frequently fractured orbital region.

Girotto et al,[365] in a review of the University of Maryland Shock Trauma Unit experience with facial trauma during 11 years, noted that 2987 of the 29,474 admitted patients, or 10.1%, sustained facial fractures and that 1338 of these fractures, or 44.8%, involved one or both orbits. Of these patients, 1240 underwent operative repair of their facial fractures. Three patients experienced postoperative complications that resulted in blindness, a total of 0.242%. They concluded that postoperative ophthalmic complications seem to be primarily mediated by indirect injury to the optic nerve and its surrounding structures. The most frequent cause of postoperative visual loss is an increase in the intraorbital pressure in the optic canal. When Girotto's data were added to the literature, blindness was attributable to the intraorbital hemorrhage in 13 of 27 patients or 48%. In 67% of the patients, they thought that visual loss was due to increased intraorbital pressure.

Stanley[331,332,592] has provided an excellent description of lateral wall fractures and their complications, including "sphenotemporal buttress" fractures,[593] which are associated with a high incidence of blindness or nerve injury. Ioannides[594] had previously indicated that nasoethmoidal fractures are associated with a high incidence of blindness (3%). MacKinnon et al[590] do not discuss the incidence of postoperative blindness after facial fracture reduction. Girotto et al[365] have an excellent summary of the literature, which demonstrated that the incidence of blindness or visual damage after orbital fracture was present but small. In this study, it was emphasized that if enough operations are done, a significant event will occur. In a comprehensive study, Wang et al[595] have described postinjury visual loss and how it was treated. They demonstrated a useful clinical algorithm, which essentially indicates that if the patient has any vision, treatment with medical-dose steroids (spinal cord-type doses) is as effective as surgery. Once visual acuity is declining in the face of medical treatment, or if visual acuity is absent, a good response to medical (steroid) treatment cannot be expected and optic nerve decompression may be justified. Chen et al[596,597] have documented that in patients with no light perception, steroids are not effective, and one should progress to surgical decompression. Blindness may occur from hypotension alone.[598]

Lacrimal System Injury

Becelli[413] has documented a 47% incidence of lacrimal obstruction after nasoethmoidal-orbital fracture, one third of which cleared spontaneously. It is noted that many of the patients were operated on initially late after the injury. External dacryocystorhinostomy was 94% successful in eliminating the obstruction. Interruption of the continuity of the lacrimal apparatus demands specific action. Most lacrimal system obstruction occurs from bone malposition or damage to the lacrimal sac or duct.[284,286,599] The most effective treatment involves satisfactory precise repositioning of the fracture segments. If transection of the soft tissue portion of the canalicular lacrimal system has occurred, it should be repaired over fine tubes with magnification.[600,601]

Intraorbital Hematoma

Intraorbital hematoma is universal in fractures; however, severe hematoma with globe or nerve compression is less common. Continuous bleeding may occur from arteries within the orbit, such as the infraorbital or the anterior or posterior ethmoidal arteries, producing an orbital compartment syndrome. A reflex vasospasm may then occur in structures providing circulation to the optic nerve. Partially lacerated arteries in particular have a tendency to continue bleeding, and in some fractures involving the medial orbital wall, a significant retrobulbar hematoma may occur. The eye appears proptotic and congested. In the face of increased orbital pressure (>15 mm Hg), reflex loss of flow in the ophthalmic artery may occur, and diminution of flow to the retina may occur because of increased intraorbital pressure. Forrest et al[602] documented that initial rises in intraocular pressure occur after orbital fracture reduction and intraorbital bone grafting, but these readjust to normal levels in $^1/_2$ hour without treatment. Usually, any displaced fractures resulting in lacerations of the periorbita decompress themselves, relieving the excess pressure from any existing hematoma. Blindness has been described as a consequence of intraorbital hematoma that occurred under firm pressure dressings or within a relatively closed orbit.[365] Hematomas within the orbit inevitably accompany fractures and are mostly diffuse rather than localized, and the management of most hematomas should be conservative. One must be careful, however, with significant hematomas or in the presence of a moderate retrobulbar hematoma to avoid a fracture reduction that greatly reduces the size of the orbit, dramatically increasing the orbital pressure. In these patients, the globe may bulge forward and become congested. The globe pressure may be easily taken at the time of fracture reduction for monitoring. Increases in globe pressure during fracture reduction have been documented by Forrest.[602]

Vision must be examined routinely before and after surgery and documented. Light pressure dressings, although necessary, should be large and well padded by soft bulky material. All patients must be frequently checked for light perception preoperatively and postoperatively. Pupillary reactivity must be assessed before and after orbital surgery and at least twice daily for the first several days. Blindness has sometimes occurred after day 1 in orbital fracture treatment.

Ptosis of the Upper Lid

True ptosis of the upper lid should be differentiated from "pseudoptosis" resulting from the downward displacement of the eyeball in enophthalmos. True ptosis is due to loss of action of the levator palpebrae superioris. This may result from injury to or dehiscence of a thin section of the tendon, transection of the levator aponeurosis, hematomas within the muscle, or damage to the superior divisions of cranial nerve III. Intramuscular hematomas may progress to fibrosis with loss of function of a portion of the levator muscle. In patients with levator aponeurosis transection, usually only a portion of the aponeurosis has been divided. These patients may be effectively treated by early repair and can be improved even by late repair. In the face of mechanical or neurogenic ptosis, a period of 6 months or more is allowed to elapse for what is presumed to be a neurogenic injury to see how much function is recovered before ptosis repair is undertaken. Ptosis in the presence of enophthalmos should not be treated until the globe position has been stabilized by enophthalmos correction. Although a ptosis procedure is usually necessary in these patients, it is usually less than anticipated after the initial repositioning of the globe.

Vertical Shortening of the Lower Lid

Vertical shortening of the lower eyelid with exposure of the sclera below the limbus of the globe in the primary position (scleral show) may result from downward and backward displacement of the fractured inferior orbital rim. In injuries that moderately comminute the inferior orbital rim, there is a tendency for the fracture segments to sink downward and posteriorly. There is also a tendency for the reconstructive surgeon to assemble comminuted rim segments in an inferior and posterior position. A straight inferior orbital rim, rather than a curved bone structure, should be sought. The septum and lower lid are "fixed length" structures and are therefore dragged downward by their tendency to adhere to the abnormally positioned orbital rim (see Fig. 66-177). Release of the septum orbitale attachment to the orbital rim and restoration of the position of the orbital rim by osteotomy may be required. If rim repositioning procedures fail, the lid position may be improved by grafts involving skin, cartilage, conjunctiva, or a combination of lid structures in the anterior or posterior lamella. Canthal repositioning may be required to adjust the tension of the lower lid and partially compensate for decreased lid elasticity. In all patients, a thorough comprehensive evaluation of the bone and soft tissue structures of the lower orbit is necessary, including an evaluation of rim position and an evaluation of whether skin, conjunctiva, or orbital septum has been lost or contracted.

Complications Involving Lid Lamellae

The problem should be defined as occurring in "anterior lid lamellae" (skin or orbicularis) or "posterior lid lamellae" (septum, lower lid retractors, and conjunctiva) areas and a plan for operative intervention developed. Only in the actual performance of the operation can the surgeon define the true nature of the problem, release the adhesions, and stabilize the lid with appropriate grafts. Re-exploration procedures generally do not elevate the lower lid by more than 3 mm. Increased recession of the supratarsal fold often accompanies vertical shortening of the lower lid. Eyelid corrective procedures must therefore be addressed individually to both the upper lid and the lower lid, with the upper lid sequenced after the lower lid. The proper canthal position should also be assessed and must be obtained.

A number of studies have demonstrated that skin-alone flaps in lower eyelid incisions are hazardous exposures in orbital trauma as they are subject to significant contracture (>40%).[89,91,100,102,603,604] Even the subciliary skin-muscle flap has a disturbing 10% to 15% temporary incidence of scleral show and ectropion.[91] This incidence is complicated by the use of titanium plates along the inferior orbital rim, which causes fibrosis in excess of that previously seen with wire reduction of inferior orbital rim fractures.[605] Proper closure of the periosteum after orbital fracture reduction not only positions the soft tissue of the cheek but also gives the lid some vertical support.[577,606,607] One

should not only close the periosteum but, before this, also refix the heavy soft tissue structure of the cheek to fixation devices along the inferior orbital rim to decrease the pull of gravity of the heavy cheek on the lower lid. Atraumatic lid dissection technique should be accomplished, and this is sometimes difficult for less experienced operators, such as residents, where dissection goes in and out of the muscle plane, shredding the orbicularis muscle. The condition of lid shortening may relate both to soft tissue contracture or inadequate support of the soft tissue and to an improper position of the inferior orbital rim. Converse[94] adopted a lower lid incision using a subtarsal division of the orbicularis muscle to reduce such complications. He postulated that partial denervation of the inferior pretarsal orbicularis oculi muscle, such as occurs with a skin-muscle flap, could be avoided by a skin-alone dissection over the pretarsal orbicularis. Careful avoidance of injury to the orbital septum also seems to decrease the incidence of lid retraction problems.

Infraorbital Nerve Sensory Loss

Infraorbital nerve sensory loss is extremely disconcerting to patients who experience it, especially initially. The area of sensory loss usually extends from the lower lid to involve the medial cheek, the lateral portion of the nose including the ala, and the ipsilateral upper lip. The anterior maxillary teeth may be involved if the branch of the infraorbital nerve in the anterior maxillary wall is involved.

Release of the infraorbital nerve from pressure of the bone fragments within the infraorbital canal may be indicated either acutely or late after fracture treatment if it has not been decompressed and the fragments demonstrate medial displacement of the infraorbital canal with impaction into the nerve. Zygomatic fractures with medial displacement are especially likely to produce complete disturbances of infraorbital nerve sensation. It should be recalled that the anterior and middle divisions of the superior alveolar nerves pass through the anterior wall of the maxilla and are thus likely to be injured in fractures that crack or crush the ipsilateral or bilateral maxilla.

The infraorbital nerve should be visualized and freed from fracture fragments in any orbital floor or zygomatic fracture exploration. Any pressure on the nerve within the bony canal should be relieved as a routine part of inferior orbital rim exploration. Because the nerve is less protected in a groove along the floor of the orbit in the middle and posterior portions before it enters the middle portion of the inferior orbital fissure, it must be avoided in orbital dissections. In the anterior part of the orbit, it is located in a canal. After blunt or contusion injury by fracture, infraorbital nerve sensation usually improves spontaneously during a 1- to 2-year period after nerve injury. Recovery may be expected to an extent after any nerve contusion; however, complete return is often not obtained. A functional result generally occurs during 1 year, however, by partial return of sensation and accommodation.

Cerebrospinal Fluid Rhinorrhea

CSF rhinorrhea occurs frequently after upper central midface, nasoethmoidal-orbital, and anterior cranial base fractures.[447] In experimental fractures in this region, isolated fractures of the nasoethmoidal-orbital region are commonly accompanied by a short longitudinal fracture in the anterior cranial fossa paralleling the cribriform plate. Such limited CSF leaks without bone displacement may be managed conservatively if there are no other indications for repair, and they almost always close spontaneously.[391,392] Repositioning of the components of the nose and orbit, which are sometimes physically distinct from the fracture, may or may not assist CSF fistula treatment. In the author's experience, it has generally not been necessary to operate on patients for control of the CSF fistula alone in the absence of other indications for neurosurgical exploration. If the patient is being explored, any CSF leak identified should be repaired. Some authors initially use antibiotic therapy for CSF fistula in an attempt to protect patients from meningitis. Antibiotic treatment in prolonged CSF fistula has not been demonstrated to reduce infection in controlled or double-blind studies because the length of time the fistula is present is long enough for the emergence of organisms resistant to the antibiotic used, which then are able to cause "superinfection."[392,608-611]

There have been occasional reports of late post-traumatic CSF rhinorrhea or late meningitis occurring 15 to 20 years after injury.[610] These patients generally have more significant fractures extending along the anterior cranial base. In the author's experience, significant anterior cranial base fractures are often accompanied by fractures of the frontal bone or frontal sinus, and many of these injuries benefit from direct dural fistula repair.

In persistent CSF rhinorrhea, radiologic evaluation[612] and metrizamide contrast-enhanced studies[611] can often document the site of the fistula. If a simple linear fracture is observed without much displacement, the leak should close spontaneously with conservative (nonoperative) treatment. The patient must be observed for signs of impending complications, such as meningitis and extradural or intradural abscess. In such patients, it is recommended that no packing or tubes be placed in the nasal area and that smoking and forced blowing of the nose be forbidden. The head of the bed should be elevated to an angle of 60 degrees, and some neurosurgeons prefer to use lumbar spinal fluid drainage to decrease the pressure in the CSF in the belief that this will assist closure of the CSF leak.

The patient should be warned against forceful blowing of the nose, especially with the nose partially obstructed, because intranasal material may in that way be forced into the intracranial cavity. If the duration of CSF rhinorrhea is more than 10 days, an operation to close the fistula should be considered. This may involve an extracranial or intracranial approach. Because of the frequent occurrence of bilateral injuries and the exposure provided by an intracranial procedure, this approach is often used by the author. Considerable success, however, has been obtained by extracranial approaches to correct localized (source documented) fistulas. Fat grafting through an intranasal and endoscopic approach has been successful. The metrizamide contrast study may delineate the area of involvement. Collins[425] stated that CSF leakage could be confirmed by the presence of glucose in amounts of more than 30 mg of glucose per 100 mL of fluid. The amount of glucose must be related to the serum concentration of glucose. The use of glucose oxidase paper is not a reliable test for glucose. As many as 75% positive reactions have been obtained when the oxidated paper test is made in patients with normal nasal secretions. Fistulas may be documented by isotope dyes placed in the lumbar or ventricular CSF spaces; they are collected on pledgets, which then can be analyzed for the presence of the radionucleotide-tagged dye. β_2-Transferrins[613] may also confirm the diagnosis, as may dye inserted into the spinal canal and collected on intranasal pledgets.

There is no question that early reduction of facial fractures in the presence of CSF rhinorrhea is one of the best methods for treatment of CSF fistula. The objective is to obtain reduction and fixation of the fractured bones to provide support for the area of dural injury and anatomic repositioning of the adjacent bone fragments. In patients in whom significant frontal fractures are present or fractures of the base of the skull are extensive, an intracranial dural repair is recommended with exposure of the anterior portions of the cranial fossa. Frequently, the dural tear not only is present along the anterior portion of the frontal fossa but also extends from the anterior cranial base along the middle cranial base of the skull. It is less likely that significant dural tears could be successfully repaired through a limited sinus or extracranial intranasal approach, and many of these extensive tears in areas of thin dura require a dural patch.

Frontobasilar Region

Fractures of the frontal bone, frontal sinus, and orbital roof areas are encountered less commonly than other facial fractures, and practitioners are therefore less familiar with the signs, diagnosis, and management of these injuries. Unlike orbital floor fractures, orbital roof fractures are not usually isolated, and they usually extend with other fractures into adjacent areas, such as the frontal bone or frontal sinus. Because of the significant energy necessary to produce a frontal bone fracture, these injuries frequently occur in the setting of severe generalized trauma of the frontal area of the skull and face in which regional and remote injuries to other organ systems accompany the fractures. The fractures usually are not isolated to the superior orbital rim but extend throughout the orbit and into the nose and midface. Complications from acute or delayed injuries to the visual system further complicate the management of these fractures, as do complications from brain and dural penetration. Complications from the sinuses also complicate the management.

The anterior cranial fossa forms the boundary between the midface and the cranial cavity. Injuries to the frontal-basilar region provide an area for interface of multiple surgical specialties. The available literature presents varying opinions regarding the type and timing of treatment, and often the literature is "specialty focused," without the broad overview necessary for perspective.

ANATOMY

The bicortical structure of the frontal bone is thick and represents one of the stronger areas of the skull. The central inferior portion of the frontal bone is weakened by the frontal sinus structures, which are often unequal in size. The frontal bone becomes unicortical at the rim of the orbit, turning posteriorly to form the orbital roof. The orbital roof is often thin and consists of compact bone, a unicortical extension of the bicortical structure of the frontal bone. At the junction of the medial and middle thirds of the superior orbital rim, a small notch or foramen is present for the supraorbital nerve and artery. About one third of the time, the nerve travels through a foramen, and about two thirds of the time, it travels in a notch. In developing exposure with a coronal incision, one must dissect the nerve free to retract the contents of the superior orbit. If the nerve is in a canal, an osteotomy of the canal is necessary to free the nerve from the superior rim, and the nerve must be dissected absolutely subperiosteally through insertion of the superior oblique muscle. The trochlea for the superior oblique muscle is located at the medial aspect of the superior orbital rim and may be detached from the bone by careful precise subperiosteal dissection. Reattachment is not required. It is in a shallow fossa just inside the rim. The orbit increases in dimension both superiorly and inferiorly just inside the rim; in dissection, the periosteal elevator must be turned to follow this enlarging orbital contour so that the periorbita is not lacerated. Lacerations of the periorbita produce troublesome prolapse of fat, which is aggravated by placement of retractors.

The orbital roof, posterior to the rim, is a thin plate of bone that separates the anterior cranial fossa from the orbital contents. It turns upward immediately behind the rim. It is thinnest in the central portion, like the orbital floor. Medially, the orbital roof becomes quite thin and is only slightly stronger than the medial portion of the orbital floor. The orbital roof also consists of the sphenoid bone, its lesser and greater wings. Posteriorly, the orbital roof slopes downward to abut the orbital portion of the zygomatic bone laterally. It joins with the ethmoid and the frontal process of the maxilla medially. The medial aspect of the frontal bone is the internal angular process, and the lateral aspect is the external angular process. The orbital roof is often extremely thin beneath a large frontal sinus, whose extent is variable. The frontal sinus may occupy only a small portion of the frontal bone, or it may extend to pneumatize almost the entire structure including the orbital roof. The floor of the frontal sinus thus forms the medial portion of the orbital roof. Radiographic confirmation of the extent of the frontal sinus on each side is important when plans are being made for the construction of a frontal bone flap or sinus exenteration in the treatment of frontobasilar fractures. The periosteum of the orbital roof is firmly adherent anteriorly at the rim but more loosely adherent posteriorly. Thus, subperiosteal hemorrhage may dissect in the superior portion of the orbit rather freely, displacing the soft tissue downward and forward. A small fossa exists at the nasal aspect of the orbital roof just behind the orbital rim for the trochlea, the superior oblique tendon. The trochlea is located approximately 4 mm behind the most anterior aspect of the rim at its medial aspect, medial to the supraorbital foramen. Medially, the supratrochlear and dorsal nasal arteries pierce the septum orbitale above and below the trochlea. The infratrochlear branch of the nasociliary nerve accompanies the arteries in this area. The supraorbital, supratrochlear, and infratrochlear nerves are branches of the ophthalmic division of the trigeminal nerve. The septum orbitale is continuous with the periosteum overlying the orbital rim, fusing inferiorly with the levator aponeurosis just above the tarsus. The superior transverse ligament of Whitnall attaches to the orbital rim temporally between the lobes of the lacrimal gland and medially to the fascia surrounding the trochlea.

The levator muscle originates just above the optic foramen near the superior oblique muscle; the latter originates just medial to the origin of the levator (Fig. 66-203). Both proceed anteriorly, beneath the periosteum of the orbital roof; the levator muscle turns inferiorly at the Whitnall ligament, and the superior oblique muscle becomes tendinous, passing through the trochlea, then passing backward to attach to the globe. The levator muscle is separated from the periorbita by a very thin layer of fat, in which the frontal

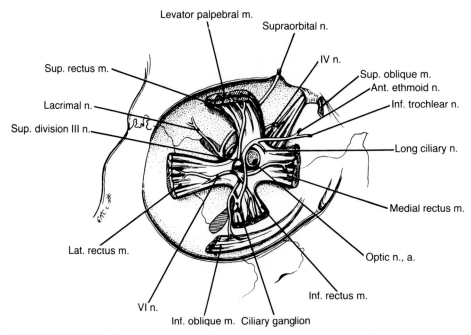

FIGURE 66-203. The contents of the superior orbital fissure and orbital apex. Note the attachments of the extraocular muscles and their innervation by the branches of cranial nerves III, IV, and VI. The sensory nerves are branches of the ophthalmic (frontal and supraorbital) divisions of the trigeminal nerve or cranial nerve V.

nerve travels. The optic foramen is a vertically ovoid anterior opening of the optic canal that measures 6 × 5 mm (Fig. 66-203). The optic nerve and ophthalmic artery, which is situated inferior and lateral to the nerve, pass through the optic canal, which enters just above and medial to the apex of the orbit. The optic canal is bounded superiorly by the greater wing of the sphenoid and inferiorly and medially by the sphenoid body. It is bounded anteriorly and medially by the posterior ethmoid cells and laterally by the bony connection between the lesser sphenoid wing and the sphenoid body.

The superior orbital fissure is formed by the greater and lesser wings of the sphenoid bone. Through the superior orbital fissure pass the superior and inferior divisions of cranial nerve III, cranial nerves IV and VI, and the ophthalmic divisions of cranial nerve V (Fig. 66-203). The dural sheaths of the optic nerve are firmly attached to the rim of the foramen and fuse with the periosteum within the canal. The nerve is suspended from the periosteum by the arachnoid. A fine vascular network accompanies the nerve through the foramen, and compression of this vascular network may account for compromised circulation to the nerve.

CLASSIFICATION AND PATTERNS

Experimental data and clinical experience indicate that fractures of the frontal skull correspond to patterns,

as do midfacial fractures, that have been organized according to the Le Fort classification. The frontal skull (so-called Le Fort IV fracture) contains thicker ridges and thinner intervening plate-like areas of bone. The thicker ridges correspond to the cranial sutures and describe a system of buttresses as in midfacial fractures. The thinner plate-like areas transilluminate. Fractures tend to extend within the thinner areas until they reach the next thicker area or buttress. Areas of the frontal skull include the temporal, the lateral frontal-orbital (extending from the supraorbital frontal bone to the coronal suture), and the central (low) frontal sinus sections (Fig. 66-204). The frontal sinus is surrounded by a semicircular buttress at its periphery. Localized fractures of the supraorbital rim occur, such as rim fractures or fractures of the external angular process of the frontal bone, which accompany high-energy zygoma fractures, but more extensive fractures usually involve one, two, or three areas of the larger sections of the frontal bone simultaneously. A common fracture pattern involves one lateral temporal-frontal-orbital area and the frontal sinus areas of the pattern, with two of the three frontal areas involved simultaneously. At lower impacts, simple linear fractures occur within a section (the weaker areas); with additional force, they extend to involve an entire sectional area with comminution and then extend to involve the adjacent section of bone.

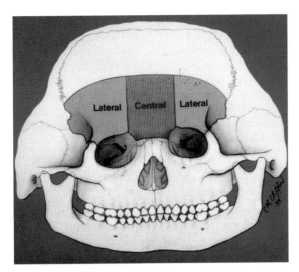

FIGURE 66-204. The three areas of the frontal skull are two lateral-temporal-orbital areas and the frontal sinus area centrally. (© Johns Hopkins University.)

Areas of weakness are described in the frontal skull, which correspond to these plate-like areas, and the weak areas are circumscribed by the cranial sutures (or buttresses). The cranial sutures are the buttresses or the "lines of strength" of the cranial vault. These correspond to the areas of strength in the Le Fort midfacial fracture classification. Fractures in the Le Fort classification occur in the lines of weakness between the areas of strength, but in the cranial vault, they occur in areas of weakness between the lines of strength. The frontal skull may be conceptualized as the Le Fort IV or frontobasilar fracture injury level. Facial injuries are often more severe on one side than on the other, and it is common to see a Le Fort IV injury superior level fracture on one side and a Le Fort III superior level injury on the other.

The dense structure of the frontal bone makes it the strongest of the bones of the face, requiring 150g per square inch[390] for the production of a fracture (see Fig. 66-194). Forces often greatly exceed the minimal force necessary for a fracture to occur. These forces in the frontal bone are four to five times the minimum required to produce fractures in the zygomatic, nasal, or mandibular subcondylar areas.

Fractures of the orbital roof may occur from either direct or indirect mechanisms. Direct roof fractures result from extension of fractures of the frontal bone, which travel through the superior orbital rim or frontal sinus and enter the orbital roof. The consistent feature is thus a fracture of the superior orbital rim. These direct fractures may either be linear, involving a single fracture of the rim and the anterior portion of the orbital roof, or involve large segments of the frontal bone, such as the lateral frontal-temporal-orbital frac-

ture (Fig. 66-204), including an entire lateral segment of the frontal bone, much of the orbital roof, the squamous portion of the temporal bone, and the frontal sinus. In larger fractures, there is greater displacement of the fragments, and the orbital roof may be comminuted in its anterior and middle sections. Comminution and severe displacement infrequently extend to involve the posterior orbit, but linear fractures may more frequently involve this area.

Indirect frontobasilar fractures can be produced in the same manner as a blowout fracture of the orbital floor. They result from a mechanism similar to that described by Smith and Regan[440] and Fujino and Makino.[614] In these injuries, a buckling force occurs that causes a fracture in an area of "least resistance." Force displacement applied in the midfrontal bone first produces an inbending in the orbital roof area. The reciprocal deformation from the impact often first occurs remote from the point of force application, such as in the orbital roof. Indirect orbital roof fractures have been reported to occur with transmission of forces from distant fracture sites, such as the nasal bones, the frontal process of the maxilla, or the caudal part of the maxillary process of the frontal bone or nasoethmoidal area, but more commonly the frontal skull. Exceptional trauma to the zygoma[375] has also been known to cause fracture lines that pass through the roof of the orbit and extend to the superior orbital fissure and optic foramen.

In a review of 1031 consecutive facial fractures, Schultz[540] found that less than 5% had supraorbital fractures. Most of these fractures resulted from automobile accidents (72%) or motorcycle accidents (14%). There is a 2:1 predominance of male patients.

SIGNS AND SYMPTOMS

The most common signs and symptoms of a fracture in the frontobasilar region are a bruise and laceration in the area of the brow or the orbit. Such a physical finding should prompt an examination for any evidence of an underlying fracture. For the orbital component of fracture, the most reliable sign is the combination of a palpebral and a subconjunctival hematoma. The palpation or the visualization of a step deformity in the rim is helpful, although it is often not apparent because of swelling and bruising. Swelling may produce upper lid ptosis from contusion, levator damage, or simply hemorrhage. In these patients, the lid should be manually opened so that the globe can be fully inspected and a proper ocular and visual examination performed to exclude globe or visual system injury.

Evaluation of the visual system is critical and should be performed as soon as the patient is stabilized. Petro et al[427] found that supraorbital fractures represented 14% of the total number of periorbital fractures but accounted for 25% of eye injuries. In their study, 50% of the patients with ocular injuries had decreased vision. The most common injury to the globe was laceration or rupture. The treatment of this complication must take precedence over other facial bone reconstructive maneuvers, even though the prognosis for vision may be poor. Retinal contusion, intraocular hemorrhage, and intraocular evidence of optic nerve damage may be present and must be documented for they have an impact on the evaluation of vision and visual potential. In particular, it is extremely important to document light perception, pupillary light reflex, and visual acuity present *before* treatment so that the treatment cannot be blamed on the visual damage produced by the fracture. If the patient is not able to cooperate for visual testing, evaluation of the pupillary response is all that is possible, but it is extremely important. Sluggishness of pupillary reaction is the first sign of optic nerve injury. A dilated pupil has no direct significance in itself with regard to optic nerve injury, as it merely indicates problems with the pupillary constrictor and its innervation. Change in reactivity to light is the important confirmation of optic nerve injury.

Evidence of paresis in a field of gaze indicates involvement of a cranial nerve or extraocular muscle. Fractures of the orbital roof commonly produce a temporary palsy of the levator muscle. They also less commonly cause a paresis of the superior rectus muscle, which can mimic incarceration of the inferior rectus muscle because the eye does not rotate upward. These two conditions must be differentiated by a thorough radiographic and clinical examination including forced duction testing. The author has not observed incarceration of a levator or superior rectus muscle in an orbital roof fracture. Fracture fragments of the roof, however, may be displaced downward, impinging on the action of these muscles. A CT scan will demonstrate bone fragments pressing into the muscles or the globe, nerves, or adnexal structures.

Hypesthesia in the distribution of the supraorbital nerve accompanies larger supraorbital fractures, especially those that involve the supraorbital foramen, and these fractures are usually the direct fractures involving the lateral frontal-temporal-orbital areas. The hypesthesia is generally temporary and usually improves with time.

Swelling in the roof of the orbit causes a downward displacement of the roof and rim of the orbit. It produces a characteristic downward and forward position of the globe (see Fig. 66-189). This is one of the most accurate clinical signs of a displaced roof fracture. The lids may not close completely over this displaced globe, resulting in corneal exposure.

Upper lid ptosis may be produced by cranial nerve damage, levator muscle contusion, or hematoma. A spectacle hematoma in the upper lid (the bruise is confined to the distribution of the orbital septum) is strong evidence of a supraorbital fracture. A high index of suspicion for a supraorbital or skull fracture should exist when lacerations involve the brow, glabella, or upper lid area or when there is significant contusion. Appropriate radiographic examination must include a carefully performed CT scan, preferably in both the axial and coronal planes, to detect small fractures.

FRONTAL LOBE AND CRANIAL NERVE INJURIES

The frontal lobe is often contused after significant supraorbital fractures, and its function and injury to it are assessed by clinical examination and CT scans. More severe brain injuries produce confusion, coma, personality change, irritability, lack of concentration, or inappropriate affect. However, many patients have few symptoms, and the initial signs may be subtle. Cranial nerve palsies exist if extension of the fractures to the cribriform plate (olfactory) and the superior orbital fissure (III, IV, V, VI) occurs (see Fig. 66-203). The silent nature of frontal lobe symptoms does not allow one to easily detect the full extent of the underlying cerebral injury on clinical examination. Significant frontal lobe contusion can occur with few if any symptoms present. Confusion, somnolence, and personality changes are the first symptoms produced. Evaluation by the Glasgow Coma Scale (see Table 66-2) documents the patient's ability to talk, move extremities, and open the eyes according to a graded response system. Lowered scores emphasize the need for precise radiologic evaluation, repeated neurologic examinations, and possibly intracranial pressure monitoring, especially if anesthesia is required. Patients with significant fractures or brain injury are at risk for rapid neurologic decompensation and require precise monitoring. The use of an intracranial pressure-monitoring device during anesthesia allows the immediate detection and treatment of any increased intracranial pressure, which may significantly alter brain perfusion or survival. Intracranial pressures of more than 20 mm Hg usually contraindicate nonemergent fracture treatment.

Fractures involving the orbital roof and anterior cranial fossa have a high frequency of dural and arachnoid lacerations, which allow CSF to leak into either the nose or the orbit. These dural fistulas also allow the passage of air inside the intracranial cavity, producing pneumocephalus. CSF leaks into the orbit (orbitorrhea) rarely cause any symptomatic problem, other than swelling, although they may be associated with meningitis if they communicate with the skin or with the nose. Meningitis is unusual after orbitorrhea. If the CSF leak communicates with the nose or sinuses,

CSF rhinorrhea exists and may be detected by examination of the fluid dripping from the patient's nose in a head-forward position. The double ring sign, explained previously, may be present when nasal secretion is examined by its absorption on a white paper towel.

The incidence of meningitis in CSF rhinorrhea ranges from 5% to 10% in those who have a CSF fistula. The frequency of meningitis increases with the duration of the leak. Although many authors favor the administration of a "prophylactic" antibiotic to protect against meningitis, it has not been demonstrated that prolonged antibiotics offer a clear advantage (see "Complications of Orbital and Nasoethmoidal-Orbital Fractures"). Any antibiotic is merely effective in eliminating a select range of bacteria, and the emergence of resistant organisms occurs quickly in multiply traumatized patients. Therefore, little long-term protection is achieved by chronic antibiotic therapy in the presence of persistent CSF fistula.

PNEUMOCEPHALUS AND ORBITAL EMPHYSEMA

Communication of the orbit and paranasal sinuses with the intracranial cavity by fracture allows the escape of air into the orbit or into the cranial cavity, producing orbital emphysema or pneumocephalus.[615] These conditions are observed in significant fractures of the frontal bone and orbital roof and resolve with reduction of the fracture, closure of the dural laceration, and healing of the sinus mucosa. There is a difference in opinion as to whether prophylactic antibiotics should be administered for these conditions on a short-term basis. Air in the orbit or within the cranium is theoretical evidence of contamination of intracranial or orbital structures with nasal or sinus organisms. It has been difficult to demonstrate, however, that the administration of antibiotics, especially on a prolonged basis, is effective in preventing infection when pneumocephalus or orbital emphysema is present. Conceptually, each of these symptoms has the same clinical significance as a CSF fistula in that it implies a communication between the nasal environment and the orbital or intracranial cavities.

ABSENCE OF THE ORBITAL ROOF AND PULSATING EXOPHTHALMOS

Fracture-dislocation or loss of the orbital roof from post-traumatic atrophy of thin bone fragments or from neurosurgical débridement after a compound skull fracture may produce the symptom of pulsating exophthalmos. Here, cerebral pulsations are transmitted directly to the globe and adnexal structures. There is usually a downward and forward displacement of the globe, which becomes exaggerated by the periodic pulsation. These symptoms are corrected by the reconstruction of the orbital roof.

CAROTID-CAVERNOUS SINUS FISTULA

Severe fractures involving both the anterior and the middle cranial fossa may result in a communication between the carotid artery and cavernous sinus,[616] which produces a syndrome of pulsating exophthalmos accompanied by severe congestion of the conjunctiva. These are rare and lethal injuries first described more than 200 years ago.[617] The syndrome is frequently accompanied by cranial nerve damage, including blindness. Its treatment is by embolization under radiographic control. Fattahi[617] has classified the lesions into four types, depending on the pattern of communication. The syndrome consists of pulsatile exophthalmos, orbital bruit, exophthalmos, chemosis, loss of vision, and cranial nerve palsies.

SUPERIOR ORBITAL FISSURE AND ORBITAL APEX SYNDROMES

Significant fractures of the orbital roof extend posteriorly to involve the superior orbital fissure and optic foramen. Involvement of the structures of the superior orbital fissure produces a symptom complex known as the *superior orbital fissure syndrome*.[545,618] This consists of partial or complete involvement of the following structures (see Fig. 66-203): the two divisions of cranial nerve III, superior and inferior, producing paralysis of the levator, superior rectus, inferior rectus, and inferior oblique muscles; cranial nerve IV, causing paralysis of the superior oblique muscle; cranial nerve VI, producing paralysis of the lateral rectus muscle; and ophthalmic division of the trigeminal nerve (V), causing anesthesia in the brow, medial portion of the upper lid, medial upper nose, and ipsilateral forehead. All symptoms of the superior orbital fissure syndrome may be partial or complete in each of the nerves. When it is accompanied by visual acuity change or blindness, the injury implies concomitant involvement of the combined superior orbital fissure (cranial nerves III, IV, V, and VI) and optic foramen (cranial nerve II). If involvement of both the optic nerve and superior orbital fissure occurs, this symptom complex is called the orbital apex syndrome (Fig. 66-205; see also Fig. 66-203).

VISUAL LOSS OR OPTIC NERVE INJURY

Visual loss is a common complication of cerebral damage or of significant facial injuries. Visual loss occurs in 6% of patients with Le Fort II and III, frontal sinus, severe zygomatic, or severe orbital fractures. Approximately 5% of patients with head trauma manifest an injury to some portion of the visual system.

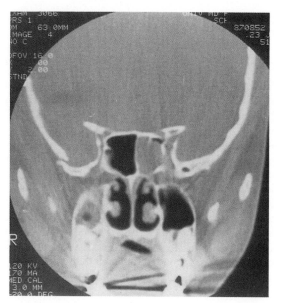

FIGURE 66-205. A coronal CT scan demonstrating a sphenoid sinus hematoma and fractures in the posterior portion of the orbit adjacent to the superior orbital fissure and optic canal. An orbital apex syndrome (symptoms of blindness and symptoms of the superior orbital fissure syndrome) was present.

About 70% of visual injuries involve the anterior visual pathways alone, with damage to the optic nerve accounting for one third of these patients. Fractures of the sphenoid bone, particularly of the body of the sphenoid, frequently accompany optic nerve and chiasmal injuries. Whereas large series of head injuries showed a 0.5% to 1.5% incidence of visual impairment, other authors demonstrated that the optic nerve is one of the most frequently injured cranial nerves, affecting 15% of survivors of *major* head injury. In an autopsy review of patients dying of acute closed head trauma, some lesions of the anterior visual pathways were present in half, and one fourth had bilateral lesions.

The mechanisms of optic nerve or visual system injury are multiple and complex and deserve careful consideration. Because of the recent early aggressive management of the trauma victim and successful control of intracranial pressure and other lifesaving therapies, there has been a significant drop in the mortality rate of patients with severe head injuries from 50% to 25%. Consideration of the visual injury demands priority, especially for these surviving patients. Of survivors of significant brain injury, 45% are capable of returning to their preinjury occupation; another 45% are able to perform a lesser job or activities of daily living. The great variety of residual visual abnormalities in this expanding survival population is currently being recorded. Assessment of visual func-

tion is often difficult in an individual with altered states of consciousness. If the vision is found to be impaired, decisions must be made about further evaluation and management based on the site of the injury. Visual impairment is defined as a visual acuity of less than 20/60, and functional blindness as less than 20/200. If less than 20% of the visual field remains, the condition of visual field restriction may be classified as blindness.

Optic Nerve Anatomy

The optic nerves are 50 mm in length and extend from the chiasm to the posterior aspect of the globe. For purposes of analysis, four segments of the optic nerve may be identified: the intracranial, the intracanalicular, the intraorbital, and the intraocular portions. The smallest portion of the optic nerve is the intraocular portion, which exits the globe nasal to and slightly above the fovea. The nerve travels through a rigidly confined scleral canal where a "watershed" area of circulation occurs between the retinal and the ciliary microcirculations in the immediate retrobulbar portion of the optic nerve. This section of the microcirculation is thus susceptible to infarction from swelling or interstitial hemorrhage within the rigid confines of the scleral canal. In addition, transmission of increased intracranial pressure into the optic nerve sheath can rupture intradural vessels and produce ischemia. A 32% incidence of intraocular hemorrhage was reported in patients with intradural hemorrhage. Preretinal hemorrhages that have broken into the vitreous through the internal limiting membrane (Terson syndrome) have been described in patients with severe cerebral trauma with intracranial hypertension.

The orbital portion of the optic nerve extends from the posterior aspect of the globe to the optic canal. It is somewhat longer than the actual straight-line distance involved and thus has a loose, slightly redundant course through the orbit. The optic nerve is covered by the dura, arachnoid, and pia mater from the brain. The nerve is surrounded by orbital fat and extraocular muscles. The central retinal artery and vein course forward in the orbit within the fat below the optic nerve. At a point 10 mm posterior to the globe, the vessels enter the optic nerve, piercing the dura mater and arachnoid. The anterior intraorbital portion of the optic nerve is vascularized by centrifugal branches of the central retinal artery, whereas the remainder of the intraorbital portion receives only pial circulation.

The intracanalicular portion of the optic nerve measures 10 mm in length and 4 mm in diameter. It traverses the optic canal, which is formed by the union of the two roots of the lesser wing of the sphenoid bone. The canal, averaging 5 to 10 mm in length and 4 to 6 mm in width, travels posterior and medially. The canal contains the ophthalmic artery as well as fibers of the sympathetic plexus with an extension of the sheaths of the meninges. The intracanalicular optic nerve is tightly fixed within the optic canal by the dura mater, which divides into two layers as it enters the orbit. One remains as the outer sheath of the optic nerve and the other becomes the orbital periosteum. The intraorbital space communicates through the optic canal and around the optic nerve to the posterior aspect of the globe.

The intracranial portion of the optic nerve is 10 mm in length. It is located in the diaphragma sellae. Immediately lateral to the optic nerve is the internal carotid artery, which gives off the ophthalmic artery just inferior to the nerve. On the ventral surface of each frontal lobe, the olfactory tract is separated from the optic nerve by the anterior cerebral and anterior communicating arteries. The intracranial portion of the optic nerve terminates at the optic chiasm.

Types of Optic Nerve Injury

From a practical standpoint, indirect injury to the optic nerve may be divided into two categories: anterior, in which ophthalmoscopic abnormalities are evident; and posterior, in which the fundus initially appears normal.[619] Anterior injury denotes involvement of the intraocular optic nerve and that portion of the intraocular segment containing the central retinal artery. In all instances, ophthalmoscopic abnormalities are visible. Central retinal artery occlusion produces an edematous retina, a pale optic disc, thread-like arterioles, and visible slugging of blood within the retinal vasculature. Traumatic ischemic optic neuropathy results in a diffusely swollen disc, with the remainder of the fundus normal in appearance.

The diagnosis of posterior indirect optic nerve injuries is based on evidence of optic nerve dysfunction and the absence of ophthalmoscopic abnormalities on initial examination and no evidence of chiasmal injury.[619] Optic disc pallor and loss of the retinal nerve fiber layer become apparent during a 4- to 8-week period. It is presumed that the lesion lies somewhere between the entry of the central retinal artery into the optic nerve and the optic chiasm. The intracanalicular portion of the optic nerve is by far the most frequent site of injury. Visual field defects may be total or partial. Partial visual field defects fall into two main categories, central scotomas and nerve fiber bundle defects.

The mechanisms of indirect optic nerve injury include complete or incomplete lacerations of the optic nerve and lesions produced by bone deformation or fracture, including those in the optic canal and those secondary to fractures of the orbital roof or of the anterior clinoid process.[619] Vascular insufficiency may be produced by either ischemia or infarction. Concussion and contusion of nerve fibers cause temporary or permanent nerve damage. Hemorrhage into the optic nerve sheath or intraneural hemorrhage also produces nerve deficits.

The degree of recovery depends on the extent of nerve damage and the mechanism of nerve injury. For example, ischemia produced by an accumulation of hematoma within the optic canal might be relieved by decompression.[620] Tearing of nerve fibers within the optic canal is not improved by decompression of the canal unless the attendant swelling produced further interference with nerve circulation. Concussion, a transient disturbance, usually recovers spontaneously, whereas contusion of the nerve is identified by a histologic structural alteration of neural tissue characterized by extravasation of blood, swelling, circulatory impairment, and perhaps cell death. The nerve lesion on histologic examination has a characteristic triangular shape with the apex internal to its base. Necrosis of some nerve fibers follows, and the ensuing visual loss is permanent.[619,621] The author has observed rare instances of partial return of optic nerve function in the visual system, mostly occurring in children.[593,622-625]

Treatment

It is obvious that multiple conditions may contribute to an "indirect" optic nerve injury. Some of these might be amenable to improvement by surgical decompression,[620] but many would not. Spontaneous improvement of impaired but not absent vision probably accounts for some of the confusion in the literature, which expresses widely divergent opinions about the advisability of decompression of the optic canal. A comparison of series in which most patients are stated to improve after surgical decompression[620] shows that only a few had no light perception whatsoever before the operations; most had "impaired vision." Most authors have noted a considerable frequency[595] of spontaneous improvement in patients with light perception or better visual acuity; therefore, this group is presumed likely to improve without surgery, and especially with megadose steroids.[55,626-629] Most authors have experienced few successes after decompression of the optic nerve for blindness.[365,586,587,630-633] Some[584,596,634-637] have experienced successes, and there has been more enthusiasm and better definition of who might favorably respond to decompression.[365] Decompression may involve the orbit (lateral canthotomy, release of orbital septum, and opening of the incisions[638-640]) or the nerve. Guidelines for decompression of the nerve are as follows:

Optic nerve decompression should not be undertaken as an elective procedure or on an unconscious patient; if the loss of vision is associated with a nonreactive pupil, and the loss occurred at the moment of impact, the procedure is probably not going to result in improvement; if the loss of vision or the loss of pupillary response to light develops after the moment of impact, the possibility of an operation improving the situation should be considered; if it cannot be determined that the loss of vision or pupillary response was delayed, a period of 4 to 6 days should elapse, and if spontaneous improvement occurs, no surgery should be undertaken. If improvement does not occur, it might be reasonable to decompress the optic canal.[619]

Currently, some authors favor a more rapid progression to decompression.[596] Most authors administer megadose steroids (spinal cord injury doses)[628,629] when an optic nerve injury is apparent with the idea that they might protect the nerve against the ischemic effects of "vicious circle" circulatory disturbances.

There are several operative approaches for optic nerve decompression. The two most commonly employed are the transorbital and transethmoid routes; others are the intranasal and intrasinus approaches as well as the transfrontal (transcranial) approach, which requires a full craniotomy and usually results in division of the olfactory tracts.

FRONTAL BONE FRACTURES

Fractures of the lower portion of the frontal bone and supraorbital and glabellar regions are less frequently encountered injuries, occurring either independently or in conjunction with nasoethmoidal or other higher facial injuries, such as the Le Fort II or III fractures. Schultz[540] noted that patients suffering supraorbital and glabellar fractures required a longer average hospital stay than did other facially injured patients irrespective of the cause of the injury.

After fracture displacement, the rim and roof of the orbit tend to flatten where they normally constitute a doubly arched structure that bows superiorly both from medial to lateral and from posterior to anterior. Thus, the fractured supraorbital roof tends to assume a flattened medial to lateral and anterior to posterior projection, which is accompanied by a lower and more forward (anterior) globe position.

The author has observed concomitant fractures of the supraorbital arch, depressed fracture of the glabellar region, and nasoethmoidal-orbital fractures in many patients. This combination of fractures commonly occurs simultaneously in the same patient.

When bone fragments are missing or not usable, the frontal cranial bone flap may be split and portions used as a bone graft. Calvarial bone grafts are also useful to reconstruct severely comminuted segments of the orbital roof, orbital floor, and medial or lateral orbital walls. They also may replace small unusable fragments of the frontal sinus walls. In the 1970s, it was fashionable to remove fractured frontal bone fragments, allowing healing of the skin against the dura to occur, and then to recall the patient for secondary cranial reconstruction a number of months after the injury

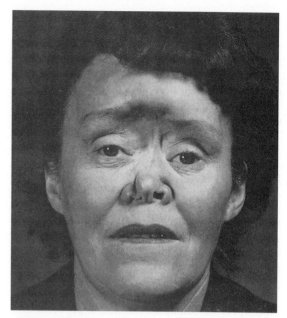

FIGURE 66-206. An example of the deformity resulting from a severe nasoethmoidal-orbital fracture and fracture of the glabellar portion of the frontal bone involving the frontal sinus. The patient suffered severe head injury and was in a coma for 72 hours; neurosurgical intervention was required for brain damage (removal of bone fragments penetrating the frontal lobes and the repair with a dural patch for CSF rhinorrhea).

(Fig. 66-206). In many of these patients, the extensive deformity of frontal bone or frontal sinus exenteration makes reconstructive surgery more difficult, and the results are inferior to early reconstruction.

Radiographic diagnosis requires axial and coronal CT scans that demonstrate the frontal and ethmoid sinuses, the frontal bone, the anterior cranial base, the middle cranial base, the orbit, the nasoethmoidal-orbital areas, the brain, and the meninges (Fig. 66-207). Only a thorough CT examination can define the extent of soft tissue, brain, and bone injury. Both bone and soft tissue windows are essential for evaluation of the cranial cavity and the brain.

Treatment nearly always involves an open reduction through either a laceration or a surgical incision. Exposure for a localized supraorbital fracture may occasionally be achieved through an appropriate laceration. Although an incision immediately above the eyebrow has been advocated, the scar, even if the incision is correctly placed, is apparent, and this approach is *never* used by the author. The scar from *any* supraorbital eyebrow incision is perceptible and is usually inferior to the aesthetic result obtained with a coronal incision. Incisions within the eyebrow produce a noticeable, hairless scar separating the upper and lower follicles of the eyebrow and are absolutely to be avoided.

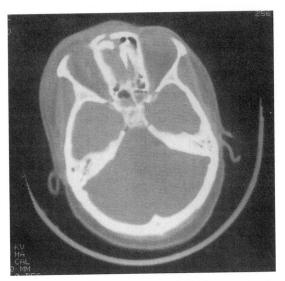

FIGURE 66-207. CT scan showing a fracture involving the cranial base and upper portion of the nasoethmoidal-orbital area. Sphenoid and ethmoid hematomas are present, implying the possibility of optic nerve damage.

This intrabrow technique is always more apparent than even a suprabrow incision.

The best technique of exposure in major fractures involving the frontal bone is the coronal incision. This allows a combined intracranial and extracranial approach, making visualization of all areas possible, including repair of dural tears, débridement of any necrotic sections of frontal lobe, and repair of the bone structures. Reduction and realignment of the fracture fragments are performed after the brain and dural injuries have been managed. Initially, fragments can be linked together with multiple interfragment wires and then stabilized by rigid fixation.

In the chainlink fence technique,[118,422,641] the bones are initially stabilized with interfragment wires linked in such a way as to achieve considerable multidirectional stability. The reconstructed bone is then placed into the defect, where it may be affixed to adjacent stable structures by junctional rigid fixation. Plate and screw fixation for frontal bone fractures may be accomplished by drill holes with a guarded burr with a stop at 4 to 5 mm; this drills just through the anterior table for 4- or 5-mm screws, avoiding penetration of the dura because the distinct shoulder stops the advance of the drill. The frontal bone flap may also provide a generous calvarial bone graft donor site, if it is split. Infection after frontal bone replacement may be diagnosed by signs of inflammation or cellulitis and drainage from the wound. CT scans, plain films, and single-photon emission computed tomographic images suggest moth-eaten and nonliving bone.[642]

FRONTAL SINUS FRACTURES

The frontal sinuses are paired structures that have only an ethmoidal anlage at birth. They have no frontal bone component initially. They begin to be detected at 3 years of age, but significant pneumatic expansion does not begin until approximately 7 years of age. The full development of the frontal sinuses is complete by the age of 18 to 20 years.[643] The frontal sinuses are lined with respiratory epithelium, which consists of a ciliated membrane with mucus-secreting glands. A blanket of mucin is essential for normal function, and the cilia beat this mucin in the direction of the nasofrontal ducts. The exact function of the paranasal sinuses is still incompletely determined. When injured, they serve as a focus for infection, especially if duct function is impaired. Their structure, however, often protects the intracranial contents from injury by absorbing energy.

The predominant form of frontal sinus injury is fracture. Fracture involvement of the frontal sinus has been estimated to occur in 2% to 12% of all cranial fractures, and severe fractures occur in 0.7% to 2% of patients with cranial or cerebral trauma.[643] Approximately one third of fractures involve the anterior table alone, and 60% involve the anterior table and posterior table or ducts. The remainder involve the posterior wall alone (Fig. 66-208). In 40% of frontal sinus fractures, there is an accompanying dural laceration.[643] Frontal sinus fractures should be characterized by description of both the anatomic location of the fractures and their displacement. Displacement of posterior wall fractures has more serious implications for dural fistula. Fractures that extend into the duct system may compromise drainage, and therefore elimination of the sinus on that basis alone may be indicated.

Diagnosis

The physical signs that accompany frontal sinus fractures include lacerations and periorbital or forehead hematomas. Lacerations, bruises, hematomas, and contusions constitute the most frequent signs. Skull fracture must be suspected if any of these signs are present. Anesthesia of the supraorbital nerve may be present. CSF rhinorrhea may occur. There may or may not be subconjunctival or periorbital ecchymoses with or without air in the orbit or intracranial cavity. In some patients, a depression may be observed over the frontal sinus, but swelling is usually predominant in the first few days after the injury, which may obscure the depression. The fractures are demonstrated on radiographic examination and may involve hematomas or air-fluid levels in the frontal sinus, which should imply the absence of duct function, especially if they persist. Small fractures may be difficult to detect, especially if they are nondisplaced. Therefore, the first presentation of a frontal sinus fracture may occasionally

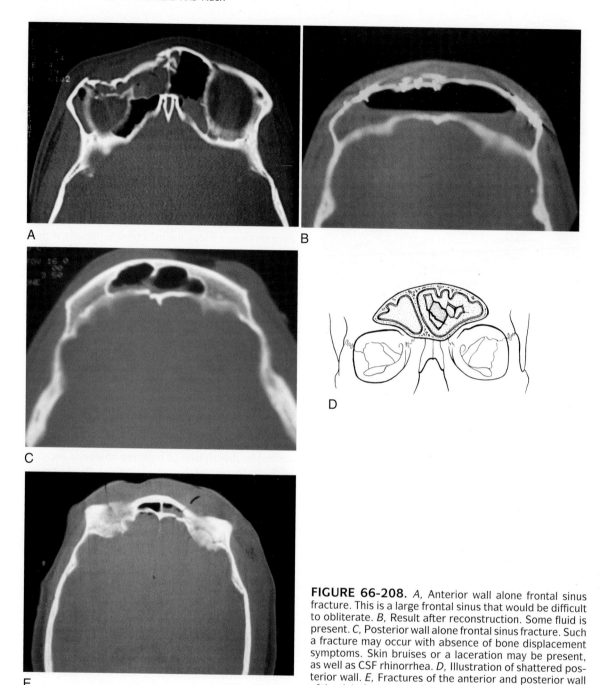

FIGURE 66-208. *A,* Anterior wall alone frontal sinus fracture. This is a large frontal sinus that would be difficult to obliterate. *B,* Result after reconstruction. Some fluid is present. *C,* Posterior wall alone frontal sinus fracture. Such a fracture may occur with absence of bone displacement symptoms. Skin bruises or a laceration may be present, as well as CSF rhinorrhea. *D,* Illustration of shattered posterior wall. *E,* Fractures of the anterior and posterior wall of the right frontal sinus. Orbital roof fractures are present.

be an infection or symptom of frontal sinus obstruction, such as mucocele or abscess formation.[644-646]

Infection in the frontal sinus may produce serious complications because of its location near the brain structures.[647] Infections include meningitis, extradural or intradural abscess, intracranial abscess, osteomyelitis of the frontal bone, and osteitis in devitalized bone fragments.[648-656]

The prevention of infectious and obstructive complications is emphasized in the management strategies proposed for frontal sinus injuries. The close communication of the intracranial venous sinus system with the mucous membrane of the frontal sinuses is a significant factor in both the production of osteomyelitis and the extension of the infectious process into the intracranial cavity, cavernous sinus, and brain substance. The development of a frontal sinus mucocele is linked to obstruction of the nasofrontal duct,[87,576,657-662] which is involved with fractures in more than one third to one half of patients with frontal sinus injury. The duct passes through the anterior ethmoidal air cells to exit adjacent to the ethmoidal infundibulum. Blockage of the nasofrontal duct[575] prevents adequate drainage of the normal mucosal secretions and predisposes to the development of obstructive epithelium-lined cysts or mucoceles. Mucoceles[663-665] may also develop when islands of mucosa are trapped by scar tissue within fracture lines and attempt to grow after the injury, producing a mucous membrane-lined cystic structure, which is obstructed. When the mucous membrane of the sinuses is eradicated in the areas except for the region of the duct, the sinus rapidly acquires a new mucosal cover by proliferation of duct mucosa. The sinus is completely obliterated only when the duct is also deprived of its lining and when the bone is burred, eliminating the foramina of Breschet,[421] in which it has been demonstrated that mucosal ingrowth occurs along veins in the walls of the sinuses.[666-668] Regrowth of mucosa can occur from any portion of the frontal sinus, especially if it is incompletely débrided, and regrowth of mucosa implies incomplete débridement. The mucosa may attach itself to the frontal lobe dura, resulting in a difficult "cleanup" problem. Investigators consider invaginations of mucosa along the channels or veins extending into the bone (foramina of Breschet) the cause of regrowth of mucosa in many patients.[421] Thus, they recommend not only stripping of the mucoperiosteum but also light burring of the surface of the bone to reduce these mucosal invaginations. This refers to a concept called the tenacity of frontal sinus mucosa espoused by Paul Donald.[421]

Treatment

In previous years, a radical removal of both bone and mucous membrane was performed, collapsing the skin against the dura. This treatment was especially favored in open fractures because of the more than theoretical potential for contamination of bone fragments (see Fig. 66-206). The patient was then referred for secondary reconstructive cranioplasty after 6 months to a year.

The indications for surgical intervention in frontal sinus fractures include depression of the anterior table, radiographic demonstration of involvement of the nasofrontal duct with presumed future nonfunction, obstruction of the duct with persistent air-fluid levels, mucocele formation, and fractures of the posterior table that are displaced and presumably have lacerated the dura.[656,669,670] Some authors recommend exploration of any posterior table fracture or any fracture in which an air-fluid level is visible. Others have a more selective approach, exploring posterior wall fractures only

if their displacement exceeds the width of the posterior table (this distance suggests simultaneous dural laceration). Simple linear fractures of the anterior and posterior sinus walls that are undisplaced are observed by many clinicians. On occasion, meningitis or evidence of a CSF fistula develops in one of these patients even if only a linear fracture involves the posterior wall. Evidence of an air-fluid accumulation is a possible sign of a CSF leak that is not escaping from the nose because of duct obstruction.

Any depressed frontal sinus fracture of the anterior wall potentially requires exploration and wall replacement in an anatomic position to prevent contour deformity. The anterior wall of the sinus may be explored by an appropriate local laceration, a coronal incision, or (recently) endoscopically. Anterior wall fragments are elevated and plated into position. When multiple fragments of the anterior wall must be removed, the mucous membrane is usually eradicated in that section. Regrowth may occur from the remainder of the sinus. If obliteration of the nasofrontal duct[49,559,660] and sinus is desired, the mucosa is thoroughly stripped, even into the recesses of the sinus, and the nasofrontal ducts are occluded with well-designed "formed-to-fit" calvarial bone plugs. If most of the posterior bony wall is intact, the cavity may be filled with either fat or cancellous bone; cancellous bone is preferred by the author. The iliac crest provides a generous source of rich cancellous bone.[565,671-673] Alternatively, the cavity may be left vacant, a process called osteoneogenesis. The cavity fills slowly with a combination of bone and fibrous tissue, but it is more frequently infected in the author's experience than are sinuses treated with cavity filling. If the posterior table is missing, no grafting need be performed for localized defects, but it is emphasized that the floor of the anterior cranial fossa should be reconstructed with bone ("cranialization"). Any involved ethmoid sinuses should be treated in the same fashion, removing abnormally injured mucosa and placing bone grafts over the duct and floor defect. Although many clinicians, especially neurosurgeons, place muscle fascia or artificial material into the duct, the author prefers cortical bone. It has been demonstrated in chronic frontal sinus infection that fat obliteration acts to prevent the regrowth of the epithelium and to fill the dead space of the sinus.[668] Fat has worked well in chronically infected sinuses, but its efficacy in the multiply fractured sinus is disputed by many individuals, including Donald.[668] Most craniofacial surgeons prefer bone, and the author prefers cancellous iliac bone for frontal sinus obliteration. The fragments of the anterior wall of the sinus may be replaced after obliteration of the sinus cavity, supplementing any bone defects by bone grafts or replacing small pieces of anterior wall bone with a larger, more contoured graft for aesthetic improvement (Figs. 66-209 and

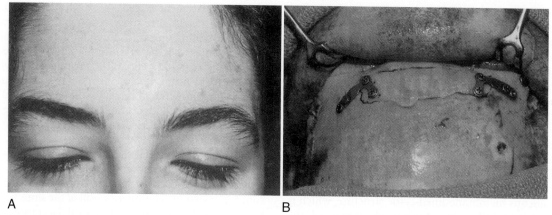

A   B

FIGURE 66-209. *A,* The result obtained after reconstruction of the frontal sinus with a bone plug. *B,* The anterior wall of the frontal sinus may be replaced with plate and screw fixation after removal of its mucosa and bone obliteration of the sinus cavity with cancellous grafting. Iliac crest cancellous bone is preferred by the author for frontal sinus obliteration.

66-210). The final brow contour is dependent on the accuracy of the rim and frontal bone reconstruction and bone resorption. In patients in whom rigid fixation is used, the fixation devices may become visible in the postoperative period as the bone resorbs away from the plate.

The orbital roof should be reconstructed primarily by thin bone grafts placed external to the orbital cavity. An intracranial exposure is often required for this orbital roof reconstruction. Primary reconstruction usually produces a more superior aesthetic result than secondary reconstruction. In cranialization, the posterior wall of the frontal sinus is removed, effectively making the frontal sinus a part of the intracranial cavity. The dead space may be filled with cancellous bone[673-676] (preferred) or left open. Any communication with the nose by the nasofrontal duct or with the ethmoid sinuses should be sealed with carefully designed bone grafts.

GALEAL FLAPS. In the treatment of extensive frontal sinus defects, a galeal flap[677,678] designed with a pedicle of the superficial temporal artery is a method proposed by Ferri et al[678] for vascularized soft tissue obliteration of frontal sinus defects (see Fig. 66-209). Frontal sinus mucosa, when damaged, has a potential to develop cysts, which erode the bone.[679] Primary and secondary cysts have a tendency to erode through the bone into the orbit or into the intracranial cavity. Several studies have demonstrated that the lining of a mucous cyst is capable of producing bone-resorbing factors, such as prostaglandin E_2 and collagenase. Bone resorption is therefore stimulated. Many authors make the point that simple stripping of mucosa is not sufficient to remove the frontal sinus mucosa, which tracks along the veins extending into bone. Remnants of mucosa may remain

stuck in tiny bone crevices. These areas can lead to regrowth of mucosa and thus to mucoceles. Current therapy requires that hidden mucosa be removed by burring of the inner table of the frontal sinus or the ethmoid sinus.

When mucoceles become infected, extradural and intracranial complications of sinusitis can occur, such as extradural abscess and meningitis. Commonly, mucoceles become colonized with group B alpha-hemolytic streptococci, *Haemophilus influenzae*, *Staphylococcus*, and *Bacteroides*. Antibiotic coverage must be sufficient to prevent intracranial infection and should include antibiotics that have CSF penetration and a broad spectrum against gram-positive, gram-negative, and anaerobic organisms. Cefuroxime and metronidazole will cover the listed organisms.

The use of artificial material to reconstruct frontal sinus defects where previous infection has occurred has a high incidence of infection, probably double the normal. Isolating the cranial defect from the nose with bone and obtaining cultures and Gram stains negative for bacteria are ways in which the area can be ensured to be sterile. Bordley[665] has concluded that the average interval between the primary injury and a frontal sinus mucocele is $7^1/_2$ years.

ENDOSCOPIC REPAIR. Endoscopically assisted repair of frontal sinus fractures[680-688] may take two forms: (1) internasal drainage of the nasofrontal duct, with or without stenting, and (2) endoscopically assisted repair through a coronal approach. Chen et al[680] have reviewed their series and have listed the criteria and effectiveness. The endoscope may be used intranasally to open the orifice of the nasofrontal duct. A stent may or may not be used for duct support. Classically, nasofrontal duct drainage procedures have not

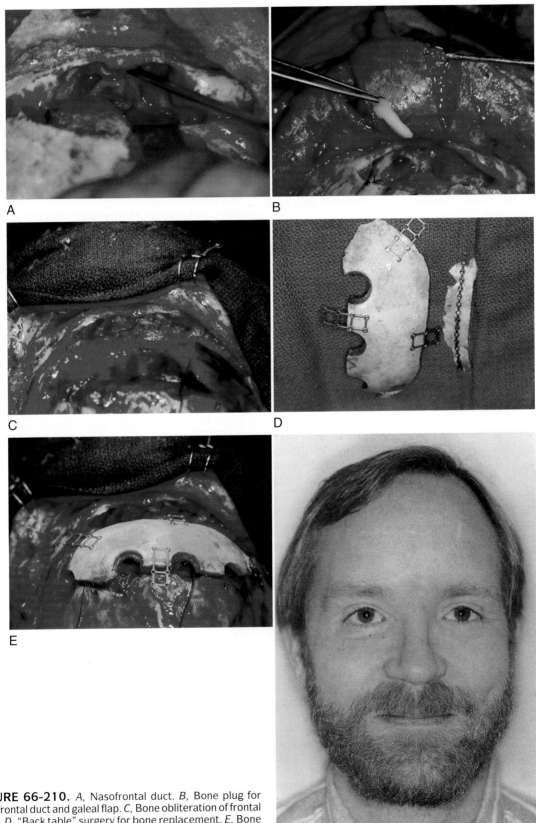

FIGURE 66-210. *A*, Nasofrontal duct. *B*, Bone plug for nasofrontal duct and galeal flap. *C*, Bone obliteration of frontal sinus. *D*, "Back table" surgery for bone replacement. *E*, Bone reconstruction and cranialization of the frontal sinus; intracranial neurosurgery. *F*, Postoperative result.

enjoyed much enthusiasm because the long-term occlusion rate exceeds 50%. The success of nasofrontal duct drainage in frontal sinus trauma is not known; only isolated reports have been presented without a large series. The technique involves cannulation of the nasofrontal duct orifices and drainage of the obstructed sinus. Conceptually, both ducts would need to be manipulated. Drainage of one hemisinus by removal of the intrasinus septum, expecting one sinus to drain the other, has not had long-term success. Presumably, this must be because of the directional nature of the intrasinus mucosal cilia. Follow-up CT scans are necessary 1 year after sinus surgery to confirm patency of the sinus. Treatment of mucoceles has been described.[687,688]

The endoscope has also been popular for aesthetic forehead procedures. It can be used in this fashion to expose the area of the frontal sinus to assist with reduction and fixation of depressed fractures isolated to the anterior wall. After the endoscope is used to establish an optical cavity, a small incision is made over the frontal sinus to assist reduction and for screwdriver placement. The fracture fragments are reduced by direct pressure with an elevator or hook placed through the counter-incision. Sometimes, the depressed fragments are locked in their depressed position by overlapping edges of fractured bone. In these patients, one fragment might have to be removed from the group to permit reduction of the others. After reduction, the fragments might be considered stable or may need stabilization by application of plates and screws. The screwdriver must be inserted through the counterincision. Plates and screws in the frontal bone should be of the lowest profile because the bone generally partially resorbs after replacement, making the fixation devices "silhouette" by standing off the plane of the resorbed bone. As of this writing, it is not feasible to treat frontal sinus fractures other than simple depressed fractures of the anterior wall with this technique.

CRANIOPLASTY. Cranioplasties may be performed with bone or artificial material (Fig. 66-211).[689] Bone cranioplasty should be performed under ideal conditions or otherwise at the time of the injury if small bone fragments need to be replaced by a larger bone graft section. Cranioplasties may be performed with hydroxyapatite cement (Fig. 66-212), methyl methacrylate[690] (Fig. 66-213), or titanium mesh (Fig. 66-214).[605,691] Brittle substances such as hydroxyapatite cement may fracture at their periphery, undergo chronic movement, and produce a foreign body reaction often colonized by *Staphylococcus epidermidis*, requiring removal. Complex reconstructions with use of CT-generated skull models with pre-formed cranioplasty sections[692] are possible, but methyl methacrylate molded at the time still has the best record of performance.

GUNSHOT WOUNDS OF THE FACE

The treatment of gunshot and shotgun wounds of the face remains controversial in that most authors advocate delayed reconstruction. Immediate reconstruction[693,694] and immediate soft tissue closure with "serial second-look" procedures have recently been advocated.[695,696] A philosophy advocating delayed closure of these difficult wounds is frequently espoused in the literature,[697,698] especially by those who have questioned the effective rehabilitation of the affected individuals, many of whom represent suicide attempts.[699] Recent experiences emphasize the safety and efficacy of

Text continued on p. 350

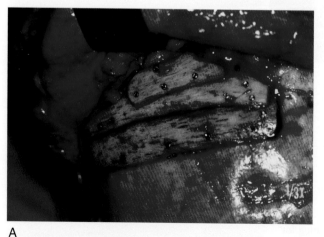

A

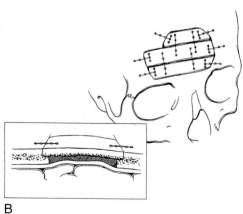

B

FIGURE 66-211. *A,* Bone cranioplasty with split ribs. *B* and *C,* Illustrations—ribs must be curved and placed under tension for proper curvature.

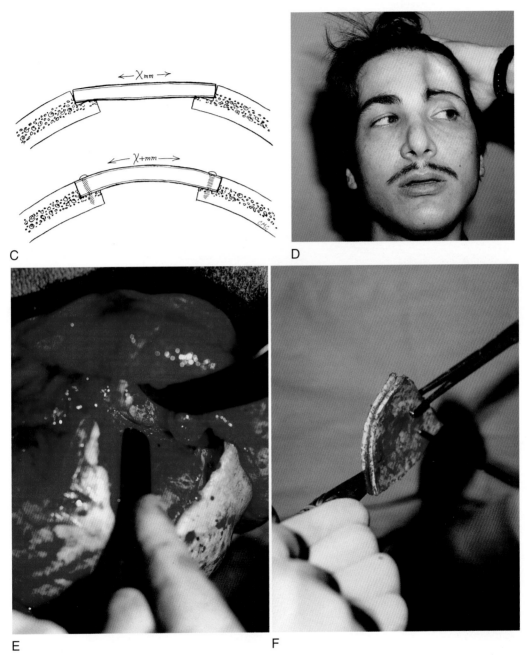

FIGURE 66-211, cont'd. *D,* Cranial defect. *E,* Defect exposed through coronal incision. *F,* Split skull
cranioplasty.
Continued

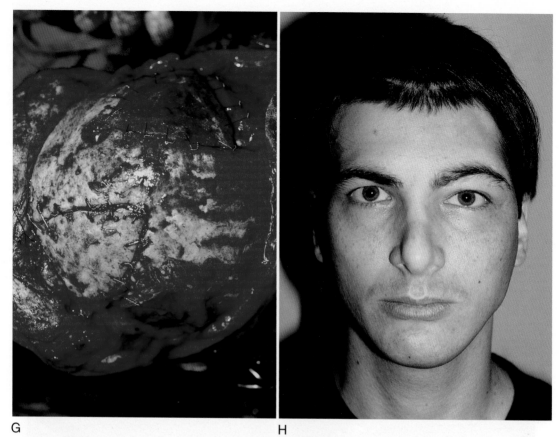

G   H

FIGURE 66-211, cont'd. *G,* Cranioplasty completed. *H,* Postoperative result. (From Crawley WA, Manson PN: Problems and complications in cranioplasty. Perspect Plast Surg 1991;5:107.)

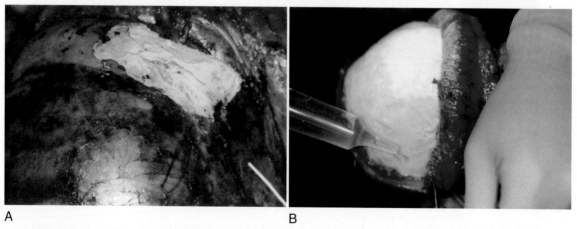

A   B

FIGURE 66-212. *A,* Hydroxyapatite cement onlay cranioplasty. *B,* Hydroxyapatite full-thickness cranioplasty over metal mesh.

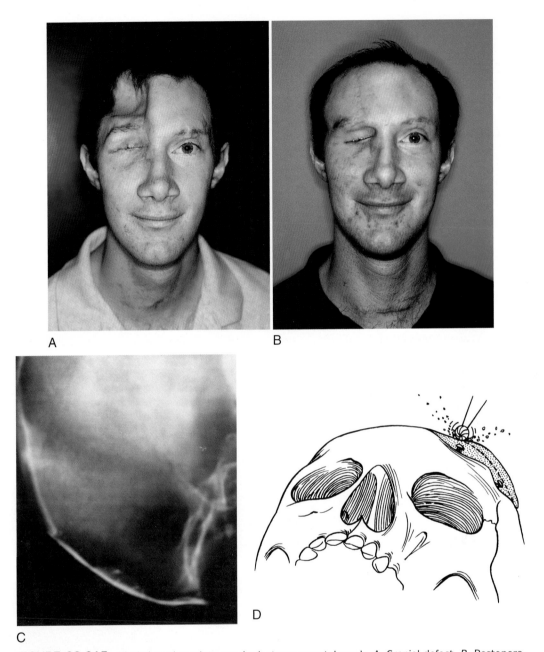

A

B

C

D

FIGURE 66-213. Methyl methacrylate cranioplasty over metal mesh. *A,* Cranial defect. *B,* Postoperative result. *C,* Radiograph. *D,* Contouring of onlay methyl methacrylate over screws by shaping bit.

Continued

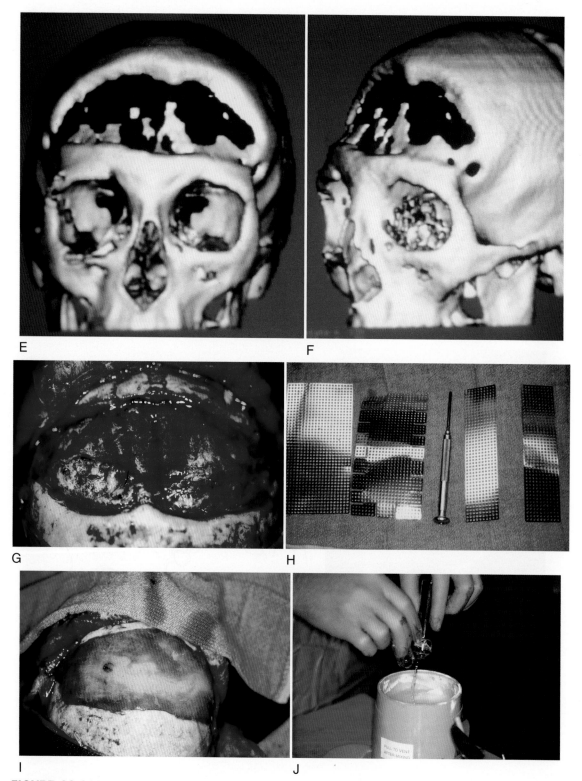

FIGURE 66-213, cont'd. *E* and *F,* Another defect. *G,* Exposure of defect. *H,* Metal mesh as a base. *I,* Methyl methacrylate over metal base. *J,* Methyl methacrylate can be mixed in a vacuum bowl connected to suction to reduce exposure of personnel to toxic fumes.

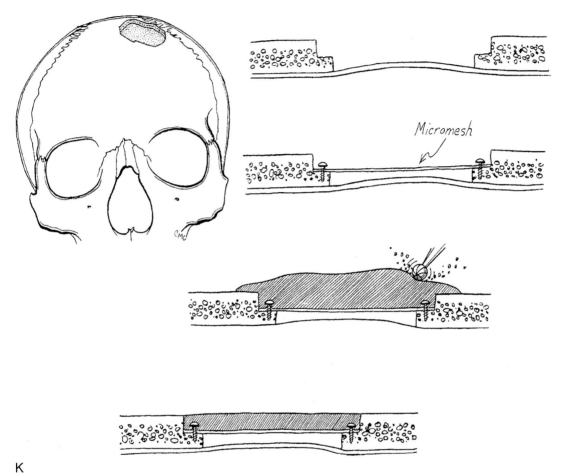

K

FIGURE 66-213, cont'd. *K,* Technique of methyl methacrylate cranioplasty—a trough cut into the edges of the defect. The mesh is anchored to the inner lip of the groove. The methyl methacrylate is used over the mesh. A flat contour is achieved. (From Crawley WA, Manson PN: Problems and complications in cranioplasty. Perspect Plast Surg 1991;5:107. From Manson P: Reoperative facial fracture repair. In Grotting J, ed: Reoperative Aesthetic and Reconstructive Plastic Surgery. St. Louis, Quality Medical Publishing, 1995:677.)

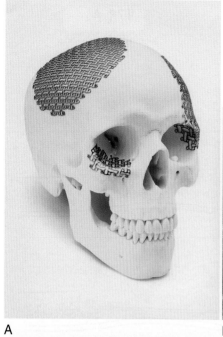

A

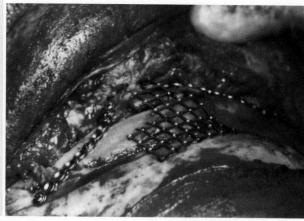

B

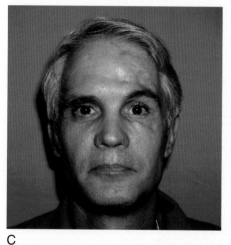

C

FIGURE 66-214. *A,* Titanium cranioplasty. *B,* Titanium mesh used to span a cranial defect. *C,* Irregular contour after primary frontal bone reconstruction. (*A* courtesy of Synthes Maxillofacial, Paoli, Pa.)

immediate soft tissue closure and bone reconstruction in an anatomically correct position. These two principles prevent soft tissue shrinkage and loss of soft tissue position and provide improved functional and aesthetic results with shorter periods of disability and an improved potential for rehabilitation, both functionally and aesthetically. When proper surgical judgment is exercised, significant complications are not increased by this emphasis on early definitive treatment, which involves primary soft tissue closure and immediate bone reconstruction and serial return to the operating room for débridement and closure.

All ballistic injuries to the face involve both soft tissue and bone injury, and many have areas of soft tissue and bone loss.[697] The degree of injury depends on the mass and the speed of the projectile. Other factors may affect the injury. The energy transmitted to the structures relates principally to the mass and speed of the projectile by the formula kinetic energy = mass × velocity^2/2 g.[700] If one doubles the velocity of a missile, one squares the kinetic energy. Mass is also important because doubling the mass doubles the kinetic energy imparted. Other factors influence tissue damage, such as tumbling of the projectile, presenting area of the missile, soft tissue drag, density of the tissue, and soft tissue distance penetrated.[701]

Ballistic injuries are classified into low-, medium-, and high-energy deposit injuries.[702,703] Low-energy deposit ballistic weapons usually involve projectiles that have a limited mass and travel at speeds of less than 1000 feet per second. These include civilian handguns, which result in limited soft tissue injury.[697] Shotgun pellets have a large mass and are considered intermediate-energy deposit projectiles. They travel at speeds of approximately 1200 feet per second and when grouped in a close distribution, at close range, are capable of causing massive injury. At a distance, the pellets are spread apart; the soft tissue injury sustained is much reduced, and bone injury is frequently avoided.[701]

Ballistic injuries often represent either assaults or suicide attempts. The pattern of injury is thus dependent on the location of the gun muzzle and the path of the projectile.[700]

In lower velocity injuries, the entrance wound of a bullet is generally a puncture hole corresponding roughly to the size of the projectile. When the bullet enters the tissue, it begins to be deflected.[701] The yaw (the angle between the axis of symmetry of the bullet and its line of flight) increases after deflection, and kinetic energy is transferred from the bullet to the tissue in all directions. The tissue continues to move outward until all energy deposited by the bullet has been absorbed. Bullets approach a sidewise orientation at 90 or 270 degrees of yaw. The maximal drag and the greatest deposit of energy occur when a bullet is moving sideways. A pistol bullet with a sidewise orientation experiences three to five times the drag it has moving point first.[701] Thus, the tissue density and resistance cause deflection and slowing of the bullet. Energy is transferred to the tissue, and tissue damage increases as the drag increases. For these reasons, the path of the injury may enlarge as the bullet travels through tissues. Exit wounds are frequently larger than entrance wounds and depend on the velocity and orientation of the bullet. Tissue damage may increase along the track of the projectile, depending on where the projectile deposits the energy. If the bullet path is short, entrance and exit wounds may be of similar size because there has been little deflection of the bullet relative to its longitudinal axis and reduced absorption of energy.

For low- and intermediate-velocity gunshot wounds, the kinetic energy imparted to the tissue is smaller. The wound produced is associated with a zone of soft tissue injury and a zone of bone injury, and there is little significant tissue loss, except in the exact path of the bullet. For high-velocity wounds, the amount of tissue injury greatly increases, and both soft tissue and bone loss are present.

In formulating a treatment plan for ballistic injuries, it is helpful to identify the entrance and exit wounds and the presumed path of the bullet and to appreciate the mass and velocity of the projectile, so that the extent of internal areas of tissue injury can be predicted.

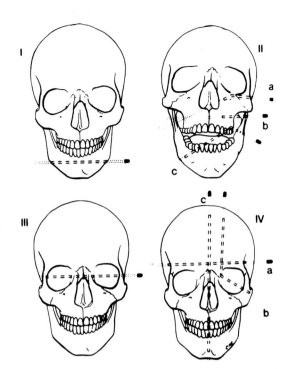

FIGURE 66-215. The four patterns of gunshot wounds of the face. Type I lower facial wounds involve the mandibular area and tongue. Type II injuries involve the lower midface and lower orbit. Type III injury is characterized by involvement of the bilateral orbit and zygomatic and temporomandibular joint areas. Type IV injury involves the frontal bone and the orbit. Two characteristics should be determined for each injury: (1) the area of soft tissue loss and (2) the area of bone loss. Fractures in the area of tissue injury are managed as routine facial fractures. Those in the area of bone loss are managed with external or internal fixation with plates and screws, which span and stabilize the bone gaps. The bullet tracks *(interrupted lines)* represent composite patterns of muscle paths. (After Clark N, Birely B, Manson PN, et al: High-energy ballistic and avulsive facial injuries: classification, patterns, and an algorithm for primary reconstruction. Plast Reconstr Surg 1996;98:583.)

Conceptually, the separate categories of soft tissue injury and bone injury and soft tissue loss and bone loss must be individually assessed (four separate components) for each injury, and the areas of each recorded. The areas of injury and the areas of loss are each precisely outlined according to a facial pattern (Fig. 66-215), which allows a plan to be developed for early and intermediate treatment of the lower, middle, and upper face.

Hollier et al[704] reviewed 121 patients with facial gunshot wounds. The gunshot wounds were multiple in one third of the patients. Overall mortality was 11%. Two thirds of the patients had a skeletal injury, and three fourths of these required surgical intervention. One fifth of patients required tracheotomy. One fifth of the patients had an intracranial injury, and half of

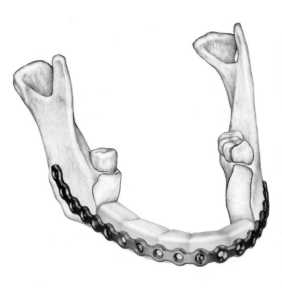

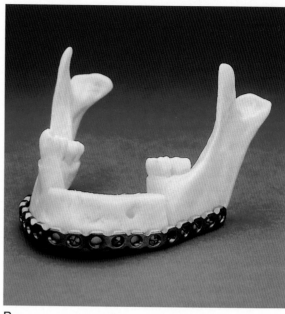

A   B

FIGURE 66-216. *A* and *B,* Scheme of attaching bone grafts to reconstruction plate. (From Clark N, Birely B, Manson PN, et al: High-energy ballistic and avulsive facial injuries: classification, patterns, and an algorithm for primary reconstruction. Plast Reconstr Surg 1996;98:583.)

those having intracranial injury required surgery. Interestingly, 14% of the patients in this series had great vessel injuries diagnosed at the time of angiography, with half of these patients requiring surgical intervention for that reason. Hollier has suggested that a Weber-Fergusson external incision be used in some patients to avoid a degloving exposure because of concern about vascularity of soft tissue in standard approaches.

Low Velocity

In general, low-velocity gunshot wounds involve little soft tissue and bone loss and have limited associated soft tissue injury outside the exact path of the bullet. It is thus appropriate that they be treated with definitive stabilization of bone and primary soft tissue closure. Limited débridement of involved soft tissue is necessary. Small amounts of bone may need to be débrided or replaced with a primary bone graft, which can be safely performed primarily in the upper face. Because of the lack of significant associated soft tissue injury, little potential for progressive death or progressive necrosis of soft tissue exists, and these injuries may be treated as "facial fractures with overlying lacerations" both conceptually and practically. Four general anatomic injury types were realized after a review of patients experiencing low-velocity gunshot wounds in the facial area (Fig. 66-215).[693]

TYPE I (LOWER FACE)

Injuries in this classification involve the tongue and the mandible (15% of facial gunshot wounds involve soft tissue alone). There is often limited loss of mandibular structures, a finding that makes closed reduction and intermaxillary fixation feasible in occasional patients. Ramus and condylar injuries are managed by a brief period of intermaxillary fixation with early mobilization. "Training" or nighttime elastics are sometimes used to maintain occlusion when mobilization of the mandible is necessary in the face of a tendency to malocclusion. One fourth of the patients sustain sufficient injury to the tongue and floor of the mouth along with marked edema to threaten the airway. Either prolonged intubation or tracheostomy should be considered. Open reduction of the fractured mandibular fragments with plate and screw fixation (Fig. 66-216) is preferred, and after a brief period of rest, the patient can be mobilized with elastic guidance.

Soft tissue loss is usually minimal in this classification. Drainage of neck and floor of mouth wounds is necessary to prevent deep space neck infection. Entrance and exit wounds are excised and closed primarily, and the internal soft tissue wound should be drained dependently. Suction drainage is preferred. Limited débridement of soft tissue should be performed along the bullet track. Drainage of the track is thought to limit infection, especially when the deep spaces of the neck are penetrated.

When open reduction is required, small fragments of bone may be débrided and plate and screw fixation used to span any bone defect. In mandibular fractures, primary nonvascularized replacement of bone fragments is accompanied by a higher incidence of infection than occurs in the upper face, and the incidence of infection after mandibular primary bone grafting (especially in the absence of intact intraoral mucosa) is significant. Primary mandibular bone grafting should in general be deferred until intact oral mucosa can be demonstrated. In some patients, a small bridge of mandibular bone is present, but secondary bone grafting may be necessary to strengthen the amount of bone present or to replace the entire bone segment that has been comminuted and partially resorbed. The decision to bone graft a mandibular defect, either primarily or secondarily, with vascularized or nonvascularized tissue depends on the ability to establish a surgically clean wound without significant intraoral communication, the size of the bone defect, and the condition of the associated soft tissue. Vascularized bone grafts would conceptually be preferred, especially if the size of the bone defect exceeds 4 cm.

TYPE II (MIDFACE)

Type II gunshot injuries involve the lower midface. The maxillary alveolus and maxillary sinuses and the lower portion of the nose and zygoma are often the only structures affected. In some patients, only a simple drainage of the maxillary sinuses is required. In other patients, open reduction and internal fixation of limited zygomatic or maxillary fractures are necessary. Injuries to the palate or to the teeth or alveolar structures may require débridement of teeth and closure of palatal or alveolar fistulas with local rotation flaps. Depending on the degree of nasal or oral swelling, airway management may be indicated. In this series,[693] no bilateral maxillary fracture produced mobility of the entire maxillary alveolus (a Le Fort type injury). No true Le Fort fractures are produced by a low-velocity gunshot wound.

TYPE III (ORBITAL)

Type III injuries involve the orbit and nasoethmoidal complex. The bullet often exits through the contralateral temporomandibular joint region. All injuries are treated by open reduction and immediate bone grafting for replacement of significant orbital bone loss for support of the orbital soft tissue. The thin structure of some of the orbital bones makes them less desirable than bone grafts for use in primary reconstruction after their crushing by a ballistic injury.

Damage to the globe is present in almost 90% of patients, with bilateral blindness in 50% and unilateral blindness in 40%. Careful ocular examination is thus imperative to detect bullet fragments in the globe

and periorbital soft tissue. Injury of the lacrimal system occurs in one third, and the disruption has been managed by primary simple intubation or repair of the lacrimal system following the principles described by Callahan.[705] Secondary reconstruction may be required in patients with severe injuries with dacryocystorhinostomy. The temporomandibular joint area may be treated by exploration and débridement. A bone gap may be left or early function permitted after débridement, or a definitive reconstruction of the area may be completed by a costal chondral graft and vascularized temporoparietal flap with postoperative mobilization in elastic guidance. Replacement of multiply comminuted segments of the original bone of the temporomandibular joint often leads to complete resorption of the replaced bone fragments with disappointing results, and costal chondral grafting is preferred. Early controlled mobilization of the mandible is indicated when reconstruction is performed by a costal chondral graft, guided by elastic traction. The patient may be replaced in occlusion each night, with daytime elastics as necessary to guide occlusal positioning.

TYPE IV (CRANIOFACIAL)

Intracranial involvement characterizes type IV injuries. The supraorbital bones, orbital roofs, frontal bone, and frontal sinus structures are involved. The need to explore simultaneous and sometimes discontinuous cranial base fractures, which are induced by reciprocal skull deformation of the impact, has been emphasized in the literature.[693] Appropriate neurosurgical débridement of dural or cerebral lacerations is important with repair of dural fistulas, elimination of the frontal sinus function by mucosal stripping, burring of the walls of the bone, bone grafting of the nasofrontal duct, and obliteration of the cavity with bone and replacement of the anterior wall. Immediate bone grafting of frontal bone defects should be performed, and calvarial bone grafts are frequently used. Globe or optic nerve injury is present in 40%, with blindness in 25% (Fig. 66-217).

Intermediate and High Velocity

Intermediate- and high-velocity ballistic injuries to the face must be managed with a specific treatment plan that involves stabilization of existing bone and soft tissue in anatomic position and maintenance of this bone and soft tissue stabilization throughout the period of soft tissue contracture and bone and soft tissue reconstruction. Wounds from intermediate- and high-energy missiles usually demonstrate areas of both soft tissue and bone loss as well as areas of soft tissue and bone injury. Usually, less loss of bone and soft tissue is present than is first suspected. It is important to

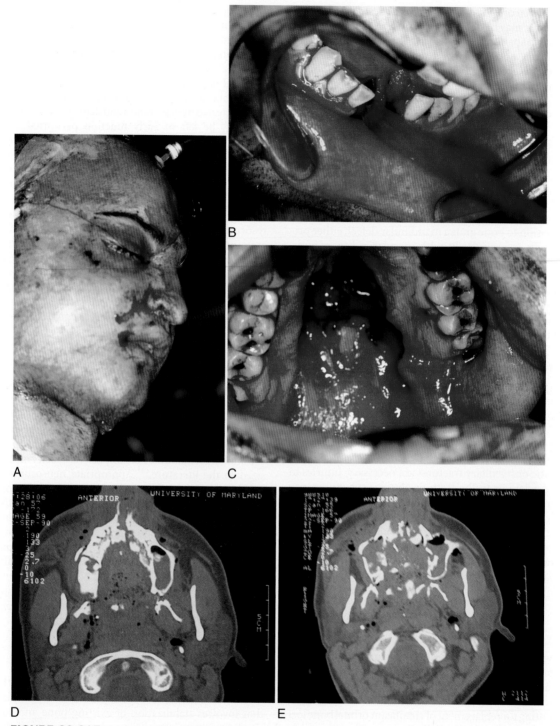

FIGURE 66-217. *A,* A craniofacial rifle wound involving the entire face (mandible, palate, midface, nasoethmoidal area, and frontal bone). *B,* Mandibular transection. *C,* Palatal injury. *D* and *E,* Radiographs of the midface and palatal injury.

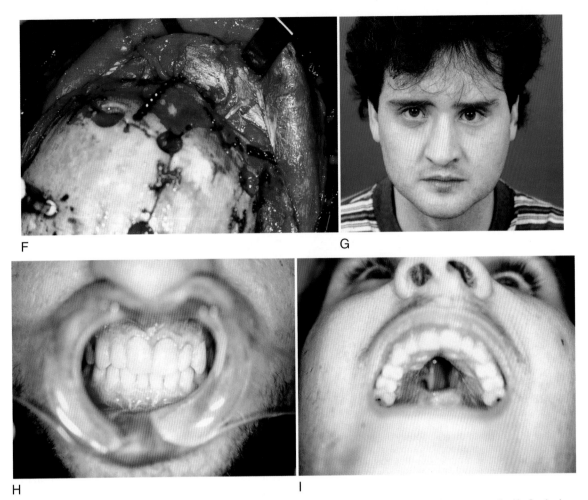

FIGURE 66-217, cont'd. *F,* Cranial and nasoethmoidal reduction. *G,* Result of one-stage repair. *H,* Occlusion. *I,* Palatal fistula was later closed with a pharyngeal flap. (From Clark N, Birely B, Manson PN, et al: High-energy ballistic and avulsive facial injuries: classification, patterns, and an algorithm for primary reconstruction. Plast Reconstr Surg 1996;98:583.)

reassemble the existing bone and soft tissue and then at intervals to carry out serial surgical débridement second-look procedures, which reopen the soft tissue to define additional areas of soft tissue necrosis, drain hematoma or developing fluid collections, and ensure bone integrity. These second-look procedures are imperative if primary reconstruction is attempted. Thus, the emphasis is on primary soft tissue "skin to skin" or "skin to mucosa" closures, with stabilization of existing bone fragments in anatomic position. Re-exploration for additional débridement occurs at 48-hour intervals or at an interval determined by the surgeon. These second-look procedures are necessary and are continued until all soft tissue loss ceases and wound hematoma and fluid collections are controlled. Pulsed lavage irrigation of the soft tissue is conducted.

In civilian practice, many of these injuries represent shotgun wounds or high-energy rifle injuries, and they often result from suicide attempts or assaults. Close-range shotgun wounds are characterized by extensive soft tissue and bone destruction. Their management depends on the anatomic area of the injury and loss, and four specific patterns of high-energy injury loss are recognized (Fig. 66-218). Hollier et al[704] have described complete free tissue transfer.

TYPE I (CENTRAL LOWER FACE)

Type I high-velocity injuries are characterized by a zone of bone loss in the central portion of the mandible and maxilla and loss of skin of the chin, lips, and lower nose, with a zone of injury extending posteriorly in the mandible and up into the central midfacial and orbital regions and possibly the brain. The zones of injury and zones of loss should each be mapped for the soft tissue and for the bone.

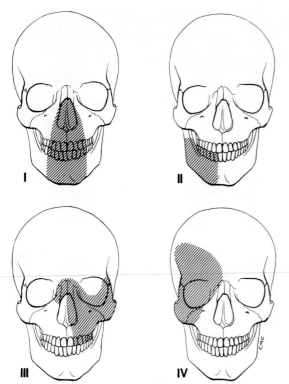

FIGURE 66-218. The four patterns of soft tissue and bone loss in shotgun injuries. The usual extent of tissue and bone injury extends far beyond the areas of soft tissue and bone loss. In these diagrams, only the areas of tissue and bone loss are shaded. I, Central mandibular and midface soft tissue and bone loss. II, Lateral mandibular soft tissue and bone loss. III, Maxillary and orbital soft tissue and bone loss. IV, Orbital and cranial soft tissue and bone loss. (After Clark N, Birely B, Manson PN, et al: High-energy ballistic and avulsive facial injuries: classification, patterns, and an algorithm for primary reconstruction. Plast Reconstr Surg 1996;98:583.)

The area of maxillary and mandibular bone loss is generally anterior and should be managed by external fixation or plate and screw fixation of the remaining portions of the mandible in anatomic position, stabilizing the bone defect. The plate and screw fixation technique may be used whether or not soft tissue cover of the plate can be provided either acutely or secondarily.

Soft tissue closure can usually be accomplished primarily in some areas, with skin to mucosa closure as one approaches the area of the soft tissue defect. Often, soft tissue closure can be accomplished primarily with some decrease in the length of the lip structures. At a secondary surgery, flap replacement of the lip structures may be performed by standard flaps for lip reconstruction, which provide the best cutaneous appearance and aesthetic result. If local flaps are not possible, a regional flap may be employed, such as a radial

forearm flap for lower lip reconstruction with a tendon to suspend it to the zygomatic body for lower lip support.

After all the soft tissue has been repaired, the maxillary and mandibular bone deficiencies may be reconstructed when no further soft tissue necrosis is seen on serial débridement and when intraoral closure is accomplished, or a free tissue transfer may be done. It is important that the anatomic position of the remaining segments of the maxilla and mandible be stabilized with combinations of rigid internal fixation and intermaxillary fixation throughout the period of soft tissue and bone reconstruction to eliminate malocclusion and to reduce the magnitude of the deformity. In extensive soft tissue loss, when primary skin and mucosa repair cannot be accomplished, skin to mucosa closure is recommended for wound closure. Exploration of the soft tissue is performed at 48-hour intervals, opening these areas to identify any devitalized tissue, to remove hematoma, to irrigate the wound, and to prepare it for secondary reconstruction. The soft tissue is completely closed after each of these procedures. Dependent drainage may be provided in the area of soft tissue closure.

Reconstruction of the mandible anteriorly is usually accomplished with a vascularized fibular graft, which may include a segment of skin for mucosal or cutaneous replacement. Two free flaps may be required in defects with significant intraoral and cutaneous defects. The maxilla may be reconstructed by a prosthesis or by a suitably designed free flap, such as a scapular or radial forearm flap.

TYPE II (LOWER LATERAL FACE)

The most frequently observed high-velocity shotgun injury is characterized by loss of a lateral mandibular segment and its surrounding soft tissue. These patients may usually be managed by primary soft tissue closure by advancement flaps from the neck and cheek after limited débridement. Nonabsorbable sutures (monofilament, nylon, or silk) should be used for intraoral closure. These sutures require removal.

The mandibular defect may be stabilized by external or internal rigid fixation, but the bones must be positioned anatomically, and the bone defect must be spanned stably. Comminuted mandibular segments are replaced into their primary position and may or may not survive, depending on infection and soft tissue vascularity. Intraoral soft tissue closure must be completed and may require a tongue flap or free flap. For small defects, the tongue may be placed over an area of mucosal loss and released secondarily. In larger defects, a free flap may be required. The mandibular bone may be reconstructed by bone grafting once intraoral soft tissue integrity has been obtained. Nonvascularized bone grafts should not be performed primarily until soft tissue stability is certain or when bone loss exceeds 4 cm. Alternatively, a free tissue transfer from the fibular area may be transplanted with a cutaneous mucosal replacement. Free flaps produce a more predictable result than nonvascularized bone grafts.

TYPE III (MIDFACE)

Type III high-velocity injuries involve the maxilla, zygoma, orbits, and maxillary sinuses. The nasoethmoidal-orbital region is always involved. When fractures are present, they are managed as routine facial fractures in the area of bone injury and as facial fractures with bone loss in the area of the bone defect. Immediate bone grafting of the orbital and nasal defects may be performed if there is enough intact mucosa and skin cover. Often, skin loss is confined to the eyelids, cheek, and nose. When skin loss prevents primary closure or when loss of maxillary sinus lining prevents coverage of existing bone fragments, an omental or muscle flap may be considered acutely for temporary vascularized coverage of bone or bone grafts. The use of omental flaps, however, does not usually prevent the necessity for a secondary free flap reconstruction with a definitive microvascular transfer involving more structured bone and soft tissue. The most significant problem existing in these injuries is the loss of sinus lining. Reconstruction performed with nonvascularized bone over a significant absence of sinus lining usually results in necrosis of the bone, cellulitis, and bone débridement. Ultimately, a larger reconstruction than what would have been required in primary replacement is then necessary, with replacement of maxillary sinus lining by a free tissue transfer. Such a free tissue transfer may be considered a component of an immediate reconstruction if serial débridement discloses no further evidence of necrosis or infection. Reconstructions of the bone are best stabilized by plate and screw fixation, and bone grafts to maxillary or orbital bone defects may be safely done if enough sinus lining or soft tissue cover is present or provided (Fig. 66-218).

In each classification, a "zone of injury" is identified where fractures are present without significant bone or soft tissue loss. Fractures in the zone of facial injury are managed as routine facial fractures. When soft tissue loss and bone loss are present, it is important to stabilize existing bone in its anatomic position until soft tissue reconstruction can be completed. The soft tissue should be closed as far as possible to stretch and maintain length and shape of the soft tissue. In some patients, it may be possible to plan a more complex reconstruction of bone and soft tissue simultaneously by a composite free tissue transfer (Fig. 66-218). Local tissue for soft tissue reconstruction, such as a local flap, ultimately provides the best cutaneous match and

aesthetic result, but it may be sufficient only for the skin and require a deeper free flap reconstruction over which the cutaneous segment is stretched. These local flaps can be rotated over free tissue transfers to improve their color and contour match.

Significant wounds of the maxillary sinus are subject to skin breakdown after primary closure under tension. When there is considerable destruction of the maxillary sinus area, consideration should be given to obliteration of this area with a free tissue transfer reconstruction, such as a muscle or an omental flap. A distant flap may be used to fill defects so that the soft tissue can be brought over a well-vascularized bed, with a vascularized or nonvascularized bone graft incorporated as appropriate. When both lining and bone in the maxillary sinus are significantly destroyed, an oral or nasal communication usually slowly erodes through the less vascularized skin unless proper lining is reconstructed. Whereas small lining defects may be able to be tolerated and heal secondarily, larger lining defects rarely provide sufficient soft tissue, and a free tissue transfer is suggested (Fig. 66-219).

Soft tissue free flap obliteration of the maxillary sinus area provides the best long-term lining. Persons who sustain significant injury to the midface should be considered candidates for arteriography to define carotid artery integrity. The emphasis remains on primary closure of soft tissue and primary reconstruction of the existing bone in its anatomic position. Nonabsorbable intraoral sutures are recommended.

TYPE IV (CRANIOFACIAL)

High-velocity type IV injuries involve the cranium and upper third of the face, including the orbit, globe, frontal bone, and frontal sinus area. They may be characterized by intracranial involvement and thus carry a worse prognosis. There may be associated injuries of the nasoethmoidal-orbital complex, frontal sinus, and zygoma. A primary reconstruction by open reduction of existing bone fragments, supplemented by bone grafting, may be performed when cutaneous covering is present and if there are no significant defects of lining or communication into the nose that cannot be closed. In general, one third of the orbit can be missing lining and the reconstruction will not be compromised. Fragments of a ruptured globe may need to be enucleated. A primary globe spacer (a ball placed in the muscle cone), followed by closure of the conjunctiva over this, is indicated. The muscles may be sutured to a "post," which may be used to mobilize a prosthesis, if the muscles can be identified. The actual soft tissue skin deficit is often less extensive in upper facial injuries, but in some of the patients, flap reconstruction of significant orbital soft tissue loss is required to "blank out" the orbital defect. This depends on individual judgment and may be determined after several "washouts"

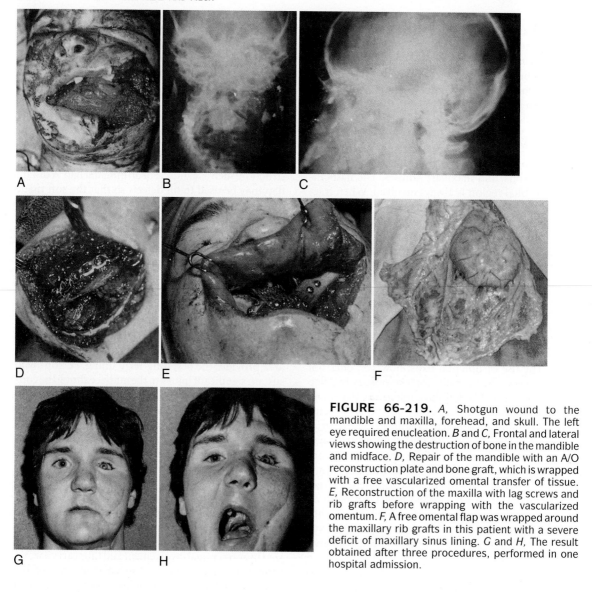

FIGURE 66-219. *A,* Shotgun wound to the mandible and maxilla, forehead, and skull. The left eye required enucleation. *B* and *C,* Frontal and lateral views showing the destruction of bone in the mandible and midface. *D,* Repair of the mandible with an A/O reconstruction plate and bone graft, which is wrapped with a free vascularized omental transfer of tissue. *E,* Reconstruction of the maxilla with lag screws and rib grafts before wrapping with the vascularized omentum. *F,* A free omental flap was wrapped around the maxillary rib grafts in this patient with a severe deficit of maxillary sinus lining. *G* and *H,* The result obtained after three procedures, performed in one hospital admission.

by the quantity of existing living soft tissue (Fig. 66-220).

Patients with gunshot or shotgun wounds of the face are often presumed to have significant soft tissue and bone injury that precludes any immediate reconstruction. In fact, although the entire zone of both soft tissue and bone loss and the zone of soft tissue injury and bone injury may be extensive, the area of actual soft tissue and bone loss is usually much more limited, with manageable tissue injury and loss in most other areas. In almost all instances, an initial primary repair in the zones of injury and stabilization on the zones of loss may be accomplished (with the exception of the mandible) safely in low-velocity injuries in all areas.[693] Primary bone grafting in the mandible is hazardous when an intact lining is not present or cannot be established. It is reasonable and effective to approach

low-velocity injuries in the same manner as comminuted facial fractures with overlying facial lacerations. Fractures in the zone of injury are managed with early immediate internal fixation, by use of plate and screw fixation. Bone grafting in the middle and upper face is successful in almost all these injuries. This treatment plan has not resulted in increased infection rates or in a dramatic increase in complications because of the washout philosophy, whereby early detection of hematoma, infection, or devitalized material is managed by serial second-look operations, when problems are taken care of before symptoms can occur. In low-velocity injuries, the lacerations and entrance and exit wounds are excised and closed after minimal débridement over a drain.

Intermediate-velocity gunshot or shotgun wounds benefit from a limited initial débridement, definitive stabilization of bone and soft tissue, and frequent second-look operations for débridement at 24- to 48-hour intervals to ensure that all soft tissue is viable and that no hematoma, abscess, or progressive tissue necrosis exists. In more extensive injuries, a larger zone of soft tissue and bone injury is defined, and the treatment can be accomplished in the usual manner as for comminuted facial fractures with overlying lacerations.

The zones of soft tissue and bone loss should also be identified. The treatment should emphasize anatomic stabilization of existing bone fragments in the correct position and early soft tissue reconstruction by local or regional flap transfer. Bone reconstruction may then proceed by either free tissue transfer or stabilization of the defect with delayed bone grafting into a clean wound. Such operative management is successful in

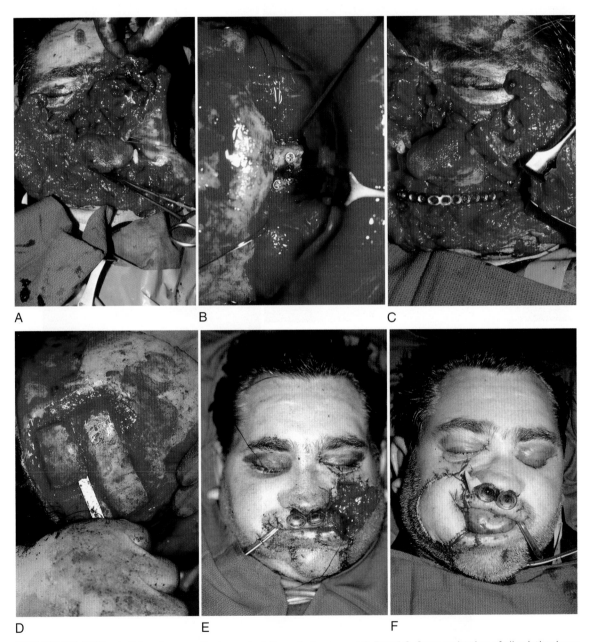

FIGURE 66-220. *A,* Extensive mandibular and midface shotgun wound. *B* and *C,* Open reduction of all existing bone and stabilization of bone defects with plate and screw fixation. The volume and shape of the skeleton are thus preserved. *D,* Calvarial bone grafts for upper midface. *E,* Cutaneous and lining defects. *F,* Free tissue transfer for soft tissue reconstruction.   *Continued*

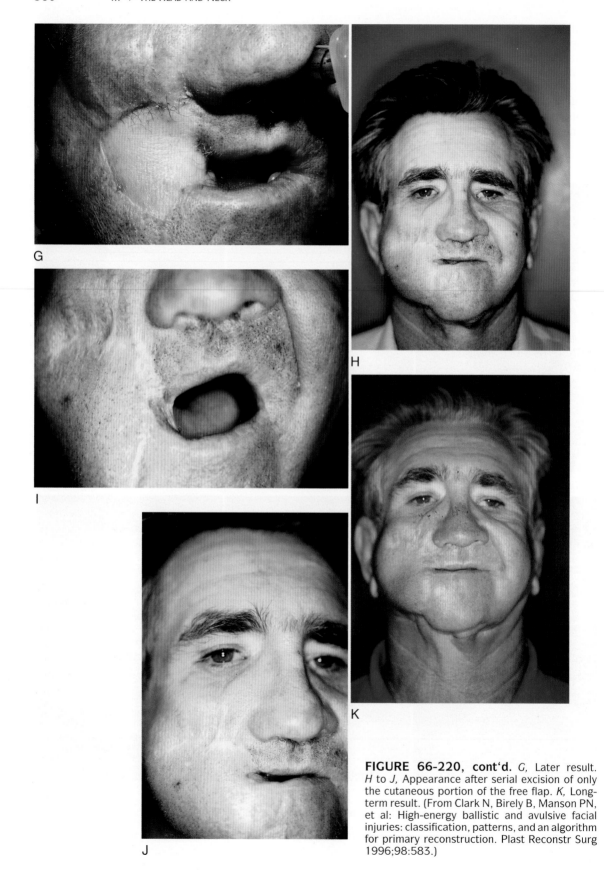

FIGURE 66-220, cont'd. *G,* Later result. *H* to *J,* Appearance after serial excision of only the cutaneous portion of the free flap. *K,* Long-term result. (From Clark N, Birely B, Manson PN, et al: High-energy ballistic and avulsive facial injuries: classification, patterns, and an algorithm for primary reconstruction. Plast Reconstr Surg 1996;98:583.)

reducing the ultimate disability of patients sustaining these injuries.

POST-TRAUMATIC FACIAL PAIN

(After Crockford[706])

Pain is a common chronic symptom after repair of facial trauma.[707-711] In the study by Girotto,[584] pain of a dysesthetic and constant quality was present in many patients after midfacial fractures. Often the patient does not volunteer that there is discomfort unless emotional agitation or stressing episodes are present. Although pain represents a common sequela of major facial injuries, most patients adapt to it; however, if it is persistent and somewhat disabling, it may result in drug addiction.[707-711] Early detection of this pattern may facilitate the chronic management of these patients.

Nerve Injuries

Nerve injuries invariably accompany facial fractures as the nerves pass through the bone in areas of weakness or foramina that are the sites of fracture, by virtue of the reduced strength of bone in these areas. Various types of nerve injuries may occur and correspond to Seddon's classification[712] of neurapraxia, axonotmesis, and neurotmesis.

It is likely that facial pain is produced by mechanisms similar to those described for peripheral nerves.[708,709,713-715] Cranial nerves may be cut, crushed, contused, or otherwise injured by facial fractures, and they can easily be injured by incisions, dissection, and attempts at bone mobilization. Traction is also a conceivable method of nerve injury. After fracture, bone proliferation and scar tissue formation may further compromise an injured nerve by compression or proliferation of bony callus. A nerve frequently subjected to injury is the inferior alveolar, passing through the mandible and exiting at the mental foramen. Most mandibular angle and body fractures result, for instance, in trauma to the inferior alveolar nerve,[141,716,717] and most zygomatic or lower orbital fractures result in trauma to the infraorbital nerve.[250] The external nasal nerve[309] may be injured as it emerges between the nasal bone and the upper lateral cartilage. If transection has not occurred, considerable recovery can be anticipated (70% to 90%), but chronic discomfort and pain may be sequelae.

The infraorbital nerve is commonly injured in orbital floor and zygomatic fractures. The zygomaticofacial and zygomaticotemporal nerves may be injured by zygoma fractures or dissection, and the injury results in pain experienced near the upper area of the cheek or in the anterior temple at the frontal process of the zygoma. The pain is persistent and sometimes can be disabling. Dissection of the zygoma over the anterior face of the malar eminence may transect the zygomaticofacial nerve,[312] which can be preserved by careful dissection, at least in immediate fracture treatment. Barclay[328] documented infraorbital nerve damage in more than 80% of fractures of the zygoma. Persistent sensory disturbance has been documented by Tajima[718] and Nordgaard,[250] frequently involving the anterior maxillary teeth. Although partial recovery of sensation usually occurs after zygomatic fracture, the recovery is usually incomplete but sufficient that the patient is asymptomatic.

The supraorbital and supratrochlear nerves are also at risk as they pass through a groove or canal in the superior portion of the orbital rim. Frontal contusions often damage these nerves, impacting them between the injuring object and the unyielding frontal bone. Coronal incisions with supraorbital nerve release also frequently damage these nerve structures. The preauricular and greater auricular nerves also may be injured by dissection from incisions for angle and ramus exposure, as can the supraorbital nerves.

Considering the nature of facial fractures, it is truly remarkable that pain is not a more prominent chronic symptom of facial injuries.[626,706,713,715] Girotto et al[584] have focused on chronic pain as a common residual; however, most patients accommodate to it without medication. In patients demonstrating fracture nonunion or malposition, one can understand how nerve function may be disturbed. Alternatively, in patients having significant fractures, it is easy to realize that the nerves have been considerably traumatized by the bone injury.[715] On histologic examination, intraneural fibrosis and intraneural disturbances have been documented after trauma to the peripheral nerves. Intraneural scarring is common; however, it has not been possible to correlate fibrosis and intraneural disturbances with the severity of clinical symptoms.[719]

Melzack and Wall[713] emphasized the distinctions between central and peripheral pain and postulated a "gate theory" that explains the neurophysiologic manifestations of pain. Neuromas or nerve entrapment obviously may produce pain by the pressure constriction of sensory axons by collagen. Peripheral nerves have been demonstrated to be inflamed and swollen several centimeters proximal to the site of significant nerve compression injury. In these patients, histologic examination confirms scar tissue between the nerve fibers. Peripheral pain, uncontrolled for several months, usually spreads centrally to become established in a self-perpetuating neuronal circuit that makes relief challenging.[706] Sympathetic fibers are responsible for modulation of this spreading pain.

The usual patient with chronic facial pain has a history of a well-defined injury that is capable of producing sensory disturbance in an anatomic distribution of a recognized sensory nerve. An occasional patient does not remember a trivial injury and presents more diagnostic difficulty.

In the great majority of patients with damage to the facial sensory nervous system,[720] there is a history of a recognizable event, with anesthesia or hypesthesia in the anatomic distribution of a cutaneous sensory nerve. Alternatively, patients with midface fractures may complain of a generalized dysesthesia.[584] The sensation may be partially recovered or be accompanied by paresthesias, which vary in frequency from occasional to persistent.[707-711]

As dysesthesias become more severe, they prevent the patient from touching the affected area.[713] The pain may be precipitated by physical or psychological stimuli. Attacks of pain may occur with response to cold, and plate sensitivity increases these symptoms. Even wind or light touching of the affected point may precipitate discomfort. Frequently, the attacks of pain are spontaneous, with no precipitating cause identifiable. The pain may spread to other areas of the face, other than the original area affected. In some patients, the skin may be discolored, having a reddish blue cast, and be cool to the touch, similar to the changes observed in Raynaud phenomenon in extremities.[713] Hyperactive vasomotor activity may simulate the "causalgia" that occurs in peripheral extremities. The onset of pain may be immediate, but in most causes, it develops as a slow, chronic sequela to the original injury. Most patients are able to relate a slow exacerbation of the pain during a period of weeks after the injury.

Recent developments bring new understanding to the physiology of pain pathways and to the complex interrelationships that neurotransmitters provide regarding the nature of chronic pain and the potential for medical intervention. Because the roots of sensory nerves transmit pain impulses in serial fashion to the brain, neurotransmitting chemicals mediate the impulses. Thus, they represent specific targets for intervention within the nervous system. Chronic pain physiology overlaps into the spheres of perception and complex biochemical mechanisms, such as the indolamine-catecholamine balance and the endogenous opioid system. These biochemical systems modulate pain and its emotional components.[707-711]

For many years, it was thought that there were no specific nerves for the mediation of pain. Pain was thought to result from overstimulation of nerve receptors. It is now postulated that small unmyelinated C fibers and A delta fibers carry pain impulses from specialized nerve endings that function as pain sensors in skin, blood vessels, muscles, and other organs.[707-711] Two types of pain have been identified, fast and slow, constituting the initial pain felt acutely by patients. The described afferent pain fibers travel to the spinal cord, where they synapse with chemical transmitters involved in the relay of neurosignals. The free nerve endings are unmyelinated and are extremely sensitive to mechanical, thermal, or chemical signals. In damaged tissue, "pain" messages may be transmitted by substances such as histamine, serotonin, and prostaglandin that are released after injuries and may make sensory nerves more excitable. The A delta and C fibers travel in discrete unmyelinated bundles of 10 to 50 nerves from visceral receptors to reach the dorsal horn. They relay their messages into one of six laminae, usually laminae one and five, and possibly four and six. In these laminae, there is a mixture of visceral and cutaneous pain signals that may serve as the basis for referred pain. Ascending fibers travel across the gray matter of the spinal cord to the lateral spinal thalamic tract and in the white matter. Descending excitatory fibers also travel from the laminae. The lateral spinal thalamic tract transmits pain signals from the dorsal horn through the medial lemnisci to the thalamus, and fibers ascend to the cerebral cortex. Synapses are involved in the medulla, the reticular activating system, the thalamus, the hypothalamus, and other parts of the limbic system. As pain evolves from an acute to a chronic state, various ancillary fiber pathways are used, and diverse areas of the brain become involved in the perception and modulation of the pain response.

Synapses are junction points between two nerves. They consist of a presynaptic portion of a nerve that transmits the incoming signal, a synaptic cleft or gap, and a postsynaptic receptor area, which is connected to another nerve cell. Neurosynaptic transmitter factors are manufactured in synaptic vesicles. The nerve electrical impulses change membrane permeability, allowing neurotransmitters to diffuse across the synaptic cleft to affect the receptor sites. These activate an area of the next nerve cell. Some chemicals mimic the action of neurosynaptic transmitters and are called agonists, occupying the same receptor site as the naturally occurring chemical. Substances that block or otherwise inhibit the production, transmission, or reception of the neurosynaptic transmitters are called antagonists.[714]

Although numerous neurotransmitter substances are known to exist, indolamines, catecholamines, and enkephalins-endorphins are compounds considered important in the psychopharmacology of chronic pain. The biogenic amines (such as norepinephrine, dopamine, and L-dopa) and the indolamines (such as serotonin) account for 2% to 5% of the neurotransmitters in the nervous system. Most biogenic amine transmitters are found in the hypothalamus, the median forebrain, and the reticular activating system. These structures, as a part of the limbic system, are believed to play an important role in the mediation and emotional perception of chronic pain. The enkephalins and endogenous pentapeptides that act on the morphine receptors within the central nervous system are also found in high concentrations within the limbic system. Specific receptors for the endogenously produced substances have been localized to the spinal cord and brain. Stimulation of areas known to be high in neurotransmitters and enkephalins produces analgesia.[707-711] The effect persists beyond the time of stimulation, indicating that enzyme induction has been involved. The compound serotonin is also associated with the activity of the enkephalins. The "pain threshold" has been raised by blocking the reuptake of serotonin with tricyclic antidepressants, such as doxepin or amitriptyline, or by augmenting the production of a precursor (L-tryptophan). Catecholamines, such as norepinephrine, are also involved in analgesia. When dopamine, a direct precursor of norepinephrine (in itself a neurotransmitter), is increased, analgesia is enhanced. If a dopamine antagonist is used, analgesia is diminished. Dopamine appears to be a component in the enkephalin-associated analgesia, and it antagonizes the activity of norepinephrine.

Of patients referred to Hendler[707-711] with a diagnosis of complex regional pain syndrome (CRPS) type I (formerly termed reflex sympathetic dystrophy), 71% of the patients were found not to have clinical and diagnostic study findings to support this diagnosis (see Chapter 195). Many of the patients had never received a sympathetic block, which is considered one of the essential diagnostic tests to confirm CRPS type I. After diagnostic evaluation, Hendler found that only 3% of the patients actually had CRPS type I exclusively, whereas 26% had a mixture of both CRPS type I and nerve entrapment syndromes. The largest category of misdiagnoses were nerve entrapment syndromes, which were verified in 96% of patients. Hendler described the "simple diagnostic framework" (Table 66-16) to assist in diagnosis. CRPS type II, formerly known as *causalgia*, needs to be recognized as a distinct entity separate from CRPS type I. Clinicians frequently assume that they are disorders of the same cause and responsive to the same treatment. CRPS type II is secondary to a partial injury to major mixed peripheral nerves caused by low- or high-velocity injury that manifests as trophic changes in the distribution of the nerve associated with extreme hypersensitivity. The pain is "diffuse and burning," and true CRPS type II *almost* always responds to sympathetic

TABLE 66-16 ✦ COMPARISON BETWEEN COMPLEX REGIONAL PAIN SYNDROME (CRPS) TYPE I AND TYPE II

Complex Regional Pain Syndrome Type II (Causalgia)

Definition	Burning pain, allodynia, and hyperpathia, usually in the hand or foot, after partial injury to a nerve or one of its branches
Site	In the region of the limb innervated by the damaged nerve, not around the entire limb
Main features	Onset is usually immediately after partial nerve injury, or it may be delayed for months
	CRPS type II of the radial nerve is very rare
	Nerves most commonly involved are the median, the sciatic and tibial, and the ulnar
	Spontaneous pain: pain described as constant, burning; exacerbated by light touch, stress, temperature change or movement of involved limb, and visual and auditory stimuli (e.g., a sudden sound or bright light, emotional disturbances)
Associated symptoms	Atrophy of skin appendages; secondary atrophic changes in bones, joints, and muscles; sensory and motor loss in structure innervated by damaged portion of nerve
Signs	Cool, reddish, clammy, sweaty skin with atrophy of skin appendages and deep structures in painful area
Laboratory findings	Galvanic skin responses and plethysmography reveal signs of sympathetic nervous system hyperactivity
	Radiographs possibly show atrophy of bone
Usual course	If untreated, the majority of patients have symptoms that persist indefinitely; spontaneous remission occurs
Relief	In the early stages of CRPS type II (first few months), sympathetic blockade plus vigorous physical therapy usually provides transient relief; repeated blocks usually lead to long-term relief
	When a series of sympathetic blocks do not provide long-term relief, sympathectomy is indicated; long-term persistence of symptoms reduces the likelihood of successful therapy
Social and physical disabilities	Disuse atrophy of involved limb; complete disruption of normal daily activities by severe pain; risk of suicide, drug abuse if untreated
Pathologic process	Partial injury to major peripheral nerve; actual cause of pain unknown; peripheral, central, and sympathetic mechanisms involved in an unexplained way
Essential features	Burning pain and cutaneous hypersensitivity with signs of sympathetic hyperactivity in portion of limb innervated by partially injured nerve

Continued

TABLE 66-16 ✦ COMPARISON BETWEEN COMPLEX REGIONAL PAIN SYNDROME (CRPS) TYPE I AND TYPE II—cont'd

Complex Regional Pain Syndrome Type I (Reflex Sympathetic Dystrophy)

Associated symptoms	Initially, there is vasodilation, with increasing temperature, hyperhidrosis, edema, and reduced sympathetic activity. Patient may also develop atrophy of skin, vasoconstriction in the appendages, and/or cool, red, clammy skin
	Disuse atrophy of deep structures possibly progresses to Sudeck atrophy of bone
	Aggravated by use of body part, relieved by immobilization; sometimes follows a herniated intervertebral disk, spinal anesthesia, poliomyelitis, severe iliofemoral thrombosis, or cardiac infarction; may appear as the shoulder-hand syndrome
	Later, vasospastic symptoms become prominent with persistent coldness of the affected extremity and pallor or cyanosis, Raynaud phenomenon, atrophy of the skin and nails and loss of hair, atrophy of soft tissues, and stiffness of joints; without therapy, these symptoms possibly persist
	Not necessary for one patient to exhibit all symptoms together; an additional limb or limbs may possibly be affected as well
Signs	Variable; may be florid sympathetic hyperactivity
Laboratory findings	In advanced cases, radiographs possibly show atrophy of bone and bone scan changes over time
Usual course	Persists indefinitely if untreated; small incidence of spontaneous remission
Relief	Sympathetic block and physical therapy; sympathectomy if long-term results not achieved with repeated blocks; may respond in early phases to high doses of corticosteroids (e.g., prednisone, 50 mg daily)
Complications	Disuse atrophy of involved limb; suicide and drug abuse if untreated; sometimes spreads to contralateral limb
Social and physical disabilities	Depression, inability to perform daily activities
Pathologic process	Unknown
Essential features	Burning pain in distal extremity usually after minor injury without nerve damage
Differential diagnosis	Local pathologic change (fracture, strain, sprain); CRPS type II post-traumatic vasospasm, nerve entrapment syndromes, radiculopathies, or thrombosis

Modified from Merskey H, Bogduk N, eds: Classification of Chronic Pain: Descriptions of Chronic Pain Syndromes and Definitions of Pain Terms, 2nd ed. Seattle, IASP Press, 1994.

CRITERIA FOR DIFFERENTIAL DIAGNOSIS OF COMPLEX REGIONAL PAIN SYNDROME TYPE I AND TYPE II

	CRPS I	CRPS II
Etiology	Any kind of lesion	Partial nerve lesion
Localization	Distal part of extremity	Any peripheral site of body
Independent from site of lesion	Mostly confined to territory of affected nerve	
Spreading of symptoms	Obligatory	Rare
Spontaneous pain	Common, mostly deep and superficial orthostatic component	Obligatory, predominantly superficial, no orthostatic component
Mechanical allodynia	Most of patients with spreading tendency	Obligatory in nerve territory
Autonomic symptoms	Distally generalized with spreading tendency	Related to nerve lesion
Motor symptoms	Distally generalized	Related to nerve lesion
Sensory symptoms	Distally generalized	Related to nerve lesion

From Hendler N: Pharmacotherapy of chronic pain. In Raj PP, ed: Practical Management of Pain. Philadelphia, Mosby, 2000.

block. The treatment often involves a number of sympathetic blocks with the expectation that longer relief might follow each subsequent block. If the response to a sympathetic block is excellent, some suggest sympathectomy.

CRPS type I is the result of minor trauma, inflammation after surgery, infection, or lacerations resulting in some degree of swelling in the affected limb; infarctions, degenerative joint disease, frostbite, and burns constitute some of these injuries. CRPS type I usually follows a minor injury and does not involve a major nerve root. Frequently, the site of the injury is the knee, ankle, or wrist, and the pain seems to get worse with cold but not with emotional upset, unlike

CRPS type II. Demineralization of the bone occurs with fibrosis of tendons and sheaths and spasms of the muscles. Dysesthesia suggests that there will be less success with sympathectomy. Hendler[707-711] suggests that the incidence of CRPS type II is 0.31 to 0.47 per 100,000, whereas the incidence of CRPS type I is between 0.46 and 0.92 per 100,000. Hendler identifies factors leading to the failure to accurately diagnose the two syndromes as confusion that exists in the literature, lack of accurate history taking, absence of a complete description of the symptoms in the history, failure to adequately appreciate that the clinical and radiologic picture of CRPS type I changes over time, ordering inappropriate tests or not ordering the appropriate tests, inability to perform the correct test, and inadequate knowledge permitting the appropriate interpretation of the various test results. He states that another reason for poor outcome is the failure to recognize that both CRPS type I and nerve entrapment syndromes coexist in the same patient. The failure to treat both, even though one has been treated properly, still leaves an input of pain to the wide-dynamic-range neurons of the spinal cord, which lowers the threshold to painful stimuli, resulting in continued hyperalgesia or allodynia. Hendler[710] has written on the pharmacologic management of pain. He also described the sympathetically maintained pain in CRPS and even the possibility of bilateral pain from sympathetic connections. He postulates three sensations associated with CRPS types I and II: (1) pain, which is a sensation usually experienced when tissue damage occurs; (2) hyperalgesia, which is an increased response to a normally painful stimulus; and (3) allodynia, which is a painful response to a normally nonpainful stimulus. These stimuli can be hot, cold, mechanical, or even chemical. The message of pain is initiated at two receptor sites: (1) a nociceptor, which is usually a free nerve ending or unmyelinated C fiber, that detects tissue damage such as temperature or chemical changes; and (2) a mechanoreceptor, which is sensitive to pressure, like a pacinian corpuscle. When tissue is damaged, it produces a primary hyperalgesia, which is a sensitivity to pain at the site of the pain; a secondary hyperalgesia is produced surrounding the zone of primary hyperalgesia in the absence of tissue damage in the second area. A sensitized nociceptor has a lower threshold to pain and produces hyperalgesia, whereas a sensitized mechanoreceptor transmits a message of pain to a normally nonpainful stimulus (i.e., allodynia). Both hyperalgesia and allodynia are the result of spinal dorsal horn body sensitization.

Treatment

Methods of pain treatment may be surgical or medical. In each patient, the effects and the treatment may be local, systemic, or central. Before a specific pain treatment is continued on a chronic basis, it must be understood that other causes of pain, such as fracture nonunion, nerve compression, or neuroma formation, have been evaluated as obvious excitatory conditions and managed specifically.

The most important responsibility of the physician is that patients developing chronic pain syndromes be recognized and given the appropriate specialized careful management that can abort the vicious circle of the pain syndromes. Patients with pain confined to a specific area of the face are relatively easy to recognize as their pain increases. A second group has diffuse pain that spreads to adjacent areas and is not confined to a specific anatomically identifiable distribution, and these patients tend to be more anxious and difficult. It is absolutely essential to incorporate a confident and understanding psychologist, psychiatrist, and pain treatment specialist as required. It is also essential to rule out causes of pain that might be alleviated by medical or surgical means and that do not have an entirely psychophysiologic basis for exacerbation. Simple treatment should be begun that may start the cycle of relief. All aggravating factors, medical, psychological, financial, and emotional, are taken into account when decisions must be made about each of these factors in the treatment plan.

NERVE BLOCKS

Diagnostic and therapeutic local nerve blocks may be performed in the anatomic distribution of an affected sensory nerve. This is one of the most helpful maneuvers to exclude anatomic isolation of pain to a specific sensory nerve. A long-acting anesthetic, such as bupivacaine (Marcaine), can be used. These injections, if effective, have prognostic value, and they indicate that the performance of successive blocks may decrease the symptomatic reaction to pain. Some individuals include a low-dose steroid in the pain injection, hoping (in this way) to decrease the cycle of inflammation and scarring in the tissue. The self-perpetuating pain cycle may be alleviated and the patient provided with much needed rest.[715] Patients with a coronal incision, who have pain in the distribution of the supraorbital nerve, may benefit from injections of both sides of the forehead at the supraorbital foramen. Pain after the neurolysis involved in the performance of the coronal incision is a common event. The relief often occurs for a longer period than may be expected from the effect of the local anesthetic alone. Bupivacaine with epinephrine is useful for prolonged anesthesia in making the injection. Some clinicians prefer to add a small amount of soluble steroid to the pain medication to decrease inflammation.[720] Crockford[706] administered small doses of a soluble steroid (Kenalog-10) to treat painful neuromas. Other clinicians consider the steroid compounds to be more active against immature than mature collagen.[309,714,720]

The emphasis should be on early detection and treatment of pain syndromes, before a pattern of narcotic addiction is established. A series of injections is usually given at biweekly to monthly intervals until sufficient relief is obtained and the vicious circle is broken. Even if a first injection does not have much activity, a second may sometimes have greater effect. In patients who demonstrate coolness or sweating of the affected area, diagnostic and therapeutic trials of sympathetic blocks (stellate ganglion blocks) are indicated. These are usually performed by anesthesiologists who supervise upper extremity pain clinic management. A course of several blocks in 2 weeks should be given. Although surgical treatment of the superior cervical sympathetic ganglion has been described, the use of serial stellate ganglion blocks is equally effective. Most clinicians have avoided more actively destructive therapies, such as phenol-alcohol block of peripheral nerves involved in post-traumatic pain, believing that these agents may contribute to further damage of the affected cutaneous nerve, with scarring and exacerbation of the pain.

Medical systemic treatment is a necessary accompaniment to any series of injections. The patient should be immediately started on a regimen consisting of minor analgesics, an antihistamine such as diphenhydramine hydrochloride (Benadryl), and a medication for sleep. Sleep is essential and may require the use of an antidepressant with a marked hypnotic effect. Some clinicians give carbamazepine (Tegretol) for its effect in trigeminal neuralgia and migraine, but the possibility of serious side effects, such as liver damage and blood dyscrasias, must be considered before resorting to its use and monitored after its application.

Some enthusiasm for the use of Botox around trigger areas of pain discomfort has recently been expressed. There have been more than anecdotal reports of its positive effect in patients with migraine headaches, for instance. The mechanism of action of Botox in pain relief is currently unknown.

SURGERY

On occasion, neurolysis of a nerve, such as might be involved in an area of fracture compression, is of value, even years after the injury. The author has decompressed the infraorbital nerve years after a zygomatic fracture, releasing the nerve completely from the foramen and extending the release into the inferior orbital fissure. This operation should always be considered in patients in whom disabling painful anesthesia exists a year or more after the injury. The decompression should be accompanied by neurolysis and freeing of compressing bone and scar tissue. Some clinicians prefer to apply a local steroid compound to the nerve at the time of surgery, presumably to decrease the inflammatory response.[720] Neurotomy has also been used to treat chronic pain, but a high recurrence rate is reported in most series. In patients in whom the symptoms mimic causalgia, a chemical block (sympathectomy) of the affected area has been employed. More complex neurosurgical procedures (such as are used in trigeminal neuralgia, where the affected nerve or its superior tracts are divided) may be successful in select patients.

Management of psychological factors[715] and a specific program of stress management are also important.

REFERENCES

1. Jones WD III, Whitaker LA, Murtagh F: Applications of reconstructive cranio-facial techniques to acute craniofacial trauma. J Trauma 1977;17:339.
2. Wolfe SA: Application of craniofacial surgical precepts following trauma and tumor removal. J Maxillofac Surg 1982;10:212.
3. Jones LT, Wobig JL: Surgery of the Eyelids and Lacrimal System. Birmingham, Ala, Aesculapius, 1976.
4. Wong L, Richtsmeier JT, Manson PN: Craniofacial growth following rigid fixation: suture excision, miniplating, microplating. J Craniofac Surg 1993;4:234.
5. Manson P, Clark N, Robertson B, et al: Subunit principles in midface fractures: the importance of sagittal buttresses, soft tissue reductions and sequencing treatment of segmental fractures. Plast Reconstr Surg 1999;103:1287.
6. Manson P, Iliff N, Robertson B: The hope offered by early surgical treatment to those patients whose blowout fractures demonstrate tight muscle restriction or true muscle incarceration. Plast Reconstr Surg 2002;109:490.
7. Manson P, ed: Maxillofacial Injuries: Secondary Management and Delayed Repair. Philadelphia, WB Saunders, 1998. Techniques in Plastic and Reconstructive Surgery; vol 5.
8. Manson PN: Facial fractures. Perspect Plast Surg 1988;2:I-36.
9. Manson PN, Crawley WA, Yaremchuk MJ, et al: Midface fractures: advantages of immediate extended open reduction and bone grafting. Plast Reconstr Surg 1985;76:1.
10. Manson PN, Su CT, Hoopes JE: Structural pillars of the facial skeleton. Plast Reconstr Surg 1980;66:54.
11. Lee R, Robertson B, Manson P: Current epidemiology of facial injuries. Semin Plast Surg 2002;16:283.
12. Lee R, Robertson R, Gamble W, Manson P: Blunt craniofacial injuries: a comprehensive analysis. J Craniofac Trauma 2000;6:7.
13. Lim LH, Lam LK, Moore MH, et al: Associated injuries in facial fractures: review of 839 patients. Br J Plast Surg 1993;46:365.
14. Altemir FH: Nasotracheal intubation in patients with facial fractures. Plast Reconstr Surg 1997;89:165.
15. Kilgo P, Osler T, Meredith W: The worst injury predicts mortality outcome the best: rethinking the role of multiple injuries in trauma outcome scoring. J Trauma 2003;55:599.
16. Yeong EK, Chen MT, Chu SH: Traumatic asphyxia. Plast Reconstr Surg 1994;93:739.
17. Fortune JB, Judkins DG, Scanzaroli D, et al: Efficacy of prehospital surgical cricothyroidotomy in trauma patients. J Trauma 1997;42:832.
18. Bernard AC, Kenady DE: Conventional surgical tracheostomy as the preferred method of airway management. J Oral Maxillofac Surg 1999;57:310.
19. Graham JS, Mulloy RH, Sutherland FR, Rose S: Percutaneous versus open tracheostomy: a retrospective cohort outcome study. J Trauma 1996;41:245.

20. Dunham CM, Barraco RD, Clark D: Guidelines for emergency tracheal intubation immediately after traumatic injury. J Trauma 2003;55:162.

21. Bynoe RP, Kerwin AJ, Parker HH: Maxillofacial injuries and life-threatening hemorrhage: treatment with transcatheter arterial embolization. J Trauma 2003;55:74.

22. Yang WG, Tsai TR, Hung CC, Tung TC: Life threatening bleeding in a facial fracture. Ann Plast Surg 2001;46:159.

23. Buchanan RT, Holtmann B: Severe epistaxis in facial fractures. Plast Reconstr Surg 1983;71:768.

24. Frable MA, El-Roman NL, Lewis A: Hemorrhagic complications of facial fractures. Laryngoscope 1974;84:2051.

25. Pearson BW, Mackenzie RG, Goodman WS: The anatomical basis of transantral ligation of the maxillary artery in severe epistaxis. Laryngoscope 1969;83:1009.

26. Shimoyama J, Kanero T, Horie IN: Initial management of massive oral bleeding after midfacial fractures. J Trauma 2003;54:332.

27. Giammanco P, Binns M: Temporary blindness and ophthalmoplegia following nasal packing. J Laryngol Otol 1970;84:631.

28. Solomons NB, Blumgart R: Severe late-onset epistaxis after Le Fort I osteotomy: angiographic localization and embolization. J Laryngol Otol 1988;102:260.

29. Gwyn PP, Carraway JJ, Horton CE, et al: Facial injuries—associated injuries and complications. Plast Reconstr Surg 1971;47:225.

30. Jeremitsky E, Omert L, Dunham CM, Protet CH: Harbingers of poor outcome the day after severe brain injury: hypothermia, hypoxia and hypotension. J Trauma 2003;54:312.

31. Healey C, Osler T, Rogers FB, Healey ML: Improving the Glasgow Coma Scale score: motor score alone is a better predictor. J Trauma 2003;54:671.

32. Lieberman JD, Pasquale MD, Garcia R, Cipolle MD: Use of admission Glasgow Coma Scale score, pupil size, and pupil reactivity to determine outcome for trauma patients. J Trauma 2003;55:437.

33. Becker DP, Miller JD, Ward JD, et al: The outcome from severe head injury with early diagnosis and intensive management. J Neurosurg 1977;97:491.

34. Gurdjian ES, Webster JE: Head Injuries: Mechanisms, Diagnosis and Management. Boston, Little, Brown, 1958:58.

35. Jane JA, Rimei RW: Prognosis in head injury. Clin Neurosurg 1982;29:346.

36. MacLeod JB, Lynn M, McKenney MG: Early coagulopathy predicts mortality in trauma. J Trauma 2003;55:39.

37. MacKenzie EJ, McCarthy ML, Ditunno JF: Using the SF-36 for characterizing outcomes after multiple trauma involving head injuries. J Trauma 2002;52:527.

38. McDonald JV: The surgical management of severe open brain injuries with consideration of the long term results. J Trauma 1980;20:842.

39. Townsend RN, Lheureau T, Protech J, et al: Timing fracture repair in patients with severe brain injury. J Trauma 1998;44:977.

40. Resnick DK, Marion DW, Carlier P: Outcome analysis of patients with severe head injuries and prolonged intracranial hypertension. J Trauma 1997;42:1108.

41. Falimirski ME, Gonzalez R, Rodriguez A, Willberger J: The need for head computed tomography in patients sustaining loss of consciousness after mild head injury. J Trauma 2003;55:1.

42. Bucholz RW, Burkhead WZ, Graham W, Petty C: Occult cervical spine injuries in fatal traffic accidents. J Trauma 1979;19:768.

43. Huelke DF, O'Day J, Mendelsohn RA: Cervical injuries suffered in automobile crashes. J Neurosurg 1981;54:316.

44. Hendey GW, Wolfson AB, Mower WR, Hoffman JR: Spinal cord injury without radiographic abnormality: results of the National Emergency X-Radiography Utilization Study in blunt cervical trauma. J Trauma 2002;53:1.

45. Diaz J, Grilman C, Morris JA, May AK: Are five plain films of the cervical spine reliable? A prospective evaluation of blunt trauma patient with altered mental status. J Trauma 2003;55:658.

46. Griffen MM, Fryberg ER, Kerwin AJ, Schinco MA: Radiographic clearance of blunt cervical spine injury: plain radiographs or computed tomography scan? J Trauma 2003;55:222.

47. Lewis VL Jr, Manson PN, Morgan RF, et al: Facial injuries associated with cervical fractures: recognition, patterns and management. J Trauma 1985;25:90.

48. Cothren CC, Moore EE, Biffl WL, et al: Cervical spine fracture patterns as predictive of blunt vertebral artery injury. J Trauma 2003;55:811.

49. Harris L, Marano GD, McCorkle D: Nasofrontal duct: CT in frontal sinus trauma. Radiology 1987;165:195.

50. Angelen J, Metzler M, Bunn P, Griffiths H: Flexion and extension views are not cost-effective in a cervical spine clearance protocol for obtunded trauma patients. J Trauma 2002;52:54.

51. Babcock JL: Cervical spine injuries: diagnosis and classification. Arch Surg 1976;111:646.

52. Lorberboym M, Gilad R, Gorin V: Late whiplash syndrome: correlation of brain SPECT with neuropsychological tests and P300 event-related potential. J Trauma 2002;52:521.

53. Harris JH: Missed cervical spinal cord injuries. J Trauma 2002;53:165.

54. Bracken MB, Shepard M, Collins W: A randomized controlled trial of methylprednisolone or naloxone in the treatment of acute spinal cord injury. N Engl J Med 1990;322:1405.

55. Gerndt SJ, Rodriguez MD, Pawlin JW, Taheri PA: Consequences of high dose steroid therapy for spinal cord injury. J Trauma 1997;42:279.

56. Manson P, Iliff N: Management of blowout fractures of the orbital floor: early repair of selected injuries. Surv Ophthalmol 1991;35:280.

57. Lee R, Robertson B, Manson P: Facial injuries: the shock trauma experience. Plast Reconstr Surg; submitted.

58. Lim LH, Lam LK, Moore H, et al: Associated injuries in facial fractures: a review of 839 patients. Plast Surg 1993;46:635.

59. Luce EA: Developing concepts and treatment of complex maxillary fractures. Clin Plast Surg 1992;19:125.

60. Gersten M, Milman AL, Lubkin V: Computerized algorithm for volumetric analysis from CT scans of the in vivo human orbit. Proceedings of the Sixth Annual Conference IEEE Engineering in Medicine and Biology Society, 1984.

61. Iliff C, Iliff W, Iliff N: Oculoplastic Surgery. Philadelphia, WB Saunders, 1979.

62. Barton FE, Berry WL: Evaluation of the acutely injured orbit. In Aston SJ, Hornblass A, Meltzer MA, Rees TD, eds: Third International Symposium of Plastic and Reconstructive Surgery of the Eye and Adnexa. Baltimore, Williams & Wilkins, 1982:34.

63. Miller GR, Tenzel RR: Ocular complications of midfacial fractures. Plast Reconstr Surg 1967;39:117.

64. Jabaley ME, Lerman M, Sanders HJ: Ocular injuries in orbital fractures: a review of 119 cases. Plast Reconstr Surg 1975;56:410.

65. Baker RS, Epstein AD: Ocular motor abnormalities from head trauma. Surv Ophthalmol 1991;35:245.

66. Lee RH, Gamble WB, Mayer MH, Manson PN: Patterns of facial laceration from blunt trauma. Plast Reconstr Surg 1997;99:1544.

67. Hussain K, Wijetunge DB, Grubnic S: A comprehensive analysis of craniofacial trauma. J Trauma 1994;17:34.

68. Putterman AM: Management of blowout fracture of the orbital floor: a conservative approach. Surg Ophthalmol 1991;35:279.

69. Rowe LD, Brandt-Zawadzki M: Spatial analysis of midfacial fractures with multidirectional and computed tomography: clinicopathologic correlates in 44 cases. Otolaryngol Head Neck Surg 1982;90:651.

70. Rowe LD, Miller E, Brandt-Zawadzki M: Computed tomography in maxillofacial trauma. Laryngoscope 1981;91:745.

71. Gentry LR, Manor WF, Turski PA, Strother CM: High-resolution CT analysis of facial struts in trauma. 1. Normal anatomy. 2. Osseous and soft tissue complications. AJR Am J Roentgenol 1983;140:523.

72. Kreipke DLK, Moss JJ Franco JM, et al: Computed tomography in facial trauma. AJR Am J Roentgenol 1984;142:1041.

73. Kassel EE, Noyek AM, Cooper PW: CT in facial trauma. J Otolaryngol 1983;12:2.

74. Luka B, Brechtelsbauer D, Gellrich N, Konig M: 2D and 3D reconstruction of the facial skeleton: an unnecessary option or a diagnostic pearl? Int J Maxillofac Surg 1995;21:99.

75. Zonneveld FW, Lobregt S, van der Meulen JC, Vaandrager JM: Three-dimensional imaging in craniofacial surgery. World J Surg 1989;13:328.

76. Ayella RJ: The face. In Ayella RJ: Radiologic Management of the Massively Traumatized Patient. Baltimore, Williams & Wilkins, 1978.

77. Finkie DR, Ringler SL, Luttenton CR, et al: Comparison of the diagnostic methods used in maxillofacial trauma. Plast Reconstr Surg 1985;75:32.

78. Chayra GA, Meador LR, Laskin DM: Comparison of panoramic and standard radiographs in the diagnosis of mandibular fractures. J Oral Maxillofac Surg 1986;44:677.

79. Wilson IF, Lokeh A, Benjamin C, et al: Contribution of conventional axial computed tomography (nonhelical) in conjunction with panoramic tomography in evaluating mandibular fractures. Ann Plast Surg 2000;45:415.

80. Wilson IF, Lokeh A, Benjamin C, et al: Prospective comparison of panoramic tomography (zonography) and helical computed tomography in the diagnosis and operative management of mandibular fractures. Plast Reconstr Surg 2001;107:1369.

81. Anastakis DS, Antonyshyn NA, Cooper PN, Yaffe MJ: Computed tomography artifacts associated with craniofacial fixation devices: an experimental study. Ann Plast Surg 1996;37:349.

82. Fiala TG, Novelline RA, Yaremchuk MC: Comparison of CT imaging artifact from craniomaxillofacial internal fixation devices. Plast Reconstr Surg 1993;92:1227.

83. Fiala TG, Paige TG, Davis TL, et al: Comparison of artifact from craniomaxillofacial internal fixation devices: magnetic resonance imaging. Plast Reconstr Surg 1994;93:725.

84. Sullivan PK, Smith JF, Rozelle AA: Cranio-orbital reconstruction: safety and image quality of metallic implants on CT and MRI imaging. Plast Reconstr Surg 1994;94:589.

85. Beer GM, Putz R, Mager K, et al: Variations in the frontal exit of the supraorbital nerve: an anatomic study. Plast Reconstr Surg 1998;102:334.

86. Knize D: A study of the supraorbital nerve. Plast Reconstr Surg 1995;96:564.

87. Satlam C, Ozer C, Guirer T: Anatomical variations in the frontal and supraorbital transcranial passages. J Craniofac Surg 2003;14:10.

88. Bales N, Baganlisa F, Schlegel G: A comparison of transcutaneous incisions used for exposure of the orbital rim and orbital floor: a retrospective study. Plast Reconstr Surg 1992;90:85.

89. Holtman B, Wray RC, Little AG: A randomized comparison of 4 incisions for orbital fractures. Plast Reconstr Surg 1981;67:731.

90. Converse JM: Discussion: A randomized comparison of 4 incisions for orbital fracture treatment. Plast Reconstr Surg 1981;67:736.

91. Heckler FR: Subciliary incision and skin muscle flap for orbital fractures. Ann Plast Surg 1983;10:309.

92. Manson PN, Iliff N: Orbital fractures. Facial Plast Surg 1988;5:243.

93. Manson P, Ruas E, Iliff N, Yaremchuk M: Single eyelid incision for exposure of the zygomatic bone and orbital reconstruction. Plast Reconstr Surg 1987;79:120.

94. Kazanjian VH, Converse J: Surgical Treatment of Facial Injuries. Baltimore, Williams & Wilkins, 1974.

95. Tessier P: The conjunctival approach to the orbital floor and maxilla in congenital malformation and trauma. J Maxillofac Surg 1973;1:3.

96. Converse JM, Firmin F, Wood-Smith D, Friedland JA: The conjunctival approach in orbital fractures. Plast Reconstr Surg 1973;52:656.

97. Soparkar CN, Patrinely J: Palpebral surgical approach for orbital fracture repair. Semin Plast Surg 2002;16:273.

98. Appling WD, Patrinely JR, Salzer TA: Transconjunctival approach vs. subciliary skin-muscle flap approach for orbital fracture repair. Arch Otolaryngol Head Neck Surg 1993;119:1000.

99. Bauman A, Ewers R: Use of the preseptal transconjunctival approach in orbit reconstruction surgery. J Oral Maxillofac Surg 2001;59:287, discussion 291.

100. Netcher DT, Patrinely JR, Peltier M, et al: Transconjunctival versus transcutaneous lower eyelid blepharoplasty: a prospective study. Plast Reconstr Surg 1995;96:1053.

101. Werther JR: Cutaneous approaches to the lower eyelid and orbit. J Oral Maxillofac Surg 1998;56:60.

102. Wray RC, Holtmann B, Ribaudo JM, et al: A comparison of conjunctival and subciliary incisions for orbital fractures. Br J Plast Surg 1977;30:142.

103. Mullins JB, Holds JB, Branham GH, Thomas JR: Complications of the transconjunctival approach. A review of 400 cases. Arch Otolaryngol Head Neck Surg 1997;123:385.

104. Westfall CT, Shore JW, Nunery WR, et al: Operative complications of the transconjunctival inferior fornix approach. Ophthalmology 1991;98:1525.

105. Alantar A, Roche Y, Maman L, Carpentier P: The lower labial branches of the mental nerve: anatomic variations and surgical relevance. J Oral Maxillofac Surg 2000;58:415.

106. Angle EH: Classification of malocclusion. Dent Cosmos 1899;41:240.

107. Gilmer TL: A case of fracture of the lower jaw with remarks on treatment. Arch Dent 1887;4:388.

108. Ivy RH: Observations of fractures of the mandible. JAMA 1922;79:295.

109. Rinehart G: Maxillomandibular fixation with bone anchors and quick release ligatures. J Craniofac Surg 1998;9:215.

110. Ellis E: Selection of internal fixation devices in mandibular fractures: how much fixation is enough? Semin Plast Surg 2002;16:229.

111. Haug RH, Street CC, Goltz M: Does plate adaptation affect stability? A biomechanical comparison of locking and non-locking plates. J Oral Maxillofac Surg 2002;60:1319.

112. Herford AS, Ellis ES: Use of locking reconstruction bone plate for mandibular surgery. J Oral Maxillofac Surg 1998;56:1261.

113. Bonanno PC, Converse JM: Primary bone grafting in management for facial fractures. N Y State J Med 1975;75:710.

114. Gruss JS, Mackinnon SE, Kasel E, Cooper PW: The role of primary bone grafting in complex craniomaxillofacial trauma. Plast Reconstr Surg 1985;75:17.

115. Gruss J: Complex craniofacial trauma: evolution of management: a trauma unit's experience. J Trauma 1990;30:377.

116. Gruss J, Phillips JH: Complex facial trauma: the evolving role of rigid fixation and immediate bone graft reconstruction. Clin Plast Surg 1989;16:93.

117. Gruss JS, Pollock RS, Phillips JH, Antonyshyn O: Combined injuries of the cranium and face. Br J Plast Surg 1989;42:385.

118. Gruss JS, Mackinnon SE: Complex maxillary fractures: role of buttress reconstruction and immediate bone grafts. Plast Reconstr Surg 1986;78:9.

119. Manson PN, Shack RB, Leonard LF, et al: Sagittal fractures of the maxilla and palate. Plast Reconstr Surg 1983;72:484.

120. Manson P, Clark N, Robertson B, Crawley W: Comprehensive management of pan facial fractures. J Craniomaxillofac Trauma 1995;11:43.
121. Kalk W, Raghoebar GM, Jansma J: Morbidity from iliac crest bone harvesting. J Oral Maxillofac Surg 1996;54:1424.
122. Zijderveld SA, ten Bruggenkate CM, van Den Bergh JP, Schulten EA: Fractures of the iliac crest after split-thickness bone grafting for pre-prosthetic surgery: report of 3 cases and review of the literature. J Oral Maxillofac Surg 2004;62:781.
123. Marx RE, Morales MJ: Morbidity from bone harvest in major jaw reconstruction: a randomized trial comparing the lateral anterior and posterior approaches to the ilium. J Oral Maxillofac Surg 1988;46:196.
124. Tessier P: Complications of facial trauma: principles of later reconstruction. Ann Plast Surg 1986;17:411.
125. Pensler J, McCarthy JG: The calvarial donor site: an anatomic study in cadavers. Plast Reconstr Surg 1985;75:648.
126. Kawamoto H: Personal communication.
127. Sullivan WG: The split calvarial donor site in the elderly: a study in cadavers. Plast Reconstr Surg 1989;84:29.
128. Ilankovan V, Jackson JT: Experience in the use of calvarial bone grafts in orbital reconstruction. Br J Oral Maxillofac Surg 1992;30:92.
129. Jackson IT, Pellett C, Smith JM: The skull as a bone graft donor site. Ann Plast Surg 1983;11:527.
130. Kline RM, Wolfe SA: Complications associated with the harvesting of cranial bone grafts. Plast Reconstr Surg 1995;95:5.
131. Young VL, Schuster RH, Harris LW: Intracerebral hematoma complicating split calvarial bone graft harvesting. Plast Reconstr Surg 1990;86:763.
132. Fischer K, Zhang F, Angel MF, Lineaweaver WC: Injuries associated with mandible fractures sustained in motor vehicle collisions. Plast Reconstr Surg 2001;108:328.
133. Ardekian L, Samet N, Shoshani Y, Taichers S: Life threatening bleeding following maxillofacial trauma. J Craniomaxillofac Surg 1993;21:336.
134. Ardekian L, Rosen D, Klein Y: Life threatening complications and irreversible damage following maxillofacial trauma. Injury 1998;29:253.
135. Lee J, Dodson T: The effect of mandibular third molar presence and position on the risk of an angle fracture. J Oral Maxillofac Surg 2000;58:394.
136. Hagan EH, Huelke DF: An analysis of 319 case reports of mandibular fractures. J Oral Surg 1961;19:93.
137. Huelke DF, Burdi AR: Location of mandibular fractures related to teeth and edentulous regions. J Oral Surg 1964;22:396.
138. Huelke DF, Burdi AR, Eyman CE: Association between mandibular fractures and site of trauma, dentition and age. J Oral Surg 1962;20:478.
139. Loukota RA, Shelton JC: Mechanical analysis of maxillofacial miniplates. Br J Oral Maxillofac Surg 1995;33:174.
140. Uglesic V, Virag M, Aljinovic N: Evaluation of mandibular fracture treatment. J Craniomaxillofac Surg 1993;21:251.
141. Behnia H, Kheradvar A, Shahrokhi M: An anatomic study of the lingual nerve in the third molar region. J Oral Maxillofac Surg 2000;58:649.
142. Dingman RO, Natvig P: Surgery of Facial Fractures. Philadelphia, WB Saunders, 1964:234.
143. Fry WK, Shepherd PR, McLeod AC, Parfitt GJ: The Dental Treatment of Maxillofacial Injuries. Oxford, Blackwell Scientific, 1942.
144. Amaratunga NA: The effect of teeth in the line of mandibular fractures on healing. J Oral Maxillofac Surg 1987;45:312, 314.
145. Schneider SS, Stern H: Teeth in the line of mandibular fractures. J Oral Surg 1971;29:107.
146. Laskin DM, Best AM: Current trends in the treatment of maxillofacial injuries in the United States. J Oral Maxillofac Surg 2000;58:207.

147. Schmidt BL, Kearns G, Gordon N, Kaban LB: A financial analysis of maxillomandibular fixation versus rigid internal fixation for treatment of mandibular fractures. J Oral Maxillofac Surg 2000;58:1206.
148. Peterson LJ: Principles of antibiotic therapy. In Tobazian RG, Goldberg MH, eds: Oral and Maxillofacial Infections, 3rd ed. Philadelphia, WB Saunders, 1994:160.
149. Chodak GW, Plaut ME: Uses of systemic antibiotics for prophylaxis in surgery: a critical review. Arch Surg 1977;112:326.
150. Zallen RD, Curry JT: A study of antibiotic usage in compound fractures. J Oral Surg 1975;33:341.
151. Chole RA, Yee J: Antibiotic prophylaxis for facial fractures: a prospective, randomized clinical trial. Arch Otolaryngol Head Neck Surg 1987;113:1055.
152. Abubaker AO, Rollert MK: Postoperative antibiotic prophylaxis in mandibular fractures: a preliminary randomized, double-blind, and placebo-controlled clinical study. J Oral Maxillofac Surg 2001;59:1415.
153. Amaratunga NA: A comparative study of the clinical aspects of edentulous and dentulous fractures. J Oral Maxillofac Surg 1988;46:3.
154. Amaratunga NA: Mouth opening after release of maxillomandibular fixation in fracture patients. J Oral Maxillofac Surg 1987;45:383.
155. Amaratunga NA: The relation of age to the immobilization period required for healing of mandibular fractures. J Oral Maxillofac Surg 1987;45:111.
156. Azman P, Manson P: Diet After Mandibular Fractures. Baltimore, Md, MIEMSS Publications, 1988.
157. Brooks M, Elkin AC, Harrison RG: A new concept of capillary circulation in bone cortex. Lancet 1961;1:1078.
158. Dingman RO, Grabb WC: Surgical anatomy of the mandibular ramus of the facial nerve based on the dissection of 100 facial halves. Plast Reconstr Surg 1962;29:2166.
159. Bolourian R, Lazow S, Berger J: Transoral 2.0 mm miniplate fixation of mandibular fractures plus 2 weeks' maxillomandibular fixation: a prospective study. J Oral Maxillofac Surg 2002;60:167.
160. Schmoker M, Von Allmen G, Tschopp HM: Application of functionally stable fixation in maxillofacial surgery according to ASIF principles. J Oral Maxillofac Surg 1982;40:457.
161. Munro IR: The Luhr fixation system for the craniofacial skeleton. Clin Plast Surg 1987;79:39.
162. Michlet FX, Dymes J, Dessus B: Osteosynthesis with miniaturized screwed plates in maxillofacial surgery. J Maxillofac Surg 1973;1:79.
163. Kruger GO: Textbook of Oral and Maxillofacial Surgery, 6th ed. St. Louis, CV Mosby, 1984.
164. Champy M, Lodde JP, Schmidt R, et al: Mandibular osteosynthesis by miniature screwed plates via a buccal approach. J Maxillofac Surg 1978;6:14.
165. Champy M, Kahn JL: Fracture line stability as a function of the internal fixation system. [discussion]. J Oral Maxillofac Surg 1995;53:801.
166. Moreno JC, Fernandez A, Ortiz JA, Montalvo JJ: Complication rates associated with different treatments for mandibular fractures. J Oral Maxillofac Surg 2000;58:273.
167. Moulton-Barrett R, Lubenstein A, Salzhaver M, et al: Complications of mandibular fractures. Ann Plast Reconstr Surg 1998;41:258.
168. Neal DC, Wagner WF, Alpert B: Morbidity associated with teeth in the line of mandibular fractures. J Oral Surg 1978;36:859.
169. Borah G, Ashmead D: Fate of teeth transfixed by osteosynthesis screws. Plast Reconstr Surg 1996;97:726.
170. Eyrich GKH, Gratz KW, Sailer HF: Surgical treatment of fractures of the edentulous mandible. J Oral Maxillofac Surg 1997;55:1081.
171. Falcone PA, Haedicke GJ, Brooks G: Maxillofacial fractures in the elderly: a comparative study. Plast Reconstr Surg 1990;83:443.

172. Mosby EL, Markle TL, Zulian MA, Hiatt WR: Technique of rigid fixation of Le Fort and palatal fractures. J Oral Maxillofac Surg 1986;44:921.

173. Zide BM: The mentalis muscle: an essential component of chin and lower lip position. Plast Reconstr Surg 2000;105:1213.

174. Ellis E III, Throckmorton GS: Facial symmetry after closed and open treatment of fractures of the mandibular condylar process. J Oral Maxillofac Surg 2000;58:719.

175. Niederdellmann H, Schilli W, Duker J, Akuamoa-Boateng E: Osteosynthesis of mandibular fractures using lag screws. Int J Oral Surg 1976;5:117.

176. Dichard A, Klotch D: Testing biomechanical strength of repairs for the mandibular angle fracture. Laryngoscope 1994;104:201.

177. Oasseri LA, Ellis E, Sinn DP: Complications of nonrigid fixation of mandibular angle fractures. J Oral Maxillofac Surg 1993;51:382.

178. Haug RH, Fattahi TT, Boltz M: A biomechanical evaluation of mandibular angle fracture plating techniques. J Oral Maxillofac Surg 2001;59:1199.

179. Shetty V, Freymuller R: Teeth in the fracture line. J Oral Maxillofac Surg 1989;47:1303.

180. Choi BH, Suh CH: Technique for applying 2 miniplates for treatment of mandibular angle fractures. J Oral Maxillofac Surg 2001;59:353.

181. Haug RH, Barber JE, Reifeis R: A comparison of mandibular angle fracture plating techniques. Oral Surg Oral Med Oral Pathol Oral Radiol Endod 1996;82:257.

182. Haug RH, Barber JE, Punjabi AP: An in vitro comparison of the effect of number and pattern of positional screws on load resistance. J Oral Maxillofac Surg 1999;57:300.

183. Manson PN: A plate is not just a plate, and a screw is not just a screw. J Craniomaxillofac Trauma 1999;5:8.

184. Ellis E III: Treatment methods for fractures of the mandibular angle. J Craniomaxillofac Trauma 1996;2:28.

185. Ellis E III, Sinn DP: Treatment of mandibular fractures using two 2.4-mm dynamic compression plates. J Oral Maxillofac Surg 1993;51:969.

186. Ellis E, Walker LR: Treatment of mandibular angle fractures with two noncompression miniplates. J Oral Maxillofac Surg 1999;52:1032.

187. Ellis E, Karas N: Treatment of mandibular angle fracture using two minidynamic compression plates. J Oral Maxillofac Surg 1992;50:958.

188. Ellis E III: Treatment of mandibular angle fractures using the AO reconstruction plate. J Oral Maxillofac Surg 1993;51:250.

189. Ellis E, Walker LR: Treatment of mandibular angle fractures with one noncompression miniplate. J Oral Maxillofac Surg 1996;54:864.

190. Niederdellmann H, Akuamoa-Boateng E: Lag-screw osteosynthesis: a new procedure for treating fractures of the mandibular angle. J Oral Surg 1981;39:938.

191. Niederdellmann H, Shetty V: Solitary lag screw osteosynthesis in the treatment of fractures of the angle of the mandibular: a retrospective study. Plast Reconstr Surg 1987;80:68.

192. Natvig P, Sicher H, Fodor PB: The rare isolated fracture of the coronoid process of the mandible. Plast Reconstr Surg 1970;46:168.

193. Cascone P, Sassano P, Spalcaccia F: Condylar fractures during growth: a follow-up of 16 patients. J Craniofac Surg 1999;10:87.

194. Hovinga J, Boering G, Stegenga B: Long-term results of nonsurgical management of condylar fractures in children. J Oral Maxillofac Surg 1999;28:429.

195. Norholt SE, Krishnan V, Sindet-Pederson S, Jensen I: Pediatric condylar fractures: a long term follow up of 55 patients. J Oral Maxillofac Surg 1993;51:1302.

196. Konstantinovic VS, Dimitrijevic B: Surgical versus conservative treatment of unilateral condylar process fractures: clinical and radiographic evaluation of 80 patients. J Oral Maxillofac Surg 1992;50:349.

197. Klotch DW, Lundy LB: Condylar neck fractures of the mandible. Otolaryngol Clin North Am 1991;24:181.

198. Choi BH, Kim KN, Kim HJ, Kim MK: Evaluation of condylar neck fracture plating techniques. J Craniomaxillofac Surg 1999;27:109.

199. Choi BH, Yoo JH: Open reduction of condylar neck fractures with exposure of the facial nerve. Oral Surg Oral Med Oral Pathol Oral Radiol Endod 1999;88:292.

200. Choi BH, Yi CK, Yoo JH: Clinical evaluation of 3 types of plate osteosynthesis for fixation of condylar neck fractures. J Oral Maxillofac Surg 2001;59:734.

201. Assael L: Open versus closed reduction of adult mandibular condyle fractures: an alternative interpretation of the evidence. J Oral Maxillofac Surg 2003;61:1333.

202. Jeter TS, Hackney F: Open reduction and rigid fixation of subcondylar fractures. In Yaremchuk M, Gruss T, Manson P, eds: Rigid Fixation of the Craniomandibular Skeleton. Boston, Butterworth-Heinemann, 1992:127.

203. Ellis E III, McFadden D, Simon P, et al: Surgical complications with open treatment of mandibular condylar process fractures. J Oral Maxillofac Surg 2000;58:950.

204. Chen CT, Lai JP, Tung TC, Chen XR: Endoscopically assisted mandibular subcondylar fracture repair. Plast Reconstr Surg 1999;103:60.

205. Lauer G, Schmelzeisen R: Endoscope-assisted fixation of mandibular condylar process fractures. J Oral Maxillofac Surg 1999;57:36.

206. Ellis E III, Moos KF, Attar A: Ten years of mandibular fractures: an analysis of 2137 cases. Oral Surg Oral Med Oral Pathol 1985;59:120.

207. Kroetsch LJ, Brook AL, Kader A, Eisig SB: Traumatic dislocation of the mandibular condyle into the middle cranial fossa: report of a case, review of the literature and a proposed management protocol. J Oral Maxillofac Surg 2001;59:88.

208. Evans G, Clark N, Manson P: Technique of costal chondral graft placement. J Craniofac Surg 1994;5:340.

209. Haug RH, Peterson GP, Goltz M: A biomechanical evaluation of mandibular condyle fracture plating techniques. J Oral Maxillofac Surg 2002;60:73.

210. Iizuka T, Lindquist C, Hallikainen D, et al: Severe bone resorption and osteoarthritis after miniplate fixation of high condylar fractures: a clinical and radiologic study of thirteen patients. Oral Surg Oral Med Oral Pathol 1991;72:400.

211. Iizuka T, Ladrach K, Geering AH, et al: Open reduction without fixation of dislocated condylar process fractures: long term clinical and radiologic analysis. J Oral Maxillofac Surg 1998;56:553.

212. Griffiths H, Townsend J: Anesthesia of the inferior alveolar and lingual nerves as a complication of a fractured condylar process. J Oral Maxillofac Surg 1999;57:77.

213. Sugiura T, Yamamoto K, Murakami K, Sugimura M: A comparative evaluation of osteosynthesis with lag screws, miniplates or Kirschner wires for mandibular condylar process fractures. J Oral Maxillofac Surg 2001;59:1161.

214. Ellis E III, Palmieri C, Throckmorton GS: Further displacement of condylar process fractures with closed treatment. J Oral Maxillofac Surg 1999;57:1307.

215. Ellis E III, Simon P, Throckmorton GS: Occlusal results after open or closed treatment of fractures of the mandibular condylar process. J Oral Maxillofac Surg 2000;58:260.

216. Ellis E III, Throckmorton GS: Bite forces after open or closed treatment of mandibular condylar process fractures. J Oral Maxillofac Surg 2001;59:389.

217. Yang WG, Chen CT, Tsay PK, Chen YR: Functional results of unilateral mandibular condylar process fractures after open and closed treatment. J Trauma 2002;52:498.

218. Baker AW, McMahon J, Moos KF: Current consensus on the management of fractures of the mandibular condyle. Int J Maxillofac Surg 1998;27:258.

219. Palmieri C, Ellis E, Throckmorton GS: Mandibular motion after closed treatment of unilateral mandibular condylar process fractures. J Oral Maxillofac Surg 1999;57:764.

220. Hammer B, Schier P, Prein J: Osteosynthesis of condylar neck fractures. A review of 30 patients. Br J Plast Surg 1997; 35:288.

221. Takenoshita Y, Ishibashi H, Oka M: Comparison of functional recovery after nonsurgical and surgical treatment of condylar fractures. J Oral Maxillofac Surg 1990;48:1191.

222. Takenoshita Y, Oka M, Tashiro H: Surgical treatment of fractures of the mandibular condylar neck. J Craniomaxillofac Surg 1989;17:119.

223. Raveh J, Vuillemin T, Ladrach K: Open reduction of the dislocated fractured condylar process: indications and surgical procedures. J Oral Maxillofac Surg 1989;47:120.

224. Raveh J, Ladrach K, Vuillemin T: Indication for open reduction of the dislocated fractured condylar process. In Worthington P, Evans J, eds: Controversies in Oral and Maxillofacial Surgery. Philadelphia, WB Saunders, 1994:173-190.

225. Worsaae N, Thorn JJ: Surgical versus nonsurgical treatment of unilateral dislocated low subcondylar process fractures: a clinical study of 52 cases. J Oral Maxillofac Surg 1994; 52:353.

226. Worsaae N, Thorn JJ: Surgical versus conservative treatment of the unilateral condylar process fracture. J Oral Maxillofac Surg 1992;50:319.

227. Silvennoinen U, Iizuka T, Oikarinen K, Lindqvist C: Analysis of possible factors leading to problems after nonsurgical treatment of condylar fractures. J Oral Maxillofac Surg 1994;52:793.

228. Haug RH, Assael L: Outcomes of open versus closed treatment of mandibular subcondylar fractures. J Oral Maxillofac Surg 2001;59:370.

229. Haug RH: Retention of asymptomatic bone plates used for orthognathic surgery and facial fractures. J Oral Maxillofac Surg 1996;54:611.

230. Zide MF, Kent JN: Indications for open reduction of mandibular condyle fractures. J Oral Maxillofac Surg 1983;41:89.

231. Zide MF: Open reduction of mandibular condyle fractures. Clin Plast Surg 1989;16:69.

232. Zide MF: Outcomes of open versus closed treatment of mandibular subcondylar fractures [discussion]. J Oral Maxillofac Surg 2001;59:375.

233. Brandt MT, Haug R: Open versus closed reduction of mandibular fractures: a review of the literature regarding the evolution of current thoughts on management. J Oral Maxillofac Surg 2003;61:1324.

234. Marciani RD, Hill O: The treatment of the fractured edentulous mandible. J Oral Surg 1979;37:569.

235. Marciani FD: Invasive management of the fractured atrophic mandible. J Oral Maxillofac Surg 2001;59:392.

236. Levine PA, Goode RL: Treatment of fractures of the edentulous mandible. Arch Otolaryngol 1982;108:167.

237. Alpert B: Discussion: Surgical treatment of the edentulous mandible. J Oral Maxillofac Surg 1997;55:1087.

238. Buchbinder D: Treatment of fractures of the edentulous mandible, 1943 to 1993: a review of the literature. J Oral Maxillofac Surg 1993;51:1174.

239. Halazonetis JA: The "weak" regions of the mandible. Br J Oral Surg 1968;6:37.

240. Kruger E, Schilli W, eds: Oral and Maxillofacial Traumatology. Chicago, Quintessence, 1982.

241. Oikarinen K, Ignatius E, Silvennoinen W: Treatment of mandibular fractures in the 1980s. J Craniomaxillofac Surg 1993;21:245.

242. Baudens JB: Fracture de la machoire inferieure. Bull Acad Med Paris 1840;5:341.

243. Robert CA: Nouveau procede de traitement des fractures de la portion alveolaire de la machoire inferieure. Bull Gen Ther 1852;42:22.

244. Obwegeser HL, Sailer HF: Another way of treating fractures of the atrophic edentulous mandible. J Maxillofac Surg 1973;1:213.

245. Zachariades N, Papavassiliou D, Triantafylou D, et al: Fractures of the facial skeleton in the edentulous patient. J Maxillofac Surg 1984;12:262.

246. Lambotte A: Chirurgie operatoire des fractures. Paris, Masson & Cie, 1913.

247. Anderson R: An ambulatory method of treating fractures of the shaft of the femur. Surg Gynecol Obstet 1936;62:865.

248. Morris JH: Biphase connector, external skeletal splint for reduction and fixation of mandibular fractures. Oral Surg 1949;2:1382.

249. Zide BM, Pfeiffer TM, Longacre MT: Chin surgery: I. Augmentation: the allures and alerts. Plast Reconstr Surg 1999;104:1843.

250. Nordgaard JO: Persistent sensory disturbances and diplopia following fractures of the zygoma. Arch Otolaryngol 1976;102:80.

251. Iizuka T, Lindqvist C, Hallikainen D, et al: Infection after rigid internal fixation of mandibular fracture: a clinical and radiographic study. J Oral Maxillofac Surg 1991;49:585.

252. Giordano AM, Foster CA, Boles LR Jr, Maisel RH: Chronic osteomyelitis following mandibular fractures and its treatment. Arch Otolaryngol 1982;108:30.

253. Phillips J, Forrest C: Le Fort fractures. In Prein J, ed: A-O Manual of Internal Fixation for Facial Injuries. New York, Springer-Verlag, 1998.

254. Punjabi AP, Thaller S: Late complications of mandibular fractures. Operative Techniques Plast Reconstr Surg 1998;5:266.

255. Cascone P, Yetrano S, Nicolai G, Fabiani F: Temporomandibular joint biomechanical reconstruction: the fluid and joint membrane. J Craniofac Surg 1999;10:301.

256. Umsteadt H, Ellers M, Muller M: Functional reconstruction of the TM joint in cases of severely displaced fractures and fracture dislocation. J Craniomaxillofac Surg 2000;28:97.

257. Ostrofsky MK, Lownie JF: Zygomatico-coronoid ankylosis. J Oral Surg 1977;35:752.

258. Serletti J, Crawley W, Manson PN: Autogenous reconstruction of the temporomandibular joint. J Craniofac Surg 1993;4:28.

259. Manson P: Facial fractures. In Grotting J, ed: Reoperative Aesthetic and Reconstructive Plastic Surgery. St. Louis, Quality Medical Publishing, 1995.

260. Manson PN: Facial bone healing and grafts: a review of clinical physiology. Clin Plast Surg 1994;21:331.

261. Winstanley RP: The management of fractures of the mandible. Br J Oral Maxillofac Surg 1994;22:170.

262. Eid K, Lynch OJ, Whitaker LA: Mandibular fractures: the problem patient. J Trauma 1976;16:658.

263. Mathog RH, Toma V, Clayman L, Wolf S: Nonunion of the mandible: an analysis of contributing factors. J Oral Maxillofac Surg 2000;58:746.

264. Haug R, Schwimmer A: Fibrous union of the mandible: a review of 27 patients. J Oral Maxillofac Surg 1994;52:832.

265. Markowitz B, Sinow JD, Kawamoto HK, et al: Prospective comparison of axial computed tomography and standard and panoramic radiographs in mandibular fractures. Ann Plast Surg 1999;42:163.

266. Dahlstrom L, Kahnberg KE, Lindhall L: 15 years follow-up on condylar fractures. Int J Oral Maxillofac Surg 1989;18:18.

267. Maloney PL, Welch TB, Doku HC: Early immobilization of mandibular fractures. J Oral Maxillofac Surg 1991;49:698.

268. Craft PD, Sargent LA: Membranous bone healing and techniques in calvarial bone grafting. Clin Plast Surg 1989;16:11.

269. Matsuo K, Hirose T, Furuta S, et al: Semiquantitative correction of posttraumatic enophthalmos with diced cartilage grafts. Plast Reconstr Surg 1989;83:429.

270. Wolfe SA, Kawamoto HK: Taking the iliac-bone graft. J Bone Joint Surg Am 1978;60:411.

271. Mathog R, Hillstrom RP, Nesi FA: Surgical correction of enophthalmos and diplopia: a report of 38 cases. Arch Otolaryngol Head Neck Surg 1989;115:169.

272. Maloney PL, Lincoln RE, Coyne CP: A protocol for the management of compound mandibular fractures based on the time from injury to treatment. J Oral Maxillofac Surg 2001;59:879.

273. Marciani RD, Haley IV, Kohn MN: Patient compliance—a factor in facial trauma repair. Oral Surg Oral Med Oral Pathol 1990;70:428.

274. Hirai H, Okumura A, Goto M, Katsuki T: Histologic study of the bone adjacent to titanium bone screws used for mandibular fracture treatment. J Oral Maxillofac Surg 2001;59:531.

275. Gutwald R, Schon R, Gellrich N, et al: Bioresorbable implants in maxillofacial osteosynthesis: experimental and clinical experience. Injury 2002;33:4.

276. Gutwald R, Schon R, Gellrich N, et al: Is there a need for resorbable implants or bone substitutes? Injury 2002;33(suppl 2):4.

277. Edwards RC, Kiely KD, Eppley B: Resorbable PLLA-PGA fixation of sagittal split osteotomies. J Craniofac Surg 1999;10:230.

278. Tatum SA, Kellman RM, Freije JE: Maxillofacial fixation with absorbable miniplates: computed tomographic follow up. J Craniofac Surg 1997;8:135.

279. Murphy RA, Birmingham KL, Okunski WJ, Wasser T: Risk factors contributing to symptomatic plate removal in maxillofacial trauma patients. Plast Reconstr Surg 2000;105:521.

280. Manor Y, Chaushu G, Taicher S: Risk factors contributing to symptomatic plate removal in orthognathic surgery patients. J Oral Maxillofac Surg 1999;57:679.

281. Stranc MF, Robertson LA: Classification of injuries to the nasal skeleton. Ann Plast Surg 1979;2:468.

282. Murray JA, Maran AG, Mackenzie IJ, Raab G: Open vs. closed reduction of the fractured nose. Arch Otolaryngol 1984;110:797.

283. Stranc MF: Primary treatment of nasoethmoid injuries with increased intercanthal distance. Br J Plast Surg 1970;23:8.

284. Stranc MF: Pattern of lacrimal injuries in nasoethmoid fractures. Br J Plast Surg 1970;23:339.

285. Gruss JS: Naso-ethmoid-orbital fractures: classification and role of primary bone grafting. Plast Reconstr Surg 1985;75:303.

286. Markowitz B, Manson P, Sargent L, et al: Management of the medial canthal tendon in nasoethmoid orbital fractures: the importance of the central fragment in treatment and classification. Plast Reconstr Surg 1991;87:843.

287. Clark GM, Wallace CS: Analysis of nasal support. Arch Otolaryngol 1970;92:118.

288. Metzinger S, Tufaro A, Davidson J, et al: The ESON classification of nasal fractures: a new system for evaluation and treatment of nasal fractures. Plast Reconstr Surg; in press.

289. Mayell MF: Nasal fractures. Their occurrence, management and some late results. J R Coll Surg Edinb 1973;18:31.

290. Rohrich RJ, Adams WP Jr: Nasal fracture management: minimizing secondary deformities. Plast Reconstr Surg 2000;106:266.

291. Rohrich R, Adams WP: Late salvage of nasal injuries. Operative Techniques Plast Reconstr Surg 1998;5:342.

292. Harrison DH: Nasal injuries: their pathogenesis and treatment. Br J Plast Surg 1979;32:57.

293. ten Koppel PG, van der Veen JM, Hein D: Controlling incision-induced distortion of nasal septal cartilage: a model to predict the effect of scoring of rabbit septa. Plast Reconstr Surg 2003;111:1948.

294. Motomura H, Muraoka M, Tetsuji Y, et al: Changes in fresh nasal bone fractures with time on computed tomographic images. Ann Plast Surg 2001;47:620.

295. Xie C, Mehendale N, Barrett D, et al: 30-year retrospective review of frontal sinus fractures: the Charity Hospital experience. J Craniomaxillofac Trauma 2000;6:7.

296. Gillies HD, Millard DR: The Principles and Art of Plastic Surgery. Boston, Little, Brown, 1957.

297. Pollack RA: Nasal trauma. Plast Surg Clin North Am 1992;19:133.

298. Pollack RA: Pathogenesis of nasal injury: structural deformation in the fresh cadaver. Personal communication.

299. Pollack RA: Septal reconstruction in 405 patients with nasal obstruction. Abstracts of the Sixty-third annual meeting of the American Association of Plastic Surgeons, Chicago, 1984:263.

300. Verwoerd CDA: Present day treatment of nasal fractures: closed versus open reduction. Facial Plast Surg 1992;8:220.

301. Burm JS, Oh SK: Indirect open reduction through cartilaginous incisions and intranasal Kirschner wire splinting in comminuted nasal fractures. Plast Reconstr Surg 1998;102:342.

302. Sear AJ: A method of internal nasal splinting for unstable nasal fractures. Ann Plast Surg 1990;24:199.

303. Yabe T, Motomura H, Muraoka M: Postoperative evaluation of nasal bone fractures using CT images and the necessity for this. Jpn Plast Reconstr Surg 1999;42:303.

304. Yabe T, Muraoka M: Double opposing V-4 hinge flap. Ann Plast Surg 2003;41:641.

305. Harshbarger RJ, Sullivan PK: Lateral nasal osteotomies: implications of bony thickness on fracture patterns. Ann Plast Surg 1999;42:365.

306. Crysdale WS, Tatham B: External septorhinoplasty in children. Laryngoscope 1985;95:12.

307. Gilbert GG: Growth of the nose and the postrhinoplastic problem in youth. Arch Otolaryngol 1958;68:673.

308. Newman H: Surgery of the nasal septum. Clin Plast Surg 1996;32:271.

309. McNeil RA: Traumatic nasal neuralgia and its treatment. Br Med J 1963;2:536.

310. Fry HJH: Interlocked stresses in human nasal septal cartilage. Br J Plast Surg 1966;19:276.

311. Fry HJH: Nasal skeleton trauma and the interlocked stresses of the nasal septal cartilage. Br J Plast Surg 1967;20:146.

312. Hwang K, Shu MS, Lee S, Chung H: Zygomaticotemporal nerve passage in the temporal area. J Craniofac Surg 2004;15:209.

313. Hwang K, Suh MS, Chung IH: Cutaneous distribution of the infraorbital nerve. J Craniofac Surg 2004;15:3.

314. Sungeil P, Lindquist C: Paresthesia of the infraorbital nerve following fracture of the zygomatic complex. Int J Oral Maxillofac Surg 1987;16:363.

315. Kersarwani A, Antonyshyn O, Mackinnon SE, et al: Facial sensibility testing in the normal and posttraumatic population. Ann Plast Surg 1989;22:416.

316. Uriens JPM, Vanderglas HW, Bosman F, et al: Information on infraorbital nerve damage from multitesting of sensory functions. Int J Oral Maxillofac Surg 1998;27:20.

317. Uriens JPM, Vanderglas HW, Bosman F, et al: Infraorbital nerve function following treatment of orbitozygomatic complete fractures: a multitest approach. Int J Oral Maxillofac Surg 1998;27:27.

318. Knight JS, North JF: The classification of malar fractures: an analysis of displacement as a guide to treatment. Br J Plast Surg 1961;13:315.

319. Yanagisawa E: Symposium on maxillofacial trauma. 3. Pitfalls in the management of zygomatic fractures. Laryngoscope 1973;83:527.

320. Hollier L, Thornton J, Pazmino P, Stal S: The management of orbitozygomatic fractures. Plast Reconstr Surg 2003;111:2386.

321. Rohrich R, Hollier LH, Watumull D: Optimizing the treatment of orbito-zygomatic fractures. Clin Plast Surg 1992;19:149.

322. Rohrich R, Mickel T: Frontal sinus obliteration: in search of the ideal autogenous material. Plast Reconstr Surg 1995;95:580.

323. Anastassou GE, Van Damme PA: Evaluation of the anatomical position of the lateral canthal ligament: clinical applications and guidelines. J Craniofac Surg 1996;7:429.

324. Whitaker LA, Yaremchuk MJ: Secondary reconstruction of posttraumatic orbital deformities. Ann Plast Surg 1990;25:440.

325. Yaremchuk M, Kim W: Soft tissue alterations associated with acute extended open reduction and internal fixation of orbital fractures. J Craniofac Surg 1992;3:134.

326. Yaremchuk M: Changing concepts in the management of secondary orbital deformities. Clin Plast Surg 1992;19:113.

327. Barclay TL: Diplopia in association with fractures of the zygomatic bone. Br J Plast Surg 1958;11:147.

328. Barclay TL: Four hundred malar-zygomatic fractures. Transactions of the International Society of Plastic Surgeons, Second Congress. Edinburgh, E & S Livingstone, 1960:259.

329. Barclay TL: Some aspects of treatment of traumatic diplopia. Br J Plast Surg 1963;16:214.

330. Antonyshyn O, Gruss JS, Kassel EE: Blow-out fractures of the orbit. Plast Reconstr Surg 1989;84:10.

331. Stanley RB, Sis BS, Frank GF, Nerd JA: Management of the displaced lateral orbital wall fractures associated with visual and ocular motility disturbances. Plast Reconstr Surg 1998;102:972.

332. Stanley RB: The temporal approach to lateral orbital wall fractures. Arch Otolaryngol Head Neck Surg 1998;114:550.

333. Furst IM, Austin P, Phardah M, Mahoney J: The use of computed tomography to define zygomatic complex position. J Oral Maxillofac Surg 2001;59:647.

334. Stanley RB Jr: Use of intraoperative computed tomography during repair of orbitozygomatic fractures. Arch Facial Plast Surg 1999;1:19.

335. Adams WM: Internal wiring fixation of facial fractures. Surgery 1942;12:523.

336. Adams WM, Adams LH: Internal wire fixation of facial fractures: a 15 year follow-up report. Am J Surg 1956;91:12.

337. Schubert W, Gear AL, Lee C, et al: Incorporation of titanium mesh in orbital and midface reconstruction. Plast Reconstr Surg 2002;110:1022.

338. Manson P, Iliff N, Robertson B: Discussion: Porous polyethylene implants in orbital reconstruction. Plast Reconstr Surg 2002;109:886.

339. Romano J, Iliff NT, Manson PN: Use of Medpor porous polyethylene implants in 140 patients with facial fractures. J Craniofac Surg 1993;4:142.

340. Byeon JH: The clinical study of Medpor in blow-out fracture treatment: one hundred patients. Korean Plast Reconstr Surg 1998;25:401.

341. Choi JC, Bstandig S, Iwamoto MA, et al: Porous polyethylene sheet implant with a barrier surface: a rabbit study. Ophthalmic Plast Reconstr Surg 1998;14:32.

342. Choi JC, Sims CD, Casanova R, et al: Porous polyethylene implant for orbital wall reconstruction. J Craniomaxillofac Trauma 1995;1:42.

343. Dingman RO, Alling CC: Open reduction and internal wire fixation of maxillofacial fractures. J Oral Surg 1954;12:140.

344. Mayer M, Manson PN: Rigid fixation in facial fractures. Philadelphia, JB Lippincott, 1991. Problems in Plastic Surgery.

345. Chen CT: Endoscopic zygomatic fracture repair. Operative Techniques Plast Reconstr Surg 1998;5:282.

346. Kobayashi S, Sakai Y, Yamada A, Ohmori K: Approaching the zygoma with an endoscope. J Craniofac Surg 1998;6:519.

347. Schmidt BL, Pogel MA, Harkin-Fael Z: The course of the temporal branch of the facial nerve in the face. J Oral Maxillofac Surg 2001;59:178.

348. Rinehart G, Marsh J, Hemmer K: Internal fixation of malar fractures: an experimental biophysical study. Plast Surg 1989;84:21.

349. Dal Santo F, Ellis E, Throckmorton GS: The effects of zygomatic complex fracture on masseteric muscle force. J Oral Maxillofac Surg 1992;50:791.

350. Davidson J, Nickerson D, Nickerson B: Zygomatic fractures: comparison of methods of internal fixation. Plast Reconstr Surg 1990;86:25.

351. Kasrai L, Hearn T, Gur F, Forrest C: A biochemical analysis of the orbital zygomatic complex in human cadavers: examination of load sharing and failure patterns following fixation with titanium and bioresorbable systems. J Craniofac Surg 1999;10:237.

352. Gosain A, Song L, Corrao M, Pintar FA: Biomechanical evaluation of titanium, biodegradable plate and screw and cyanoacrylate glue fixation systems in craniofacial surgery. Plast Reconstr Surg 1998;101:582.

353. Manson PN, Solomon G, Paskert JP, et al: Compression plates in midface fractures. Plast Surg Forum 1986;9:265.

354. Rohrich RJ, Watumull D: Comparison of rigid plate versus wire fixation in the management of zygomatic fractures: a long-term follow-up clinical study. Plast Reconstr Surg 1995;96:570.

355. O'Hara D, Delvecchio D, Bartlett S, Whitaker L: The role of microfixation in malar fractures: a quantitative biophysical study. Plast Reconstr Surg 1996;97:345.

356. Rohner D, Tay A, Meng CW, et al: The sphenozygomatic suture as a key site for osteosynthesis of the orbitozygomatic complex in panfacial fractures: a biochemical study in cadavers based on clinical practice. Plast Reconstr Surg 2002;110:1463.

357. Brown JB, Fryer MP, McDowell F: Internal wire-pin immobilization of jaw fractures. Plast Reconstr Surg 1949;4:30.

358. Ellis E, Ghali GE: Lag screw fixation of anterior mandible angle fractures. J Oral Maxillofac Surg 1991;49:234.

359. Manson P, Markowitz B, Mirvis S, et al: Toward CT-based facial fracture treatment. Plast Reconstr Surg 1990;85:202.

360. Stanley RB Jr, Mathog RH: Evaluation and correction of the combined orbital trauma syndrome. Laryngoscope 1983;93:856.

361. Manson PN: Computed tomography use in repair of orbitozygomatic fractures. Arch Facial Plast Surg 1999;1:25.

362. Hammer B, Kunz C, Schramm A, et al: Repair of complex orbital fractures: technical problems, state-of-the-art solutions and future perspectives [review]. Ann Acad Med Singapore 1999;28:687.

363. Natvig P: Personal communication, 1962.

364. Stajcic Z: The buccal fat pad in the closure of oro-antral communications. J Craniomaxillofac Surg 1992;20:193.

365. Girotto J, Gamble B, Robertson B, et al: Blindness following reduction of facial fractures. Plast Reconstr Surg 1998;102:1821.

366. Ketchum LD, Ferris B, Masters FW: Blindness in midface fractures without direct injury to the globe. Plast Reconstr Surg 1976;55:187.

367. Perino KE, Zide MF, Kinnebrew MC: Late treatment of malunited malar fractures. J Oral Maxillofac Surg 1980;42:20.

368. Kawamoto HK Jr: Late posttraumatic enophthalmos: a correctable deformity? Plast Reconstr Surg 1982;69:423.

369. Manson PN, Iliff N: Surgical anatomy of the orbit. In Marsh J, ed: Current Therapy in Plastic and Reconstructive Surgery. Philadelphia, BC Decker, 1989:117.

370. Lund K: Fractures of the zygoma: a follow up study of 62 patients. J Oral Surg 1975;29:557.

371. Stuzin JM, Wagstrom L, Kawamoto HK, et al: The anatomy and significance of the buccal fat pad. Plast Reconstr Surg 1990;85:29.

372. Francel T, Birely B, Ringleman P, Manson PN: The fate of plates and screws after facial fracture reconstruction. Plast Reconstr Surg 1992;90:505.

373. Rowe NL, Killey HC: Fractures of the Facial Skeleton, 2nd ed. Baltimore, Williams & Wilkins, 1968.

374. Stanley RB Jr: The zygomatic arch as a guide to reconstruction of comminuted malar fractures. Arch Otolaryngol 1989;115:1459.

375. Vondra J: Fractures of the Base of the Skull. London, Peter Nevill, 1965.
376. Naham AM: The biomechanics of facial bone trauma. Laryngoscope 1975;85:140.
377. Crawley W, Azman P, Clark C, et al: The edentulous Le Fort fracture. J Craniofac Surg 1997;8:298.
378. Rudderman R, Mullen R: Biomechanics of the facial skeleton. Clin Plast Surg 1992;19:11.
379. Naham AM: The biomechanics of maxillofacial trauma. Clin Plast Surg 1975;2:59-67.
380. Kuepper RC, Harrington WF: Treatment of midfacial fractures at Bellevue Hospital Center, 1955-1976. J Oral Surg 1977;35:420.
381. Hendrickson M, Clark N, Manson P: Sagittal fractures of the maxilla: classification and treatment. Plast Reconstr Surg 1998;101:319.
382. Le Fort R: Etude experimentale sur les fractures de la machoire superieur. Rev Chir Paris 1901;23:208, 360, 479.
383. Manson PN: Some thoughts on the classification and treatment of Le Fort fractures. Ann Plast Surg 1986;17:356.
384. Wells MD, Oishi D, Sengezer M: Sagittal fractures of the palate: a new method of treatment. Can J Plast Surg 1995;3:87.
385. Romano JJ, Manson PN, Mirvis WE, et al: Le Fort fractures without mobility. Plast Reconstr Surg 1990;85:355.
386. Morgan BD, Maden DK, Bergerot JP: Fractures of the middle third of the face—a review of 300 cases. Br J Plast Surg 1972;25:147.
387. Manson P, Glassman D, Vander Kolk C, et al: Rigid stabilization of sagittal fractures of the maxilla and palate. Plast Reconstr Surg 1990;85:711.
388. Park S, Ock JJ: A new classification of palatal fractures and an algorithm to establish a treatment plan. Plast Reconstr Surg 2001;107:1669.
389. Sturla F, Abnsi D, Buquet J: Anatomical and mechanical considerations of craniofacial fractures: an experimental study. Plast Reconstr Surg 1980;66:815.
390. Swearingen JJ: Tolerances of the human face to crash impact. Report from the Office of Aviation Medicine, Federal Aviation Agency, July 1965.
391. Bell R, Dierks E, Homer L, Potter B: Management of cerebrospinal fluid leak associated with craniomaxillofacial trauma. J Oral Maxillofac Surg 2004;62:676.
392. Raaf J: Post-traumatic cerebrospinal fluid leaks. Arch Surg 1967;95:648.
393. Morley TP, Hetherington RF: Traumatic cerebrospinal fluid rhinorrhea and otorrhea, pneumocephalus and meningitis. Surg Gynecol Obstet 1957;104:88.
394. Haug RH, Prather J, Bradrick JP, et al: The morbidity associated with fifty maxillary fractures treated by closed reduction. Oral Surg Oral Med Oral Pathol 1992;73:659.
395. Cohen S, Leonard D, Markowitz B, Manson PN: Acrylic splints for dental alignment in complex facial injuries. Ann Plast Surg 1993;31:406.
396. Kelly K, Manson PN, Vander Kolk C, Markowitz B: Sequencing treatment in midface fractures. J Craniofac Surg 1990;1:168.
397. Kelley P, Klebuc M, Hollier L: Complex midface reconstruction: maximizing contour and bone graft survival utilizing periosteal free flaps. J Craniofac Surg 2003;14:779.
398. Manson P, Clark N, Robertson B, Crawley W: Comprehensive management of pan-facial fractures. J Craniofac Trauma 1995;1:43.
399. Gruss J: Advances in craniofacial fracture repair. Scand J Plast Reconstr Surg Hand Surg Suppl 1995;27:67.
400. Rohrich R, Shewmake K: Evolving concepts of craniomaxillofacial trauma management. Clin Plast Surg 1992;19:1.
401. Ferraro JW, Berggren RB: Treatment of complex facial fractures. J Trauma 1973;13:783.
402. Welsh LW, Welsh JJ: Fractures of the edentulous maxilla and mandible. Laryngoscope 1976;86:1333.
403. Manson P: Complications of facial fractures. In Goldwyn R, Cohen S, eds: Complications in Plastic Surgery. New York, Lippincott-Raven, 2001:489-513.
404. Mauriello JA, Fiore PM, Kotch M: Dacryocystitis: late complication of orbital floor fracture repair with implant. Ophthalmology 1987;94:248.
405. Manson PN: Facial fractures. In Goldwyn R, Cohen S, eds: The Unfavorable Result in Plastic Surgery—Avoidance and Treatment, 3rd ed. Philadelphia, Lippincott Williams & Wilkins, 2001:489-520.
406. O'Sullivan ST, Snyder BJ, Moore MH, David DJ: Outcome measurement of the treatment of maxillary fractures: a prospective analysis of 100 consecutive cases. Br J Plast Surg 1999;52:519.
407. McCoy FJ, Chandler RA, Magnan CG Jr, et al: An analysis of facial fractures and their complications. Plast Reconstr Surg 1962;29:381.
408. Zins JE, Whitaker LA: Membranous vs. endochondral bone complications for craniofacial reconstruction. Plast Reconstr Surg 1983;72:778.
409. Tong L, Buchman SR: Facial bone grafts: contemporary science and thought. J Craniomaxillofac Trauma 2000;6:31.
410. Schmitz JP, Hollinger JO: The critical size defect as an experimental model for craniomandibulofacial nonunions. Clin Orthop 1986;205:299.
411. Sarnat BG, Gans BJ: Growth of bones: methods of assessing and clinical importance. Plast Reconstr Surg 1952;52:263.
412. Reynolds JR: Late complications vs. method of treatment in a large series of mid-facial fractures. Plast Reconstr Surg 1978;61:871.
413. Becelli R, Renzi G, Mannino G: Posttraumatic obstruction of the lacrimal pathways: a retrospective analysis of 58 consecutive nasoethmoid orbital fractures. J Craniofac Surg 2004;15:29.
414. Zapala J, Bartkowski AM, Bartkowski SB: Lacrimal drainage system obstruction: management and results in 70 patients. J Craniomaxillofac Trauma 1992;20:178.
415. MacGillivray RF, Stevens MR: Primary surgical repair of traumatic lacerations of the lacrimal canaliculi. Oral Surg Oral Med Oral Pathol Oral Radiol Endod 1996;81:157.
416. Stanley RB Jr, Nowak GM: Midface fractures: importance of angle of impact to horizontal craniofacial buttresses. Otolaryngol Head Neck Surg 1985;93:186.
417. Denny A, Celik N: A management strategy for palatal fractures: a 12-year review. J Craniofac Surg 1999;10:49.
418. Sargent LA, Fulks KW: Reconstruction of internal orbital fractures with Vitallium mesh. Plast Reconstr Surg 1991;88:31.
419. Manson P, Iliff N, Vander Kolk C, et al: Rigid fixation of orbital fractures. Plast Reconstr Surg 1990;86:1103.
420. Glassman RD, Manson PN, Petty P, et al: Techniques for improved visibility and lid protection in orbital explorations. J Craniofac Surg 1990;1:69.
421. Donald PJ: The tenacity of frontal sinus mucosa. Otolaryngol Head Neck Surg 1979;87:557.
422. Munro IR, Chen YR: Radical treatment for fronto-orbital fibrous dysplasia; the chain link fence. Plast Reconstr Surg 1981;67:719.
423. Crikelair GF, Rein JM, Potter GD, Cosman B: A critical look at the "blowout" fracture. Plast Reconstr Surg 1972;49:374.
424. Barkowski SB, Krzystkowa KM: Blowout fracture of the orbit: diagnostic and therapeutic considerations, and results in 90 patients treated. J Maxillofac Surg 1982;10:155.
425. Collins A, McKellar G, Momnsour F: Orbital injuries: a historical overview. Oral Maxillofac Surg Clin North Am 1993;5:409.
426. Gruss JS, Hurwitz JJ: Isolated blow in fracture of the lateral orbit causing globe rupture. Ophthalmic Plast Reconstr Surg 6:221:1990.
427. Petro J, Tooze FM, Bales CR, Baker CR: Ocular injuries associated with periorbital fractures. J Trauma 1970;19:730.

428. Holt GR, Holt SE: Incidence of ocular injuries in facial fractures: an analysis of 727 cases. Otolaryngol Head Neck Surg 1983;91:276.

429. Poon A, McCluskey PJ, Hill DA: Eye injuries in patients with major trauma. J Trauma 1999;46:494.

430. Wachler BSB, Hold JB: The missing muscle syndrome in blowout fractures: an indication for surgery. Ophthalmic Plast Reconstr Surg 1998;14:17.

431. Soll DB, Polly BJ: Trapdoor variety of blowout fracture of the orbital floor. Am J Ophthalmol 1965;60:269.

432. Egbert JE, May K, Kersten RC, Kulwin DR: Pediatric orbital floor fracture: direct extraocular muscle involvement. Ophthalmic Plast Reconstr Surg 2000;107:1875.

433. Gola R, Nerini A, Jallut Y: A fracture trap, the trapdoor fracture of the orbital floor. Ann Chir Plast 1982;27:322.

434. Kersten RC: Blowout fracture of the orbital floor with entrapment caused by isolated trauma to the orbital rim. Am J Ophthalmol 1987;103:215.

435. Jordan DR, Allen LH, White J, et al: Intervention within days for some orbital floor fractures: the white-eyed blow-out fracture. Ophthalmic Plast Reconstr Surg 1998;14:379.

436. Sires BS, Stanley RB, Levine LM: Oculocardiac reflux caused by orbital floor fracture: an indication for urgent repair. Arch Ophthalmol 1998;116:955.

437. Kestenbaum A: Applied Anatomy of the Eye. New York, Grune & Stratton, 1963:161-191, 239-248.

438. Smith RR, Blount RL: Blowout fractures of the orbital roof with pulsating exophthalmos, blepharoptosis and superior gaze paresis. Am J Ophthalmol 1971;71:1052.

439. Catone GA, Morrissette MP, Carlson ER: Retrospective analysis of untreated orbital blowout fractures. J Oral Maxillofac Surg 1988;46:1033.

440. Smith B, Regan WF Jr: Blowout fracture of the orbit: mechanism and correction of internal orbital fracture. Am J Ophthalmol 1957;44:733.

441. Pfeiffer RL: Traumatic enophthalmos. Arch Ophthalmol 1943;30:718.

442. Erling B, Iliff N, Robertson B, Manson B: "Footprints" of the globe: a practical look at the mechanism of orbital blowout fracture, with a revisit to the work of Raymond Pfeiffer. Plast Reconstr Surg 1999;103:1313.

443. Koornneef L: New insights in the human orbital connective tissue: result of a new anatomical approach. Arch Ophthalmol 1977;95:1269.

444. Callahan MA: Fixation of the medial canthal structures: evolution of the best method. Ann Plast Surg 1983;11:242.

445. Yoshioka N, Tominaga Y, Motomura H, Muraoka M: Surgical treatment for greater sphenoid wing fracture (orbital blow-in fracture). Ann Plast Surg 1999;42:87.

446. Bernard RW, Matusow GR, Bonnano PC: Blow-in fracture causing exophthalmos. N Y State J Med 1978;78:652.

447. Lighterman I, Reckson C: "Blow-in" fracture of the orbit. Ann Plast Surg 1979;3:572.

448. Alqurainy IA, Stassen LF, Dutton GN, et al: Diplopia following midfacial fractures. J Oral Maxillofac Surg 1988;46:3.

449. Alqurainy IA, Stassen LF, Dutton GN, et al: The characteristics of midfacial fractures and the association with ocular surgery: a prospective study. J Oral Maxillofac Surg 1991;29:302.

450. Koornneef L: Current concepts on the management of blowout fractures. Ann Plast Surg 1982;9:185.

451. Millman AL, Lubkin V, Gersten M: Three-dimensional reconstruction of the orbit from CT scans and volumetric analysis of orbital fractures: its role in the evaluation of enophthalmos [editorial]. Adv Ophthalmic Plast Reconstr Surg 1987;6:265.

452. Lisman RD, Smith BC, Rodgers R: Volkmann's ischemic contracture and blowout fractures. Adv Ophthalmic Plast Reconstr Surg 1987;7:117.

453. Millman AL, Della Rocca RC, Spector S: Steroids and orbital blowout fractures: a new systematic concept in medical management and surgical decision-making. Adv Ophthalmic Plast Reconstr Surg 1987;6:291.

454. Putterman A: An interview: Dr. Allen Putterman on the subject of blowout fractures of the orbital floor. Ophthalmic Plast Reconstr Surg 1985;1:73.

455. Lang W: Traumatic enophthalmos with retention of perfect acuity of vision. Trans Ophthalmol Soc Engl 1889;9:44.

456. Smith B: The discovery of blowout fracture of the orbit. Adv Ophthalmic Plast Reconstr Surg 1987;6:193.

457. Lagrange F: Les fractures de l'orbite per les projetiles de guerre. Paris, Masson & Cie, 1917.

458. Linhart WO: Emphysema of the orbit: a study of 7 cases. JAMA 1943;123:89.

459. Fujino T, Sato TB: Mechanism, tolerance limit curves and theoretical analysis in blowout fractures in two and three dimensional orbital wall models. Proceedings of the Third International Symposium on Orbital Disorders. The Hague, W Junk, 1978:240-247.

460. Takizawa H, Sugiura K, Baba M, et al: Structural mechanics of the blowout fracture: computer simulation of orbital deformation by the finite element method. Neurosurgery 1988;22:1053.

461. McCord CD, Putnam JR, Ugland DN: Pressure-volume orbital measurements comparing decompression approaches. Ophthalmic Plast Reconstr Surg 1985;1:55.

462. Parsons GS, Mathog RH: Orbital wall and volume relationships. Arch Otolaryngol Head Neck Surg 1988;114:743.

463. Fries R: Some problems in therapy of traumatic enophthalmos. Mod Probl Ophthalmol 1975;14:637.

464. Stabile JR, Trekel SM: Increase in intra-orbital volume obtained by decompression in dried skulls. Ophthalmology 1983;95:327.

465. Pearl RM: Enophthalmos correction: principles guiding proper treatment. Operative Techniques Plast Reconstr Surg 1998;5:352.

466. Roncevic R, Stajcic Z: Surgical treatment of post-traumatic enophthalmos: a study of 72 patients. Ann Plast Surg 1994;32:288.

467. Hawes MJ, Dortzbach RK: Surgery on orbital floor fractures: influence of time of repair and fracture size. Ophthalmology 1985;90:1066.

468. Dolynchuk V, Tadjalle H, Manson P: Orbital volumetric analysis: clinical application in orbitozygomatic injuries. J Craniomaxillofac Trauma 1996;2:56.

469. Stahlnecker M, Whitaker L, Herman G, Katowitz J: Evaluation and secondary treatment of post-traumatic enophthalmos. Presented at the American Association of Plastic Surgeons, Coronado Beach, Calif, April 29, 1985.

470. Raskin E, Millman A, Lubkin U: Prediction of late enophthalmos by volume analysis of orbital fracture. Ophthalmic Plast Reconstr Surg 1998;14:19.

471. Yab K, Tijima S, Imai K: Clinical application of a solid three-dimensional model for orbital wall fractures. J Craniomaxillofac Surg 1993;21:275.

472. Pearl RM: Prevention of enophthalmos: a hypothesis. Ann Plast Surg 1990;25:132.

473. Pearl RM: Surgical management of volumetric changes in the bony orbit. Ann Plast Surg 1987;19:349.

474. Schubert W, Quillopa N, Shons AR: A study of orbital anatomy and volume for the correction of enophthalmos. Surg Forum 1990;41:597.

475. Grivas A: Evaluation of post-traumatic orbital deformity by computed tomography: volume determinations and "three-dimensional" surface reconstructions [master's thesis]. Baltimore, Johns Hopkins University, 1984.

476. Bite U, Jackson IT, Forbes GS, Gehring D: Orbital volume measurements using three-dimensional CT imaging. Plast Reconstr Surg 1985;75:502.

477. Manson PN, Grivas A, Rosenbaum A, et al: Studies on enophthalmos: II. The measurement of orbital injuries and their treatment by quantitative computed tomography. Plast Reconstr Surg 1986;77:203.

478. Jin HR, Shin SG, Chao MJ, Chai YS: The relationship between the extent of fracture and the degree of enophthalmos in isolated blowout fractures of the medial orbital wall. J Oral Maxillofac Surg 2000;58:657.

479. Waterhouse N, Lyne J, Urdang M, Garey L: An investigation into the mechanism of blow-out fractures. Br J Plast Surg 1999;52:607.

480. Fujino T: Mechanism of orbital injuries in automobile accidents. Automotive Crash Injury Research of the Cornell Aeronautical Laboratory, Buffalo, NY, 1963.

481. Phalen JJ, Baumel JJ, Kaplan PA: Orbital floor fractures: a reassessment of pathogenesis. Nebr Med J 1990;75:100.

482. Fujino T: Experimental "blowout" fracture of the orbit. Plast Reconstr Surg 1974;54:81.

483. Fujino T: Mechanism of the orbital blowout fracture. Jpn J Plast Surg 1974;17:427.

484. Jones E, Evans JN: "Blowout" fractures of the orbit: an investigation into their anatomical basis. J Laryngol Otol 1967;81:1109.

485. Green RP, Peters DR, Shore JW: Force necessary to fracture the orbital floor. Ophthalmic Plast Reconstr Surg 1990; 6:211.

486. Fan X, Li J, Zhu J: Computer-assisted orbital volume measurement in the surgical correction of late enophthalmos caused by blowout fractures. Ophthalmic Plast Reconstr Surg 2003;19:207.

487. Burm JS, Chung CH, Oh SJ: Pure orbital blowout fracture: new concepts and the importance of the medial orbital wall. Plast Reconstr Surg 1999;103:1439.

488. Brown MS, Ky W, Lisman RD: Concomitant ocular injuries with orbital fractures. J Craniomaxillofac Trauma 1999;5:41.

489. Tong L, Bauer RJ, Buchman SR: A current 10-year retrospective survey of 199 surgically treated orbital floor fractures in a nonurban tertiary care center. Plast Reconstr Surg 2001;108:612.

490. Raflo GT: Blow-in and blow-out fractures of the orbit: clinical correlations and proposed mechanisms. Ophthalmic Surg 1984;15:114.

491. Wojno TH: The incidence of extraocular muscle and cranial nerve palsy in orbital floor blowout fractures. Ophthalmology 1987;94:682.

492. Rubin MM: Trochlear nerve palsy simulating an orbital blowout fracture. J Oral Maxillofac Surg 1992;50:1238.

493. Rutman MS, Harris GJ: Orbital blowout fracture with ipsilateral fourth nerve palsy. Am J Ophthalmol 1985;100:343.

494. Mathog RH, Archer KF, Nesi F: Post-traumatic enophthalmos and diplopia. Otolaryngol Head Neck Surg 1989;94:69.

495. Lyon DB, Newman SA: Evidence of direct damage to extraocular muscles as a cause of diplopia following orbital trauma. Ophthalmic Plast Reconstr Surg 1989;5:81.

496. Cahan M, Fischer B, Iliff N, et al: Less common orbital fracture patterns: the role of computed tomography in the management of depression of the inferior oblique origin and lateral rectus involvement in blow-in fractures. J Craniofac Surg 1996;7:449.

497. Clifford CM: Supporting ligaments of the globe [master's thesis]. Baltimore, Johns Hopkins University, 1982.

498. Manson PN, Clifford CM, Su CT, et al: Mechanisms of global support and post-traumatic enophthalmos: I. The anatomy of the ligament sling and its relation to intramuscular cone orbital fat. Plast Reconstr Surg 1986;77:193.

499. Manson P, Iliff N: Management of blowout fractures of the orbital floor: early repair of selected injuries. In Worthington T, ed: Controversies in Oral Surgery. Philadelphia, WB Saunders, 1993:235-250.

500. Hammerschlag SB, Hughes S, O'Reilly GV, et al: Blow-out fractures of the orbit. Radiology 1983;145:487.

501. Hammerschlag SB, Hughes S, O'Reilly GV, Weber AL: Another look at blowout fractures of the orbit. AJR Am J Roentgenol 1982;139:133.

502. Linberg J: Orbital compartment syndromes following trauma. Adv Plast Reconstr Surg 1987;6:51.

503. Smith B, Lisman RD: Volkmann's contracture of the extraocular muscle following blowout fracture. Plast Reconstr Surg 1984;74:200.

504. Iliff N, Manson P, Katz J, et al: Mechanisms of extraocular muscle injury in orbital fractures. Plast Reconstr Surg 1999;103:787.

505. Metz HS, Scott WE, Madson E, Scott AB: Saccadic velocity and active force studies in blowout fractures of the orbit. Am J Ophthalmol 1974;8:655.

506. Fells P: Acute enophthalmos. Trans Ophthal Soc UK 1982;102:88.

507. Mathog RH: Relationship between the extent of fracture and blow out fractures of the medial orbital wall. J Oral Maxillofac Surg 2000;58:620.

508. Manson P, Iliff N: Posttraumatic orbital repositioning. In Keating RF, Stewart WB: An Atlas of Orbitocranial Surgery. London, Martin Dunitz, 1999:108-201.

509. Hemprich A, Breier T: Secondary correction of traumatogenic enophthalmos with auto- and alloplastic implants. Rev Stomatol Chir Maxillofac 1993;94:37.

510. Manson PN, Lazarus RB, Morgan R, Iliff N: Pathways of sympathetic innervation to the superior and inferior (Muller's) tarsal muscles. Plast Reconstr Surg 1986;78:33.

511. Pearl RM, Vistnes LM: Orbital blowout fractures: an approach to management. Ann Plast Surg 1978;1:267.

512. Koornneef L, Zonneveld FW: Orbital anatomy. The direct scanning of the orbit in three phases and their bearings on the treatment of mobility disturbances of the eye after orbital "blowout" fractures. Acta Morphol Neerl Scand 1985;23:229.

513. Pieramici D, Au Eong KG, Sternberg P, Marsh MJ: The diagnostic significance for classifying mechanical injuries of the eye (globe) in open-globe injuries. J Trauma 2003;54:750.

514. Burm JS, Oh SJ: Direct local approach through a W-shaped incision in moderate or severe blow-out fractures of the medial orbital wall. Plast Reconstr Surg 2001;107:920.

515. Boush GA, Lemke BN: Progressive infraorbital nerve hypesthesia as a primary indication for blowout fracture repair. Ophthalmic Plast Reconstr Surg 1994;10:271.

516. Hakelius L, Ponten B: Results of immediate and delayed surgical treatment of facial fractures with diplopia. J Maxillofac Surg 1973;1:150.

517. Converse JM, Smith B: Enophthalmos and diplopia in fracture of the orbital floor. Br J Plast Surg 1957;9:265.

518. Converse JM, Smith B, Obear MF, Wood-Smith D: Orbital blowout fractures: a ten year survey. Plast Reconstr Surg 1967;39:20.

519. Emery JM, Noorden GK, Sclernitzauer DA: Orbital floor fractures: long term follow up of cases with and without surgical repair. Trans Am Acad Ophthalmol Otolaryngol 1971;75:802.

520. Putterman AM, Stevens T, Urist MJ: Nonsurgical management of blowout fractures of the orbital floor. Am J Ophthalmol 1974;77:232.

521. Chen CT, Chen YR: Application of the endoscope in orbital fractures. Semin Plast Surg 2002;16:241.

522. Sandler N, Carran R, Ochs M, Beatty R: The use of maxillary sinus endoscopy in the diagnosis of orbital floor fractures. J Oral Maxillofac Surg 1999;57:399.

523. Lee C, Stiebel M, Young DM: Cranial nerve III region of the traumatized facial skeleton: optimizing repairs with the endoscope. J Trauma 2001;48:423.

524. Saunders CJ, Whetzel TP, Stokes RB, et al: Transantral endoscopic orbital floor exploration: a cadaver and clinical study. Plast Reconstr Surg 1999;900:575.

525. Woog J, Harstein M, Gliklich R: Paranasal sinus endoscopy and orbital fracture repair. Arch Ophthalmol 1998;116:688.

526. Kakibuchi M, Fukazawa K, Fukuda K: Combination of transconjunctival and endonasal-transantral approach in the repair of blowout fracture involving the orbital floor. Br J Plast Surg 2004;57:37.

527. Mun GH, Song YH, Bang SI: Endoscopically assisted transconjunctival approach in orbital medial wall fractures. Ann Plast Reconstr Surg 2002;49:337, discussion 344.

528. Shorr N, Baylis HI, Goldberg RA: Transcaruncular approach to the orbit and orbital margin. Ophthalmology 2000;102:1459.

529. Dingham RO, Grabb WC: Costal cartilage homografts preserved by irradiation. Plast Reconstr Surg 1961;28:562.

530. Milauskas AT: Diagnosis and Management of Blowout Fractures of the Orbit. Springfield, Ill, Charles C Thomas, 1969.

531. Hammer B: Orbital Fractures: Diagnosis, Operative Treatment and Secondary Correction. Bern, Switzerland, Hoegrefe & Huber, 1995.

532. Prasad SS: Blowout fracture of the medial wall of the orbit. In Bleeker GM, Lyle TK, eds: Proceedings of the Second International Symposium on Orbital Disorders, vol 14. Basel, Karger, 1975.

533. Jackson IT: Classification and treatment of orbito-zygomatic and orbito-ethmoid fractures: the place of bone grafting and plate fixation. Clin Plast Surg 1989;16:77.

534. Dodick JM, Galin MA, Littleton JT, Sod LM: Concomitant medial wall fracture and blowout fracture of the orbit. Arch Ophthalmol 1971;85:273.

535. Flanagan JC, McLachlan DL, Shannon GM: Orbital roof fractures: neurological and neurosurgical considerations. Ophthalmology 1980;87:325.

536. Jeanette YM, Henry CV: Supraorbital roof fracture: a formidable entity with which to contend. Ann Plast Reconstr Surg 1997;38:223.

537. Stranc MF, Gustavson EH: Plastic surgery: primary treatment of fractures of the orbital roof. Proc R Soc Med 1973;66:303.

538. Messinger A, Radkowski MA, Greenwald MJ, Pensler JM: Orbital roof fractures in the pediatric populations. Plast Reconstr Surg 1989;84:213.

539. Rougier J, Freidel C, Freidel M: Fractures of the orbital roof and ethmoid region. In Bleeker GM, Lyle TK, eds: Proceedings of the Symposium on Orbital Fractures. Amsterdam, Excerpta Medica, 1969.

540. Schultz RC: Supraorbital and glabellar fractures. Plast Reconstr Surg 1970;45:227.

541. Miller SH, Lung RJ, Davis TS, et al: Management of fractures of the supraorbital rim. J Trauma 1978;18:507.

542. Patell P, Bauer B: Supraorbital fractures in children. Operative Techniques Plast Reconstr Surg 1998;5:275.

543. Manson PN, Iliff NT: Fractures of the orbital roof. In Hornblass A, ed: Oculoplastic, Orbital and Reconstructive Surgery, vol 2. Baltimore, Williams & Wilkins, 1990:1139.

544. Kurzer A, Patel MP: Superior orbital fissure syndrome associated with fractures of the zygoma and orbit. Plast Reconstr Surg 1979;64:715.

545. Zachariades N, Vairaktaris E, Papavassiliou D: The superior orbital fissure syndrome. J Maxillofac Surg 1985;13:125.

546. Converse JM: Orbital and naso-orbital fractures. In Tessier P, Callahan A, Mustardé JC, Salyer KE, eds: Symposium on Plastic Surgery in the Orbital Region. St. Louis, CV Mosby, 1976:79.

547. Converse JM, Smith B: Naso-orbital fractures (symposium: midfacial fractures). Trans Am Acad Ophthalmol Otolaryngol 1963;67:622.

548. Dingman RO, Grabb WC, O'Neal RM: Management of injuries of the naso-orbital complex. Arch Surg 1969;98:566.

549. Converse JM, Smith B: Naso-orbital fractures and traumatic deformities of the medial canthus. Plast Reconstr Surg 1966;38:147.

550. Converse JM, Smith B, Wood-Smith D: Deformities of the midface resulting from malunited orbital and naso-orbital fractures. Clin Plast Surg 1975;2:107.

551. Converse JM, Smith B, Wood-Smith D: Orbital and naso-orbital fractures. In Converse JM, ed: Reconstructive Plastic Surgery, 2nd ed, vol 2. Philadelphia, WB Saunders, 1977:748-793.

552. Tessier P, Guiot G, Rougerie J, et al: Cranio-naso-orbito-facial osteotomies. Hypertelorism. Ann Chir Plast 1967;12:103.

553. Mulliken JB, Kaban LB, Evans CA, et al: Facial skeletal changes following hypertelorism correction. Plast Reconstr Surg 1986;62:7.

554. Markowitz B, Manson P, Yaremchuk M, et al: High-energy orbital dislocations: the possibility of traumatic hypertelorism. Plast Reconstr Surg 1991;88:20.

555. Evans G, Manson PN, Clark N: Identification and management of minimally displaced nasoethmoidal orbital fractures. Ann Plast Surg 1995;35:469.

556. Paskert JP, Manson PN: The bimanual examination for assessing instability in nasoethmoid orbital fractures. Plast Reconstr Surg 1989;83:165.

557. Stimac GK, Sundsten JW, Prothero JF, et al: Three-dimensional contour surfacing of the skull, face and brain from CT and MR image and from anatomic motions. AJR Am J Roentgenol 1988;151:807.

558. Stanley RB: Management of complications of frontal bone and frontal sinus fractures. Operative Techniques Plast Reconstr Surg 1998;5:296.

559. Stanley RB, Becker TS: Injuries of the nasofrontal orifices in frontal sinus fractures. Laryngoscope 1987;97:728.

560. Remmler D, Denny A, Gosain A, Subichin S: Role of 3-dimensional computed tomography in the assessment of naso-orbital-ethmoid fractures. Ann Plast Surg 2000;44:553.

561. Mafee MF, Pruzansky S, Corrales MM, et al: CT in the evaluation of the orbit and the bony interorbital distance. AJNR Am J Neuroradiol 1986;7:265.

562. Spiessl B, Schroll K: Naso-ethmoidal injuries. Osterr Z Stomatol 1973;70:2.

563. Sargent LA: Acute management of nasoethmoid orbital fractures. Operative Techniques Plast Reconstr Surg 1998;5:213.

564. Cruse CW, Blevins PK, Luce EA: Naso-ethmoid-orbital fractures. J Trauma 1980;20:551.

565. Stanley RB: Management of frontal sinus fractures. Facial Plast Surg 1998;5:231.

566. Boutros S, Bernard R, Galiano R, et al: The temporal sequence of periosteal attachment after evaluation. Plast Reconstr Surg 2003;111:1942.

567. Lipziger L, Manson PN: Nasoethmoid-orbital fractures. Clin Plast Surg 1992;19:167.

568. Anderson RL: The medial canthal tendon branches out. Arch Ophthalmol 1977;95:2051.

569. Robinson TJ, Stranc MF: The anatomy of the medial canthal ligament. Br J Plast Surg 1970;23:1.

570. Rodriguez RI, Zide BM: Reconstruction of the medial canthus. Clin Plast Surg 1988;15:255.

571. Zide BM, Jelks G: Surgical Anatomy of the Orbit. New York, Raven Press, 1985:2-9, 59-65.

572. Zide BM, McCarthy JG: The medial canthus revisited—anatomical basis for canthopexy. Ann Plast Surg 1983;11:1.

573. Converse JM, Cole G, Smith B: Late treatment of blowout fracture of the floor of the orbit. Plast Reconstr Surg 1961;29:183.

574. Manson P: Secondary treatment of nasoethmoid. Seventh International Symposium on Craniofacial Fractures. Milan, Monduzzi Editore, 2000.

575. May M: Nasofrontal-ethmoid injuries. Laryngoscope 1977;87:948.

576. May N: Nasofrontal duct in frontal sinus trauma. Arch Otolaryngol 1970;12:534.

577. Wolfe SA: Treatment of posttraumatic orbital deformities. Clin Plast Surg 1988;15:225.

578. McQueen CT, DiRuggerio DL, Campbell JP: Orbital osteology: a study of surgical landmarks. Laryngoscope 1995;105:783.

579. Mauriello JA: Inferior rectus muscle entrapped by Teflon implant after orbital floor fracture repair. Ophthalmic Plast Reconstr Surg 1990;6:218.

580. Heitsch M, Mohr C: Blindness as a complication following surgical orbital floor revision. Consequences for the surgical procedures [in German]. Fortschr Kiefer Gesichtschir 1991;36:152.

581. Kohn R: Lacrimal obstruction after migration of an orbital floor implant. Ophthalmology 1976;82:934.

582. Biesman BS, Hornblass A, Lisman R, Kazlas M: Diplopia after surgical repair of orbital floor fractures. Ophthalmic Plast Reconstr Surg 1996;12:9.

583. Millman AL, Della Rocca RC, Spector S, et al: Steroids and orbital blowout fractures—a new systematic concept in medical management and surgical decision-making. Adv Ophthalmic Plast Reconstr Surg 1987;6:291.

584. Girotto J, MacKenzie E, Fowler C, et al: Long term physical impairment and functional outcomes following complex facial fractures. Plast Reconstr Surg 2001;108:312.

585. Miller GR: Blindness developing a few days after a midfacial fracture. Plast Reconstr Surg 1968;42:384.

586. Converse JM, Smith B: Reconstruction of the floor of the orbit by bone grafts. Arch Ophthalmol 1950;44:1.

587. Nicholson DH, Guzak SW: Visual loss complicating repair of orbital floor fractures. Arch Ophthalmol 1971;86:369.

588. Wilkins RB, Havins WE: Current treatment of blowout fractures. Ophthalmology 1982;89:464.

589. Lederman IR: Loss of vision associated with surgical treatment of zygomatic-orbital floor fracture. Plast Reconstr Surg 1981;68:94.

590. MacKinnon CA, David DJ, Cooter RD: Blindness and severe visual impairment in facial fractures: an 11 year review. Br J Plast Surg 2002;55:1.

591. Anderson RL, Panje WR, Gross CE: Optic nerve blindness following blunt forehead trauma. Ophthalmology 1992;89:445.

592. Stanley RB: Management of severe frontobasilar skull fractures. Otolaryngol Clin North Am 1991;24:139.

593. Funk GE, Stanley RB, Becker TS: Reversible visual loss due to impacted lateral wall fractures. Head Neck Surg 1987;113:87.

594. Ioannides C, Freihofer HP: Fractures of the frontal sinus: classification and implications for surgical treatment. Am J Otolaryngol 1999;20:273.

595. Wang B, Robertson B, Girotto J, et al: Posttraumatic optic neuropathy: a review of 61 patients. Plast Reconstr Surg 2001;107:1655.

596. Yang WG, Chen CT, Tsay RK, et al: Outcomes for traumatic optic neuropathy—surgical vs. nonsurgical treatment. Ann Plast Surg 2004;52:36.

597. Lo LJ, Hung KF, Chen YR: Blindness as a complication of a Le Fort I osteotomy for maxillary distraction. Plast Reconstr Surg 2002;109:668.

598. Vallejo A, Lorenta J, Bas ML: Blindness due to anterior ischemic neuropathy in a burn patient. J Trauma 2002;53:139.

599. Gruss JS, Hurwitz JJ, Ink NA, Kasei E: The pattern and incidence of nasolacrimal injury in nasoethmoid orbital fractures: the role of delayed assessment and dacryocystorhinostomy. Br J Plast Surg 1985;38:116.

600. Anderson RL, Edwards JJ: Indications, complications and results with silicone stents. Ophthalmology 1979;86:1474.

601. Whelham RAN: The lacrimal system. In Mustardé JC, ed: Repair and Reconstruction in the Orbital Region. Edinburgh, Churchill Livingstone, 1991:299.

602. Forrest CR, Khairallah E, Kuzon W: Intraocular and intraorbital compartment pressure changes following orbital bone grafting: a clinical and laboratory study. Plast Reconstr Surg 1999;104:48.

603. Lacy MF, Pospisil OA: Lower blepharoplasty post-orbicularis approach to the orbit—a prospective study. Br J Oral Maxillofac Surg 1987;25:398.

604. Pospisil OA, Fernando TD: Review of the lower blepharoplasty incision as a surgical approach to the zygomatic orbital fractures. Br J Maxillofac Surg 1984;22:261.

605. Heissler E, Fischer FS, Bolouri S, et al: Custom-made cast titanium implants produced with CAD/CAM for the reconstruction of cranium defects. Int J Oral Maxillofac Surg 1998;27:334.

606. Phillips J, Gruss J, Wells M: Periorbital suspension of lower eyelid and cheek following subciliary exposures of facial fractures. Plast Reconstr Surg 1991;88:145.

607. Wolfe SA, Davidson J: Avoidance of lower lid contraction in surgical approaches to the lower orbit. Operative Techniques Plast Reconstr Surg 1998;5:201.

608. Dagi TF, Meyer FB, Poletti CA: The incidence and prevention of meningitis after basilar skull fractures. Am J Emerg Med 1983;1:295.

609. Schneider RC, Thompson JM: Chronic and delayed traumatic cerebrospinal rhinorrhea as a source of recurrent attacks of meningitis. Ann Surg 1957;145:517.

610. Levin S, Nelson KE, Spies HW, Lepper MH: Pneumococcal meningitis: the problem of the unseen cerebrospinal fluid leak. Am J Med Sci 1972;264:319.

611. Schaefer SD, Diehl JT, Briggs WH: The diagnosis of CSF rhinorrhea by metrizamide CT scanning. Laryngoscope 1980; 90:871.

612. Lund VJ, Savy L, Lloyd G, Howard D: Optimum imaging and diagnosis of cerebrospinal fluid rhinorrhea. J Laryngol Otol 2000;114:988.

613. Nandapalan V, Watson ID, Swift AC: Beta$_2$-transferrin and cerebrospinal fluid rhinorrhea. Clin Otolaryngol Allied Sci 1996;21:251.

614. Fujino T, Makino K: Entrapment mechanisms and ocular injury in orbital blowout fracture. Plast Reconstr Surg 1980;65:571.

615. Jacobs JB, Perky MS: Traumatic pneumocephalus. Laryngoscope 1980;90:515.

616. Cahill DW, Rao KC, Ducker TD: Delayed carotid-cavernous fistula and multiple cranial neuropathy following basal skull fracture. Surg Neurol 1980;16:17.

617. Fattahi T, Brandt MT, Jenkins WS, Steinberg B: Traumatic carotid-cavernous fistula: pathophysiology and treatment. J Craniofac Surg 2003;14:240.

618. Zachariades N: The superior orbital fissure syndrome: report of a case and review of the literature. Oral Surg 1982;53:237.

619. Kline LB, Morawetz RB, Swaid SN: Indirect injury of the optic nerve. Neurosurgery 1984;14:756.

620. Fukado Y: Results in 400 cases of surgical decompression of the optic nerve. In Bleeker GM, Lyle TK, eds: Proceeding of the Second International Symposium on Orbital Disorders. Basel, Karger, 1975.

621. Lessel S: Indirect optic nerve trauma. Arch Ophthalmol 1989;107:382.

622. McCarney DL, Char DH: Return of vision after 36 hours of postoperative blindness. Am J Ophthalmol 1985;100:602.

623. Wolin MJ, Lavin PJM: Spontaneous visual recovery from traumatic optic neuropathy after blunt head injury. Am J Ophthalmol 1990;109:430.

624. Knox BE, Gates GA, Berry SM: Optic nerve decompression via the lateral facial approach. Laryngoscope 1990;100:458.

625. Ishikawa A, Okabe H, Nakagawa Y, Kiyosawa M: Treatment and followup of traumatic optic neuropathy. Neuro-ophthalmology 1996;13:175.

626. Spoor TC, Hartel WC, Lensink DB, Wilkinson MJ: Treatment of traumatic optic neuropathy with corticosteroids. Am J Ophthalmol 1990;110:665.

627. Spoor TC, McHenry JG: Management of traumatic optic neuropathy. J Craniomaxillofac Trauma 1996;2:14.

628. Seiff S: High dose corticosteroids for treatment of vision loss due to indirect injury to the optic nerve. Ophthalmic Surg 1990;21:389.

629. Seiff SR: Trauma and the optic nerve. Ophthalmol Clin North Am 1992;5:839.

630. Chen YR, Fischer DM: Discussion: Blindness as a complication of Le Fort osteotomies: the role of atypical fracture patterns and distortion of the optic canal. Plast Reconstr Surg 1998;102:1422.

631. Weymuller EA Jr; Blindness and Le Fort III fractures. Ann Otol Rhinol Laryngol 1984;93:2.

632. Volpe N, Lessel S, Kline L: Traumatic optic neuropathy diagnosis and management. Int Ophthalmol Clin 1991;31:142.

633. Liu D: Blindness after blow-out fracture repair. Ophthalmic Plast Reconstr Surg 1994;10:206.

634. Chou PI, Sadun AA, Chen YC, et al: Clinical experiences in the management of traumatic optic neuropathy. Neuro-ophthalmology 1996;16:325.

635. Li KK, Teknos TN, Lai A, et al: Traumatic optic neuropathy: result in 45 consecutive surgically treated patients. Otolaryngol Head Neck Surg 1999;120:5.

636. Li KK, Teknos TN, Lai A, et al: Extracranial optic nerve decompression: a 10-year review of 92 patients. J Craniofac Surg 1999;10:454.

637. Rubin PAD, Bilyk JR, Shore JW: Management of orbital trauma: fractures, hemorrhage and traumatic optic neuropathy. Focal points. Am Acad Ophthalmol 1997;12:1.

638. Mine S, Yamakami I, Yamaura A, et al: Outcome of traumatic optic neuropathy. Comparison between surgical and nonsurgical treatment. Acta Neurochir 1999;141:27.

639. Lipkin AF, Woodson E, Miller RH: Visual loss due to orbital fracture: the role of early reduction. Arch Otolaryngol Head Neck Surg 1987;113:81.

640. Levin L, Beck R, Joseph M, et al: The treatment of traumatic optic neuropathy. Ophthalmology 1999;106:1268.

641. Gruss JS, Bubak PJ, Egbert M: Craniofacial fractures: an algorithm to optimize results. Clin Plast Surg 1992;19:195.

642. Strumas N, Antonyshyn O, Caldwell CB, Mainprize J: Multimodality imaging for precise location of craniofacial osteomyelitis. J Craniofac Surg 2003;14:215.

643. Sataloff RT, Sariego J, Myers DL, Richter HJ: Surgical management of frontal sinus. Neurosurgery 1984;15:593.

644. Schenck NL: Frontal sinus disease. III. Experimental and clinical factors in failure of the frontal osteoplastic operation. Laryngoscope 1975;85:76.

645. Luce EA: Frontal sinus fractures: guidelines to management. Plast Reconstr Surg 1987;80:500.

646. Peri G, Chabannes J, Menes R, et al: Fractures of the frontal sinus. J Maxillofac Surg 1981;9:73.

647. Remmler D, Boles R: Intracranial complications of frontal sinusitis. Laryngoscope 1980;90:1814.

648. Hybels RL, Newman MH: Posterior table fractures of the frontal sinus: I. An experimental study. Laryngoscope 1977;87:171.

649. Heckler FR: Discussion of frontal sinus fractures: guidelines to management. Plast Reconstr Surg 1987;80:509.

650. Gerbino G, Roccia F, Benech A, Caldarelli C: Analysis of 158 frontal sinus fractures: current surgical management and complications. J Craniomaxillofac Surg 2000;28:133.

651. Jacobs JB: 100 years of frontal sinus surgery. Laryngoscope 1997;107:1.

652. Rohrich R, Hollier L: Management of frontal sinus fractures: changing concepts. Clin Plast Surg 1992;19:219.

653. Lynch RC: The technique of a radical frontal sinus operation which has given me the best results. Laryngoscope 1921;31:1.

654. Manolidis S: Management of frontal sinus trauma. Semin Plast Surg 2002;16:261.

655. Manolidis S: Frontal sinus injuries: associated injuries and surgical management of 93 patients. J Oral Maxillofac Surg 2004;62:882.

656. Wallis A, Donald J: Frontal sinus fractures: a review of 72 cases. Laryngoscope 1998;98:593.

657. Freeman SB, Bloom ED: Frontal sinus stents. Laryngoscope 2000;110:1179.

658. Weber R, Draf W, Kratzsch B, et al: Modern concept of frontal sinus surgery. Laryngoscope 2001;111:137.

659. Weber C, Draf W, Kahle G, Kind M: Obliteration of the frontal sinus: state of the art and reflections on new material. Rhinology 1999;37:1.

660. Heller EM, Jacobs JB, Holliday RA: Evaluation of the nasofrontal duct in frontal sinus fractures. Otolaryngol Head Neck Surg 1989;11:46.

661. McLaughlin LB, Rehl RM, Lanza D: Clinically relevant frontal sinus anatomy and physiology. Otolaryngol Clin North Am 2001;34:1.

662. Mickel TJ, Rohrich R, Robinson J: Frontal sinus obliteration: a comparison of fat, muscle and bone and spontaneous osteogenesis in the cat model. Plast Reconstr Surg 1995;95:586.

663. Smoot C, Bowen D, Lappert D: Delayed development of an ectopic frontal sinus mucocele after pediatric cranial trauma. J Craniofac Surg 1995;6:327.

664. LaRossa DD, Noone RB, Jackson P: Facial deformity after frontal sinus mucocele: single stage surgical correction. Plast Reconstr Surg 1977;60:917.

665. Bordley JE, Bosley W: Mucoceles of the frontal sinus: causes and treatment. Ann Otol Rhinol Laryngol 1973;82:696.

666. Donald PJ: Frontal sinus ablation by cranialization. Arch Otolaryngol 1982;108:142.

667. Donald PJ, Bernstein L: Compound frontal sinus injuries with intracranial penetration. Laryngoscope 1978;88:225.

668. Donald PJ, Ettin M: The safety of frontal sinus fat obliteration when sinus walls are missing. Laryngoscope 1986;96:190.

669. Wolfe SA, Johnson P: Frontal sinus injuries: primary care and management. Plast Reconstr Surg 1988;82:781.

670. Burstein F, Cohen S, Hudgins R, Boydston W: Frontal basilar trauma: classification and treatment. Plast Reconstr Surg 1997;99:1314.

671. Kakibucci M, Fukada K, Yamada N: A simple method of harvesting a thin iliac bone graft for reconstruction of the orbital wall. Plast Reconstr Surg 2003;111:961.

672. Gosain A, Song L, Capel CC, et al: Biomechanical and histological alteration of facial recipient bone after reconstruction with bone and alloplastic implants: a one-year study. Plast Reconstr Surg 1998;101:1561.

673. Shumrick KA, Smith CP: The use of cancellous bone for frontal sinus obliteration and reconstruction of bony defects. Arch Otolaryngol Head Neck Surg 1994;120:1003.

674. Kay PP: Frontal sinus fractures: to obliterate or not to obliterate outlook. Plast Surg 1989;9:6.

675. Wilson BC, Davidson B, Corey JD: Comparison of complications following frontal sinus fractures managed with exploration with or without obliteration over 10 years. Laryngoscope 1988;98:516.

676. Petruzzelli GJ, Stankiewicz JA: Frontal sinus obliteration with hydroxyapatite cement. Laryngoscope 2002;112:32.

677. Disa J, Robertson B, Metzinger S, Manson P: Transverse glabellar flap for obliteration/isolation of the nasofrontal duct from the anterior cranial base. Ann Plast Surg 1996;36:453.

678. Ferri J, Bordure P, Huet P, Faure A: Usefulness of the galea flap in treatment of extensive frontal bone defects: a study of 14 patients. J Craniofac Surg 1995;6:164.

679. Mendians AD, Marks SC: Outcome of frontal sinus obstruction. Laryngoscope 1999;109:1495.

680. Chen DJ, Chen CT, Chen YR, Feng GM: Endoscopically assisted repair of frontal sinus fracture. J Trauma 2003;55:378.

681. Graham HD, Spring P: Endoscopic repair of frontal sinus fractures: case report. J Craniomaxillofac Trauma 1996;2:82.

682. Gross WE, Gross CW, Becker D: Modified transnasal endoscopic Lothrop procedure as an alternative to frontal sinus obliteration. Otolaryngol Head Neck Surg 1995;113:427.

683. Lappert PW, Lee JW: Treatment of an outer table frontal sinus fracture using endoscopic reduction and fixation. Plast Reconstr Surg 1998;102:1642.

684. Onishi K, Osaki M, Maruyama Y: Endoscopic osteosynthesis for frontal bone fracture. Ann Plast Reconstr Surg 1998; 40:650.

685. Lee D, Brody R, Har-El G: Frontal sinus outflow anatomy. Am J Rhinol 1997;11:283.

686. Oerko D: Endoscopic surgery of the frontal sinus without external approach. Rhinology 1989;27:119.

687. Har-El G: Endoscopic management of 108 sinus mucoceles. Laryngoscope 2001;111:2131.

688. Har-El G: Transnasal endoscopic management of frontal mucocele. Otolaryngol Clin North Am 2001;34:243.

689. Rish BL, Dillon JD, Meirowsky AM, et al: Cranioplasty: a review of 1030 cases of penetrating head injury. Neurosurgery 1979;4:381.

690. Manson PN, Crawley WA, Hoopes JE: Frontal cranioplasty: risk factors and choice of cranial vault reconstructive material. Plast Reconstr Surg 1986;76:888.

691. Wong L, Manson P: Rigid mesh fixation for alloplastic cranioplasty. J Craniofac Surg 1994;5:265.

692. Chang P, Parker T, Patrick C, Miller M: The accuracy of stereolithography in planning craniofacial bone replacement. J Craniofac Surg 2003;14:164.

693. Clark N, Birely B, Manson PN, et al: High-energy ballistic and avulsive facial injuries: classification, patterns, and an algorithm for primary reconstruction. Plast Reconstr Surg 1996;98:583.

694. Gruss JS, Phillips JH: An early definitive bone and soft tissue reconstruction of major gunshot wounds of the face. Plast Reconstr Surg 1991;87:436.

695. Robertson, Manson B, Manson P: The importance of serial débridement and second look procedures in high-energy ballistic and avulsive facial injuries. Operative Techniques Plast Reconstr Surg 1998;5:236.

696. Robertson B, Manson P: High-energy ballistic and avulsive injuries: a management protocol for the next millennium. Surg Clin North Am 1999;79:1489.

697. Kihtir T, Ivatury RR, Simon RJ, et al: Early management of civilian gunshot wounds to the face. J Trauma 1993; 35:569.

698. May M, West JW, Heeneman H, et al: Proceedings: Shotgun wounds to the head and neck. Arch Otolaryngol 1973;98:373.

699. Williams CN, Cohen M, Schultz RC: Immediate and long-term management of gunshot wounds to the lower face. Plast Reconstr Surg 1988;892:433.

700. Lindsey D: The idolatry of velocity, or lies, damn lies, and ballistics. J Trauma 1980;20:1968.

701. Fackler ML: Wound ballistics: a review of common misconceptions. JAMA 1988;259:2730.

702. Goodman JM, Kalsbeck J: Outcome of self-inflicted gunshot wounds of the head. J Trauma 1965;5:636.

703. Goodstein WA, Stryker A, Weiner LJ: Primary treatment of shotgun injuries to the face. J Trauma 1979;19:961.

704. Hollier L, Grantcharova EP, Kattash M: Facial gunshot wounds: a 4-year experience. J Oral Maxillofac Surg 2001;59:277.

705. Callahan MA: Silicone intubation for lacrimal canaliculi repair. Ann Plast Surg 1979;2:355.

706. Crockford DA: Posttraumatic facial pain. In Converse JM, ed: Reconstructive Plastic Surgery, 2nd ed. Philadelphia, WB Saunders, 1977:741.

707. Hendler H: The anatomy and psychopharmacology of chronic pain. J Clin Psychiatry 1982;43:15.

708. Hendler N: Complex regional pain syndrome. Type I and II. In Weiner RS: Pain Management. New York, CRC Press, 2002.

709. Hendler N: Differential diagnosis of complex regional pain syndrome. Type I. Pan Arab J Neurosurg 2002;6:1.

710. Hendler N: Pharmacological management of pain. In Raj PP: Practical Management of Pain, 3rd ed. St. Louis, CV Mosby, 2000:chapter 12.

711. Hendler N, Berguson C, Morrison C: Overlooked physical diagnoses in chronic pain patients involved in litigation, part II. Psychosomatics 1996;37:509.

712. Seddon HJ: Three types of nerve injury. Brain 1943;66:237.

713. Melzack R, Wall PD: Pain mechanisms: a new theory. Science 1965;150:971.

714. Wilson ME: The neurological mechanisms of pain: a review. Anesthesia 1974;29:407.

715. Speculand B, Goss AN, Hallett E, Spence ND: Intractable facial pain. Br J Oral Surg 1979;17:166.

716. Tams J, Van Loon JP, Otten B, Bos RRM: A computer study of biodegradable plates for internal fixation of mandibular angle fractures. J Oral Maxillofac Surg 2001;59:404.

717. Tams J, Van Loon JP, Rozema FR: A three dimensional study of loads across the fracture for different sites in the mandible. Br J Oral Maxillofac Surg 1997;55:693.

718. Tajima S: Malar bone fractures: experimental fractures on the dried skull and clinical sensory disturbances. J Maxillofac Surg 1977;5:150.

719. Collins WF: Physiology of pain. In Youmans JR, ed: Neurological Surgery, 2nd ed, vol 2. Philadelphia, WB Saunders, 1982.

720. Pataky PE, Graham WP III, Munger BL: Terminal neuromas treated with triamcinolone acetonide. J Surg Res 1973;14:36.

Pediatric Facial Injuries

CRAIG R. DUFRESNE, MD ✦ PAUL N. MANSON, MD

DEVELOPMENTAL MALFORMATIONS OF THE FACIAL
SKELETON
    Postnatal Growth of the Face
    Postnatal Growth of the Mandible
    Postnatal Growth of the Nasomaxillary Complex

CLINICAL EXAMINATION

RADIOLOGIC EVALUATION

EMERGENCY TREATMENT

PRENATAL, BIRTH, AND INFANT INJURIES

BATTERED CHILD SYNDROME

SOFT TISSUE INJURIES

DOG BITES

FACIAL FRACTURES
    Etiology
    Incidence

Alveolar Fractures
Mandibular Fractures
The Ability of the Dentofacial Structures to
    Accommodate Malocclusion
Condylar Fractures
Midfacial Fractures
Zygomatic and Orbital Fractures
Nasal and Naso-orbital Fractures
Frontal Bone and Frontal Sinus Fractures
Supraorbital Fractures
Compound, Multiple, and Comminuted Midfacial
    Fractures
Rigid Fixation and Growth
Translocation of Plates
Resorbable Fixation

COMPLICATIONS OF PEDIATRIC FACIAL TRAUMA

THE ROLE OF RESTRAINTS IN VEHICULAR SAFETY

Facial injuries in children are considered separately because of special problems that arise in their treatment and management.[1-6] Children are subject to injuries and trauma similar to adult types.[7] However, facial injuries are much less common in children, particularly during the first 5 years of life. In children, 95% of fractures occur after the age of 5 years. By the age of puberty, the frequency and the pattern of maxillofacial injuries begin to parallel those seen in adults. The principles for treatment of facial trauma in children are basically the same as those in adults. However, the techniques must be modified by certain anatomic, physiologic, and psychological factors specifically related to childhood and growth, and the timing of treatment must be early.

The automobile is responsible for a large number of deaths and severe injuries in childhood.[8,9] Both pedestrian and motor vehicle accidents are seen as a result of the automobile.[10] Children younger than 5 years account for 2% to 3% of automobile occupant deaths.[11] Children younger than 14 years account for approximately 6% of automobile deaths. Of children between the ages of 5 and 14 years who are injured in automobile collisions, only 56% were actual occupants of the automobiles.[1,8,9,12] Pediatric patients also demonstrate a significantly higher percentage of associated injuries (73%) compared with adults (58%). A greater number of cranial injuries have been documented in the pediatric population (55%) than in adults (39%).[13,14] With the use of air bags, car seats, and seat belts, there is significantly less facial trauma to motor vehicle occupants, with a resultant decrease in incidence of facial fractures.[15,16] However, the abuse of alcohol by adults continues to contribute to accidents that harm children.[17]

Other causes of accidents in children extend over a wide range from falls to thermal burns. In the Fairfax Hospital year 2000 experience,[18] 3252 trauma patients were seen, of which 11.3% were pediatric (14 years or younger). The leading cause of injury in children was falls (accounting for 36%), followed by motor vehicle accidents (25%), pedestrians (12%), bicycles (10%), motorcycle injuries (1%), and other types of injuries (16%). Athletic activities are responsible for facial injuries in older children. Baseball injuries account for 2% to 8% of the emergency department visits per year. Of the estimated 162,000 visits to the emergency department that will occur for patients between 5 and 14 years of age, approximately 26% are fractures and 37% are contusions and abrasions. The vast canine population in the United States subjects children to dog bites that often result in considerable soft tissue disorganization and loss and (less commonly known) a specific incidence of facial fractures.[19]

Soft tissue injuries and fractures may require special therapeutic techniques because of the difficulties in obtaining the cooperation of young children. Another important aspect of facial injuries in children is the potential for late effects on growth and facial development. A post-traumatic facial deformity in the child may be the result not only of the displacement of bone structures caused by the fracture but also of faulty or arrested development (growth) stemming from the injury.[20-24] Developmental malformations seen in young adolescents and adults are often secondary to early childhood injuries. A statement should always be made to the parents of a child, preferably in writing, that maldevelopment of growth may result from facial fractures despite adequate treatment, particularly in injuries involving the nasomaxillary complex and the condylar region of the mandible in children younger than 5 years. Such statements are an essential medicolegal precaution.

DEVELOPMENTAL MALFORMATIONS OF THE FACIAL SKELETON

Some facial developmental malformations may be attributed to trauma in early childhood. Trauma may have a deleterious effect on the growth and development of facial bone structure in postnatal life similar to that of a defective gene during prenatal development. In many patients, it is difficult to ascertain whether the disturbances occurred before or after birth. Koltai et al[20-23] have thoroughly reviewed the effects of the trauma on growth; many result in subtle alterations, but more substantial growth restriction may occur.

Postnatal Growth of the Face

Knowledge of craniofacial growth has been determined by a variety of methods (see Chapter 66).[25] The cross-sectional approach requires the use of large numbers of skulls of varying ages.[26,27] Early growth of the face is rapid. At 3 months, the face is less than half the size of that of an adult (approximately 40%). At 2 years, it has reached approximately 70%; and at 5.5 years, it attains approximately 80% of adult size.[25,28-31]

The proportions of the face change markedly during the period of postnatal growth (Fig. 67-1 and Table 67-1). The skull at birth presents a relatively large cranial portion and a small facial component compared with an adult skull. The cranial-to-facial proportions are 8:1 at birth, but they fall to 4:1 by 5 years of age and 2:1 in the adult (Figs. 67-2 to 67-6).[25,28-31] These changes are due to two factors: the actual

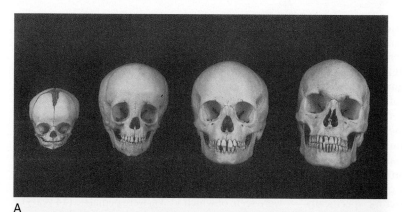

A

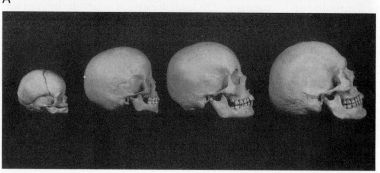

B

FIGURE 67-1. Series of skulls showing changes in the size of the face as well as the position of the face in relation to the cranium. Growth of the face is associated with growth of the jaws and eruption of the teeth. *A,* Frontal view. *B,* Lateral view. (From Dufresne CR, Manson PN: Pediatric facial trauma. In McCarthy JG, ed: Plastic Surgery. Philadelphia, WB Saunders, 1990:1142.)

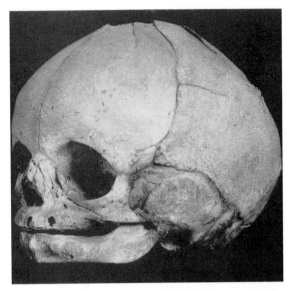

FIGURE 67-2. Skull of an infant in the first year of life. (From Dufresne CR, Manson PN: Pediatric facial trauma. In McCarthy JG, ed: Plastic Surgery. Philadelphia, WB Saunders, 1990:1142.)

growth of the face; and a modification of proportions, which brings forth characteristics distinguishing the adult faces of men from those of women and establishes distinctive adult individual features.[25]

The overall facial skeleton is relatively small at birth. The nasal cavity and paranasal sinuses are also small. The nasal cavities are as wide as they are high. The piriform aperture is broad at its lower border, and the floor of the nasal cavities is on a level slightly below that of the lower rim of the orbit in a horizontal line

TABLE 67-1 ✦ TABLE OF FACIAL GROWTH

	Onset (yr)	Maximum Growth (yr)	Growth Complete (yr)
Cranium	0	1-2	10
Nose	5	10-14	16
Orbit	0	1-2	7
Frontal sinus	5	8-16	20
Maxillary sinus	5	10-12	14
Maxilla	5	8-12	16
Mandible	1-4	8-14	20

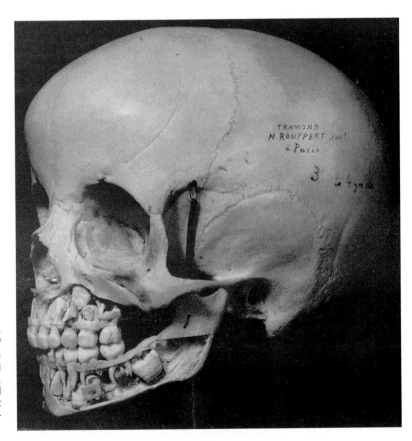

FIGURE 67-3. Skull of a 3-year-old child showing the position of the permanent (secondary) teeth in relation to the deciduous (primary) dentition. (From Dufresne CR, Manson PN: Pediatric facial trauma. In McCarthy JG, ed: Plastic Surgery. Philadelphia, WB Saunders, 1990:1142.)

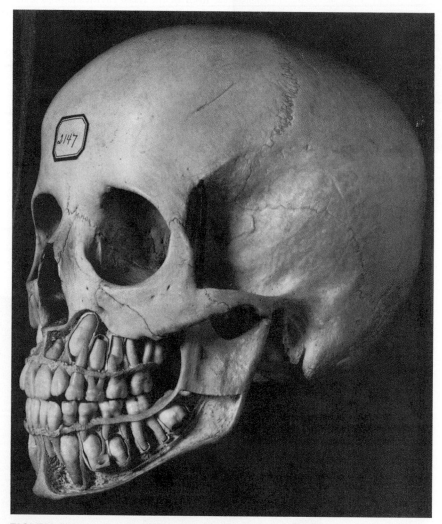

FIGURE 67-4. Skull of a child in the seventh year showing the position of the permanent teeth in relation to the deciduous dentition. (From Dufresne CR, Manson PN: Pediatric facial trauma. In McCarthy JG, ed: Plastic Surgery. Philadelphia, WB Saunders, 1990:1142.)

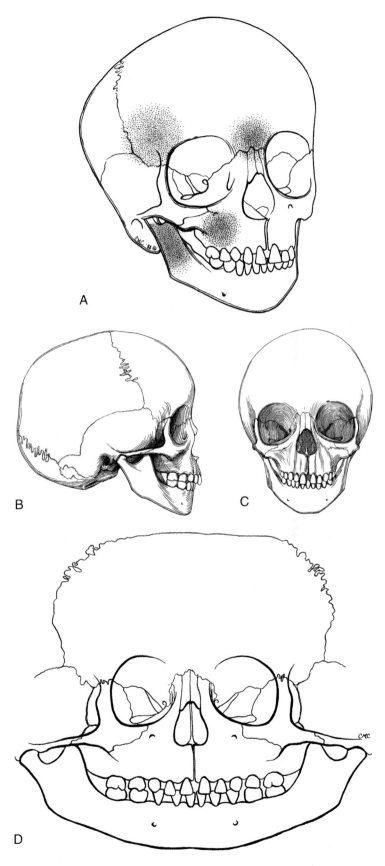

FIGURE 67-5. *A,* Mandibular pattern of growth. *B* and *C,* A child's skull. *D,* Pan face diagram of a child's face and skull.   *Continued*

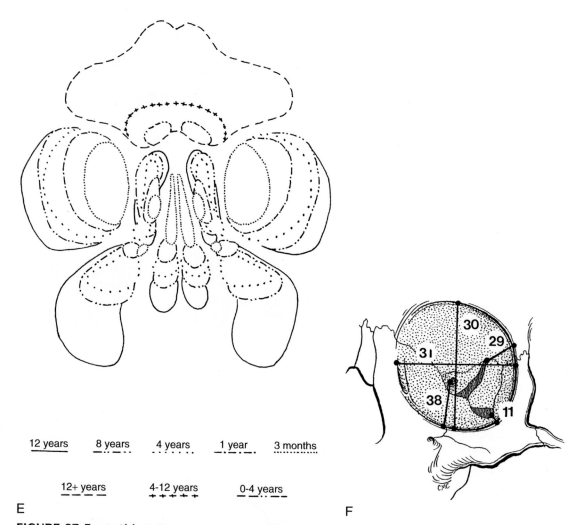

12 years   8 years   4 years   1 year   3 months

12+ years   4-12 years   0-4 years

E   F

FIGURE 67-5, cont'd. *E,* Sinus development. *F,* Orbital dimension of a child.

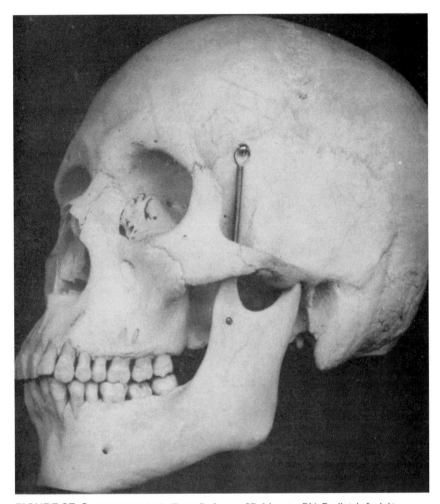

FIGURE 67-6. The adult skull. (From Dufresne CR, Manson PN: Pediatric facial trauma. In McCarthy JG, ed: Plastic Surgery. Philadelphia, WB Saunders, 1990:1142.)

passing approximately through the two infraorbital foramina (Fig. 67-7).[25,28-31]

Children are further characterized from adults in that the nose and sinuses are essentially a single structure, the sinuses being small or absent. The ethmoid and maxillary sinuses begin to invaginate from the nasal cavity in the second trimester. They first present as separate recesses, with the ethmoid sinuses later growing into a honeycomb of cells. The growth of the maxillary sinus parallels that of the face. The maxillary sinuses are narrow in the newborn and not sufficiently developed to reach the area beneath the orbit. The sinuses slowly increase in size and become large after the age of 5 years.[32,33] During the first year, the medial and lateral dimensions have reached beneath the orbit but no farther laterally than the infraorbital foramina. During the third and fourth years, the mediolateral dimensions of the maxillary sinus increase considerably. By 5 years of age, they extend to a point lateral to the infraorbital canal. The floor of the maxillary sinus remains above the level of the floor of the nose in the child up to the age of 8 years. It is only after the eruption of the permanent dentition in the twelfth year and the development of the alveolar process that the maxillary sinus descends below the level of the floor of the nose. Eruption of the permanent maxillary teeth determines the inferior growth of the maxillary sinus and therefore the level of the sinus floor. The floor is at the level of the inferior meatus by the age of 8 years and reaches the level of the nasal floor by the age of 10 to 12 years. The maxillary sinus is fully developed by the age of 16 years.[25,32,34,35]

The frontal sinus develops as invaginations from the nose during the second trimester. It can be distinguished from the ethmoid sinuses after the age of 5 years. The sinus reaches adult size by late puberty. The frontal sinuses are seldom symmetric and vary greatly

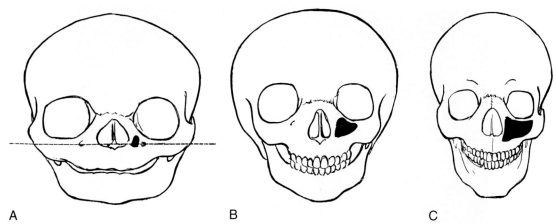

A   B   C

FIGURE 67-7. The skull at birth *(A)*, at 5 years *(B)*, and in the adult *(C)*. The skull is drawn with the same vertical dimension to show the relative size increases of the maxillary sinus. Note the progressive increase in the size of the maxillary sinus, extending laterally beyond the infraorbital foramen *(B)* and descending below the level of the floor of the nose *(C)* after eruption of the permanent teeth. (From Kazanjian VH, Converse JM: The Surgical Treatment of Facial Injuries, 3rd ed. Baltimore, Williams & Wilkins, 1974.)

in size and shape. On occasion, they may be absent. The lining of the sinus cavities is respiratory mucous membrane that is continuous with the mucosal lining of the nasal cavity. Fractures may impair sinus drainage by blocking the sinus ostia or interfering with the ciliary function of mucosa. Retained secretion, mucocele, or abscess may occur under these conditions and may require drainage procedures.[32,33,35]

In the early years of life, the cranium is large in comparison with the size of the facial bones. A major increase in cranial size occurs in the first two years. The first 6 months of life is characterized by a period of generalized rapid growth, followed by a slower period of growth from 6 months to 4 years. The increase in the vertical dimension of the face is due in part to the development and eruption of the dentition. In the newborn, the crown portions of the upper and lower teeth and the alveolar process do not contribute to the vertical height, as the teeth have not erupted. A rapid phase of growth characterizes the period from 4 to 7 years, and this rapid growth phase is followed by a slower period of growth from 9 to 15 years. From 15 to 19 years, another period of rapid growth is observed. The facial bones continue to grow until the age of 21 years in the male, but at different rates according to the area of the face. Much of the growth, however, is complete well before the teenage period. The orbits, for example, have usually attained their full adult size by the age of 7 years and are similar in dimension to the adult orbits by 2 years of age. The palate and maxilla have achieved two thirds of adult size by the age of 6 years. In contrast, the nasal bones show major growth in the adolescent period. A major proportion of cranial growth is complete by the age of 2 years. From birth to 10 years, the brain triples in size and is 90% of its final size

by the age of 10 years. From birth, the cranium increases four times to its adult size, whereas the facial skeleton increases 12 times to obtain its adult proportions.[25,28-31,36,37]

Increase in facial height is greater in the middle third of the face than in the lower third.[38] The increase in the anteroposterior direction is greater in the lower jaw than in the upper jaw. The face also widens more in the lower jaw than in the upper jaw.[39]

At birth, the proportion of the nasal fossa occupied by the ethmoid bone is twice the height of the maxillary portion. During childhood, the growth of the maxillary portion is accelerated, approximating the ethmoidal portion at the seventh year when adult proportions are obtained. The growth of the maxillary portion of the nasal fossa is due in part to the increase in size of the maxillary sinus and to the eruption of the dentition and the supporting alveolar processes. Changes in the maxilla and mandible result in characteristic changes of profile.[25,28-31,36,37,39]

The peak rate of growth in the head and upper face occurs between 3 and 5 years. After this period, growth proceeds slowly, but an acceleration occurs again between years 8 and 12. Growth greatly diminishes after the age of 15 years. Growth of the nose is complete near the age of 12 to 14 years (Fig. 67-8). From a surgical standpoint, however, one may consider the growth of the nose complete at approximately the age of 16 years. Minor changes occur throughout life.[40,41] Facial growth is restricted after premaxillary resection (see Table 67-1).[42]

Postnatal Growth of the Mandible

The mandible is the facial bone most frequently involved in post-traumatic developmental malfor-

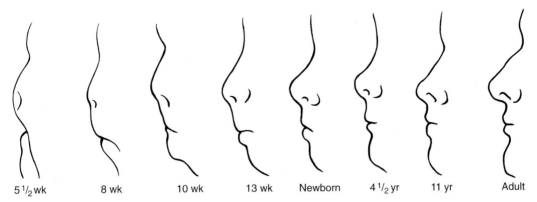

| 5 1/2 wk | 8 wk | 10 wk | 13 wk | Newborn | 4 1/2 yr | 11 yr | Adult |

FIGURE 67-8. Series of profile outlines of the face from 5.5 weeks to adulthood. (After Peter and Schaefer. From Dufresne CR, Manson PN: Pediatric facial trauma. In McCarthy JG, ed: Plastic Surgery. Philadelphia, WB Saunders, 1990:1142.)

mations.[16] Embryologically, the dorsal portion of the first mandibular arch grows forward beneath the developing orbital region to the olfactory area, forming the maxillary process. As a result of this formation, the mesenchymatous condensation that gives origin to the first pharyngeal arch becomes convex, and part of the dorsal portion becomes chondrified, forming a small cartilaginous mass that represents the pterygoquadrate bar of lower vertebrates. The remaining ventral and much larger portion of the pharyngeal arch chondrifies to form Meckel cartilage.[25]

The posterior extremities of the pterygoquadrate bar of Meckel cartilage articulate with each other. The intermediate portion of Meckel cartilage retrogresses and its sheath becomes ligamentous, forming the anterior ligament of the malleus and the sphenomandibular ligament. The dorsal portion, in contact with the pterygoquadrate cartilage, becomes recognizable as a definitive cartilaginous rudiment of the malleus, whereas the ventral portion is involved in development of the incus (Fig. 67-9).[39]

Later in development, two membranous bones are laid down on the outer side of Meckel cartilage. The most anterior of these membranous bones, which appears early, is related to the lateral aspect of the ventral portion of the cartilage and forms the mandible. At first it is a small covering of membranous bone. However, by growth and extension, it soon surrounds Meckel cartilage, except at its anterior extremity, where endochondral ossification occurs. Upward growth forms the mandibular ramus at the posterior end of the developing mandible. This portion of the mandible comes into contact with the squamous portion of the temporal bone to form the temporomandibular joint, in which a fibrocartilaginous articular disk develops. Part of the ramus of the mandible is transformed into cartilage before cartilage ossification occurs.[25,39,43-48]

In mammals, as in many other vertebrates, arches of the membranous bone are laid down lateral to the cartilages of the first pharyngeal arch and in the substance of the maxillary and mandibular processes. In the maxillary process of each side, four such ossification areas form the premaxilla, maxilla, and zygomatic and squamous portion of the temporal bones.[25]

The mandible, small at birth, is destined to grow both by bone growth and by development of the alveolar process, which accompanies development of the teeth (see Figs. 67-2 to 67-6).[49] The recognition of condylar growth centers showed that the forward projection of the mandible is a consequence of this posterior growth. Elongation of the mandible involves continuous addition of bone at each condyle and along the posterior border of the ramus. Posterior appositional growth is only one of many movements associated with total mandibular growth, as all the different portions of the bone participate in the growth process. In addition to the centers of growth, increase in size is the result of surface apposition; the local contours of the mandible are constantly undergoing changes as a result of remodeling, resorptive, and depository activities.[25,39,43,44,47,48]

Growth of the condyle is the result of endochondral ossification in the epiphysis. Microscopic examination of human material shows chondrogenic, cartilaginous, and osseous zones. The condyle is capped by a narrow layer of a vascular fibrous tissue, which contains connective tissue cells and a few cartilage cells. The inner layer of this covering is chondrogenic, giving rise to hyaline cartilage cells that form the second or cartilaginous zone. Destruction of the cartilage and ossification around the cartilage scaffolding can be seen in the third zone. The cartilage of the head of the mandible is not similar to the epiphyseal cartilage of the long bone; it differs from articular cartilage in that the free surface

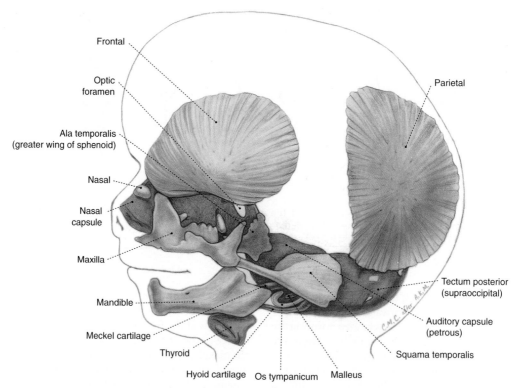

Frontal

Optic
foramen

Parietal

Ala temporalis
(greater wing of sphenoid)

Nasal

Nasal
capsule

Maxilla

Mandible

Tectum posterior
(supraoccipital)

Meckel cartilage

Auditory capsule
(petrous)

Thyroid

Squama temporalis

Hyoid cartilage   Os tympanicum   Malleus

FIGURE 67-9. Lateral aspect of a model of the skull of an 80-mm human embryo. (Based on Hertwig's model, from Kolmann's Handatlas, 1970. From Hamilton WJ, Boyd JD, Mossman HW: Human Embryology. Baltimore, Williams & Wilkins, 1945.)

bordering the articular spaces is covered by fibrous tissue. Trauma plays a particularly important role in the condylar articular cartilage; it may result in mandibular hypoplasia (Fig. 67-10), particularly if the trauma occurs before the age of 5 years (Fig. 67-10B).[39,43,44,47,48]

Postnatal Growth of the Nasomaxillary Complex

The skeleton of the midface area is formed from membranous bone, with the exception of the nasal cartilaginous capsule. These bones grow in a complex manner in a variety of regional directions. Numerous anatomists have studied the growth and development of the nasomaxillary complex. The anteroposterior growth of the nasomaxillary complex is related in utero and also after birth to the growth of the cranial base cartilages and their synchondroses. The intersphenoidal and the septoethmoidal synchondroses show evidence of activity until adulthood. At birth, the nasal septum is continuous with the cartilages of the cranial base. Around the first year, the perpendicular plate of the ethmoid starts to ossify from the nasoethmoidal center. At 3 years of age, there is bone union between the ethmoidal and the vomer bones. The bone

structures of the nasomaxillary areas follow a complex process of growth.[25,39,46]

There is not only a forward and downward growth of the maxilla but also a constant remodeling of its multiple regional parts. The main steps in development include a displacement away from the cranial base, a posterior enlargement corresponding to the lengthening of the dental arch, and an anterior resorption of the malar region. The nasal vaults grow forward and laterally, and the descent of the premaxillary area occurs by resorption on the superior and anterior surface of the nasal spine and by bone deposition on the inferior surface.[25,28-31,50-54]

Considerable controversy has arisen over the role of the septum in the growth of the nasomaxillary complex and the implications of trauma in abnormal growth of the area. The midfacial area is formed of membranous bone, with the exception of the cartilaginous nasal capsule. Some authors consider the septum to be the driving force in the growth of the midfacial area.[30,51,52] Others think that the role of the nasal septum in growth is of lesser importance.[46] According to Moss,[39,43,44,47] facial growth is controlled by a functional matrix that comprises the nonskeletal elements of the face, including spaces, muscles, and soft tissue. Langford et al[55,56] have documented rapid

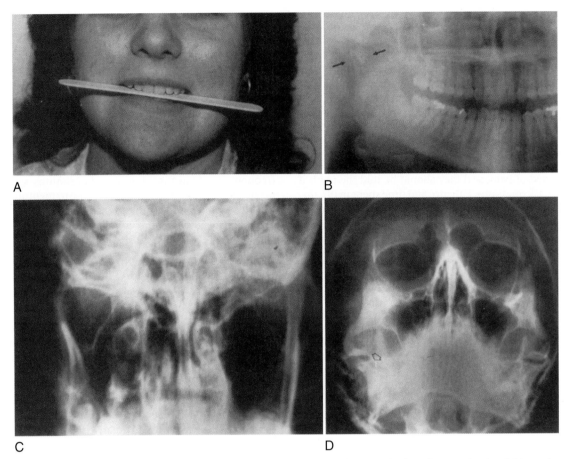

FIGURE 67-10. *A,* A 20-year-old woman showing asymmetric facial growth after she sustained a right condylar fracture at the age of 5 years. Right maxillary growth was affected, resulting in an occlusal cant and a 15-mm height difference between the rami. *B,* Panoramic radiograph showing a shortened, deformed right condyle. *C,* Plain film revealing asymmetry of the rami and condyles. *D,* Waters view demonstrating the malformation of the right ramus and condyle. (From Dufresne CR, Manson PN: Pediatric facial trauma. In McCarthy JG, ed: Plastic Surgery. Philadelphia, WB Saunders, 1990:1142.)

growth of the maxilla in the periods 0 to 5 years, 5 to 11 years, and after 15 years. The maxilla grows steadily at the age of 5 years and has reached 53% of its volume at 15 years. There is an accelerated rate of growth from 5 to 11 years of age, which corresponds to the growth of the permanent dentition. From 11 to 15 years of age, the rate of growth slows.

Others have concluded that the maxilla drifts forward as part of an overall genetic and environmental pattern of growth, and bone is laid down in the sutures and on the maxillary tuberosity. The maxilla is thought to be more easily influenced in its growth than is the mandible.[25,57,58]

The role of trauma in the interference of growth and development of the midfacial area seems to be difficult to determine. When one compares other facial areas, namely, the mandible, one finds considerable disparity between the extent of the damage suffered by the condylar area and the extent of the ensuing maldevelopment. In some patients, a fracture of the condylar area may heal with complete restoration of anatomic form without interference with growth and development. In other patients, with injuries that seem to be minor, damage results in mandibular hypoplasia. In some patients, mandibular hyperplasia may occur after injury. Much depends on the extent of the damage to the condylar cartilage, and subsequent skeletal and occlusal changes can be noted after an injury to this structure (see Fig. 67-10).[3,21-23,51,52,59-67]

CLINICAL EXAMINATION

The clinical examination of children is often difficult. Pediatric patients are frequently unable or unwilling to provide a history, and the parents may or may not be present to add detailed information. Children are often uncooperative and become easily frightened and apprehensive. The fear and anxiety of the parents is transmitted to the child, and the clinical examination can be difficult in the absence of cooperation. If the parents are contributing to the anxiety of the child, they should be removed from the examination area. Such decisions regarding child, parent, and physician interaction are based on the physician's ability to deliver optimal evaluation and treatment. The proper assessment of a particular child and the management of his or her parents demand an individual evaluation, considerable patience, some psychiatric qualifications, and a gentle but firm determination. Children should be warned of pain, and they should be told the truth if they ask questions. Patience and time spent in obtaining their confidence can be helpful. However, they often remain unwilling to cooperate, and the examination must then proceed. Sedation may be necessary in patients in whom the observation of a head injury is not a concern, and general anesthesia may sometimes be required for adequate examination and treatment.

Injuries outside the facial region are observed in 60% of patients with pediatric trauma. Skull fractures and cervical spine injuries accompanying facial fractures are frequent in childhood.[68] The identification of a head injury may be difficult because the subtle symptoms of a cerebral injury are not easily distinguished from the emotional reaction to the accident.[1,3,69-79]

The clinical examination consists of an orderly inspection of all facial areas, including observation, palpation, and a functional examination.[80] Areas in which lacerations or bruises are present are identified as specific areas of concern. Frequently, an underlying fracture is present. An orderly palpation of all bone surfaces should be performed by beginning in the skull and forehead areas; the rims of the orbits and the nose are palpated to identify any evidence of tenderness, irregularity, and "step" or "level" discrepancies in the surface bone structure. Crepitus may be present, particularly over a nasal or orbital rim fracture. The examination is continued over the zygomatic arches, the cheeks, and the surface of the mandible. An intraoral examination is performed to demonstrate loose teeth and to identify intraoral lacerations or hematomas. Lateral pressure on the mandibular and maxillary dental arches is necessary to determine instability or pain in fractures involving the midline of the mandible or maxilla. A common fracture is a "sagittal" fracture of the palate and maxilla. The fracture may easily be missed in the absence of a mucosal laceration if the segments of the maxilla are not examined for lateral instability as well as for anteroposterior movement. The presence of avulsed, loose, or missing teeth should signal the possibility of a significant fracture of the mandible or maxilla.[81-85]

A cooperative child may even be examined for such conditions as double vision. A visual acuity may be recorded and visual fields assessed. The child may volunteer that mandibular motion is painful or that the "bite" is not correct. Such details help provide additional evidence of fracture and point to the anatomic location that requires further examination and radiologic evaluation.

In a series of 1385 pediatric patients presenting to a hospital emergency department with soft tissue injuries, Zerfowski and Bremerich[86] found that 24% of the patients had dental trauma, 8% had sustained fractures, and 90% of the injuries were minor. Falls, altercations, and motor vehicle accidents were the most frequent mechanisms of injury. Lacerations were located in the central "falling zone" (nose to mentum); the most common fracture was that of the mandible, and 80% of the mandible fractures involved the condyle.

RADIOLOGIC EVALUATION

Historically, the standard radiologic evaluation consisted of specific views including Caldwell, Waters, submentovertex, Towne, and lateral skull. The quality of films is directly proportional to the child's cooperation. Frightened and apprehensive children move during the examination and produce blurring of the radiograph. In children, the bone structures are sufficiently cancellous that fracture lines are difficult to observe.[81-83,85] These conditions complicate the radiographic evaluation of pediatric fractures.

Failure to confirm a suspected fracture on radiography should not always deter treatment. Clinical judgment should overrule other considerations. The advent of computed tomographic (CT) scanning has improved the radiologic diagnosis of mid and upper facial fractures and has replaced the use of plain films (Table 67-2).[87] Fractures of the condyle are well demonstrated,[88] as are the extent and pattern of fractures of the horizontal portion of the mandible. Fractures of the frontal area, orbit, and maxilla are precisely demonstrated, although the examination may require sedation (Fig. 67-11). In addition, concomitant brain injury can be evaluated by combining facial and cranial CT scans in a single examination. Greenstick (incomplete) and nondisplaced fractures are not as easily identified in CT scans. The one partial exception to the lack of value of plain radiographs and general utility of the CT scan is the Panorex examination of the mandible, which does require the cooperation of the patient. A CT scan is often more revealing than even a Panorex examination for vertical mandible fractures.

Sedation should generally be avoided because it confuses the neurologic examination. CT scans should be interpreted in the light of normal values.[89,90]

Nimkin[91] has summarized the imaging criteria when child abuse is suspected so clinicians can recognize the pattern and symptoms as child abuse (see "Battered Child Syndrome"). Rib fractures correlate with

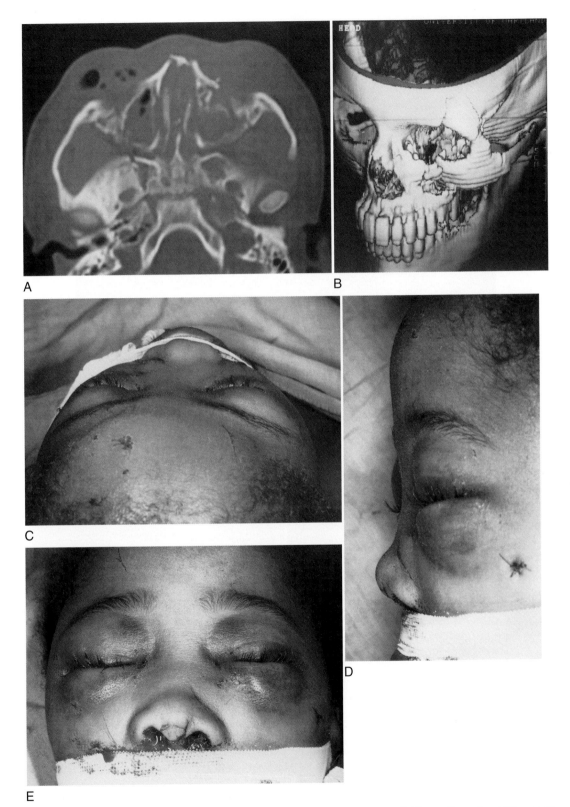

FIGURE 67-11. *A,* CT scan of a child with nasoethmoidal-orbital fractures. *B,* Three-dimensional CT scan of nasoethmoidal-Le Fort fracture. *C* to *E,* Flattened interorbital area and midface.   *Continued*

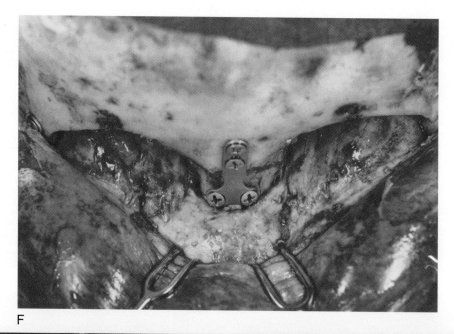

F

G   H

FIGURE 67-11, cont'd. *F,* Open reduction with transnasal fixation of canthal ligament-bearing medial orbital rims. *G,* Immediate improvement in profile. *H,* Postoperative result.

TABLE 67-2 ✦ TABLE OF RADIOLOGIC STUDIES

	Plain Radiography	Computed Tomography
Skull	Posteroanterior and lateral skull	Axial and coronal view Bone and soft tissue windows
Frontal sinus	Posteroanterior and lateral skull	Axial and coronal views
Zygoma	Caldwell, Waters Submentovertex	Axial and coronal views Bone and soft tissue windows
Nose	Nasal bones	Axial and coronal views
Orbit	Caldwell, Waters Orbital foramen	Axial and coronal views Bone and soft tissue windows
Nasoethmoid	Waters, Caldwell Lateral face	Axial and coronal views Bone and soft tissue views
Maxilla	Waters, Caldwell Lateral face	Axial and coronal views
Mandible, horizontal	Posteroanterior mandible Lateral obliques Occlusal, Panorex	Axial and coronal views
Mandible, vertical	Townes, lateral obliques Condyle, temporomandibular joints Panorex	Axial and coronal views

nonaccidental trauma in children younger than 3 years with a correlation of 95%.[92] A CT scan should always be obtained in significant facial trauma, and a Panorex examination should be added in mandibular trauma (Fig. 67-12). Head injury patients should not be sent unmonitored to radiographic examination, and sedation under anesthetic supervision may be necessary in some patients.

The management of major injuries in children challenges the clinician to achieve a rapid, accurate alignment of facial bone fragments to minimize functional disturbances and to permit maximal future growth and development.[69,93]

Children are often subjected to injuries from falls and accidents. The frequency of fractures is small, however, and children's bones, which are soft and resilient, are protected by both anatomic and environmental factors. The larger cancellous-to-cortical structural ratio makes the bones bend and resist injury. The incomplete (greenstick) fracture is common (Fig. 67-13), and this fracture is difficult to see in CT scans and plain radiographs. Children have a smaller face-to-head size ratio and thus have protection for their faces by the protrusion of the frontal skull.[72] The soft tissues are proportionately thicker in children and thus provide for more padding.[81-83] Posnick[78,94] found that boys (60%) were involved in more accidents and falls than were girls (37%). Children aged 6 to 12 years were the largest group involved in traffic accidents. Pedestrian injuries and falls were the most common injuries, in that order, and together accounted for 88% of the facial fractures studied. Mandible (34%) and orbital (23%) fractures predominated over midface fractures, which were found in 7% of patients. Plain films are not presently of much use. A CT scan should be obtained in all suspected fractures, with the addition of a Panorex examination in mandible fractures.

EMERGENCY TREATMENT

The control of hemorrhage, the provision of an adequate airway, and the prevention of aspiration are the major considerations that demand emergency management in facially injured children. In young children, the dimensions of the trachea and pharynx are small, and they can easily be obstructed by blood clots, mucus, fractured teeth, or foreign objects. Provision of an adequate airway is initiated by the removal of such material from the oropharynx. Obstruction of the hypopharynx may be relieved simply by forward traction on the tongue or mandible. Tracheostomy is not usually necessary in children, and protection of the airway can be achieved by orotracheal or nasotracheal intubation.[95-97] Intubation should be accomplished for airway obstruction and when bleeding threatens aspiration.

Pediatric endotracheal tubes are not cuffed (Table 67-3), and thus material from the oropharynx may enter the trachea around the tube. A throat pack helps protect the trachea from aspiration and is essential in anyone with nasal or oral bleeding and is preferred in all patients. The small size of the trachea makes

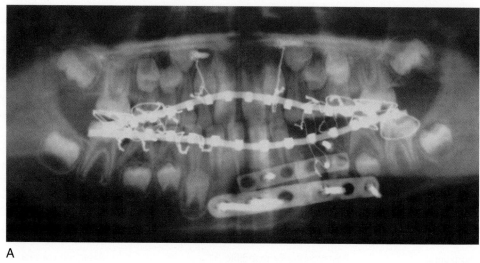

A

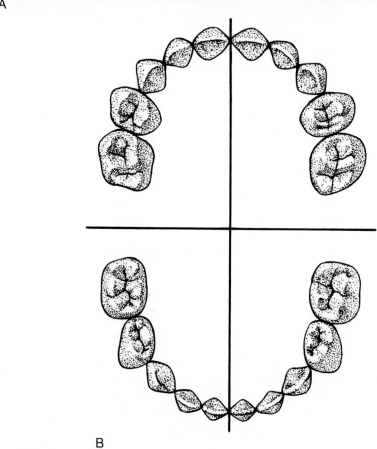

B

FIGURE 67-12. *A,* Panorex examination of a child with mandibular fractures repaired with upper and lower plates. Intermaxillary fixation was stabilized with skeletal wires. *B,* Pediatric dentition.

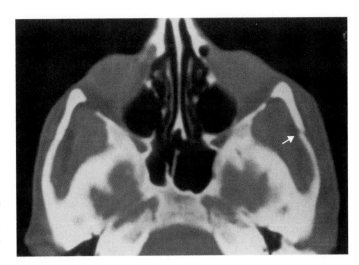

FIGURE 67-13. Example of a greenstick, nondisplaced zygoma fracture *(arrow)* on CT scan. (From Dufresne CR, Manson PN: Pediatric facial trauma. In McCarthy JG, ed: Plastic Surgery. Philadelphia, WB Saunders, 1990:1142.)

obstruction by retained mucous secretions a constant threat, even in the face of endotracheal intubation. Appropriate airway management with humidification, suction, and mucolytic agents is required. Tracheostomy complications or decannulation problems

TABLE 67-3 ♦ PEDIATRIC ENDOTRACHEAL TUBES

Tube Size for Intubation by Age

Age	Tube Size Internal Diameter
Premature (<2.5 kg)	2.5 mm
Birth (term)	3.0 mm
6 months	3.5 mm
12 months	4.0 mm
18-24 months	4.5 mm
>24 months	age/4 + 4.5 mm

Lip → Trachea Distance

Newborn	
1 kg	7 cm
2 kg	8 cm
3 kg	9 cm
1 year	10-11 cm
2-10 years	12 cm + age/$^1/_2$

Laryngoscope Blades

Premature	Miller 00 or 0
Birth	Miller 0
0-6 months	Miller 1
6-24 months	Miller 2
>24 months	Miller 2

From Lebowitz PW, Newberg LA, Gillette MT: Clinical Anesthesia Procedures of the Massachusetts General Hospital. Boston, Little, Brown, 1982. Modified from Johns Hopkins Anesthesia Handbook.

occur in half of those who undergo the procedure, and virtually all the complications occur in patients younger than 5 years. Complications include pneumothorax, emphysema, bleeding, infection, tracheal erosion or stenosis, occlusion of the cannula, displacement of the tube, and difficulty in decannulation.[95,96] The prolonged use of an endotracheal tube permits the development of tracheal stenosis by excess pressure and necrosis. Stenosis is minimized by attention to hygiene and positioning and possibly by the use of stents and corticosteroids in appropriate patients who have sustained a tracheal injury.

The blood volume of children is small, and significant circulatory compromise occurs with the loss of 20% or less of total blood volume. The blood volume is 90 mL/kg before the age of 1 year. Hemorrhage from lacerations associated with closed fractures must be treated immediately. The control of significant hemorrhage from cutaneous lacerations may usually be achieved with digital pressure. Precise identification of the bleeding vessel before ligation facilitates the avoidance of facial nerve injury. For significant nasopharyngeal hemorrhage from closed maxillofacial fractures, nasopharyngeal packing is used. Intranasal tamponade is generally successful in the management of profuse nasopharyngeal hemorrhage associated with severe facial fractures. A posterior pack is placed in the back of the nose through the mouth and pulled into place with strings led through the nose.[68,98] Alternatively, small Foley catheter balloons can be inflated in the nasopharynx after a catheter has been passed through each nostril and then pulled anteriorly and secured so that they form an obturator of the posterior choanae. Anterior packing is placed within the recesses of the nasal cavity to provide the pressure necessary to tamponade the hemorrhage. The packing materials are better tolerated if they are soaked with antibiotic-impregnated ointments. In patients with injuries to the cranial base, care should be taken that the packing is not inadvertently placed intracranially.[98] Initial control of bleeding should be obtained in the admission area and is best accomplished with the patient intubated. Children have restricted airway space; anterior-posterior nasal packs should not be used without anesthesia, intubation, and control of the airway with monitoring in the intensive care unit.

Aspiration is frequent with significant injuries of the mandible and maxilla and contributes to rapid respiratory obstruction or impairment of respiratory gas exchange. In the series of McCoy et al[70,99] and Posnick,[78,79,94] aspiration was found to be the most frequent complication. Aspiration can be prevented by intubation and the use of a pharyngeal pack; it can also be minimized by frequent oronasopharyngeal suctioning when the use of an endotracheal tube is undesirable. The prolonged use of an endotracheal tube often results in the complication of tracheal stenosis. Tracheal stenosis can be minimized by appropriate attention to size, detail of positioning, and possibly the use of steroids. Radiographic studies of the airway can be used to identify patients with a constriction of the tracheal lumen. Those in whom tracheal narrowing is identified are treated with bronchoscopy, removal of granulation tissue, systemic steroids, and a tracheal stent for the acute tracheal intubation injury.[70,78,94,95,97,99,100]

PRENATAL, BIRTH, AND INFANT INJURIES

Intrauterine compression is thought to be the cause of some prenatal deformities, although evidence of this type of injury has never been substantiated. Anecdotal reports have described instances in which positioning or crowding of multiparous siblings resulted in facial deformities.

Birth injuries may result from prolonged labor with difficult passage through the birth canal and delivery by obstetric forceps. Most of the injuries due to obstetric forceps are minimal, and recovery usually takes place without residual deformity. Infant and child skulls are pliable because of the segmental arrangement, flexibility, resilience, and relative softness of the bones. The bones develop as a loosely joined system in the matrix surrounding the brain. They are separated by fontanels and sutures and covered by thin fibrous sheaths. These characteristics explain the malleability of the cranial and facial bones and the fact that they are subject to distortion in crushing injuries, which may have developmental repercussions.[36]

Fractures of the skull are occasionally encountered, usually after forcible attempts at delivery, although they may occur spontaneously. There are two presentations, an appearance of a shallow groove and an elliptical or round depression posterior to the coronal suture. The shallow groove is common and has few sequelae. The depression, without surgical revision, results in death in more than 50% of patients secondary to increased intracranial pressure or hemorrhage.[36] However, this observation was made before the use of CT scans, and this phenomenon has not been noted by the authors. Presumably, this occurred from a depressed skull fracture with an epidural hematoma or possibly from a sagittal sinus injury. A CT scan evaluates the location and extent of hematoma and brain parenchymal injury.

Deviation of the septum or nose has been attributed to forced deflection of the nose during birth.[101] More severe injuries have been attributed to forceps compression of the soft tissues and bones of the face. This may cause permanent facial scars or osseous deformities in the region of the zygomatic arch and temporomandibular joint, which may result in temporomandibular ankylosis with developmental hypoplasia of the mandible. The lack of development of the mastoid process at birth and the subcutaneous position of the seventh cranial nerve predispose to facial paralysis by pressure from delivery forceps. Such injuries are observed when the posterior blade of the forceps places pressure over the stylomastoid foramen where the seventh nerve exits. Spontaneous recovery in a few days is the general rule,[36] but permanent paralysis has also occurred with some frequency.

Injuries to the eye or its adnexa, such as damage to the extraocular musculature, may be caused by intraorbital hemorrhage. Linear fractures with little if any displacement have been observed in which healing occurs without treatment. Newborns have been observed with separation of the halves of the mandible at the symphysis following placement of the surgeon's finger in the baby's mouth for manipulation to deliver the baby.[20-23]

Injury to the sternocleidomastoid muscle may occur, particularly during a breech delivery with lateral hyperextension. There may be a tear of the muscle or fascia, resulting in a hematoma and eventual cicatricial torticollis deformity.[102] If it is not corrected or released, the contracture of the muscle may lead to craniofacial asymmetry (deformational frontal plagiocephaly).[103,104] Steroid injections into the areas of the contracture and muscle stretching have been used for constructive therapy.[103,104]

It has long been suspected that infants fall much more frequently than is generally known. Of 536 infants involved in the study sponsored by the National Safety Council, 47.5% fell from a high place such as an adult bed, a crib, or an infant dressing table during their first year of life. Some 10% of the infants in the study suffered cranial, intracranial, and facial injuries. Facial trauma occurring in such falls in infants, although it does not often result in fractures because of the elasticity of the neonatal bones, may be sufficient to induce developmental malformations of the face observed in later years.[101,105,106]

BATTERED CHILD SYNDROME

The Third National Incidence Study of Child Abuse and Neglect[107] estimated that 2,815,600 children are harmed or endangered by their caretakers annually. Three children die each day of abuse or neglect, and 51% of the fatalities are caused by physical abuse. An estimated 2000 children die annually in the United States of the inflicted injuries. Children who are younger than 2 years are particularly at risk. Other risk factors for child abuse include prematurity, physical disability, low birth weight, and low socioeconomic level. Males, twins, and stepchildren are particularly at risk.

The battered and abused child may present in several ways.[87,108-110] The astute clinician must identify indications of physical abuse that should raise suspicion. Physical indications of child abuse include bruises and welts, burns, lacerations and abrasions, skeletal injuries, head injuries, and internal injuries. Craniofacial, head, face, and neck injuries occur from child abuse in more than half of patients.

Bruises and welts, when they are associated with abuse, will often be seen on an infant, especially around the facial area.[72,73] Bruises may also be seen on the posterior side of the body and trunk, hidden by clothing. Suspicion should be aroused if the bruises appear to have an unusual pattern that reflects the use of an instrument or if there is an indication of human bite marks. Clustered bruises indicate repeated contact with a hand or an instrument. Other suspicious signs are bruises at various stages of healing with fresh ones being noted in nearly contiguous areas. The abuse may result in contusions or lacerations of the tongue, buccal mucosa, palate, gingiva, or frenulum; fractured, displaced, or avulsed teeth; facial bone fractures; or bruising or scarring at the corners of the mouth.

Bite marks are lesions that may indicate abuse to a child. Bite marks should be suspected when ecchymoses, abrasions, or lacerations are found in an elliptical or ovoid pattern, particularly if there is a central area of ecchymoses.

Burns may also be indicative of child abuse and may not be related to accidental trauma. Immersion-type burns are suggested when hot liquid is placed around the arms or legs, such as a "stocking-type burn" or a "donut burn" in the area of the buttocks or genitalia. Cigarette burns are also indicative of child abuse, as are rope burns, which indicate confinement around the arms or legs. Other types of injuries, such as dry burns, indicate that the child may have been forced to sit on a hot surface or has had a hot implement applied to the skin.

Lacerations to the face, particularly the lip, eye, or any other portion of the infant's face, such as tears in the gum tissue, may be caused by force-feeding. Any laceration or abrasion to the external genitalia should raise concerns about child abuse.

Caffey,[111,112] more than 50 years ago, was the first to describe the association of unexplained subdural hematomas and long bone fractures in infants that was later termed the battered child syndrome. Radiographic imaging of the skeleton still remains a primary tool in documenting child abuse in infants and children (Fig. 67-14). Skeletal injuries, such as those to the metaphyseal region or corner fractures of long bones, a splintering of the end of the bone that is caused by twisting and pulling, are indicative of abuse. Epiphyseal separation at the center of the bone from the rest of the shaft can also be caused by twisting and pulling actions. Periosteal elevation and detachment of the periosteum from the shaft of the bone are

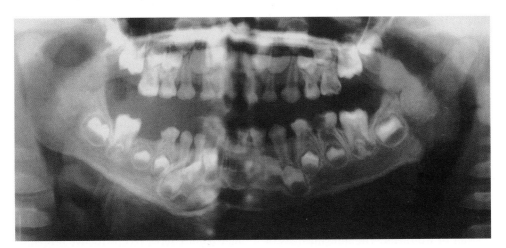

FIGURE 67-14. Fractures may result from nonaccidental trauma (child abuse).

associated with hemorrhaging from the periosteal shaft and are also associated with either blunt trauma or twisting.

Internal injuries, such as duodenal or jejunal hematomas, blood clots in the duodenum or small intestine due to kicking or hitting in the midline of the abdomen, rupture of the vena cava, and peritonitis, may result from trauma by kicking and hitting. Such trauma should always be suspected in a young child, particularly when associated injuries are noted.

One of the most common causes of neurologic dysfunction in children is secondary to head trauma or head injury. Head trauma may account for as much as 43% of all deaths of children between the ages of 5 and 9 years.[107] Unlike in adults, the majority of head traumas seen in children are due to reasons other than motor vehicle accidents. Between 55% and 65% of head injuries in younger children are results of falling accidents. Child abuse accounts for an unsubstantiated but probably significant percentage of head injuries in children younger than 2 years. In older children and adolescents, sports-related accidents cause many head injuries. In adolescents 15 years and older, motor vehicle accidents account for a larger portion of head injuries. In younger children, absence of hair or hemorrhaging beneath the scalp is associated with vigorous hair pulling. Subdural hematomas are associated with shaking and striking the young child. Retinal hemorrhages and detachments are also associated with the "shaken baby" syndrome.[111,112] More violent trauma may result in mandibular and nasal fractures, which should always alert the clinician.[91]

The plasticity of the pediatric skeleton tolerates blunt trauma readily, but the presence of a rib fracture correlates with child abuse with a frequency of 95% in children younger than 3 years and 100% when a history of absence of other factors is added.[92] Children with nonaccidental trauma were more likely to have multiple rib fractures (5.9 per child). Of 51 children with nonaccidental trauma, 29% had rib fractures as their only skeletal sequela of nonaccidental trauma; 78% of the rib fractures were either posterior (43%) or lateral (35%). Oblique radiographic views increase the sensitivity of detection.[92] It is difficult to absolutely pinpoint the etiology of the trauma in some circumstances, and the combination of clinical, physical, psychosocial, and historical information appears most predictive.[11,113,114]

SOFT TISSUE INJURIES

Maxillofacial soft tissue trauma and injuries in the pediatric population range from contusions and abrasions to massive avulsive injuries. As with any injury, the return to normal function and appearance is the paramount aim of treatment. The fundamentals of management of such injuries are similar to those in adults. Débridement of tissues should be restricted to devitalized tissue. Careful cleaning and irrigation of wounds should be performed to remove dirt and any foreign material. On occasion, a stiff nylon or wire brush, needle, or No. 11 blade is required to remove small embedded particles that would result in tattooing of the soft tissues.[5,32,49,115]

Contusions and ecchymosis usually require only symptomatic treatment.[5] When these are combined with a hematoma, drainage may have to be performed. In the "currant jelly" stage, a hematoma can most easily be drained by incision. After further liquefaction, aspiration may be performed. Hematomas of the external ears present special problems; if not evacuated, they organize into residual subcutaneous and perichondrial scar tissue and result in the "cauliflower ear" deformity.[68,116]

Lacerations may be of the simple, beveled, torn, burst, or stellate type.[115] Repair should be undertaken after the tissue has been cleaned and débrided and the foreign bodies have been removed. Most wound edges should be débrided conservatively but adequately. Suturing should be in layers and must be meticulous. When lacerations through soft tissue containing cartilage are being repaired, as in the ear or nose, stabilizing stitches with absorbable material should be used to stabilize the cartilage in its proper place, followed by a layered closure. Quilting sutures prevent reaccumulation of hematoma. Lacerations in special regions of the face require particular attention to realignment of the anatomy (e.g., the vermilion border of the lips, eyelid margin, and eyebrows). The eyebrow should never be shaved because regrowth may not occur.[84,117]

Soft tissue wounds in children heal rapidly and therefore benefit from definitive primary treatment. Children's fractures generally heal in half the time of fractures in adults.[6,106] Lacerations properly repaired at an early age will become less conspicuous with the passage of time. Pediatricians often advise parents to wait until the child has reached adolescence before secondary scar repair is accomplished. This advice must be individualized because many scars repaired in infancy and childhood are inconspicuous or hardly visible in adolescence.[117] Revision in the adolescent period is likely to result in a hypertrophic scar, often worse than in the remote injury. The hypertrophic scar is a frequent result of surgical incisions in adolescence.

Cheek and mandibular margin wounds tend to heal with considerable hypertrophic scarring, a common event in children. These discouraging results sometimes benefit from surgical revision, with avoidance of absorbable suture material, but the possibility of scar persistence and even further deformity should be mentioned to the parents. Densely scarred areas may require serial reconstructive procedures. Dense restrictive scars may interfere with bone growth,

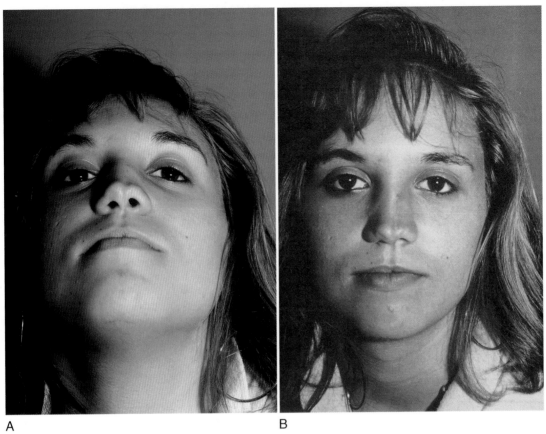

A   B

FIGURE 67-15. *A*, A 14-year-old girl struck in the nose at the age of 5 years, which resulted in a hematoma. *B*, Untreated, the hematoma deformed the nasal tip, with a contracture and fibrosis of the left side of the nose.

particularly in the area of the chin and mandible (Fig. 67-15).[84,117]

Loss of soft tissue of the face by avulsion or thermal burns is remedied by skin transplantation. Defects of the nose are adequately repaired in some patients with composite auricular grafts, which show a good success rate in children. Subtotal or total loss of the nose is rare.[117] Larger defects of the nose need forehead flap reconstruction.

Intraoral lacerations are usually sutured precisely to prevent contamination. Lacerations of the tongue are sutured in several layers to reduce the chance of hematoma formation. When a major salivary gland duct is lacerated, both ends must be located and a suture anastomosis performed. If the parotid duct is lacerated, the distal end is usually first found by placement of a probe or a catheter (22-gauge angiocatheter sleeve) through the oral opening after the sphincter has been dilated with a pediatric punctum dilator. The tube used for duct irrigation may also be anchored at the duct orifice and used as a stent for the duct anastomosis. The stent is left in place for 2 weeks, if possible, and removed. It has not been determined

whether leaving the stent in place improves the success of the anastomosis. After repair of the duct, soft tissue is closed in individual layers, a maneuver that reduces the potential for dead space and fistula formation and helps avoid the formation of a sialocele. A dependent or suction drain may be used. If a fistula develops, it may be treated by aspiration, pressure dressings,[84,117] or placement of a suction drain.

If branches of the facial nerve are divided, the nerve should be repaired primarily if the wound is clean and the laceration relatively sharp. In more destructive injuries, such as avulsions or gunshot wounds, nerve repair is usually performed secondarily with nerve grafts. The traditional rule was that facial nerve injuries should be repaired surgically if they occur posterior to a vertical line drawn through the lateral canthus. Presently, injuries occurring anterior to this line should be repaired if the branches can be located.[68,117,118]

Soft tissue hematomas may result in disturbance of a growth center or fibrosis, inhibiting facial growth. Hematomas should be drained because pressure necrosis or thinning of the surrounding structures, such as the skin, may occur. If they occur over cartilage, hematomas can result in septal necrosis, exporation, or distortion, as in a cauliflower ear or nasal septum (see Fig. 67-15).[24] Growth may be restricted after injury, and the parents should be advised that either hard or soft tissue injury may cause late disturbances.

DOG BITES

Approximately 600,000 dog bites require hospital treatment, and estimates suggest that more than 2,000,000 occur every year in the United States.[19,110] Children are the most common victims of dog bite injuries, and most of the dogs responsible belong to the household of the victim. Male dogs of the chow and German shepherd species are the most likely to be involved.[19]

In the United States, 44,000 facial injuries occur in children each year from dog bites. Approximately 1% of facial dog bite injuries require hospitalization. The overall infection rate is below 10%; *Pasteurella multocida* is the most commonly cultured organism, identified in more than 50% of the infections. *Staphylococcus* was involved in 20% and *Streptococcus* in 15%. Antibiotics are recommended (dicloxacillin, clindamycin) because débridement is usually incomplete. Although few of the patients included in the report sustained facial fractures, they are more common than is suspected and probably occur in 2% to 5% of facial dog bites.[19] Appropriate awareness of the possibility and the appropriate use of a CT scan are indicated. Most facial dog bites, or human bites, should be primarily closed with drains or "second-look" washout procedures used for avulsive injuries (Figs. 67-16 and 67-17).[119,120]

FACIAL FRACTURES

Etiology

The etiology of fractures in children is directly related to the age of the child. In the infant, falls, toy injuries, and animal bites are common. One should also be aware of the battered baby syndrome, in which lacerations (particularly in the frenulum of the upper lip), facial or skull fractures, and cervical spine and cerebral injuries can be observed.[111,112,116,121-123] Falls from heights are frequent in infants.[124] Vehicular trauma (sustained in a motor vehicle or on a bicycle), athletic injuries, sporting accidents, and injuries occurring from airborne objects are often observed in children older than 5 years. Unrestrained children in motor vehicles (guest passenger injuries) are a frequent problem. Boys are subject to injury more than girls are in almost all age groups after 5 years. In infants, falls are frequent after they have begun to walk and occur from strollers, baby seats, and dressing tables before that time.[12,112] Birth injuries frequently dislocate the nasal septum[24] or injure the facial nerve[57] or temporomandibular joint.[36,125,126]

The history of the injury may indicate the mechanism and direction of force of the injury and may provide clues for the focus of the clinical examination. Such symptoms may include swelling, pain, and numbness in a cranial nerve distribution; a visual disturbance consists of diminished vision, double vision, or inability to open the eyelid. Nasal or oral bleeding, tooth displacement, difficulty in eating, malocclusion, decreased excursion of the jaw, bruising, and ecchymosis point to a skeletal injury. Exophthalmos or enophthalmos may be present. A cerebrospinal fluid (CSF) leak may indicate involvement of the cranial

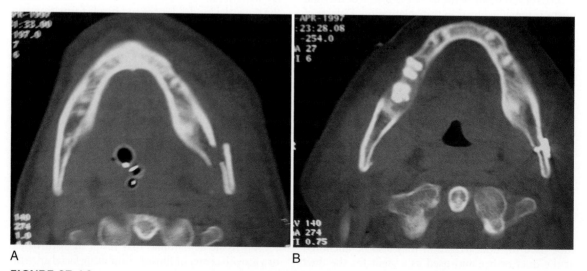

A   B

FIGURE 67-16. *A,* This patient sustained multiple facial lacerations and an angle mandible fracture from a dog bite. The angle fracture was treated with open reduction and rigid fixation. *B,* Appearance after fixation.

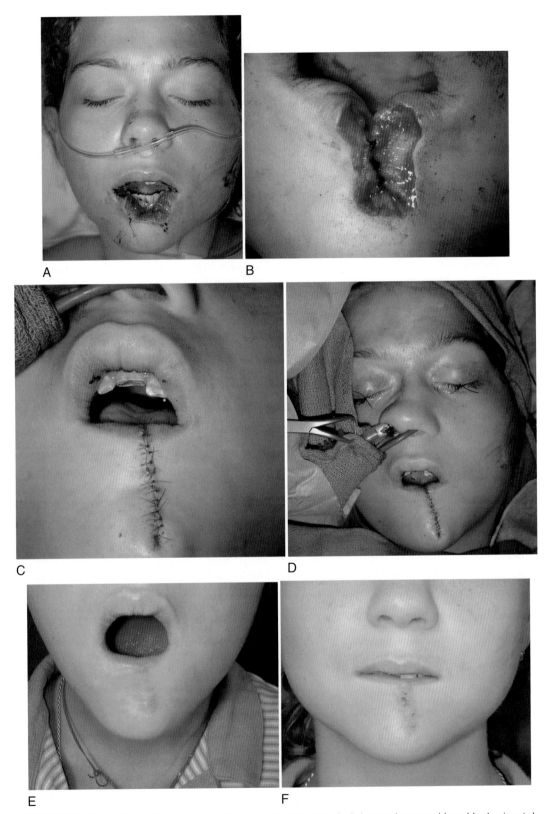

FIGURE 67-17. *A,* Loss of central lower lip from dog bite. *B* to *D,* Primary closure achieved by horizontal lip shortening and advancement. *E* and *F,* Appearance after repair.

base. Subcutaneous emphysema is seen in the periorbital area when air enters the tissues from fractures of the nose, orbit, or sinuses.

Incidence

Fractures of the facial bones are less frequent in children than in adults. Except in large medical centers, the total experience of any surgeon managing facial fractures in children is limited.

During their early years, children live in a protected environment under close parental supervision. The resilience of the developing bone, the short distance of the fall, and the thick overlying soft tissue enable the child to withstand forces that in the adult would result in dislocated fractures rather than the greenstick fractures seen most frequently in children. The tooth-to-bone ratio in the developing mandible is comparatively high, and the bone has more elastic resistance. The rudimentary paranasal sinuses, the large cartilaginous growth centers, and the small volume ratio between the jaws and the cranium are factors providing additional protection to the facial bone structures.

The incidence of facial bone fractures in children varies according to different reports. In a series of mandibular fractures reviewed by Kazanjian and Converse[127] and also in those of Posnick[78,79,94] and Shand,[128] children between 4 and 11 years of age represent approximately 10% of the group. In a series reported by Panagopoulos,[129] fractures of facial bones in children represented only 1.4% of the entire series. Pfeifer,[130] in a review of 3033 patients with facial bone fractures, noted that 4.4% had occurred in children from birth to 10 years; in the age group extending to 14 years, the incidence was 11%, and in the age group from 11 to 20 years, the incidence was 10.6%. Bamjee et al[77] found that 8% of injuries were in children.

Rowe[85,131-134] summarized his data by stating that 1% of all facial fractures occur before the sixth birthday, and a total of 5% occur in children younger than 12 years. Approximately 1 in 10 fractures in children younger than 12 years involves the midfacial skeleton. Rowe[85,131-134] noted that midfacial fractures are uncommon before the age of 8 years.

One of the principal causes cited for the rarity of fractures of the facial skeleton in children is the large size of the cranium in relation to the facial skeleton. McCoy et al[70] and Posnick,[78,79,94] in an analysis of 1500 patients with facial fractures, described 86 children, of whom 35 (40.8%) had associated skull fractures.

Facial fractures are infrequent before the age of 5 years but become more common up to the age of 10 years, when the frequency, pattern, and distribution of fractures tend to parallel those observed in adults. The two peaks of fracture incidence in children are in the 5- to 8-year and the 10- to 12-year age groups.

Around the age of 5 years, children enter school and are exposed to a new life style with participation in contact sports. They are subject to physical acts of violence, such as fighting. Sports and bicycle activities are no longer under close parental supervision, and an increasing frequency of accidents is observed. In the early teenage years, the adventuresome spirit and energy again dominate activity and are unsuppressed by concerns about the consequences of actions. In comparison, infants and preschool children are protected by their parents and constantly supervised, and as a result, few significant facial fractures are observed.[49,81,85,106]

The incidence of fractures of the midface and frontal region varies with the series reported, with the society or country surveyed, and with the characteristics of practice of the reporting author. Nasal fractures and alveolar fractures of the maxilla, for example, are the two most common midfacial injuries.[72,73,78,79,94,106] Both are frequently managed on an outpatient basis and often escape hospital recordkeeping. Thus, the low incidence of midfacial fractures usually reflects only the group admitted to the hospital.[72,73,78,79,94]

The period of childhood includes birth to the ages of 14 to 16 years. Several authors have indicated that the proportion of facial injuries observed in children accounts for 5% of the total of facial fractures observed (Table 67-4). In general, 1% of these injuries are observed in the 0- to 5-year age group. Midfacial fractures are uncommon (Table 67-5), with no such injury reported by Kaban et al[73] in their series of 109 children or by other authors.[20-23,72,135,136] Hall[71] found a 6% incidence of middle third fractures. Rowe[131] reported that 0.2% of facial injuries in children are midfacial fractures. At the Johns Hopkins Hospital, a 10-year survey was completed and included 300 patients admitted to the pediatric trauma center each year. Less than 5% of these patients had a facial fracture (Table 67-6). Soft tissue injuries were frequent and usually were lacerations or contusions. However, more than 60% of these patients admitted to the hospital had a significant head injury. The protection of the facial

TABLE 67-4 ✦ FACIAL FRACTURES OBSERVED IN CHILDREN (%)*

Panagopoulos (1957)	1.4
Pfeifer (1966)	4.4
Rowe (1968, 1969)	5
Converse (1979)	10
McCoy et al (1966)	6
Bamjee (1996)	8

*Percentages reflect proportion of pediatric facial fractures in the total number of facial fractures observed.

From Dufresne CR, Manson PN: Pediatric facial trauma. In McCarthy JG, ed: Plastic Surgery. Philadelphia, WB Saunders, 1990:1142.

TABLE 67-5 ✦ MIDFACIAL AND MAXILLARY ALVEOLAR FRACTURES

Author	Midfacial (%)	Maxillary Alveolar (%)
MacLennan (1956)	0.25	
Rowe (1968, 1969)	0.2	
Hall (1972)	6	
Kaban et al (1977)	0	3
Converse (1979)	10	
Fortunato et al (1982)	13	2
Reil and Kranz (1982)	16.5	9.5
Ramba (1985)	8	22
Ferreira (2005)	4.6	19.4

Percentages reflect proportion of pediatric facial fractures in the total number of facial fractures observed.

Modified from Dufresne CR, Manson PN: Pediatric facial trauma. In McCarthy JG, ed: Plastic Surgery. Philadelphia, WB Saunders, 1990:1142.

bones achieved by the smaller face-to-head size ratio and the resilient soft bone structure are emphasized by these statistics. In most series of patients, fractures of the nasal bones and mandible account for the majority of injuries (Table 67-7). As previously mentioned, the statistics do not reflect the true incidence of the anterior dental-alveolar fracture and the nasal fracture, which are usually managed without hospital admission on an outpatient basis (see Table 67-5).[137] Penetrating facial trauma is not common,[80] accounting for 1% to 2% of injuries; 28% of boys and 16% of girls sustained some type of dentoalveolar injury.[137]

Alveolar Fractures

In the young child, teeth may be dislodged from a segment of the alveolar bone subjected to labial, buccal, or lingual displacement (Fig. 67-18).[137] The fragments of bone can frequently be molded into alignment, and the teeth survive if they are adequately supported for several months by an arch bar or orthodontic support.

TABLE 67-6 ✦ THE JOHNS HOPKINS SERIES OF PEDIATRIC TRAUMA ADMISSIONS

	Total Admissions 3010		Facial Fractures 158			
Age	0-3¹/₂ yr 11.8%	4-7 yr 23.7%	8-11 yr 26.7%	12-16 yr 37.6%		
Etiology	Motor vehicle accident 49.5%	Physical violence 21.7%	Sports 15%	Miscellaneous 13.7%		
Fracture	Mandible 31.6%	Nasal 26.7%	Orbital 22.7%	Zygomatic 7.9%	Frontal 2.9%	Le Fort 2.7%
	Le Fort fractures by type					
	Le Fort I	1.9%				
	Le Fort II	0.9%				
	Le Fort III	1.9%				

Modified from Dufresne CR, Manson PN: Pediatric facial trauma. In McCarthy JG, ed: Plastic Surgery. Philadelphia, WB Saunders, 1990:1142.

TABLE 67-7 ✦ DISTRIBUTION (%) OF PEDIATRIC FACIAL FRACTURES

Author	Mandible	Nasal	Orbital	Zygomatic	Le Fort
Hall (1972)	20	60			6
Bales et al (1972)	64.8		5.4	8	16.2
Reil and Kranz (1976)	87		2	4.5	6.5
Kaban et al (1977)	35	50.4	17.4	5.5	0
Adekeye (1980)	86	5.3		5.3	2.7
Schultz and Meilman (1980)	14	64		15.5	6.5
Fortunato et al (1982)	55		20	9	13
Ramba (1985)	65	5.8	7	17	8
Ferreira (2005)	49		3.1	24	5

Modified from Dufresne CR, Manson PN: Pediatric facial trauma. In McCarthy JG, ed: Plastic Surgery. Philadelphia, WB Saunders, 1990:1142.

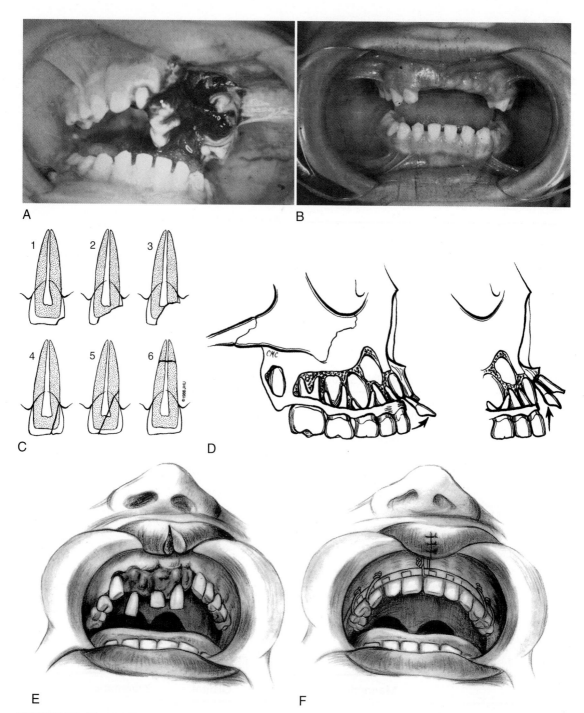

FIGURE 67-18. Maxillary alveolar fracture with dislocation and avulsion of several teeth. *A,* Preoperative appearance. *B,* Postoperative healing after removal of the deciduous teeth, replacement of the alveolar bone, and suture of the soft tissues. *C* and *D,* Illustrations of tooth replacement. *E* and *F,* Subluxation and replacement.

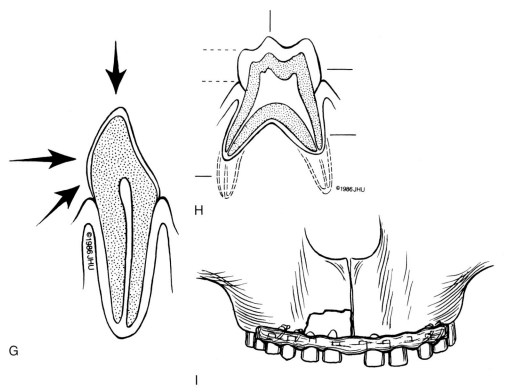

FIGURE 67-18, cont'd. *G,* Types of tooth injuries (intrusion, displacement). *H,* Structure of tooth. *I,* Splinting of alveolar fracture. (*A* and *B* from Dufresne CR, Manson PN: Pediatric facial trauma. In McCarthy JG, ed: Plastic Surgery. Philadelphia, WB Saunders, 1990:1142.)

An acrylic splint is good support. Skeletal wires (Fig. 67-19) may be used to support arch bars. In the child with incompletely developed tooth roots, teeth may regain their blood supply and survive (Fig. 67-18C to F). In some instances, if treatment is begun within an hour and root canal therapy is instituted, a tooth can be replanted with success. If the teeth are fractured and the alveolar structures hopelessly damaged so they cannot retain tooth structures, it is best to remove the teeth, trim the irregularities of the alveolar process, and suture the soft tissues over the retained injured bone. Bone fragments should not be dissected from the attached soft tissue if possible. These loose bone fragments, if covered with soft tissue, often survive as grafts (Fig. 67-18E and F).[5,59,60,62-65,115,137,138]

Fractured crowns of teeth without exposure of the pulp should be protected by dental methods because they can usually be restored successfully. If the crown of the tooth is fractured and dental pulp exposed, the prognosis may be good if the tooth is capped or a partial pulpectomy is performed. This type of therapy is most successful in the tooth with an open apex. However, even in the more fully developed tooth, pulpectomy and root canal treatment may be effective in saving

the tooth structures. Fracture of the root near the base of the crown usually requires extraction. If teeth can be retained only a few months, they may be useful in maintaining space until prosthetic replacement can be provided. Damage to the permanent tooth buds may result in deformed tooth structures, false eruption, or irregular arrangement of the erupting teeth in the dental arch.[59,60,63,115,137]

Dental injuries have traditionally been divided into those that involve deciduous teeth and those that involve permanent dentition. Injuries to deciduous dentition may occur between the ages of 1 and $2\frac{1}{2}$ years when children are learning to walk. Owing to the relative softness of the premaxilla at this age, the most common injury is one of displacement of the upper incisors. This may result in an intrusion of the tooth into the premaxilla, a loosening or partial dislocation with lingual or buccal displacement, or a total tooth avulsion.[3,5,59,60,62-65,128,138]

Intruded teeth frequently re-erupt in the subsequent weeks and may reach full eruption in 4 to 6 months. In a child younger than $2\frac{1}{2}$ years with incomplete root formation, intruded teeth may retain normal vitality after re-eruption. In children older than $2\frac{1}{2}$ or 3 years,

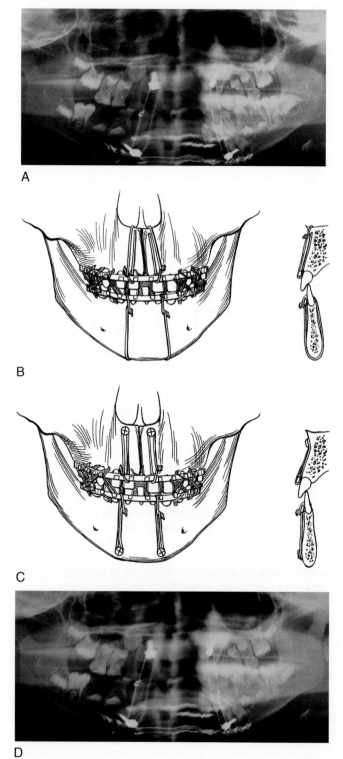

A

B

C

D

FIGURE 67-19. *A*, Skeletal wires should frequently be employed in children's dentition. *B*, Wire loops. *C*, Wires to screws. *D*, Wires to screws in Panorex.

calcific degeneration and necrosis of pulp are common sequelae to the re-eruption of intruded teeth after root formation is mature.[59,60,64,65]

Elaborate methods for fixation of injured deciduous teeth are contraindicated. Partially dislocated deciduous teeth should be reoriented intraorally if they are sufficiently stable (Fig. 67-18E and F). Otherwise, they should be extracted, followed in some instances by placement of a space maintainer. The future of partially dislocated teeth is related to the maturity of the dental root at the time of injury. The capacity of teeth, particularly those with an open apex, to retain viability is considerable, given immobilization for 3 to 4 weeks and the prevention of infection. Total avulsion of deciduous teeth is less common than are other forms of displacement, but it results in the greatest damage to the overlying permanent teeth.[62,63]

Fractures of the crown and roots of the deciduous teeth are comparably rare and far less common than fractures in the permanent teeth. Fractured crowns with exposed dentin but without pulpal involvement should be protected until definitive dental restoration can be completed. An extensive crown fracture invariably involves the pulp, and the tooth should be extracted. Root fractures, particularly those involving the coronal portions of the root, also require extraction of the tooth. Surgical removal of the apical portions of the fractured deciduous tooth roots is necessary to prevent interference in the eruption of the permanent teeth. Fractures in the apical portions of the root usually heal uneventfully.[63,64,134]

Trauma to the deciduous teeth, because of the close anatomic relationships between the apices of the primary and the permanent teeth, may result in damage to the developing permanent dentition. The prevalence of such developmental disturbances ranges from 12% to 69%.[63-65,106,139]

In one review of 103 patients with traumatized permanent dentition, white or yellow-brown discoloration of the enamel was observed in 23%, and discoloration of the teeth and enamel associated with circular enamel hypoplasia was observed in 12%.[64] Other morphologic disturbances, such as crown dilaceration, late root angulation, and partial or complete arrested root formation, were found in 6% of patients. Disturbances in the permanent dentition were less frequent in patients whose injury occurred after they reached 4 years of age.[133,139-141]

Subluxation of permanent teeth with the associated alveolar bone is treated by repositioning and splinting according to conventional methods. The teeth frequently become nonvital and require root canal therapy and root canal filling at a later date, particularly when the root formation is complete at the time of injury. If complete avulsion of the permanent tooth occurs when the root is immature and the apex widely open, the tooth should be reimplanted and stabilized

in the socket within a few minutes of injury (Fig. 67-18C and D).[139-141] In these instances, the prognosis for pulp revitalization, revascularization, reinnervation, and continued root formation is good. Reimplantation of a complete avulsion when root formation is mature, especially when the avulsion is more than 30 minutes old, invariably leads to pulp necrosis and root resorption. The resorption may be an exceedingly slow process, however, taking 10 years or more. Reimplantation in such patients should include pulp removal, pulp space restoration, and splinting.[72,85,86,132-134,137]

Mandibular Fractures

The mandible is a complex bone consisting of horizontal components. Fractures tend to occur in the weak portions and tend to be multiple as often as single. Fracture can be compound intraorally more frequently than extraorally, and most compound fractures occur in the tooth-bearing horizontal portion of the mandible. The weak portions change with growth and development to simulate those of the adult.

Predisposition to greenstick or incomplete fractures in developing bone is attributed to two factors. The first is subcutaneous tissue, mainly adipose tissue, which increases rapidly in thickness during the 9 months after birth. At the age of 5 years, the subcutaneous layer is actually only half as thick as in a 9-month-old infant. The second factor is the resilience of the developing bone. The line of differentiation between cortical bone and medullary bone is not sharply defined, and the resilience of the young bone explains the higher frequency of greenstick fractures in children. When fractures occur, as in the body of the mandible, there is often a considerable degree of displacement.[60] The fracture lines tend to be long and oblique, extending downward and forward from the upper border of the mandible. The obliquity of the fracture line is different from that observed in the adult, in whom the direction of the fracture line is usually downward and backward.[5,21,32,84,142]

Before the eruption of the permanent or secondary dentition, the developing follicles occupy most of the body of the mandible. For avoidance of injury to the tooth buds of the permanent dentition (see Figs. 67-3 and 67-18), this anatomic characteristic must be considered if interosseous fixation is to be employed. The wires must be placed near the lower border of the mandible. The roots of the deciduous teeth are gradually being resorbed, and between the ages of 5 and 9 years (a period of mixed dentition), because of the frequent absence of teeth and the poor retentive shape of the crowns of the deciduous teeth, it is more difficult to use the dentition for fixation as in ligation of arch bars.[20,72,84,115,117,128,129]

The teeth cannot be employed for fixation in the treatment of mandibular fractures in young infants in whom the teeth are unerupted or only partly erupted. These fractures are best treated by open reduction with small rigid fixation devices, such as the 1.3, 1.5, or 2.0 systems. Care is taken in placement to avoid the developing dentition. Unicortical screws and proper plate placement are required. Alternatively, and considerably more cumbersome, an impression of the mandible can be taken under light anesthesia and an acrylic splint fabricated. After realignment of the fragments, the splint is placed over the mandibular arch, lined with softened dental compound for conformity adjustment, and maintained in position by screws or circummandibular wires.[72,73,94,143,144] This type of reverse monomaxillary fixation was formerly adequate in selected patients, but it has been almost completely replaced by plate and screw fixation.[23,79]

Intermaxillary fixation is obtained by the assistance of skeletal wires to support and stabilize arch bars.[145] These are anchored to screws placed to avoid tooth buds. Transalveolar wiring above the apices of the teeth can be used in the older child after the eruption of the secondary dentition. After 10 years of age, however, the dentition may be adequate for standard intermaxillary dental fixation.[23,72,73,117,143,144]

During the period when the deciduous dentition is being replaced by the permanent dentition, particularly in the period between the ages of 6 and 12 years, some difficulty may be experienced in obtaining interdental fixation. Skeletal wires are useful in this age group (see Fig. 67-19).[146-148]

In older children in whom the dentition is more retentive, various types of fixation may be employed. A band and arch appliance can be employed if the teeth permit retention of the appliance (Fig. 67-20). Skeletal wires aid in stabilizing the arch bars. Direct interosseous fixation of arch bars, with placement of the skeletal wire near the lower border of the mandible to avoid injury to the tooth buds, is of considerable assistance in maintaining fixation when only deciduous teeth are present.[23] The interosseous wires may be placed through an intraoral approach after the mandible is degloved (Fig. 67-20D). A circumferential

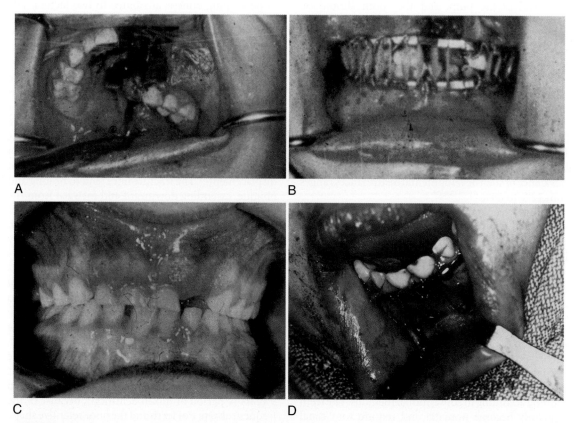

A

B

C

D

FIGURE 67-20. Compound maxillary fracture with displacement of fragments and avulsion of the teeth. *A,* Preoperative appearance. *B,* After reduction, the fractured segments were replaced, the remaining teeth were stabilized with an arch bar, and intermaxillary fixation was established. Note the skeletal wire reinforcing the lower arch bar. *C,* Satisfactory result with survival of the fragments and avulsed teeth. *D,* Placement of skeletal wire to stabilization screws in the maxilla. (*A* to *C* from Dufresne CR, Manson PN: Pediatric facial trauma. In McCarthy JG, ed: Plastic Surgery. Philadelphia, WB Saunders, 1990:1142.)

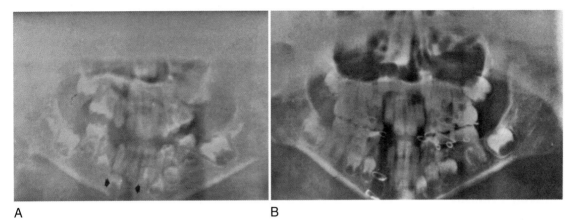

FIGURE 67-21. *A,* Preoperative panoramic radiograph of a parasymphyseal mandibular fracture and alveolar fractures in a child. *B,* Treatment included open reduction and stabilization with wire fixation. Note the proximity of the secondary tooth follicles. (From Dufresne CR, Manson PN: Pediatric facial trauma. In McCarthy JG, ed: Plastic Surgery. Philadelphia, WB Saunders, 1990:1142.)

wire around the mandible is another but more traumatic method of reinforcing the fixation established by arch bars; it can be employed after exposure of the ends of the fractured bone intraorally by the degloving procedure.[23,72,84,117,127,149]

Fractures of the mandible, like those of other facial bones, must be recognized and treated early in children because of the rapid reparative process.[23] The loose and displaced bone fragments become adherent to one another within 3 or 4 days after injury. Soon, partially healed fragments become difficult to manipulate and must be loosened under general anesthesia and even by osteotomy before reduction of the fracture is possible (Figs. 67-21 to 67-23).[150]

Minor degrees of malunion and malocclusion may be tolerated in the growing facial bones and mandible because of the corrective adjustments that take place with the erupting teeth under normal masticatory

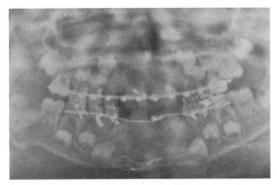

FIGURE 67-22. Panoramic radiographic view of a reduced symphyseal fracture stabilized with wire fixation and arch bars. (From Dufresne CR, Manson PN: Pediatric facial trauma. In McCarthy JG, ed: Plastic Surgery. Philadelphia, WB Saunders, 1990:1142.)

stresses.[117,151-153] Demianczuk et al[154] and Lehman[67] both argue for aggressive anatomic reduction of fractures to reduce deformity. Demianczuk et al[154] found that 22% of children 4 to 7 years and 17% of children 8 to 11 years needed orthognathic surgery to correct disturbances of growth after trauma. Lehman[67] has even found that condyle dislocations are best treated with operative intervention.[66,67] Limited mouth opening is related to age but may follow any fracture, particularly fractures involving the temporomandibular joint.[155]

The Ability of the Dentofacial Structures to Accommodate Malocclusion

Numerous statements in the literature indicate that practitioners need not be as concerned about accurate occlusion in young children as in adults because there is considerable "adaptive and remodeling potential" in the process of growing of the alveolar structures, eruption of the secondary dentition, and remodeling of the teeth.[2,156] Although there is considerable ability in the adaptive potential of eruption of the secondary dentition and the growth of the alveolar structures to accommodate minor degrees of malocclusion, the literature fails to document the success of this process. These statements were proffered at a time when accurate open reduction was impossible because of the inability of wires or splints to achieve a three-dimensional stable fixation with reliable stability. With the open approaches preferred today and with the precision afforded by three-dimensionally stable plate and screw fixation, there seems to be no reason to tolerate less than anatomic reduction including accurate occlusal stability. Therefore, precise restoration of the original anatomy and occlusion should be accomplished for all displaced and unstable fractures.[21,24,154,157] Effects on growth are definite and might possibly be minimized by precise alignment and fixation.

Winzenburg[158] and Imola[149] have also reviewed the effects of rigid fixation on craniofacial growth after fracture treatment, as has Demianczuk et al.[154] In general, rigid fixation has a 3% to 5% potential growth restriction. A 5% growth restriction is generally anticipated when rigid fixation is used in developmental periods.[159]

Condylar Fractures

The condylar articulation with the base of the skull is a complex ginglymoarthrodial joint that permits rotation and forward motion of the condyle onto the anterior lip of the glenoid fossa as the jaw opens (Fig. 67-24A). The joint surfaces are lined with cartilage (Fig. 67-24B), and a disk of fibrocartilage is suspended between the joint surfaces. Condylar fractures and "crush" injuries may result in growth deformity in the mandible, but it is more likely with a condylar fracture. In older children, the condylar areas thin with growth and represent a weak point considered

more susceptible to greenstick or complete fracture (Fig. 67-24C).

The articular disk may also be bruised, torn, or dislocated, impairing joint motion. Hematoma may occur within the joint, resulting in fibrosis and ankylosis (Fig. 67-24D to F). Splinters of cartilage may be produced that heal with partial obliteration of the joint spaces, reducing the ability of the joint to function (ankylosis).

CHARACTERISTICS

Fractures of the condylar head in young patients tend to splinter the head (Fig. 67-24G). Many believe that these should be treated with early motion, with or without consideration for guided elastic traction. More frequently, condylar fractures involve the neck or, in older children, the subcondylar area (Fig. 67-24H and I). Treatment depends on the degree of displacement, the amount of bone contact, the characteristics of override or overlap of fracture fragments, and the pressure of malocclusion.

Fractures of the condylar neck may be complete or incomplete (greenstick) and may be characterized by

Text continued on p. 417

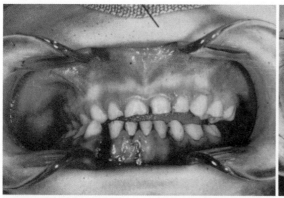

A

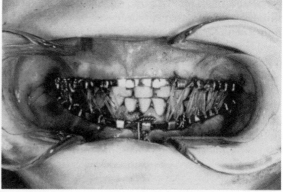

B

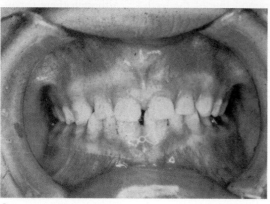

C

FIGURE 67-23. Band and arch appliance. *A,* Compound fracture of the mandible between the right deciduous lateral incisor and cuspid tooth. *B,* Closed reduction with arch bar fixation and a circumferential wire around the symphysis of the mandible to stabilize the lower arch bar. Note the circumferential wire twisted at the top of the arch bar. *C,* Occlusion of the teeth 2 years later.

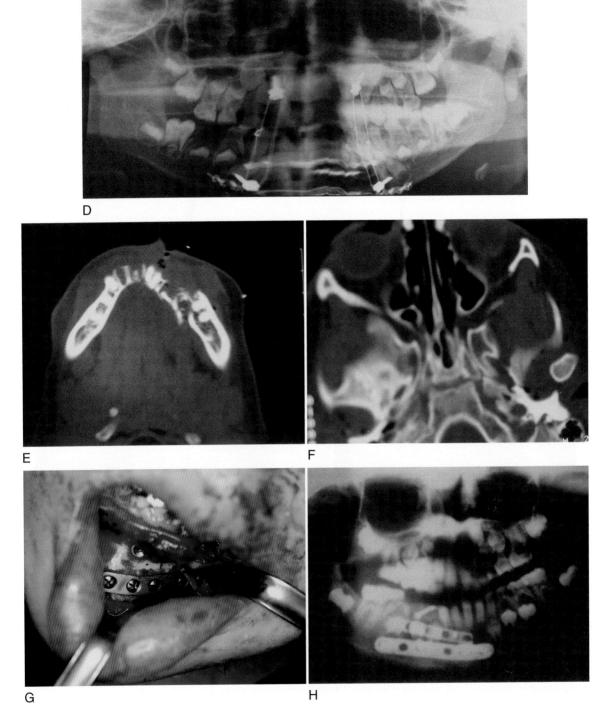

FIGURE 67-23, cont'd. *D,* Skeletal wires for arch bar stabilization. *E* and *F,* Comminuted symphysis and condylar head fracture. *G,* Open reduction with plate and screw fixation. *H,* Panorex view. (*A* to *C* from Dufresne CR, Manson PN: Pediatric facial trauma. In McCarthy JG, ed: Plastic Surgery. Philadelphia, WB Saunders, 1990:1142.)

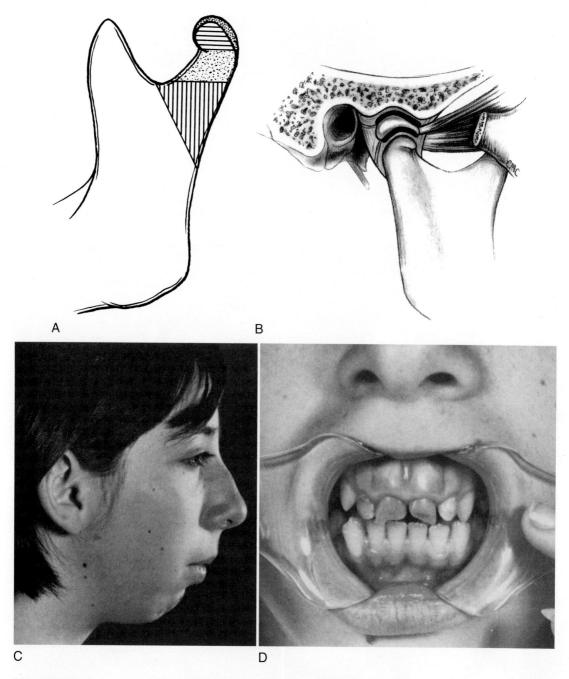

FIGURE 67-24. *A,* Units of the condyle (head, neck, subcondyle) of the mandible in a young child. *B,* Structures of the temporomandibular joint. *C,* A typical mandibular deformity resulting from condylar injury in early childhood is an underdeveloped mandible with temporomandibular ankylosis. *D,* Maximal opening (1 to 2 mm) achieved by the patient. Note the hygienic status of the teeth.

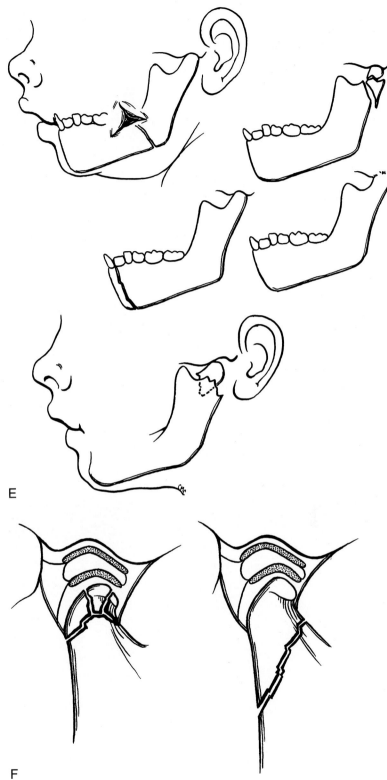

FIGURE 67-24, cont'd.
E, Common combinations of condyle fractures and fractures capable of inducing condylar dislocation. Ankylosis *(center, right)* may involve bone or be generated by fibrous scar tissue. *F,* Condylar deformities after fracture: *left,* comminuted head fracture; *right,* subcondylar fracture.

Continued

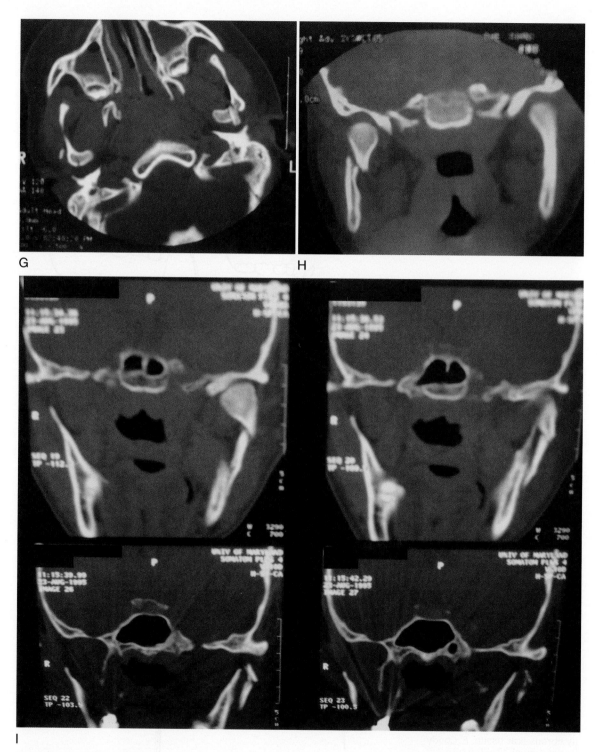

FIGURE 67-24, cont'd. *G,* High condylar head fractures (teeth closed). *H,* Condylar neck fracture. *I,* Subcondylar fracture. (*C* and *D* from Dufresne CR, Manson PN: Pediatric facial trauma. In McCarthy JG, ed: Plastic Surgery. Philadelphia, WB Saunders, 1990:1142.)

the degree of angulation between fragments (more angulation equals more deviation of the distal mandible and more ramus shortening) and the degree of override or overlapping of the fragments (Fig. 67-24F). Greenstick fractures heal quickly, whereas dislocated fractures without bone contact or with override heal slowly with potential malocclusion. The condyle may also be dislocated from the fossa, and it is usually found medial to the joint in the pterygoid fossa. The issues in adults have involved which types of deviation and dislocation benefit from open reduction because closed reduction is unable to reduce the displacement completely. Placement of the patient in intermaxillary fixation in occlusion does reposition the distal fragment, but the proximal fragment may be repositioned only with open reduction and fixation.

RESTITUTIONAL REMODELING

The condyle area in young individuals is capable of restitutional remodeling. It is not uncommon for individuals to generate a new condylar head (albeit blunted) after a complete dislocation. As the child grows older, the potential for restitutional remodeling decreases, and the child cannot re-form parts but only repair fractures.

The issues have centered about the ability to restitutionally remodel the condyle, the functional and growth results related to the degree of fracture displacement or dislocation, and the benefits of open versus closed reduction. Most experienced surgeons believe that the young (<5 years) should frequently be managed with closed reduction and an initial period of intermaxillary fixation followed by guided elastic traction, whereas the older child with significant severe derangement should be considered for open reduction.

Condylar cartilage is first noted during prenatal life at the 12th week. Large vascular channels appear during the 20th week of fetal life and persist until the second or third year of postnatal life, when they progressively diminish in size. During this period, the neck of the condyle begins to progressively increase in length, eventually to form the long, slender condylar neck of the adult. During the first 3 years of postnatal life, the condyle is short and thick and thus less susceptible to fracture; however, it is more vulnerable to a crushing injury because of its vascular trabecular structure. The crushing results in intra-articular and periarticular hemorrhage and scattered osteogenesis, and progressive ossification may result in temporomandibular ankylosis. Early or immediate motion is thought to minimize the ankylosis complication.[71,141,160-162]

Before the age of 5 years, the condylar neck is less developed, and the bone tissues are soft and more susceptible to the crush type of injury. After the age of 5 years, the condyle will, in all probability, fracture at

the neck. The crush type of injury may also be associated with condylar cartilage damage, which may be the predominant component of a blunt injury. Because the condylar cartilage is one of several factors contributing to mandibular growth, mandibular hypoplasia may result when the cartilage is injured. The degree of deformity seems to be inversely proportional to the age at which the injury is sustained. The younger the patient at the time of injury, the more severe is the deformity.[129,132,163,164]

There seems therefore to be a distinct difference in the results of a crushing injury in early childhood and a fracture of the condylar neck in later childhood. Whereas the crushing injury and the damage to the condylar cartilage, as emphasized by Walker,[165,166] may result in developmental arrest, the deformity arising from the condylar neck fractures, when it is treated by simple intermaxillary fixation, is almost always limited or self-corrected. Even the advisability of intermaxillary fixation in fractures of the condylar neck in children has been questioned by some authors, who observed spontaneous recovery of function, form, and occlusion in children with unilateral or bilateral condylar neck fractures treated by early motion and no immobilization.[133] Despite these observations from nonoperative treatment, intermaxillary fixation for an initial period of rest in normal occlusion is recommended when the child cannot voluntarily establish or maintain normal occlusion. Release of fixation must be followed by close observation of the occlusion and institution of intermittent or constant elastic traction in patients with deviation after release of intermaxillary fixation. If a child can repeatedly bring the mandible into proper occlusion after a subtle, essentially nondisplaced or greenstick fracture, a trial of observation and soft diet without either open reduction or intermaxillary fixation is warranted with continued close observation of the occlusion. Range of motion should ultimately exceed 40 mm (Fig. 67-24D).[55]

Condylar fractures that involve the bone of the neck of the condyle are often of the greenstick (incomplete) variety and are not usually accompanied by disturbances of the temporomandibular joint. Fortunately, most fractures in the condylar area of the mandible in children are not followed by ankylosis or growth disturbance.[141,143,156,167-169]

Fractures or injuries to the articular surfaces or internal anatomy (disks, ligaments, joint spaces) of the temporomandibular joints should be suspected in all children who have suffered a severe blow to the chin. Radiographic studies may demonstrate fractures of one or both mandibular condyles with or without displacement. Impacted fractures are common and are subtle. Nondisplaced ramus and condylar fractures are sometimes even difficult to confirm on CT scan, and treatment should proceed on the suspicion of a fracture. Condylar fractures and injuries should always be viewed with concern in the young child because of the possibility of secondary growth disturbances resulting from damage to the condylar growth centers (Fig. 67-24).[170] Injuries to the articular surface of the joint may result in hemarthrosis with cicatricial organization and ankylosis. These potential problems should always be considered and discussed with the parents in injuries of this type.[148,160-162,171]

Temporomandibular ankylosis may follow injury to the soft tissue of the condylar articulation. Often, there is no or only a vague history of injury, and radiologic examination is unremarkable. Months later, limitation of motion of the mandible may develop as a result of partial ankylosis. A progressive straightening of the neck of the condyle is observed after fractures in which bone contact between the fragments has been maintained.[130,140,141] Pfeifer[130] noted that in fracture-dislocation with loss of contact between the fragments, there was a shortening of the ramus on the affected side and asymmetry of the mandibular arch. In these patients, resorption of the condyle was observed, followed by the formation of a new joint with a shorter, flatter condylar head. Ankylosis did not occur in any of these patients, although deviation on opening of the mouth, due to shortening of the ramus and dysfunction of the lateral pterygoid muscle, was frequently observed. Advancement of the mandible,[172] genioplasty, or both may be required.

DISLOCATED CONDYLAR FRACTURES: EVIDENCE FOR OPEN REDUCTION

Lehman[67] discussed some unresolved controversial issues for pediatric mandibular fractures including the long-term impact of trauma and surgery on the growing pediatric mandible, the use of intermaxillary fixation in the mixed dentition, the use of rigid fixation, and the lack of long-term studies documenting outcome. Sixty percent of his pediatric mandible fractures involved the condyle, a higher percentage than in adults. Not all pediatric mandible fractures can be grouped together because the mandible is constantly growing and the dentition is evolving. As the mandible enlarges and becomes more rigid, the pattern of fractures changes and becomes similar to that observed in adults. The management of the condylar fracture (including the dislocated condyle in young children) may be approached with surgery or conservative treatment. Lehman maintains that there are a growing group of surgeons who think that operative treatment is indicated in the dislocated condyle, especially in the older child. Lehman points out that the condyle of the mandible articulates with temporal bone and glenoid fossa. This joint has certain unique anatomic features. Both joints must function in harmony, and certain movements are influenced by the teeth. The meniscus, located between the condyle and the glenoid fossa, separates the joint into upper and lower regions. On opening, the condyle moves as a hinge initially and then glides forward as the mandible completes its full range of motion. The joint is surrounded by a capsule that fuses with the meniscus in the lateral aspect of the condylar neck. The meniscus acts as a flexible cushion and moves with the condylar head on opening (Fig. 67-24A and B).[67]

The lateral pterygoid muscle has two heads that function separately. The inferior head inserts into the anterior aspect of the condylar neck and assists in opening the mouth. The smaller superior head attaches to the joint capsule and meniscus. In dislocated fractures of the condyle, the condylar head is displaced medially by the pull of the inferior portion of the lateral pterygoid muscle. The condyle may penetrate through the medial aspect of the joint capsule, and the meniscus is usually displaced with the condyle (Fig. 67-25). The condylar head itself has an elliptical shape, and each side may be different. The medial-lateral dimension of the condyle is almost twice that of the anterior-posterior dimension. Before the age of 5 years, the condylar neck is short and not well developed, rendering the neck less susceptible to fracture. However, because of the trabecular vascular channels of bone, it is more vulnerable to crush injuries. Crushing injuries may result in intra-articular and periarticular hemorrhage that can become calcified and lead to ankylosis.[66,67] Topazian[173] noted that 30% of patients with temporomandibular joint ankylosis had a history of childhood trauma.

The crushing type of injury may also cause damage to the condylar cartilage.[169] Because the condylar cartilage is a factor in condylar growth, hypoplasia of the condylar head may occur. Many isolated hypoplasias of the mandible, excluding hemifacial microsomia, can be related to undiagnosed condylar fractures in childhood. After 5 years of age, the condylar neck increases in length to eventually form the anatomic shape seen in adults. During the early period of maturation, fractures are frequently of the greenstick varieties; as the bone matures, the pattern of the fractures becomes similar to that of the adult mandible. As this pattern of fracture changes, so does the dentition. As the mixed dentition evolves into the permanent dentition, crush-type injuries occurring in the deciduous dentition are less frequent than fractures of the neck. Dislocated fractures may occur in all age groups and with any type of dentition. The mandible is the most frequently fractured bone of the facial skeleton in children with the exception of the nasal bones.[66,67]

Traditionally, condylar fractures are divided into two groups, intracapsular and extracapsular, as they relate to the joint capsule and the joint. Extracapsular fractures may be further subdivided into condylar neck and subcondylar fractures. The condylar neck fractures may be further subdivided into dislocated and nondislocated varieties of fracture. The small subset of dislocated fractures are Lehman's source of controversy. Lehman[66,67] treated 87% of condylar fractures conservatively. For intracapsular fractures, the "conservative" treatment consisted of early motion and pain medication. Nondislocated neck fractures were treated by a soft diet and pain medication or a short period of intermaxillary fixation (2 to 4 weeks). Lehman's method of intermaxillary fixation was arch bars with or without the use of skeletal wires. Of 77 patients described by Lehman, 10 had dislocated fractures and had open reduction and fixation with a wire, pin, or plate (13%). Lehman used a preauricular approach and recommended drilling a screw into the condylar head to allow it to be levered back into the fossa. In this maneuver, the pterygoid muscle is sometimes detached. Lehman points out that the displaced meniscus must also be repositioned. Lehman's "more aggressive" surgical approach was precipitated by treatment of a condylar dislocation conservatively 20 years ago; the patient (after treatment) had a lateral

and anterior open bite and an inability to reach centric occlusion. In his experience, dislocated fractures do not "re-form" a condyle after the age of 7 years; however, the authors have radiographic evidence of condyles re-forming in younger individuals (Fig. 67-26; see also Fig. 67-25). Lehman's patient required a costal chondral graft and ramus osteotomy for restoration of function and occlusion.

Lehman's paper focuses on several patients in whom reconstitution did not occur and who therefore required costal chondral grafting. A major problem resulting from treatment of dislocated condyle fractures by closed reduction is early dysfunction with an inability to consistently achieve centric occlusion, which may also lead to late arthritic changes. Hoopes et al[167] reported that 93% of patients with condylar fractures had good results with conservative treatment but readvocated a postauricular approach to the condyle for dislocated head fractures in the older child or teenager. Georgiade[82,83] stated that all dislocated fractures of the condyle result in some future type of malfunction and malocclusion if nonoperative treatment

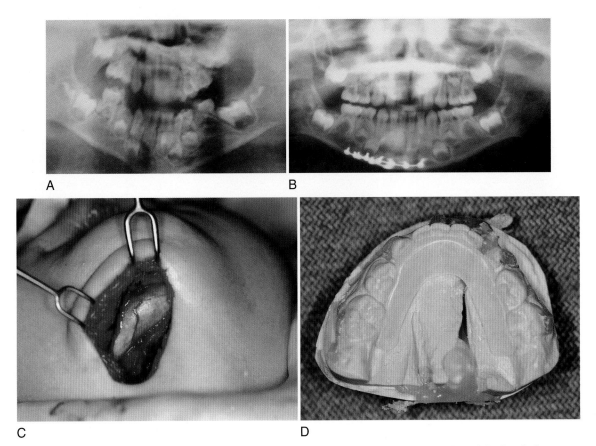

A

B

C

D

FIGURE 67-25. *A,* Condylar fracture-dislocation in a child. *B,* Re-formation of a blunted condylar head after treatment with closed reduction and maxillomandibular fixation. *C,* Fracture of parasymphysis in the child. *D,* Preparation of a lingual splint to key the reduction. *Continued*

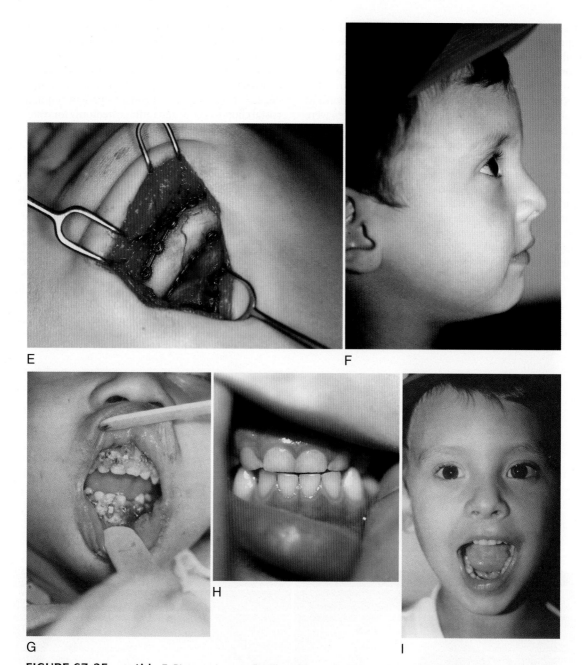

FIGURE 67-25, cont'd. *E,* Plate and screw fixation of fracture with small plates and monocanthal screws to avoid tooth roots. *F,* Patient's profile. *G,* Range of motion. *H,* Occlusion. *I,* Range of mandible in early postoperative period.

alone is used. It is difficult to observe pediatric patients on a long-term basis, which may account for the presumption in many studies of "good function" in this group of patients.

Midfacial Fractures

Midfacial fractures in children up to the age of 12 years constitute less than 5% of all facial fractures.[131,174] Because of the higher degree of elasticity of the facial bones, the absence of sinus development, and the lesser degree of development of the midfacial skeleton in relation to the cranial area, midfacial fractures in children are less frequent than in adults. Iizuka et al[175] found, in decreasing frequency, that maxillary alveolar, zygoma, and Le Fort fractures were common in face injuries observed from the ages of 13 to 15 years. No Le Fort fracture was observed in a child younger than 6 years. Maxillary, naso-orbital, and orbital blowout fractures can occur. In young children submitted to an unusually strong traumatic force, frontal bone and telescoping naso-orbital fractures can be associated with the midfacial fractures.[85]

The typical Le Fort lines of fracture are rarely seen in young children's fractures. Low maxillary or Le Fort I types of fracture are not common until after the age of 10 years because of the incomplete development of the facial sinus structures. Pyramidal or Le Fort II fractures are seen more commonly and sometimes even unilaterally. The patients frequently present with a split palate from weakness (incomplete fusion) of the midpalatal suture (Fig. 67-27). Problems with fixation are similar to those encountered in the

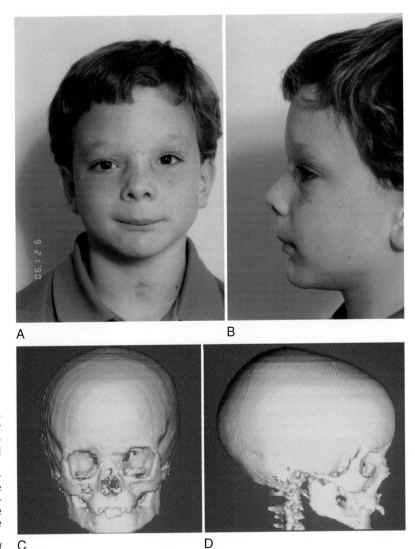

FIGURE 67-26. *A and B,* A 4-year-old child involved in a motor vehicle accident with nasoethmoidal-orbital fractures, closed head trauma, and coma for 1 month. The bilateral condylar fractures initiated shortening of the lower face. *C to E,* Three-dimensional CT skull films reveal the skeletal and particularly the mandibular deformities.

Continued

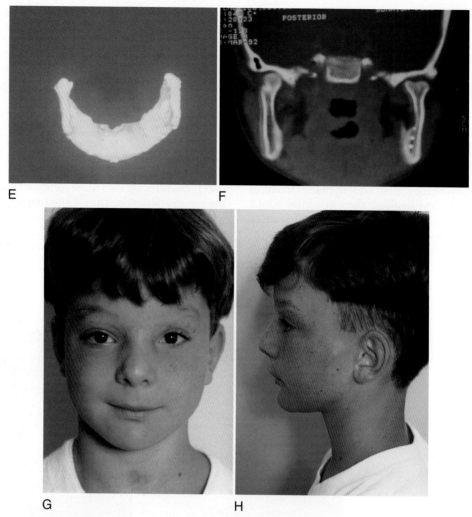

FIGURE 67-26, cont'd. *F,* Bilateral grafts were used for the reconstruction of the rami. Radiographs demonstrate the reconstruction. *G* and *H,* Postoperative appearance with better facial relationships and proportion.

treatment of mandibular fractures because of the presence of poorly retentive teeth. In addition, alveolar fractures are associated with tooth loosening, luxation, avulsion, and fracture, particularly of the anterior teeth, which are especially exposed to injury. A dental fixation appliance (orthodontic bands, acrylated arch bar, cable arch, arch, or acrylic splint) may be attached to the remaining teeth and, in the older child, to the selected erupted permanent teeth (see Figs. 67-23 and 67-27).[176,177] In general, fixation is accomplished with splints, arch bars, and skeletal wires.

Careful internal interfragment wiring is less stable than plate and screw fixation as a means of internal fixation. In the young child, skeletal wires may be unsatisfactory because the bone is soft and the wire, when it is placed under tension, may cut through the bone.

"Skeletal" internal wire fixation to the edges of the piriform aperture (either a drill hole or a screw), which consists of thicker and stronger bone, is the preferred method.[127]

Rapid fabrication of an acrylic splint or acrylated arch bar may be achieved in the operating room with a quick-curing acrylic resin when extensive tooth loss has occurred. Such a splint stabilizes the space for the dentition. Fractures of the midface are provisionally positioned by initial intermaxillary fixation[117,127] and then stabilized by internal fixation (plating) to stable bony skeletal structures. Open reduction and fixation of a Le Fort II fracture may be accomplished with a gingival buccal sulcus, bilateral inferior orbital rim, and coronal incision as required. The upper incision (coronal) is sometimes not necessary. The utility of the use of resorbable plates is under study; 1.3-mm plates are recommended.

Even when they are properly reduced, midfacial fractures may eventually lead to a midfacial retrusion, deformity, or asymmetry because of the injury to the growth centers of the maxilla and nasal septum.[20,24] With maxillary growth, there is not only a forward and downward component but also a concomitant remodeling of the multiple regional parts. The development includes a displacement away from the cranial base, a posterior enlargement corresponding to lengthening of the dental arch, and an anterior resorption in the malar region. The nasal vaults grow forward and laterally; descent of the premaxillary area occurs by resorption on the superior and anterior surface of the nasal spine, promoting bone deposition on the inferior surface. It is fortunate that this complex developmental scenario is seldom interrupted by maxillary fracture in childhood.[3,50,84,100,142,178] Young children (<5 years) with severe midface

fractures are most susceptible to maxillary retrusion.[72,73]

Incomplete reduction and immobilization of maxillary fractures, however, is the most frequent cause of malunion with elongation or malreduction of the facial height and malocclusion in the pediatric age group. Malunion is best prevented by immediate exploration and open reduction and rigid fixation of the fractured segments. Intermaxillary fixation should be used for 1 to 2 weeks and then the occlusion observed after release. The timing of the reduction becomes critical, however, because bone healing occurs rapidly. Remobilization of a malunited maxillary fracture in children is extremely difficult 2 to 3 weeks after injury, as opposed to remobilization of a similar fracture in adults.[49,100] New unfavorable fracture lines may result from forceful attempts to mobilize a partially healed fracture, and direct osteotomy at the Le Fort II level, for instance, is preferred. The callus stimulated by partial bone union obstructs the establishment of

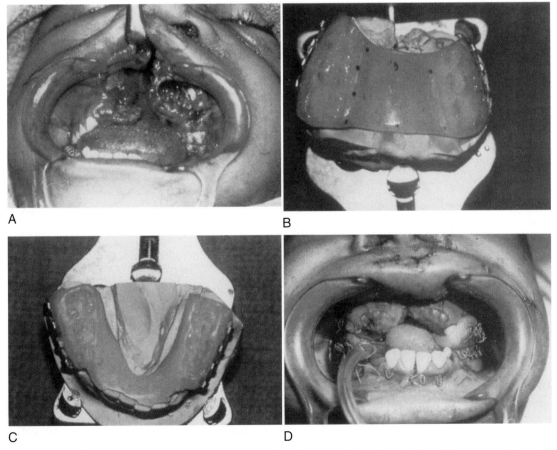

A   B

C   D

FIGURE 67-27. *A*, A 7-year-old child with multiple facial fractures including a Le Fort II fracture, split palate, nasoethmoidal-orbital fracture, right zygomatic fracture, and dentoalveolar fractures. *B*, After model surgery to realign the split palatal fractures by a splint, the occlusal splint is fabricated. *C*, Mandibular splint. *D*, Appearance of the child after open reduction of the facial fractures and insertion of the occlusal splints.   *Continued*

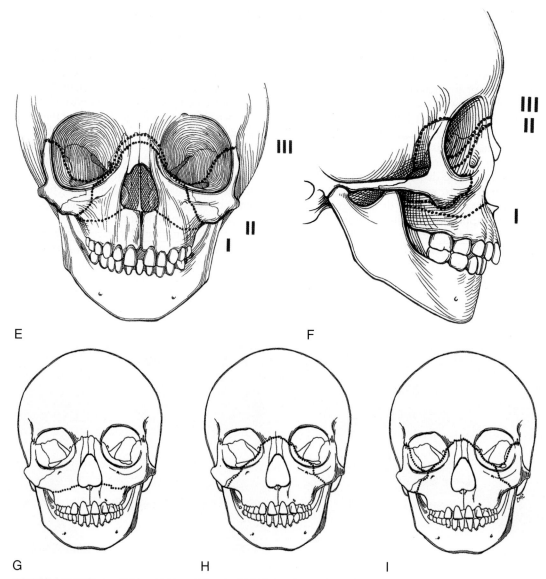

FIGURE 67-27, cont'd. *E* and *F*, Types of Le Fort fractures. *G*, Le Fort I fracture. *H*, Le Fort II fracture. *I*, Le Fort III fracture. (*A* to *D* from Dufresne CR, Manson PN: Pediatric facial trauma. In McCarthy JG, ed: Plastic Surgery. Philadelphia, WB Saunders, 1990:1142.)

normal occlusion and may have to be removed from the fracture line before correct repositioning can be accomplished.

Zygomatic and Orbital Fractures

Zygomatic fractures are rare in younger children and most commonly occur in the older child.[20,179,180] Considerable force is required to fracture the resilient zygoma of the young child, and the fracture usually takes the form of a fracture-dislocation. Lack of complete union at the zygomaticofrontal suture also explains the infrequency of this type of fracture.

Treatment is similar to that of adult zygomatic fractures[176,177] and includes three anterior incisions for most fractures to explore the zygomaticofrontal suture, infraorbital rim, and maxillary alveolar process for alignment and fixation (Fig. 67-28).

The incidence has been reported as 4.7% for pure pediatric zygomatic fractures and 16.3% for zygomatic fracture with a significant orbital component.[70,99,100] In another series, the incidence of zygomatic fracture necessitating operative treatment was only 0.3%.[85,132] Malar complex fractures with asymmetry and flattening of the eminence or fractures of the orbital rims with a palpable step-off deformity must be corrected

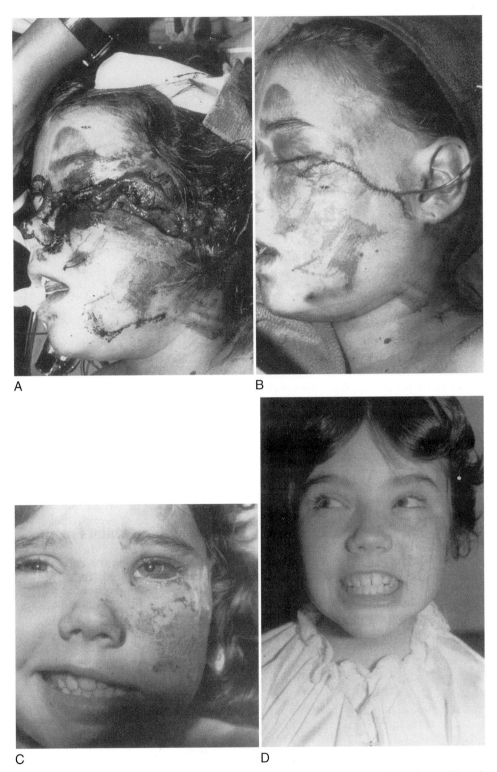

A   B

C   D

FIGURE 67-28. *A,* A 7-year-old child after severe trauma to the left side of the face, with avulsion of soft tissues, open zygomatic fracture, and avulsion of the buccal branches of the facial nerve. *B,* Appearance at completion of open reduction and fixation of the zygomatic fracture, repair of the facial nerve, and approximation of the soft tissues. *C,* Early postoperative view demonstrating facial weakness and edema. *D,* One-year follow-up demonstrating return of facial nerve function and satisfactory restoration of facial symmetry.   *Continued*

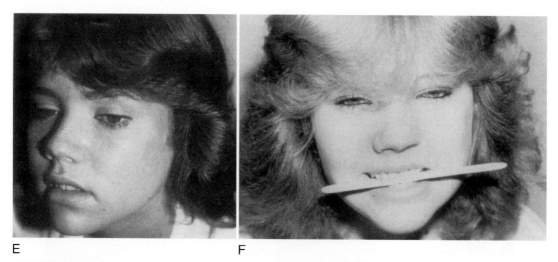

E   F

FIGURE 67-28, cont'd. *E,* Seven-year follow-up showing return of function and satisfactory facial symmetry. *F,* Ten-year follow-up showing slight growth reduction in the zygomatic area. (From Dufresne CR, Manson PN: Pediatric facial trauma. In McCarthy JG, ed: Plastic Surgery. Philadelphia, WB Saunders, 1990:1142.)

accurately within the first 5 to 7 days to avoid later dysfunction and deformity. Unlike the situation in the adult, after this type of fracture has healed, it is not as amenable to correction by refracturing or bone grafting because of the association of tooth buds in the middle and inferior maxilla.[181,182]

Depressed malunited zygomatic fractures vary in their severity. There is often a residual hypesthesia of the upper lip, nose, and anterior maxillary teeth and some retrusion or flatness of the cheek. The lateral canthus may be displaced inferiorly, giving an antimongoloid slant to the palpebral fissure. In addition, the inferior displacement of the fracture may impinge the zygoma against the coronoid process of the mandible, resulting in restricted mandibular movement or, less commonly, an open bite.[85,134,183]

Orbital fractures in older children are observed after automobile accidents and are often characterized by a separation of the zygomaticofrontal junction and the lateral orbital wall, with downward displacement of the orbital floor. This type of unilateral craniofacial detachment is more frequent in the child than is the Le Fort III bilateral craniofacial dysjunction.

The major mass of the zygoma forms the malar eminence, and it has five principal attachments to adjacent structures: the frontal bone, the zygomatic arch, the medial maxilla at the infraorbital rim, the maxillary alveolus inferiorly, and the greater wing of the sphenoid within the orbit. Fractures of the zygoma always involve the orbital floor, with the exception of fractures isolated to the zygomatic arch. The infraorbital nerve is usually involved in its exit from the upper anterior maxillary wall adjacent to the infraorbital rim. The diagnosis of an orbital fracture is suggested by the presence of periorbital and subconjunctival

hematomas and by hypesthesia in the distribution of the infraorbital nerve. The "orbital" fracture is frequently a fracture-dislocation of the zygoma.[84,117,184] If the zygoma is dislocated inferiorly, the lateral canthus, attached to the zygoma at Whitnall tubercle, is displaced inferiorly, causing an antimongoloid slant to the palpebral fissure. A step-off or inferior orbital rim level discrepancy may be palpable on the infraorbital rim or at the zygomaticofrontal suture. Tenderness may be present over these areas. A hematoma is often noted in the upper buccal sulcus, and zygomatic fractures are usually accompanied by unilateral epistaxis, which occurs from bleeding within the fractured maxillary sinus. Depending on the extent of the orbital floor involvement, there may be extraocular muscle dysfunction, which results in diplopia. Young children tend to get "trap-door" fractures of the orbital floor, which need urgent release if they are accompanied by true muscle incarceration. Difficulty in chewing or moving the jaw or mild occlusal discrepancies of a temporary nature are secondary to swelling in the area of the zygomatic arch, with interference in excursion of the coronoid process of the mandible. Isolated zygomatic arch fractures are usually bowed inward. After resolution of the swelling, a depression is seen in the lateral cheek in the preauricular area.[84,117,184] Medial displacement of the complete zygoma narrows the orbital volume, producing exophthalmos.[185]

The radiographic evaluation of a zygomatic fracture formerly consisted of Waters and Caldwell views to assess the displacement (Fig. 67-29). The Waters view defines the infraorbital rim and lateral wall of the maxillary sinus; the orbital floor is also visualized. The Caldwell view assesses displacement at the

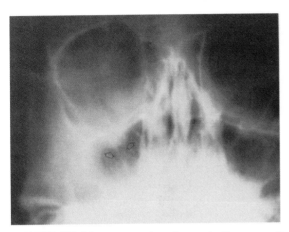

FIGURE 67-29. Waters view demonstrating a small blowout fracture with herniation of the orbital contents into the maxillary sinus (the teardrop sign). (From Dufresne CR, Manson PN: Pediatric facial trauma. In McCarthy JG, ed: Plastic Surgery. Philadelphia, WB Saunders, 1990:1142.)

zygomaticofrontal suture.[186] Posterior displacement of the malar eminence and depression of the zygomatic arch are assessed through submentovertex skull films or axial CT scans.[176,177,180,186]

A CT examination is presently obtained routinely in any patient in whom a maxillary or orbital fracture is suspected. Plain radiographs in children are difficult to interpret, and the identification of fracture lines may be impossible. Plain films do not display the bones, soft tissues, and contents of the orbit with the same accuracy and detail as can be obtained with a CT examination (Fig. 67-30).[79,87,123]

The indications for open reduction are deformity, cheek retrusion, enophthalmos, persistent diplopia, vertical malposition of the globe, retrusion of the malar eminence, and anesthesia or hypesthesia in the infraorbital nerve distribution.[34,106,178,184] These symptoms can, however, occur with a medially displaced zygomatic fracture. Significant fracture fragment displacement that is evident on radiographic examination is treated by open reduction and rigid fixation at the zygomaticofrontal suture and the infraorbital rim.[81,187] The infraorbital rim and the zygomaticofrontal suture may be exposed through a subciliary incision with a skin-muscle flap.[188,189] The lateral canthus may be detached to expose the zygomaticofrontal suture through this incision. This approach provides a wide exposure of the zygoma and orbital floor and leaves a barely perceptible scar. Alternatively, the lateral portion of an upper lid blepharoplasty incision provides zygomaticofrontal suture exposure. After zygomatic fracture reduction, 1.3-mm plates and screws may be used to obtain stability.

The intraoral visualization of the zygomaticomaxillary junction through an upper gingival buccal sulcus incision may permit proper alignment and reduction of the zygoma with this approach alone in medially impacted large-fragment (greenstick) fractures at the zygomaticofrontal suture. The anterior face of the zygoma is exposed, the zygoma is reduced, and the continuity of the orbital floor is confirmed with an endoscopic evaluation through the maxillary sinus. If the orbital floor fracture produces a lack of globe support, a lower eyelid incision may be added to provide inferior orbital reconstruction. In adults, placement of plates is routine at the Le Fort I level; however, caution should be exercised in children because of the presence of unerupted permanent teeth. In young children, the maxillary sinus is not fully developed and the bone is soft. Caution must be observed when screws are tightened so that the screw is not overtightened through the soft cancellous bone. As previously emphasized, fractures of the zygoma usually are not seen in small children because of the incomplete development of the maxillary sinus. The bone structure of the midface must be weakened by development of the sinus for the typical fracture lines to occur.[34,117,187]

The orbital floor is explored routinely as part of the operative treatment of the displaced zygomatic fracture when it is indicated on the basis of CT scan (Fig. 67-31). Many fractures of the orbital floor in children are linear and will be accurately repositioned by

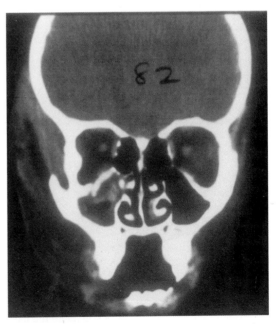

FIGURE 67-30. Coronal CT view of an orbital floor fracture entrapping the inferior rectus muscle between the two fractured segments. (From Dufresne CR, Manson PN. Pediatric facial trauma. In McCarthy JG ed: Plastic Surgery. Philadelphia, WB Saunders Company, 1990:1142.)

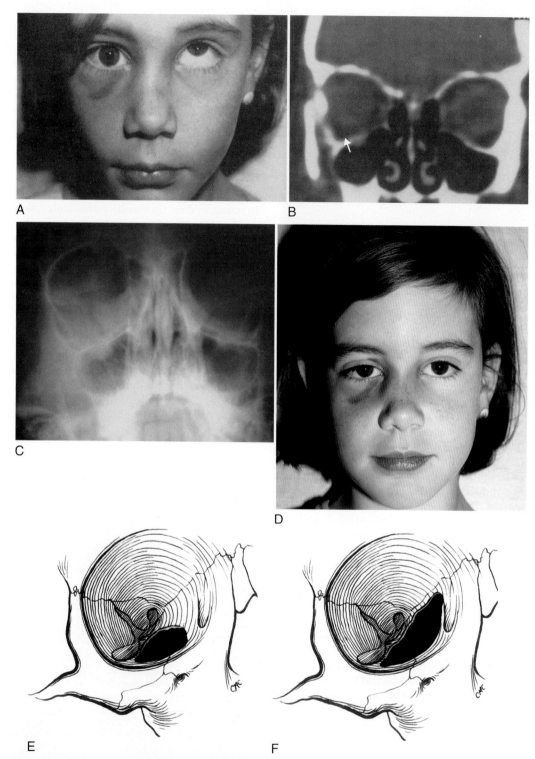

FIGURE 67-31. *A,* Appearance of an 8-year-old girl who sustained a blow to the right eye with entrapment of the inferior rectus muscle. Note the limitation of upward gaze. *B,* Coronal CT view demonstrated entrapment of the inferior rectus muscle in a linear fracture along the orbital floor *(arrow).* Urgent release is required if the function of the muscle is to be preserved. *C,* Plain radiograph of entrapped muscle. *D,* The patient in *C* with a "white-eyed blowout fracture." *E,* Large orbital floor fracture. *F,* Combination floor and medial wall fracture. (*A* and *B* from Dufresne CR, Manson PN: Pediatric facial trauma. In McCarthy JG, ed: Plastic Surgery. Philadelphia, WB Saunders, 1990:1142.)

TABLE 67-8 ✦ ORBITAL FLOOR RECONSTRUCTIVE MATERIALS

	Advantages	Disadvantages
Bone		
Rib	Vascularized, bending memory	70% resorption
Calvaria*	Vascularized	50% resorption
Iliac	Vascularized	70% resorption
Alloplastic		
Silicone	Smooth surface	Not vascularized
Polyethylene		
Supramid MEDPOR	Smooth surface	Not vascularized
	Porous, ingrowth of soft tissue, bending memory	Soft tissue adherence
Barrier MEDPOR	Porous on one side, smooth surface on the other side; bending memory	Not vascularized on the smooth side
Titanium	Bending memory	Generates soft tissue fibrosis

*May not be able to be harvested before the age of 4 years.

alignment of the major buttresses of the zygoma and orbital rim. Depending on the integrity of the floor, a MEDPOR or Supramid plate of 0.6- to 0.8-mm thickness can be used to cover a bone defect; it should be anchored (screwed) to the floor or rim to prevent displacement (Table 67-8). Linear orbital fractures are usually aligned with reduction of the orbital rim, and an implant is not required. The orbital dissection should progress until all the edges of the orbital defect are completely identified, so that the entire area of the defect may be spanned by the reconstructive material. A split rib graft or a graft from the inner table of the iliac crest may be harvested. Care should be taken to spare the superior cartilaginous lip of the iliac crest in children; in young children, the cartilaginous lip is not only a growth center but also of the wrong consistency for reduction. If the child is old enough, a thin split calvarial graft may be taken[190] (see "Calvarial Bone Grafting"). A Tessier rib contour forceps may be used to shape the graft to the exact curvature desired for orbital wall reconstruction. Bone grafts may be secured with a screw or plate if desired. A rapid, efficient method is to anchor the graft by a "lag" or "tandem" screw to the zygoma.[147,191]

Malunited zygomatic fractures commonly occur either because of an unstable or inadequate reduction or because periorbital and cheek edema obscure the bone displacement so that reduction is not attempted.[192] On occasion, the fracture may have been adequately reduced, but pressure or a subsequent blow to the face again moves the fragments out of position. Some authors report a 10% to 20% incidence of malalignment in reduction of zygomatic fractures.[81,187] Dingman[187] noted that complications are more common with conservative (closed) reduction of the fracture and advocated open reduction.

Zygomatic-coronoid ankylosis may occasionally follow a severe zygomatic or Le Fort fracture, especially if a deep laceration penetrates the temporalis muscle. It is usually managed by intraoral coronoidectomy.[34,147,191,193,194] The coronoid process may or may not be fractured if a lateral blow is sustained. The ankylosis may be bone or scar tissue, and it may be from the zygomatic arch or body of the zygoma or orbit to the mandible. The complication is especially frequent after open injuries and gunshot wounds.

Koltai[20] examined the pattern and frequency of orbital fractures in children. Interestingly, the most frequent fracture observed was that of the orbital roof (14 of 40 patients); 10 children had fractures of the orbital floor, 14 children had mixed fractures of the floor medial walls, and 2 children had fractures of the medial orbital wall (see Fig. 67-31). The mean age of the children with roof fractures was 5 years, and the mean age of the children with other orbital fractures was 12 years. As expected, orbital roof fractures had a significantly greater likelihood of associated neurocranial injuries. Pensler[190] has also identified the orbital roof fracture as a possible contributor to pulsating exophthalmos. Others identify the orbital roof fracture as likely to yield inferior and anterior globe positional change (Fig. 67-32).[195] This "blow-in" fracture can occur with either supraorbital or zygomatic fractures.[185] These fractures reduce the volume of the orbit, resulting in exophthalmos.

BLOWOUT FRACTURES

The etiology of "pure" orbital blowout fractures in children, unassociated with zygomatic fracture, is similar to that in adults.[196] They are caused by the patient's being struck in the orbital region with a ball or another child's fist or by trauma received in automobile accidents.[197] The maxillary sinus is small in the young child. The floor of the orbit is concave, dipping downward behind the rim of the orbit, an anatomic characteristic that can mislead the surgeon into an erroneous diagnosis of orbital floor collapse

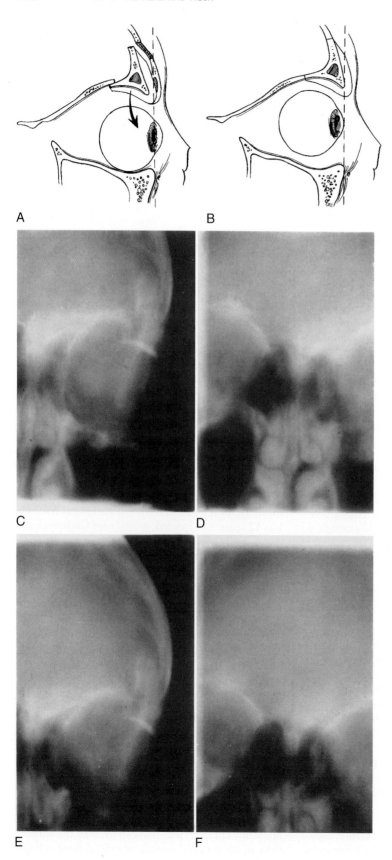

FIGURE 67-32. *A,* Orbital roof fracture compromising orbital volume. The fracture represents the lateral temporal-orbital fracture with exophthalmos and inferior globe displacement. *B,* Normal orbit and globe. *C* to *F,* Plain radiographs of a patient with a displaced supraorbital fracture.

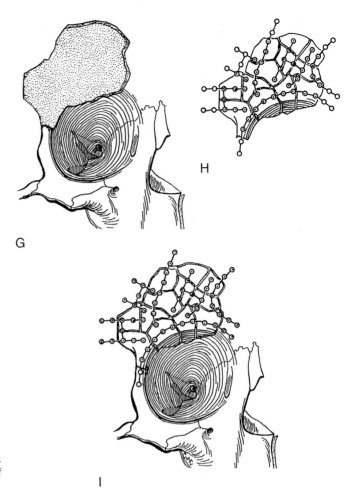

FIGURE 67-32, cont'd. *G to I,* Stabilization of a supraorbital fracture with plates of the mucosystem. (See also Fig. 67-48.)

on plain radiographic films. Despite the small size of the maxillary sinus, orbital contents escape through the fractured floor and may cause enophthalmos (see Fig. 67-31).[117,147,194]

Restoration of the continuity and position of the orbital floor and the shape of the orbit is the method of treatment, as in the adult. Comminuted orbital fractures in children should be carefully reconstructed as soon as possible because the bone fragments consolidate rapidly in a malaligned position. Release of the entrapped orbital contents from the area of the blowout fracture is followed by floor reconstruction with bone or alloplastic implants (see Table 67-8). Reconstruction is usually followed by rapid return of complete oculorotary movements. Children seem to have rapid recuperative abilities after a blowout fracture, usually achieving a functional range of asymptomatic extraocular muscle activity. Proper positioning and selection of these floor replacement structures prevent adhesions between the globe, the periorbital fat, the inferior rectus and inferior oblique muscles, and the orbit floor.[147,191,194]

Diplopia and enophthalmos are complications that may follow various types of orbital floor fractures (see Fig. 67-31). Diplopia is usually present immediately after injury but may occur with resolution of the swelling. Later, enophthalmos becomes a more obvious sign. Injury to and entrapment of the periorbita may cause inflammation, fibrosis, and atrophy, with muscle adherence to the orbital walls, fibrosis of the muscles or their restraining ligaments, and impairment of muscle function. Herniated, entrapped, ecchymotic orbital fat and muscle may undergo necrosis. Fracture expansion of the orbital floor increases orbital volume and makes the eye appear small through the mechanisms of enophthalmos.

Loss of vision may develop from postoperative orbital hemorrhage, trauma to the optic nerve, central retinal artery occlusion, or thrombosis of the orbital veins. The superior orbital fissure syndrome (paralysis of cranial nerves III, IV, VI, and frontal sensory V) also occurs after trauma. When it is accompanied by visual loss (cranial nerve II), it is called the orbital apex syndrome.[198] To prevent the complication of blindness, every effort should be made in a fracture reduction to avoid excessive pressure or tension on the globe and periorbita. Hematoma in the retrobulbar region should be avoided. Alloplastic material must be stabilized in a position that avoids pressure in the area of the optic nerve when placement is far posterior within the orbit.[178,184,199]

Complete correction of late enophthalmos caused by a healed, enlarged, and depressed bony orbit can occasionally be accomplished by simple procedures, such as alloplastic or bone graft supplementation of the orbital floor and sidewalls. Complete relocation and recontouring of the entire involved bony orbit by total osteotomy, such as an orbital dystopia procedure or less commonly marginal osteotomies with supplemental bone grafts, are usually required to correct such deformities.[147,191,194,199] Relocation of the lateral and medial canthal ligaments is sometimes also required.

TRAP-DOOR FRACTURES OF THE ORBIT IN CHILDREN

Children are susceptible to a specific type of orbital fracture. The presence of spongy bone, which rebounds quickly, and the absence of the adult sinus development[200,201] produce linear bone fractures, which may "trap" an extraocular muscle as the bone rebounds, closing on the slower soft tissue. In adults, the traditional blowout fracture contuses but does not usually trap the muscle. In general, fracture traps the extraocular muscle fibrous ligament system, but the muscle is seldom truly itself incarcerated. In children, true muscle entrapment probably occurs 5% to 10% of the time in blowout fractures.[118] These patients lose the ability to look upward, and the muscle is tightly incarcerated. Some patients have pain, nausea, and vomiting on looking upward, indications of true muscle incarceration. A number of authors have now shown that tight incarceration of the muscle itself or of the musculofibrous ligament system should be released early to improve results (summarized in reference 118). One must especially consider the incarcerated muscle, which is often able to be diagnosed on CT scan, as justifying urgent treatment (see Figs. 67-30 and 67-31B). These patients often present with the "white-eyed blowout" and "missing muscle" syndromes because of their lack of significant periorbital ecchymosis and the "pinching" of the muscle out of the orbit. Some authors have recommended that in release of the muscle, it should not be tugged on, but an opening should be made into the maxillary sinus through a nonfractured portion of the floor and the intervening floor excised until the muscle is able to be easily released from the enlarged hole into the sinus.[202]

Emphasis has also been placed on the Kawamoto "shave" (thin) cranial bone graft as a technique for orbital wall reconstruction. This is a thin piece of cranial bone that has attached periosteum; it makes an excellent orbital wall replacement because it is more bendable than brittle, full-thickness calvarial bone. It makes sense that early release would allow the muscle to recover maximally from being "scissored" in the fracture. After a delay of 2 weeks, full muscle recovery may not be achieved; it has been the authors' experience that operating after 2 weeks all too frequently produces minimal muscle excursion. Others have recommended high-dose steroids as being protective in muscle recovery. Grant et al[200] and the discussion by Manson[118] indicate that patients with tight restriction of the extraocular muscles or those with true muscle incarceration must be distinguished from the majority of patients with more benign blowout fractures in which muscle contusion can be safely observed.[135,203,204]

Nasal and Naso-orbital Fractures

Fractures of the nasal skeleton in children are more frequent than fractures of the maxilla and zygoma.[24,205-214] In the early years of childhood, the nasal skeleton is proportionally more cartilaginous than bone,[215] and the diagnosis of nasal fracture is clinical rather than from plain radiographs.[205,206] The nasal bones in children may separate in the midline along an open suture line.[216] The "open book" type of fracture, with overriding of the nasal bones over the frontal processes of the maxilla, is a characteristic of significant fractures of the nasal bones in children.[117,207,208,217] As with other types of childhood facial injuries, but more so in nasal injuries, a complicating factor is that growth and development may be affected even after accurate diagnosis and adequate treatment (Fig. 67-33).[65,210,218]

The first 5 years of postnatal life are years of rapid facial growth. After a period of moderately active growth, a second period of rapid growth occurs between the ages of 10 and 15 years. Growth of the nasomaxillary complex may be affected by trauma during the early postnatal years and may be more frequent than generally expected. Such injuries, as well as those suffered during delivery, may explain nasal deviation and nasomaxillary hypoplasia that have no other apparent cause.[24,40,41,219]

The diagnosis of nasal injury in a young child is more difficult and may require general anesthesia to permit careful intranasal and extranasal skeletal inspection and palpation. Despite the occasional lack of benefit, radiographic CT examination is a prerequisite for diagnostic and medicolegal purposes to document injury to the adjacent bony skeleton.

The nasal bones are formed on the surface of the cartilaginous capsule, and there is considerable overlap between the upper lateral cartilages and the nasal bones. The upper lateral cartilages may be detached from the undersurface of the nasal bones because of

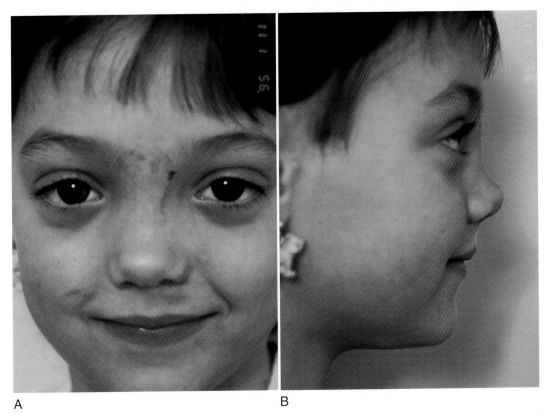

A   B

FIGURE 67-33. *A,* A 5-year-old child involved in a motor vehicle accident with a severe nasal fracture and collapse of the nasal septum. *B,* Lateral profile demonstrates loss of nasal projection.

the relatively loose attachment in the child and may collapse in conjunction with a fracture of the septum. A hematoma may form within the septum or between the lateral cartilages and the undersurface of the nasal bones. It should be evacuated through an appropriate incision.[214,220] An important distinction between adult and pediatric nasal fractures is that the nasal bones are not fused in children until adolescence, so that they may fracture individually. Greenstick or incomplete fractures are common in children and require that the fracture be completed for stability after reduction. Incomplete fractures will slip back into a displaced position.

Fractures and dislocation of the septal cartilage are universal in fractures of the nasal bones, but they may occur independently with injuries of the distal cartilaginous nose (see Fig. 67-33). Hematoma of the septum, a collection of blood between the cartilage and the mucoperichondrium caused by rupture of the abundant vasculature of the area, is manifested as a bluish red bulging in the vestibule of the nasal fossa. One should be aware of the child who cannot breathe through the nose after a nasal injury.[187] Septal hematoma may rarely be caused by a traumatic bending of the septal cartilage without fracture or dislocation. Hematoma of the septum is always a serious complication in children, not only because of the nasal obstruction that results from fibrous thickening of the septum but also because of the possibility of collapse of the dorsum (saddle deformity) with loss of septal cartilage support through pressure necrosis from hematoma or abscess.[117,214,220]

Special care should be taken to drain any septal hematoma. A straight or L-shaped incision, extending through the mucoperiosteum over the vomer, is made along the floor of the nose and extended vertically upward through the mucoperichondrium over the septal cartilage. The flap of mucous membrane is raised and the hematoma evacuated. The dependent position of the incision ensures drainage and thus prevents a recurrent collection of blood. Septal quilting sutures of plain gut on a short, straight 4-0 needle prevent recurrence of the hematoma. When the septal framework is fractured, the hematoma may collect bilaterally on both sides of the septal cartilage. A portion of the septal cartilage can be removed so that the two areas of hematoma communicate; alternatively, a bilateral septal incision through the mucoperichondrium provides dependent drainage and prevents recurrence of the hematoma.[117] Bilateral incisions should not be made over each other or a septal perforation might occur.

Treatment of nasal bone fractures in children is similar to that in adults. Under general anesthesia, an elevator is placed in the nasal fossa, and the fractured fragments of nasal bones and the frontal processes of the maxilla are elevated. Outfracture of each side should be completed separately with the instrument in each nasal fossa, followed by infracture by digital remolding. Realignment is obtained by external manual manipulation. The septum, if it is fractured, is straightened with an Asch forceps; and if they are dislocated, the upper lateral cartilages are realigned and repositioned. Suturing or interosseous fixation is preferred for stability in open injuries. A splint is placed over the nose for 5 to 7 days. Intranasal packing is often necessary, in conjunction with the external splint, to assist in the support and alignment of the bony and cartilaginous fragments.[214,220]

Nasal bone fractures heal rapidly in children, frequently with overgrowth of bone. Slight bone distortion and hypertrophic callus are common. These sequelae of fracture healing result in a widening of the bony dorsum of the nose and a nasal "hump" or bending of the nose.[221] Children who have suffered comminuted nasal bone fractures may show developmental deformities years later,[207] even though they received adequate treatment after the accident. The possibility of late changes and growth disturbance as a result of the fracture must be discussed with the family from a medicolegal viewpoint. The deformities may include deviation and thickening of the septum, flattening of the nasal dorsum, widening of the bony nasal skeleton by hypertrophic callus, and varying degrees of nasomaxillary hypoplasia (see Fig. 67-33).[101,209,214,220]

One should not hesitate to realign the nasal pyramid or septum by osteotomy in children who have suffered an injury resulting in an incomplete fracture that is malunited, producing deviation or nasal obstruction.[40,41] The risk of further impairment of growth is minimal because the growth potential has already been affected by the initial trauma. The deformity, characterized by depression of the dorsum and widening of the nasal bridge, may require correction for psychological as well as functional reasons. A costal cartilage or bone graft may be needed, with the understanding that further definitive surgery will be required during adolescence when nasal growth has been completed.[24,117,184,222]

NASOETHMOIDAL FRACTURES

Nasal-orbital fractures in which the bone structures of the nose are pushed backward into the interorbital space along with the medial orbital rims and walls frequently occur in automobile accidents and are treated by open reduction, interfragment wiring, and rigid fixation techniques supplemented by bone and cartilage grafts.[78,184] The coronal incision provides optimal exposure for these fractures, which also require inferior orbital rim and gingival buccal sulcus exposures. Open reduction may prevent the sequelae of traumatic telecanthus, saddle nose deformity, and lacrimal apparatus obstruction. Nasoethmoidal-orbital fractures are always associated with blowout fractures of the orbital floor and medial orbital walls and fractures of the orbital rims.[147,181,182,191,194]

Nasoethmoidal-orbital fractures may result from a direct severe blow to the frontal, glabellar, or upper nasal region or accompany frontal bone or high Le Fort II or III fractures. The nasal components of the nasoethmoidal-orbital fracture are usually laterally and posteriorly displaced (Fig. 67-34). Nasoethmoidal-orbital fractures are characterized by retrusion and flattening of the nasal pyramid and an increase in the columella-lip angle with loss of distal septal support. Telecanthus exists when the interorbital distance exceeds the length of a palpebral fissure and additionally age-specific values of the intercanthal distances are available.[223] The fracture is not isolated to the nose but involves the medial portion of the orbital rims and extends into the ethmoidal sinuses, orbital floors, and medial portions of the infraorbital rims on one or both sides, depending on the extent of the injury (Fig. 67-35). A small laceration is frequently present over the nasal bridge or forehead area. Epistaxis may be severe. The finding of bilateral periorbital hematoma signals not only the fracture of the nose and orbit but also the possibility of a fracture continuing into the anterior cranial fossa. Greenstick or incomplete nasoethmoidal-orbital fractures or fractures with minimal displacement may be missed unless a high index of suspicion is present when patients with trauma to the frontonasal area are examined. Partial fractures are usually incomplete (greenstick fractures) at the nasofrontal suture.[49,68,117,183]

The radiographic evaluation consists of a CT scan (Fig. 67-36). Thin cuts should be taken through the area of interest, namely, the medial orbital rim.[176] Axial and coronal sections and bone and soft tissue windows are prepared for analysis.

Fractures that complete isolation of the medial orbital rim with its attached medial canthal ligament characterize the fully developed nasoethmoidal-orbital injury and permit the potential for canthal ligament migration and instability. The necessity for a precise physical examination to determine mobility of this "central" (or canthal ligament-containing) fragment cannot be overemphasized. Tenderness over the medial orbital rim should signal the possible presence of a nasoethmoidal-orbital fracture. A CSF leak or pneumocephalus may also be present.[117,224] A bimanual test for mobility of the medial orbital rim may be performed

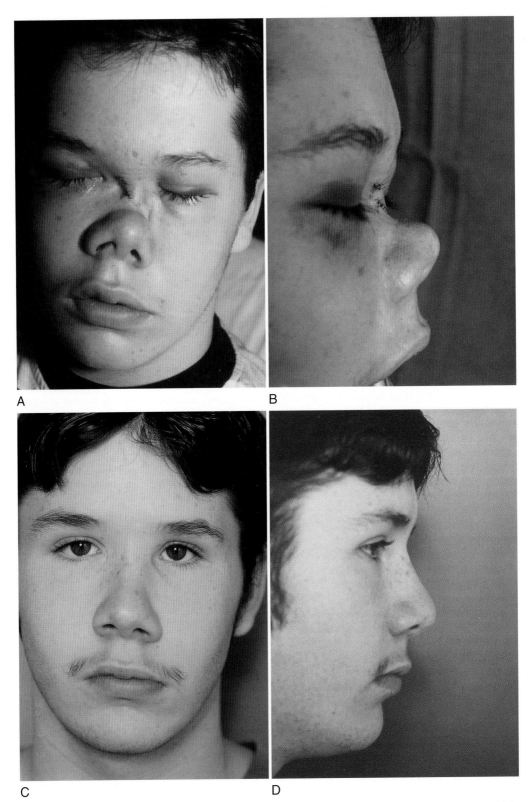

FIGURE 67-34. *A* and *B*, A 14-year-old boy who struck the dashboard of the car in a motor vehicle accident; he sustained a severe nasoethmoidal-orbital fracture with collapse of the nasal structures. *C* and *D*, After open reduction and internal fixation of the nasoethmoidal-orbital fracture and primary bone graft of the nasal bridge.

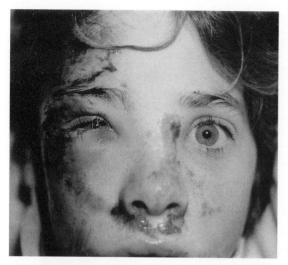

FIGURE 67-35. A 12-year-old child who sustained a right-sided unilateral nasoethmoidal-orbital fracture and a frontal bone fracture. Note the unilateral right-sided telecanthus. (From Dufresne CR, Manson PN: Pediatric facial trauma. In McCarthy JG, ed: Plastic Surgery. Philadelphia, WB Saunders, 1990:1142.)

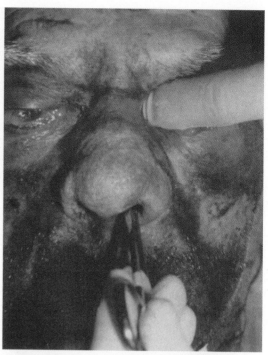

FIGURE 67-37. Bimanual examination for confirmation of a nasoethmoidal-orbital fracture. A clamp is placed intranasally directly under the frontal process of the maxilla, and the bone is moved between an external palpating finger and the clamp. Care must be taken not to misdiagnose a nasal fracture as a nasoethmoidal-orbital fracture. The palpating finger should be placed deeply over the canthal tendon. (From Dufresne CR, Manson PN: Pediatric facial trauma. In McCarthy JG, ed: Plastic Surgery. Philadelphia, WB Saunders, 1990:1142.)

by inserting a clamp into the nose and pressing the tip intranasally against the medial orbital rim opposite the canthal ligament (Fig. 67-37).[225] Pressing a finger against the external surface of the canthal ligament, one can move the fractured medial orbital rim frag-

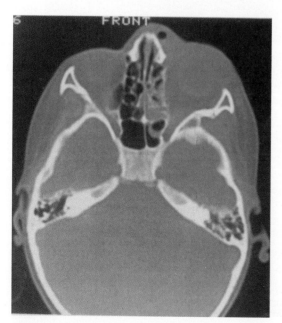

FIGURE 67-36. Fracture of the left zygoma extending to the greater wing of the sphenoid with a left-sided nasoethmoidal-orbital fracture. (From Dufresne CR, Manson PN: Pediatric facial trauma. In McCarthy JG, ed: Plastic Surgery. Philadelphia, WB Saunders, 1990:1142.)

ment between the clamp and the index finger. Any mobility of the canthal ligament-bearing fragment signals the necessity for an open reduction. One fourth of nasoethmoidal-orbital fractures demonstrated on CT scan are not sufficiently mobile or displaced to require open reduction in children.

Nasoethmoidal-orbital fractures often accompany other frontal bone or facial fractures. A linear fracture may extend superiorly into the frontal bone, a common condition in children. In adults, fractures of the frontal sinus and supraorbital area frequently accompany a nasoethmoidal-orbital injury. Nasoethmoidal-orbital fractures often accompany high Le Fort II and III fractures and are often unilateral. In summary, one should suspect the presence of a nasoethmoidal-orbital fracture when there are severe nasal fractures with anteroposterior displacement, lacerations of the frontal and nasal areas, or bilateral periorbital ecchymoses. Traumatic telecanthus may be observed in the immediate postinjury period in severely displaced fractures, but it often develops more slowly during a period of a week to 10 days in those fractures demonstrating less comminution.[70,81,171] In the eyelid traction test,[191] lateral movement of the medial canthal ligament occurs when traction is applied to the lower eyelid. This test is seldom useful for the evaluation of these injuries because it only confirms the worst injuries, whereas the bimanual examination is extremely accurate (see Fig. 67-37).

If the patient's neurologic condition is stable, the injuries should be treated by definitive open reduction if any mobility or displacement is present. A Richman screw is used to monitor the intracranial pressure if anesthesia is required in the presence of a significant head injury (Fig. 67-38).[74,213] The open reduction consists of an exposure of the frontal bone, orbits (upper, medial, and inferior aspects), nose, and infraorbital areas through coronal and bilateral lower eyelid and gingival buccal sulcus incisions. The entire framework of the nasoethmoidal-orbital area is exposed in a subperiosteal plane. Multiple drill holes are placed to link each bone fragment initially by wires to the adjacent fragment of the orbital rims, proceeding from intact bone to intact bone. Frequently, the

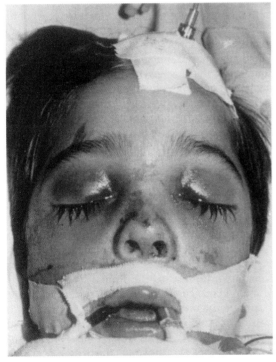

FIGURE 67-38. A young child after severe frontal-temporal-orbital fracture and a greenstick nasoethmoidal-orbital fracture. The need for ventricular pressure monitoring (Richman screw) to detect increased cerebral pressure for edema and possible herniation was evident on admission. (From Dufresne CR, Manson PN: Pediatric facial trauma. In McCarthy JG, ed: Plastic Surgery. Philadelphia, WB Saunders, 1990:1142.)

open reduction extends from the frontal bone to the upper portion of the Le Fort I level. The Le Fort I area is exposed through gingival buccal sulcus incisions. After the fragments have been provisionally linked with wires, "junctional" rigid fixation is completed; bone grafts are placed to complete the continuity of the medial and inferior orbital walls. The rim fragments are held in reduction and the wires tightened.

The most important principle in the treatment of nasoethmoidal-orbital fractures is to restore the proper intercanthal distance by a transnasal reduction of the medial orbital rims. The transnasal wires are placed through bone behind the canthal ligament on the posterior edge of the medial orbital rim fragment above and behind the lacrimal fossa and led to the other side so that the distance between the medial orbital rims is limited by the tightening of the two wires. It is not necessary to detach the medial canthal ligament to accomplish a transnasal reduction in the usual nasoethmoidal-orbital fracture. In fact, the architecture of the canthus and the intercanthal distance are improved if the canthal ligament is not detached from the medial orbital insertion during the bone reduction. A bone graft may be used to reconstitute nasal height, to provide a smooth nasal dorsum, or to improve distal septal support. It is fixed in cantilever fashion with lag screws or anchored with a plate at the glabella area.[100,117,184,224] When the canthal ligament has been avulsed in the injury or inadvertently detached in the reduction or dissection, or if the canthus must be stripped to reduce a medial orbital rim where the fracture or comminution extends beneath the canthal ligament insertion, the canthus must be reapproximated to the bone in the position of the transnasal reduction by a separate set (for each canthus) of transnasal wires connected to a suture placed in the canthus by a small external incision over the medial eyelid commissure at the insertion of the canthus to the tarsal plates (Fig. 67-39).

Nasoethmoid fractures undisplaced at the junction of the frontal process of the frontal bone may be treated with lower eyelid and gingival sulcus approaches alone. A coronal incision may be avoided. One third to one half of nasoethmoid fractures may usually be so managed.

A fracture in the base of the anterior cranial fossa adjacent to the cribriform plate always accompanies significant nasoethmoidal-orbital injuries. In early childhood, the anterior cranial bone is cartilaginous with only an anlage of frontal sinus development. Isolated basal frontal sinus fractures have not been routinely treated by frontal sinus manipulation or ablation, and most patients do not demonstrate late problems with mucocele formation[226] or nasofrontal duct obstruction.[35] These patients need long-term follow-up, however, to exclude sinus obstruction or mucocele. Basal skull fractures are also frequently

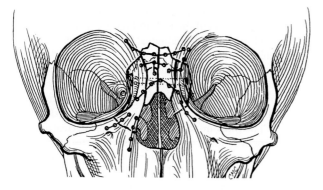

FIGURE 67-39. Scheme for open reduction and internal fixation of a nasoethmoidal fracture with and without reattachment of the canthal ligament. Dotted lines are for transnasal sinus and for canthal attachment wires.

accompanied by contusion of the frontal and temporal lobes.[27]

Fractures of the supraorbital rim or comminuted frontal bone or frontal sinus fractures are managed as described in the following section. The lacrimal system usually is not transected in the absence of lacerations near the medial canthus or avulsion of the ligament from the bone, which are less common situations. Late lacrimal obstruction occurs in 5% of patients having an open nasoethmoidal reduction, is usually located in the nasolacrimal duct, and may be treated by dacryocystorhinostomy.[193]

Frontal Bone and Frontal Sinus Fractures

Patients with head injuries should be evaluated by neurologic examination, CT scan, and Glasgow coma scale (Table 67-9).[74,122] The survival outcome of severe head injury is better in children (as far as survival and function are concerned) than in adults.[227-232] The prognosis, however, for memory, intellect, and mental function may not be as satisfactory.[233] These findings may reflect the peculiar sensitivity of the childhood nervous system.[105,234] There is high incidence of diffuse swelling and low incidence of mass lesions. It is important to keep the intracranial pressure below 20 mm Hg.[213] Flaccidity, absence of a gag reflex, lack of oculovestibular stimulation, and abnormal respiratory pattern carry the worst prognosis.

The frontal skull in children is more prominent than the face, and thus linear skull fractures are frequent.[104,235] Many times, the fracture line is vertical and linear and extends into the orbit near the supraorbital foramen. A CT scan evaluates displacement and the need for open reduction in closed injuries. In open injuries, débridement is necessary to ensure the absence of significant contamination.[229] Neurosurgical criteria for open reduction of skull fractures include significant skeletal displacement, presence of an accompanying dural tear, intracranial or extracranial hematoma, CSF leak, pneumocephalus, and frontal lobe contusion with mass effect. A CSF leak may exit the wound or may be manifested as CSF rhinorrhea. In patients with epistaxis, it may be difficult to document rhinorrhea for several days. Although the cranial base is cartilaginous in the central anterior sections in small children, it heals quickly. Fracture lines in cartilage are not seen in radiographs. In adult fractures, fracture lines are clearly seen in CT scans. Fractures in bone may not be visualized in plain radiographs. Frequently, the only sign of a closed skull fracture may be a contusion or bruise in the forehead area or, in basal skull fractures, an upper eyelid "spectacle" hematoma. There may be accompanying lacerations and, less commonly, depressions from displaced bone fragments. The radiographic examination is a craniofacial CT scan for precise evaluation of the frontal bone, frontal sinus, orbit, and brain.

Treatment consists of broad exposure of the frontal bone, orbital rims, all fracture sites, and frontal lobes through a coronal incision (Figs. 67-40 and 67-41). Localized incisions or lacerations do not provide the access or flexibility that open treatment often requires. The fractured area is exposed with subperiosteal dissection, and the fracture fragments are repositioned or removed for evaluation of the dura. A precise débridement is performed, and any dural lacerations are closed after evacuation of epidural hematoma. Injuries to the frontal lobe are appropriately managed by removal of devitalized bone. The bone fragments are cleared of any remnants of missing or unstable frontal sinus mucosa by thorough removal and light burring of the walls. A light abrasive burr is used to remove any traces of frontal sinus mucosa from the frontal sinus bony walls. The bone fragments are replaced and stabilized with rigid fixation. The primary replacement of frontal bone fragments is usually successful in children, and the risk of infection is lower than in adults. Replacement of frontal bone fragments avoids late cranioplasty, and

TABLE 67-9 ✦ GLASGOW COMA SCALE

Eye Opening (total points: 4)

Spontaneous	4
To voice	3
To pain	2
None	1

Verbal Response (total points: 5)

Older Children		*Infants and Young Children*	
Oriented	5	Appropriate words; smiles, fixes, and follows	5
Confused	4	Consolable crying	4
Inappropriate	3	Persistently irritable	3
Incomprehensible	2	Restless, agitated	2
None	1	None	1

Motor Response (total points: 6)

Obeys	6
Localizes pain	5
Withdraws	4
Flexion	3
Extension	2
None	1

Clinical Stage

1	*2*	*3*	*4*	*5*
Lethargic	Combative	Comatose	Comatose	Comatose
Follows commands	Inconsistent following of commands	Occasional response to commands	Responds only to pain	No response to pain
Pupils reactive	Pupils sluggish	Eyes may deviate	Weak pupillary response	No pupillary response
Breathing normal	May hyperventilate	Irregular breathing	Very irregular breathing	Requires mechanical ventilation
Normal muscle tone	Reflexes inconsistent	Decorticate posturing	Decerebrate posturing	Absent tendon reflexes—flaccid

Modified from Teasdale G, Jennett B: Assessment of coma and impaired consciousness. Lancet 1974;2:81.

primary reconstruction of the frontal skull is usually safe.[236-238]

The frontal-temporal-orbital fracture consists of the lateral superior rim and roof of the orbit and anterior portion of the squamous temporal bone in young children and results in inferior and anterior globe displacement because of the constricted orbital volume. Repositioning (if the temporal aspect of the fracture is near the middle meningeal artery) must be performed with the awareness that the levering of the fracture without a craniotomy may be accompanied by a rapidly developing epidural hematoma.

The frontal sinus usually is not developed to any significant extent until the teenage years. Frontal sinus fractures may involve the anterior and posterior walls or the nasofrontal duct singly or simultaneously.[239] Management depends on extent of displacement and involvement of surrounding structures.[117,162,176,240,241] Frontal sinus fractures demonstrating significant displacement involving the anterior or posterior walls are treated by thorough removal of mucous membrane, light abrasion of the surface of the bony frontal sinus cavity to eliminate the microscopic invaginations (along the foramina of Breschet) of the mucous membrane, and replacement of the

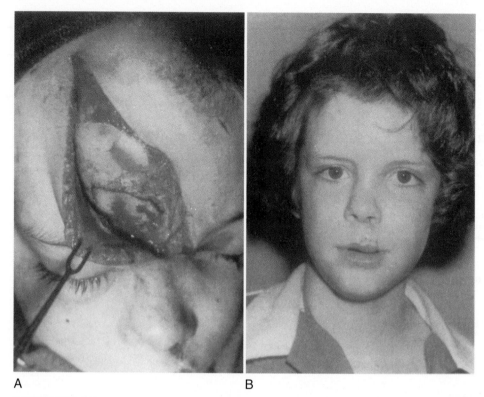

A   B

FIGURE 67-40. *A,* Appearance of a 9-year-old boy with a soft tissue avulsion, a frontal bone fracture, and a left unilateral nasoethmoidal-orbital fracture. *B,* One year after treatment, with evidence of mild telecanthus and facial asymmetry. (From Dufresne CR, Manson PN: Pediatric facial trauma. In McCarthy JG, ed: Plastic Surgery. Philadelphia, WB Saunders, 1990:1142.)

anterior frontal sinus wall bone fragments. The cavity may be obliterated by a cancellous bone graft. Most craniofacial surgeons prefer to fill cancellous bone graft material into the exenterated frontal sinus cavity. Bone plugs are used to seal the nasofrontal duct area from communication with the nose. Conceptually, a cavity left open becomes filled by a fibrous bony material over time even if no material is placed to fill the frontal sinus cavity. This treatment (osteoneogenesis) is not preferred because it has a higher incidence of infection than duct and sinus obliteration with bone. Fractures of the frontal sinus that are not displaced but that demonstrate persistent air-fluid levels should be managed by "elimination," frontal sinus exploration through a coronal incision with removal of the mucous membrane, bone graft plugging of the nasofrontal duct, and obliteration of the cavity with bone graft. Significantly displaced fractures of the anterior wall alone of the frontal sinus are managed by open reduction of that wall alone. Elimination or obliteration of the sinus is not necessary in patients with an isolated fracture. The mucous membrane may be locally débrided or removed as necessary; full sinus ablation may not be

required unless the function of the duct is compromised. Linear undisplaced anterior wall fractures without significant persistent fluid accumulation (indicating nasofrontal duct obstruction) may be managed by observation alone. Posterior wall frontal sinus fractures are treated as depressed skull fractures, with repair of the dura and appropriate assessment of the frontal lobe, especially if the displacement exceeds the thickness of the bone of the posterior wall. Undisplaced posterior wall fractures may be carefully observed, but meningitis, intracranial abscess, and sinus obstruction are possibilities in any posterior wall injury.[242]

"GROWING" SKULL FRACTURES

An unusual phenomenon called pseudogrowth of skull fractures may occur in children.[243] The skull fractures radiographically and clinically seem to enlarge slowly during a period of 1 to 6 months after the fracture.[244] A palpable bone defect with protrusion of the meninges develops in some patients and requires bone replacement. In other patients, the pseudogrowth of skull fractures can be seen on radiographic study

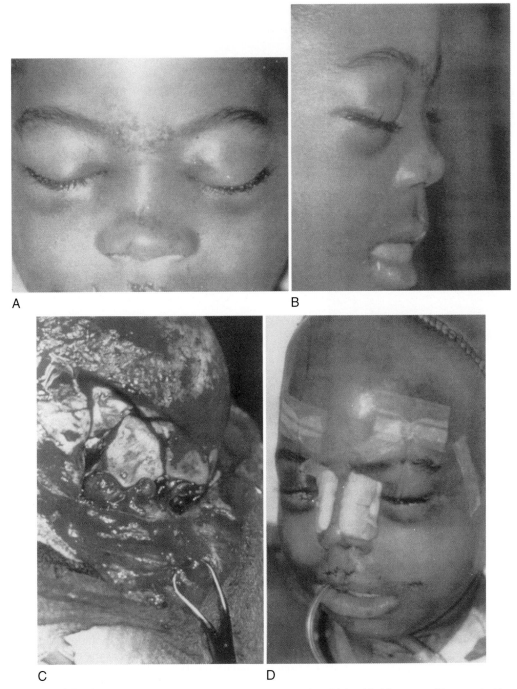

FIGURE 67-41. A young child with severe bilateral nasoethmoidal-orbital fracture with comminution of the frontal bone and telecanthus. *A,* Frontal view. *B,* Lateral view. *C,* Intraoperative view showing a comminuted frontal and nasoethmoid complex. *D,* Immediate postoperative appearance with nasal splints in place. Note the bicoronal and bilateral subciliary incisions. The eyelids are occluded and suspended to the forehead with Frost sutures.

Continued

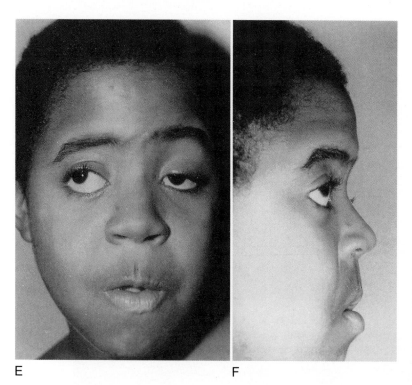

FIGURE 67-41, cont'd. *E,* Follow-up frontal view demonstrating satisfactory facial symmetry and nasal profile. However, the extraocular muscles require balancing. *F,* Follow-up lateral view. (From Dufresne CR, Manson PN: Pediatric facial trauma. In McCarthy JG, ed: Plastic Surgery. Philadelphia, WB Saunders, 1990:1142.)

(Fig. 67-42). The defect may not always be identifiable clinically by palpation. The radiographic appearance is not a guide to treatment. It is the clinical examination of the integrity of the skull that dictates the need for calvarial reconstruction.[190,243-245] In some patients, the phenomenon is due to dural laceration with expansion of the remainder of the meninges and brain through the dural defect, with pressure causing bone resorption. Repair requires at least dural repair and possibly bone reconstruction, depending on the age of the patient (determines efficiency of periosteal reformation of bone). Some authors recommend routine radiographic follow-up 1 year after any skull fracture to document any pseudogrowth.[244]

Havlik et al[246] summarized the problem of growing skull fractures and their craniofacial equivalents. They found an incidence of 0.6% to 2% in skull fractures. The contributing factors were a craniofacial bone defect, a dural tear, and an expanding intracranial process, which could be either growth or a condition such as hydrocephalus. All of the children were younger than 2 years. In the authors' experience, approximately one patient a year is seen with this problem, and approximately 100 pediatric skull trauma patients are seen a year. A skull film is routinely taken 1 year after a skull fracture managed nonoperatively to make sure a growing skull fracture is not present. Patients with growing skull fractures are managed by resection of the meningeal cyst and

dural repair. The cause of the problem may be the lack of dural repair, allowing brain penetration, which produces further bone resorption. Havlik et al[246] described "rarefaction and thickening" as a product of the pressure in the absence of the bone-forming capability of the dura. They noted that destruction of brain from pressure at the edges of such defects may be possible.

CALVARIAL BONE GRAFTING

Koenig et al[247] analyzed scans of 96 children and determined that split cranial bone grafting can be performed cautiously after the age of 3 years. In terms of the ability to split the skull, their recommendation was that in situ cranial bone grafting should not be performed before the age of 9 years. Their regression (Fig. 67-43) and probit (Fig. 67-44) models indicate the range and mean of their data. They also described the value of a preoperative CT scan to determine calvarial thickness. At the age of 3 years, for instance, 20% of children did not have a diploic space demonstrated on CT scan, and the skull was less than 50% of its adult thickness. They did not recommend in situ splitting of the cranial bone before the thickness of the parietal region is 6.0 mm; this normally occurs at about 9 years of age. The adult calvarial bone graft anatomy was analyzed by Pensler and McCarthy[190] in 1985 (see Chapter 66).

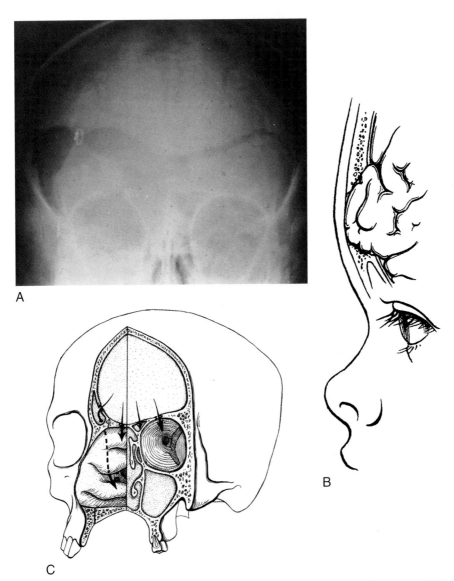

FIGURE 67-42. *A,* Young infant who sustained a frontal bone fracture that resulted in pseudogrowth after wire fixation. *B,* Mechanism for pseudogrowth of skull fracture by brain pressure. *C,* Common sites of spinal fluid leaks.

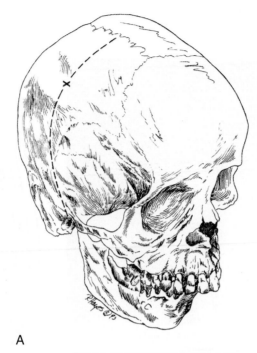

A

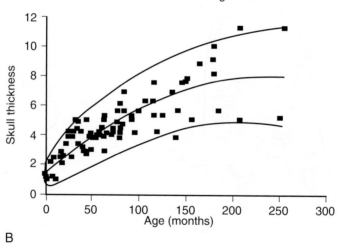

B

FIGURE 67-43. *A,* Skull thickness was measured by Pensler and McCarthy[190] at the point shown. The point is two thirds of the distance from the external auditory meatus to the sagittal suture. *B,* Regression curve for thickness versus age. (From Pensler J, McCarthy JG: The calvarial donor site: an anatomic study in cadavers. Plast Reconstr Surg 1985;75:648.)

PRESENCE OF DIPLOIC SPACE WITH AGE

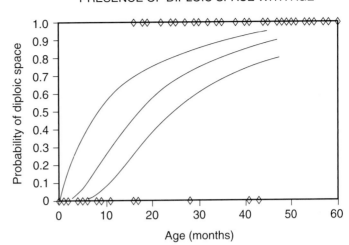

FIGURE 67-44. Probit model analysis for presence or absence of diploic space versus natural log of age. Each diamond represents one patient and indicates age and presence (1) or absence (0) of a diploic space. The central line is the probit estimate for the probability of a diploic space. The outer lines reflect the 95% confidence interval for the probability estimate. (From Pensler J, McCarthy JG: The calvarial donor site: an anatomic study in cadavers. Plast Reconstr Surg 1985;75:648.)

Supraorbital Fractures

Supraorbital fractures involve the superior portion of the orbital rim and orbital roof.[185,248-252] These fractures either may be localized, involving small fragments of the superior orbital rim alone, or may extend to involve much of the lateral portion of the frontal bone and entire two thirds of the lateral frontal and temporal (supraorbital) area (Figs. 67-45 and 67-46). This more extensive supraorbital fracture is known as the lateral frontal-temporal-orbital fracture.[253]

Supraorbital fractures may be diagnosed by identifying a depression, step, or level discrepancy in the contour of the supraorbital rim. A spectacle hematoma is present. Hypesthesia may be present in the distribution of the supraorbital nerve. The roof of the orbit

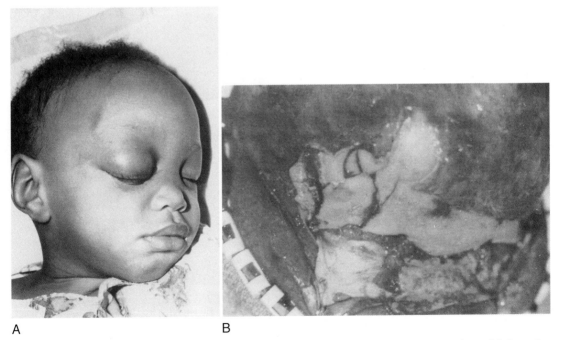

A   B

FIGURE 67-45. *A,* A 3-year-old who sustained a severe right-sided supraorbital fracture after a fall down the stairs. *B,* Intraoperative view showing the extent and comminution of the frontal-temporal-orbital fracture. (*B* from Dufresne CR, Manson PN: Pediatric facial trauma. In McCarthy JG, ed: Plastic Surgery. Philadelphia, WB Saunders, 1990:1142.)

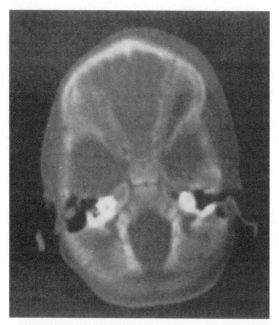

FIGURE 67-46. CT scan of a young child who sustained a right-sided supraorbital fracture. (From Dufresne CR, Manson PN: Pediatric facial trauma. In McCarthy JG, ed: Plastic Surgery. Philadelphia, WB Saunders, 1990:1142.)

Lacerations should not be extended because this maneuver results in unnecessary visible scarring. The bone fragments are replaced in proper position, and each is connected to adjacent intact bone, stabilized with rigid fixation or interfragment wires. If a bone graft is necessary to restore continuity in the supraorbital rim or orbital roof, it should be thin and may be placed superior to the edges of the adjacent intact orbital roof (within the intracranial cavity). Frontal lateral-temporal-orbital fractures require neurosurgical exposure and treatment of epidural hematoma, brain injury, or dural lacerations.[176,177]

Whenever a supraorbital fracture or globe injury is suspected, a thorough visual screening examination must be performed. The basic visual screening examination consists of an evaluation of visual acuity; confrontation fields, extraocular motion, pupil size and reactivity, and diplopia assessment; examination of the anterior and posterior chambers; and determination of intraocular pressure. The muscle involved in the production of diplopia may be identified by determining the field in which the diplopia is produced.[176,177] This may be accomplished by analysis of the CT scan and a forced duction examination. The necessity of operative intervention, which is often required in orbital floor fractures, is uncommon for diplopia alone in supraorbital fractures.

is generally involved and depressed inferiorly. The depression of the roof pushes the globe inferiorly and anteriorly, and the patient demonstrates exophthalmos and inferior globe displacement (Figs. 67-47 and 67-48). Paralysis of the levator muscle may produce a partial or complete ptosis. The patient may be unable to rotate the eye upward because of direct muscle contusion or involvement of the motor nerves in the superior orbital fissure. Severe fractures extending into the superior orbital fissure may produce a superior orbital fissure syndrome (Fig. 67-49). When it is complete, the syndrome produces paralysis of all the extraocular muscles, complete ptosis, and anesthesia in the ophthalmic division of the trigeminal nerve. When the fracture extends to the optic foramen, the orbital apex syndrome may be produced, consisting of the superior orbital fissure syndrome and blindness.[147,184,193,194,198]

Radiographic evaluation of the supraorbital fracture consists of a CT scan with axial and coronal sections.[254] A craniofacial CT scan is mandatory for the evaluation of the brain and orbit or for the exact determination of the pattern of the frontal and orbital fractures and their displacement.[147,194]

Open reduction of a supraorbital fracture may rarely be accomplished through a cutaneous laceration, but a coronal incision is usually required.

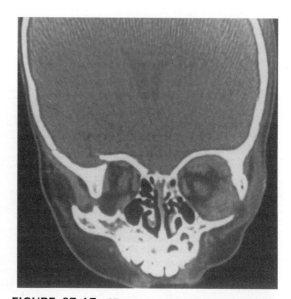

FIGURE 67-47. CT cross section demonstrating the mechanism by which a frontal-temporal-orbital fracture results in an ipsilateral exophthalmos. The lateral orbital wall compression results in reduced volume of the orbit, and the orbital contents are pushed anteriorly. (From Dufresne CR, Manson PN: Pediatric facial trauma. In McCarthy JG, ed: Plastic Surgery. Philadelphia, WB Saunders, 1990:1142.)

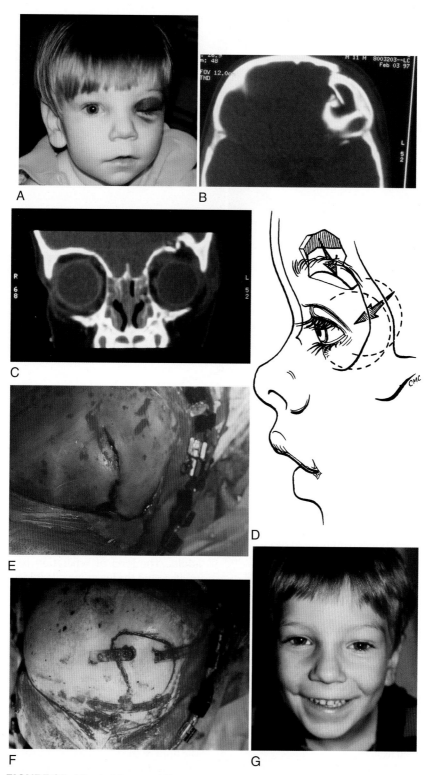

FIGURE 67-48. *A,* A 2-year-old boy who fell from a second-story balcony with trauma to the frontal area; he sustained a supraorbital fracture and dural tears. Also evident is left orbital proptosis and ecchymosis. *B* and *C,* Displacement of the orbital rim and frontal bone. *D,* Diagram of mechanism of deformity. *E,* The orbital-frontal fracture. *F,* The repaired dural and frontal bone with absorbable plates. *G,* The 2-year follow-up with no adverse sequelae of growth.

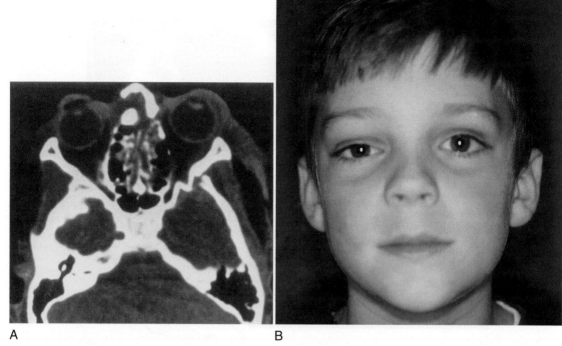

A   B

FIGURE 67-49. *A,* Frontal-temporal-orbital fracture that has resulted in collapse and compression of the structures of the superior orbital fissure (superior orbital fissure syndrome). Note the irregularities of the greater wing of the sphenoid. *B,* Deformity of right eye from nonreduced supraorbital fracture. (*A* from Dufresne CR, Manson PN: Pediatric facial trauma. In McCarthy JG, ed: Plastic Surgery. Philadelphia, WB Saunders, 1990:1142.)

Compound, Multiple, and Comminuted Midfacial Fractures

In trauma of particularly severe violence, lacerations with partial avulsion of the soft tissues and multiple fractures of the facial bones require serial surgical procedures to prevent facial disfigurement (Fig. 67-50 and Table 67-10).[94,255-257]

TABLE 67-10 ✦ PRINCIPLES FOR MANAGEMENT OF COMPLEX CRANIAL-ORBITAL FRACTURES

Accurate assessment of the deformity
Early reconstruction
Complete exposure of the involved craniofacial skeleton
Accurate anatomic reduction of the fracture fragments
Use of rigid internal fixation
Autogenous cranial bone grafting
Follow-up should include serial photographs, three-dimensional computed tomographic imaging, and cephalometric analysis to study growth.

From Denny AD, Rosenberg MW, Larson DL: Immediate reconstruction of complex cranioorbital fractures in children. J Craniofac Surg 1993;4:8.

Partly or nearly totally avulsed flaps of soft tissue and loose comminuted bone fragments should be preserved and replaced. The blood supply of the face (particularly in children) is generally adequate for tissue survival and for prevention of infection.

Maxillary fractures in children are classified as in adults. The level of separation between the upper midface and the lower maxilla is identified and forms the basis for the Le Fort maxillary classification.[13] The common terminology is consistent with that described by Le Fort. The Le Fort I or horizontal maxillary fracture separates the maxillary alveolus from the remainder of the upper midfacial skeleton. The fracture lines run horizontally from the base of the piriform aperture and extend across the nasomaxillary and zygomaticomaxillary buttresses. These fractures are infrequent in young children because of the absence of the maxillary sinuses. With the development of the permanent dentition, the tooth buds disappear and the floor of the maxillary sinus reaches the level of the floor of the nose. This alteration in bone configuration with permanent dentition weakens the bone structure at the Le Fort I level significantly and predisposes to the occurrence of a Le Fort I fracture.[81,84,117] This is the predominant shape of the fracture fragment in young children.

The Le Fort II or pyramidally shaped central midface segment is separated from the adjacent zygomatic portions of the facial skeleton. The maxillary alveolus, medial orbit, and nose thus move as a single segment.[81,117]

The Le Fort III fracture, or craniofacial dysjunction, separates the facial bones from the cranial skeleton through the orbits. The highest fracture lines extend from the zygomaticofrontal junction across the lateral orbit and orbital floor and either enter the nasoethmoid area to cause a dysjunction of the nose from the frontal bone or comminute the nasoethmoid area to produce a nasoethmoidal-orbital fracture. Le Fort III fractures are rarely a single fragment and usually exist as comminuted combinations of lesser Le Fort fragments, such as unilateral or bilateral zygomatic fractures and a Le Fort II fracture. The superior level of the fracture observed is usually higher (in terms of Le Fort classification) on one side than on the other. It is common, for example, to see a Le Fort III superior level fracture on one side with a Le Fort II superior level fracture on the other. In this

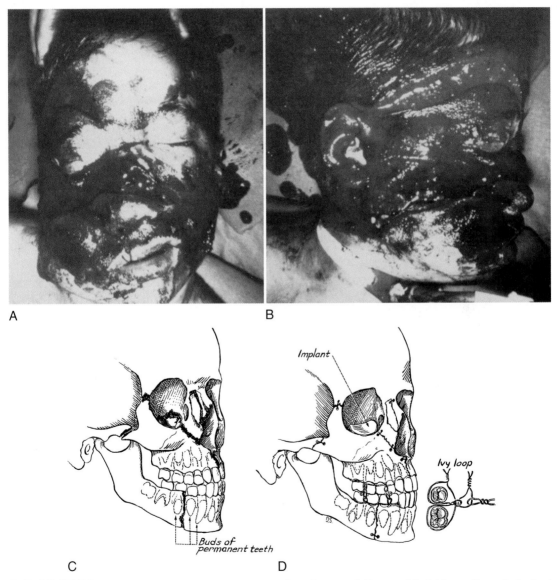

A B

C D

FIGURE 67-50. A 5-year-old boy struck by a descending elevator. *A,* Extent of facial lacerations. *B,* Avulsed flaps of soft tissue. He also sustained partial lacerations of the buccal branches of the facial nerve and division of Stensen duct. *C,* Sites of fractures. *D,* The orbital blowout fracture was repaired by a Silastic implant. Other fractures were treated by realignment and internal fixation with plates and screws. *Continued*

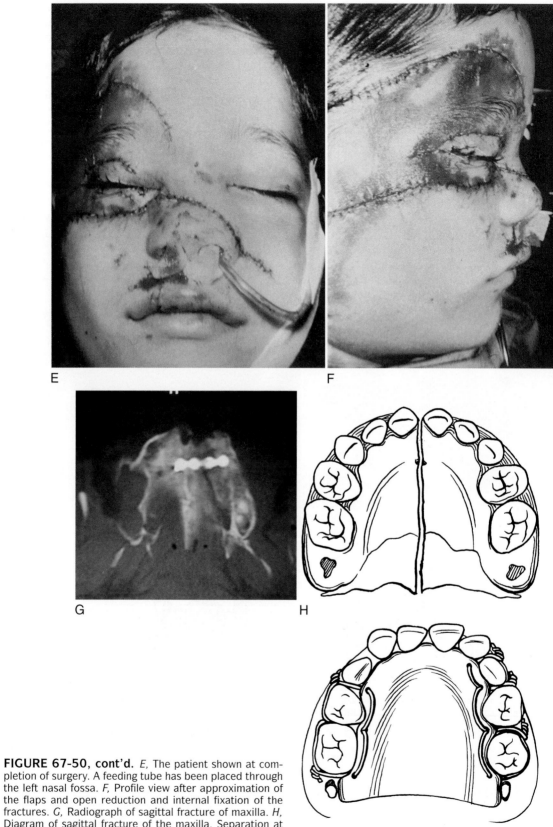

FIGURE 67-50, cont'd. *E,* The patient shown at completion of surgery. A feeding tube has been placed through the left nasal fossa. *F,* Profile view after approximation of the flaps and open reduction and internal fixation of the fractures. *G,* Radiograph of sagittal fracture of maxilla. *H,* Diagram of sagittal fracture of the maxilla. Separation at the midline. *I,* Treatment with a lingual splint.

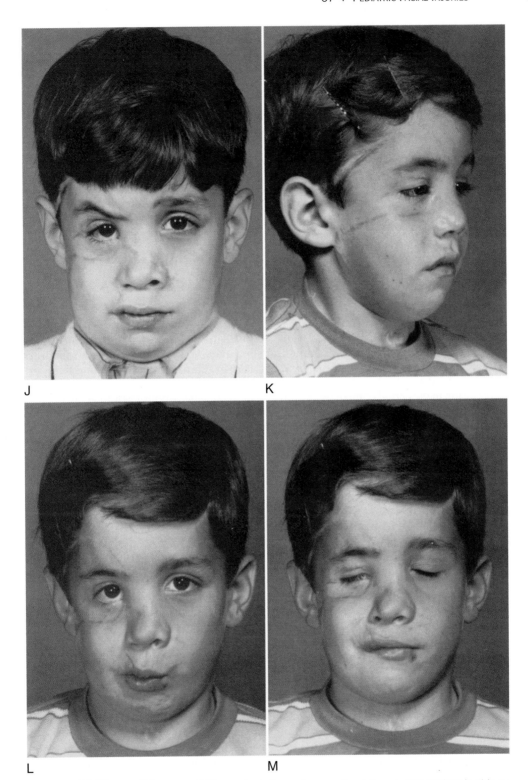

J   K

L   M

FIGURE 67-50, cont'd. *J* and *K,* The patient shown 1 year after injury. *L,* The patient is able to whistle without associated movements of the eyelids. *M,* When the patient closes his eyelids, associated movement of the right upper lip is noted. This is from "crossed innervation" by regrowth of facial nerves into other branches. (*A* to *F* and *J* to *M* from Dufresne CR, Manson PN: Pediatric facial trauma. In McCarthy JG, ed: Plastic Surgery. Philadelphia, WB Saunders, 1990:1142. *H* from Hendrickson M, Clark N, Manson PN, et al: Palatal fractures: classification, patterns, and treatment with rigid internal fixation. Plast Reconstr Surg 1998;101:319.)

situation, the fractured fragments consist of a Le Fort II segment carrying the maxillary dentition accompanied by a zygomatic fracture on the Le Fort III side. A single-fragment Le Fort III fracture can be suspected when bilateral periorbital ecchymoses are accompanied by slight occlusal abnormalities.[81,117] These fractures produce a subtle disturbance of occlusion and are easily missed or overlooked. The maxilla is not mobile; thus, the fracture is incomplete, and the displacement can be minimal.

The midpalatal suture running sagittally does not complete ossification until the end of the second decade of life. It is thus common to see a hemipalatal fracture dividing the maxillary alveolus in segments. Hemi-Le Fort fractures may also accompany the split palatal fractures. A palatal fracture is often suggested by an accompanying laceration of the lip, alveolus, or palate. A palatal fracture may be documented on a CT scan or on plain films of the palate taken with an occlusal dental radiograph (Fig. 67-50G).[147,191]

The diagnosis of a Le Fort fracture is usually confirmed by maxillary mobility or malocclusion. In rare instances, because of greenstick fracture or impaction, the maxilla is not mobile, but a malocclusion can be observed. It may be difficult to confirm a minor malocclusion in the period of mixed dentition. Accompanying fractures, such as zygomatic, orbital, and nasoethmoidal-orbital fractures, are commonly associated with Le Fort fractures; the Le Fort III fracture usually consists of the upper fractures in association with a mobile maxillary alveolus at the Le Fort I or II level. If no primary treatment is rendered for several days, the midface is usually elongated and retruded. The maxilla drops downward, especially posteriorly, and an anterior open bite is present. Profuse nasopharyngeal bleeding usually accompanies a Le Fort fracture. Facial swelling may be massive and impressive and is usually bilateral. A CSF leak may accompany high Le Fort II or III fractures, and pneumocephalus may be present if the fractures extend to the cranial base.[117,147,191,194]

The radiographic evaluation of a Le Fort fracture consists of a CT scan in axial and coronal planes. Bone and soft tissue windows are prepared for precise evaluation of the orbits, nasoethmoid, and maxillary areas.

The treatment of Le Fort fractures consists of placing the patient in intermaxillary fixation in occlusion. Open reduction and rigid fixation are performed at all of the levels of fracture (see Chapter 66). A unicortical screw placement system may be required to avoid the teeth. The maxilla is usually stable within 2 to 4 weeks in children. In patients with a split palate, open reduction with small plates and screws is performed in the palatal vault and at the piriform margin in addition to the four maxillary buttresses. Alternatively, a palatal acrylic splint should be placed to ensure the precise relationship of the halves of the maxillary

alveolus. Dental impressions are taken and stone models are prepared. The models are sectioned at the sites of the fracture and repositioned. A splint is made to fit the repositioned model. It may be necessary to retain a splint longer than 4 weeks if mobility is demonstrated in the fracture of the palate after release of intermaxillary fixation.[81,117,177,182]

Open reduction and plating are preferred for the treatment of upper facial fractures involving the orbit and nasoethmoidal-orbital area, as described in previous sections on zygoma, nasoethmoidal-orbital, and orbital floor fracture treatment. The vertical buttresses of the mid and upper face are restored by plate and screw fixation.[177,182] In general, exposure of the lower fractures at the Le Fort I level is performed for rigid fixation of the fractured areas. Care must be taken to avoid screw penetration of tooth buds. Soft tissue replacement onto the reassembled craniofacial skeleton and closure of the soft tissue in layers are especially important.[154,258]

Open reduction eliminates the need for suspension wires in midface fracture treatment, but arch bars may require support with piriform aperture or skeletal wires in patients with missing teeth, primary or mixed dentition, or alveolar fractures. The difficulty of ligating deciduous teeth to an arch bar is secondary to the bulbous shape of the crowns of the primary teeth. The fact that the roots are shallow or incomplete allows the teeth to be easily extracted. In the period of mixed dentition, the resorbing root structure makes extrusion more likely. In some patients, the arch bar may be incorporated into a lingual or palatal splint, which assists stability, if alveolar fractures are present. Acrylic may also be applied to the arch bars for additional stability. Splints, where necessary, are secured with skeletal wires or with screws to basal bone of the palate or the piriform aperture. Wires to screws placed in the lower portions of the mandible basal bone (versus circummandibular wires) are used to stabilize the arch bars.

The treatment of combined maxillary and mandibular fractures involves ligation of arch bars to the maxillary and mandibular dentition and stabilization of these arch bars with skeletal wires attached to screws in basal bone (See Fig. 67-19C). The bars are used to place the patient in occlusion, with the teeth in proper relationship and in maximal intercuspation. Open reduction of the fractures is performed with rigid fixation. The intermaxillary fixation relationship is held for 2 to 4 weeks for soft tissue rest and until fracture healing has occurred or the patient is considered stable in terms of the rigid fracture fixation, which permits no further movement. For many patients, 2 weeks of maxillary rest in intermaxillary fixation in occlusion is followed by release of intermaxillary fixation with elastic guidance and frequent observation of the occlusion. More complicated fractures, such as comminuted maxillary, split palate, panfacial, and alveolar fractures, may require intermaxillary fixation for a more prolonged period. Patients released from intermaxillary fixation should be watched at least weekly for proper occlusal relationship until they are considered stable (at least 4 weeks). Because children heal more quickly than adults do, the period of intermaxillary fixation rarely exceeds 3 or 4 weeks in total. Intermaxillary fixation screws may be used but are less stable and have almost no options for postoperative occlusal adjustment. Complications result from intermaxillary fixation screws when proper positioning is not provided by multiple occlusal contacts.

The care of the patient in intermaxillary fixation with fractures involving the occlusion must include intermittent observation of the occlusal relationship and permit the adjustment of wires or elastic traction, as indicated.[259] The use of a splint in the presence of an alveolar fracture or missing teeth may prevent fracture segment tipping or collapse with reduction in the height necessary for the dentition. Overriding or telescoping of the segments of the dentition occurs when teeth are missing and may be prevented by a splint with an "occlusal stop" to provide for the missing dentition. The range of mandibular excursion should exceed 35 mm after therapy and ideally should approach 45 to 55 mm.[176]

Growth after midface osteotomies or fractures may be restricted[93,159,260]; this usually follows severe midface fractures sustained in young (<5 years) individuals. Growth after mandibular fractures may be impaired.[261-265] Demianczuk et al[154] noted that children younger than 4 years or older than 12 years rarely required orthognathic surgery to correct facial growth disturbances after mandibular fracture (which accounted for 14% of children's fractures). In contrast, 22% of children aged 4 to 7 years and 17% of children aged 8 to 11 years required orthognathic surgery to correct growth disturbances. The condyle was the most common site of mandibular fracture, and condylar fractures led to facial asymmetry most frequently. These are unusual data, but the thoroughness of the study implies that they are correct.

Rigid Fixation and Growth

Considerable study has involved the long-term effects of "rigid fixation" devices that are retained on the growing cranial maxillofacial skeleton. At least eight studies have documented that both rigid fixation and surgical manipulation have effects on growth that are proportional to the amount of surgical manipulation and hardware application, which are maximally seen when such manipulation occurs during a period of rapid craniofacial growth. In some of these studies, the surgical manipulations were not performed at the maximum period of growth.[78,146,266-278]

The growth of a bone is a complex process consisting of deposition and remodeling. In the maturing facial skeleton, multiple centers of remodeling and growth are present. The most rapid growth is usually seen in utero, but there are other growth spurts that vary in rate according to the anatomic area of the facial skeleton considered. The frontal cranium, for instance, has an earlier growth spurt than the condylar area (see Table 67-1). Some investigators believe that growth represents a composite interaction between facial soft tissues and bone.[43-46] Remodeling and growth occur as a complex process that can be affected by multiple soft tissue or bone processes, such as a soft tissue scar within an affected region. Excision of a bone area such as a suture does not produce as significant a disturbance as premature closure does. Most studies have shown mild (4% to 9%) differences in growth after miniplate fixation.[146,272,273] Lesser (2% to 3%) degrees of growth restriction were seen as a result of wire fixation. Two studies have shown that growth restriction is less with resorbable plates than with titanium but slightly more prominent than with wires. Most investigators have noted contralateral overgrowth opposite the side on which growth is restricted. Most investigators also think that the growth restriction is not as important as proper stable three-dimensional positioning and that the stability of reduction is far more important than possible growth restrictions.

At present, correlation of the results from animal models with the response in humans does not exist. Although some individuals have advocated abandoning miniplate and screw fixation in children, most others think that the stability and positional control afforded by plate and screw fixation far outweigh any potential adverse effect on growth, although this theory has not been able to be confirmed with precision in the human system. It would make sense to support the tentative conclusion that smaller plates and screws, which provide sufficient rigid internal fixation without as much tension, should be used. Routine plate removal, although advocated by some, is not recommended by most investigators. Plates and screws have greatly improved position control and maintenance of expansion of the facial skeleton. Their use is therefore still indicated, although a 5% growth restriction can be observed when growing structures are plated experimentally. Soft tissue damage on removal of plate and screw devices also is not a reason to avoid their use. Schweinfurth and Koltai,[23] in an excellent monograph on the biology of pediatric facial fractures, summarize the studies showing that patients with pediatric fractures have a small but defined degree of hypoplasia compared with unfractured peers. Children with a history of nasomaxillary fractures, studied during adolescence, were found to have elevation of the anterior palatal plane, reduction in the length of the premaxilla and nasal spine, decreased nasal projection, and modifications in the occlusal plane of the mandible. Rigid fixation, however, can also improve surgical results by providing increased survival of bone grafts.[270,271]

Translocation of Plates

Translocation of plates can occur after application in the growing skull. The plates may be found inside the calvaria; or in the cranium, the plates may translate to the inner surface of the calvaria and be found in or on the dura. This phenomenon has been observed in patients undergoing reoperation with congenital cranial deformities, particularly syndromic craniofacial surgery,[268,279] and has not been described in patients with facial injury.

Resorbable Fixation

Problems reported with metal plates and screws have included restriction of craniofacial growth, bone resorption secondary to stress shielding, increased incidence of infection, extrusion, palpability, and cold sensitivity. Investigators have also been concerned about metalosis, or migration of metal degradation products occurring through the process of fretting corrosion.[158,180,280] Conceptually, biodegradable rigid fixation can easily eliminate a majority of these problems because the material provides adequate fixation for a finite interval corresponding to the time of bone repair.[278,281-283] Biodegradable plate and screw systems are now offered and consist of polyglyconate and polylactate; they have been proved to be successful in the cranium and areas where light fixation strength is required. They are beginning to be used in the mandible, but because of the contamination with oral flora in many mandibular fractures, clinical applications in this area have been restricted. Suuronen et al[280] have done extensive laboratory and clinical investigation of biodegradable bone plates and screws. Similarly, Turvey et al[284] found that the use of self-reinforced polylactite bone plates and screws to stabilize elective maxillary and mandibular osteotomies has been favorable on short-term observation; 3% of the patients experienced problems that resulted in immediate loosening of the bone screws. Edwards et al[285] used resorbable devices for genioplasty, and they have been enthusiastic supporters of this method of fixation.

Kumar et al[281] have advocated bioresorbable plates and screws in pediatric craniofacial surgery. Only 1 of 22 patients exhibited unsatisfactory wound healing or local inflammation. They found resorbable plates to provide satisfactory fixation, and they were not visible through the skin. Two patients had plates that were palpable at the 4-month follow-up. One patient, with repair of a blowout fracture of the orbit with resorbable mesh, had redness and swelling over the wound site 2 weeks postoperatively with resolution 4 weeks postoperatively. This early experience suggests that resorbable fixation, although it is an option for pediatric craniofacial surgery patients in the cranium, might be more susceptible to inflammation in the orbit. Whether dissolvable plates and screws represent the standard of care could be debated. Koltai et al[22] found rigid fixation with titanium to have advantages over traditional wire techniques. Of 62 children treated, 1 child required plate removal; 18 of the 62 had rigid fixation. There was one patient with sinusitis who required ethmoidectomy and maxillary antrostomy, and another patient who had perioperative sinusitis required antibiotics.

Imola et al[149] have also studied resorbable plate fixation in pediatric craniofacial surgery with an emphasis on long-term outcome. They observed 57 patients in whom resorbable plates and screws were used for fixation. Anatomic union and uncomplicated bone healing occurred in 96% of the patients. Plate extrusion or exposure occurred in 4%. These results were comparable to metal osteosynthesis, and costs were similar to existing metal fixation systems. Others have found more cost and increased inflammatory complications. Cost-benefit comparisons of metallic and absorbable plates are not supported in the authors' experience because resorbable systems are several times the cost. Imola[149] reported that success in fracture treatment in segmental repositioning and "low-stress" non-load-bearing areas of the middle and upper craniofacial skeleton proved this technique represented an advance in pediatric craniofacial surgery because plate removal would no longer be necessary. Extensive positive experience with resorbable fixation has been reported.[280,284-288] Others have noted problems of abscess formation, palpability, granuloma formation, slow resorption, redness, and infection. The authors generally prefer titanium fixation on the basis of familiarity, stability, cost, and extremely reliable performance with buttress stabilization.

COMPLICATIONS OF PEDIATRIC FACIAL TRAUMA

Multiple types of complications may follow pediatric facial trauma.[289] Pulmonary complications include aspiration of stomach contents; gastric dilation occurs in more than 25% of children in some series.[70,95,97,99] Some authors note that tracheostomy does not prevent this complication and suggest that a cuffed tube should consequently be employed. Early evacuation of the stomach contents by nasogastric tube is indicated as a preoperative or preanesthesia and postoperative or postanesthesia measure.[70,99] Sinus complications are potentially serious because of the proximity of the eye and brain.[290] Mucoceles[291,292] also follow frontal sinus fractures[293] and may produce mass lesions invading the orbit or brain.

Ocular injuries, damage to the lacrimal system, and CSF rhinorrhea are observed in children and must receive the same consideration that these complications require in the adult patient.[176] Nonunion occurs infrequently. Malunion is frequent in fractures undergoing late or closed reduction. Osteomyelitis (which at one time was a serious complication of fractures) is rarely seen with modern antibiotic therapy.[117,176]

Underdevelopment, maldevelopment, malocclusion, and ankylosis are all potential complications that can occur with facial trauma, particularly in facial bone fractures in those younger than 5 years.

Complications from facial fracture treatment occur in 10% to 20% of patients and relate to the organ system injured and the efficacy of treatment. Dental problems include delayed eruption of teeth, malformed teeth, loss of permanent teeth, and damage to tooth bud follicles.[294] Cystic or malignant degeneration of a tooth bud has not been observed. Tooth buds in the line of fracture usually survive with a 20% incidence of deformation of the crown.[59,65,295]

Other complications from orbital trauma include double vision, reduction in visual acuity, and lacrimal system obstruction. These result from scar tissue formation to the extraocular musculature and to the lacrimal drainage system.

CSF rhinorrhea is managed as in adults with primary repair of the dural tear at the time of the bone or brain surgery or delayed repair at 1 to 3 weeks if the CSF leak does not cease spontaneously.[98,296,297] Preoperative evaluation of the CSF leak by metrizamide or radionucleotide scan facilitates documentation of the location of the injury[298] and surgical repair. Late CSF leaks presenting months or years after the injury are unusual but almost always require surgical repair. Posttraumatic facial deformities are complications that may result from injuries to bone or soft tissue structures, uncorrected displacement of structures, or arrested development of growth centers or skeletal structures.[40,104,299-302] Overall, most children grow and develop normally after injury. However, some developmental malformations in adolescents and adults occasionally are the result of early trauma. Patients younger than 5 years with severe trauma to the mandibular condylar head or the nasoethmoid area seem most likely to develop skeletal growth disturbances.

THE ROLE OF RESTRAINTS IN VEHICULAR SAFETY

Murphy et al[15,16] examined 412 pediatric injuries for age and use of restraint systems. A Pennsylvania law requires that all children younger than 4 years be restrained by an infant seat or car seat appropriate for their age and weight. Of the 412 injuries, 17 patients were restrained with a car seat and 121 were wearing a seat belt; 30 children sustained facial fractures, and 50 children suffered facial lacerations. There is a statistically significant increase in the incidence of facial fractures with increasing age of the child. Of the facial fractures, 70% of the patients 5 to 12 years of age and 90% of patients 13 to 15 years of age were unrestrained. The authors concluded that despite legislation mandating the use of restraints, a large proportion of children involved in motor vehicle collisions were unrestrained. There also seemed to be a direct relationship between the age of the child and the incidence of facial fractures.

Holland et al[5] described a series of 46 children with 59 facial fractures presenting during a 4-year period. The mean age was 10 years. Motor vehicle, pedestrian, and cyclist injuries accounted for 63%. In 7 of the patients involved in motor vehicle accidents, the injury was sustained either in a front seat passenger or as a result of inappropriate restraints for age and size. In all but one patient, the presence of a fracture was associated with an overlying laceration, abrasion, or significant soft tissue edema. Facial CT was performed in 38 children, and all results were abnormal. Operative intervention was required for a facial fracture in 26 patients. Associated injuries of the head and limbs were common. Plain radiologic assessment only by a pediatric clinician led to diagnostic delay in 9 of the children. The study emphasized the importance of facial CT in diagnosis.

Arbogast[303] commented on the head and brain injury consequences of inappropriate seat belt use by children and thought that these mechanisms might also place a child at risk for facial fracture; 92 children were identified as suffering from fractures of the facial bones, representing 0.07% of all children in crashes. Among restrained children with facial fractures, patients inappropriately restrained were at a 1.6-fold higher risk of significant injury than were those appropriately restrained for their age. The investigators reported that excessive head excursion resulting from suboptimal torso restraint caused facial impact, resulting in the facial injuries described. They concluded that the potential for disfigurement associated with these facial injuries may strongly encourage parents to promote prevention and may provide additional motivation for proper restraint. They emphasized that appropriate infant restraints and placement of children in the rear seat are important precautions for the pediatric population.

Grisoni et al[304] evaluated pediatric air bag injuries of children in the front passenger seat. They seemed to be at greater risk of trauma from air bag deployment. The charts of children treated at three regional pediatric trauma centers in Ohio were evaluated; 27 children aged 1 month to 12 years sustained air

TABLE 67-11 ✦ PRINCIPLES FOR MANAGEMENT OF PEDIATRIC CRANIOFACIAL INJURIES

Maintain a high index of suspicion for maxillofacial injury in the pediatric patient, especially when multiple trauma exists.

In addition to careful physical examination, use CT scanning liberally on a routine basis, even for apparently trivial injuries.

Give consideration to "observation only" for minimally displaced fractures.

Respect the functional matrix and employ the least invasive surgical approach that will access the fracture and allow stable reduction to be achieved.

Employ methods of fixation that adequately stabilize the facial skeleton without rigidly immobilizing long segments.

If rigid internal stabilization is necessary, in the form of conventional plate and screw fixation, give consideration to interval removal.

Microplates appear to provide enough stability so that their use can be advocated whenever possible.

Avoid the use of alloplastic materials, especially in the very young patient.

Use bone grafts sparingly except in instances in which inlay reconstruction is necessary or onlay reconstruction is required to maintain soft tissue support.

Be aware of the pediatric dentition and avoid iatrogenic injury to evolving teeth and tooth buds.

From Bartlett SP, DeLozier JB 3rd: Controversies in the management of pediatric facial fractures. Clin Plast Surg 1992;19:245.

bag–related injuries, and 61% of the patients were girls. All crashes were at reported speeds of less than 45 mph, and 64% were head-on collisions. There were no significant differences between head, ocular and facial, and extremity fractures and numbers of deaths. Abdominal organ injury was exclusive to the restrained group. Decapitation occurred only among unrestrained children. These data indicate that air bags with or without proper safety restraints can lead to morbidity in children with respect to the abdomen. These data also emphasize that proper use of restraints is important in minimizing children's facial trauma. Margolis[17] has also related alcohol to the cause of children's injuries in motor vehicle accidents.

CONCLUSION

Facial injuries in children should be diagnosed early and precisely treated. Although some controversy exists in regard to exposure and fixation, Bartlett and DeLozier[106] have described 10 key principles in the management of craniofacial fractures in pediatric patients (Table 67-11). The necessity of documenting injuries was stressed thoroughly, including methods of treatment for observation of patients serially and detection of growth disturbances. There is good evidence that early definitive treatment minimizes deformity and maximizes function. In addition, evidence suggests that the invasive treatment described in this text does not produce growth disturbances and that the best long-term results are often produced by early open reduction and fixation of significant fractures.

REFERENCES

1. Adekeye EO: Pediatric fractures of the facial skeleton: a survey of 85 cases from Kaduna, Nigeria. J Oral Surg 1980;38:355.
2. Anderson PJ: Fractures of the facial skeleton in children. Injury 1995;26:47.
3. Bales CR, Randall P, Lehr HB: Fractures of the facial bones in children. J Trauma 1972;12:56.
4. Haller JA: Life-threatening injuries in children: what have we learned and what are the challenges? Bull Am Coll Surg 1995;80:9.
5. Holland AJ, Broome C, Steinberg A, Cass DT: Facial fractures in children. Pediatr Emerg Care 2001;17:157.
6. Manson PN, Vander Kolk CA, Dufresne CR: Facial injuries. In Oldham K, Faglia R, Colombani P, eds: Surgery of Infants and Children. Philadelphia, Lippincott-Raven, 1997:429.
7. Ramba J: Fractures of the facial bones in children. Int J Oral Surg 1985;14:472.
8. Agran PF, Dunkle DE: Motor vehicle occupant injuries to children in crash and noncrash events. Pediatrics 1982;70:993.
9. Agran PF, Dunkle DE, Winn DG: Motor vehicle childhood injuries caused by noncrash falls and ejections. JAMA 1985;253:2530.
10. Peng RY, Bongard FS: Pedestrian versus motor vehicle accidents: an analysis of 5,000 patients. J Am Coll Surg 1999;189:343.
11. Williams AF: Children killed in falls and motor vehicles. Pediatrics 1981;68:576.
12. Burdi AR, Huelke F, Snyder RG, Lowry AH: Infants and children in the adult world of automobile safety design: pediatric and anatomical considerations in design of child restraints. J Biomech 1969;1:167.
13. Gussack GS, Lutterman A, Rodgers K, et al: Pediatric maxillofacial trauma: unique features in diagnosis and treatment. Laryngoscope 1987;97:925.
14. Ellis E, Scott K: Assessment of patients with facial fractures. Emerg Med Clin North Am 2000;18:1.
15. Murphy RX, Birmingham KL, Okunski WJ, Wasser T: The influence of airbag and restraining devices on the patterns of facial trauma in motor vehicle collisions. Plast Reconstr Surg 2000;105:516.
16. Murphy RX, Birmingham KL, Okunski WJ, Wasser T: Influence of restraining devices on patterns of pediatric facial trauma in motor vehicle collisions. Plast Reconstr Surg 2001;107:34.
17. Margolis LH, Foss RD, Tolbert WG: Alcohol and motor vehicle-related deaths of children as passengers, pedestrians, and bicyclists. JAMA 2000;28:2245.
18. Dufresne CR: Unpublished data.
19. Tu A, Girotto A, Singh N, et al: Facial fractures from dog bite injuries. Plast Reconstr Surg 2002;109:1259.
20. Koltai P, Amjad I, Meyer D, Feustel P: Orbital fractures in children. Arch Otol Head Neck Surg 1995;121:1375.
21. Koltai PJ, Rabkin D: Management of facial trauma in children. Pediatr Clin North Am 1996;43:1253.
22. Koltai PJ, Rabkin D, Hoehn J: Rigid fixation of facial fractures in children. J Craniomaxillofac Trauma 1995;1:32.
23. Schweinfurth JM, Koltai PJ: Pediatric mandibular fractures. Facial Plast Surg 1998;14:31.
24. Xie C, Mehendale N, Barrett D, et al: 30-year retrospective review of frontal sinus fractures: the Charity Hospital experience. J Craniomaxillofac Trauma 2000;6:7.

25. Enlow DH: Handbook of Facial Growth, 2nd ed. Philadelphia, WB Saunders, 1982.

26. Johnson HA: A modification of the Gillies' temporalis transfer for the surgical treatment of lagophthalmos of leprosy. Plast Reconstr Surg 1962;30:378.

27. Harwood-Nash DC: Fractures of the petrous and tympanic parts of the temporal bone in children: a tomographic study of 35 cases. Am J Roentgenol 1970;110:598.

28. Scott JH: The analysis of facial growth from fetal life to adulthood. Angle Orthod 1963;33:110.

29. Scott JH: The cartilage of the nasal septum. Br Dent J 1953;95:37.

30. Scott JH: Further studies on the growth of the human face. Proc R Soc Med 1959;52:263.

31. Scott JH: Growth at facial sutures. Am J Orthod 1956;42:381.

32. Bernstein L: Maxillofacial injuries in children. Otol Clin North Am 1969;2:397.

33. Bernstein L: Pediatric sinus problems. Otol Clin North Am 1971;4:126.

34. Fearon B, Edmonds B, Bird R: Orbito-facial complications of sinusitis in children. Laryngoscope 1979;89:947.

35. Brook I, Friedman EM: Intracranial complications of sinusitis in children. Ann Otol Rhinol Laryngol 1982;91(pt 1):41.

36. Hellman LM, Pritchard JA, eds: William's Obstetrics, 14th ed. New York, Appleton-Century-Crofts, 1971.

37. Hellman M: The face in its developmental career. In The Human Face: A Symposium. Philadelphia, Dental Cosmos, 1935.

38. Siegel MI: Mechanisms of early maxillary growth. J Oral Surg 1976;34:106.

39. Moss ML, Rankow R: The role of the functional matrix in mandibular growth. Angle Orthod 1968;38:95.

40. Ortiz-Monasterio F, Olmedo A: Corrective rhinoplasty before puberty: a long-term follow-up. Plast Reconstr Surg 1981; 68:381.

41. Muller D: Long-term results after rhinoplasty of nose trauma in childhood. Laryngol Rhinol Otol 1983;62:116.

42. Hellquist R: Facial skeleton growth after periosteal resection. Scand J Plast Reconstr Surg Hand Surg Suppl 1972;10:1.

43. Moss ML: The primacy of functional matrices in orofacial growth. Dent Pract Dent Rec 1968;19:65.

44. Moss ML, Salentijn L: The primary role of functional matrices in facial growth. Am J Orthod 1969;55:566.

45. Moss ML: Vertical growth of the human face. Am J Orthod 1964;50:359.

46. Moss ML, Bromberg BE, Song JC, et al: The passive role of nasal septal cartilage in mid-facial growth. Plast Reconstr Surg 1968;41:536.

47. Moss ML, Salentijn L: The capsular matrix. Am J Orthod 1969;56:474.

48. Moss ML, Young RW: A functional approach to craniology. Am J Phys Anthropol 1960;18:281.

49. Mustarde JC: Facial injuries in children. In Mustarde JC, ed: Plastic Surgery in Infancy and Childhood. Philadelphia, WB Saunders, 1971:178.

50. Sarnat BG: The face and jaws after surgical experimentation with the septovomeral region in growing and adult rabbits. Acta Otolaryngol Suppl (Stockh) 1970;268:1.

51. Sarnat BG, Gans BJ: Growth of bones: methods of assessing and clinical importance. Plast Reconstr Surg 1952;9:140.

52. Sarnat BG, Gans BJ: Growth of bones: methods of assessing and clinical importance. Plast Reconstr Surg 1952;52:263.

53. Sarnat BG, Wexler MR: Growth of the face and jaws after resection of the septal cartilage in the rabbit. Am J Anat 1966; 118:755.

54. Sarnat BG, Wexler MR: Rabbit snout growth after resection of central linear segments of nasal septal cartilage. Acta Otol 1967;63:467.

55. Langford R, Sgourus S, Natarajan K, et al: Maxillary volume growth in childhood. Plast Reconstr Surg 2003;111:1591.

56. Langford R, Sgourus S, Natarajan K, et al: Maxillary volume growth in craniosynostosis. Plast Reconstr Surg 2004;111:598.

57. May M, Fria TJ, Blumenthal F, Curtin H: Facial paralysis in children: differential diagnosis. Otolaryngol Head Neck Surg 1981;89:841.

58. Shapiro PA, Kokvich VG, Hohl TH: The effects of early LeFort I osteotomies on craniofacial growth of juvenile *Macaca nemestrina* monkeys. Am J Orthod 1981;79:49.

59. Andreasen JO: Fracture of the alveolar process of the jaw. A clinical and radiographic follow-up study. Scand J Dent Res 1970;78:362.

60. Andreasen JO: Luxation of permanent teeth due to trauma. Scand J Dent Res 1970;78:273.

61. Andreasen JO: Etiology and pathogenesis of traumatic dental injuries. A clinical study of 1,298 cases. Scand J Dent Res 1970;78:439.

62. Andreasen JO: Treatment of fractured and avulsed teeth. J Dent Child 1971;28:29.

63. Andreasen JO, Andreasen FM: Essentials of Traumatic Injuries of the Teeth, 2nd ed. St. Louis, Mosby, 2000.

64. Andreasen JO, Ravn JJ: The effect of traumatic injuries to primary teeth on their permanent successors. II. A clinical and radiographic follow-up study of 213 teeth. Scand J Dent Res 1971;79:284.

65. Andreasen JO, Sundstrom B, Ravn JJ: The effect of traumatic injuries to primary teeth on their permanent successors. I. A clinical and histologic study of 117 injuries to permanent teeth. Scand J Dent Res 1971;79:219.

66. Lehman JA Jr, Saddawi ND: Fractures of the mandible in children. J Trauma 1976;16:773.

67. Ziccardi VB, Ochs MW, Braun TW, Malave DA: Management of condylar fractures in children: review of the literature and case presentations. Compend Contin Educ Dent 1995;16(9):874.

68. Reil B, Kranz S: Traumatology of the maxillofacial region in childhood. J Maxillofac Surg 1976;4:197.

69. Freid MG, Baden E: Management of fractures in children. J Oral Surg 1954;12:129.

70. McCoy FJ, Chandler RA, Crow ML: Facial fractures in children. Plast Reconstr Surg 1966;37:209.

71. Hall RK: Facial trauma in children. Aust Dent J 1974;19:336.

72. Kaban LB: Diagnosis and treatment of fractures of the facial bones in children 1943-1993. J Oral Maxillofac Surg 1993; 51:722.

73. Kaban LB, Mulliken JB, Murray JE: Facial fractures in children: an analysis of 122 fractures in 109 patients. Plast Reconstr Surg 1977;59:15.

74. Mayer T, Matlak ME, Johnson DG, Walker ML: The modified injury severity scale in pediatric multiple trauma patients. J Pediatric Surg 1980;15:719.

75. Tanaika N, Uchide N, Suzuki K: Maxillofacial fractures in children. J Craniomaxillofac Surg 1993;21:289.

76. McGraw L, Cole RR: Pediatric maxillofacial trauma: age related variations in injury. Arch Head Neck Surg 1990;116:41.

77. Bamjee Y, Lownie JF, Cleaton-Jones PE, Lownie MA: Maxillofacial injuries in a group of South Africans under 18 years of age. Br J Oral Maxillofac Surg 1996;34:298.

78. Posnick JC: The role of plate and screw fixation in the treatment of pediatric facial fractures. In Gruss JS, Manson PM, Yaremchuk MJ, eds: Rigid Fixation of the Craniomaxillofacial Skeleton. Stoneham, Mass, Butterworth, 1992:396.

79. Posnick J, Wells M, Pron GE: Pediatric facial fractures: evolving patterns of treatment. J Oral Maxillofac Surg 1993;51:836, discussion 844.

80. Goldman JL, Ganzel TM, Ewing JE: Priorities in the management of penetrating maxillofacial trauma in the pediatric patient. J Craniomaxillofac Trauma 1996;2:52.

81. Dingman RO, Natvig P: Facial fractures in children. In Dingman RO, Natvig P: Surgery of Facial Fractures. Philadelphia, WB Saunders, 1964:311.

82. Georgiade NG, Pickrell KL: Treatment of maxillofacial injuries in children. J Int Coll Surg 1967;27:640.

83. Georgiade NG, Pickrell KL, Douglas W, Altarug F: Extraoral pinning of displaced condylar fractures. Plast Reconstr Surg 1956;18:383.

84. Converse JM: Facial injuries in children. In Mustarde JC, ed: Plastic Surgery in Infancy and Childhood. Edinburgh, Churchill Livingstone, 1979.

85. Rowe NL, Williams JC: Children's fractures. In Rowe NL, Williams JC: Maxillofacial Injuries. New York, Churchill Livingstone, 1985:538.

86. Zerfowski M, Bremerich A: Facial trauma in children and adolescents. Clin Oral Investig 1998;2:120.

87. Tsai RY, Zee CS, Apthorp JS, Dixon GH: Computed tomography in child abuse head trauma. J Comput Tomogr 1980;4:277.

88. Chacon GE, Dawson KH, Myall RW, Beirne OR: A comparative study of 2 imaging techniques for the diagnosis of condylar fractures in children. J Oral Maxillofac Surg 2003;61:668.

89. Waitzman AA, Posnick JC, Armstrong DC, Pron GE: Craniofacial skeletal measurements based on computer tomography: I. Accuracy and reproducibility. Cleft Palate Craniofac J 1992; 29:112.

90. Waitzman AA, Posnick JC, Armstrong DC, Pron GE: Craniofacial skeletal measurements based on computer tomography: II. Normal and growth trends. Cleft Palate Craniofac J 1992; 29:129.

91. Nimkin K, Kleinman PK: Imaging of child abuse. Radiol Clin North Am 2001;39:4.

92. Barsness KA, Cha ES, Bensard DD, et al: The positive predictive value of rib fractures as an indicator of nonaccidental trauma in children. J Trauma 2003;45:1107.

93. Freihofer HP Jr: Results of osteotomies of the facial skeleton in adolescence. J Maxillofac Surg 1977;5:267.

94. Posnick JC: Management of facial fractures in children and adolescents [review]. Ann Plast Surg 1994;33:442.

95. Oliver P, Richardson JR, Clubb RW, Flake CA: Tracheotomy in children. N Engl J Med 1962;276:631.

96. Bridges CP, Ryan RF, Longenecker CG, Vincent RW: Tracheostomy in children: a twenty year study at Charity Hospital in New Orleans. Plast Reconstr Surg 1966;37:117.

97. Othersen HB Jr: Intubation injuries of the trachea in children. Management and prevention. Ann Surg 1979;189:601.

98. Rasmussen PS: Acute traumatic liquorrhea. Acta Neurol Scand 1965;41:441.

99. McCoy FJ, Chandler RA, Magnan CG, et al: An analysis of facial fractures and their complications. Plast Reconstr Surg 1962;29:381.

100. McCoy FJ: Late results in facial fractures. In Goldwyn RM, ed: Long-term Results in Plastic and Reconstructive Surgery, vol II. Boston, Little, Brown, 1980:484.

101. Jazbi B: Subluxation of the nasal septum in the newborn: etiology, diagnosis and treatment. Otolaryngol Clin North Am 1977;10:125.

102. Keith A, Campion C: A contribution to the mechanism of growth of the human face. Int J Orthod 1922;8:607.

103. Roemer FJ: Relation of torticollis to breach delivery. Am J Obstet Gynecol 1954;68:1146.

104. Bruneteau RJ, Mulliken JB: Frontal plagiocephaly: synostotic, compensational or deformational. Plast Reconstr Surg 1992;89:21.

105. Lindenberg R, Fisher RS, Dunlacher S, et al: The pathology of the brain in blunt head injuries of infants and children. Proceedings, 2nd International Congress of Neuropathology, vol 1. Amsterdam, Excerpta Medica, 1955:477.

106. Bartlett SP, DeLozier JB 3rd: Controversies in the management of pediatric facial fractures. Clin Plast Surg 1992;19:245.

107. Sedlak AJ, Broadhurst DD: The Third National Incidence Study of Child Abuse and Neglect (NIS-3). Washington, DC, US Department of Health and Human Services, 1996.

108. American Academy of Pediatrics: Oral and dental aspects of child abuse and neglect. Policy Statement. Pediatrics 1999; 104:348.

109. American Academy of Pediatrics: Guidelines for evaluation of sexual abuse in children: subject review. Pediatrics 1999; 103:186.

110. Wolff KD: Management of animal bite injuries of the face: experience with 94 patients. J Oral Maxillofac Surgery 1998;56:838.

111. Caffey J: Multiple fractures in the long bones of infants suffering from chronic subdural hematoma. AJR Am J Roentgenol 1946;56:163.

112. Caffey J: The whiplash shaken infant syndrome: manual shaking by the extremities with whiplash-induced intracranial and intraocular bleedings, linked with residual permanent brain damage and mental retardation. Pediatrics 1974;54:396.

113. Worlock P, Stower M, Barbor P: Patterns of fractures in accidental and nonaccidental injury in children. Br Med J 1986; 293:100.

114. American Academy of Pediatrics: When inflicted skin injuries constitute child abuse. Pediatrics 2002;110:644.

115. Haug RH, Foss J: Maxillofacial injuries in the pediatric patient. Oral Surg Oral Med Oral Pathol Oral Radiol Endod 2000; 90:126.

116. Tate RJ: Facial injuries associated with the battered child syndrome. Br J Oral Surg 1971;9:41.

117. Converse JM, Dingman RO: Facial injuries in children. In Converse JM, ed: Reconstructive Plastic Surgery. Philadelphia, WB Saunders, 1977:794.

118. Manson PN, Iliff N, Robertson B: Discussion: trapdoor fracture of the orbit in a pediatric population. Plast Reconstr Surg 2002;109:490.

119. Datubo-Brown DD: Human bites of the face with tissue loss. Ann Plast Surg 1988;21:322.

120. Hallock GG: Dog bites of the face with tissue loss. J Craniofac Trauma 1996;2:49.

121. Silverman FN: The roentgen manifestations of unrecognized skeletal trauma in infants. Am J Roentgenol Radium Ther Nucl Med 1953;69:413.

122. Teasdale G, Jennett B: Assessment of coma and impaired consciousness. Lancet 1974;2:81.

123. Cohen RA, Kaufman RA, Myers PA, Towbin RB: Cranial computed tomography in the abused child with head injury. AJR Am J Roentgenol 1986;146:97.

124. Kravits H, Driessen G, Gomberg R, Korach A: Accidental falls from elevated surfaces in infants from birth to one year of age. Pediatrics 1969;44(suppl):869.

125. Moffett B: The morphogenesis of the temporomandibular joint. Am J Orthod 1966;52:401.

126. Steinhauser EW: The treatment of ankylosis in children. Int J Oral Surg 1973;2:129.

127. Kazanjian VH, Converse JM: The Surgical Treatment of Facial Injuries, 3rd ed. Baltimore, Williams & Wilkins, 1974.

128. Shand JM, Heggie AA: Maxillofacial injuries at the Royal Children's Hospital of Melbourne: a five year review. Ann R Australas Coll Dent Surg 2000;15:166.

129. Panagopoulos AP: Management of fractures of the jaws in children. J Int Coll Surg 1957;28:806.

130. Pfeifer G: Kieferbruche im Kindesalter und ihre Auswirkungen auf das Wachstum. Fortschr Kiefer Gesichtschir 1966;11:43.

131. Rowe NL: Fractures of the facial skeleton in children. J Oral Surg 1968;26:505.

132. Rowe NL: Fractures of the jaws in children. J Oral Surg 1969;27:497.

133. Rowe NL: Injuries to teeth and jaws. In Mustarde JC, ed: Plastic Surgery in Infancy and Childhood. Philadelphia, WB Saunders, 1971.

134. Rowe NL, Winter GB: Traumatic lesions of the jaws and teeth. In Mustarde JC, ed: Plastic Surgery in Infancy and Childhood. Philadelphia, WB Saunders, 1971:154.

135. Oji C: Fractures of the facial skeleton in children: a survey of patients under the age of 11 years. J Craniomaxillofac Surg 1998;26(5):322-325.

136. Sherick DG, Buchman SR, Patel PP: Pediatric facial fractures: analysis of differences in subspecialty care. Plast Reconstr Surg 1998;102:28.

137. Vanderas AP, Papagiannoulis L: Incidence of dentofacial injuries in children: a 2-year longitudinal study. Endod Dent Traumatol 1999;15:235.

138. Roed-Petersen B, Andreasen JO: Prognosis of permanent teeth involved in jaw fractures. Scand J Dent Res 1970;78:343.

139. Berkowitz R, Ludwig S, Johnson R: Dental trauma in children and adolescents. Clin Pediatr 1980;19:166.

140. MacLennan WD: Fractures of the mandible in children under the age of six years. Br J Plast Surg 1956;9:125.

141. MacLennan WD, Simpson W: Treatment of fractured mandibular condylar processes in children. Br J Plast Surg 1965;18:423.

142. Dawson RIG, Fordyce GL: Complex fractures of the middle third of the face and their early treatment. Br J Surg 1953;41:254.

143. Graham GG, Peltier RJ: Management of mandibular fractures in children. J Oral Surg 1960;18:416.

144. Dansforth HB: Mandibular fractures: use of acrylic splints for immobilization. Laryngoscope 1969;79:280.

145. Hagan EH, Huelke DF: An analysis of 319 case reports of mandibular fractures. J Oral Surg 1961;19:93.

146. Manson PN: Commentary on long-term effects of rigid fixation on the craniofacial skeleton. J Craniofac Surg 1991;2:69.

147. Manson PN, Shack RB, Leonard LG, et al: Sagittal fractures of the maxilla and palate. Plast Reconstr Surg 1983;72:484.

148. Khosla M, Boren W: Mandibular fractures in children and their management. J Oral Surg 1971;29:16.

149. Imola MJ, Hamlar DD, Shao W, et al: Resorbable plate fixation in pediatric craniofacial surgery: long-term outcome. Arch Facial Surg 2001;3:79.

150. Thoren H, Iizuka T, Hallikainen D, et al: Different patterns of mandibular fractures in children: an analysis of 220 fractures in 157 patients. J Craniomaxillofac Surg 1992;20:292.

151. Nahabedian MY, Tufaro A, Manson PN: Improved mandible function after hemimandibulectomy, condylar head preservation, and vascularized fibular reconstruction. Ann Plast Surg 2001;46(5):506.

152. Phillips J, Gruss J, Wells M: Periosteal suspension of the lower eyelid and cheek following subciliary exposure of facial fractures. Plast Reconstr Surg 1991;88:145.

153. Ferreira PC, Amarante J, Silva P, et al: Retrospective study of 1251 maxillofacial fractures in children and adolescents. Plast Reconstr Surg 2005;115(6):1500.

154. Demianczuk AN, Verchere C, Phillips JH: The effect on facial growth of pediatric mandibular fractures. J Craniofac Surg 1999;10:323.

155. Landtwing K: Evaluation of the normal range of vertical mandibular opening in children and adolescents with special reference to age and stature. J Maxillofac Surg 1978;6:157.

156. Anderson MF, Ailing CC: Subcondylar fractures in young dogs. Oral Surg 1985;19:263.

157. Fernandez JR: A three-dimensional numerical simulation of mandible fracture reduction with screwed miniplates. J Biomech 2003;36:329.

158. Winzenburg SM, Imola MJ: Internal fixation in pediatric maxillofacial fractures. Facial Plast Surg 1998;14:45.

159. Washburn MC, Schendel SA, Epker BN: Superior repositioning of the maxilla during growth. J Oral Maxillofac Surg 1982;40:142.

160. Blevins C, Gore RJ: Fractures of the mandibular condyloid process: results of conservative treatment in 140 patients. J Oral Surg 1961;19:392.

161. Boyne PJ: Osseous repair and mandibular growth after subcondylar fractures. J Oral Surg 1967;25:300.

162. Fortunato MA, Fielding AF, Guernsey LH: Facial bone fractures in children. Oral Surg 1982;53:225.

163. Profitt WR, Vig KW, Turvey TA: Early fractures of the mandibular condyles: frequently an unsuspected cause of growth disturbances. Am J Orthod 1980;78:1.

164. Lee CY, McCullon C III, Blaustein DI, Mohammadi H: Sequelae of unrecognized, untreated mandibular condylar fractures in the pediatric patient. Ann Dent 1993;52:5.

165. Walker RV: Traumatic mandibular condylar fracture dislocations: effect on growth in the *Macaca* rhesus monkey. Am J Surg 1960;100:850.

166. Walker DG: The mandibular condyle: fifty cases demonstrating arrest in development. Dent Pract 1957;7:160.

167. Hoopes JE, Wolfort FG, Jabaley ME: Operative treatment of fractures of the mandibular condyle in children using the post-auricular approach. Plast Reconstr Surg 1970;46:357.

168. Cascone P, Sassano P, Spallaccia F, et al: Condylar fractures during growth: follow-up of 16 patients. J Craniofac Surg 1999;10:87.

169. Lindahl L, Hollender L: Condylar fractures of the mandible: a radiographic study of remodeling processes in the temporomandibular joint. Int J Oral Surg 1977;6:153.

170. Norholt S, Krishnan V, Sindet-Pedersen S, Jensen I: Pediatric condylar fractures: a long-term follow-up study of 55 patients. J Oral Maxillofac Surg 1993;51:1302.

171. James D: Maxillofacial injuries in children. In Rowe NL, Williams JI, eds: Maxillofacial Injuries, vol I. London, Churchill Livingstone, 1985:538.

172. Huang CS, Ross RB: Surgical advancement of the retrognathic mandible in growing children. Am J Orthod 1982;82:89.

173. Topazian RG: Etiology of ankylosis of the temporomandibular joint. J Oral Surgery 1961;22:227.

174. Morgan BD, Madan DK, Bergerot JP: Fractures of the middle third of the face—a review of 300 cases. Br J Plast Surg 1972;25:147.

175. Iizuka T, Thoren H, Annino DJ Jr, et al: Midfacial fractures in pediatric patients. Frequency, characteristics, and causes. Arch Otolaryngol Head Neck Surg 1995;121:1366.

176. Schultz RC, Meilman J: Facial fractures in children. In Goldwyn RM, ed: Long-term Results in Plastic and Reconstructive Surgery. Boston, Little, Brown, 1980.

177. Schultz RC: Pediatric facial fractures. In Kernahan DA, Thompson HG, Bauer BS, eds: Symposium on Pediatric Plastic Surgery. St. Louis, CV Mosby, 1982.

178. Iida S, Matsuya T: Paediatric maxillofacial fractures: their aetiological characters and fracture patterns. J Craniomaxillofac Surg 2002;30:237.

179. Denny AD, Rosenberg MW, Larson DL: Immediate reconstruction of complex cranioorbital fractures in children. J Craniofac Surg 1993;4:8.

180. Triana RJ Jr, Shockley WW: Pediatric zygomatico-orbital complex fractures: the use of resorbable plating systems. A case report. J Craniomaxillofac Trauma 1998;4:32.

181. Manson PN, Hoopes JE, Su CT: Structural pillars of the facial skeleton: an approach to the management of Le Fort fractures. Plast Reconstr Surg 1980;66:54.

182. Manson PN, Crawley WA, Yaremchuk MJ, et al: Midface fractures: advantages of immediate extended open reduction and bone grafting. Plast Reconstr Surg 1985;76:1.

183. Riefkohl R, Georgiade N: Facial fractures in children. In Serafin D, Georgiade N, eds: Pediatric Plastic Surgery. St. Louis, CV Mosby, 1984.

184. Converse JM: Orbital and naso-orbital fractures. In Tessier P, Callahan A, Mustarde JC, Salyer KE, eds: Symposium on Plastic Surgery in the Orbital Region, vol 12. St. Louis, CV Mosby, 1976:79.

185. Gruss JS: Orbital roof fractures in the pediatric population. Plast Reconstr Surg 1989;84:217.

186. Roberts F, Shopfner CE: Plain skull roentgenograms in children with head trauma. Am J Roentgenol Radium Ther Nucl Med 1972;114:230.

187. Dingman RO: Symposium: malunited fractures of the zygoma. Repair of the deformity. Trans Am Acad Ophthalmol Otolaryngol 1953;57:889.

188. Manson P, Ruas E, Iliff N: Single eyelid incision for exposure of the zygomatic bone and orbital reconstruction. Plast Reconstr Surg 1987;79:120.

189. Glassman RD, Manson PN, Petty P, et al: Techniques for improved visibility and lid protection in orbital explorations. J Craniofac Surg 1990;1:69.

190. Pensler J, McCarthy JG: The calvarial donor site: an anatomic study in cadavers. Plast Reconstr Surg 1985;75:648.

191. Manson PN, Clifford CM, Su CT, et al: Mechanisms of global support and posttraumatic enophthalmos. I. The anatomy of the ligament sling and its relation to intramuscular cone orbital fat. Plast Reconstr Surg 1986;77:193.

192. Tessier P, Callahan A, Mustarde JC, Salyer KE, eds: Symposium on Plastic Surgery in the Orbital Region, vol 12. St. Louis, CV Mosby, 1976:67.

193. Furnas DW: Emergency diagnosis of the injured orbit. In Tessier P, Callahan A, Mustarde JC, Salyer KE, eds: Symposium on Plastic Surgery in the Orbital Region, vol 12. St. Louis, CV Mosby, 1976.

194. Manson PN, Grivas A, Rosenbaum A, et al: Studies on enophthalmos: II. The measurement of orbital injuries and their treatment by quantitative computed tomography. Plast Reconstr Surg 1986;77:203.

195. Manson PN, Iliff N: Orbital roof fractures. In Hornblass A, ed: Oculoplastic, Orbital, and Reconstructive Surgery. Baltimore, Williams & Wilkins, 1989.

196. Baker SM, Hurwitz JJ: Management of orbital and ocular adnexal trauma. Ophthalmol Clin North Am 1999;12:3.

197. Mizuno A, Nakamura T, Kanabata T, et al: Blow-out fracture of the orbit in 4 children. Int J Oral Surg 1985;14:284.

198. Zachariades N: The superior orbital fissure syndrome. Review of the literature and report of a case. Oral Surg 1982;53:237.

199. Furnas J: The eyelid traction test to detect instability in nasoethmoid fractures. Plast Reconstr Surg 1973;52:315.

200. Grant J, Patrinely J, Weiss A, et al: Trapdoor fracture of the orbit in a pediatric population. Plast Reconstr Surg 2002:109:480.

201. Bansagi ZC, Meyer DR: Internal orbital fractures in the pediatric age group. Ophthalmic Plast Reconstr Surg 2000; 107:829.

202. Iliff N, Manson P, Katz R, Rever L: Mechanisms of extraocular muscle injury in orbital fractures. Plast Reconstr Surg 1999;103:1313.

203. Converse JM, Smith B, Obear MF, Wood-Smith D: Orbital blow-out fracture: a ten-year survey. Plast Reconstr Surg 1967;29:20.

204. Putterman AM, Stevens T, Urist MJ: Nonsurgical management of fractures of the orbital floor. Am J Ophthalmol 1974;77:232.

205. Crysdale WS, Tatham B: External septorhinoplasty in children. Laryngoscope 1975;95:12.

206. Crysdale WS, Walker PJ: External septorhinoplasty in children: patient selection and surgical technique. J Otolaryngol 1994;23:28.

207. Dommerby H, Tos M: Nasal fractures in children—long-term results. ORL J Otorhinolaryngol Relat Spec 1985;47:272.

208. East CA, O'Donaghue G: Acute nasal trauma in children. J Pediatr Surg 1987;22:308.

209. Gilbert GG: Growth of the nose and the septo-rhinoplastic problem in youth. Arch Otolaryngol 1958;68:673.

210. Fry H: Nasal skeletal trauma and the interlocked stresses of the nasal septal cartilage. Br J Plast Surg 1967;20:146.

211. Grymer LF, Gutierrez C, Stokstead P: The importance of nasal fractures during differential growth periods on the nose. J Laryngol Otol 1985;99:741.

212. Grymer LF, Gutierrez C, Stokstead P: Nasal fractures in children: influence on the development of the nose. J Laryngol Otol 1985;99:735.

213. Miller JD, Becker DP, Ward JD, et al: Significance of intracranial hypertension in severe head injury. J Neurosurg 1977; 47:503.

214. Tucker CA: Management of early nasal injuries with long-term follow-up. Rhinology 1984;22:45.

215. Stolsted P, Schonsted-Madsen V: Traumatology of the newborn's nose. Rhinology 1979;17:77.

216. Stacher FJ, Bryarly RC, Shockley WW: Management of nasal trauma in children. Arch Otolaryngol 1984;11:190.

217. Winters HP: Isolated fractures of the nasal bones. Arch Chir Neerl 1967;19:159.

218. Walker PJ, Crysdale WS, Farkas LG: External septorhinoplasty in children: outcome and effect on growth of septal excision and reimplantation. Arch Otolaryngol Head Neck Surg 1993;119:984.

219. Mayell MJ: Nasal fractures: their occurrence, management and some later results. J R Coll Surg Edinb 1973;18:31.

220. Stucker FJ Jr, Bryarly C, Shockley WW: Management of nasal trauma in children. Arch Otolaryngol 1984;110:190.

221. O'Neal R, Dodenhoff R, McClatchey K: The role of perichondrium in modifying curved cartilage: an experimental study. Ann Plast Surg 1987;19:343.

222. Converse JM, Campbell RM: Bone grafts in surgery of the face. Surg Clin North Am 1954;34:365.

223. Morin JD, Hill JC, Anderson JE, Grainger RM: A study of growth in the interorbital region. Am J Ophthalmol 1963;56:895.

224. Markowitz B, Manson PN, Margent L, et al: Management of the medial canthal tendon in nasoethmoid orbital fractures—the importance of the central fragment in treatment and classification. Plast Reconstr Surg 1991;87:843.

225. Paskert J, Manson P: The bimanual examination for assessing instability in nasoethmoid orbital fractures. Plast Reconstr Surg 1989;83:165.

226. Bordley JE, Bosley WR: Mucoceles of the frontal sinus: causes and treatment. Ann Otol Rhinol Laryngol 1973;82:696.

227. Hendrick EB: The use of hypothermia in severe brain stem lesions in childhood. Arch Surg 1959;79:362.

228. Hendrick EB, Harwood-Nash DC, Hudson AR: Head injuries in children: a survey of 4465 consecutive cases at the Hospital for Sick Children. Clin Neurosurg 1964;11:46.

229. Gruszkiewicz J, Doron Y, Peyser E: Recovery from severe craniocerebral injury and brain stem lesions in childhood. Surg Neurol 1973;1:197.

230. Bruce DA, Alavi A, Bilaniuk L, et al: Diffuse cerebral swelling following head injuries in children: the syndrome of "malignant brain edema." J Neurosurg 1981;54:170.

231. Bruce DA, Schut L, Bruno LA, et al: Outcome following severe head injuries in children. J Neurosurg 1978;48:679.

232. Luce E: Frontal sinus fractures: guidelines to management. Plast Reconstr Surg 1987;80:500.

233. Berger MS, Pitts LH, Lovely M, et al: Outcome from severe head injury in children and adolescents. J Neurosurg 1985;62:194.

234. Levin HS, Eisenberg HM, Wigg NR, Kobayashi K: Memory and intellectual ability after head injury in children and adolescents. Neurosurgery 1982;11:668.

235. Arnaud E, Renier D, Marchac D: Development of the frontal sinus and glabellar morphology after frontocranial remodeling. J Craniofac Surg 1994;5:81.

236. Carrington KW, Taren JA, Kahn EA: Primary repair of compound skull fractures in children. Surg Gynecol Obstet 1960;110:203.

237. Gillingham FJ: Neurosurgical experiences in northern Italy. Br J Surg War Surg Suppl 1947;1:81.

238. Lyerly JG: The treatment of depressed fractures of the skull with special reference to the cranial defect. Am Surg 1957;23:1115.

239. Weber SC, Cohn AM: Fracture of the frontal sinus in children. Arch Otolaryngol 1977;103:241.

240. Rohrich RJ, Hollier LH: Management of frontal sinus fractures. Clin Plast Surg 1992;19:219.

241. Wright ML, Hoffman HT, Hoyt DB: Frontal sinus fractures in the pediatric population. Laryngoscope 1992;102:1215.

242. Parker GS, Tanie TA, Wilson JF, Fetter TW: Intracranial complications of sinusitis. South Med J 1989;82:563.

243. Goldstein FP, Rosenthal SA, Garancis JC, et al: Varieties of growing skull fractures in childhood. J Neurosurg 1970;33:25.

244. Manson PN, Carson B: Commentary on growing skull fractures. J Craniofac Surg 1995;6:111.

245. Sekhar LN, Scarff TB: Pseudogrowth of skull fractures in childhood. Neurosurgery 1980;6:285.

246. Havlik R, Sutton L, Bartlett S: Growing skull fractures and their craniofacial equivalents. J Craniofac Surg 1995;6:103.

247. Koenig WJ, Donovan JM, Pensler J: Cranial bone grafting in children. Plast Reconstr Surg 1995;95:1.

248. Ioannides C, Freihoffer HPM, Braset I: Trauma of the upper third of the face. J Maxillofac Surg 1984;12:255.

249. Matras H, Kunderna H: Combined craniofacial fractures. J Maxillofac Surg 1980;8:82.

250. Messinger A, Radkowski MA, Greenwald MJ, Pensler JM: Orbital roof fractures in the pediatric population. Plast Reconstr Surg 1989;84:213.

251. Moore MH, David DJ, Cooter RD: Oblique craniofacial fractures in children. J Craniofac Surg 1990;1:4.

252. Moran WB: Nasal trauma in children. Otolaryngol Clin North Am 1977;10:95.

253. Hirano A, Tsuneda K, Nisimura G: Unusual fronto-orbital fractures in children. J Craniomaxillofac Surg 1991;19:81.

254. Mauriello JA, Lee HJ, Nguyen L: CT of soft tissue injury and orbital fractures. Radiol Clin North Am 1999;37:1.

255. Hove C, Koltai P, Eames F, Cacace A: Age related changes in the pattern of midfacial fractures in children: a chronographic analysis. Presented at the 14th annual meeting of the American Society of Pediatric Otolaryngology, 1999.

256. Howes SH, Dowling PJ: Triage and initial evaluation of the oral facial emergency. Emerg Med Clin North Am 2000;18:3.

257. Mouzakes J, Koltai P: The biology of pediatric fractures. Facial Plast Surg Clin North Am 1998;6:487.

258. Manson P, Clark N, Robertson B: Subunit principles in midface fractures: the importance of sagittal buttresses, soft tissue reductions, and sequencing of segmental fractures. Plast Reconstr Surg 1999;103:1287.

259. Thaller SR, Mabourakh S: Pediatric mandible fractures. Ann Plast Surg 1991;26:511.

260. Wolford LM, Schendel SA, Epker BN: Surgical-orthodontic correction of mandibular deficiency in growing children. J Maxillofac Surg 1979;7:61.

261. Ranta R, Ylipaavalniemi P: The effect of jaw fractures in children on the development of permanent teeth and the occlusion. Proc Finn Dent Soc 1973;69:99.

262. Waite DE: Pediatric fractures of the jaw and facial bones. Pediatrics 1973;51:551.

263. Rock WP, Brain DJ: The effects of nasal trauma during childhood upon growth of the nose and midface. Br J Orthod 1983;10:38.

264. Sanders B: Pediatric Oral and Maxillofacial Surgery. St. Louis, CV Mosby, 1979.

265. Thaller SR, Huang V: Midfacial fractures in the pediatric population. Ann Plast Surg 1992;29:348.

266. Bachmayer DI, Ross RB, Munro IR: Maxillary growth following LeFort III advancement surgery in Crouzon, Apert, and Pfeiffer syndromes. Am J Orthod Dentofacial Orthop 1986; 90:420.

267. Bergland O, Borchgrevink H: The role of the nasal septum in midfacial growth in man elucidated by the maxillary development in certain types of facial clefts: a preliminary report. Scand J Plast Reconstr Surg 1974;8:42.

268. Goldberg D, Bartlett S, Yu J, et al: Critical review of microfixation in pediatric craniofacial surgery. J Craniofac Surg 1995;6:301.

269. Laurenzo JF, Canady JW, Zimmerman B, et al: Craniofacial growth in rabbits: effects of midfacial surgical trauma and rigid plate fixation. Arch Otolaryngol Head Neck Surg 1995;121:556.

270. Lin KY, Bartlett SP, Yaremchuk MJ, et al: An experimental study of the effects of rigid fixation on the developing craniofacial skeleton. Plast Reconstr Surg 1991;87:229.

271. Lin K, Bartlett S, Yaremchuk M, et al: The effect of rigid fixation on the survival of onlay bone grafts. Plast Reconstr Surg 1990;86:449.

272. Wong L, Dufresne CR, Richtsmeier JT, Manson PN: The effect of rigid fixation on the growth of the neurocranium. Plast Reconstr Surg 1991;88:395.

273. Wong L, Richtsmeier JT, Manson PN: Craniofacial growth following rigid fixation: suture excision, miniplating and microplating. J Craniofac Surg 1993;4:234.

274. Marschall M, Chidyllo S, Figueroa A, Cohen M: Long-term effects of rigid fixation on the growing craniofacial skeleton. J Craniofac Surg 1991;2:63.

275. Resnick, JL, Kinney BM, Kawamoto HK: The effect of rigid internal fixation on cranial growth. Ann Plast Surg 1990; 25:372.

276. Yaremchuk MJ, Fiala TG, Barker F, Ragland R: The effects of rigid fixation on craniofacial growth of rhesus monkeys. Plast Reconstr Surg 1994;93:1.

277. Polley J, Figueroa A, Hung KF, et al: Effect of rigid microfixation on the craniomaxillofacial skeleton. J Craniofac Surg 1995;6:132.

278. Eppley BL, Platis JM, Sadove AM: Experimental effects of bone plating in infancy on craniomaxillofacial skeletal growth. Cleft Palate Craniofac J 1993;30:164.

279. Papay F, Hardy S, Morales L, et al: "False" migration of rigid fixation appliances in pediatric craniofacial surgery. J Craniofac Surg 1995;6:309.

280. Suuronen R, Kallela I, Lindqvist C: Bioabsorbable plates and screws: current state of the art in facial fracture repair. J Craniofac Trauma 2000;6:19.

281. Kumar AV, Staffenberg DA, Petronio JA, Wood RJ: Bioabsorbable plates and screws in pediatric craniofacial surgery: a review of 22 cases. J Craniofac Surg 1997;8:97.

282. Eppley BL, Sadove AM: Resorbable coupling fixation in craniosynostosis surgery: experimental and clinical results. J Craniofac Surg 1995;6:455.

283. Eppley BL, Prevel CD, Sadove AM, et al: Resorbable bone fixation: its potential role in craniomaxillofacial trauma. J Craniomaxillofac Trauma 1996;2:56.

284. Turvey T, Bell R, Tejera T, Proffit W: The use of self-reinforced biodegradable bone plates and screws in orthognathic surgery. J Oral Maxillofac Surg 2002;60:59.

285. Edwards RC, Kiely KD, Eppley BL: Resorbable fixation techniques for genioplasty. J Oral Maxillofac Surg 2000;58:269.

286. Eppley BL, Sadove AM: Effects of resorbable fixation on craniofacial growth: modification of plate size. J Craniofac Surg 1994;5:110.

287. Eppley BL, Sadove AM, Havlik RJ: Resorbable plate fixation in pediatric craniofacial surgery: a two-year experience. Plast Reconstr Surg 1997;100:1.

288. Landes C, Kreiner S: Resorbable plate osteosynthesis of sagittal split osteotomies with major bone movement. Plast Reconstr Surg 2003;111:1828.

289. Mathog RH, Rosenberg Z: Complications in the treatment of facial fractures. Otolaryngol Clin North Am 1976;9:533.

290. Manson PN, Hoopse JE, Chambers RG, Jacques DA: Algorithm for nasal reconstruction. Am J Surg 1979;138:528.

291. Lund JV: Anatomical considerations in the etiology of frontal sinus mucoceles. Rhinology 1987;25:83.

292. Lund JV, Milroy CM: Frontal ethmoidal mucoceles: a histopathological analysis. J Laryngol Otol 1991;105:921.

293. Smoot EC, Bowen DG, Lappert P, Ruiz J: Delayed development of an ectopic frontal sinus mucocele after pediatric cranial trauma. J Craniofac Surg 1995;6:327.

294. Gelbier S: Injured anterior teeth in children. A preliminary discussion. Br Dent J 1967;123:331.

295. Schneider SS, Stern M: Teeth in the line of mandibular fractures. J Oral Surg 1971;29:107.

296. Grote W: Traumatische Liquorfisteln im Kindes und Jugendalter. Z Kinderchir Grenzgeb 1966;3:11.

297. Caldicott WJ, North JB, Simpson DA: Traumatic cerebrospinal fluid fistula in children. J Neurosurg 1973;38:1.

298. Schneider RC, Thompson JM: Chronic and delayed traumatic cerebrospinal rhinorrhea as a source of recurrent attacks of meningitis. Ann Surg 1957;145:517.

299. Munro IR: The effect of total maxillary advancement on facial growth. Plast Reconstr Surg 1978;62:751.

300. Osterhout DK, Vargervik K: Maxillary hypoplasia secondary to midfacial trauma in childhood. Plast Reconstr Surg 1987;80:491.

301. Precious DS, Delaire J, Hoffman CD: The effects of nasomaxillary injury on future facial growth. Oral Surg 1988;66:525.

302. Precious DS, McFadden LR, Fitch SJ: Orthognathic surgery for children. Int J Oral Surg 1985;14:466.

303. Arbogast KB, Durbin DR, Kallan MJ, et al: The role of restraint and seat position in pediatric facial fractures. J Trauma 2002;52:693.

304. Grisoni ER, Pillai SB, Volsko TA, et al: Pediatric airbag injuries: the Ohio experience. J Pediatr Surg 2000;35:160.

Endoscopic Facial Fracture Management: Techniques

CHEN LEE, MD, MSc, FRCSC
✦ CHRISTOPHER R. FORREST, MD, MSc, FRCSC

GENERAL CONSIDERATIONS
    Historical Considerations and Advances in
      Management
    Established Operative Techniques
    Problems with Established Techniques: The
      Undesirable Outcome
    Adjunctive and Alternative Procedures
    Minimal Access and Endoscopic Techniques

"BAILOUT" STRATEGIES
APPLICATION IN SPECIFIC ANATOMIC REGIONS
    Condylar Neck of the Mandible
    Symphysis of the Mandible
    Zygomatic Arch
    Anterior Wall of the Frontal Sinus
    Internal Orbit
EVOLVING APPLICATIONS AND FUTURE DIRECTIONS

GENERAL CONSIDERATIONS

The fundamentals of facial fracture repair are similar to the principles of orthopedic surgery of the long bones. The objective of fracture management is anatomic restoration of displaced bone fragments to their native premorbid position with application of fixation to stabilize the reduction until osseous union takes place. Whereas these objectives are common to both specialties, fractures of the face must uphold another defining distinction—surgical repair of the facial skeleton must be accomplished with as few surgical stigmata as possible. Unfavorable outcome and stigmata may result from residual skeletal malreduction; loss of normal soft tissue to bone relationships with malpositioning of aesthetically sensitive soft tissue landmarks[1]; and incisional sequelae, such as scarring, eyelid ectropion, dysesthesia, alopecia, and nerve palsy (Fig. 68-1).

Conservative management of facial fractures with closed reduction and external splints generally yields an unacceptably high rate of skeletal malreduction. Appropriate application of principles of wide surgical exposure and rigid anatomic fracture repair has largely resolved problems of inadequate skeletal reduction for most anatomic regions of the injured face. These established techniques of facial fracture repair necessitate direct access incisions and extensive soft tissue dissections.[2-5] Associated iatrogenic sequelae have been attributed to the surgical access.

An anatomically perfect skeletal reconstruction marred by disfiguring facial scar and soft tissue ptosis is deflating for the surgeon and undeserved for the patient.

Minimally invasive and endoscopic techniques are the most recent additions to the surgical armamentarium. Their use in certain surgical situations has been supported by improved outcomes for patients with a simultaneous decrease in overall costs of patient care. These benefits were realized only after extensive product development and ample surgical training. As an example of its acceptance, competence with the endoscope has become a requirement for completion of general surgery training.

Craniofacial surgeons are only beginning to realize the potential applications and benefits of minimal access and endoscopic techniques. For the past 5 years, endoscope-assisted minimal access techniques have been applied to different regions of the craniofacial skeleton and the treatment of fractures of the orbital floor,[6-8] orbital-zygomatic complex,[9-13] and mandible,[14-18] but to date, they have not revolutionized the management of these injuries. There are several reasons for this. Minimal access techniques by their very nature involve smaller incisions and do not allow extensive exposure. As the result of technical limitations with the current instrumentation, these techniques are not easier to apply than the traditional methods. This means longer operating times and increasing levels of frustration for the operating

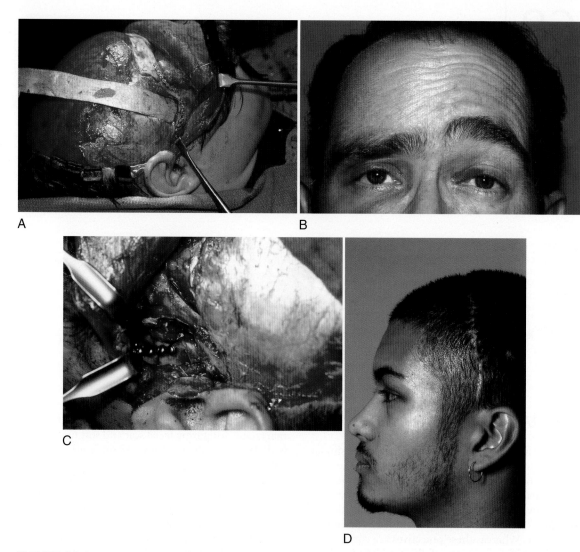

FIGURE 68-1. *A,* Traditional open coronal incision requires extensive dissection for access to the upper facial skeleton. *B,* Injury to the frontal branch of cranial nerve VII will result in an ipsilateral frontalis palsy. *C,* Open repair of the condyle is a technical challenge requiring an extensive dissection and risks transection of the main trunk of the facial nerve. *D,* Scarring with alopecia after coronal access for facial fracture repair can be apparent in young men with short hairstyles. (From Lee C, Stiebel M, Young DM: Cranial nerve VII region of the traumatized facial skeleton: optimizing fracture repair with the endoscope. J Trauma 2000;48:423-431, discussion 431-432.)

surgeon. In addition, endoscopic instrumentation represents additional costs that treating institutions may not be willing to afford. Finally, swelling and hemorrhage make the techniques of minimal access surgery sometimes difficult to apply. At present, the technique of minimal access surgery represents a refinement of the traditional methods that can be rewarding to those dedicated to the pursuit of improving the outcome of patients with facial trauma. This chapter details the evolution of novel "cutting edge" applications. It is hoped that application of these techniques will bring about a decrease in the morbidity associated with the treatment of facial fractures and stimulate those who

are seeking to improve surgical outcomes to continue the search for excellence. New and novel applications of these techniques will depend on the development of improved instrumentation.

Historical Considerations and Advances in Management

The management of facial fractures has undergone many changes during the last 2 decades. Historically, the absence of powerful, accurate imaging tools delayed any sort of intervention until a proper external evaluation of facial contour, deformity, and function could be performed. In some instances, such as with orbital fractures, deformity might not even be apparent to external observation until several weeks after the initial trauma. This delay in intervention often gave rise to technical difficulties with surgical repair because of early osseous union of malpositioned bone fragments and soft tissue contracture. The advent of computed tomographic (CT) imaging provided physicians with an extraordinarily precise method to determine fracture malalignment of facial injuries.[19] With this tool, fractures can be detected early and repaired immediately—even when physical examination is impaired by early facial swelling.

An improved understanding of bone healing, the greater availability of antibiotics, and the introduction of internal skeletal fixation have contributed to the development of surgical techniques with improved efficacy and outcomes. Work by Manson[19-21] and Gruss[2,4,22,23] in the early 1980s revolutionized the approach to treatment of facial fractures by introducing the concepts of anatomic reduction, rigid internal fixation, and primary bone grafting employing the techniques of wide exposure. However, apart from the development of smaller fixation systems, bioresorbable plates and screws,[24,25] and new bone substitutes,[26,27] relatively little has been done to improve the outcome of patients sustaining significant facial trauma until recently.

Established Operative Techniques

Fracture management in the new millennium consists of an orderly stepwise approach. Radiographic imaging is of such sophistication and importance that fracture topography of the injured facial skeleton must be precisely mapped out and studied to design an efficacious surgical strategy. Incisions are strategically placed. The intervening soft tissues are elevated in a subperiosteal plane. Surgical access to the underlying bone is directly achieved by retraction of the soft tissue envelope. Fracture disorder is overcome by a planned orderly sequence of operative steps. It is critical to use the uninjured stable bone as the foundation on which to rebuild the facial skeleton. Therefore, reduction and fixation commence from uninjured facial bone. Exacting repair is a priority at functional subunits of the orbit, dental occlusion, and nasal root. Fractures extending across multiple anatomic subunits are converted to more simplified fracture patterns. The subunit principle of fracture repair is most applicable to complex panfacial injuries in which the upper facial orbital-nasal root regions are anatomically reconstructed independent of the lower facial dental occlusal unit—the upper and lower facial regions are then unified much like a simple Le Fort I fracture repair. During wound closure, meticulous attention to restoration of the normal anatomic bone to soft tissue relationship is equally important for the overall success of the repair.

Problems with Established Techniques: The Undesirable Outcome

Undesirable outcome after repair of a facial fracture may be categorized into residual skeletal malreduction, soft tissue malpositioning, or incisional sequelae.

RESIDUAL SKELETAL MALREDUCTION

Residual skeletal malreduction may result from either inadequate primary fracture reduction or insufficient stabilization with secondary fracture displacement. Elegant studies have improved our understanding of the complex load-bearing characteristics of the facial skeleton. The acquired knowledge has been incorporated into the design and technique of implant placement to minimize the likelihood of malreduction from inadequate stability.[28] Manson[3] and Gruss[2] have popularized a philosophy of anatomic fracture reduction and rigid repair in a single surgical stage. Surgical access is achieved by camouflaged incisions to widely deglove the injured facial skeleton. Meticulous application of this philosophy of anatomic fracture repair has dramatically reduced the incidence of skeletal malreduction in most regions of the injured face.[29] Despite these gains with conventional techniques, anatomic repair of the internal bony orbit[30-32] and condyle[33,34] of the mandible remains a challenge. Established techniques yield inconsistent outcomes, and anatomic repair has been elusive in these subunits of the face.

The bony orbit houses the fragile ocular globe and delicate muscles that precisely motor the eye. Small volume discrepancies as a result of blowout fracture of the orbital walls can cause significant degrees of enophthalmos. Whereas the treatment philosophy in the orbit is to reconstruct the three-dimensional skeletal form anatomically, the limited space and proximity of fragile ocular structures predispose to technical problems with accurate repair. Minimal access techniques can potentially improve the fidelity of repair at this technically challenging site.

In contrast, most condylar fractures are managed by inaccurate closed methods (Fig. 68-2). Treatment philosophy differs in that malreduction is anticipated. Therapy is focused on adaptation to a biomechanically disadvantaged structure through forced functional rehabilitation. Conventional methods of open surgical condylar fracture repair have not been popular because of the difficult access, facial scarring, and risk of facial nerve transection. Alternative endoscopic techniques are introduced in this chapter. These techniques are evolving and have the potential to become the

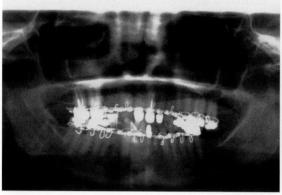

A

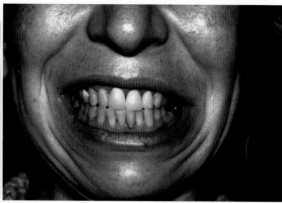

B

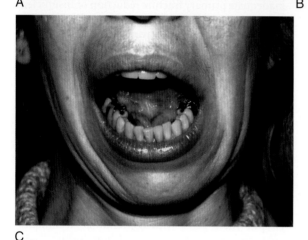

C

FIGURE 68-2. This 44-year-old woman was assaulted. She sustained unilateral left subcondylar and right angle mandibular fractures. *A*, Despite tight maxillomandibular fixation, the left subcondylar fracture remains malreduced with a shortened ramus and persistent dislocation of the condyle out of the fossa. *B*, One year after conservative treatment with maxillomandibular fixation. Multiple dental procedures have been performed to improve the malocclusion. *C*, On dynamic jaw motion, the chin point deviates to the shortened mandibular side. The patient also complains of hypermobility and popping of the normal contralateral temporomandibular joint. (From Lee C: Subcondylar fracture of the mandible: an endoscopic-assisted technique. Operative Techniques Plast Reconstr Surg 1998;5:287-294.)

standard by which anatomic fracture repair of the condyle will be achieved.

SOFT TISSUE MALPOSITIONING

Phillips et al[1] were first to recognize that extensive degloving of the facial skeleton for fracture exposure might yield malpositioning of aesthetically sensitive soft tissue landmarks. The resulting soft tissue derangements may be more disfiguring than the untreated original skeletal deformity. Even if the fracture is anatomically repaired, insufficient attention to re-establishment of normal soft tissue to bone attachments may yield deformities such as temporal hollowing from failure to repair the deep temporal fascia at a repaired zygomatic arch, an antimongoloid cant to the palpebral fissure from disinsertion of the lateral canthus, and sagging of the malar prominence with deepened nasolabial folds from ptosis of the cheek soft tissues. These deformities are prevented by resuspension of critical soft tissue landmarks with suture approximation often to strategically sited drill holes in the facial skeleton. By necessity, these critical steps are always at the end of the surgical procedure when the surgical team is tired and the tissue landmarks are difficult to identify because of the intense edema. Frequently, errors of omission or technique and intense swelling may cause subsequent loss of the normal soft tissue to bone relationships. Minimal access methods of fracture repair require less dissection and undermining. The likelihood of soft tissue displacement is minimized, thereby simplifying the operative step of soft tissue resuspension.

INCISIONAL SEQUELAE

Each subregion of the facial skeleton can be accessed from one or more of the four traditional surgical incisions. The coronal scalp incision offers access to the zygomatic arch, frontal sinus, nasal root, and upper orbit (see Fig. 68-1). The lower eyelid incision yields access to the lower orbit and upper maxilla. Oral upper and lower sulcus incisions offer access to maxilla and anterior mandible. Posterior cutaneous facial incisions, such as the Risdon, preauricular, and retromandibular, give access to the ramus and condylar process of the mandible.

With the exception of the oral sulcus incisions, each of these traditional incisions is associated with undesirable outcomes. The coronal incision can result in increased blood loss, injury to the frontal branch of the facial nerve, loss of sensation posterior to the incision, and scar alopecia. The lower eyelid incision is often associated with lid malpositioning and ectropion. Posterior facial incisions for access to the mandible result in visible facial scarring, and the facial nerve is at risk for injury at the mandibular branch or even the main trunk. Minimal access procedures must be designed to have an inherently lower risk of these incisional sequelae to be of value to the practicing surgeon.

Adjunctive and Alternative Procedures

Techniques established during the last 2 decades have vastly improved the results of facial fracture repair. Instead of despair from permanent facial disfigurement, we now strive to achieve a perfect fracture reconstruction in a single operative step. Implementation of effective therapy is contingent on preoperative surgical planning with use of high-resolution CT images of the facial skeleton. This diagnostic information is used to plan the operative surgical access. However, the ultimate accuracy of the repair depends greatly on the surgeon's skill in realigning the spatially displaced bone fragments of the injured face. Presently, the intraoperative process of fracture reduction is subjective and highly dependent on the ability of the surgeon to cognitively rebuild "normal." This is a challenge even in experienced hands. Therefore, new adjunctive technologies have been emerging to streamline and enhance the fidelity of facial fracture repair.[35,36] These techniques offer greatest potential benefit in management of complex comminuted facial fractures. Furthermore, less experienced and training surgeons may also benefit from the better spatial orientation provided by surgical navigation and stereotactic systems.

Earlier stereotactic systems required preoperative computed images of the face to be acquired with an externally referenced head frame.[37] At surgery, the head frame had to be reapplied to permit intraoperative correlation with the previously acquired radiographic images. This method of external registration with a head frame had the advantage of being inexpensive but was too cumbersome for practical use. Instead, operative navigation and guidance systems designed for extirpative intracranial tumor surgery have been adapted for use in craniofacial skeletal surgery.[35,36] External registration is achieved with a frameless stereotactic system that combines three-dimensional computer-assisted imaging with a hand-guided, position-sensing, articulated probe in the operative field. The instrumentation permits direct interactive visualization of preoperatively acquired CT image data in the operating room. By orienting the surgeon to an exact location throughout the procedure, the stereotactic viewing probe has been found to be useful in defining intraorbital anatomy, in determining ocular globe position, and in delineating margins for tumor ablation. Excellent anatomic spatial correlation can be obtained because the probe tip position is accurate to 2 mm. Despite positive attributes, stereotactic viewing is based on the preoperatively acquired radiologic images. Current navigation systems are incapable of displaying real-time changes of mobile fractured bone segments of the face during an operative repair. Therefore, intraoperative validation of the repair has not been possible with these surgical guidance systems.

Preoperative high-resolution computed images of the fractured facial skeleton are indispensable in establishment of diagnosis and conception of an effective surgical plan (Fig. 68-3). At surgery, visual fracture realignment and the surgeon's familiarity with anatomic landmarks are the most common means by which the adequacy of repair can be judged. Postoperative CT imaging is currently the most accurate method to evaluate the adequacy of repair. Unfortunately, the post hoc nature of this method of validation greatly impedes our capacity to intervene for outcomes that are found to be less than desired. To empower the surgeon, Stanley[38] has proposed the intraoperative acquisition of CT images of the repaired facial bones so that corrective revisions can be performed without delay. In his clinical study, a mobile CT scanner was employed in the operating room to evaluate the surgical repair of a series of orbitozygomatic complex fractures. At surgery, patients under general anesthesia and still in the sterile field were placed into a radiolucent head holder and interfaced with the mobile scanner. Approximately 20% of the treated patients demonstrated persistent malreduction. The newly acquired operative CT images were then used to guide the corrective revision without delay. All malreductions were substantially improved. Correction of persisting malreduction at the time of acute repair, rather than during costly and more difficult delayed revisions, is an unrealized benefit of intraoperative CT scans. Furthermore, in selected cases, it may be possible to reduce the degree of soft tissue dissection by limiting direct fracture repair to only the most displaced sites and using the scanner to indirectly validate the reduction at undissected fracture sites. Unfortunately, the high cost of the specialized equipment, prolonged operative time, and increased need for specialized personnel are considerable drawbacks to this adjunctive technique.

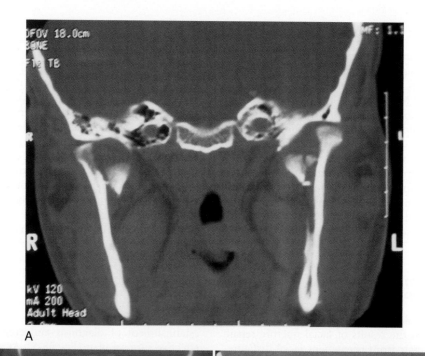

A

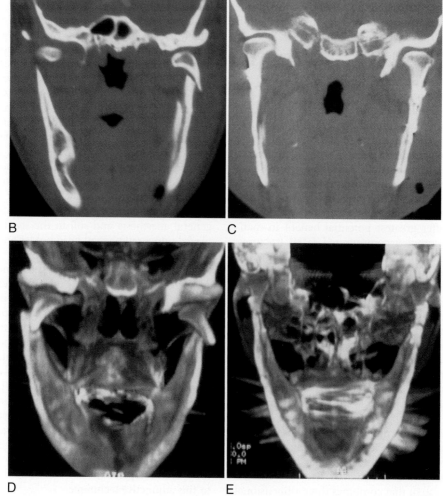

B

C

D

E

FIGURE 68-3. High-resolution CT images are necessary to delineate the size and position of the fractured proximal condylar pole. Intracapsular and comminuted injuries were considered a contraindication to endoscopic repair. A, Coronal CT images demonstrate bilateral intracapsular fractures of the mandible. The small size and medial location of the proximal fragment are unfavorable conditions for operative repair. Whereas coronal images demonstrate in one plane the degree of mandibular shortening, a substantial review of the entire set of images is necessary to delineate the spatial topography of the fracture. B and C, Coronal images before and after repair in a patient treated with endoscopic techniques. These particular coronal images show improvement but remain inconclusive as to the exact severity of the injury and effectiveness of the repair. D, Three-dimensional reformatted image clearly demonstrates that both condyles were initially dislocated medially out of the articulating fossa. This preoperative image more easily demonstrates the spatial topography of the fracture, facilitating operative repair. The image demonstrates bilateral extracapsular fractures. The left condylar neck fracture is more favorable for repair because the condyle laterally overrides the ascending ramus at the fracture interface. The right condylar neck fracture is medially overridden and hidden by the superiorly telescoped ramus; repair is technically possible but much more challenging with this medial spatial orientation at the fracture site. The right condylar fracture must first be delivered into a lateral position before reduction and fixation can be accomplished. E, Three-dimensional postoperative image confirms relocation, and accurate fracture repair was bilaterally possible by an endoscope-assisted technique.

Minimal Access and Endoscopic Techniques

Better outcomes for patients justify the use of the endoscope in surgery. For universal acceptance, surgery with the endoscope must be cost-effective, be quicker than standard techniques, and result in decreased morbidity of patients. It was only after extensive product development and ample training periods that such goals were realized. As a testament to its acceptance, competence with the endoscope has become a requirement for anyone today training in the field of general surgery.

Plastic surgeons are at the same threshold that pioneering general surgeons faced when they initially brought the endoscope into the operating room. Just as with laparoscopic surgery in previous years, plastic surgeons need to justify the benefits an endoscope would bring to the existing surgical armamentarium. Herein, many of the minimal access techniques described represent refinements of technique based on conventional established methods of management. In addition, plastic surgeons are in the exciting position of having the opportunity to use the endoscope on injuries that were previously not treated with surgery. The reader is introduced to a rapidly evolving novel methodology of facial fracture management.

DEFINITION

Minimally invasive operative techniques use limited and well-hidden incisions in anatomically distant sites to remotely treat pathologic structures. An optical cavity adjacent to the site of the pathologic process is necessary for visualization and to accommodate purposeful movement to treat the pathologic condition surgically. Specialized equipment, such as endoscopy, fluoroscopy, and robotics, is often required to enhance visualization and to increase the precision of purposeful movement to compensate for the lack of direct access, absence of tactile feedback, and loss of visual depth.

AESTHETICS TO RECONSTRUCTION: EVOLUTION OF MINIMAL ACCESS TECHNIQUES

Whereas endoscopic technology has been the standard of care for many orthopedic, urologic, and general surgical procedures for some time, it has only been during the past 5 years that the minimal access techniques have been adopted for facial rejuvenation surgery, allowing smaller incisions, limited dissection, and shorter recovery times.[39-49] In the management of patients with facial fractures, it is unlikely that morbidity associated with the injury pattern will decrease. However, improvement of morbidity associated with the treatment of these injuries may represent a potential area for progress. Therefore, the increasing popularity of endoscopic technology and minimal access techniques in facial rejuvenation surgery has inspired individuals to develop novel applications in patients with facial trauma. Surgical techniques, applications of endoscopic technology, and indications and contraindications are presented.

DEVELOPMENT OF TECHNIQUES, ACCESS, AND EXPOSURE: CADAVER TO CLINICAL STUDIES

It is hoped that application of minimal access techniques in the management of patients with facial fractures will decrease morbidity and maintain the standard of care that has been established with the traditional techniques of open reduction and internal fixation. To this end, most techniques have been conceived and evaluated in the cadaver laboratory before introduction into clinical practice. The principles of endoscope-assisted techniques for the treatment of facial fractures involve adequate visualization, manipulation of fracture fragments, proper instrumentation, and appropriate fixation with the development and maximization of the optical cavity. The process of endoscope-assisted fracture repair can be divided into three common operative steps: surgical access by use of remote portals, establishment and retention of an optical cavity, and fracture repair by remote portal manipulation of reduction and application of fixation.

Surgical access through anatomically remote portals requires specialized instrumentation to transfer purposeful digital motion from the surgeon's hand to the actual site of the fracture to be repaired. Freedom of hand motion is significantly impaired, much like a bottleneck through which instruments must pass to effect purposeful movement. Therefore, strategic placement of two or more access portals is recommended to achieve triangulation and bimanual transfer of focused hand motion at the fracture site.

Unlike the natural cavities of the abdomen and thorax, the optical cavity surrounding a facial fracture must be surgically made by dissection of a soft tissue pocket of sufficient dimensions to permit functional viewing and work within the cavity. With exception of the paranasal sinuses, retention of the cavity requires mechanical retraction of the dissected soft tissue pocket. Whereas the natural cavity of the paranasal sinuses does not require retention, its limited working space significantly impairs surgical manipulation. The paranasal sinus cavity has room to admit an endoscope and only one dissecting instrument, effectively reducing the operator's functionality to the equivalent of a single-handed surgeon.

Finally, fracture repair is achieved by reduction and fixation through remote access portals. This step has proved challenging. The surgeon must remotely use instruments to manipulate the fracture into a reduced position. Proximal and distal fracture fragment control is a requirement. After reduction is achieved, temporary stability is necessary to permit an effective transition to rigid internal fixation.

The safety and feasibility of endoscope-assisted fracture repair of the condylar neck of the mandible,[50-53] zygomatic arch,[11] frontal sinus,[8,54,55] and inferior orbital wall[6,8] have been developed and studied in fresh cadaver heads. These exploratory cadaver dissections have been crucial preliminary steps necessary before incorporation into clinical practice.

Surgical repair of condylar neck fractures of the mandible is technically challenging. The main trunk of cranial nerve VII lies directly over the neck of the mandibular condyle; its more distal nerve divisions travel superficial to the parotid gland and masseter muscle. Established external techniques of repair leave visible facial scars and risk transection of the facial nerve. Intraoral techniques minimize these risks but have historically yielded insufficient visibility and access. Lee et al[51] used cadaver dissections to evaluate an endoscope-assisted intraoral technique of rigid repair of condylar neck fractures. For safe development of an optical cavity centered over the condylar neck, dissections in the cadaver heads were simplest

with an intraoral buccal sulcus incision over the oblique line of the mandible. The optical cavity for endoscope placement was made by elevating the soft tissues in a subperiosteal plane from the entire lateral ramus of the mandible. Condylar neck plate fixation was experimentally performed in eight cadaver heads. Subsequent facial nerve dissections demonstrated anatomic continuity in all miniplate repairs of the experimental condylar neck fractures. Furthermore, reduction and miniplate fixation were feasible for extracapsular fractures of the condylar process of the mandible. Independently, Troulis et al[52,53] developed an extraoral endoscopic method of accessing the ramus of the mandible through a 1.5-cm incision at the angle of the mandible. Using this access incision as the main endoscopic portal, they have developed innovative methods of osteotomy, condylectomy, and fracture repair.

Lee at al[11] used six fresh cadaver heads to determine whether aesthetically acceptable remote access incisions and natural tissue planes could be dissected to develop an internal optical cavity for fracture repair of the zygomatic arch. A unilateral depressed comminuted malar arch fracture was experimentally made. The contralateral arch was not violated to permit an anatomic comparison of the fracture repair with the normal uninjured side. Endoscope-assisted zygomatic arch fracture repair involved removal of the fractured segments of the arch, ex vivo application of fixation, and anatomic replacement by use of periauricular and lateral orbital access incisions. After repair of the fractured arch, the integrity of the frontal branch of the facial nerve was anatomically inspected by dissecting out its course from the stylomastoid foramen to the frontalis muscle. The adequacy of fracture repair was determined by stripping all soft tissues from the facial skeleton and comparing the repaired zygomatic arch with the contralateral uninjured side. Excellent fracture reduction was demonstrated in all cadaver skulls. The repaired comminuted arch demonstrated symmetry with the contralateral uninjured arch. Facial nerve dissections demonstrated complete frontal branch continuity in all specimens.

Forrest[8] has developed an endoscope-assisted technique of anatomic repair of fractures of the anterior wall of the frontal sinus. Using fresh cadaver heads and a surgical approach similar to that for aesthetic endoscopic brow lifts, he was able to demonstrate that fractures of the anterior wall of the frontal sinus can be effectively repaired without a coronal incision. Strong[56] revisited this cadaver model and used the endoscope to place a fast-curing hydroxyapatite bone paste to camouflage displaced fractures of the anterior wall of the frontal sinus. The deformities were effectively camouflaged, and fracture manipulation was not required. This is a proposed alternative to anatomic repair of the fractured anterior wall of the frontal sinus.

Saunders et al[6] have used fresh cadaver heads to extensively study blowout fractures of the inferior orbital wall. Transantral endoscopy of the maxillary sinus was used as a diagnostic aid to determine the size and precise location of the bone ledges of traumatic orbital floor defects. Experimental blowout fractures in six fresh cadaver heads were evaluated endoscopically through the maxillary antrum. In the cadaver, the orbital floor and the course of the infraorbital nerve were easily identified. Transantral orbital floor exploration allowed precise determination of the size and location of the orbital floor fracture and the presence of entrapped periorbita. They recommend transantral use of the endoscope as a diagnostic tool to identify patients who would benefit from a traditional lower lid method of orbital floor repair. Furthermore, a transantral endoscopic orbital floor defect may assist in precise identification of the posterior shelf for implant placement.

TECHNOLOGY AND INSTRUMENTATION

Commercially designed equipment for facial fracture repair is not yet widely available. Most instruments used for this purpose have been adapted from endoscopic sets designed for paranasal sinus endoscopy and aesthetic soft tissue surgery of the brow and face (Fig. 68-4). Maintenance of the optical cavity is an important step in all endoscopic procedures. An endoscope-mounted retractor has aided most techniques described in this chapter. The endoscope-mounted retractor facilitates the procedure by simultaneously maintaining the optical cavity and stabilizing the orientation of the field. For the purpose of fracture repair, the authors have found the commercially available 4-mm endoscope-mounted retractor* to be widely effective in maintaining the optical cavity for a wide variety of facial fractures. Similarly, the 4-mm-diameter 30-degree angled rigid endoscope commonly packaged in sinus endoscopy sets of most operating rooms has been effective at visually imaging a variety of facial fractures. The endoscopic image is captured and displayed with a video system. Preferably, a three-chip camera, xenon light source, and camera converter are used to capture a high-fidelity image and project it to a video display. Tools used for fracture reduction and fixation have been adapted from standard commercial titanium implants designed for conventional facial fracture repair. Research and product development are active. Design-specific tools will soon be commercially available to facilitate these challenging procedures.

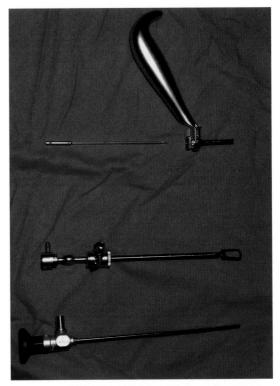

FIGURE 68-4. The optical cavity is maintained by mechanical retraction of soft tissues. Instruments adapted from endoscopic aesthetic brow lift sets can be helpful. The 4-mm endoscope-mounted retractor and 4-mm-diameter, 30-degree angled scope are especially useful for fracture repair. (From Lee C, Mankani MH, Kellman RM, Forrest CR: Minimally invasive approaches to mandibular fractures. Facial Plast Surg Clin North Am 2001;9:475-487.)

ACQUISITION OF SKILLS

Surgeons are traditionally trained to harmonize their stereoscopic vision, proprioceptive hand positioning, and tactile sensory response of tissues to surgical manipulation. These sources of sensory input are then integrated to generate a motor response to achieve purposeful and highly specific surgical actions toward a therapeutic endpoint. However, the sources of sensory input are intrinsically different in minimally invasive procedures. Stereoscopic vision is replaced with a two-dimensional electronic image without depth perception. The tactile feedback from tissue manipulation is altered. Furthermore, fixed surgical portals significantly restrict and impede the surgeon's hand motion. At times, it can bear semblance to working with chopsticks down a narrow bottleneck. Therefore, a new set of surgical skills must be acquired to gain endoscopic proficiency. Synthetic skulls with silicone soft tissue

---

*Isse dissector-retractor, Karl Storz, Tuttlingen, Germany.

envelopes* have been specifically designed to simulate the restricted soft tissue access expected with minimal access procedures. Preliminary training on synthetic models and fresh cadaver heads is a necessary step to acquire proficiency with endoscopic skills to repair facial fractures.

GENERAL INDICATIONS AND CONTRAINDICATIONS

Exuberant enthusiasm for new techniques must not eclipse good clinical judgment. Most techniques of facial fracture repair (traditional and endoscopic methods) have been designed to manage fractures in the mature facial skeleton. Caution should be exercised in managing facial injuries in the pediatric population. Surgical intervention may alter future growth and must be factored into the overall management algorithm.

Endoscopic techniques are still evolving. Presently, these techniques are challenging and often require longer operative times. This is likely to change with greater experience and better instruments. Associated head injury with increased intracranial pressure and unstable cervical spinal injury are unfavorable anesthetic risks and should be considered contraindications to minimally invasive facial surgery.

Preoperative high-resolution CT scans must be meticulously examined to aid in surgical planning. Some fractures, such as intracapsular condylar fractures of the mandible, are technically not amenable to endoscopic repair. Unnecessary endoscopic exploration can be avoided by accurately delineating these fracture patterns on the preoperative CT images.

"BAILOUT" STRATEGIES

Minimally invasive and endoscope-assisted techniques of facial fracture repair are still evolving. The skills necessary to become proficient differ substantially from those of traditional surgery. These techniques are challenging, and the learning curve is steep. The cumulative experience gained with these techniques is presently insufficient for abandonment of traditional techniques to be recommended. It is more logical to acquire proficiency with traditional methods of facial fracture repair before embarking on the acquisition of skills to perform these novel minimally invasive techniques. Should insurmountable difficulties be encountered with an endoscopic fracture repair, the surgeon must have the resourcefulness and ability to implement a change of surgical strategy to achieve therapeutic goals by established traditional surgical methods of fracture repair.

---

*Synthes Maxillofacial, West Chester, Pa.

APPLICATION IN SPECIFIC ANATOMIC REGIONS

Condylar Neck of the Mandible

Approximately 20% to 30% of mandibular fractures involve the condylar region.[57] Fracture displacement in this region results in shortening of the posterior mandibular height and an abnormally postured condyle.[58] The shortened posterior mandibular height reduces the radius of rotation in the ipsilateral mandible, restricts jaw opening, and predisposes to unpleasant chin point deviation seen on dynamic jaw motion. The abnormally postured condyle negatively affects the normal translation movement of the condylar head in the glenoid fossa, resulting in asynchronous motion and greater loads on the contralateral normal temporomandibular joint. These anatomic abnormalities combine to produce a biomechanically disadvantaged mandible with increased risk of oromasticatory dysfunction, unappealing loss of aesthetic chin projection, deviant jaw motion, potential for hypermobility, and late internal joint derangement of the contralateral normal temporomandibular joint (see Fig. 68-2).

Whereas the treatment paradigm for most facial fractures now includes open anatomic rigid repair, most mandibular condylar neck fractures continue to be managed by closed methods. Acute fracture management by conservative maxillomandibular fixation rarely achieves anatomic fracture reduction. Forced functional adaptation and neuromuscular rehabilitation to the altered condylar mechanics may restore dental occlusion.[34] However, the mandible remains anatomically disadvantaged, and patients often complain of residual loss of chin projection, deviant jaw motion, and hypermobility of the contralateral normal temporomandibular joint.[57-59] These findings are most apparent when the dentition is in slight repose or when there are insufficient posterior occluding teeth to prevent posterior collapse of the shortened mandible (see Fig. 68-2). Silvennoinen et al[60] have prospectively observed a cohort of patients with unilateral condylar neck fractures treated with closed techniques and reported a 39% incidence of mandibular dysfunction.

Attempts to improve functional and aesthetic outcomes for patients with condylar neck injuries have led to complicated open surgical procedures (see Fig. 68-1).[61-64] Although these operations typically produced good reductions, the difficulty in fracture exposure demands extraordinary surgical skill and the use of visible facial incisions, and the facial nerve is placed at risk for transection. Open surgical repair has not been popular. Many practicing surgeons reserve this technique for the most severely disrupted condylar injuries.[65]

Significant shortcomings exist for most established methods of closed and open repair of condylar neck fracture. Deficiencies primarily result from inadequate fracture reduction or from the stigmata of the surgical access. To address both of these limitations, a minimally invasive, endoscopically assisted method of rigid anatomic repair of the fractured condylar neck has been developed.[66-69] By use of endoscopic visual enhancement with an intraoral method of fracture reduction and rigid fixation, the disadvantages traditionally associated with open condylar fracture repair have been minimized. More important, anatomic fracture reduction with restoration of normal condylar mechanics and immediate jaw motion can be reliably achieved with most adult extracapsular noncomminuted condylar neck fractures. Premorbid oromasticatory function, aesthetic chin projection, and dynamic jaw motion can be achieved with minimal risks. Endoscopic condylar neck fracture repair has been efficacious at functional, aesthetic, and radiographic restoration of the mandible without postoperative maxillomandibular fixation.

INDICATIONS AND CONTRAINDICATIONS

Most centers have restricted the application of minimally invasive repair to compliant adult patients with acute condylar neck fractures. Injuries must demonstrate significant radiographic displacement in association with varying degrees of malocclusion, dysfunctional jaw motion, and loss of the aesthetic jaw line. Among pediatric patients, there is a potential for deleterious effects on mandibular development because growth largely originates from the condylar poles. Therefore, closed conservative methods have been favored in management of pediatric patients.[34,70,71]

PREOPERATIVE RADIOGRAPHS

Radiographic imaging is critical to evaluate the location, degree of comminution, and spatial orientation of the fracture (see Fig. 68-3). Fine-cut axial and coronal CT images of the mandible as well as three-dimensional reformatted images of the fractures are useful in the surgical planning.[72] These images are used to identify the relative position of the condylar pole to the ascending ramus. Among most adult condylar neck fractures, the proximal condylar pole lies lateral to the ascending ramus at the fracture interface.[73] A lateral override is considered a favorable position for endoscopic repair because the lateral surface of the fractured condylar pole can be expeditiously exposed and reduced. Medial override, in which the proximal condylar pole lies medial to the ascending ramus at the fracture site, is a far more challenging fracture repair. The pterygomasseteric muscle forces act to telescope the ascending ramus over the lateral surface of the proximal condyle, severely reducing visibility of the proximal pole.

TECHNIQUE

The endoscopic technique of subcondylar fracture repair employs an intraoral subperiosteal dissection to expose the ascending ramus and lateral surface of the extracapsular proximal condylar fracture fragment. Anatomic fracture reduction relies heavily on endoscopic visual fracture alignment. Rigid screw and plate fixation is then placed transbuccally by use of a percutaneous trocar. Postoperative maxillomandibular fixation is not necessary, and recovery of normal jaw motion is usually achieved by the eighth postoperative week. Compared with established open surgical methods, this dissection is simpler with insignificant visible scarring and minimal risk of facial nerve transection. Because the dissection is limited to the extracapsular lateral subcondylar region, the vascularity of the condyle remains unimpeded, minimizing the risk of late ischemic condylar remodeling.

Up to three operative portals are necessary to visualize, reduce, and rigidly fix a displaced condylar neck fracture (Fig. 68-5; see also Fig. 68-4). The first portal is obtained through an oral buccal sulcus incision over the oblique line of the mandible. This approach permits elevation of the soft tissues from the entire lateral ramus of the mandible; the subperiosteal dissection also forms the endoscope's optical cavity. The second portal is placed anterior to the lobule of the auricle. This 3-mm-long incision allows manipulation of the proximal condylar pole by the trocar cannula and facilitates the application of percutaneous screws for fixation. An optional third portal, also measuring 3 mm, can be placed at the angle of the mandible, permitting introduction of a narrow-diameter periosteal elevator for further mobilization of the proximal condylar pole. The third portal can also serve as an alternative endoscope insertion point to provide a better viewing angle of the fracture along the posterior border of the mandible.

The optical cavity is maintained by transoral placement of the endoscope-mounted, guarded retractor. Visibility of the proximal condylar segment is enhanced by rotation of the angled viewing surface of the endoscope toward the fracture. The presence of a medial or lateral override is verified. In fractures with an unfavorable medial override, the condylar pole must be manipulated into a lateral position (Fig. 68-6). The patient is then placed into temporary maxillomandibular fixation with elastic rubber bands to facilitate the reduction. The proximal condylar segment can then be maneuvered into a reduced position by the end of a transbuccally placed trocar. The fracture plate is positioned through the intraoral incision. Fixation screws are placed through the trocar positioned at the second portal.

A blenderized diet should be prescribed postoperatively for 6 weeks. The patient should be allowed to

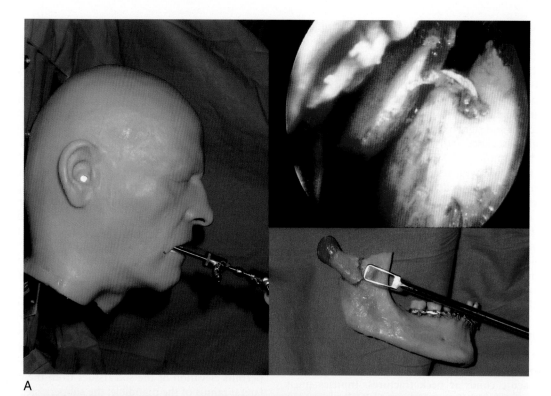

A

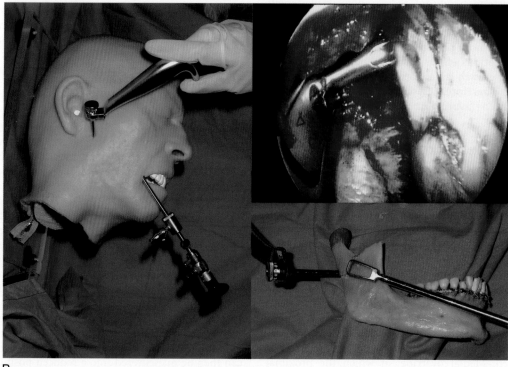

B

FIGURE 68-5. Up to three operative portals are necessary to visualize, reduce, and rigidly fix a displaced condylar neck fracture. This technique is most favorable for laterally overridden condylar fractures of the mandible. *A,* The first portal is made through an oral buccal sulcus incision over the oblique line of the mandible. Subperiosteal dissection of the soft tissue envelope at the lateral ramus establishes the endoscope's optical cavity. *B,* A second portal anterior to the lobule of the auricle is used for trocar access to manipulate the proximal condylar pole and to place percutaneous screws for fixation.

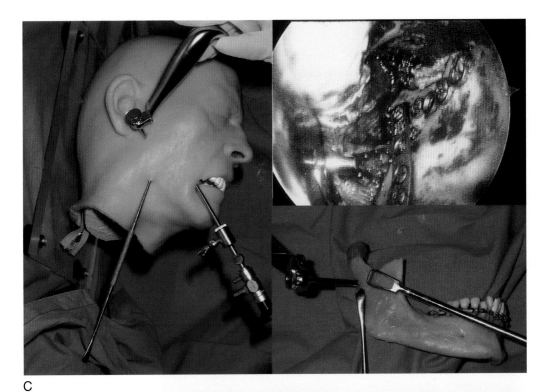

C

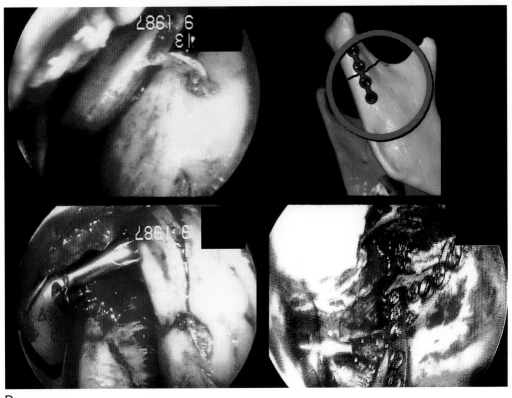

D

FIGURE 68-5, cont'd. *C,* An optional third portal can be placed at the angle of the mandible, permitting introduction of a narrow-diameter periosteal elevator for further mobilization of the proximal condylar pole. The third portal can also serve as an alternative point for endoscope insertion and may provide a better view of the fracture along the posterior border of the mandible. *D,* Only a limited region of the condyle is endoscopically visible. The degree of preoperative preparation and anatomic familiarity correlate positively with the ease of the procedure.

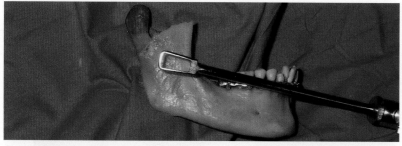

A

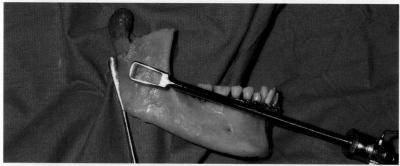

B

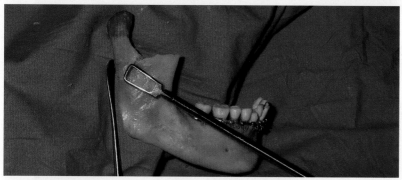

C

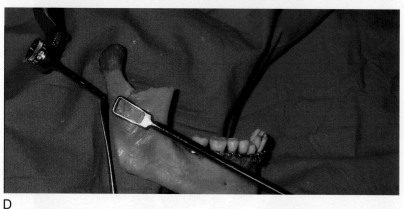

D

FIGURE 68-6. *A,* Medial override fracture topographic positions at the condylar neck of the mandible are especially difficult to reduce because the ascending ramus of the mandible obscures the surgeon's access to manipulate the proximal fracture fragment. *B,* This is usually resolved by using the third portal to deliver the condyle to a lateral site to facilitate surgical reduction. *C,* The procedure often necessitates a conversion of the fracture displacement to a more favorable lateral override before application of fixation. *D,* Maintaining fracture reduction during the transition to rigid fixation is much more difficult with a medial override. Plate application to the proximal condylar pole to facilitate fracture reduction is sometimes necessary.

freely mobilize the jaw during waking hours but maintain maxillomandibular fixation with light elastic rubber bands at night. Jaw opening exercises are commenced in the fourth postoperative week.

Alternatively, an extraoral endoscope-assisted technique has been independently reported for condylar fracture repair.[17,18] The extraoral techniques have been described with a 1- to 2-cm incision at the mandibular angle as the primary portal for surgical access. Because the angle of the scope follows the posterior border of the mandible, visualization is more favorable along the posterior border of the mandible and condylar unit. Troulis and Kaban[18] have also used this external access portal to perform endoscopically assisted condylectomies. The visible facial incision and risk of marginal mandibular branch palsy of the facial nerve are significant disadvantages. Nevertheless, the external technique has great versatility with potential to refine difficult procedures involving complex osteotomies and reconstructive procedures for the ramus and condyle of the mandible.

RESULTS AND COMPLICATIONS

An anatomically accurate repair almost always yields a passively perfect restoration of the dental occlusion with normal midline jaw motion and jaw line appearance. Interincisal jaw opening usually exceeds 40 mm by the eighth postoperative week (Fig. 68-7). In most cases, anatomic rigid realignment of the displaced condylar pole is achieved (Figs. 68-8 to 68-10). The risk of facial nerve transection is low. Nevertheless, temporary traction palsy of the facial nerve has been reported after an overzealous retraction of the cheek soft tissues.

TIPS AND PEARLS

The endoscopic method of subcondylar fracture reduction relies heavily on visual fracture alignment; fixation necessitates sufficient extracapsular bone length for placement of fixation plate and screws. Therefore, in dealing with the technical feasibility of endoscopic repair, the following fracture considerations merit review: condylar head malpositioning, fracture location, fracture comminution, and displacement at the fracture site.

CONDYLAR HEAD MALPOSITIONING. Approximately 80% of adult subcondylar fractures present with a condyle that sags in the fossa and is flexed in the anterior-posterior direction. Unlike pediatric fractures, only 10% to 20% of adult fractures show medial subluxation or dislocation of the condylar head out of the fossa.[73] The malpositioned condylar head exacerbates the deviant jaw motion because of an absence or delayed activation of ipsilateral condylar head translation. Condylar head malpositioning does not alter the technical difficulty of endoscopic repair.

FRACTURE LOCATION. Intracapsular fractures are not amenable to endoscopic repair. Although intracapsular fractures are susceptible to late degenerative joint changes, there is usually minimal loss of posterior mandibular height with these fractures. Such patients typically demonstrate normal chin projection and minimal jaw deviation. High subcondylar fractures can be approached with endoscopy, provided there is sufficient extracapsular proximal bone length to manipulate visual reduction and place two screws for miniplate fixation.

FRACTURE COMMINUTION. Endoscopic fracture repair relies heavily on visual fracture alignment and interfragmentary contact. A high degree of comminution at the fracture line must be considered a contraindication to this technique. Minor degrees of fracture comminution affecting only a portion of the fracture line can be approached with endoscopy.

DISPLACEMENT AT THE FRACTURE SITE. This is the single most important variable that determines the technical feasibility and difficulty of endoscopic subcondylar fracture repair. In adult patients, loss of posterior mandibular height is most often due to override displacement of the proximal condylar fracture fragment on the ascending ramus.[74] In pediatric fractures, loss of mandibular height more often is due to a transversely oriented greenstick fracture in the subcondylar region with condylar head subluxation. Endoscopic subcondylar fracture repair is particularly satisfying to perform in patients presenting with a transverse or lateral override of the proximal condylar fracture fragment over the ascending ramus. The high incidence of lateral override in adult fractures (>90% in our center) makes this endoscopic technique particularly effective. In contrast, the medial override subcondylar fracture has been especially difficult to repair. Contraction of the pterygomasseteric muscle sling at the angle of the mandible telescopes the ascending ramus proximally. Fractures with medial override displacement are extremely difficult to repair because the telescoped ascending ramus obscures the visual access to the lateral surface of the proximal condylar fragment. Furthermore, controlled manipulation of the condylar fragment is greatly impaired from the physical obstruction produced by the telescoped ramus. Because established methods of open subcondylar fracture repair involve lateral proximal fragment exposure and manipulation, surgical repair of injuries with topographic medial override displacement at the fracture site would be technically difficult regardless of the surgical approach employed. Fortunately, the medial override fracture displacement represents only a minority of adult subcondylar fractures. At present, the degree of technical difficulty should be carefully considered before one embarks

Text continued on p. 485

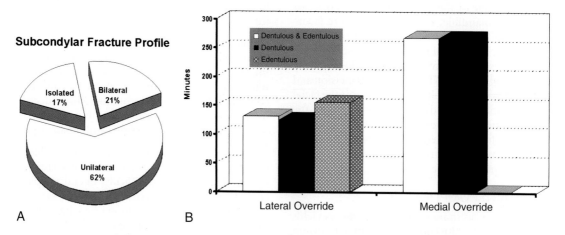

Mandible: Operative Time

Subcondylar Fracture Profile

Maximal Interincisal Jaw Opening

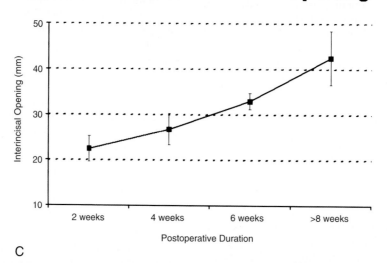

C

FIGURE 68-7. *A,* In our population, the majority of patients with an endoscopically treated extracapsular condylar neck fracture also had concomitant open surgical repair at other sites of fracture within the mandible. *B,* Operative times were least for patients with occluding dentition and lateral fracture override. Endoscopic repair of medial override fractures was the most difficult and required the longest surgical times. *C,* Most dentate patients recovered a normal range of jaw opening within 8 weeks of endoscopic condylar fracture repair. (*B* and *C* from Lee C, Mueller RV, Lee K, Mathes SJ: Endoscopic subcondylar fracture repair: functional, aesthetic, and radiographic outcomes. Plast Reconstr Surg 1998;102:1434-1443.)

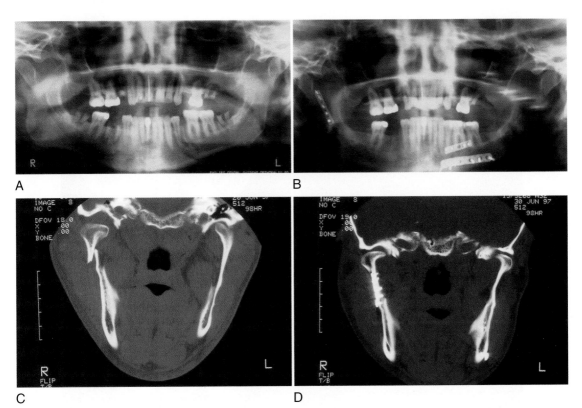

FIGURE 68-8. A 32-year-old man was assaulted, sustaining unilateral right subcondylar and left parasymphyseal mandibular fractures. *A,* Preoperative Panorex shows the typical flexion of the right proximal condylar fracture fragment and shortening of the posterior mandibular height. *B,* Postoperative Panorex shows anatomic restoration of the mandible. *C,* Preoperative high-resolution coronal CT image shows the topographic lateral override fracture displacement in the right subcondylar region and shortening of the posterior mandibular height. *D,* After endoscopic subcondylar fracture repair, the anatomic restoration of the condylar position and mandibular height is evident. Note the high extracapsular reach of the fixation hardware.   *Continued*

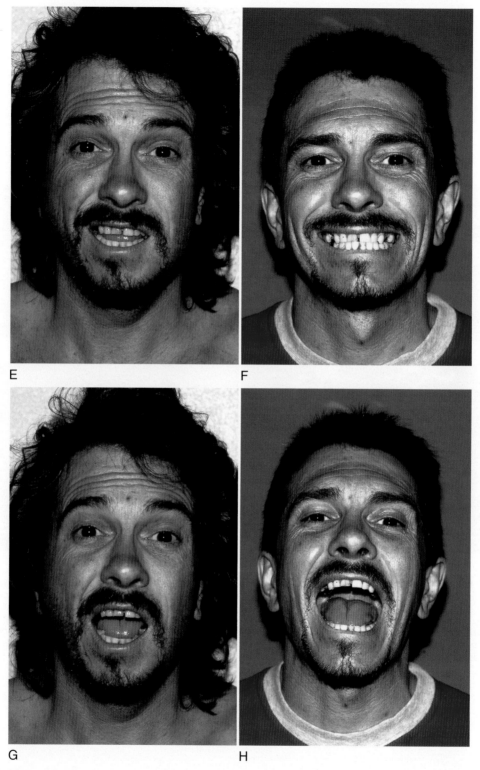

FIGURE 68-8, cont'd. *E* and *F,* The occlusion is restored. *G,* Preoperative photograph demonstrates chin point deviation to shortened right subcondylar fracture side on jaw opening. *H,* One year after endoscopic repair of the right subcondylar fracture and traditional rigid plate fixation of the left parasymphyseal fracture. Maximal interincisal jaw opening exceeds 40 mm and is midline. (*C, D, G,* and *H* from Lee C: Subcondylar fracture of the mandible: an endoscopic-assisted technique. Operative Techniques Plast Reconstr Surg 1998;5:287-294.)

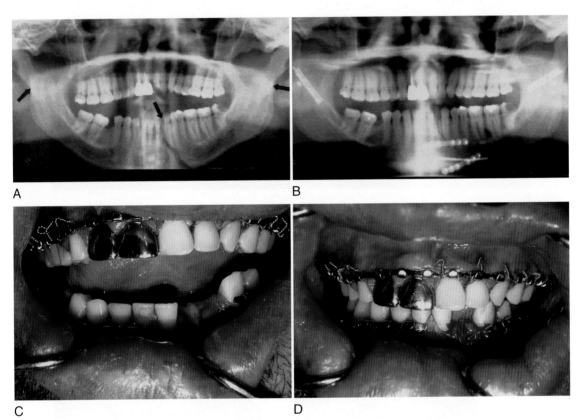

FIGURE 68-9. *A,* Bilateral mandibular subcondylar and left parasymphyseal fractures were present on preoperative Panorex radiograph. *B,* Panorex 8 weeks after surgery. *C,* Preoperative occlusion shows traumatic loss of the mandibular lateral incisor, anterior open bite, and collapse of the mandibular arch. *D,* Immediate postoperative occlusion is anatomically correct.

Continued

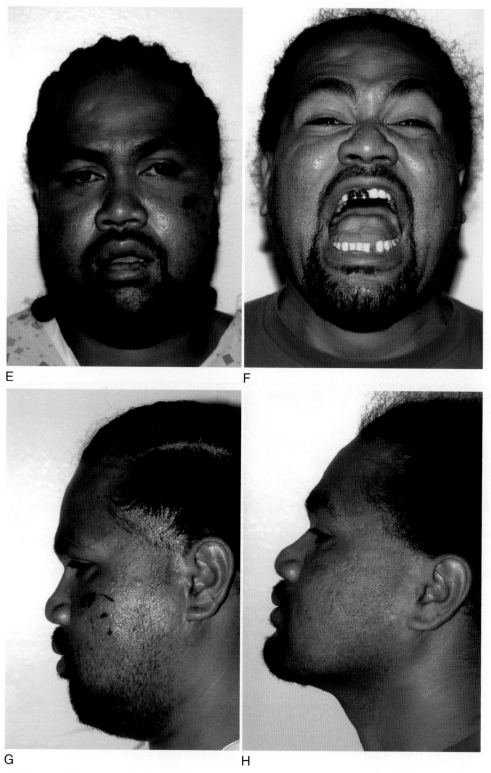

FIGURE 68-9, cont'd. *E,* Preoperative frontal view demonstrates a widened lower third of the face. *F,* Frontal view 8 weeks after surgery. *G,* Preoperative lateral view demonstrates the loss of the anteroposterior chin projection and weak jaw line. *H,* Lateral view 8 weeks after surgery. (From Jacobovicz J, Lee C, Trabulsy PP: Endoscopic repair of mandibular subcondylar fractures. Plast Reconstr Surg 1998;101:437-441.)

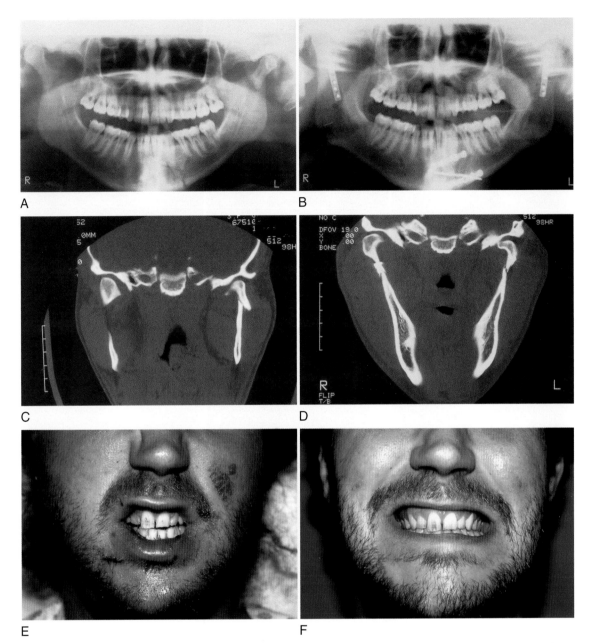

FIGURE 68-10. This 24-year-old man sustained injuries in a fall from a great height. Bilateral subcondylar and symphyseal mandibular fractures were present. *A* and *B,* Panorex radiographs preoperatively and postoperatively demonstrated that endoscopic repair was feasible. *C* and *D,* High-resolution coronal CT image demonstrated that mid-high left subcondylar fracture with lateral override and low right lateral override subcondylar fracture were well reduced. *E* and *F,* Malocclusion has resolved with treatment. *Continued*

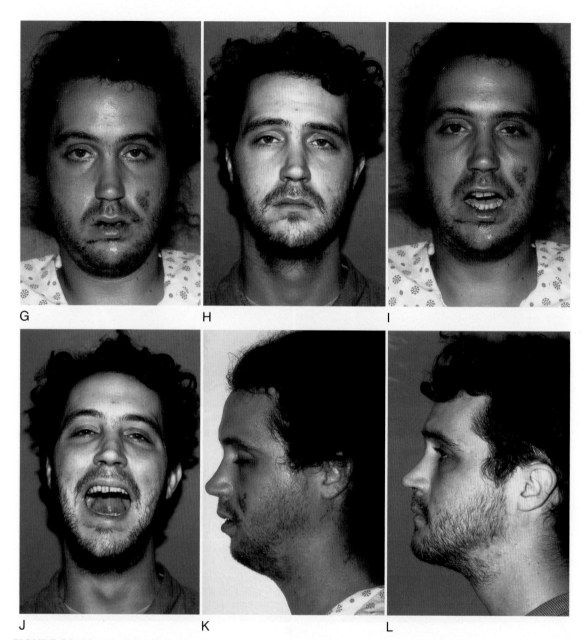

FIGURE 68-10, cont'd. *G* to *J,* Preoperative frontal photographs demonstrate widened lower face and deep labio-mental groove from loss of jaw projection. Three months after bilateral endoscopic subcondylar fracture repair and traditional rigid fixation of the symphyseal fracture, the patient reports that his jaw function and facial contours are restored to normal. *K* and *L,* Preoperative lateral facial view shows loss of chin projection and unpleasant jaw and neck contours in this patient with bilateral condylar fractures. Postoperative chin point and jaw line improved after bilateral endoscopic repair without postoperative maxillomandibular fixation. (*A* to *D* from Lee C, Mueller RV, Lee K, Mathes SJ: Endoscopic subcondylar fracture repair: functional, aesthetic, and radiographic outcomes. Plast Reconstr Surg 1998;102:1434-1443.)

on surgical repair of a subcondylar fracture with medial override fracture displacement.

GROWTH CONSIDERATIONS. Displaced subcondylar fractures in the growing mandible of a pediatric patient differ substantially from those in adults. In children, fractures tend to be greenstick and transversely oriented, and they have a high incidence of medial condylar head dislocation. Although technically feasible, surgical repair may compromise mandibular growth and is contraindicated. Furthermore, pediatric mandibular growth may accommodate and even normalize condylar malpositions from a malunited subcondylar fracture. In contrast, adults have very little capacity for anatomic self-correction of malunited fractures. Because most subcondylar fractures are amenable to endoscopic repair with minimal risks, anatomic fracture repair should be carefully considered in all adult patients with displaced subcondylar fractures.

ASSOCIATED FRACTURES. Fractures of the mandible remote from the injured condylar region must first be treated with open reduction and rigid internal fixation to restore the mandibular arch. Preliminary rigid restoration of the mandibular arch form facilitates the controlled manipulation and reduction of the highly mobile and unstable subcondylar fracture fragments.

MAXILLOMANDIBULAR FIXATION. The isolated use of maxillomandibular fixation rarely reduces a displaced subcondylar fracture. However, the use of maxillomandibular fixation as an adjunctive intraoperative guide greatly facilitates accurate fracture repair. In subcondylar fracture reduction, tight wire maxillomandibular fixation will often lock the displaced condylar fragment in a malreduced position. To permit fracture manipulation while the occlusion is held stable, rubber band anterior maxillomandibular fixation has been especially effective in our hands. Operative correction of the collapsed posterior mandibular height can be achieved by temporary creation of a posterior open bite to distract and elongate the collapsed subcondylar fracture site. This is effectively accomplished by placing a 3-mm wedge in the posterior occlusion while the anterior dentition is held in tight rubber band maxillomandibular fixation. The proximal condylar fragment can then be endoscopically guided into a visual reduction. Removal of the posterior occlusal wedge will then permit the rubber band traction to impact the fractured bone ends together, temporarily enhancing stability through interfragmentary friction. The minimal degree of stability achieved from interfragmentary friction facilitates the application of rigid plate fixation.

EDENTULOUS MANDIBLE. Endoscopic repair of the edentulous mandible with a subcondylar fracture can be technically challenging. The absence of occluding dentition interferes with endoscopic control and stabilization of the highly mobile fracture fragments. Even after an adequate endoscopic operative repair, the absence of posterior occluding dentition places greater strain on the fixation hardware and predisposes to hardware failure in the edentulous jaw. In comparison, the posterior dental occlusion of a dentulous jaw will partially absorb and shield the hardware from the vertical pterygomasseteric muscle compressive forces at the subcondylar region. The repair can be somewhat protected in the edentulous jaw by placement of more durable hardware, early use of preexisting partial dentures, or fabrication of posterior splints to absorb compressive forces.

Symphysis of the Mandible

Displaced fractures of the parasymphysis and symphysis may be treated by a variety of techniques that follow the standard principles of open reduction and internal fixation with either plates and screws or lag screws.[75-80] However, these methods involve wide exposure for adequate access with subperiosteal dissection extending well beyond the fracture site to facilitate fixation. Possible sequelae include increased risk of blood loss, lower lip muscle dysfunction, difficulty with oral hygiene and nutrition, devascularization of bone segments, and traction injuries on the mental nerve.

A modification of the traditional open methods for the surgical management of anterior mandibular fractures is proposed with the principles of minimal access surgery. This technique involves small incisions with transmucosal or percutaneous lag screw fixation with minimal soft tissue stripping. Lag screw fixation represents the most efficient method of achieving static interfragmentary compression with maximum stability and a minimum amount of implant material. Although applications have been described for mandibular angle[81-83] and condylar neck fractures, the region of the symphysis and parasymphysis represents the area where lag screw fixation may be most easily and efficiently applied. Potential advantages include shorter operative time, economic savings, decreased morbidity (swelling, scarring, mental nerve and lower lip muscle dysfunction), and improvement in functional rehabilitation. Minimal access techniques for the fractured symphysis represent a logical effort to increase the patient's comfort and to minimize costs. It is hoped that application of minimal access techniques will decrease the morbidity associated with open reduction but at the same time maintain the standard of care associated with internal fixation techniques.

INDICATIONS AND CONTRAINDICATIONS

This technique incorporates the use of lag screws introduced through small incisions transmucosally or percutaneously after anatomic reduction of the fracture and relies on accurate preoperative radiologic assessment of the fracture pattern and location.[15,68] This technique is indicated for any favorable fracture in the anterior mandibular arch that could achieve osteosynthesis with lag screw fixation and is dependent on the use of an interdental bridle wire or dental arch bar as a tension band. Success depends on selection of patients. Important parameters include fracture location, degree of comminution, condition of occluding dentition, type of fixation, and timing of the repair. Noncomminuted linear fractures are favorable to this minimally invasive approach. Optimal patients have excellent occluding dentition adjacent to the fracture line; this helps guide the fracture reduction. Fracture stabilization at the inferior border of the mandible is usually achieved through percutaneous or transmucosal application of a single lag screw. Fractures through the anterior symphyseal arch, which can be stabilized with lag screw fixation, are candidates for this minimally invasive technique. To minimize the accumulation of interfragmentary debris that can impede fracture reduction, repairs should be completed within 48 hours of the injury. Contraindications include unfavorable fracture patterns (long oblique, comminuted, flat mandibular plane), poor dental support for maintenance of an arch bar due to missing or loose teeth, inability to determine the fracture pattern preoperatively, and operator inexperience.

PREOPERATIVE RADIOGRAPHS

Accurate radiologic visualization of the fracture is mandatory and may be obtained with either Panorex or CT scan to identify the exact location and orientation of the fracture. Care is taken to identify the location of the mental foramina and any low-lying tooth roots on the radiograph. Because the technique of lag screw fixation is unforgiving, strict attention to detail and assessment of mandibular fracture pattern are crucial.

TECHNIQUE

Arch bars are first placed on the mandibular dentition in a segmental fashion. Free manipulation of the fracture mandibular segments is possible only if the arch bar does not bridge the fractured dental segments. An interdental bridle wire reduces and stabilizes the fracture segments at the occlusal border of the mandible. Maxillomandibular fixation is gently applied with care taken not to overtighten the fixation—this avoids flaring and fracture distraction at the inferior border of the mandible.[84] A large bone clamp is then placed transmucosally to compress the fracture space and to prepare the bone for the lag screw application. Two 1-cm vertical incisions are made equidistant from the fracture down to the periosteum at the site of the lag screw insertion. A minimal amount of periosteal

stripping is performed to facilitate drilling of two partial-thickness buccal cortex holes, and a large towel clip is engaged and applied across the fracture to produce satisfactory compression and reduction (Fig. 68-11). Alternatively, fixation can be passed transcutaneously through a trocar puncture site (Fig. 68-12). Just before application of fixation, mandibular angle flare is prevented by manual compression of the mandibular rami medially to ensure that the lingual cortices at the site of the fracture are in contact and appropriate facial width is established. After this, the lag screw is introduced across the fracture site in the usual fashion with use of a standard tissue guard. The principles of lag screw fixation dictate the placement of a gliding hole equidistant from a fixation hole with respect to the fracture edge. Access for fixation can be achieved through either a percutaneous or transmucosal puncture. Ideally, the screw is placed at right angles to the fracture plane. A gliding hole is made in the proximal cortex and is best placed close to the midline to facilitate retraction and to angle the drill, which must be oriented along the inferior border of the mandible away from dental tooth roots and mental nerves. After this, the fixation hole is drilled; the length of screw is measured and then introduced, producing static interfragmentary compression and satisfactory fixation of the fracture. Only one screw is usually necessary, although two may be applied. After fixation, maxillomandibular fixation should be released to confirm the stability of the repair and the adequacy of occlusion. Care is taken to ensure that no distraction along the superior alveolar border of the mandible has occurred with formation of a diastema between the teeth adjacent to the fracture site.

Fracture stability at the occlusive border can be enhanced with either adjustments to the interdental bridle wire or conversion of the segmentally applied arch bar to a single unit that crosses the fracture. The incisions are closed with absorbable suture, and two to four light dental elastics are applied to maintain premorbid occlusion and to counteract muscle spasm. An on-table plain radiograph or postoperative Panorex confirms the position of the screw. Postoperative management consists of light dental elastic intermaxillary fixation for 1 to 2 weeks, diligent oral hygiene, and a soft "no-chew" diet for 6 weeks. Arch bar removal is performed at 5 to 6 weeks postoperatively under neuroleptic anesthesia.

RESULTS AND COMPLICATIONS

This technique has been successfully employed in patients presenting with facial fractures isolated to the mandible (Fig. 68-13). Although a prospective study comparing this with traditional techniques is not yet available, avoidance of a large degloving incision along the anterior mandible was noted to be

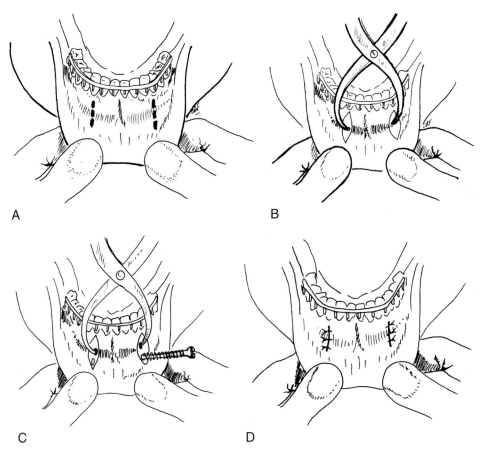

FIGURE 68-11. Schematic representation of transmucosal lag screw technique for fixation of parasymphyseal or symphyseal mandibular fracture. *A,* After restoration of the normal mandibular arch with arch bar and dental wire fixation, two vertical 1-cm incisions are marked equidistant from the fracture site and infiltrated with vasoconstrictor. *B,* Incisions are taken down to the periosteum, and a limited dissection is undertaken to facilitate drilling of monocortical holes for application of a large towel clip. Wide dissection is not performed, and the periosteal attachments over the fracture site are maintained. The fracture is reduced, intermaxillary fixation is achieved, the towel clip is applied, and the fracture site is compressed. *C,* The position of the lag screw is marked; after the gliding and fixation holes are drilled, a screw of the appropriate length is introduced, and fixation of the fracture is secured. Care must be taken to ensure visualization of the exit site of the screw. *D,* The incisions are closed with absorbable suture, and occlusion is checked. (From Forrest CR: Application of minimal-access techniques in lag screw fixation of fractures of the anterior mandible. Plast Reconstr Surg 1999;104:2127-2134.)

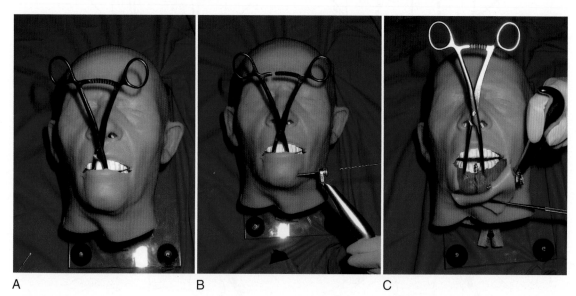

A   B   C

FIGURE 68-12. Alternative fracture stabilization at the inferior border of the mandibular symphysis with percutaneous application of the lag screw. *A,* The upper border of the mandible is stabilized with interdental wiring. A large bone clamp is then placed transmucosally to compress the fracture space and to prepare the bone for the lag screw application. *B,* Access for fixation can be achieved through a percutaneous trocar puncture. *C,* Fixation with a single 2.4-mm-diameter screw is achieved with orientation along the inferior border of the mandible away from dental tooth roots and mental nerves. (From Lee C, Mankani MH, Kellman RM, Forrest CR: Minimally invasive approaches to mandibular fractures. Facial Plast Surg Clin North Am 2001;9:475-487.)

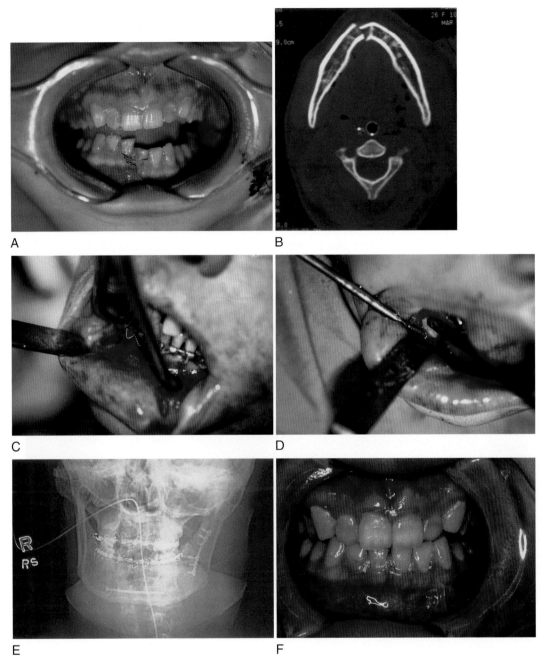

FIGURE 68-13. A 27-year-old woman after a motor vehicle accident with displaced fractures of the left angle and symphyseal region. *A,* Intraoperative view demonstrating displaced fracture exiting between the right and left lower central incisors. A dental wire was placed to provide a temporary reduction. *B,* Preoperative axial CT scan demonstrating fracture pattern. *C,* After limited subperiosteal dissection, monocortical holes are drilled to allow application of a large towel clip and compression and reduction of the fracture. Gliding and fixation holes are drilled in the usual fashion. *D,* After measurement of the appropriate length, lag screw fixation is achieved. *E,* Postoperative radiograph demonstrating position of screw. A small bone fragment is noted on the inferior mandibular border next to the head of the screw. *F,* Final result at 6 months with satisfactory restoration of occlusion and minimal intraoral lower buccal sulcus scarring. (From Forrest CR: Application of minimal-access techniques in lag screw fixation of fractures of the anterior mandible. Plast Reconstr Surg 1999;104:2127-2134.)

associated with decreased postoperative swelling and scarring, improved dental hygiene, better nutrition and communication, and decrease in recovery time. Other theoretical advantages include decreased chance for traction injury of the mental nerve, less probability of lower lip muscle dysfunction, maintenance of vascular supply to the bone due to less periosteal disruption, minimal amount of implant material, and decrease in operative time. In addition, the ability to use the arch bar as a tension band obviates the need for application of a monocortical miniplate along the alveolar border, which may become symptomatic or require removal once mandibular healing has been achieved. Finally, a comparison of implant material cost suggests that a single lag screw plus arch bar and wires provides a significant cost saving compared with a minimum six-hole mandibular plate plus tension band, arch bar, and dental wires.

An unusual complication has been reported.[15] A 1.5-cm length of a 1.8-mm-diameter drill bit broke off in the right body of the mandible during drilling of the fixation hole (Fig. 68-14). The procedure was successfully completed with use of the lag screw technique by changing the orientation of the drill. Because removal would entail a mandibular corticotomy, the drill bit was left in situ and the patient informed. With

a follow-up of more than 1 year, the patient has not experienced any significant problems related to the drill bit, nor is there any radiologic finding that suggests adverse tissue reaction to the retained drill bit. This unusual complication may occur whenever a lag screw technique is employed and is not thought to be unique to the modifications described herein.

TIPS AND PEARLS

Enthusiasm for this technique must be tempered with attention to the strict indications to which it may be applied. Fractures along flat mandibular planes (mandibular body) or long oblique and comminuted fracture patterns do not lend themselves to satisfactory fixation with lag screw techniques. Similarly, because this technique relies on the use of the arch bar as a tension band, inability to provide adequate support along the alveolar border because of missing or broken teeth should be viewed as a contraindication. However, this technique may prove useful in the surgical treatment of edentulous mandibular fractures where a tension band is not necessary and periosteal stripping of thin atrophic mandible may bring about avascular necrosis of the bone segments.[85,86] Finally, operator inexperience and uncertainty about the

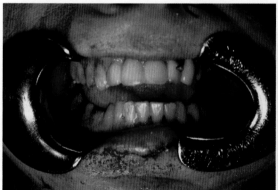

A

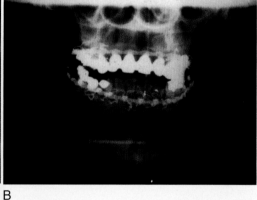

B

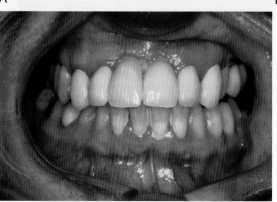

C

FIGURE 68-14. A 45-year-old woman after a motor vehicle accident; she had bilateral condylar neck and symphyseal fractures. *A,* Intraoperative view of occlusion before application of arch bars and placement of a single lag screw through a combination of a small submental laceration and intraoral mucosal incision. *B,* Postoperative radiograph demonstrating satisfactory bone alignment; a 1.8-mm-diameter segment of a broken drill bit in the right mandibular body is adjacent to the inferior alveolar canal and was left in situ. *C,* Final result at 12 months demonstrating minimal intraoral scarring and satisfactory restoration of premorbid occlusion. Mobility of the right lateral incisor was noted before application of arch bars and accounts for the small diastema seen adjacent to the right mandibular canine. No problems related to the retained drill bit have been encountered. Mental nerve sensation was not affected.

fracture pattern are indications for application of traditional open methods of plate and screw osteosynthesis. Application of lag screw fixation in fracture management is technically challenging and unforgiving, and strict adherence to protocol is required to prevent technical failure. The technique described relies on precise diagnosis and assessment of the fracture pattern to arrive at the choice of fixation technique. Inadequate radiologic visualization and inaccurate assessment of the nature of the fracture may result in suboptimal fixation, displacement, and postoperative malocclusion.

Avoidance of a wide approach with transmucosal or percutaneous lag screw fixation may cause difficulties in fracture reduction if a significant amount of time is allowed to pass before surgery is performed. Clinical experience has demonstrated that the fracture site becomes filled with soft tissue within 24 hours after the injury. Wide exposure of the fracture site allows the surgeon to facilitate anatomic reduction by distraction of the bone segments and débridement of the fracture site. This is not possible with the technique described, and therefore advantage in achieving a satisfactory reduction is provided by early (<24 hour) surgical intervention whenever possible. It was thought that inability to visualize reduction at the fracture site may be compensated for by careful assessment of the alignment of the dental arch.

Strict adherence to the principles of lag screw fixation dictates that a single screw will allow rotation of bone fragments. Although it would be simple to introduce a second screw for fixation, rotational deformity across the site of fracture was not noted to be a problem in any of the patients treated. The architecture of the anterior mandible, fracture pattern, indications for application of this technique, careful compression of the fracture by a large towel clip, and use of the arch bar may have helped prevent this theoretical problem. In situations in which multiple fractures of the mandible were present, consideration was given to restoration of the dental arch first.

Technical problems related to instrumentation resulted in breakage of the distal end of the drill bit with a retained fragment reported in one patient (see Fig. 68-14). Long drill bits are flexible and subject to bending when they encounter the inner surface of distal cortex at an oblique angle. Modification of instrumentation with the development of a combined reduction forceps and drill guide is currently being implemented to help prevent this problem.

Long oblique and comminuted fractures are not usually favorable for lag screw fixation. Because application of this technique relies on the arch bar to act as a tension band, adequate dentition must be present. Loose or lost teeth adjacent to the fracture site may necessitate the use of traditional open methods with placement of a superior border, monocortical miniplate to act as the tension band and to prevent splaying as the result of compressive forces applied along the inferior border of the mandible. In the edentulous mandible, a tension band is not necessary for obvious reasons.

Zygomatic Arch

The zygomatic arch is a key landmark to anatomic repair of complex orbitozygomatic and Le Fort III facial fractures.[4,5] Its anatomic repair can enhance the overall accuracy of the fracture reduction as well as augment the stability of repair in complex midfacial fractures.[87] Historically, arch exposure has necessitated a coronal scalp incision and thus suffers from its associated disadvantages. These include increased risk of blood loss, alopecia, loss of sensation posterior to the incision, and hollowing of the temporal fossa. Furthermore, proximity of the frontal branch of the facial nerve to the arch predisposes it to transection. With surgical endoscopy and limited access incisions, these undesirable risks associated with surgical fixation of the arch can be minimized.

INDICATIONS AND CONTRAINDICATIONS

The criteria for endoscopic arch repair are essentially the same as for traditional coronal repair. An anatomically repaired zygomatic arch can improve the accuracy of reduction and enhance the stability of repair to complex fractures of the orbitozygomatic and midface regions of the facial skeleton.

ISOLATED ARCH. Seldom is it necessary to repair an isolated fracture to the zygomatic arch. A robust temporal fat pad will often camouflage minor isolated fracture displacements of the arch. On occasion, endoscopic arch repair is indicated in the patient with isolated severe fracture disruption of the arch. These patients usually have a diminutive temporal fat pad and delicate soft tissue envelope.

COMPLEX ZYGOMA. Low-energy orbitozygomatic fractures rarely require repair of the arch. With low-energy injuries, direct fracture repair is accomplished at the zygomaticomaxillary, inferior orbital rim, and zygomaticofrontal fracture sites. Arch repair is technically demanding and unnecessary with low-energy zygomatic fractures, for which direct techniques already yield consistent results. Gruss et al[4] have used the zygomatic arch as a key landmark in the anatomic restoration of facial width and projection in orbitozygomatic fractures with comminution, loss of anteroposterior projection, and telescoping or lateral bowstringing of the arch. The corresponding patterns of arch disruption that should be considered for repair include major lateral arch displacement, posterior telescoped arch, and severe medial arch displacement (Fig. 68-15). Surgical reduction without fixation (e.g., Gillies arch elevation) may improve the depressed fracture displacement of a medialized and posteriorly telescoped arch. However, the laterally displaced arch does not favorably respond to elevation because it is already lateralized and will only become more displaced with elevation. Lateral arch displacement is an indication for surgical reduction and fixation.

LE FORT III. These fractures are usually high energy in nature and require stabilization of the midface to the cranium. Therefore, arch repair is warranted to enhance midface fracture reduction and stability. Endoscope-assisted arch repair is preferable as long as a coronal incision is not required for concomitant procedures, such as cranial bone graft harvest or repair of nasoethmoidal fractures.

TECHNIQUE

Arch repair is usually a single component of a more complicated Le Fort III or complex zygomatic fracture repair. This technique describes the endoscopic component of an arch repair (Figs. 68-16 and 68-17). Two minimally invasive access incisions are used to expose the zygomatic arch endoscopically: a preauricular incision at the anterior margin of the helical crus extending superiorly to approximately 2 cm above the auricle and a transverse 1-cm incision at the lateral orbital region in a skin crease superior to the lateral canthal region. For an adequate optical cavity to be made for endoscopic viewing, the scalp extension of the preauricular incision is used to expose the deep temporal fascia. An optical cavity is made superiorly by use of a periosteal elevator to dissect superficial to the surface of the deep temporal fascia. Under optical endoscopic magnification, the dissection is carried in this plane down to the arch. To prevent postoperative temporal hollowing, the temporal fat pad is not violated. The frontal branch of the facial nerve is not routinely visualized. Once the upper border of the arch is reached, the overlying periosteum is incised, and the dissection is carried in a subperiosteal plane to expose the entire midfacial arch. Fracture reduction and fixation then proceed by sequential reduction and plating of fractures with screws passed through a percutaneous trocar.

Kobayashi et al[9] have described an alternative method of endoscopic fracture repair at the zygomatic arch with use of incisions in the temporal scalp and intraoral sites. Although this has the advantage of less visible scarring, the precise placement of fixation plates and screws is exceedingly difficult from these access sites remote from the arch. A preauricular skinfold is preferred for endoscopic access to the zygomatic arch for repair.

FIGURE 68-15. Major arch disruptions in which surgical fixation should be considered. The rationale for arch repair is either to enhance the anatomic reduction or to increase the stability of a complex repair to the upper facial skeleton. *A,* Major lateral arch displacement. *B,* After endoscopic repair. *C,* Posterior telescoping of the arch with severe loss of malar projection. *D,* After endoscopic repair. *E,* Major medial arch displacement. *F,* After endoscopic repair. (From Lee CH, Lee C, Trabulsy PP, et al: A cadaveric and clinical evaluation of endoscopic assisted zygomatic fracture repair. Plast Reconstr Surg 1998; 101:333-345.)

RESULTS AND COMPLICATIONS

Endoscopic arch repair has proved to be a versatile technique that can easily be integrated into more complicated operative protocols for repair of Le Fort III and complex zygomatic fractures (Figs. 68-18 to 68-20).[7,10,11,51] Endoscope-assisted arch reduction and fixation enhanced the accuracy and stability of complex midfacial and orbitozygomatic fractures without the need for a coronal incision. By avoidance of dissection in the temporal fat pad, hallowing seldom occurred. Approximately 25% of patients demonstrated temporary frontalis muscle palsy after endoscopic fracture repair. All cases of frontalis palsy recovered spontaneously and completely.

Anterior Wall of the Frontal Sinus

The treatment of anterior table frontal sinus fractures by endoscope-assisted minimal access techniques represents a significant and definitive advantage over the traditional methods using a bicoronal incision. Theoretically, the lack of a coronal scar and scalp numbness should decrease morbidity of patients, but a comparative outcome study has yet to be performed. Care must be taken, however, not to compromise the conversion to a traditional open technique if access to the floor is necessary or if the sinus requires obliteration. Given the current state of instrumentation available, it is not possible to remove all sinus mucosa adequately. Minimal access techniques have been strictly limited in the frontal sinus to treatment of anterior table fractures, assessment of the nasofrontal drainage system, and burring of the sinus to remove residual mucosa in the recesses of the sinus, especially with extensions toward the lateral orbital region. The last is done by a traditional coronal technique, but use of the endoscope in this manner obviates the need for a supraorbital osteotomy for access. This approach is technically demanding.

Text continued on p. 503

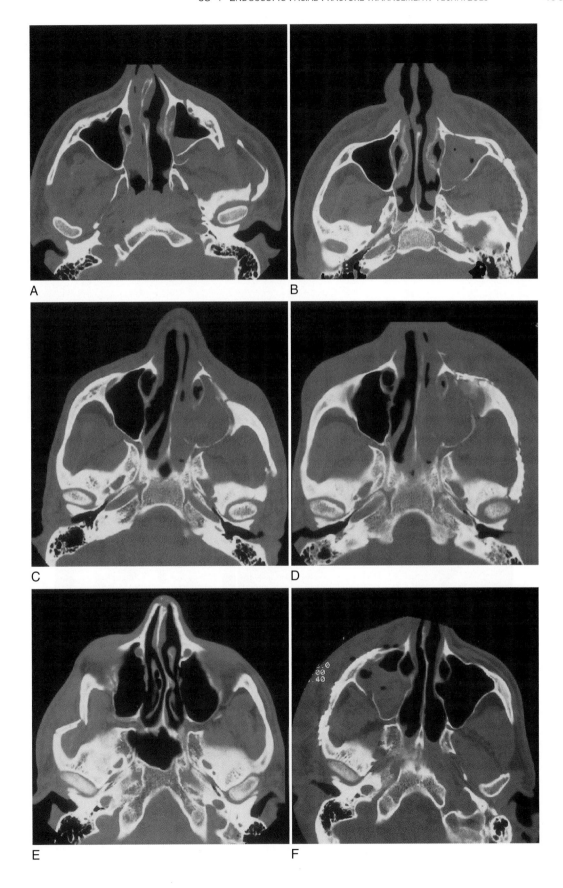

A

B

C

D

E

F

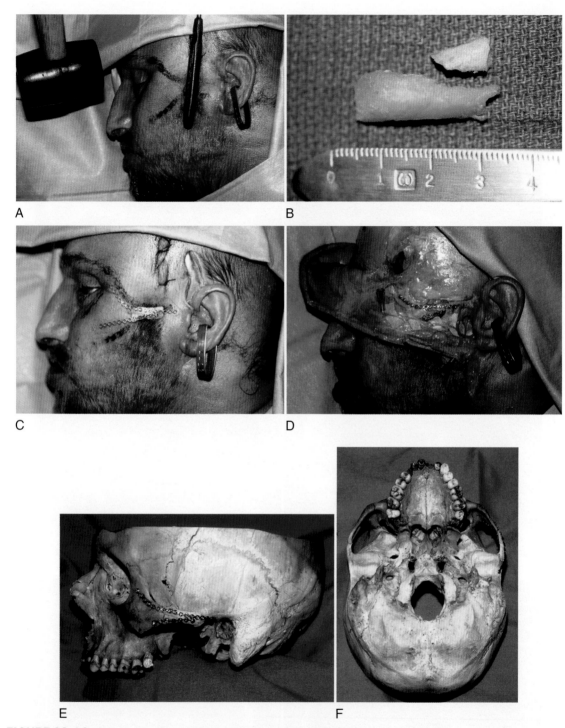

FIGURE 68-16. Endoscopic arch repair was first evaluated in a fresh cadaver head. Surgical access involved a preauricular incision at the anterior margin of the helical crus extending 2 cm superior to the auricle and a 1-cm transverse incision at the lateral orbital region in a skin crease superior to the lateral canthal region. *A,* A unilateral fracture of the zygomatic arch was made by striking an 8-ounce rubber mallet onto a metallic rod. *B,* The comminuted arch was dissected free under endoscopic guidance. *C,* A mini-adaptation plate was contoured and applied to the free arch segment on a side table. *D,* After endoscopic reduction and fixation of the arch, the frontal branch of the facial nerve was dissected out. The nerve was found to be anatomically intact in all dissections. *E,* Soft tissues were stripped from the skull. Lateral view of the repair demonstrates an anatomic restoration of the fractured arch. *F,* The repaired arch was found to be symmetric with the uninjured contralateral side. (From Lee CH, Lee C, Trabulsy PP, et al: A cadaveric and clinical evaluation of endoscopic assisted zygomatic fracture repair. Plast Reconstr Surg 1998;101:333-345.)

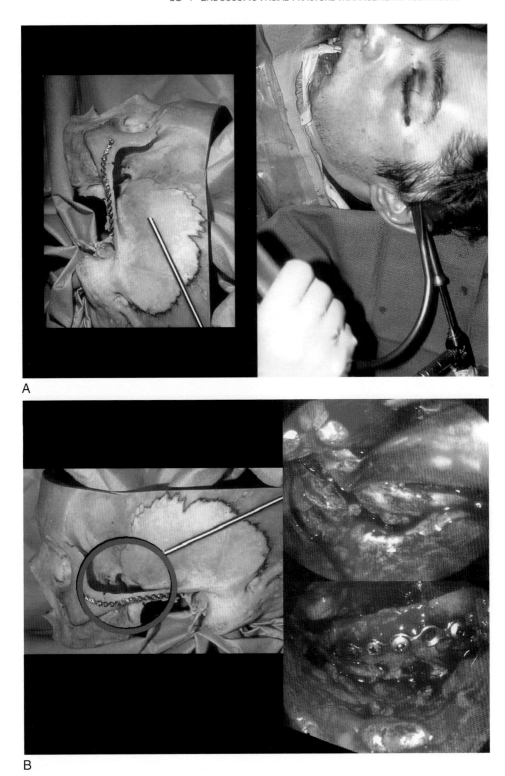

FIGURE 68-17. Endoscopic arch repair was integrated into the clinical armamentarium for use as an alternative to a coronal incision. *A,* An endoscope-mounted retractor is placed through a preauricular incision for access to the arch. *B,* Endoscopic images of a fractured arch before repair and after reduction and fixation. (From Lee CH, Lee C, Trabulsy PP, et al: A cadaveric and clinical evaluation of endoscopic assisted zygomatic fracture repair. Plast Reconstr Surg 1998;101:333-345.)

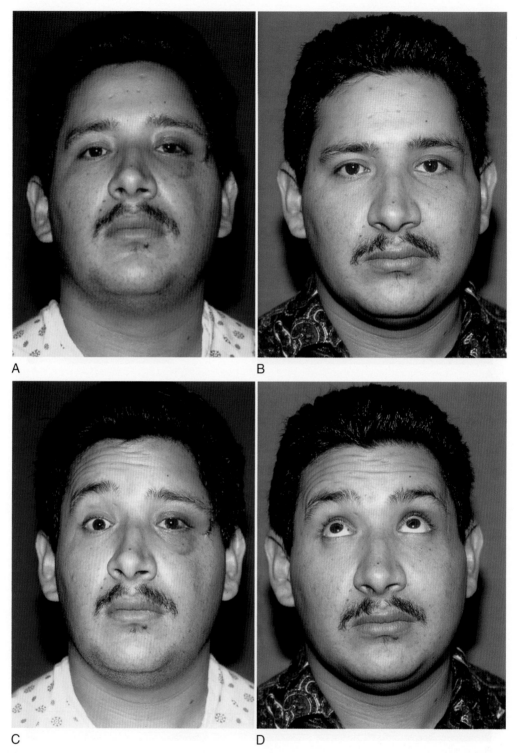

FIGURE 68-18. Clinical photographs of the patient in Figure 68-15. *A* and *C*, Preoperative frontal views demonstrate the clinical loss of frontal cranial nerve VII function. *B* and *D*, No exploration of the nerve was performed. Spontaneous frontal cranial nerve VII recovery took place after surgery, attesting to the anatomic preservation of nerve continuity with this endoscopic technique.

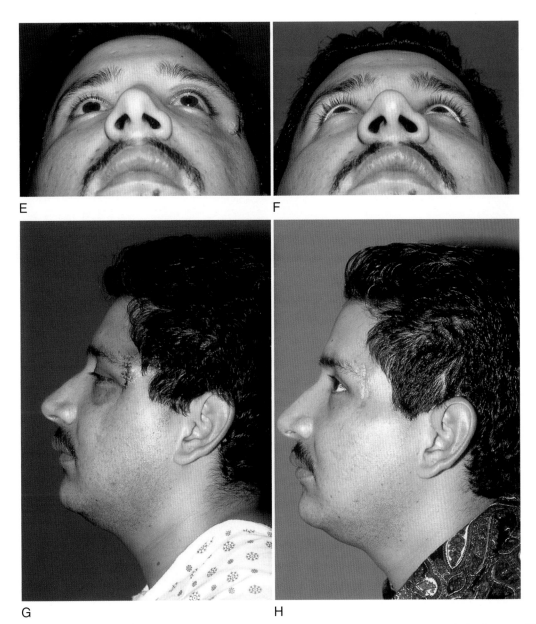

FIGURE 68-18, cont'd. *E* to *H,* Facial proportions are improved after anatomic repair of the facial fracture. (From Lee CH, Lee C, Trabulsy PP, et al: A cadaveric and clinical evaluation of endoscopic assisted zygomatic fracture repair. Plast Reconstr Surg 1998;101:333-345.)

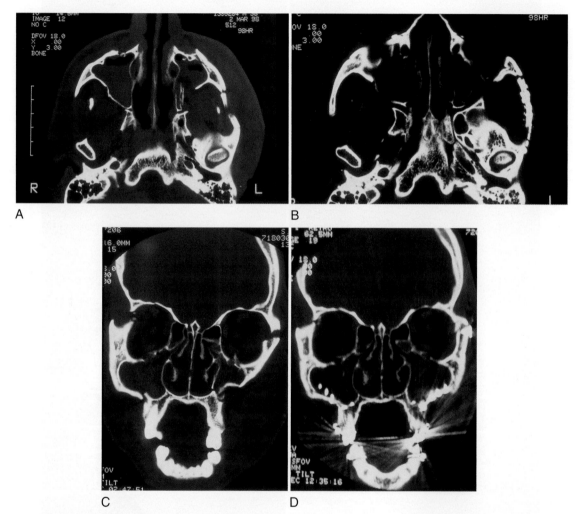

FIGURE 68-19. A moderate-energy facial impact with resulting left-sided Le Fort III facial fracture treated with endoscopic arch repair to enhance the stability of the maxilla. *A* and *B*, Axial CT images before and after repair. *C* and *D*, Coronal CT images before and after repair.

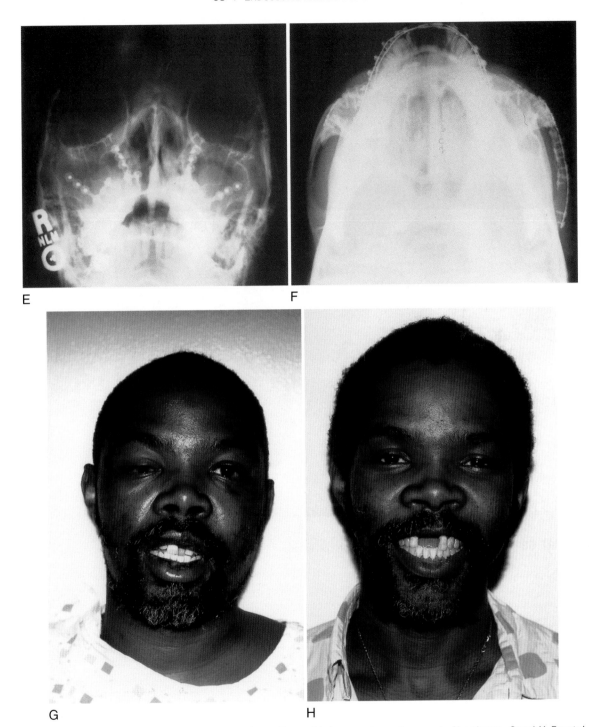

FIGURE 68-19, cont'd. *E* and *F,* Postoperative radiographic images show placement of hardware. *G* and *H,* Frontal view shows postoperative correction of the malocclusion. Note that the single central incisor was traumatized and extracted. *Continued*

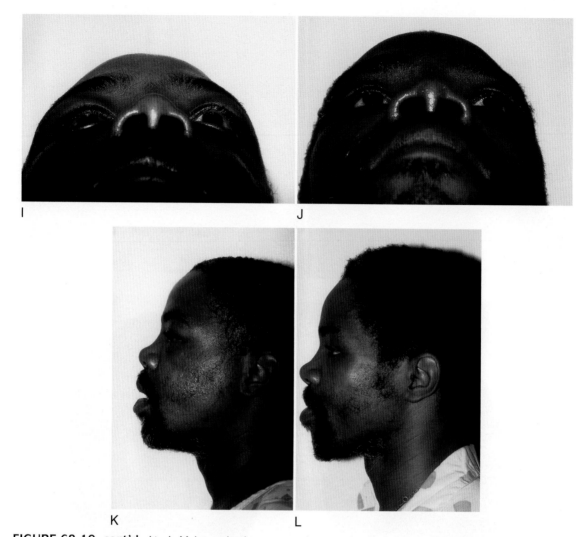

I   J

K   L

FIGURE 68-19, cont'd. *I* to *L,* Malar projection corrected.

FIGURE 68-20. A high-energy motor vehicle accident facial impact with resulting right-sided Le Fort III fracture, split palate, and blowout fracture of the right orbital floor treated by endoscope-assisted repair of the arch and transantral titanium mesh repair of the right orbital floor without a lower eyelid incision. *A* and *B,* Fracture pattern drawn on plastic skull. *C* to *F,* CT images before and after repair. Postoperative images show placement of hardware as well as the location of the orbital titanium mesh.

Continued

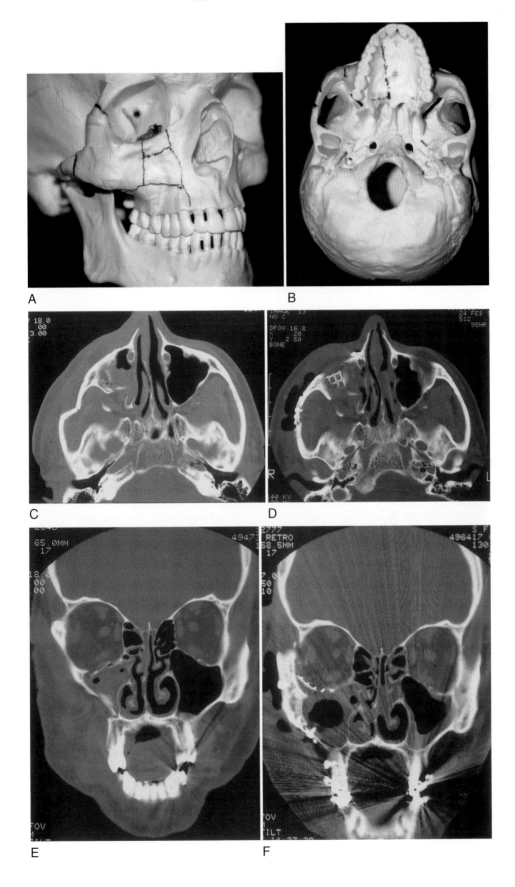

A

B

C

D

E

F

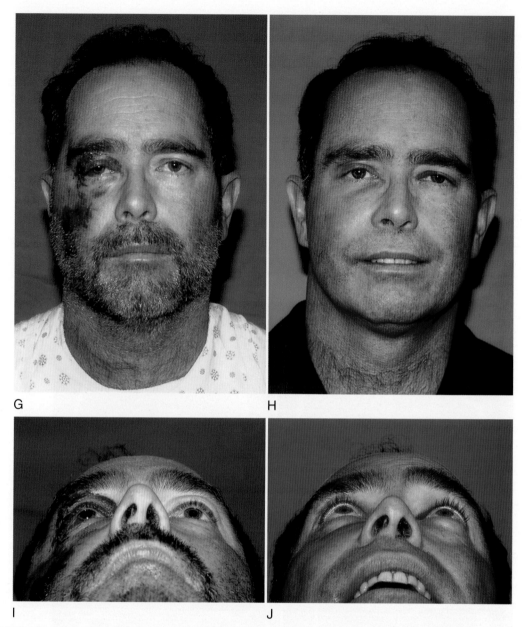

FIGURE 68-20, cont'd. *G* to *L*, Preoperative and postoperative facial images with improvement of occlusion and facial contour and good right globe projection. (From Lee C, Jacobovicz J, Mueller RV: Endoscopic repair of a complex midfacial fracture. J Craniofac Surg 1997;8:170-175.)

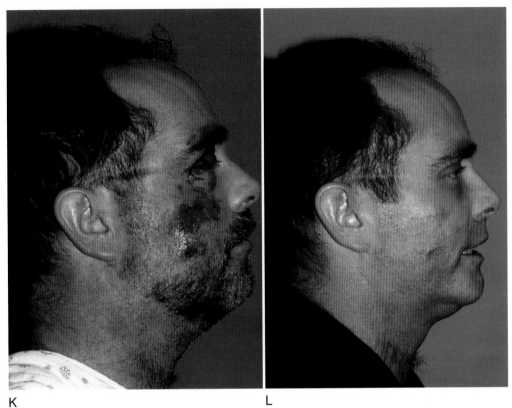

K   L

FIGURE 68-20, cont'd.

INDICATIONS AND CONTRAINDICATIONS

Endoscopic techniques were employed in patients presenting with acute frontal sinus fractures involving the anterior table only.[8,88] Contraindications to this approach included displaced posterior table fractures, compound injuries, and cerebrospinal fluid leakage or any other injuries that required a craniotomy.

TECHNIQUE

Access to the frontal sinus is achieved through three small (5-mm) incisions along the anterior hairline with additional incisions made in the medial brow region or superior portion of the naso-orbital valley (Fig. 68-21). Wide subperiosteal dissection is performed down to the level of the supraorbital rim and across to the nasofrontal suture. Visualization of the neurovascular bundles ensures preservation. Placement of retraction sutures along the forehead may enhance the optical cavity (Fig. 68-22). Visualization is best achieved with the 30-degree endoscope, but a 70-degree endoscope may be used for visualization of the floor of the frontal sinus. Microplates are introduced through the incisions, manipulated into place, and fixed percutaneously by small stab incisions over the glabellar region or in

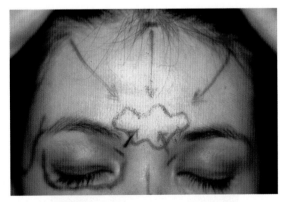

FIGURE 68-21. Access to the frontal sinus can be achieved through a series of hairline incisions for viewing and manipulation in addition to incisions in the medial brow or naso-orbital valley for bone fragment and microplate manipulation and percutaneous screw fixation. (From Forrest CR: Application of endoscope-assisted minimal-access techniques in orbitozygomatic complex, orbital floor, and frontal sinus fractures. J Craniomaxillo-fac Trauma 1999;5:1-13.)

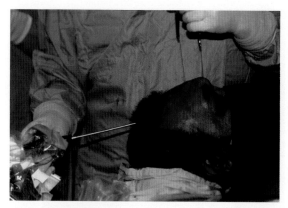

FIGURE 68-22. Traction sutures used to establish a satisfactory optical window.

expression lines (Fig. 68-23). Uses of the endoscope included reduction and fixation of anterior table fractures, evaluation of the nasofrontal duct, removal of frontal sinus septum to permit drainage, and removal of sinus mucosa.

RESULTS AND COMPLICATIONS

Incisions in the medial brow and naso-orbital valley have not proved to be cosmetically a problem. Current problems with this approach, which include disimpaction and manipulation of bone fragments, transcutaneous placement of screws, and plate placement, have resulted in increased operative times. A theoretical alternative for anterior table fractures is the use of titanium mesh as an onlay over the displaced bone fragments or application of bone paste through a long cannula to ensure appropriate contour restoration in the management of established post-traumatic deformities.[56]

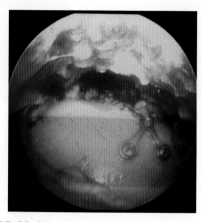

FIGURE 68-23. Microplates in situ after reduction of anterior table fracture fragments.

Internal Orbit

CT images of the orbit are of such accuracy that significant orbital floor blowout defects can be confidently diagnosed without invasive techniques. Endoscopy of the orbital floor may be of diagnostic benefit in cases in which the information from original CT scans is no longer valid because of an intervention; for example, after repair of an orbitozygomatic fracture, an orbital floor defect may become apparent only after reduction of the displaced zygomatic bone. Under these circumstances, transantral endoscopic viewing of the orbital floor can be of substantial diagnostic benefit. Sandler et al[89] were able to use the endoscope under local anesthesia to evaluate the roof of the maxillary antrum in patients with suspected orbital floor injuries. Their study demonstrated that with use of local anesthesia, orbital floor blowout fractures could be detected with a high degree of specificity.

INDICATIONS AND CONTRAINDICATIONS

Transantral endoscopic inspection of the orbital floor is useful in diagnosis of significant defects in patients who have not been suitable for coronal CT scans or after reduction of the zygoma. It may also serve as an assist device in delineating the posterior ledge of a substantial orbital floor defect. With increased experience, the possibility of routine transantral orbital floor repair without an eyelid incision exists for selected single-wall defects.

TECHNIQUE

The maxillary antrum has been used as an optical cavity for inspection of the orbital floor. Access to the orbital floor was achieved through the maxillary sinus, preferably through a Caldwell-Luc approach or intranasally with a small antrostomy under the uncinate process of the inferior turbinate (Fig. 68-24). Forrest[8] described a provocative test to evaluate the integrity of the orbital floor (Figs. 68-25 to 68-27). Digital depression of the globe posteriorly into the orbit while the endoscope was in place demonstrated herniation of periorbital tissue into the antrum through the defect in the orbital floor. This was coined a positive "pulse test" result. Less commonly, repair of single-wall defects in the orbital floor has been reported without an eyelid incision. Such an undertaking would require substantial endoscopic experience and familiarity with microanatomy to avoid ocular injury as well as to achieve adequate surgical repair.

RESULTS AND COMPLICATIONS

The maxillary antrum is anatomically ideal as an optical cavity for visualization of the orbital floor. Application of endoscopic technology in the management of orbital floor fractures could be considered

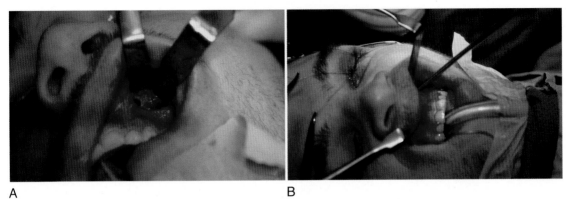

FIGURE 68-24. Access to the orbital floor through an upper buccal sulcus incision with small antrostomy *(A)* and introduction of the 30-degree endoscope *(B)*. (From Forrest CR: Application of endoscope-assisted minimal-access techniques in orbitozygomatic complex, orbital floor, and frontal sinus fractures. J Craniomaxillofac Trauma 1999;5:1-13.)

minimal access only if it afforded the opportunity to avoid a lower lid incision. To date, this has not been routinely attempted. Instead, most endoscopic surgeons have been using transantral viewing of the orbital floor as a diagnostic and surgical assist instrument. Endoscopic visualization of the orbital floor through a transantral approach has proved valuable in establishing the diagnosis by the pulse test, releasing entrapped periorbital tissue, identifying the posterior ledge of the orbital floor defect, and ensuring appropriate positioning after orbital floor reconstruction with bone graft or alloplastic material (Figs. 68-28 and 68-29). The pulse test has been most useful in

diagnosis of significant orbital floor defects in patients who have not been suitable for coronal CT scans or after reduction of the zygoma. No patient in our series with a negative pulse test result (i.e., absence of herniation of the periorbital soft tissues into the maxillary antrum) developed late enophthalmos. In this way, endoscopic assistance represents a refinement of the traditional approach to orbital floor fractures and theoretically should produce improved outcome compared with the standard techniques.

Saunders et al[6] performed anatomic analysis of the orbital floor and concluded that anterior orbital floor defects may be amenable to reconstruction by a

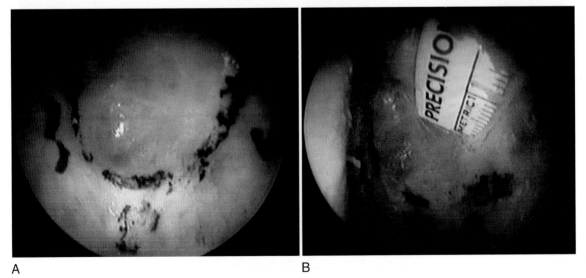

FIGURE 68-25. Endoscopic view of the orbital floor in cadaver specimen before *(A)* and after *(B)* an orbital floor defect is made. The medial (M) and lateral (L) walls of the maxillary antrum are marked for reference. (From Forrest CR: Application of endoscope-assisted minimal-access techniques in orbitozygomatic complex, orbital floor, and frontal sinus fractures. J Craniomaxillofac Trauma 1999;5:1-13.)

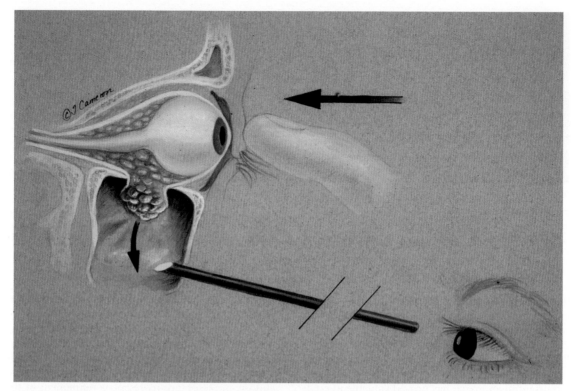

FIGURE 68-26. The pulse test to determine orbital floor integrity. When significant (>1 cm^2) orbital floor defects exist, retropulsion of the globe will result in fat herniation into the maxillary antrum, which is easily visualized with a 30-degree endoscope. (From Forrest CR: Application of endoscope-assisted minimal-access techniques in orbitozygomatic complex, orbital floor, and frontal sinus fractures. J Craniomaxillofac Trauma 1999;5:1-13.)

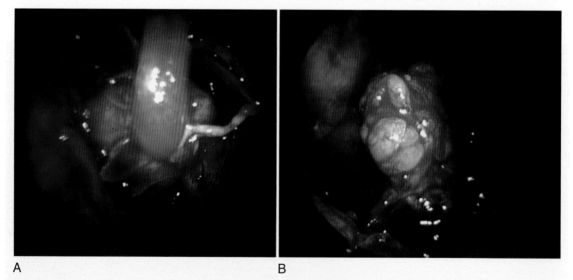

A   B

FIGURE 68-27. Endoscopic images of orbital floor defects showing herniation of periorbital fat around the infraorbital nerve *(A)* and with digital retropulsion of the globe demonstrating a positive pulse test result *(B)*.

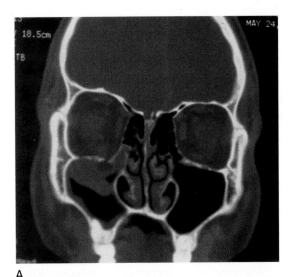

A

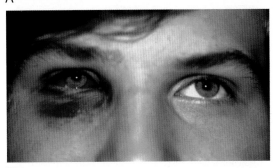

B

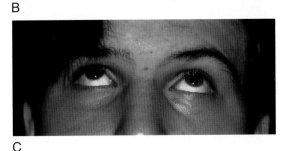

C

FIGURE 68-28. *A,* CT scan demonstrating "trap-door" orbital floor fracture with entrapment of periorbital soft tissue in the fracture site. *B* and *C,* Clinical photographs of patient before endoscopic release of periorbital tissue demonstrating limitation of superior gaze and 3 months after surgery.

transantral approach. Mohammad et al[90] have confirmed that reconstruction of orbital floor defects by a transantral approach is feasible in cadavers but acknowledged that significant technical difficulties exist. Currently, the problems relate to inadequate instrumentation for manipulation and difficulties with visualization due to hemorrhage and risk of globe injury.

Transantral repair of an orbital floor defect by use of titanium mesh without a lower eyelid incision has

been reported in an isolated instance as a component of a midfacial fracture repair by Lee et al.[7] To date, Stanley[91] has the largest experience with transantral repair of single-wall defects confined to the orbital floor. In his series, repair of the floor without an eyelid incision is routinely attempted with moderate success reported. In his preliminary report, no ocular injuries have been described. Failed transantral repairs were converted to traditional transconjunctival lower eyelid access with use of the scope as an assist device.

EVOLVING APPLICATIONS AND FUTURE DIRECTIONS

The latter part of the 20th century will be known for the rapid evolution of new surgical principles and methodology in the field of plastic and reconstructive surgery. Advances in the field of imaging and a better understanding of the anatomy of the facial skeleton resulted in the development of miniature fixation appliances and allowed the development of the principles of open reduction and internal fixation for the sophisticated surgical management of facial fractures. This chapter outlines the current state of the art in the area of minimal access surgery and endoscopic applications in facial trauma with the expectation that morbidity of patients will be decreased without compromise in care. Current limitations relate to visualization technology and instrumentation. However, with innovation, imagination, and demand, it is expected that these hurdles will be overcome and the envelope will be expanded. For the practicing surgeon with an interest in facial trauma, continued refinement of these techniques will provide improvement in results and decreased morbidity of patients. It is likely that future applications of these techniques will be developed in the fields of robotic and remote-operator surgery.

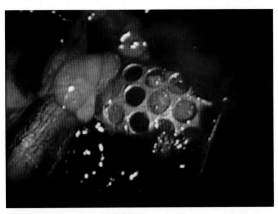

FIGURE 68-29. Endoscopic image of bone graft construct in situ, confirming adequate position.

REFERENCES

1. Phillips JH, Gruss JS, Wells MD, Chollet A: Periosteal suspension of the lower eyelid and cheek following subciliary exposure of facial fractures. Plast Reconstr Surg 1991;88:145-148.
2. Gruss JS, Phillips JH: Complex facial trauma: the evolving role of rigid fixation and immediate bone graft reconstruction. Clin Plast Surg 1989;16:93-104.
3. Markowitz BL, Manson PN: Panfacial fractures: organization of treatment. Clin Plast Surg 1989;16:105-115.
4. Gruss JS, Van Wyck L, Phillips JH, Antonyshyn O: The importance of the zygomatic arch in complex midfacial fracture repair and correction of posttraumatic orbitozygomatic deformities. Plast Reconstr Surg 1990;85:878-890.
5. Stanley RB Jr: The zygomatic arch as a guide to reconstruction of comminuted malar fractures. Arch Otolaryngol Head Neck Surg 1989;115:1459-1462.
6. Saunders CJ, Whetzel TP, Stokes RB, et al: Transantral endoscopic orbital floor exploration: a cadaver and clinical study. Plast Reconstr Surg 1997;100:575-581.
7. Lee C, Jacobovicz J, Mueller RV: Endoscopic repair of a complex midfacial fracture. J Craniofac Surg 1997;8:170-175.
8. Forrest CR: Application of endoscope-assisted minimal-access techniques in orbitozygomatic complex, orbital floor, and frontal sinus fractures. J Craniomaxillofac Trauma 1999;5:1-13.
9. Kobayashi S, Sakai Y, Yamada A, Ohmori K: Approaching the zygoma with an endoscope. J Craniofac Surg 1995;6:519-524.
10. Lee CH, Lee C, Trabulsy PP: Endoscopic-assisted repair of a malar fracture. Ann Plast Surg 1996;37:178-183.
11. Lee CH, Lee C, Trabulsy PP, et al: A cadaveric and clinical evaluation of endoscopic assisted zygomatic fracture repair. Plast Reconstr Surg 1998;101:333-345.
12. Chen CT, Lai JP, Chen YR, et al. Application of endoscope in zygomatic fracture repair. Br J Plast Surg 2000;53:100-105.
13. Honda T, Nozaki M, Isono N, Sasaki K: Endoscope-assisted facial fracture repair. World J Surg 2001;25:1075-1083.
14. Lee C, Mueller RV, Lee K, Mathes SJ: Endoscopic subcondylar fracture repair: functional, aesthetic, and radiographic outcomes. Plast Reconstr Surg 1998;102:1434-1443.
15. Forrest CR: Application of minimal-access techniques in lag screw fixation of fractures of the anterior mandible. Plast Reconstr Surg 1999;104:2127-2134.
16. Chen CT, Lai JP, Tung TC, Chen YR: Endoscopically assisted mandibular subcondylar fracture repair. Plast Reconstr Surg 1999;103:60-65.
17. Schmelzeisen R, Lauer G, Wichmann U: Endoscope-assisted fixation of condylar fractures of the mandible [in German]. Mund Kiefer Gesichtschir 1998;2(suppl 1):S168-S170.
18. Troulis MJ, Kaban LB: Endoscopic approach to the ramus/condyle unit: clinical applications. J Oral Maxillofac Surg 2001;59:503-509.
19. Manson PN, Markowitz B, Mirvis S, et al: Toward a CT-based facial fracture treatment. Plast Reconstr Surg 1990;85:202-212.
20. Manson PN, Hoopes JE, Su CT: Structural pillars of the facial skeleton: an approach to the management of Le Fort fractures. Plast Reconstr Surg 1980;66:54-61.
21. Manson PN, Crawley WA, Yaremchuk MJ, et al: Midface fractures: advantages of immediate extended open reduction and bone grafting. Plast Reconstr Surg 1985;76:1-12.
22. Gruss JS, Mackinnon SE: Complex maxillary fractures: role of buttress reconstruction and immediate bone grafts. Plast Reconstr Surg 1986;78:9-22.
23. Antonyshyn OM, Gruss JS, Galbraith DJ, Hurwitz JJ: Complex orbital fractures: a critical analysis of immediate bone graft reconstruction. Ann Plast Surg 1989;22:220-235.
24. Eppley BL, Prevel CD: Nonmetallic fixation in traumatic midfacial fractures. J Craniofac Surg 1997;8:103-109.
25. Eppley BL, Sadove AM, Havlik RJ: Resorbable plate fixation in pediatric craniofacial surgery. Plast Reconstr Surg 1997;100:1-7.
26. Amarante MTJ, Constantinescu MA, O'Connor D, Yaremchuk MJ: Cyanoacrylate fixation of the craniofacial skeleton: an experimental study. Plast Reconstr Surg 1995;95:639-646.
27. Constantino PD, Friedman CD, Jones R, et al: Experimental hydroxyapatite cement cranioplasty. Plast Reconstr Surg 1992;90:174-185.
28. Rudderman RH, Mullen RL: Biomechanics of the facial skeleton. Clin Plast Surg 1992;19:11-29.
29. Klotch DW, Gilliland R: Internal fixation vs. conventional therapy in midface fractures. J Trauma 1987;27:1136-1145.
30. Pearl RM: Prevention of enophthalmos: a hypothesis. Ann Plast Surg 1990;25:132-133.
31. Pearl RM: Surgical management of volumetric changes in the bony orbit. Ann Plast Surg 1987;19:349-358.
32. Pearl RM: Treatment of enophthalmos. Clin Plast Surg 1992;19:99-111.
33. Hall MB: Condylar fractures: surgical management. J Oral Maxillofac Surg 1994;52:1189-1192.
34. Walker RV: Condylar fractures: nonsurgical management. J Oral Maxillofac Surg 1994;52:1185-1188.
35. Demianczuk AN, Antonyshyn OM: Application of a three-dimensional intraoperative navigational system in craniofacial surgery. J Craniofac Surg 1997;8:290-297.
36. Bernstein MP, Caldwell CB, Antonyshyn OM, et al: Spatial and temporal registration of CT and SPECT images: development and validation of a technique for in vivo three-dimensional semiquantitative analysis of bone. J Nucl Med 2000;41:1075-1081.
37. Fialkov JA, Phillips JH, Gruss JS, et al: A stereotactic system for guiding complex craniofacial reconstruction. Plast Reconstr Surg 1992;89:340-345, discussion 346-348.
38. Stanley RB Jr: Use of intraoperative computed tomography during repair of orbitozygomatic fractures. Arch Facial Plast Surg 1999;1:19-24.
39. Isse NG: Endoscopic facial rejuvenation: endoforehead, the functional lift. Case reports. Aesthetic Plast Surg 1994;18:21-29.
40. Ramirez OM: Endoscopic techniques in facial rejuvenation: an overview. Part I. Aesthetic Plast Surg 1994;18:141-147.
41. Ramirez OM: Endoscopic full facelift. Aesthetic Plast Surg 1994;18:363-371.
42. Ramirez OM: Endoscopic subperiosteal browlift and facelift. Clin Plast Surg 1995;22:639-660.
43. Daniel RK, Tirkanits B: Endoscopic forehead lift. Aesthetics and analysis. Clin Plast Surg 1995;22:605-618.
44. Vasconez LO, Core GB, Oslin B: Endoscopy in plastic surgery. An overview. Clin Plast Surg 1995;22:585-589.
45. Paige KT, Eaves F, Wood RJ: Endoscopically assisted plastic surgical procedures in the pediatric patient. J Craniofac Surg 1997;8:164-168.
46. Papay FA, Stein JM, Dietz JR, et al: Endoscopic approach for benign tumor ablation of the forehead and brow. J Craniofac Surg 1997;8:176-180.
47. Weiss DD, Robson CD, Mulliken JB: Transnasal endoscopic excision of midline nasal dermoid from the anterior cranial base. Plast Reconstr Surg 1998;102:2119-2123.
48. Song IC, Pozner JN, Sadeh AE, Shin MS: Endoscopic-assisted recontouring of the facial skeleton: the forehead. Ann Plast Surg 1995;34:323-325.
49. Park DH, Lee JW, Song CH, et al: Endoscopic application in aesthetic and reconstructive facial bone surgery. Plast Reconstr Surg 1998;102:1199-1209.
50. Sandler NA, Andreasen KH, Johns FR: The use of endoscopy in the management of subcondylar fractures of the mandible: a cadaver study. Oral Surg Oral Med Oral Pathol Oral Radiol Endod 1999;88:529-531.
51. Lee C, Stiebel M, Young DM: Cranial nerve VII region of the traumatized facial skeleton: optimizing fracture repair with the endoscope. J Trauma 2000;48:423-431, discussion 431-432.

52. Troulis MJ, Perrott DH, Kaban LB: Endoscopic mandibular osteotomy, and placement and activation of a semiburied distractor. J Oral Maxillofac Surg 1999;57:1110-1113.

53. Troulis MJ, Nahlieli O, Castano F, Kaban LB: Minimally invasive orthognathic surgery: endoscopic vertical ramus osteotomy. Int J Oral Maxillofac Surg 2000;29:239-242.

54. Forrest CR, Antonyshyn OM: Endoscopic approaches in the management of facial fractures [abstract]. Can J Plast Surg 1995;3:17A.

55. Forrest CR: Endoscopic repair of frontal sinus and orbital-zygomatic complex fractures. In Whitaker LA, ed: Craniofacial Surgery: Proceedings of the Seventh International Congress of the International Society of Craniofacial Surgery. Bologna, Italy, Monduzzi Editore, 1997:213-214.

56. Strong EB: Endoscopic management of frontal sinus fractures. Presented at the Endoscopic Management of the Craniomaxillofacial Skeleton Symposium sponsored by AO/ASIF North America, San Diego, Calif, November 17-18, 2001.

57. Lindahl L: Condylar fractures of the mandible. I. Classification and relation to age, occlusion, and concomitant injuries of teeth and teeth-supporting structures, and fractures of the mandibular body. Int J Oral Surg 1977;6:12-21.

58. Krenkel C: Biomechanics and Osteosynthesis of Condylar Neck Fractures of the Mandible. Chicago, Quintessence Publishing, 1994.

59. Lindahl L: Condylar fractures of the mandible. III. Positional changes of the chin. Int J Oral Surg 1977;6:166-172.

60. Silvennoinen U, Raustia AM, Lindqvist C, Oikarinen K: Occlusal and temporomandibular joint disorders in patients with unilateral condylar fracture. A prospective one-year study. Int J Oral Maxillofac Surg 1998;27:280-285.

61. Ellis E III, Dean J: Rigid fixation of mandibular condyle fractures. Oral Surg Oral Med Oral Pathol 1993;76:6-15.

62. Hammer B, Schier P, Prein J: Osteosynthesis of condylar neck fractures: a review of 30 patients. Br J Oral Maxillofac Surg 1997;35:288-291.

63. Sargent LA, Green JF Jr: Plate and screw fixation of selected condylar fractures of the mandible. Ann Plast Surg 1992;28:235-241.

64. Mokros S, Erle A: Transoral miniplate osteosynthesis of mandibular condyle fractures—optimizing the surgical method [in German]. Fortschr Kiefer Gesichtschir 1996;41:136-138.

65. Zide MF, Kent JN: Indications for open reduction of mandibular condyle fractures. J Oral Maxillofac Surg 1983;41:89-98.

66. Lee C: Subcondylar fracture of the mandible: an endoscopic-assisted technique. Operative Techniques Plast Reconstr Surg 1998;5:287-294.

67. Lauer G, Schmelzeisen R: Endoscope-assisted fixation of mandibular condylar process fractures. J Oral Maxillofac Surg 1999;57:36-39, discussion 39-40.

68. Lee C, Mankani MH, Kellman RM, Forrest CR: Minimally invasive approaches to mandibular fractures. Facial Plast Surg Clin North Am 2001;9:475-487.

69. Jacobovicz J, Lee C, Trabulsy PP: Endoscopic repair of mandibular subcondylar fractures. Plast Reconstr Surg 1998;101:437-441.

70. Norholt SE, Krishnan V, Sindet-Pedersen S, Jensen I: Pediatric condylar fractures: a long-term follow-up study of 55 patients. J Oral Maxillofac Surg 1993;51:1302-1310.

71. Lindahl L, Hollender L: Condylar fractures of the mandible. II. A radiographic study of remodeling processes in the temporomandibular joint. Int J Oral Surg 1977;6:153-165.

72. Schimming R, Eckelt U, Kittner T: The value of coronal computer tomograms in fractures of the mandibular condylar process. Oral Surg Oral Med Oral Pathol Oral Radiol Endod 1999;87:632-639.

73. Lindahl L: Condylar fractures of the mandible. IV. Function of the masticatory system. Int J Oral Surg 1977;6:195-203.

74. Silvennoinen U, Iizuka T, Oikarinen K, Lindqvist C: Analysis of possible factors leading to problems after nonsurgical treatment of condylar fractures. J Oral Maxillofac Surg 1994;52:793-799.

75. Ellis E III: Use of lag screws for fractures of the mandibular body. J Oral Maxillofac Surg 1996;54:1314-1316.

76. Niederdellmann H, Shetty V: Lag screws in mandibular fractures. In Yaremchuk MJ, Gruss JS, Manson PN, eds: Rigid Fixation of the Craniomaxillofacial Skeleton. Toronto, Butterworth-Heinemann, 1992:187-194.

77. Niederdellmann H, Shetty V: Principles and technique of lag screw osteosynthesis. In Yaremchuk MJ, Gruss JS, Manson PN, eds: Rigid Fixation of the Craniomaxillofacial Skeleton. Toronto, Butterworth-Heinemann, 1992:22-27.

78. Prein J, Rahn B: Scientific and technical background. In Prein J, ed: Manual of Internal Fixation in the Cranio-Facial Skeleton. New York, Springer-Verlag, 1998:1-50.

79. Schilli W: Mandibular fractures. In Prein J, ed: Manual of Internal Fixation in the Cranio-Facial Skeleton. New York, Springer-Verlag, 1998:57-94.

80. Spiessel B: Internal Fixation of the Mandible. New York, Springer-Verlag, 1998:45-51.

81. Ellis E III, Ghali G: Lag screw fixation of anterior mandibular angle fractures. J Oral Maxillofac Surg 1991;49:234-243.

82. Ellis E III, Walker LR: Treatment of mandibular angle fractures using one compression miniplate. J Oral Maxillofac Surg 1996;54:864-871.

83. Iizuka T, Lindqvist C: Rigid internal fixation of fractures in the angular region of the mandible: an analysis of factors contributing to different complications. Plast Reconstr Surg 1993;91:265-271.

84. Ellis E III, Tharanon W: Facial width problems associated with rigid fixation of mandibular fractures: case reports. J Oral Maxillofac Surg 1992;50:87-94.

85. Luhr HG, Reidick T, Merten HA: Results of treatment of fractures of the atrophic edentulous mandible by compression plating: a retrospective evaluation of 84 consecutive cases. J Oral Maxillofac Surg 1996;54:250-254.

86. Thaller SR: Fractures of the edentulous mandible: a retrospective review. J Craniofac Surg 1993;4:91-94.

87. Gruss JS: The role of microfixation in malar fractures: a quantitative biophysical study [discussion]. Plast Reconstr Surg 1996;97:351.

88. Shumrick KA, Ryzenman JM: Endoscopic management of facial fractures. Facial Plast Surg Clin North Am 2001;9:469-474.

89. Sandler NA, Carrau RL, Ochs MW, Beatty RL: The use of maxillary sinus endoscopy in the diagnosis of orbital floor fractures. J Oral Maxillofac Surg 1999;57:399-403.

90. Mohammad JA, Warnke PH, Shenaq SM: Endoscopic exploration of the orbital floor: a technique for transantral grafting of floor blow-out fractures. J Craniomaxillofac Trauma 1998;4:16-19.

91. Stanley RB Jr: Endoscopic management of orbital fractures. Presented at the Endoscopic Management of the Craniomaxillofacial Skeleton Symposium sponsored by AO/ASIF North America, San Diego, Calif, November 17-18, 2001.

Endoscopic Mandible Fracture Management: Techniques

Reid V. Mueller, MD

SCOPE OF THE PROBLEM

EVALUATION

ANATOMY

CLINICAL EXAMINATION

DIAGNOSTIC STUDIES
Computed Tomography
Panoramic Tomography
Standard Radiography

TREATMENT
Treatment Goals
Nonsurgical Versus Surgical Management
Algorithm for Surgical Treatment
Surgical Technique

OUTCOMES

THE FUTURE

Few aspects of mandible fracture management generate more controversy than the management of condylar process fractures. The majority of these fractures have traditionally been managed with closed techniques. Proponents of closed treatment point to a large body of literature suggesting that most patients do well after a period of maxillomandibular fixation (MMF) followed by physiotherapy and training elastics. Whereas acceptable outcomes have usually been achieved with closed treatment, clinicians advocating open reduction argue that the failure of MMF to restore anatomy leads to condylar deformity, mandibular dysfunction, and facial asymmetry. Open approaches have been reserved for certain specific circumstances,[1,2] which many regard as too restrictive given modern techniques. Eager for better and more predictable outcomes, some have turned to open reduction with rigid fixation, and recent work reveals comparable if not superior results with the open approach.[3-15]

Proponents of endoscopic approaches to condylar process fractures have strived to accomplish anatomic reduction and rigid fixation equivalent to those of traditional open approaches while eliminating much of the morbidity that concerns critics of open treatment. When applied to favorable fractures, endoscope-assisted treatment combines the best of open and closed treatments. In the final analysis, it seems clear that we should ask ourselves not whether condylar process fractures should be treated open or closed but rather what the best treatment of this particular fracture is on the basis of the patient's age, the fracture's geometry, and the patient's informed preference.

SCOPE OF THE PROBLEM

Condylar process fracture, one of the most common mandible fractures, accounts for 25% to 50% of all mandible fractures with widespread variation in incidence on the basis of age, geographic location, and socioeconomic level of the population (Table 69-1).[16-30] The predominant etiology varies according to the study population. In adults, automobile accidents and interpersonal violence are the most common causes; sporting accidents, work-related incidents, and falls account for the remainder.[16,18-20,30,31] The majority of mandible fractures occur in 20- to 30-year-old men.[19,30]

At least 48% of condylar process fractures have been associated with other mandible fractures, and half of these are in the symphysis and the parasymphyseal regions. Most condylar process fractures are unilateral (84%); of these, 72% are subcondylar, 19% condylar neck, and 9% intracapsular. When condylar fractures are bilateral, they are more likely to be the result of falls and traffic accidents; of these, 38% are subcondylar, 36% condylar neck, and 26% intracapsular.[20,30] Up to 90% of subcondylar fractures show lateral override of the proximal fragment.[32]

EVALUATION

All patients with significant facial trauma, especially those with mandible fractures, should receive an initial evaluation of airway, breathing, circulation, and concomitant cervical and other facial fractures. The association between facial injuries and cervical spine injuries has been well documented. Approximately 10%

of those with facial fractures have a cervical spine injury; 18% of those with cervical spine injuries have a maxillofacial injury.[33,34] Once the patient has had a thorough trauma evaluation and been appropriately resuscitated and other injuries have been tended to, evaluation of the mandible fracture can proceed.

Evaluation of condylar fractures for possible endoscopic repair is no different from that of any other fracture; however, particular attention must be paid to the geometry of the condylar fracture, for that will dictate the likelihood of success by the endoscopic approach. The appeal and difficulty of endoscopy are a result of limited surgical incisions. Restricted access and visualization inherent in endoscopic procedures demand better preoperative imaging and clearer understanding of the fracture before repair is attempted.

ANATOMY

In 1977, Lindahl[31] described a system that classified fractures according to the anatomic location of the fracture, the relationship of the condylar segment to the mandibular segment, and the relationship of the condylar head to the condylar fossa. These relationships are the basis for selection of fractures for endoscopic repair.

In discussing condylar process fractures, proximal is defined as toward the condylar head, and distal is toward the mandibular angle. Fractures of the condylar process are classified into three broad groups (Fig. 69-1). Intercondylar fractures involve the condylar head and are proximal to the insertion of the joint capsule. Fractures of the neck occur just distal to the joint capsule

TABLE 69-1 ✦ INCIDENCE OF CONDYLAR FRACTURES AS A PERCENTAGE OF TOTAL MANDIBLE FRACTURES

Author	Year	Incidence of Condylar Fracture (%)
Chalmers[21]	1947	8.0
Kromer[22]	1953	25.0
Ekholm[23]	1961	27.7
Schuchardt and Metz[24]	1966	25.0
Rowe[25]	1968	35.6
Tasanen and Lamberg[26]	1976	32.4
Larsen and Nielsen[16]	1976	37.0
van Hoof et al[18]	1977	47.0
Olson et al[27]	1982	52.4
Hill et al[17]	1984	49.0
Andersson et al[28]	1984	40.0
Ellis et al[19]	1985	29.0
Haug et al[29]	1990	21.0
Silvennoinen et al[20]	1992	52.4
Marker et al[30]	2000	41.0

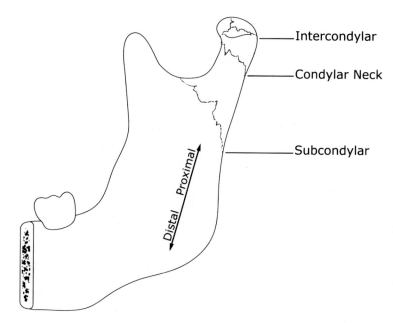

FIGURE 69-1. Three broad groups of condylar fractures are intercondylar, involving the condylar head proximal to the insertion of the joint capsule; neck, just distal to the joint capsule at the thin and slightly constricted portion of the bone; and subcondylar, typically extending from the lowest point of the sigmoid notch obliquely toward the posterior border of the ascending ramus.

at the thin and slightly constricted portion of the bone. Subcondylar fractures account for the remainder and typically extend from the lowest point of the sigmoid notch obliquely toward the posterior border of the ascending ramus. Subcondylar fractures are frequently further characterized into high or low subcondylar fractures, indicating that the fracture is relatively proximal or distal, respectively. This subclassification is useful because it correlates with the difficulty of exposure and hardware fixation. The lower the fracture, the easier the exposure and the more bone stock available to apply fixation hardware. Intracapsular and neck fractures are not amenable to endoscopic treatment because there is insufficient room on the proximal fragment to apply the fixation hardware.

Displacement is a measure of the distance between and relationship of the fracture fragments. Most fractures will have some degree of fracture displacement with overlap of the proximal and distal fragments. The overlapping of fragments results in shortening of the ascending ramus, premature posterior dental contact, and resultant anterior open bite.

Approximately 90% of subcondylar fractures are such that the proximal fragment is lying lateral to the distal fragment. This is defined as *lateral override*. Those fractures with the proximal fragment located medial to the distal fragment are said to have *medial override* (Fig. 69-2). This distinction is important in assessing the applicability of the endoscopic approach. All endoscopic approaches to the ascending ramus create an optical cavity on the lateral surface of the ascending ramus. Secondary ports through cheek trocar and submandibular or intraoral incisions allow the introduction of instruments; however, the access is largely

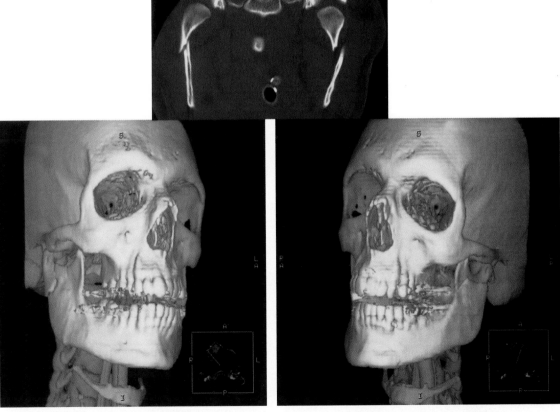

Lateral Override   Medial Override

FIGURE 69-2. The upper coronal CT and lower three-dimensional reconstructions show bilateral subcondylar fractures. The fracture on the left shows lateral override of the proximal fragment, whereas the fracture on the right shows medial override. The lateral override fracture is amenable to endoscopic repair; the medial override fracture would prove more difficult.

limited to the lateral surface. Therefore, the ability to manipulate medially displaced proximal fragments (medial override) is severely restricted.

The orientation of the proximal fragment can be further defined by describing the angulation of the fragment in a coronal plane and the sagittal plane. The superior head of the lateral pterygoid originates from the infratemporal crest and inferior aspect of the lateral surface of the greater wing of the sphenoid. The inferior head originates from the lateral surface of the lateral pterygoid plate. The muscle passes horizontally backward and laterally to insert on the anterior neck of the condyle and the anterior margin of the articular disk.[35] After a fracture of the ascending ramus, the pull of the lateral pterygoid forces the proximal fragment into a flexed posture; in other words, the distal aspect of the proximal fragment is displaced anteriorly in a sagittal plane. If there is any disruption of the joint capsule, the lateral pterygoid will displace the condylar head medially, causing angulation in the coronal plane. Reduction of a fracture requires correction of the displacement caused by the lateral pterygoid.

Dislocation describes the relationship of the condylar head to the glenoid fossa (Fig. 69-3). A *nondisplaced* condylar head is in the normal relationship to the glenoid fossa. *Displacement* of the condyle is sometimes used to describe a condylar head that remains within the glenoid fossa but demonstrates some alteration of the joint space. A *dislocated* condyle lies completely outside the glenoid fossa and must include rupture of the joint capsule. The lateral capsule is much stronger than the medial capsule; therefore, lateral dislocation is rare. Anterior and medial dislocation is much more common because of the weakness of the medial capsule and pull of the lateral pterygoid muscle.

The retromandibular vein and maxillary artery are situated posteriorly and medially with respect to the ascending ramus. In exposing the ascending ramus and condylar neck, these vessels may be injured as the periosteum along the posterior border of the mandible is elevated to create an optical cavity. Care must be taken to stay in the subperiosteal plane because injury to these vessels will cause significant bleeding that will obscure the visual field and severely impede surgical progress. The use of a 6-mm stop bit drill will prevent inadvertent injury on drilling through the condylar process.

The facial nerve trunk crosses the proximal portion of the condylar neck and may be subject to trauma from transbuccal trocars and retraction. The marginal

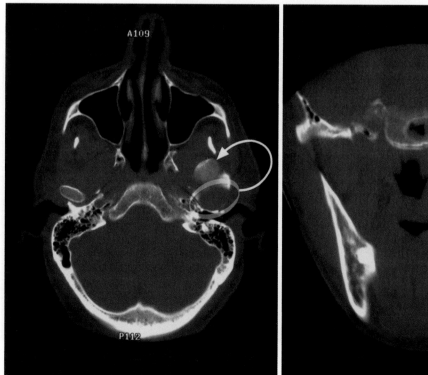
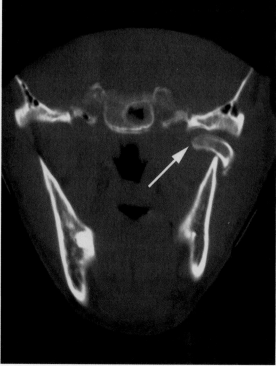

FIGURE 69-3. The axial CT image *(left)* shows a dislocated subcondylar fracture with the head displaced anteromedially out of the glenoid fossa. The coronal CT image *(right)* shows the angulation of the proximal head in a coronal plane due to the forces of the lateral pterygoid muscle.

mandibular branch of the facial nerve travels anteriorly and parallel to the inferior border of the mandible. Posterior to the facial artery, the mandibular branch passes superior to the inferior border of the mandible 81% of the time and passes in an arch within 1 cm of the inferior border of the mandible in the other 19%.[36] Anterior to the facial artery, the nerve is always superior to the border of the mandible. For this reason, a submandibular incision should be located 2 cm below the mandibular border to allow a margin of safety.

CLINICAL EXAMINATION

Trauma evaluation and resuscitation should be completed before maxillofacial evaluation. Once the patient is stabilized and other more serious injuries have been treated, attention can be directed toward evaluation of the face and in particular the mandible. The history will often be consistent with mandibular trauma and may give some clue as to the nature of the ultimate fracture. For example, a blow to the chin with a fist often produces a unilateral subcondylar fracture associated with a parasymphyseal fracture, whereas a high-energy impact to the chin in a high-speed motor vehicle accident produces bilateral condylar neck fractures.

The following findings on examination are suggestive of a condylar fracture.

MALOCCLUSION. Any change in occlusion is highly suggestive of a mandible fracture. Patients are keenly aware of minute changes in occlusal relationship and will report that their "teeth fit together differently" or "feel funny." The patient's assessment of the occlusion is sensitive; however, it is nonspecific. A careful clinical examination may reveal further evidence of fracture. Premature posterior contact and anterior open bite are often associated with unilateral or bilateral condylar neck fractures.

PAIN OR SWELLING. Tenderness to palpation over the condyle or ascending ramus is often exacerbated with mandibular motion.

CLICKING OR CREPITATION. The patient may report a clicking sound or crunching sound with movement of the mandible as fracture fragments rub against one another close to the ear.

EXTERNAL EVIDENCE OF FACIAL TRAUMA. The patient often has external bruising, abrasions, or laceration at the site of impact. This gives the surgeon a sense of the nature and direction of the antecedent injury.

FACIAL ASYMMETRY. Patients with a displaced subcondylar fracture have shortening of the ascending ramus, resulting in facial asymmetry and ipsilateral chin point deviation with jaw opening. Patients with bilateral subcondylar fractures may exhibit bilateral loss of facial height.

ANESTHESIA OR DYSESTHESIA OF THE LOWER LIP. Although this may occur from simple lower lip contusion, it is usually a sign of ipsilateral mandibular fracture with injury to the inferior alveolar nerve. This may be a result of a mandibular body fracture in which the nerve is encased in bone, or it may be the result of a subcondylar fracture with medial override of the proximal fragment. As the condylar and mandibular segments overlap, the proximal fragment can impinge on the nerve as it enters the medial surface of the mandibular ramus.

DIAGNOSTIC STUDIES

The goal of diagnostic studies in patients with suspected mandible fractures is identification of any fracture to determine the fracture's geometry, which will direct subsequent treatment. Panoramic tomography is currently the informal "gold standard" by virtue of its simplicity and projection of the entire mandible on a single film. The accuracy of panoramic tomography for the diagnosis of mandible fractures has been reported as 92%, compared with 66% for standard mandibular series. Panoramic tomography detected 88% of fractures compared with 77% by nonhelical computed tomography (CT).[37,38] Creasman et al[39] found plain radiography to have better sensitivity (89%) than nonhelical axial CT (64%). A comparison of modern helical CT and panoramic tomography reported a sensitivity of 100% for helical CT versus 86% for panoramic tomography.

The utility of various imaging methods for patients thought to have condylar process fractures favors those methods that image the condylar process well and enable evaluation of the relationship between the condylar and mandibular fracture fragments. Helical CT scan is the single most informative radiographic test for making this determination; however, incomplete availability of modern helical CT scanners maintains a role for panoramic tomography. The trend in mandibular imaging in North America is toward axial and coronal helical CT with three-dimensional reconstructions; the bias in Europe remains plain radiography mandible series combined with panoramic tomography.

Analysis of current imaging methods and clinical correlation suggest that the studies for imaging of suspected condylar process fractures in order of utility are (1) helical CT, (2) panoramic tomography, (3) Towne view (oblique anterior-posterior frontooccipital view), (4) oblique lateral view, and (5) posterior-anterior view.

Computed Tomography

The accuracy of modern helical CT has surpassed that of panoramic tomography in the detection of mandibular fractures. Earlier studies reported lower sensitivity of nonhelical CT compared with plain radiography, especially for nondisplaced fractures of the posterior mandible.[39] Nonhelical CT has also been reported to have reduced sensitivity in the detection of angle fractures compared with both plain radiography and coronal CT.[38] Many of the limitations of nonhelical CT have been overcome with the advent of helical CT scanning. Using 1-mm collimated images (with a pitch of two) and 1-mm axial images reconstructed on every second image, Wilson et al[40] compared helical CT with panoramic tomography in detecting 73 mandibular fractures in 42 consecutive patients and correlated the results with known surgical findings. Helical CT detected 100% of the fractures, whereas panoramic tomography detected only 86%. In six missed fractures, the surgical management was altered by the additional information provided from the CT scan. In one patient, the nature of a dental root fracture was better seen on panoramic tomography.

Axial head CT scans are routinely obtained during initial evaluation of many trauma patients with head injuries. If there is any suspicion of maxillofacial injury, the entire face and mandible should be imaged at the same setting as the brain scan. It is frequently impossible to obtain true coronal CT scans during the initial evaluation because cervical spine precautions preclude appropriate positioning for the coronal scans. In this case, coronal re-formations can be computed from the axial data set, or true coronal images can be obtained at a later date when the patient has been stabilized.

If it is technically possible, both axial and coronal images with three-dimensional reconstructions from the axial data set should be obtained. The coronal scans provide the best information about the configuration of the ascending ramus and condyle; the axial images are best suited to evaluation of fractures of the anterior mandible. Modern postacquisition processing of the axial image data sets can generate three-dimensional reconstructions of the mandible from any virtual vantage point. This furnishes a clear mental picture of the fracture configuration without the sometimes inaccurate "mind's eye" mental reconstruction with which anyone who relies on standard images is familiar. The three-dimensional reconstructions improve the surgeon's understanding of the relationship between fracture fragments but are not useful for detection of nondisplaced fractures. Mathematical smoothing of the image obscures fine detail otherwise present in the two-dimensional images. This is a byproduct of interpolation between axial images to generate the three-dimensional polygonal mesh that

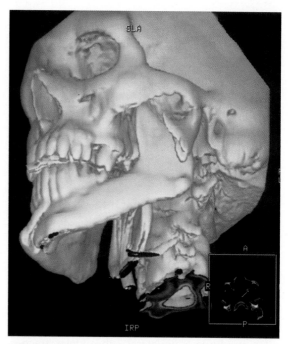

FIGURE 69-4. A three-dimensional CT reconstruction showing a left-sided low subcondylar fracture with lateral override of the proximal fragment and a symphyseal fracture.

is subsequently rendered into the final image. Despite the inevitable smoothing, the ability to view the mandible from any virtual position gives the surgeon an unparalleled appreciation of the fracture (Fig. 69-4).

Panoramic Tomography

Panoramic tomography has the advantage of being a relatively inexpensive, simple technique that can image the entire mandible on a single film (Fig. 69-5). It enables evaluation of the relationship between the fracture line and teeth that may require extraction or other dental treatment in the course of therapy. An understanding of the relative position of the condyle to the glenoid fossa in an anterior-posterior direction and the degree of flexion posture of the condyle is readily acquired. The panogram is not helpful in assessing whether there is medial or lateral override of the proximal fragment of a subcondylar fracture. Panoramic tomography with a Panorex machine requires that the patient sit in an upright position during image acquisition. For many polytrauma patients, this is not possible. A zonogram with a Zonarc machine is obtained with the patient in a supine position, broadening applications in trauma patients not able to sit. In many institutions, panoramic tomography units are located in

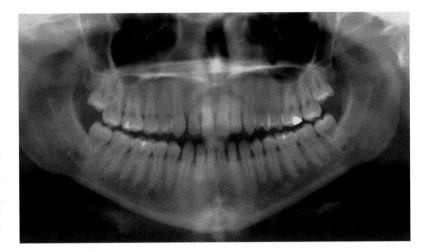

FIGURE 69-5. This panoramic tomogram shows a noncomminuted left subcondylar fracture. These images give good information about possible condylar dislocation but no hint of whether there is medial or lateral override of the proximal fragment.

dental facilities and are not part of routine radiology services, which further restricts access on weekends and evenings. It is preferable to obtain a panogram if possible before surgery. However, surgery should not be delayed if a panogram cannot be obtained owing to concomitant injury or availability issues.

Standard Radiography

The standard mandible series in most institutions consists of a Towne (oblique anterior-posterior fronto-occipital) view, two oblique lateral views, and a posterior-anterior view. When evaluated by an experienced physician, they can surpass panoramic tomography in diagnostic accuracy.[38] Chayra et al[37] compared the sensitivity of a standard mandible series with panographic tomography in detecting mandibular fractures and found that the panoramic tomogram had a high accuracy in detecting all types of mandible fracture (92% versus 66%) except fractures of the ramus, for which the images were of comparable value. Whereas standard radiographs have a role in the diagnosis of patients with suspected mandibular fractures, the compression of three-dimensional structures into two-dimensional images limits their utility in clarifying the important fracture relationships of subcondylar fractures. In regard to condylar process fractures, the Towne view gives the most information about condylar dislocation, fracture displacement, and override of the proximal fragment. At many institutions, the availability of helical CT scanning and panoramic tomography has virtually abolished the routine application of standard radiography.

TREATMENT

Treatment Goals

Treatment of condylar process fractures may be deemed successful if five basic criteria are met: (1)

restoration of premorbid occlusion, (2) pain-free jaw opening with 40 mm or more of interincisal opening, (3) good excursion of the jaw in all directions, (4) good facial and jaw symmetry, and (5) minimal morbidity (e.g., no injury to facial nerve branches, good-quality hidden scars, no anesthetic complications). Most authors would agree that closed techniques are simpler to perform, and in general we should strive for the simpler of several otherwise equal treatments. The more difficult question is under what specific circumstances is the closed, traditional open, or endoscopic approach the best treatment option.

Nonsurgical Versus Surgical Management

ARGUMENT AGAINST CLOSED TREATMENT

Closed treatment of mandibular fractures with MMF has a long and successful history but is not without significant morbidity. The best results have been achieved in skeletally immature children, in whom condylar remodeling can often restore condylar anatomy to nearly normal even with little or no fracture reduction. Despite almost miraculous condylar remodeling in children, the outcomes have not been uniform, and a significant percentage suffer long-term occlusal and functional problems.[41-45] Few studies exist that compare similar fractures treated by open versus closed methods. Most studies show equal or better functional outcomes after open treatment despite the fact that more severely injured patients tended to undergo open treatment (Table 69-2).[3-6,9,11,13,14,46-48] Patients treated with an open approach had better restoration of condylar anatomy, less facial height loss and asymmetry, and faster recovery of jaw motion. Some studies have shown less chronic pain after the open approach. In general, long-term functional results were similar. The most important long-term complication of closed

TABLE 69-2 ✦ COMPARISON OF OPEN VERSUS CLOSED TREATMENT OF CONDYLAR PROCESS FRACTURES

Author	Year	Closed Treatment	Open Treatment	Treatment Selection Method	Summary of Findings
de Amaratunga[3]	1987	55	55	Surgeon selection based on fracture	Patients treated with maxillomandibular fixation had decreased interincisal opening at 1, 3, and 6 months postoperatively
Konstantinovic and Dimitrijevic[9]	1992	54	26	Not stated	Radiographic evidence of better condylar position after open treatment; no difference in clinical parameters (interincisal opening, deviation, protrusion)
Worsaae and Thorn[14]	1994	28	24	Randomized by day of admission	Higher incidence of malocclusion, mandibular asymmetry, impaired masticatory function, and pain in closed treatment group
Widmark et al[46]	1996	13	22	Historical control	After 12 months, patients treated open tended to have less pain, slightly better interincisal opening
Palmieri et al[11]	1999	74	62	Patient choice	Patients treated open had better condylar mobility despite greater initial fracture displacement in the open treatment group
Moreno et al[47]	2000	136	96	Surgeon selection based on fracture	No difference in complication rates; complication rate correlated with fracture severity
Ellis et al[6]	2000	77	65	Patient choice	Patients treated closed had a greater percentage of malocclusion despite greater initial fracture displacement in the open treatment group
Ellis and Throckmorton[5]	2000	81	65	Patient choice	Patients treated closed had a greater percentage of facial asymmetry characterized by loss of facial height on the side of the injury
Throckmorton and Ellis[13]	2000	74	62	Patient choice	Patients treated open regained mandibular mobility faster than did those treated closed; those treated closed continued to have reduced excursion toward the fracture for 3 years
Ellis and Throckmorton[4]	2001	91	64	Patient choice	Maximum voluntary bite forces not significantly different; neuromuscular adaptations to the fracture occurred in both groups
Haug and Assael[48]	2001	10	10	Institutional protocol	No differences in outcomes for range of motion, occlusion, facial contour, motor or sensory function; the open treatment was associated with perceptible scars, the closed treatment with chronic pain

treatment is persistent malocclusion, which is reported in up to 28% of patients.[14,49,50]

In assessing the shortcomings of closed treatment, the significant independent morbidities associated with MMF are often overlooked because of the surgical simplicity of its application. All synovial joints will suffer some degradation in mobility with immobilization, and the temporomandibular joint is no exception. Studies in rhesus monkeys have demonstrated loss of inner incisal opening and maximal stimulated bite force after MMF,[51,52] and comparisons of patients with condylar neck fractures randomized to open versus MMF treatment have demonstrated that after MMF, patients have decreased range of motion necessitating long periods of physiotherapy to regain their premorbid function.[6,14] Many patients find MMF uncomfortable, and those with dementia or psychiatric diagnosis may simply not tolerate the procedure. It is difficult to maintain good oral hygiene with MMF; orthodontic treatment must be delayed during the period of MMF, and those with seizure disorders or alcoholism are at risk for aspiration and death.

ARGUMENT AGAINST OPEN TREATMENT

All surgical approaches for the open treatment of condylar fractures require some kind of facial incision, and nearly all will result in a perceptible scar[48]; up to 4% report an unsightly scar.[6] Proximity of the facial nerve to the condylar neck compromises access to the fracture segment and makes the dissection tedious. Efforts to improve surgical access may result in either a direct facial nerve injury or a traction injury during retraction. The risk of permanent facial nerve injury reported in 21 different series of open approaches comprising 455 patients averages 1%; the risk of transient palsy ranges from 0% to 46% with a mean of 12%.[2,8,9,12,14,26,46,53-65] Perforation of the auditory canal has been reported in up to 10% of preauricular approaches; however, significant auditory canal stenosis was not seen.[62] Transient wound drainage attributed to salivary fistulas has been reported in 2.3% of open approaches.[66] These usually resolved with antisialagogues and occlusive pressure dressings. Intraoperative bleeding, infection, and Frey syndrome have been reported infrequently.

Dissatisfaction with the morbidity of external incision approaches to the condylar process inspired some to approach the condylar process through an intraoral incision. The intraoral approach obviates many of the aforementioned morbidities associated with standard open incisions. Many low subcondylar fractures can be addressed with this approach; however, high subcondylar fractures and neck fractures cannot be treated because of inadequate visualization. Even with adequate visualization, significant technical hurdles must be overcome to stabilize and control the proximal condylar fragment and to apply fixation to the fracture. This is especially true in high condylar neck fractures and those in which the condyle is displaced medially out of the fossa.

RATIONALE FOR ENDOSCOPIC APPROACH

Open approaches to condylar neck fractures have not found broader application outside the traditional indications set forth by Zide and Kent[2] in 1983 because of technical demands of the open approach, external scar, fear of facial nerve injury, and the belief that a closed approach is adequate. Most surgeons accept, on an intellectual level, that fracture reduction and rigid fixation with restoration of anatomy is a laudable goal if it can be achieved without undue morbidity. For most surgeons, the risk and demands of an external approach have not warranted its use for routine condylar neck fractures. The endoscopic approach described here has the potential to reduce morbidity by limiting scar, reducing the risk to the facial nerve, and eliminating the need for MMF, all the while embracing the accepted advantages of anatomic reduction and rigid fixation. The reduction in morbidity associated with endoscopic reduction may well expand the indications for reduction and rigid fixation in the future.

Algorithm for Surgical Treatment

Patients with condylar process fractures are selected for endoscopic reduction and fixation on the basis of age, location of fracture, degree of comminution, direction of proximal fragment displacement, dislocation of condylar head, concomitant medical or surgical illness, and, importantly, choice of the patient (Table 69-3). The guidelines put forth by Zide and Kent[2] in 1983 for open treatment of condylar fractures form a starting point for surgical decision-making; however, their relative indications should be broadened in the

TABLE 69-3 ✦ CONTRAINDICATIONS TO ENDOSCOPIC REDUCTION AND RIGID FIXATION OF MANDIBULAR CONDYLE FRACTURES

Absolute	Intercondylar fractures
	Condylar neck fractures without sufficient room for two fixation screws
	Any patient with medical illness or other serious injury who may be harmed by a longer surgical procedure or extended general anesthetic
Relative	Child younger than 12 years
	Comminuted fracture
	Medial override of the proximal fragment
	When a simpler method is equally effective

context of current surgical technique and decreased morbidity when an endoscopic approach is used.

AGE

There is consensus that most fractures in children are best treated with MMF. This belief is not entirely founded on solid science, and some endoscopic enthusiasts have successfully used endoscopy to assist in fracture reduction for severely displaced fractures with or without rigid fixation. Endoscopy can be used in selected cases if conditions would otherwise favor the traditional open approach.

LOCATION OF FRACTURE

Fracture within the joint capsule and fractures of the condylar neck are not amenable to endoscopic repair because the proximal fragment will not afford sufficient room to accommodate at least two screws of a 2.0 plate. Most subcondylar fractures will have enough length on the proximal fragment distal to the joint capsule to accommodate two or three screws (Fig. 69-6).

DEGREE OF COMMINUTION

High-energy comminuted fractures are a relative contraindication for endoscopic repair and should not be attempted by the inexperienced endoscopic surgeon (Fig. 69-7). During reduction, the anterior and

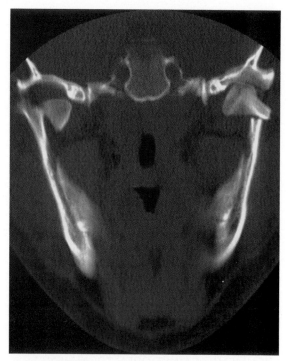

FIGURE 69-6. A coronal CT image showing an intercondylar fracture on the patient's right (our left) and a high subcondylar fracture on the left. The intercondylar fracture is not amenable to endoscopic repair; the subcondylar fracture is high but appears to have sufficient room for two fixation screws.

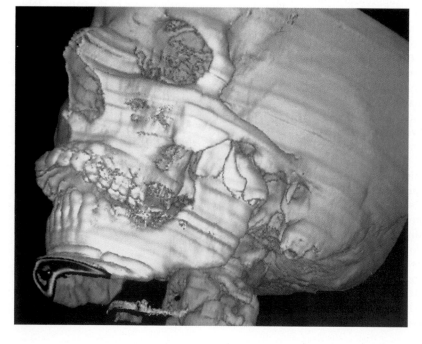

FIGURE 69-7. A three-dimensional CT reconstruction showing a severely comminuted subcondylar fracture with a dislocated condylar head. This is a challenging fracture to repair endoscopically and should be treated endoscopically only by an experienced surgeon.

posterior border of the fracture line is used as an anatomic landmark to assess accurate reduction. Comminuted fractures often have fracture fragments that involve the border and thereby obscure the landmarks. Microcomminution will obscure the interdigitation of small irregularities along the fracture line that ordinarily assist in precise reduction. Unfortunately, the visual limitations of endoscopy make reliable assessment of reduction challenging in the face of comminution.

DIRECTION OF PROXIMAL FRAGMENT DISPLACEMENT

Fractures with lateral displacement of the proximal fragment are the most favorable for endoscopic repair. The proximal fragment is much easier to control in abutting the lateral surface of the distal fragment, and reduction is achieved with medially directed pressure through a cheek trocar. When the proximal fragment is located medially, it is difficult to control and is partially hidden behind the distal fragment (see Fig. 69-2). The mechanics needed for control and reduction of these fractures require some experience with the technique, and they should be reserved for those with some endoscopic experience.

DISLOCATED CONDYLAR HEAD

Fractures associated with nondislocated condylar heads are the most favorable for endoscopic repair. A displaced condylar head without true dislocation can usually be relocated into anatomic position easily, but those fractures with dislocation of the condylar head are more challenging.

CONCOMITANT MEDICAL OR SURGICAL ILLNESS

Any patient with medical illness or other serious injury who may be harmed by a longer surgical procedure or

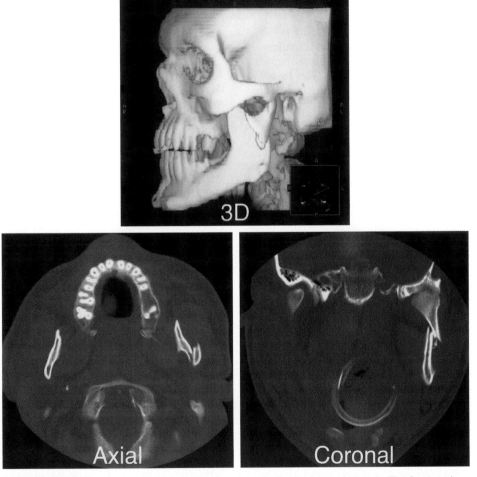

FIGURE 69-8. These CT scans show an ideal fracture for endoscopic repair. The fracture is a noncomminuted low subcondylar fracture with lateral override of the proximal fragment and no dislocation of the condylar head.

extended general anesthetic should not undergo endoscopic repair. Patients with even mild coagulopathies present difficulties from persistent bleeding that may obscure the limited visual field.

PREFERENCE OF THE PATIENT

When no absolute or relative contraindications exist for endoscopic repair, every patient has the right to choose the treatment after a discussion of the risks, benefits, and alternatives. Patients need to understand that the data regarding open versus closed treatment of condylar fractures are imperfect but that functional outcomes in general are at least as good as if not better than with open approaches. They should clearly understand the risks of traditional open approaches, including significant scar (especially dark-skinned individuals) and facial nerve injury. They should also understand that endoscopy can offer reduced morbidity and good outcomes but that no long-term data are yet available.

THE IDEAL PATIENT

The perfect patient for endoscopic fracture repair is one with a noncomminuted subcondylar fracture with minimal lateral displacement of the proximal fragment and a nondislocated condylar head (Fig. 69-8). A surgeon interested in starting to perform endoscopic reduction and fixation of subcondylar fractures should seek out a fracture of this description.

Surgical Technique

The patient is nasally intubated, with the nasotracheal tube secured and directed over the forehead in the midline. Penicillin G (2 million units intravenously) is given before the procedure. Some surgeons, in an effort to reduce postoperative swelling, administer dexamethasone (16 mg intravenously) as a single preoperative dose.[67] If it is not otherwise contraindicated, mildly hypotensive anesthesia will reduce bleeding and improve visualization. A discussion with the anesthesiologist about the desire for hypotensive anesthesia and the timing of pharmacologic paralysis should take place before the operation to avoid later confusion and possible complication. The endoscope video monitor is located at the head of the bed slightly toward the contralateral shoulder. The surgeon stands on the ipsilateral side and the assistant on the contralateral side (Fig. 69-9).

The operation begins with the application of arch bars and treatment of other associated mandible fractures. Precise reduction and fixation of the other fractures will restore the dental arch and make reduction of the condylar segment more straightforward.

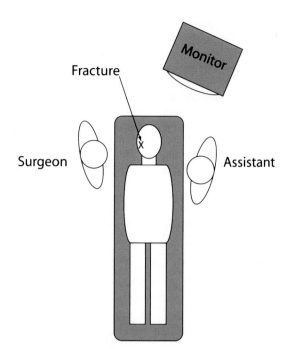

FIGURE 69-9. Arrangement of the surgeon, assistant, and endoscopic video monitor in relation to a fracture.

After the other fractures have been addressed, MMF is released and replaced with elastic MMF. Elastic MMF should be tight enough to maintain proper occlusal relationships but not so tight as to prevent distraction of the fracture when downward traction is applied to the angle of the mandible.

INTRAORAL APPROACH

The intraoral incision site and the lateral aspect of the mandible and condylar region are injected with a 1 : 200,000 epinephrine solution 10 minutes before the incision is made. A 2-cm intraoral incision along the anterior border of the ascending ramus is carried down to periosteum with electrocautery (Fig. 69-10). The approach is much like that used for transoral vertical ramus osteotomy. A subperiosteal dissection is used to elevate the masseteric attachments and to liberate the pterygomasseteric sling from the posterior and inferior ramus. Wide subperiosteal dissection allows increased mobility of the soft tissue envelope and improved visualization by virtue of a larger optical cavity. It is important that the dissection be strictly subperiosteal to avoid bleeding that will quickly obscure the endoscopic view. Hypotensive anesthesia will help minimize bleeding; however, if bleeding should occur from the retromandibular vein, it is best to pack gauze into the wound, apply external pressure, and wait 5 to 10 minutes—the bleeding will usually stop.

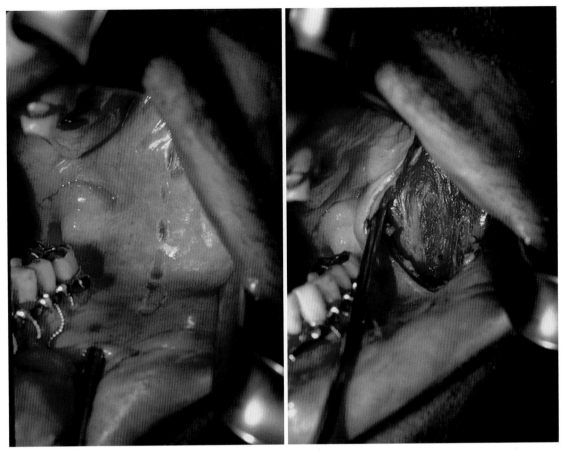

FIGURE 69-10. Location of the intraoral incision along the anterior border of the ascending ramus. After the incision is made with electrocautery, a subperiosteal dissection of the lateral ascending ramus and condylar process is undertaken.

A 4-mm 30-degree endoscope fitted with an endoscopic brow sheath is inserted into the optical cavity (Fig. 69-11). With the endoscope in one hand and a periosteal elevator in the other, the subperiosteal dissection is carried proximally. The assistant may hold the endoscope while the surgeon uses the periosteal elevator and suction to continue the dissection proximally to reveal the condylar fragment. A common mistake is inadvertent dissection under (or medial to) the proximal fragment. This occurs because of a failure to appreciate the degree of lateral override and coronal plane angulation of the proximal fragment. Once the proximal fragment is identified, the subperiosteal dissection continues on the lateral surface up to the joint capsule or a sufficient distance to place the fixation hardware (Fig. 69-12).

The endoscope is transferred into a specialized retractor that is a modification of a LeVasseur-Merrill retractor (Fig. 69-13). This retractor has been designed with a window in the blade that assists with mainte-nance of the optical cavity, stabilization of the endoscope, and ease of use for less experienced camera operators. If this retractor is not available, the endoscope may be mounted with an endoscopic brow sheath, and a large Obwegeser-type retractor may be placed into the intraoral incision and directed superiorly and laterally to assist in maintaining the optical cavity.

SUBMANDIBULAR APPROACH

A 1.5-cm incision is made 1.5 to 2 cm below the angle of the mandible to avoid the marginal mandibular branch of the facial nerve. The dissection is carried down to bone and then extended superiorly in a subperiosteal plane. Wide exposure of the entire lateral surface of the mandibular ramus will increase the optical cavity and improve visualization. As in the intraoral approach, dissection in a subperiosteal plane will minimize bleeding. A 4-mm 30-degree endoscope with

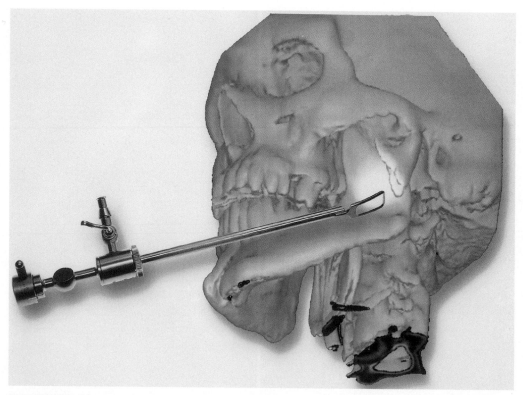

FIGURE 69-11. A 4-mm 30-degree endoscope fitted with an endoscopic brow lift sheath approaches the fracture through the intraoral incision in a subperiosteal plane.

an endoscopic brow sheath is inserted into the incision and the remainder of the subperiosteal dissection, and identification of the fracture is completed. An angled Obwegeser-type retractor may be placed into the incision and directed superiorly to assist in maintaining the optical cavity. If the submandibular incision is made, either instrumentation or endoscope may be inserted. Excellent visualization (especially of the posterior border) is achieved with this approach, but risk of noticeable facial scarring should not be overlooked. Although the submandibular port is advocated for fracture management,[68,69] this port is not generally used because of unacceptable scarring.

PLACEMENT OF CHEEK TROCAR

Once the fracture is exposed, a cheek trocar is passed through the cheek directly opposite the fracture at the posterior border of the mandible. This point can be identified by placing a finger into the intraoral incision and, after palpation of the fracture, transferring the point to the external cheek. At this time, it is important that the patient not be paralyzed. Once the absence of paralysis has been confirmed with the anesthesiologist, a 4-mm stab incision is made in the cheek. A small clamp is passed into the intraoral incision by use of spreading dissection. During this maneuver, the face is observed for any sign of facial nerve stimulation. If stimulation is seen, the clamp should be redirected. A transbuccal cheek trocar is then passed along the same path, again watching for any sign of facial nerve stimulation.

REDUCTION OF THE FRACTURE

If a submandibular incision has been used, a hole is drilled at the mandibular angle and a wire passed to facilitate downward traction during fracture reduction. Others have passed percutaneous wires affixed to a screw placed through the intraoral incision, whereas others have simply placed a perforating towel clamp on the mandibular angle.

Appreciation of the position of the condylar fragment will shed light on maneuvers needed to reduce the fracture. The proximal fragment is typically situated with a lateral override and in a flexed posture. At this point in the operation, pharmacologic muscle relaxation will assist in the reduction by paralyzing the lateral pterygoid and masseter muscles. The initial maneuver to reduce the fracture is distraction of the mandibular angle downward by the assistant while the surgeon pushes the condyle back into

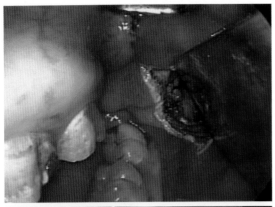

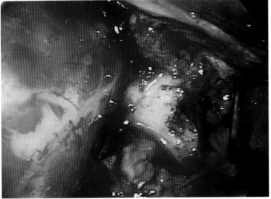

FIGURE 69-12. Endoscopic view of the initial incision and the subsequent dissection of the optical cavity in a subperiosteal plane to reveal the proximal condylar fragment. Note the angulation of the proximal fragment.

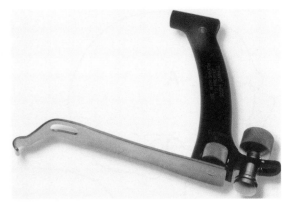

FIGURE 69-13. This retractor (a modification of a LeVasseur-Merrill retractor) has a hole in the blade to accommodate transbuccal trocar instruments, a hook to engage the posterior border of the mandible, and an attachment for a 4-mm endoscope.

APPLICATION OF RIGID FIXATION

Fractures are stabilized with standard five- or six-hole 2.0 craniofacial zygoma dynamic compression plates.* This particular plate is thin and malleable enough that in situ self-contouring is possible, yet it is strong enough that plate failures are rare. The plate is affixed with at least two 6-mm screws on either side of the fracture. The plate is temporarily mounted on a plate delivery device with a hinge mechanism that allows precise positioning of the plate (Fig. 69-16). Others have simply delivered the plate into the wound on a long clamp or dangling from a suture. The plate should be positioned with at least two holes on either side of the fracture along the posterior border of the mandible.

The cheek trocar is used to engage the plate, usually in the proximal hole. A 1.5-mm drill with a 6-mm stop is used, followed by 6-mm 2.0 screws through the cheek trocar. The plate can then be rotated into final position parallel to the posterior border of the mandible, and any other hole can be affixed with another screw. If the plate delivery device is used, a locking screw is disengaged, and the device is removed.

Before fixation is completed, the reduction is checked. The anterior and posterior borders of the fracture are inspected for anatomic alignment. In non-comminuted fractures, this is usually straightforward; however, a fracture with even slight comminution will be difficult to assess. The submandibular approach is especially suited for inspection of the posterior border of the mandible, and if any question exists about the

reduction using the combination of cheek trocar and periosteal elevator inserted into the intraoral or submandibular incisions (Fig. 69-14). Persistent medially directed pressure on the condylar fragment with the cheek trocar is maintained until the fracture is reduced. The downward traction on the angle can then be released. Interfragmentary friction will frequently hold the fracture in reduction without pressure from the cheek trocar.

If the reduction is not stable and the fracture has sufficient obliquity, a temporary lag screw may be placed to hold the reduction while plate fixation is applied. The cheek trocar is situated near the distal aspect of the proximal fragment after reduction is achieved. The reduction is maintained with medially directed pressure from the trocar while a 1.5-mm hole is drilled through the trocar followed by a 6-mm 2.0 screw. An alternative is to secure the fixation hardware to the proximal fragment and use the plate as a handle to move the proximal fragment into reduction (Fig. 69-15).

*Synthes, Paoli, PA 19301.

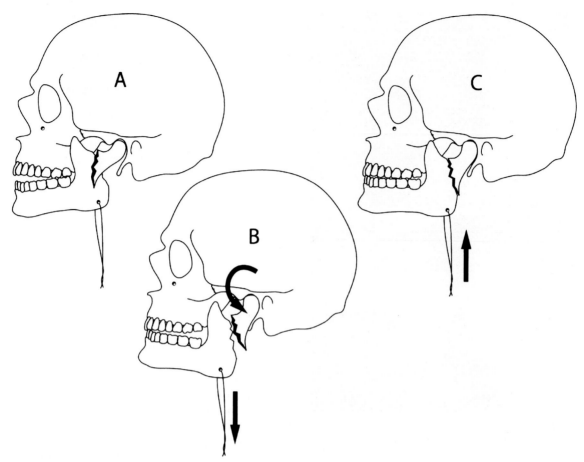

FIGURE 69-14. The maneuvers needed for reduction are shown above. *A,* Initial configuration. *B,* Distraction of the fracture by a downward pull on the mandibular angle and rotation of the proximal fragment out of a flexed posture. *C,* Final reduction after release of downward pull on the angle. The fracture will often be stable in this configuration by virtue of interfragmentary friction.

alignment at the posterior border, the endoscope is inserted into the submandibular incision to confirm reduction. If reduction is not acceptable, one screw may be removed and the fragments repositioned. Once reduction has been confirmed, the remaining screws are placed through the cheek trocar. If possible, a second plate should be placed.

REDUCTION OF THE DIFFICULT FRACTURE

Surgeons early in their experience with endoscopic repair should restrict themselves to noncomminuted fractures with lateral override of the proximal fragment and no dislocation of the condyle. In attempting reduction of a dislocated condyle, medially directed pressure on the distal aspect of the condylar fragment may not bring the condyle into reduction. In these situations, other techniques are needed to reduce the

fracture. One technique that has been used is lateral pressure on the medial surface of the condylar head with concomitant medial pressure on the distal aspect of the condylar fragment. Others have applied the fixation hardware to the proximal fragment and used the plate as a handle to bring the condyle upright. A threaded fragment manipulator used as a joystick has the greatest utility in reducing these fractures.

The threaded fragment manipulator is essentially a 2.0-mm self-drilling, self-tapping 10-cm-long steel screw on a stick that can be affixed to a standard handle (Fig. 69-17). It is passed in the same manner as the cheek trocar into the optical cavity. A "suture boot" is placed over the threads as it is passed through the cheek to reduce the risk of facial nerve injury. After insertion into the optical cavity, the suture boot is removed with an endoscopic grabber. The fixation plate is placed over the proximal fragment, and the threaded

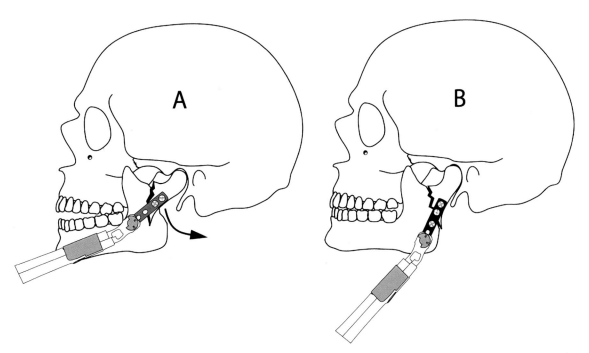

FIGURE 69-15. The proximal fragment may be rotated into reduction with the aid of an affixed 2.0 plate. Here the plate is attached to the hinged plate delivery device.

fragment manipulator is screwed into the condyle through the most proximal hole (Fig. 69-18). The manipulator acts as a joystick to manipulate the fracture into reduction. This method has the unique ability to apply lateral traction on the condylar head during reduction to bring a medially dislocated head upright.

The next screw is placed into the distal fragment, followed by the second hole on the proximal fragment. Once at least one screw on either side of the fracture has been secured, the threaded fragment manipulator can be safely detached from the condyle without fear of loss of reduction.

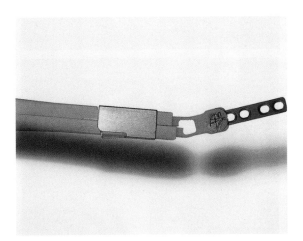

FIGURE 69-16. Plate delivery device. A five- or six-hole 2.0 plate is attached with a locking screw to this delivery device that is hinged to allow positioning of the plate. After the plate is affixed to the mandible, the plate is released from the device with a quarter turn of the locking screw.

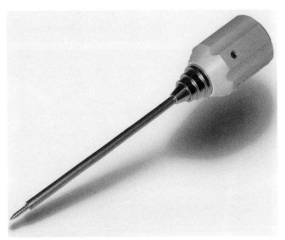

FIGURE 69-17. The threaded fragment manipulator is a long self-drilling, self-tapping steel screw that can be used as a joystick to bring the fracture into reduction after it is passed through the cheek and secured to the proximal fragment.

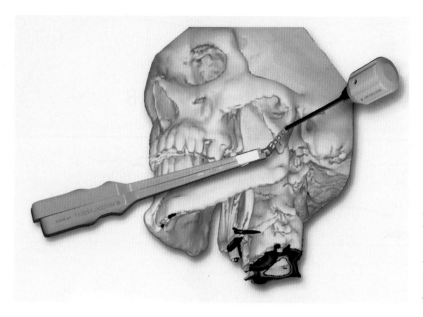

FIGURE 69-18. A threaded fragment manipulator is placed through the proximal hole of the plate and attached to the condylar fragment. After the manipulator is used as a joystick to obtain reduction, screws are placed proximal and distal to the fracture, and the manipulator is removed.

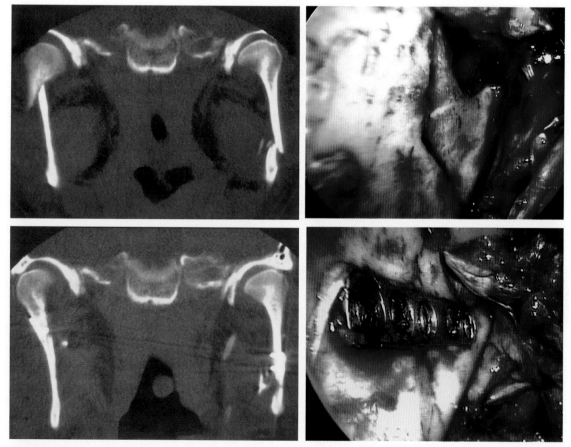

FIGURE 69-19. The panels on the left show preoperative and postoperative coronal CT scans of a patient with bilateral subcondylar fractures. The panels on the right show an endoscopic view of the fracture after initial endoscopic reduction and after final reduction and fixation. Note the anatomic alignment of the posterior border.

CONFIRMING REDUCTION

Careful inspection of the anterior and posterior borders of the fracture will confirm proper reduction (Fig. 69-19). Any comminution will make assessment of the reduction more difficult. If the condyle was dislocated preoperatively and there is any uncertainty about the reduction, a cross-table intraoperative lateral cephalogram should be obtained (Fig. 69-20). Submandibular placement of the endoscope is helpful in assessing the accuracy of reduction but is not desirable if facial scarring is to be avoided. The elastic MMF is released and the fixation is inspected while the mouth is opened and closed to confirm stable fixation. MMF is not needed postoperatively. The intraoral incision is closed with absorbable suture, and a single fast-absorbing 5–0 gut suture is placed in the cheek trocar wound. No drains are used.

POSTOPERATIVE MANAGEMENT

Patients are maintained with a soft diet for 6 weeks. Perioperative antibiotic therapy consists of penicillin VK, 500 mg by mouth every 6 hours for 5 days; however, recent data have not shown any benefit in the reduction of postoperative infections.[70] Patients are instructed in postsurgical physiotherapy, and any patient who is unable to easily reproduce normal occlusal relationships will have elastics placed. A postoperative panoramic tomogram to confirm reduction of the fracture and anatomic location of the condylar head in the glenoid fossa should be obtained (Fig. 69-21).

BAILOUT STRATEGY

Reduction and fixation occasionally will not be possible with an endoscopic approach. A bailout strategy should be planned and discussed with the patient before any procedure. Some patients, when presented with the alternatives, will elect a standard open approach; others will be content with MMF.

OUTCOMES

Lee et al[32] published their initial series of 22 fractures in 20 patients and reported 43-mm interincisal jaw opening after 8 weeks, with restoration of premorbid occlusion and radiographic evidence of anatomic reduction in 21 of 22 fractures. Patients were pleased with the aesthetic restoration of their chin projection, jaw line, and symmetric midline movement of the chin point on jaw opening. Late radiographs showed stable fixation, good bone healing, and no condylar resorption. Other smaller reports have described encouraging results with minimal morbidity,[68,71-75] but good prospective data are not yet available.

The author has collected data on 45 fractures in 39 patients; 43 of 45 fractures had anatomic reduction, whereas 2 fractures in patients with high-energy severely comminuted fractures were inadequately reduced and required a second endoscopic procedure for reduction. Interincisal opening has averaged 42 mm after 8 weeks (Fig. 69-22). The operative time has been decreasing as experience is gained. The average operative time for exposure, reduction, and fixation of the subcondylar fracture is 116 minutes (Fig. 69-23). This last figure is deceiving because more challenging fractures are now being attempted. The average time for simple noncomminuted fractures with lateral override is about 70 minutes. There was one late plate fracture without functional detriment to the patient. One transient frontal branch palsy was observed. All patients have been pleased with the cosmetic outcome.

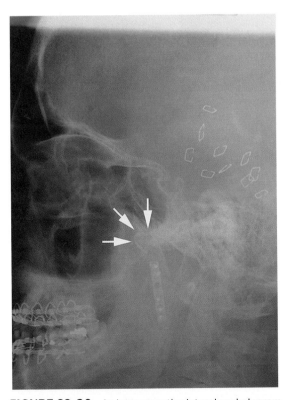

FIGURE 69-20. An intraoperative lateral cephalogram obtained during endoscopic repair of a severely comminuted fracture (see Fig. 69-7). Reduction is difficult to judge in comminuted fractures because the anterior and posterior borders are often indistinct. In this case, the intraoperative cephalogram led to removal of the fixation and another reduction of the fracture.

THE FUTURE

A randomized multicenter prospective trial is planned to compare MMF, standard open, and endoscopic

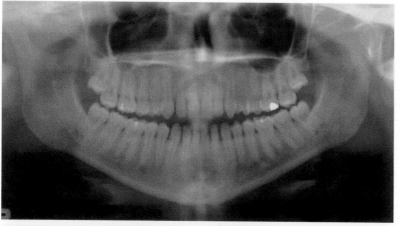

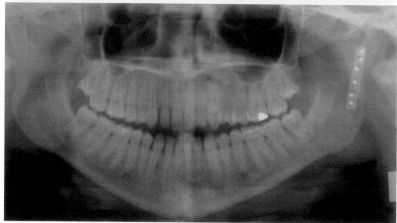

FIGURE 69-21. Top image shows preoperative panoramic tomogram with left subcondylar fracture. The bottom panel shows a postoperative image with good anatomic reduction.

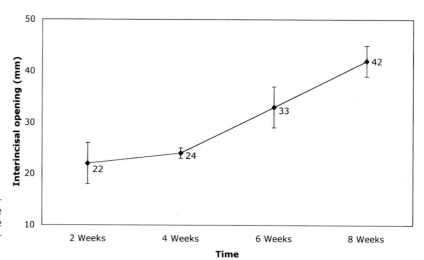

FIGURE 69-22. Mean interincisal jaw opening ± SEM of the last 45 subcondylar fractures the author has treated endoscopically.

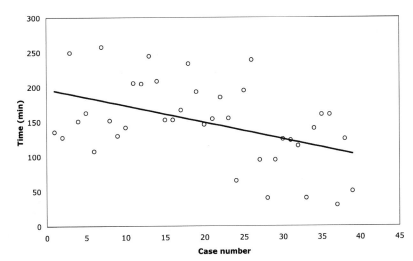

FIGURE 69-23. Operative time to expose, reduce, and apply rigid fixation of the last 45 subcondylar fractures the author has treated endoscopically.

treatment of subcondylar fractures. Good data along with long-term follow-up will allow evidence-based surgical decision-making and treatment. It is hoped that continued technical refinements in technique, equipment, and case selection will allow the endoscopic approach to give our patients the best possible treatment of their fractures.

REFERENCES

1. Zide MF: Open reduction of mandibular condyle fractures. Indications and technique. Clin Plast Surg 1989;16:69.
2. Zide MF, Kent JN: Indications for open reduction of mandibular condyle fractures. J Oral Maxillofac Surg 1983;41:89.
3. de Amaratunga NA: Mouth opening after release of maxillomandibular fixation in fracture patients. J Oral Maxillofac Surg 1987;45:383.
4. Ellis E 3rd, Throckmorton GS: Bite forces after open or closed treatment of mandibular condylar process fractures. J Oral Maxillofac Surg 2001;59:389.
5. Ellis E 3rd, Throckmorton G: Facial symmetry after closed and open treatment of fractures of the mandibular condylar process. J Oral Maxillofac Surg 2000;58:719.
6. Ellis E 3rd, Simon P, Throckmorton GS: Occlusal results after open or closed treatment of fractures of the mandibular condylar process. J Oral Maxillofac Surg 2000;58:260.
7. Jeter TS, Van Sickels JE, Nishioka GJ: Intraoral open reduction with rigid internal fixation of mandibular subcondylar fractures. J Oral Maxillofac Surg 1988;46:1113.
8. Klotch DW, Lundy LB: Condylar neck fractures of the mandible. Otolaryngol Clin North Am 1991;24:181.
9. Konstantinovic VS, Dimitrijevic B: Surgical versus conservative treatment of unilateral condylar process fractures: clinical and radiographic evaluation of 80 patients. J Oral Maxillofac Surg 1992;50:349.
10. Lachner J, Clanton JT, Waite PD: Open reduction and internal rigid fixation of subcondylar fractures via an intraoral approach. Oral Surg Oral Med Oral Pathol 1991;71:257.
11. Palmieri C, Ellis E 3rd, Throckmorton G: Mandibular motion after closed and open treatment of unilateral mandibular condylar process fractures. J Oral Maxillofac Surg 1999;57:764.
12. Raveh J, Vuillemin T, Ladrach K: Open reduction of the dislocated, fractured condylar process: indications and surgical procedures. J Oral Maxillofac Surg 1989;47:120.
13. Throckmorton GS, Ellis E 3rd: Recovery of mandibular motion after closed and open treatment of unilateral mandibular condylar process fractures. Int J Oral Maxillofac Surg 2000;29:421.
14. Worsaae N, Thorn JJ: Surgical versus nonsurgical treatment of unilateral dislocated low subcondylar fractures: a clinical study of 52 cases. J Oral Maxillofac Surg 1994;52:353.
15. Worsaae N, Thorn JJ: Surgical versus non-surgical treatment of unilateral dislocated fractures of the lower mandibular condyle [in Danish]. Ugeskr Laeger 1995;157:3472.
16. Larsen OD, Nielsen A: Mandibular fractures. I. An analysis of their etiology and location in 286 patients. Scand J Plast Reconstr Surg 1976;10:213.
17. Hill CM, Crosher RF, Carroll MJ, et al: Facial fractures—the results of a prospective four-year-study. J Maxillofac Surg 1984;12:267.
18. van Hoof RF, Merkx CA, Stekelenburg EC: The different patterns of fractures of the facial skeleton in four European countries. Int J Oral Surg 1977;6:3.
19. Ellis E 3rd, Moos KF, el-Attar A: Ten years of mandibular fractures: an analysis of 2,137 cases. Oral Surg Oral Med Oral Pathol 1985;59:120.
20. Silvennoinen U, Iizuka T, Lindqvist C, et al: Different patterns of condylar fractures: an analysis of 382 patients in a 3-year period. J Oral Maxillofac Surg 1992;50:1032.
21. Chalmers JLC: Fractures involving the mandibular condyle: a post-treatment survey of 120 cases. J Oral Surg 1947;5:45.
22. Kromer H: The closed and open reduction of condylar fractures. Dent Rec 1953;569.
23. Ekholm A: Fractures of condyloid process of the mandible: a clinical, pantomographic and electromyographic study. Suomen Hammaslaakariseuran Toimituksia 1961;57:9.
24. Schuchardt K, Metz HJ: Injuries of the facial skeleton. Mod Trends Plast Surg 1966;2:62.
25. Rowe NL: Fractures of the facial skeleton in children. J Oral Surg 1968;26:505.
26. Tasanen A, Lamberg MA: Transosseous wiring in the treatment of condylar fractures of the mandible. J Maxillofac Surg 1976;4:200.
27. Olson RA, Fonseca RJ, Zeitler DL, et al: Fractures of the mandible: a review of 580 cases. J Oral Maxillofac Surg 1982;40:23.

28. Andersson L, Hultin M, Nordenram A, et al: Jaw fractures in the county of Stockholm (1978–1980). I. General survey. Int J Oral Surg 1984;13:194.

29. Haug RH, Prather J, Indresano AT: An epidemiologic survey of facial fractures and concomitant injuries. J Oral Maxillofac Surg 1990;48:926.

30. Marker P, Nielsen A, Bastian HL: Fractures of the mandibular condyle. Part 1. Patterns of distribution of types and causes of fractures in 348 patients. Br J Oral Maxillofac Surg 2000;38:417.

31. Lindahl L: Condylar fractures of the mandible. I. Classification and relation to age, occlusion, and concomitant injuries of teeth and teeth-supporting structures, and fractures of the mandibular body. Int J Oral Surg 1977;6:12.

32. Lee C, Mueller RV, Lee K, et al: Endoscopic subcondylar fracture repair: functional, aesthetic, and radiographic outcomes. Plast Reconstr Surg 1998;102:1434.

33. Lewis VL Jr, Manson PN, Morgan RF, et al: Facial injuries associated with cervical fractures: recognition, patterns, and management. J Trauma 1985;25:90.

34. Gwyn PP, Carraway JH, Horton CE, et al: Facial fractures—associated injuries and complications. Plast Reconstr Surg 1971;47:225.

35. Gray H: Gray's Anatomy, 30th American ed. Clemente C, ed. Philadelphia, Lea & Febiger, 1985.

36. Dingman RO, Grabb WC: Surgical anatomy of the mandibular ramus of the facial nerve based on the dissection of 100 facial halves. Plast Reconstr Surg 1962;29:266.

37. Chayra GA, Meador LR, Laskin DM: Comparison of panoramic and standard radiographs for the diagnosis of mandibular fractures. J Oral Maxillofac Surg 1986;44:677.

38. Markowitz BL, Sinow JD, Kawamoto HK Jr, et al: Prospective comparison of axial computed tomography and standard and panoramic radiographs in the diagnosis of mandibular fractures. Ann Plast Surg 1999;42:163.

39. Creasman CN, Markowitz BL, Kawamoto HK Jr, et al: Computed tomography versus standard radiography in the assessment of fractures of the mandible. Ann Plast Surg 1992;29:109.

40. Wilson IF, Lokeh A, Benjamin CI, et al: Prospective comparison of panoramic tomography (zonography) and helical computed tomography in the diagnosis and operative management of mandibular fractures. Plast Reconstr Surg 2001;107:1369.

41. Feifel H, Risse G, Opheys A, et al: Conservative versus surgical therapy of unilateral fractures of the collum mandibulae—anatomic and functional results with special reference to computer-assisted 3-dimensional axiographic registration of condylar paths [in German]. Fortschr Kiefer Gesichtschir 1996;41:124.

42. Guven O, Keskin A: Remodelling following condylar fractures in children. J Craniomaxillofac Surg 2001;29:232.

43. Hovinga J, Boering G, Stegenga B: Long-term results of non-surgical management of condylar fractures in children. Int J Oral Maxillofac Surg 1999;28:429.

44. Kellenberger M, von Arx T, Hardt N: Results of follow-up of temporomandibular joint fractures in 30 children [in German]. Fortschr Kiefer Gesichtschir 1996;41:138.

45. Strobl H, Emshoff R, Rothler G: Conservative treatment of unilateral condylar fractures in children: a long-term clinical and radiologic follow-up of 55 patients. Int J Oral Maxillofac Surg 1999;28:95.

46. Widmark G, Bagenholm T, Kahnberg KE, et al: Open reduction of subcondylar fractures. A study of functional rehabilitation. Int J Oral Maxillofac Surg 1996;25:107.

47. Moreno JC, Fernandez A, Ortiz JA, et al: Complication rates associated with different treatments for mandibular fractures. J Oral Maxillofac Surg 2000;58:273.

48. Haug RH, Assael LA: Outcomes of open versus closed treatment of mandibular subcondylar fractures. J Oral Maxillofac Surg 2001;59:370.

49. Silvennoinen U, Iizuka T, Oikarinen K, et al: Analysis of possible factors leading to problems after nonsurgical treatment of condylar fractures. J Oral Maxillofac Surg 1994;52:793.

50. Silvennoinen U, Raustia AM, Lindqvist C, et al: Occlusal and temporomandibular joint disorders in patients with unilateral condylar fracture. A prospective one-year study. Int J Oral Maxillofac Surg 1998;27:280.

51. Ellis E 3rd, Carlson DS: The effects of mandibular immobilization on the masticatory system. A review. Clin Plast Surg 1989;16:133.

52. Ellis E 3rd, Dechow PC, Carlson DS: A comparison of stimulated bite force after mandibular advancement using rigid and nonrigid fixation. J Oral Maxillofac Surg 1988;46:26.

53. Silvennoinen U, Iizuka T, Pernu H, et al: Surgical treatment of condylar process fractures using axial anchor screw fixation: a preliminary follow-up study. J Oral Maxillofac Surg 1995;53:884.

54. Chossegros C, Cheynet F, Blanc JL, et al: Short retromandibular approach of subcondylar fractures: clinical and radiologic long-term evaluation. Oral Surg Oral Med Oral Pathol Oral Radiol Endod 1996;82:248.

55. Kallela I, Soderholm AL, Paukku P, et al: Lag-screw osteosynthesis of mandibular condyle fractures: a clinical and radiological study. J Oral Maxillofac Surg 1995;53:1397.

56. Pereira MD, Marques A, Ishizuka M, et al: Surgical treatment of the fractured and dislocated condylar process of the mandible. J Craniomaxillofac Surg 1995;23:369.

57. Koberg WR, Momma WG: Treatment of fractures of the articular process by functional stable osteosynthesis using miniaturized dynamic compression plates. Int J Oral Surg 1978;7:256.

58. Mikkonen P, Lindqvist C, Pihakari A, et al: Osteotomy-osteosynthesis in displaced condylar fractures. Int J Oral Maxillofac Surg 1989;18:267.

59. Takenoshita Y, Oka M, Tashiro H: Surgical treatment of fractures of the mandibular condylar neck. J Craniomaxillofac Surg 1989;17:119.

60. Iizuka T, Lindqvist C, Hallikainen D, et al: Severe bone resorption and osteoarthrosis after miniplate fixation of high condylar fractures. A clinical and radiologic study of thirteen patients. Oral Surg Oral Med Oral Pathol 1991;72:400.

61. Krenkel C: Axial "anchor" screw (lag screw with biconcave washer) or "slanted-screw" plate for osteosynthesis of fractures of the mandibular condylar process. J Craniomaxillofac Surg 1992;20:348.

62. MacArthur CJ, Donald PJ, Knowles J, et al: Open reduction-fixation of mandibular subcondylar fractures. A review. Arch Otolaryngol Head Neck Surg 1993;119:403.

63. Eckelt U, Hlawitschka M: Clinical and radiological evaluation following surgical treatment of condylar neck fractures with lag screws. J Craniomaxillofac Surg 1999;27:235.

64. Hammer B, Schier P, Prein J: Osteosynthesis of condylar neck fractures: a review of 30 patients. Br J Oral Maxillofac Surg 1997;35:288.

65. Anastassov GE, Rodriguez ED, Schwimmer AM, et al: Facial rhytidectomy approach for treatment of posterior mandibular fractures. J Craniomaxillofac Surg 1997;25:9.

66. Ellis E 3rd, McFadden D, Simon P, et al: Surgical complications with open treatment of mandibular condylar process fractures. J Oral Maxillofac Surg 2000;58:950.

67. Weber CR, Griffin JM: Evaluation of dexamethasone for reducing postoperative edema and inflammatory response after orthognathic surgery. J Oral Maxillofac Surg 1994;52:35.

68. Troulis MJ, Kaban LB: Endoscopic approach to the ramus/condyle unit: clinical applications. J Oral Maxillofac Surg 2001;59:503.

69. Troulis MJ, Nahlieli O, Castano F, et al: Minimally invasive orthognathic surgery: endoscopic vertical ramus osteotomy. Int J Oral Maxillofac Surg 2000;29:239.

70. Abubaker AO, Rollert MK: Postoperative antibiotic prophylaxis in mandibular fractures: a preliminary randomized, double-blind, and placebo-controlled clinical study. J Oral Maxillofac Surg 2001;59:1415.

71. Schmelzeisen R, Lauer G, Wichmann U: Endoscope-assisted fixation of condylar fractures of the mandible [in German]. Mund Kiefer Gesichtschir 1998;2(suppl 1):S168.

72. Chen CT, Lai JP, Tung TC, et al: Endoscopically assisted mandibular subcondylar fracture repair. Plast Reconstr Surg 1999;103:60.

73. Lauer G, Schmelzeisen R: Endoscope-assisted fixation of mandibular condylar process fractures. J Oral Maxillofac Surg 1999;57:36.

74. Lee C, Stiebel M, Young DM: Cranial nerve VII region of the traumatized facial skeleton: optimizing fracture repair with the endoscope. J Trauma 2000;48:423.

75. Sandler NA: Endoscopic-assisted reduction and fixation of a mandibular subcondylar fracture: report of a case. J Oral Maxillofac Surg 2001;59:1479.

Temporomandibular Joint Dysfunction

Stephen A. Schendel, MD, DDS ✦ Andrew E. Turk, MD

ANATOMY

TEMPOROMANDIBULAR JOINT DYSFUNCTION
    Myofascial Problems
    Inflammation of the Capsule and Ligaments
    Internal Derangement of the Joint
    Condyle and Bone Problems
    Congenital and Developmental Abnormalities
    Condylar Fractures
    Osteoarthritis
    Rheumatoid Arthritis

HISTORY AND PHYSICAL EXAMINATION
    Oral Examination
    Diagnostic Imaging

MEDICAL OCCLUSAL MANAGEMENT

SURGICAL MANAGEMENT
    Temporomandibular Joint Arthroscopy
    Open Arthrotomy
    Surgical Management of Specific Disorders

The causes of temporomandibular pain can include masticatory dysfunction, myofascial pain syndromes, atypical facial pain, and temporomandibular joint (TMJ) abnormalities. These conditions can make diagnosis and treatment extremely difficult in this group of patients. Differential diagnosis of pain resulting from neuritic, neuralgic, vascular, and temporomandibular origin complicates management even further. The principles discussed in this chapter assist the plastic and reconstructive surgeon in diagnosis and management of TMJ dysfunction.

ANATOMY

The mandibular bone allows rotational and translational movement through the TMJ. The mandibular condyle articulates with the squamous portion of the temporal bone at the TMJ. The blood supply to the mandible is through the inferior alveolar artery and the muscle and gingival attachments.[1] The myohyoid muscle, which elevates the tongue, attaches to the medial surface of the mandible. The geniohyoid muscles insert onto the genial tubercles and, with the anterior belly of the digastric muscle, depress and retract the mandible (Fig. 70-1).

The muscles that elevate or protrude the mandible are the masseter, temporalis, medial, and lateral pterygoid muscles (Fig. 70-2). The inferior portion of the lateral pterygoid muscle inserts onto the neck of the condyle, which helps protrude the mandible when it is contracting. The superior portion of the lateral pterygoid muscle inserts on the fibrous capsule and meniscus of the TMJ, stabilizing the meniscus during the movement of the mandible. All these muscles are innervated by cranial nerve V. The TMJ articular surfaces are lined with fibrocartilage, an avascular fibrous connective tissue that contains cartilage cells. This differs from other synovial joints that are lined with hyaline cartilage.

The articular disk is a dense fibrous connective tissue structure that separates the joint into two spaces.[2] The upper joint space volume of 1 mL extends from the glenoid fossa to the articular eminence. The lower joint space volume of 0.5 mL begins above the insertion of the lateral pterygoid muscle anteriorly and then spreads out over the condyle. The articular disk is an avascular, noninnervated fibrous sheet with some cartilaginous component. The pars gracilis is the thin central zone. The anterior band or pes meniscus is superiorly attached to the articular eminence and superior belly of the lateral pterygoid. Inferiorly, the anterior band attaches to the condyle by a synovial membrane along the attachment of the lateral pterygoid muscle. The posterior band is highly innervated and vascularized tissue, a bilaminar zone or retromeniscal pad (Fig. 70-3). The upper layer of the bilaminar zone attaches to the tympanic plate of the temporal bone; the lower runs from the posterior meniscus to the neck of the condyle.

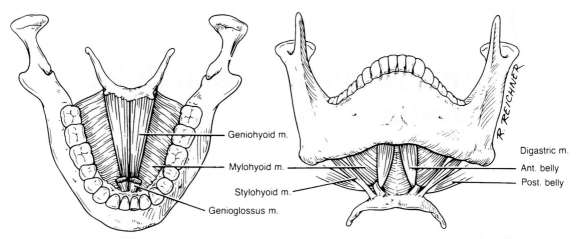

FIGURE 70-1. Muscles of the floor of the mouth and suprahyoid region: depressors of the anterior mandible. (From Georgiade N, ed: Textbook of Plastic Maxillofacial Surgery, 2nd ed. Baltimore, Williams & Wilkins, 1992.)

The hinge movement of the mandible is completed in the inferior joint space (ginglymus), and translation is followed in the superior joint space (arthrodial). The retromeniscal or retrodiskal pad is believed to be the origin of pain in TMJ dysfunction. If there are abnormal loading forces on the joint surfaces as a result of disk disease, this can lead to TMJ disorders.[3-5]

The condyles are elliptical, measuring 20 mm medial to lateral and 10 mm anteroposterior. The fibrous joint capsule attaches to the condyle inferiorly and the zygomatic arch superiorly.[3] It is reinforced anteriorly and laterally by the temporomandibular ligament. The blood supply arises from the superficial temporal vessels and branches of the masseteric artery through the sigmoid notch of the mandible. The auriculotemporal,

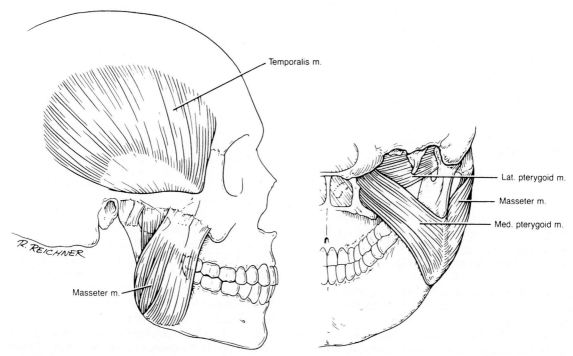

FIGURE 70-2. Muscles of mastication. (From Bessette RW, Jacobs JS: Temporomandibular joint dysfunction. In Aston SJ, Beasley RW, Thorne CHM, eds: Grabb and Smith's Plastic Surgery. Philadelphia, Lippincott-Raven, 1997.)

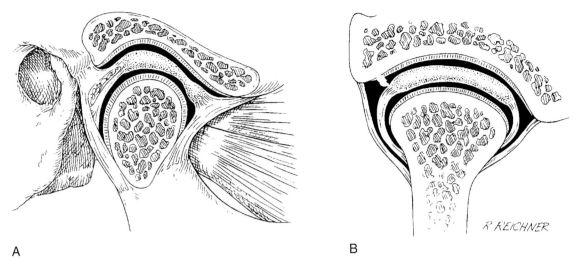

A   B

FIGURE 70-3. *A,* Temporomandibular joint in sagittal section demonstrates the concave configuration of the articular disk, bilaminar posterior attachment, and insertion of the external pterygoid on the disk and condylar head. *B,* Temporomandibular joint in coronal section demonstrates the position of the disk over the convexity of the condylar head and the separate attachments of the disk on the condyle in distinction from the capsule. (From Bessette RW, Jacobs JS: Temporomandibular joint dysfunction. In Aston SJ, Beasley RW, Thorne CHM, eds: Grabb and Smith's Plastic Surgery. Philadelphia, Lippincott-Raven, 1997.)

masseteric, and deep temporal branches of the trigeminal nerve supply innervation to the TMJ.[1]

TEMPOROMANDIBULAR JOINT DYSFUNCTION

Myofascial Problems

The cause of myofascial pain and dysfunction is usually related to the masticatory muscles. Myofascial pain and dysfunction were first described by Laskin[6,7] and are characterized by a limited range of motion, aching pain, and severe tenderness on palpation of the muscles. Certain trigger points within the masticatory muscles refer the pain. Producing an ache in the jaw, the masseter muscle is the most common. Next most common is pain in the temporalis muscle, producing pain in the side of the head. The lateral pterygoid muscle can generate an earache or pain behind the eye. Medial pterygoid involvement causes pain on swallowing or stuffiness in the ear.

The limitation of mandibular movement in myofascial pain and dysfunction usually correlates with the amount of pain. The etiology can be overclosure, occlusal prematurity, bruxism, and severe anxiety. Each of these leads to spasms of the masticatory muscles, focusing pain around the TMJ.

Breaking the cycle of spasm is the key to the management of myofascial pain and dysfunction. Occlusal splint therapy can guide the dental occlusion to relax the muscle system. Other treatment includes drug therapy, such as nonsteroidal anti-inflammatory drugs, muscle relaxants, antidepressants, Botox, and local anesthetics for diagnostic blocks.[8] Physical therapy with modalities of heat, massage, diathermy, ultrasound, and biofeedback is also indicated in these patients. Any question about disk disease warrants magnetic resonance imaging (MRI) in these patients.

Inflammation of the Capsule and Ligaments

Zide describes posterior capsulitis involving the neurovascular bilaminar zone and the posterior capsular ligament. Such inflammation can be due to acute trauma or infection causing the retrodiskal tissues to become edematous. He describes physical tests to make the diagnosis of posterior capsulitis.[9]

Sprain of the capsular ligaments from malocclusion or trauma usually heals in several weeks. Chronic sprain can lead to stretching of the ligaments.[9] Medical occlusal treatment usually addresses these conditions.

Internal Derangement of the Joint

The existence of a natural progression of internal derangement of the TMJ is well documented.[10] In early stage I derangement, the patient complains of clicking on opening and closing of the jaw (Fig. 70-4 and Table 70-1). The problem is secondary to anterior disk displacement. The oral excursion and lateral movements of the jaw should be within the normal range.

In stage II, the patient begins to complain of intermittent limitation of jaw movement. Internal derangement is due to anterior disk displacement with

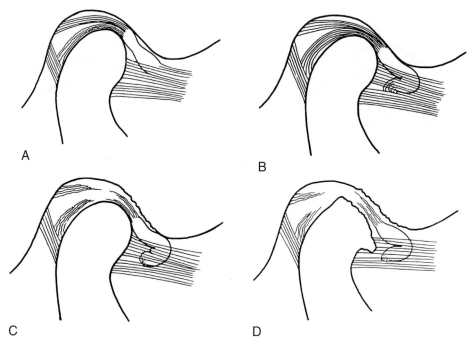

FIGURE 70-4. Stages in the classic progression of internal derangement of the temporomandibular joint. *A,* Internal joint derangement secondary to anterior disk displacement with reduction (intermittent locking may occur). *B,* Anterior disk displacement without reduction. *C,* Perforation of the bilaminar zone. *D,* Osteoarthrosis. (From Thomas M, ed: Arthroscopy of the Temporomandibular Joint. Philadelphia, WB Saunders, 1991.)

TABLE 70-1 ✦ STAGING OF INTERNAL DERANGEMENT OF TEMPOROMANDIBULAR JOINT

Stage	Clinical	Imaging	Surgical
I Early	Painless clicking No restricted motion	Slightly forward disk Normal osseous contours	Normal disk form Slight anterior displacement Passive incoordination (clicking)
II Early/intermediate	Occasional painful clicking Intermittent locking Headaches	Slightly forward disk Early disk deformity Normal osseous contours	Anterior disk displacement Thickened disk

III
Intermediate
	Frequent pain
	Joint tenderness,
	  headaches
	Locking
	Restricted motion
	Painful chewing
		Anterior disk displacement
		Moderate to marked disk
		  thickening
		Normal osseous contours
			Disk deformed and displaced
			  anteriorly
			Variable adhesions
			No bone changes

IV
Intermediate/late
	Chronic pain, headache
	Restricted motion
		Anterior disk displacement
		Marked disk thickening
		Abnormal bone contours
			Degenerative remodeling of bone
			  surfaces
			Osteophytes
			Adhesions, deformed disk without
			  perforation

V
Late
	Variable pain
	Joint crepitus
	Painful function
		Anterior disk displacement
		  with disk perforation and
		  gross deformity
		Degenerative osseous changes
			Gross degenerative changes of disk
			  and hard tissues; disk perforation
			Multiple adhesions

From Wilkes CH: Internal derangements of the temporomandibular joint: pathological variations. Arch Otolaryngol Head Neck Surg 1989;115:469.

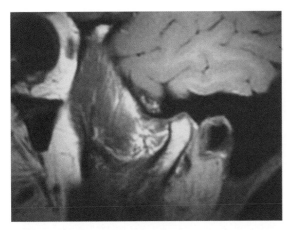

FIGURE 70-5. MRI demonstrating an anteriorly displaced disk that is malformed in the closed position. There is also flattening of the anterior superior condylar head.

reduction and intermittent locking. Pain is common at this stage and localized over the TMJ. In stage III, the patient has a chronic limitation of opening less than 25 to 30 mm. The mandible deviates to the affected side on opening and with protrusive movements. The internal derangement is without disk reduction and is an acute closed lock.

Chronic internal derangement without disk reduction (stage IV) results in injury to the retrodiskal tissue. Pain may diminish because of fibrous changes occurring in the retrodiskal tissue.[11] Limited mouth opening is common here as the disk blocks full condylar translation (Fig. 70-5). This condition responds well to TMJ arthroscopy and release of adhesions and joint lavage.[12,13] In stage V, remodeling of the temporal and condylar bone components occurs.

The management of stage I or stage II is nonoperative except for arthroscopy. Such treatment includes occlusal splint therapy, allowing the normal disk condylar relationships to be re-established. Those with later stage disease require aggressive intervention; the surgical alternatives are discussed subsequently with TMJ arthrotomy and reconstruction of the joint.

Condyle and Bone Problems

A noninflammatory disorder, osteoarthrosis, involves a cycle of condylar cartilage breakdown and repair. In addition to the condylar articular cartilage, it can involve the synovial membrane and subchondral bone. Initial cartilage degeneration or chondromalacia is seen in the early stages of osteoarthrosis. Further cartilage destruction can lead to focal bone denudation.

A late, progressive stage of osteoarthrosis leads to denudation of the subchondral bone. Gross alterations of the bone can be detected with radiographs in this

stage. They include sclerosis of the subchondral bone, osteophytic lipping, cyst formation, flattening of the condyle, and decreased height of the ramus (Fig. 70-6).[14] Chronic anterior disk displacement is associated with posterior superior condylar resorption seen as flattening and loss of bone in this area.

Idiopathic condylar resorption can also occur in either juvenile or adult individuals. In both forms, there is a diminished condylar head. In the juvenile form, the exact cause is unknown and is multifactorial but leads to decreased mandibular growth and a class II malocclusion. The adult form can follow orthognathic surgery of the mandible or disk displacement. Both types are self-limited and are treated conservatively until the condition stabilizes. Surgery may then be indicated.[15,16]

Congenital and Developmental Abnormalities

Hypoplasia of the condyle is discussed elsewhere in this text (see Chapter 91). However, developmental abnormalities include coronoid hypertrophy, condylar hyperplasia, and osteochondromas.

Limitation of mandibular motion can be due to enlarged coronoid processes. It may impinge on the zygomatic arch, causing pain and trismus. For severe, incapacitating pain and limitation in mandibular movement, a coronoidectomy can be performed by an intraoral approach. The coronoid process should be removed from the sigmoid notch obliquely to the anterior notch of the mandible.[17] Coronoid hypertrophy has also been reported in Möbius syndrome.[18]

Condylar hyperplasia and osteochondromas of the condyle can cause growth disturbances and malocclusion. Such developmental disease can cause significant disturbance in the TMJ mechanism. The treatment of such disorders is discussed in Chapter 90.

Condylar Fractures

A history of condylar fractures can lead to subsequent pain and limitation of the TMJ (see Chapter 66). Intracapsular fractures are usually treated by closed techniques, although serious dysfunction is found in 33% of patients. Condylar fractures without loss of vertical height do the best in terms of function.[19] Diagnostic imaging is helpful in locating the bony, internal derangement or other soft tissue abnormalities in these patients. The usual displacement of the condylar head is medial and anterior out of the glenoid fossa due to pull of the lateral pterygoid muscle (Fig. 70-7). Open reduction of subcondylar fractures is recommended when there is a loss of vertical height, significant condylar dislocation or displacement into the middle cranial fossa, and bilateral condylar fractures. Endoscopic

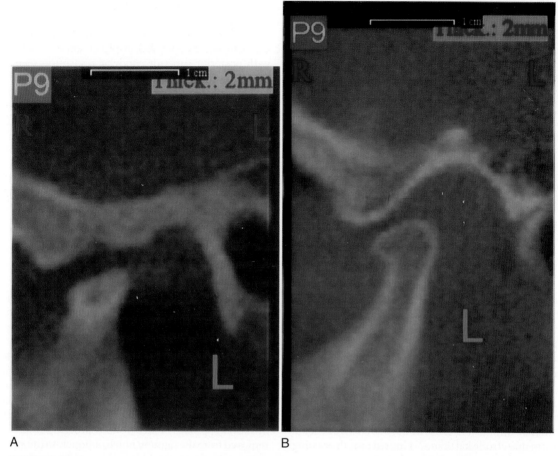

A   B

FIGURE 70-6. *A,* Tomography in the open position with severe osteoarthritic changes of the condylar head and almost total loss of the condyle. This causes vertical posterior facial collapse, open bite deformity, and mandibular retrusion. *B,* The normal condyle in the same patient.

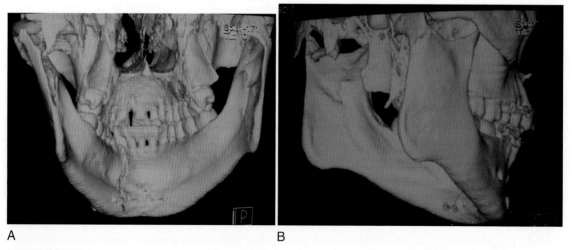

A   B

FIGURE 70-7. *A* and *B,* Three-dimensional computed tomogram of a patient with bilateral subcondylar fractures with anterior medial dislocation of the fractured segments.

reduction has now become common in the treatment of subcondylar fractures to avoid some of the morbidity associated with other open techniques. The surgical approach is either intraoral through a ramus incision or extraoral through a small Risdon-type incision.[20,21]

Osteoarthritis

Osteoarthritis is a chronic noninflammatory disease that characteristically affects the articular cartilage of synovial joints; it is associated with remodeling of the underlying subchondral bone and development of a secondary synovitis. It is the most common disease affecting the TMJ. It has a gradual onset. Usually, only one side is affected. The radiographic change is subchondral bone sclerosis in the condyle. Severe stages of this disease can cause a bone cyst within the condyle.[22] Treatment frequently involves drug therapy, occlusal appliance therapy, physical therapy, and, when it is most severe, surgery.

Rheumatoid Arthritis

Rheumatoid arthritis is a chronic inflammatory disease that primarily affects the periarticular structures, such as the synovial membrane, capsule, tendons, and ligaments. More than 50% of patients with rheumatoid arthritis have involvement of the TMJ during the course of their disease.[22,23] When the TMJ is involved, patients relate a dull aching pain in the preauricular area, muscle tenderness, poor range of jaw motion, clicking, and TMJ stiffness in the morning.

Progression of the disease includes condylar resorption and fibrous and bony ankylosis (Fig. 70-8). The

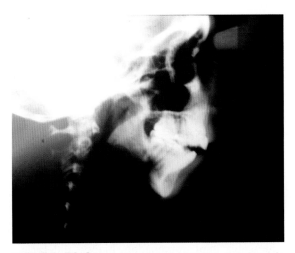

FIGURE 70-8. In rheumatoid arthritis, the condyle becomes smaller and the relationship with the fossa mismatched, resulting in retrusion of the mandible and development of an anterior open bite.

classic malocclusion is caused by loss of the height of the condyles. Juvenile rheumatoid arthritis affects patients before the age of 16 years. Up to 40% of children with juvenile rheumatoid arthritis have involvement of the TMJ.[24] Defective development of the mandible leads to micrognathia. MRI can delineate disk destruction, condylar bone erosion, and cartilaginous thinning. The radiographs of the TMJ include loss of joint space and condylar resorption with anterior subluxation of the condyle.

The treatment goals in rheumatoid arthritis are pain relief, reduction of inflammation, maintenance of function, and prevention of further deformity. This treatment may include drug therapy, occlusal appliance, physical therapy, and dental and surgical procedures of the TMJ and mandible. Most surgery is reserved for correction of joint ankylosis and severe malocclusion.

HISTORY AND PHYSICAL EXAMINATION

A patient may describe the pain's originating from the TMJ, preauricular area, or surrounding masticatory muscles. In addition, the discomfort may radiate from the ear, teeth, or neck area. The onset of pain in the morning is often due to nocturnal bruxism, grinding of teeth, in which constant pain after jaw function suggests intracapsular joint disease. Patients with TMJ dysfunction relate a triad of preauricular pain, clicking or grinding noises from the TMJ, and poor mandibular movement.[25]

Some patients may describe noises in the joint associated with daily jaw movement. Such clicking may be benign solitary clicks, which occur in 40% of the normal population. When there is anterior subluxation of the disk with jaw opening, condylar contact results in a click. A reciprocal click occurs as the disk subluxes when the condyle repositions into the glenoid fossa. The abnormal joint surfaces lead to a grinding or crepitus from the joint. Closed lock is a sudden irreducible anterior subluxation of the disk, limiting mandibular motion. Other reasons for limited excursion of the jaw may be local muscle dysfunction, bony or fibrous ankylosis of the joint, and blocking of the coronoid process by the zygoma.

Before the oral evaluation, a complete physical examination is required. The examination of the patient with TMJ pain centers on the head, neck, and TMJ. The facial examination includes any soft tissue asymmetry or skeletal deformities. Examination of the cranial nerves I through XII is performed to exclude any central nervous system disorders. The ear canals and tympanic membrane are examined to rule out primary benign or malignant diseases. Similarly, the oral tissues are evaluated for mucosal lesions, swellings, periodontal disease, alveolar process abnormalities, and evidence of cheek or lip biting.

Oral Examination

The teeth are examined for caries, mobility of teeth, absent teeth, prosthetics, molar impactions, supraerupted teeth, malocclusion, and displacement of the mandible during contact of the teeth. The incisor relationship is important to delineate overbite, overjet, or open bite, all of which can contribute to the TMJ symptoms. Palpation of the area of the TMJ can detect clicking or crepitus. Joint sounds must be determined as popping, clicking (reciprocal or nonreciprocal), or crepitations.

Palpation of the TMJ can detect swelling, tenderness, and joint sounds. Auscultation can be more sensitive in determining the type of joint sounds. The masticatory and cervical muscles must also be excluded as areas of tenderness or spasm. The presence or absence of pain, intensity of pain, location of pain, and referred pain must be documented.

The TMJ range of motion should be measured. Any pain or deviation to the left or right on opening is noted. The normal interincisor opening distance is 40 to 50 mm. The lateral jaw movement is at least 10 mm on each side of the incisor midline. Any restriction of the interincisal range of motion at opening, lateral restriction, deviation on opening, and development of new anterior open bite can be indicators of the degree of joint involvement.[9] At this point, diagnostic imaging is required.

Diagnostic Imaging

The most common conventional radiographic technique for diagnostic imaging of the TMJ is the transcranial projection. It depicts the TMJ with the glenoid fossa, articular tubercle, and condyle. Tomography provides sectional images in the sagittal or coronal views, usually taken in the open and closed positions. This modality demonstrates bone disease and range of condylar motion but provides no information on soft tissue disease. One study showed that up to 85% of patients with TMJ disease had normal tomographic findings.[26]

The evaluation of the TMJ soft tissue and disk has traditionally been with contrast arthrography. Arthrography can be performed as either single-contrast lower compartment[27] or dual-space contrast arthrotomography.[28] TMJ arthrography is highly reliable in determining disk disease but has mostly been replaced now by MRI, which provides information similar to these techniques. MRI visualizes soft tissue directly and is noninvasive. It can also give information about the swelling and inflammation in the joint.[29]

With abnormal findings, MRI commonly detects anterior, anterior medial, and anterior lateral displacement of the disk. In sagittal images, the disk is anterior to the condyle in the closed mouth position.

Furthermore, MRI may provide insight into the bone marrow abnormalities of the condyle. If the central area of the condyle has a low signal, this may suggest a pathologic condyle consistent with avascular necrosis.

Computed tomography (CT) is useful to evaluate bone abnormalities, bony ankylosis, and acute traumatic injuries to the head and neck areas. Otherwise, CT of the disk is difficult. The advantages of MRI over CT include absence of ionizing radiation, fewer artifacts from dense bone and metal clips, imaging in multiple planes, and good detail of the soft tissues.

The first step in imaging of a patient with TMJ pain and dysfunction is a plain film or tomography. The next modality should be arthrography or MRI, focusing on the soft tissue and disk. For postsurgical imaging, MRI is the best choice.[30] Traumatic or osseous deformities are best visualized by CT and especially three-dimensional reformatting of the images.

MEDICAL OCCLUSAL MANAGEMENT

The goal of medical management is to break the cycle of pain and anxiety in myofascial pain and dysfunction. The common area in which to begin is the dental occlusion. With a fabricated occlusal splint, the mandible can be guided along a path to relax the neuromuscular system that is strained during premature contact of the teeth and remove pressure from the joint area. This treatment is combined with nonsteroidal anti-inflammatory drugs and a soft diet. With occlusal therapy, resolution of myofascial pain and dysfunction is a realistic goal. If pain is exacerbated by splinting, however, internal derangement of the disk should be ruled out with an MRI examination.

Many factors can affect the success of occlusal appliance therapy. The insertion and adjustment of the appliance and compliance of the patient are examples. The various types of occlusal splints are the muscle relaxation appliance, the anterior bite plate, and the soft appliance. The choice of the splint depends on the patient's history, physical examination findings, and needs and the cause of the myofascial pain and dysfunction.

SURGICAL MANAGEMENT

Temporomandibular Joint Arthroscopy

The arthroscope enables the surgeon to perform endoscopic joint examination, biopsy, and lavage. McCain et al[31] found that more than 90% of patients with internal derangement treated through arthroscopy had reduced symptoms and improved jaw function.

In addition to the arthroscope, a high-intensity light source, video camera, and monitor are required. The instrumentation varies, but blunt and sharp trocars and cannulas are used for joint entry. Fluids used for joint lavage include lactated Ringer solution. Measured landmarks for TMJ entry have been reported.[32] The point of entry is along a line from the tragus to the lateral canthus of the eye. The site is 10 mm anterior to the tragus and 2 mm inferior to the line. Use of these landmarks will help prevent complications involving the temporal branch of the facial nerve and the auriculotemporal branch of the trigeminal nerve. A 27-gauge needle is inserted at the posterior entry point to insufflate the TMJ with irrigating fluid. After the superior compartment of the joint is distended, the arthroscope is inserted through the same entry (the single-portal technique). A double-portal technique requires another cannula placed anteriorly so that the scope and the surgical instruments can be interchanged, alternating the inflow and outflow portals.

Joint lavage or arthrocentesis, lysis of adhesions, and disk manipulation can then be achieved. It is important to increase the mobility of the disk to help improve joint function, so lysis of adhesions and opening of the anterior recess on the anterior slope of the eminence are essential.[14]

Open Arthrotomy

Open arthrotomy allows an open view and examination of the joint.[13,17,31,33] The preauricular approach is most common. The most important structure at risk during surgery is the frontal branch of the facial nerve. Staying on the deep white temporalis fascia during dissection will prevent such injury, remembering that it splits about an inch above the zygomatic arch. The subfascial technique is one method; the skin incision is carried to the deep temporal fascia, cutting the fascia at its split to allow subperiosteal exposure.[13]

Instead of the subfascial method, an alternative is to continue inferiorly over the arch to the parotid-masseteric fascia. After the fascioperiosteal layer is bared over the arch to the level of the articular eminence, an incision is made at midarch with a vertical extension reflecting the periosteum inferiorly.[34] Such a suprafascial approach has a higher risk of injury to the facial nerve.

Surgical Management of Specific Disorders

ANKYLOSIS

The type of ankylosis can be intra-articular or extra-articular. The fusion at the articular level may be fibrous or bony in nature.[35] Patients with ankylosis develop poor oral hygiene, dental caries, and abscesses. In juvenile rheumatoid arthritis, mandibular growth and facial development are reduced; surgery is sometimes required to correct the dentofacial deformities.

Extra-articular ankylosis may be due to enlargement of the muscles of mastication, the facial nerve, or the coronoid process. The common causes of intra-articular ankylosis are trauma, infection, and juvenile rheumatoid arthritis. These lead to the deterioration of disk and bone elements. A fibrous union narrows the joint space, leading to bone fusion. The diagnostic modalities for ankylosis of the TMJ include tomography and CT scanning. These studies can delineate types of ankylosis and allow the physician to choose the optimal therapy. CT with three-dimensional reformatting is especially useful.

Surgical treatment of the common ankyloses includes several areas: condylectomy, gap arthroplasty, and interpositional arthroplasty. For patients with early ankylosis, condylectomy is performed. It is technically difficult to release the fused elements of the condylar head at the joint space delineating the glenoid fossa, and thereby it has lost favor as a treatment.[30]

A gap arthroplasty involves removal of bone at or below the joint level without interposition of any material. Often, there is high recurrence of the ankylosis as well as production of an open bite deformity.[36] In patients with severe disease, placement of alloplastic or autogenous materials after resection of the condyle is the favored surgical approach. The interposition of materials is used to maintain vertical height and to restore a functional joint. A commonly used alloplast has been silicone rubber[37] to produce a pseudoarticulation.

Autogenous replacement of the resected condyle to prevent reankylosis includes dermis, fat, fascia lata, and muscle. The costochondral graft harvested from the contralateral sixth rib is the optimal approach to reconstruction and is the preferred technique.[38] Autologous condylar reconstruction is preferred in the growing patient and young adult, in whom a prosthetic implant will probably wear out at some point and need to be replaced.[39] The patient needs aggressive physical therapy to maintain motion of the reconstructed joint space.[37]

Total TMJ reconstruction has proved safe and effective in long-term management of selected patients (Fig. 70-9). The prosthesis should be custom fitted; computer-aided design and manufacturing technology has proved beneficial in this area.[40]

AVASCULAR NECROSIS

Avascular necrosis is rare. The causes include trauma and complications of TMJ surgery. The classic symptoms are severe pain and decreased range of motion of the jaw. MRI is an important imaging modality for

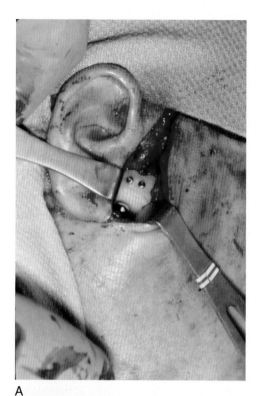

A

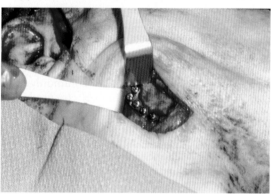

B

FIGURE 70-9. *A* and *B,* Total joint prosthesis requires reconstruction of both the glenoid fossa and condylar elements.

detecting devascularization of the condyle. The management of patients with severe disease is surgical débridement of the necrotic condyle and reconstruction with autogenous tissue.

DISLOCATIONS

Acute dislocations result from the condyle's extending anteriorly beyond the articular eminence. If spontaneous reduction does not occur, manual reduction with a muscle relaxant or anesthesia is often needed. The surgeon places downward force along the inferior

border of the mandible while moving the jaw posterior to slide the condyle into the fossa.

BONE LOSS OF THE CONDYLE

The bone loss of the condyle can be reconstructed with regenerative bone. McCarthy[41] has shown that the mandible has the ability to form new bone under the influences of osteodistraction. The effect on the TMJ has been shown to be significant remodeling changes.[42] The rate of distraction and its effect on producing new bone without TMJ pain are also of importance in reconstruction of the mandible.[43] However, there is a potential for reconstructing a new condylar bony head or neocondyle with this technique.[42]

REFERENCES

1. Boyer CC, Williams TW, Stevens FH: Blood supply of the temporomandibular joint. J Dent Res 1964;43:224.
2. Dixon AD: Structure and functional significance of the intraarticular disc in the human temporomandibular joint. J Oral Surg 1962;15:48.
3. Chonkas NC, Sicher H: Structure of the temporomandibular joint. Oral Surg Oral Med Oral Pathol 1960;13:1203.
4. Bell WH: Surgical Correction of Dentofacial Deformities: New Concepts. Philadelphia, WB Saunders, 1985.
5. Dautrey J, Pepersack J: Functional surgery of the temporomandibular joint. Clin Plast Surg 1981;9:591.
6. Laskin DM: Etiology of the pain-dysfunction syndrome. J Am Dent Assoc 1969;79:147.
7. Laskin DM: Diagnosis and etiology of myofascial pain and dysfunction. Oral Maxillofac Surg Clin North Am 1995;7:73.
8. Syrop SB: Pharmacologic management of myofascial pain and dysfunction. Oral Maxillofac Surg Clin North Am 1995;7:87.
9. Turk AE, Schendel SA: Pain in the jaw joint: diagnosis and treatment. In Harris ED, Genovese MC, eds: Primary Care Rheumatology. Philadelphia, WB Saunders, 2000:227-233.
10. Friction J, Schellhas KP, Braun BL, et al: Joint disorders: derangements and degeneration. In Friction J, Kroening R, Hathaway K, eds: TMJ and Craniofacial Pain. St. Louis, Ishiyaku Euro America, 1988:85-130.
11. Scapino R: Histopathology associated with malposition of the human temporomandibular joint disc. Oral Surg 1983;55:382.
12. Dimitroulis G: A review of 56 cases of chronic closed lock treated with temporomandibular joint arthroscopy. J Oral Maxillofac Surg 2002;60:519.
13. Reston JT, Turkelson CM: Meta-analysis of surgical treatments for temporomandibular articular disorders. J Oral Maxillofac Surg 2003;61:3.
14. Bronstein SL, Thomas M: Arthroscopy of the Temporomandibular Joint. Philadelphia, WB Saunders, 1991.
15. Arnett GW, Milam SB, Gottesman L: Progressive mandibular retrusion–idiopathic condylar resorption. Part I. Am J Orthod Dentofacial Orthop 1996;110:8.
16. Arnett GW, Milam SB, Gottesman L: Progressive mandibular retrusion–idiopathic condylar resorption. Part II. Am J Orthod Dentofacial Orthop 1996;110:117.
17. Kreutziger KL: Surgery of the temporomandibular joint. I. Surgical anatomy and surgical incisions. Oral Surg Oral Med Oral Pathol 1984;58:637.
18. Turk AE, McCarthy JG, Nichter LS, Thorne CH: Moebius syndrome: the new finding of hypertrophy of the coronoid process. J Craniofac Surg 1999;10:93.
19. Hlawithschka M, Eckelt U: Assessment of patients treated for intracapsular fractures of the mandibular condyle by closed techniques. J Oral Maxillofac Surg 2002;60:784.

20. Sandler NA: Endoscopic-assisted reduction and fixation of a mandibular subcondylar fracture: report of a case. J Oral Maxillofac Surg 2001;59:1479.

21. Schon R, Schramm A, Gellrich N, Schmelzeisen R: Follow-up of condylar fractures of the mandible in 8 patients at 18 months after transoral endoscopic-assisted open treatment. J Oral Maxillofac Surg 2003;61:49.

22. Akerman S, Kopp S, Nilner M, et al: Relationship between clinical and radiologic findings of the temporomandibular joint in rheumatoid arthritis. Oral Surg Oral Med Oral Pathol 1988;66:639.

23. Laskin DM: Diagnosis of pathology of the temporomandibular joint: clinical and imaging perspectives. Radiol Clin North Am 1993;31:135.

24. Larheim TA, Hoyeraal HM, Starbrun AE, et al: The temporomandibular joint in juvenile rheumatoid arthritis: radiographic changes related to clinical and laboratory parameters in 100 children. Scand J Rheumatol 1982;11:5.

25. Bessette RW, Jacobs JS: Temporomandibular joint dysfunction. In Aston SJ, Beasley RW, Thorne CHM, eds: Grabb and Smith's Plastic Surgery. Philadelphia, Lippincott-Raven, 1997:247-271.

26. Stanson AW, Baker HL: Routine tomography of the temporomandibular joint. Radiol Clin North Am 1976;14:105.

27. Farrar WB, McCarty WL Jr: Inferior joint space arthrography and characteristics of condylar paths in internal derangements of the TMJ. J Prosthet Dent 1979;41:548.

28. Westesson PL: Double-contrast arthrotomography of the temporomandibular joint: introduction of an arthrographic technique for visualization of the disc and articular surfaces. J Oral Maxillofac Surg 1983;41:163.

29. Schellhas KP, Wilkes CH, Fritts HM, et al: Temporomandibular joint: MR imaging of internal derangements and postoperative changes. AJNR Am J Neuroradiol 1987;8:1093.

30. Greenberg SA, Jacobs JS, Bessette RW: Temporomandibular joint dysfunction: evaluation and treatment. Clin Plast Surg 1989;16:707.

31. McCain JP, Sanders B, Koslin MG, et al: Temporomandibular joint arthroscopy. J Oral Maxillofac Surg 1992;50:926.

32. Holmlund A, Hellsing G: Arthroscopy of the temporomandibular joint. Int J Oral Surg 1985;14:169.

33. Kreutziger KL: Surgery of the temporomandibular joint. I. Surgical anatomy and surgical incisions. Oral Surg Oral Med Oral Pathol 1984;58:637.

34. Zide BM: The temporomandibular joint. In McCarthy JG, ed: Plastic Surgery. Philadelphia, WB Saunders, 1990:1475-1513.

35. Freedus M, Zitoc W, Doyle P: Principles of treatment for temporomandibular ankylosis. J Oral Surg 1975;33:757.

36. Topazian RG: Comparison of gap and interposition arthroplasty in the treatment of temporomandibular ankylosis. J Oral Surg 1966;24:405.

37. Gallagher DM, Wolford LM: Comparison of Silastic and Proplast implants in the temporomandibular joint after condylectomy for osteoarthritis. J Oral Maxillofac Surg 1982;40:627.

38. Munro IR, Chen YR, Park BY: Simultaneous total correction of temporomandibular ankylosis and facial asymmetry. Plast Reconstr Surg 1986;77:517.

39. Mercuri LG, Anspach WE III: Principles for the revision of total alloplastic TMJ prostheses. Oral Maxillofac Surg 2003; 32:353.

40. Mercuri LG, Wolford LM, Sanders B, et al: Long-term follow-up of the CAD/CAM patient fitted total temporomandibular joint reconstruction system. J Oral Maxillofac Surg 2002;60:1440.

41. McCarthy JG, Schreiber J, Karp N, et al: Lengthening of the human mandible by gradual distraction. Plast Reconstr Surg 1992;89:1.

42. Stelnicki EJ, Stucki-McCormick SU, Rowe N, McCarthy JG: Remodeling of the temporomandibular joint following mandibular distraction osteogenesis in the transverse dimension. Plast Reconstr Surg 2001;107:647.

43. Schendel SA, Heegaard JH: A mathematical model for mandibular distraction osteogenesis. J Craniofac Surg 1996;7:465.

Acquired Cranial Bone Deformities

MICHAEL J. YAREMCHUK, MD

ANATOMY OF THE SKULL

CRANIOPLASTY
    Timing of Surgery
    Technique of Cranioplasty
    Choice of Material for Cranioplasty

Computer-Aided Design/Computer-Aided
    Manufacture
    Microvascular Composite Tissue Transplantation

TEMPORAL HOLLOWING

Acquired cranial bone deformities are most often the result of trauma or extirpation for tumor. Although careful physical examination is paramount in the preoperative evaluation, computed tomographic or magnetic resonance imaging is performed in most cases to provide optimal definition of the real or anticipated defect and the status of the adjacent neurologic structures. Computer-generated reformatting of two-dimensional computed tomographic data can provide a three-dimensional digital image of the skull defect (Fig. 71-1).

Knowledge of plastic surgical concepts and techniques used to reconstruct major defects of the skull is necessary for management of acquired cranial deformities. Successful reconstruction of acquired cranial bone deformities requires facility with bone carpentry and the use of alloplastic materials. Equally important to a successful outcome is adherence to basic principles of wound healing: adequate débridement, obliteration of dead space, and tension-free closure with well-vascularized tissues.

ANATOMY OF THE SKULL

The calvaria has three distinct layers in the adult: the hard internal and external laminae and the cancellous middle layer or diploë. The adult bony vault has an average thickness of about 7 mm but varies considerably across areas and individuals.[1] Skull thickness lessens considerably in the elderly. The thickest area is usually the occipital, and the thinnest is the temporal.

The calvaria is covered with periosteum on both the outer and inner surfaces. On the inner surface, it fuses with the dura to become the dura's outer layer.

Unlike in other areas of the skeleton and perhaps because of the lack of functional stresses on the skull, the periosteum of the skull seems to have little osteogenic potential in the adult. Therefore, the loss or removal of the calvaria requires its replacement if its location is important from a protective or aesthetic standpoint.

The frontal bone is aesthetically the most important calvaria because only a small portion of it is concealed by hair-bearing scalp. In addition, it forms the roof and portions of the medial and lateral walls of the orbit. Displaced frontal fractures may therefore cause visible deformity or globe malposition. The frontal bone also includes the frontal sinuses, which are paired structures that lie between the inner and outer lamellae of the frontal bone. The lesser thickness of the anterior wall of the frontal sinus makes this area more susceptible to fracture than the adjacent temporo-orbital areas.

CRANIOPLASTY

Cranioplasty may become necessary when primary repair or bone replacement is not appropriate during acute-phase treatment. Eradication of infection may require removal of bone flaps used in elective procedures or bone fragments replaced immediately after trauma. The resultant deformity is reconstructed after the clinical infection has been treated and the area remains clinically infection free.

As is true of acute craniomaxillofacial reconstruction, the reconstructive goals in cranioplasty are to provide protection of the brain and to restore the preinjury appearance. In addition, speech problems and

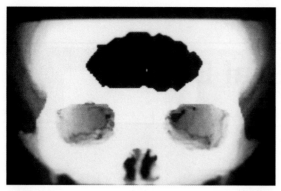

FIGURE 71-1. A three-dimensional image computer generated from two-dimensional computed tomographic data of the post-traumatic frontal defect. (From Yaremchuk MJ, Rubin JP: Surgical repair of major defects of the scalp and skull. In Schmidek HH, ed: Operative Neurosurgical Techniques, 4th ed. Philadelphia, WB Saunders, 1999.)

hemiparesis may improve by cranial reconstruction if the defect is large enough to allow the scalp to exert direct pressure on the brain.[2-5] Skull defects of greater than 2 or 3 cm should be considered for repair. However, this decision varies with location. Even small defects in the frontal area can be disturbing to the patient and therefore can be considered for repair. Small defects of the temporal and occipital areas, which are covered by thick muscle, are usually not reconstructed.

Timing of Surgery

The incidence of infection is influenced by the timing of cranioplasty. A significant reduction in incidence of infection has been shown when 1 year is allowed to elapse between the initial injury or infection and the subsequent reconstruction.[6-8]

A review of the literature shows that a history of infection increases the incidence of infection after cranioplasty an average of 14% and that cranioplasty in the frontal area causes twice the incidence of infection than that in all other areas (5%).[9,10] In reviewing their experience of 42 post-traumatic reconstructions of frontal defects in which both bone and acrylic were used, Manson et al[6] found that the material employed was not as important as the timing of reconstruction (more than 1 year after infection), communication between the cranial vault reconstruction and sinus cavities, and residual ethmoidal or frontal sinus inflammatory disease. These data are consistent with the author's clinical observations. Delay of cranioplasty is preferred for, ideally, 1 year after control of infection to treat all sinus disease before reconstruction and to eradicate communication between the sinus cavities and the reconstruction. Mucocele formation is avoided by removing all sinus mucosa from the frontal sinus and

preventing its ingrowth through the nasofrontal ducts. Burring the inner table with a high-speed drill removes all mucosal invaginations that follow bridging veins into bone.[11] Occluding the nasofrontal duct with custom-fit bone plugs prevents mucosal ingrowth from the nose. A further mechanical barrier between the nose and the intracranial compartment and potential cranioplasty can be accomplished with nonvascularized grafts of fat, bone, or muscle.[12,13] Large communications between the sinuses and the anterior cranial fossa, which may be the case after massive trauma requiring frontal sinus cranialization or after cranium-based tumor removal, require placement of a vascularized barrier for effective isolation. A galeal frontalis flap, if available and adequate, or a free tissue transfer may be required.

Technique of Cranioplasty

Before cranioplasty, compromised areas of scalp overlying the proposed reconstruction are revised and residual frontal or ethmoidal sinus disease is eliminated. At surgery, the patient is positioned so that a panoramic view of the skull and, if appropriate, the upper face can be draped into the field. This position allows the surgeon to mimic the contralateral anatomy and to avoid unnatural transitions. Preinjury photographs may be helpful in certain situations. A skull model should be available to aid in the design of complex curvatures and landmarks.

Old scars are usually incised for exposure, and the skull flap is removed carefully from the underlying dura and brain. Any dural tears are repaired. Resecting the bone edge to identify normal dura and establishing a plane of dissection may be necessary.

The exposed bone edge is saucerized by removal of the outer table with rongeurs or a high-speed burr. This lip prevents the implant from slipping into the defect and provides a ledge for subsequent fixation.

Choice of Material for Cranioplasty

Both autogenous bone and alloplastic materials are used to reconstruct the skull. Bone is employed when there is potential for sinus communication, with a history of recurrent infection, or when overlying soft tissues are compromised. Otherwise, in adults, most reconstructions are performed with alloplastic materials.

Acquired cranial deformities are rare in infants and young children. Treatment is usually deferred until late childhood or adolescence when cranial growth is nearly complete. The choice of reconstructive materials is determined by adult criteria and the surgeon's preference.

Methyl Methacrylate. The most commonly used alloplastic material for skull reconstruction is methyl methacrylate. Methyl methacrylate reconstruction is technically less demanding than reconstruction with autogenous bone and avoids bone donor site morbidity. The contour of this substance is stable. It is radiolucent and therefore does not affect postoperative radiologic imaging. It is unaffected by temperature and is strong. Because it is encapsulated by the host rather than incorporated by surrounding soft tissues, methyl methacrylate is believed by some to be more susceptible to infection and late complications.[6,14]

Cranioplasty kits are available that contain a single dose of 30 g of powdered polymer and 17 mL of liquid monomer. The elements are mixed with a spatula in a bowl. The mixing should be conducted under ventilation so that the person mixing is not overcome by fumes. Mixing takes about 30 seconds. The bowl is then covered to avoid evaporation of the monomer. Doughing time varies with the temperature and is about 5 minutes at 72°F.

Shaping of the plastic implant is usually performed by placing the doughy mixture in a plastic sleeve provided in the cranioplasty kit (Fig. 71-2). The sleeve containing the still pliable implant mixture is placed onto the skull defect and molded by digital compression. The molding process occurs under continuous irrigation to avoid thermal damage to the dura and brain. A molding time of 6 to 8 minutes is usual. The exothermic polymerization process is allowed to take place away from the surgical field.

Some surgeons place a wire mesh into the skull defect (Fig. 71-3). Methyl methacrylate is then cured directly on the mesh. This technique allows more risk for burn damage to the dura during the exothermic reaction, which unlike in the sleeve technique takes place in the surgical field. However, data from Manson et al[6] show that temperature rises less than 3°C when the implant is continuously irrigated. Stelnicki and Ousterhout[15] developed an in situ model to quantify the effects of saline irrigation on acrylic curing temperature with varying implant thickness. They concluded that in situ polymerization of acrylic implants with saline irrigation is safe if the implant is 6 mm or less in thickness.

Complex curvatures, particularly in the supraorbital area, are formed by adding material to an initial construct. Final adjustments can be made with a contouring burr on a high-speed drill. The implants may be fixed with wires or, more simply and rapidly, with microscrews. The screws are used to fix the position of the implant in one of two ways. In both techniques, the implant must overlie intact skull. Screws may be driven through the acrylic and into underlying bone before it is completely hardened. Another technique, particularly useful in augmenting contour depressions, is first to place the screw in the area to be augmented, leaving the head and two or three threads above the bone surface. The acrylic is then poured over the screw so that it is incorporated in the construct (Fig. 71-4).

The plate may be perforated to allow the dura to be tented up to it. This method lessens the potential for epidural collection. Perforations in the implant also allow drainage and soft tissue ingrowth, which also aids in implant fixation.

BONE CRANIOPLASTY. Bone is championed by many plastic surgeons because it becomes revascularized to varying extents by the host and therefore is less susceptible to infection and late complications. It has the disadvantages of requiring a donor site, being technically demanding to perform, exhibiting variable resorption, and therefore being prone to irregular contour. Bone donor sites include ribs and calvaria.

Split ribs are useful when large defects are to be reconstructed and calvarial bone is in short supply. Split ribs are usually fitted into a shelf made in the adjacent intact skull. In the past, an interlocking "chain link" technique[16] was used for stabilization; now most craniofacial surgeons use a combination of plates and screws to make a stable construct (Fig. 71-5). The plates are bent to the appropriate shape and are fixed to a stable anatomic point. The grafts are then attached to the plates with screws. Titanium has become a popular material for craniofacial plates because of its high strength and decreased artifact on computed tomographic and magnetic resonance imaging studies compared with stainless steel or cobalt chromium (Vitallium).[17-19]

Calvarial bone is the preferred donor site of most craniofacial surgeons because it is in the surgical field and the donor site is painless. Because there is great variability in the thickness of the skull at any given point, and because there is no clinically useful correlate between skull thickness and age, sex, or weight,[1] a coronal computed tomographic image in the area to be harvested is obtained to look for the presence of a diploic space before cranial bone graft harvest is attempted. Although it is shown to be safe in the hands of trained, experienced surgeons, cranial bone graft harvest can have significant complications, including dural tear with bleeding, cerebrospinal fluid leak, and meningitis.[20,21]

The calvarial bone is harvested in two ways. The outer table may be harvested from the intact skull. The parietal area usually serves as the donor site because this area is usually accessible, and the donor site contour deformity is hidden by the patient's hair (Figs. 71-6 and 71-7). A clinical example of a frontal defect repaired with calvarial bone harvested from the outer table demonstrates the effectiveness of cranial bone for reconstruction with avoidance of donor site deformity (Fig. 71-8).

Another technique for harvesting of cranial bone is to perform a craniotomy with harvest of a full-thickness piece of skull of appropriate size and curvature. The inner table is split from the outer table

Text continued on p. 555

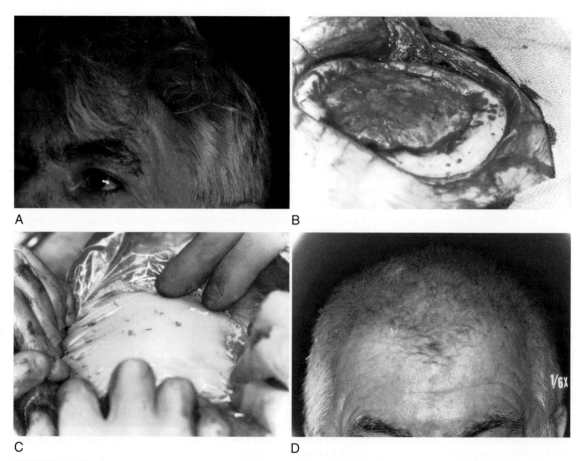

A

B

C

D

FIGURE 71-2. Acrylic cranioplasty by plastic sleeve molding technique. *A,* Preoperative appearance. *B,* Intraoperative view of right frontoparietal defect. *C,* Molding of methyl methacrylate to defect. *D,* Postoperative result. (From Yaremchuk MJ, Rubin JP: Surgical repair of major defects of the scalp and skull. In Schmidek HH, ed: Operative Neurosurgical Techniques, 4th ed. Philadelphia, WB Saunders, 1999.)

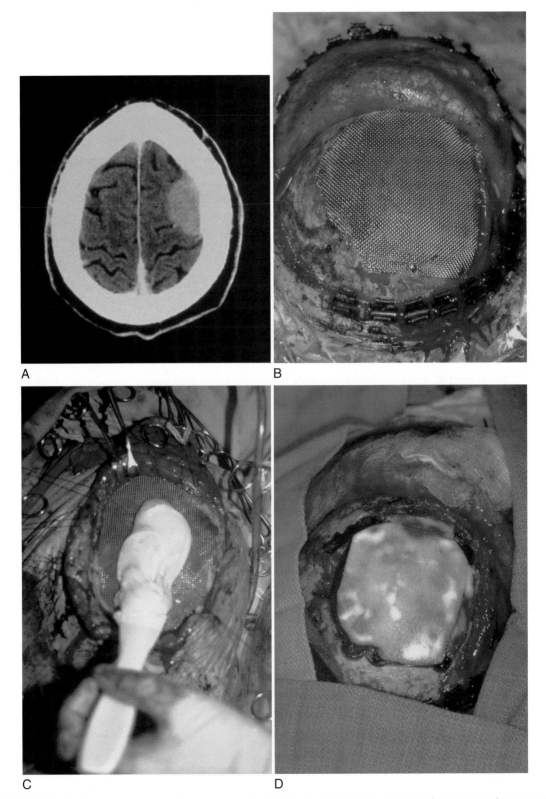

FIGURE 71-3. Acrylic cranioplasty by mesh-only technique. *A,* Preoperative computed tomogram shows menin-gioma requiring skull resection and subsequent cranioplasty. *B,* Intraoperative view of titanium mesh spanning defect. *C,* Methyl methacrylate being spread over metallic template. *D,* Acrylic polymerizing on mesh.   *Continued*

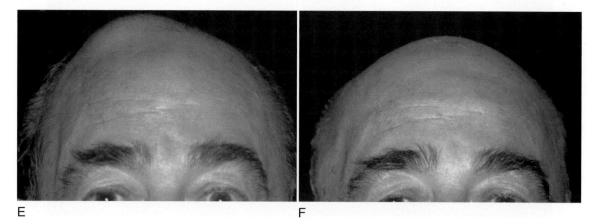

E   F

FIGURE 71-3, cont'd. *E,* Preoperative frontal view. *F,* Postoperative frontal view.

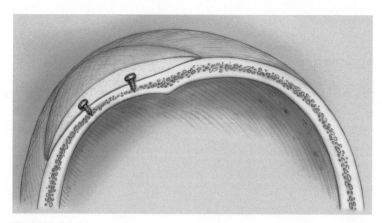

FIGURE 71-4. Diagrammatic representation of screw stabilization of acrylic onlays. A titanium screw purchases the outer table of the skull in area of defect. The screw head is left above the skull surface. Acrylic is spread over the screw head to incorporate the construct and to prevent movement of the implant.

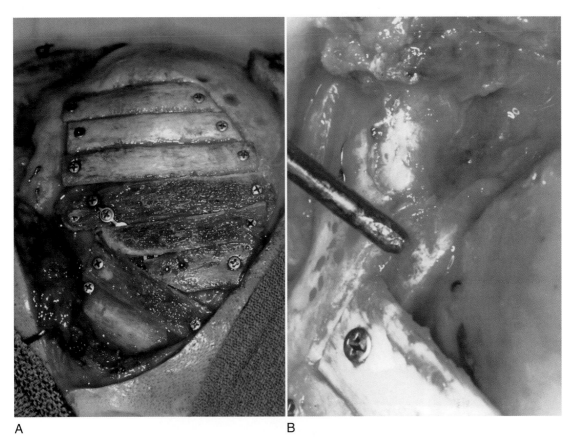

A   B

FIGURE 71-5. An example of split rib cranioplasty of right frontotemporal area stabilized with plates and screws. *A,* Completed reconstruction. *B,* Close-up view during reconstruction shows metal suction apparatus pointing to ledge made by removal of outer table at edge of defect. This allows a ledge for rib graft and ease of screw fixation. (From Yaremchuk MJ, Rubin JP: Surgical repair of major defects of the scalp and skull. In Schmidek HH, ed: Operative Neurosurgical Techniques, 4th ed. Philadelphia, WB Saunders, 1999.)

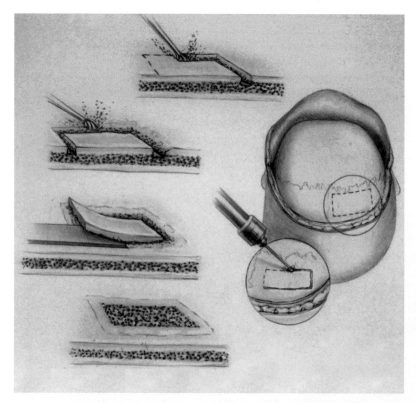

FIGURE 71-6. Diagrammatic representation of outer table calvarial bone harvest. Most often, the temporal or occipital areas are chosen. The midline is avoided to preclude possible damage to the sagittal sinus. With a small contouring burr, a trough is made through the outer table to the diploë. Sharp, thin osteotomes are then used to split the outer table from the inner table. Visualizing an edge of the osteotome at all times helps control depth and angle of bone penetration.

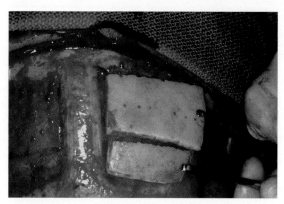

FIGURE 71-7. Clinical example of outer table harvest.

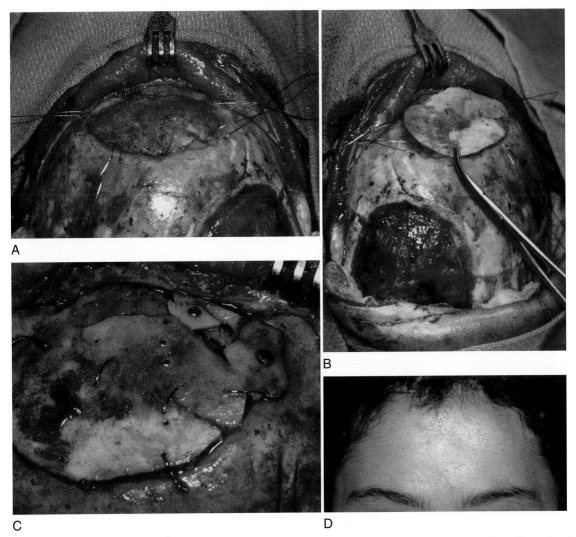

FIGURE 71-8. Frontal cranioplasty performed with outer table cranial bone. (Figure 71-1 shows three-dimensional computed tomogram of frontal defect.) *A,* Intraoperative coronal view of defect. *B,* Intraoperative view shows both donor site and graft in position. *C,* Close-up view of outer table graft harvest stabilized with screws. The supraorbital rim was augmented with onlay grafts. *D,* Postoperative appearance. (From Yaremchuk MJ, Rubin JP: Surgical repair of major defects of the scalp and skull. In Schmidek HH, ed: Operative Neurosurgical Techniques, 4th ed. Philadelphia, WB Saunders, 1999.)

(Fig. 71-9). A simple way to do this is with the aid of the Midas Rex drill* and the C-1 bit (Fig. 71-10). This thin bit is placed in the diploë between the two skull cortices. The outer cortex can be replaced, and the inner cortex is used for reconstruction of the defect. Most often, microplates and screws are used to stabilize this reconstruction.

Other Materials. Porous polyethylene† has recently been used for the reconstruction of skull defects. This inert material is porous, allowing soft tissue ingrowth. It has good strength yet is contourable and can be stabilized with plates and screws. Various-sized implants are available.

Hydroxyapatite is a ceramic biomaterial composed of calcium phosphate. It can be manufactured synthetically or formed by chemically converting the naturally porous calcium carbonate skeleton of marine coral. Hydroxyapatite cement has been shown to be osteoconductive, but only minimal direct bone or vascular ingrowth occurs because of the implant's extremely small pore size.[22-25] Any bone ingrowth that occurs is a direct turnover of hydroxyapatite

---

*Midas Rex Pneumatic Tools, Fort Worth, Texas.
†MEDPOR, Porex Surgical, Newnan, Georgia.

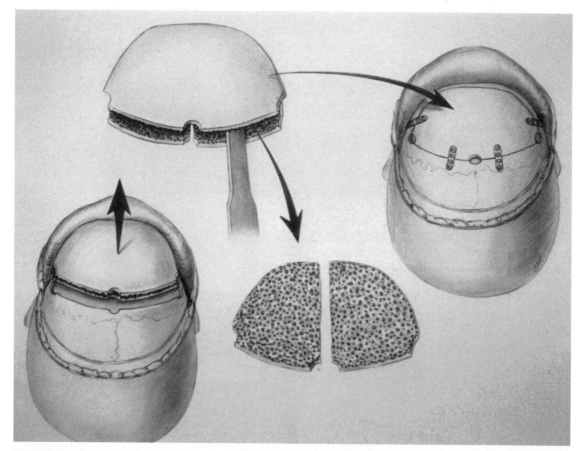

FIGURE 71-9. Schematic representation of inner table harvest after craniotomy. The outer table is returned to the donor site.

to bone at the periphery of the implant. Implant volume is thought to remain stable because the implant remains largely avascular. Three forms of hydroxyapatite have been used for facial skeletal reconstruction. Block hydroxyapatite has been used as relatively small interposition grafts.[26] It is extremely brittle, making it difficult to contour. Granular hydroxyapatite has been used as an onlay for orbitocranial defects. The problems with this material included slow cement consolidation and unpredictable volume restoration.[27] A powdered form of hydroxyapatite became available in 1996.* When it is mixed with water, the powder becomes a paste that is easily applied to regular surfaces. The paste sets in approximately 20 minutes. Because of its low flexural resistance, it is recommended for use as an onlay material to improve contour. It has been used with metallic mesh to reconstruct defects. The appropriate role of this alloplastic material in cranial vault reconstruction will be determined by careful clinical evaluation.[28]

Computer-Aided Design/ Computer-Aided Manufacture

Computed tomographic imaging of skull defects provides digitized information that can be transferred to design software. Data describing the contour along the edge of the defect and the surface characteristics of the normal cranium surrounding the defect can be used to design a custom-fit implant. The electronic data describing the newly designed prosthesis are then used by a computer-controlled manufacturing system to make a wax model, which is then cast, or to directly mill raw material into the finished implant (Fig. 71-11).[29-31]

Microvascular Composite Tissue Transplantation

Microvascular composite tissue transplantation can be invaluable to the success of certain cranial vault

*Bone Source, Leibinger Corp., Carrollton, Texas.

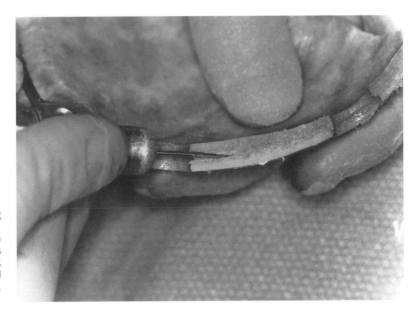

FIGURE 71-10. Bone flap being split with Midas Rex drill and C-1 bit. (From Yaremchuk MJ, Rubin JP: Surgical repair of major defects of the scalp and skull. In Schmidek HH, ed: Operative Neurosurgical Techniques, 4th ed. Philadelphia, WB Saunders, 1999.)

reconstructions. It is useful when there is a history of infection, compromised soft tissues, dead space after brain loss, or large communication between the sinuses and intracranial cavity.

The most frequently used free tissue transfer for the reconstruction of acquired cranial deformities is the rectus abdominis myocutaneous flap,[32] which is used for reconstruction after cranium-based tumor extirpation. Its well-vascularized bulk is used to isolate the intracranial cavity from sinus remnants after tumor removal. The soft tissue component may be included to reconstruct accompanying cutaneous defects. Its anterior location allows flap harvest to

proceed simultaneously with tumor extirpation, therefore reducing operative time.[33]

The latissimus dorsi is a large flat muscle. The latissimus dorsi muscle flap is ideal for resurfacing large defects of the scalp and calvarium.

The omental free tissue transfer is particularly useful for the reconstruction of acquired cranial deformities. The rich, interconnecting vascular network of the omentum allows it to conform to almost any three-dimensional wound requirement, providing both coverage and dead space obliteration (Figs. 71-12 and 71-13). It also has the advantage of providing an extremely long vascular pedicle that

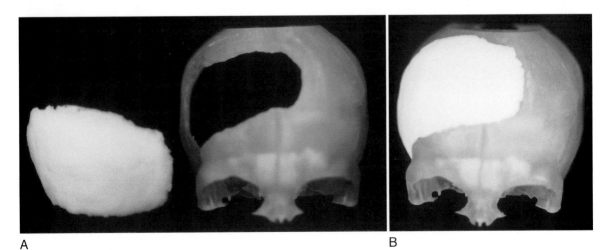

A   B

FIGURE 71-11. A three-dimensional model of a skull defect with a polyethylene implant generated by computer-aided design and manufacture. *A,* Adjacent to the skull. *B,* Fit into the defect.

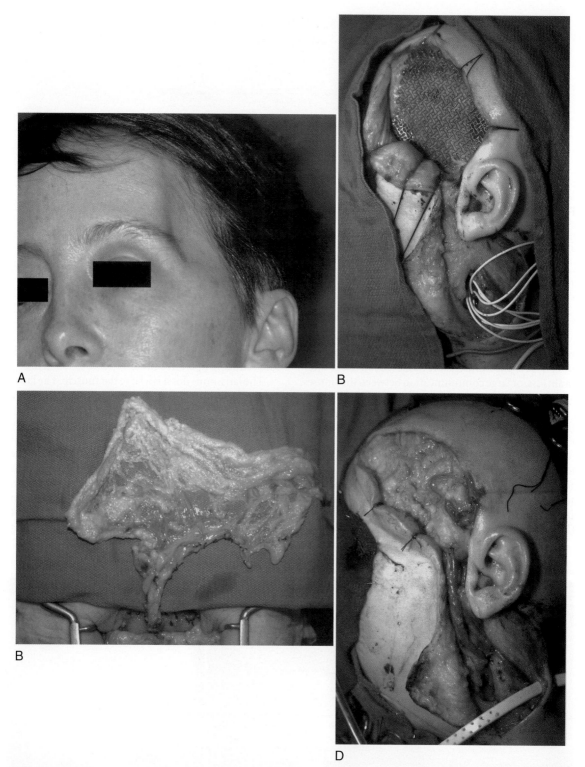

FIGURE 71-12. A 45-year-old woman underwent a temporal craniotomy for a cerebral aneurysm repair. The bone flap was lost because of infection. An acrylic cranioplasty and then a hydroxyapatite cranioplasty were lost to infection. One year after the second failed cranioplasty, a skull reconstruction was performed with titanium metal and a free omental transfer. *A,* Preoperative appearance. *B,* Intraoperative view shows mesh in place. Vessel loops surround vessels of external carotid and external jugular systems. *C,* Omentum at harvest. *D,* Omentum used to obliterate dead space between scalp and brain. Gastroepiploic vessels were anastomosed to neck vessels.

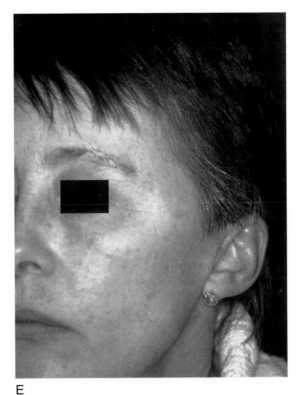

E

FIGURE 71-12, cont'd. *E,* Postoperative appearance.

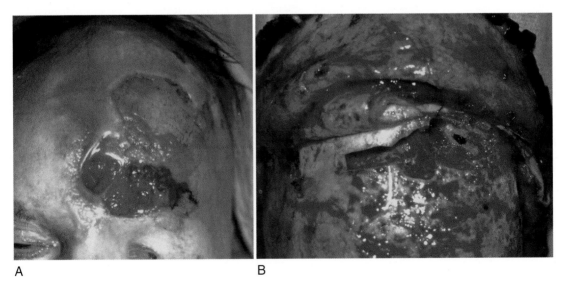

A B

FIGURE 71-13. A 26-year-old man suffered 60% body surface area burns including fourth-degree burns to his frontal area with loss of the anterior table of the frontal sinus. Omentum was used to obliterate the frontal sinus and to provide coverage for a cranial bone cranioplasty and exposed frontal bone. The omentum was covered with split-thickness skin grafts. *A,* Preoperative appearance. *B,* View from above after bicoronal incision is used for exposure. The frontal sinus mucosa was exenterated.

Continued

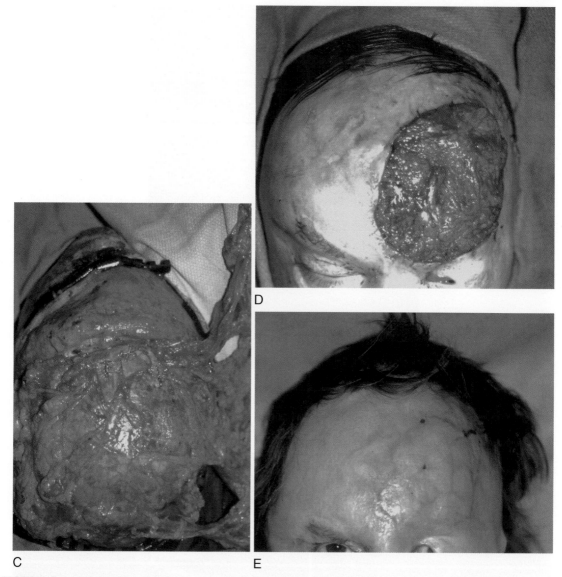

FIGURE 71-13, cont'd. *C,* Coronal view showing cranial bone cranioplasty. An arcade of omentum was used to obliterate the frontal sinus. The rest of the omentum will cover the cranioplasty and exposed frontal bone. *D,* Reconstruction before skin graft coverage of omentum. *E,* Postoperative result.

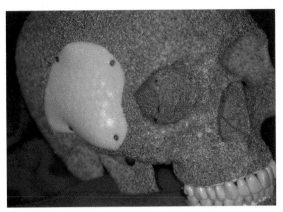

FIGURE 71-14. Porous polyethylene implant used to correct temporal hollowing due to temporalis muscle disinsertion and atrophy during frontotemporal craniotomy.

allows microvascular anastomoses to the neck vessels.[33,34]

TEMPORAL HOLLOWING

Disinsertion and reattachment of the temporal muscle lead to its atrophy. The subsequent loss of volume of this muscle may result in a visible depression in the temporal area. Alloplastic materials can be used to augment the volume of the temporal muscle and thereby restore contour. The alloplastic materials can be placed behind the muscle or between the muscle and the overlying soft tissues. Porous polyethylene implants are available in shapes specifically

designed for this application. They are modified as appropriate during the surgery (Figs. 71-14 and 71-15).[35]

SUMMARY

Reconstruction of acquired deformities of the skull requires that the plastic surgeon have access to computerized imaging techniques for perioperative evaluation and the availability of neurosurgical consultation and collaboration. The surgeon must have facility with bone carpentry, use of alloplastic materials, and rigid fixation techniques. Successful, long-lasting reconstruction also requires that the

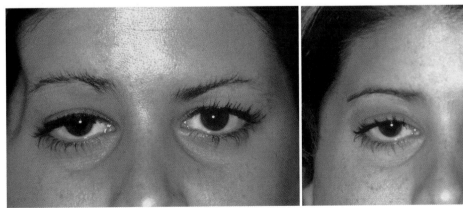
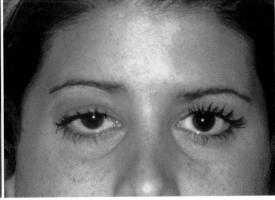

A   B

FIGURE 71-15. Clinical example of porous polyethylene implant used to correct temporal hollowing in a 25-year-old woman. *A*, Preoperative appearance. *B*, Postoperative appearance after stabilization of custom-carved porous polyethylene implant to zygomatic arch and lateral orbital rim with titanium microscrews.

surgeon abide by the basic tenets of soft tissue reconstruction: the obliteration of dead space and tension-free closure with well-vascularized tissues.

REFERENCES

1. Pensler J, McCarthy JG: The calvarial donor site: an anatomic study in cadavers. Plast Reconstr Surg 1985;75:648.
2. Grantham EG, Landis HP: Cranioplasty and posttraumatic syndrome. J Neurosurg 1948;5:19.
3. Carmichael FA: The reduction of hernia cerebri by tantalum cranioplasty. A preliminary report. J Neurosurg 1945;2:379.
4. Tabaddor K, LaMorgese J: Complication of a large cranial defect. Case report. J Neurosurg 1976;44:506.
5. Stula D: The problem of "sinking skin-flap syndrome" in cranioplasty. J Craniomaxillofac Surg 1982;10:142.
6. Manson PN, Crawley WA, Hoopes JE: Frontal cranioplasty: risk factors and choice of cranial vault reconstructive material. Plast Reconstr Surg 1986;77:888.
7. Hammon WM, Kempe LG: Methyl methacrylate cranioplasty: 13 years experience with 417 patients. Acta Neurochir 1971;25:69.
8. Rish BL, Dillon JD, Meirowsky AM, et al: Cranioplasty: a review of 1030 cases of penetrating head injury. Neurosurgery 1979;4:381.
9. White JC: Late complications following cranioplasty with alloplastic plates. Ann Surg 1948;128:743.
10. Woolf JI, Walker AE: Cranioplasty. Int J Surg 1945;81:1.
11. Donald PJ: The tenacity of the frontal sinus mucosa. Otolaryngol Head Neck Surg 1971;87:557.
12. Mickel TJ, Rohrich RJ, Robinson JB Jr: Frontal sinus obliteration: a comparison of fat, muscle, bone and spontaneous osteoneogenesis in a cat model. Plast Reconstr Surg 1995;95:586.
13. Rohrich RJ, Mickel TJ: Frontal sinus obliteration: in search of the ideal autogenous material. Plast Reconstr Surg 1995;95:580.
14. Wolfe SA: Discussion in: Manson PN, Crawley WA, Hoopes JE: Frontal cranioplasty: risk factors and choice of cranial vault reconstructive material. Plast Reconstr Surg 1986;77:901.
15. Stelnicki EJ, Ousterhout DK: Prevention of thermal tissue injury induced by the application of polymethylmethacrylate to the calvarium. J Craniofac Surg 1996;7:192.
16. Munro IR, Guyuron B: Split-rib cranioplasty. Ann Plast Surg 1981;7:341.
17. Fiala TGS, Paige KT, Davis TL, et al: Comparison of artifact from craniomaxillofacial internal fixation devices: magnetic resonance imaging. Plast Reconstr Surg 1994;93:725.
18. Saxe AW, Doppman JL, Brennan MF: Use of titanium surgical clips to avoid artifacts seen on computed tomography. Arch Surg 1982;117:978.
19. Fiala TGS, Novelline FA, Yaremchuk MJ: Comparison of CT imaging artifacts from craniomaxillofacial internal fixation devices. Plast Reconstr Surg 1993;92:1227.
20. Fearon JE: A magnetic resonance imaging investigation of potential subclinical complications after in situ cranial bone graft harvest. Plast Reconstr Surg 2000;105:1935.
21. Kline RM Jr, Wolfe SA: Complications associated with the harvesting of cranial bone grafts. Plast Reconstr Surg 1995;95:5.
22. Constantino PD, Friedman CD, Jones K, et al: Experimental hydroxyapatite cement cranioplasty. Plast Reconstr Surg 1992;90:174.
23. Burstein FD, Cohen SR, Hudgins R, et al: The use of hydroxyapatite cement in secondary craniofacial reconstruction. Plast Reconstr Surg 1999;104:1270.
24. Constantino PD, Friedman CD, Jones K, et al: Hydroxyapatite cement: I. Basic chemistry and histologic properties. Arch Otolaryngol Head Neck Surg 1991;117:379.
25. Constantino PD, Friedman CD, Jones K, et al: Hydroxyapatite cement: II. Obliteration and reconstruction of the cat frontal sinus. Arch Otolaryngol Head Neck Surg 1991;117:385.
26. Rosen HM: Porous, block hydroxyapatite as an interpositional bone graft substitute in orthognathic surgery. Plast Reconstr Surg 1989;83:985.
27. Burstein FD, Cohen SR, Hudgins R, Boydston W: The use of porous granular hydroxyapatite in secondary orbitocranial reconstruction. Plast Reconstr Surg 1997;100:869.
28. Matic D, Phillips JH: A contraindication for the use of hydroxyapatite cement in the pediatric population. Plast Reconstr Surg 2002;110:1.
29. Wehmoller MW, Eufinger H, Kruse D, Massberg W: CAD by processing of computed tomography data and CAM of individually designed prostheses. Int J Maxillofac Surg 1995;24:90.
30. Eufinger H, Wehmoller MW, Machtens E, et al: Reconstruction of craniofacial bone defects with individual alloplastic implants based on CAD/CAM manipulated CT-data. J Craniomaxillofac Surg 1995;23:175.
31. Ono I, Gunji H, Kaneko F, et al: Treatment of extensive cranial bone defects using computer-designed hydroxyapatite ceramics and periosteal flaps. Plast Reconstr Surg 1993;92:819.
32. Taylor GI, Corlett RS, Boyd, JB: The versatile deep inferior epigastric (inferior rectus abdominis) flap. Br J Plast Surg 1984;37:330.
33. Thomson JG, Restifo RJ: Microsurgery for cranial base tumors. Clin Plast Surg 1995;22:563.
34. Barrow DL, Nahai F, Tindall GT: The use of the greater omentum vascularized free flaps for neurosurgical disorders requiring reconstruction. J Neurosurg 1984;60:305.
35. Lacy J, Antonyshyn O: Use of porous high-density polyethylene implants in temporal contour reconstruction. J Craniofac Surg 1993;4:74.

Acquired Facial Bone Deformities

S. Anthony Wolfe, MD ✦ Maria Teresa Rivas-Torres, MD
✦ Omer Ozerdem, MD

ACCESS INCISIONS
    Coronal Incisions
    Lower Eyelid Incisions
    Intraoral Incisions
BONE GRAFTS
    Soft Tissue Cover

TREATMENT OF SPECIFIC DEFECTS
    Cranium
    Nose
    Nasoethmoid Area
    Orbitozygomatic Region
    Maxilla
    Mandible
    Chin

The various causes of acquired deformities of the facial skeleton include trauma (vehicular, ballistic, and other types), infection, and surgical and radiotherapeutic treatment of neoplasia. The surgical treatment of these acquired deformities has changed radically during the past 3 decades because of the development of the subspecialty of craniofacial surgery. Craniofacial surgery developed almost entirely from the work of Paul Tessier, who revolutionized facial skeletal surgery with his seminal work regarding treatment of congenital malformations, such as Crouzon disease,[1] Apert syndrome,[2] Treacher Collins-Franceschetti syndrome, vertical orbital dystopias, and orbital hypertelorism.[3-8] As a new generation of plastic surgeons learned Tessier's methods, they also learned the basic principles[9] of his approach, which include the following:

- Complete subperiosteal exposure of the areas of interest of the facial skeleton can be obtained through coronal, lower eyelid, or intraoral incisions.
- If a portion of the craniofacial skeleton is not in its proper position, it is better to move it to its proper position and fix it there as rigidly as possible with interposed autogenous bone grafts to provide consolidation of the structure.[10] Onlay "camouflage" grafts are to be avoided because they do not provide a three-dimensional correction of the entire deformity.
- Only fresh autogenous bone grafts—obtainable in whatever amount for whatever size defect from the ribs,[11] the anterior and posterior ilium,[12] the tibia,[11] and particularly the skull[11]—should be used. There is little if any place for bone substitutes, whether alloplastic materials or cadaver bone,[13] in craniofacial reconstruction.
- If the structure is not present to be moved, it can be either constructed in situ or constructed and then moved.
- The once forbidden boundary zone between the cranial cavity and the midface can safely be transgressed if proper care is taken in its reconstruction. Regular and frequent collaboration between the plastic surgical and neurosurgical members of a craniofacial team decreases the risks of a transcranial approach.
- Other members of a craniofacial team, such as ophthalmologists and orthodontists, will need to be called on in the treatment of acquired deformities, just as for congenital malformations.

ACCESS INCISIONS

Access to the facial skeleton is provided through coronal, lower eyelid, and intraoral incisions. The following paragraphs deal with important factors involved in the proper techniques for these incisions. If they are improperly done, subsequent operations may be made much more difficult.

Coronal Incisions

Coronal incisions should be made far back from the anterior hairline, almost at the vertex. An anterior cutback from the area behind the ear into the sideburn in front of the ear allows the coronal flap to be

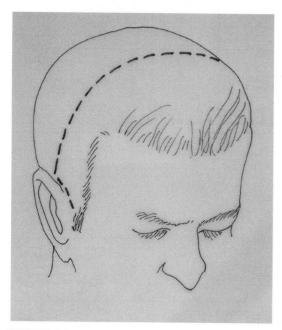

FIGURE 72-1. Coronal incision.

turned forward without tension. Incisions close to or along the anterior hairline can be noticeable, and it may be difficult or impossible to improve these scars and areas of alopecia. Once a coronal incision has been made, the same incision should be used again. A scalp with multiple scars may greatly complicate later reconstruction. A hemicoronal incision with an extension onto the forehead is a neurosurgical relic of the past and should be discarded. A standard coronal incision is not more difficult to make. Under the coronal incision, the dissection is usually supraperiosteal down to the supraorbital ridges, where it becomes subperiosteal. The temporalis muscle must be respected, and if it is elevated, it should be resutured to the lateral orbital rim and anterior temporal crest, and posteriorly to the posterior portion of the coronal incision, so that it is put back with its original tension. The superficial temporal fascia is generally divided to get back down to the deeper temporal fascia on the way to the zygomatic arch and malar areas and should be resuspended at the time of closure. After the temporal muscle has been sutured back into position under proper tension, a suture is taken (from beneath the coronal incision) near the lateral canthal raphe and passed through the temporal aponeurosis to reposition the lateral canthus properly (Fig. 72-1).

Lower Eyelid Incisions

Lower eyelid incisions can be made through the conjunctiva[14] or through the lower eyelid.[15] If a cutaneous approach is used, it should be lower in the eyelid, beneath the tarsal plate, rather than in the immediate subciliary area.[16]

Intraoral Incisions

Upper buccal sulcus incisions should have an adequate inferior cuff for subsequent closure; the infraorbital nerve should be protected, and protrusion of the buccal fat pad is avoided if possible. Lower buccal sulcus incisions provide good exposure to almost all of the mandible, except for the area just beneath the mental nerves and the condyle. Even the condyle can be visualized through the intraoral incision if endoscopic equipment is available.[17]

BONE GRAFTS

The key element to success in moving or replacing portions of the facial skeleton lies in the liberal and exclusive use of fresh autogenous bone grafts. Paul Tessier has written a treatise on harvesting of bone grafts, combining his experience during a 50-year practice with that of a number of his trainees who have been active in craniofacial surgery. The group experience of more than 20,000 bone graft harvestings from rib, tibia, ilium, and cranium was examined for complications, and a number of technical points were given to make harvesting of bone grafts easy, rapid, and safe.[18]

Soft Tissue Cover

The success of free bone grafts depends on the intimate contact of well-vascularized soft tissues both above and below the grafts. This means that areas between bone grafts must be filled in with other graft material and hematoma formation prevented by fastidious hemostasis and adequate postoperative drainage. Where soft tissues are inadequate because of the original trauma or radiotherapy, they must be replaced with good soft tissue before bone grafts can be expected to do well.

Given adequate exposure, an acceptable amount of autogenous bone grafts, and the means to provide rigid fixation, the correction of deformities in various areas of the facial skeleton should proceed smoothly.

TREATMENT OF SPECIFIC DEFECTS
Cranium

Cranial defects in children younger than $1^1/_2$ or even 2 years often spontaneously ossify and do not require treatment. In the authors' experience, the youngest patient with a cranial bone that can be successfully split ex vivo is between 3 and 4 years. If there are reasons that cranial bone cannot be used, split rib grafts can be used from about the age of 4 to 5 years, depending on the size of the patient. Good results can be obtained with split rib, but because of its quality and proximity, cranial bone is the material of choice for most cranioplasties.[19] Alloplastic materials should not be used in children as a primary reconstructive option. If the cranial defect has been corrected with autogenous bone grafts and all reconstructive work is complete, for minor surface irregularities present a year or so later, small amounts of alloplastic material such as Norian, BoneSource, or hydroxyapatite materials that are applied in soft state and molded before they set to a final hard state can reasonably be used.

In adults, small defects such as burr hole sites that are far from the frontal sinus may also be corrected with these materials. Near the frontal sinus, only autogenous bone should be used.[20] If there is a full-thickness cranial defect near the frontal sinus, the sinus should be cranialized; if the posterior wall of the sinus is intact and the nasofrontal duct appears to be blocked, all mucosa should be removed from the sinus and the sinus filled with autogenous cancellous grafts (Fig. 72-2).[21]

The preferred donor area for cranial grafts is the right parietal area in right-handed patients[22]; when larger grafts are required, the craniotomy can be extended anteriorly beyond the coronal suture and posteriorly into the occipital region. If additional bone is required, the other parietal region can be taken. When large cranial defects are present, the harvested bone should be slightly larger in dimension than the area to be corrected. Even segments that are 12 cm or more in diameter can be split through the diploic space to give two segments the dimensions of the donor segment. The inner table is replaced in the donor area and fixed with interosseous wires at the level of the original skull. A defect several millimeters in width will be present, varying with the thickness or kerf of the craniotome blade. This defect is placed posteriorly and filled in with small bone chips, slivers, and bone dust and covered with a pericranial flap.[23] The bone graft for the defect is tailored exactly to the defect. On occasion, it is good to enlarge the defect slightly by burring back to healthy bone. Fixation with wires, not mini-plates, is preferred (Figs. 72-3 and 72-4).

The most commonly encountered tumor of the fronto-orbital area is fibrous dysplasia, either monostotic or polyostotic,[24] and if possible, all of the involved bone should be excised and reconstructed with split cranial bone grafts.[25-27] If the orbital roof and optic canal are involved, this bone should be excised and the optic nerve unroofed. If both optic nerves are involved, only one side should be unroofed at the first operation because there is some risk to vision with this procedure, albeit slim. However, leaving the optic nerves encased in fibrous dysplasia also carries a considerable risk.[28] The orbital roof does not need to be completely reconstructed, and at least 10 to 12 mm of orbital roof is left free of bone over the optic nerve to avoid any possibility of compression from a bone graft (Fig. 72-5).

Neurofibromatosis, or von Recklinghausen disease, has a characteristic form of involvement of the orbitopalpebral area. The eye may be involved to the extent that it loses vision, and there is an enlargement of the orbit and superior orbital fissure and optic canal. Treatment consists of a radical reduction of orbital contents and eyelids and reconstruction of a properly situated orbital cavity. If the eye is extensively involved, a better result will be obtained by removing it and placing an ocular prosthesis. The condition is progressive until early adulthood, and repeated operations may often be required to correct deterioration of the result (Fig. 72-6).

Nose

When the nasal dorsum needs to be elevated or the nose significantly lengthened, bone[29] is preferred over cartilage. Bone consolidates to underlying and adjacent bone, and if a second procedure is required, it is much easier to perform it over a bone graft than over a cartilage graft. In most instances, there is no justification for use of any alloplastic materials in the nose, given that bone,[30] cartilage,[31] and fascia[32] are so easy to harvest and become incorporated into the patient's tissues and vascularized, often resulting in permanent resistance to infection. Rib[33] and iliac bone have their advocates. Both of these donor areas provide perfectly acceptable material; however, calvarial bone is preferred[34] because it is easily available in a nearby area, can be tailored and fixed better than rib and hip, results in a relatively painless donor area, and leaves a scar covered by hair. Again, the right parietal area is usually the preferred donor area, although the occipital region is also acceptable because it has the thickest bone of the skull.

If one is not using a coronal incision for other reasons, nasal bone grafts can be harvested through a 10-cm longitudinal incision. The dimensions of the desired graft are scored on the skull with an oscillating saw, and the edges around this are chipped off with a sharp osteotome and preserved. Once the diploic space is reached, thin curved osteotomes are used to separate the outer table segment. The chips that were removed with the osteotome are placed back on the donor area, covered by Gelfoam and a pericranial flap. Overnight drainage with a Hemovac is generally a wise precaution. Replacement of the bone chips helps prevent a palpable donor defect and preserve the strength of the skull. An open rhinoplasty approach makes it possible to separate the alar cartilages and

Text continued on p. 573

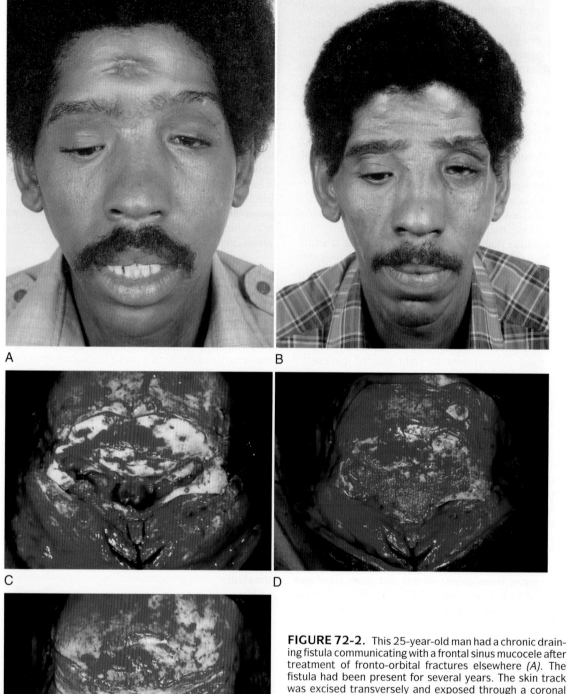

A

B

C

D

E

FIGURE 72-2. This 25-year-old man had a chronic drain-ing fistula communicating with a frontal sinus mucocele after treatment of fronto-orbital fractures elsewhere *(A)*. The fistula had been present for several years. The skin track was excised transversely and exposed through a coronal incision in the large frontal sinus extending almost from lateral orbital rim to lateral orbital rim *(C)*. All mucosa was meticulously removed with a small burr, sharp periosteal elevators, and small curets. The entire sinus cavity was then filled with fresh autogenous iliac cancellous bone *(D)* and covered with a pericranial flap *(E)*. The wound healed without difficulty, and the patient is shown 6 years later *(B)* without having had any further surgery. Fresh, cancellous bone is the best material to use for obliteration of the frontal sinus, even with chronic infection as was the situation here.

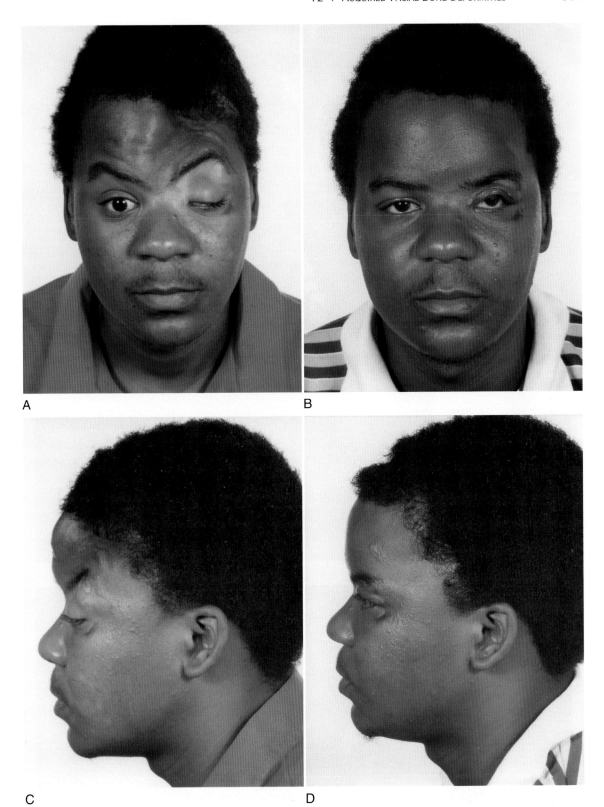

FIGURE 72-3. This 23-year-old was shot through the right frontal region and has extensive débridement of the left frontal bone, supraorbital ridge, and orbital roof (*A* and *C*). He is shown after a split cranial bone cranioplasty, reconstruction of the orbital roof and supraorbital ridge, and subsequent ptosis correction by reattachment of the levator muscle to the tarsal plate (*B* and *D*).   *Continued*

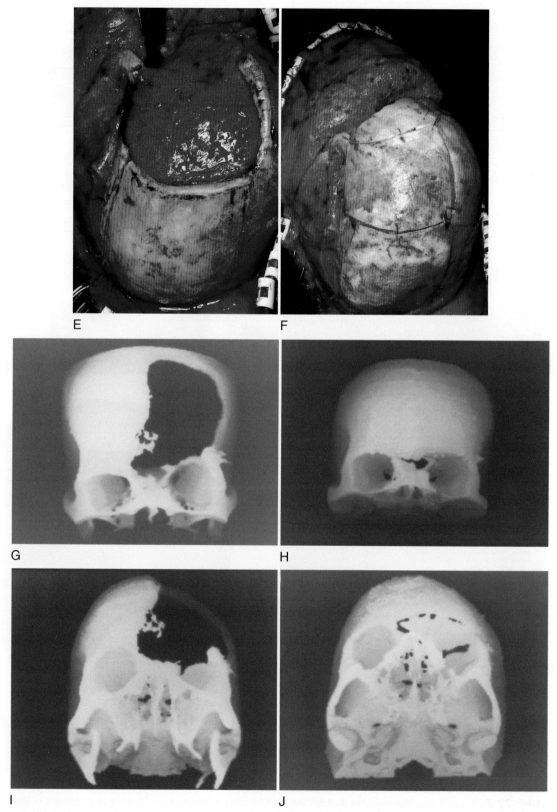

FIGURE 72-3, cont'd. All bone reconstruction should be complete before the fine details of soft tissue repair are addressed (*E* to *J*). (From Wolfe SA, Berkowitz S: Plastic Surgery of the Facial Skeleton. Boston, Little, Brown, 1989.)

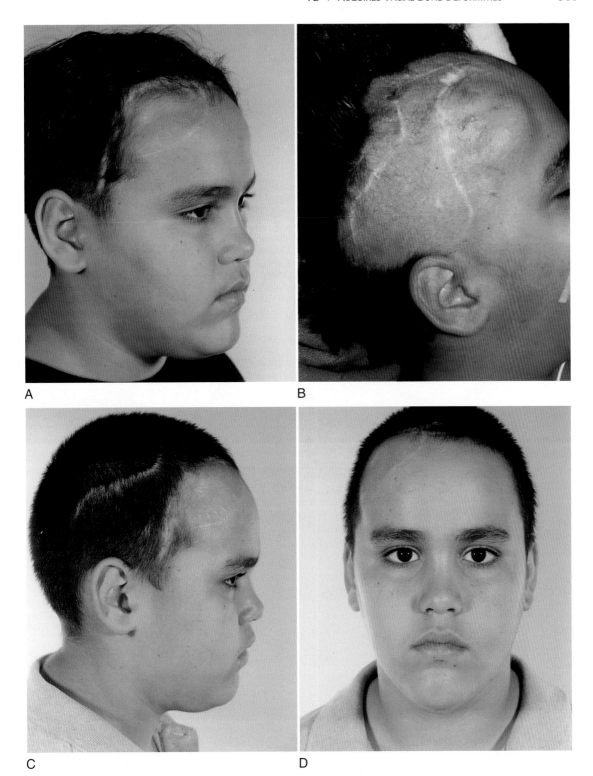

FIGURE 72-4. This 12-year-old boy was in an automobile accident in Cuba and sustained an open right frontal fracture. The original laceration is apparently the sweeping scar from near the midpoint of the anterior hairline to a point above the right sideburn *(A)*. A subsequent neurosurgical procedure was performed through an incision just along the right anterior hairline, and yet another procedure was performed through a more posterior incision *(B)*. Through one of these incisions, an attempt was made to correct the cranial defect with an alloplastic material that had to be removed because of infection. The cranial defect was approached through an anterior hairline incision that extended into a more posterior coronal incision on the left side.   *Continued*

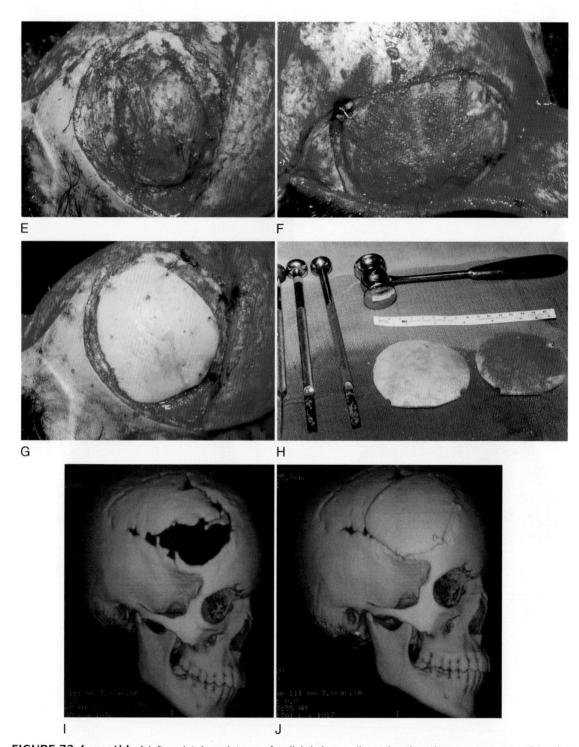

FIGURE 72-4, cont'd. A left parietal craniotomy of a slightly larger dimension than the measurements of the right frontal cranial defect was performed *(E),* and the cranial flap was split (ex vivo) into two segments through the diploic space *(H).* The outer table segment was used for the frontal defect after precise trimming *(F),* and the inner table segment was placed back in the donor area *(G, I,* and *J).* Healing was uneventful *(C* and *D).* There are two important lessons to be learned from this patient. First, use a posterior coronal incision, and use it for all subsequent procedures. Second, use autogenous cranial bone for cranioplasties whenever possible.

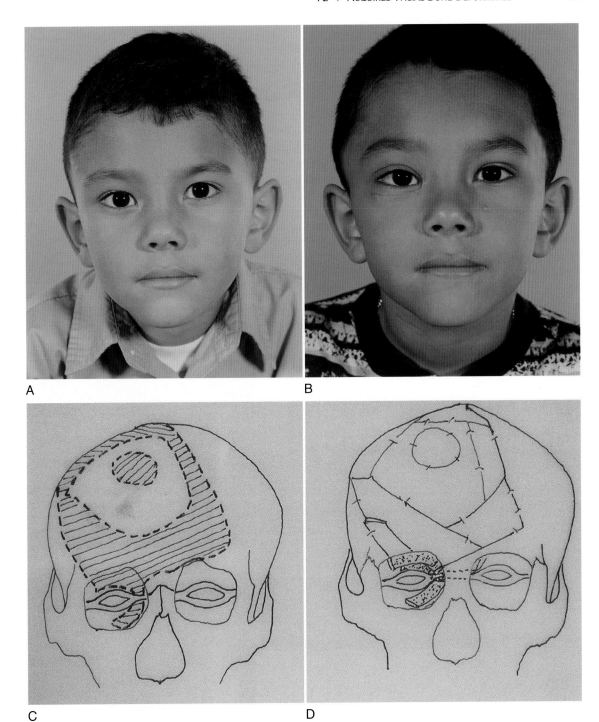

FIGURE 72-5. The mother of this 5-year-old noticed a distortion of the right side of his face *(A)*. A computed tomographic scan showed involvement of almost the entire frontal bone, the right orbital roof, the medial orbital wall, and a portion of the orbital floor *(F and G, next page)*. The optic canal on the right was completely encased with thick, dysplastic bone, with the characteristic appearance of fibrous dysplasia. All of the abnormal bone was removed from the frontal area and orbital floor *(C)*. The orbital roof was removed and the optic nerve unroofed. Some of the dysplastic bone was left in the cranial base medial and posterior to the optic canal.   *Continued*

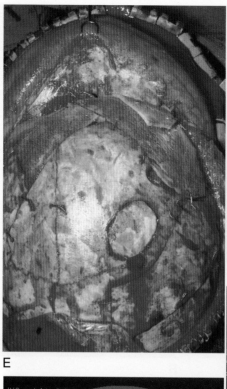

E

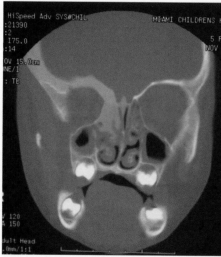

F

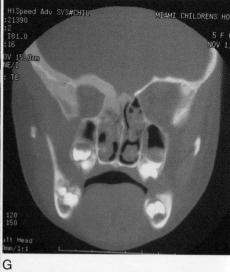

G

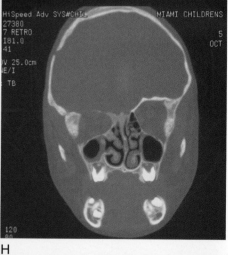

H

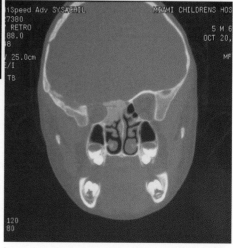

I

FIGURE 72-5, cont'd. All of the missing bone was reconstructed with split cranial bone (*D* and *E*), except for the posterior 10 to 12 mm of the orbital roof, where bone grafts were not placed for fear of making contact with the optic nerve. He is shown postoperatively after some burring of his infraorbital rim *(B)*. Note the correction of the hypoglobus with proper reconstruction of the orbit. The upper computed tomographic scans are preoperative (*F* and *G*), and the lower scans show cuts through the same region with the absence of bone in the posterior portion of the orbit extending back to the opened optic canal (*H* and *I*).

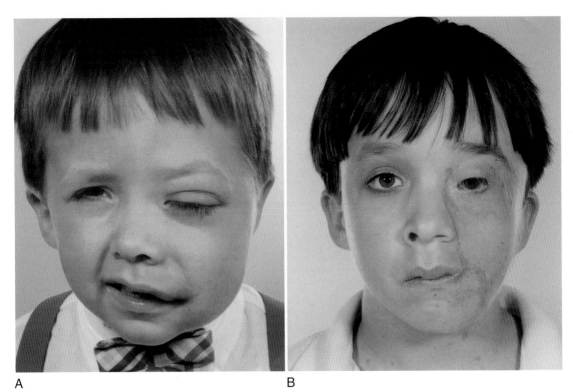

A B

FIGURE 72-6. A 5-year-old patient with left orbitopalpebral neurofibromatosis and involvement of cheek with left facial palsy *(A)*. The eye was extensively involved and had no light perception; it was therefore removed and an ocular prosthesis placed. He is shown 4 years later after a number of procedures, including transcranial elevation of the left orbit, resection of the lateral portion of the involved eyelids, transnasal medial canthopexy, and resection of portions of the cheek and suspension of the corner of the mouth to the left zygoma *(B)*. This is a progressive condition that often continues until the late teens; repeated procedures are often required.

then sew them over the nasal bone graft, which should not press into the nasal tip.

Bone grafts for a depressed dorsum are simply placed into an appropriate pocket after dissection of the skin alone. If they are placed through an intranasal approach, it is good to use intracartilaginous incisions so that the nasal closure sutures can pass through mucosa and cartilage, which minimizes the chances of exposure of the bone graft. In general, the bone graft is not rigidly fixed in place; care must be taken that the posterior portion of the bone graft is flat to avoid shifting of the graft. Making bilateral nasal vestibular incisions also helps provide an appropriate pocket so that the graft will remain in the center of the nose. If a graft does shift in the postoperative period, it can often be repositioned and maintained with SteriStrips. If it stubbornly resists this approach, a percutaneous K-wire can be placed under local anesthesia and maintained in position until consolidation of the bone graft occurs (Fig. 72-7).

If substantial lengthening (>1 cm) of the nose is required, such as in Binder syndrome[35] or post-

traumatic nasal foreshortening, dissection of the skin alone is not sufficient. The lining needs to be lengthened as well. Tessier has shown that considerable lengthening can be obtained, even in congenitally short noses, by dissecting the lining from beneath the nasal bones all the way back to the pharynx.[36] Another approach is to purposely section the lining (and bone) at the nasofrontal area, as in a Le Fort III osteotomy.[37] The undersurface of the bone graft may be exposed to the nasal cavity, but healing proceeds uneventfully, as it does in a Le Fort III, over bone grafts exposed to the maxillary sinus with a Le Fort I, and over orbital floor bone grafts (Figs. 72-8 and 72-9).

This type of procedure would not be applicable to the contracted, foreshortened nose that is associated with sustained cocaine use. Here the lining is either altogether absent or chronically granulating and infected. Before a nasal bone graft can be added, nasal lining must be provided by bringing in tissue from other areas, such as nasolabial, forehead, or buccal sulcus flaps.[38]

Text continued on p. 580

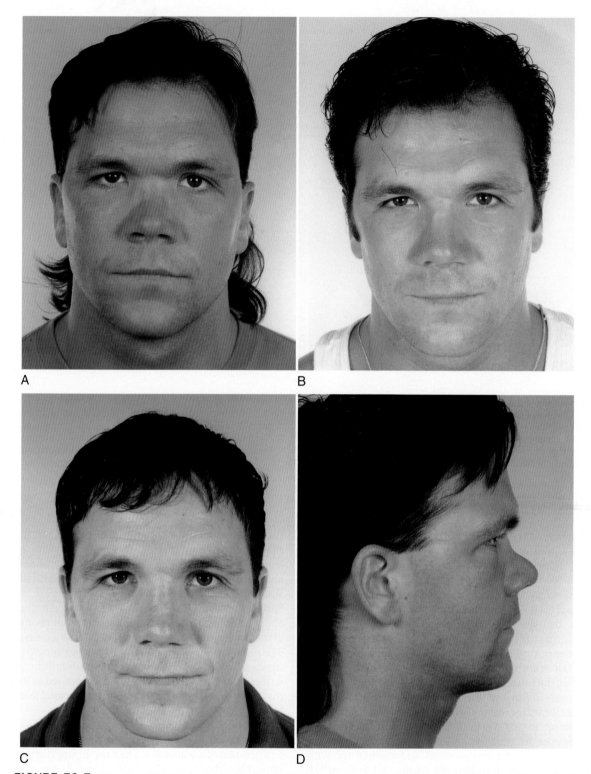

FIGURE 72-7. This is a 30-year-old ex-professional football player with a saddle nose deformity after multiple fractures (*A* and *D*). He is shown the day after his operation (under local anesthesia) with his companion *(G)*, 1 year postoperatively (*B* and *E*), and 6 years postoperatively (*C* and *F*).

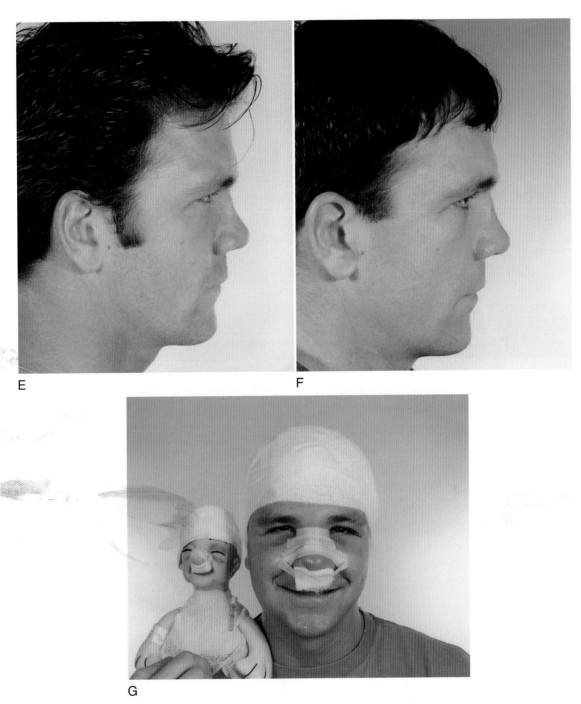

E

F

G

FIGURE 72-7, cont'd. There has been little if any resorption of the bone graft.

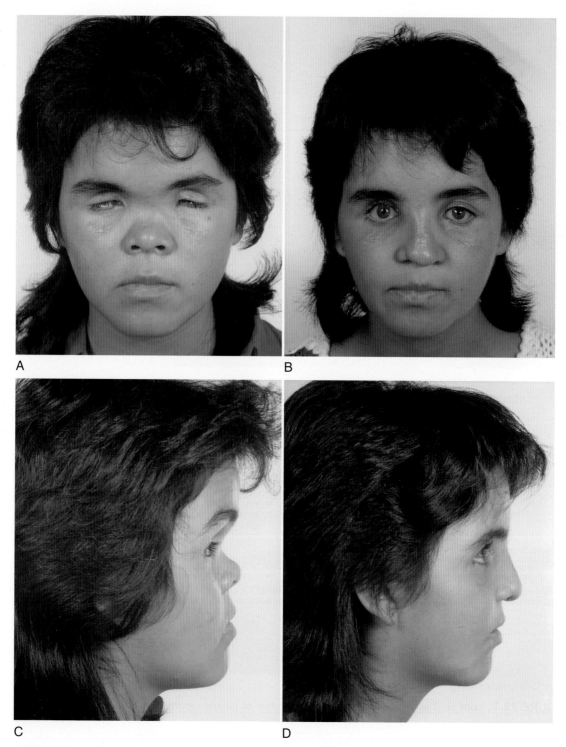

FIGURE 72-8. This 17-year-old girl was involved in a vehicular accident in South America (*A* and *C*). She was treated with wire traction from the zygomas to a head cap of some sort. Both globes were severely damaged, and she was blind. She is shown 6 months after a complete subperiosteal dissection of the orbital cavities and midface through coronal, intraorbital, and lower eyelid incisions, with mobilization of all malpositioned segments, extensive bone grafting with both iliac and cranial bone, and rigid fixation. The nasal lengthening was accomplished by sectioning of the contracted lining at the Le Fort III level and placement of an iliac bone graft in the created gap and as a dorsal graft along with a conchal cartilage graft to the nasal tip. The class III malocclusion was also corrected. In the postoperative photographs (*B* and *D*), she has ocular prostheses (cosmetic cover shells).

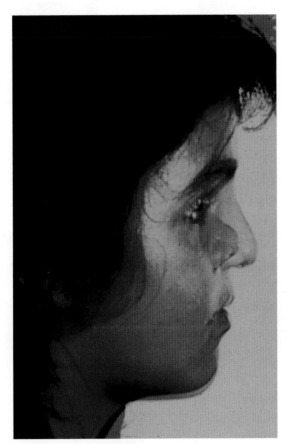

E

FIGURE 72-8, cont'd. The computer-generated overlay of her preoperative and postoperative photographs shows the degree of true nasal lengthening *(E)*. (From Wolfe SA, Berkowitz S: Plastic Surgery of the Facial Skeleton. Boston, Little, Brown, 1989.)

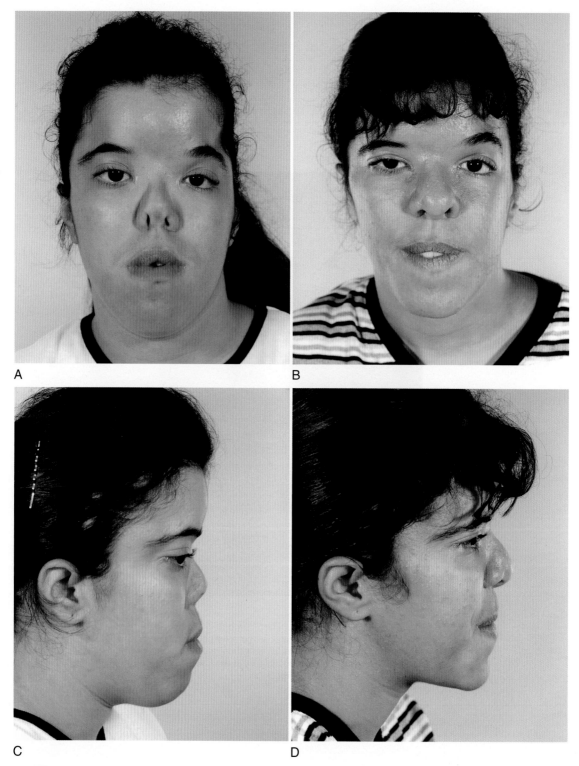

FIGURE 72-9. This patient, initially seen at the age of 13 years, had a transcranial correction of orbital hypertelorism a number of years previously; a postoperative infection caused loss of a portion of her glabella and probably the nasal bone graft (*A, C, E,* and *G*). The initial operation consisted of dissection of both orbital cavities through coronal and lower eyelid incisions, extensive dissection of nasal skin and lining through an open (columellar base) approach, and iliac bone grafting to glabellar and supraorbital defects and the nose.

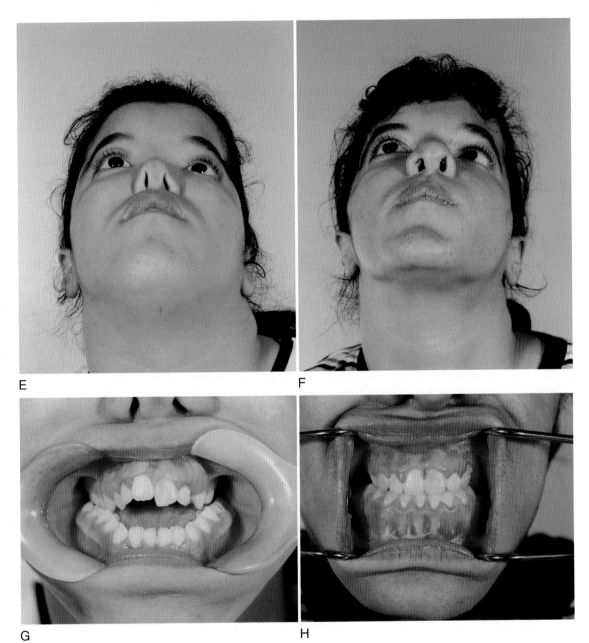

FIGURE 72-9, cont'd. A conchal cartilage graft was also placed in the nasal tip. After completion of presurgical orthodontic treatment, her open bite was corrected by Le Fort I impaction and maxillary expansion, bilateral sagittal splits of the mandibular rami, and reduction-advancement genioplasty. She is shown at age 15 years after completion of treatment (*B, D, F,* and *H*).

Nasoethmoid Area

Acute naso-orbital-ethmoid fractures are difficult to deal with, but after they have consolidated in malposition, they are even more difficult. In both situations, the best approach to correction of the telecanthus is to move the bone fragments attached to the medial canthal tendons into proper position rather than to detach the tendons and perform a transnasal medial canthopexy.[39,40] Some overcorrection of these medial wall segments is desirable, as in the correction of orbital hypertelorism. A circling wire can be passed around the segments with use of a curved awl. In late reconstructions, the dissection must be extensive, often with coronal, lower eyelid, and buccal sulcus incisions. The displaced segments must be delineated and osteotomized, moved into proper position, and kept there with appropriate stable fixation, which generally means miniplates or microplates and screws.[41] A nasal bone graft is also usually required (Fig. 72-10).

Orbitozygomatic Region

Acute isolated fractures of the zygomatic arch require an open approach if they cannot be reduced percutaneously. A coronal incision gives access for reduction and plating of the fracture or harvesting of bone grafts if necessary.

Orbitozygomatic fractures vary considerably in their presentation, depending on the vector and force of the causative injury. Lesser injuries may result in nondisplaced fractures of the zygoma with minimal disruption of the orbital floor. In this instance, no treatment other than follow-up observation is necessary. If one has underappreciated the extent of the orbital floor fracture, late enophthalmos is a possible sequel, but because it is relatively easily corrected,[42] one certainly does not have to operate on questionable fractures simply because of the possibility of late enophthalmos. This approach was advocated by some when it was thought that enophthalmos could not be corrected.[43,44]

Greater forces cause greater disruption, and because of the elastic nature of bone, the extent of bone displacement during the injury may be much greater than the displacement seen when the patient first presents. Severe late enophthalmos may develop after orbitozygomatic fractures. If one has treated dysthyroid exophthalmos by valgus displacement of the zygoma and opening of the periorbita to allow fat extrusion into the paranasal sinuses, one may obtain a posterior movement of the globe of 6 to 8 mm,[45-47] which is much less than the 10 to 15 mm of enophthalmos seen in some patients after trauma. This would indicate that the tearing of soft tissues during the original fracturing process is a great deal more than the surgeon can accomplish during orbital expansion for Graves disease.[48]

Nevertheless, if one puts the orbital framework into proper position with rigid fixation and repairs the internal orbital defects with autogenous bone grafts, enophthalmos will not result. Reduction of an orbitozygomatic fracture in which the zygomatic body has been displaced away from the globe can usually be accomplished in the first week after the fracture simply by removing callus in the fracture lines and grasping solid segments of bone with bone clamps. When the zygoma has been displaced by the injury toward the globe, proptosis or at least lack of enophthalmos may be present when the patient is first seen. In some instances, it may not be possible to reduce the fracture even by exerting considerable force on the bone clamps; in these instances, one must be prepared to perform an osteotomy through the fracture lines with an osteotome or reciprocating saw to be able to reduce the fracture.

Most fractures that are seen after a delay of 3 weeks or more will have consolidated and will require refracture by osteotomy and repositioning. Coronal, lower eyelid, and buccal sulcus incisions are used in most of these patients to provide good access for the osteotomies and also to allow the surgeon to fully appreciate the internal orbital anatomy, both of the medial orbital wall and of the lateral orbital wall. The sphenoidal portion of the lateral orbital wall should be perfectly aligned. A positioning wire is then placed through the frontozygomatic suture, and finally the inferior orbital rim is aligned. A wire is usually all that is needed for the frontozygomatic suture, and a small plate is placed to stabilize the inferior orbital rim. The zygomatic buttresses[49,50] should be checked through the upper sulcus incision and fixed in proper position with a larger plate. Finally, the zygomatic arch is plated, and one should have exposure of the normal side (if one is present) to check the exact shape of the normal zygomatic arch. If the arches are fractured on both sides, recall that they should be fairly straight (and not bowed), which will provide proper projection of the midface.

POST-TRAUMATIC ENOPHTHALMOS

Post-traumatic enophthalmos can result either from isolated defects of the orbital floor and medial orbital wall, in which there is herniation of orbital contents into the maxillary and ethmoidal sinuses, or from displaced orbitozygomatic fractures, in which there is herniation of orbital contents into the paranasal sinuses.[51] If there is even a slight displacement of the zygoma from its proper position, it should be osteotomized and properly positioned. Autogenous bone grafts are used to replace missing or displaced portions of the internal orbit.[52-54] In the presence of a seeing eye, post-traumatic enophthalmos can be completely corrected in most instances if the bony orbit is completely reconstructed and all of the orbital contents returned to the orbital cavity.[55] Overcorrection by several millimeters

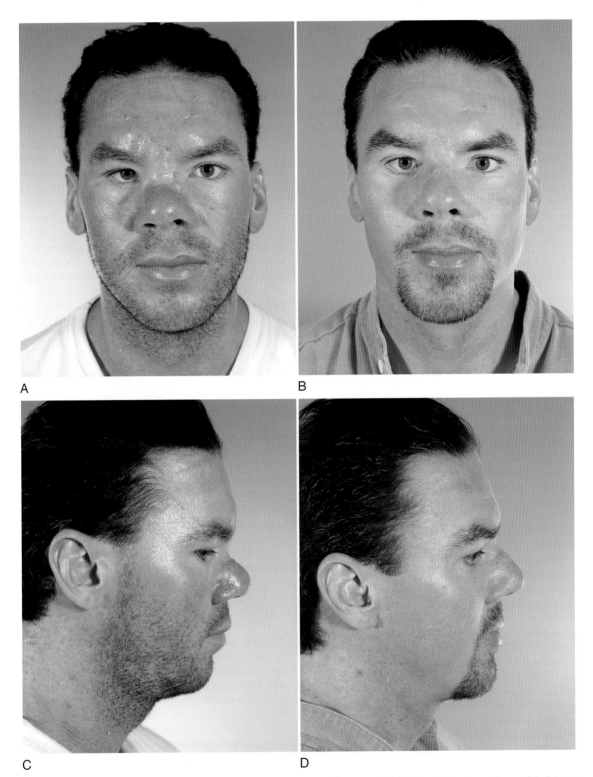

A

B

C

D

FIGURE 72-10. This 32-year-old man sustained a compound naso-orbital-ethmoid fracture, for which he was treated elsewhere several months before (*A* and *C*). He is shown a little more than a year after exploration of both orbits through coronal and lower eyelid incisions, extensive dissection of the nasal skin cover and lining, cranial bone grafts to both orbital floors and the right medial wall, right transnasal medial canthopexy, and dacryocystorhinostomy (*B* and *D*).

in both the vertical and sagittal directions should be performed to compensate for operative swelling.

In patients with inadequate late correction of enophthalmos, even if it is mild, a coronal and sagittal computed tomographic scan will show a few areas where further bone grafting can provide a complete correction. If this is performed, the residual enophthalmos will be corrected. When one is performing secondary bone grafting such as this, it is important to bear in mind that the orbital cavity may not have any areas of egress because all of the communications into paranasal sinuses have been closed off with bone grafts. Bringing a small drain (such as a TLS drain) from the orbital floor out through the sideburn area will lessen the possibility of a volume and pressure increase due to hematoma (Figs. 72-11 to 72-15).[56]

THE IRRADIATED ORBIT

Irradiation of the orbit in early childhood, such as for retinoblastoma, will result in a small orbit and often restriction of growth of the temporal fossa. If a seeing eye is still present, one can deal with the temporal fossa defect with a soft tissue flap, most efficiently by composite tissue transplantation. The orbit itself should not be altered. If the eye is absent and the orbit small, an orbital expansion can be performed to give an orbit of normal dimensions.[57] This is followed by socket reconstruction and placement of an ocular prosthesis.

The overall approach for secondary correction of displaced facial bone segments is the same as for primary correction: have adequate exposure, put the segments into proper position and keep them there with appropriate rigid fixation, and liberally use autogenous bone grafts for any residual bone defects. The main difference is that the soft tissue dissection is often much more difficult because of scarring and contraction of the soft tissue envelope over the malpositioned facial bone segments. Sharp periosteal elevators are essential to proper, clean elevation of periosteum. The buccal fat pad and other soft tissue elements of the midface may have prolapsed into the maxillary sinus through defects in the anterior maxillary wall, and these must be completely retrieved. Autogenous bone grafts are used to recreate the anterior maxillary wall and to keep the soft tissues in their proper place. As noted previously, the dissected midfacial tissues are suspended to the temporal aponeurosis, and a lateral canthopexy is performed. This maneuver has been appropriated into aesthetic surgery as in the so-called subperiosteal face lift.

Maxilla

If maxillary fractures have not received proper treatment primarily, they may require late treatment.

Again, the approach is to section the displaced bone segment and move it to a proper position, fix it there rigidly, and use autogenous bone grafts as required. It is not uncommon for a Le Fort I fracture to be treated by intermaxillary fixation with a satisfactory occlusal result but a shortened midface. This occurs if the maxillary buttresses have all been fractured and the maxilla jammed upward until bone contact occurs.[58] The deformity can be prevented if a primary reconstruction of the buttresses is carried out at the primary repair.[55,59,60] Correction of the late deformity requires sectioning of the maxilla at the Le Fort I level, mobilization of the maxilla, and intermaxillary fixation. If the maxilla-mandible complex in intermaxillary fixation is allowed to find its own position in the lightly anesthetized unparalyzed patient, this position represents the degree of lengthening desired. The two sides of the sectioned maxilla can now be plated in this position; adequate amounts of autogenous bone grafts are essential to the consolidation of the maxilla in its new position (Fig. 72-16).

MAXILLARY TUMORS

In the past, a Weber-Ferguson incision has often been routine for removal of both benign and malignant tumors of the maxilla. Unless skin is going to be resected for oncologic reasons, a hemimaxillectomy can easily be performed through an intraoral approach alone. The resultant defect was traditionally treated with a split-thickness skin graft, and the patient was eventually fitted with an obturator attached to the remaining teeth that would support the soft tissues of the cheek. There are still voices heard against primary maxillary reconstruction, just as they were heard several decades ago against primary mandibular reconstruction. The criticism of primary reconstruction was that the reconstruction might mask a potential tumor recurrence. With the current availability of high-resolution imaging provided by computed tomographic scans and magnetic resonance imaging, direct incision of a maxillary defect is not necessary for tumor surveillance. Primary reconstruction of maxillary tumors should be undertaken just as primary reconstruction is routinely done for mandibular ablation with the same criteria for success. No reconstruction of either jaw can be considered complete without a proper dental reconstruction. At present, this means osseointegrated implants placed in adequate bone stock to allow normal chewing and mastication of a normal diet.[61]

MAXILLARY RECONSTRUCTION

The same dissection previously described for traumatic deformities can be employed for either primary or secondary reconstruction of maxillary defects

Text continued on p. 594

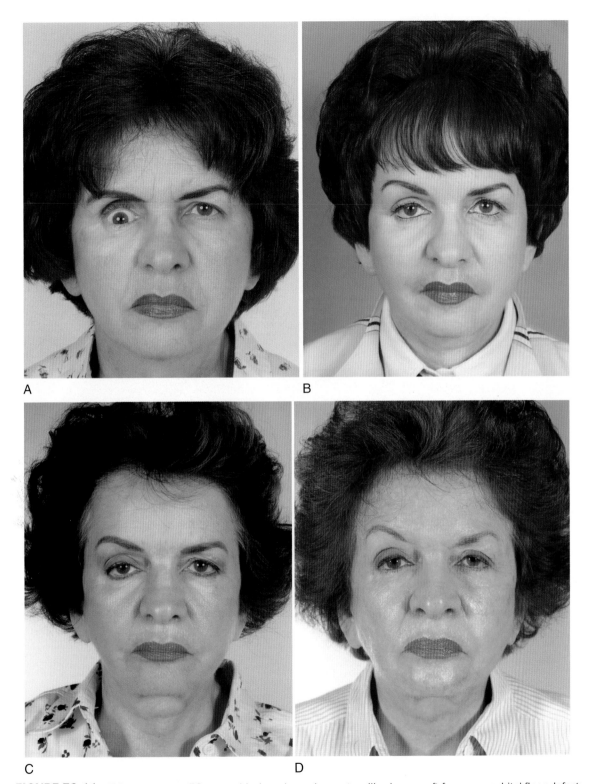

FIGURE 72-11. This woman was 56 years old when she underwent an iliac bone graft for a pure orbital floor defect that was responsible for a profound (13.5 mm) enophthalmos and hypoglobus *(A)*. She is shown 1 year *(B)*, 10 years *(C)*, and 17 years *(D)* postoperatively. There was perhaps some slight undercorrection that can be appreciated on the first postoperative photograph *(B)*, where the upper palpebral sulcus on the right is deeper than on the left. There does not seem to be any further deterioration of the result with time. She has had no other surgery in the interim other than a face lift.   *Continued*

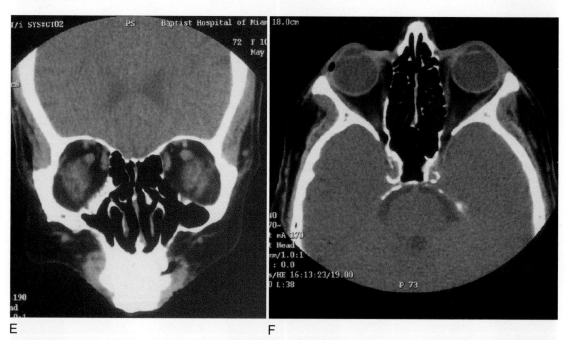

FIGURE 72-11, cont'd. A careful evaluation of coronal and sagittal computed tomographic scans (*E* and *F*) indicates where further bone can be added to the right orbit, but this was not done because the patient was pleased with the result. (From Wolfe SA, Berkowitz S: Plastic Surgery of the Facial Skeleton. Boston, Little, Brown, 1989.)

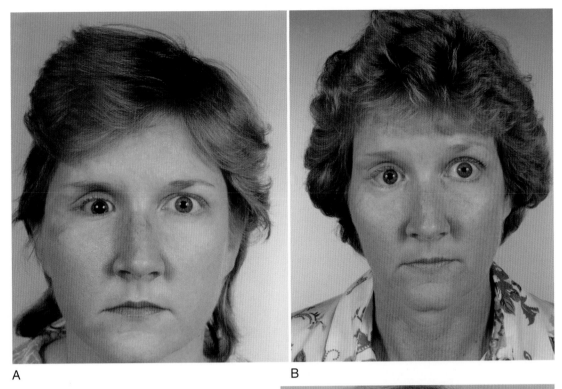

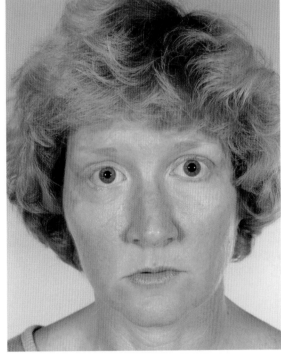

FIGURE 72-12. This woman was 32 years old when an osteotomy and repositioning of the right zygoma were performed along with an iliac bone graft *(A)*. An undercorrection was noted 6 years later *(B, D,* and *F)*. A computed tomographic evaluation showed a persistent small defect in the posterior medial orbital wall as well as an enlargement of the inferior orbital fissure; the addition of a small amount of cranial bone corrected the persistent enophthalmos completely. *Continued*

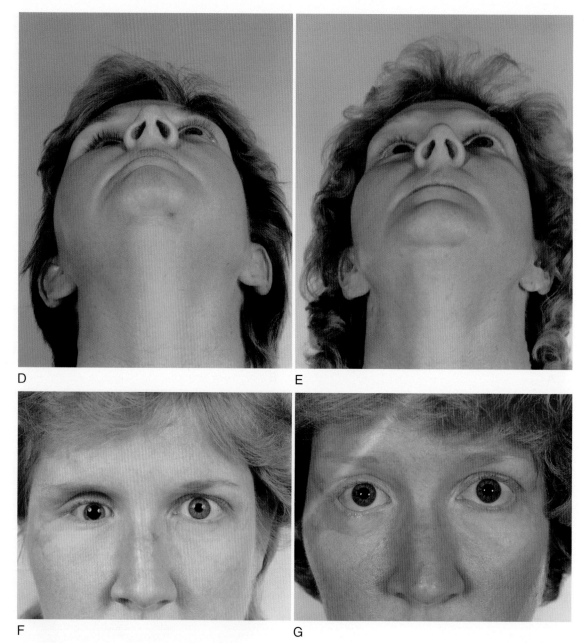

FIGURE 72-12, cont'd. She is shown 4 years after the second operation and 10 years after the first operation (*C, E,* and *G*).

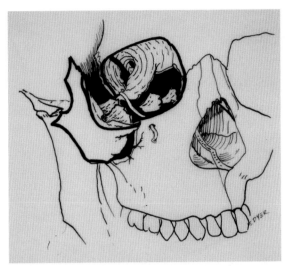

H

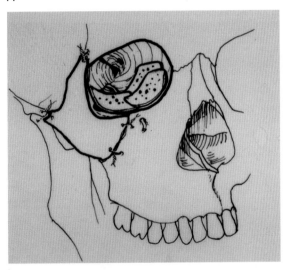

I

FIGURE 72-12, cont'd. Two operations are sometimes required to provide a complete correction, as in this patient (*H* and *I*).

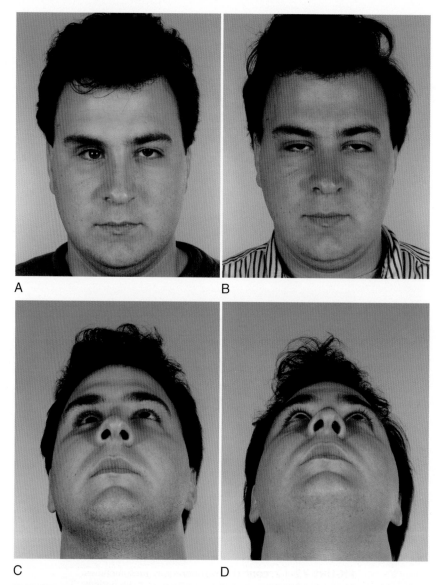

FIGURE 72-13. This 28-year-old man was struck in the right eye during a mugging on the Paris Metro. He related that several radiologic examinations were performed, and he was told that no fractures were noted. When he was first seen 6 months later, a significant right enophthalmos was present (*A* and *C*).

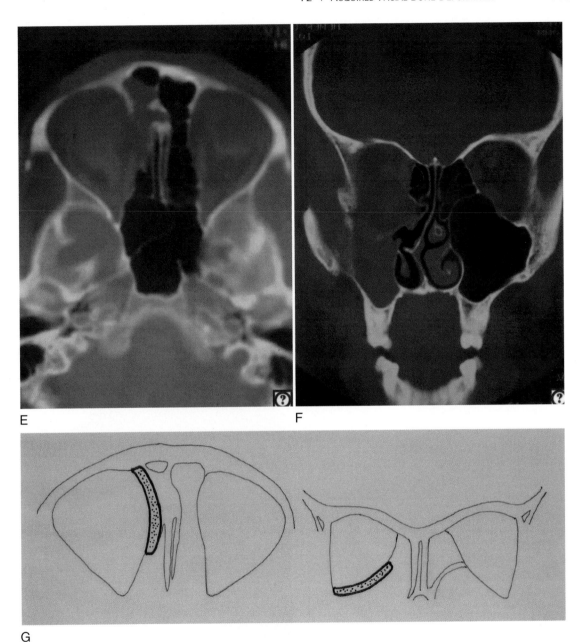

E

F

G

FIGURE 72-13, cont'd. Computed tomographic scans showed substantial fractures of the medial orbital wall and orbital floor (*E* and *F*). These types of fractures could easily be missed on routine radiologic examinations. For this reason, there is little use in ordering them. If there is enough clinical suspicion of anything other than an isolated zygomatic arch fracture, one should go directly to the computed tomographic scan. The patient is shown 3 months after cranial bone grafts to the medial orbital wall and orbital floor (*G*), with the globe in the desired position (*B* and *D*).

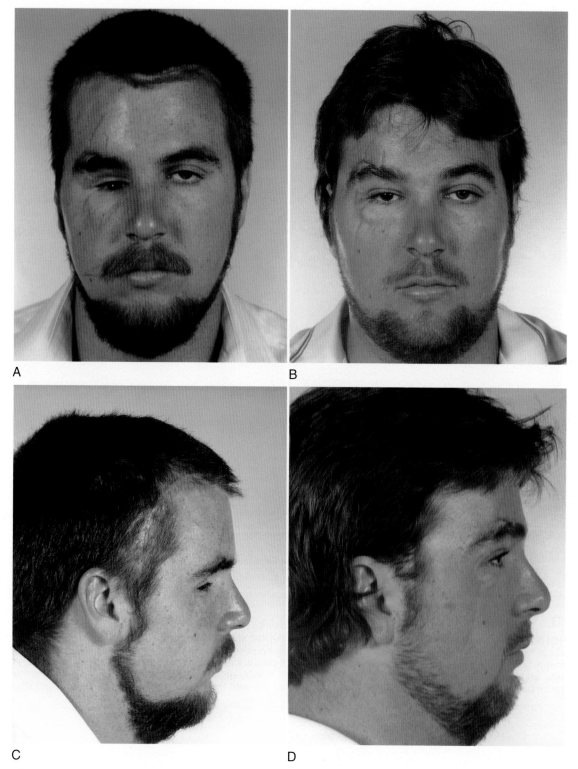

FIGURE 72-14. This 23-year-old man suffered major right orbitocranial fractures several years previously in a vehicular accident. A defect of most of the right frontal bone had been reconstructed with methyl methacrylate. There was profound enophthalmos and hypoglobus of the right eye, which still retained some vision (*A* and *C*).

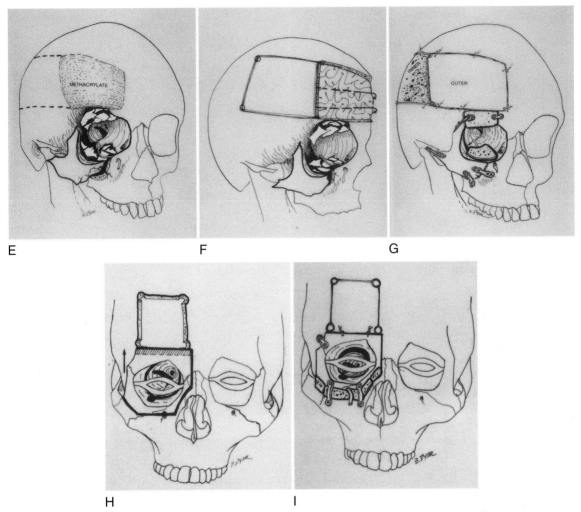

E   F   G

H   I

FIGURE 72-14, cont'd. In the initial operation, the alloplastic material was removed *(E),* and the frontal defect was reconstructed with split cranial bone. Major reconstructive orbital surgery is not recommended if there is any alloplastic material in the region of the periorbital sinuses. At the same time, refracture and repositioning of the right zygoma were performed *(F)* along with cranial bone grafting of the medial orbital wall and orbital floor defects *(G).* This corrected the enophthalmos, but the patient was left with a considerable persistent hypoglobus. This was treated as a true vertical orbital dystopia, with an intracranial elevation of the entire—now intact—orbital cavity. The medial canthal tendon was left attached to bone and was elevated with the orbit *(H* and *I).* The patient is shown 3 years after the second operation *(B* and *D).*

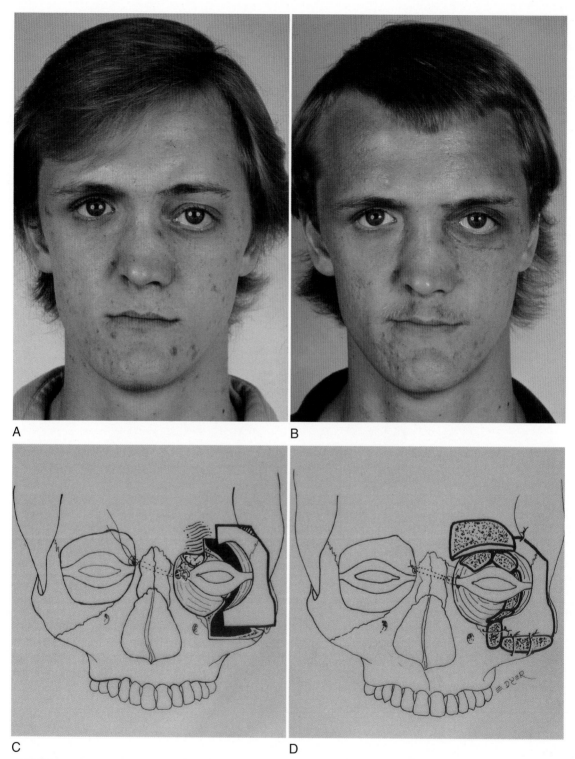

FIGURE 72-15. In this post-trauma patient, one can see a hypoglobus without enophthalmos *(A)*. The orbital roof had been pushed into the orbital cavity, resulting in a slight proptosis. The globe was elevated by an osteotomy and repositioning of the zygoma, elevation of the orbital roof, and bone grafting of the orbital floor along with a transnasal medial canthopexy *(B to D)*. The canthopexy shows that the canthal tendon is brought through a drill hole in the medial orbital wall just above and posterior to the lacrimal fossa and tied over a toggle on the contralateral side. (From Wolfe SA, Berkowitz S: Plastic Surgery of the Facial Skeleton. Boston, Little, Brown, 1989.)

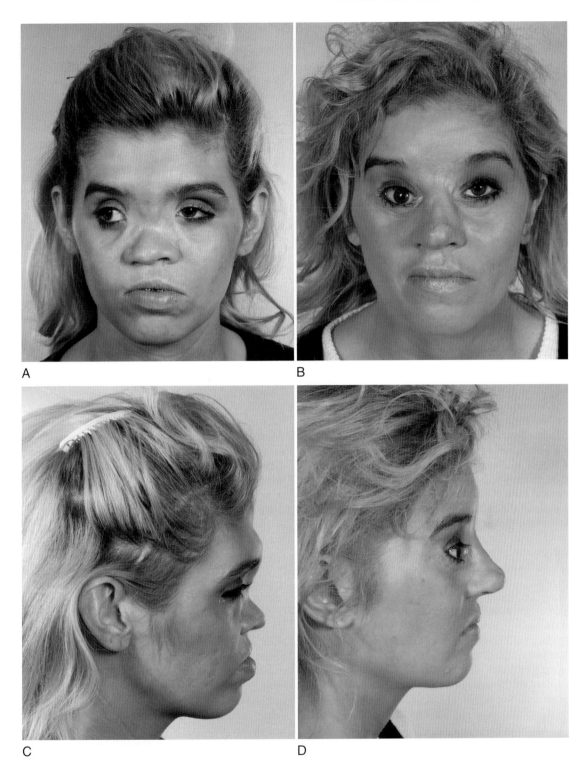

A   B

C   D

FIGURE 72-16. This girl was 17 years old when she was first seen (*A, C,* and *E*). She had been involved in a major automobile accident a year earlier. A craniotomy had been performed for a cerebrospinal fluid leak, and her facial fractures were plated by a surgeon who, it turned out, had taken a course at which the senior author had been a faculty member. Unfortunately, a number of errors were made. The maxilla, although plated, was plated in malposition because buttress reconstruction had not been performed and the maxilla was foreshortened. Gruss has coined the term OIF for patients like this in whom plating has been performed but without the necessary reduction (the R of ORIF).

Continued

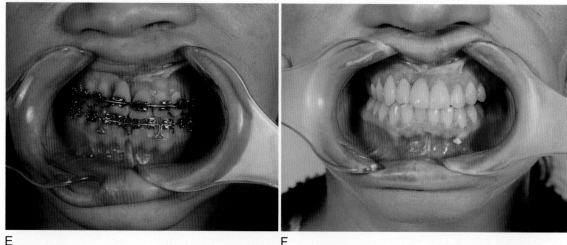

E   F

FIGURE 72-16, cont'd. Also, even though many of the fractures were plated, no bone grafting was performed, which allowed the telescoping contraction of soft tissues, particularly the nose. She is shown postoperatively after a number of operations including an exchange of cranial flaps to reconstruct her forehead, nasal lengthening as described earlier, transnasal medial canthopexies, Le Fort I osteotomy with interpositional bone grafting to provide maxillary lengthening, and Abbe flap. She is shown 8 years postoperatively (*B, D,* and *F*), having satisfactorily delivered a healthy baby. Almost 10 years after her injury, she developed meningitis, which was of uncertain relation to her original injury because there was no further cerebrospinal fluid leak.

subsequent to removal of maxillary tumors by use of the temporalis muscle.[62] In the initial coronal dissection, mobilization of the temporalis muscle is carried out to its posterior extent, which is often 5 cm or more posterior to the upper portion of the ear. The zygomatic arch is completely dissected, and the muscle is dissected from the lateral orbital wall deep into the temporal fossa. The zygomatic arch and a portion of the body of the zygoma are removed, and the muscle flap (which is usually about half of the muscle) is brought into the oral cavity after finger dissection enlarges the passage. A hemimaxillary defect can easily be closed with this muscle flap. The muscle does not need to be covered by mucosa or skin grafted because it is rapidly covered by mucosa naturally. There needs to be an alveolar defect, either lateral or anterior, to easily bring in the muscle flap. If the alveolar ridge is intact, it is difficult to bring in a muscle flap because it involves making a hole through the anterior maxillary wall or bringing the muscle behind the maxillary tuberosity. For large central palatal defects that cannot be closed by local palatal flaps, a microsurgical solution is preferred. The flap of choice is the radial forearm flap.[63]

After complete healing of the soft tissue palatal repair, a bony alveolar ridge can be reconstructed with iliac bone grafts or microvascular osseous flaps (fibular or parascapular flaps are the most common).[64-66] After the bone repair is well consolidated, osseointegrated implants can be placed to accept a denture and finish the reconstruction (Fig. 72-17).

Mandible

In-continuity defects of the mandible less than 3 to 4 cm in length covered by healthy soft tissue can be corrected with free bone grafts[67,68] (iliac[69] and cranial[70] represent the bone grafts of choice) and rigid fixation with miniplates. An adequate amount should be present (20 mm or more) in the vertical dimension in tooth-bearing areas for placement of osseointegrated implants.

If defects involve the alveolus alone, either in the maxilla or in the mandible, getting enough bone for implants to take as a free graft may be difficult. If enough bone is present to permit a horizontal osteotomy, distraction osteogenesis will provide the best result because the gingiva will come up with the distracted bone and one can easily overcorrect the bone defect. Overcorrection may cause premature contact at the apex of the (now overcorrected) deficiency, with overeruption of the posterior molar teeth.

Although in-continuity defects of the mandible longer than 5 cm can be dealt with by free nonvascularized bone grafts,[71] these larger defects are better corrected with microvascular transplantation of osseous flaps, particularly when the overlying soft tissues are less than optimal in condition or have been irradiated. The fibular free flap is ideal for longer defects because it can be repeatedly osteotomized and bent to any desired shape; the iliac free flap is well suited for anterior defects. The lesser amount of bone available in the radial forearm and scapular free flaps makes them less desirable choices (Fig. 72-18).

Text continued on p. 599

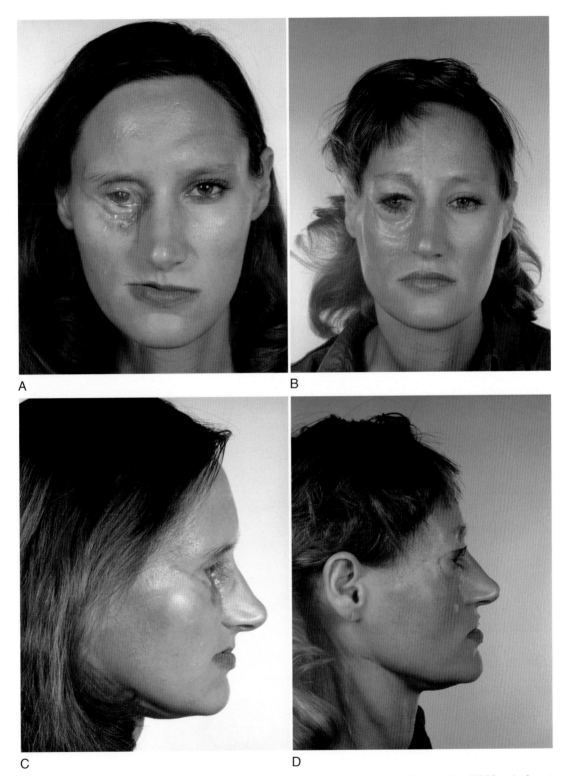

A

B

C

D

FIGURE 72-17. This 29-year-old woman had undergone a hemimaxillectomy and more than 7000 rad of postoperative irradiation for a neuroesthesioblastoma (*A* and *C*). Shortly after the initial preoperative photograph was taken, her right eye spontaneously perforated and she underwent an evisceration (removal of all of the orbital contents down to periosteum). *Continued*

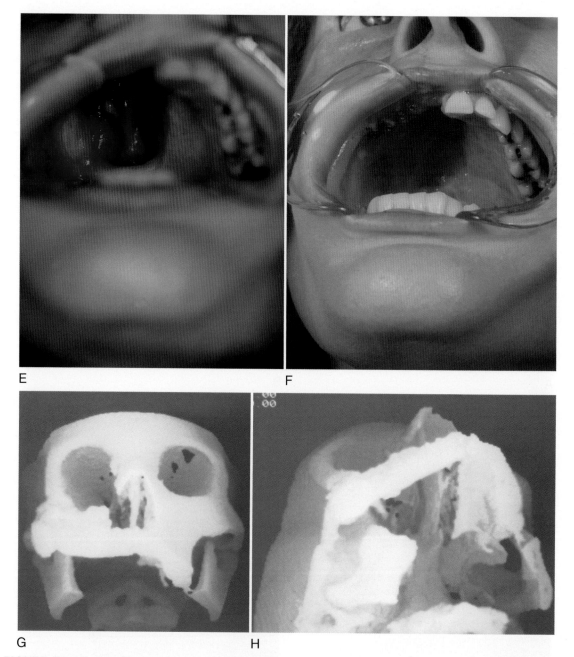

FIGURE 72-17, cont'd. At the initial operation *(G to I)*, a temporalis muscle flap was used to close the palatal defect *(E)*; the radiation-damaged skin of the lower eyelid and cheek was resected and a skin graft placed over the temporalis muscle.

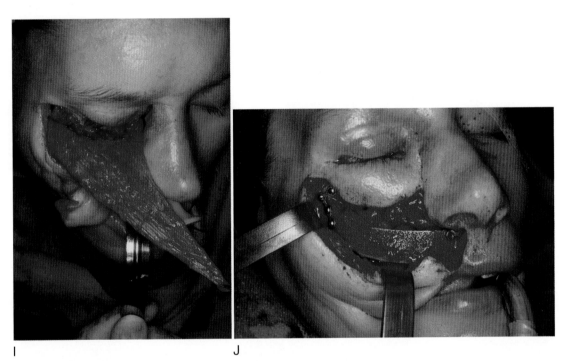

I   J

FIGURE 72-17, cont'd. At a subsequent operation *(J)*, an iliac bone graft was placed from alveolar ridge to ptery-goid region, well nourished by the underlying temporalis muscle; the lower eyelid was reconstructed with a forehead flap. Osseointegrated implants have been placed in the maxillary bone graft, and this portion of her reconstruction has been completed *(F)*. A second forehead flap has been required for the lower eyelid reconstruction; she currently has a socket that will accept a prosthesis, but the result (so far) is such that she still prefers to wear an epiprosthesis *(B* and *D)*. (From Wolfe SA, Berkowitz S: Plastic Surgery of the Facial Skeleton. Boston, Little, Brown, 1989.)

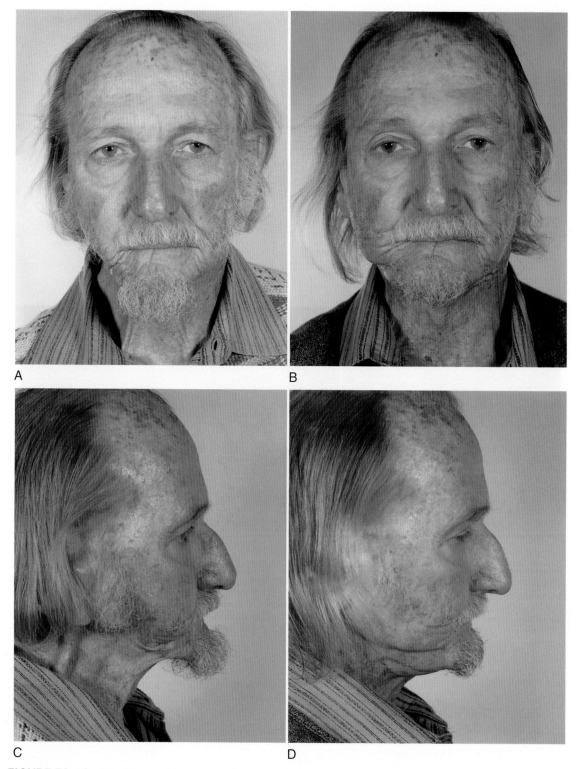

FIGURE 72-18. This 65-year-old man several years earlier had undergone a right radical neck dissection and partial right mandibulectomy, followed by radiotherapy for squamous carcinoma of the floor of the mouth (*A* and *C*).

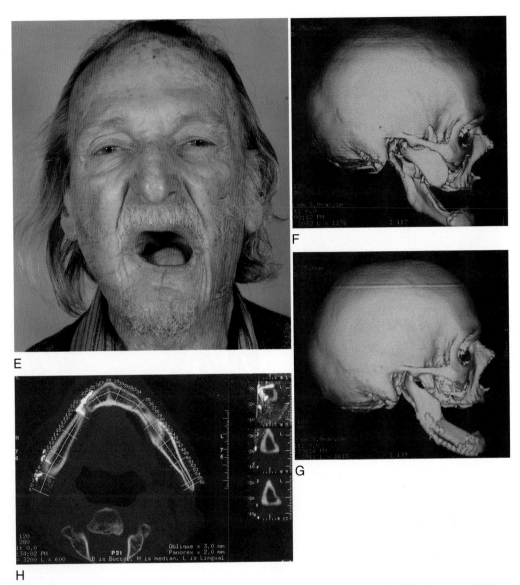

FIGURE 72-18, cont'd. He is shown after a microvascular transfer of a vascularized fibular segment. The condylar segment had been rotated upward and inward by pull of unopposed masticatory muscles *(F)*. A coronoidectomy was performed to enable the condylar segment to be positioned properly relative to the rest of the mandible *(G and H)*. He is shown about 6 months postoperatively *(B, D, and E)*, before placement of an osseointegrated implant into maxilla and mandible.

Chin

The most common reason for osseous procedures on the chin for acquired deformities has been an unfortunate outcome from a chin implant. Many of the patients have indeed had a number of chin implants, with removal, replacement, and often removal again, for reasons of infection and displacement.[72] Under these circumstances, an osseous genioplasty[73] should be performed,[74-76] rather than trying again with an alloplastic material. The capsule that forms around the implant should be removed to allow the osseous expansion to keep the soft tissue envelope properly stretched. In some patients, a proper diagnosis had not been made in the first place, and the corrective procedure may need to provide proper correction of the original deformity, such as lengthening the chin for a congenital shortness (Figs. 72-19 and 72-20).

Rarely, if the chin has had many previous operations and there is not adequate bone stock for an osseous genioplasty, a microvascular osteocutaneous free flap may provide the only solution (Fig. 72-21).

Text continued on p. 605

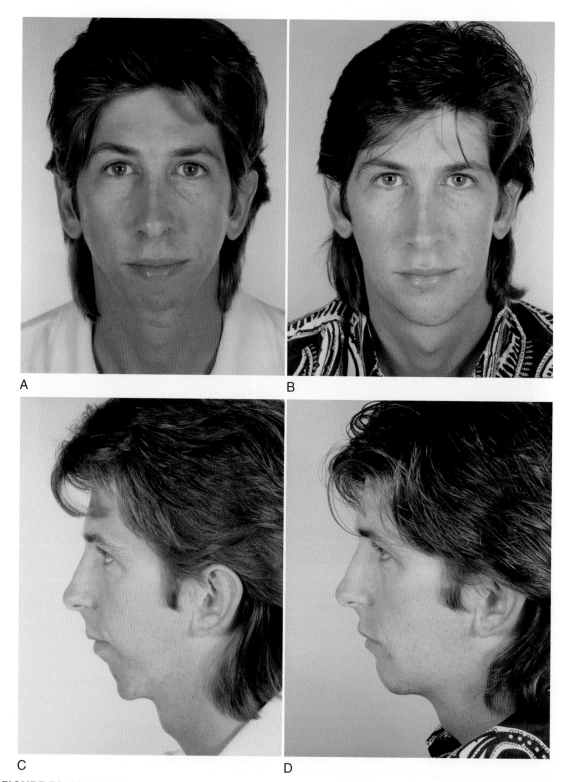

A

B

C

D

FIGURE 72-19. This 30-year-old man had had five different chin implants (*A* and *C*), the last one being a long "wrap-around" model placed below the lower border of his mandible. As with the others, he was displeased with the result of this one. He is shown after removal of the implant and a "jumping genioplasty" (*B* and *D*). If he wished further projection of the chin, after an interval of 6 months or so, a sliding advancement genioplasty could be done through the previous genioplasty. Chin implants are appropriate for mild degrees of retrogenia, but severe retrogenia, chins requiring vertical or lateral alteration, and failures of previous chin implants should be treated with osseous genioplasties.

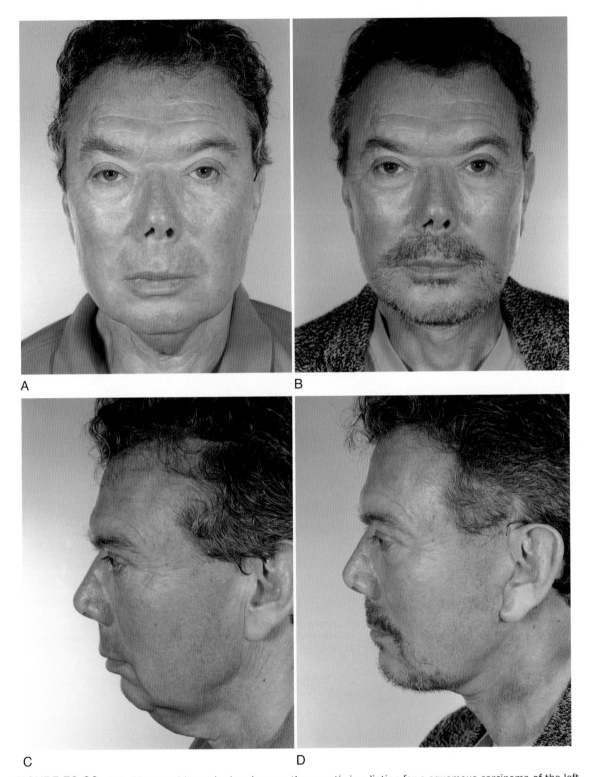

FIGURE 72-20. This 63-year-old man had undergone therapeutic irradiation for a squamous carcinoma of the left floor of the mouth (*A*, *C*, and *E*).

Continued

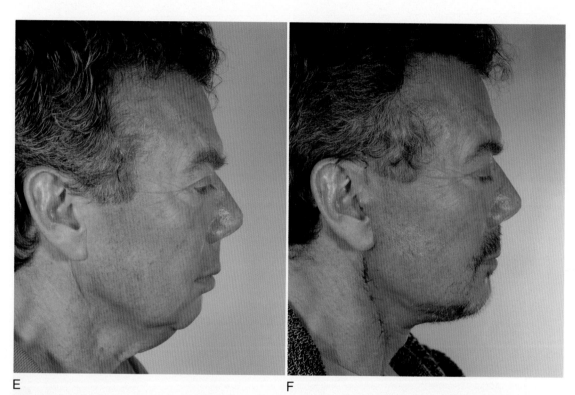

E   F

FIGURE 72-20, cont'd. He had a vertical scar on the right side of the neck extending from the earlobe almost to the external notch *(E)*. He is shown 1 week after a sliding advancement genioplasty, meloplasty, and submental lipectomy (*B, D,* and *F*). On the right side, the vertical neck scar rather than the usual retroauricular incision was used because of blood supply considerations *(F)*. A sliding genioplasty, which is a well-vascularized myo-osseous flap, is preferable to a chin implant in a patient who has received high-dose irradiation to the chin area.

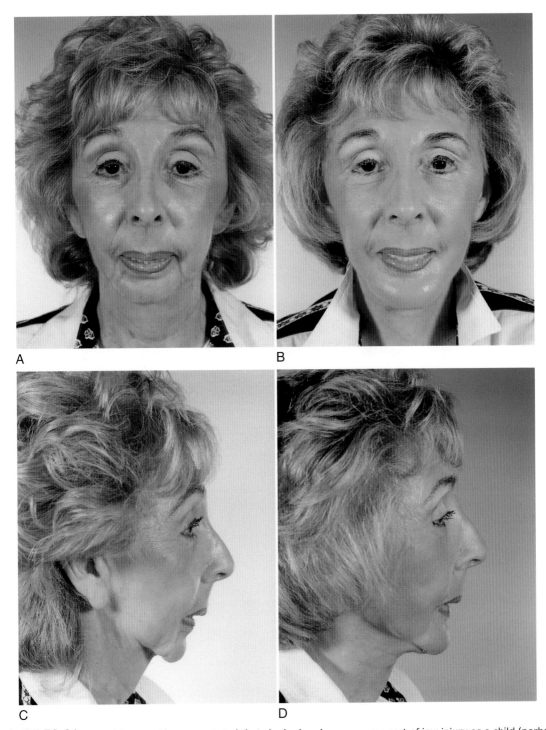

FIGURE 72-21. This 67-year-old woman stated that she had undergone some sort of jaw injury as a child (perhaps condylar fractures) and had been treated, among others, by Dr. Robert Ivy in Philadelphia and Dr. Varaztad Kazanjian in Boston. In total, she had undergone more than 26 operations in attempts to construct a chin. Segments of block hydroxyapatite had been successfully placed along the mandibular body, but all of the chin implants had to be removed because of infection or intraoral exposure (*A* and *C*). She had only a thin segment of bone connecting the parasymphyseal areas, and the intraoral soft tissues were thin and scarred; it was thought that they would not provide adequate coverage for any type of conventional genioplasty. After considerable explanation to the patient and her husband, the decision was made to go ahead with the only method that could most likely provide her with a chin: microsurgical reconstruction with use of an iliac osteocutaneous free flap.   *Continued*

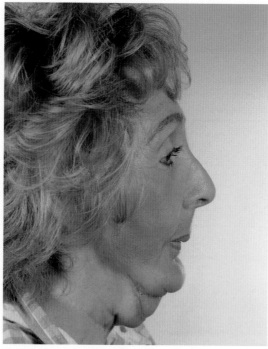

E

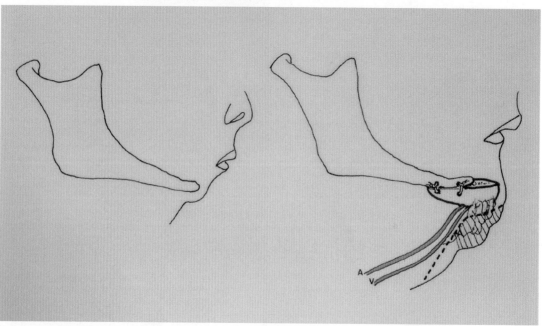

F

FIGURE 72-21, cont'd. The U-shaped segment of iliac bone was attached to the inferior border of what remained of her native symphysis, and a skin paddle and soft tissue attachments were transferred with the bone segment *(F)*. She is shown a month after the operation, with the skin paddle in place *(E)*, and a year after the original operation, following defatting of the pedicle and removal of the skin island *(B and D)*.

REFERENCES

1. Tessier P: Dysostoses cranio-faciales. Transactions of the Fourth International Congress of Plastic and Reconstructive Surgery, Rome, 1967. Amsterdam, Excerpta Medica, 1969.

2. Tessier P: Osteotomies totales de la face: syndrome de Crouzon, syndrome d'Apert, oxycephalies, turricephalies. Ann Chir Plast 1967;12:273.

3. Tessier P: Experience in the treatment of orbital hypertelorism. Plast Reconstr Surg 1974;53:4.

4. Tessier P: Orbital Hypertelorism. Scand. J. Plast Reconstr Surg 1972;6:135.

5. Tessier P, Guiot G, Rougier J, et al: Osteotomies cranio-naso-orbitales: hypertelorisme. Ann Chir Plast 1967;12:103.

6. Tessier P: Present status of craniofacial surgery. Presented at International Course on Craniofacial Surgery, Italian Society of Plastic Surgery, Rome, March 10, 1982.

7. Tessier P: Present status and future prospects of cranio-facial surgery. Transactions of the 7th International Congress of Plastic and Reconstructive Surgery, Cartgraf, Campinas, Brazil, 1979.

8. Tessier P: State of the Art Address: The current and future status of craniofacial surgery. Presented at VIII International Congress of Plastic Surgery, Montreal, Canada, June 1983.

9. Wolfe SA: The influence of Paul Tessier on our current treatment of facial trauma, both in primary care and in the management of late sequelae. Clin Plast Surg 1997;24:515-518.

10. Shenk RK: Histologie der Primaren Knochenheilung. Fortschr Kiefer Gesichtschir 1975;19:8.

11. Wolfe SA: Autogenous bone grafts versus alloplastic materials. In Wolfe SA, Berkowitz S: Plastic Surgery of the Facial Skeleton. Boston, Little, Brown, 1989:25-38.

12. Wolfe SA, Kawamoto HK: Taking the iliac-bone graft. J Bone Joint Surg Am 1978;60:411.

13. Epker BN, Friedlaender L, Wolford L, West R: The use of freeze-dried bone in middle-third facial advancements. J Oral Surg 1976;42:278.

14. Tessier P: The conjunctival approach to the orbital floor and maxilla in congenital malformation and trauma. J Maxillofac Surg 1973;1:3.

15. Holtman B, Wray RC, Little AG: A randomized comparison of four incisions for orbital fractures. Plast Reconstr Surg 1981;67:731.

16. Manson PN, Ruas E, Iliff N, Yaremchuck M: Single eyelid incision for exposure of the zygomatic bone and orbital reconstruction. Plast Reconstr Surg 1987;79:120.

17. Park DH, Lee JW, Song CH, et al: Endoscopic application in aesthetic and reconstructive facial bone surgery. Plast Reconstr Surg 1998;102:1199.

18. Tessier P: Introduction to oto-mandibular dysplasias or "20 years after." Ann Chir Plast Esthet 2001;46:381.

19. Wolfe SA: Cranial defects. In Wolfe SA, Berkowitz S: Plastic Surgery of the Facial Skeleton. Boston, Little, Brown, 1989: 692.

20. White JC: Late complications following cranioplasty with alloplastic plates. Ann Surg 1948;128:743.

21. Wolfe SA, Johnson P: Frontal sinus injuries: primary care and management of late complications. Plast Reconstr Surg 1988; 82:781.

22. Pensler J, McCarthy JG: The calvarial donor site: an anatomic study in cadavers. Plast Reconstr Surg 1985;75:648.

23. Wolfe SA: Utility of pericranial flaps. Ann Plast Surg 1978;1:146.

24. Albright F, Butler AM, Hampton AO, Smith P: Syndrome characterized by osteitis fibrosa disseminata, areas of pigmentation and endocrine dysfunction, with precocious puberty in females: report of five cases. N Engl J Med 1937;216:727.

25. Munro IR, Chen Y: Radical treatment for fronto-orbital fibrous dysplasia: the chain-link fence. Plast Reconstr Surg 1981;67: 719.

26. Derome P, Tessier P: Reconstruction of the anterior cranial base for benign orbitocranial tumors. In Tessier P, Rougier J, Hervouet F, et al, eds: Plastic Surgery of the Orbit and Eyelids. Wolfe SA, trans. New York, Masson, 1981:103-106.

27. Edgerton M: Discussion of "radical treatment for fronto-orbital fibrous dysplasia." Plast Reconstr Surg 1981;67:730.

28. Papay FA, Morales L Jr, Flaharty P, et al: Optic nerve decompression in cranial base fibrous dysplasia. J Craniofac Surg 1995;6:5, discussion 11.

29. Gruss JS: Fronto-naso-orbital trauma. Clin Plast Surg 1982;9:577.

30. Wheeler ES, Kawamoto HK, Zarem HA: Bone grafts for nasal reconstruction. Plast Reconstr Surg 1982;69:9.

31. Emery BE, Stucker FJ: The use of grafts in nasal reconstruction [review]. Facial Plast Surg 1994;10:358.

32. Leaf N: SMAS autografts for the nasal dorsum. Plast Reconstr Surg 1996;97:1249.

33. Chait LA, Becker H, Cort A: The versatile costal osteochondral graft in nasal reconstruction. Br J Plast Surg 1980;33: 179.

34. Jackson IT, Smith J, Mixter RC: Nasal bone grafting using split skull grafts. Ann Plast Surg 1983;11:533.

35. Binder DH: Dysostosis maxilla-nasalis, ein arhinencephaler Missbildungskomplex. Dtsch Zahnarztl Z 1962;6:438.

36. Tessier P, Tulasne JF, Delaire J, Resche F: Treatment of Binder's maxillonasal dysostosis [author's transl; in French]. Rev Stomatol Chir Maxillofac 1979;80:363.

37. Wolfe SA: Lengthening the nose: a lesson from craniofacial surgery applied to post-traumatic and congenital deformities. Plast Reconstr Surg 1994;94:78.

38. Millard DR Jr: Reconstructive rhinoplasty. In Millard DR Jr: A Rhinoplasty Tetralogy. Boston, Little, Brown, 1996:482-490.

39. Markowitz BL, Manson PN, Sargent L, et al: Management of the medial canthal tendon in nasoethmoid orbital fractures: the importance of the central fragment in classification and treatment. Plast Reconstr Surg 1991;87:843.

40. Leipziger LS, Manson PN: Nasoethmoid orbital fractures: current concepts and management principles. Clin Plast Surg 1992; 19:167.

41. Lovaas G: Microplate fixation of extended osteotomies for correction of the difficult nose. Presented at Facial Injury State of the Art Management Symposium, Chicago, April 1991.

42. Wolfe SA: Application of craniofacial surgical precepts in orbital reconstruction following trauma and tumor removal. J Maxillofac Surg 1982;10:212.

43. Putterman AM: Management of blow out fractures of the orbital floor III. The conservative approach. Surv Ophthalmol 1991;35:292.

44. Dingman R: Discussion. In Tessier P, Callahan A, Mustarde J, Salyer K, eds: Symposium on Plastic Surgery in the Orbital Region. St. Louis, Mosby, 1976:122.

45. Wolfe SA: Exophthalmos. In Wolfe SA, Berkowitz S: Plastic Surgery of the Facial Skeleton. Boston, Little, Brown, 1989: 549-574.

46. Stark B, Olivari N: Treatment of exophthalmos by orbital fat removal. Clin Plast Surg 1993;20:285, discussion 290.

47. Tessier P: Expansion chirurgicale de l'orbite: les orbites trop petites; exophthalmies basedowiennes; exorbitisme des dysostoses cranio-faciales; atresies orbitaires des jeunes enuclees; tumeurs orbitaires. Ann Chir Plast 1969;14:207.

48. Wolfe SA: Modified three-wall orbital expansion to correct persistent exophthalmos or exorbitism. Plast Reconstr Surg 1979;64:448.

49. Manson PN, Iliff NT: Orbital fractures. Facial Plast Surg 1988;5:243.

50. Manson PN, Hoopes JE, Su CT: Structural pillars of the facial skeleton: an approach to the management of Le Fort fractures. Plast Reconstr Surg 1980;66:54.

51. Lang W: Traumatic enophthalmos with retention of perfect acuity of vision. Trans Ophthalmol Soc UK 1889;9:41.

52. Wolfe SA: Correction of a persistent lower lid deformity caused by a displaced orbital floor implant. Ann Plast Surg 1979;2:448.

53. Wolfe SA: Correction of a lower eyelid deformity caused by multiple extrusions of alloplastic orbital floor implants. Plast Reconstr Surg 1981;68:429.

54. Gillies H, Millard DR Jr: The Principles and Art of Plastic Surgery. Boston, Little, Brown, 1957.

55. Wolfe SA: Posttraumatic orbital deformities. In Wolfe SA, Berkowitz S: Plastic Surgery of the Facial Skeleton. Boston, Little, Brown, 1989:572-624.

56. Forrest CR, Khairallah E, Kuzon WM Jr: Intraocular and intraorbital compartment pressure changes following orbital bone grafting: a clinical and laboratory study. Plast Reconstr Surg 1999;104:48.

57. Jackson IT, Carls F, Bush K, et al: Assessment and treatment of facial deformity resulting from radiation to the orbital area in childhood. Plast Reconstr Surg 1996;98:1169, discussion 1180.

58. Gruss JS, Mackinnon SE: Complex maxillary fractures: role of buttress reconstruction and immediate bone grafts. Plast Reconstr Surg 1986;78:9.

59. Manson PN, Crawley WA, Yaremchuk MJ, et al: Midface fractures: advantages of immediate open reduction and bone grafting. Plast Reconstr Surg 1985;76:1.

60. Gruss JS: Naso-ethmoid-orbital fractures: classification and role of primary bone grafting. Plast Reconstr Surg 1985;75:303.

61. Eriksson E, Branemark PI: Osseointegration from the perspective of the plastic surgeon. Plast Reconstr Surg 1994;93:626.

62. Wolfe SA: Use of temporal muscle for closure of palatal defects. Presented at 66th Annual Meeting of American Association of Plastic Surgeons, Nashville, Tenn, May 3-6, 1987.

63. Futran ND, Haller JR: Considerations for free-flap reconstruction of the hard palate. Arch Otolaryngol Head Neck Surg 1999;125:665.

64. Foster RD, Anthony JP, Sharma A, Pogrel MA: Vascularized bone flaps versus nonvascularized bone grafts for mandibular reconstruction: an outcome analysis of primary bony union and endosseous implant success. Head Neck 1999;21:66.

65. Laure B, Van Hove A, Aboumoussa J, et al: The fibular free flap. Anatomy and technique for removal [in French]. Rev Stomatol Chir Maxillofac 2000;101:147.

66. Martin D, Pistre V, Pinsolle V, et al: The scapula: a preferred donor site for a free flaps or pedicles transfer [in French]. Ann Chir Plast Esthet 2000;45:272.

67. Ivy RH, Eby JD: Maxillofacial Surgery, part 2, vol 110. Medical Department, US Army in the World War (Surgery). Washington, DC, US Government Printing Office, 1924:462.

68. Gillies HD: Plastic Surgery of the Face. London, Oxford Medical Publications, 1920:177-189.

69. Blocker TG, Stout RA: Mandibular reconstruction World War II. Plast Reconstr Surg 1949;4:153.

70. Wolfe SA, Berkowitz S: The use of cranial bone grafts in the closure of alveolar and anterior palatal clefts. Plast Reconstr Surg 1983;72:659.

71. Tessier P: The scope of craniofacial surgery. Presented at the 8th International Congress of Plastic and Reconstructive Surgery, Montreal, June 29, 1983.

72. Hoffman S: Loss of a Silastic chin implant following a dental infection. Ann Plast Surg 1981;7:484.

73. Hinds EC, Kent JN: Genioplasty: the versatility of horizontal osteotomy. J Oral Surg 1969;27:690.

74. Wider TM, Spiro SA, Wolfe SA: Simultaneous osseous genioplasty and meloplasty. Plast Reconstr Surg 1997;99:1273.

75. Spear SL, Mausner ME, Kawamoto HK Jr: Sliding genioplasty as a local anesthetic outpatient procedure: a prospective two-center trial. Plast Reconstr Surg 1987;80:55.

76. Cohen SR, Mardach OL, Kawamoto HK Jr: Chin disfigurement following removal of alloplastic chin implants. Plast Reconstr Surg 1991;88:62, discussion 67.

Scalp Reconstruction

MARK D. WELLS, MD

ANATOMY

SCALP DISORDERS
  Cicatricial Alopecia
  Aplasia Cutis Congenita
  Physical Trauma and Burns
  Infection
  Neoplasms

EVALUATION OF THE DEFECT

RECONSTRUCTIVE OPTIONS
  Primary Closure
  Split-Thickness Skin Grafting
  Local Flaps
  Tissue Expanders

Distant Flaps
Microvascular Composite Tissue Transplantation
Scalp Replantation

HAIR RESTORATION
  Hair Cycle
  Etiology of Hair Loss
  Classification of Hair Loss Patterns
  Medical Treatment
  Surgical Treatment
  Hair Transplantation
  Scalp Reduction
  Tissue Expansion
  Scalp Flaps

ANATOMY

The scalp extends anatomically from the supraorbital margin anteriorly to the superior nuchal line posteriorly. Laterally, it extends to a line drawn through the frontal process of the zygoma, across the zygomatic arch to the prominence of the mastoid process. The scalp classically consists of five layers. These layers can easily be remembered by the mnemonic SCALP (Fig. 73-1). The layers are the skin, subcutaneous tissue, aponeurosis and muscle, loose areolar tissue, and pericranium.[1,2]

The outermost layer of the scalp consists of the skin and subcutaneous tissue. Because there is not a natural cleavage plane between the two layers, they should be considered together. Contained within this layer are hair follicles, sweat glands, and fat cells. Connective tissue fibers within the subcutaneous layer connect the skin to the underlying musculoaponeurotic layer, providing firm fixation.

Underneath the subcutaneous tissue is the galea aponeurotica, or musculoaponeurotic layer. The galea consists of fibrous tissue that extends from the frontalis muscle anteriorly to the occipitalis muscle posteriorly (Fig. 73-2). Laterally, the galea continues as the temporoparietal fascia or superficial temporal fascia.[3] The galea and temporoparietal fascia are highly vascularized tissues. Both structures have found utility in many reconstructive procedures about the head and neck. The fascial layer of the galea extends anteriorly into the face as the superficial musculoaponeurotic system as outlined by Mitz and Peyronie[4] and later modified by Jost.[5]

The muscle components of this layer consist of the paired frontalis and occipitalis muscles as well as the auricular muscles laterally. The frontalis muscles originate from the galea and insert into the dermis at the level of the superciliary arch. Anteriorly, the frontalis blends with the procerus, corrugator supercilii, and orbicularis oculi. The paired occipitalis muscles take origin from the superior nuchal line and mastoid, inserting onto the galea. There are three auricular muscles on each side of the scalp, the anterior auricular, superior auricular, and posterior auricular muscles. They originate from the temporalis fascia and mastoid bone and insert into the pericranium of the external ear. Superiorly, they blend with the superficial temporal fascia.

Under the galea is a loose areolar layer of tissue known as the subgaleal fascia. The subgaleal fascia is thin over the vertex of the skull and becomes progressively thicker in the temporoparietal region. This layer has a rich blood supply that can be elevated as a separate vascularized layer of tissue.[6,7]

The deepest layer of the scalp is the pericranium. This is the periosteal layer of the calvaria. This thick collagenous layer has a rich blood supply and is firmly attached to the skull in the region of the sutures. The use of pericranial flaps as a reconstructive option has been well described in the literature.[8]

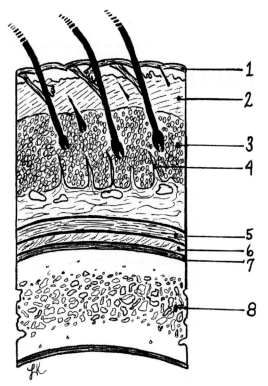

FIGURE 73-1. Anatomy of the scalp and cranium: 1, epidermis; 2, dermis; 3, subcutaneous fat; 4, fibrous septa; 5, galea aponeurotica; 6, subgaleal tissue; 7, pericranium; 8, calvaria.

In the temporal-parietal region, there are four distinct fascial layers with anatomic significance (Fig. 73-3). The most superficial fascial layer is the temporoparietal fascia or superficial temporal fascia. This layer is a lateral extension of the galea. It is closely applied to the overlying skin and subcutaneous fascia and is difficult to dissect. Unless care is taken, it is easy to damage the overlying hair follicles, resulting in temporal alopecia.[9-11]

Deep to the superficial temporal fascia is the subgaleal fascia. This layer is well developed and easily dis-

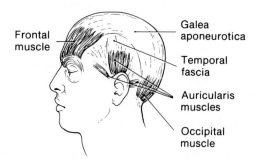

FIGURE 73-2. Muscle anatomy of the scalp. (From Vallis CP: Hair replacement surgery. In McCarthy JG, ed: Plastic Surgery. Philadelphia, WB Saunders, 1990:1514.)

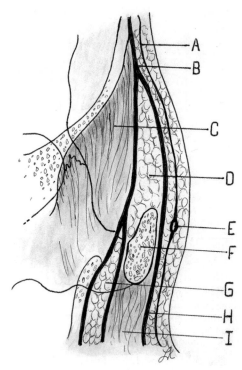

FIGURE 73-3. Cross section of the temporal region at the level of the zygomatic arch showing the relationship of the frontal branch of the facial nerve to superficial and deep temporal fascia. A, temporoparietal fascia; B, deep temporal fascia splitting at the line of fusion; C, superficial temporal fat pad; D, temporalis muscle; E, frontal branch of the facial nerve; F, zygomatic arch; G, deep temporal fat pad from the buccal fat; H, parotid-masseteric fascia; I, masseter muscle.

sected. Contained within this layer are the superficial temporal artery and the frontal branch of the facial nerve. Under the subgaleal fascia is the superficial temporal fat pad. Numerous large perforating veins course through this layer, making dissection somewhat difficult. Under the temporal fat pad lies the deep temporal fascia. It is a thick fascial layer overlying the temporalis muscle. Superiorly, it fuses with the pericranium. Inferiorly, at the level of the superior orbital margin, the temporal fascia splits into two layers. The superficial layer attaches to the lateral border of the zygomatic arch. The deep layer fuses with the medial aspect of the arch. There is a small amount of fat between the layers. Dissection in this layer allows reflection of the bicoronal flap without injury to the frontal branch of the facial nerve as it passes over the arch of the zygoma.[12]

Between the temporalis fascia and the muscle fiber of the temporalis muscle is a thin layer of fat. It is continuous inferior with the buccal fat pad of the midface. The temporalis muscle originates from the temporal fossa and inserts onto the coronoid process of the mandible. It is supplied by two deep temporal branches

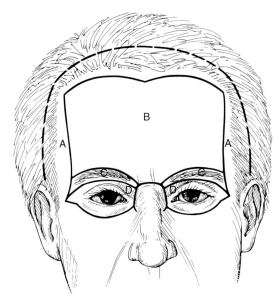

FIGURE 73-4. Diagrammatic representation of the aesthetic units of the periorbital, forehead, and temporal regions of the scalp. A, temporal unit; B, forehead unit; C, brow unit; D, periorbital unit.

of the internal maxillary artery, the middle and deep temporal arteries.

The forehead is an aesthetic unit of the face (Fig. 73-4). It can be subdivided into five subunits: one central, two temporal, and two eyebrow units. The position of the hairline and eyebrows must be taken into account in planning forehead reconstruction.[13] The muscles of the forehead are innervated by the frontal branch of the facial nerve (Fig. 73-5). The branch emerges from the parotid gland 2.5 cm anterior to the tragus. The nerve ascends over the central portion of the zygomatic arch, passing 1.5 cm lateral to the lateral

orbital rim to innervate the frontalis muscles on their deep surfaces. The occipitalis muscle is supplied by the posterior auricular branch of the facial nerve. This branch originates with the facial nerve as it exits the stylomastoid foramen. The temporalis muscle is supplied by the posterior and anterior deep temporal nerves, which are branches of the trigeminal nerve.

The supratrochlear and supraorbital nerves, branches of the first division of the trigeminal nerve, provide sensation to the forehead and anterior scalp. In the temporal region, the zygomaticotemporal nerve, a branch of the second division of the trigeminal nerve, supplies sensation. The auriculotemporal nerve provides additional innervation anterior to the ear. The occipital nerves supply the posterior scalp sensation.

The scalp has a rich vascular plexus supplied by branches of both the internal and external carotid arteries (Fig. 73-6). The supraorbital and supratrochlear arteries are terminal branches of the internal carotid artery and supply the anterior scalp and forehead. The superficial temporal, postauricular, and occipital arteries are branches of the external carotid artery. These vessels supply the lateral and posterior aspects of the scalp. The extensive interconnections between each of the angiosomes allows replantation of the entire scalp based on a single donor vessel. The venous system parallels the arterial supply (Fig. 73-7). There are numerous interconnections between the veins in the scalp and forehead, eventually draining into the internal and external jugular veins.

The lymphatic network of the scalp is unique in that there are no lymph nodes and therefore no barriers to lymphatic flow. The lymphatic system is primarily subcutaneous. The lymph vessels drain toward the parotid gland, the preauricular region, and the upper neck as well as to the occipital area. Skin cancers of the scalp tend to spread by local extension rather than through lymphatic or vascular channels. This lack of lymphatic or vascular spread reflects unique tumor biology of scalp neoplasms.[14]

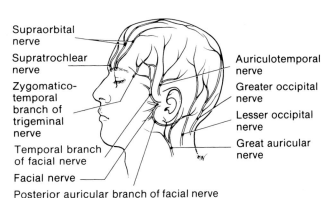

FIGURE 73-5. The nerve (motor and sensory) supply of the scalp. (From Vallis CP: Hair replacement surgery. In McCarthy JG, ed: Plastic Surgery. Philadelphia, WB Saunders, 1990:1514.)

Supraorbital nerve
Supratrochlear nerve
Zygomatico-temporal branch of trigeminal nerve
Temporal branch of facial nerve
Facial nerve
Posterior auricular branch of facial nerve
Auriculotemporal nerve
Greater occipital nerve
Lesser occipital nerve
Great auricular nerve

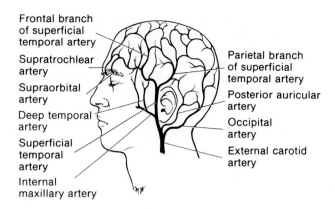

Frontal branch
of superficial
temporal artery

Supratrochlear
artery

Supraorbital
artery

Deep temporal
artery

Superficial
temporal
artery

Internal
maxillary artery

Parietal branch
of superficial
temporal artery

Posterior auricular
artery

Occipital
artery

External carotid
artery

FIGURE 73-6. The arterial supply of the scalp. (From Vallis CP: Hair replacement surgery. In McCarthy JG, ed: Plastic Surgery. Philadelphia, WB Saunders, 1990:1514.)

SCALP DISORDERS

Cicatricial Alopecia

Cicatricial alopecia is characterized by scarring of the skin with loss of hair. The area of alopecia can vary from a linear scar to large areas of the entire scalp. Etiologic mechanisms of cicatricial alopecia are listed in Table 73-1.[15,16]

Aplasia Cutis Congenita

This condition was first reported in 1776. Since that time, some 500 patients with this condition have been described in the literature.[17] In infants, the patient is born with a cutaneous defect resembling an eschar or newly formed scar of the skin. The scalp is the most

common location for aplasia cutis congenita. It is involved in 65% of all patients presenting with the disease. In older children, there is usually a hairless patch within the scalp resembling an atrophic scar. The defect is always near the midline over the vertex. Less frequently, the lesions are found on the arms, knees, trunk, lower limbs, and face. In some children, there are associated defects of the calvaria and dura.

The etiology of the malformation remains unclear. Hypotheses include a malformation of the neural tube or mechanical disruption of the skin in utero. Vascular accidents, direct pressure, and amnionic bands have been advanced as etiologic factors. Most of the instances of this disorder appear to be sporadic; however, several patients within families have been described. Chromosomal disorders have also been linked with the condition. Maternal intake of medication and perinatal viremia have also been evoked as possible etiologic mechanisms.[18]

Wound treatment in patients with superficial ulceration is generally conservative, with regular dressing

FIGURE 73-7. Venous drainage of the scalp. A, anterior auricular vein; B, supratrochlear vein; C, supraorbital vein; D, superficial temporal vein; E, posterior auricular vein; F, occipital vein; G, internal jugular vein; H, exterior jugular vein.

TABLE 73-1 ✦ ETIOLOGY OF CICATRICIAL ALOPECIA

Congenital
Aplasia cutis congenita
Acquired
Trauma
Physical
Burns
Thermal
Electrical
Chemical
Radiation
Infections
Localized
Systemic

changes.[19] Larger defects, especially with underlying bone defects, are susceptible to infection, meningitis, sagittal sinus thrombosis, and hemorrhage. The potential for a fatal outcome is greatest in the first month of life. This period is when the eschar cracks and starts to separate. In these deeper lesions, dural reconstruction, cranioplasty, and flap reconstruction may prove lifesaving.[20,21]

Physical Trauma and Burns

Scar may occur in the scalp from traumatic lacerations or avulsions that are repaired primarily or allowed to heal by secondary intention. Postsurgical alopecia may result from surgical flaps or skin grafts applied for removal of benign and malignant tumors. The resultant defect may be large or small, depending on the size of the tumor.

Thermal injury to the scalp may result in large areas of skin loss and necrosis.[22] Scald burns of hot water, coffee, and grease account for the majority of scalp injuries in children. Direct thermal injury by flame causes more scalp burns in adults. The depth of the burn determines the ultimate area of hair and scalp loss. Second-degree burns can result in alopecia by thermal injury to hair follicles. Hair loss can occur even though the skin goes on to heal by re-epithelialization. Deeper third-degree burns can destroy the subcutaneous layer, necessitating the use of skin grafts to effect closure. In fourth-degree injuries, the necrosis extends to periosteum or bone. Avascularity of these wounds dictates a more complex method of reconstruction.[23,24]

Electrical burns of the scalp are less common than thermal injuries. Electrical wounds are more localized and often show deeper destruction.[25] If the periosteum is intact, the wound can be débrided and skin grafts applied. For full-thickness injuries, the bone is débrided and the dura covered with a flap. Alternatively, in dire situations, skin grafts can be applied directly to the dura and secondary calvarial reconstruction entertained later.

Contact of the scalp with toxic chemicals can result in tissue loss and alopecia. Industrial chemicals and occasionally concentrated cosmetic solutions for hair dyeing, bleaching, and straightening may damage the scalp and hair follicles.[26]

Exposure to ionizing radiation can result in temporary or permanent alopecia. Heavily irradiated wounds are more susceptible to minor trauma and infection. Necrosis can extend down to the underlying calvaria or brain.[27,28] In general, wide débridement of all nonviable tissue is recommended. These wounds are not favorable sites for local procedures such as skin grafts, direct closure, or local flaps because of the relative avascularity of the wounds. Free muscle flaps, transplanted by microsurgical technique, are generally chosen because of their ability to fight off infection and to change the ischemic biology of the wound.[29,30] Luce[31] has recommended preservation of the bone and coverage with well-vascularized tissue if the skull is not grossly necrotic. If osteomyelitis is present, the bone is removed and the defect similarly resurfaced. Secondary cranioplasty is deferred for 3 to 6 months.

Infection

Systemic granulomatous diseases, such as leprosy and lupus vulgaris, can result in permanent alopecia. Other diseases, like lichen planus and lupus erythematosus, can attack the scalp and result in scarring. Localized folliculitis and perifolliculitis can result in hair loss as well. Localized pyogenic infection can result in scalp necrosis. Viral diseases, such as herpes and varicella, have caused scalp scarring and hair loss. Fungal infections, such as kerion and favus, can result in cicatricial alopecia.[32,33]

Neoplasms

The differential diagnosis of a subcutaneous nodule of the scalp is legion. Most lesions of the scalp will be benign. Primary malignant tissues of the scalp are most frequently epithelial in origin, although tumors from adnexal and connective tissue elements also occur.[34] Approximately 2% of epithelial tumors of the skin are located on the scalp. Basal cell cancer predominates, followed by squamous cell tumors and malignant melanoma. Other primary tumors that may occur on the scalp are sarcomas (fibrosarcoma, dermatofibrosarcoma, malignant fibrous histiocytoma, angiosarcoma, leiomyosarcoma, and rhabdomyosarcoma), lymphomas, adenocarcinomas, and primary adnexal cancers. The scalp is a common repository for metastatic tumors, most likely because of its rich vascularity.

As with the majority of skin cancers, cumulative sun exposure and fair skin are risk factors. Approximately 65% of the tumors occur in men. The majority of skin cancers occur in hair-bearing skin rather than in bald areas as one would intuitively expect. About half the tumors occur in the temporal region, followed by the postauricular and occipital areas.[14]

There are varieties of premalignant conditions of the scalp that predispose to the development of malignancy. Nevus sebaceus of Jadassohn is a yellow plaque that develops in the scalp of children. At puberty, the lesion often becomes nodular. Basal cell carcinoma develops in 5% to 7% of the patients with nevus sebaceus. In rare instances, squamous cell carcinoma and apocrine carcinomas have developed in these lesions.[35,36]

Nevoid basal cell carcinoma syndrome is an autosomal dominant condition associated with the development of multiple basal cell carcinomas. Associated findings include odontogenic jaw cysts, mental retardation, calcification of the falx cerebri, skeletal abnormalities, and palmar and plantar pits.[37,38]

Of all melanomas, 20% originate in the head and neck. Of these tumors, 12% to 30% involve the scalp.[39-41] Giant congenital compound nevus in children is thought to be a precursor lesion for malignant melanoma, although the transformation rate is variably debated. The risk for melanomatous transformation has been reported to range from 2% to 42%. The treatment of choice is usually prophylactic excision and reconstruction.

Dysplastic nevi are also thought to be a risk factor for the development of melanoma. These lesions may arise spontaneously or in association with familial dysplastic nevus syndrome. Dysplastic nevi are usually larger than ordinary melanocytic nevi, measuring between 5 and 15 mm. They exhibit variability in color and shape and often have irregular borders.[42]

The presence of a chronic burn scar of the scalp increases the likelihood for development of a Marjolin ulcer or squamous cell carcinoma within the confines of the wound. These can be aggressive tumors with an increased propensity to metastasize early to regional lymph nodes.[43]

Xeroderma pigmentosum is an autosomal recessive disorder characterized by intolerance of the skin to ultraviolet light. It is due to inability of the individuals affected with this disorder to repair damage induced by sunlight to their DNA. Normally, damaged segments of DNA are excised and replaced with new sequences of bases. In xeroderma pigmentosum, there is inadequate excision because of a deficiency of DNA endonuclease that initiates the excision process. These patients develop multiple epithelial malignant neoplasms at an early age, most frequently in sun-exposed parts of the body. Tumors include squamous cell carcinoma, basal cell carcinoma, and rarely fibrosarcoma. In about 3% of patients with xeroderma pigmentosum, malignant melanoma develops. Treatment involves sun avoidance and skin protection with sunscreens.[44]

The treatment of choice for a malignant neoplasm of the scalp is generally surgical excision. Irradiation is usually less effective, especially in large lesions, but it may be indicated in debilitated patients who are poor operative risks. The scalp's thick galeal layer offers a natural barrier to vertical growth of cutaneous malignant neoplasms. Once penetrated, the areolar tissue in the subgaleal plane offers little resistance to lateral spread. The periosteum of the scalp and outer cortex of the skull also provide an effective barrier to tumor invasion. Once violated, however, tumor can spread in the diploic space and through perforating channels to the dura.[45,46]

Basal cell carcinomas of the scalp are usually slowly progressive. The tumors usually spread radially for an extended period before developing a vertical phase. Metastatic spread to regional lymph nodes is extremely unusual.

Squamous cell tumors present as ulcerative or fungating masses of the scalp. They often spread extensively radially before penetrating deeply. Regional lymph node metastasis occurs in 17% of patients with squamous cell carcinoma of the scalp. Neck dissection is indicated only with clinically positive disease.

The abundant vascular supply and rich lymphatic plexuses of the scalp allow easy radial extension of melanomas. Melanomas of the scalp are aggressive and often difficult to control. Radial extension and metastatic spread to regional lymph nodes are more common than is penetration into the deeper tissues of the scalp. The width of excision is based on the thickness of the melanoma. Superficial melanomas less than 1 mm thick can be treated with 1-cm margins. Intermediate and deep melanomas are excised with 2- and 3-cm margins, respectively. Sentinel lymph node mapping is indicated in patients with clinically negative nodes who are thought to be at increased risk for nodal metastasis. This determination is based on the thickness of the primary tumor. Lymph from the scalp drains toward the parotid gland, preauricular and postauricular areas, upper neck, and occiput. Regional lymph node dissections are indicated for clinically positive nodal disease or lymphatic basins that are positive after sentinel lymph node biopsy.[47-49]

Mohs micrographic surgery has been used on the scalp. Cure rates for basal cell carcinoma treated by this technique are 99%. Cure rates decrease with larger and deeper tumors. Indications for use of the technique include scar carcinomas, morpheaform or sclerosing basal cell carcinoma, and squamous tumors with aggressive features such as perineural invasion. Clinically suspected bone invasion is a contraindication to the technique.[50,51]

EVALUATION OF THE DEFECT

When scalp and forehead reconstruction is considered, several factors are important in development of a treatment plan. Obviously, the size and depth of the defect are critical in the evaluation of the patient. However, one must also consider the effect the reconstruction might have on nearby mobile structures, such as the hairline and brow. If periosteum has been lost and there is bone exposure, flap reconstruction must be considered in lieu of skin grafting because of relative avascularity of the wound bed. If a bone defect is present, consideration should be given to cranioplasty. Cranial reconstruction can be accomplished primarily when the wound conditions are optimal or as a delayed procedure if there is concern about infection or the viability of the overlying skin. Prior irradiation or scarring may limit reconstructive options. The relative inelasticity of the scalp often necessitates larger flaps to distribute tension and to maximize the vascularity of the construct.

Whenever possible, Millard's principle of replacing like tissue with like should be invoked.[52] If hair-bearing tissue has been lost, it is best reconstructed with surrounding scalp tissue. Gonzalez-Ulloa's concept of aesthetic subunits of the face should be considered when cosmetically critical areas, such as the forehead, are reconstructed.[53] Consideration should be given to excision of entire subunits and repair of the defect as a unit. This allows the placement of incisions in cosmetically superior positions, avoiding the "patchwork" effect that results when only portions of the subunit have been excised and repaired.[54]

RECONSTRUCTIVE OPTIONS
Primary Closure

Hosts of techniques have been advocated over the years to restore the integrity of the scalp after traumatic loss or resection for malignant lesions. For small lesions (<3 cm), primary closure can often be effected.[55,56] If tension is excessive, wide undermining and advancement are often possible. The rich blood supply of the scalp often makes closure under tension possible with a relatively low incidence of necrosis. Some surgeons have advocated scoring of the underlying galea as a method of decreasing tension on the repair. The use of this technique may result in a significant decrease in blood supply to the overlying skin.[57]

Split-Thickness Skin Grafting

Primary split-thickness skin grafting may be used when the medical condition of the patient precludes larger, more complex procedures. Alternatively, it can be combined with staged procedures, such as tissue expansion, to provide temporary wound coverage. A necessary prerequisite for the technique is adequate vascularity of the underlying bed. Preservation of cranial periosteum or the underlying subcutaneous tissues of the scalp allows successful revascularization of the graft. Exposure of the underlying bone generally requires resurfacing with vascularized flap tissue. Alternatively, multiple drill holes can be placed in the outer cortex, allowing the wound to granulate during several weeks with dressing changes. Interval split-thickness skin grafting can be performed when the bed appears satisfactory. Long-term stability of this type of coverage tends to be a problem.[14,31]

The primary advantage of split-thickness skin grafting for scalp reconstruction is its technical simplicity. The downside is the cosmetically inferior appearance of the skin graft compared with a scalp reconstructed with hair-bearing tissue. In addition, skin grafts may prove unstable in hostile wound environments, such as in a patient who has received previous irradiation to the recipient bed.

Local Flaps

Hosts of local tissue rearrangements have been employed in scalp reconstruction (Fig. 73-8). These have included transposition, advancement, and rotation flaps used singly or in combination. Component tissue elements of the scalp, such as skin, muscle, galea, and pericranium, can be separated from one another and used to resurface a variety of adjacent soft tissue defects.

Avulsions of non-hair-bearing skin of the forehead can be treated by use of the crane principle.[52] This involves rotating a hair-bearing scalp flap over the exposed bone. The donor defect is covered with a temporary split-thickness graft. Several weeks later, the flap is elevated, leaving a layer of vascularized tissue over the donor defect. The previous split-thickness skin graft is excised, and the hair-bearing flap is returned to its original anatomic position. The forehead is then resurfaced with a full-thickness graft or sheet of thick split graft.

Larger flaps with broad bases are generally preferable to smaller flaps, given the thickness of the scalp and its relative noncompliance. If a named vessel (e.g., the superficial temporal, occipital, and supraorbital vessels) can be included with the flap, the surviving length is often improved. Smaller peripheral defects can often be closed with one flap. Scalps with central or vertex wounds often require multiple flaps to effect closure. Orticochea[58] published his four-flap scalp reconstructive technique based on known vascular territories of the scalp (Fig. 73-9). He expanded these flaps by dividing the galea perpendicular to the direction of advancement. He subsequently modified the technique into a three-flap reconstruction in 1971 (Fig. 73-10).[59] Defects as large as 30% of the cranium can be closed by this technique. Arnold[57] stressed the need to divide the galea with extreme care and magnification to avoid injury to the underlying blood supply. In his opinion, narrow flaps, even those based on named vessels, are more likely to suffer from vascular compromise and necrosis.

When a large scalp flap is rotated, the dissection should be subgaleal, preserving the underlying periosteum. This layer may prove to be an invaluable recipient bed for a skin graft if primary closure of the donor site of the transposed flap is not possible. A large dog-ear is often formed at the point of rotation of the flap. The temptation to revise the dog-ear primarily should be resisted. This maneuver will often narrow the vascular pedicle of the transposed flap, resulting in necrosis of the most distal and often the most critical portion of the construct. A dog-ear will often flatten

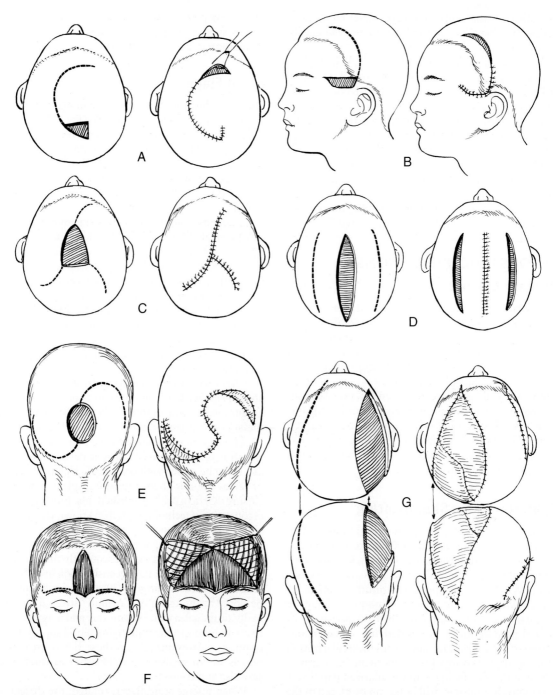

FIGURE 73-8. Some techniques for the closure of scalp defects. *A* and *B*, Rotation flaps. *C*, Gillies' tripod technique (1944). *D*, Bipedicled flaps. *E*, Double opposing rotation flaps. If complete closure cannot be obtained, split-thickness skin grafts are applied over the pericranium to cover the remaining exposed areas. *F*, Kazanjian and Converse's crisscross incisions through the frontalis muscle or the galea aponeurotica to distend the flaps and achieve closure of the defect. *G*, A large flap transposed over a lateral scalp defect. The residual defect is covered with a split-thickness skin graft over the pericranium. (From Marchac D: Deformities of the forehead, scalp, and cranial vault. In McCarthy JG, ed: Plastic Surgery. Philadelphia, WB Saunders, 1990:1538.)

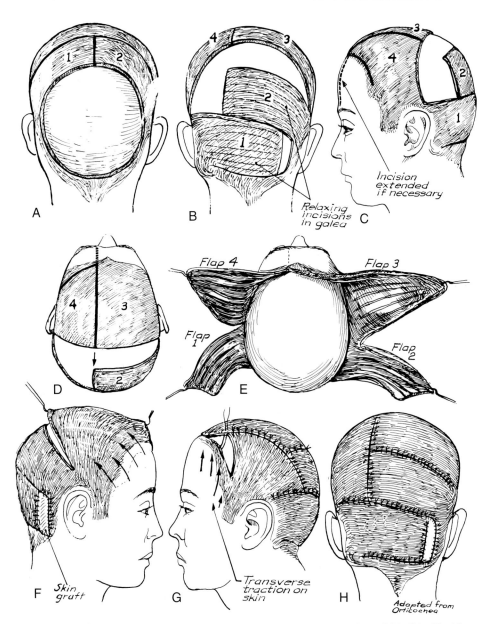

FIGURE 73-9. Four-flap technique, which is particularly applicable in a child. (Modified from Orticochea M: New three-flap scalp reconstruction technique. Br J Plast Surg 1971;24:84. Copyright 1971, with permission from The British Association of Plastic Surgeons.)

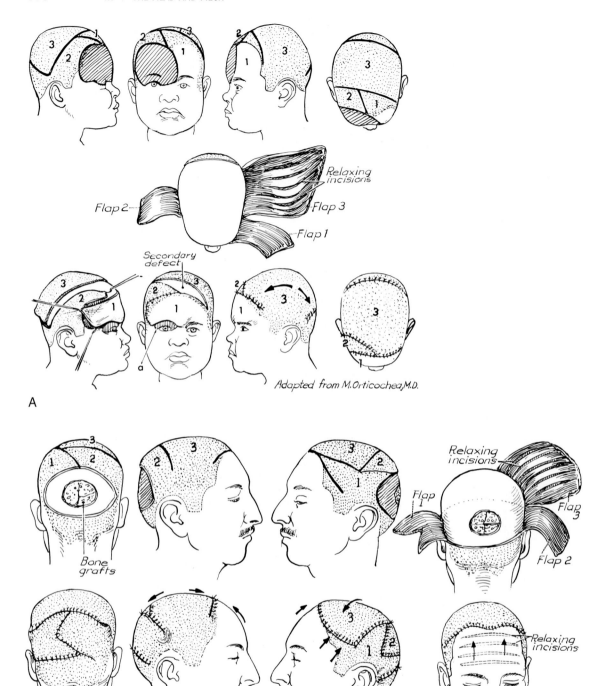

FIGURE 73-10. *A,* Development of the three-flap technique. It is preferable to cut flaps 1 and 2 at an angle as shown. The secondary defect that results after juxtaposition of flaps 1 and 2 is smaller than the primary one. *B,* The three flaps have been mobilized. Parallel incisions have been made in the aponeurosis of the large flap (3) transverse to the longitudinal axis of the skull. Flaps 1 and 2 are sutured in juxtaposition but without tension because their pedicles are narrow. (Modified from Orticochea M: New three-flap scalp reconstruction technique. Br J Plast Surg 1971;24:184. Copyright 1971, with permission from The British Association of Plastic Surgeons.)

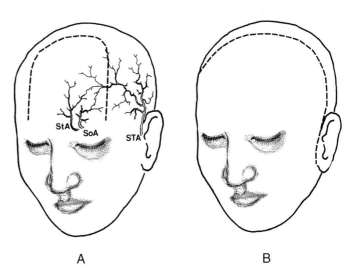

FIGURE 73-11. *A,* Branches of the superficial temporal artery (STA), supraorbital artery (SoA), and supratrochlear artery (StA) provide the blood supply of anterior galeal or galeoperitoneal flaps. *B,* A bicoronal scalp incision maximizes the length of the reconstructive galeal-pericranial flaps; it may be extended laterally to the preauricular area for an anterolateral approach to the cranial base. (Modified from Snyderman CH, Janecka IP, Sekhar LN, et al: Anterior cranial base reconstruction: role of galeal and pericranial flaps. Laryngoscope 1990;100:607.)

with time or can be revised later if it does not. Excessive tension should be avoided because it will inhibit healing and increase the likelihood of necrosis of the flap tip.

A drain is used postoperatively to prevent fluid accumulation under the transposed flaps. Care should be taken not to apply a tight pressure dressing to the scalp; this will often result in flap necrosis. If necessary, a halo device is temporarily inserted into the cranium to prevent direct pressure on the flaps from the weight of the head with the patient in the recumbent position.[60]

Advantages of scalp flaps include excellent cosmesis, replacement of hair-bearing defects with hair-bearing scalp, one donor site, and technical simplicity of the procedure. Potential drawbacks include the relative lack of scalp mobility and the potential to displace mobile structures, such as an eyebrow or hairline, if the flap is not properly planned.

Component separation of the scalp has been described by a number of authors to close small defects on the scalp. The layers of the scalp are delaminated, providing vascularized tissue to cover adjacent areas of bone exposure. Examples include galeal flaps, osteogaleal flaps, and temporoparietal fascial flaps.

Galeal flaps have proved to be an extremely useful source of vascularized tissue in craniofacial surgery. The galeal flap is commonly based on a named scalp vessel or combination of vessels to provide a reliable flap that can often cross the midline. When they are elevated with the frontalis muscle of the forehead, these flaps have proved invaluable in repair of defects in the anterior cranial base (Figs. 73-11 and 73-12). Galeal flaps have the advantage of an excellent blood supply with minimal donor site morbidity. The thin, supple nature of the flaps allows them to conform to complex three-dimensional defects.[61-64]

The temporoparietal fascial flap has found its greatest utility in ear reconstruction. However, it can be taken alone or with bone to repair a variety of craniofacial problems. The flap's vascular pedicle is based on the superficial temporal artery and vein (Fig. 73-13). The artery bifurcates into an anterior and

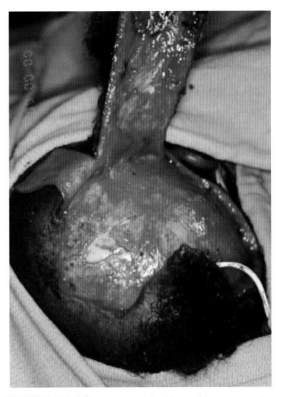

FIGURE 73-12. Bicoronal incision with preservation of the galeal frontalis flap for obliteration of a proposed defect in the anterior cranial fossa after resection of a meningioma.

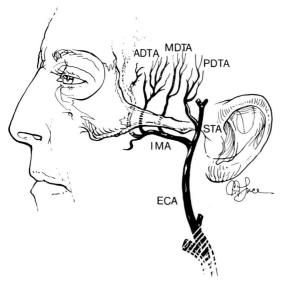

FIGURE 73-13. The superficial and deep temporal arterial system. The superficial temporal artery (STA) is a terminal branch of the external carotid artery (ECA), and the deep temporal artery is a branch of the internal maxillary artery (IMA). Note the terminal branches of these two systems, which make up the deep temporal artery. ADTA, anterior deep temporal artery; MDTA, middle deep temporal artery; PDTA, posterior deep temporal artery. (From McCarthy JG, Cutting CB, Shaw WW: Vascularized calvarial flaps. Clin Plast Surg 1987;14:40.)

posterior branch to supply the majority of the parietal region of the skull. Care should be taken to avoid inclusion of the anterior branch in the flap design. The frontal branch of the facial nerve runs close to this vessel. Injury can result in brow ptosis and unilateral forehead paralysis postoperatively. The plane of dissection between the overlying skin and the superficial temporal fascia is often difficult. Guiding the plane of dissection too superficially can result in damage to overlying hair follicles. The consequence can be postoperative alopecia. Despite these disadvantages, the flap is useful in reconstructive procedures. It has a reliable blood supply with an inconspicuous donor site. The flap is elastic and thin, and it is able to conform snugly to a variety of defects.[9-12] When it is used with underlying calvaria, it can provide a source of vascularized cranial bone for reconstruction of defects in the orbital and facial skeleton.

The subgaleal fascia is an ultrathin vascularized structure between the overlying galea and the underlying periosteum of the skull. This areolar layer receives its own blood flow from perforating vessels from the overlying galea. This delicate layer allows the movement of the galea on top of the pericranium. On the superficial and deep surfaces of this tissue is an areolar layer consisting of blood vessels and nerves. Between these two structures is a central lamina of collagenous tissue. With some difficulty, this layer can

be dissected free between the galea and periosteum. A cuff of galea is often preserved at the perforating vessel to prevent inadvertent injury to the vascular pedicle. The delicate nature of the flap allows its coaptation to complex three-dimensional structures such as the ear.[7] Alternatively, it can be raised with the underlying periosteum as a turnover flap to provide vascularized coverage for denuded calvaria.[8]

The temporalis fascia is a direct lateral extension of the scalp periosteum (Fig. 73-14).[65] This structure obtains its blood supply from the middle temporal artery, a branch of the superficial temporal artery. Thus, a composite flap of superficial temporal fascia and temporalis fascia can be isolated on the same vascular leash. By separation of the two fascial structures, the overall surface areas of the flap can be increased.

The temporalis muscle takes origin from the temporal fossa on the lateral portion of the skull. It passes under the zygomatic arch to insert on the coronoid process of the mandible. It receives its blood supply from the paired deep temporal arteries, which are branches of the internal maxillary artery. The surface of the muscle will require grafting if it is used to resurface a cutaneous or intraoral surface because there are no direct perforators to the overlying skin. The muscle has found its greatest utility in orbital reconstruction.[66-68] However, by release of the origin of the muscle, it can be rotated to fill defects that are more distant. Although the functional loss of one temporalis muscle is minimal, a cosmetically significant temporal hollow often remains after transfer of the muscle. This can often be camouflaged by insertion of one of the commercially available temporal implants into the resultant donor defect.[69]

Tissue Expanders

Tissue expansion is particularly useful in scalp reconstruction because it provides the surgeon with the

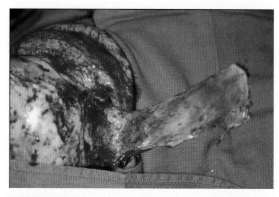

FIGURE 73-14. The temporalis fascia is a direct lateral extension of the scalp periosteum. It can be elevated with the temporalis muscle to obliterate defects in the anterior and middle cranial fossa.

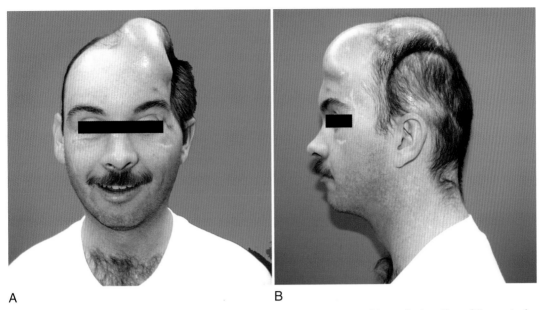

FIGURE 73-15. *A* and *B*, Insertion of tissue expanders to reconstruct a skin-grafted portion of the posterior scalp. Expansion allows the operator to replace missing tissue with a tissue of similar quality and thickness.

opportunity to replace missing tissue with a tissue of similar quality and thickness (Fig. 73-15).[24,70,71] The technique increases the amount of locally available tissue, preserves sensation, and maintains hair follicles and adnexal structures. In addition, tissue expansion produces a delay phenomenon, increasing the vascularity of the expanded flap.[72] Defects up to 50% of the scalp can be reconstructed without an appreciable change in hair density. The timing of expansion often depends on the etiology of the defect. If the lesion to be removed is benign, it is often possible to expand adjacent to the lesion primarily. In traumatic wounds or malignant processes, the wound is excised and closed temporarily with a skin graft or flap. Tissue expansion is initiated once there is stable coverage. Austad[73] advocates against tissue expansion in acute injuries because of the risk of contamination and implant exposure.

Care should be taken to map out vascular territories on the scalp preoperatively around the margin of the defect. The proposed flap should be designed on the scalp before the implantation of the expander. This will maximize flap length and avoid scars that could jeopardize flap vascularity. Placement of insertion incisions at the margin of the skin-grafted defect risks exposure of the implant. It is better to make a radial incision with respect to the point of highest tension of the expander remote from the defect. Endoscopy-assisted dissection gives adequate visualization of the pocket and ensures hemostasis.[74] Intuitively, one might assume that the most efficient plan for coverage of the scalp defect is the formation of an advancement flap

from the expanded tissue. However, Joss[75] noted that advancement flaps waste tissue at both ends of the flap. The tissue incorporated into these dog-ears can more efficiently be distributed over the defect by designing a rotation or transposition flap.

One of the major disadvantages of tissue expansion is the length of time it takes to expand the adjacent scalp. Expansion periods of 2 to 3 months are not uncommon. The goal is to establish a flap that is 50% longer and wider than the calculated need. The flap length can be estimated by measuring the distance over the dome of the implant and subtracting the base diameter of the expander. Another disadvantage is the requirement for two procedures, one to insert the expander and the second to remove the implant and develop flaps to rotate into the defect.

Tissue expansion of the scalp is not without problems. Complication rates as high as 48% have been described. Common problems include hematoma, implant exposure, infection, flap necrosis, alopecia, and wide scars. Pressure from the expander can deform the cranial vault. This may require burring of the calvaria to improve contour. This effect is more pronounced in children. However, unlike in adults, bone ridges from expanders in children often correct spontaneously during several months.[73,76]

Distant Flaps

More reliable pedicled regional musculocutaneous flaps and free tissue transfers have replaced multiple-staged tubed skin flaps. Regional musculocutaneous flaps include the trapezius, pectoralis major, latissimus dorsi, and splenius capitis flaps. All are useful flaps, but the respective arc of rotation does not permit the repair of vertex defects. Free tissue transplantation has proved more useful for massive defects of the cranial vault.

The pectoralis major musculocutaneous flap has proved to be useful for head and neck reconstruction for the past 25 years. With adequate mobilization, the muscle can reach temporal and mastoid regions of the skull. Inclusion of the rectus fascia and transection of the clavicle can extend the arc of rotation of the flap. The donor defect leaves a minimal functional deficit. The flap can be somewhat bulky if a skin paddle is included. Breast distortion may occur if the musculo-cutaneous option is used in women.[77-79]

Both the pedicled and free variants of the latissimus dorsi flap are useful for scalp reconstruction. By passage of the muscle through the axilla, defects in the orbit and temporal bone can be repaired. Risks include brachial plexus injury and axillary vessel injury.[80-82] Larger defects (Fig. 73-16) are best treated with micro-surgical techniques.[83]

The trapezius muscle receives its blood supply from the transverse cervical, dorsal scapular, and occipital arteries. Some blood flow is additionally obtained from the paraspinal perforators. Two flaps have been described, a transverse flap based on the upper portion of the muscle and a vertical flap consisting of middle and inferior fibers of the trapezius.[84,85] The transverse design may result in shoulder drop. It should be used only in individuals with previous sacrifice of the spinal accessory nerve. This flap is most useful for temporal and neck coverage. The vertical flap design has minimal functional consequence and is the more useful for scalp reconstruction. By design of a skin island between the spine and the scapula, defects of the occipital region can be reached. The donor site can often be closed primarily.[86-88]

The splenius capitis muscle receives its blood supply from the occipital, transverse cervical, and ver-tebral arteries. By basing the muscle superiorly on the occipital artery, defects of the neck and occiput can be covered.[89]

Microvascular Composite Tissue Transplantation

For extensive defects of the skull, local and regional flaps are often inadequate. Free tissue transplantation is the best solution because of the lack of dependence on a fixed point of rotation and reliability. In experi-enced hands, survival rates in excess of 90% have been described. Wide varieties of flap types have been described in the literature, each with its advantages and disadvantages. The most common transplants are the latissimus, scapular, radial forearm, and omental flaps.[29,30,90,91] Recipient vessels have included the superficial temporal artery and vein as well as multi-ple different branches of the external carotid vascula-ture (Fig. 73-17). Selection of the flap should be based on the amount of tissue required to cover the defect as well as the length of the vascular pedicle. Long vein grafts should be avoided, if possible, because the inci-dence of perioperative thrombosis of the flap is increased.

The skin-grafted latissimus is particularly useful in massive defects of the skull. It has a long vascular pedicle, which often allows primary anastomosis in the neck. The intermuscular blood supply of the latissimus allows the muscle to be split into two distinct musculocutaneous flaps for coverage of complex three-dimensional defects. If additional muscle is required, the serratus anterior and scapular flaps can be carried on the subscapular vascular pedicle.

Free hair-bearing flaps have been described in the literature. A temporo-occipital scalp flap can be ele-vated on the superficial temporal artery and vein.[92,93] The flap can be transplanted to the contralateral side and anastomosed to the temporal vessels, providing coverage on the alopecic side. Advantages include a one-stage hair-bearing reconstruction with hair of normal direction and density. A preliminary tissue expansion phase can ensure that the donor site is closed primarily.

Scalp Replantation

The first successful microsurgical replantation of the scalp was described in 1976.[94] Since that time, replan-tation has been the treatment of choice for complete or nearly complete avulsions of the scalp. There is no other method of scalp reconstruction that can match the results from replantation. Avulsions usually result from entanglement of long hair in moving machin-ery, applying an oblique shearing force to the scalp. Other causes have included dog bites, motor vehicle accidents, farm tractors, and boat motors. Scalp avul-sions follow a predictable pattern, depending on the force applied and on the amount and location of hair. Scalp avulsions occur in the loose areolar layer between the galea and the periosteum. If the force is extensive, shearing will occur until it reaches the fascial attach-ments of the thinnest portion of the skin in the supra-orbital, temporal, auricular, and occipital regions. The temporal tears often include the superior portion of the ear, probably because of galeal insertions into the superior auricular muscles. Blood loss is often exten-sive. Fluids and blood products should be replaced vigorously (Fig. 73-18).

Because of the avulsive nature of the injury, resec-tion of damaged vessels and primary vein grafting are often required. Vein grafts are a necessary

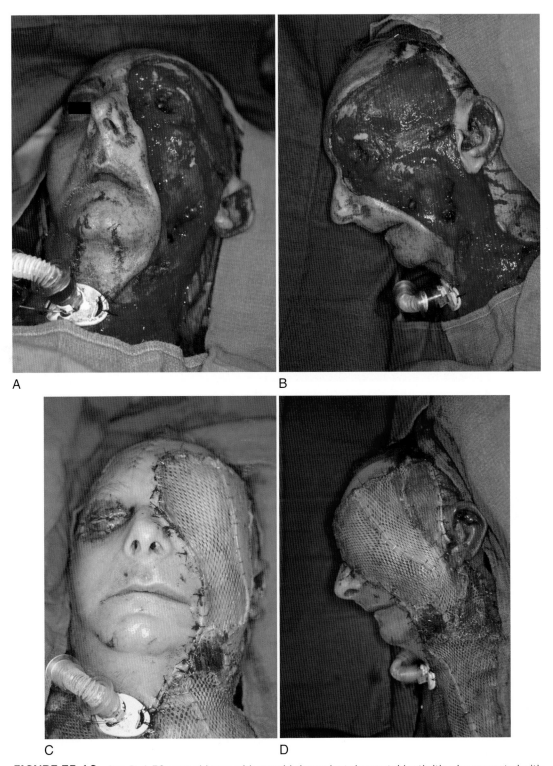

FIGURE 73-16. *A to D,* A 58-year-old man with steroid-dependent rheumatoid arthritis who presented with a necrotizing infection of the head and neck. After serial débridement and enucleation of the left eye, coverage was effected with a combination of a free latissimus muscle flap and pectoralis muscle flap with skin graft.

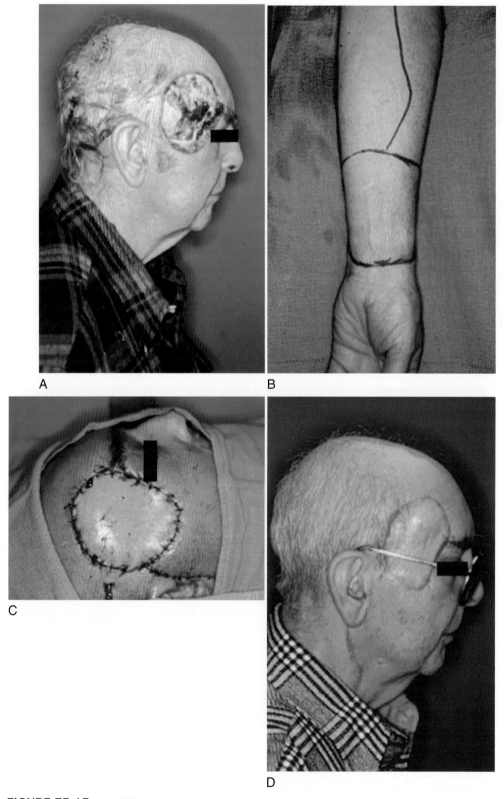

FIGURE 73-17. *A,* A 72-year-old man after Mohs resection of an invasive squamous cell carcinoma of the temporal fossa. *B,* Outline of a radial forearm flap on the nondominant forearm. *C* and *D,* Early and late postoperative result with use of the branches of the external carotid and jugular vein as recipient vessels.

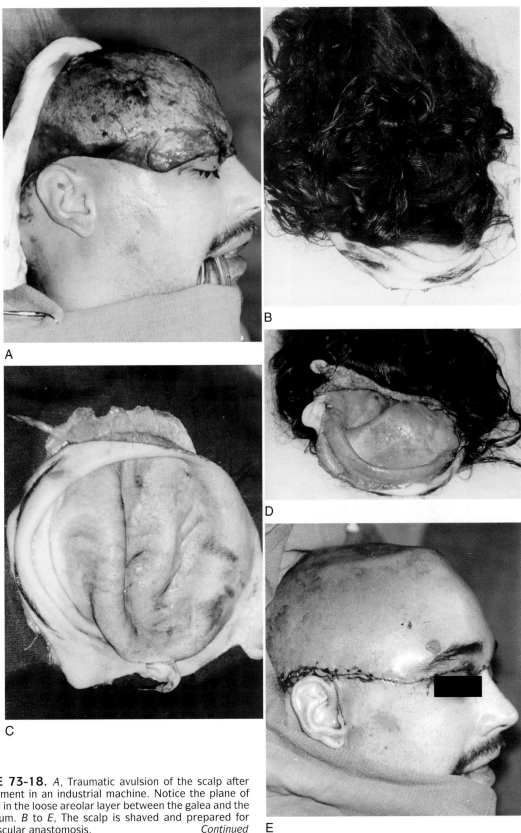

FIGURE 73-18. *A*, Traumatic avulsion of the scalp after entanglement in an industrial machine. Notice the plane of cleavage in the loose areolar layer between the galea and the periosteum. *B* to *E*, The scalp is shaved and prepared for microvascular anastomosis. *Continued*

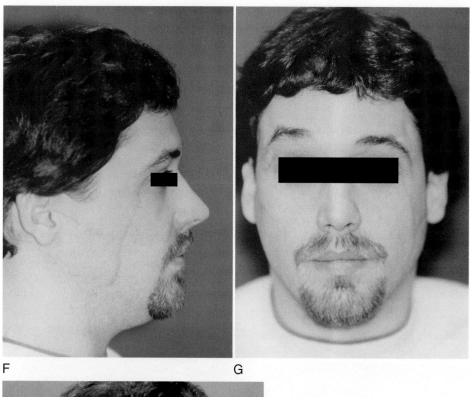

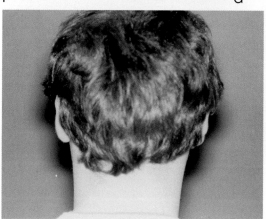

FIGURE 73-18, cont'd. *F*, Late postoperative result showing lush hair growth. *G* and *H*, No other method of reconstruction can replace hair-bearing scalp, eyebrows, and portions of ear and forehead musculature in one procedure.

precondition to perform microvascular repair out of the zone of injury. To minimize the ischemic interval and to aid in the identification of suitable veins, the arterial repair is completed first. Most commonly, the superficial temporal artery has been used for microsurgical repair. One superficial temporal artery is capable of ensuring the survival of the entire scalp (Fig. 73-19). The occipital, supraorbital, and postauricular vessels have also been used. Microvascular clips should be placed on draining veins to prevent blood loss while the venous circulation is re-established. At

least two venous repairs should be attempted to prevent flap congestion and subsequent venous insufficiency.[95-98]

Contraindications to replantation of the scalp are few. These include hemodynamic instability of the patient and a severely macerated amputated part with multiple segmental injuries. Concomitant severe life-threatening injuries that prohibit a lengthy operation are an obvious contraindication. Every attempt should be made to replant the scalp if possible. No other method of reconstruction can replace hair-bearing

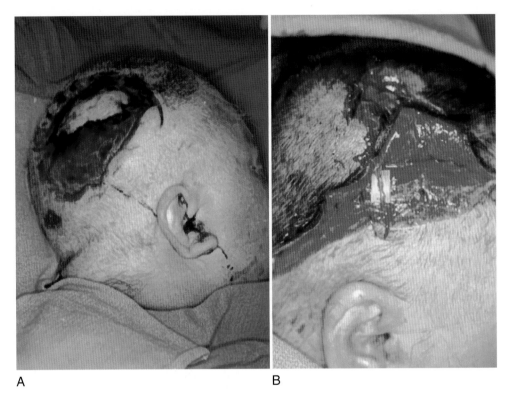

FIGURE 73-19. *A,* A 28-year-old man who sustained a full-thickness scalp avulsion after being ejected through an automobile window. *B,* Preparation of the superior temporal artery and vein for microvascular anastomosis.

scalp, eyebrows, and portions of ear and forehead musculature in one procedure.

HAIR RESTORATION

Hair Cycle

On average, each human scalp has about 140,000 hairs. Scalp hair grows 0.35 mm/day. However, this rate can be affected by age, nutrition, pregnancy, and environmental factors. There are two types of hair, vellus and terminal. Vellus hair is short and uncolored. Terminal hair is long, brittle, and colored.

The visible hair shaft is composed of keratin, the end product of growth of the hair matrix. The matrix of all hair follicles undergoes cycles of growth and degeneration. The hair cycle has three phases: the growth phase (anagen), the resting phase (catagen), and the shedding phase (telogen). At any give time, about 90% of human hairs are in the growing phase. The growing phase of human scalp hair is about 1000 days; catagen lasts 2 to 3 weeks, and telogen lasts a few months.[99,100]

Etiology of Hair Loss

The etiology of male pattern baldness is related to androgen metabolism, genetic predisposition, and age.

About 30% of men show some element of balding by their mid-30s; this increases to 60% by the age of 60 years. At 20 years of age, hair density is 615 follicles/cm². By 50 years, this number has dropped to 485 follicles/cm². Bald scalps usually have less than 300 follicles/cm², generating only vellus hairs.

Men castrated before puberty do not develop male pattern hair loss. If they are treated with testosterone early in life, they develop hair loss patterns similar to those of age-matched controls. Blood levels of testosterone are similar in balding and nonbalding men. Testosterone, secreted by the testis, is the principal androgen circulating in the plasma in men. Androgenic alopecia appears to be dependent on the action of serum dihydrotestosterone (Fig. 73-20). Testosterone is converted to dihydrotestosterone by the enzyme 5α-reductase. Dihydrotestosterone may be a more potent androgen than testosterone because it binds more tightly to androgen receptors within the cell. It is thought to be the hormone responsible for male pattern baldness. Balding follicles have higher concentrations of 5α-reductase activity than do nonbalding follicles. The mechanism by which dihydrotestosterone causes baldness within the cell is not understood. It has been suggested that dihydrotestosterone has an inhibitory effect on cyclic adenosine

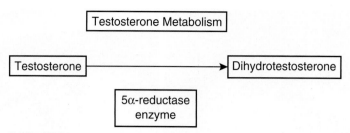

FIGURE 73-20. Testosterone is converted to dihydrotestosterone by the enzyme 5α-reductase. Dihydrotestosterone may be a more potent androgen than testosterone because it binds more tightly to androgen receptors within the cell. It is thought to be the hormone responsible for male pattern baldness. Balding follicles have higher concentrations of 5α-reductase activity than do nonbalding follicles. The mechanism by which dihydrotestosterone causes baldness within the cell is not understood.

monophosphate within the hair follicle. This effect is thought to result in shortening of the hair cycle and an increased transition of anagen hairs into telogen hairs and later into miniaturized hairs.

The relationship between hair loss and genes is probably multifactorial or polygenic. It is likely that several genes combined with genetic factors are responsible for hair loss.

Classification of Hair Loss Patterns

Norwood's classification[101] of male pattern baldness is probably the most commonly used today (Fig. 73-21). Type I is minimal recession of the anterior hairline. Type II is frontotemporal recession that does not extend more than 2 cm from a line drawn in the coronal plane from each external auditory meatus. Type III is deep temporal recession within 2 cm of the midcoronal line. Type III vertex is type III recession with associated balding in the vertex. Type IV is more severe frontal recession than type III with vertex involvement. There is a moderately dense bridge of hair-bearing tissue that separates the area of frontal balding from the vertex. Type V is similar to type IV in that the vertex and frontotemporal recession regions remain separate. However, the band of hair-bearing tissue separating the two regions is sparse, and the bald areas are increased in size. In type VI, there is a loss of the bridge of hair-bearing tissue between the frontal region and the vertex. A narrow horseshoe of hair-bearing tissue that begins just anterior to the ear and extends low occipitally characterizes type VII.

There is an A variant of male pattern alopecia. This pattern is characterized by progressive recession of the anterior hairline without simultaneous development of associated vertex alopecia.

Male pattern baldness is uncommon in women unless a virilizing disease affects them. Most commonly, these patients have associated hirsutism and acne. A thorough endocrinologic workup is in order. Female baldness is characterized by incomplete coronal hair loss with diffuse thinning of hair. There is a general decrease in density of the hair, without any particular pattern. Ludwig[102] classifies this into three types: I, mild; II, moderate; and III, severe. There may be sparing of the occipital region, making surgical correction possible.

There are three options in the treatment of male pattern baldness: medical treatment, surgical therapy, and a hairpiece.

Medical Treatment

Minoxidil (Rogaine) is an antihypertensive drug that was found to cause hypertrichosis as a side effect of treatment. When minoxidil is applied as a topical 2% solution twice daily to individuals with hair loss, 8% have dense regrowth, 31% have moderate regrowth, 36% have minimal regrowth, and 25% have no regrowth. It was able to halt further hair loss in the majority of patients. Regrown hairs fall out 4 to 6 months after use is terminated. The drug is not as effective in patients with extensive areas of baldness (Norwood types V to VII). The mechanism of action of the drug is unknown, but it is thought to exert its effect by producing a local vasodilatory effect on the follicular epithelium.[103,104]

Finasteride (Propecia) is a 5α-reductase inhibitor. It was originally used in the treatment of benign prostatic hypertrophy under the trade name Proscar in a dosage of 5 mg/day. Given at a dose of 1 mg/day, the drug was found to decrease hair loss and to improve hair density. Finasteride has been shown to reverse the conversion of terminal hairs to vellus hairs. It also promotes the conversion of hair follicles to the anagen phase. The drug is contraindicated in women and children. It may cause genital abnormalities in the developing male fetus. About 2% of men have

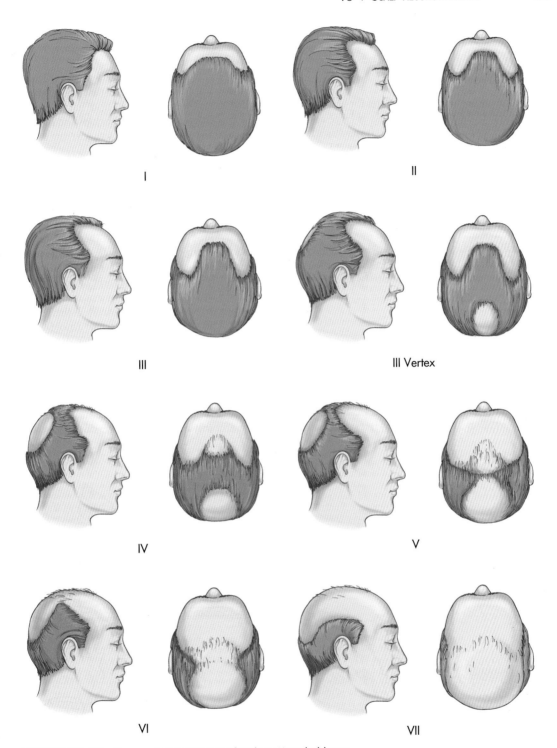

FIGURE 73-21. Norwood classification of male pattern baldness.

sexual side effects that necessitate termination of therapy.[105-107]

Surgical Treatment

Not all patients are suitable candidates for hair restoration surgery. If the area of baldness is large and the available donor site hair is limited, it may be impossible to achieve an aesthetically acceptable result. Younger individuals with thinning hair but a family history of significant hair loss are also problematic. Future hair loss should be anticipated and donor sites preserved. Reconstruction should be directed at restoration of the frontal hairline rather than random distribution of grafts over the scalp or vertex.

Surgical reconstruction is broadly classified into hair transplantation as free grafts, direct excision, flap reconstruction, and scalp expansion by a variety of techniques.

Hair Transplantation

Orentreich[108] is attributed with development of the multiple punch graft technique for the treatment of androgenic alopecia. Round composite grafts were harvested from the temporo-occipital region and transplanted into the recipient holes established in the frontal region and the vertex. He established the concept of donor site dominance of the lower parieto-occipital region in maximizing hair growth after hair transplantation.

The punch graft technique was complicated by a "cornrow" or "doll's hair" look that was most obvious in the frontal hairline. In addition, harvesting of multiple punch grafts from the back of the head proved on occasion to result in extensive scarring and wasted precious donor material.

The trend in modern hair transplantation surgery is to use smaller hair-follicle units. Although it is much more labor-intensive, minigraft (1 to 2.5 mm) and micrograft (<1.5 mm) reconstruction has resulted in superior aesthetic results.[109-111]

The donor site is selected in the fringe area of the temporo-occipital region (Fig. 73-22). Donor hair is trimmed to a length of 2 to 3 mm before elliptical strip removal under local anesthesia. The strip can be removed with a No. 10 blade or a multiple-blade knife separated by spacers. The donor site is then closed primarily. The strip is "bread loafed" into 1-mm slices with a razor blade. The slices are then dissected under magnification to yield grafts varying from one hair to as many as four hairs per graft.

The most difficult aspect of hair transplantation is to construct a natural hairline. The hairline should not be excessively low in the midline and include a moderate amount of temporal recession. The hairline is

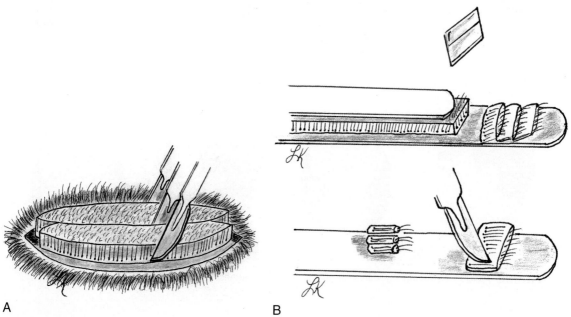

A   B

FIGURE 73-22. Hair transplantation by a minigraft (1 to 2.5 mm) or micrograft (<1.5 mm). The donor site is selected in the fringe area of the temporo-occipital region. *A,* Diagrammatic representation of a multiple-blade knife harvesting strips of donor hair from the occipital donor site. It is important to keep the angle of the blade parallel to the hair follicles to prevent injury to the donor grafts. *B,* The strip is "bread loafed" into 1-mm slices with a razor blade. The slices are then dissected under magnification to yield grafts varying from one hair to as many as four hairs per graft.

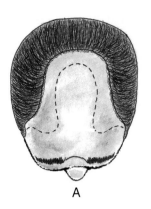
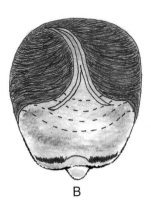

FIGURE 73-23. Scalp reduction. *A,* A horseshoe incision is made around the margin of the hair-bearing scalp. The scalp is undermined inferiorly both occipitally and temporally in the subgaleal plane. The flaps are transposed superiorly and medially to delineate the amount of bald scalp to be excised. *B,* After two or three serial excisions, the amount of residual alopecic scalp requiring free grafting is significantly reduced.

A   B

actually a transition zone rather than a fixed point on the scalp. The finest hairs are located most anteriorly, blending to coarser hairs posteriorly. This transition zone should be duplicated; single-hair grafts are placed most anteriorly, followed by two- and three-hair grafts as one progresses posteriorly.

The graft recipient sites have been made in the bald scalp with a variety of different instruments, including needles, blades, punches, and lasers. The angle of each slit should be made carefully to re-establish the patient's original hair pattern. In general, this is forward in the frontal and middle scalp. More posteriorly, the radial whorl in the crown should be duplicated. Grafts are implanted into the recipient holes, ensuring that the epidermal surface of the graft is flush with the scalp. A pressure dressing is applied overnight. The patient is allowed to shampoo the next day.

During the next 3 to 4 weeks, the hair enters the phase of telogen and begins to fall out. Regrowth usually occurs at 3 months from the time of surgery. Complications of the procedure include temporary swelling and pain. Numbness of the scalp is often noted after the procedure. It tends to improve with time. Infection is a relatively rare complication. Poor graft take, graft compression, and pitting around the grafts can occasionally be noted. Pitting is due to excessive seating of the graft below the epidermal surface of the scalp. Hypertrophic scarring and spreading of the donor site scar have been described.

Scalp Reduction

This technique was popularized by the Unger brothers in 1978 as a means of decreasing the area of bald scalp to improve the donor-to-recipient ratio in patients undergoing a hair transplantation procedure.[112,113] The original technique involved excision of a longitudinal ellipse of skin from the central portion of the scalp (Fig. 73-23). Problems with the technique included stretchback of the scar and a slot formation

in the posterior scalp due to the abnormal direction of the hairs of the advanced flaps. Frechet[114] has described a flap to correct this problem and to establish the normal whorl pattern over the vertex of the skull. Numerous modifications of this technique have evolved by excision of various patterns of tissue from the central and lateral scalp. Wide undermining past the galea into the nape of the neck and supra-auricular and postauricular areas has been performed to recruit more hair-bearing skin to the vertex. Risks have included scarring, flap necrosis, and hair loss due to diminished vascularity of the flaps.[115]

Tissue Expansion

Tissue expansion has been reported for the treatment of male pattern baldness. It has the advantage of providing tissue that matches the scalp in color, texture, and hair-bearing characteristics. Tissue expansion can be used as an adjunct to scalp reduction techniques or incorporated into various flap designs. The process of expansion enhances the vascularity of the overlying scalp, allowing the design of more reliable flaps to cover the balding regions. Anderson[116] has described combining tissue expansion with a Juri flap to provide frontal hairline reconstruction. He has subsequently modified his flap design to reconstruct large areas of alopecia. His expanded bilateral advancement transposition flaps allow two-staged reconstruction of the frontal hairline. Advantages include more ideal hair direction, formation of a temporal recession, and smaller dog-ear than with the expanded Juri flap. His expanded triple advancement transposition flap modification is similar to the bilateral advancement transposition flap but adds a third expanded occipital transposition flap to repair the occiput.

Disadvantages of tissue expansion include the obvious cosmetic deformity the patient experiences during the period of expansion. This often extends for 2 to 3 months. The need for two procedures and the potential for implant infection and flap necrosis should be carefully explained to the patient before embarking on this course of treatment.

Frechet[117] developed an ingenious modification of the scalp expansion concept. Scalp extenders consist of two parallel strips of silicone elastomer with rows of hooks attached to each end. The device is stretched, and hooks are inserted onto the undersurface of the galea. By a process of continuous nonvolumetric expansion, hair-bearing scalp is generated over the vertex of the skull. The device is usually inserted at the time of initial scalp reduction surgery. At 4 to 6 weeks, the device can be removed, allowing a second more extensive scalp reduction procedure. A major advantage is the lack of cosmetic deformity during the tissue expansion process.

Scalp Flaps

The main advantage of using flaps to treat male pattern baldness is the ability to establish hair of normal density in previous regions of alopecia in one stage. Growth of the hair is immediate, without the intervening stage of telogen that follows hair transplantation procedures. The transposed hair has a superior density compared with most grafting techniques.

Juri[118,119] first popularized the use of the temporoparieto-occipital flap in scalp reconstruction. This hair-bearing transfer is based on the parietal branch of the superficial temporal artery. To ensure survival of the tip of the flap, two preliminary delay procedures are carried out before transposition. Flaps as long as 28 cm based on a 4-cm pedicle have been described. One week after the second delay, the flap is elevated and transposed to the frontal hairline. The anterior scalp incision should be beveled anteriorly to allow hair from the flap to grow up through the incision line. This apparently softens the abrupt appearance of the anterior hairline. For areas of more extensive baldness, a second flap can be performed a month later and transposed behind the first flap.

Several authors have described modifications of the flap. Nordstrom[120] was able to narrow the pedicle of the flap to 2 cm by including the vascular supply of the retroauricular artery with the superficial temporal vessels. He described only two patients who experienced flap necrosis in 55 flaps without use of a preliminary surgical delay.

Fleming and Mayer[121] have modified their temporoparietal flap to improve the frontal hairline. The design of the superior portion of the flap is irregular, resulting in the illusion of a less abrupt frontal hairline. A frontotemporal recession is established, preventing the development of an ape-like hairline.

A number of serious complications have followed flap transposition. These include flap necrosis and donor site dehiscence. Less serious problems have included poor hairline design, abrupt transition from bald to hair-bearing scalp, hairline scars, and donor site alopecia. In addition, the direction of hair within the flap is different from that of normal scalp hair. Instead of being oriented anteriorly, the flap hair is directed posteriorly. A patient may experience problems with hair styling if the hair is combed forward or laterally. However, if normal hair density is a patient's priority, no other method of alopecia correction approaches flap reconstruction.

ACKNOWLEDGMENTS

I would like to thank Linda Knapp, RN, of Crystal Plastic Surgeons for her assistance with the artwork and Roderick Jordan, MD, of MetroHealth Medical Center of Cleveland for kindly providing some patient photographs for this chapter.

REFERENCES

1. Mustoe TA, Corral CJ: Soft tissue reconstructive choices for craniofacial reconstruction. Clin Plast Surg 1995;22:543-554.
2. Ortiz MF: Surgical anatomy of the scalp. Plast Reconstr Surg 1992;90:335-336.
3. Tremolada C, Candiani P, Signorini M, et al: The surgical anatomy of the subcutaneous facial system of the scalp. Ann Plast Surg 1994;32:8-14.
4. Mitz V, Peyronie M: The superficial musculo-aponeurotic system (SMAS) in the parotid and cheek area. Plast Reconstr Surg 1976;58:80-88.
5. Jost G, Levet Y: Parotid fascia and face lifting: a critical evaluation of the SMAS concept. Plast Reconstr Surg 1984;74:42-51.
6. Tolhurst DE, Carstens MH, Greco RJ, et al: The surgical anatomy of the scalp. Plast Reconstr Surg 1991;87:603-612.
7. Carstens MH, Greco RJ, Hurwitz DJ, et al: Clinical applications of the subgaleal fascia. Plast Reconstr Surg 1991;87:615-626.
8. Lai CS, Lin SD, Chou CK, et al: The subgalea-periosteal turnover flap for reconstruction of scalp defects. Ann Plast Surg 1993;30:267-271.
9. Batchelor J, McGuinness A: Microvascular anatomy of the galeal and temporoparietal fascia. Plast Reconstr Surg 1996;97:1085.
10. Brent B, Byrd HS: Secondary ear reconstruction with cartilage grafts covered by axial, random, and free flaps of temporoparietal fascia. Plast Reconstr Surg 1983;72:141-152.
11. Tellioglu AT, Tekdemir I, Erdemli EA, et al: Temporoparietal fascia: an anatomic and histologic reinvestigation with new potential clinical applications. Plast Reconstr Surg 2000;105:40-45.
12. Stuzin JM, Wagstrom L, Kawamoto HK, et al: Anatomy of the frontal branch of the facial nerve: the significance of the temporal fat pad. Plast Reconstr Surg 1989;83:265-271.
13. TerKonda RP, Sykes JM: Concepts in scalp and forehead reconstruction. Otolaryngol Clin North Am 1997;30:519-539.
14. Minor LB, Panje WR: Malignant neoplasms of the scalp. Etiology, resection, and reconstruction. Otolaryngol Clin North Am 1993;26:279-293.
15. Headington JT: Cicatricial alopecia. Dermatol Clin 1996;14:773-782.
16. Whiting DA: Cicatricial alopecia: clinico-pathological findings and treatment. Clin Dermatol 2001;19:211-225.
17. Evers ME, Steijlen PM, Hamel BC: Aplasia cutis congenita and associated disorders: an update. Clin Genet 1995;47:295-301.
18. Kruk-Jeromin J, Janik J, Rykala J: Aplasia cutis congenita of the scalp. Report of 16 cases. Dermatol Surg 1998;24:549-553.

19. Yilmaz S, Apaydin I, Yenidunya O, et al: Conservative management of aplasia cutis congenita. Dermatol Surg 1997;23:402-403.

20. Kim CS, Tatum SA, Rodziewicz G: Scalp aplasia cutis congenita presenting with sagittal sinus hemorrhage. Arch Otolaryngol Head Neck Surg 2001;127:71-74.

21. Islamoglu K, Ozgentas E: Aplasia cutis congenita of the scalp: excessive bleeding and reconstructive problems. Ann Plast Surg 2001;47:213-214.

22. Felman G: Post-thermal burn alopecia and its treatment using extensive horizontal scalp reduction in combination with a Juri flap. Plast Reconstr Surg 1994;93:1268-1273.

23. Cooper RL, Brown D: Pretransfer tissue expansion of a scalp free flap for burn alopecia reconstruction in a child: a case report. J Reconstr Microsurg 1990;6:339-343.

24. Zuker RM: The use of tissue expansion in pediatric scalp burn reconstruction. J Burn Care Rehabil 1987;8:103-106.

25. Luce EA, Hoopes JE: Electrical burn of the scalp and skull. Case report. Plast Reconstr Surg 1974;54:359-363.

26. Boucher J, Raglon B, Valdez S, et al: Possible role of chemical hair care products in 10 patients with face, scalp, ear, back, neck and extremity burns. Burns 1990;16:146-147.

27. Di Meo L, Jones BM: Surgical treatment of radiation-induced scalp lesions. Br J Plast Surg 1984;37:373-378.

28. Kim YH, Aye MS, Fayos JV: Radiation necrosis of the scalp: a complication of cranial irradiation and methotrexate. Radiology 1977;124:813-814.

29. Shen Z: Reconstruction of refractory defect of scalp and skull using microsurgical free flap transfer. Microsurgery 1994;15:633-638.

30. Lutz BS, Wei FC, Chen HC, et al: Reconstruction of scalp defects with free flaps in 30 cases. Br J Plast Surg 1998;51:186-190.

31. Oishi SN, Luce EA: The difficult scalp and skull wound. Clin Plast Surg 1995;22:51-59.

32. Jackson JM, Callen JP: Scarring alopecia and sclerodermatous changes of the scalp in a patient with hepatitis C infection. J Am Acad Dermatol 1998;39(pt 2):824-826.

33. Stephens CJ, Hay RJ, Black MM: Fungal kerion—total scalp involvement due to *Microsporum canis* infection. Clin Exp Dermatol 1989;14:442-444.

34. Frentz G, Sorensen JL, Flod K: Non melanoma skin cancer of the scalp. On the etiology. Acta Derm Venereol 1989;69:142-146.

35. Beer GM, Widder W, Cierpka K, et al: Malignant tumors associated with nevus sebaceous: therapeutic consequences. Aesthetic Plast Surg 1999;23:224-227.

36. Jang IG, Choi JM, Park KW, et al: Nevus sebaceous syndrome. Int J Dermatol 1999;38:531-533.

37. Gorlin RJ: Nevoid basal cell carcinoma syndrome. Dermatol Clin 1995;13:113-125.

38. Mirowski GW, Liu AA, Parks ET, et al: Nevoid basal cell carcinoma syndrome. J Am Acad Dermatol 2000;43:1092-1093.

39. Benmeir P, Baruchin A, Lusthaus S, et al: Melanoma of the scalp: the invisible killer. Plast Reconstr Surg 1995;95:496-500.

40. Shumate CR, Carlson GW, Giacco GG, et al: The prognostic implications of location for scalp melanoma. Am J Surg 1991;162:315-319.

41. Hudson DA, Krige JE: Results of 3 cm excision margin for melanoma of the scalp. J R Coll Surg Edinb 1995;40:93-96.

42. Tucker MA, Greene MH, Clark WH Jr, et al: Dysplastic nevi on the scalp of prepubertal children from melanoma-prone families. J Pediatr 1983;103:65-69.

43. Bartle EJ, Sun JH, Wang XW, et al: Cancers arising from burn scars. A literature review and report of twenty-one cases. J Burn Care Rehabil 1990;11:46-49.

44. Mitra S, Narasimharao KL, Pathak IC: Xeroderma pigmentosa. J Indian Med Assoc 1983;81:204-205.

45. Lang NP, Kendrick JH, Flanigin H, et al: Surgical management of advanced scalp cancer. Head Neck Surg 1983;5:299-305.

46. Schaefer SD, Byrd HS, Holmes RE: Forehead and scalp reconstruction after wide-field resection of skin carcinoma. Arch Otolaryngol 1980;106:680-684.

47. Thompson JF: The Sydney Melanoma Unit experience of sentinel lymphadenectomy for melanoma. Ann Surg Oncol 2001;8(suppl):44S-47S.

48. Uren RF, Thompson JF, Howman-Giles R: Sentinel lymph node biopsy in patients with melanoma and breast cancer. Intern Med J 2001;31:547-553.

49. Chao C, McMasters KM: Update on the use of sentinel node biopsy in patients with melanoma: who and how. Curr Opin Oncol 2002;14:217-220.

50. Becker GD, Adams LA, Levin BC: Secondary intention healing of exposed scalp and forehead bone after Mohs surgery. Otolaryngol Head Neck Surg 1999;121:751-754.

51. Snow SN, Stiff MA, Bullen R, et al: Second-intention healing of exposed facial-scalp bone after Mohs surgery for skin cancer: review of ninety-one cases. J Am Acad Dermatol 1994;31(pt 1):450-454.

52. Millard DR: The crane principle for the transport of subcutaneous tissue. Plast Reconstr Surg 1969;43:451-462.

53. Gonzalez-Ulloa M: Regional aesthetic units of the face. Plast Reconstr Surg 1987;79:489-490.

54. Burget GC, Menick FJ: The subunit principle in nasal reconstruction. Plast Reconstr Surg 1985;76:239-247.

55. Cox AJ III, Wang TD, Cook TA: Closure of a scalp defect. Arch Facial Plast Surg 1999;1:212-215.

56. Ritchie AJ, Rocke LG: Staples versus sutures in the closure of scalp wounds: a prospective, double-blind, randomized trial. Injury 1989;20:217-218.

57. Arnold PG, Rangarathnam CS: Multiple-flap scalp reconstruction: Orticochea revisited. Plast Reconstr Surg 1982;69:605-613.

58. Orticochea M: Four flap scalp reconstruction technique. Br J Plast Surg 1967;20:159-171.

59. Orticochea M: New three-flap reconstruction technique. Br J Plast Surg 1971;24:184-188.

60. Wooden WA, Curtsinger LJ, Jones NF: The four-poster halo vest for protection of a microvascular free-tissue transfer reconstruction of the scalp. Plast Reconstr Surg 1995;95:166-167.

61. Jackson IT, Adham MN, Marsh WR: Use of the galeal frontalis myofascial flap in craniofacial surgery. Plast Reconstr Surg 1986;77:905-910.

62. Sharma RK, Kobayashi K, Jackson IT, et al: Vascular anatomy of the galeal occipitalis flap: a cadaver study. Plast Reconstr Surg 1996;97:25-31.

63. Fukuta K, Potparic Z, Sugihara T, et al: A cadaver investigation of the blood supply of the galeal frontalis flap. Plast Reconstr Surg 1994;94:794-800.

64. To EW, Pang PC, Chan DT, et al: Subcranial anterior skull base dural repair with galeal frontalis flap. Br J Plast Surg 2001;54:457-460.

65. Hirase Y, Kojima T, Hirakawa M: Secondary ear reconstruction using deep temporal fascia after temporoparietal fascial reconstruction in microtia. Ann Plast Surg 1990;25:53-57.

66. Cordeiro PG, Wolfe SA: The temporalis muscle flap revisited on its centennial: advantages, newer uses, and disadvantages. Plast Reconstr Surg 1996;98:980-987.

67. Hanasono MM, Utley DS, Goode RL: The temporalis muscle flap for reconstruction after head and neck oncologic surgery. Laryngoscope 2001;111:1719-1725.

68. Yucel A, Yazar S, Aydin Y, et al: Temporalis muscle flap for craniofacial reconstruction after tumor resection. J Craniofac Surg 2000;11:258-264.

69. Watanabe K, Miyagi H, Tsurukiri K: Augmentation of temporal area by insertion of silicone plate under the temporal fascia. Ann Plast Surg 1984;13:309-319.

70. Antonyshyn O, Gruss JS, Zuker R, et al: Tissue expansion in head and neck reconstruction. Plast Reconstr Surg 1988;82:58-68.

71. Wieslander JB: Repeated tissue expansion in reconstruction of a huge combined scalp-forehead avulsion injury. Ann Plast Surg 1988;20:381-385.

72. Austad ED, Pasyk KA, McClatchey KD, et al: Histomorphologic evaluation of guinea pig skin and soft tissue after controlled tissue expansion. Plast Reconstr Surg 1982;70:704-710.

73. Austad ED: Contraindications and complications in tissue expansion. Facial Plast Surg 1988;5:379-382.

74. Serra JM: Retractor with mobile endoscope. Plast Reconstr Surg 1997;100:529-531.

75. Joss GS, Zoltie N, Chapman P: Tissue expansion technique and the transposition flap. Br J Plast Surg 1990;43:328-333.

76. Antonyshyn O, Gruss JS, Mackinnon SE, et al: Complications of soft tissue expansion. Br J Plast Surg 1988;41:239-250.

77. Ariyan S: The pectoralis major myocutaneous flap. A versatile flap for reconstruction in the head and neck. Plast Reconstr Surg 1979;63:73-81.

78. Liu R, Gullane P, Brown D, et al: Pectoralis major myocutaneous pedicled flap in head and neck reconstruction: retrospective review of indications and results in 244 consecutive cases at the Toronto General Hospital. J Otolaryngol 2001;30:34-40.

79. Palmer JH, Batchelor AG: The functional pectoralis major musculocutaneous island flap in head and neck reconstruction. Plast Reconstr Surg 1990;85:363-367.

80. Hayden RE, Kirb SD, Deschler DG: Technical modifications of the latissimus dorsi pedicled flap to increase versatility and viability. Laryngoscope 2000;110:352-357.

81. Prakash PJ, Gupta AK: The subscapular approach in head and neck reconstruction with the pedicled latissimus dorsi myocutaneous flap. Br J Plast Surg 2001;54:680-683.

82. Freedlander E: Brachial plexus cord compression by the tendon of a pedicled latissimus dorsi flap. Br J Plast Surg 1986;39:514-515.

83. Tanaka Y, Miki K, Tajima S, et al: Reconstruction of an extensive scalp defect using the split latissimus dorsi flap in combination with the serratus anterior musculo-osseous flap. Br J Plast Surg 1998;51:250-254.

84. Yang D, Morris SF: Trapezius muscle: anatomic basis for flap design. Ann Plast Surg 1998;41:52-57.

85. Panje WR: Myocutaneous trapezius flap. Head Neck Surg 1980;2:206-212.

86. Lynch JR, Hansen JE, Chaffoo R, et al: The lower trapezius musculocutaneous flap revisited: versatile coverage for complicated wounds to the posterior cervical and occipital regions based on the deep branch of the transverse cervical artery. Plast Reconstr Surg 2002;109:444-450.

87. Mathes SJ, Stevenson TR: Reconstruction of posterior neck and skull with vertical trapezius musculocutaneous flap. Am J Surg 1988;156:248-251.

88. Ozbek MR, Kutlu N: Vertical trapezius myocutaneous flap for covering wide scalp defects. Handchir Mikrochir Plast Chir 1990;22:326-329.

89. Elsahy NI, Achecar FA: Use of the splenius capitis muscle flap for reconstruction of the posterior neck and skull in complicated Arnold-Chiari malformation. Plast Reconstr Surg 1994;93:1082-1086.

90. Hussussian CJ, Reece GP: Microsurgical scalp reconstruction in the patient with cancer. Plast Reconstr Surg 2002;109:1828-1834.

91. McLean DH, Buncke HJ Jr: Autotransplant of omentum to a large scalp defect, with microsurgical revascularization. Plast Reconstr Surg 1972;49:268-274.

92. Ohmori K: Hair transplantation with microsurgical free scalp flap. J Dermatol Surg Oncol 1984;10:974-978.

93. Harii K, Omori K, Omori S: Hair transplantation with free scalp flaps. Plast Reconstr Surg 1974;53:410-413.

94. Miller GD, Anstee EJ, Snell JA: Successful replantation of an avulsed scalp by microvascular anastomoses. Plast Reconstr Surg 1976;58:133-136.

95. Bickel KD: Microsurgical replantation of the avulsed scalp. Plast Reconstr Surg 1997;99:2105.

96. Cheng K, Zhou S, Jiang K, et al: Microsurgical replantation of the avulsed scalp: report of 20 cases. Plast Reconstr Surg 1996;97:1099-1106.

97. Thomas A, Obed V, Murarka A, et al: Total face and scalp replantation. Plast Reconstr Surg 1998;102:2085-2087.

98. Nahai F, Hurteau J, Vasconez LO: Replantation of an entire scalp and ear by microvascular anastomoses of only 1 artery and 1 vein. Br J Plast Surg 1978;31:339-342.

99. Sawaya ME: Regulation of the human hair cycle. Curr Probl Dermatol 2001;13:206-210.

100. Courtois M, Loussouarn G, Hourseau C, et al: Hair cycle and alopecia. Skin Pharmacol 1994;7:84-89.

101. Norwood OT: Male pattern baldness: classification and incidence. South Med J 1975;68:1359-1365.

102. Ludwig E: Classification of the types of androgenetic alopecia (common baldness) occurring in the female sex. Br J Dermatol 1977;97:247-254.

103. Katz HI: Topical minoxidil: review of efficacy and safety. Cutis 1989;43:94-98.

104. Clissold SP, Heel RC: Topical minoxidil. A preliminary review of its pharmacodynamic properties and therapeutic efficacy in alopecia areata and alopecia androgenetica. Drugs 1987;33:107-122.

105. McClellan KJ, Markham A: Finasteride: a review of its use in male pattern hair loss. Drugs 1999;57:111-126.

106. Whiting DA: Advances in the treatment of male androgenetic alopecia: a brief review of finasteride studies. Eur J Dermatol 2001;11:332-334.

107. Cather JC, Lane D, Heaphy MR Jr, et al: Finasteride—an update and review. Cutis 1999;64:167-172.

108. Orentreich N: Hair transplantation: the punch graft technique. Surg Clin North Am 1971;51:511-518.

109. Unger WP: The history of hair transplantation. Dermatol Surg 2000;26:181-189.

110. Stough D, Whitworth JM: Methodology of follicular unit hair transplantation. Dermatol Clin 1999;17:297-306.

111. Norwood O, Limmer BL: Advances in hair transplantation. Adv Dermatol 1999;14:89-113.

112. Unger MG: Scalp reduction. Clin Dermatol 1992;10:345-355.

113. Unger MG, Unger WP: Management of alopecia of the scalp by a combination of excisions and transplantations. J Dermatol Surg Oncol 1978;4:670-672.

114. Frechet P: A new method for correction of the vertical scar observed following scalp reduction for extensive alopecia. J Dermatol Surg Oncol 1990;16:640-644.

115. Brandy DA: Circumferential scalp reduction. The application of the principles of extensive scalp-lifting for the improvement of scalp reduction surgery. J Dermatol Surg Oncol 1994;20:277-284.

116. Anderson RD: The expanded "BAT" flap for treatment of male pattern baldness. Ann Plast Surg 1993;31:385-391.

117. Frechet P: Scalp extension. J Dermatol Surg Oncol 1993;19:616-622.

118. Juri J: Use of parieto-occipital flaps in the surgical treatment of baldness. Plast Reconstr Surg 1975;55:456-460.

119. Juri J, Juri C: Temporo-parieto-occipital flap for the treatment of baldness. Clin Plast Surg 1982;9:255-261.

120. Nordstrom RE: One variety of a long, nondelayed temporo-parieto-occipital flap. J Dermatol Surg Oncol 1988;14:755-761.

121. Fleming RW, Mayer TG: New concepts in hair replacement. Arch Otolaryngol Head Neck Surg 1989;115:278-279.

Reconstruction of the Auricle

BURTON D. BRENT, MD

CONGENITAL DEFORMITIES
    History of Auricular Reconstruction
    Anatomy
    Practical Embryology and Understanding the
        Middle Ear Problem
    Etiology
    Diagnosis
    Associated Deformities
    Complete Microtia (Hypoplasia)
    Methods of Microtia Repair
    First Stage of Reconstruction
    Other Stages of Auricular Construction
    Variations in Total Ear Reconstruction Technique

Secondary Reconstruction
Bilateral Microtia
The Constricted Ear
Cryptotia
The Prominent Ear
ACQUIRED DEFORMITIES
    Replantation of the Amputated Auricle
    Deformities without Loss of Auricular Tissue
    Deformities with Loss of Auricular Tissue
    Partial Auricular Loss
    Specific Regional Defects
    Tumors of the Auricle

CONGENITAL DEFORMITIES

Total auricular reconstruction with autogenous tissues is one of the greatest technical feats a reconstructive surgeon may encounter. Whereas an inherent understanding of sculpture and design influences one's surgical success, strict adherence to basic principles of plastic surgery and tissue transfer is of equal importance.

During the years, ear reconstruction has stimulated the imagination of many surgeons who have provided countless contributions. Various techniques that have stood the test of time are documented, and guidelines for management of a variety of ear deformities are provided.

History of Auricular Reconstruction

Ear reconstruction was first referred to in the *Sushruta Samhita*,[1] which suggested a cheek flap for repair of the earlobe. As early as 1597, Tagliacozzi described repair of both upper and lower ear deformities with retroauricular flaps.[2] In 1845, Dieffenbach described repair of the ear's middle third with an advancement flap (see Fig. 74-55)[3]; this may occasionally have application today. This early work focused mainly on traumatic deformities. However, by the end of the 19th century, surgeons began to address congenital defects—particularly prominent ears.[4]

The origin of microtia repair had its significant beginnings in 1920, when Gillies[5] buried carved costal cartilage under mastoid skin, then separated it from the head with a cervical flap. Ten years later, Pierce[6] modified this method by lining the new sulcus with a skin graft and building the helix with a tubed flap. In 1937, Gillies[7] repaired more than 30 microtic ears with use of maternal ear cartilage; these were found to progressively resorb.[8] Experiencing the same frustration as others,[9-12] Steffensen[13] used preserved rib cartilage to produce excellent results but later reported progressive resorption of the same cartilage frameworks.[14]

A major breakthrough came in 1959, when Tanzer[15] rekindled use of autogenous rib cartilage, which he carved in a solid block. His excellent results have persisted during the years.[16] In an effort to circumvent large operations, Cronin[17] introduced silicone ear frameworks but found that like other inorganic implants (e.g., polyethylene, nylon mesh, Marlex, polyester net, and Teflon), they suffered a high incidence of extrusion.[18,19] Initially, Cronin[20] minimized this problem by providing fascia lata or galeal and fascial flaps for extra autogenous rim coverage, but when he found later that the alloplastic frames still extruded, he discontinued this practice.

In spite of some investigators' enthusiasm with MEDPOR frameworks,[21,22] these foreign substances seem to encounter the same problems that have plagued silicone. Most recently, a patient came to my consultation with an infected sinus track that had been draining from her MEDPOR implant for 2 years; another patient presented with three separate exposed areas of MEDPOR in his reconstructed ear. On the other hand, an autogenous ear framework in a microtia patient is rarely or never lost; only one has been lost from trauma in a patient with poor compliance to postoperative instructions.[23] To date, more than 70 of my reconstructed ears have survived major trauma.

For many years, there has been considerable interest in development of a "prefabricated" framework from autogenous cartilage to circumvent the necessity of fabricating an ear framework during a prolonged reconstructive procedure and to attempt to eliminate the variability of the surgeon's artistry in providing a realistic ear framework from rib cartilage. Young[24] and Peer[25] first conceived the idea of framework prefabrication before the actual auricular reconstruction in the 1940s. This innovative technique was accomplished by means of "diced" pieces of autogenous rib cartilage that were placed in a fenestrated two-piece, ear-shaped Vitallium mold, which in turn was banked in the patient's abdominal wall. After several months, they retrieved the banked mold, opened it, and harvested the framework of cartilage chips, which had united by connective tissue that had grown through the mold's openings. However, the results were not consistent, perhaps because contraction of the fibrous tissue surrounding the multiple cartilage islands distorted the resultant framework.

Interest in this prefabrication concept has been rekindled through modern "tissue engineering" techniques in which cartilage cells are grown in the laboratory and seeded on a synthetic, biodegradable ear form that is then implanted beneath the skin of a mouse.[26] The early results are interesting, but the trial work is not being carried out under the same conditions as in a clinical human ear reconstruction—the investigators' frameworks are being placed under the *loose skin* of an animal's back, whereas in human ear repair, the new framework must be placed underneath *snug skin* just in front of the hairline in the ear region.

Although these new laboratory studies are intriguing, unless a firm, substantial three-dimensional framework can be produced from *autogenous* tissues, it is likely to suffer the same consequences of frameworks created by Young's and Peer's method, that is, flattening out under the restrictive, two-dimensional skin envelope under which the framework must be placed to complete the ear reconstruction. The other obvious limitation of prefabricated ear frameworks is the difficulty in accommodating the great variation in size and shape that must be produced to match the opposite, normal ear. In sculpting directly from rib cartilage, these limitations do not exist because the surgeon develops the required specific size and shape each time.

However, there has long been an interest in development of a living prefabricated ear framework. Research has begun[27] to explore the possibilities of

bioengineering *firm, autogenous* cartilage frameworks to see whether some of the limitations can be overcome.[28] Autogenous costal cartilage is grown in varying-sized molds made from "idealized" frameworks that are sculpted and cast; but to fill these molds with chondrocytes obtained by digesting a *large* volume of rib cartilage would merely be reproducing Young's and Peer's work by newer technology. The goal is to exploit the technology by using a *small* piece of cartilage (perhaps obtained by biopsy from the microtia patient at age 3 to 4 years, when neochondrogenic potential is high), then to efficiently extract the chondrocytes, to expand them in culture, and to infuse them into the ideal matricial substrate within the ideal ear framework mold for that specific patient. Once generated to satisfaction, the engineered framework would be "banked" under the patient's hairless periauricular skin as the first reconstructive surgical phase. For this technique to be successful, the major problems that must be overcome are replicating sufficient chondrocytes from a small cartilage sample (25 to 50 million cells/mL are needed for neocartilage formation in a construct, and the ear mold volume is about 5 mL) and the ability of those chondrocytes to regenerate *firm* cartilage matrix so that the engineered framework can withstand the pressure caused by the constraints of a two-dimensional skin cover that is taut, inelastic, and restrictive.

Until tissue engineering evolves beyond these problems, sculpted autogenous rib cartilage remains the most reliable material that produces results with the least complications.[16,23,29-33] Furthermore, rib cartilage provides the most substantial source for fabricating a total ear framework. Although contralateral conchal cartilage has been used for this purpose,[34,35] it seems best to reserve auricular cartilage for repair of partial ear defects, for which considerably less tissue bulk is needed.

Anatomy

The ear is difficult to reproduce surgically because it is composed of a complexly convoluted frame of delicate elastic cartilage that is surrounded by a fine skin envelope (Fig. 74-1). The denuded cartilage framework conforms almost exactly to the ear's surface contours except for its absence in the earlobe, which consists of fibrofatty tissue rather than cartilage. In most microtic vestiges, the presence of this lobule tissue is a valuable asset in the repair (see Fig. 74-8). When the lobule is lost in total ear avulsions, it is best recreated by shaping the bottom of the carved ear framework to resemble the lobe.

The ear's rich vascular supply comes from the superficial temporal and posterior auricular vessels, which can nourish a nearly avulsed ear even on surprisingly narrow tissue pedicles. The sensory supply

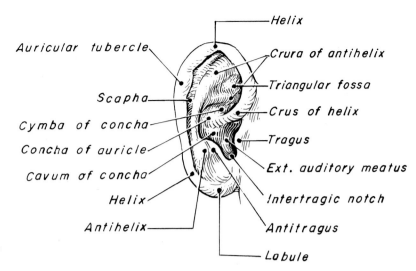

Helix

Crura of antihelix

Triangular fossa

Crus of helix

Tragus

Ext. auditory meatus

Intertragic notch

Antitragus

Labule

Auricular tubercle

Scapha

Cymba of concha

Concha of auricle

Cavum of concha

Helix

Antihelix

FIGURE 74-1. Anatomy of the auricle.

is chiefly derived from the inferiorly coursing great auricular nerve. Upper portions of the ear are supplied by the lesser occipital and auriculotemporal nerves, whereas the conchal region is supplied by a vagal nerve branch.

Understanding this anatomy facilitates blocking of the ear with local anesthetic solution (Fig. 74-2). First, the great auricular nerve is blocked by injecting a wheal

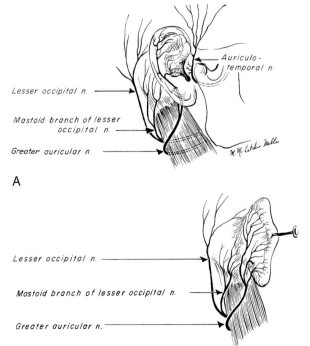

Auriculo-temporal n.

Lesser occipital n.

Mastoid branch of lesser occipital n.

Greater auricular n.

A

Lesser occipital n.

Mastoid branch of lesser occipital n.

Greater auricular n.

B

FIGURE 74-2. Sensory nerve supply of the auricle.

underneath the lobule. After awaiting its effect, one continues injecting upward along the auriculocephalic sulcus, around the top of the ear and down to the tragus. Finally, the vagal branch can be anesthetized without discomfort by traversing the conchal cartilage with a needle placed through the already anesthetized auriculocephalic sulcus to raise a wheal of solution just behind the canal.

Practical Embryology and Understanding the Middle Ear Problem

At consultation, parents of a microtic infant are usually most concerned with the hearing problem. They believe either that the child is completely deaf on the affected side or that hearing can be restored by merely opening a hole in the skin. Because these are misconceptions, the physician can do much to alleviate parents' anxieties by fundamentally explaining ear embryology. Because the human ear's receptive (inner) portion is derived from different embryologic tissue than the conductive (external and middle) portion (Fig. 74-3), the inner ear is rarely involved in microtia, and these patients have at least some hearing in the affected ear. The problem is conduction, which is blocked by the malformed middle and external ear complex. Typically, these patients have a hearing threshold of 40 to 60 dB on the affected side. By comparison, normal function allows us to hear sounds beginning between 0 and 20 dB.

Tissues of both the middle ear and external ear are derived chiefly from the first (mandibular) and second (hyoid) branchial arches. The auricle itself is formed from six "hillocks" of tissue that lie along these arches and can first be seen in the 5-week embryo (Figs. 74-4 and 74-5).[36-38] On the other hand, the inner ear first

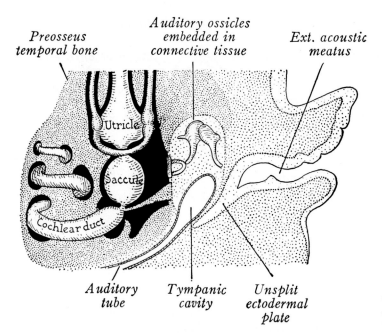

FIGURE 74-3. Partly schematic section of the ear in a 3-month embryo. (From Arey LB: Developmental Anatomy, 6th ed. Philadelphia, WB Saunders, 1954.)

appears at 3 weeks and is derived from tissues of distinctly separate ectodermal origin. Perhaps this explains why it is usually spared the developmental mishap that almost invariably involves the middle ear of microtic patients. Refinements in radiographic technique (polytomography and computed tomography scans) have only occasionally demonstrated dysplasia and hypoplasia of the inner ear.[39,40] Inner ear abnormalities are found in approximately 10% of microtia and atresia patients, but the abnormalities are usually slight (e.g., a dilatation of the lateral semicircular canal). Interestingly, in evaluating approximately 1500 microtic cases during a 25-year period, the author has seen only three patients

who were totally deaf. Remarkably, these were patients with unilateral microtia who had no family history of microtia. Because of their normal inner ear, even patients with bilateral microtia usually have serviceable hearing with use of bone-conductive hearing aids to overcome the transmission block. If they are referred to an audiologist so that aids can be used as soon as possible, these patients usually develop normal speech. There is no point in waiting several months. Hearing aids should be applied within weeks of birth. Because these bone-conductive aids are cumbersome and label the child "different" from his or her peers, it is optimal to correct the hearing deficit surgically to eliminate the aids. However, surgical correction of this conductive problem is difficult because the middle ear beneath the closed skin is not normal.

Exploration involves one's cautiously avoiding the facial nerve while drilling a canal through solid bone. One must usually provide a tympanum with tissue grafts; the distorted or fused ossicles may be irreparable. Because skin grafts do not take well on the drilled bony canal, chronic drainage is a frequent complication and meatal stenosis is common. Finally, unless the surgeon can close the functional difference between the repaired and normal ear to within 15 to 20 dB (an elusive feat in most surgeons' hands), binaural hearing will not be achieved. However, in the hands of a competent otologist with a large volume of experience, restoration of middle ear function surgically can be rewarding—even if only one ear is involved.[41-43]

Because many microtia patients do well without middle ear surgery—eight of nine patients have

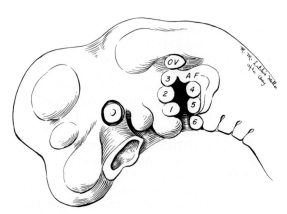

FIGURE 74-4. Development of the auricle in a 5-week human embryo: 1 to 6, elevations (hillocks) on the mandibular and hyoid arches; ov, otic vesicle. (After Arey.)

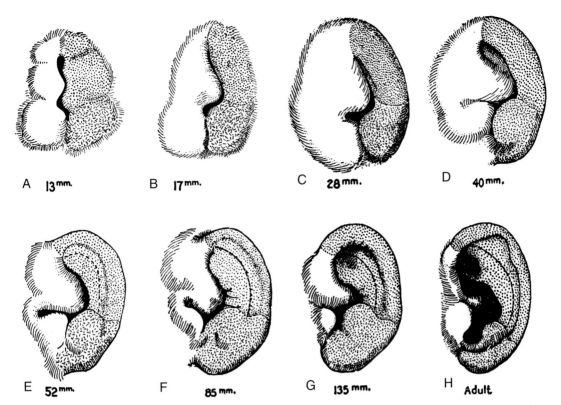

A   13 mm.   B   17 mm.   C   28 mm.   D   40 mm.

E   52 mm.   F   85 mm.   G   135 mm.   H   Adult

FIGURE 74-5. The retardation of growth of the auricular component of the mandibular arch and the expansion and forward rotation of the component of the hyoid arch. (After Streeter; from Patten M: Human Embryology, 3rd ed. New York, McGraw-Hill, 1968.)

unilateral microtia, and they are born "adjusted" to the monaural condition—most surgeons presently believe that potential gains from middle ear surgery in unilateral microtia are outweighed by potential risks and complications of the surgery itself and that this surgery should be reserved for children with bilateral microtia. It is the author's conviction that if the otologic surgeon is not comfortable with the unilateral cases, he or she should certainly not be operating on patients with bilateral microtia either.

When middle ear surgery is contemplated, a team approach must be planned with an experienced, competent otologist. In these patients, the auricular construction should precede the middle ear surgery; once an attempt is made to "open the ear," the virgin skin is scarred, which compromises a satisfactory auricular construction. In the future, implantable acoustic devices may offer a solution for these patients.

Etiology

INCIDENCE

According to an extensive study conducted by Grabb,[44] microtia occurs once in every 6000 births. The occurrence is estimated at 1 in 4000 in Japanese and as high as 1 in 900 to 1200 births in Navajo Indians.[45]

HEREDITARY FACTORS

In a superb study conducted by Rogers,[46] morphologic, anatomic, and genetic interrelationships were shown to exist between microtia, constricted ears, and protruding ears. In this thorough investigation, he demonstrated that these deformities are interrelated and can be hereditary.

Preauricular pits and sinuses and a combination of pits, preauricular appendages, cupping deformity, and deafness are hereditarily dominant.[1,47] Both dominant and recessive characteristics have been revealed in deafness associated with several auricular abnormalities.[48] Ear deformities frequently recur in families of mandibulofacial dysostosis (Treacher Collins syndrome).[49] In the author's experience, these are frequently constricted ear deformities, an abnormality that is known to be hereditary.[11,50-52] Hanhart[51] found a severe form of microtia associated with a cleft or high palate in 10% of family members studied, and Tanzer[53] found that approximately 25% of his 43 microtia patients had relatives with evidence of the first and second branchial arch syndrome (craniofacial microsomia); microtia was present in four instances.

In 4.9% of the author's 1000 microtia patients, family histories revealed that major auricular deformities occurred within the immediate family (i.e., parents, siblings, aunts, uncles, or grandparents).[23] When "distant" relatives were included, the percentage jumped up to 10.3%. In 6% of the patients, preauricular skin tags or minor auricular defects were observed in the immediate family. This number also rose to 10.3% when all relatives were included. Immediate family members of 1.2% of patients had normal auricles but underdeveloped jaws or facial nerves.[23]

In a thorough, intensive survey of 96 families of their 171 microtic patients, Takahashi and Maeda[54] ruled out chromosome aberrations and concluded that inheritance must be multifactorial and that the recurrence risk is 5.7%. In previous studies, others have found multifactorial inheritance between 3% and 8% in first-degree relatives. If a couple has two children with microtia, the risk of recurrence in future offspring is thought to be as high as 15%.

SPECIFIC FACTORS

McKenzie and Craig[55] and Poswillo[56] theorized that the cause of developmental auricular abnormalities is in utero tissue ischemia resulting from either an obliterated stapedial artery or a hemorrhage into the local tissues. This speaks in favor of the deformity's arising from a mishap during fetal development rather than from a hereditary source. In support of this, the author has treated 12 microtia patients who have an *identical* twin with normal ears.[23] Only one set of the author's identical twin patients have had concordance for outer ear deformities. Of interest is that each of these male twins with microtia also had signs and symptoms of pyloric stenosis within 2 days of each other and were operated on at 6 weeks of age.

The occurrence of deafness and occasional microtia resulting from rubella during the first trimester of pregnancy is well known. Also, certain drugs during this critical period may be causative; the author has seen at least three cases of microtia that resulted from the mother's ingestion of the tranquilizer thalidomide.[57,58] Isotretinoin has also been cited as causing ear deformities when it is ingested during the first trimester.[59] In the author's series, several mothers had been unaware of this problem and had used this drug to control acne. Other medications that reportedly cause microtia are clomiphene citrate[60] and retinoic acid.[61]

Diagnosis

CLASSIFICATION

Rogers[46] noted that one could classify most types of auricular hypoplasia in a descending scale of severity.

TABLE 74-1 ✦ CLINICAL CLASSIFICATION OF AURICULAR DEFECTS (TANZER)

Anotia
Complete hypoplasia (microtia)
  With atresia of external auditory canal
  Without atresia of external auditory canal
Hypoplasia of middle third of auricle
Hypoplasia of superior third of auricle
  Constricted (cup and lop) ear
  Cryptotia
  Hypoplasia of entire superior third
Prominent ear

This corresponds to Streeter's depiction of embryologic patterns of auricular development.[38] Rogers divides developmental ear defects into four groups: microtia; lop ear, that is, folding or deficiency of the superior helix and scapha; "cup" or constricted ear, with a deep concha and deficiency of the superior helix and antihelical crura; and the common prominent or protruding ear.

Using a system that correlates with embryologic development, Tanzer classifies congenital ear defects according to the approach necessary for their surgical correction (Table 74-1).[62]

Associated Deformities

As discussed previously, embryologic development dictates that the microtic ear is usually accompanied by middle ear abnormalities. In full-blown, classic microtia, one usually finds canal atresia and ossicular abnormalities. The middle ear deformity may range from diminished canal caliber and minor ossicular abnormalities to fused, hypoplastic ossicles and failure of mastoid cell pneumatization.

Because the auricle develops from tissues of the mandibular and hyoid branchial arches, it is not surprising that a significant percentage of microtic patients exhibit deficient facial components that originate from these embryologic building blocks. These deformities are compiled under "hemifacial microsomia" (first and second branchial arch syndrome) (Fig. 74-6), and an obvious facial asymmetry was noted in 35% of the author's 1000 microtia patients.[23] The most complete genetic expression of this condition includes defects of the external and middle ear; hypoplasia of the mandible, maxilla, zygoma, and temporal bones; macrostomia and lateral facial clefts; and atrophy of facial muscles and parotid gland.[44,63,64] Furthermore, Brent[23] found that 15% of his 1000 patients had paresis of the facial nerve. Dellon et al[65] have shown that the palatal muscles are rarely spared in this syndrome.

Urogenital tract abnormalities are increased in the presence of microtia,[66] particularly when the patient

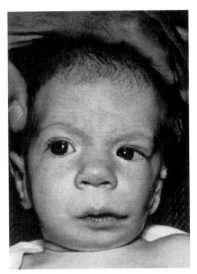

FIGURE 74-6. Patient with unilateral craniofacial microsomia (first and second branchial arch syndrome) displaying microtia; macrostomia; hypoplasia of the zygoma, maxilla, and mandible; and soft tissue hypoplasia.

is afflicted with other manifestations of the first and second branchial arch syndrome (Table 74-2).[67]

Complete Microtia (Hypoplasia)

CLINICAL CHARACTERISTICS

Microtia varies from the complete absence of auricular tissues (anotia) to a somewhat normal but small ear with atretic canal. Between these extremes, one finds an endless variety of vestiges, the most common being a vertically oriented sausage-shaped nubbin (Figs. 74-7 and 74-8; see also Fig. 74-26). Microtia is nearly twice as frequent in boys as in girls, and the right-left-bilateral ratio is roughly 6:3:1 (Table 74-3).[23,29,68]

In most instances, the microtic lobule is displaced superiorly to the level of the opposite, normal side, although incomplete ear migration occasionally leaves it in an inferior location. Approximately one third to half the patients exhibit gross characteristics of

TABLE 74-2 ✦ DEFORMITIES ASSOCIATED WITH MICROTIA*

Branchial arch deformities
  Obvious bone and soft tissue deficit, 36.5%
    Family perceives it as "significant," 49.4%
  Overt facial nerve weakness, 15.2%
    Of these, more than one branch involved, 42.6%
Macrostomia, 2.5%
Cleft lip and/or palate, 4.3%
Urogenital defects, 4.0%
Cardiovascular malformations, 2.5%
Miscellaneous deformities, 1.7%

*Author's series of 1000 patients.

hemifacial microsomia, although Converse et al[69,70] have demonstrated tomographically that skeletal deficiencies exist in all cases. Whatever the deformity, the author has been impressed with its potential for psychological havoc among the entire family, varying from the patient's emotional insecurity to the parents' deep-seated guilt feelings.

GENERAL CONSIDERATIONS

During the initial consultation, it is imperative to realistically describe to the patient and family the technical limitations involved in surgical correction of microtia and to outline alternative methods of managing each individual's particular deformity. The author strongly favors autogenous rib cartilage for auricular construction. Although its use necessitates an operation with significant morbidity of the patient, it must be noted that unlike a reconstruction using alloplastic materials, a successful construction with autogenous tissue is less susceptible to trauma and therefore eliminates a patient's overcautious concern during normal activities.

The age at which an auricular construction should begin is governed by both psychological and physical considerations. Because the body image concept usually begins forming around the age of 4 or 5 years,[71] it would be ideal to begin construction before the child enters school and is psychologically traumatized by peers' cruel ridicule. However, surgery

TABLE 74-3 ✦ MICROTIA: AUTHOR'S SERIES OF 1000 PATIENTS

	Patients		Total No. of Ears			
Right	582	(58.2%)	582	Boys	631	(63.1%)
Left	324	(32.4%)	324	Girls	369	(36.9%)
Bilateral	94	(9.4%)	188			
	1000	100.0%	1094		1000	100.0%

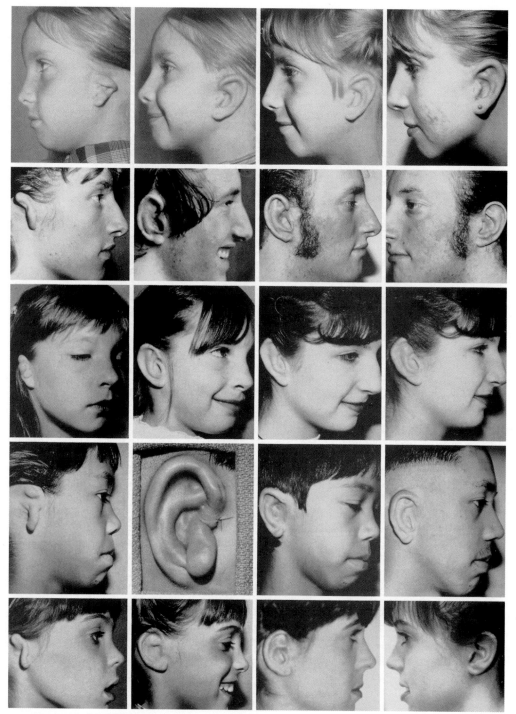

FIGURE 74-7. Long-term stability of ears constructed with autogenous rib cartilage grafts. First patient, an 8-year-old girl with microtia shown preoperatively and then at 1, 4, and 12 years postoperatively. Second patient, a 13-year-old boy shown preoperatively, at 1 year, and at 10 years postoperatively, comparing both ears. Third patient, a 6-year-old girl shown preoperatively and then at 1 and 8 years postoperatively; ear growth is particularly obvious in this patient. Fourth patient, an 8-year-old boy shown preoperatively and immediately after cartilage grafting and then at 2 and 8 years postoperatively. Fifth patient, a 6-year-old girl shown preoperatively, at 1 year, and at 12 years postoperatively, comparing both ears. (From Brent B: Auricular repair with autogenous rib cartilage grafts: two decades of experience with 600 cases. Plast Reconstr Surg 1992;90:355.)

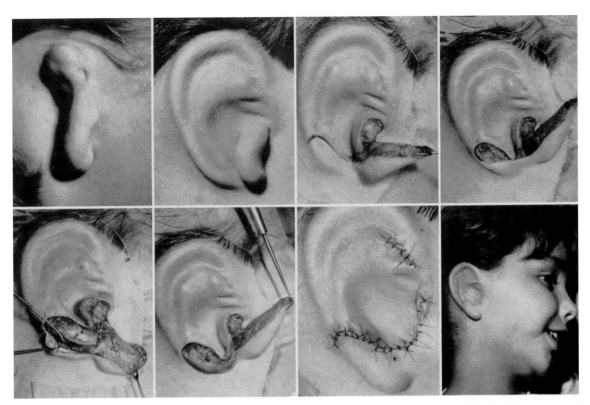

FIGURE 74-8. Lobule transposition. *Above, left,* The microtic vestige. *Above, left center,* The healed ear several months after framework insertion. *Above, right center,* By incision around it, the lobule has been mobilized as an inferiorly based flap; an incision has been made at the proposed superior inset margin. *Above, right, through below, left center,* The skin overlying the lower ear region has been loosened and slid under the elevated framework's tip to surface the "floor" beneath it. Note that connective tissue has been carefully preserved over the cartilaginous tip. *Below, right center,* The lobule has been filleted and wrapped around the framework tip in a two-layered wound closure; the former lobule site is closed, and the vestigial tissue is excised from the triangular fossa region. *Below, right,* The healed repair. (From Brent B: Auricular repair with autogenous rib cartilage grafts: two decades of experience with 600 cases. Plast Reconstr Surg 1992;90:355.)

should be postponed until rib growth provides substantial cartilage to permit a quality framework fabrication.

In the author's experience with more than 1500 microtia patients from age 1 month to 62 years, the patients and their families consistently stated that their psychological disturbances rarely began before age 7 years and usually became overt from ages 7 to 10 years. The family is anxious to have the ear repaired as soon as possible, but it is important for the surgeon to wait until it is technically feasible. There usually is enough rib cartilage to serve as the sculpting medium by 6 years of age, allowing ear reconstruction; however, if the patient is small for age or the opposite, normal ear is large, it is prudent to postpone the surgery for several years. The optimal age to begin is about 8 years. At this age, the child is more aware of the problem and usually wants it resolved as much as the family does. The child can also be more cooperative than a younger child during the postoperative care phase.

At age 6 years, the normal ear has grown to within 6 or 7 mm of its full vertical height,[72] which permits one to construct an ear that will have reasonably constant symmetry with the opposite normal ear. In his follow-up mail survey, Tanzer[16,73] found that an ear constructed from autogenous rib cartilage grows at the same rate as the normal ear, with the possible exception of patients operated on at 6 to 7 years of age, in whom he noted that 50% of the ears lagged several millimeters behind in growth; the roles played in the growth of his patients' surgically constructed ears by soft tissues and by cartilage have not been determined. In evaluation of "lay" data from my first 500 unilateral microtia patients operated on between the ages of 5 and 10 years with a minimum 5-year follow-up (76 patients),[29] 48% of the constructed ears grew at an even pace with the opposite, normal ear; 41.6% grew several millimeters larger; and 10.3% lagged several millimeters behind the normal side. From the limited number of long-term patients in this age group (it is particularly difficult to get patients and their families to fly out for a visit once the surgical repair is complete), most constructed ears have grown, and many of these have not only kept up with the little residual growth in the opposite ear but have *slightly* overgrown.[29] Few have shrunk, softened, or lost their detail (see Fig. 74-7). On the basis of these observations, one should try to match the opposite side during the preoperative planning session, regardless of age. There is certainly no reason to construct the ear larger, as some investigators have previously thought, and one might even consider making the framework several millimeters smaller in the youngest patients, in whom normal, in situ costal cartilage can be expected to exceed normal auricular cartilage growth.

Methods of Microtia Repair

STAGING THE AURICULAR CONSTRUCTION

The cartilage graft is the "foundation" of an auricular construction, and as in construction of a house, it should be built and well established under ideal conditions before further stages or refinements are undertaken. By implanting the cartilage graft as the first surgical stage, one takes advantage of the optimal elasticity and circulation of an unviolated, virgin skin "pocket." For these reasons, the author prefers to avoid initial lobule transposition or vestige division; the resulting scars cannot help but inhibit the circulation and restrict the skin's elasticity, which in turn diminishes its ability to safely accommodate a three-dimensional cartilage graft. In the author's experience, it seems easier both to judge the earlobe's placement and to "splice" the lobule correctly into position with reference to a well-established, underlying framework. Although Tanzer transposed the lobule simultaneously with implantation of the cartilage graft in the last three patients of his clinical practice[74] and Nagata routinely does this in his technique,[32] the author finds that there is far less risk of tissue necrosis and that it is far more accurate to transpose the lobule as a secondary procedure (see Fig. 74-8).[75-77] One can safely transpose the lobe and simultaneously elevate the ear from the head with skin graft if the earlobe vestige is short because its small wound closure will not compromise the ear's anterior circulation (see Fig. 74-16).[23,29]

During the third stage, the ear is separated from the head and surfaced on its underside with a skin graft to create an auriculocephalic sulcus.

In general, the fourth stage combines tragus construction, conchal excavation, and simultaneous contralateral otoplasty, if indicated. By combination of these procedures, tissues that are normally discarded from an otoplasty can be employed advantageously as free grafts in the tragus construction.

PREOPERATIVE CONSULTATION

During the initial consultation, surgical expectations and psychological considerations should be discussed with the patient and the family, emphasizing goals of the reconstruction. Although costal cartilage can be carved to form a delicate framework, the volume and projection of the furnished three-dimensional framework are limited by the two-dimensional skin flap under which it is placed. Furthermore, because the retroauricular-mastoid skin that covers the framework is somewhat thicker than normal, delicate anterolateral auricular skin, it blunts the details of a carved framework. It is important for these limitations to be stressed to patient and family, lest they have unrealistic expectations of what can or cannot be produced by surgery. Hence, the plastic surgeon's aim is to achieve accurate representation, that being to provide an acceptable facsimile of an ear that is the proper size, in the proper position, and properly oriented to other facial features.

During the consultation, surgical discomforts and inconveniences should be described, including the expected chest pain, duration of dressings, and limited activities for 4 to 6 weeks. Finally, risks and possible complications of the surgery are discussed thoroughly. These include pneumothorax, cartilage graft loss secondary to infection, skin flap necrosis, and hematoma. It should be stressed that with proper precautions, these risks are comparatively less severe than the emotional trauma associated with an absent ear.

PLANNING, PREPARATION, AND CORRELATION WITH THE CORRECTION OF OTHER FACIAL DEFICIENCIES

The result of a total ear reconstruction depends not only on a surgeon's meticulous surgical technique but on careful preoperative planning. It is essential that one practice carving techniques on a volume of human cadaver cartilage before any live-patient application. An acrylic or plaster replica of a normal ear serves as an excellent model for practice carvings.

During the patient's second office consultation, preoperative study photographs are obtained and an x-ray film pattern is traced from the opposite, normal ear. This pattern is reversed, and a framework pattern is designed for the new ear (Fig. 74-9). After sterilization, these patterns serve as guidelines for framework fabrication at the time of surgery.

The reconstructed ear's location is predetermined by first noting the topographic relationship of the opposite, normal ear to facial features and then duplicating its position at the proposed reconstruction site. First, one compares the vestige's height from the front view with that of the opposite, normal ear. From the

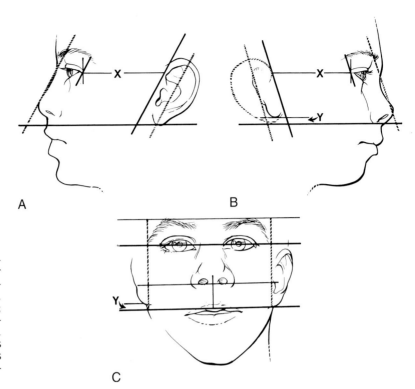

FIGURE 74-9. *A to C,* Preoperative determination of auricular location. The ear's axis is positioned to match the opposite side, roughly parallel to the nasal profile; the helical root is positioned equidistant from the lateral canthus. The reversed auricular pattern is traced 6 mm below the lobule, as determined by frontal measurement.

side, it should be noted that the ear's axis is roughly parallel to the nasal profile.[35,78] Finally, one notes and records the distance between the lateral canthus and the normal ear's helical root.

The ear's location is established in the office by first taping the reversed film pattern to the proposed construction site and then adjusting its position until it is level to and symmetric with the opposite normal ear. The pattern is traced on the head, noting the ear's axial relation to the nose, its distance from the lateral canthus, and its lobule's position, which is usually superiorly displaced. The ear's new position is straightforward and easy to plan in a pure microtia, but much more difficult when severe hemifacial microsomia exists. Not only are the heights of the facial halves asymmetric, but the anteroposterior dimensions of the affected side are foreshortened as well. In these patients, one best plans the new ear's height by lining it up with the normal ear's upper pole— its distance from the lateral canthus is somewhat arbitrary.

In pure microtia, the vestige-to-canthus distance mirrors the helical root-to-canthus distance of the opposite, normal side. However, in patients with severe hemifacial microsomia, the vestige is much closer to the eye. If one places the new ear's anterior margin at the vestige site, the ear appears too close to the eye;

if one uses the measured distance of the normal side as a guide, the ear looks too far back on the head. In these patients, it is best to compromise by selecting a point halfway between these two positions.

When both auricular construction and bone repairs are planned, integrated timing is essential. Most often the family pushes for the ear repair to begin first, which helpfully ensures the auricular surgeon unscarred skin. The craniomaxillofacial surgeon argues that by going first, the facial symmetry will be corrected, thus making ear placement easier.[79] This is unnecessary when the described guidelines are followed.

If the bone work is done first, it is imperative that scars be peripheral to the proposed auricular site. When a coronal incision is used to approach the upper face or to harvest cranial bone grafts, special care must be taken so that the scar does not precariously lie over the future region of the upper helix.

First Stage of Reconstruction

Almost invariably, the author's first-stage "foundation" in correction of microtia is fabricating and inserting the cartilaginous ear framework. As discussed previously, scars can be a significant handicap; the author rarely employs a preliminary procedure.

OBTAINING THE RIB CARTILAGE

Rib cartilages are obtained en bloc from the side contralateral to the ear being constructed to use natural rib configuration. The rib cartilages are removed through a horizontal or slightly oblique incision made just above the costal margin. After division of the external oblique and the rectus muscles, the film pattern is placed on the exposed cartilages to determine the necessary extent of rib resection.

The helical rim is fashioned separately with cartilage from the first free-floating rib (Fig. 74-10). Excision of this cartilage facilitates access to the synchondrotic region of ribs six and seven, which supplies a sufficient block to carve the framework body. Extraperichondrial dissection is preferable in obtaining an unmarred specimen. One can significantly decrease well-documented chest deformities[80,81] by preserving even a minimal rim of the upper margin of the sixth rib cartilage where one obtains the basic shape of the ear (see Fig. 74-10). This precautionary measure retains a tether to the sternum so that the rib does not flare outward to distort the chest as the child grows. If the synchondrotic region seems inadequate in width, one can compensate for framework width by bowing the helix away from the

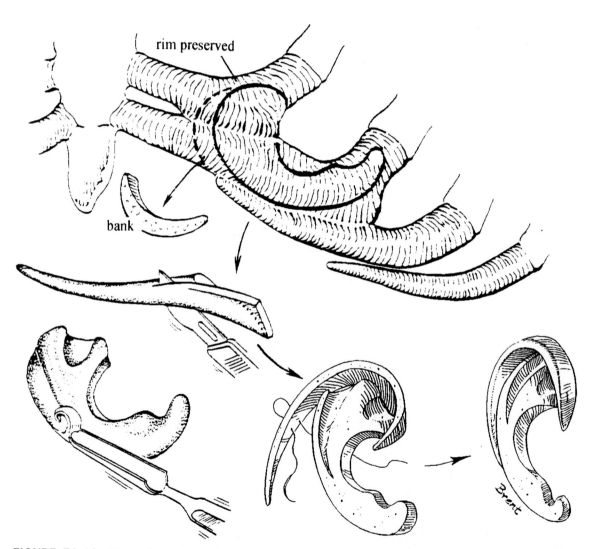

FIGURE 74-10. Rib cartilage harvest for ear framework fabrication. Note that the upper border of the sixth cartilage is preserved; this will help prevent subsequent chest deformity as the child grows. The entire "floating cartilage" will be used to create the helix. To produce the acute flexion necessary to form the helix, the cartilage is deliberately warped in a favorable direction by thinning it on its outer, convex surface. The thinned helix is affixed to the main sculptural block with horizontal mattress sutures of 4–0 clear nylon; the knots are placed on the framework's undersurface.

framework body (the "expansile" design),[82] rather than violating the sixth rib margin and sacrificing chest wall integrity.

In cases in which the delicate pleura is entered during this dissection, there is no great reason for concern because a leak in the lung has not been produced. However, when a pleural tear is discovered, a rubber catheter is inserted well into the chest through the pleural opening; the chest wound is then closed in layers by the assistant while the surgeon fabricates the framework, thus conserving operative time. When skin closure is complete, the catheter is attached to suction, the lung is expanded, and the catheter is rapidly withdrawn. As a final precaution, every patient receives a portable upright chest radiograph in the operating room.

FRAMEWORK FABRICATION

In fabricating an ear framework, the surgeon's aim is to exaggerate the helical rim and the details of the antihelical complex (Fig. 74-11). This is achieved with

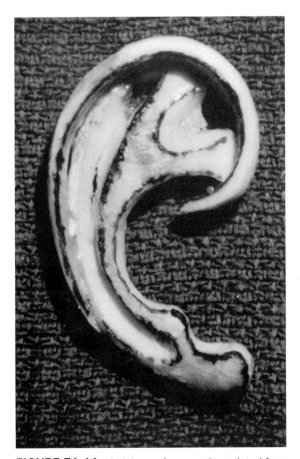

FIGURE 74-11. A right ear framework, sculpted from autogenous rib cartilage as illustrated in Figure 74-10.

scalpel blades and rounded woodcarving chisels. To minimize possible chondrocytic damage, the use of power tools for sculpting is strictly avoided—one should keep in mind that cartilage sculpting differs from basic woodcarving in that a good long-term result ultimately depends on living tissue.

The basic ear silhouette is carved from the previously obtained cartilage block (see Fig. 74-10). It is necessary to thin little if any of the basic form for a small child's framework, but it is essential for framework fabrication in most older patients. When thinning is necessary, care is taken to preserve the perichondrium on the lateral, outer aspect of the framework to facilitate its adherence ("take") and subsequent nourishment from surrounding tissues.

Because warping must be taken into consideration,[83] one sculpts and thins the cartilage to cause a deliberate warping in a favorable direction. This allows one to produce the acute flexion necessary to form a helix, which is fastened to the framework body with horizontal mattress sutures; the knots are buried on the frame's undersurface.

FRAMEWORK MODIFICATIONS IN OLDER PATIENTS

Adult rib cartilages are often fused into a solid block, which invites one to sculpt the ear framework in one piece—not unlike doing a woodcarving (Fig. 74-12). In my experience, this is advantageous because adult cartilage is often calcified; it is difficult if not impossible to create a separate helix that will bend without breaking. If a one-piece carving produces insufficient helical projection, one can detach the helix and slide it up the framework body to augment the protrusion of the rim. This improved contour is maintained by reattaching the helix to the framework with several permanent sutures (Fig. 74-13).

FRAMEWORK IMPLANTATION

A cutaneous pocket is formed with meticulous technique to provide an adequate recipient vascular covering for the framework. Because several hours can lapse during the rib removal and framework fabrication, the auricular region is prepared and scrubbed just before the cutaneous pocket is made. If two surgeons well versed in ear reconstruction are working together, one can develop the cutaneous pocket while the other finishes the cartilage sculpture.

Through a small incision along the back side of the auricular vestige, a thin flap is raised by sharp dissection, with care taken to preserve the subdermal vascular plexus. To evaluate the flap's vascular status and to ensure accurate hemostasis, epinephrine-containing solutions are avoided. With great care, one dissects the skin from the gnarled, native cartilage remnant, which then is excised and discarded. Finally,

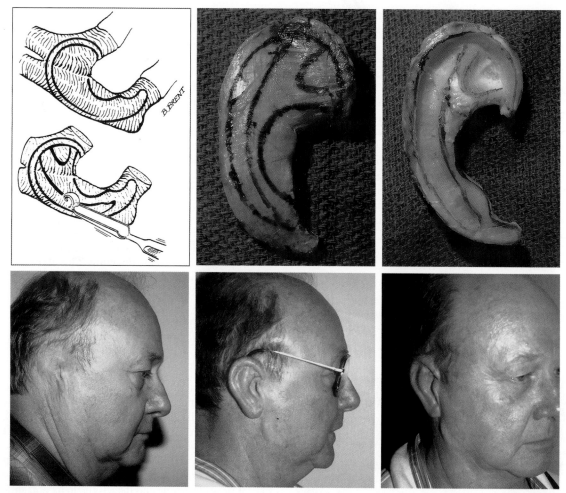

FIGURE 74-12. Framework modifications in the adult patient. *Above, left,* When a solid, fused cartilage block is encountered, the framework is sculpted in one piece. *Above, center,* Cartilage block marked for carving. *Above, right,* Completed framework sculpted from the block. *Below, left,* A 60-year-old man with traumatic total ear loss. *Below, center and right,* Result achieved with a one-piece sculpture from a fused cartilage block, 1 year postoperatively. Simulation of the absent earlobe was achieved by sculpting its likeness in the framework's inferior pole. (From Brent B: Technical advances in ear reconstruction with autogenous rib cartilage grafts: personal experience with 1200 cases. Plast Reconstr Surg 1999;104:319.)

the pocket is completed by dissecting a centimeter or two peripherally to the projected framework markings (Fig. 74-14).

Insertion of the framework into the cutaneous pocket takes up the valuable skin slack that was made when the native cartilage remnant was removed. The framework displaces this skin centrifugally in an advantageous posterosuperior direction to displace the hairline just behind the rim. This principle of anterior incision and centrifugal skin relaxation, introduced by Tanzer,[15] not only permits advantageous use of the hairless skin cover but also preserves circulation by avoiding incisions and scars along the helical border.

Although Tanzer[15,84] initially suggested the use of bolster sutures to coapt the skin flap to underlying framework, the author finds it far safer to do this with suction, which simultaneously prevents fluid collection and minimizes the risk of flap necrosis along the helical margin. Silicone catheters are used to attain skin coaptation by suction, or perforated drains are fashioned from infusion catheters with the needles inserted into rubber-topped vacuum tubes (see Fig. 74-14), the tubes being retained on a rack to observe changes in quantity and quality of drainage. Although a dressing is applied that accurately conforms to the convolutions of the newly formed auricle, firm pressure is dangerous and unnecessary and must be avoided.

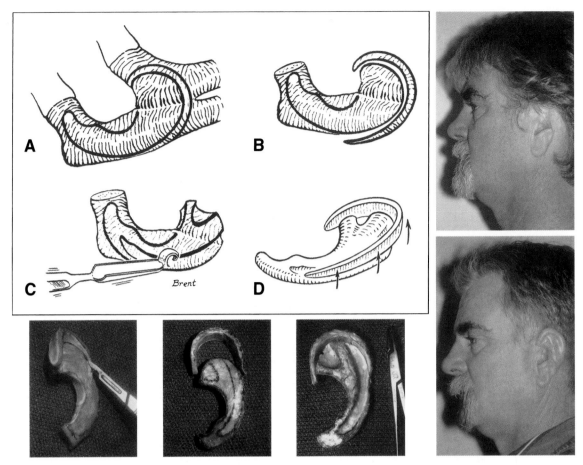

FIGURE 74-13. Maximizing rim projection in adult patient with sliding helical advancement. *Above, left: A and B,* Harvesting fused rib cartilage block and separating the inflexible helical portion; *C,* sculpting body of framework; *D,* sliding and reattaching the helix to maximize its projection. *Above, right,* A 50-year-old man with ear loss from a dog bite. *Below, left, second from left, and third from left,* Construction of the framework by use of the technique illustrated in the drawings. *Below, right,* The completed repair. This patient had his hairline "idealized" by laser treatment before the rib cartilage graft (see Fig. 74-22). (From Brent B: Technical advances in ear reconstruction with autogenous rib cartilage grafts: personal experience with 1200 cases. Plast Reconstr Surg 1999;104:319.)

Hemostasis and skin coaptation are provided by the suction drain.[17,29,75,77]

IMMEDIATE POSTOPERATIVE CARE AND MANAGEMENT OF COMPLICATIONS

The new ear's convolutions are packed with petrolatum gauze, and a bulky, noncompressive dressing is applied. Because the vacuum system provides both skin coaptation and hemostasis, pressure is unnecessary and contraindicated. The first day, the tubes are changed by the ward nurses every few hours, then every 4 to 6 hours thereafter or when a tube is one-third full. Although the patient leaves the hospital in several days, the drains remain in place another 2 to 3 days until the test tubes contain only drops of serosanguineous drainage. Postoperatively, the ear is checked and the protective head dressing is changed several times. The protective head dressing is removed after about 12 days.

Attentive postoperative management is imperative for a successful ear reconstruction that remains unhampered by disastrous complications. The newly constructed auricle is scrutinized frequently and carefully for signs of infection or vascular compromise. Early infection is usually manifested by neither auricular pain nor fever but through local erythema, edema, subtle fluctuation, drainage, or a combination of these. Hence, frequent observations and the immediate institution of aggressive therapy can deter an overwhelming infection. Immediately when an infection is suspected, an irrigation drain is introduced below the flap, and continuous antibiotic drip irrigation is

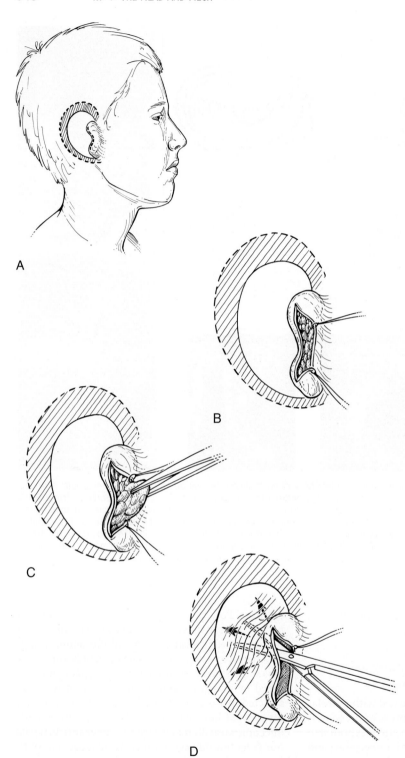

A

B

C

D

FIGURE 74-14. *A* to *F,* The cutaneous "pocket." The vestigial native cartilage is excised and then a skin pocket is created. To provide tension-free accommodation of the framework, the dissection is performed well beyond the proposed auricular position. With use of two silicone catheters, the skin is coapted to the framework by means of vacuum tube suction.

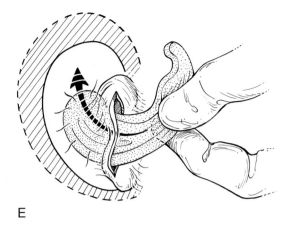

E

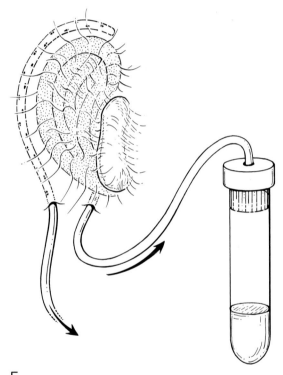

F

FIGURE 74-14, cont'd.

becomes evident, appropriate steps must be taken without delay. Although at times a small local flap may be required to cover exposed cartilage, small localized ulcerations may heal with good local wound care. Wound care consists of continuous coverage with antibiotic ointment to prevent cartilage desiccation and restraints to prevent the patient from lying on the ear during sleep. However, major skin flap necrosis merits a more aggressive approach if the framework is to be salvaged. The necrotic skin is excised early, and the framework is covered by transposition of a local skin flap or by use of a small fascial flap and skin graft.

POSTOPERATIVE ACTIVITIES AND CARE

Once it is initially healed, no specific care is necessary for an ear constructed with autogenous tissues. To avoid flattening of the helical rim, the patient is instructed to sleep on the opposite side. A soft pillow ensures protection if the patient should sleep on the affected site.

Two weeks postoperatively, the patient may return to school; however, running and sports are discouraged an additional 3 weeks while the chest wound heals. This is the case in any major surgical procedure where wound strength is essential.

The ear itself withstands trauma well because it, like the opposite, normal ear, houses a framework of autogenous cartilage. To date, the author has witnessed numerous traumatic episodes in reconstructed ears (e.g., baseball and soccer blows, a bee sting, and a dog bite). They have all healed well.[29] For these reasons, no conspicuous, protective headgear is recommended, except in sports such as football and wrestling, in which such equipment is used routinely.

Other Stages of Auricular Construction

Major stages in auricular construction subsequent to the initial framework implantation are lobule rotation, separation of the ear with a skin graft, deepening of the concha, and formation of a tragus. These stages can be planned independently or in various combinations, depending on which best achieves the desired end result.

ROTATION OF THE LOBULE

The author prefers to perform earlobe transposition as a secondary procedure because it seems easier both to judge placement of the earlobe and to splice the lobule correctly into position with reference to a well-established, underlying framework. Although the author has occasionally transposed the lobule simultaneously with implantation of the cartilage graft, it is safer and far more accurate to transpose the lobule as a secondary procedure.

begun. Appropriate adjustments are made in both the antibiotic drip irrigation and in the systemic therapy when sensitivities are available from the initial culture. Cronin[17] has salvaged Silastic-frame reconstructions impressively by this technique, and the author has had success in managing the rare infection in cartilage graft reconstructions.

Skin flap necrosis results from excess tension in an inadequate-sized pocket, tight bolster sutures, or damage to the subdermal vascularity during the flap dissection. This complication is best avoided by meticulous technique; however, once skin necrosis

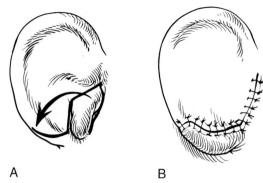

A   B

FIGURE 74-15. Total ear construction, stage 2: lobule transposition. *A,* Healed stage 1 repair and proposed lobule transposition. The appropriate lobule position will be de-epithelialized to receive the transposed earlobe. *B,* Completed procedure. The lobule has been transposed as an inferiorly based flap.

The "rotation" or repositioning of this normal but displaced structure is accomplished essentially by Z-plasty transposition of a narrow, inferiorly based triangular flap (Fig. 74-15). Nagata[32] and Firmin[30,85] transpose the earlobe and use skin from the lobule's posterior surface to line the framework's tragal strut during the first-stage surgery. This does produce an excellent tragal appearance, but the price paid is greater risk of skin necrosis and earlobes that are at times compromised in appearance and often unable to accommodate earrings. This problem is no small issue for young female patients, who often submit to surgery with eventual earlobe piercing as their highest priority.[23] If the lobe vestige is short so that a substantial skin bridge can be preserved above it during its transposition, one can safely move the earlobe while simultaneously separating the auricle from the head to form the auriculocephalic sulcus[23,29] and preserve sufficient posterior earlobe skin to permit the use of earrings (Fig. 74-16).

TRAGAL CONSTRUCTION AND CONCHAL DEFINITION

One can form the tragus, excavate the concha, and mimic a canal in a single operation. This is accomplished by placing a thin elliptical chondrocutaneous composite graft beneath a J-shaped incision in the conchal region (Fig. 74-17).[75,77] The main limb of the J is placed at the proposed posterior tragal margin; the crook of the J represents the intertragal notch. Extraneous soft tissues are excised beneath this tragal flap to deepen the concha; this excavated region looks quite like a meatus when the newly constructed tragus casts a shadow on it.

It is advantageous to harvest the composite graft from the normal ear's anterolateral conchal surface because of its ideal shape and the paucity of subcutaneous tissue between the delicate anterolateral skin and adjacent cartilage. This technique is particularly ideal when a prominent concha exists in the normal donor ear; closure of the donor site facilitates an otoplasty, which often is needed to gain frontal symmetry.

An alternative method consists of design of the tragus as an integral strut of the original framework during its initial fabrication. A small piece of rib cartilage is first fastened to the frame to simulate the antitragal eminence. The strut is thinned on one side, then curved around and affixed by its distal tip with a clear nylon suture that stretches across to the frame's crus helix. The result is a delicate tragus that flows naturally from the main framework through an arched intertragal notch (Fig. 74-18). This method of tragus construction is particularly advantageous in bilateral microtia, where there is no source for special composite tissue grafts. Nagata also creates the tragus with an extra cartilage piece attached to his main framework (see Fig. 74-23) and lines it with skin from the earlobe vestige during the first stage of surgery.

Another option for tragus construction in bilateral microtia is the modified Kirkham method, which consists of an anteriorly based conchal flap doubled on itself.[11]

DETACHING THE POSTERIOR AURICULAR REGION

Auricular separation with skin grafting is used solely to eliminate the cryptotic appearance by defining the ear through formation of a sulcus. This procedure will not project a framework that has been carved with insufficient depth.

The posterior auricular margin is defined by separating the ear from the head and covering its undersurface with a thick split-skin graft. This should not be attempted until the edema has markedly subsided and the auricular details have become well defined. When this occurs, an incision is made several millimeters behind the rim, with care taken to preserve a protective connective tissue layer on the cartilage framework. The retroauricular skin is then advanced into the newly created sulcus so that the only graft requirement is on the ear's undersurface. A medium split-thickness skin graft is harvested from a hidden region (usually underneath the bathing suit area) and sutured to the wound, with the sutures left long; these are tied over a bolster to tamponade the graft to the recipient bed (Fig. 74-19).

Greater projection of the auricle can be obtained by placing a wedge of rib cartilage behind the elevated ear, but this must be covered with a tissue flap for the skin graft to take over the cartilage. Nagata[32] accomplishes this with an axial flap of temporoparietal fascia

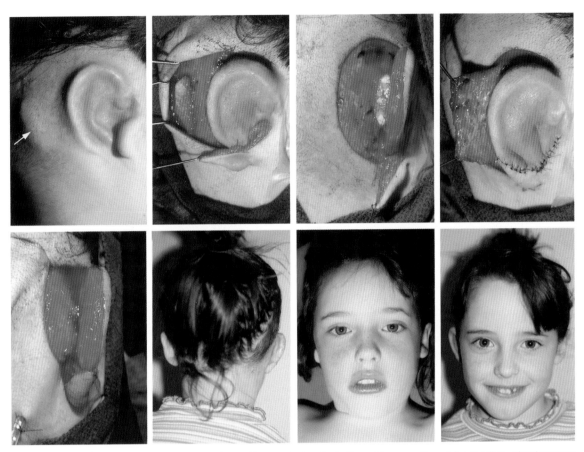

FIGURE 74-16. Augmenting ear projection with a scalp-banked rib cartilage graft and fascial flap; simultaneous earlobe transposition. *Above, left,* Healed first-stage repair of a microtic ear. Note banked rib cartilage behind the ear framework *(arrow). Above, second from left,* Stage 2: retroauricular scalp undermined to retrieve banked cartilage; earlobe transposition begun. *Above, second from right,* Banked cartilage wedged behind the elevated ear to augment its projection; lobule suspended on the inferior pedicle. *Above, right,* Retroauricular fascial flap raised; earlobe transposition complete. *Below, left,* Fascial flap turned over the cartilage wedge to provide a nourishing cover for skin graft. *Below, second from left,* Complete skin graft "take" on the elevated ear. *Below, second from right,* Preoperative view of the patient. *Below, right,* Healed postoperative appearance. (From Brent B: Technical advances in ear reconstruction with autogenous rib cartilage grafts: personal experience with 1200 cases. Plast Reconstr Surg 1999;104:319.)

(Fig. 74-20). However, use of that fascial flap is not without a certain morbidity, and this fascia should be reserved for significant traumatic and secondary reconstruction cases in which there is no other option for their solution.[29] Like Firmin[85] and Weerda,[86] the author prefers instead to cover the cartilage wedge with a turnover "book flap" of occipitalis fascia from behind the ear (see Fig. 74-16).[23] When this cartilage-wedging technique is used, there is no need to subject the patient to a second uncomfortable chest operation to harvest rib cartilage anew, as does Nagata.[87] Instead, an extra piece of cartilage can be banked underneath the chest incision during the initial first-stage procedure. When the wedge is needed during the elevation procedure, it can easily be retrieved by incising through the original chest scar. Alternatively, this cartilage wedge is banked underneath the scalp, just posterior to the main

pocket where the completed ear framework is placed (see Fig. 74-16).[23] This site is particularly advantageous in that one can more conveniently retrieve the nearby banked cartilage when later lifting the new ear from the head; furthermore, this scalp site seemingly provides better nourishment for the banked cartilage than does the subcutaneous chest region.

When harvesting this cartilage wedge material during the first-stage procedure, I split the cartilage in situ, which allows a wider portion of cartilage to be obtained to achieve maximum projection of the ear. This technique consists of shaving the outer cartilage from the rib and deliberately violates Gibson's balanced cross-sectional principles,[83] causing the cartilage wedge to warp into an ideal shape for the posterior conchal wall that it will form (Fig. 74-21). This method of tissue

Text continued on p. 656

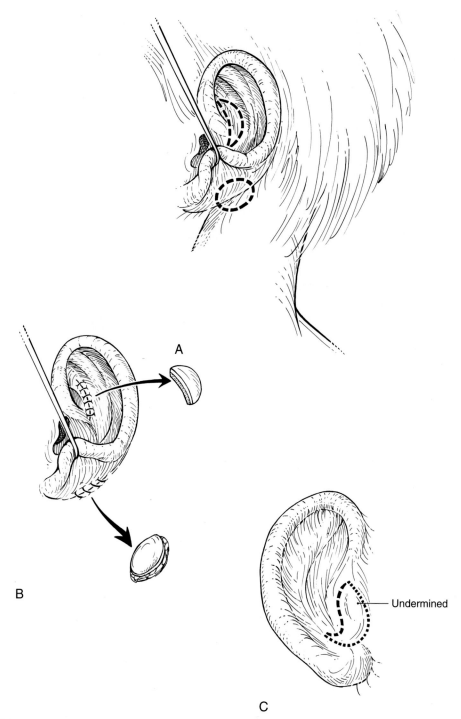

FIGURE 74-17. *A* to *H,* Stage 4, tragus construction and conchal excavation. Harvested from the opposite normal ear's conchal region, a chondrocutaneous composite graft is placed under a thin J-shaped flap to form the tragus. Before the floor of the tragal region is surfaced with a full-thickness skin graft (FTSG) harvested from behind the opposite earlobe, extraneous soft tissues are excised to deepen the region.

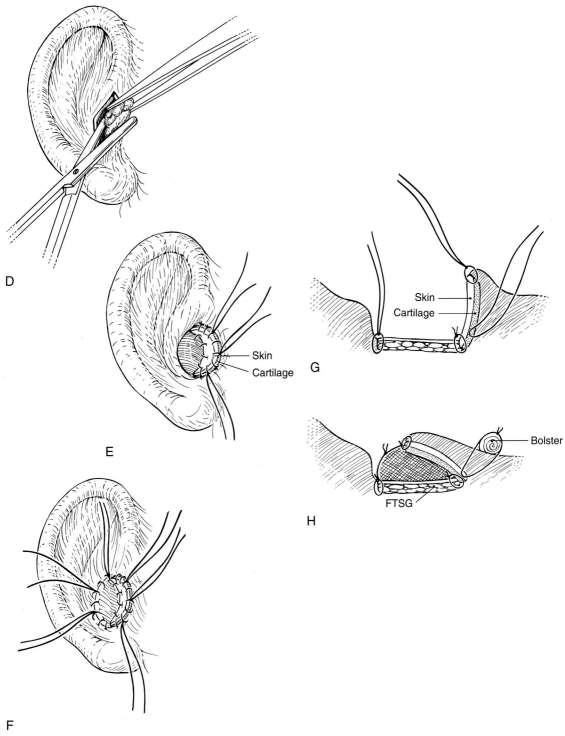

D

E

Skin
Cartilage

F

G

Skin
Cartilage

H

Bolster

FTSG

FIGURE 74-17, cont'd.

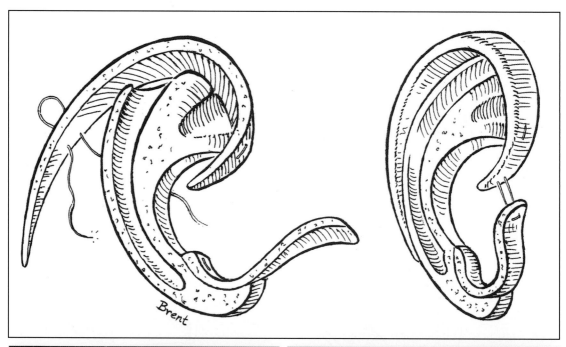

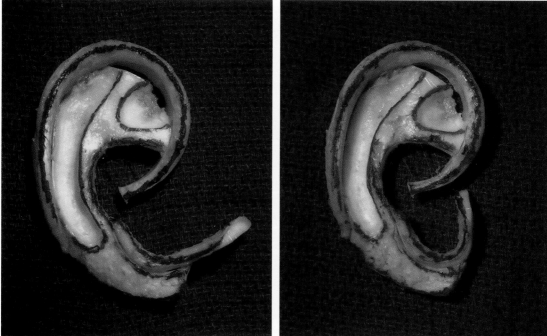

FIGURE 74-18. Ear framework fabrication with integral tragal strut. *Above,* Construction of the frame. The floating cartilage creates a helix, and a second strut is arched around to form the antitragus, intertragal notch, and tragus. This arch is completed when the tip of the strut is affixed to the crus helix of the main frame with horizontal mattress suture of clear nylon. *Below,* Actual framework fabrication with the patient's rib cartilage. (From Brent B: Technical advances in ear reconstruction with autogenous rib cartilage grafts: personal experience with 1200 cases. Plast Reconstr Surg 1999;104:319.)

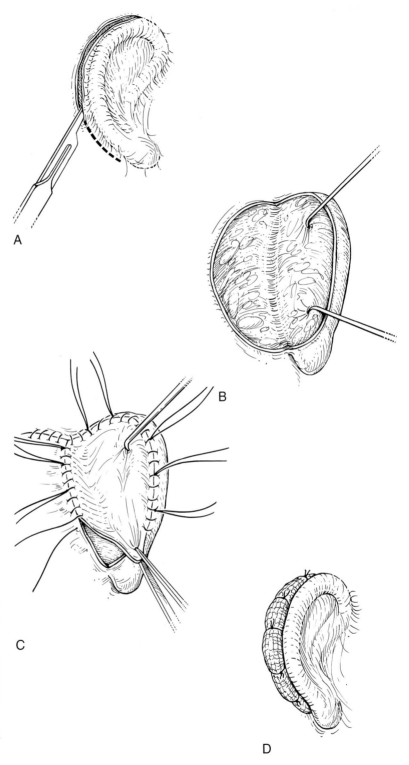

FIGURE 74-19. *A to D,* Stage 3, separating the surgically constructed ear from the head with skin graft. An incision is made several millimeters peripheral to the surgically constructed ear, and the auricle is sharply elevated from its fascial bed. The scalp is advanced to the newly created sulcus both to decrease graft requirements and to hide the graft by limiting its placement mostly to the ear's undersurface. Long silk sutures are tied over a bolus dressing.

harvest leaves the inner cartilage lamella intact, once again maximizing chest wall integrity and minimizing deformity.

MANAGING THE HAIRLINE

Low hairline is one of the most common and troublesome problems in auricular construction. Because the normal hairline is usually lower than the apex of a normal ear, and sometimes considerably lower in microtia, insertion of the framework beneath the periauricular skin often places hair on a portion of the new auricle. In trying to avoid hairy skin over the superior helix, the surgeon may be tempted to place the ear too low. Another complication arises when the framework is displaced anteriorly by the hairline, which acts as a constricting band at the juncture between the thin, hairless retroauricular skin and the thick scalp skin. This can be avoided by limiting the anterior dissection of the cutaneous pocket and by checking the framework's position before closing the incision.

Historically, Letterman and Harding[88] used a "scalp roll" and free skin graft to provide a hairless skin cover; however, this new cover lacks the elasticity of virgin skin. Instead, the author usually first implants the framework and later eradicates any undesirable hair. This can be done with electrolysis, by laser, or by replacing the follicular skin with a graft.[29] Before placement of an ear framework, if one predicts a tight pocket and a hairline that will cover half the new ear, a primary fascial flap may be considered.[89]

Dealing with this unwanted hair depends on how much ear is actually involved. If hair is limited to the helix, electrolysis or clipping is clearly the method of choice. If hair covers a third or more of the ear, the ear is often resurfaced with a skin graft[29] (with or without a fascial flap). Regardless of hair quantity, it is ideal to eradicate the hair by nonsurgical means, which eliminates a "patchwork" appearance and preserves the normal aesthetic and protective qualities of the local skin. Such a depilatory method would be even better if it simultaneously thinned the follicle-containing scalp skin to provide the new ear with finer skin coverage. Perhaps in the future both of these goals will be achieved without surgery.

In recent years, lasers have become useful adjuncts for treating the skin and its appendages.[90] In treatment of axillary hidradenitis with the laser, it has been found that not only is the condition improved by elimination of the apocrine sweat glands,[91] but by reduction of the bulk these epidermal appendages constitute, the skin also becomes finer and softer.[92] By virtue of the same principle, I am hopeful that significant reduction of the hair follicles may likewise alter the scalp skin so that when it does cover a portion of the ear framework, it will be somewhat thinner and

finer, resulting in enhanced detail of the completed ear.

Although it is still not consistently producing permanent results at this writing, laser treatments can favorably alter hair growth to make it both finer and slower. Furthermore, as contrasted to needle electrolysis, patients can tolerate laser treatment of much larger areas during a given session. The two schools of treatment concentrate on targeting the melanin (and thus the heavily pigmented follicles) within the depth of the dermis[93] versus targeting only the follicles by loading

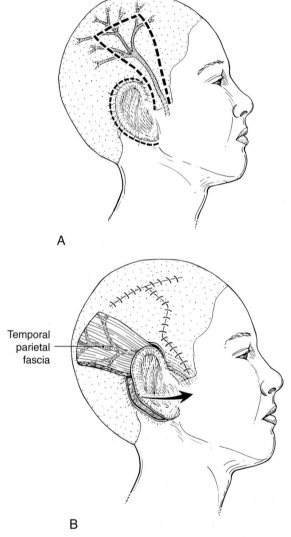

A

B

Temporal parietal fascia

FIGURE 74-20. *A to E,* Separating and projecting the surgically constructed ear, Nagata technique. The surgically constructed ear is separated from the head at the second stage. Projection is supplemented by wedging a piece of rib cartilage (harvested anew from the chest), then covering it with a temporal vessel–containing fascial flap and skin graft.

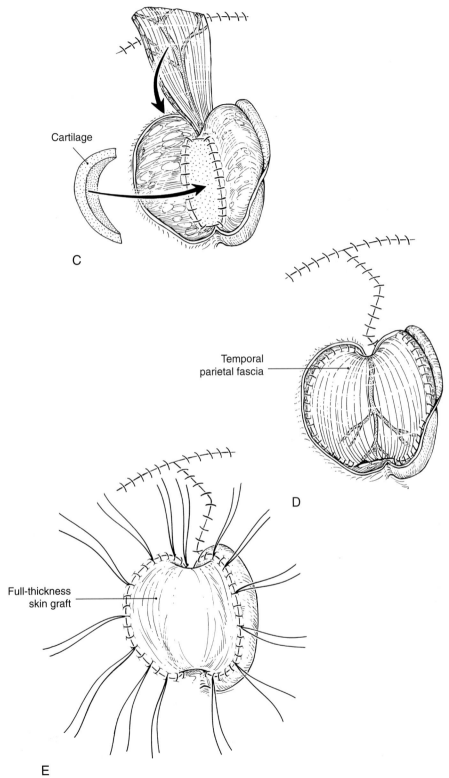

Cartilage

C

Temporal
parietal fascia

D

Full-thickness
skin graft

E
FIGURE 74-20, cont'd.

them with carbon particles through a gel transport medium and then focusing the laser on the carbon.[94,95] The trick is to deliver enough energy density through the laser to destroy the hair follicles without damaging the skin, which causes scarring or hypopigmentation. Presently, laser treatments decrease hair density and texture so that only a few "maintenance treatments" are needed per year. Laser technology continues to improve with such advances as better coolant techniques, which permit a higher fluence of energy to be delivered safely. Soon, it should consistently be possible to achieve permanent hair removal without injurious side effects to the surrounding skin.[96] It is my vision to "pre-treat" ear reconstruction patients with the laser and thus create the ideal hairline *before* initiating the surgical ear repair (Fig. 74-22). To aid the laser technician (who often may be at a great distance from my practice), a template is provided that makes it easy to precisely relocate the exact target area during the serial treatments (see Fig. 74-22).[23]

Variations in Total Ear Reconstruction Technique

Numerous variations in technique have evolved during the years and will continue to emerge. One of the current popular variations is the Nagata technique, in which the ear reconstruction is accomplished in two stages.[32,87] In this method, the cartilage framework implantation, tragus construction, and lobule transposition are performed in the first stage; the ear is separated from the head at the second stage with a block of cartilage (harvested by entering the chest for a second time), which is covered by a fascial flap and skin graft.

Although this eliminates several stages of surgery, all the soft tissue manipulation in the initial stage dramatically increases the risk of tissue necrosis; the complication rate with this procedure is 14% (by contrast, the author's technique has experienced a complication rate of less than 0.25% during the past 1000 cases). This combination of procedures also sacrifices the earlobe quality by lining the tragus with the lobe's valuable back-side skin. In the author's opinion, the final appearance and quality of the earlobe are far more important than forming a tragus during the initial first stage.

Because the Nagata technique produces the antihelical complex by wiring an extra piece of cartilage to the base block (Fig. 74-23), the ears produced are thick, and more rib cartilage is needed and excised from the chest with attendant chest wall donor deformity.[80,81] The numerous wire sutures that are used to apply these two pieces together (as well as to attach the helix) are placed on the lateral cartilage surfaces and lie precariously under the thin auricular integument (see Fig. 74-23), and thus they bear great risk of frequent

extrusion through the skin.[97] Tanzer reported wire extrusions in 20 of his 44 cases,[53] and he used one fourth as many sutures per ear as does Nagata.

To achieve ear projection, the Nagata technique uses the superficial temporal vessel–containing fascial flap in every case (see Fig. 74-20), with its attendant scalp scar and its risk of hair thinning in the donor site.[29] Because Nagata enters the chest again (to obtain the cartilage wedge) during this procedure, the patient is subjected to a second uncomfortable operation.

Finally, the Nagata technique does not address frontal symmetry of the two ears, and for the technique to deal with this and to be complete, a third stage is really required.[97] In the author's technique, the symmetry is dealt with during the tragus construction when the grafts for the tragus are harvested from the opposite ear (see Fig. 74-17). This allows one to adjust the donor ear to the reconstructed ear and to achieve frontal symmetry; by doing this as the final stage, the healed final position of the elevated ear has occurred so one knows where to set the opposite ear during the tragus construction so that symmetry can be accomplished.

The Nagata technique has produced some interesting and useful variations in ear reconstruction and continues to evolve.[30,85] Other variations will emerge as the quest for improved ear reconstruction continues.

FIGURE 74-21. Augmenting ear projection with split cartilage graft and retroauricular turnover fascial flap. *Above,* Broad cartilage wedge harvested by splitting rib cartilage. Chest wall integrity is maintained by preserving inner cartilage lamella; the harvested outer lamella predictably warps to favorably shape the posterior conchal wall wedge. *Second row, left,* Splitting the rib cartilage in situ. *Second row, center,* Outer cartilage lamella predictably begins to warp. *Second row, right,* The harvested wedge. Note preserved inner cartilage lamella of the chest wall. The curved cartilage graft is banked subcutaneously until needed for projecting the surgically constructed ear. *Third row,* Scheme of separating the surgically constructed ear from the head, placing the projection-maintaining cartilage wedge and covering it with turnover flap of retroauricular fascia, then applying split-skin graft. *Below, left,* Projection of elevated ear augmented with the banked split-cartilage graft. Note how the purposeful warp has remained and produced an ideal shape for the new posterior conchal wall *(inset).* This particular graft had been subcutaneously banked beneath the original chest incision. *Below, second from right,* The fascial flap turned over the cartilage wedge, before skin graft is applied. *Below, right,* The healed repair. Note maintenance of projection and auriculocephalic sulcus. (From Brent B: Technical advances in ear reconstruction with autogenous rib cartilage grafts: personal experience with 1200 cases. Plast Reconstr Surg 1999;104:319.)

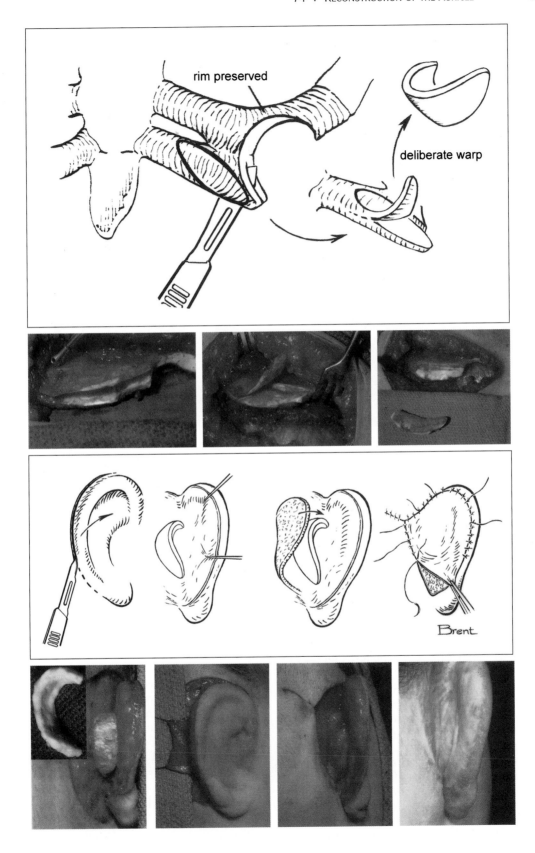

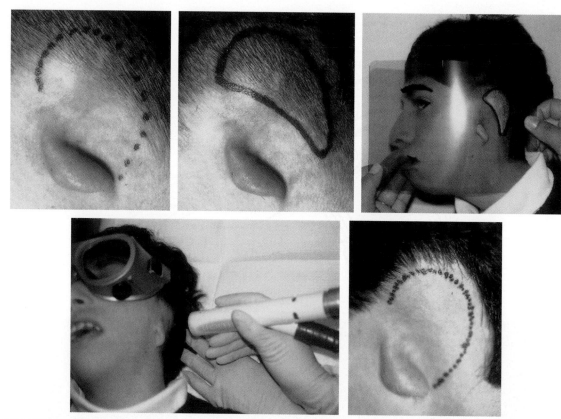

FIGURE 74-22. "Hairline idealization" by presurgical laser treatment. *Above, left,* Microtia with typical low hairline, which would cover the upper portion of the proposed auricular construction. *Above, center,* Crescent-shaped area designated for laser de-epilation before embarking on surgical ear repair. *Above, right,* Film template to aid in relocating the exact crescent during serial laser treatments. Note aids in applying the template: cut-out area slips over vestige; eyebrow, lateral canthus, and oral commissure are marked on film. *Below, left,* The laser treatment in progress. *Below, right,* The same microtia after several laser treatments. The hairline is now ideal, and surgical construction of the ear will begin. (From Brent B: Technical advances in ear reconstruction with autogenous rib cartilage grafts: personal experience with 1200 cases. Plast Reconstr Surg 1999;104:319.)

Secondary Reconstruction

The difficulties in surgically constructing an ear are substantiated by the often disheartening result that emerges despite the surgeon's persistent efforts. Discouragingly, at times the end result bears no resemblance to an auricle, other than for its location. Furthermore, the scars that result from multiple procedures may extend the defect well beyond the original deformity. The impact of such failures is emotionally devastating to the patient and proportionately frustrating for the surgeon.

Tanzer[98] managed secondary reconstruction by first excising the scar and skin grafting the defect, then waiting for the graft to mature before implanting a new cartilage framework. However, this approach is often beset with compromises in that skin-grafted tissues have limited elasticity as a cutaneous pocket, and a detailed framework with depth cannot be

introduced without significant tension. Furthermore, deeply scarred tissue beds may be so severely damaged that this approach is not even possible, and, seemingly, the patient is left with no solution to the problem.

In an effort to resolve this skin coverage impasse, Brent and Byrd[89] implemented a more optimal method for secondary ear reconstruction: excision of the entire auricular scar area and immediate placement of a sculpted autogenous rib cartilage graft, which is covered with a temporoparietal fascial flap and skin graft (Figs. 74-24 and 74-25).

Bilateral Microtia

Although relatively rare, bilateral microtia frequently afflicts patients with such conditions as Treacher Collins–Franceschetti syndrome, bilateral craniofacial

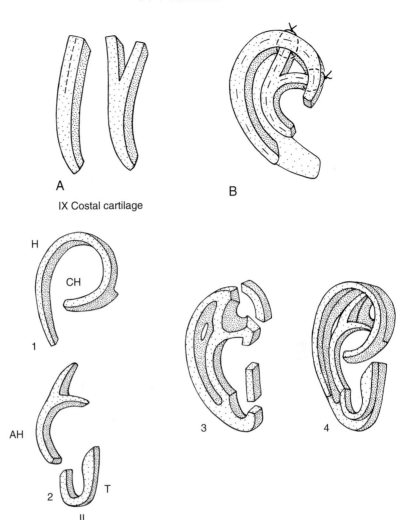

IX Costal cartilage

FIGURE 74-23. Ear framework fabrication with appliqué of cartilage components. *Above* (*A* and *B*), Spina first applied a separate antihelical complex to the base block in 1971. (Redrawn from Spina V, Psillakis JM: Total reconstruction of the ear in congenital microtia. Plast Reconstr Surg 1971;48:349.) *Below,* Nagata revived Spina's technique and added his own modifications. The numerous wire sutures used in this method lie precariously under the thin auricular skin. H, helix; CH, crus of helix; AH, antihelix; T, tragus. (Redrawn from Nagata S: Modification of the stages in total reconstruction of the auricle. Plast Reconstr Surg 1994;93:221.) See text.

microsomia, and other uncommon craniofacial malformations (see Chapter 103). The reconstructive principles for management of bilateral microtia are the same as for the unilateral deformity.

For optimal function and aesthetics in bilateral microtia, one must plan to integrate surgical procedures so that one does not compromise the other. In these cases, the auricular construction must precede the middle ear surgery; once an attempt is made to "open" the ear, chances of obtaining a satisfactory auricular repair are severely compromised because the invaluable virgin skin has been scarred.

In bilateral microtia, cartilage graft procedures are performed on each side several months apart because each hemithorax contains sufficient cartilage for only one good ear framework. Simultaneous bilateral reconstruction necessitates bilateral chest wounds with attendant splinting and respiratory distress. Furthermore,

the first auricular repair might be jeopardized on turning the head to do the second side. For these reasons, it is preferable to perform the first stage of each ear on separate occasions.

Several months after the second cartilage graft, both earlobes are transposed during a single procedure. Once this stage is healed, one can either separate the ears from the head with skin grafting or pursue the middle ear surgery. Nine of 10 patients with microtia have only unilateral involvement, and most do well without middle ear surgery because they are born "adjusted" to their monaural condition.

To ensure that the gains of middle ear surgery outweigh the risks and complications of the procedure itself, this surgery is reserved for cases in which the patient is highly motivated and there is favorable radiologic evidence of middle ear development. Then, it must be thoughtfully planned in a "team approach"[23]

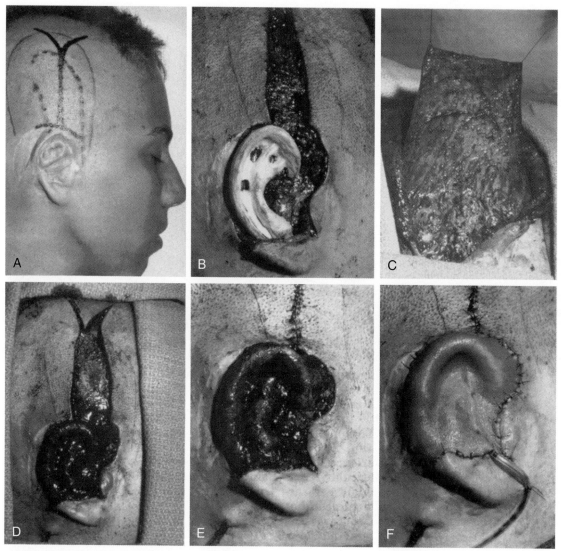

FIGURE 74-24. Ear reconstruction with autogenous rib cartilage surfaced by a skin graft–covered temporoparietal fascial flap. *A,* A patient with a scarred auricular region. Doppler vessels, the flap extent, and the Y-shaped incision are indicated. *B,* Scar excision, framework fabrication, and scalp dissection are begun. *C,* Raising a fascial flap that contains the superficial temporal vessels. *D,* Fascial flap draped over the ear framework. *E,* Scalp wound sutured. *F,* Skin graft applied over the fascia-covered ear framework. (From Brent B, Byrd HS: Secondary ear reconstruction with cartilage grafts covered by axial, random, and free flaps of temporoparietal fascia. Plast Reconstr Surg 1983;72:141.)

with an otologist who is competent and well experienced in atresia surgery.

In the team approach, the plastic surgeon initiates the procedure by lifting the ear from its bed while carefully preserving connective tissue on the framework's undersurface. Then the otologist proceeds, first drilling a bony canal, completing the ossiculoplasty, and then repairing the tympanum with a temporal fascial graft. Finally, the plastic surgeon resumes by excising soft tissues to exteriorize the meatus through the conchal region and harvesting a skin graft, which the otologist uses to line the new canal and complete the repair (Fig. 74-26).

The Constricted Ear

Tanzer has applied "constricted ear" to a group of ear anomalies in which the encircling helix seems tight, as if constricted by a purse string (Fig. 74-27). Once loosely termed cup or lop ears, these deformities collectively have helical and scaphal hooding and varying degrees of flattening of their antihelical complexes.

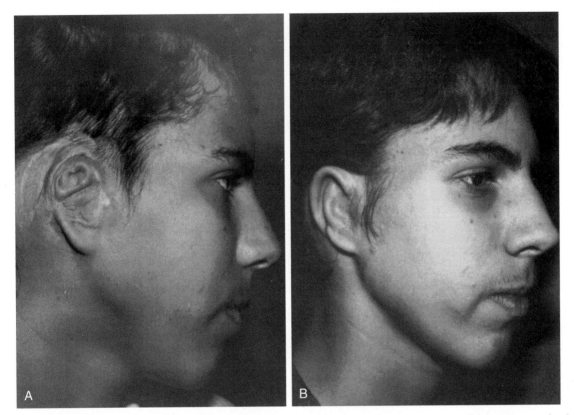

FIGURE 74-25. Secondary ear reconstruction with a rib cartilage graft surfaced with a superficial temporoparietal fascial flap and skin graft. *A,* A patient with a scarred auricular region after multiple failed procedures. *B,* Result achieved in one surgical stage with rib cartilage graft and fascial flap by the techniques outlined in Figure 74-24.

Although Tanzer gave these ears a numerical classification that corresponds to each deformity's severity,[62] in practical surgical terms, one needs to determine whether the ear can be repaired by reshaping the existing tissues or whether skin coverage or the supporting cartilage must be supplemented.

One must individualize constricted ear repairs for each specific ear deformity. If helical lidding is the main defect and the height discrepancy is minimal, the overhanging tissue can merely be excised. At times, the cartilage lid can be used as a "banner flap" to increase ear height (Fig. 74-28). Moderate height discrepancies necessitate augmentation of the cartilage height by modifying the ipsilateral ear cartilage[99,100] or employing contralateral conchal cartilage grafts.[76] The key to repair of these moderate deformities is to visualize the defective cartilage armature, which is possible only after one "degloves" the skin envelope (Figs. 74-29 and 74-30).

When constriction is severe enough to produce a height difference of 1.5 cm, one must add both skin and cartilage and essentially correct the deformity as if it were a formal microtia (Fig. 74-31).

Cryptotia

Cryptotia is an unusual congenital deformity in which the upper pole of the ear cartilage is buried beneath the scalp (Fig. 74-32). The superior auriculocephalic sulcus is absent but can be demonstrated through gentle finger pressure. This has stimulated Japanese physicians to correct this deformity nonsurgically[101] because it occurs in Japan as frequently as 1 in 400 births.[102]

This nonsurgical procedure is accomplished through application of an external conforming splint. If the splint is applied before 6 months of age, it may successfully mold a permanent retroauricular sulcus.[103] Tan et al[104] have successfully applied such nonsurgical splinting techniques for constricted ears as well (Fig. 74-33). Yotsuyanagi et al[105] have successfully employed these nonsurgical methods to correct a variety of ear deformities in children older than neonates.

Surgical repairs entail addition of skin to the deficient retroauricular sulcus by skin grafts and Z-plasties, V-Y advancement flaps,[106] or rotational flaps.[103]

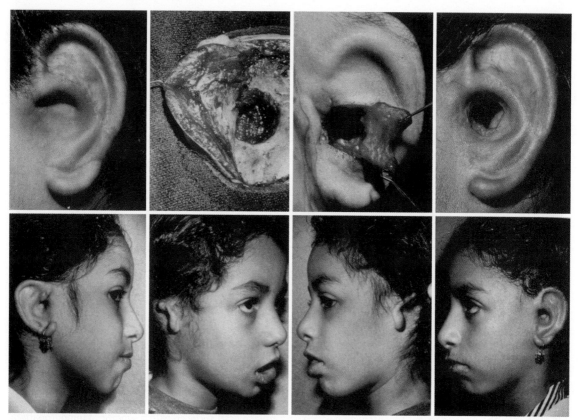

FIGURE 74-26. Team approach to bilateral microtia. *Above, left,* Initial auricular repair, after framework placement and lobule transposition. *Above, left center,* Team approach to middle ear. The plastic surgeon lifts constructed auricle from bed, taking care to preserve connective tissue on cartilage framework; next, the otologic surgeon drills bony canal and completes middle ear repair. *Above, right center,* The plastic surgeon then raises a conchal skin flap and removes intervening soft tissues to exteriorize canal. *Above, right,* With use of the flap to circumvent atresia by breaking up contractual forces, it is dropped into the introitus of the canal, which is skin grafted to complete the repair. Alternatively, the skin flap could have been based anteriorly and doubled on itself for a Kirkham tragal construction. *Below, center,* Preoperative views of the same bilateral microtia patient. *Below, left and right,* Bilateral results of the external and middle ear team repair. (From Brent B: Auricular repair with autogenous rib cartilage grafts: two decades of experience with 600 cases. Plast Reconstr Surg 1992;90:355.)

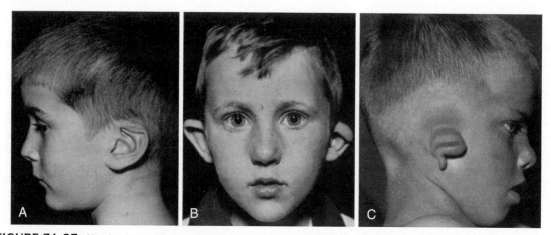

FIGURE 74-27. Varying types of constricted ears. *A,* Involvement of the helix only. *B,* Involvement of the helix and scapha (left auricle). *C,* Severe cupping deformity coupled with incomplete migration of the auricle.

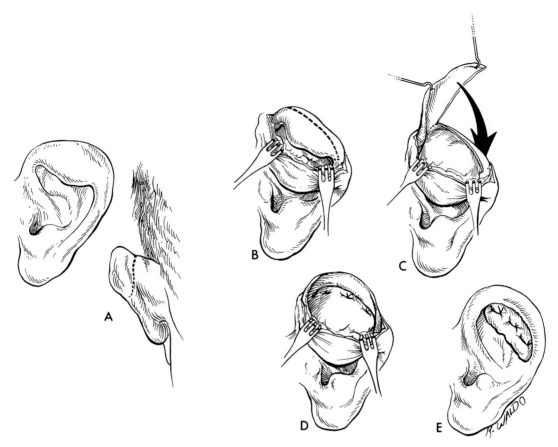

FIGURE 74-28. Correction of grade I ear constriction. *A,* The incision for exposure of the skeletal deformity. *B,* The deformed cartilage has been filleted from its soft tissue cover. The line of detachment of the angulated segment is marked. *C,* The deformed cartilage is lifted on a medially based pedicle and rotated into an upright position. *D,* The repositioned cartilage is sutured to the scapha. *E,* The skin is redraped, and the helical sulcus is maintained by through-and-through sutures tied over gauze pledgets. (From Tanzer RC, Edgerton MT, eds: Symposium on Reconstruction of the Auricle. St. Louis, CV Mosby, 1974:141.)

When a cartilage deformity accompanies the skin deficiency, various remodeling techniques are needed to facilitate the repair.[102,107]

The Prominent Ear

PATHOLOGY

During the third month of gestation, the auricle's protrusion increases; by the end of the sixth month, the helical margin curls, the antihelix forms its fold, and the antihelical crura appear. Anything that interferes with this process produces prominent ears.

The most common deformity arises from the antihelix's failing to fold. This widens the conchoscaphal angle as much as 150 degrees or more (Fig. 74-34), which flattens the superior crus and, in severe forms, the antihelical body and inferior crus. In extreme cases, the helical roll may be absent, which produces a flat, shell-like ear with no convolutions.

Producing protrusion of the ear's middle third, conchal widening may occur as an isolated deformity or in conjunction with antihelical deformities described before. This abnormality is usually bilateral and is frequently noted in siblings and the parents.

TREATMENT

In repair of prominent ears, symmetry is most important and, paradoxically, may be more difficult to achieve in unilateral than in bilateral cases. The repaired ear convolutions should appear smooth and unoperated on. The most lateral point of the completed repair should be between 1.7 and 2.0 cm from the head, and the helix should be visible behind the antihelical body when one sees the ears from the frontal view.[108]

To attain these goals, a great number of techniques have been described, many of which produce

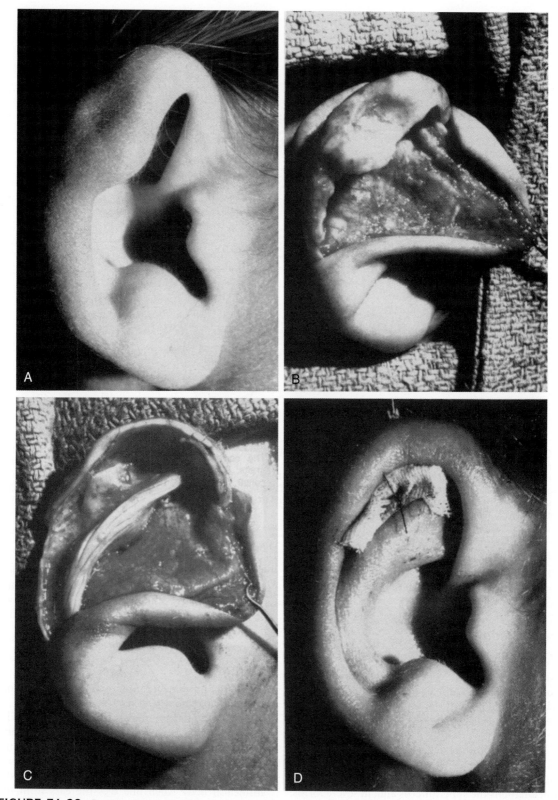

FIGURE 74-29. Repair of a moderately constricted ear. *A,* Preoperative appearance. *B,* "Degloving" the ear to expose the distorted cartilage. *C,* The cartilage is expanded, the antihelix is formed, and a contralateral conchal cartilage graft repairs the deficient upper third. *D,* Skin redraped to complete the repair. See Figure 74-30*B*. (From Brent B: The correction of microtia with autogenous cartilage grafts. II. Atypical and complex deformities. Plast Reconstr Surg 1980;66:13.)

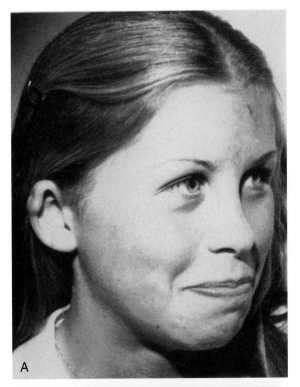

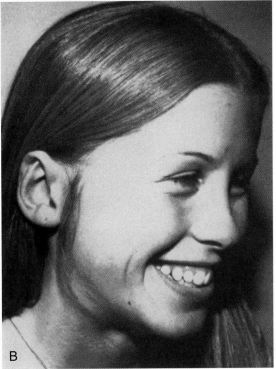

FIGURE 74-30. Repair of a moderately constricted ear by the technique shown in Figure 74-29. (From Brent B: The correction of microtia with autogenous cartilage grafts. II. Atypical and complex deformities. Plast Reconstr Surg 1980;66:13.)

acceptable results. However, the author recommends that the surgeon direct efforts toward correcting the specific problem areas of each individual ear rather than following a routine "cookbook recipe."

If the upper third of the ear protrudes because of an absent or weak antihelix, one must form an exaggerated antihelix. If the middle third is too prominent, one must recess the concha by either cartilage excision or suture fixation.[109] Finally, if the lobule protrudes, one must either resect or reposition the cartilaginous tail of the cauda helicis[110] or excise retrolobular skin.

CONCHAL ALTERATION

Dieffenbach[3] is credited with the first otoplastic attempt in 1845. This consisted of his excising skin from the auriculocephalic sulcus and then suturing conchal cartilage to the mastoid periosteum.

In addition to narrowing the auriculocephalic sulcus, Ely[4] (1881) and others excised a strip of conchal wall, a procedure that is attributed to Morestin[111] in 1903. This old method of tacking back the concha to mastoid periosteum has been revived throughout the years (Fig. 74-35).[109,112-115]

Also, one can correct the wide concha by excising a cartilaginous ellipse beneath the antihelical body. This may create a redundant skinfold, which then may require excision.

RESTORING OF THE ANTIHELICAL FOLD

Luckett (1910) first conceptualized that prominent ears result from the antihelix's failure to fold. He restored this fold by excising a crescent of medial skin and cartilage (Fig. 74-36).[116] The majority of subsequent otoplasty procedures have focused on making a smoother antihelix than is produced by employing Luckett's sharp cartilage-breaking technique.[108,117-119]

ALTERING THE MEDIAL CARTILAGE SURFACE

To permit its smooth molding, one can recontour the scaphal cartilage by a number of techniques. McEvitt[120] and Paletta[113] weakened the scapha with multiple parallel cuts; Converse et al[121] used burr abrasion.

Becker,[122,123] Converse,[121] and Tanzer[124] used parallel cuts and permanent sutures to form a smooth, cornucopia-like antihelix (Fig. 74-37). Advantageously, this cartilage tube encases substantial scar to lock the cartilage into position and prevent recurrence of deformity.

Reviving a long-forgotten suggestion of Morestin,[111] Mustarde[125,126] formed the antihelix by inserting permanent mattress sutures through the cartilage without using any actual cartilage incisions. The author finds this technique particularly useful in the pliable ear

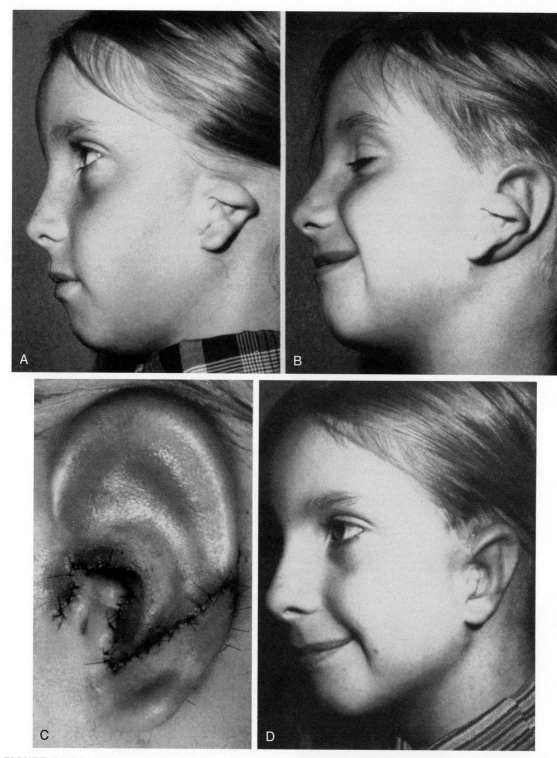

FIGURE 74-31. Repair of severe ear constriction by the classic microtia technique. *A,* A patient with a severely constricted ear. *B,* Appearance after insertion of total ear framework of rib cartilage. *C,* Use of the vestige to form the earlobe and tragus. *D,* Final result after separation from the head with a skin graft. (From Brent B: The correction of microtia with autogenous cartilage grafts. II. Atypical and complex deformities. Plast Reconstr Surg 1980;66:13.)

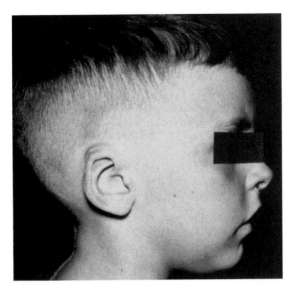

FIGURE 74-32. Cryptotia.

cartilage of children. Surgeons who criticize this technique mention recurrence of the deformity, presumably because the sutures tear through the cartilage. I have circumvented this technical problem by hydrodissecting the anterolateral skin from the cartilage with saline injected through a 30-gauge needle just before passing each permanent suture. This has worked well in preventing recurrent deformities (Fig. 74-38).

ALTERING THE LATERAL CARTILAGE SURFACE

Exploiting cartilage's tendency to warp when one surface is cut,[83] Chongchet[127] scored the anterior scaphal cartilage with multiple cartilage cuts to roll it back and form an antihelix. While Chongchet did this under direct vision using a scalpel, Stenstrom[128] produced the same effect by using a short-tined rasp instrument to "blindly" score the antihelical region through a posterior stab incision near the cauda helicis. The lateral cartilage surface has also been morselized or abraded under direct vision through a lateral incision.[129]

Finally, Kaye[130] advocates an otoplasty method that combines both lateral cartilage scoring and fixation with permanent sutures. He accomplishes both of these maneuvers through minimal incisions (Fig. 74-39).

ACQUIRED DEFORMITIES

Total auricular reconstruction in the acquired deformity presents special problems not encountered in microtia. These merit separate consideration.

The lack of skin coverage is much more critical than in microtia; an existing meatus precludes use of the anterior incision, and extra skin, as usually gained by removing the crumpled microtic cartilage, is not available. This factor compounds the previously mentioned hairline problem. If one can use the existing skin, the cutaneous pocket is best developed by incisions above or below the proposed auricular site. If the local tissues are heavily scarred or restrict the surgeon

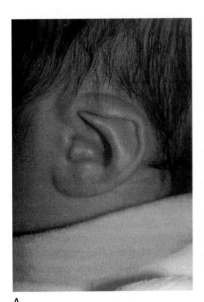
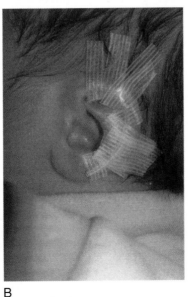
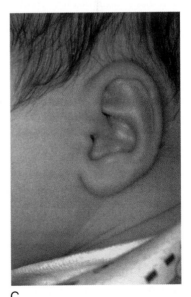

A   B   C

FIGURE 74-33. *A,* Neonate with lop ear. *B,* Custom splint used to correct helical fold. *C,* Follow-up photograph taken 2 months after completion of 10 weeks of splinting. (From Tan ST, Abramson DL, MacDonald DM, Mulliken JB: Molding therapy for infants with deformational auricular anomalies. Ann Plast Surg 1997;38:263.)

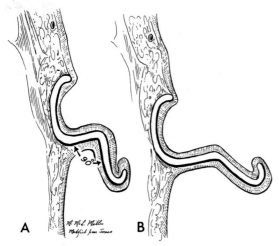

FIGURE 74-34. *A,* Cross section of a normal ear. *B,* Prominent ear resulting from an increased conchoscaphal angle.

from developing an ample skin pocket, the repair must be supplemented with fascial flap coverage (see Figs. 74-24 and 74-25).[89] Skin expanders have also been employed to stretch the covering skin but bear risks of extrusion and scar capsule formation.

Replantation of the Amputated Auricle

Replantation of amputated segments of the auricle was practiced in the 17th century. Cocheril[131] cites the memoirs of Strafford written during the reign of the English king Charles I. To punish Puritan and colonist opposition to the regime, the victim's ear was frequently nailed to a wooden post and then amputated. Three of these many victims have been specifically documented: Burton, a minister in the government; Prynne, a lawyer; and Bartwick, a physician.[131] Prynne had earlier published a book that was considered offensive to the queen and consequently had his ears amputated. When he appeared before the Tribunal a second time, the presiding judge was surprised to see Prynne with two normal-appearing ears. Prynne's ears were exposed but showed the signs of mutilation. Having been condemned to have his ears amputated a second time, Prynne retrieved the amputated ears, hoping to have them sutured back to their original site as had been done previously. No information is available about the fate of Burton's ears. We know that Bartwick's wife collected his amputated ears and placed them carefully into a handkerchief, hoping to have them replanted. All this took place between 1630 and 1640.

Cocheril cites many examples of successful replantations during the 19th century and states, "It is difficult to doubt the good faith of these authors: the prestige attached to their names; the clarity of their reports; the official approval given to their reports should suffice to consider them as veracious. The vascularity of the auricle, the rapid healing of wounds of this structure, the fact that the vessels remain gaping, ready to receive nourishing fluid—all mitigate in favor of the veracity of the reports." The only information missing in all of these reports is the size of the amputated parts.

To the modern plastic surgeon, choosing a salvage procedure is influenced by the size of the amputated

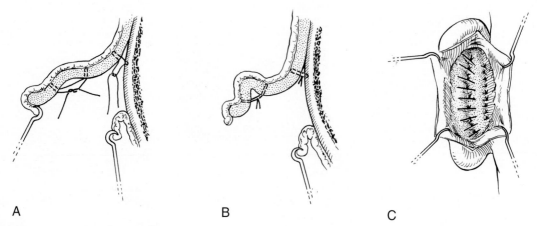

FIGURE 74-35. Technique of reducing prominence by conchomastoid sutures. *A,* Cross section of the auricle showing placement of the sutures to reduce the conchomastoid angle and to restore the antihelical fold. *B,* Correction of the prominence. *C,* View of the medial surface of the auricular cartilage after correction of the prominence. (From Spira M, McCrea P, Gerow F, Hardy B: Analysis and treatment of the protruding ear. Transactions of the 4th International Congress of Plastic Surgery. Amsterdam, Excerpta Medica, 1969.)

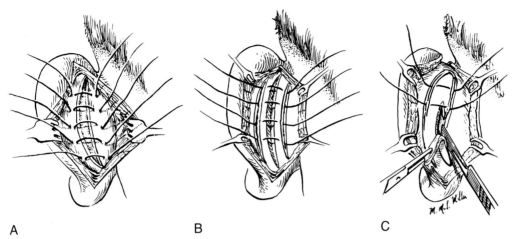

FIGURE 74-36. Evolution of the tubing principle for correction of prominent ears. *A*, Luckett; *B*, Barsky; *C*, Becker.

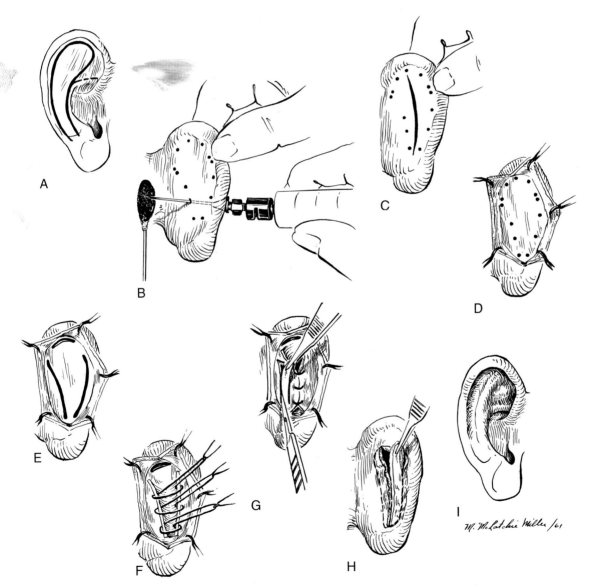

FIGURE 74-37. Complete corrective otoplasty (Tanzer modification of Converse procedure).

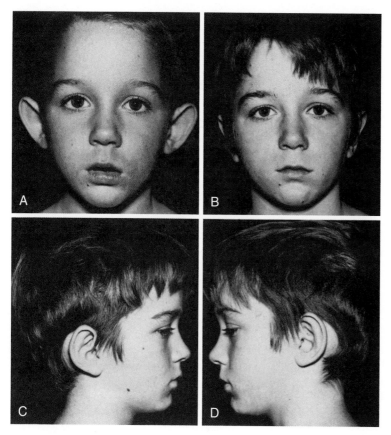

FIGURE 74-38. *A,* Prominent ears characterized by wide conchae and lack of antihelical folds. Previous treatment of the cartilage by mattress sutures resulted only in recurrence. *B* to *D,* Correction by cartilage tubing to form an antihelical fold and elliptical excision of excess concha.

portion; the condition of the tissues of the amputated segment; and the condition of the stump and surrounding tissues, particularly in the retroauricular area. A clean-cut amputation gives the surgeon a better chance for success. When the ear and its surrounding tissues are mangled and avulsed and bone is exposed, the reconstruction is difficult if not insurmountable. Small amputated segments are replaced as composite grafts with some hope of success. Larger amputated segments and subtotal amputation require further consideration.

REPLANTATION OF AURICULAR TISSUE ATTACHED BY A NARROW PEDICLE

Because an ear is richly vascularized and has major vessels extending through its periphery, one can successfully replace the partly avulsed auricular tissue even though the remaining attachment is tenuous (Fig. 74-40).

REPLANTATION OF AURICULAR TISSUE AS A COMPOSITE GRAFT

Even when the piece of auricle is large, the completely detached ear tissue may survive when replaced as a composite graft, although few successful cases have been reported in the plastic surgery literature (Figs. 74-41 and 74-42).[132-134]

REPLANTATION OF AURICULAR CARTILAGE

Because a cartilaginous framework is difficult to reproduce, the salvage and use of denuded auricular cartilage were recommended by numerous surgeons.[135-138] Various techniques have been employed to preserve cartilage from an avulsed ear. The skin may be removed and the cartilage buried in an abdominal pocket,[139] buried in a cervical pocket,[140] or placed under the skin of the retroauricular area.[141] The orthotopic cartilage replantation can be employed only if regional cutaneous tissues are in good condition.

Although logical, the author finds this procedure futile; the flimsy ear cartilage almost invariably flattens beneath the snug, discrepant two-dimensional skin cover. Furthermore, when amputated ear cartilage has been "banked" in the retroauricular region, it hampers later reconstructive attempts by producing an irregular, amorphous structure that is adherent to the overlying regional skin.

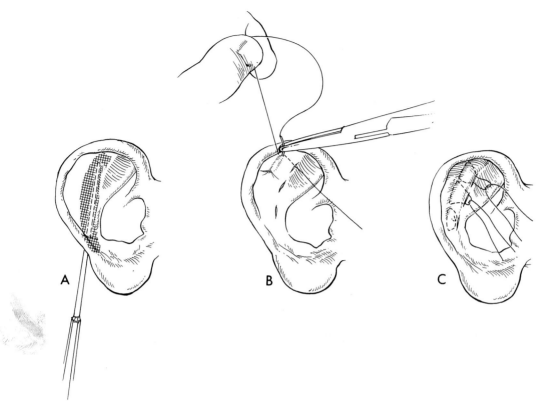

FIGURE 74-39. The Kaye method to correct flattening of the antihelix. *A,* A subperichondrial tunnel is made on the lateral surface of the cartilage through a medial incision near the cauda helicis; a sharp-tined instrument produces curling by multiple vertical striations. *B* and *C,* The proper amount of antihelical roll is maintained by several mattress sutures introduced through tiny incisions along the conchal crest and carried across the antihelical fold through holes in the skin. (From Kaye BL: A simplified method for correcting the prominent ear. Plast Reconstr Surg 1967;40:44. Copyright © 1967, The Williams & Wilkins Company, Baltimore.)

REPLANTATION OF THE DERMABRADED AMPUTATED AURICLE

Mladick et al[142] and Mladick and Carraway[143] have advocated first dermabrasion and then reattachment of the amputated ear to its stump. The reattached ear is then buried in a subcutaneous postauricular pocket, which allows revascularization through the exposed dermis of the dermabraded auricle (Fig. 74-43). Several weeks later, the ear is exteriorized by blunt dissection from its covering flap, which is allowed to slide behind the helical rim. At this time, the subcutaneous attachments of the medial auricular surface are left intact. The exposed raw auricular surface is dressed, and epithelialization begins within several days.

Rather than separate the medial auricular attachments from their bed several weeks later to allow spontaneous re-epithelialization as Mladick originally suggested, the author thinks it is safer to wait several months before separating the ear frame from the head.

At that time, one can skin graft the new retroauricular sulcus as in a classic ear reconstruction.

REPLANTATION OF THE AMPUTATED AURICLE ON REMOVAL OF POSTAURICULAR SKIN AND FENESTRATION OF CARTILAGE

Almost invariably, the replantation of large composite parts is doomed to fail,[144] unless one increases the vascular recipient area. Instead of employing dermabrasion to achieve this, Baudet[145] removed the skin from the postauricular portion of the amputated part, fenestrated the cartilage, and placed the auricular segment into a raw area established by raising a flap of retroauricular-mastoid skin (Fig. 74-44). The cartilaginous windows allowed direct contact of the auricular skin with the recipient site, thus facilitating its revascularization. Although some distortion of the superior helical border occurred (Fig. 74-45), the result was satisfactory.

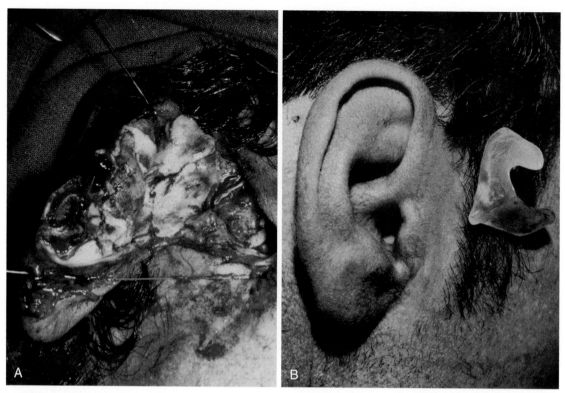

FIGURE 74-40. Repair of a major auricular avulsion. *A,* The avulsed ear remains attached by a narrow pedicle, which maintains its viability; the canal is transected. *B,* Result after repair of the canal and maintenance of an acrylic mold for 4 months.

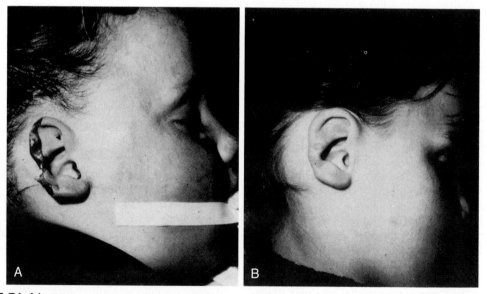

FIGURE 74-41. Replantation of auricular tissue as a composite graft. *A,* Loss of a portion of the scapha and helix resulting from a dog bite. *B,* The amputated segment was retrieved and sutured in position as a composite graft, with this result 2 years later. (Patient of Dr. Andries Molenaar.)

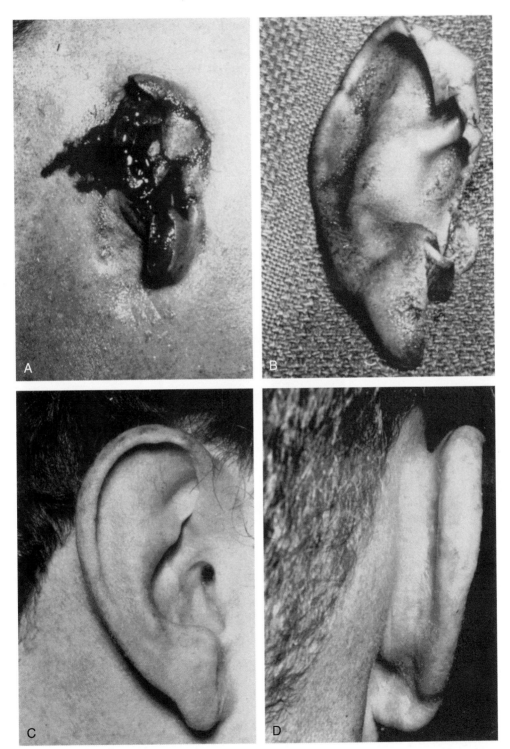

FIGURE 74-42. Replantation of a totally amputated auricle as a composite graft. *A,* The stump of the amputated auricle $5^1/_2$ hours after the accident. *B,* The amputated part includes the pinna, the earlobe, and part of the concha. *C* and *D,* The final result after reattachment. (From Clemons JE, Connelly MV: Reattachment of a totally amputated auricle. Arch Otolaryngol 1973;97:269.)

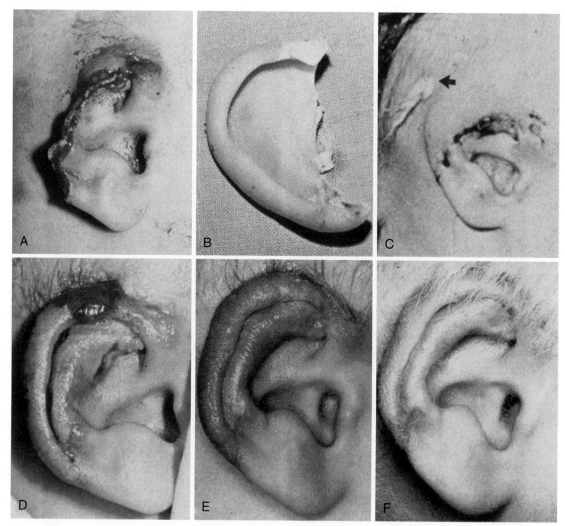

FIGURE 74-43. Reattachment of the severed auricle by dermabrasion and subcutaneous "pocketing." *A*, The amputated stump. *B*, The severed part. *C*, The dermabraded reattached part is buried in a postauricular pocket; a traction suture *(arrow)* from the helix flattens out the auricle to gain better apposition of the tissues. *D*, The ear has been exteriorized and is almost completely epithelialized (see text for details); one granulating area is seen at the superior margin. *E*, One month after injury, the ear has a red flush over the reattached segment. *F*, Appearance at 5 months. (From Mladick R, Carraway J: Ear reattachment by the modified pocket principle. Plast Reconstr Surg 1973;51:584. Copyright © 1973, The Williams & Wilkins Company, Baltimore.)

REPLANTING THE EAR CARTILAGE AND IMMEDIATELY COVERING IT WITH A FASCIAL FLAP AND SKIN GRAFT

In selected cases in which the wounds are clean, the scalp is intact, and the patient's general condition is stable, one might be tempted to remove the amputated ear's skin and to cover the filleted cartilage immediately with a fascial flap and skin graft. Because poor results in filleted ear cartilages that have been subcutaneously banked are frequently observed, it is preferable to use Baudet's fenestration technique initially and to reserve the fascia for secondary reconstruction should this effort fail.

MICROSURGICAL EAR REPLANTATION

Although there have been several reports of successful microsurgical replantation of ears,[146,147] this procedure tends to fail because of such small vessels within the amputated ear. Therefore, what initially appears to be a successful replantation often fails as venous congestion ensues. However, such cases have been salvaged by application of leeches to the congested replant.[148]

With this in mind, the author believes that one should accomplish the anastomosis end-to-side in the temporal vessels rather than sacrificing them for an end-to-end repair. An axial-pattern fascial flap is

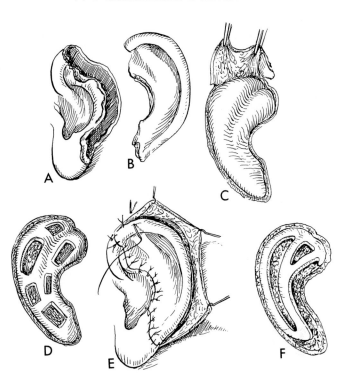

FIGURE 74-44. Replantation of the amputated auricle after removal of the posteromedial auricular skin and fenestration of the cartilage (after Baudet[145]). *A* and *B*, The extent of the amputation. *C*, Skin removed from the medial aspect of the amputated part. *D*, Windows cut through the cartilage. *E*, Reattachment of the amputated part; the denuded portion of the auricle is applied against the raw surface in the auriculomastoid area. *F*, Technique of fenestration suggested by Brent to prevent the deformity seen in Figure 74-45*D*.

preserved for a future reconstruction should the replant fail.

Deformities without Loss of Auricular Tissue

IRREGULARITIES IN CONTOUR

The most common traumatic auricular deformities without actual tissue loss result from faulty approximation of full-thickness lacerations, which manifest the helical border's distortion and notching.

Meticulous approximation of sutures is essential in primary repair of lacerations or in secondary repair of maladjusted tissues. Z-plasties, stepping, halving, and dovetailing of cartilage edges and soft tissue wounds are important measures in preventing recurrence of contour irregularities.

OTOHEMATOMA: "CAULIFLOWER EAR"

Frequently found in pugilists, this deformity results from a direct blow or excessive traction that produces a hemorrhage. Blood collects between the perichondrium and cartilage, which produces a fibrotic clot that thickens and obliterates the ear's convolutions. This is similar to the process that produces thickening of the septal cartilage, which is frequent in boxers and wrestlers.

Immediately after hematoma has occurred, one must drain the blood clots and serum. Whereas mere needle aspiration is followed almost invariably by recurrent fluid collection, a small incision will permit evacuation of the hematoma under direct vision. The incision should be long enough to permit retraction, inspection, and application of a large suction tip for the aspiration of blood clots. Conforming, compressive gauze bolsters are placed on either side of the auricle and are maintained for 7 to 10 days by horizontal mattress sutures (4–0 nylon) that traverse the bolsters as well as the ear.

Late treatment of the cauliflower ear deformity consists of carving out the thickened tissue to improve the auricular contour. Exposure is obtained by raising a skin flap through carefully placed incisions. After the carving is completed, similar dressings must be applied to ensure coaptation of the soft tissues to the cartilaginous framework and to prevent hematoma.

STENOSIS OF THE EXTERNAL AUDITORY CANAL

The concha is elongated inward by the external auditory canal through an opening, the meatus, through which lacerations may extend and ultimately produce stenosis.

Whenever possible, one must carefully suture circular lacerations involving the canal and keep the canal packed tightly during the healing period. A small, prosthetic appliance should be prepared to keep the canal open. This is made by taking an impression with dental

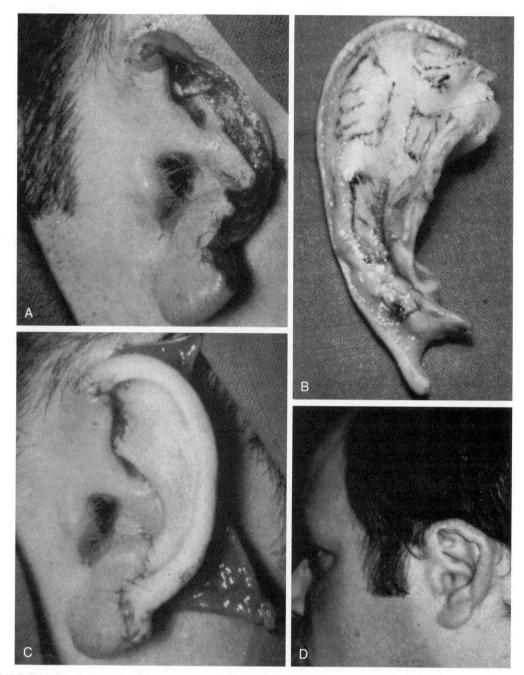

FIGURE 74-45. Replantation of the amputated auricle after removal of the posteromedial auricular skin and fenestration of the cartilage. *A,* Appearance of the stump of the amputated auricle. *B,* The denuded medial aspect of the cartilage; the outlines of the windows to be cut through the cartilage are indicated. *C,* The auricle immediately after reattachment. *D,* Final appearance. (Courtesy of Dr. J. Baudet.)

compound and creating a perforated mold of acrylic resin. This prosthetic support should be worn for 3 or 4 months until the tendency toward stenosis disappears (Fig. 74-46).

Cicatricial stenosis of the external auditory meatus and canal is remedied by Z-plasties of the cicatricial bands.[149] In severe stenosis, when the meatus is closed and the canal is filled with scar tissue, the cicatricial tissue must be excised; the skin defect is repaired by means of the skin graft inlay technique, for which a full-thickness retroauricular graft is uniquely suitable. To facilitate this grafting, one should take two

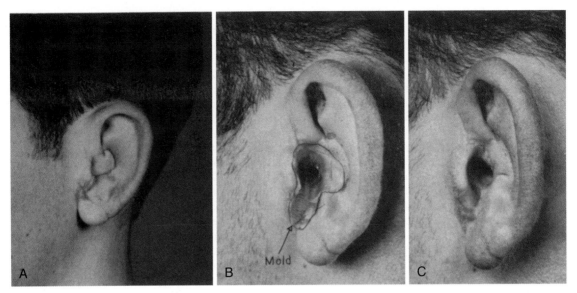

FIGURE 74-46. Traumatic stenosis of the external auditory canal. *A,* Stenosis of the external auditory canal resulting from laceration. *B,* Acrylic mold worn after skin grafting. *C,* Result obtained; the canal remains patent. (From Converse JM: Reconstruction of the auricle. Plast Reconstr Surg 1958;22:150. Copyright © 1958, Williams & Wilkins Company, Baltimore.)

impressions of the canal with dental compound. One impression serves to apply the graft firmly within the canal until the skin graft has taken; the other impression is duplicated in clear acrylic and should be worn by the patient for a period of 3 or 4 months to counteract the tendency for secondary contraction of the graft and subsequent stenosis (see Fig. 74-46). A detail worth noting is to prepare the mold in such a manner that the mold's distal portion itself fills the concha; this precaution ensures prosthesis stability.

Deformities with Loss of Auricular Tissue

These deformities may result from loss of skin, loss of cartilage, or full-thickness loss of auricular tissue.

LOSS OF AURICULAR SKIN

Auricular trauma that results only in a skin loss is usually secondary to burns. Loss of retroauricular skin results in adhesions between the ear and the mastoid region, whereas skin loss from the anterolateral surface may cause forward folding of the ear. When a burn destroys the skin, the cartilage becomes involved also, the result being a full-thickness defect of the auricle (see Chapter 65 for early treatment of the burned ear). However, partial-thickness burns that are adequately treated may heal with only varying degrees of contraction and thinning of the helical border.

FULL-THICKNESS DEFECTS OF THE AURICLE

For purposes of classification, full-thickness defects of the ear may be divided into six groups: defects of the upper third, middle third, and lower third; partial and total loss; and loss of the lobule (or lobe) of the ear.

MAJOR AURICULAR LOSS AFTER TRAUMA

Loss of a major portion of the auricle or of the entire ear itself may result from a razor slash, flying glass, gunshot wound, flame or radiation burns, and human or dog bites. Complete traumatic loss of the auricle is an unusual occurrence, for a portion of the concha and the external auditory canal are usually preserved even in cases of severe injury. When a large portion of the auricle or the entire ear has been destroyed, a number of obstacles must be surmounted in successive stages. These include (1) a suitable skin covering devoid of hair follicles; (2) a framework of cartilage to maintain the upright position of the reconstructed auricle and to represent its characteristic convolutions; and (3) a covering of skin for the posteromedial aspect of the auricular framework after it is raised from the mastoid area. Additional "retouching" procedures may be necessary to achieve a satisfactory repair of the reconstructed auricle.

THE SKIN COVERING

The presence of supple and well-vascularized skin is a sine qua non for success in auricular reconstruction. The quality of the residual local soft tissues varies in traumatic defects. When amputation of the auricle is by means of a clean-cut laceration, the local residual skin remains relatively unscarred and thus may be used. Likewise, minimally scarred skin after healed partial-thickness burns may be of sufficiently good quality to avoid skin grafting. To the contrary, if the auricle has been avulsed, destroyed by a burn, or injured by a gunshot, the area may show multiple linear or surface scars, thus necessitating excision and replacement with a skin graft before the auricular reconstruction begins. Should this be necessary, a full-thickness graft from the contralateral retroauricular region or supraclavicular area is most suitable for this purpose, although if this is not available, a thick split graft will suffice. It is essential that the skin overlying a cartilage graft have an adequate blood supply and be sufficiently loose to permit insertion of a good three-dimensional framework. Therefore, the skin graft must be allowed to mature for a number of months before cartilage replacement.

At times, the local skin will be irreparably scarred or grafts will mature inadequately to permit framework placement without supplementing the soft tissue cover. Under these circumstances, one must employ a fascial flap.[89] First, all heavy scars and unusable tissues are excised while great care is taken to preserve the temporal vessels, which may be entangled in the traumatically scarred tissues. Rib cartilage is then harvested, and a framework is sculpted as for correction of a virgin microtia (see Figs. 74-10, 74-11, 74-18, and 74-23). Finally, the fascial flap is raised.

To realize how large a fascial flap is needed for adequate coverage, one must first assess the periauricular skin. At times, the scar excision will be so extensive that total fascial flap coverage of the framework is necessary. However, at other times, the framework's lower portion can be "pocketed" beneath available skin, and therefore only a variable portion of the upper framework will need fascial flap coverage.

In using this fascial flap, one must be familiar with the course of the superficial temporal vessels. The artery remains beneath the subcutaneous tissue and within the temporoparietal fascia until a point approximately 12 cm above the anterosuperior auriculocephalic attachment. Here the artery emerges superficially and interlinks with the subdermal vascular plexus.[150] Consequently, this is the limit of fascial vascular domain; continued distal dissection would interrupt the fascial circulation.

After the vessels are first mapped with a Doppler probe, exposure to the fascia is gained through a Y-shaped incision that extends superiorly above the proposed auricular region. The dissection begins just deep to the hair follicles and continues down to a plane where subcutaneous fat adheres to the temporoparietal fascia. Because initial identification of this plane can be difficult, care must be taken to damage neither the follicles nor the underlying axial vessels. Although tedious, once the scalp dissection is accomplished, the inferiorly based temporoparietal fascial flap is raised easily from the underlying deep fascia that envelops the temporalis musculature.

Subsequently, the fascial flap is first draped over the framework (see Fig. 74-24) and then coapted to it by means of suction by a small infusion catheter. The flap is then affixed to the peripheral skin in a "vest-under-pants" fashion to secure a tight closure. Finally, a patterned thick split-skin graft is sutured on top of the fascia-covered framework. The new ear's convolutions are then packed with petrolatum gauze; last, a head dressing is applied.

AURICULAR PROSTHESES

The auricular prosthesis should be reserved for instances in which surgical reconstruction is impractical or contraindicated or when an experienced surgeon is unavailable. For the most part, an auricular prosthesis has no practical value for children and is worthwhile for older persons who have undergone ablative cancer surgery or who have extensive burns. Even so, many adults find them undesirable after a short trial experience; there is always a constant fear of the prosthesis becoming dislodged at embarrassing moments and the psychological discomfort of wearing an "artificial part." The innovation of osseointegrated percutaneous implants has offered a solution to the retention of ear prostheses.[151]

Additional problems that arise from local skin irritation from the adhesive glue frequently necessitate discontinuance of the prosthesis for a time, which in turn causes the patient further embarrassment. Furthermore, obvious color contrast calls attention to the prosthetic ear in climatic changes when the prosthetic part remains a constant color while the surrounding skin varies as the patient passes from indoor to outdoor environmental surroundings.

When an auricular prosthesis has been elected for the younger patient, a trial period should ensue, with the realization that surgical reconstruction may be desired later. It is wise to avoid preliminary excision of the microtic lobule or other remnants merely to "gain an improved surface for adherence of the prosthesis," as has been advocated. Should the patient desire surgical reconstruction later, which has often been my experience, the missing lobule, shortage of skin, and existing scar become a significant handicap.

Partial Auricular Loss

Most auricular deformities encountered in everyday practice are acquired partial defects. They present the surgeon with an unlimited variety of unique problems. Reconstruction is influenced by the etiology, location, and nature of each residual deformity.

USE OF RESIDUAL TISSUES

In management of acute auricular trauma, initial meticulous reapproximation of tissues and appropriate wound care will greatly facilitate the reconstructive task ahead. Likewise, the innovative use of residual local tissues in a post-traumatic deformity will greatly simplify the reconstruction and contribute to a pleasing outcome.

STRUCTURAL SUPPORT

Contralateral Conchal Cartilage

A variety of tissues are available to provide the structural support required for an auricular reconstruction. Although the quantity of cartilage needed to fabricate a total ear framework necessitates the use of costal cartilage, often one is not compelled to employ this tissue in a small, partial auricular reconstruction. Because it is often possible to use an auricular cartilage graft, which is obtained most frequently from the contralateral concha under local anesthesia, the correction of partial losses is less extensive than the procedure to correct total auricular losses. Auricular cartilage, used as an orthotopic graft in ear reconstruction, is superior to costal cartilage in that it provides a delicate, flexible, thin support.

The conchal cartilage graft can be obtained by a posteromedial incision, as described by Adams[152] and Gorney,[35] or through an anterolateral approach, which the author uses more frequently. The anterolateral approach, performed through an incision several millimeters inside the posterior conchal wall–inferior crus contour line, is a simple method of obtaining a precise graft with direct visual exposure.[153]

Ipsilateral Conchal Cartilage

In certain partial reconstructions, it is more advantageous to employ an ipsilateral rather than a contralateral conchal cartilage graft. However, it is imperative that an intact antihelical strut be present to permit removal of an ipsilateral conchal cartilage graft without subsequent collapse and further deformity of the ear.

An ipsilateral conchal cartilage graft is particularly advantageous when a retroauricular flap is being raised to repair a major defect in the helical rim. Elevation of the flap provides the required conchal cartilage exposure without the necessity of an additional incision, and removal of this cartilage graft subsequently lowers the ear closer to the mastoid region. In effect, this produces a relative gain in length, thus enabling the flap to cover the cartilage graft once it is spliced onto the rim and eliminating the need for a skin graft in the flap's donor bed.

Furthermore, the ipsilateral concha may be used occasionally as a composite flap of skin and cartilage (Fig. 74-47). This innovative technique, proposed by Davis,[34] is applicable to defects of the auricle's upper third and again should be employed only when the antihelical support remains intact.

Composite Grafts

Small to moderate-sized defects may be repaired with composite grafts from the unaffected ear, particularly if it is large and protruding.[152,154-156] A wedge-shaped composite graft of less than 1.5 cm in width is resected from the scapha and helix of the unaffected ear and transplanted to a clean-cut defect on the contralateral ear (Fig. 74-48). The success rate of composite grafts can be enhanced by removing a portion of the skin and cartilage, thus converting part of the "wedge" to a full-thickness skin graft, which is readily vascularized by a recipient advancement flap mobilized from the loose retroauricular skin.[157] A strut of the helical cartilage is preserved within the graft for contour and support (Fig. 74-49).

Despite a slight inclination toward shrinkage after transplantation, the composite graft offers a simple and expeditious reconstructive technique for partial auricular defects.

Specific Regional Defects

HELICAL RIM

Acquired losses of the helical rim may vary from small defects to major portions of the helix. Small defects usually result from tumor excisions or from minor traumatic injuries and are best closed by advancing the helix in both directions as described by Antia and Buch[158] (Fig. 74-50). The success of this excellent technique depends first on totally freeing the entire helix from the scapha by an incision in the helical sulcus that extends through the cartilage but not through the skin on the ear's back surface. Second, the posteromedial auricular skin is undermined, dissecting just superficial to the perichondrium until the entire helix is hanging as a chondrocutaneous component of the loosely mobilized skin (Fig. 74-50C and D). Extra length can be gained by a V-Y advancement of the crus helix (Fig. 74-50E), and surprisingly large defects can be closed without tension.

Although this technique was originally described for upper third auricular defects (Fig. 74-51),[158] the author has found that it is even more effective for middle third defects and is equally applicable in repair of earlobe losses.[157] Reconstruction of larger helical

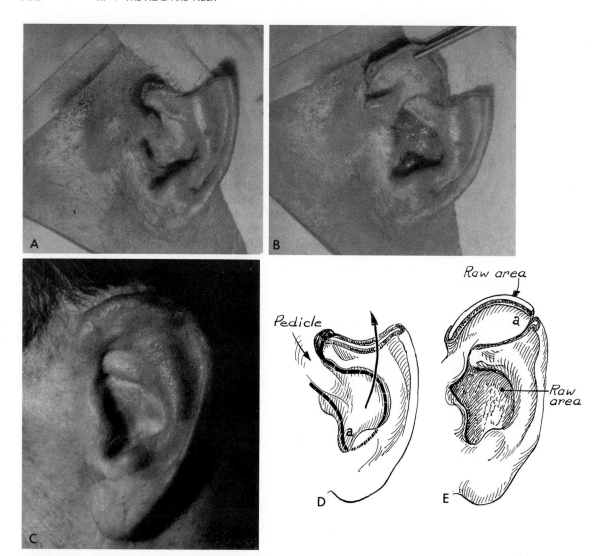

FIGURE 74-47. Upper auricular defect repaired with a composite flap of conchal skin and cartilage. *A*, The defect. *B*, The composite conchal flap elevated. *C*, The final appearance. *D* and *E*, Diagram of the procedure indicating the incisions and the raw surfaces to be grafted. The anterior cutaneous pedicle (crus helicis) maintains the blood supply. (After Davis.[34])

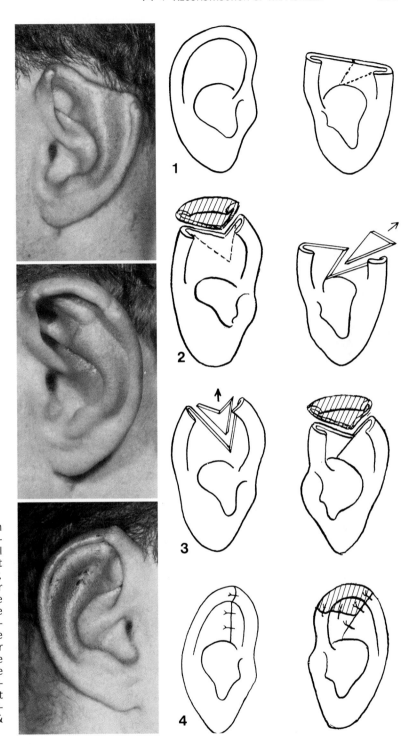

FIGURE 74-48. Reconstruction of an auricular defect with a composite graft from the contralateral ear. *Left: above,* an auricular defect resulting from a human bite; *center,* appearance of the ear 3 years after reconstruction with a composite graft; *below,* appearance of the donor ear 14 days after the surgical procedure. *Right,* The sequence of repair, top to bottom; the donor ear is at the left, and the defective ear being reconstructed is on the right. (From Nagel F: Reconstruction of a partial auricular loss. Plast Reconstr Surg 1972;49:340. Copyright © 1972, The Williams & Wilkins Company, Baltimore.)

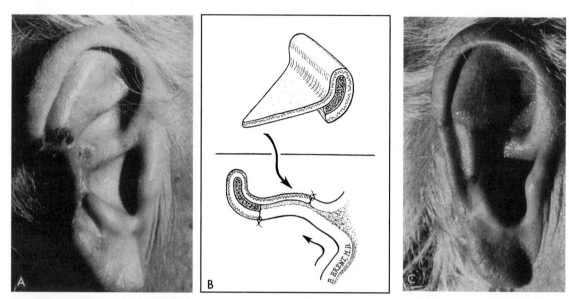

FIGURE 74-49. Enhancement of composite graft revascularization by decreasing "composite bulk." *A*, Auricular defect with residual chondrodermatitis. *B*, The bulkiness of the composite graft is decreased by removing the posteromedial auricular skin and cartilage while preserving a cartilage strut in the helical rim. A retroauricular flap is advanced to serve as a recipient bed for the remaining anterolateral cutaneous portion of the wedge-shaped graft. *C*, The final result.

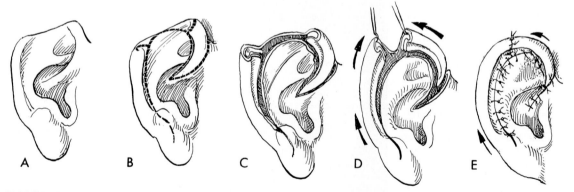

FIGURE 74-50. Helical defect repaired by advancement of auricular skin cartilage. *A*, Defect of the upper portion of the auricle. *B*, Lines of incisions through skin and cartilage. *C*, The incisions completed; note the downward extension into the earlobe. *D*, The skin-cartilage flaps mobilized. *E*, The repair completed. (After Antia NH, Buch VI: Chondrocutaneous advancement of flap for the marginal defect of the ear. Plast Reconstr Surg 1967;39:472. Copyright © 1967, The Williams & Wilkins Company, Baltimore.)

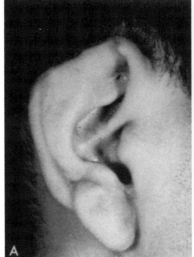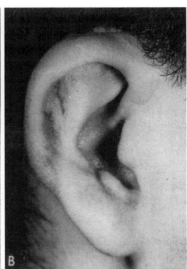

FIGURE 74-51. *A,* Traumatic defect of the superior helical region. *B,* Repair by helical advancement as illustrated in Figure 74-50. (After Antia NH, Buch VI: Chondrocutaneous advancement of flap for the marginal defect of the ear. Plast Reconstr Surg 1967;39:472. Copyright © 1967, The Williams & Wilkins Company, Baltimore.)

defects requires a more sophisticated procedure that recreates the absent rim with use of an auricular cartilage graft covered by an adjacent flap as previously described in the text. Although advancement flaps of local soft tissues have also been employed to provide helical contour, the author finds that these flaps often suffer a disappointing long-term result unless a strut of cartilage has been incorporated into the repair (Figs. 74-52 and 74-53).

Another sophisticated method of helical reconstruction is the use of thin-caliber tubes that can successfully form a fine, realistic helical rim when meticulous technique is used in conjunction with careful case selection (Fig. 74-54). Minor burns often destroy the helical rim yet leave the auriculocephalic sulcus skin intact, thus providing a superb site for tube construction[159] and minimizing tube migration, risk of failure, and secondary deformity.

UPPER THIRD AURICULAR DEFECTS

Upper third defects may be reconstructed by five major methods. Minor losses are usually confined to the rim and are repaired either by helical advancement, as previously described (see Fig. 74-50), or by a readily accessible preauricular flap.

Intermediate losses of the upper third are repaired with a banner flap, as described by Crikelair,[160] which is based anterosuperiorly in the auriculocephalic sulcus. This flap should be used in conjunction with a small cartilage graft to ensure a good long-term result.

Major losses in the superior third are most successfully reconstructed with a contralateral conchal cartilage graft as classically described by Adams.[152] In using this technique, it is imperative that the cartilage graft

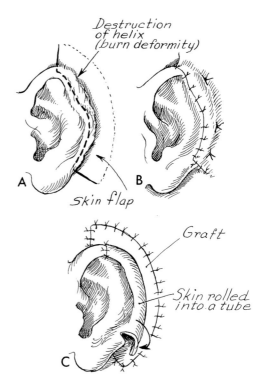

FIGURE 74-52. Technique for restoring the helical margin. *A,* Outline of the incisions for an advancement flap from the retroauricular area. *B,* The advancement flap sutured in position. *C,* In a second stage, the pedicle of the advancement flap has been sectioned, the flap rolled into a tube, and the resulting defect covered by a split-thickness skin graft. See results produced in Figure 74-53. (After Padgett and Stephenson, 1948.)

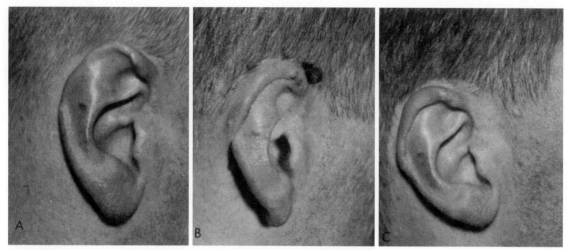

FIGURE 74-53. Helical reconstruction with a postauricular flap, as illustrated in Figure 74-52. *A,* Acquired loss of the helical rim. *B,* The postauricular flap in position over the auricular margin. *C,* The completed reconstruction, after division of the flap. (From Lewin M: Formation of the helix with a postauricular flap. Plast Reconstr Surg 1950;5:452. Copyright © 1950, The Williams & Wilkins Company, Baltimore.)

be anchored to the cartilaginous remnant of the helical root by means of a suture placed through a small incision at that point. This prevents the cartilage graft from "drifting" and ensures helical continuity.

Should the existing skin be unfavorable for this technique, the entire concha may be rotated upward as a chondrocutaneous composite flap on a small anterior pedicle of the crus helix.[34] This is a technically demanding procedure, and it is restricted to individual instances in which a large concha exists (see Fig. 74-47).

MIDDLE THIRD AURICULAR DEFECTS

Major middle third auricular defects are usually repaired with a cartilage graft that is either covered by an adjacent skin flap (Fig. 74-55) or inserted by Converse's tunnel procedure (Fig. 74-56).[161] Conditions may occasionally favor a specially prepared composite graft as described previously (see Fig. 74-49).

The tunnel procedure[161] is an effective technique for moderate-sized defects of the auricle (Fig. 74-57),

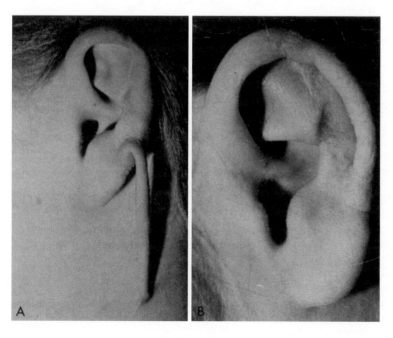

FIGURE 74-54. Helical restoration with a fine-caliber tube flap. *A,* Migration of the supraclavicular tube flap to the ear with helical loss. *B,* Completion of the helical reconstruction; note the splice of the superior junction by a Z-plasty.

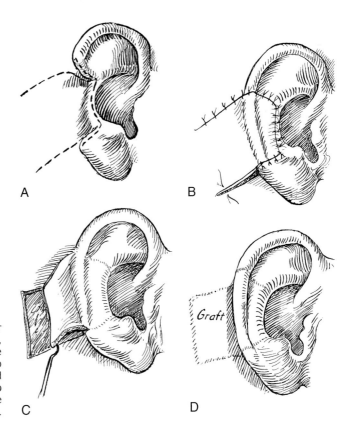

FIGURE 74-55. Dieffenbach's technique for reconstruction of the middle third of the auricle, drawn from his description (1829-1834). *A,* The defect and the outline of the flap. *B,* The flap advanced over the defect. *C* and *D,* In a second stage, the base of the flap is divided and the flap is folded around the posteromedial aspect of the auricle. A skin graft covers the scalp donor site.

and in major defects it has the advantage of preserving the retroauricular sulcus (Fig. 74-58). In employing this technique, one presses the auricle against the mastoid area and draws an ink line on the skin in this area, keeping the line parallel and adjacent to the edge of the auricular defect (Fig. 74-58*C*). Incisions are made through the skin along the ink line and also through the edge of the auricular defect (Fig. 74-58*D*). The medial edge of the auricular incision is sutured to the anterior edge of the mastoid skin incision (Fig. 74-58*E* and *F*). A cartilage graft is then placed in the soft tissue bed and is joined to the edges of the auricular cartilage defect (Fig. 74-58*H*). The mastoid skin, which has been undermined, is advanced to cover the cartilage graft, and the edge of this skin flap is sutured to the lateral edge of the auricular skin (Fig. 74-58*I*). A healing and vascularization period of 2 or 3 months is permitted; during this period, the cutaneous tunnel behind the auricle must be cleaned with cotton-tipped applicators. The auricle is detached in a second stage, and the resulting elliptical raw areas on the ear and mastoid region are grafted (Figs. 74-58*J* and 74-59).

Middle third auricular tumors are excised and closed either by wedge resection with accessory triangles or by helical advancement, as previously described.

LOWER THIRD AURICULAR DEFECTS

Lower third losses that encompass more than earlobe tissue are an especially complex challenge and must include a cartilage graft to provide the support necessary to ensure long-term contour.

Although Preaux[162] has described an impressive technique for repairing lower third defects by means of a superiorly based flap doubled on itself, the author finds that contour and support are provided and maintained with less risk by primarily inserting a contralateral conchal cartilage graft subcutaneously in the proposed site of reconstruction.

ACQUIRED EARLOBE DEFORMITIES

Traumatic clefts and keloids that result from ear piercing are the most common acquired defects of the earlobe. Cleft earlobes, usually occurring from the dramatic extraction of earrings, can be repaired most efficiently by means of Pardue's ingenious adjacent flap, which is rolled into the apex of the wedge repair, thus maintaining a track lined with skin that permits further use of earrings (Fig. 74-60).[163]

Another common occurrence in everyday practice is the earlobe keloid, which heretofore has been treated with varying degrees of success with irradiation and steroid injections.[164,165] Because there is strong evidence

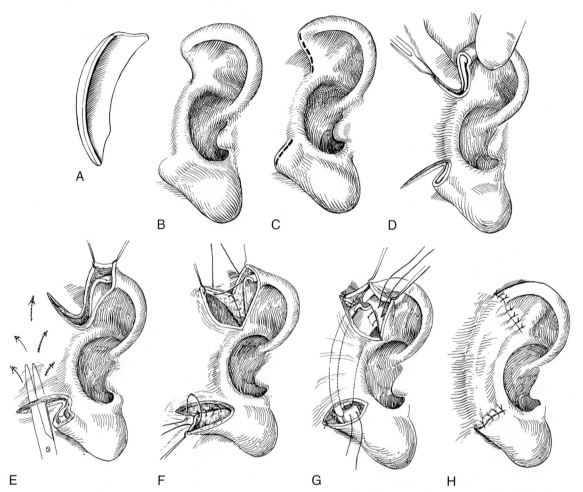

FIGURE 74-56. Repair of a defect of the middle third of the auricle: the tunnel procedure. *A,* Carved costal carti-lage graft. *B,* The defect. *C,* Incisions through the margins of the defect. *D,* Incisions through the edge of the defect are extended backward through the skin of the mastoid area. *E,* The skin of the mastoid area is undermined between the two incisions. *F,* The medial edge of the incision at the border of the auricular defect is sutured to the edge of the postauricular incision. A similar type of suture is placed at the lower edge of the defect. *G,* The cartilage graft is placed under the skin of the mastoid area and anchored to the auricular cartilage with sutures. *H,* Suture of the skin incision. (From Converse JM: Reconstruction of the auricle. Plast Reconstr Surg 1958;22:150, 230. Copyright © 1958, The Williams & Wilkins Company, Baltimore.)

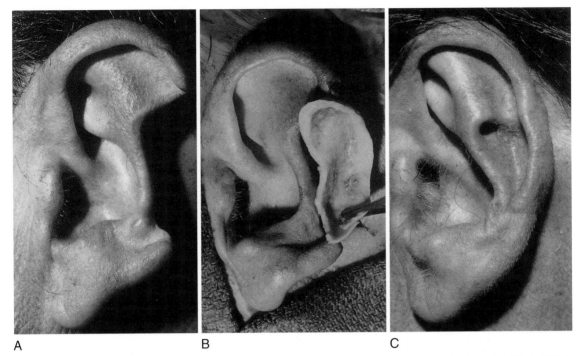

A   B   C

FIGURE 74-57. Partial auricular reconstruction with conchal cartilage graft, as illustrated in Figure 74-56. *A,* Middle third postsurgical defect. *B,* Conchal cartilage graft from contralateral ear. *C,* Result obtained by tunnel procedure of Converse. Secondary procedures will be necessary to release the ear and to improve helical contour. (From Brent B: The versatile cartilage autograft: current trends in clinical transplantation. Clin Plast Surg 1979;6:163.)

that pressure plays an important role in keloid therapy,[166,167] a light pressure-spring earring device may be worth a trial in reducing postexcisional recurrence of earlobe keloids.[168]

Construction of an earlobe is rarely required in congenital microtia because the lobe is formed by the repositioning of auricular remnants. However, a portion of the lobe or the entire lobe may be missing in traumatic deformities of the ear, and a variety of techniques for its reconstruction have been proposed. As early as 1907, effective techniques were innovated to repair earlobes with local flap tissues.[169] Since then, numerous methods have been developed (Figs. 74-61 to 74-65).[170-172]

Tumors of the Auricle

BENIGN TUMORS

Sebaceous cysts of the auricle are often treated improperly or neglected. Most often, one finds them on the medial aspect of the ear, particularly in the lobe, and these should be excised in toto during the quiescent period through the medial surface of the lobule to minimize deformity.

The most common auricular lesion is actinic keratosis, which occurs, as does carcinoma, in outdoor workers with fair complexions. Other benign auricular lesions, such as granuloma pyogenicum, beryllium granuloma, verruca contagiosa, verruca senilis, cylindroma, nevus, papilloma, lipoma, lymphangioma, leiomyoma, and chondroma, should be surgically excised. Keloid of the earlobe is common; the treatment of this lesion is discussed elsewhere.

MALIGNANT TUMORS

More than 5% of skin cancers involve the auricle.[173] Most of these are cutaneous, usually basal cell or squamous cell carcinomas. A lesser percentage are malignant melanoma.

When first seen, the cartilage is involved by direct extension in about one third of the cutaneous carcinomas of the auricle. For this reason, and because cartilage is an excellent barrier to the tumor's spreading, it is thought that the cartilage must be included in the surgical excision.[174]

The cervical lymph nodes are rarely involved in basal cell carcinoma of the auricle but are involved in approximately one third of all squamous cell carcinomas and malignant melanomas.

The majority of these malignant lesions are on the helical rim and can be eradicated with a wedge excision, or a helical advancement, as previously described. Many of the tumors on the lateral and medial

Text continued on p. 695

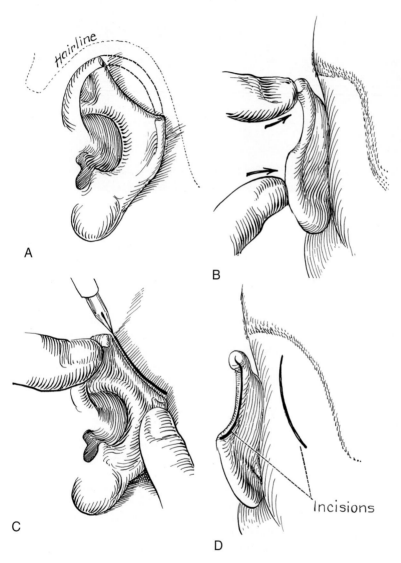

A

B

C

D

Incisions

FIGURE 74-58. Repair of a posterosuperior auricular defect by the tunnel procedure of Converse. *A,* The portion of the ear to be restored. *B,* The auricle is pressed against the mastoid process. *C,* An ink outline is traced on the skin overlying the mastoid process, parallel to the edge of the auricular defect. *D,* Incisions are made along the edge of the defect and through the skin of the mastoid area.

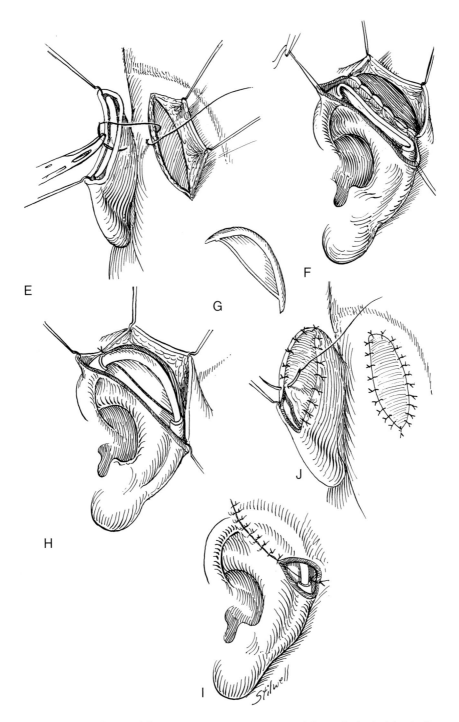

FIGURE 74-58, cont'd. *E,* Suture of the medial edge of the auricular incision to the anterior edge of the mastoid incision. *F,* The suture has been completed. *G,* Costal cartilage graft. *H,* The costal cartilage graft has been embedded. *I,* The skin of the mastoid area is advanced to cover the cartilage graft. *J,* In a second stage, the auricle is separated from the mastoid area, and full-thickness retroauricular grafts from the contralateral ear cover the defects. (From Converse JM: Reconstruction of the auricle. Plast Reconstr Surg 1958;22:150, 230. Copyright © 1958, The Williams & Wilkins Company, Baltimore.)

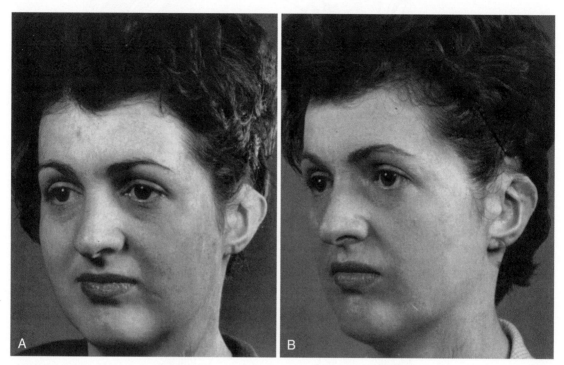

FIGURE 74-59. A superior auricular defect resulting from a burn. *A,* Preoperative appearance. *B,* The result obtained by the tunnel procedure shown in Figure 74-58. (From Converse JM: Reconstruction of the auricle. Plast Reconstr Surg 1958;22:150, 230. Copyright © 1958, The Williams & Wilkins Company, Baltimore.)

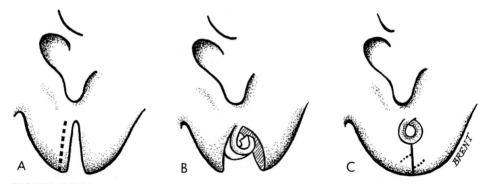

FIGURE 74-60. Repair of an earlobe cleft with preservation of the perforation for an earring. *A,* A flap is prepared by a parallel incision on one side of the cleft; the other side is "freshened" by excision of the margin. *B,* The flap is rolled in to provide a lining for preservation of the earring track. *C,* Closure is completed; a small Z-plasty may be incorporated. (After Pardue.[163])

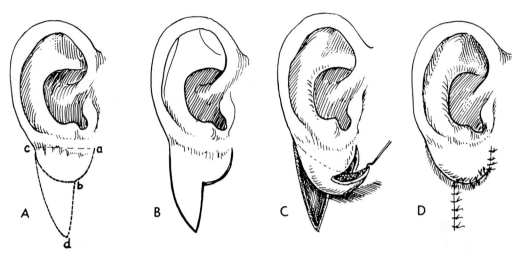

FIGURE 74-61. Reconstruction of the earlobe. *A,* The curved line *abc* outlines the proposed earlobe as measured on the unaffected contralateral auricle. A vertical flap is outlined; line *bd* is equal in length to line *ab,* and *cd* is equal to *ca. B,* Incisions are made through the outlined skin and subcutaneous tissue. *C,* The vertical flap is raised from the underlying tissue as far upward as the horizontal line *ac,* and the apex of the flap is sutured to point *a. D,* The operation completed. (After Zenteno Alanis.[172])

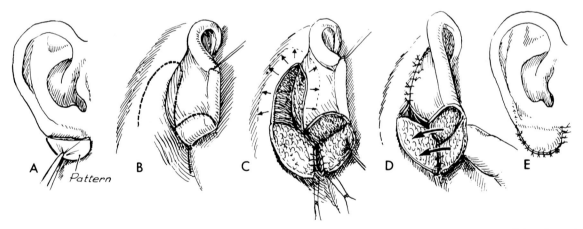

FIGURE 74-62. Reconstruction of the earlobe by a two-flap technique (Converse). *A,* The pattern of the planned earlobe. *B,* The pattern has been placed on the posteromedial aspect of the auricle and an outline made. The outline of the second flap from the retroauricular area is also shown; note the line of the vertical incision for insertion of the lobe. *C,* Each of the flaps is sutured to an edge of the vertical incision, thus anchoring the new earlobe. *D,* The two flaps are sutured to each other. *E,* The operation completed. (From Kazanjian and Converse.)

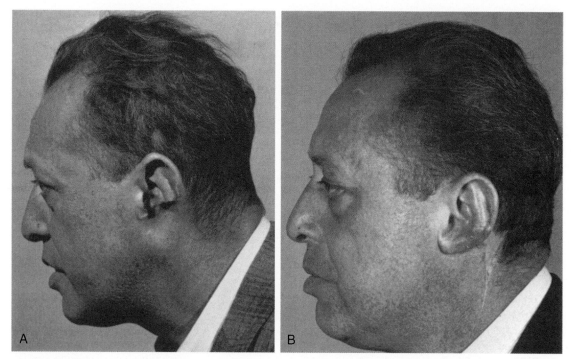

FIGURE 74-63. *A*, Loss of the lower part of the auricle. *B*, The result obtained with a flap based on the mastoid process and folded on itself. Note the scar of the approximated edges of the flap's donor site. (Patient of Dr. Cary L. Guy.)

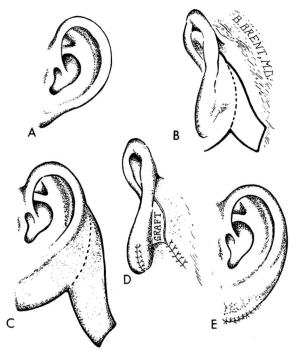

FIGURE 74-64. Construction of an earlobe with a reverse contoured flap. *A*, The earlobe deficiency. *B*, An auriculomastoid flap outlined. *C*, The elevated flap hanging as a curtain from the inferior auricular border. *D*, The flap folded under and sutured and the mastoid defect closed. A small graft is placed over the auricular donor defect. *E*, The completed earlobe, exaggerated by one third to allow for shrinkage. (From Brent B: Earlobe reconstruction with an auricular-mastoid flap. Plast Reconstr Surg 1976;57:389. Copyright © 1976, The Williams & Wilkins Company, Baltimore.)

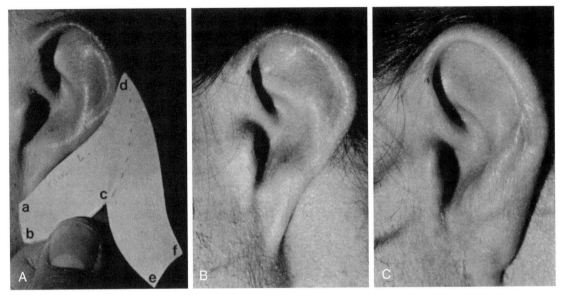

FIGURE 74-65. Earlobe reconstruction. *A,* The reverse contour pattern, in which *ab* is equal to *ef, bc* to *ce,* and *ad* to *df. B,* Congenital deficiency of lobular tissue. *C,* Completed construction by the technique illustrated in Figure 74-64. (From Brent B: Earlobe reconstruction with an auricular-mastoid flap. Plast Reconstr Surg 1976;57:389. Copyright © 1976, The Williams & Wilkins Company, Baltimore.)

auricular surfaces can be treated adequately by excision and subsequent skin grafting or by local flap coverage. Others require definitive reconstructive procedures previously detailed in this chapter. Radiation therapy is of no value in managing recurrences and metastases and is poorly tolerated by the auricle.

When the cancer is large and includes cartilaginous invasion, one must totally excise the ear with surrounding soft tissue. Radical resection of the cervical lymph nodes in continuity with resection of the involved auricle should be performed. In patients with lymph node metastases, one must resect the ear and all cervical lymph nodes. Melanomas require early radical intervention. At times, one's only hope of effecting a cure in auricular cancer includes resection of the temporal bone.[175-177]

Patients requiring total auricular ablation are usually older and generally are not candidates for total auricular reconstruction. A prosthesis is often preferred, but if total ear reconstruction is indicated, it is advisable that reconstruction be postponed until the threat of recurrence is well past.

REFERENCES

1. Bhishagratna KKL: An English Translation of the Sushruta Samhita. Calcutta, Wilkins Press, 1907.
2. Tagliacozzi G: De Curtorum Chirurgia per Insitionem. Venice, Gaspare Bindoni, 1597.
3. Dieffenbach JF: Die operative Chirurgie. Leipzig, FA Brockhaus, 1845.
4. Ely ET: An operation for prominence of the auricles. Arch Otolaryngol 1881;10:97.
5. Gillies H: Plastic Surgery of the Face. London, H. Frowde, Hodder & Stoughton, 1920.
6. Pierce GW: Reconstruction of the external ear. Surg Gynecol Obstet 1930;50:601.
7. Gillies H: Reconstruction of the external ear with special reference to the use of maternal ear cartilages as the supporting structure. Rev Chir Structive 1937;7:169.
8. Converse JM: The absorption and shrinkage of maternal ear cartilage used as living homografts: follow-up report of 21 of Gillies' patients. In Converse JM, ed: Reconstructive Plastic Surgery, 2nd ed. Philadelphia, WB Saunders, 1977:308.
9. Brown JB, Cannon B, Lischer CE, et al: Surgical substitution for losses of the external ear: simplified local flap method of reconstruction. Surg Gynecol Obstet 1947;84:192.
10. Dupertuis SM, Musgrave RM: Experiences with the reconstruction of the congenitally deformed ear. Plast Reconstr Surg 1959;23:361.
11. Kirkham HJD: The use of preserved cartilage in ear reconstruction. Ann Surg 1940;11:896.
12. Potter EL: A hereditary ear malformation transmitted through five generations. J Heredity 1937;28:255.
13. Steffensen WH: Comments on total reconstruction of the external ear. Plast Reconstr Surg 1952;10:186.
14. Steffensen WH: Comments on reconstruction of the external ear. Plast Reconstr Surg 1955;16:194.
15. Tanzer RC: Total reconstruction of the external ear. Plast Reconstr Surg 1959;23:1.
16. Tanzer RC: Microtia—a long-term follow-up of 44 reconstructed auricles. Plast Reconstr Surg 1978;61:161.
17. Cronin TD: Use of a Silastic frame for total and subtotal reconstruction of the external ear: preliminary report. Plast Reconstr Surg 1966;37:399.
18. Curtin JW, Bader KF: Improved techniques for the successful silicone reconstruction of the external ear. Plast Reconstr Surg 1969;44:372.
19. Lynch JB, Pousti A, Doyle J, Lewis S: Our experiences with Silastic ear implants. Plast Reconstr Surg 1972;49:283.

20. Cronin TD: Use of a Silastic frame for reconstruction of the auricle. In Tanzer RC, Edgerton MT, eds: Symposium on Reconstruction of the Auricle. St. Louis, CV Mosby, 1974:33.

21. Bresnick SD, Reinsch RF: Reconstructive techniques for salvage of the Medpore ear reconstruction. Presented at Ear Reconstruction '98: Choices for the Future, Chateau Lake Louise, Canada, March 5, 1998.

22. Wellisz T: Reconstruction of the burned external ear with a Medpore porous polyethylene pivoting helix framework. Plast Reconstr Surg 1993;91:811.

23. Brent B: Technical advances in ear reconstruction with autogenous rib cartilage grafts: personal experience with 1200 cases. Plast Reconstr Surg 1999;104:319.

24. Young F: Cast and precast cartilage grafts. Surgery 1944;15:735.

25. Peer LA: Reconstruction of the auricle with diced cartilage grafts in a vitallium ear mold. Plast Reconstr Surg 1948;3:653.

26. Cao Y, Vacanti JP, Paige KT, et al: Transplantation of chondrocytes utilizing a polymer-cell construct to produce tissue-engineered cartilage in the shape of a human ear. Plast Reconstr Surg 1997;100:297.

27. Ting V, Sims CD, Brecht LE, et al: In vitro prefabrication of human cartilage shapes using fibrin glue and human chondrocytes. Ann Plast Surg 1998;40:413.

28. Saadeh PB, Brent B, Longacre M, et al: Human cartilage engineering: chondrocyte extraction, proliferation, and characterization for construct development. Ann Plast Surg 1999;42:509.

29. Brent B: Auricular repair with autogenous rib cartilage grafts: two decades of experience with 600 cases. Plast Reconstr Surg 1992;90:355.

30. Firmin F: Ear reconstruction in cases of typical microtia. Personal experience based on 352 microtic ear corrections. Scand J Plast Reconstr Hand Surg 1998;32:35.

31. Fukuda O: The microtic ear: survey of 180 cases in 10 years. Plast Reconstr Surg 1974;53:458.

32. Nagata S: Modification of the stages in total reconstruction of the auricle. Plast Reconstr Surg 1994;93:221.

33. Osorno G: Autogenous rib cartilage reconstruction of congenital ear defects: report of 110 cases with Brent's technique. Plast Reconstr Surg 1999;104:1951.

34. Davis J: Reconstruction of the upper third of the ear with a chondrocutaneous composite flap based on the crus helix. In Tanzer RC, Edgerton MT, eds: Symposium on Reconstruction of the Auricle. St. Louis, CV Mosby, 1974:247.

35. Gorney M, Murphy S, Falces E: Spliced autogenous conchal cartilage in secondary ear reconstruction. Plast Reconstr Surg 1971;47:432.

36. Arey LB: Developmental Anatomy, 7th ed. Philadelphia, WB Saunders, 1974.

37. His W: Zur Entwickelung des Acusticofacialisgebiets beim Menschen. Arch Anat Phys Anat Suppl 1899.

38. Streeter GL: Development of the auricle in the human embryo. Carnegie Contrib Embryol 1922;14:111.

39. Nauton R, Valvassori G: Inner ear anomalies: their association with atresia. Laryngoscope 1968;78:1041.

40. Reisner K: Tomography in inner and middle ear malformations: value, limits, results. Radiology 1969;92:11.

41. Jahrsdoerfer RA, Yeakley JW, Hall JW III, et al: High-resolution CT scanning and auditory brain stem response in congenital aural atresia: patient selection and surgical correlation. Otolaryngol Head Neck Surg 1985;93:292.

42. Jahrsdoerfer RA, Hall JW III: Congenital malformations of the ear. Am J Otol 1986;7:267.

43. Jahrsdoerfer RA, Yeakly JW, Aguilar EA, et al: Grading system for the selection of patients with congenital aural atresia. Am J Otol 1992;13:6.

44. Grabb WC: The first and second branchial arch syndrome. Plast Reconstr Surg 1965;36:485.

45. Aase JM, Tegtmeier RE: Microtia in New Mexico: evidence for multifactorial causation. Birth Defects 1977;13:113.

46. Rogers B: Microtia, lop, cup and protruding ears: four directly inherited deformities? Plast Reconstr Surg 1968;41:208.

47. Wildervanck LS: Hereditary malformations of the ear in three generations: marginal pits, preauricular appendages, malformations of the auricle and conductive deafness. Acta Otolaryngol 1962;54:553.

48. Konigsmark BW: Hereditary deafness in man. N Engl J Med 1969;281:713.

49. Rogers B: Berry-Treacher Collins syndrome: a review of 200 cases. Br J Plast Surg 1964;17:109.

50. Erich JB, Abu-Jamra FN: Congenital cup-shaped deformity of the ears: transmitted through four generations. Mayo Clin Proc 1965;40:597.

51. Hanhart E: Nachweis einer einfach-dominanten, unkomplizierten sowie einer unregelmassig-dominanten, mit Atresia auris, Palatoschisis und anderen Deformationen-verbundenen Anlage zu Ohrmuschel-Verkummerung (Mikrotie). Arch Julius Klaus-Stift 1949;24:374.

52. Kessler L: Beobachtung einer über 6 Generationen einfach-dominant vererbten Mikrotie 1. Grades. HNO 1967;15:113.

53. Tanzer RC: Total reconstruction of the auricle: the evolution of a plan of treatment. Plast Reconstr Surg 1971;47:523.

54. Takahashi H, Maeda K: Survey of familial occurrence in 171 microtia cases. Jpn J Plast Surg 1982;15:310.

55. McKenzie J, Craig J: Mandibulo-facial dysostosis (Treacher Collins syndrome). Arch Dis Child 1955;30:391.

56. Poswillo DE: The pathogenesis of the first and second branchial arch syndrome. Oral Surg 1973;35:302.

57. Jorgensen MB, Kristensen HK, Buch NH: Thalidomide-induced aplasia of the inner ear. J Laryngol Otol 1964;78:1095.

58. Mundrick K: Handbuch Hals- Nasen- Ohrenheilkunde, vol III, pt 1. Stuttgart, Thieme, 1965:668.

59. Jahn AF, Ganti K: Major auricular malformations due to Accutane (isotretinoin) Laryngoscope 1987;97:832.

60. Jahrsdoerfer RA: Causative agents in microtia-atresia. Discussion at Microtia-Atresia Support Group; Manhattan Day School, New York, NY; November 2, 1997.

61. Lammer EJ, Chen DJ, Hoar RM, et al: Retinoic acid embryopathy. N Engl J Med 1985;313:837.

62. Tanzer RC: The constricted (cup and top) ear. Plast Reconstr Surg 1975;55:406.

63. Longacre JJ, de Stefano GA, Holmstrand KE: The surgical management of first and second branchial arch syndromes. Plast Reconstr Surg 1963;31:507.

64. May H: Transverse facial clefts and their repair. Plast Reconstr Surg 1962;29:240.

65. Dellon AL, Claybaugh GL, Hoopes JE: Hemipalatal palsy and microtia. Ann Plast Surg 1983;10:475.

66. Longenecker CG, Ryan RF, Vincent RW: Malformations of the ear as a clue to urogenital anomalies: report of six additional cases. Plast Reconstr Surg 1965;35:303.

67. Taylor WC: Deformity of ears and kidneys. Can Med Assoc J 1965;93:107.

68. Ogino Y, Yoshikawa Y: Plastic surgery for the congenital anomaly of the ear. Keisei Geka 1963;6:79.

69. Converse JM, Horowitz SL, Coccaro PJ, Wood-Smith D: The corrective treatment of the skeletal asymmetry in hemifacial microsomia. Plast Reconstr Surg 1973;52:221.

70. Converse JM, Wood-Smith D, McCarthy JG, et al: Bilateral facial microsomia. Plast Reconstr Surg 1974;54:413.

71. Knorr NJ, Edgerton MT, Barbarie M: Psychologic factors in the reconstruction of the ear. In Tanzer RC, Edgerton MT, eds: Symposium on Reconstruction of the Auricle. St. Louis, CV Mosby, 1974:187.

72. Farkas LG: Growth of normal and reconstructed auricles. In Tanzer RC, Edgerton MT, eds: Symposium on Reconstruction of the Auricle. St. Louis, CV Mosby, 1974:24.

73. Tanzer RC: Correction of microtia with autogenous costal cartilage. In Tanzer RC, Edgerton MT, eds: Symposium on Reconstruction of the Auricle. St. Louis, CV Mosby, 1974:47.

74. Tanzer RC: Microtia. Clin Plast Surg 1978;5:317.

75. Brent B: The correction of microtia with autogenous cartilage grafts: I. The classic deformity. Plast Reconstr Surg 1980; 66:1.

76. Brent B: The correction of microtia with autogenous cartilage grafts: II. Atypical and complex deformities. Plast Reconstr Surg 1980;66:13.

77. Brent B: Total auricular construction with sculpted costal cartilage. In Brent B, ed: The Artistry of Reconstructive Surgery. St. Louis, CV Mosby, 1987:113-127.

78. Broadbent TR, Mathews VI: Artistic relationships in surface anatomy of the face. Plast Reconstr Surg 1957;20:1.

79. Lauritzen C, Munro IR, Ross RB: Classification and treatment of hemifacial microsomia. Scand J Plast Reconstr Surg 1985;19:33.

80. Ohara K, Nakamura K, Ohta E: Chest wall deformities and thoracic scoliosis after costal cartilage graft harvesting. Plast Reconstr Surg 1997;99:1030.

81. Thomson HG, Kim TY, Ein SH: Residual problems in chest donor sites after microtia reconstruction: a long-term study. Plast Reconstr Surg 1995;95:961.

82. Brent B: Ear reconstruction with an expansile framework of autogenous rib cartilage. Plast Reconstr Surg 1974;53:619.

83. Gibson T, Davis W: The distortion of autogenous cartilage grafts: its cause and prevention. Br J Plast Surg 1958;10:257.

84. Tanzer RC: An analysis of ear reconstruction. Plast Reconstr Surg 1963;31:16.

85. Firmin F: Controversies in autogenous auricular reconstruction. Presented at Ear Reconstruction '98: Choices for the Future, Chateau Lake Louise, Canada, March 4, 1998.

86. Weerda, H: Discussion of personal technique. In Panel by Brent B: Solving problems in autogenous auricular reconstruction. Presented at Ear Reconstruction '98: Choices for the Future, Chateau Lake Louise, Canada, March 5, 1998.

87. Nagata S: Two-stage total auricular reconstruction with autogenous costal cartilage. Presented at Ear Reconstruction '98: Choices for the Future, Chateau Lake Louise, Canada, March 4, 1998.

88. Letterman GS, Harding RL: The management of the hairline in ear reconstruction. Plast Reconstr Surg 1956;18:199.

89. Brent B, Byrd HS: Secondary ear reconstruction with cartilage grafts covered by axial, random, and free flaps of temporoparietal fascia. Plast Reconstr Surg 1983;72:141.

90. Wheeland RG: Laser-assisted hair removal. Dermatol Clin 1997;15:469.

91. Dalrymple JC, Monaghan JN: Treatment of hidradenitis suppurativa with the carbon dioxide laser. Br J Surg 1987;74:420.

92. Sasaki G: Personal communication, 1998.

93. Lask G, Elman M, Slatkine M, et al: Laser-assisted hair removal by selective photothermolysis. Preliminary results. Dermatol Surg 1997;23:737.

94. Littler CM: Laser hair removal in a patient with hypertrichosis lanuginosa congenita. Dermatol Surg 1997;23:705.

95. Nanni CA, Alster TS: Optimizing treatment parameters for hair removal using a topical carbon-based solution and 1064-nm Q-switched neodymium:YAG laser energy. Arch Dermatol 1997;133:1546.

96. Dierickx CC, Grossman MC, Farinelli WA, Anderson RR: Permanent hair removal by normal-mode ruby laser. Arch Dermatol 1998;134:837.

97. Brent B: Discussion of Nagata S: Modification of the stages in total reconstruction of the auricle. Plast Reconstr Surg 1994;93:267.

98. Tanzer RC: Secondary reconstruction of the auricle. In Tanzer RC, Edgerton MT, eds: Symposium on Reconstruction of the Auricle. St. Louis, CV Mosby, 1974:238.

99. Cosman B: Repair of moderate cup ear deformities. In Tanzer RC, Edgerton MT, eds: Symposium on Reconstruction of the Auricle. St. Louis, CV Mosby, 1974:118.

100. Cosman B: Repair of the constricted ear. In Brent B, ed: The Artistry of Reconstructive Surgery. St. Louis, CV Mosby, 1987:99.

101. Matsumoto K: The characteristics of cryptotia and its therapy. Jpn J Plast Reconstr Surg 1977;20:563.

102. Ohmori S, Matsumoto K: Treatment of cryptotia, using Teflon string. Plast Reconstr Surg 1972;49:33.

103. Torikai T: Anatomy of the auricular muscles and its application to surgical treatment of cryptotia. Jpn J Plast Reconstr Surg 1982;25:46.

104. Tan ST, Abramson DL, MacDonald DM, Mulliken JB: Molding therapy for infants with deformational auricular anomalies. Ann Plast Surg 1997;38:263.

105. Yotsuyanagi T, Yokoi K, Urushidate S, Sawada Y: Nonsurgical correction of congenital auricular deformities in children older than early neonates. Plast Reconstr Surg 1998;101:907.

106. Fukuda O: Otoplasty of cryptotia. Jpn J Plast Surg 1968;11:117.

107. Washio H: Cryptotia—pathology and repair. Plast Reconstr Surg 1973;52:648.

108. McDowell AJ: Goals in otoplasty for protruding ears. Plast Reconstr Surg 1968;41:17.

109. Furnas DW: Correction of prominent ears by concha-mastoid sutures. Plast Reconstr Surg 1968;42:189.

110. Webster GV: The tail of the helix as a key to otoplasty. Plast Reconstr Surg 1969;44:455.

111. Morestin H: De la reposition et du plissement cosmetiques du pavillon de l'oreille. Rev Orthop 1903;14:289.

112. Owens N, Delgado DD: The management of outstanding ears. South Med J 1955;58:32.

113. Paletta F, Ship A, Van Norman R: Double spring release in otoplasty for prominent ears. Am J Surg 1963;106:506.

114. Spira M, McCrea R, Gerow FJ, Hardy SB: Analysis and treatment of the protruding ear. Transactions of the Fourth International Congress of Plastic Surgery. Amsterdam, Excerpta Medica, 1969:1090.

115. Stark RB, Saunders DE: Natural appearance restored to the unduly prominent ear. Br J Plast Surg 1962;15:385.

116. Luckett WH: A new operation for prominent ears based on the anatomy of the deformity. Surg Gynecol Obstet 1910;10:635.

117. Cloutier AM: Correction of outstanding ears. Plast Reconstr Surg 1961;28:412.

118. Erich JB: Surgical treatment of protruding ears. Eye Ear Nose Throat Monthly 1958;37:390.

119. Straith RE: Correction of the protruding ear. Plast Reconstr Surg 1959;24:277.

120. McEvitt WG: The problem of the protruding ear. Plast Reconstr Surg 1947;2:481.

121. Converse JM, Nigro A, Wilson FA, Johnson N: A technique for surgical correction of lop ears. Plast Reconstr Surg 1955;15:411.

122. Becker OJ: Surgical correction of the abnormally protruding ear. Arch Otolaryngol 1949;50:541.

123. Becker OJ: Correction of the protruding deformed ear. Br J Plast Surg 1952;5:187.

124. Tanzer RC: The correction of prominent ears. Plast Reconstr Surg 1962;30:236.

125. Mustarde JC: The correction of prominent ears using simple mattress sutures. Br J Plast Surg 1963;16:170.

126. Mustarde JC: The treatment of prominent ears by buried mattress sutures: a ten-year survey. Plast Reconstr Surg 1967;39:382.

127. Chongchet V: A method of anthelix reconstruction. Br J Plast Surg 1963;16:268.

128. Stenstrom SJ: A "natural" technique for correction of congenitally prominent ears. Plast Reconstr Surg 1963;32:509.

129. Ju DMC, Li C, Crikelair GF: The surgical correction of protruding ears. Plast Reconstr Surg 1963;32:283.

130. Kaye BL: A simplified method for correcting the prominent ear. Plast Reconstr Surg 1967;40:44.

131. Cocheril RC: Essai sur la restauration du pavillon de l'oreille [these pour le Doctorat en Medecine]. Lille, L. Danel, 1894.

132. Clemons JE, Connelly MV: Reattachment of a totally amputated auricle. Arch Otolaryngol 1973;97:269.

133. Gifford GH: Replantation of severed part of an ear. Plast Reconstr Surg 1972;49:202.

134. McDowell F: Successful replantation of severed half of ear. Plast Reconstr Surg 1971;48:281.

135. Conway H, Neumann CG, Golb J, et al: Reconstruction of the external ear. Ann Surg 1948;128:226.

136. Greeley PW: Reconstruction of the external ear. US Naval Med Bull 1944;42:1323.

137. Musgrave RH, Garrett WS: Management of avulsion injuries of the external ear. Plast Reconstr Surg 1967;40:534.

138. Suraci AJ: Plastic reconstruction of acquired defects of the ear. Am J Surg 1944;66:196.

139. Sexton RP: Utilization of the amputated ear cartilage. Plast Reconstr Surg 1955;15:419.

140. Conroy CC: Salvage of an amputated ear. Plast Reconstr Surg 1972;49:564.

141. Bonanno PC, Converse JM: Reconstruction of the ear. In Kazanjian VH, Converse JM, eds: Surgical Treatment of Facial Injuries, 3rd ed. Baltimore, Williams & Wilkins, 1974:1292.

142. Mladick RA, Horton CE, Adamson JE, Cohen BI: Pocket principle: a new technique for reattachment of a severed ear part. Plast Reconstr Surg 1971;48:219.

143. Mladick RA, Carraway JH: Ear reattachment by modified pocket principle. Plast Reconstr Surg 1973;51:584.

144. Grabb WC, Dingman RO: The fate of amputated tissues of the head and neck following replacement. Plast Reconstr Surg 1972;49:28.

145. Baudet J, Tramond P, Goumain A: A new technic for the reimplantation of a completely severed auricle [in French]. Ann Chir Plast 1972;17:67.

146. Juri J, Irigaray A, Juri C, et al: Ear replantation. Plast Reconstr Surg 1987;80:431.

147. Pennington DG, Lai MF, Pelly AD: Successful replantation of a completely avulsed ear by microvascular anastomosis. Plast Reconstr Surg 1980;65:820.

148. Mutimer K, Banis JC, Upton J: Microsurgical reattachment of totally amputated ears. Plast Reconstr Surg 1987;79:535.

149. Steffensen WH: Method of correcting atresia of ear canal. Plast Reconstr Surg 1946;1:329.

150. Byrd HS: The use of subcutaneous axial fascial flaps in reconstruction of the head. Ann Plast Surg 1980;4:191.

151. Albrektsson T, Branemark PI, Jacobsson M, Zelistrom A: Present clinical applications of osseointegrated percutaneous implants. Plast Reconstr Surg 1987;79:721.

152. Adams WM: Construction of the upper half of the auricle utilizing a composite concha cartilage graft with perichondrium attached on both sides. Plast Reconstr Surg 1955;16:88.

153. Brent B: The versatile cartilage autograft: current trends in clinical transplantation. Clin Plast Surg 1979;6:163.

154. Day HF: Reconstruction of the ears. Boston Med Surg J 1921;185:146.

155. Nagel P: Reconstruction of a partial auricular loss. Plast Reconstr Surg 1972;49:340.

156. Pegram M, Peterson R: Repair of partial defects of the ear. Plast Reconstr Surg 1956;18:305.

157. Brent B: The acquired auricular deformity. A systemic approach to its analysis and reconstruction. Plast Reconstr Surg 1977;59:475.

158. Antia NH, Buch VI: Chondrocutaneous advancement flap for the marginal defect of the ear. Plast Reconstr Surg 1967;39:472.

159. Steffanoff DN: Auriculo-mastoid tube pedicle for otoplasty. Plast Reconstr Surg 1948;3:352.

160. Crikelair GF: A method of partial ear reconstruction for avulsion of the upper portion of the ear. Plast Reconstr Surg 1956;17:438.

161. Converse JM: Reconstruction of the auricle. Plast Reconstr Surg 1958;22:150, 230.

162. Preaux J: A simple procedure for reconstruction of the lower part of the auricle [in French]. Ann Chir Plast 1971;16:60.

163. Pardue AM: Repair of torn earlobe with preservation of the perforation for an earring. Plast Reconstr Surg 1973;51:472.

164. Cosman B, Wolff M: Bilateral earlobe keloids. Plast Reconstr Surg 1974;53:540.

165. Ramakrishnan KM, Thomas KP, Sundararajan CR: Study of 1,000 patients with keloids in South India. Plast Reconstr Surg 1974;53:276.

166. Ketchum LD, Cohen IK, Masters FW: Hypertrophic scars and keloids. A collective review. Plast Reconstr Surg 1974;53:140.

167. Snyder GB: Button compression for keloids of the lobule. Br J Plast Surg 1974;27:186.

168. Brent B: The role of pressure therapy in management of earlobe keloids: preliminary report of a controlled study. Ann Plast Surg 1978;1:579.

169. Gavello P: Quoted by Nelaton C, Ombredanne L: Les autoplasties. Paris, G. Steinheil, 1907.

170. Brent B: Earlobe construction with an auriculomastoid flap. Plast Reconstr Surg 1976;57:389.

171. Guerrero-Santos J: Correction of hypertrophied earlobes in leprosy. Plast Reconstr Surg 1970;46:381.

172. Zenteno Alanis S: A new method for earlobe reconstruction. Plast Reconstr Surg 1970;45:254.

173. Arons MD, Sadin RC: Auricular cancer. Am J Surg 1971;122:770.

174. Lewis JS: Cancer of the ear. Laryngoscope 1960;70:551.

175. Hoopes JE: Reconstruction of the auricle after tumor resection. In Tanzer RC, Edgerton MT, eds: Symposium on Reconstruction of the Auricle. St. Louis, CV Mosby, 1974:232.

176. Mladick RA, Horton CE, Adamson JE, Carraway JH: The core resection for malignant tumors of the auricular area and subjacent bones. Plast Reconstr Surg 1974;53:281.

177. Parsons H, Lewis JS: Subtotal resection of the temporal bone for cancer of the ear. Cancer 1954;7:995.

Forehead Reconstruction

MAHESH H. MANKANI, MD ◆ STEPHEN J. MATHES, MD

ANATOMY
    Boundaries, Subunits, and Skin
    Tissue Layers
    Vascularity and Innervation
GENERAL PRINCIPLES
    Defect Size, Location, and Depth
RECONSTRUCTIVE OPTIONS
    Direct Wound Edge Approximation

Closure by Secondary Intention
Skin Grafting
Local Flaps
Skin Expansion
Distant Flaps
Microvascular Composite Tissue Transplantation
    and Flap Prefabrication
Eyebrow Reconstruction

The forehead has dual anatomic roles; it is both the anterior portion of the cranium and the superior portion of the face. As a result, it has both functional and aesthetic significance. It provides soft tissue coverage and protection of the cranium, and it makes critical contributions to facial appearance and expression. The location of the eyebrows, the height of the anterior hairline, and the smoothness of the skin can all convey youth and attractiveness. Expression is modulated by the frontalis, procerus, and corrugator muscles, which act to animate the eyebrows.

The operative goals in forehead reconstruction are appropriate to most repairs. In general, the reconstruction should achieve stable coverage with tissues that are functionally and aesthetically appropriate to the area. Additional goals specific to the forehead include

- reconstruction of the anterior forehead with non–hair-bearing skin of similar color and quality;
- provision of a smooth, consistent forehead surface;
- proper positioning and shape of the eyebrows;
- preservation of a smooth, continuous anterior hairline;
- new scar placement along natural skin lines, including transverse scars in the anterior forehead and vertical scars in the glabella or along the boundaries of hair-bearing areas (e.g., the hairline, above the eyebrow); and
- stable skin and soft tissue to support reconstruction of underlying bone defects or to support hair transplants for eyebrow reconstruction.

ANATOMY

Boundaries, Subunits, and Skin

The forehead is bounded by the eyebrows inferiorly, the frontal hairline superiorly, and the anterior temporal hairline laterally. Deep to the skin of the forehead lie the frontalis muscle and the frontal bone. The forehead is divided into the following subunits (Fig. 75-1): anterior region, bilateral pretemporal regions, bilateral eyebrows, bilateral suprabrow or supra-eyebrow regions, and glabellar region.

The anterior region makes up the majority of the forehead. Its skin is smooth and elastic in youth. By the sixth decade, transverse furrows and wrinkles are evident and are more pronounced with activation of the frontalis muscle. This skin increasingly relaxes. Prolonged sun exposure and smoking can contribute to visible skin damage in this area and can directly influence the quality of the reconstructive result.

The pretemporal region, which is immediately anterior to the temporal hairline, comprises the most lateral portion of the forehead. It extends inferiorly to the level of the eyebrows.

Eyebrow position and shape differ between the genders. The eyebrows are ideally located over the supraorbital ridges in men. In women, they are ideally located slightly superior to this point.

As with the anterior region of the forehead, the glabella experiences greater laxity with age. Activity of the procerus and corrugator muscles contributes to pronounced vertical wrinkles. Glabellar skin is slightly thinner and more pliable than the skin slightly superior to it.[1]

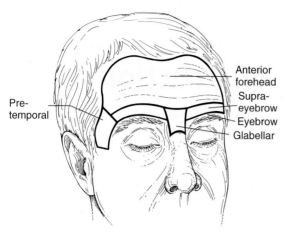

FIGURE 75-1. Forehead divisions.

Pre-temporal

Anterior forehead

Supra-eyebrow

Eyebrow

Glabellar

As in aesthetic brow surgery, care must be taken to appreciate anatomic relationships and distances. The eyebrows can be properly placed in relationship to the superior orbital rim; they should lie at the rim in men and slightly above it in women. In addition, they can be placed in relationship to the pupil; the distance from midpupil to the superior edge of the eyebrow is 2.5 cm. In turn, the anterior hairline should lie 5 cm above the superior edge of the eyebrows.[2]

Tissue Layers

The layers of the forehead and scalp are similar. From superficial to deep, they include skin, subcutaneous tissue, epicranius aponeurosis or muscle, loose areolar tissue, and pericranium (Fig. 75-2). The skin of the forehead differs from scalp in its thinness and the absence of hair follicles. The subcutaneous layer is relatively thin and undergoes little variation with overall weight gain; however, it thins with increasing age. Within it is a rich vascular plexus, responsible for the blood supply to the skin. The epicranius aponeurosis is a tough membranous sheet overlying the calvaria and is often termed the galea aponeurosis. This aponeurosis is the tendinous portion of the epicranius, or occipitofrontalis, muscle. It is continuous with the superficial temporal fascia as well as with the superficial musculoaponeurotic system (SMAS) of the face. The anterior portion of the epicranius is the frontalis muscle; the posterior portion is the occipitalis muscle. The loose areolar layer allows mobility of the overlying skin relative to the deeper pericranium. The pericranium is densely adherent to the underlying calvaria but can be dissected free of the bone with relative ease.

The dominant muscle of the forehead is the frontalis. This broad bilateral muscle originates from the epicranius aponeurosis at a line anterior to the vertex. It inserts into the skin and subcutaneous tissues near the eyebrows and therefore has no bone attachments. The frontalis acts to elevate the eyebrows, and it is also responsible for transverse wrinkles in the forehead during frowning. The ability of each unilateral frontalis muscle to function independently contributes to the wide spectrum of facial expression.

At its insertion, the frontalis interdigitates with fibers of the procerus and corrugator supercilii muscles. The procerus is vertically oriented and inserts into the skin over the glabella. When activated, it produces transverse wrinkles in the glabella. The corrugator muscles are oriented from upper lateral to lower medial and also insert into the glabellar skin, where they correspondingly produce vertical wrinkles. In addition to serving as mediators of facial expression, these muscles help achieve a squint and thus serve to reduce glare in bright sunlight.

Vascularity and Innervation

The skin of the forehead is as well perfused as the scalp because of its rich arterial plexus, consisting of the supratrochlear, supraorbital, and superficial temporal arteries (Fig. 75-3). The bilateral supratrochlear and supraorbital arteries traverse foramina of the same name to enter the forehead just superior to the eyebrows. Both vessels are terminal branches of the

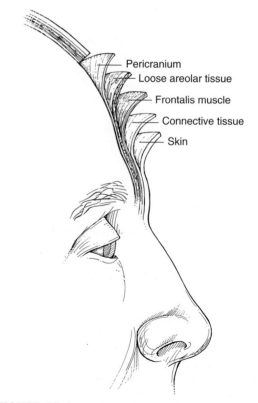

Pericranium

Loose areolar tissue

Frontalis muscle

Connective tissue

Skin

FIGURE 75-2. Anatomy of the scalp.

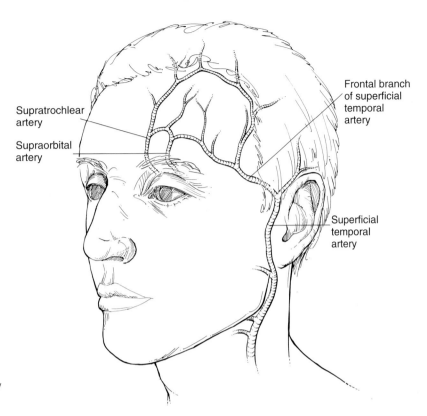

FIGURE 75-3. Arterial supply of the scalp.

internal carotid artery. They cross the plane of the frontalis muscle to lie in the subcutaneous tissues of the anterior forehead, where they freely anastomose with each other. These interconnections allow the rich variety of forehead flaps. A limited number of branches from these arteries cross the loose areolar layer to the underlying pericranium, therefore providing a limited contribution to frontal bone and pericranial vascularity. The anterior branch of the superficial temporal artery, a terminal branch of the external carotid artery, begins approximately 2 cm above the zygomatic arch, courses anteriorly at the level of the anterior temporal hairline, and retains anastomotic connections with the supraorbital and supratrochlear arteries.

Motor innervation of the frontalis, procerus, and corrugator muscles is through the frontal branch of cranial nerve VII (Fig. 75-4). The nerve exits the superficial lobe of the parotid gland to cross the zygomatic arch at its middle third. The nerve lies along the superficial surface of the arch within the temporoparietal or superficial temporal fascia. From here it enters the frontalis muscle above the orbital rim. The nerve lies inferior and parallel to the anterior branch of the superficial temporal artery.[3] Its course can be described by a line extending from the anterior border of the lobule of the ear to a point just lateral to the lateral border of the eyebrow.[1] As a result, reconstruction of the forehead in a plane superficial to the frontalis muscles or superficial

temporal fascia should spare the frontal branch of cranial nerve VII.

Sensation of the forehead arises from the bilateral supraorbital and supratrochlear nerves, each a terminal branch of the ophthalmic division of cranial nerve V. Sensation of the pretemporal region arises from the zygomaticotemporal nerve, a branch of the maxillary division of cranial nerve V.

GENERAL PRINCIPLES

Wounds of the forehead must be prepared for closure in a manner similar to other portions of the body. They must be devoid of overt infection, including cellulitis. Should cellulitis or abscess exist, it must be treated with antibiotics and drainage, respectively. The wound margins and base must be viable. In the fresh wound, areas of questionable viability may benefit from a second-look operation rather than immediate excision. This staged excision may preserve more tissue than would otherwise have been left after an immediate excision. In the mature wound, areas of necrosis must be excised back to a viable margin. The presence of granulation tissue at the margin or base is not a necessary precursor to closure. However, any compromise of the vascularity of the wound margins, such as that seen after radiation therapy, must be acknowledged and incorporated into the treatment plan.

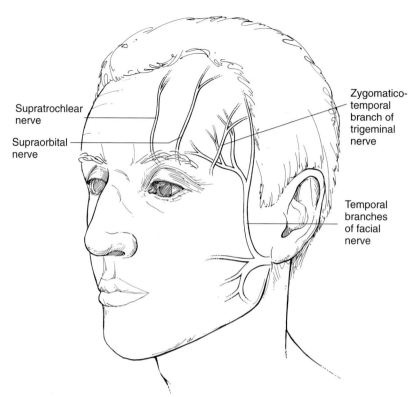

Supratrochlear
nerve

Supraorbital
nerve

Zygomatico-
temporal
branch of
trigeminal
nerve

Temporal
branches
of facial
nerve

FIGURE 75-4. Innervation of
the scalp.

Specific clinical problems bear mentioning. Trauma resulting in forehead injury must be addressed systemically, with care taken to confirm integrity of the cervical spine, cranial contents, frontal bone, and frontal sinus. This requires completion of a focused clinical history and physical examination. Radiologic studies, including plain radiographs and computed tomographic scans, may be necessary to evaluate these areas properly in the presence of either a suggestive history or examination.

For defects secondary to cancer extirpation, the margins and base of the defect should be clear of disease before the reconstruction is initiated. Adequacy of margins is based on both a wide-margin resection and careful histologic examination of the paraffin-embedded operative margins. Invasive squamous cell carcinoma may also require partial bone resection for adequate margins to be established. Reliance solely on frozen sections before reconstruction is fraught with uncertainty, given the minute chance that subsequent examination of the permanent sections may change the diagnosis.

Defect Size, Location, and Depth

Defect size, location, and depth are important considerations in determining the appropriate closure technique. Small defects are amenable to direct approx-

imation of the wound margins, as long as extensive mobilization of surrounding tissues does not result in deformity of the anterior hairline, eyebrows, and upper eyelids. Such deformities can include lateral displacement or focal elevation of the eyebrows, disruption of the anterior hairline, and elevation of the upper eyelids resulting in exposure of the ocular globe.

Large defects present their own challenges. When they are large enough to encompass more than half the forehead, reconstruction of the entire forehead as a single aesthetic unit should be considered. Such en bloc reconstructions can extend from the superior border of the eyebrows to the anterior hairline. Should the defect include a portion of the eyebrows, consideration should be given to preservation of the fully intact eyebrow while the eyebrow already partially or completely lost is reconstructed. Patients with extensive forehead burn scarring are likely to have concomitant loss of the entire eyebrow and involvement of the upper eyelids. Reconstruction of these structures should be included in the operative plan.

Defect location is important because it affects or involves structures at the margins of the forehead, including the anterior hairline and eyebrows. Reconstruction of hair-bearing areas in combination with glabrous areas requires recruitment of two different skin types, and this correspondingly increases the complexity of the approach. Wound location is of less concern in older patients, whose skin laxity and relative redundancy reduce the likelihood of tension, and therefore adjacent tissue deformation, across the closure.

Correct assessment of wound depth is important because the tissue at the base of a deep wound may not carry the vasculature necessary to support the reconstruction, and reconstruction of a deep wound may leave the patient with a contour defect if it is not appropriately addressed. Wounds extending as deep as calvaria or pericranium typify these two challenges.

RECONSTRUCTIVE OPTIONS

The options available for forehead reconstruction are typical of those used elsewhere in the body (Table 75-1). The most appropriate reconstructive choice for a particular patient depends on the patient's problem, the overall clinical condition, and the patient's desires in terms of outcome. These can best be determined after a careful history has been obtained, a clinical examination has been completed, and expectations have been fully discussed with the patient.

Direct Wound Edge Approximation

Coaptation of the wound edges is the simplest and most direct method of obtaining immediate wound closure. It is most appropriate for elliptical defects that are oriented transversely in the anterior portion of the forehead, parallel to lines of relaxation. Under such circumstances, the resultant scar will parallel or even lie within a natural wrinkle, and the natural laxity of the skin may preclude the need for undermining to achieve a tension-free closure. For success, the transverse dimension of the defect can be as long as the full width of the forehead; however, the wound must have a limited vertical height.

Direct closure can be used with vertically oriented wounds, but in so doing, the practitioner may forego its advantages. By necessity, the transverse dimension will need to be short to avoid undue skin tension, and the vertical scar can be prominent.

Unilateral wounds that are close to either the anterior hairline or eyebrows may be addressed by skin edge approximation only if care is taken not to distort either of these structures.

Advantages of this technique include the relative rapidity of the closure, the ability to complete it in one stage, and the absence of additional scars in the forehead. It can be used to close full-thickness defects, including those extending to the cranium. Among its disadvantages is its inappropriateness for wounds that are long in the transverse dimension and for some unilateral wounds adjacent to the eyebrows. However, is some instances, direct wound approximation can yield excellent results.

Closure by Secondary Intention

Closure by secondary intention is a technique with limited clinical applications in the forehead. It is most appropriate for small lesions, such as 3- to 4-mm punch biopsy wounds. In addition, it should be considered for those patients with a large defect who are unable to tolerate a larger operative procedure. This technique is also commonly used for closure of the median forehead flap donor site where direct closure is not possible. Aided by the process of wound contraction, the resultant scar is acceptable and is superior to the closure achieved primarily with skin grafting. Of greatest advantage to the patient is the absence of an operation and any additional scars resulting from additional procedures. For most patients, immediate closure is preferred to avoid the long lag period until healing is complete.

Skin Grafting

There are limited indications for skin grafting of the forehead. It is most appropriate for small partial-thickness defects, of less than 2 cm in diameter, that are not amenable to direct reapproximation or local flap coverage. Such wounds can be covered with a split-thickness, unmeshed graft. The supraclavicular area provides the optimum donor site from the standpoint of color match, although it leaves the patient with an additional, visible scar.[4] Full-thickness grafts can be used to minimize a contour deformity. Compared with split-thickness skin grafts, they provide better skin quality, undergo less contraction, and experience less discoloration over time (Table 75-2).[5]

Whereas a skin graft can be used over any region of the forehead, it is best used near the hairline or eyebrows, locations where other techniques may distort normal anatomy. The main advantages of skin grafts are the relative rapidity of the procedure, minimal operative morbidity, and high likelihood of success. The greatest disadvantages include a second operative site with potential donor site morbidity and difficulty in achieving good color and texture matches. Over time, skin grafts may appear shiny, exhibit less pliability than native skin, and leave the patient with a visible depression at the graft site.

Skin grafting requires a vascularized base, which may include dermis, subcutaneous tissues, or pericranium. Should cranium lie at the base of the wound, several techniques have been described for establishing a graftable surface. Historically, the outer table of the cranium was burred, exposing a granulating cancellous bone surface on which split-thickness skin grafts could be placed. Such skin is fixed to bone, has no pliability, and has an unnatural contour.[6] Alternatively, a periosteal flap can be rotated from underneath

TABLE 75-1 ◆ FOREHEAD RECONSTRUCTIVE OPTIONS

	Advantages	Limitations	Appropriate Defect Size and Shape	Bone Viability at Wound Base	Contour Quality	Tissue Pliability	Tissue Stability	Appearance
Direct wound edge approximation	Rapid operative time One-stage procedure Absence of additional scars	Difficult for wounds close to the anterior hairline or eyebrows	For elliptical transverse defects with a limited vertical height	Can cover bone denuded of periosteum	Excellent	Pliability increases with time	Excellent	Excellent
Closure by secondary intention	Nonoperative No additional scarring	Long healing time Possible distortion of surrounding structures	3- to 4-mm punch biopsy wounds Medial forehead flap donor sites	Necessitates viable bone at base	Adequate	Poor to adequate	Adequate	Adequate Skin is occasionally thin and shiny
Skin grafting	Minimizes distortion of surrounding structures High likelihood of success Rapid operative time	Donor site scar, usually at supraclavicular fossa	Small, partial-thickness defects, <2 cm diameter	Necessitates viable bone and periosteum at base May first necessitate transfer of a periosteal flap to support the graft	May become depressed over time	Adequate	Adequate	Poor to adequate Over time, skin appears shiny and depressed

Local flap	Rapid operative time One-stage procedure	Flap donor site scar	5 mm to 3 cm in size	Can cover bone denuded of periosteum	Excellent	Excellent	Excellent	Very good
Distant flaps	Entire forehead can be reconstructed without use of microvascular composite tissue transplantation	Significant donor defect	Entire forehead can be reconstructed as a unit	Can cover bone denuded of periosteum	Adequate Can be bulky	Excellent	Excellent	Very good
Skin expansion	Uses adjacent forehead skin, minimizing additional donor defects Excellent appearance	Staged procedures Transient deformity during expansion Risk of expander loss or infection	Subtotal forehead defects	Can cover bone denuded of periosteum	Very good	Excellent	Excellent	Excellent
Microvascular composite tissue transplantation	Single-stage reconstruction for entire forehead Can provide a functional reconstruction	Complex procedure Long operative time Risk of flap loss	Total forehead defects	Can cover bone denuded of periosteum	Adequate Can be bulky	Excellent	Excellent	Very good
Flap prefabrication	Can theoretically provide for the design of complex flaps incorporating novel combinations of tissue elements	Complex staged procedures	Total forehead defects	Can cover bone denuded of periosteum	Adequate Can be bulky	Excellent	Excellent	Very good

TABLE 75-2 ✦ SKIN GRAFT OPTIONS

	Split-Thickness Skin Grafts	Full-Thickness Skin Grafts
Advantages	Rapid graft take and high likelihood of wound closure in 1 stage	Very good color and texture match with normal forehead skin
Limitations	Sizable donor site scar	Longer healing interval and greater chance of graft loss than with split-thickness skin grafts; limited donor site material
Appropriate defect size and shape	Partial-thickness defects	Partial-thickness defects
Contour quality	Will only minimally correct contour irregularities, as in depressed wound beds	Can correct contour irregularities in depressed wound beds
Graft pliability	Adequate	Good
Graft stability	Adequate	Good
Graft appearance	Poor to adequate	Very good
Graft contraction	Moderate	Minimal to moderate
Technique used to harvest graft	Tangential excision at intraepidermal level	En bloc sharp excision of combined epidermis and dermis
Length of operative time	Brief	Brief
Technique used to close donor site	Wound left open and allowed to re-epithelialize	Direct closure by re-approximation of skin edges
Donor site comfort	Significant discomfort for the patient during first 2-3 postoperative days	Minimal
Donor site appearance	Significant scar, usually hypopigmented or hyperpigmented	Linear scar
Comment	These grafts should not be meshed because meshing will create obvious contour irregularities. They should instead be minimally perforated (pie-crusted) to minimize hematomas and seromas.	Full-thickness grafts offer better texture and color match and contract less than split-thickness grafts do.

the edge of the wound to cover the exposed cranium, which can then be covered with a split-thickness skin graft.[7] These flaps can be based anteriorly, anterolaterally, or posterolaterally, and they are reported to have a maximal length-to-width ratio of 1.5:1. They should be handled with care and are extremely sensitive to desiccation and excessive pressure. Defects as large as 7 cm in diameter and rectangular defects measuring 8 × 4 cm have been closed successfully in this manner.

The crane principle[8] can be used to surface bare bone (Fig. 75-5).[6] The crane principle involves placing a flap on a wound for a short time, returning it to its location, and leaving behind a layer of tissue at the recipient site for a skin graft. A scalp flap, elevated just deep to the galea, can be transferred to the forehead. The galea can also be incised to provide more length. Three weeks later, at the second stage, the flap is elevated in the subcutaneous plane and returned to its donor site, leaving galea and subcutaneous tissue at the forehead site. These can be closed with a split-thickness skin graft from a supraclavicular site. The advantages include minimal donor site morbidity, formation of a smooth pliable bed in the forehead, and adequate color matching with use of supraclavicular skin. This technique is rarely used because it requires two operative stages and the possibility of additional procedures to achieve an optimum appearance.

TECHNICAL CONSIDERATIONS

Split-Thickness Skin Grafting

Skin grafts for reconstruction of the forehead are best obtained from the supraclavicular area; this skin most closely matches the forehead skin in color and texture. Split-thickness grafts from the supraclavicular area are best obtained with a Weck dermatome. This is a hand-powered device that most closely resembles a small barber's razor. Its size makes it particularly suitable for harvesting of small grafts, even as modest as 1 cm².

The supraclavicular area is prepared for harvest by converting its concavity into a convexity; this minimizes the relative prominence of the clavicle and anterior border of the trapezius muscle, which can constrain the movement of the dermatome. This change in contour can best be accomplished by a subdermal injection of 10 to 30 mL of either plain saline or saline with epinephrine (1:1,000,000 concentration). Care should be taken to ensure that only injectable saline, rather than saline for irrigation, is used.

Graft thickness is determined by both the dermatome guard (0.01 inch is recommended for this

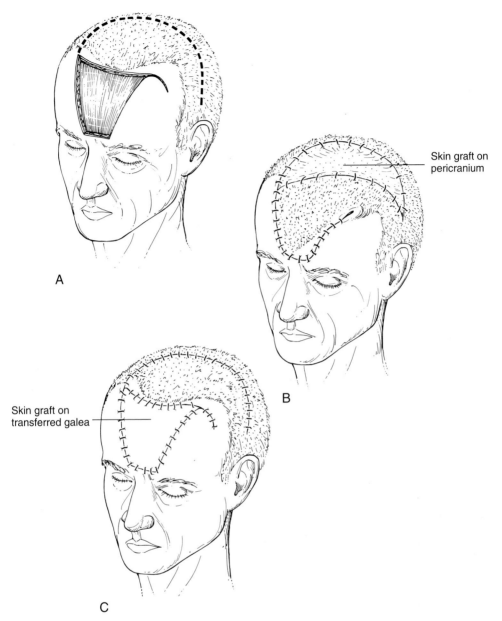

FIGURE 75-5. *A to C,* Flap based on the crane principle.

purpose) and the pressure applied by the operator, such that greater pressure will result in a thicker graft.

The skin grafts used in forehead reconstruction should never be meshed; a meshed graft will retain its cobblestone appearance long after it has healed. The three main advantages attributable to meshing either are not necessary in this area or can be approximated with other techniques. First, stretching of a meshed graft to cover a larger wound can be avoided by harvesting the bilateral supraclavicular areas simultaneously. Second, easy egress of serum and blood from beneath the graft can be accomplished by

pie-crusting, or perforation of the graft with minute stab wounds at the time of placement; these usually heal without a visible scar. Third, meshed graft conformation to an uneven wound bed contour is rarely necessary in the forehead, which usually has a smooth convex shape.

Skin grafts can be secured to the recipient site with fine nonabsorbable sutures. The grafts should be further secured with a tie-over bolster dressing; this consists first of one layer of petroleum-impregnated gauze, followed by a thick layer of cotton fluffs, and last by 2-0 nylon sutures tied to the margins of the wound. All dressings and sutures can be removed on the fifth postoperative day.

The split-thickness skin graft donor site can be dressed with petroleum-impregnated gauze, which can be allowed to dry to the wound. It will fall off when healing is complete.

Full-Thickness Skin Grafting

Full-thickness skin grafts from the supraclavicular area can be harvested by excision of an elliptical area of epidermis and dermis. The donor site can be closed directly in two layers with monofilament absorbable suture in the subcutaneous plane and separately as a subcuticular running stitch. As with the split-thickness graft in the forehead, it should be left unmeshed and secured to the wound bed with fine non-absorbable sutures and a tie-over bolster dressing.

Local Flaps

Local flaps are the mainstays of forehead reconstruction. Because they come from adjacent forehead skin, they provide excellent color and texture match. Proper selection of the patient and flap can minimize donor site morbidity as well as scarring. These operations are limited in scope and can be completed with use of local anesthesia. They are most appropriate for wounds of limited size, from 5 mm to 3 cm in diameter, although the Worthen flap can cover more sizable defects.[9] Care should be taken to minimize additional scarring adjacent to the site of closure, some of which may be perpendicular to the transverse skin lines.

Flap choices include rotation flaps, the largest of which, the Worthen, extends across the width of the forehead to close a lateral forehead or suprabrow defect (Fig. 75-6).[9] Rhomboid, dual rhomboid, banner, and bilobed are the majority of random flaps in this region (Fig. 75-7).[10,11] Bilateral temporal artery V-Y fasciocutaneous advancement flaps, used to close the full width of the brow, have also been described.[12] Pedicled flaps based on the combination of bilateral supratrochlear and supraorbital vessels can be advanced laterally to close lateral forehead defects.[13] Likewise, island flaps based on either supratrochlear or supraorbital vessels may be used to close defects near the eyebrow without distortion. Central forehead defects may be closed with shutter flaps, based superiorly or inferiorly and extending as far laterally as the temporal hairline. The donor site can be closed with a split-thickness skin graft, although with proper handling of the paired flaps, direct closure of the donor sites is readily achieved (Fig. 75-8).[14]

TECHNICAL CONSIDERATIONS

The greatest challenge facing the novice plastic surgeon in designing local flaps in the forehead is deciding on the direction from which the flap should be rotated. This orientation of the flap in turn determines the orientation of the donor site scar.

The classic rhomboid flap is used to close rhomboid-shaped defects whose internal angles are 120 degrees and 60 degrees. The long axis of the defect should be oriented perpendicular to the lines of skin tension. The axis of the flap will lie parallel to one of the sides of the defect, and the tip of the flap will lie along a line parallel to the short axis of the defect. Once the flap is transposed, this will result in a donor site scar that lies parallel to the lines of skin tension. In the middle of the forehead and in the suprabrow area, the donor site scar should lie parallel to the horizontal skin tension lines. At the lateral edges of the forehead, as in the pretemporal area, the donor site scar should lie parallel to the anterior temporal hairline (Fig. 75-9).

Bilobed flaps are useful for closing circular defects. The secondary flap should lie parallel to skin tension lines. In the middle of the forehead and in the suprabrow area, the donor site scar for the secondary flap should lie parallel to the horizontal skin tension lines. At the lateral edges of the forehead, as in the pretemporal area, the donor site scar for the secondary flap should lie parallel to the anterior temporal hairline (Fig. 75-10).

Shutter flaps can be based superiorly or inferiorly. Inferiorly based flaps, perfused by the supraorbital vessels, are appropriate for midline defects. The limits of the flap are the anterior and pretemporal hairline; the flap should be incised outside the hair-bearing scalp to preclude hairline distortion. The dissection of the flaps should extend just deep to the dermis, but not into the frontalis muscle fascia, to minimize danger to the frontal branch of the facial nerve. The flaps can be transposed to the midline and secured with fine nonabsorbable suture. The donor site can be closed directly if temporal scalp can be elevated and mobilized anteriorly. Alternatively, the donor site can be closed with a skin graft, which can subsequently be serially excised.

An additional issue facing the surgeon is the safe and effective depth of the incision and dissection. In general, the incision for the donor flap should extend down to the level of the loose areolar tissue, just deep to the dermis. This allows safe elevation of the flap without risk of injury to the frontal branch of the facial nerve. When the defect is near the anterior temporal hairline, it is important to draw out the anticipated course of this nerve to minimize the opportunity for nerve injury or transection during flap elevation. The course of the frontal branch can be described by a line extending from the anterior border of the lobule of the ear to a point just lateral to the lateral border of the eyebrow.[1] Inadvertent division of the nerve leads to immediate paralysis of the ipsilateral brow.

Text continued on p. 713

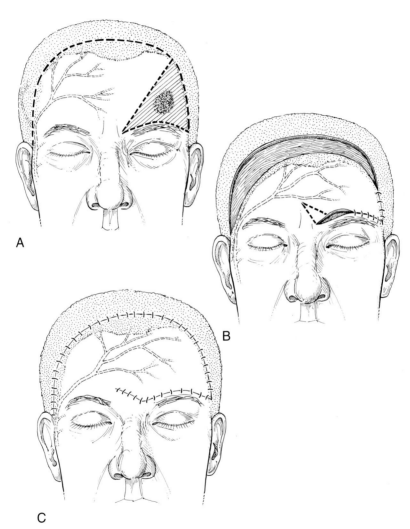

FIGURE 75-6. *A* to *C*, Worthen flap.

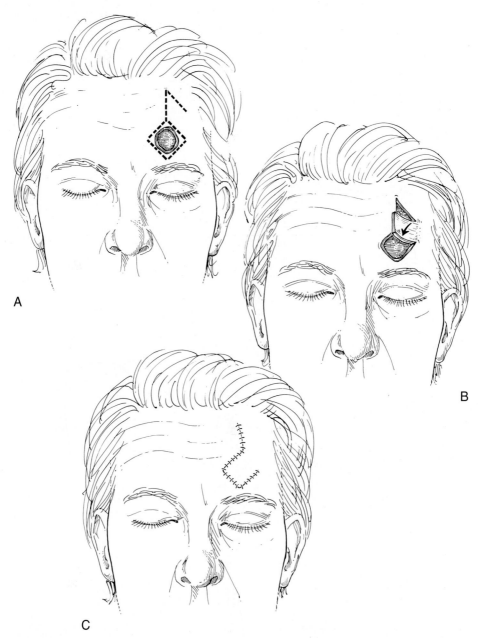

FIGURE 75-7. *A* to *C*, Rhomboid flap.

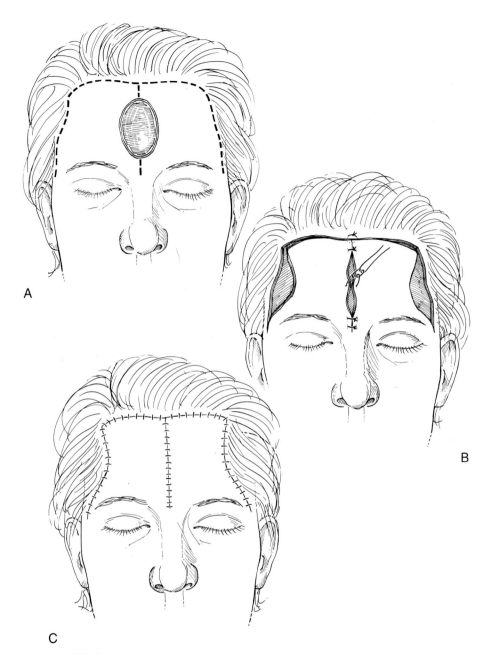

A

B

C

FIGURE 75-8. *A to C,* Shutter flap.

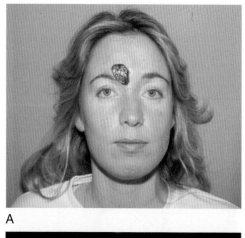

A

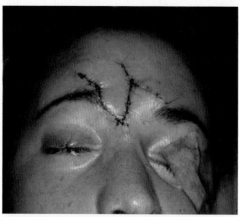

B

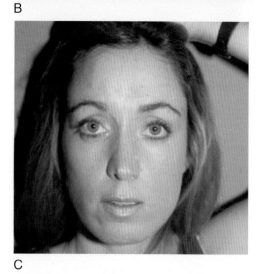

C

FIGURE 75-9. Local flaps for forehead defect closure. *A,* Defect after micrographic resection of basal cell carcinoma. *B,* Rhomboid flap with donor site on glabellar region avoids malposition of eyebrow. *C,* Postoperative view at 6 months demonstrates defect closure with acceptable donor site closure.

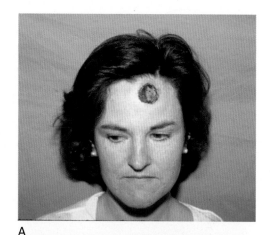

A

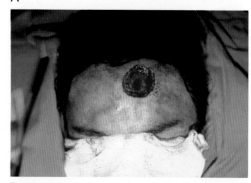

B

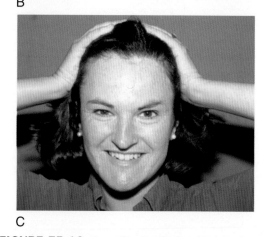

C

FIGURE 75-10. Local flap for forehead defect closure. *A,* After excision of basal cell carcinoma with midline defect in young patient. *B,* Bilateral temporal artery fasciocutaneous flaps are designed with planned rotation-advancement for closure of midline defect. *C,* Six-month postoperative view reveals defect closure with donor site scar at hairline.

Skin Expansion

Skin expansion allows the recruitment of otherwise inadequate, adjacent forehead skin to reconstruct significant but subtotal defects. The expanded skin has a color, texture, and thinness similar to that which was lost. The use of expanded skin minimizes scars in the donor site. In addition, expanded flaps are more resistant to infection than are random cutaneous flaps.[15] Central defects can be closed by expanding bilateral normal forehead skin on each side.[16] Alternatively, the contralateral forehead can be expanded to close a suprabrow wound.[16,17] The pedicled supratrochlear flap can be pre-expanded before transfer to a contralateral defect.[18]

Selection of an optimum skin expander can distinguish a complicated reconstruction from a relatively effortless one. Expanders are available in many sizes and shapes and may have an incorporated filling port or a remote filling port connected to the expander by Silastic tubing (see "Technical Considerations") (Fig. 75-11). Some prefer incorporated ports to remote ports in this region because tenting of the expanding forehead-scalp may obscure a distant filling port. However, most expanders used in the head and neck region have a distant filling port. When expanders with incorporated ports are used, there is a higher risk of implant puncture during repeated inflations. In addition, the incorporated fill ports are most often located over the center of the expander. The skin over the fill port is therefore stretched more than the skin at the periphery of the expander, putting it at greater risk for injury. Repeated trauma to the expanding

skin flap through needle sticks may injure the flap[19] and even lead to expander exposure. Placement of the expander in a plane superficial to the fascia of the frontalis muscle minimizes injury to the frontal branch of cranial nerve VII; however, the simultaneous expansion of skin and frontalis muscle in the forehead generates sensate cutaneous cover and innervated muscle for the restoration of forehead expresson.[20]

The expander can be placed nearly collapsed to facilitate skin closure, and expansion can begin as an outpatient procedure once the incision has healed, typically within 2 weeks. The scalp or forehead skin can be expanded every week to 2 weeks. The expander should be injected with sufficient saline to cause the patient a mild degree of discomfort and a sensation of tightness over the expander. At this point, only enough saline to restore comfort should be removed from the expander; this should equal 1 to 5 mL of volume. Confirm the patient's ability to work and sleep comfortably in the days that follow each injection and titrate subsequent injections to the patient's tolerance for discomfort. Expansion should progress until the expander has reached its full fill volume (approximately 6 to 8 weeks),[21] at which point expander removal and flap advancement can be scheduled. Waiting 2 to 3 weeks after the goal volume is achieved to remove the expanders is sometimes desirable because this allows the skin to soften. At the time of surgery, after expander removal, the patient should be preoperatively marked to establish the boundaries of the forehead. This is especially critical in establishing the anterior or pretemporal hairline. During the

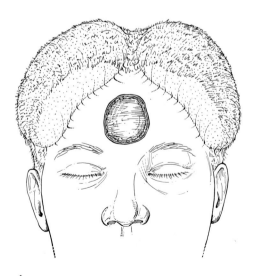

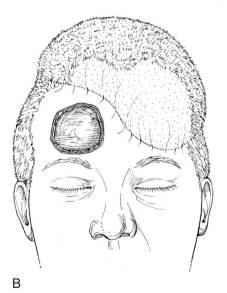

A   B

FIGURE 75-11. *A* and *B,* Tissue expanders in place. Expanded skin will be used for subsequent forehead reconstruction.

procedure, the expanded skin will then be advanced only as far as necessary to complete the reconstructive aims of the operation (Figs. 75-12 and 75-13; see also Fig. 75-24).

The greatest cost associated with skin expansion in this area mirrors that seen with skin expansion elsewhere—it requires staged procedures, and it leaves the patient with a transitory deformity during the expansion phase.

TECHNICAL CONSIDERATIONS

Expanders are available in various shapes and sizes to provide the maximal surface area of desired tissue, and custom-made expanders can be manufactured when unique situations are encountered. The single self-sealing filling port may be incorporated into the body of the expander, or it may be connected to the body of the expander by silicone tubing (distant injection

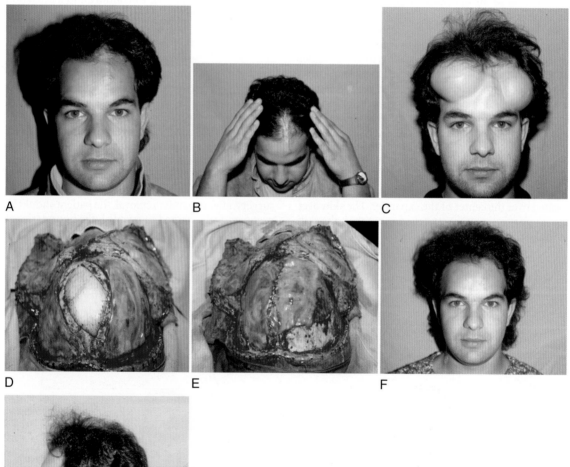

FIGURE 75-12. Tissue expansion for anterior scalp and forehead defect. *A* and *B*, Preoperative anterior and lateral views reveal traumatic alopecia at hairline and depressed scar due to underlying cranial defect. *C*, Tissue expanders inserted to allow advancement of forehead and frontal scalp at time of cranioplasty and scar revision. *D*, Methyl methacrylate used for cranioplasty. *E*, Periosteal flap was used to cover the cranioplasty site. *F* and *G*, Postoperative view at 1 year demonstrates stable coverage over the cranioplasty site and removal of forehead and scalp scar. Expander flaps were closed over defect with tension and provided restoration of forehead and scalp.

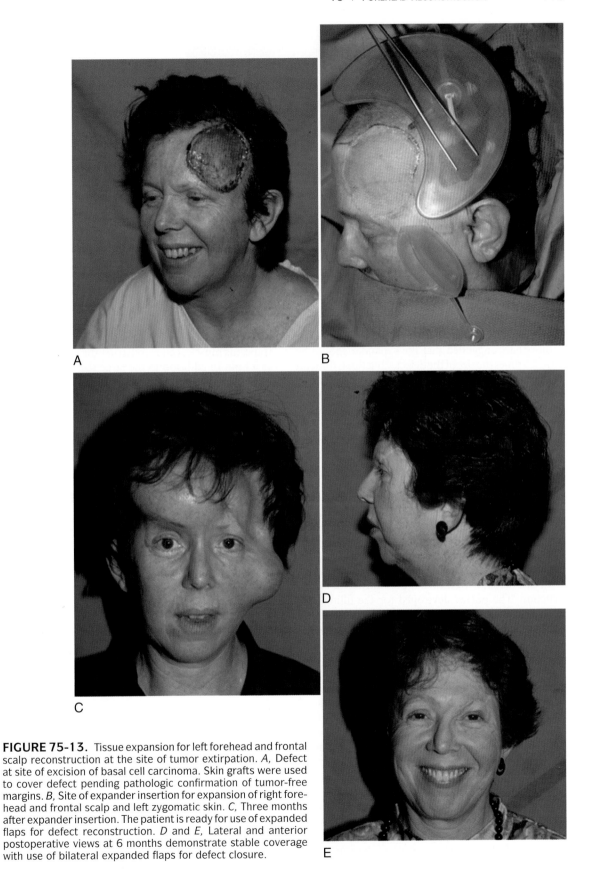

FIGURE 75-13. Tissue expansion for left forehead and frontal scalp reconstruction at the site of tumor extirpation. *A,* Defect at site of excision of basal cell carcinoma. Skin grafts were used to cover defect pending pathologic confirmation of tumor-free margins. *B,* Site of expander insertion for expansion of right forehead and frontal scalp and left zygomatic skin. *C,* Three months after expander insertion. The patient is ready for use of expanded flaps for defect reconstruction. *D* and *E,* Lateral and anterior postoperative views at 6 months demonstrate stable coverage with use of bilateral expanded flaps for defect closure.

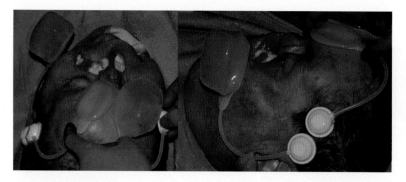

FIGURE 75-14. Various types of tissue expanders are available in numerous sizes and shapes. Expanders shown have distant filling ports often used for head and neck reconstruction. (Photograph courtesy of Malcolm Lesavoy, MD.)

port) (Fig. 75-14). The remote port may be placed subcutaneously away from the body of the expander, or it may be passed externally. For expansion in the forehead, multiple expanders with volumes ranging from 200 to 400 mL with distant injection ports are recommended.

In general, the diameter of the expander should be approximately the same size as the defect. Some authors have suggested that the expander should be up to 2.5 times the size of the defect,[22] but this is difficult to accommodate in the head and neck area. Blunt dissection for development of the pocket is recommended to preserve the longitudinal blood supply.[23] The dissected pocket should be large enough to accommodate the expander comfortably with the edge of the expander approximately 2 cm away from the suture line.[9] To assess the adequacy of pocket dissection, one should inject the fill port with approximately 50 mL of sterile isotonic sodium chloride solution and allow the expander to unroll. If the pocket is not large enough to accommodate expansion comfortably, further dissection should be performed.

When using an expander with a distant filling port, one should consider the comfort of the patient as well as the ease of removing the filling port during the reconstruction. The pocket developed for the filling port should be just large enough to insert the port but not tight enough to necrose the overlying skin. Pockets that are too large may allow the port to flip over and become unusable. The tubing that connects the filling port should not be too taut; this may cause it to rupture during the filling process as both the expander and the port are rapidly fixed in position by scar formation.[9]

The danger of tissue expansion is thinning of the overlying skin flap to the point that exposure may occur. Imminent implant exposure may be treated by removal of the expansion solution, allowing the overlying skin to heal; proceed with reconstruction, taking advantage of the available expanded skin. Although the available skin may not be adequate for the entire reconstruction to be accomplished, partial success may be better in some instances than loss of the entire flap. Implant exposure necessitates immediate

surgery, taking advantage of whatever available expanded tissue is present. In these situations, the patient may choose to undergo a second series of expansions once the wound is healed.[9]

Distant Flaps

Flaps from distant donor sites, including the scalp and trapezius muscle, can reconstruct the entire forehead as a unit. In addition to the large size, such flaps are well vascularized, allowing coverage of deep hard tissue defects, including cranium and bone graft. In patients who cannot tolerate the rigors associated with microvascular composite tissue transplantation, these flaps can provide a less complex alternative. However, the utility of these flaps is to some degree balanced by their cost.

Few distant non-hair-bearing flaps will reach the forehead. Although the three- and four-flap technique developed by Orticochea[24,25] will reach the forehead, these flaps are primarily used for hair-bearing defects (Figs. 75-15 and 75-16). However, the principle of these flaps can be used for superior and lateral forehead defects. Frequently, such defects require hair replacement to restore the hairline as well as forehead coverage. The two anterior flaps may be located at the temporal hairline and transposed to the central forehead with the posterior flap (three-flap technique), or bilateral posterior flaps (four-flap technique) may be used for the donor defect and areas of unstable scalp skin. In some instances, the donor defect from the scalp flap is likely to require split-thickness skin graft coverage.

The vertical pedicled trapezius musculocutaneous flap may be used in forehead reconstruction (Fig. 75-17). This flap is vascularized by the descending branch of the transverse cervical artery and vein, a branch of either the thyrocervical trunk or subclavian artery and vein. For elevation of the flap, an incision is made between the posterior base of the neck and the cephalad margin of the skin island. An additional incision is then made on the lateral edge of the planned skin island. The superficial surface of the trapezius muscle is identified above and lateral to the skin island over the scapula. The muscle is identified at the edge of the skin island, and the deep surface of the middle and lower thirds of the muscle are separated from the chest wall and rhomboid muscles. The medial skin island is incised, and the fibers of origin of the muscle from the vertebral column are divided to the level of the superior scapula. To reach the forehead, the muscle is divided from its fibers of origin on the vertebral column, and the dissection continues laterally toward the acromioclavicular joint as required for an adequate arc of rotation. Direct donor site closure is recommended because a noticeable contour deformity may develop if skin grafts are placed on the exposed rhomboid muscles. Shoulder immobilization postoperatively will help reduce tension on the donor site closure.[26] Use of the vertical musculocutaneous trapezius muscle flap leaves the patient with a posterior vertical trunk donor scar.

TECHNICAL CONSIDERATIONS

The key to the three- and four-flap technique developed by Orticochea is galeal incisions that release the flap and increase the arc of rotation (Figs. 75-18 and 75-19). Excessive tension in closing must be avoided. This flap is contraindicated if prior traumatic lacerations and blunt trauma have injured the blood supply. Vascular patency (especially temporal or occipital arteries) of the flap can usually be confirmed by Doppler examination.[26]

For the vertical pedicled trapezius musculocutaneous flap procedure, the patient should be placed into a lateral decubitus position, with the face and hemithorax prepared as a single operative field. A vertical skin paddle matching the defect and lying over the medial muscle should be identified preoperatively and marked. The skin and muscle are elevated as a unit and transposed to the forehead recipient area. Passage of the flap through a neck tunnel is not recommended to avoid constriction of the flap base. Instead, the flap is tubed at its base and will require delayed flap base division and inset (Fig. 75-20).[26]

In patients who have undergone radical neck dissection or radiation therapy, the anterior ascending and posterior descending branches of the transverse cervical artery may be divided or injured. Selective arteriography should be performed preoperatively in these patients to confirm patency of the transverse artery before surgery.[26]

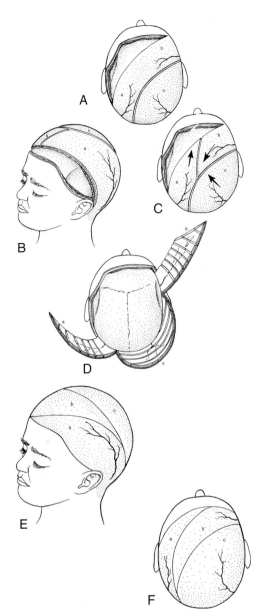

FIGURE 75-15. Three-flap scalp expansile technique. *A,* Bipedicle flap oriented parallel (a-b) to defect on left temporal frontal scalp. *B* and *C,* Bipedicle flap divided to form two flaps. Flap based on occipital artery (a) will advance to interior scalp; flap based on parietal branch of superficial temporal artery (b) will advance to posterior scalp; flap based on contralateral occipital artery (c) will close donor defect as an advancement flap. *D,* Parallel incisions through galea at 2- to 3-cm intervals allow flap expansion without interruption of vascular pedicles superficial to galeal layer. *E,* Hairline position restored and donor site defect closed. *F,* Inset and donor site closure. (From Mathes SJ, Nahai F: Reconstructive Surgery: Principles, Anatomy, and Technique. Edinburgh, Churchill Livingstone, 1997.)

Microvascular Composite Tissue Transplantation and Flap Prefabrication

Free tissue transplantation is sometimes thought of as a procedure of last resort because of its complexity.

Text continued on p. 723

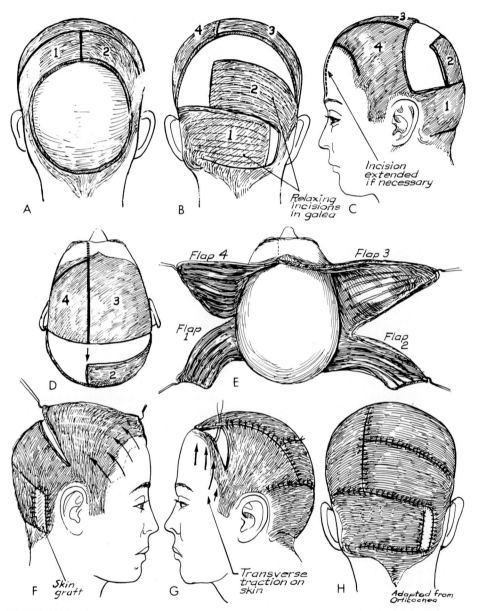

FIGURE 75-16. Four-flap scalp reconstruction technique, which is particularly useful in children. (Modified from Orticochea M: Four-flap scalp reconstruction technique. Br J Plast Surg 1967;20:159.)

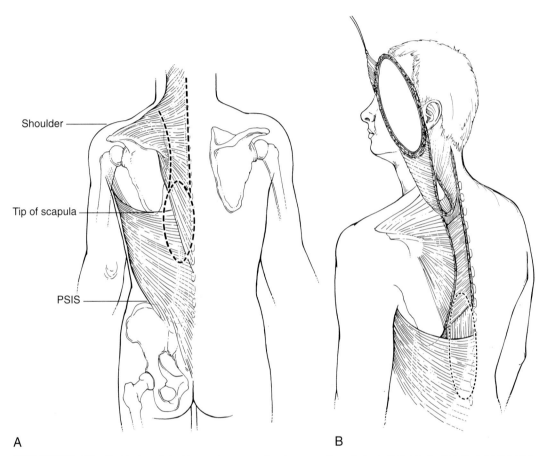

Shoulder

Tip of scapula

PSIS

A   B

FIGURE 75-17. Vertical pedicled trapezius musculocutaneous flap. *A,* An incision is made between the posterior base of the neck and the cephalad margin of the skin island. An additional incision is then made on the lateral edge of the planned skin island. PSIS, posterior superior iliac spine. *B,* The muscle is identified above and lateral to the skin island over the scapula. The medial skin island is incised, and the fibers of origin of the muscle from the vertebral column are divided to the level of the superior scapula. With release of the superior muscle fibers, the point of rotation will be in the posterior midneck. The flap will then reach the upper third of the face and forehead.

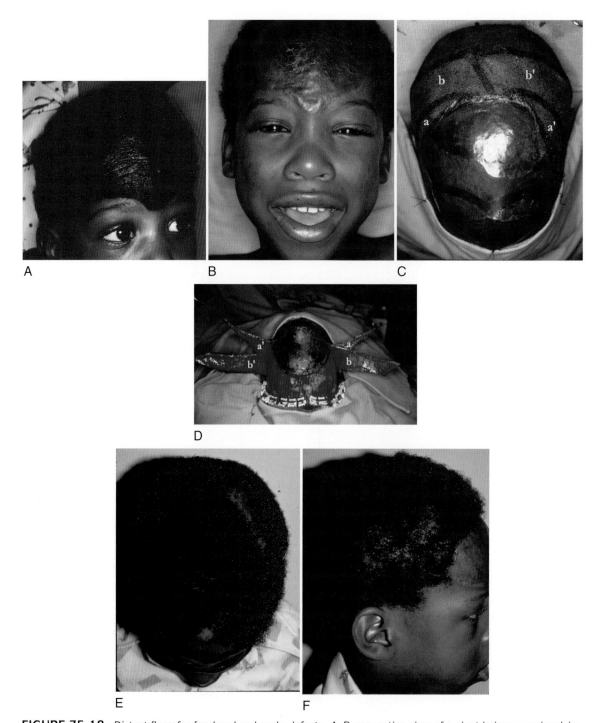

FIGURE 75-18. Distant flaps for forehead and scalp defects. *A,* Preoperative view of a giant hairy nevus involving the forehead and scalp. *B,* Nevus is resected with skin grafts for immediate defect coverage. *C,* Design of four-flap expansile technique (a, a'—frontal flap based on the frontal branches of the temporal vessels; b, b'—posterior parietal flap based on postauricular and temporal vessels). *D,* Four flaps are elevated. The patient is now in the supine position. Galeal incisions are oriented perpendicular to the long axis of the flap to expand the flap's arc of rotation. *E* and *F,* Postoperative anterior and lateral views demonstrate coverage of forehead defect and restoration of hair-bearing frontal scalp with tumor site closures.

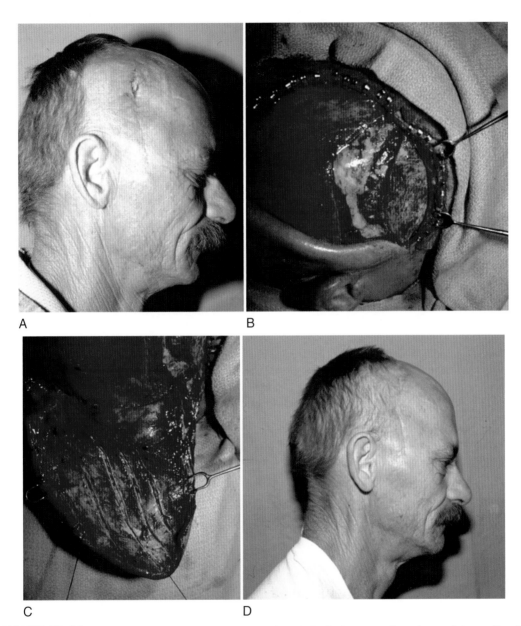

A

B

C

D

FIGURE 75-19. Distant flaps for forehead reconstruction. *A,* Radiation necrosis at the craniotomy site with exposed, nonviable cranial bone. *B,* Débridement of nonviable bone flap. *C,* Temporal parietal flap evaluated. Note galeal incisions. *D,* Postoperative view at 8 months demonstrates use of scalp advancement flap for closure of frontal-temporal defect.

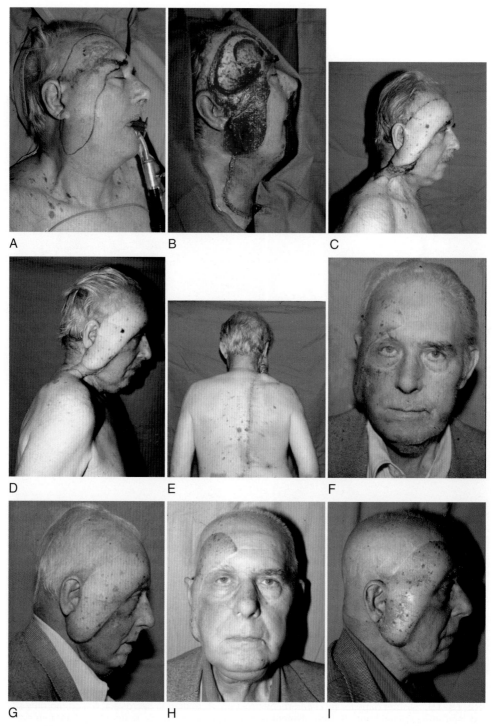

FIGURE 75-20. Distant flap for reconstruction of forehead defect—trapezius musculocutaneous flap. *A,* Preoperative resections for angiosarcoma included forehead resection, total parotidectomy, and neck dissection for lymphadenectomy. *B,* Extirpation defect includes lateral third of forehead, frontal bone, and midface (note: facial nerve preserved). *C* and *D,* Vertical trapezius musculocutaneous flap inset (note: base of flap is skin grafted with planned division and inset of flap at 6 weeks). *E,* Posterior view showing donor scar on trunk from flap. *F* and *G,* Early postoperative anterior and lateral views of flap during radiation therapy for tumor control. *H* and *I,* Postoperative views 6 weeks after completion of radiation therapy (note: stable coverage provided by trapezius musculocutaneous flap for forehead and face reconstruction).

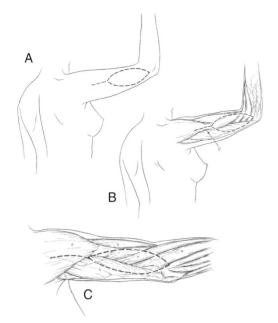

FIGURE 75-21. *A* to *C,* Lateral arm flap. Dominant pedicle: radial collateral artery (D). b, biceps; d, deltoid; e, extensor carpi radialis longus; h, brachioradialis; r, brachialis; t_1, lateral head of triceps; t_2, long head of triceps. (From Mathes SJ, Nahai F: Reconstructive Surgery: Principles, Anatomy, and Technique. Edinburgh, Churchill Livingstone, 1997.)

Nevertheless, defects of the entire forehead are sometimes best managed by this method. A number of flaps have been effectively used, including the latissimus dorsi musculocutaneous flap,[27,28] radial forearm fasciocutaneous flap,[16,27,29] groin fasciocutaneous flap,[29] and lateral arm fasciocutaneous flap (Figs. 75-21 to 75-23).[29] The superficial inferior epigastric artery (SIEA) fasciocutaneous flap is preferred over the groin fasciocutaneous flap, since the SIEA flap offers a longer and more consistent vascular pedicle. Disadvantages associated with these procedures center on the extended operative time and risk of flap failure. Characteristics, indications, and uses of these flaps are based on several factors (Table 75-3).

In addition to providing coverage, free flaps can confer function in the forehead area. Functional reconstruction of the frontalis muscle with a free, thinned gracilis musculocutaneous flap has succeeded in conferring eyebrow motion.[30] Consistent with other functional muscle transplantations, it is critical to place the transplanted muscle under appropriate tension at the time of placement.

Free flap prefabrication represents an exciting combination of tissue engineering techniques and microsurgical transplantation and allows the incorporation of heterotopic tissue elements into a composite tissue. As an example, Khouri[31] desired to transfer shoulder skin to the forehead because it matched the forehead skin in both color and texture. Since the intended flap lacked adequate size as well as a pedicle, he placed a free radial forearm fascial flap beneath the shoulder skin and vascularized the flap by the cervical vessels. Simultaneously, he placed a tissue expander deep to the flap and steadily expanded the overlying skin and flap during the next 3 months. The fully expanded capsulofasciocutaneous flap, measuring 9×20 cm, was then transferred to the forehead as a unit. It was revascularized by the temporal vessels without the need for interpositional vein grafts. Although successful, the reconstruction required multiple operative procedures, two sets of microvascular anastomoses, and division of the patient's radial artery. Whereas prefabrication cannot be considered a primary reconstructive option at this time, it is hoped that improvements in technique will increase its practicality in difficult problems.

Eyebrow Reconstruction

The eyebrows are essential to facial expression; their loss alone can give the impression of a mask-like face.[32] Consequently, eyebrow reconstruction should be considered an integral portion of any forehead reconstruction.

The eyebrows are unique among hair-bearing areas in the body for a variety of reasons; the hair is notable for its thinness, the complicated pattern of direction, and the acute angle between hair shaft and skin.[33] Each of the hairs is of small diameter, has a short length, and grows slowly. The orientation of the hairs changes on the basis of their location within the eyebrow (Fig. 75-24). Hairs in the medial and lower eyebrow grow in a superolateral direction; those in the lateral and upper regions grow in an inferolateral direction.[33] As a result, hair transplants that do not conform to these orientations can appear odd.

Reconstruction of the partial eyebrow, as seen after resection of a small tumor with diameter equivalent to the eyebrow height, is often best managed by local flaps with the remaining portion of that eyebrow.[33,34] Use of the contralateral eyebrow is rarely justified, given the difficulty in hiding a donor site deformity.[33] Local flaps include transverse advancement flaps, with or without Burow triangles, and V-Y advancement flaps. Similarly, the double-Z rhombic technique can be used to collapse the eyebrow in a horizontal direction, leaving its vertical dimension intact (see Fig. 75-9).[35]

Reconstruction of the entire eyebrow is more of a problem. Options center on three categories of repair and include hair plug transplants, hair strip grafts, and pedicled scalp flaps. Each method has its indications and advantages (Table 75-4).

Text continued on p. 728

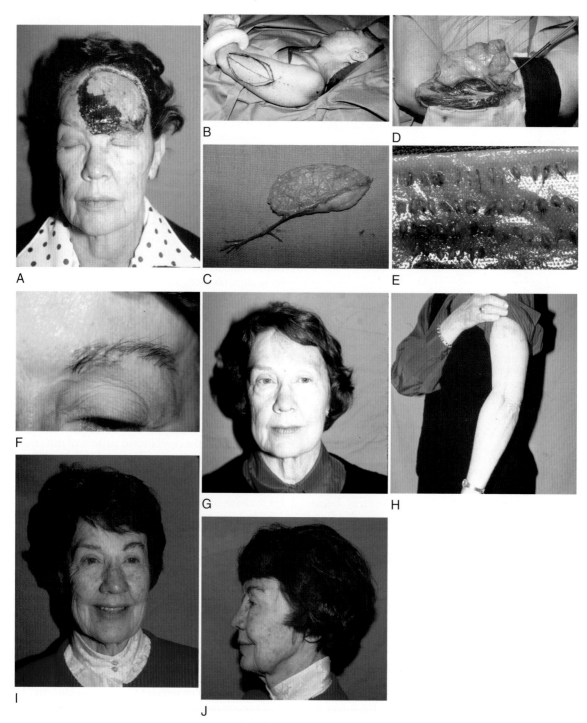

FIGURE 75-22. Microvascular composite tissue transplantation for extensive forehead defect. *A,* Defect after excision of squamous cell carcinoma involving 50% of the forehead. Temporary skin graft was used for defect coverage pending pathologic confirmation of adequate tumor-free margins. *B,* Design of lateral arm fasciocutaneous flap. *C,* Anatomic specimen (latex injected) demonstrates vascular pedicle, radial collateral arteries, and associated venae comitantes. *D,* Flap elevation; note location of septocutaneous pedicle at the lateral intermuscular septum. *E,* Single hair follicle grafts provide for eyebrow reconstruction. *F,* Close-up view of reconstructed brow. *G,* Anterior postoperative view demonstrates stable coverage at flap inset site. The flap has been debulked by suction-assisted lipectomy. *H,* Redundant skin on the lateral upper arm allows direct donor site closure. *I* and *J,* One-year postoperative view demonstrates stable coverage with use of lateral arm flap for major forehead reconstruction.

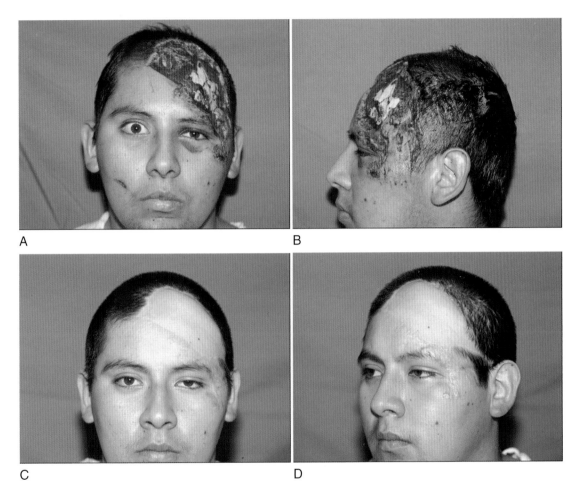

A

B

C

D

FIGURE 75-23. Microvascular composite tissue transplantation followed by scalp tissue expansion for an extensive forehead defect. *A* and *B*, Defect involving 30% of the forehead after a motor vehicle accident. *C* and *D*, Postoperative views after reconstruction with a radial forearm flap. *Continued*

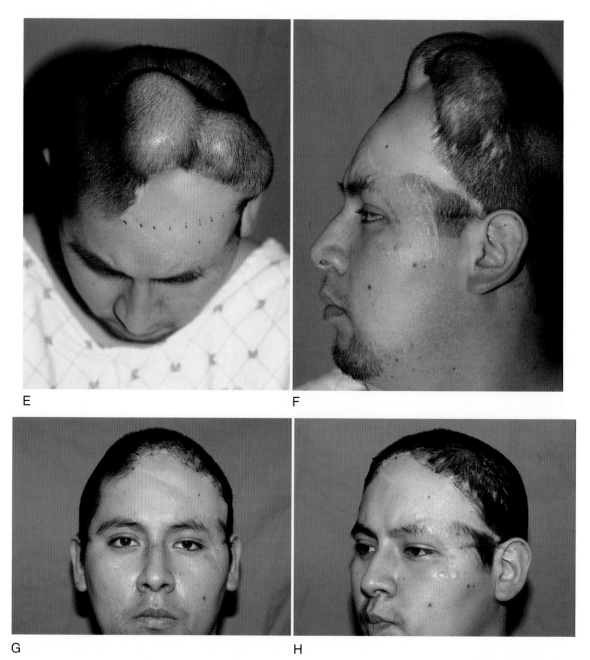

E

F

G

H

FIGURE 75-23, cont'd. *E* and *F,* Paired tissue expanders allow advancement of hair-bearing scalp to reconstruct anterior hairline. *G* and *H,* Reconstructed hairline is improved but still elevated relative to the contralateral side.

TABLE 75-3 ✦ MICROVASCULAR COMPOSITE TISSUE TRANSPLANTATION OPTIONS

	Lateral Arm Fasciocutaneous	Radial Forearm Fasciocutaneous	Latissimus Myocutaneous	SIEA Fasciocutaneous
Vascular anatomy	Radial collateral artery	Radial artery	Thoracodorsal artery	Superficial inferior epigastric artery
Pedicle length/ arterial diameter	7 cm/2.5 mm	20 cm/2.5 mm	8 cm/2.5 mm	4-6 cm/1-1.5 mm
Vein grafts?	May be necessary	Unlikely to be necessary	May be necessary	May be necessary
Dimension	8 × 15 cm	10 × 40 cm	25 × 35 cm	15 × 30 cm
Thickness	Varies by patient	Varies by patient	Muscle flap: 0.8 cm Myocutaneous flap: varies by patient	Varies by patient
Appearance	Flat, pliable skin	Flat, pliable skin	Flat, fan-shaped muscle	Flat, relatively thick skin
Donor site closure	Direct closure for defects < 6 cm wide	Direct closure for defects < 2 cm wide	Direct closure for defects < 10 cm wide	Direct closure possible for all sizes of flaps
Advantages	Thin, pliable, relatively hairless flap Donor and recipient sites can undergo simultaneous operation	Thin, pliable, relatively hairless, with a long pedicle Donor and recipient sites can undergo simultaneous operation	Large flap	Large flap Donor and recipient sites can undergo simultaneous operation
Limitations	Short pedicle, which may require vein graft In overweight or older patients, flap may require defatting	Donor site requires skin grafting	Thick and therefore ill-suited to match forehead contour Will likely require defatting at a subsequent stage Short pedicle Patient may need to be repositioned for flap placement Harvest may result in functional deficit	Potentially thick and therefore may be ill-suited to match forehead contour Will likely require defatting at a subsequent stage Short pedicle, which may require vein graft

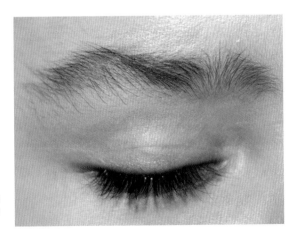

FIGURE 75-24. The eyebrow hair follicle direction is specific to its location in the eyebrow, as seen in this 10-month-old boy.

TABLE 75-4 ✦ EYEBROW RECONSTRUCTION OPTIONS

	Single Follicles	Hair Plugs	Composite Grafts	Superficial Temporal Parietal Flaps
Hair density	Can be modulated	Can be modulated	Can be overly dense	Can be overly dense
Follicle direction	Determined by surgeon	Determined by surgeon	Dependent on follicle direction in donor site	Dependent on follicle direction in donor site
Donor site	Hair-bearing scalp	Hair-bearing scalp	Hair-bearing scalp	Hair-bearing scalp overlying the superficial temporal artery
Recipient site	Requires a well-vascularized, minimally scarred bed	Requires a well-vascularized, minimally scarred bed	Requires a well-vascularized, minimally scarred bed	Appropriate for poorly vascularized wound beds
Complexity of procedure	Simple but tedious	Simple	Simple	Mildly complex
Single vs. multiple stages	Multiple, to achieve sufficient hair density	Multiple, to achieve sufficient hair density	Single	Single stage if flap is tunneled. Two stages if a tubed flap is employed

Hair plug transplantation is a low-morbidity procedure (Fig. 75-25). These transplants are most appropriate where the skin underlying the eyebrow is unscarred and of normal thickness and character. It is most difficult in burn scar beds.[36] Hair plugs of appropriate thickness can be harvested from the scalp, although this hair is usually far from ideal given its far greater thickness and faster growth rate than that needed for the eyebrow.[34] Nonetheless, these hairs are usually abundant, and their loss is easily camouflaged by well-placed incisions. Hair plugs can be placed at the desired acute angle relative to the skin (Fig. 75-26).[33] Multiple procedures are often required to achieve a sufficiently normal hair density. In addition, patients must periodically trim the fast-growing transplant hairs to maintain length parity with the contralateral normal eyebrow.

Free composite grafts of hair-bearing skin, also referred to as hair strip grafts, are a faster method of delivering hair follicles to the recipient site (Fig. 75-

27). Like hair plug transplants, these grafts require a well-vascularized, minimally scarred bed to survive. Hair-bearing scalp is the most common donor site and offers a set of hairs and follicles that are uniformly oriented but often overly dense.[34] Survival of these grafts is less than that of hair plugs because of the larger volume of tissue transferred. Survival can be optimized by removal of residual galea aponeurosis and as much fat as possible while still leaving the follicles intact.[36] Nonetheless, multiple procedures may be necessary to achieve a complete eyebrow.

Where the eyebrow bed is insufficiently vascularized to support free grafts or hair plugs, pedicled scalp flaps provide a safe alternative. The donor site for such flaps should be properly oriented and placed to ensure that the hairs grow in the same direction as eyebrow hairs. Inattention to these details can lead to a hairbrush-appearing eyebrow.[37] In male patients, the scalp donor site should be away from expected areas of male pattern baldness because any tendency toward

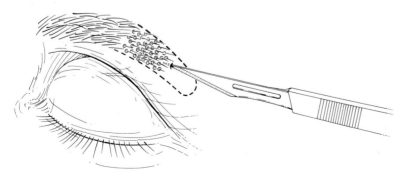

FIGURE 75-25. Eyebrow reconstruction by single-follicle "hair plug" implantation.

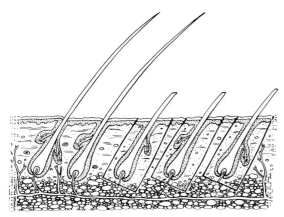

FIGURE 75-26. Hair plugs placed at desired acute angle relative to the skin.

alopecia will travel with the flap.[38] The postauricular temporoparietal region, perfused by a branch of the superficial temporal artery, is a popular donor site for these reasons (Fig. 75-28).[36]

Prefabrication techniques can also be applied to eyebrow reconstruction.[39] Where no pedicle exists beneath a desired patch of scalp donor flap, a pedicle of inferior epigastric artery and vein can be anastomosed to the superficial temporal artery and vein, with the end of the pedicle beneath the flap. After 2 weeks,

the flap can be transferred to the eyebrow region as a pedicled flap.

Eyebrow defects can present a significant challenge to the plastic surgeon. Judicious use of these techniques can minimize the deformity.

TECHNICAL CONSIDERATIONS

Single-follicle hair transplants are first harvested from hair-bearing scalp as strips of full-thickness skin and subcutaneous tissue encompassing 10 to 30 follicles (see Fig. 75-22E and F). The donor site should first undergo trimming of the hair, such that a 3- to 5-mm stubble of hair remains. This hair serves as a handle for manipulating the follicle, and it provides a guide to the orientation of the follicle within the skin. Each skin strip is subdivided with a sharp scalpel into segments of tissue, each of which includes a single follicle; each tissue segment will measure approximately 1 mm in width. The recipient site should consist of a pliable, well-vascularized bed with sufficient thickness to support the depth of the follicle. With a No. 11 scalpel blade, a set of deep, narrow stab incisions is made in the recipient bed. Care should be taken to orient the axis of the incisions along the intended direction of the follicle (Fig. 75-29). With the aid of fine tweezers or jeweler's forceps, an individual follicle is then placed directly into each incision. If incisions are made inadvertently long, two or three follicles can be placed in a single incision.

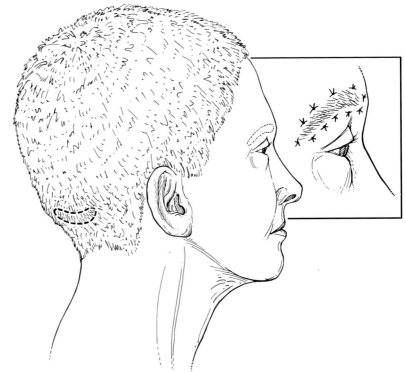

FIGURE 75-27. Free composite graft of scalp used for eyebrow reconstruction.

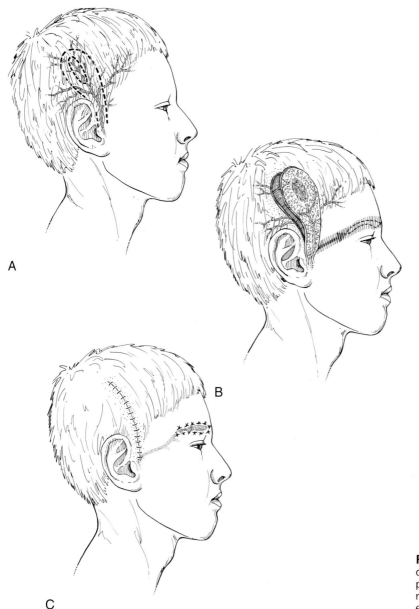

A

B

C

FIGURE 75-28. *A* to *C*, Pedicled scalp flap placed in the postauricular temporoparietal region for reconstruction of the eyebrow.

Once the recipient site has healed and a significant portion of postoperative swelling has subsided, the procedure can be repeated. At the second and subsequent stages, new incisions are placed between previously placed follicles. Care should be taken to avoid injury to older follicle transplants.

Hair plug placement is generally faster but may offer the surgeon less direct control over follicular direction. Harvest of plugs can be accomplished with one of two techniques. First, a strip of skin can be harvested as described before, and the strip is subdivided into segments incorporating two to five follicles. Alternatively, a 2-mm dermal punch can be used to harvest a set of cores of skin, each core encompassing two to five follicles. At the recipient site, plug grafts can be placed into minute incisions that have been oriented along the intended direction of hair growth.

SUMMARY

Because the forehead protects the anterior portion of the cranium and also animates the superior portion of the face, reconstructive considerations should be both functional and aesthetic. The majority of forehead defects occur after surgical removal of a skin

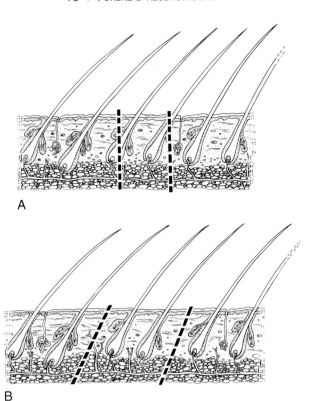

FIGURE 75-29. Single-follicle hair transplants are first harvested as strips of full-thickness skin and subcutaneous tissue from the hair-bearing scalp. Each strip is divided into segments of tissue that contain a single follicle. Care should be taken to orient the axis of the incisions along the intended direction of the follicle. *A,* Parallel incision. *B,* Vertical incision.

malignant neoplasm; however, defects may also be due to trauma, congenital defects, or infections. A number of options for both functional and aesthetic repair of these defects are available. The key to optimal forehead reconstruction is maximal preservation of nerves, consideration of the cosmetic subunits during operative planning, and placement of scars in skin-relaxed tension lines or hair-bearing boundaries (e.g., hairline, above the eyebrow).

REFERENCES

1. Jackson IT: Local Flaps in Head and Neck Reconstruction. St. Louis, CV Mosby, 1985.
2. McKinney P, Mossie RD, Zukowski ML: Criteria for the forehead lift. Aesthetic Plast Surg 1991;15:141-147.
3. Stuzin JM, Wagstrom L, Kawamoto HK, et al: Anatomy of the frontal branch of the facial nerve: the significance of the temporal fat pad. Plast Reconstr Surg 1989;83:265-271.
4. Edgerton MT, Hansen FC: Matching facial color with split thickness skin grafts from adjacent areas. Plast Reconstr Surg 1960;25:455-464.
5. Coleman DJ: Use of expanded temporal flaps to resurface the skin grafted forehead. Br J Plast Surg 1987;40:171-172.
6. Hamilton R, Royster HP: Reconstruction of extensive forehead defects. Plast Reconstr Surg 1971;47:421-424.
7. Terranova W: The use of periosteal flaps in scalp and forehead reconstruction. Ann Plast Surg 1990;25:450-456.
8. Millard DR: The crane principle for the transport of subcutaneous tissue. Plast Reconstr Surg 1969;43:451-462.
9. Worthen EF: Repair of forehead defects by rotation of local flaps. Plast Reconstr Surg 1976;57:204-206.
10. Sutton AE, Quatela VC: Bilobed flap reconstruction of the temporal forehead. Arch Otolaryngol Head Neck Surg 1992;118:978-982, discussion 983-984.
11. Yenidunya MO: Axial pattern bilobed flap for the reconstruction of the midline forehead defects. Plast Reconstr Surg 1999;103:737.
12. Gruber S, Papp C, Maurer H: Case report. Reconstruction of damaged forehead with bilateral fasciocutaneous temporal V-Y-advancement island flaps. Br J Plast Surg 1999;52:74-75.
13. Okada E, Maruyama Y: A simple method for forehead unit reconstruction. Plast Reconstr Surg 2000;106:111-114.
14. Levine NS, Sahl WJ, Stewart JB: The "shutter flap" for large defects of the forehead. Ann Plast Surg 1996;36:425-427.
15. Barker DE, Dedrick DK, Burney RE, et al: Resistance of rapidly expanded random skin flaps to bacterial invasion. J Trauma 1987;27:1061-1065.
16. Di Giuseppe A, Di Benedetto G, Stanizzi A, et al: Skin expansion versus free forearm flap in forehead reconstruction. Microsurgery 1996;17:248-253.
17. Fan J, Yang P: Versatility of expanded forehead flaps for facial reconstruction. Case report. Scand J Plast Reconstr Surg Hand Surg 1997;31:363-363.
18. Iwahira Y, Maruyama Y: Expanded unilateral forehead flap (sail flap) for coverage of opposite forehead defect. Plast Reconstr Surg 1993;92:1052-1056.
19. Antonyshyn O, Gruss JS, Mackinnon SE, Zuker R: Complications of soft tissue expansion. Br J Plast Surg 1988;41:239-250.
20. Antonyshyn O, Gruss JS, Zuker R, Mackinnon SE: Tissue expansion in head and neck reconstruction. Plast Reconstr Surg 1988;82:58-68.
21. van Aalst JA, McCurry T, Wagner J: Reconstructive considerations in the surgical management of melanoma. Surg Clin North Am 2003;83:187-230.
22. van Rappard JH, Molenar J, van Doorn K: Surface-area increase in tissue expansion. Plast Reconstr Surg 1988;82:833-839.

23. Radovan C: Tissue expansion in soft-tissue reconstruction. Plast Reconstr Surg 1984;74:482-492.

24. Orticochea M: New three-flap scalp reconstruction technique. Br J Plast Surg 1971;24:184-188.

25. Orticochea M: Four-flap scalp reconstruction technique. Br J Plast Surg 1967;20:159-171.

26. Mathes SJ, Nahai F: Reconstructive Surgery: Principles, Anatomy, and Techniques. Edinburgh, Churchill Livingstone, 1997.

27. Earley MJ, Green MF, Milling MA: A critical appraisal of the use of free flaps in primary reconstruction of combined scalp and calvarial cancer defects. Br J Plast Surg 1990;43:283-289.

28. Eufinger H, Wehmoller M, Scholz M, et al: Reconstruction of an extreme frontal and frontobasal defect by microvascular tissue transfer and a prefabricated titanium implant. Plast Reconstr Surg 1999;104:198-203.

29. Weinzweig N, Davies B, Polley JW: Microsurgical forehead reconstruction: an aesthetic approach. Plast Reconstr Surg 1995;95:647-651.

30. Sasaki K, Nozaki M, Nada Y, et al: Functional reconstruction of forehead with microneurovascular transfer of attenuated and broadened gracilis muscle. Br J Plast Surg 1998;51:313-316.

31. Khouri RK, Ozbek MR, Hruza GJ, et al: Facial reconstruction with prefabricated induced expanded (PIE) supraclavicular skin flaps. Plast Reconstr Surg 1995;95:1007-1015, discussion 1016-1017.

32. McConnell CM, Neale HW: Eyebrow reconstruction in the burn patient. J Trauma 1977;17:362-366.

33. Kasai K, Ogawa Y: Partial eyebrow reconstruction using subcutaneous pedicle flaps to preserve the natural hair direction. Ann Plast Surg 1990;24:117-125.

34. Goldman GD: Eyebrow transplantation. Dermatol Surg 2001;27:352-354.

35. Cedars MG: Reconstruction of the localized eyebrow defect. Plast Reconstr Surg 1997;100:685-689.

36. Ziccardi VB, Lalikos JF, Sotereanos GC, et al: Composite scalp strip graft for eyebrow reconstruction: case report. J Oral Maxillofac Surg 1993;51:93-96.

37. Dzubow LM: Basal-cell carcinoma of the eyebrow region. J Dermatol Surg Oncol 1984;10:609-614.

38. Juri J: Eyebrow reconstruction. Plast Reconstr Surg 2001; 107:1225-1228.

39. Hyakusoku H: Secondary vascularised hair-bearing island flaps for eyebrow reconstruction. Br J Plast Surg 1993;46:45-47.

Reconstruction of the Periorbital Adnexa

S. Anthony Wolfe, MD ✦ Maria Teresa Rivas-Torres, MD
✦ Omer Ozerdem, MD

PRIORITIES FOR RECONSTRUCTION
    Bony Orbit
    Eyelids
    Canthal Attachments
    Eyelid Muscles

SPECIFIC DIAGNOSES AND TREATMENTS
    Exophthalmos
    Orbital Exenteration and Transcranial Orbitectomy
    Socket Reconstruction

The soft tissue structures attaching to, filling, and surrounding the bony orbital cavity are collectively called the periorbital adnexa. These include the upper and lower eyelids with their inner and outer lamellae, the muscles responsible for opening and closing the eyelids, the medial and lateral canthal attachments of the eyelids to bone, and the lacrimal drainage system.

PRIORITIES FOR RECONSTRUCTION

The orbital cavity is home to our most specialized sense organ, the eye, and all reconstructive surgery in this area must have as its first priority provision of protective coverage of the cornea with a lubricating mucosal surface. Once protective coverage of the cornea has been accomplished, one can proceed at a more leisurely pace in planning a strategy for subsequent reconstruction.

The overall sequencing, although there will be exceptions, is as follows:

1. Correction of any abnormalities of the bony orbit, including enophthalmos if it is present.
2. Provision of adequate inner and outer lamellae of the eyelids.
3. Proper positioning of the medial and lateral canthi.
4. Establishment of eyelid opening and closing and restoration of lacrimal drainage.

Bony Orbit

Correction of abnormalities of the bony orbit, including enophthalmos, is presented in Chapter 72.

Eyelids

In the presence of a seeing eye, mucosal lining must be adequate to cover and protect the cornea and extend into cul-de-sacs or fornices. The levator muscle, if it is present, must attach to a tarsal plate in the upper eyelid. There needs to be a tarsal plate, or cartilaginous tarsal replacement, for support of the lower lid.

Chondromucosal grafts from the nasal septum, upper lateral nasal cartilage,[1] and split palatal mucosal grafts are commonly used materials for the inner lamella. If they are available, chondromucosal grafts from the nasal septum and upper lateral cartilage are preferred. Free buccal mucosal grafts are a poor choice because of their propensity for marked contraction.

Skin cover for the upper eyelid can come from the contralateral upper lid if smaller amounts are required. An excellent material for skin in the upper lids, if larger amounts are required, is a medium-thickness (0.015 to 0.016 inch) split graft from the upper, inner arm. This is an area that provides a good color match and is usually devoid of hair, even in hirsute men. Full-thickness grafts, except from the contralateral upper lid, are too thick for the upper lid. Thicker split grafts or thinner full-thickness grafts (such as postauricular) are used for the lower eyelid, where support rather than suppleness is more important (Figs. 76-1 to 76-3).

For defects of less than 25% of the upper and lower eyelid, a lateral canthotomy alone will allow satisfactory closure of the eyelid. After any wedge resection of a portion of an eyelid, the gray line, the lash line, and the tarsal plate should be carefully sutured separately.

Text continued on p. 738

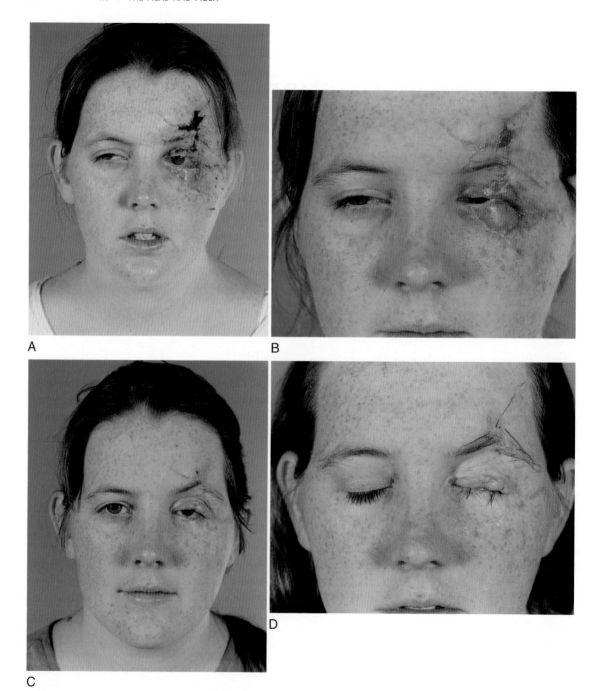

FIGURE 76-1. *A,* This 18-year-old woman is shown approximately 2 weeks after an automobile accident. She sustained open fractures of the supraorbital ridge and zygoma. *B,* Because of the poor condition of the soft tissues, a tarsorrhaphy was performed to provide corneal protection, and the soft tissues were allowed to heal during the next 6 weeks. With the tarsorrhaphy still in place, osteotomies and repositioning of the zygoma were then performed, with cranial bone grafting of the orbital floor and supraorbital ridge defects. After another 6 weeks, the tarsorrhaphy was then divided along with a medium split-thickness skin graft (from the upper, inner arm) to the upper lid. *C* and *D,* She is shown 6 months after the accident and will require further revisional work of the eyebrow and upper eyelid.

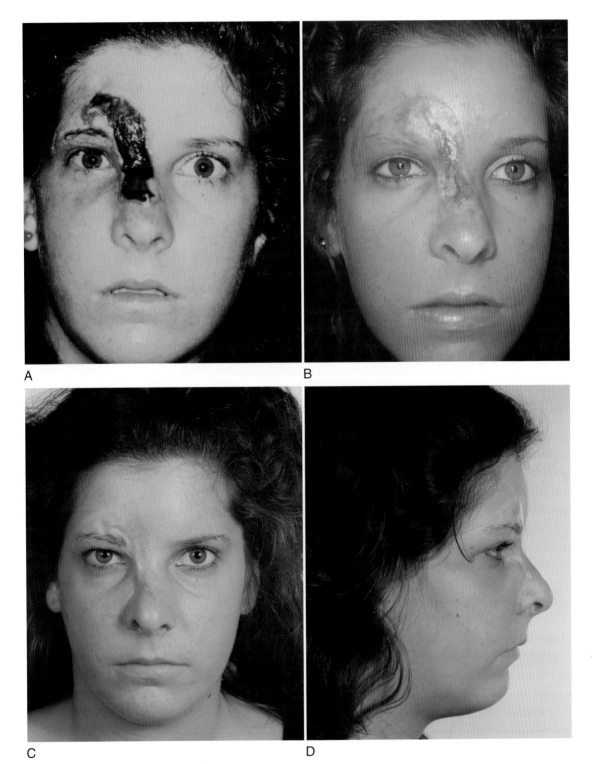

A

B

C

D

FIGURE 76-2. This woman was 19 years old when she was first seen (*C* and *D*), approximately 1 year after a boating accident in which a portion of her forehead, medial canthal area, root of eyebrow, and dorsum of nose had been sliced off. The initial photographs (*A* and *B*), provided by the patient, show a black eschar soon after the injury and the degree of secondary healing several months later with a small area of exposed nasal bone. At the first operation, the scar above the brow was excised *(G, next page),* and the right side of the forehead, based laterally, was rotated down *(H).*

Continued

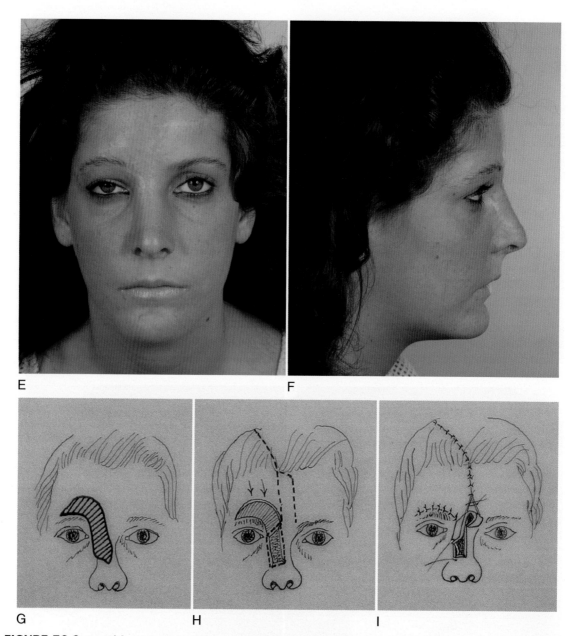

E

F

G

H

I

FIGURE 76-2, cont'd. At the same time, a paramedian forehead flap based on the left epitrochlear vessels was used to reconstruct the dorsal nasal aesthetic unit, with the flap inset along both nasal sidewalls and at the supratip area *(I)*. The forehead flap was subsequently divided and inset at the level of the nasion. A genioplasty was also performed at the second operation. *E* and *F,* She is shown 2 years after the two operations.

FIGURE 76-3. *A,* This 55-year-old woman sustained multiple facial, chest, and extremity lacerations when she was run over by a motorboat propeller. She lost light perception in the left eye and received her initial treatment by a surgeon who transposed a glabellar flap to the left medial canthal area. This is a poor choice of flap for this area, so the flap was returned to the forehead. A medial canthopexy with split-thickness skin graft (upper, inner arm) was performed to the left upper eyelid along with a cranial bone graft to the nose. *B,* The left cheek was advanced in to join the aesthetic unit along the left nasal sidewall. *C to G,* A tongue flap and Abbe flap were performed to reconstruct the missing portions of the left lip. The left eye was enucleated by an ophthalmologist after a failed conjunctival flap, and split palatal grafts were then performed to extend the upper and lower sulcus so that an eye prosthesis could be fitted.

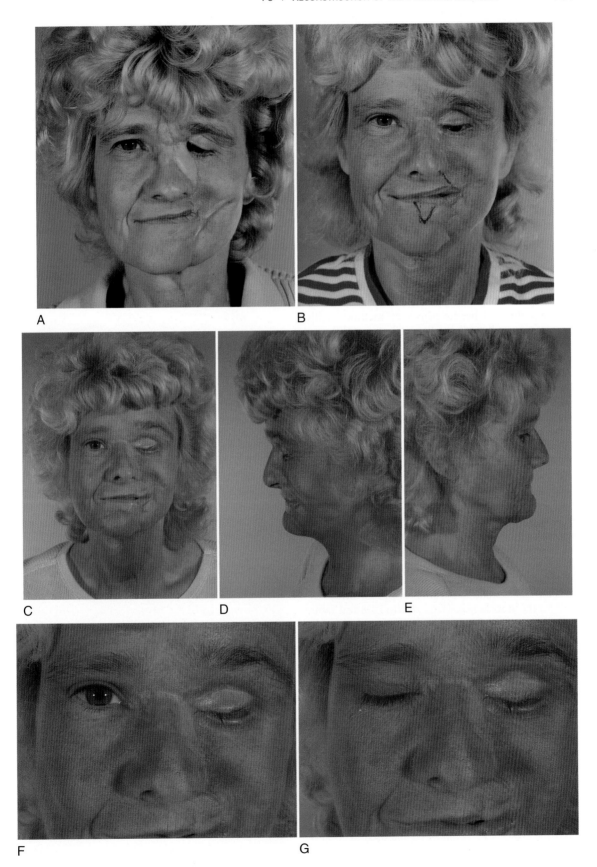

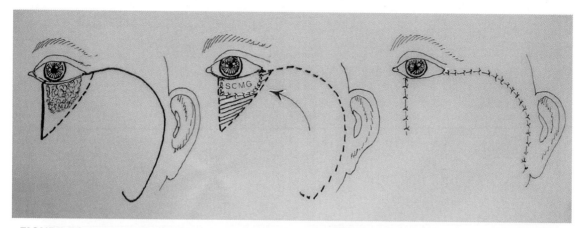

FIGURE 76-4. Mustardé lateral rotation flap. SCMG, septal chondromucosal graft.

For defects of more than 25% of the upper eyelid, up to the entire upper eyelid, reconstruction is best performed by the Mustardé method,[2] with use of a narrowly pedicled flap of lower eyelid in a two-stage procedure. At the same time, the lower eyelid is then reconstructed. An external incision is based on the size of the defect. If 50% to 60% of the eyelid is missing and the defect is located laterally, a Mustardé cheek flap (or the Tenzel variation[3]) can be rotated in for the outer lamella, and a septal chondromucosal graft is used for the inner lamella. The rigidity of the septal cartilage is essential for support of the eyelid with this method (Figs. 76-4 and 76-5).

For total or nearly total defects of the lower eyelid, the nasojugal flap of Tessier[4] with an upper lateral nasal chondromucosal graft is an excellent method because of the vascularity of the flap. It can be firmly suspended to the lateral canthus. It is important that the base of the flap be taken above the level of the lateral canthus. With a 50% to 60% defect of the medial portion of the lid, it is preferable to use this flap for the skin replacement and a smaller chondromucosal graft for the inner lamella (Figs. 76-6 to 76-8 and Table 76-1).

Canthal Attachments

Medial and lateral canthopexies can often be performed along with the procedures listed in the preceding section (osseous and eyelid). If the bone structures are in the proper position, the medial canthus is best

Text continued on p. 743

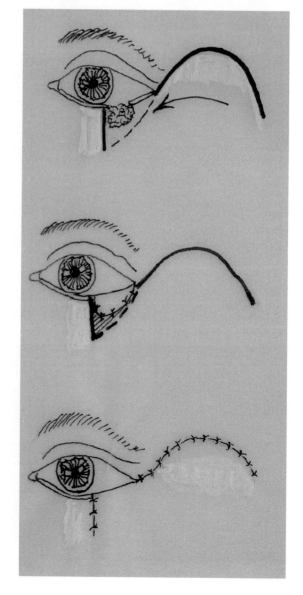

FIGURE 76-5. The Tenzel procedure is a more limited form of a Mustardé flap. A rotation flap is brought in from the tissue adjacent to the upper lid and used to cover a chondromucosal graft.

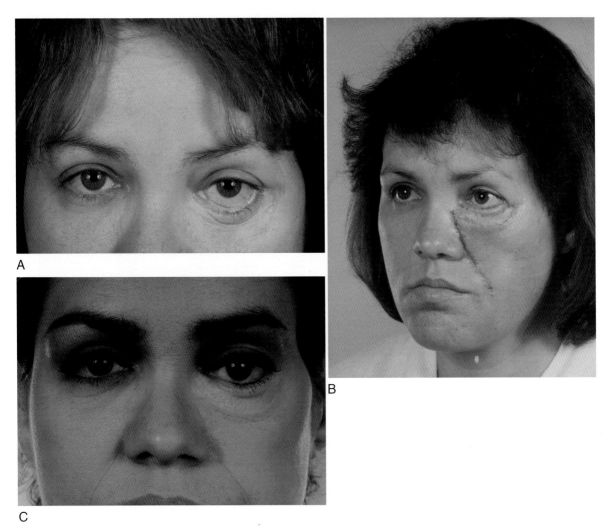

FIGURE 76-6. This 36-year-old woman was struck in the face by a jet ski while lying on the beach. Le Fort I and left orbital zygomatic fractures resulted, and an exploration of the left orbit was performed elsewhere through a subciliary incision. For unknown reasons, the fracture was not reduced. She underwent a Le Fort I osteotomy and reduction of the left orbital fracture. The orbit was explored through the previous subciliary incision, and the soft tissues of the cheek were suspended to the infraorbital rim along with a Frost suture suspension of the lower eyelid. *A,* Subsequent attempts to correct the ectropion with lateral canthopexy and temporalis muscle flap and a full-thickness skin graft were unsuccessful. *B,* A nasojugal flap, as used for total lower eyelid reconstruction, was the only remaining option. *C,* The postoperative photograph was taken 4 years after the original injury, and she shows slight persistent laxity in the lower eyelid that would benefit from a lateral canthopexy.

TABLE 76-1 ✦ ALGORITHM FOR RECONSTRUCTION OF FULL-THICKNESS EYELID DEFECTS

	Defect Size	Treatment
Upper lid	≤¹/₄	Primary closure ± lateral canthotomy
	>¹/₄	Abbe/Mustardé switch
Lower lid	Marginal <8 mm	Kolner or Hughes (transconjunctival from upper lid)
	≤¹/₄	Primary closure ± lateral canthotomy
	Lateral half	Mustardé or Tenzel flap with chondromucosal graft (septum, split palate, upper lateral nasal cartilage)
	Medial half	Nasojugal flap of Tessier with chondromucosal graft
Both lids		Forehead flap with chondromucosal or split palatal graft

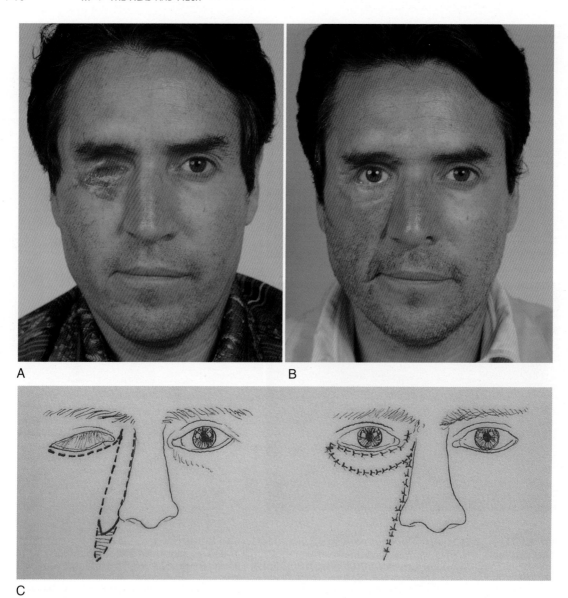

A

B

C

FIGURE 76-7. *A,* This 40-year-old man lost his right eye and much of his right lower eyelid in an automobile accident in South America. *B,* He is shown 6 months after a single operation consisting of a right nasojugal flap *(C)* and septal chondromucosal graft. He has been fitted with an ocular prosthesis.

FIGURE 76-8. *A,* This 82-year-old woman had a lesion of the left lower eyelid that had been present for some indeterminate time. No biopsy had been done. Clinically, it was consistent with a basal cell carcinoma, with pearly, elevated edges. It was explained to the patient that this was very likely a skin cancer and that a biopsy specimen would be taken and examined by frozen section. If the biopsy confirmed the diagnosis, all involved tissue would be removed until tumor-free margins were obtained. It was also explained that an appropriate reconstruction would be performed that might require suturing her eyelids together for a number of weeks. *B* and *C,* The operative photographs show that approximately 85% of the transverse dimension of the eyelid was involved and removed. The resection extended approximately 1 cm beyond the lateral canthus and to the inferior extent of the conjunctival cul-de-sac. It was thought that the most appropriate method of reconstruction would be to use a tarsoconjunctival flap from the upper eyelid with a full-thickness skin graft. The operative photographs show design of the flap *(D),* leaving several millimeters of tarsus in the upper eyelid *(E* and *F),* adequately mobilizing the tarsoconjunctival segment by dissection with a cotton-tipped applicator *(G),* precisely suturing the tarsus to the remaining medial tarsus and the lateral canthus *(H),* and covering the skin deficit with a full-thickness skin graft (preauricular, defatted as much as possible) *(I).*   *Continued*

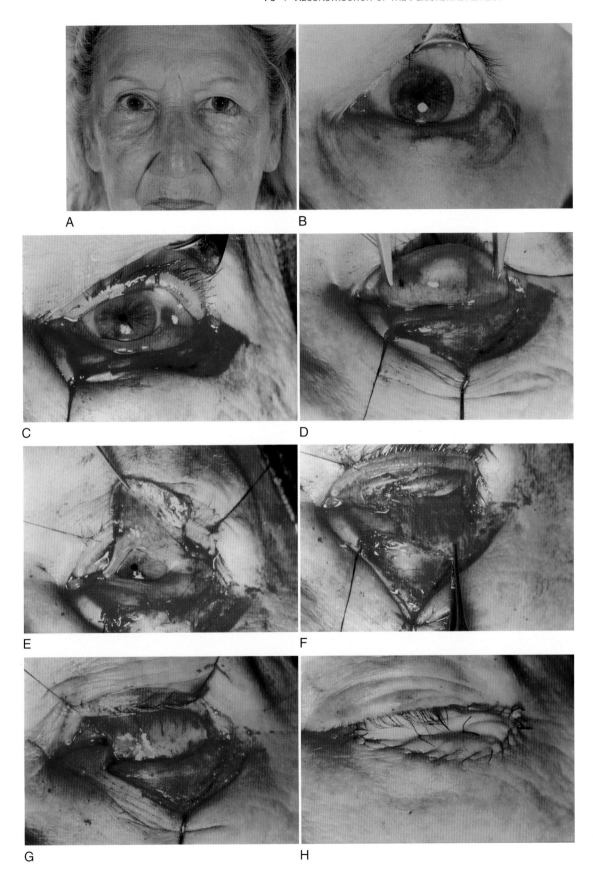

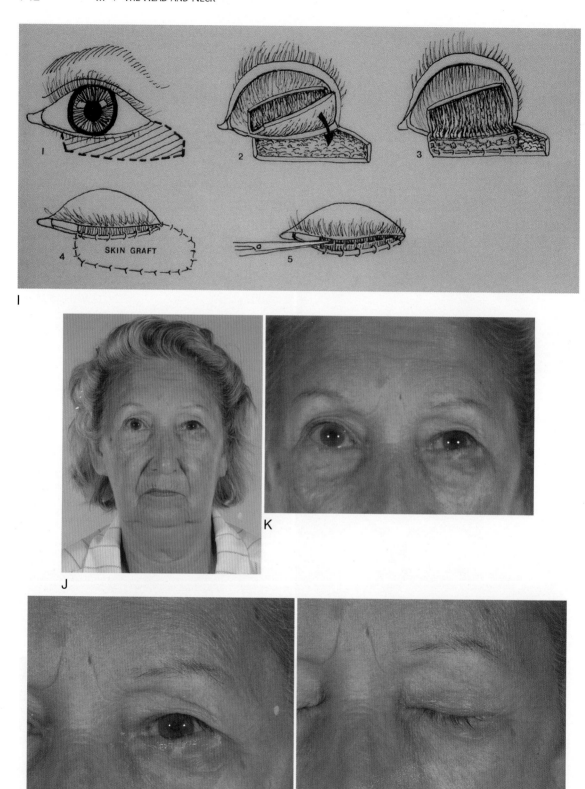

FIGURE 76-8, cont'd. The flap was divided at 3¹/₂ weeks, with care being taken to have a little extra conjunctiva up over the skin graft anteriorly to prevent contact of the skin graft with the cornea. *J* to *M,* The donor area of the upper lid, after division of the pedicle, was allowed to heal secondarily.

TABLE 76-2 ✦ CANTHOPEXY METHODS

Medial canthopexy	Canthal tendon and orbital wall are present	Fixation of canthus to medial orbital wall with canthopexy wires that are passed through transnasal hole
	Medial orbital wall is absent	Canthopexy wires are fixed to reconstructing bone graft
	Canthal tendon has been destroyed	Staged reconstruction with a split tendon graft
Lateral canthopexy	Coronal incision is present	Fixation of canthus to temporal aponeurosis
	Tightening is necessary	Canthus is sutured to superolateral orbital rim through upper blepharoplasty incision
	Greater degree of lower eyelid laxity is present	Lateral canthotomy and fixation of tarsus to lateral orbital rim after de-epithelialization and demucosalization
	Severe lid laxity is present	Pennant canthoplasty through lateral orbital rim

corrected by a transnasal medial canthopexy. This is far preferable in most instances to fixation to a screw. The transnasal medial canthopexy, as developed by Tessier,[5] is such an important procedure in periorbital soft tissue reconstruction that it deserves specific attention (Table 76-2).

TRANSNASAL MEDIAL CANTHOPEXY

An external incision just over the canthus provides the best exposure of the glistening white fibers of the canthal tendon, which should be clearly visualized. If there is a subtarsal lower lid incision, it can be extended vertically quite close to the canthus. Periosteal and orbital septal attachments of the upper and lower eyelids should be completely free all the way to the lateral canthus so that the medial canthus can easily be displaced in all directions. A swaged-on 2-0 wire suture is passed twice through the canthal tendon. A hole is made with a 3- to 4-mm sharp perforating canthopexy awl (similar to an icepick). This hole can be higher on the nasal dorsum of the contralateral side and should be carried out at the desired location of the medial canthus determined from the position of the contralateral medial canthus (if normal) or 1 or 2 mm above and posterior to the lacrimal fossa. If a dacryocystorhinostomy is also performed, it should be done before completion of the canthopexy. Completing the two procedures simultaneously complicates matters, and it may be a reasonable tactic to postpone the dacryocystorhinostomy to another day. In fact, if the medial canthus is in the proper position, many patients with lacrimal obstruction will not be bothered by epiphora (Fig. 76-9).

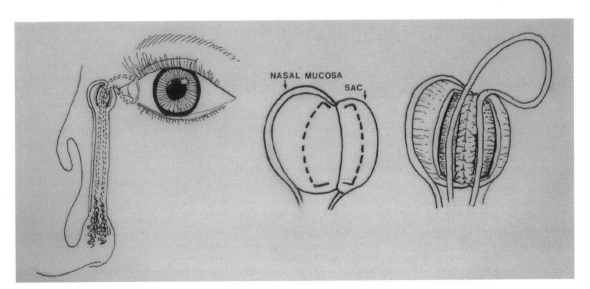

FIGURE 76-9. Diagram of a dacryocystorhinostomy. If there is a blockage between the sac and the nasal mucosa with a dilated sac, a large hole is burred out over the nasal mucosa, and two flaps developed from the nasal mucosa and the sac are then sutured behind the silicone tubing. The skin and other tissues are closed over the defect. It is generally not possible to obtain mucosal coverage of both the posterior and anterior walls.

A wire loop is passed through the transnasal hole to retrieve the canthopexy wires. If any thick scar tissue is present between the canthus and the nasal bone, this should be thoroughly removed. It is a good idea to suture the medial portion of the eyelid incision before tightening the canthopexy wires. This should be done by pulling firmly on the canthopexy wires so the tendon is brought well into the hole in the bone. Fixation of the wires is performed by twisting them over a toggle made of tightly twisted wire or any other wire strut.[5] If the medial orbital wall is absent, the tendon should be brought through a hole in the reconstructing bone graft. Once the soft tissue closure is complete, several nylon sutures can be passed through with use of a Keith needle or a K-wire driver, penetrating through the nose just above the canthus. These sutures are tied over petrolatum gauze to maintain the depth of the naso-orbital hollow (Fig. 76-10).

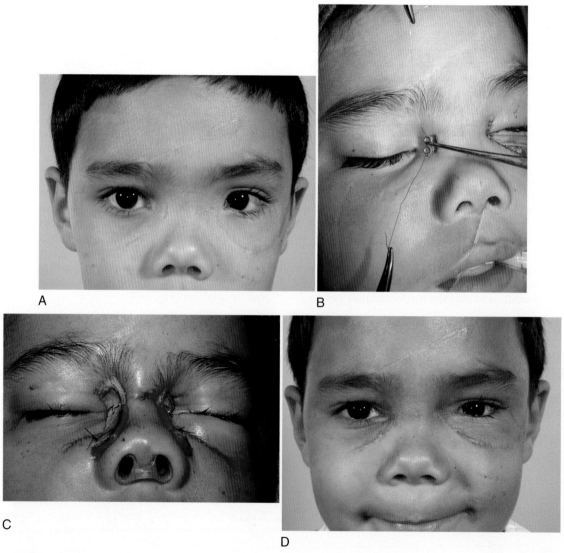

FIGURE 76-10. *A,* This 6-year-old boy was bitten by a pit bull and had multiple facial lacerations and avulsion of the medial canthal tendons on both sides. He has had previous surgery, but the canthopexy has not held properly. *B,* Dacryocystorhinostomy and transnasal medial canthopexy were performed. The previous medial canthal incisions were extended into the previous scars in the inferomedial eyelid area. The medial canthal tendon was dissected out on both sides and a hole made superior and posterior to the lacrimal fossa. A 4-0 canthopexy wire was passed transnasally and used to fix the medial canthal tendon. This wire was tightened over a two-hole plate on the opposite side. *C,* Other wires had also been passed through the canthopexy hole, and then transcutaneously these transnasal wires were tightened over lead plates made for the canthal hollow on each side and padded with Adaptic. *D,* Patient seen after 1 month.

If the medial canthal tendon has been destroyed, a useful tactic is to perform a preliminary procedure in which a tendon graft (palmaris longus,[6] short toe extensor) is split into a Y, and the two thinner limbs are placed over the medial portions of the upper and lower tarsal plates. Several months later, the thicker portion of the tendon is exposed and used as a medial canthal tendon (Fig. 76-11).

The transnasal medial canthopexy is an excellent procedure, but even a good canthopexy cannot provide a result superior to maintaining the canthus on its original bone attachment and moving the bone segment. In patients with acute fractures, canthal bone attachments should be restored whenever possible. A good transnasal medial canthopexy always looks a bit sharper than the softly curved attachment of a normal medial canthus. Also, a transnasal canthopexy, even if it is well done, can be subject to some long-term relapse.

LATERAL CANTHUS

The lateral canthus deserves special attention as well. A lateral canthopexy can be performed from beneath a coronal incision. It is a routine part of the closure of a craniofacial dissection carried out through a coronal incision to resuture the superficial temporalis fascia to the underlying temporal aponeurosis. This suspends the soft tissues of the cheek and, to a certain extent, the lateral canthus. A skin hook can be used to snag the fibers of the lateral canthal raphe nearer to the lateral canthus itself. A suture is passed through this tissue, then sutured through the temporal aponeurosis to place the lateral canthus in its desired position (snugly tied). When a tight canthopexy is performed by this method, patients should be warned that they may be troubled by the tightness and blurred vision for several weeks.

If one is not using a coronal incision, there are a variety of lateral canthopexy methods that can be performed through eyelid incisions. In order of increasing strength and complexity, they are the following:

1. Tightening of the lateral canthus through an upper blepharoplasty incision. This approach has been around for years but has been refined and succinctly described by Jelks,[7,8] who calls the procedure an inferior retinacular repair. The lateral canthal attachments to the lateral orbital rim are lysed, and a double-armed permanent suture (4-0 Supramid) is passed through the inferior retinaculum of the lateral canthal raphe. Both sutures are passed from inside the superolateral orbital rim through periosteum and tied. This procedure is most often used in aesthetic surgery for mild senile laxity of the lower eyelid. One should aim to position the lateral

canthus at the upper border of the pupil (Fig. 76-12).

2. If there is a greater degree of horizontal laxity of the lower eyelid (a negative "snap test" result), a lateral canthotomy can be combined with de-epithelialization and demucosalization of the tarsus. The tarsus is then sutured to the lateral orbital rim as described before. This procedure is often used to treat ectropion that develops with facial paralysis in association with lid loading by a gold weight to aid in upper lid closure. There may be some unsightly overhang of upper lid skin associated with this procedure that requires judicious trimming (Fig. 76-13).

3. Finally, there is the "pennant" canthoplasty originally described by Edgerton.[9] In this procedure, which gives the strongest canthopexy, a strip of de-epithelialized skin and muscle is developed that extends 12 to 15 mm laterally from the lateral canthus. After extensive freeing of all periosteal attachments, the de-epithelialized flap is passed through a 3- to 4-mm hole in the superolateral rim and sutured to the temporal aponeurosis (Figs. 76-14 and 76-15).

CHEMOSIS

After any extensive periorbital dissection, particularly in the correction of enophthalmos when bone grafts are added to the orbit or tight medial and lateral canthopexies are performed, substantial conjunctival edema, or chemosis, may develop and herniate through the palpebral fissure in an unsightly but benign manner. Chemosis may be prevented by the use of symblepharon conformers, which are thin acrylic ocular conformers with a central hole to avoid contact with the cornea. These are removed after 5 to 7 days. Once chemosis has become established, multiple nicks in the edematous conjunctiva are made with a No. 11 blade, and either a symblepharon conformer is inserted or the eyelids are closed by temporary tarsorrhaphy sutures until the chemosis subsides.

Eyelid Muscles

There are two sets of muscles in the upper and lower eyelids, one for opening and one for closing. Closing of the eyelids is provided by the orbicularis oculi muscle innervated by the facial nerve. The muscle has different portions with different functions; the portion overlying the tarsal plates is responsible for blinking, a rapid and regular eyelid movement that provides continuous lubrication of the cornea. In planning eyelid incisions, this portion of the orbicularis muscle should be left undisturbed. Other portions of the orbicularis oculi muscle extend well beyond the superior and inferior orbital rims and

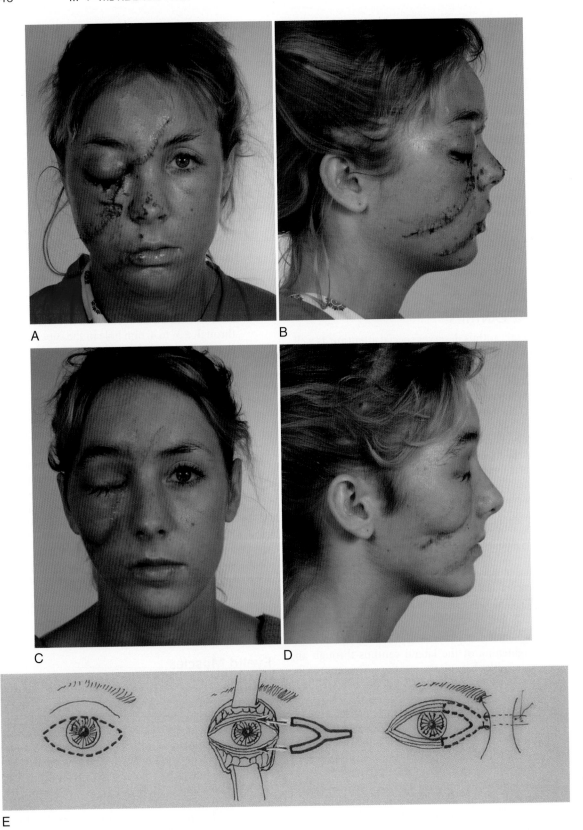

FIGURE 76-11. *See legend on opposite page.*

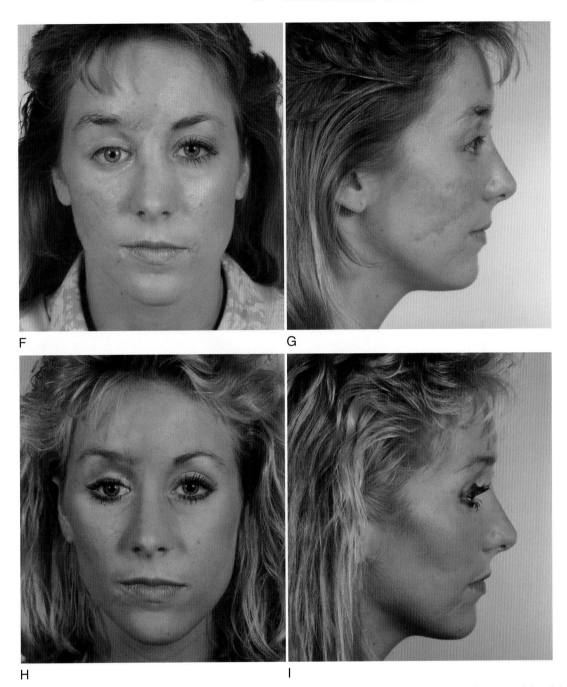

F   G

H   I

FIGURE 76-11. *A* and *B,* This 19-year-old woman was seen several days after a compound fracture of the right orbit and maxilla. Her right globe had ruptured and was enucleated at the first operation, at which time extensive bone grafting (iliac) was performed to the right orbital floor and medial orbital wall; the right side of the frontal sinus was stripped of mucosa and packed with cancellous bone. *C* and *D,* The displaced zygoma was reduced and wire osteosynthesis performed at the frontozygomatic, infraorbital rim, and maxilla. Because the medial canthal tendon had been partially destroyed by the original injury, a palmaris longus tendon graft was split into a Y, with the two thinner limbs tacked down over the upper and lower tarsal plates at a second operation *(E).* Several months later, the medial canthal area was re-explored; the wider, base portion of the Y was used to perform a transnasal medial canthopexy *(F* and *G)* that can be noted to be approximately 1.5 mm higher than the normal left side. *H* and *I,* Scar revisions and dermabrasion were also performed for scars of the right cheek and chin. She is shown with a right ocular prosthesis in place 3 years after the original injury. The canthal reconstruction would not have been possible if the bone graft of the medial orbital wall had not been performed at the first operation. (From Wolfe SA, Berkowitz S: Plastic Surgery of the Facial Skeleton. Boston, Little, Brown, 1989.)

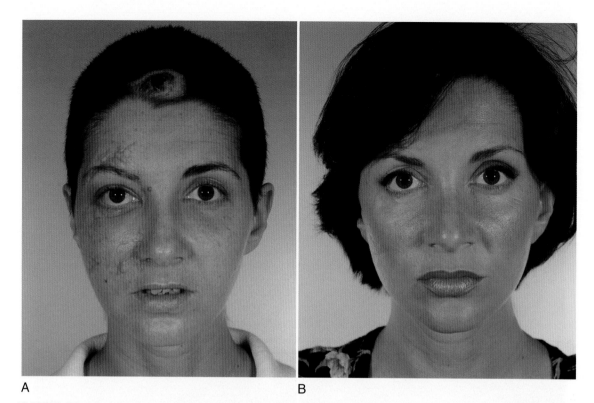

A   B

FIGURE 76-12. *A,* This 31-year-old model was sitting in a sidewalk café in Rome when a motor scooter suddenly veered off the street and struck her in the face, causing a number of facial and scalp lacerations and a right orbital fracture. The fracture was reduced and plated appropriately through a right subtarsal skin incision. When first seen approximately 3 weeks after the accident, she showed some lower lid retraction and healing lacerations of the scalp, right forehead, and cheek. *B,* She is shown a year after a right lateral canthopexy with an upper lateral nasal chondromucosal graft to the right lower eyelid, excision of the area of post-traumatic alopecia with a scalp flap, and scar revision and dermabrasion of the facial scars. This is the type of lower eyelid incision preferred by the authors because it is rarely associated with lower lid retraction.

provide the slower eyelid movement of a squint or forced closure. In some situations in which the portion of the orbicularis near the lower part of the upper eyelid has been lost either from trauma or by overzealous resection in aesthetic blepharoplasty and eyelid closure has been lost, a section of the still functioning upper portion of the orbicularis can be transposed inferiorly to provide better eyelid closure. When there is no function whatsoever of the orbicularis oculi, as is the case in facial paralysis, and facial nerve function cannot be re-established, a number of methods have been developed to help provide eyelid closure. In the past, springs,[10] elastic silicone slings,[11] and magnets[12] have been proposed, but none of these methods provided satisfactory long-term closure. Upper lid loading, with either a full-thickness graft[4] or a gold weight,[13] provides a more satisfactory solution. The gold weight method is the most commonly used (Table 76-3).

Commercially available gold weights come in 5-, 10-, and 15-g sizes. One can try one of the weights by

taping it to the lower midportion of the upper lid and checking to see whether the patient can satisfactorily open and close the eyelid. The weight that seems the best can be inserted under local anesthesia. A transverse incision is made 12 to 14 mm from the lid margin, and dissection is carried down beneath the orbicularis muscle to the tarsal plate. The weight is sutured to the tarsal plate through the holes in the plate. Care should be taken to ensure that the weight is centered above the midportion of the cornea. The eyelid incision is closed in layers.

The opposite situation, overactivity of the orbicularis oculi muscle, is encountered in the condition called essential blepharospasm. Here the patient involuntarily and continually squints, a distressing situation. This was one of the first conditions to be treated by botulinum toxin, and this remains the treatment of choice.[14]

Opening of the eyelids is provided by the third nerve innervated by the levator palpebrae superioris and to a lesser extent by the lower lid retractors.

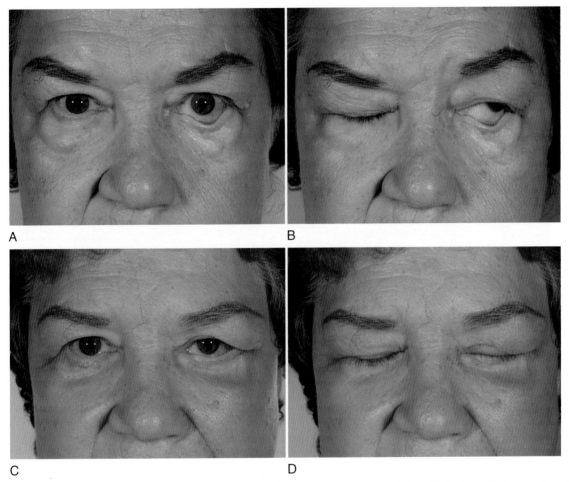

FIGURE 76-13. *A* and *B*, A 65-year-old woman who had a long-standing left facial paralysis due to Bell palsy. *C* and *D*, She is shown before and after an upper lid loading with a gold weight and a lateral canthopexy.

TABLE 76-3 ✦ TREATMENT OF PROBLEMS OF EYELID MUSCLES

Lagophthalmia	Lower portion of palpebral orbicularis is lost	Intact upper orbicularis is transposed inferiorly
	No function of orbicularis is detected	Upper lid loading (full-thickness graft or gold weight; no springs, elastic silicone slings, or magnets)
Essential blepharospasm		Botulinum toxin or surgical excision of orbicularis muscle
Ptosis of upper eyelid	Function of levator muscle is present	Shortening and reattachment of muscle
	Muscle function is absent	Frontalis sling or transfer of frontalis muscle
Eyelid spasm, retraction		Levator recession with temporalis fascia spacer for upper lid
		Recession of lower lid with a spacer graft (split palatal) in conjunction with lateral canthopexy

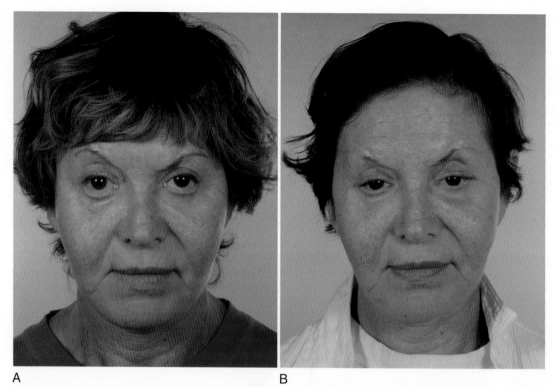

A   B

FIGURE 76-14. *A*, This 65-year-old woman originally had upper and lower lid blepharoplasties and developed an ectropion of the right lower lid. Several operations, including a full-thickness skin graft, failed to correct the ectropion. She was thought to have a moderate degree of proptosis of both eyes, which makes correction of an ectropion difficult. She is shown postoperatively after expansion of both orbital cavities by lowering of the orbital floors and lateral canthopexies with the pennant procedure. This type of firm canthopexy made it possible to remove the previously placed skin graft entirely. *B*, She is shown 2 years postoperatively.

Underfunction or nonfunction of the levator muscle causes a ptosis of the upper eyelid. If any function of the levator muscle is present, shortening or reattachment of the muscle to the tarsal plate should be attempted. If no function is present, the only recourse is to use the forehead levators to provide eyelid opening by either a frontalis sling or transfer of the frontalis muscle.[15] If there is no forehead motion and no levator function, there is currently no solution available. The patient must be left with the ptosis. If the eyelid does not close completely, a central tarsorrhaphy should be done to protect the cornea.

Overfunction of the eyelid opening muscles occurs in the eyelid spasm and retraction associated with the dysthyroid ophthalmopathy of Graves disease. If this condition occurs without significant exophthalmos, levator recession can be carried out for the upper lid, and a spacer graft (upper lateral chondromucosal or split palatal) may be performed along with recession of the lower eyelid retractor in conjunction with lateral canthopexy.

SPECIFIC DIAGNOSES AND TREATMENTS

Exophthalmos

Exophthalmos should be differentiated from exorbitism. In exophthalmos, there is a normal orbital cavity and an increase in orbital contents. In exorbitism, the contents are normal and the container is small (e.g., Crouzon disease). Exophthalmos can be caused by orbital tumors, "pseudotumor" (an inflammatory process of unknown origin), and Graves disease.

The precise cause of exophthalmos associated with Graves disease is unknown but is thought to be autoimmune because a round cell infiltrate is often found in the enlarged eye muscle and engorged orbital fat. In many instances, exophthalmos develops after the treatment of hyperthyroidism with radioiodine, thyroidectomy, or propylthiouracil.

Surgery should generally be avoided in the acute or "wet" phase of dysthyroid exophthalmopathy; steroids and occasionally radiotherapy provide control

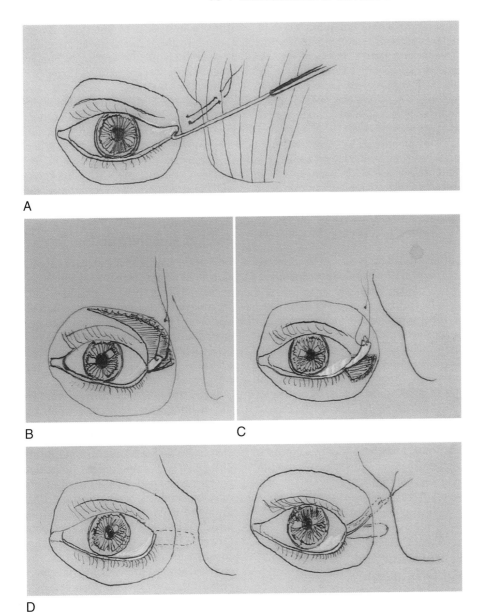

FIGURE 76-15. Four types of canthopexy. *A,* Through a coronal incision, the lateral canthal raphe can be grasped with a skin hook; a suture placed through the coronal incision is then sutured to the temporal aponeurosis. *B,* Through an upper eyelid incision, an inferior retinacular suture is taken through the upper lid incision and sutured inside the lateral orbital rim (Jelks). *C,* If the lower lid is more lax, a lateral canthotomy can be performed and a portion of the tarsus de-epithelialized and used in a similar fashion. *D,* A pennant canthoplasty (Edgerton) involves de-epithelialization of a strip of skin including some muscle based at the lateral canthus, which is then brought through a drill hole through the lateral orbital rim and sutured to the temporal aponeurosis.

of the acute situation. When the condition has stabilized, there are a number of treatments to improve both the protrusion and staring appearance of the eyeball as well as the corneal irritation. When eyelid retraction is the primary problem, levator recession is the best approach. This alone will mask a certain degree of exophthalmos without changing globe position.

Exophthalmos is quantitated by measuring from the most posterior portion of the lateral orbital rim to the most anterior surface of the cornea with an exophthalmometer (either a simple clear ruler or a Hertel exophthalmometer). A normal measurement for white individuals is 16 to 18 mm; normal readings may be slightly higher in African Americans and Asians.

The actual protrusion of the globe can be corrected by expansion of the orbital cavity or removal of orbital contents. The orbital cavity can be expanded by a Le Fort III minus Le Fort I procedure[16] or by a valgus osteotomy of the malar bone[17,18] and centrifugal expansion into the maxillary, ethmoidal, and on occasion frontal sinuses. Olivari[19] has shown that some correction of globe protrusion can be attained by extensive removal of intraconal orbital fat. The most efficient correction of the protruding eye is by extensive removal of intraconal orbital fat. The most efficient correction of the protruding eye by bone surgery is provided by the sagittal expansion of a Le Fort III, but some patients may not be candidates for this approach (the procedure alters the nose). In severe instances of exophthalmos, neither bone expansion nor fat removal provides enough expansion, and it is preferable in these patients to use both approaches (Figs. 76-16 and 76-17).

Orbital Exenteration and Transcranial Orbitectomy

When highly malignant tumors such as adenoid cystic carcinoma of the lacrimal gland and malignant melanoma are present in the orbit, or when basal or squamous carcinoma invades the orbit, subperiosteal removal of the eye and all orbital contents or of the entire bony orbit with all of the orbital contents is indicated. Orbital exenteration leaves a raw orbital cavity that can be treated with a split skin graft alone. However, filling the orbital cavity with a portion of the temporalis muscle that is then covered with a full-thickness skin graft provides a considerably less disfiguring result.[20] With the availability of magnetic resonance imaging, concern about tumor recurrence is no longer an excuse for performing an extensive procedure with a potentially disfiguring result. The temporalis muscle can be transposed through a fenestration in the lateral orbital wall, but it is much easier to remove a portion of the anterior lateral orbital rim and bring the muscle

directly into the orbit anteriorly. If a patient wishes, an epiprosthesis can be made; insertion of osseointegrated implants into remaining bone will help with retention of the prosthesis and avoid the need for skin glues (Figs. 76-18 to 76-20).[21]

If removal of the entire orbital cavity and its contents is indicated, a frontal craniotomy is performed; the orbital roof and any other portions needing to be removed are taken out en bloc. A larger portion of the temporalis muscle is brought in to cover the anterior cranial fossa defect, and then either a full-thickness skin graft or a scalp flap is used to provide skin cover.

Socket Reconstruction

One of the most difficult areas in surgical reconstruction of the orbital soft tissues is dealing with contracted sockets in which an ocular prosthesis cannot be placed. In congenital microphthalmia, a few surgeons have performed bone expansion followed by eyelid reconstruction and socket grafting and have been able to fit an ocular prosthesis. Most of the results obtained, including those of the authors, are considered mediocre.[22]

In an acquired deformity, if there is a contracted socket along with mutilated, nonmoving eyelids, the patient is probably better off wearing a patch or an epiprosthesis. If the orbit has been previously irradiated, such as for retinoblastoma in childhood, the problems are compounded. In patients in whom the eyelids and remaining orbital contents are retracted into the orbit, sectioning of the orbital contents at the optic nerve level and placement of temporalis muscle posteriorly will allow the contents to move forward. At a later date, one can attempt to establish adequate fornices behind the eyelids with thick split- or full-thickness grafts. Skin grafts are used because an adequate amount of mucosa (except perhaps from the pharynx) cannot be obtained in most instances. Free mucosal grafts have a strong propensity to contract as well.

Even with an extensive dissection well beyond the orbital rims, a skin-grafted socket will lose a substantial portion of the re-established fornices with healing. This wound contraction is particularly true of the lower fornix. One may attempt to fix a solid methyl methacrylate conformer to the inferior orbital rim with a titanium screw, but even this has been unsuccessful in maintaining an adequate lower fornix to allow placement of an ocular prosthesis. It may well be that the best approach is to use vascularized skin, such as with a radial forearm flap, when there would be no likelihood of contraction. Like craniofacial surgery for congenital malformation, these difficult reconstructions are best handled in a few specialized

Text continued on p. 762

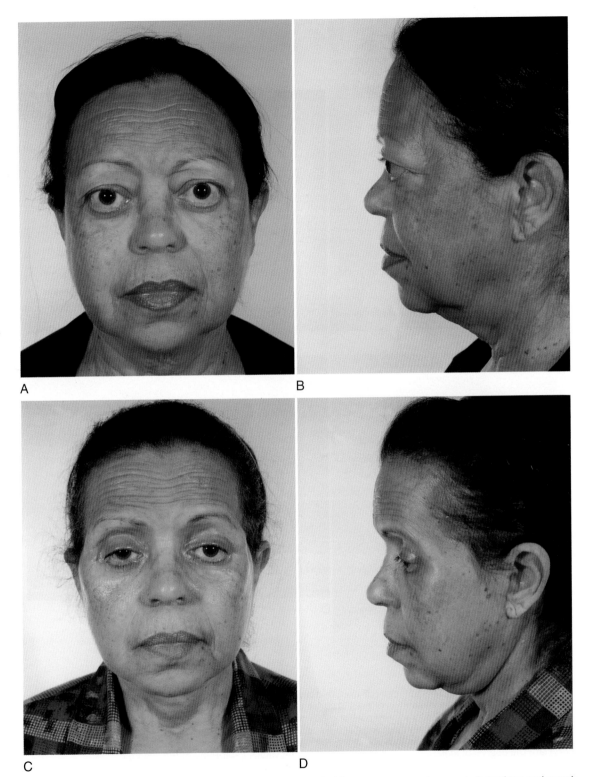

FIGURE 76-16. *A* and *B,* This 65-year-old woman presented with severe recurrent corneal ulcerations and exophthalmos after treatment many years previously for hyperthyroidism. *C* and *D,* She is shown 1 year after a three-wall orbital expansion with valgus movement of the zygoma and lateral orbital wall, removal of much of the orbital floor and medial orbital floor, and removal of intraconal orbital fat. She is shown postoperatively with a mild ptosis that was purposely not corrected because she still had an unstable although improved corneal situation. One can note the substantial posterior movement of the globe on the lateral photograph *(D).*

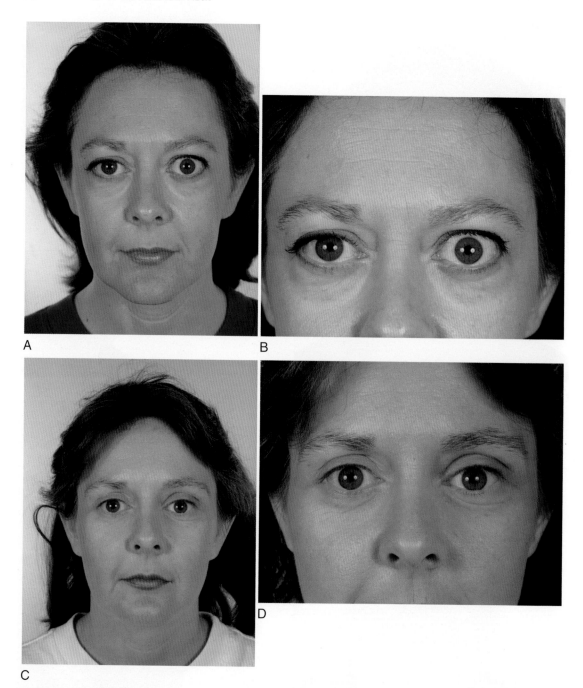

FIGURE 76-17. *A* and *B,* This 33-year-old woman developed asymmetric exophthalmos after treatment of hyperthyroidism. She is shown after expansion of both orbital cavities by three-wall orbital expansion with valgus movement of the zygoma and lateral orbital wall, removal of much of the orbital floor and medial orbital floor, and removal of intraconal orbital fat from both sides but substantially more from the left. *C* and *D,* At a second operation, a lengthening of the levator muscle was performed on the left side with interposition of a temporalis fascia graft. One can appreciate the degree of malar augmentation provided by the valgus osteotomy of the zygoma.

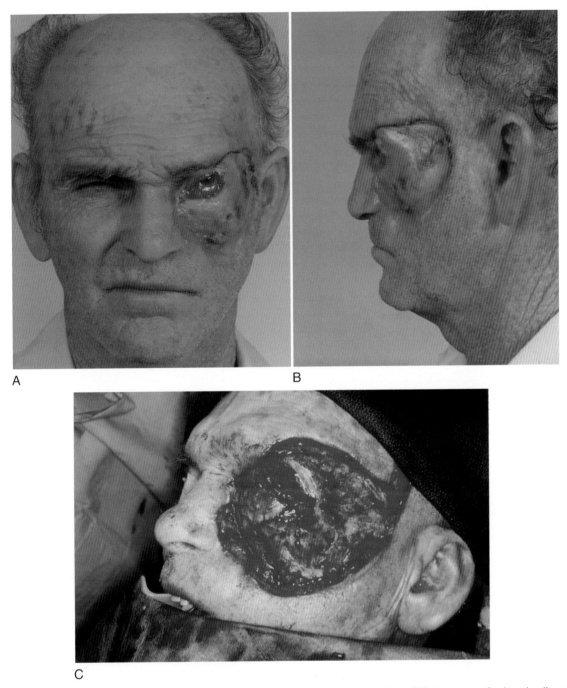

FIGURE 76-18. *A* and *B,* This 61-year-old man was first seen after completion of Mohs surgery for basal cell carcinoma involving both upper and lower eyelids. Because there were no remaining eyelids present, he was considered a medical emergency and was operated on the day after the initial photograph. *C,* A large split palatal graft (almost the entire hard palate) was taken and sutured to the remnants of upper and lower conjunctiva.   *Continued*

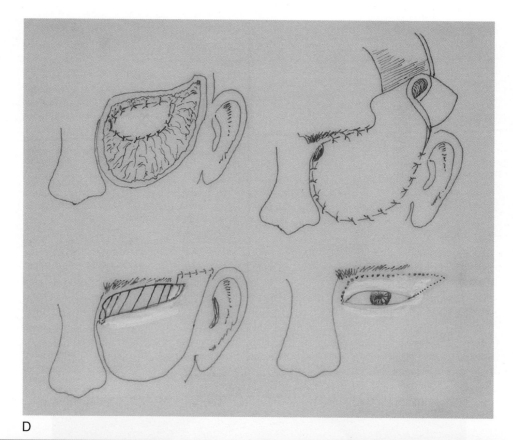

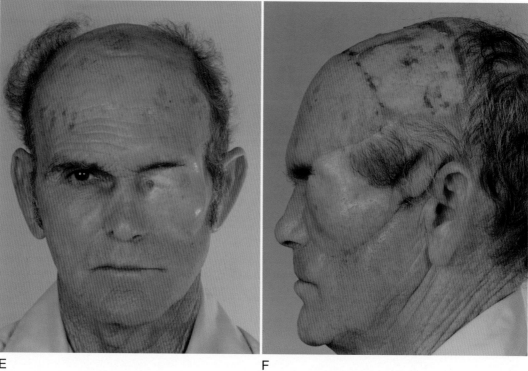

FIGURE 76-18, cont'd. *D,* A large scalp flap was then taken that also covered the entire malar area. *E* and *F,* A small opening was left centrally to provide for drainage. Before the flap was split, the upper lid portion was radically thinned and covered with a medium-thickness skin graft from the upper, inner arm.

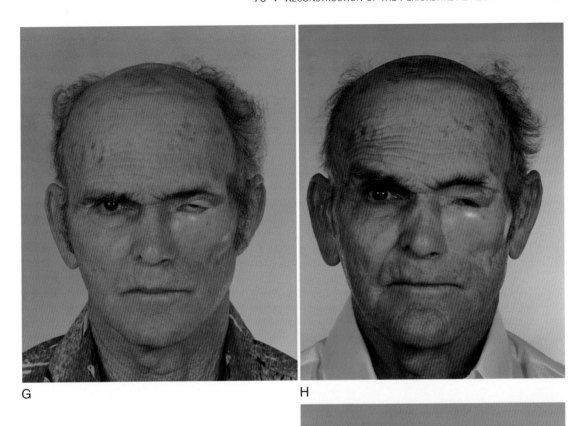

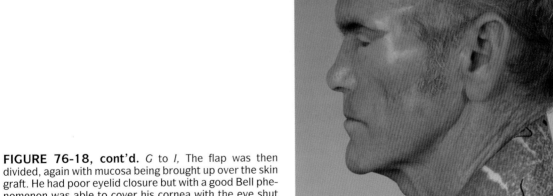

FIGURE 76-18, cont'd. *G* to *I*, The flap was then divided, again with mucosa being brought up over the skin graft. He had poor eyelid closure but with a good Bell phenomenon was able to cover his cornea with the eye shut and had useful vision in the eye. (From Wolfe SA, Berkowitz S: Plastic Surgery of the Facial Skeleton. Boston, Little, Brown, 1989.)

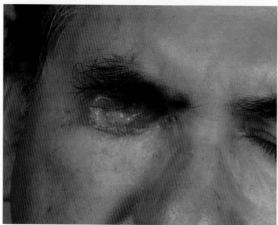

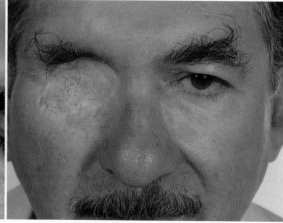

A

B

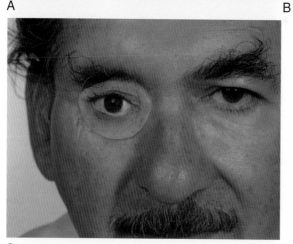

C

FIGURE 76-19. *A,* This 53-year-old man presented with a neglected skin cancer of the eyelids that had invaded the eye, a good example of a so-called rodent ulcer. *B,* After frozen section confirmation of the diagnosis of basal cell carcinoma, an orbital exenteration was performed and a temporal muscle flap was transposed into the orbital cavity and covered with a full-thickness skin graft. *C,* Postoperatively, he was fitted with an epiprosthesis that was held in place with tissue glue. If the glue is unsatisfactory, osseointegrated implants can be placed into the superior and inferior orbital rims to provide a firmer hold of the epiprosthesis. Like all patients with only one seeing eye, this patient was urged to always wear protective glasses, which if lightly tinted would improve the final result.

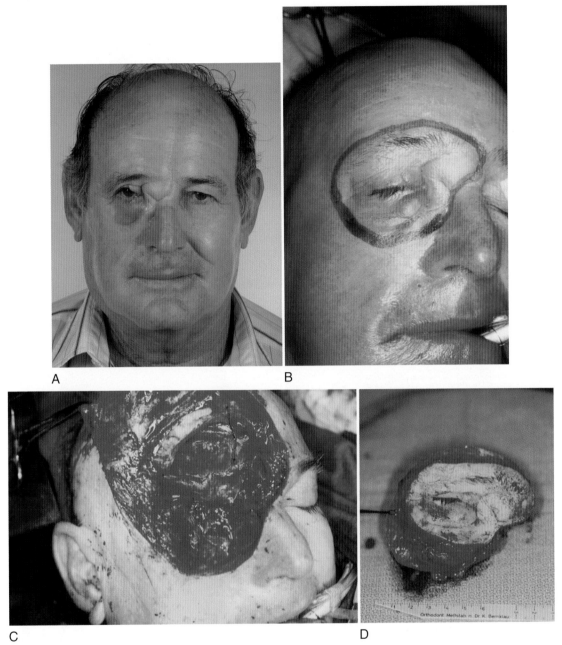

A   B

C   D

FIGURE 76-20. *A,* This 62-year-old man was referred after excision of a malignant melanoma of the right lower eyelid. Several attempts at eyelid reconstruction had been made, including a midline forehead flap. A right radical neck dissection had been performed for palpable adenopathy; a number of nodes in the specimen were positive for melanoma. A computed tomographic scan showed what appeared to be considerable tumor in the right orbit. *B* to *D,* A wide excision of both eyelids and the eyebrow, the forehead flap, and an in-continuity transcranial total orbitectomy (back to the optic foramen) were performed.   *Continued*

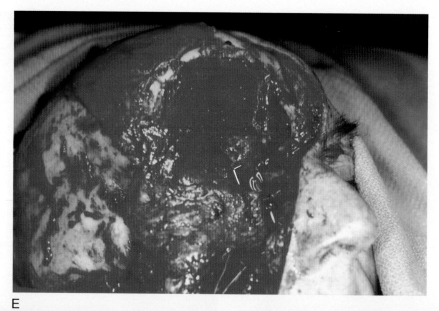

E

F   G

FIGURE 76-20, cont'd. *E,* A temporalis muscle flap was used to cover the cranial base, and the right hemiscalp was rotated down to cover the orbit. *F* and *G,* Although this was envisaged as a "toilet procedure" to control local tumor growth, to the authors' surprise the patient is alive and well 8 years after the procedure and is wearing an epiprosthesis that attaches to his glasses.

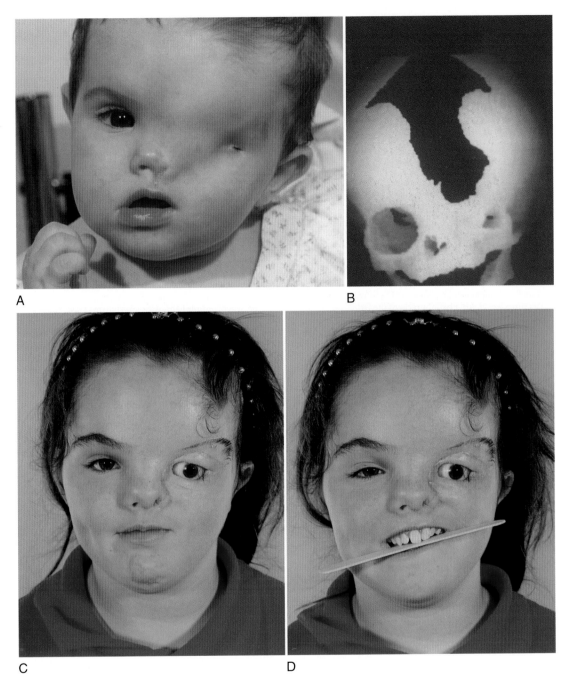

FIGURE 76-21. *A* and *B,* This child was born with a cranial defect and an encephalocele, left hemiarrhinia, and microphthalmia. There is no left nasal airway and only a minuscule left orbital cavity. She is shown postoperatively after numerous procedures that included a transcranial approach to correct the encephalocele and fix the cranial defect, formation of a left orbital cavity, and nasal reconstruction and temporalis muscle transfer followed by skin grafting to the socket. The eyebrow graft was done by another surgeon and requires frequent trimming. *C,* The abnormal hair pattern extending up along the lines of her facial cleft has not yet been corrected. *D,* Even though she has an eye prosthesis, the result still must be considered mediocre. Further surgery will be done later to straighten her jaws.

units with a team who regularly work together. The multidisciplinary team for socket reconstruction should consist of a plastic or oculoplastic surgeon, an ophthalmologist, an ocularist, a surgeon adept at placing osseointegrated implants, and a maxillofacial prosthetician (Fig. 76-21).

REFERENCES

1. Tessier P: The ectropions. In Tessier P, Rougier J, Hervouet F, et al, eds: Plastic Surgery of the Orbit and Eyelids. Wolfe SA, trans. New York, Masson, 1981:307-327.
2. Mustardé JC: Reconstruction of the upper lid. In Mustardé JC: Repair and Reconstruction in the Orbital Region, 3rd ed. Edinburgh, Churchill Livingstone 1991:191-232.
3. Tenzel RR, Stewart WB: Eyelid reconstruction by the semicircle flap technique. Ophthalmology 1978;85:1164-1169.
4. Tessier P: Eyelid reconstruction or blepharopoesis. In Tessier P, Rougier J, Hervouet F, et al, eds: Plastic Surgery of the Orbit and Eyelids. Wolfe SA, trans. New York, Masson, 1981:335-355.
5. Tessier P: Orbitonasal dislocations (OND). In Tessier P, Rougier J, Hervouet F, et al, eds: Plastic Surgery of the Orbit and Eyelids. Wolfe SA, trans. New York, Masson, 1981:58-73.
6. Bachelor EP, Jobe RP: The absent lateral canthal tendon: reconstruction using a Y graft of palmaris longus tendon. Ann Plast Surg 1980;5:362-368.
7. Jelks GW, Glat PM, Jelks EB, Longaker MT: The inferior retinacular lateral canthoplasty: a new technique. Plast Reconstr Surg 1997;100:1262-1270.
8. Glat PM, Jelks GW, Jelks EB, Wood M, et al: Evolution of the lateral canthoplasty: techniques and indications. Plast Reconstr Surg 1997;100:1396-1405.
9. Marsh JL, Edgerton MT: Periosteal pennant lateral canthoplasty. Plast Reconstr Surg 1979;64:24-29.
10. Morel-Fatio D, Lalardrie JP: Use of a counter-spring in the treatment of certain types of palpebral ptosis [in French]. Ann Chir Plast 1968;13:170-174.
11. Arion HG: Dynamic closure of the lids in paralysis of the orbicularis muscle. Int Surg 1972;57:48-50.
12. Muhlbauer WD, Segeth H, Viessmann A: Restoration of eyelid function in facial paresis by implantation of permanent magnets [in German]. In Hohler H, ed: Plastische und Wiederherstellungs-Chirurgie. Stuttgart, Schattauer, 1975:157-164.
13. Jobe R: Lid loading with gold for upper lid paralysis. Plast Reconstr Surg 2000;106:735-736.
14. Anderson RL, Patel BC, Holds JB, Jordan DR: Blepharospasm: past, present, and future. Ophthal Plast Reconstr Surg 1998;14:305-317.
15. Beard C: Advancements in ptosis surgery. Clin Plast Surg 1978;5:537-545.
16. Wolfe SA: Exophthalmos. In Wolfe SA, Berkowitz S: Plastic Surgery of the Facial Skeleton. Boston, Little, Brown, 1989:549-574.
17. Tessier P: Expansion chirurgicale de l'orbite: les orbites trop petites; exophthalmies basedowiennes, exorbitisme des dysostoses cranio-faciales; atresies orbitaires des jeunes enuclees; tumeurs orbitaires. Ann Chir Plast 1969;14:207.
18. Wolfe SA: Modified three-wall orbital expansion to correct persistent exophthalmos or exorbitism. Plast Reconstr Surg 1979;64:448-455.
19. Olivari N: Transpalpebral decompression of endocrine ophthalmopathy (Graves' disease) by removal of intraorbital fat: experience with 147 operations over 5 years. Plast Reconstr Surg 1991;87:627-641.
20. Cordeiro PG, Wolfe SA: The temporalis muscle flap revisited on its centennial: advantages, newer uses, and disadvantages. Plast Reconstr Surg 1996;98:980-987.
21. Jackson IT, Tolman DE, Desjardins RP, Branemark PI: A new method for fixation of external prostheses. Plast Reconstr Surg 1986;77:668-672.
22. Wolfe SA: Orbital expansion. Clin Plast Surg 1978;5:513-515.

Subacute and Chronic Respiratory Obstruction

CHRISTOPHER B. GORDON, MD ✦ ERNEST K. MANDERS, MD

OBSTRUCTIVE DISORDERS IN THE PEDIATRIC PATIENT
    Nasopharyngeal Obstruction
    Oropharyngeal Anomalies
    Laryngeal, Tracheal, and Thoracic Airway Anomalies
    Pediatric Malignant Neoplasms in Airway
      Obstruction
    Pediatric Vascular Anomalies and Hemangiomas

Obstructive Sleep Apnea
Craniofacial Anomalies
OBSTRUCTIVE SLEEP APNEA IN THE ADULT PATIENT
    Diagnosis and Treatment Criteria
    Treatment of Sleep Apnea

OBSTRUCTIVE DISORDERS IN THE PEDIATRIC PATIENT

Nasopharyngeal Obstruction

Breathing disorders in the pediatric population are most commonly related to congenital malformations of the nose, nasopharynx, and craniofacial skeleton. These range from clinically benign disorders, such as a deviated septum, to life-threatening abnormalities that may require urgent surgical correction or tracheostomy, such as choanal atresia or profound micrognathia (Fig. 77-1). Recognition of breathing disorders requires attention to physical examination findings because the infant and small child will not communicate the problem verbally. Most infants are obligate nose breathers, so significant obstruction of the nasal airflow manifests as neonatal respiratory distress. This period of nose breathing is variable but usually lasts for the first 6 months of life. Depending on the degree of obstruction and the degree to which the infant is an obligate nose breather, the symptoms may range from mild hypopnea, relieved by crying, to apnea, cyanosis, failure to thrive, and even death. Some estimates based on the physics of airflow and the anatomy of the infant nasopharynx suggest that there is a nearly fourfold increase in nasal airway resistance in this age group.[1,2]

Several anatomic points of obstruction affect infants and young children. Deformities of the external nares are uncommon and can range from nasal agenesis (arrhinia) to malposition of the lower lateral cartilages, causing obstruction of the antrum. There is no effective method of rhinometry in infants, so diagnosis is by physical examination and flexible endoscopy. This can be performed without sedation in an unstable child, and young infants tolerate nasoendoscopy well.

Beginning with the first portion of the nasal respiratory tract, obstruction at the piriform in children is an uncommon anomaly that is referred to as congenital nasal piriform aperture stenosis. This relatively newly described diagnosis refers to an overgrowth of the bones at the nasal inlet. The resulting clinical syndrome is that of newborn cyanosis with episodic relief that coincides with crying. There is frequent respiratory distress accompanying nursing.[3] This can resemble choanal atresia if careful endoscopy and computed tomography (CT) are not performed. Interestingly, 60% of these patients have a single central megaincisor. There are also frequent anomalies of the pituitary, suggesting that this may represent a forme fruste of holoprosencephaly.[4]

The most significant of the nasopharyngeal malformations is choanal atresia. This is an anatomic abnormality of the posterior nasal passages and choanae in which the palatal bone, vomer, pterygoids, and maxillary wall form an atresia plate that obstructs the nasal sinus. Prevalence is estimated to be 1 in 6000 to 8000 live births. Newer reports suggest that bony atresia represents approximately 30% of the cases, and the remainder are a combination of bony and membranous atresia.[5,6] This disorder is associated with the CHARGE spectrum of anomalies. This acronym is used to describe a syndrome that presents with colobomas, heart disorders, atresia, retardation, genitourinary anomalies, and ear anomalies including deafness. The

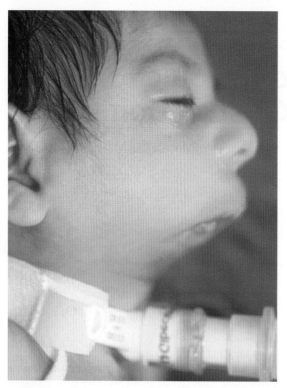

FIGURE 77-1. Profound micrognathia requiring tracheostomy.

syndrome is of unknown cause, but there is speculation, based on advanced paternal age and a small but real incidence of familial CHARGE syndrome, that there is a genetic basis for the syndrome. The proposed mechanism is developmental field arrest involving neural crest and neural tube structures. Bilateral choanal atresia and male sex were both linked with mortality in a large review of the syndrome.[7]

The classic presentation of the patient with bilateral choanal atresia is with cyanosis that is improved on crying. This indicates a nasal obstruction and merits a diagnostic work-up. Air movement or lack thereof is documented by fogging of a mirror held under the nares. Next, flexible endoscopy is used to examine the choana and to assess the obstruction. Infants tolerate nasoendoscopy well, and no sedation is routinely needed. CT scanning is the preferred method of imaging the nasopharynx to plan a surgical correction. Before surgery, enteral feeding is recommended, but this should be through an orogastric tube because a nasogastric tube combined with routine suctioning may cause respiratory embarrassment.

The surgery for choanal stenosis may be accomplished with a variety of methods. Historically, a blind puncture was performed through the nasal vestibule, but that method has been largely abandoned. There

was a period in which transpalatal surgery was popular, but this has fallen into disfavor owing to the negative effect on subsequent midfacial growth. Currently, most surgeons use rigid endoscopes in conjunction with high-speed burrs to remove the atresia plate.[8] The airway is then stented and permitted to heal for several months to minimize the chance for restenosis.

Septal deformities are uncommon in the young child but can result from birth trauma or forceps delivery. If the septal deviation is significant enough to cause respiratory distress, prompt closed reduction should be undertaken. If there is no impact on breathing, septal repositioning may be deferred until the child is older and better able to tolerate anesthesia. In older children, this may require an open surgical approach to the septum to achieve airway goals. Previous concerns about subsequent facial growth are beginning to change; several authors have reported acceptable long-term results after open septoplasty. Standard endonasal and external rhinoplasty approaches have been used with minimal morbidity.[9,10]

Septoplasty has also been used to treat nasal obstruction successfully in unilateral cleft nasal deformity. The cleft patient has a widely patent airway before lip closure. In rare cases, severe septal deviation associated with wide clefts may cause postoperative airway obstruction and sleep apnea. Conservative septoplasty with cartilage conservation may correct this deformity with less risk to facial growth patterns than by traditional submucous resection.[11] Primary cleft rhinoplasty permits repositioning of the lower lateral cartilages and minimizes collapse of the external nasal valve. This can be accomplished through the rotation-advancement flap incisions, with use of small Fomon scissors to free the cartilages from the overlying skin. The accessory chain should be freed from the piriform on the cleft side to prevent webbing of the vestibule with subsequent airway obstruction. Tajima or McComb sutures should be used to reposition the alar cartilages and close the dead space, recreating the alar groove.[12,13] Studies have correlated the severity of unrepaired cleft nasal deformity with nasal obstructive symptoms and rhinomanometry findings and support the concept of primary cleft rhinoplasty as a functional as well as aesthetic procedure.[14]

Arrhinia and hemiarrhinia are rare congenital disorders in which there may be complete agenesis of the nasal structures (Fig. 77-2). These patients typically present with respiratory distress. Treatment is complex but involves resection of a portion of the abnormal maxilla, followed by lining with skin grafts. The nasal skeleton is usually formed with costochondral cartilage grafting, turndown local flaps for lining, and forehead flaps for coverage.[15] The lacrimal apparatus is usually present but does not empty into the sinuses, so Jones tube placement is warranted to avoid later infection or chronic epiphora.

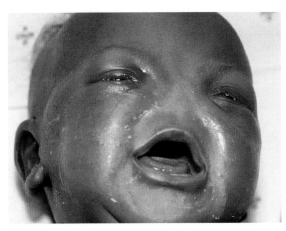

FIGURE 77-2. Arrhinia. (Case of Dr. Wolfgang Losken.)

Turbinate hypertrophy is uncommon in young children but has been associated with other pathologic processes in the paranasal sinuses. Nearly half of children who underwent endoscopy for congenital nasolacrimal duct obstruction also had hypertrophy of the inferior turbinates. It appears that outlet obstruction of the duct may be caused by hypertrophic inferior turbinates. Although it is not routinely advised for treatment of nasolacrimal duct obstruction, one group reported that inferior turbinate fracture led to resolution of obstruction in all 52 patients whose probe, irrigation, and intubation procedures had failed.[16,17]

Although rare, pediatric nasal tumors can present with airway obstruction. The most common nasal mass in the infant is a lacrimal duct cyst. This is caused by terminal blockage of the nasolacrimal duct and can present as a large cystic mass that can obstruct the entire nasal airway. These congenital dacryocystoceles may extend into the nasopharynx and often cause respiratory distress. If the lesion is bilateral, it may precipitate emergency surgery for decompression. The current surgical procedure of choice is endoscopic marsupialization after CT or magnetic resonance confirmation of the diagnosis. The use of Crawford tubes or pigtail catheters may prevent recurrence if there is upper lacrimal involvement.[18,19] In the neonatal period, other masses can include nasal dermoid cysts, dentigerous cysts, incisive canal or nasoalveolar cysts, and mucous cysts. In later infancy, nasal obstruction is sometimes a symptom of cystic fibrosis, with mucous cysts and nasal polyps obstructing the sinuses.[20-22]

Any congenital midline nasal mass should be regarded as having a possible central nervous system connection. The embryology of this region suggests that there is a normal outcropping of dura mater in the prenasal region. If there is faulty closure of the anterior neuropore, this diverticulum may persist along the foramen cecum, cribriform plate, or sphenoethmoid complex. This may be contiguous with the nasal skin in the form of a nasal pit or a larger and more developed herniation of the nasopharynx, including meningocele, meningoencephalocele, and nasal glioma (Fig. 77-3). Nasal pits frequently have cilia or hair protruding from the ostium, and there may be a caseous material coming from the track. These pits may represent the ostium of a dermal sinus, which can track to the deep structures of the nasopharynx along the cranial base. These are part of a continuum of anomalies that represent fusion defects of the region of the fonticulus frontalis of the developing embryo.

The nasal dermoid cyst, a benign ectodermal cyst, has an epithelial lining and contains other adnexal tissues that may contain elements of all three embryonic germ layers. These are thought to represent residual portions of the dural diverticulum that become trapped extracranially. Although they usually contain a homogeneous, cheesy material, they may rarely contain hair, teeth, or other more mature tissues. They occur infrequently in the nose; in the aerodigestive tract, they are more common in the oral cavity. Treatment of nasal dermoids is complete excision to prevent recurrence from residual epithelial tissues.[23]

Nasal gliomas are also developmental tumors that represent ectopic central nervous system tissues. They occur when portions of the developing brain are trapped by the developing cranium and become extracranial in the region of the nasofrontal suture, foramen cecum, or cribriform. They consist of disordered astrocytes and gliosis and are not thought to have malignant potential. Nonetheless, they can recur locally and may be more extensive than physical examination would suggest. Because they may have an intracranial connection, a team approach is merited. Some groups report that 20% of nasal gliomas have a patent connection to the central nervous system.[24]

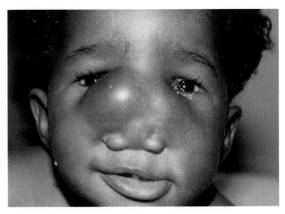

FIGURE 77-3. Nasoethmoid meningoencephalocele. (Case of Dr. Wolfgang Losken.)

The frequency of finding intracranial connections in congenital midline masses is such that any lesion that appears to come from the superomedial portion of the nasopharynx merits a careful work-up. Lesions of the medial portion of the middle turbinate are especially suspicious. CT or magnetic resonance imaging should precede any attempt at biopsy or resection of these lesions because a cerebrospinal fluid leak or meningitis can complicate these procedures. Any of these may present with nasal obstruction, so the diagnosis may be difficult to confirm until imaging is performed. Especially in the setting of cleft palate, a basilar encephalocele may obstruct the bulk of the nasopharynx.[25] This can require urgent tracheostomy before definitive treatment of the lesion.

Encephaloceles can sometimes be diagnosed by eliciting a Valsalva maneuver because the lesions bulge with increased venous pressure. The Furstenberg test, consisting of manual obstruction of the jugular vessel, may cause enlargement of the lesion as well. There may also be visible pulsations. These may occasionally present with epistaxis or clear rhinorrhea. Therefore, in this clinical presentation, careful examination is advisable. In the setting of large midline defects, such as frontonasal dysplasia or orbital hypertelorism, the accompanying encephaloceles can also cause airway obstruction. This is best managed on a case by case basis because these complex anomalies require multispecialty care.

Other causes for obstruction of the nasopharynx include teratoma, hamartoma, craniopharyngioma, and other rare lesions.[26,27] Teratomas are solid germ cell tumors that include all three types of tissue in the germ layers of the developing embryo (endoderm, mesoderm, and ectoderm). In contrast to dermoid tumors, in which the elements remain primarily undifferentiated, there are mature elements of all three tissue types in the teratoma. Head and neck teratomas represent only 5% of all neonatal teratomas; the majority are found in the lumbosacral region.

Congenital teratomas of the nasopharynx are not uncommon, representing approximately half of all head and neck teratomas.[28] They may be large lesions, occupying the nasopharynx and occasionally even the bulk of the oropharynx. They may be sessile or polypoid, or they may present with a more homogeneous, confluent appearance. Cervical teratomas may bulge into the airway as well and cause airway compromise. These larger lesions are relatively easy to diagnose with ultrasound examination in the prenatal period, and this may permit a team approach for a safe delivery, airway control, and appropriate surgical management of the mass with relative safety.[29] These may grow to spectacular size and completely obstruct the airway. We recently participated in the care of a child with a massive nasopharyngeal teratoma that was diagnosed prenatally. The child was delivered by cesarean section and placed on placental circulatory bypass to permit the surgeons to perform a tracheostomy before beginning to ventilate the patient (Fig. 77-4). Currently, these tumors are not thought to frequently undergo malignant transformation, but some authors recommend screening with alpha-fetoprotein determinations and CT scans to rule out recurrence.[30]

Congenital hamartomas are also tumors that represent disordered differentiation of embryologic tissue but are usually composed of mature cells and tissues that are common to their place of origin. There can be cells of all three germ layers, but a single tissue type usually predominates. They are rare in the nasopharynx but can present as obstructing masses in both children and adults. A series of hamartomas of the head and neck described a wide variety of lesions that include chondroid, mucosal, and vascular tissue types. The tissue type most commonly found is ectodermal in origin and is described as ciliated respiratory epithelium with glandular and fibrofatty elements. The differential diagnosis includes inverted papillomas, angiofibromas, and pharyngeal bursa. The treatment is excision, which is usually easily accomplished because these lesions tend to be well circumscribed.[31]

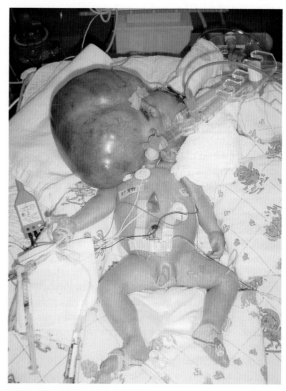

FIGURE 77-4. Teratoma obstructing the airway. The infant underwent tracheostomy at delivery by cesarean section on "placental bypass" before the umbilical cord was divided.

Craniopharyngiomas are pathologically and histologically benign epithelial tumors of the central nervous system that behave in an aggressive fashion and have a high recurrence rate. They rarely invade the nasopharynx but have been described to cause nasal obstruction. They are usually treated with an intracranial approach but can be treated with a transnasal-transsphenoidal approach as well. Facial translocation has been useful in certain cases for access to the skull base.

Oropharyngeal Anomalies

The most common neoplasms of the airway are hemangiomas and vascular malformations, which are discussed in a later section. These are followed by mucoceles, which may be found anywhere in the airway from the nasopharynx to the glottis. They are cystic masses caused by obstruction of salivary glands; they are pseudocysts of the minor salivary glands. They do not have an epithelial lining and are not encapsulated. When found in the floor of the mouth as a sequela of obstruction of the sublingual gland duct, they are called ranulas. These present as glossy white or bluish, rounded masses in the floor of the mouth. They can become large and extend into the neck; these are called plunging ranulas, and excision can be risky because of proximity to the lingual and hypoglossal nerves. Excision or marsupialization is the treatment of choice, but total excision is preferred if it can be performed without placing neurovascular structures at risk.

Lingual thyroid is an uncommon condition in which the embryonic thyroid gland does not descend into the neck through the foramen cecum at the tongue base. It may present as a mass at the tongue base that is firm and nontender, and it may obstruct the airway. It is wise to confirm the location of all thyroid tissue with radionuclide scanning before surgical resection because the lingual thyroid may represent the only thyroid tissue in the child. If this is the case, excision is contraindicated. The mass can be reduced by the use of oral thyroid replacement. Only with ongoing airway obstruction should this be resected, and thought should be given to autotransplantation to avoid a lifetime of thyroid replacement therapy.[32] Resection can be through a tongue-splitting approach, with endoscopy, or with carbon dioxide laser.

Another uncommon congenital oral anomaly is the thyroglossal duct cyst. These cysts represent residual epithelium-lined tracks that trace the path of descent of the thyroid. They can be found anywhere in the paramedial region of the neck but are usually found in the midline, with a connection to the hyoid bone. Whereas these typically present in the neck, they may become large enough to obstruct the airway. There are reports in the literature of thyroglossal duct remnants causing death by obstruction in a "ball-valve" fashion. Resection of these lesions is carried out through the neck by use of the Sistrunk procedure. The track is dissected, and excision is performed en bloc with a portion of the hyoid bone to prevent recurrence. Meticulous neck dissection techniques and careful preservation of neurovascular structures are critical.

Macroglossia, or congenital enlargement of the tongue, is uncommon and should be differentiated from glossoptosis, in which micrognathia causes a normal-sized tongue to protrude and potentially to obstruct the upper airway. The most common causes of macroglossia are congenital vascular malformation and hemangioma, which are discussed in detail in the next section. It may also be seen in hypothyroidism and amyloidosis, but rarely of a degree to cause airway compromise. Macroglossia is seen in Beckwith-Wiedemann syndrome, which is a congenital metabolic disorder (mucopolysaccharidosis) consisting of macroglossia, hypoglycemia, omphalocele, and organomegaly (Fig. 77-5). Airway obstruction has been reported in this group, but some authors believe that tongue reduction through a midline wedge resection should be reserved for those patients in whom malocclusion, articulation errors, or aesthetic concerns

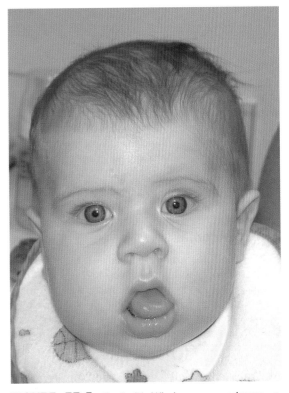

FIGURE 77-5. Beckwith-Wiedemann syndrome, a mucopolysaccharidosis characterized by macroglossia. (Case of Dr. Wolfgang Losken.)

are more important. The airway obstruction may be effectively treated in the other group with tonsillectomy and adenoidectomy.[33]

Another common cause of macroglossia is Down syndrome. There is debate about the nature of the "enlargement," and some authors attribute the problem to poor muscle tone. There are several reports of successful treatment of macroglossia in Down syndrome by glossectomy, with adequate speech and feeding and correction of airway obstruction. This is always through a midline approach to avoid injury to the neurovascular bundles that are located bilaterally.[34]

Adenoidal hypertrophy has been implicated in chronic airway obstruction in older children. The adenoidal tissue of the posterior nasopharynx does not typically play a role in neonatal airway disease. The hypertrophy of tonsillar and adenoidal tissue does not appear until after the first year of life. Adenotonsillar hypertrophy remains the most common cause of pediatric sleep apnea, and the benefits of tonsillectomy with adenoidectomy for the treatment of apnea are well documented. Indeed, the growth spurt that is seen after this procedure has been the focus of several studies. Previously, this was thought to be a metabolic phenomenon related to the work of breathing. Elimination of airway obstruction was thought to decrease calorie expenditure and to promote growth. Recent work has suggested that deranged sleeping patterns in obstructive sleep apnea cause a reduction in the insulin-like growth factor 1 and insulin-like growth factor-binding protein 3 levels during sleep. These levels were shown to normalize after surgery. This shows a clear link between growth hormone secretion and sleep apnea in growing children with tonsilloadenoidal hypertrophy.[35] Further investigation is warranted to refine this finding and to compare the results with other methods of airway management. This may represent a biochemical marker to follow the management of sleep apnea because it may be a sensitive mechanism compared with physiologic parameters of obstructed breathing.

Laryngeal, Tracheal, and Thoracic Airway Anomalies

In the neonate or young child, chronic or intractable signs of upper airway obstruction may be misleading. Because viral laryngotracheobronchitis is the most common cause of stridor in children, there is a tendency to treat empirically and to assume that chronic low-grade stridor is a manifestation of superimposed bacterial infection. Subglottic hemangioma is a relatively common entity, and failure to respond to medical management is an indication for diagnostic endoscopy. Other causes of chronic cough in this population include vascular rings. Plain films can document midline trachea, which is an abnormal finding

in infants. Subsequent work-up can reveal a double aortic arch in a significant percentage of these patients.

In the supraglottic larynx, the most common cause of obstruction is laryngomalacia. Some authors cite laryngomalacia as the single most common cause of congenital stridor. The patients present with inspiratory stridor and feeding problems. Laryngomalacia is a congenital flaccidity of the cartilage and mucosa of the supraglottic structures, including the epiglottis, arytenoids and arytenoepiglottic folds, and surrounding mucosa. These tissues prolapse into the laryngeal inlet during inspiration, causing stridor. The presentation can be insidious, with slowly progressive obstruction of the supraglottic airway, or it can be striking, with need for urgent airway control. There may be positional changes, and there may be increasingly noisy respiration with supine position, with agitation, or during sleep. Edema of the mucosa may play a role in the process, so treatment of gastroesophageal reflux should precede any contemplated surgery because a significant portion of the population may improve with medical reflux therapy.

Approximately 20% of patients will require surgical management; the remainder respond to continuous positive-pressure ventilation devices, oxygen, and supportive measures. Most patients will gradually improve as the cartilages become more mature, and most have normalized their airway by the age of 2 years.

Diagnosis is made by endoscopy, and diagnosis is more accurate with awake endoscopy to maintain normal muscle tone in the airway. There is a characteristic "omega"-shaped collapse of the epiglottis during inspiration. There may be prolapse of the cuneiform cartilages into the airway, and there can be nearly complete obstruction of the glottis in severe cases. Treatment remains controversial, although there is a trend toward endoscopic excision of the arytenoepiglottic folds and redundant epiglottic tissue as a less invasive first-line therapy in those whose conservative management fails.[36] More aggressive procedures include epiglottopexy with suture stabilization of the epiglottis to the pharyngeal wall; epiglottoplasty, in which the epiglottis is actually partially divided; and combined procedures to manage subglottic stenosis simultaneously, such as cricoid split procedures with anterior cartilage grafting to enhance the airway caliber.

Discussion of the merits of each of these procedures is beyond the scope of this chapter, but most authors believe that syndromic or neurologically impaired patients have less improvement of their airway with arytenoepiglottoplasty than do other patients and may require other methods of maintaining the airway. In severe cases, prolonged tracheostomy may be required. Also, overaggressive resection, fixation, or division of the epiglottis may produce chronic aspiration that can further aggravate the airway patency. This represents one of the difficult issues in airway management. There is some interest in aortopexy for severe cases. This is accomplished by suspending the aortic arch and a portion of the ascending aorta to the sternum with sutures. If this is unsuccessful or technically difficult, the trachea may be stented with rib grafts. This has been successful in small series of patients with refractory tracheomalacia in whom decannulation was not possible previously.[37]

The glottis itself is occasionally involved in pediatric airway obstruction. Most commonly, there may be vocal cord paralysis. This is usually idiopathic and self-limited, and only a few children require treatment for this condition. If there is bilateral paralysis, there may be significant biphasic stridor requiring airway management. The patient with unilateral paralysis presents with hoarseness or a weak cry but rarely with frank airway obstruction. In the patient with bilateral paralysis, tracheostomy is sometimes needed. Diagnosis is made with endoscopy. Glottic webs are congenital tissue bands of the anterior glottis that may occasionally cause reduction of the airway, but they are not usually symptomatic. Those larger webs that do cause symptoms present with aphonia and variable stridor. If 50% of the glottic airway is affected by the web, most authors believe that they merit treatment.[38] They may be resected with carbon dioxide laser assistance.

Other causes of the paralysis must be investigated, such as neuromuscular disorders, birth trauma, central nervous system abnormalities (Chiari malformation), and thoracic anomalies. Patients with neuromuscular disorder often require chronic tracheostomy. In contrast to earlier thinking that brainstem dysfunction in neonates and young infants with Chiari II malformations is congenital and therefore uncorrectable, there have been some promising results with early surgery. Those infants with hydrocephalus or Chiari malformation may recover completely if they are diagnosed early. By the time bilateral vocal cord paralysis and severe central hypoventilation are diagnosed, meaningful recovery may be unlikely. Early decompression of the brainstem is critical in maintaining function.[39] The pathophysiologic mechanism is probably compression of the vagal nerve roots in the brainstem as the brainstem or cerebellum herniates through the foramen magnum.

Laryngeal cysts are air-filled blind passages of the laryngeal wall. They may extend from the laryngeal saccule and infiltrate substantial portions of the surrounding tissues. They may arise anteriorly and extend to the false vocal fold and arytenoepiglottic fold or through the thyrohyoid membrane. They present with symptoms of stridor and feeding problems, similar to other laryngeal pathologic processes.

Saccular cysts may mimic laryngeal cysts but are typically a form of mucocele and do not have an ostium into the airway. Both may be treated with endoscopic marsupialization, but saccular cysts are best treated with an open transcervical approach with excision of the cyst wall to minimize recurrence.

A rare lesion of the larynx is the laryngeal cleft. It is a defect of the posterior laryngeal wall that communicates with the esophagus. There are several types of clefts, and they may extend along some or all of the larynx and trachea. This anomaly causes aspiration and stridor. Diagnosis is with endoscopy, although they may be incidentally discovered with an esophagogram that shows nonanatomic passage of gastric contents into the trachea. Treatment is with a multilayered closure of the intervening tissue planes.

Subglottic stenosis is a serious congenital anomaly that consists of a deformed, diminutive cricoid cartilage. There may be associated soft tissue hyperplasia and edema, and there is an acquired form caused by scarring in the subglottis after prolonged intubation or tracheostomy. The clinical presentation is inspiratory or biphasic stridor with a characteristic barking cough. The diagnosis is confirmed by demonstration of narrowing of the subglottis on rigid endoscopy, and the failure to pass a 4-mm rigid endoscope into the trachea is considered diagnostic. Treatment of the congenital form is with anterior cricoid split, in which cartilage grafts are used to enlarge the cartilaginous ring in the area of narrowing, or by a more ambitious laryngotracheal reconstruction with use of multiple cartilage grafts. This is a large surgery with significant morbidity, and salvage surgery is difficult. Some groups have had success with cricotracheal resection for salvage after laryngotracheal reconstruction. The results are promising, and this is being investigated as a primary treatment of laryngotracheal stenosis.[40]

FOREIGN BODY

The problem of foreign body aspiration has received intense scrutiny in the United States as efforts to "child-proof" toys and inform parents have multiplied. Nonetheless, foreign body aspiration is a common cause of emergency surgical procedures. It remains the most common cause of accidental death in infants. The most commonly aspirated items remain food items that form airway-sized pieces, such as hot dogs, nuts, hard candy, grapes, seeds, and eggshells. Children should not be allowed to have nuts or seeds until their dentition permits adequate chewing at 4 to 5 years of age. Non-foodstuff objects were more varied, but the single most common cause of fatal aspiration in the child remains the toy balloon.[41]

Once aspiration has taken place, removal of the foreign body by a ventilating bronchoscope with the appropriate forceps should be attempted in the operating room with a tracheostomy set at hand. Great care should be taken to not push the foreign object farther into the airway. Radiographs are of some diagnostic and planning help, but because many foreign bodies are radiolucent, prompt operative intervention remains the first-line therapy. At the level of the glottis, extraction may be difficult. Tracheotomy may be performed to permit ventilation and may also be used as a port from which to manipulate the object from below to permit extraction. The tracheotomy may then be allowed to close immediately, barring any other reason to maintain a surgical airway.

FACIAL TRAUMA

A pediatric facial fracture can rarely cause airway compromise. Le Fort fractures are less common in children, ostensibly because of the elasticity of the bones, and infrequently cause airway obstruction. In contrast, the pediatric mandible is frequently fractured, often in the subcondylar position. In young children, these are often managed with nonsurgical methods, such as intermaxillary fixation. Growth disturbances are common after these fractures, but orthognathic surgery is rarely needed after conservative management of these injuries. The exception is in the mixed dentition stage, when approximately 20% of children required surgical management of crossbite and asymmetry.[42] The bilateral subcondylar fracture is a special case because loss of posterior facial height may cause airway impingement. Therefore, some authors advocate a surgical approach to these cases to avoid airway emergencies in the perioperative period. This may avoid asymmetry and provide early mobilization, assisting with oral rehabilitation.[43] Tracheostomy for trauma is uncommon in this age group because fiberoptic techniques have improved to the point that most patients can be intubated.[44]

INFECTIOUS CAUSES OF AIRWAY OBSTRUCTION

The most common cause of upper airway obstruction in the pediatric population is infectious pharyngotonsillitis. This is typically caused by group A beta-hemolytic *Streptococcus pyogenes*. The complicated case can progress to peritonsillar abscess or quinsy, which is classically described as causing drooling, a "hot potato voice," and localized tenderness near the deep pharyngeal structures affected. In cases that required surgical drainage for airway compromise, there is a different bacterial spectrum, with *Haemophilus influenzae* predominating. This may be confirmed only with core biopsy because surface swabs do not always correlate with the deep flora in these infections.[45]

Ludwig angina involves an infection of the sublingual space that may track along fascial planes and through the submandibular space to involve the entire anterior neck, floor of mouth, and oropharynx. When this occurs, rapid airway compromise may ensue. This necrotizing infection was first described by Ludwig in 1836, and his account remains an accurate description of the clinical syndrome. He described a "woody" edema that accompanied a rapidly spreading cellulitis of the neck. Other symptoms included lingual edema, erythema of the surrounding skin, trismus, and high fever.[46] This syndrome is thankfully uncommon but may be associated with dental extractions in adolescents. Treatment is surgical and should include fiberoptic intubation with the surgeon standing by in case of need for a surgical airway. In addition to surgical exploration and drainage, antibiotics (typically penicillin and clindamycin) are administered to include anaerobic coverage.

Another surgical emergency in the pediatric population is bacterial epiglottitis. The usual agent is type b *H. influenzae*, but other bacterial agents may cause the syndrome as well. The clinical presentation is that of a toxic-appearing child, in a characteristic posture, with stridor, drooling, and sore throat. Previous *H. influenzae* type b immunization does not confer long-term immunity in a significant portion of patients. Radiographs may show the epiglottis to be enlarged and protruding into the airway in the classic "thumb sign." This is a true emergency when minutes count, and even simple radiographic imaging may be too time-consuming to be safely performed in this setting.

Another common cause of airway obstruction at the level of the glottis is respiratory papillomatosis. Human papillomavirus is a subgrouping of the family of DNA viruses that cause epithelial infections in humans. There is considerable variation among the subtypes and predispositions of the types for disease. Those that affect the respiratory mucosa include types 6 and 11. These are both also common to genital condylomas, and there is evidence that perinatal transmission is the most common method of contraction. The infection usually becomes symptomatic in the preschool years, manifesting as hoarseness and stridor. There is often a history of being delivered to a primigravida with active genital disease. The diagnosis is made by endoscopic examination, and treatment can be performed simultaneously. Any part of the respiratory epithelium can be affected, so panendoscopy is recommended. Most authors think that the disease becomes self-limited with the passage of time, so laser ablation is thought to control the symptomatic patient until the lesions involute spontaneously. There may be a role for antiviral agents, but there is no consensus about timing, route of delivery, or duration of treatment. Tracheostomy should be avoided in these patients, and laser ablation should be conservative to avoid stenosis of the airway.

PEDIATRIC GASTROESOPHAGEAL REFLUX DISEASE

Gastroesophageal reflux (GER) is a well-known clinical entity that is often undertreated and plays a significant role in pediatric airway disease. All infants have a degree of GER, which is considered to be the retrograde flow of gastric contents into the esophagus. The reflux may range from benign postprandial vomiting in early infancy to chronic esophagitis, failure to thrive, and chronic airway disease. Current research suggests that GER plays a role in several significant airway issues, and it has been implicated in both acute life-threatening events (ALTEs) and sudden infant death syndrome (SIDS). It probably causes or plays a role in laryngitis, stridor, and chronic pulmonary disease. The early research in GER focused on potential vagal mediation of reflux and subsequent asthma. Further work showed that there was a subgroup of patients whose only symptoms were respiratory, and this was confirmed in children. Indeed, serious GER-related airway compromise is more common in children, and they are less likely to complain of classic reflux symptoms, such as eructation and heartburn. Therefore, GER must be considered in the differential diagnosis in many of the pediatric airway diseases.

Many practitioners believe that GER improves as soon as the infant begins to eat solid food. This is true in more than half of patients, but a small portion of the patients with GER require ongoing treatment. If GER is left untreated, there is a 5% mortality in chronic pediatric GER. There is a body of evidence that implicates lower esophageal sphincter relaxation in chronic GER. Acidic gastric contents are able to escape the stomach and cause microaspiration, chemical pneumonitis, true aspiration, and airway reactivity. Because children swallow less than adults do during sleep, they are less protected against the effects of GER during sleep. In turn, the resulting esophagitis can decrease the protective swallow response to a reflux event.

The most common site of reflux injury is the glottis. The symptoms of reflux laryngitis include cough, hoarseness, and stridor. The effects are potentiated in children with laryngomalacia because they are more susceptible to development of negative pressures sufficient to cause reflux. This causes a vicious circle that can result in chronic edema, scarring, and even obliteration of the airway.

Asthma is also exacerbated by GER. Through a similar mechanism, the negative pressures developed in the patient with asthma are sufficient to cause reflux of gastric contents. Chronic asthma leads to chronic GER, and many of the medicines used to treat pediatric asthma cause an exacerbation of GER by reducing lower esophageal sphincter tone. Aspiration of gastric contents is a powerful stimulator of bronchospasm, chronic bronchial inflammation, and even scarring of the airway.

The role of GER in obstructive sleep apnea is currently the focus of intense investigation. The infant responds to regurgitation not with cough but with apnea. The more frequent the regurgitation, the more prolonged the apnea, and the more potentially severe the sequelae. This is thought to be mediated by laryngeal chemoreceptors through the superior laryngeal nerve and causes apnea with bradycardia, hypotension, swallowing, and arousal with termination of the apneic event.[47] If the apnea is so severe that hypoxia results, arousal may not reliably occur, with potentially life-threatening results.

ALTEs are severe apneic events with cyanosis, gagging, and loss of normal muscle tone. These are documented risk factors for SIDS, and 4% of children with ALTE go on to die of SIDS. There is a significant proportion of children who have had an ALTE, up to 90% in some series, who have documented reflux. Interestingly, the duration of these episodes of reflux seems to correlate with the severity of the apneic event. Further, data suggest that GER may play the major role in ALTEs in otherwise healthy babies. Infants who have a high rate of reflux episodes are at a 9% annual risk of dying of SIDS. The authors also correlated these with infants with the same severe reflux pattern who underwent antireflux surgery and found that there were no deaths in the surgical group.

Any child who is thought to have reflux should undergo a screening evaluation. The milk scan is a measure of all reflux events and has the advantage of detecting the neutral or basic pH reflux that is missed by a pH probe test. The "gold standard" is panendoscopy with esophageal biopsy. This can histologically confirm reflux that is not visually apparent and should be performed in all microlaryngobronchoscopy when there is a question of reflux. In addition, the bronchoalveolar lavage fluid should be sent for examination to test for lipid-laden macrophages. This is diagnostic of GER with a high degree of sensitivity.

Medical treatment should include H_2 blockers like ranitidine, then prokinetic agents such as metoclopramide, along with dietary modifications. Surgery is usually reserved for those cases in which medical therapy is ineffective. Most authors today perform the Nissen procedure, and current trends are toward the endoscopic Nissen fundoplication in the pediatric population.

Pediatric Malignant Neoplasms in Airway Obstruction

Lymphoma is the most common malignant neoplasm of childhood. It infrequently involves the airway, but the trachea and bronchi can be extrinsically compressed by a primary mediastinal tumor, resulting in respiratory symptoms. These lesions progress rapidly and can decrease the airway caliber by 35% to 93% by some estimates.[48] Patients typically present with stridor, orthopnea, and dyspnea. Most of these tumors are managed with medical therapies, and surgery is frequently palliative. Non-Hodgkin lymphoma may affect the larynx and can be confused with chronic allergic epiglottitis or croup. Biopsy of the affected tissues and CT imaging help distinguish this from benign conditions. These lesions are manageable by radiation and chemotherapy, so early diagnosis is critical to successful management. They are more common in the immunodeficient patient, and those with human immunodeficiency virus infection are at risk for lymphoma. Rarely, these may affect the tissues of Waldeyer ring. The patients may present with dysphagia, oropharyngeal airway obstruction, and speech alteration. There may be tonsillar fossa tumor as well. Excisional biopsy is suggested for asymmetric tonsillar lesions, and these should be sent fresh to permit the use of immunohistochemical typing. Once the diagnosis is confirmed, referral for metastatic work-up and staging should be made to a center where pediatric oncologic management is centralized.

The most common malignant neoplasm of childhood is rhabdomyosarcoma, which represents 50% of childhood sarcomas; it is also the most common sarcoma of the head and neck in children. These neoplasms can occur anywhere in the aerodigestive tract and often present as a painless mass. With involvement of the oral cavity, they may occur in the tongue, cheek, and soft palate. They grow rapidly and may bleed, ulcerate, or obstruct the oropharynx. Those in the nasopharynx and paranasal sinuses typically present with obstructive symptoms. There may be increased stridor at night. There may be Horner syndrome with those that involve the cranial nerves, and metastasis at the time of diagnosis is common. Regional adenopathy is uncommon in these malignant neoplasms. Although the primary treatment is currently multimodal, surgery has a role in controlling local disease and may lower radiation requirements. These tumors are usually embryonal in the younger age group (4 to 8 years) and alveolar in older children. The embryonal rhabdomyosarcomas have a 90% 5-year survival rate; the alveolar type is more aggressive, with only 55% 5-year survival. Rare malignant neoplasms like hemangiopericytoma, mucoepidermoid carcinoma, and adenoid cystic carcinoma may present in the oropharynx or nasopharynx. They may occasionally masquerade as hemangiomas or vascular anomalies, so magnetic resonance or CT imaging and careful examination are warranted.

An uncommon neoplasm of the young infant is the melanotic neuroectodermal tumor of infancy. It typically appears as an anterior maxillary tumor with facial swelling and may go on to obstruct the nasal inlet. On examination, a pigmented, firm mass of the alveolar ridge and nasal spine region may be seen. Excision is usually curative, although there may be dental anomalies that require later management. Other malignant neoplasms of the aerodigestive system in childhood are rare and beyond the scope of this chapter.

Pediatric Vascular Anomalies and Hemangiomas

A wide spectrum of vascular lesions affect the head and neck during infancy and childhood. Mulliken et al[49] presented the first coherent scheme that organized these tumors into distinct classifications based on history and growth characteristics. The most common vascular tumor of childhood is the hemangioma. This is a characteristic lesion that can affect any part of the body but is most commonly found in the head and neck (Fig. 77-6A). Girls are more commonly affected than are boys in a 3:2 ratio, and most are single lesions.[50] The incidence is more common in premature infants of less than 1000 g birth weight.[51] The natural history of these lesions is that of early, rapid proliferation.

Hemangiomas typically appear as small macular lesions that are bright red, blanch with pressure, and have well-defined borders. They are usually invisible at birth, progressing to become nodular, soft tissue masses during weeks to months. They may remain in the subdermal region, in which case they have a more bluish tint, or they may invade the dermis and subcutaneous tissue, assuming a characteristic "strawberry" red color. On physical examination, the mass is rubbery, is fairly firm to palpation, and rapidly refills. There is often ulceration, especially of the lips, which can cause feeding difficulties in the infant. Within the oral cavity and sinuses, the lesions can involve large areas of mucosa and have a more diffuse appearance. These may infrequently involve the bones. It is also uncommon that they cause significant skeletal deformity, in contrast to the vascular malformations.

There may be an element of substantial vascular channels in larger lesions, but the tumors are typically composed of masses of thin-walled, endothelium-lined channels that are confluent and not separated by intervening connective tissue or organized structure comparable to normal veins or arteries. Some of the cells grow without forming recognizable vascular lumens. These cells are thought to be hormone responsive, and an unknown angiogenic stimulus causes the endothelial cells to outgrow normal patterns. There are measurably elevated levels of basic fibroblast growth factor in the blood stream, which may be a factor in the growth phase of the lesions. In addition, insulin-like growth factor 2 has been shown to cause vascular sprouting in explanted hemangioma tumors in vitro.[52]

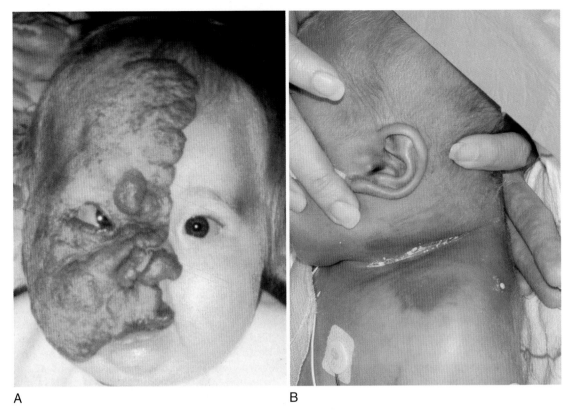

A   B

FIGURE 77-6. *A,* A large cervicofacial hemangioma. (Case of Dr. Wolfgang Losken.) *B,* Infant with vascular anomaly and Kasabach-Merritt syndrome. (Case of Dr. Wolfgang Losken.)

These lesions are usually benign, and more than half will have spontaneously resolved by 5 years of age; more than 70% resolve by the age of 7 years. Treatment is controversial and can involve systemic steroids, interferon alfa, intralesional steroids, laser therapy, surgical debulking, and embolization, in various combinations. Those lesions of immediate concern are those that obstruct the oropharynx or subglottis. Bleeding into the airway is uncommon but must be considered. In children with a subglottic hemangioma, there is biphasic stridor that progresses as the tumor grows. There may be sleep apnea and growth disturbance as the hemangioma progresses. These hemangiomas are more commonly posteriorly based and are visible on endoscopy as compressible masses in the subglottis. Biopsy is not recommended because bleeding may be difficult to control. In more than half of infants with subglottic hemangioma, there is a visible cutaneous hemangioma of the head and neck region. Any child with a cervicofacial hemangioma and stridor must be examined for subglottic hemangioma; failure to consider this possibility before any intubation attempt may cause loss of control of the airway.

In large cervicofacial lesions, there can be platelet trapping in the interstices of the vessels. This is known as Kasabach-Merritt syndrome, after its original description by these authors in 1940 (Fig. 77-6*B*). This serious phenomenon occurs in the early, rapid growth phase, and intralesional bleeding or necrosis in a hemangioma can be an early warning sign of the phenomenon. If there are hemorrhages or petechial lesions around a cervicofacial hemangioma, this diagnosis must be considered. With significant platelet trapping, there may be profound thrombocytopenia, with platelet levels as low as 2000 to 40,000 cells/mL. Fibrinogen is progressively consumed, causing prolongation of the prothrombin and partial thromboplastin times. Systemic or visceral hemorrhage with shock, airway obstruction, and death is common.

In cervicofacial hemangioma complicated by the Kasabach-Merritt syndrome, respiratory distress due to airway compression and high-output heart failure can also be present. This intravascular disseminated coagulation can be initially treated by aspirin, ticlopidine, and corticosteroids but often requires more aggressive treatment with superselective embolization and interferon alfa-2a. Some authors advocate irradiation of the primary hemangioma, but there is little consensus over this treatment. Early intervention before development of the coagulopathy seems to be the only reliable method of preventing serious complication or death. The incidence of mortality with this syndrome has been shown to be up to 77.4% in untreated patients and 27% in treated patients.[53]

If treatment is required, the first agent is often systemic corticosteroid. Those that progress or do not respond may require surgical treatment. The treatment of airway hemangiomas may be performed with pulsed carbon dioxide laser in those patients who do not respond to medical therapy. Laryngoscopy is performed, and the lesion is removed or debulked as appropriate. Circumferential treatment of the subglottis is avoided to prevent subsequent stenosis. Tracheostomy is reserved for those patients in whom these modalities are unsuccessful.[4] Interferon alfa-2a is a newer modality that has been effective in the treatment of aggressive hemangiomas, especially those with associated platelet trapping. There have been significant reports of morbidity associated with this drug, including prolonged fever, malaise, neutropenia, anemia, and spastic paralysis of unknown etiology. Until further clinical research of side effects is completed, this treatment is probably best reserved for large, refractory lesions. Conventional surgery may also be carried out in selected patients. There is a subset of well-circumscribed or involuting hemangiomas in which direct excision may be performed with safety. The pulsed dye laser is especially useful in controlling the cutaneous and mucosal aspects of the cervicofacial hemangioma, and there are few reports of significant morbidity with this modality.

VASCULAR MALFORMATIONS

Vascular malformations of the head and neck are distinct from hemangiomas in several ways. They represent congenital anomalies of the vasculature and may fall into several categories. These include capillary vascular malformation or "port-wine stain," a characteristic lesion that presents in the distribution of the trigeminal nerve; venous malformations, in which there are larger, chiefly venous channels that show dilatation and are lined with normal endothelium; and lymphangiomas, which are chiefly lymphatic channels. These last lesions are frequently called cystic hygromas in the head and neck, but that terminology is giving way to the more descriptive lymphatic vascular malformation. Mixtures of all of the types are the rule, and the terms are used to describe the predominant character of the vessels in the lesion. None of these lesions undergoes hyperplasia as hemangiomas do. There may be slow, progressive dilatation of the vascular components in response to pressure gradients, but there is no cellular proliferation of the component cells.

These lesions may be found in virtually any tissue of the head and neck but are common in the lips, tongue, cheeks, and muscle. There is also commonly bone involvement that may lead to bone hypertrophy. These lesions are all typically soft and compressible and refill slowly. They tend to grow proportionately to the child and often undergo growth with puberty, infection, or trauma. Complete surgical extirpation is difficult because the borders of these lesions are often indistinct, and they may infiltrate important nerves and vessels. There is characteristic expansion with venous obstruction, and this may be exploited to aid in clinical diagnosis. Gentle Valsalva or jugular compression may cause the lesions to expand. Craniofacial bone involvement is common. There may be dental involvement as well.

Venous and mixed vascular malformations tend to grow slowly and not expand beyond the local region. Bleeding, pain, and facial asymmetry may be associated with these lesions. Often, phleboliths form in the dilated channels and can be visualized on radiographs. Treatment is based on clinical bleeding or airway obstruction. These mixed or venous lesions are often treatable with sclerotherapy, which consists of injection of 95% ethanol or a detergent (2% sodium dodecyl sulfate) into the lesions. This causes scarring and local obstruction of the vascular channels, eventually resulting in reduction in size. There may be necrosis, prolonged edema, renal toxicity, and even extravasation with blindness if the sclerosing agent reaches the ophthalmic circulation. Therefore, these procedures may ideally be performed with imaging guidance and in several smaller stages to avoid morbidity. Older techniques of excision and grafting are giving way to minimally invasive approaches.

Lymphatic vascular malformations, on the other hand, grow slowly and may present with obstruction of the oropharynx. They are more common in the anterior and posterior triangles of the neck, frequently distorting adjacent structures. These lymphatic tumors may bleed, cause pain, become infected, or ulcerate. Progression is often marked by the appearance of cutaneous or mucosal vesicles. There may be macrocheilia, macroglossia, and macrodontia. These may produce slowly progressive airway compromise, requiring intervention. These lesions can present with isolated macroglossia without other cutaneous or mucosal signs, and the appearance of the petechiae and vesicles may be delayed for years. Macroglossia may therefore merit an examination by magnetic resonance imaging to assess the surrounding structures for vascular anomalies.

Lymphatic vascular malformations have often been grouped into invasive or noninvasive varieties. The type I or noninvasive variety is most common in the neck and has macrocystic characteristics. The type II or infiltrative lesions are diffuse and can be found in any part of the head and neck. Treatment is largely supportive. Surgery can exacerbate the lesions and should be reserved for those lymphatic vascular malformations that cause airway compromise or severe functional compromise.

Serial injection, sclerotherapy, and radiation therapy are unnecessary and may cause further progression. If necessary, surgical excision is preferable.[54] These procedures may be extensive and require meticulous dissection of nerves and great vessels. These lesions tend to drain lymphatic fluid for a prolonged time, often requiring closed suction drainage for weeks to prevent accumulation. Therefore, some surgeons have advocated the use of the carbon dioxide laser to resect intraoral and supraglottic lesions to help minimize postoperative drainage. This laser cuts tissue and theoretically seals the open vessel ends more effectively than diathermy. Those portions that involve mucosa may be amenable to neodymium:yttrium-aluminium-garnet laser treatment. This laser penetrates into the superficial portion of the mucosa and coagulates the vessels without destroying the integrity of the overlying mucosa. Therefore, a judiciously staged approach with the neodymium:yttrium-aluminium-garnet laser may delay the onset of intraoral manifestations.[55]

Hemorrhage into a previously stable lymphatic vascular malformation has been well described and may present as stridor and new-onset swelling. Those lesions that are aggressive and likely to obstruct the airway most often do so within the first year of life. Most commonly, rapid swelling in a cervicofacial lymphatic vascular malformation represents infection and should be treated with intravenous antibiotics, airway protection, and occasionally surgical drainage or later debulking.

Arteriovenous malformations are the most dangerous of all the vascular anomalies of the head and neck. These are high-flow lesions that are interconnections between venous and arterial systems. They are most commonly found intracranially but may be encountered anywhere in the body. They may present in childhood as space-occupying lesions of the airway and have a tendency to grow slowly. These lesions may be true congenital anomalies with connections between the low-pressure venous circulation and the arterial circulation, or they may form after trauma to adjacent vessels creates an artificial shunt between the two limbs of the circulatory system. They present as a bluish or reddish blush with pulsations and a palpable thrill in larger lesions. Bruits are common, and they are usually readily distinguishable from the other types of lesions. Because of the redundant connections in the vasculature, these lesions may rapidly expand and extend beyond the original limits of their borders. They may not become symptomatic until quite large, and

heart failure may be one of the first symptoms of this high-flow shunt. Other symptoms can include throbbing pain, pulsatile tinnitus, and even palpable thrill. These lesions present with pain, bleeding, or ulceration. Subsequent work-up often demonstrates bone destruction. Radiologic examination should include magnetic resonance angiography, and arteriography is useful in identifying involved vessels. All identifiable branches should be identified and included in the extirpation. Nonetheless, despite this aggressive treatment regimen, recurrence is common, and death from hemorrhage or airway obstruction is common.

If surgery is contemplated, it must be curative. Any residual arteriovenous malformation will shunt to surrounding vessels and escape the area of local resection. These lesions are best treated by preoperative embolization or sclerotherapy, followed closely by wide extirpation, similar to the treatment of aggressive neoplasms. If resection is incomplete, recurrence with distant invasion is the rule. There is no efficacy to ligation of "feeding vessels" without radical surgical extirpation. This actually exacerbates the problem and may precipitate symptomatic extension into other anatomic regions.[56,57]

Obstructive Sleep Apnea

Obstructive sleep apnea is a phenomenon that describes airway obstruction with apnea or transient interruption of breathing. There are three types of apnea: obstructive, mixed, and central apnea. Central apnea is defined as lack of respiratory effort during the apnea episode. Obstructive apnea describes ongoing respiratory effort in the face of airway blockage. Mixed apnea is a combination of the other two types. In young infants, there is significant variation in the patterns of breathing. There is a phenomenon called periodic breathing in which there may be normal breathing for a time, followed by a short apneic episode; these are repetitive and by convention happen at least three times in succession. This is a normal phenomenon in young and preterm infants. Clinically significant apneas in this age group are those that cause desaturation below 80%, cause bradycardia, or last longer than 20 seconds.

In children and adults, the normal breathing parameters change, and the apnea index is used to measure the severity of apnea. This is defined as the number of apneas of more than 10 seconds in duration per hour of sleep. There is more frequent apnea in younger children, but the episodes are typically shorter, so the apnea index remains approximately 0.1. Hypopnea, or periods of inadequate ventilation or partial obstruction, is also common in this age group. There is no consensus on the measurement of hypopnea, so some authors advocate following capnometry and oxygen saturation as more reproducible measures of apnea. Any end-tidal carbon dioxide above 50 mm

Hg or oxygen saturation less than 90% merits further work-up.

Gastroesophageal reflux has been repeatedly shown to be a major cause of sleep apnea in infants and young children. Micrognathia, craniofacial anomalies, chronic nasal obstruction, laryngotracheal disease, obesity, and neurologic disorders have been implicated in apneic breathing episodes. The severity of the obstruction corresponds to the physiologic changes that ensue. Mild apnea may cause only mild bradycardia, systolic hypertension, diastolic hypotension, and deranged sleep patterns. More severe obstruction may predispose the child to cerebral hypoxia during a significant portion of the sleep cycle, cor pulmonale, and even death. There is substantial evidence that links obstructive sleep apnea with ALTEs and SIDS.

Diagnosis is made with polysomnography, careful observation during sleep, and measurement of chest wall impedance. The respiratory trace from this study with electrocardiographic data is called a pneumocardiogram. Because there may be respiratory effort without air movement, modern thermistor monitors with oximetry and capnometry are preferred. If there are no data regarding reflux, a pH probe may be combined with the sleep study. Some authors advocate lateral cephalograms to evaluate airway patency, and cookie swallows may help document reflux, aspiration, and possible thoracic anomalies. Once obstructive sleep apnea is documented, panendoscopy is the next step in diagnosis. If there is an anatomic reason for airway obstruction, aggressive management is indicated because the morbidity of untreated obstructive sleep apnea is significant.

Some authors advocate medical treatment with theophylline or caffeine to stimulate the respiratory drive. Caffeine is the currently preferred agent because it has fewer side effects and a longer duration. Reflux should be treated with H_2 blockers, proton pump blockade, and sometimes promotility agents before surgical reflux procedures such as a Nissen fundoplication.

Feeding may be difficult in these infants, and gastrostomy may be contemplated until the cause of the obstructive sleep apnea can be controlled. In severe cases, tracheostomy may be warranted. In many patients in whom the apnea is attributable to congenital craniofacial anomalies or micrognathia, surgery to advance the midface or mandible may offer an alternative to long-term tracheostomy.

Craniofacial Anomalies

MICROGNATHIA

Congenital micrognathia represents another common reason for upper airway obstruction in the neonatal population (Fig. 77-7). The most common micrognathia "syndrome" is the Pierre Robin sequence, a clinical entity consisting of the triad of micrognathia, cleft palate, and glossoptosis. It is not in itself a genetic syndrome but a clinical description that comprises several possible diagnoses. Estimates of incidence suggest that 1 in 8500 babies are affected with Pierre Robin sequence.[58] Of these children, up to 80% have a genetically recognizable craniofacial syndrome that causes the anomaly.[59] First described by Pierre Robin in 1923, the Robin triad is referred to as a sequence

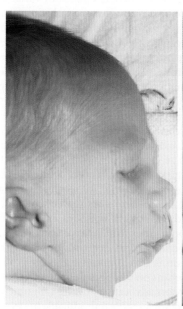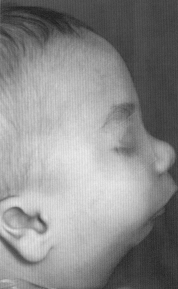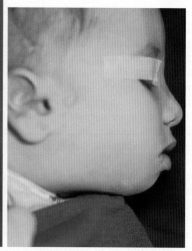

FIGURE 77-7. Micrognathia with airway obstruction requiring distraction osteogenesis.

because some authors think that the palatal cleft results from the interference by the retropositioned tongue with the fusion of the palatal shelves.[60] This sequence of events has not been universally accepted. Other theories favor an orofacial cleft mechanism for the triad.[61] Mild cases of obstruction due to Pierre Robin sequence can be managed by lateral or prone positioning of the infant to prevent the posterior prolapse of the tongue that can precipitate airway obstruction. If this is unsuccessful, the next intervention should be placement of a nasogastric or orogastric tube. These must function more by maintaining the tongue in an anterior position than as actual airways because they function well even when obstructed with secretions. Actual nasal trumpets and hard plastic oral airways are more difficult to manage; they require careful and frequent inspection of the surrounding soft tissue to prevent pressure necrosis. Special bottles, such as the Haberman or Mead-Johnson devices, are useful in feeding the infant with Pierre Robin sequence, in whom both the airway compromise and cleft palate cause difficulties in feeding.

If these maneuvers are unsuccessful, consideration is frequently given to tracheostomy. Infants cannot simultaneously swallow and breathe as adults do. Their response to transient airway obstruction during feeding in the supine or seated position is unpredictable and can precipitate an episode of frank apnea. The cough reflex does not develop until later.[62] The lip-tongue adhesion procedure consists of creating a small raw surface on the lower lip and tongue, usually with opposing flaps that are then sutured together. The concept was designed to maintain the tongue in an anterior position, but there is controversy about its current role in the management of Pierre Robin sequence.[63] Tracheostomy has remained the mainstay of management in severe cases when other methods have failed. The establishment of a safe airway must be of paramount importance.

Nevertheless, distraction osteogenesis has vaulted onto the scene in the management of congenital micrognathia and may well be supplanting other methods of treating these infants. By osteotomizing the mandible and gradually lengthening the bones, all of the floor of mouth musculature and the hyoid bone are advanced together. Early results in infants are promising. The patient typically remains intubated for several days during the distraction sequence and is extubated once a safe degree of advancement has been achieved.[64] There is significant morbidity associated with neonatal tracheostomy, ranging from infection to subglottic stenosis. In addition, the cost of maintaining a child with a tracheostomy is considerable. Social issues, delayed speech and language development, and parental acceptance may all play a role in the evolution of treatment for severe micrognathia. One of the authors (C.B.G.) has performed more than

50 mandibular distraction procedures in infants, with minor morbidity (Fig. 77-8). These patients were offered distraction as an alternative to tracheostomy or as an attempt to achieve decannulation in those whose conventional decannulation protocols failed. Of these patients, only seven either required ongoing tracheostomy or failed decannulation after mandibular distraction. These children had normalization of growth curves and facial growth patterns, and there was even resolution of gastroesophageal reflux in more than a third of patients. Further investigation is warranted to verify these results.

Special mention must be made of the role of pharyngeal flaps in the care of the cleft child. After cleft palate repair, a substantial percentage of infants go on to develop velopharyngeal insufficiency. The most effective method of treating this is to design a superiorly based pharyngeal flap, which is sutured to the soft palate, forming a nearly obstructing soft tissue bridge between the oropharynx and the nasopharynx. Only the two small lateral ports permit nasal airflow. This greatly improves the quality of speech but can be risky in the infant with Pierre Robin sequence, in whom the airway is compromised. In a prospective study of pharyngeal flaps in patients with cleft palate, more than 90% still had obstructive sleep apnea, regardless of technical details of flap surgery. This airway obstruction was more severe in the population of younger patients. In Pierre Robin sequence, six of seven children who underwent pharyngeal flap required flap takedown for subsequent obstructive apnea.[65,66]

Hemifacial microsomia is a common congenital anomaly of the head and neck. It is a form of the ocular-auricular-vertebral spectrum of anomalies that include microtia, Goldenhar syndrome, and oculoauriculofrontonasal syndrome. Hemifacial microsomia is a common anomaly, occurring in approximately 1.4 per 10,000 births in the United States. There is hypoplasia of both hard and soft tissues of the face, and the deformity may be both unilateral and bilateral, although unilateral cases are much more common. There is variable mandibular micrognathia, compensatory maxillary changes, and frequent obstructive sleep apnea. This was the first disorder to be treated with mandibular distraction, and distraction has become the most common treatment for this anomaly.

Crouzon syndrome is the most common of the craniofacial dysostosis syndromes. It is autosomal dominant and has widely variable clinical manifestations. It is characterized by coronal suture synostosis, midface hypoplasia, and varying degrees of obstructive sleep apnea. Vigilance must be taken to examine the eyes carefully because elevated intracranial pressure, papilledema, and even blindness can ensue. These patients have severe brachycephaly, and the midface impinges on the posterior pharyngeal wall. Previous management included tracheostomy and craniofacial

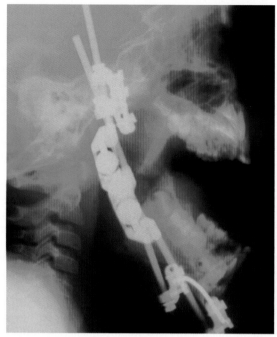
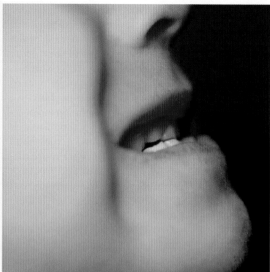

FIGURE 77-8. Distraction procedure with follow-up picture of occlusion.

advancements, although midface distraction techniques are promising in reducing relapse and maintaining airway patency.

Apert syndrome is another rare craniofacial dysostosis syndrome. The craniofacial anomaly is similar to that of Crouzon syndrome, with severe midfacial hypoplasia, turribrachycephaly, exophthalmos, polysyndactyly, and cleft palate. Other accompanying disorders include conductive hearing loss, elevated intracranial pressure, and strabismus. The midfacial hypoplasia is more profound than in Crouzon syndrome, and airway issues become critical in early life. In both Crouzon and Apert syndromes, single mutations in the gene encoding fibroblast growth factor are involved. The management is evolving but typically involves a monobloc or bipartition procedure. More authors are embracing distraction to achieve the formidable advances that may be required in the correction of the cranial vault and midfacial pathologic processes. Secondary micrognathia of the mandible may be noted, and several groups are performing mandibular distraction in conjunction with midfacial advancement to maintain occlusion and to improve airway patency.

In mild cases or when distraction must be delayed, there is a role for continuous positive airway pressure, tonsillectomy and adenoidectomy, and antireflux therapy. The definitive treatment remains the correction of the bone deformity.

Other rare syndromes with midfacial hypoplasia include Carpenter, Pfeiffer, Saethre-Chotzen, Jackson-Weiss, and Baller-Gerold syndromes, among others. Management of respiratory issues is similar for all of these syndromes.

Treacher Collins syndrome (mandibulofacial dysostosis) is a rare syndrome that involves hypoplasia of the mandible and malar regions bilaterally. Some authors prefer to describe the defect as a bilateral Tessier craniofacial cleft of type 6-8. There are colobomas with occasional cranial deformities. Bilateral microtia is common. There is invariably a degree of micrognathia, and there may be severe micrognathia with extreme maxillary hyperplasia. This may require urgent management in the neonatal period. The success of distraction in this group for airway management has all but replaced conventional orthognathic surgery. Nager syndrome is a similar disorder in which there are additional limb anomalies, such as preaxial radial deficiencies with hypoplastic thumbs. There may also be genitourinary, spinal, pelvic, and lower extremity deformities. Intelligence is normal in both of these deformities, so early bone advancement and decannulation or avoidance of tracheostomy may have a salutary effect on social and emotional development, speech, and language.

TREATMENT OF AIRWAY OBSTRUCTION BY DISTRACTION OSTEOGENESIS

There are dozens of techniques for the treatment of obstructive sleep apnea. Of the nonsurgical techniques, several are simple and reliable. The plastic surgeon is frequently confronted with a young infant with congenital micrognathia, sleep apnea, and failure to thrive. Traditionally, these children were treated first with positioning. The glossoptosis associated with micrognathia is often amenable to lateral or prone positioning while the child sleeps. Some of these children cannot tolerate feeding in a supine position without obstructing. If these maneuvers are insufficient, a soft rubber nasal trumpet may help maintain a more anterior tongue position. This must be done with caution because any nasal cannula can cause pressure necrosis of the nasal alae. Alternatively, a pediatric orogastric tube can be placed with similar effect. The infant must be carefully observed to rule out ongoing obstruction and to ensure sufficient calorie intake and weight gain. The long-term effects of even mild apnea can include right-sided heart failure, growth impairment, and developmental delay. If these measures are unsuccessful, surgical management is indicated.

Surgical management can conveniently be divided into soft and hard tissue techniques. The soft tissue techniques involve either reduction of a portion of the oropharyngeal airway, such as uvulopalatopharyngoplasty, or suspension procedures, which can include lip-tongue adhesion, hyoid suspension, tongue suspension, or a combination of these procedures.[67] Tongue base traction is a relatively noninvasive technique that uses suspension sutures in the floor of the mouth to maintain a forward tongue position.[68] For many years, the standard treatment of obstructive sleep apnea for congenital micrognathia was lip-tongue adhesion with secondary division when the mandible had grown sufficiently to permit normal feeding and sleeping. These procedures are relatively well tolerated, but there is no single soft tissue technique that reliably prevents the airway obstruction associated with congenital micrognathia. They all improve breathing mechanics, but none is a definitive treatment.

The hard tissue techniques involve bone advancement of some or all of the anterior mandible to treat sleep apnea. These techniques have the advantage of directly treating the cause of the apnea in many patients, namely, micrognathia. Orthognathic surgery, with combinations of sagittal split osteotomies and Le Fort I osteotomies in skeletally mature patients, is successful in improving sleep apnea.[69] Other novel osteotomies have been devised to advance a portion of the mandible to bring the floor of mouth musculature forward. These include sliding genioplasty, mortised genioplasty, and "genioglossus" advancement procedures, discussed in more detail later.[70,71] Several technical reasons have limited the acceptance of distraction in the skeletally immature patient, namely, the position of the tooth buds and the course of the inferior alveolar nerve. Traditional osteotomies have also been reported to cause significant growth disturbance in children. With the advent of distraction

osteogenesis procedures, the indications for bone advancement have begun to change.[72]

Distraction osteogenesis is a method for osteotomy and gradual elongation of bones. It was introduced by Alexander Codivilla[73] near the turn of the 20th century for the treatment of shortened limbs. This concept was reintroduced by Ilizarov in the 1960s as a means of correcting post-traumatic defects of the long bones. These advances provided the scientific basis for a reliable way to apply these techniques in the craniofacial skeleton.[74]

There was no report of use of these techniques in the craniofacial skeleton until Snyder et al[75] described a method of mandibular lengthening in a canine model in 1973. Building on this work, McCarthy[76] modified the technique and described the first human cases of mandibular distraction in 1992. Concurrently, Molina and Ortiz Monasterio[77] assembled a significant series of cases demonstrating the wide clinical application of these concepts in syndromic patients. Since then, these techniques have been applied to a wide variety of problems in craniofacial surgery, with little standardization.[78]

One area of consensus is the applicability of the techniques for elongation of the pediatric mandible. Multiple authors have advocated the use of distraction for the treatment of obstructive sleep apnea. Distraction has become the de facto standard of care for treatment of many types of congenital micrognathia and is becoming increasingly more common in adult surgery.[79,80] Compared with traditional osteotomies and advancement procedures, distraction has several advantages that may lead to its supplanting these procedures entirely. Specifically, the sagittal split osteotomy and mandibular advancement with screw fixation has been used for many years to improve the patency of the upper airway. Variants of this technique, first introduced by Obwegeser, are effective in the treatment of obstructive sleep apnea in adults.[81]

In severe micrognathia, nonsurgical methods of growth enhancement and conservative measures have had mixed success in management of the pediatric airway.[82,83] Therefore, in severe upper airway obstruction, treatment has included tracheostomy, continuous positive-pressure ventilation during sleep, tonsillectomy with adenoidectomy, and hyoid suspension. Some groups have had success with epiglottopexy and epiglottoplasty. These two procedures have sometimes led to chronic aspiration, scarring, or deranged swallowing, so they have not been widely embraced as first-line treatment.

Further, severe obstructive sleep apnea is known to be associated with gastroesophageal reflux.[84] This is often treated with long-term medication or Nissen fundoplication and may even require chronic tracheostomy to protect the lung from the deleterious effects of ongoing aspiration. Chronic apnea has been associated with permanent right-sided heart failure, developmental and growth disturbance, and even intellectual impairment. Tracheostomy has been the gold standard for treatment of severe micrognathia, but that can entail years of expensive enteral feeding and tracheostomy care before sufficient mandibular growth is attained for decannulation.[85] The impact of long-term tracheostomy on oromotor development, speech, and social interaction has been well studied, and the effects cannot be overstated. The costs associated with treatment of long-term tracheostomy, reflux, and associated disorders are also significant. In the United States, chronic tracheostomy in infants often entails intensive home nursing care or placement in a chronic care facility. Therefore, a safe alternative for early mandibular advancement has long been sought.

Mandibular distraction can reduce the need for additional airway procedures by restoring normal mandibular morphologic features. By fashioning osteotomies at the mandibular angle and distracting the mandibular body forward, the surgeon can leave the floor of mouth musculature attached to the mandible (Fig. 77-9). Subsequent distraction of the segment carries this soft tissue forward, improving glossoptosis and prolapse of the epiglottis into the airway. No data are available to dictate how much bone advancement is required to correct a given degree of micrognathia and maintain a patent airway. Neither is it known how much relapse is to be expected, nor how subsequent mandibular growth will be affected. These questions must be answered to permit distraction to gain widespread acceptance as the most effective treatment of upper airway obstruction associated with micrognathia.

Many mandibular distractors are available, both internal and external types. External distractors were the first to be introduced and are still the most popular

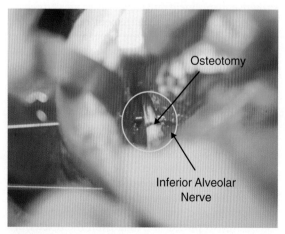

FIGURE 77-9. Osteotomy for distraction osteogenesis.

devices. These typically comprise a frame of bilateral articulating threaded bars that support pins entering the mandible percutaneously. As the activation screw is turned, the fragments are slowly distracted apart. Typically, one turn of the distraction screw moves the pins 0.5 or 1.0 mm to simplify distraction management. The area of bone growth between the fragments is replaced with osteoid or callus (Fig. 77-10). This callus calcifies and matures into bone during a period of weeks to months.

There are some single-vector devices on the market, but they do not permit management of the shape of the bony callus growth during distraction. Multivector devices have the ability to control varus-valgus, angulation, and vertical and sagittal advancement. The surgeon may therefore simultaneously correct for nonparallelism and occlusal concerns and mimic the normal growth of the mandible during the distraction period.

Internal mandibular distractors are similar in concept to the external devices, but they are miniaturized to permit placement in a subperiosteal pocket adjacent to the osteotomy. They are typically located along the buccal cortex of the mandibular angle. Osteotomies are usually performed through intraoral exposure. The activation screw is brought out percutaneously or intraorally through the buccal mucosa. There may be some advantage to these designs. First, as distraction proceeds, there is no "pin tracking" scar. Acceptance by patients is good, and there is no intimidating external hardware. There is little loss of mechanical advantage with the short lever arm of the device adjacent to the bone.

Distraction has rapidly supplanted conventional methods of mandibular advancement in the pediatric population and is making inroads in the adult literature as well. Virtually all congenital micrognathia syndromes can be managed effectively. In older children, the surgeon often uses a modified sagittal split or vertical osteotomy, or even an external corticotomy, to avoid damage to the inferior alveolar nerve. In infants, the nerve courses medially to the mandibular ramus and enters the body medial and mesial to the retromolar region of the body. This permits the surgeon to perform a full osteotomy with less risk to the inferior alveolar nerve.[86,87]

Of the congenital syndromes, the most frequent cause of micrognathia is hemifacial microsomia, a part of the ocular-auricular-vertebral family of deformities. In addition to cervical spine deformities, renal anomalies, and other less common deformities, there is underdevelopment of both the mandibular ramus and condyle. In more severe cases, there can be microtia, global soft tissue hypoplasia of the first and second branchial arch structures, occasional facial nerve palsy, and a progressive deformity that appears to be related to maxillary growth compensation. Pruzansky devel-

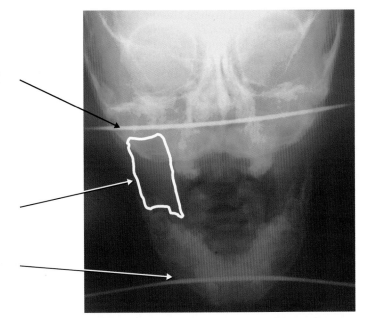

Superior pin placement

Distraction callus

Inferior pin placement

FIGURE 77-10. Generation of callus at the site of osteotomy.

oped the grading scale that has gained widespread acceptance. Grade I cases have hypoplasia of the condyle and fossa. Grade II deformities have a more significant deficiency of the ramus with variable soft tissue hypoplasia. In grade III cases, there is complete absence of the ramus and condyle. Before distraction techniques, the typical treatment plan included conventional orthognathic procedures for patients with grade I and grade II deformities and costochondral grafts for reconstruction of the mandibular ramus for patients with grade III deformities.[88] In some centers, reconstruction of the temporomandibular joint was also performed. These techniques have significant morbidity, including donor site discomfort, potential overgrowth or distortion of the rib graft, ankylosis of the neocondyle, and scarring.

Currently, the most common treatment method for hemifacial microsomia is external mandibular distraction. The surgeon typically places an external, multivector device that is affixed to four threaded Steinmann pins placed percutaneously through the mandible adjacent to the site of planned osteotomy. These are bicortical pins that avoid the trajectory of the inferior alveolar nerve and the tooth buds. The mandible is then dissected from an intraoral approach and osteotomized near the mandibular angle. After adjustment of the device, there is often a latent period of several days before distraction is begun. Distraction rates range from 1 to 3 mm/day, with younger patients receiving more rapid distraction. In neonates, rates have been reported up to 4 mm daily. To date, there is no consensus about exact timing, rate of distraction, or

even pin placement. Complications include nerve and tooth bud injury, scarring, open bite, device loosening or hardware failure, and pin track infection. There is a growing group of authors who perform bilateral osteotomies to help minimize changes to the temporomandibular joint of the affected side, permitting a more modest change in the relationship of the condyle to the skull base.

Pierre Robin sequence is the most common nonsyndromic cause of micrognathia. This sequence can be associated with a number of congenital syndromes but is most frequently idiopathic or associated with Stickler syndrome. It consists of micrognathia, glossoptosis with airway obstruction, and cleft palate. There is a wide spectrum of deformity, but severely affected patients often require tracheostomy, lip-tongue adhesion, and prolonged vigilance for sleep apnea. The treatment of these infants has been revolutionized by distraction. Multiple authors have published preliminary reports describing effective treatment of the micrognathia by distraction osteogenesis.[89-92] Rapid distraction sequences of up to 4 mm/day have been presented, permitting the use of endotracheal intubation as a temporizing measure in conjunction with rapid distraction. After several days of distraction, the infants can usually be safely extubated, continuing with nasogastric or orogastric feeding until the device is removed.[93]

At Children's Hospital of Pittsburgh, the aerodigestive team evaluates the infant with micrognathia. Radiographic studies include three-dimensional CT scans of the craniofacial structures and cephalograms.

Polysomnography with pH probe is also used to evaluate the severity of sleep apnea. The pH probe permits evaluation of reflux, which must be treated concurrently to maximize the chances of decannulation or avoidance of tracheostomy. The otolaryngologist performs diagnostic endoscopy of the nasopharynx, oropharynx, glottic structures, and trachea. If there was no previous pH probe, esophageal biopsy is performed. If micrognathia is thought to be the cause of the apnea, mandibular distraction is performed.

The authors prefer external devices for this application because the long distractions (up to 75 mm) needed in some cases cannot be performed with the current generation of internal devices. Another concern is the lack of safe locations for pin placement. The soft bone of the infant mandible is not robust enough to support threaded screws for much time. Many authors have reported device displacement after a short distraction sequence. This is secondary to rapid resorption of the bone around the screws affixing the distractor to the bone. Therefore, the authors have developed a technique that uses two smooth Steinmann pins placed in parallel in a through and through fashion (Fig. 77-11). The superior pin traverses the superior rami and the oropharynx, and the inferior pin traverses the menton. A single vector must be used because there is no three-point fixation to permit vector management. After generation of a robust callus, the new bone is manipulated to close the bite and restore normal anatomic features. For the inferior pin, a 5/64-inch smooth Steinmann pin is placed percutaneously just inferior to the tooth buds and just posterior to the mental nerve in the anterior mandible. Superiorly, the transpharyngeal pin is placed as high along the mandibular ramus as possible.

There are multiple benefits to the two-pin or "shish kebab" technique. Virtually all forms of fixation loosen before the desired distraction is completed. With the transfacial pins, the device may loosen and slide to and fro, but it cannot become completely dislodged unless the mandible fractures. Screws, on the other hand, virtually always pull out before completion of distraction in this age group. Another advantage is the wide spacing of the pins. There is little scarring associated with pin tracking.

The anatomy of the infant mandible is ideally suited to this technique. There is an area just distal and inferior to the canine tooth bud that is devoid of other vital structures. This is the location for the anterior pin. The inferior alveolar nerve enters the mandible mesial and medial to the retromolar area of the mandibular angle. There is no distinctive lingula or condyle. Instead, the nerve enters directly into the bone without coursing through the ramus at all. Superiorly, there is no true subcondylar area that would be vulnerable to fracture. All of the ramus is anterior to the carotid and velum. Therefore, this two-pin technique is reliably and safely performed in young infants and is also useful in older children. The osteotomy is performed in a mild sagittal orientation, near the mandibular angle, adjacent to the neurovascular bundle. This is easily carried out through a standard oral buccal sulcus incision.

An added benefit of the flexible pins is being able to predict when premature callus consolidation is occurring. There is increased pain and bowing of the pins associated with this phenomenon. The surgeon can return to the operating room with knowledge of the location of the bundle. Therefore, a blind osteotomy near the distal or posterior aspect of the new callus

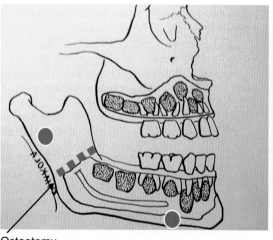

Osteotomy

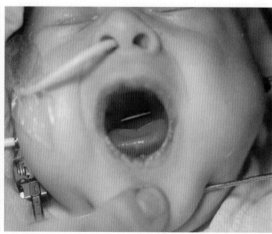

FIGURE 77-11. Placement of two Steinmann pins for mandibular distraction.

permits continued distraction without early termination because of early consolidation. In more than 50 cases of mandibular distraction in the first 18 months of life, all but 6 patients either avoided tracheostomy or were successfully decannulated. There were no open bites, which is a common complication of conventional distraction; scarring was minimal, and there were no distraction failures.[94]

Neonates are usually left intubated and observed in the intensive care unit for 3 to 5 days until repeated microlaryngobronchoscopy demonstrates that extubation can be performed. The child is observed in stepdown until there are no further apneas or bradycardias of significance. The mandible is overcorrected in a sagittal sense, planning on a certain amount of relapse. This is followed by device removal, callus manipulation to close the bite, and slight sagittal overcorrection with a stable occlusion (Fig. 77-12). This permits a certain amount of relapse. The soft callus is stable enough to support mastication and suckling but allows the pterygomasseteric sling to tend to close the bite and maintain normal intermaxillary relationships until the callus matures during the next several weeks. Repeated imaging studies demonstrate the stability of the bony

regenerate. Lateral cephalograms show the epiglottis and tongue base and permit mandibular growth to be observed over time. Sleep studies should be repeated to confirm correction of sleep apnea.

These basic techniques are widely applicable to pediatric micrognathias of a wide variety. Although the details of timing, hardware preferences, and long-term stability remain to be worked out, it is clear that mandibular distraction is rapidly evolving into the treatment of choice for obstructive sleep apnea in children. This may eventually apply to the adult with micrognathia as well.

Midface Distraction

Obstructive sleep apnea is frequently associated with craniofacial syndromes and is particularly common in the craniofacial dysostoses with associated midfacial hypoplasia, such as Crouzon and Apert syndromes.[95] The neonate is an obligate nose breather, and infants with these syndromes typically present with obstructive apnea. Many require tracheostomy to control the airway. Although there are many factors involved in the apnea, a major factor is narrowing of the nasopharynx related to the midfacial stenosis.

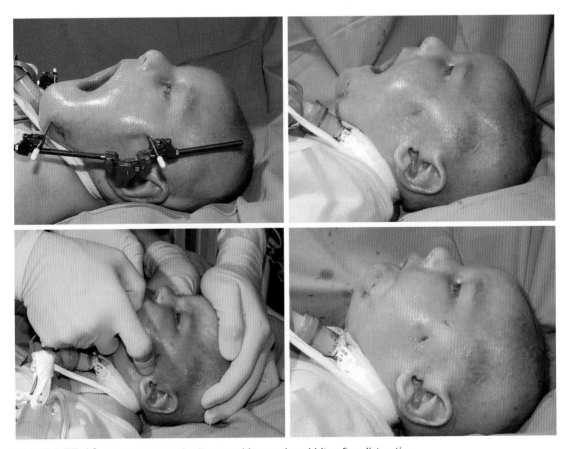

FIGURE 77-12. Manipulation of callus to achieve a closed bite after distraction.

Previous recommendations from major craniofacial centers advocated tracheostomy to prevent serious morbidity or death in the syndromic craniosynostoses.[96] The use of traction to maintain the position of the midface has been well known for more than a century. Midface fractures were treated with traction for decades preceding the current era of distraction. Delaire introduced a reverse-pull orthopedic appliance to assist facial growth in the midface without the use of osteotomies. The Delaire mask is a commonly used device in dentistry and is also used to assist in distraction of the midface.[97,98] Tessier reported on the use of neurosurgical halos with outriggers to provide traction to the midface. Polley and Figueroa[99] applied this type of device to midfacial distraction with excellent stability and proof of concept.

Advancement of the midface by more than 10 to 12 mm with conventional techniques has been held to be unstable. Distraction osteogenesis is gaining acceptance as a more stable and predictable technique for larger advances.[100,101] The unpredictability and morbidity of conventional Le Fort III advancement have led to a reluctance to use this osteotomy if lesser procedures will suffice. Not until the advent of distraction has the relapse been controlled, permitting correction of severe midfacial retrusion that was not amenable to Le Fort I procedures. In addition, this has the added advantage of increasing the nasopharyngeal space compared with other midfacial procedures. Several groups have embraced this procedure as an answer to the craniofacial syndromes.[102]

Ortiz Monasterio introduced an advancement of the entire frontofacial segment in a monobloc. This procedure is often criticized for tendency for relapse, infection, and technical difficulty. A variant of this procedure, the facial bipartition, is used to treat concomitant hypertelorism.[103] These new bone distraction techniques permit the surgeon to advance these segments with less morbidity and superior management of aesthetics, relapse, and airway obstruction.[104-108]

The authors' preferred method for midface advancement is integrated distraction of either the Le Fort III or monobloc segment with a "finishing" Le Fort I osteotomy that may be distracted or fixated, depending on skeletal analysis. This hybrid procedure permits even more aggressive advancements in syndromic craniosynostoses. In several cases, the combined procedures have attained more than 50 mm of advancement at the anterior nasal spine. Sleep apnea resolves during early distraction. It appears that even with only 2 years of follow-up, this is a definitive procedure for many forms of midfacial hypoplasia-associated apnea. Future work is being planned to perform these large procedures with a minimally invasive approach.[109]

After frontofacial advancements of such magnitude, there is often a skeletal malocclusion. The mandible is often relatively hypoplastic as well, but it was not typically treated in the past in light of the difficulty of achieving stable midfacial advancement. Several authors now advocate mandibular advancement to completely correct the bone abnormalities in these syndromes. These radical combined procedures are effective in treating sleep apnea. Further work will be needed to elucidate the preferred treatment plans for these complex cases.

Internal midface distractors are not unlike internal mandibular distractors. These typically consist of distractor screws with threaded bases that are affixed to the midface on one end and to the cranial base at the other. The distractors are placed subperiosteally along the lateral orbit and brought out in the scalp. Distraction is carried out in a fashion similar to that with the external devices. These early devices are constantly improving and are likely to evolve rapidly into tiny, easily placed internal distractors.

The era of distraction osteogenesis has radically changed the surgical treatment of obstructive sleep apnea. The ease with which new bone can be formed and manipulated may herald the end of the need for many of the soft tissue procedures that have traditionally been used to treat apnea. These are exciting developments that promise to transform the lives of these previously difficult to manage patients.

OBSTRUCTIVE SLEEP APNEA IN THE ADULT PATIENT

Adults may suffer airway obstruction from large turbinates, displaced nasal septum, large tonsils, neck infections and epiglottitis, trauma, and malignant neoplasms. Most of the causes of obstruction seen in childhood will have been diagnosed and treated by adulthood. The spectrum of malignant neoplasms is different from those of children, particularly in the case of oropharyngeal and laryngeal squamous cell carcinoma. Among adults, obstructive sleep apnea is a problem of increasing numbers as the North American population becomes progressively more overweight. The prevalence of this disorder and its importance in management of patients hospitalized for other problems demand that plastic surgeons be aware of how to diagnose and treat the condition.

Diagnosis and Treatment Criteria

Obstructive sleep apnea may be defined as cessation of tidal flow for at least 10 seconds with a continued paradoxical chest wall motion. The diagnosis of clinical obstructive sleep apnea is made when there are more than 5 obstructive apneas per hour or more than 10 hypopneas per hour. No more than 25% of the apneas should be central or mixed according to these strict diagnostic criteria. An obstructive hypopnea was originally defined as greater than 50% fall in tidal flow for at least 10 seconds; there is persistent chest wall motion during this period of reduced flow. More recently, a significant hypopnea has been defined as a 30% decrease in airflow with persistent chest wall motions accompanied by a 4% desaturation of hemoglobin.[110]

More than 30 apneas per night are considered the threshold to allow the diagnosis of sleep apnea syndrome (Table 77-1). Apneas are considered significant if they are more than 10 seconds in duration and if they are accompanied by a cardiac arrhythmia.[111-113] Longitudinal studies have now demonstrated that an apnea-hypopnea index (the sum of apneas and hypopneas occurring per hour) of more than 5 events per hour of sleep is associated with a significantly higher incidence of cardiovascular disease.[110]

During normal sleep, young adults normally descend into the third stage of sleep that is known as REM or rapid eye movement sleep. Sleep apnea, however, is characterized by continued arousal due to obstruction of breathing. The time spent in deep sleep stages two, three, and four is therefore very much reduced (Fig. 77-13). It is also frequently interrupted.

This disordered sleep leads to daytime symptoms characterized by daytime sleepiness including discrete sleep attacks. Patients with significant apnea often report that they are extremely sleepy during the day and may even fall asleep while eating breakfast. They complain of excessive fatigue, early morning headaches, and impaired alertness and coordination. Driving is especially dangerous, and patients with unrecognizable sleep apnea may be discovered among those who present in the emergency department after motor vehicle accidents. In addition, there may be behavioral changes leading to less sociability and the formation of negative impressions on behalf of those around the patient with sleep apnea.

TABLE 77-1 ♦ CRITERIA FOR DIAGNOSIS OF OBSTRUCTIVE SLEEP APNEA

History	Daytime somnolence
	Difficulty staying awake while driving
	Trouble staying asleep, awaking tired
	Loud snoring, gasping, snorting
	Moves around, flails, displacing bedding
	Movement in sleep with self-arousal
	Cessation of inspiration observed by others
	Morning occipital headache
	Essential hypertension
	Enuresis
Physical examination	Often obese, although not always
	Large tonsils, retrusive mandible
	Large, long uvula
	Status pharyngeal flap without tonsillectomy
	Large tongue, especially in acromegaly
	Elevated blood pressure
	Rarely cyanosis from desaturation
Laboratory tests	Diagnostic sleep recordings
	More than 5 apneas per hour (cessation of flow for at least 10 sec)
	More than 10 obstructive hypopneas per hour (at least >50% fall in tidal flow for at least 10 sec with persistent respiratory effort; or more recently, >30% reduction in airflow with chest motion continuing and at least 4% decrease in hemoglobin saturation)
	30 apneas per night or apnea-hypopnea index >5 per hour
	Appearance of cardiac arrhythmias with desaturation
	Room air arterial gases: desaturation with hypercapnia
	Echocardiography: right ventricular enlargement with elevated pulmonary artery pressure

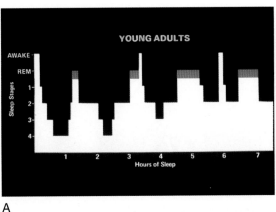

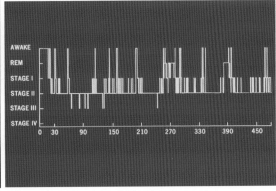

A   B

FIGURE 77-13. *A*, A normal sleep profile with time spent in sleep stage III. *B*, A disordered sleep pattern with little time spent in stage III because of obstructive sleep apnea.

Nocturnal symptoms include loud snoring, snorting, and gasping. The apnea episodes with continued exhortatory effort might be alarming to bed partners. The patients often present the appearance of respiratory distress. There are frequent body movements including frequent turning and flailing of the arms, and this can be a source of great consternation to bed partners. The respiratory effort and the neuromuscular movement associated with the effort to relieve the airway obstruction may lead to diaphoresis and even enuresis.

Patients with obstructive sleep apnea are often obese. They may have elevated blood pressure and otherwise unexplained cor pulmonale. The cor pulmonale in the obese patient may present as a large edematous pannus with a peau d'orange change in the skin. There can be large lymphocele-like masses protruding from the posteromedial thighs just above the knees (Fig. 77-14). It is notable that these patients usually have normal findings on upper airway examination while awake.

The pathogenesis of cor pulmonale is important because right-sided heart failure represents a significant health risk for the patient. Patients who are desaturated have an elevated pulmonary artery pressure in response. A PO_2 of less than 55 mm Hg and a PCO_2 of more than 47 mm Hg should prompt evaluation for elevated right pulmonary pressure and right-sided heart failure.[114] The elevated pulmonary artery pressure requires more work of the right ventricle, which may dilate and prove inadequate with decompensation. Increasing right ventricular pressure leads to high atrial pressure and accompanying high venous pressure, causing the engorged veins and the lymphedema of the abdominal pannus and the lower extremities. When stressed after a major operation, the heart may not be capable of handling the venous return, thereby producing a high systemic venous pressure. This leads to massive fluid loss in wounds. A panniculectomy in a patient with right-sided heart failure can lead to such enormous fluid loss that it will be virtually impossible to maintain adequate intravascular volume and plasma composition. Patients with large wounds and right-sided heart failure can die of this complication.

Diagnostic methods include an interview with the bed partner, a sleep laboratory evaluation, a 24-hour cardiac monitoring for those patients for whom it is deemed advisable, a clinical laboratory assessment, an upper airway examination, and a consultation among the medical team members (most often pulmonologists and cardiologists) caring for these patients. On physical examination, these patients may appear perfectly normal when they are awake. However, on nasal pharyngoscopy, the experienced observer will note that there are frequently numerous rugous folds in the hypopharynx as if the camera were looking down the space between loosely closed fingers and the palm when a fist is made. One does not typically see a collapse of the airway while the patient is awake, however (Fig. 77-15).

There are a number of general admonitions to share with the patients, and one is that they should avoid all central nervous system depressants. This is important for the anesthesia team and treating surgeons in the operative and postoperative periods. All pharyngeal abnormalities should be corrected; hypertrophic tonsils, retrusive mandibles, and extraordinarily long uvulas should be corrected surgically. If the means of reducing airway resistance are not successful, the gold standard for treatment of obstructive sleep apnea is tracheostomy (Table 77-2). This effectively bypasses the obstruction and restores a normal airway with pulmonary artery hemoglobin saturation, a reduction of pulmonary artery pressure, compensation of the right side of the heart if it was failing, and a remarkable change in the level of alertness in the wakeful patient.

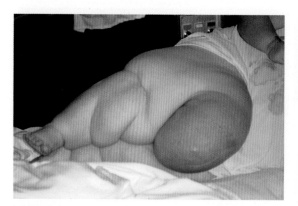

FIGURE 77-14. Massive lymphocele on thigh of patient with right-sided heart failure. Blood gas analysis on room air showed PO_2 of 38 mm Hg and PCO_2 of 72 mm Hg.

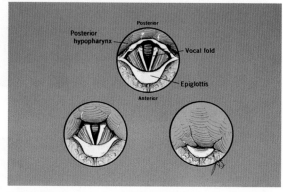

FIGURE 77-15. Appearance of the airway in obstructive sleep apnea with posterior collapse during obstructive episodes.

TABLE 77-2 ✦ STRATEGIC APPROACH TO THE TREATMENT OF SLEEP APNEA

Continuous positive airway pressure or bilevel positive airway pressure	Least invasive, but compliance is an issue
Uvulopalatopharyngoplasty (UPP)	50% of patients cured
Tongue advancement with sling	Variable results
Tongue and hyoid advancement	With UPP, may avoid tracheostomy
Two-jaw orthognathic surgery	Major surgery
Tracheostomy	The gold standard for relief of obstruction

On occasion, there are underlying medical or systemic disorders that require astute diagnosis and treatment. Among these one can list acromegaly and muscular dystrophy.[115] Cranial nerve palsies seldom result in obstructive sleep apnea.

Treatment of Sleep Apnea

Treatment may be divided between medical and surgical approaches. The medical treatment attempted in the past included medroxyprogesterone, tricyclic antidepressants, γ-hydroxybutyrate, acetazolamide, strychnine, oxygen, and weight loss. It is seldom that a medical treatment is successful. Weight loss in particular has proved difficult for most patients.

Of greatest success are continuous positive airway pressure and bilevel positive airway pressure. In our center, continuous positive airway pressure has largely been supplanted by bilevel positive airway pressure or bimodal pharyngeal airway pressure. In these treatment alternatives, a patient wears a mask strapped to the face, and airway pressure determined to be adequate to relieve the obstruction by holding the airway open while the patient is supine is delivered to the airway. This increase in pressure holds the hypopharynx open and relieves obstructed breathing. It is effective for some patients. Studies of continuous positive airway pressure, however, have demonstrated that most patients do not comply with the treatment 50% of the time, which means they are untreated half the time. This will allow the persistence of medical abnormalities, including hypertension and daytime sleepiness.

Other nonsurgical treatments include nasopharyngeal intubations, the tongue-retaining device that moves that mandible forward slightly and holds the mouth open, and instructions to the patients that sticky food and fluids and alcohol should be avoided in the hours before sleep.

Many patients will unfortunately require surgical treatment of sleep apnea. Some are not adequately treated with continuous positive airway pressure or bilevel positive airway pressure, and many patients among those who might be adequately treated cannot tolerate wearing a mask and the necessity of sleeping with it in place. When deciding on the best approach for relief of airway obstruction for a given patient, the surgeon should explain to the patient that every reduction in airway resistance leads to an improvement. The first intervention may not adequately relieve the obstruction, but when it is coupled with a second intervention, a significant relief may be obtained and the continuous positive airway pressure may be eliminated. The patient should be instructed that there is a treatment ladder to solve the problem of airway obstruction and sleep apnea. The lowest rung is typically a uvulopalatopharyngoplasty, and options ascend from here through various steps to the final gold standard for treatment, namely, tracheostomy.

The surgical treatment should correct the anatomic obstruction. This should include relief of nasal obstruction when necessary. Other alternatives include uvulopalatopharyngoplasty, tonsillectomy and adenoidectomy, tongue advancement, tongue reduction, fascial sling for tongue advancement, orthognathic surgery, and, last, tracheostomy (see Table 77-2).

UVULOPALATOPHARYNGOPLASTY

Uvulopalatopharyngoplasty was popularized by Fujita.[116] In this operation, the redundant uvula and the excess mucosal folds of the soft palate are removed (Fig. 77-16). The mucosa of the anterior and posterior tonsillar pillars is also typically removed, and tonsillectomy is performed if there are clinically detectable tonsils.

One might ask why this works. To understand why, one must consider the side view of the patient. The soft palate and uvula normally descend behind the tongue. Indeed, we have described patients whose uvula was so long that it actually entered the laryngeal inlet. This was directly observed under nasopharyngeal endoscopy. When the patient is relaxed and especially when the patient is recumbent, the soft tissue of the uvula and soft palate are lying behind the tongue. Here they function like a plug, just like the stem of a needle valve. By reducing this soft tissue, one effectively opens the valve and allows the passage of air. It has been demonstrated that the continual stretching with inspiration causes the hypertrophy of the muscular uvula. This further complicates the problem. It is as if the constant stretching is causing a tissue expansion and hypertrophy, which only worsens the problem.[117] Uvulopalatopharyngoplasty may be curative.

Relief may not be absolute. Uvulopalatopharyngoplasty should then be considered an important adjunct

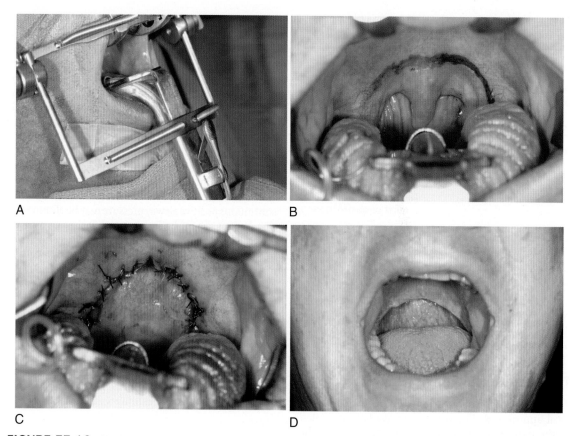

FIGURE 77-16. Uvulopalatopharyngoplasty. *A,* The Dingman retractor in place on the tongue. *B,* The marking on the soft palate and anterior tonsillar pillars. *C,* After excision of the soft palate and the anterior tonsillar pillars. *D,* The late result of the operation.

to other treatments. It is not a substitute for tracheostomy in cases of severe desaturation and right-sided heart decompensation.

Uvulopalatopharyngoplasty will benefit two of three patients in the early postoperative period. It is an excellent treatment for excessive snoring. It is always indicated for uvular prolapse into the larynx when this has been demonstrated or when it is suspected. Long-term studies have demonstrated that approximately 50% of patients are clinically cured in 2 years after the surgery.[118] Interestingly, when the cohort of treated patients were observed, some of those patients whose treatment initially failed had open airways and were cured of sleep apnea at the later evaluation.

The operation is conducted today in one of several ways. It is a straightforward procedure that may be performed with direct electrocautery or a laser ablation in the outpatient setting. Radiofrequency tissue destruction has also been used. It is possible to anesthetize the uvula and the soft palate under direct vision with the patient's mouth open. One of these ablative techniques can then be used to reduce the soft tissue.

The operative techniques with general anesthesia afford a better exposure and allow more extensive removal of excessive tissue. For this to be carried out, the patient is placed on an operating room table with a roll under the shoulder. The neck is extended, and a Dingman retractor is placed in the mouth with the tongue blade centered over the endotracheal tube positioned over the middle of the tongue. The Dingman retractor is opened to expose the oral cavity. Because many of these patients have large tongues, it sometimes requires a few minutes to maneuver the tongue, balancing its bulk so that the tube rests right in the middle and so holds it out of the way. The operator should take care to see that the tongue is not pressed against the mandibular incisors, potentially making it ischemic and leading to swelling later. The markings are made across the soft palate about 1 cm or so above the highest arc of the mucosa adjacent to the uvula. It is possible to turn the forceps in one hand so that the round end is used as a probe. One can usually see the point at which the mucosa thins as it passes over the edge of the palatal musculature. One can feel this as the end of the forceps is passed across the hard palate over the muscle of the soft palate and then over the hanging velum of mucosa adjacent to the uvula. The markings for the incision are extended down onto the anterior tonsillar pillar. If there is a tonsil present, this is noted, and the proper instruments for a tonsillectomy are moved to the field. The area for incision is injected with 1% lidocaine containing epinephrine 1:100,000 for hemostasis.

Now the mucosa is incised from the anterior tonsillar pillar across the soft palate, across the base of the uvula, and down the other side in a mirror image fashion. A sharp pointed scissor is now brought to the field. The uvula is grasped and placed under tension, and the scissor is passed through the mucosal incision and through the posterior mucosa of the soft palate; this is repeated on the other side of the uvula. Scissors are then inserted with one blade in either of the perforations just made, and the muscular uvula is transected sharply. Now it may be of advantage to transect the specimen. On one side of the uvula or the other, one then picks up the mucosa and dissects with the scissors, removing the excess mucosa down to the tonsillar fossa. If there is palpable tonsil present, one now proceeds to perform a tonsillectomy. The mucosa is grasped with a forceps, and a Fisher dissecting tool is used to gently move the muscle of the anterior tonsillar pillar away from the tonsil. The tonsil is delivered outward from its fossa on its inferior vascular pole and is then encircled by a snare; electrocautery is then applied to cauterize the inferior pole vessels as the snare is tightened. The tonsil's vasculature is divided, and the tonsil is delivered. Redundant mucosa on the posterior tonsillar pillar can now be excised sharply with the scissor. The same routine is carried out on the other side, and then both sides are inspected for hemostasis. Electrocautery is used when necessary to gain good hemostasis. The open wound is now closed with interrupted 3-0 sutures of absorbable material.

The operator will immediately observe the increase in size of the airway after this closure is complete. The operation is not complete, however, without the passage of the nasopharyngeal airway and its being secured to the membranous septum with a suture. It has been our custom to have the patients sleep the first night with this in place and then, finding that he or she has done well, removing it the next morning.

By and large, patients do well. They report that they have difficulty with speaking and swallowing for 1 week after surgery, but this rapidly resolves. There is neither change in voice nor velopharyngeal incompetence. A rare patient notes that there may be some escape of drinking water into the nasopharynx when the patient bends over to drink from a low-lying water fountain. Overall, pharyngeal function is unaffected by the operation, and the airway may be greatly improved.

If the patient reports transient regurgitation of food and fluid into the nasopharynx in the first week, this calls for reassurance. The regurgitation is simply due to the patient's being reluctant to fully move the soft palate because of pain. As soon as this pain resolves, the swallowing will be normal.

The role of the tongue in sleep apnea is still somewhat difficult to ascertain, but it does appear that the tongue is a major contributor to obstruction. If a patient has had uvulopalatopharyngoplasty and continues to have persistent obstruction, the next thing to suggest is that the patient employ a dental device that holds the mouth open and advances the jaw slightly so that the tongue is moved forward and the oral airway is held open at night. This can result in successful treatment of sleep apnea in those patients for whom uvulopalatopharyngoplasty has not been adequate.

TONGUE ADVANCEMENT

Tongue advancement may be of value for infants with micrognathia, for adults with retrusion, for patients whose uvulopalatopharyngoplasty fails, and for avoidance or reversal of tracheostomy. The tongue may be advanced in one of several ways. One may use a fascial sling, which has been described for infants by Puckett et al.[119] One can perform sliding window genioplasty and hyoid suspension, orthognathic surgery such as sagittal split ramus osteotomy, or sagittal split ramus osteotomy with simultaneous maxillary advancement.[120,121]

Fascial Tongue Sling

The fascial tongue sling begins with harvesting of a strip of fascia lata of approximately 20 cm in length in the adult (Fig. 77-17). This gives plenty of length to allow passage of the fascia and ready tying of a fascial knot to fix the fascia to the mandible. The fascial sling is designed to the specifications of 20 cm long and 0.5 cm or more wide. To insert the fascial sling, one makes an incision in the submental crease. The mandible is exposed at the symphysis. A long fine curved hemostat is then inserted through the musculature of the base of the tongue to a point at or below the circumvallate papilla of the posterior tongue. The index finger is placed on this area and advances the hemostat to it. When the clamp reaches this point, one creates a stab wound in the mucosa of the tongue and the hemostat emerges. One end of the fascia is now passed to the hemostat, which is withdrawn, delivering the fascia to the anterior wound.

Now the clamp is passed with the curve of the hemostat positioned opposite the original pass. One goes through the other side of the base of the tongue, passing the snap 1 or 2 cm from the midline to the exit site already established. When the snap emerges, the other

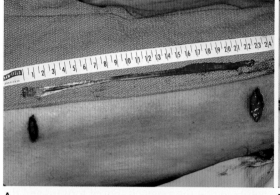

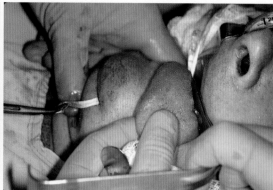

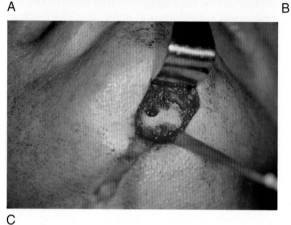

FIGURE 77-17. Designing a fascial sling for the tongue. *A,* Harvest of a fascial strip. *B,* Passing the strip through the tongue. *C,* Tying the fascial strip through a hole at the symphysis.

fascial end is delivered into the open tip of the snap, and the fascia is drawn into the tongue so that it is not visible below the musca. The mucosal stab wound can now be closed with a chromic stitch.

The symphysis is now drilled so that there is a hole adequate to allow passage of the one end of the fascia. The fascia is drawn somewhat tight, and a half-hitch is tied with the operator's index finger lying on the posterior tongue where the closure sutures are palpable. The fascial strips should be pulled tight and held snug when the operator feels the groove in the posterior tongue lift off the index finger. The fascia can now be secured to itself by completing the knot and by reinforcing this knot with permanent sutures.

The fascial sling is not at all evident when the submental incision is closed. The tongue itself is not advanced. It is important to understand this. What happens can be demonstrated to the patient by holding a tie in one's hand. The end is extended to the patient as if it were a tongue. One then demonstrates by pushing with a finger how one makes a groove in the more vertical posterior tongue when the sling is inserted. The tongue itself is not advanced, but it is the groove that opens the airway when the patient is recumbent (Fig.

77-18). This has not interfered with glutition or speech in any of our patients.

Sliding Window Genioplasty and Hyoid Suspension

This operation can actually reverse tracheostomy in patients who have been dependent on this option for treatment of sleep apnea. The operation consists of two parts, a tongue advancement and a hyoid suspension, either of which may be performed first (Fig. 77-19).

The operation is begun with an incision in the submental crease. One enters the plane just above the digastric muscles and follows this down to the hyoid. Infiltration of 1% lidocaine with epinephrine 1:100,000 before this dissection is helpful. The anterior face of the hyoid is exposed, and then a right-angled clamp is inserted underneath the sternohyoid, omohyoid, and thyrohyoid muscles. These are divided with electrocautery. The anterior belly of the digastrics and the stylohyoid attachments are divided laterally. This allows a significant elevation of the hyoid.

Now one drills two holes on either side of the midline of the hyoid. Through each hole, a strand of wire is drawn; the suspension material is placed right to its posterior aspect. By advancing the genio-tubercle forward, one moves the base of the muscle forward, thereby advancing the entire tongue. Once again, it is the base of the tongue that is advancing. The tip of the tongue does not visibly advance with this procedure.

To advance the geniotubercle, one inscribes a rectangle on the center of the symphysis. It is about 2 cm in transverse diameter and 1 cm in vertical dimension. It should lie below the roots of the central incisors. One can get an idea of proper placement by looking at the undersurface of a native mandible. One can also palpate the geniotubercle with a finger. It can also be located with a probing needle if necessary.

The bone is now cut with a saw, and a towel clip is used to lift the rectangle up and forward. It is turned 90 degrees, thereby holding it fast in the advanced position; because the symphysis is thick here, there will be at least 1 cm of advancement.

The outer table of the symphysis is excised at this point, giving a lower profile to the remaining piece of symphysis that is holding the genioglossus muscle forward. The piece of outer table is now bisected and placed in the defect on either side of the inner table that has been turned 90 degrees. This construct is now secured with a wire suture or plate so that it is secure in its new orientation. One now closes the wound, and the operation is complete.

Nelson Powell first described this operation, which has proved surprisingly effective even in severe cases of obstructive sleep apnea. In an evaluation of our patients in whom this technique was used, five of seven patients with tracheotomies for whom this operation was performed had improvement that was significant enough to allow reversal of their tracheostomies.

The effect of the hyoid suspension and the sliding window genioplasty can be verified with radiographs of the neck. These should be obtained in the upright position and then with the patient supine. The supine radiograph will demonstrate significant opening of the airway with advancement of the posterior tongue.

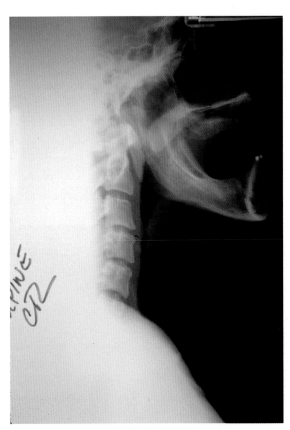

FIGURE 77-18. Radiograph demonstrating fascial restraint of the tongue with the patient in the supine position.

underneath, and the wire is tightened securely. It has been our custom to use the rolled edge of a sheet of Marlex. This is incorporated into the tissues well, and it has been employed with the thought that should it ever fatigue or break, there would be a fibrous sleeve to perpetuate the suspension. Fascia lata could also be used. The strips can now be drawn through the incision, and one can repeatedly demonstrate in the operating room a significant advancement of the hyoid with gentle traction. At this junction, drill holes are placed through the caudal border of the symphysis, and the strands are drawn through and secured with wire ligatures. This moves the hyoid up and forward, but it does predispose the patient to several days of aspiration. This can be overcome with careful counseling so the patient sips slowly and cautiously and eats food that is pureed at the beginning of the postoperative period.

The second portion of the procedure rests on the anatomic realization that the genioglossus muscle originates on a spur on the internal surface of the symphysis. It branches out with multiple strands that go through the body of the tongue from the anterior base

TRACHEOSTOMY

It must be said that although many patients fear it, tracheostomy is the gold standard for relief of sleep apnea. Only those physicians who have never treated patients with severe sleep apnea could doubt that tracheostomy is the preferred treatment of the most advanced forms of this condition. Tracheostomy is revitalizing. The response of the patient is absolutely magnificent. Weight loss almost invariably follows tracheostomy, and it can be massive. In patients who have right-sided heart failure, the weight loss with or without the use of diuretics may exceed 100 pounds. The greatest weight loss in our experience was 136

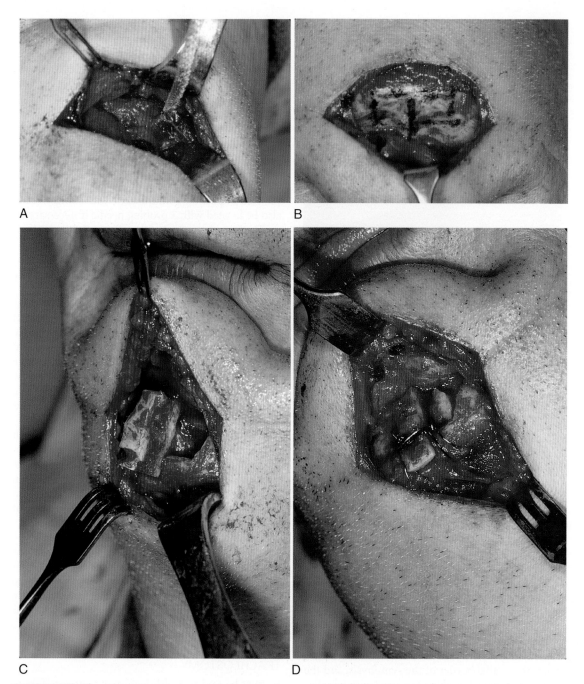

FIGURE 77-19. Hyoid suspension and genioglossus tubercle advancement of the tongue. *A*, Exposure of the hyoid bone with muscle releases and attachment of straps of Marlex. *B*, Rectangular osteotomies in the symphysis. *C*, Moving the bone forward with a 90-degree turn of the segment. *D*, Symphysis with bone and hyoid straps secured.

pounds within 10 days of tracheostomy. This occurred because the reversal of right-sided heart failure allowed a significant mobilization of fluid with subsequent diuresis.

For the patient with a PO_2 of 38 mm Hg and a PCO_2 of 72 mm Hg on room air, a tracheostomy is typically required. Preoperative evaluation with an echocardiogram will reveal an elevated pulmonary pressure and a dilated right ventricle. A patient such as this should not have major surgery without having a tracheostomy performed first and a period for cardiac recovery from right-sided heart failure (see Fig. 77-

14). It was the patient with these gas values who lost 136 pounds in just 10 days after tracheostomy.

Tracheostomy should be performed with a local anesthesia with the anesthesia staff standing by. It is usually necessary for the surgeon to remind the anesthesia staff, especially residents involved in the care of patients with sleep apnea, that these patients should not receive any sedation. Arrhythmias have been observed in patients with sleep apnea who were unwittingly sedated before their surgeries. With 10 mL of 1% lidocaine with epinephrine, one can obtain adequate local anesthesia to allow smooth and rapid tracheostomy for these patients.

It has also been our custom to avoid use of standard Jackson or Shiley tracheostomy tubes or even the more modern Bevona tubes. We have preferred instead to place a Montgomery cannula, which is a simple silicone tube (Fig. 77-20). The Montgomery cannula has two flanges on its innermost end, which are angled at 27 degrees to the horizontal. This is the typical angle from the vertical of the trachea in the neck. The flanges therefore lie on the anterior tracheal wall and support the tube in position. The tube fits tightly, and numerous patients have been able to swim with the tube in place. Patients are told that they should not dive in and that they should not swim in an area where their feet do not touch bottom with the neck out of the water. The Montgomery cannula is particularly successful because there is virtually no drainage and no air escape. It requires little or no daily care. Patients can shower without water entering the airway.

We have used Jackson tubes, Olympic tubes, and Shiley tubes in addition to the Montgomery cannula. Our conviction is that the Montgomery cannula is by far superior. The Jackson tube is a time-honored device. It is available everywhere. It is easily cleaned and easily replaced. It is reliable. It is nonreactive, and several sizes are available. It is, however, uncomfortable. There is odor and drainage, and it requires a tie around the neck. Water enters the trachea in the shower, and speech may be complicated by air escape; the irritation of the tube in the airway may cause coughing.

The Teflon Olympic tube does not require ties. It is comfortable and has an inner cannula that is easy to clean. It is easily closed with an obturator and easily changed. However, odor is a major problem. The Teflon is permeable and porous enough to allow bacterial growth, and drainage is sometimes a problem. Granulation tissue frequently forms along the anterior lip of the tracheostomy stoma, and displacement is not uncommon. There are retaining feet that lift outward with insertion of the inner cannula to help hold the tube in the trachea. With long-term use, these can fatigue and rarely break. Only two lengths are available. There is an obturator that closes the cannula. The obturator is worn during the day, and at night a hollow cannula is inserted. As these two devices (obturator and cannula) are inserted, they spread the feet to help stabilize the tube. This tube does not have a beveled edge, however, and it therefore projects into the airway. The fact that only two lengths are available also limits its adaptability. It did serve some patients well, however, its chief advantage being its low profile at the level of the stoma.

The Montgomery tube is a simple design. It maximizes the airway and need not be removed. It can be removed weekly and even daily, however, if so desired. Patients can learn to take this tube out, clean it in the sink, and return it to its correct position. The length can be adjusted with scissors. It is comfortable, and most patients adapt very well indeed.

The tracheostomy operation is conducted with an incision approximately two finger spaces above the suprasternal notch. The incision need only be approximately 3 cm long at the most. The skin is retracted to expose the subcutaneous fat, and then the operation is a shared venture between the surgeon and the assistant. Initially, each holds a pair of double hooks in the left hand and spreads with a hemostat in the right hand. The two operators spread at right angles to each other. This will carry them through the subcutaneous soft tissues down to the strap muscles, which are separated in a similar fashion in the midline. When this is accomplished, an Army-Navy retractor is inserted on each side and the wound is spread widely. This separates the strap muscles and exposes the thyroid. The thyroid is now visualized, and a right-angled clamp is placed underneath the superior isthmus. The isthmus is dissected off the trachea, and then a right-angled clamp is placed with its tip projecting caudally on one side; a mirror image application of another right-angled clamp is carried out on the other side. The thyroid isthmus is split between these two right-angled clamps, and a permanent suture is placed as a suture ligature around the stump

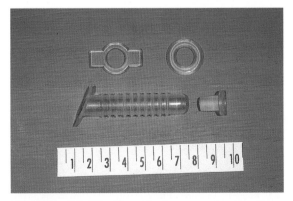

FIGURE 77-20. The Montgomery tracheostomy cannula.

of divided thyroid. This is continued until the isthmus is divided and the anterior trachea is exposed nicely.

At this juncture, a special tool, the Montgomery trephine tool, is brought to the field (Fig. 77-21). It has a barrel with a toothed tip. This is applied firmly to the anterior tracheal wall. A cannula with a smooth cutting edge on the other end and an adaptor for suction tubing is inserted into the stabilized outer cannula. The outer cannula is positioned first to involve the second tracheal ring, leaving the first intact. The cutting sleeve is now passed into the positioning cannula and twisted against the trachea until the trachea is entered and the disk is aspirated into the suction line. The Montgomery cannula is now brought to the field and is grasped with a curved hemostat and simply inserted under direct vision. Both feet must be in the trachea. It is then pulled forward until it is seated properly. A single stitch placed on either side of the cannula serves to close the skin incision. The tube should not be plugged because this will lead to subcutaneous emphysema. We routinely leave the tube unplugged for 3 days.

There is a retaining washer that may be placed over the tube. If it is placed on the cannula, it should not initially be placed down to skin level. There will be some swelling, and with projection of the patient's neck, the tube can be dislodged if the retaining washer is placed at skin level. It is therefore best to position it higher away from the skin.

The patient is instructed to cover the end of the tube with the finger to speak. The operator can demonstrate this to the patient, and indeed this is reassuring for the patient.

This operation goes extremely well and is quick as well as virtually painless for the patient. At the conclusion, the patient is usually watched in the hospital for 2 days before discharge to home. In the hospital, the patient is taught how to clean the tube with a cotton-tipped applicator. Some patients are issued ear curets to scrape away crust on the inside when necessary. There are wire loop ear curets and also solid ear curets. The solid ear curets are preferred because the metal of the wire loop may fatigue and break.

The gratitude of patients receiving tracheostomies is one of the most satisfying observations that the surgeon will encounter in practice. Lives are literally transformed for the better by the simple act of inserting a tracheostomy into a patient who is severally compromised by obstructive sleep apnea.

The aftercare is simple. Tubes are normally left in place for a good 6 weeks before patients are taught how to remove the tube and change it. The short-term tube has ridges that circle the tube almost down to the intertracheal portion. The long-term silicone cannulas have a smooth portion that occupies most of the space below the skin level. These are therefore much easier to remove and replace in the home setting.

It is extremely important to counsel the patient that whenever he or she is going to sleep, even to nap, the cannula should be unplugged. The plugs are typically attached to a retaining ring so that they are close at hand and ready for reinsertion with awakening. Medical personnel who care for the patient must be instructed that at the time of anesthesia, the tube need not be removed. The endotracheal tube can easily pass by the Montgomery cannula, and this can be observed directly with a flashlight if anyone so wishes. The tube should be plugged during the course of the anesthesia. Afterward, in recovery, it is absolutely essential that the tube be unplugged. During the period of recovery from general anesthesia, airway obstruction is common unless the tracheostomy is open.

It is possible to place a Montgomery cannula in a patient with a thick fatty neck. In some patients, however, it will be of advantage to reduce the subcutaneous fat with a suction lipectomy. This reduces the large roll that may descend over the tracheostomy tube. By reducing this fat, one can obtain a much better result for the patient. This can be done under local anesthesia before the insertion of the tracheostomy. It can even be carried out afterward also.

Early recognition and treatment of sleep apnea are most valuable and will greatly benefit the patient. It is a gratifying experience for the surgeon, too, because lives can literally be saved through this intervention. There is an enormous benefit in terms of quality of life as well. Those surgeons choosing to work with pulmonologists and internists in the diagnosis and care of patients with significant obstructive sleep apnea will find this work a great delight.

REFERENCES

1. Rouge JC, Lacourt G: Effects of nasogastric intubation on respiratory resistance and work in newborn and premature infants [in French]. Ann Anesthesiol Fr 1975;16(spec no 1):101-104.

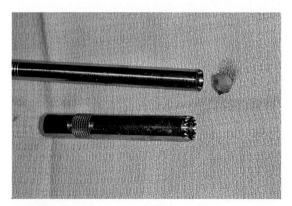

FIGURE 77-21. The Montgomery trephine tool with a 6-mm-diameter disk of anterior tracheal wall.

2. Lacourt G, Polgar G: Interaction between nasal and pulmonary resistance in newborn infants. J Appl Physiol 1971;30:870-873.

3. Losken A, Burstein FD, Williams JK: Congenital nasal pyriform aperture stenosis: diagnosis and treatment. Plast Reconstr Surg 2002;109:1506-1511, discussion 1512.

4. Johnson PJ, Rydlund K, Hollins RR: Congenital nasal pyriform aperture stenosis. Plast Reconstr Surg 1999;103:1696-1699.

5. Nemechek AJ, Amedee RG: Choanal atresia. J La State Med Soc 1994;146:337-340.

6. Harris J, Robert E, Kallen B: Epidemiology of choanal atresia with specific reference to CHARGE association. Pediatrics 1997;99:363-367.

7. Tellier AL, Cormier-Daire V, Abadie V, et al: CHARGE syndrome: report of 47 cases and review. Am J Med Genet 1998;76:402-409.

8. Keller JL, Kacker A: Choanal atresia, CHARGE association, and congenital nasal stenosis. Otolaryngol Clin North Am 2000;33:1343-1351, viii.

9. Koltai PJ, Hoehn J, Bailey CM: The external rhinoplasty approach for rhinologic surgery in children. Arch Otolaryngol Head Neck Surg 1992;118:401-405.

10. Healy GB: An approach to the nasal septum in children. Laryngoscope 1986;96:1239-1242.

11. Josephson GD, Levine J, Cutting CB: Septoplasty for obstructive sleep apnea in infants after cleft lip repair. Cleft Palate Craniofac J 1996;33:473-476.

12. Byrd HS, Salomon J: Primary correction of the unilateral cleft nasal deformity. Plast Reconstr Surg 2000;106:1276-1286.

13. McComb H: Treatment of the unilateral cleft lip nose. Plast Reconstr Surg 1975;55:596-601.

14. Anastassov GE, Joos U, Zollner B: Evaluation of the results of delayed rhinoplasty in cleft lip and palate patients. Functional and aesthetic implications and factors that affect successful nasal repair. Br J Oral Maxillofac Surg 1998;36:416-424.

15. Meyer R: Total external and internal construction in arhinia. Plast Reconstr Surg 1997;99:534-542.

16. Wesley RE: Inferior turbinate fracture in the treatment of congenital nasolacrimal duct obstruction and congenital nasolacrimal duct anomaly. Ophthalmic Surg 1985;16:368-371.

17. Yagci A, Karci B, Ergezen F: Probing and bicanalicular silicone tube intubation under nasal endoscopy in congenital nasolacrimal duct obstruction. Ophthalmic Plast Reconstr Surg 2000;16:58-61.

18. Hepler KM, Woodson GE, Kearns DB: Respiratory distress in the neonate. Sequela of a congenital dacryocystocele. Arch Otolaryngol Head Neck Surg 1995;121:1423-1425.

19. Righi PD, Hubbell RN, Lawlor PP Jr: Respiratory distress associated with bilateral nasolacrimal duct cysts. Int J Pediatr Otorhinolaryngol 1993;26:199-203.

20. Bloom DC, Carvalho DS, Dory C, et al: Imaging and surgical approach of nasal dermoids. Int J Pediatr Otorhinolaryngol 2002;62:111-122.

21. Wesley RK, Scannell T, Nathan LE: Nasolabial cyst: presentation of a case with a review of the literature. J Oral Maxillofac Surg 1984;42:188-192.

22. Gysin C, Alothman GA, Papsin BC: Sinonasal disease in cystic fibrosis: clinical characteristics, diagnosis, and management. Pediatr Pulmonol 2000;30:481-489.

23. Bratton C, Suskind DL, Thomas T, Kluk EA: Autosomal dominant familial frontonasal dermoid cysts: a mother and her identical twin daughters. Int J Pediatr Otorhinolaryngol 2001;57:249-253.

24. Verney Y, Zanolla G, Teixeira R, Oliveira LC: Midline nasal mass in infancy: a nasal glioma case report. Eur J Pediatr Surg 2001;11:324-327.

25. Shimizu T, Kitamura S, Kinouchi K, Fukumitsu K: A rare case of upper airway obstruction in an infant caused by basal encephalocele complicating facial midline deformity. Paediatr Anaesth 1999;9:73-76.

26. Cohen AF, Mitsudo S, Ruben RJ: Nasopharyngeal teratoma in the neonate. Int J Pediatr Otorhinolaryngol 1987;14:187-195.

27. Cheddadi D, Triki S, Gallet S, et al: Neonatal rhinopharyngeal obstruction due to craniopharyngioma [in French]. Arch Pediatr 1996;3:348-351.

28. Coppit GL 3rd, Perkins JA, Manning SC: Nasopharyngeal teratomas and dermoids: a review of the literature and case series. Int J Pediatr Otorhinolaryngol 2000;52:219-227.

29. Sagol S, Itil IM, Ozsaran A, et al: Prenatal sonographic detection of nasopharyngeal teratoma. J Clin Ultrasound 1999;27:469-473.

30. April mm, Ward RF, Garelick JM: Diagnosis, management, and follow-up of congenital head and neck teratomas. Laryngoscope 1998;108:1398-1401.

31. Wenig BM, Heffner DK: Respiratory epithelial adenomatoid hamartomas of the sinonasal tract and nasopharynx: a clinicopathologic study of 31 cases. Ann Otol Rhinol Laryngol 1995;104:639-645.

32. Minuto FM, Fazzuoli L, Rollandi GA, et al: Successful autotransplantation of lingual thyroid: 37-year follow-up. Lancet 1995;346:910.

33. Rimell FL, Shapiro AM, Shoemaker DL, Kenna MA: Head and neck manifestations of Beckwith-Wiedemann syndrome. Otolaryngol Head Neck Surg 1995;113:262-265.

34. Morgan WE, Friedman EM, Duncan NO, Sulek M: Surgical management of macroglossia in children. Arch Otolaryngol Head Neck Surg 1996;122:326-329.

35. Nieminen P, Lopponen T, Tolonen U, et al: Growth and biochemical markers of growth in children with snoring and obstructive sleep apnea. Pediatrics 2002;109:e55.

36. Loke D, Ghosh S, Panaese A, Bull PD: Endoscopic division of the aryepiglottic folds in severe laryngomalacia. Int J Pediatr Otorhinolaryngol 2001;60:59-63.

37. Bullard KM, Scott Adzick N, Harrison MR: A mediastinal window approach to aortopexy. J Pediatr Surg 1997;32:680-681.

38. Milczuk HA, Smith JD, Everts EC: Congenital laryngeal webs: surgical management and clinical embryology. Int J Pediatr Otolaryngol 2000;52(1)1-9.

39. Pollack IF, Kinnunen D, Albright AL: The effect of early craniocervical decompression on functional outcome in neonates and young infants with myelodysplasia and symptomatic Chiari II malformations: results from a prospective series. Neurosurgery 1996;38:703-710.

40. Hartley BE, Rutter MJ, Cotton RT: Cricotracheal resection as a primary procedure for laryngotracheal stenosis in children. Int J Pediatr Otorhinolaryngol 2000;54:133-136.

41. Lifshultz BD, Donoghue ER: Deaths due to foreign body aspiration in children: the continuing hazard of toy balloons. J Forensic Sci 1996;41:247-251.

42. Demianczuk AN, Verchere C, Phillips JH: The effect on facial growth of pediatric mandibular fractures. J Craniofac Surg 1999;10:323-328.

43. Landa L, Gordon CB, Kathju S, Sotereanos G: Open reduction of condylar fracture: a long-term follow-up. J Oral Maxillofac Surg; in press.

44. Kaban LB: Diagnosis and treatment of fractures of the facial bones in children 1943-1993. J Oral Maxillofac Surg 1993;51:722-729.

45. Brodsky L, Moore L, Stanievich J: The role of *Haemophilus influenzae* in the pathogenesis of tonsillar hypertrophy in children. Laryngoscope 1988;98:1055-1060.

46. Spitalnic SJ, Sucov A: Ludwig's angina: case report and review. J Emerg Med 1995;13:499-503.

47. Silva AB: Airway manifestations of pediatric gastroesophageal reflux disease. In Wetmore RF, Muntz HR, McGill TJ, eds: Pediatric Otolaryngology. New York, Thieme, 2000:619.

48. Azizkhan RG, Dudgeon DL, Buck JR, et al: Life-threatening airway obstruction as a complication to the management of mediastinal masses in children. J Pediatr Surg. 1985;20:816-822.

49. Mulliken JB, Glowacki J: Hemangiomas and vascular malformations in infants and children: a classification based upon endothelial characteristics. Plast Reconstr Surg 1982;69:412-422.

50. Mulliken JB: A biologic approach to cutaneous vascular anomalies. Pediatr Dermatol 1992;9:356-357.

51. Amir J, Metzker A, Krikler R, Reisner SH: Strawberry hemangioma in preterm infants. Pediatr Dermatol 1986;3:331-332.

52. Ritter MR, Dorrell MI, Edmonds J, et al: Insulin-like growth factor 2 and potential regulators of hemangioma growth and involution identified by large-scale expression analysis. Proc Natl Acad Sci USA 2002;99:7455-7460.

53. Lopriore E, Markhorst DG: Diffuse neonatal haemangiomatosis: new views on diagnostic criteria and prognosis. Acta Paediatr 1999;88:93-97.

54. DeLuca L, Guyuron B, Najem RW: Management of an extensive cervicofacial lymphovenous malformation of the maxillofacial region. Ann Plast Surg 1996;36:644-648.

55. Hartl DM, Roger G, Denoyelle F, et al: Extensive lymphangioma presenting with upper airway obstruction. Arch Otolaryngol Head Neck Surg 2000;126:1378-1382.

56. Kaban LB, Mulliken JB: Vascular anomalies of the maxillofacial region. J Oral Maxillofac Surg. 1986;44:203-213.

57. Coleman CC Jr: Diagnosis and treatment of congenital arteriovenous fistulas of the head and neck. Am J Surg 1973;126:557-565.

58. Bush PG, Williams AJ: Incidence of the Robin anomalad (Pierre Robin syndrome). Br J Plast Surg 1983;36:434-437.

59. Prows CA, Bender PL: Beyond Pierre Robin sequence. Neonatal Netw 1999;18:13-19.

60. Robin P: A fall of the base of the tongue considered as a new cause of nasopharyngeal respiratory impairment: Pierre Robin sequence, a translation. 1923 [classical article]. Plast Reconstr Surg 1994;93:1301-1303.

61. Ricks JE, Ryder VM, Bridgewater LC, et al: Altered mandibular development precedes the time of palate closure in mice homozygous for disproportionate micromelia: an oral clefting model supporting the Pierre-Robin sequence. Teratology 2002;65:116-120.

62. Thacht BT: Maturation and transformation of reflexes that protect the laryngeal airway from liquid aspiration from fetal to adult life [review]. Am J Med 2001;111(suppl 8A):69S-77S.

63. Cruz MJ, Kerschner JE, Beste DJ, Conley SF: Pierre Robin sequences: secondary respiratory difficulties and intrinsic feeding abnormalities. Laryngoscope 1999;109:1632-1636.

64. Ortiz Monasterio F, Drucker M, Molina F, Ysunza A: Distraction osteogenesis in Pierre Robin sequence and related respiratory problems in children. J Craniofac Surg 2002;13:79-83.

65. Abramson DL, Marrinan EM, Mulliken JB: Robin sequence: obstructive sleep apnea following pharyngeal flap. Cleft Palate Craniofac J 1997;34:256-260.

66. Liao YF, Chuang ML, Chen PK, et al: Incidence and severity of obstructive sleep apnea following pharyngeal flap surgery in patients with cleft palate. Cleft Palate Craniofac J 2002;39:312-316.

67. Aragon SB: Surgical management for snoring and sleep apnea. Dent Clin North Am 2001;45:867-879.

68. Karakasis DT, Michaelides CM, Tsara V: Mandibular distraction combined with tongue-base traction for treatment of obstructive sleep apnea syndrome. Plast Reconstr Surg 2001;108:1673-1676.

69. Turnbull NR, Battagel JM: The effects of orthognathic surgery on pharyngeal airway dimensions and quality of sleep. J Orthod 2000;27:235-247.

70. Li KK, Riley RW, Powell NB, Troell RJ: Obstructive sleep apnea surgery: genioglossus advancement revisited. J Oral Maxillofac Surg 2001;59:1181-1184, discussion1185.

71. Hendler BH, Costello BJ, Silverstein K, et al: A protocol for uvulopalatopharyngoplasty, mortised genioplasty, and maxillomandibular advancement in patients with obstructive sleep apnea: an analysis of 40 cases. J Oral Maxillofac Surg 2001;59:892-897, discussion 898-899.

72. Bell RB, Turvey TA: Skeletal advancement for the treatment of obstructive sleep apnea in children. Cleft Palate Craniofac J 2001;38:147-154.

73. Codivilla A: On the means of lengthening in the lower limbs, the muscles and tissues which are shortened through deformity. Am J Orthop Surg 1905;2:353-369.

74. Ilizarov GA, Devyatov AA, Keamerin VK: Plastic reconstruction of longitudinal bone defects by means of compression and subsequent distraction. Acta Chir Plast 1980;22:32-41.

75. Snyder CC, Levine GA, Swanson HM, et al: Mandibular lengthening by gradual distraction. Plast Reconstr Surg 1973;51:506-508.

76. McCarthy JG, Schreiber J, Karp N, et al: Lengthening of the human mandible by gradual distraction. Plast Reconstr Surg 1992;89:1-10.

77. Molina F, Ortiz Monasterio F: Mandibular elongation and remodeling by distraction: a farewell to major osteotomies. Plast Reconstr Surg 1995;96:825-840.

78. Swennen G, Schliephake H, Dempf R, et al: Craniofacial distraction osteogenesis: a review of the literature. Part 1. Clinical studies. Int J Oral Maxillofac Surg 2001;30:89-103.

79. Li KK, Powell NB, Riley RW, Guilleminault C: Distraction osteogenesis in adult obstructive sleep apnea surgery: a preliminary report. J Oral Maxillofac Surg 2002;60:6-10.

80. Cohen SR, Burstein FD, Williams JK: The role of distraction osteogenesis in the management of craniofacial disorders [review]. Ann Acad Med Singapore 1999;28:728-738.

81. Aragon SB: Surgical management of snoring and sleep apnea [review]. Dent Clin North Am 2001;45:867-879.

82. Huertas D, Ghafari J: New posteroanterior cephalometric norms: a comparison with craniofacial measures of children treated with palatal expansion. Angle Orthod 2001;71:285-292.

83. Mattick CR, Chadwick SM, Morton ME: Mandibular advancement using an intraoral osteogenic distraction technique: a report of three clinical cases. J Orthod 2001;28:105-114.

84. Cohen SR, Simms C, Burstein FD, Thomsen J: Alternatives to tracheostomy in infants and children with obstructive sleep apnea. J Pediatr Surg 1999;34:182-186.

85. Figueroa A, Glupker TJ, Fitz MG, BeGole EA: Mandible, tongue, and airway in Pierre Robin sequence: a longitudinal cephalometric study. Cleft Palate Craniofac J 1991;28:425-434.

86. Mandell DL, Yellon RF, Bradley JP, et al: Mandibular distraction for micrognathia and severe upper airway obstruction. Arch Otolaryngol Head Neck Surg 2004;130(3):344-348.

87. Molina F, Ortiz Monasterio F: Mandibular elongation and remodeling by distraction: a farewell to major osteotomies. Plast Reconstr Surg 1995;96:825-840.

88. Kaban LB, Moses MH, Mulliken JB: Surgical correction of hemifacial microsomia in the growing child. Plast Reconstr Surg 1988;82:9-19.

89. Cohen SR, Burstein FD, Williams JK: The role of distraction osteogenesis in the management of craniofacial disorders. Ann Acad Med Singapore 1999;28:728-738.

90. Rodriguez JC, Dogliotti P: Mandibular distraction in glossoptosis-micrognathic association: preliminary report. J Craniofac Surg 1998;9:127-129.

91. Cohen SR, Simms C, Burstein FD: Mandibular distraction osteogenesis in the treatment of upper airway obstruction in children with craniofacial deformities. Plast Reconstr Surg 1998;101:312-318.

92. Judge B, Hamlar D, Rimell FL: Mandibular distraction osteogenesis in a neonate. Arch Otolaryngol Head Neck Surg 1999;125:1029-1032.

93. Denny AD, Talisman R, Hanson PR, Recinos RF: Mandibular distraction osteogenesis in very young patients to correct airway obstruction. Plast Reconstr Surg 2001;108:302-311.

94. CB Gordon, MD; BV Heil, MD; T Chang, MD; XP Reyna Radriguez, DDS; F Ortiz Monasterio, MD; Personal communication.

95. Edwards TJ, David DJ, Martin J: Aggressive surgical management of sleep apnea syndrome in the syndromal craniosynostoses. J Craniofac Surg 1992;3:8-10, discussion 11.

96. Lauritzen C, Lilja J, Jarlstedt J: Airway obstruction and sleep apnea in children with craniofacial anomalies. Plast Reconstr Surg 1986;77:1-6.

97. Delaire JP, Verdon J, Lumineau A, et al: Quelques résultats des tractions extra-orales à appui fronto-mentonnier dans le traitement orthopédique des malformations maxillo-mandibulaires de class III et des séquelles osseuses des fentes labio-maxillaires. Rev Stomatol Chir Maxillofac 1972;73:633.

98. Staffenberg DA, Wood RJ, McCarthy JG, et al: Midface distraction advancement in the canine without osteotomies. Ann Plast Surg 1995;34:512-517.

99. Polley JW, Figueroa AA: Management of severe maxillary deficiency in childhood and adolescent through distraction osteogenesis with an external, adjustable, rigid distraction device. J Craniofac Surg 1997;8:181.

100. Guerrero CA: Maxillary intraoral distraction osteogenesis. In Arnaud E, Diner PA, eds: Proceedings, 3rd International Congress on Cranial and Facial Bone Distraction Processes, Paris, France, June 14-16, 2001. Bologna, Italy, Monduzzi Editore, 2001:381-387.

101. Altuna G, Walker DA, Freeman E: Surgically assisted rapid orthodontic lengthening of the maxilla in primates—a pilot study. Am J Orthod Dentofac Orthop 1995;107:531-536.

102. Ko EW, Figueroa AA, Guyette TW, et al: Velopharyngeal changes after maxillary advancement in cleft patients with distraction osteogenesis using a rigid external distraction device: a 1-year cephalometric follow-up. J Craniofac Surg 1999;10:312-320, discussion 321-322.

103. Cohen SR, Boydston W, Hudgins R, Burstein FD: Monobloc and facial bipartition distraction with internal devices. J Craniofac Surg 1999;10:244-251.

104. Meling TR, Tveten S, Due-Tonnessen BJ, et al: Monobloc and midface distraction osteogenesis in pediatric patients with severe syndromal craniosynostosis. Pediatr Neurosurg. 2000;33:89-94.

105. Polley JW, Figueroa AA, Charbel FT, et al: Monobloc craniomaxillofacial distraction osteogenesis in a newborn with severe craniofacial synostosis: a preliminary report. J Craniofac Surg 1995;6:421-423.

106. Nadal E, Dogliotti PL, Rodriguez JC, Zuccaro G: Craniofacial distraction osteogenesis en bloc. J Craniofac Surg 2000;11:246-251, discussion 252-253.

107. Cohen SR: Craniofacial distraction with a modular internal distraction system: evolution of design and surgical techniques. Plast Reconstr Surg 1999;103:1592-1607.

108. Cohen SR, Boydston W, Burstein FD, Hudgins R: Monobloc distraction osteogenesis during infancy: report of a case and presentation of a new device. Plast Reconstr Surg 1998;101:1919-1924.

109. Levine JP, Rowe NM, Bradley JP, et al: The combination of endoscopy and distraction osteogenesis in the development of a canine midface advancement model. J Craniofac Surg 1998;9:423-432.

110. Meoli AL, Casey KR, Clark RW, et al: Hypopnea in sleep-disordered breathing in adults. Sleep 2001;24:469-470.

111. Cadieux RJ, Manders EK, Manfredi RL, et al: Uvulopalatopharyngoplasty as a treatment of obstructive sleep apnea precipitated by uvular prolapse. Ann Plast Surg 1987;19:566.

112. Piccirillo JF, Thawley SE: Sleep-disordered breathing. In Cummings CW, Krause CJ, Schuller DE, et al, eds: Otolaryngology and Head and Neck Surgery. St. Louis, Mosby, 1998:1546-1571.

113. Walker RP: Snoring and obstructive sleep apnea. In Bailey BJ, Calhoun KH, Derkay CS, et al, eds: Head and Neck Surgery-Otolaryngology, vol 1, 3rd ed. Philadelphia, Lippincott Williams & Wilkins, 2001:579-597.

114. Sugarman HJ: Obesity. In Wilmore DW, Cheung LY, Harken AH, et al, eds: ACS Surgery: Principles and Practice. New York, WebMD, 2002:1005.

115. Cadieux RJ, Kales A, McGlynn TJ, et al: Sleep apnea precipitated by pharyngeal surgery in a patient with myotonic dystrophy. Arch Otolaryngol 1984;110:611-613.

116. Fujita S, Conway W, Zorick F, et al: Surgical correction of anatomic abnormalities in obstructive sleep apnea syndrome: uvulopalatopharyngoplasty. Otolaryngol Head Neck Surg 1981;89:923.

117. Stauffer JL, Buick MK, Sharkey FF, et al: Morphology of the uvula in obstructive sleep apnea. Am Rev Respir Dis 1989;140:724-728.

118. Vgontzas AN, Manders EK, Bixler EO, et al: Long-term efficacy of uvulopalatopharyngoplasty for sleep apnea. In Beigel A, Lâopez Ibor, et al (eds): Past, Present, and Future of Psychiatry: IX World Congress of Psychiatry, vol II. Singapore, World Scientific, 1994:832-836.

119. Puckett CK, Pickens J, Reinisch JF: Sleep apnea in mandibular hypoplasia. Plast Reconstr Surg 1982;70:213-216.

120. Powell NB, Guilleminault C, Riley RW, Smith L: Mandibular advancement and obstructive sleep apnea syndrome. Bull Eur Physiopathol Respir 1983;19:607.

121. Riley R, Powell N, Guilleminault C: Current surgical concepts for treating obstructive sleep apnea syndrome. J Oral Maxillofac Surg 1984;18:237.

Lower Third Face and Lip Reconstruction

MALCOLM ALAN LESAVOY, MD ✦ ANDREW D. SMITH, MD

LIP RECONSTRUCTION
   Anatomy
   Classification of Lip Defects
   Reconstruction

CHEEK RECONSTRUCTION
   Anatomy
   Reconstruction

LIP RECONSTRUCTION

Lip deformities have many causes, and most can be categorized as either congenital or acquired. The most frequently seen congenital deformity is cleft lip (see Volume IV). Acquired deformities can arise from traumatic or neoplastic etiologies. The following discussion focuses on reconstruction of the lip as a result of acquired defects from traumatic injury and neoplastic resection.

Anatomy

The lip provides oral competence and is basically controlled by the orbicularis oris muscle. The orbicularis oris muscle is composed of horizontal muscle fibers that start at the modiolus, insert into the opposite philtral column of the upper lip, and act to compress or purse the lips. Oblique fibers run from the commissure to the anterior nasal septum and nasal floor and act to evert the upper lip.

The major elevators of the upper lip are the levator labii superioris, zygomaticus major, and levator anguli oris (Fig. 78-1). The zygomaticus major extends from the zygomatic arch at the zygomaticofrontal suture line and inserts on the modiolus.

The paired mentalis muscles produce elevation and protrusion of the central portion of the lower lip. In patients who have lip incompetence, these muscles can become hypertrophic, and these patients must voluntarily close the lower lip to the upper lip in repose. This action causes the chin to dimple and produces an obtuse and nonprotruding chin. This type of chin is characteristic in long face syndrome, in which the maxilla has an elongated vertical dimension.

Other muscles that act on the lower lip include the depressor labii inferioris (quadratus) and the depressor anguli oris (triangularis). The depressor labii inferioris originates on the lower border of the mandible, and the fibers interdigitate with the orbicularis medially. This muscle acts to displace the lower lip inferiorly. The depressor anguli oris arises just inferior to the depressor labii inferioris and inserts on the modiolus. It helps pull the angle of the mouth inferiorly and laterally in conjunction with the platysma.

The rich blood supply to the upper and lower lips is derived from the facial artery (Fig. 78-2). The superior and inferior labial arteries travel within the orbicularis muscles, close to the mucosal margin. Lymphatic drainage from the lips is primarily to the submandibular and submental nodes.

Innervation of the lip muscles is derived from the buccal and marginal mandibular rami of the facial nerve, cranial nerve VII. The marginal mandibular branches supply the depressors; the buccal branches innervate the orbicularis oris. Sensory innervation of the upper lip is from the trigeminal nerve, cranial nerve V, infraorbital nerve (V2); the lower lip is innervated by the mental nerve (V3).

Classification of Lip Defects

Defects of the lip may be classified according to three locations: upper lip, lower lip, and lip commissure. In addition, lip defects may be classified as partial (involving only skin or mucosa) or full thickness, which involves both skin and muscle (with or without mucosal involvement).[1,2]

For the plastic surgeon, the size of the defect is often the most important consideration because it is usually

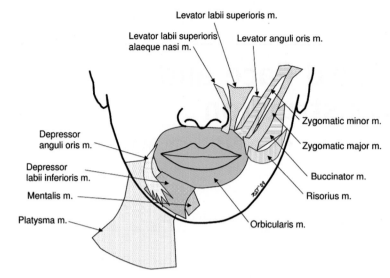

FIGURE 78-1. Perioral musculature. Elevators are shown on the right and depressors on the left. (From Krunic AL, Weitzul S, Taylor RS: Advanced reconstructive techniques for the lip and perioral area. Dermatol Clin 2005;23:43.)

a strong indicator as to the optimal method of reconstruction. Therefore, a defect of approximately 30% of the upper or lower lip can be reconstructed with primary closure because of the great elasticity of the lips. Smaller defects involve 30% or less of the upper or lower lip, whereas larger defects involve 30% or more of one or both of the lips. If a horizontal defect is greater than 30% of the lip, tissue must be added (or "shared") from the opposite normal lip to reconstruct the deformity. For example, if there has been a 50% loss of upper lip, 25% of the lower lip can be used for reconstruction of the upper lip. In this way, both lips will have less than the 30% deformity. If, however, there is a major horizontal loss and 30% or less of the opposite normal lip will not add up to 70% (greater than 60% loss), other adjacent or distant flaps may be needed for lip reconstruction.[3] Total upper or lower defects may involve loss of one or both lips from trauma or resection.

Reconstruction

The lips and eyelids can be compared anatomically in that the upper lip (like the upper eyelid) is the more important structure, as far as contour is concerned. In eyelid reconstruction, the lower eyelid may be used for reconstruction of the upper eyelid. The opposite is not true, that is, the upper eyelid should not be used to share the reconstruction of the lower eyelid. The lower eyelid may be subsequently reconstructed from local cheek skin.

The upper lip gently protrudes beyond the anterior projection of the lower lip. For this reason, the lower lip is minimally hidden by the overhanging upper lip, and it is a subtle dimension that should be kept in mind. This dimension is most important in reconstruction of the oral commissure. The lower lip will share and give its tissue for upper lip and commissure reconstruction (specifically the vermilion), and sub-

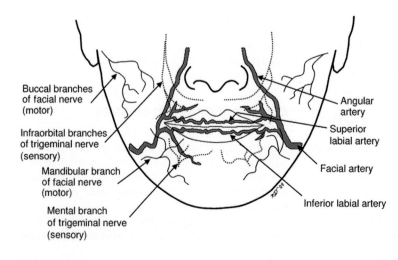

FIGURE 78-2. Arteries and nerves supplying the perioral region. (From Krunic AL, Weitzul S, Taylor RS: Advanced reconstructive techniques for the lip and perioral area. Dermatol Clin 2005;23:43.)

sequently, the lower lip vermilion and fullness will be reconstructed from local buccal mucosa advancement.

The importance of the lower lip and its contribution to the oral stoma is that, functionally, it maintains oral secretions to prevent drooling and acts as a dam. If the patient has an optimal aesthetic outcome of the lower lip but it does not function correctly as a dam or a competent oral sphincter, the reconstructive outcome is not sufficient. Both cosmesis and functionality must be given due consideration in both upper and lower lip reconstruction.

It is not uncommon for the uninitiated physician in the emergency department to state that a lip laceration has produced "missing tissue." It is incumbent on the reconstructive surgeon to understand the function of the orbicularis oris muscle and that if it is completely divided, retraction away from the wound will give the appearance of missing tissue. Reapproximation of the muscle in full-thickness defects will allow closure of the wound. One must also keep in mind that if there truly is avulsed tissue of the upper or lower lip, one can still directly reapproximate and successfully join wound edges when up to 30% of the lip is missing.

Although there are various techniques for reconstruction of the upper or lower lip, the plastic surgeon must always keep functionality and durability in mind. In reconstruction of the lips, one of the most important aspects of both these qualities is lining. Although one can devise various techniques of constructing a beautiful lip on the operating table, without adequate lining, the tissue will contract and become diminutive over time.

The oral stoma and lips are extremely vital portions of an individual's face and personality that provide visual contact to our fellow man and convey feelings and emotions at a glance. When one is speaking, the listener frequently stares at one's lips. Not only are lips important to the reception of speech, but they are also extremely important in the formation of speech. The task of the reconstructive surgeon is to maintain this important piece of anatomy and to construct a lip that has the function of feeding and competency of the oral stoma. At times, this can be an almost impossible task, but with ingenuity, imagination, and thought, the reconstruction of the lips can be a most rewarding and beneficial experience for all concerned.

FULL-THICKNESS SKIN GRAFTS

For reconstruction of selected, shallow cutaneous defects that do not involve the lip vermilion or have only minor encroachment, full-thickness skin grafts may be used (Figs. 78-3 and 78-4). Care must be taken with skin grafts to ensure that the repair does not appear "patched" and unnatural. Choose donor sites for full-thickness grafts that are inconspicuous and easily closed

primarily. Full-thickness skin grafts are more suitable in women than in men. In men, the upper lip, but also the lower lip, requires hair. Hairless skin becomes noticeable as the beard grows in the adjacent skin by the end of the day. In men, a wedge excision or lip-switch flap is a more appropriate reconstructive choice.

Full-thickness skin grafts are also used in patients with lip retraction or mucosal contour defects secondary to cicatricial retraction. Release and replacement with full-thickness skin grafts may yield an excellent result (Fig. 78-5).

VERMILION RECONSTRUCTION

When patients sustain smaller partial-thickness defects as a result of trauma, whether the defect is in a vertical position or encompasses not only the vermilion but also the mucocutaneous border, appropriate interrupted sutures at definitive landmarks should be placed after wound excision and débridement have been accomplished. One should not start suturing a wound of this type from either end. The surgeon must first be certain that the white roll and mucocutaneous or vermilion border are aligned. The orbicularis oris muscle can then be approximated so that competency of the oral stoma is maintained and splinting of the cutaneous and mucosal portions of the wound is accomplished. Good muscle approximation will prevent future cutaneous scar widening because of the appropriate decrease in horizontal skin tension.

For reconstruction of tumor resections, incisions that cross the vermilion border should do so at a 90-degree angle (Fig. 78-6). The white roll should be marked and approximated precisely. A 1-mm discrepancy in alignment is noticeable at conversational distance. Defining anatomic boundaries of the vermilion is therefore critical in performing surgical resection or subsequent reconstruction of the vermilion.

Vermilion flaps, as described by Gillies and Millard,[4] can be used for horizontal loss of vermilion, both in trauma and to fill insufficient bulk in cleft lip deformities, as described by Kawamoto.[5] For reconstruction of large amounts of vermilion, when opposing lip vermilion cannot be shared, a mucosal apron flap, as described by Gillies and Millard,[4] is useful (Fig. 78-7). In this instance, the buccal mucosa of the opposing lip can be a donor flap based on the "normal" vermilion, and the donor defect can be skin grafted. Obviously, one cannot reconstruct the entire apron for a period of 7 to 10 days unless nasal gastric feeding is accomplished. Lateral ports can be maintained, and after division of the central apron, two small mucosal aprons can be constructed for the lateral ports.

Premalignant lesions or carcinoma in situ will occasionally require a total vermilionectomy or a so-called lip-shaving procedure. Reconstruction can then be accomplished by several methods, including a

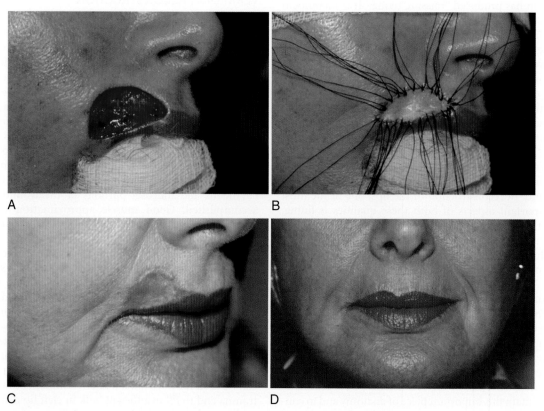

FIGURE 78-3. *A,* Full-thickness skin defect of upper lip. *B,* Full-thickness skin graft to right upper lip, "replacing kind with kind." *C,* Maturing full-thickness skin graft. *D,* Final result with good contour.

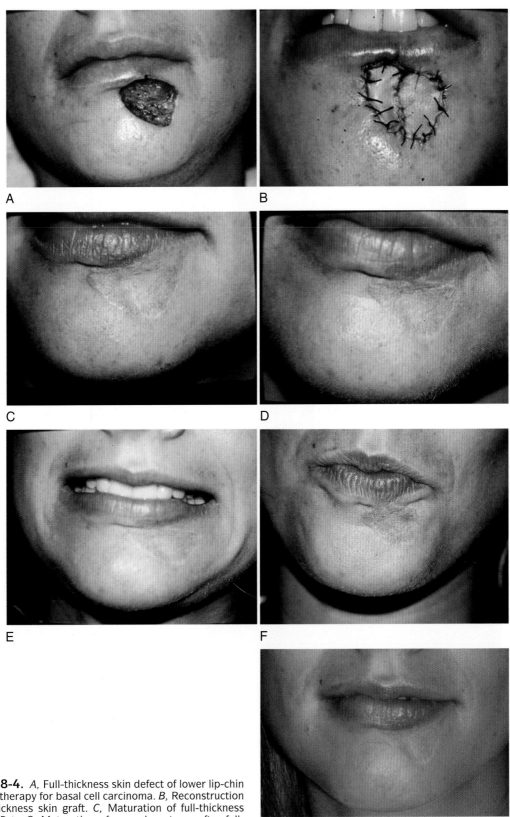

FIGURE 78-4. *A,* Full-thickness skin defect of lower lip-chin from Mohs therapy for basal cell carcinoma. *B,* Reconstruction with full-thickness skin graft. *C,* Maturation of full-thickness skin graft. *D* to *G,* Maturation of normal anatomy after full-thickness skin graft.

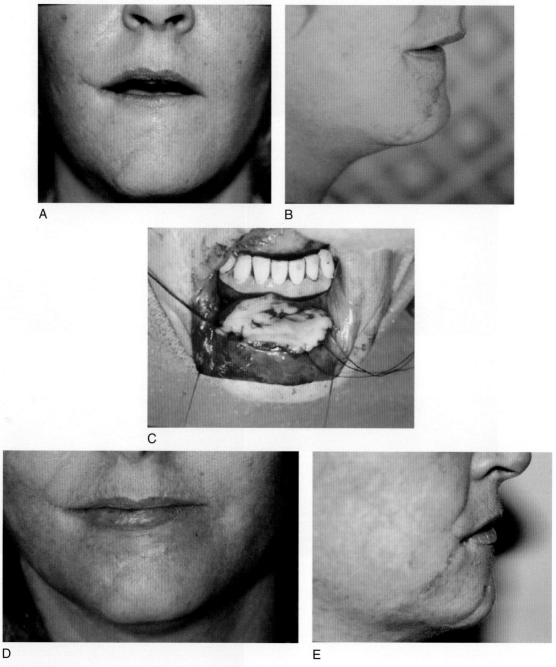

FIGURE 78-5. *A* and *B*, Traumatic retraction of lower lip. *C*, Release of contracted and retracted horizontal lower lip mucosal scar and reconstruction with full-thickness skin graft. *D* and *E*, Excellent contour of lower lip in relationship to upper lip.

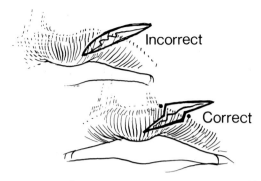

FIGURE 78-6. Skin-vermilion excisions. Every effort should be made to cross the skin-vermilion border at a 90-degree angle. (From Zide BM: Deformities of the lips and cheeks. In McCarthy JG, ed: Plastic Surgery. Philadelphia, WB Saunders, 1990:2009.)

bipedicled flap to advance intraoral mucosa and to resurface the vermilion, with a skin graft at the donor site. An incisional release at the labial sulcus may be used to advance the mucosa anteriorly (Fig. 78-8).[6] Other reconstructive methods can use adjacent buccal or tongue mucosa to resurface the vermilion.[7-10] Tongue flaps need to remain attached for 2 weeks before division and usually are a last option because of poor color and texture match. Palatal mucosal full-thickness skin grafts may also be used and are best suited to the area behind the wet line of the vermilion (see "Flap Reconstruction").

DIRECT CLOSURE AND WEDGE EXCISION

Direct closure of lip defects is possible because of the tremendous distensibility of the three elements of the lip (skin, orbicularis oris muscle, and buccal mucosa), provided the defect involves 30% or less of the lip tissue. Direct closure must, however, be accomplished in layers after sharp débridement. If more than 30% of the lip tissue is missing, direct closure may not be possible and more extensive reconstructive methods must be used.[3]

Traumatic wounds of the lips may be complicated by through-and-through lacerations of jutting teeth. Technically, the inner border of the lips is that of the firm and nongiving teeth. If an object subsequently strikes a direct blow to the lips, the soft tissue between (lips) may sustain severe damage from this bony inner border. For that reason, the human lip is in great jeopardy from blunt trauma. Frequently, the lacerations are not incurred by the offending object (e.g., fist, pool cue) but by the teeth (Fig. 78-9). The treating surgeon must keep in mind the tremendous bacterial content of the human mouth and understand that this type of laceration must be considered a "human bite" with appropriate treatment.

If through-and-through lacerations of the lip are produced by jutting teeth, total excision of the wound margins, copious irrigation, and careful direct closure can be accomplished under local anesthesia. The definitive closure should always maintain appropriate landmarks of the lips so that the orbicularis muscle approximation is accomplished and good skin cover is maintained. If the laceration is through-and-through to the buccal mucosa, loose approximation or even nonclosure of the oral mucosa can frequently be accomplished for appropriate drainage. The administration of tetanus toxoid and penicillin is almost always appropriate in these patients with these types of injuries.[3]

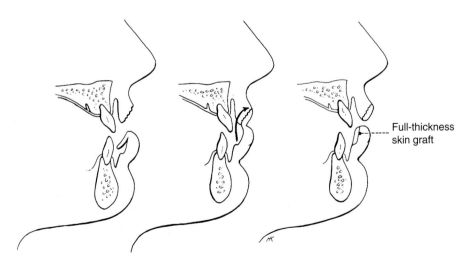

Full-thickness skin graft

FIGURE 78-7. Vermilion apron. (From Lesavoy MA: Lip deformities and their reconstruction. In Lesavoy MA, ed: Reconstruction of the Head and Neck. Baltimore, Williams & Wilkins, 1981:95.)

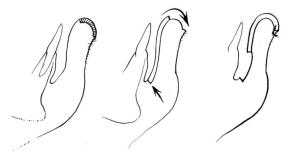

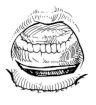

FIGURE 78-8. The usual vermilionectomy involved excision and primary closure without undermining. Wilson and Walker[6] modified the procedure with an incision release in the sulcus (bipedicled flap) to reduce some of the problems associated with simple approximation of the wound. (From Zide BM: Deformities of the lips and cheeks. In McCarthy JG, ed: Plastic Surgery. Philadelphia, WB Saunders, 1990:2009.)

Louis[11] is credited with the first wedge excision and direct suture closure in 1768. In 1955, Webster[12] reported his experience with vertical wedge excision for the treatment of lip lesions. For superficial defects of the upper lip, he described a vertical lip excision with primary closure. For full-thickness defects, he described a full-thickness excision including a peri-alar crescent. Closure is obtained by advancement of a lateral cheek flap. Smaller lip defects can be excised and closed by a simple V-shaped wedge excision closure (Figs. 78-10 to 78-13). In men, philtral distortion may be concealed with a mustache (Fig. 78-14). In some instances, it may be necessary to include a V-Y

Text continued on p. 812

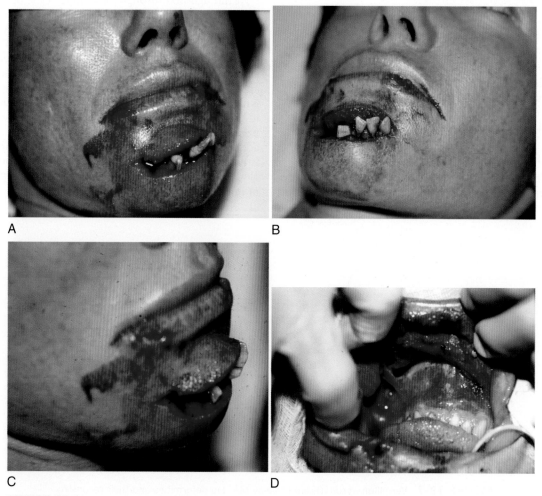

FIGURE 78-9. *A to C,* Traumatic laceration of lower lip gingival sulcus with penetration of teeth. *D,* Intraoral lower lip and gingival buccal sulcus view of traumatic laceration with intact left mental nerve.

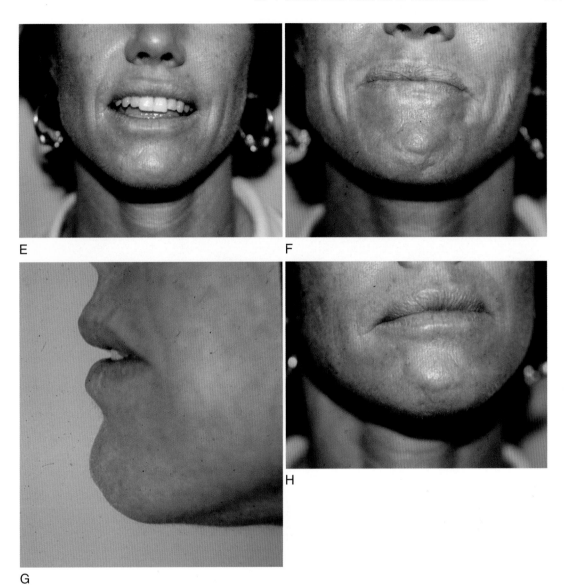

E

F

G

H

FIGURE 78-9, cont'd. *E* to *H,* Excellent healing after dental stabilization and débridement of all three layers of the wound, with excellent contour and animation.

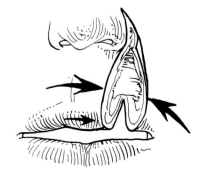

FIGURE 78-10. Transformation of defect into V-wedge excision. (From Zide BM: Deformities of the lips and cheeks. In McCarthy JG, ed: Plastic Surgery. Philadelphia, WB Saunders, 1990:2009.)

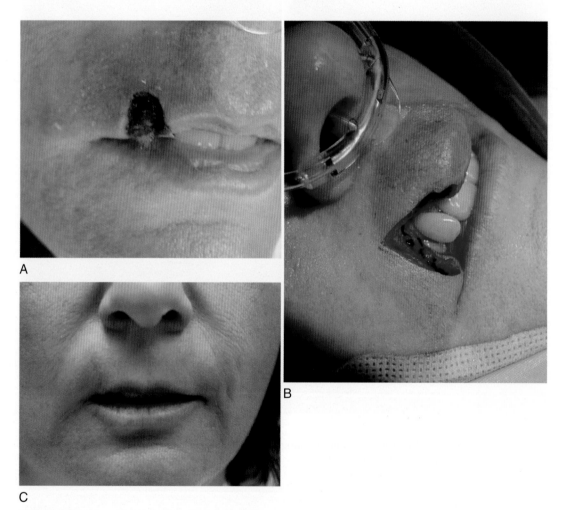

FIGURE 78-11. *A,* Full-thickness defect of upper lip after Mohs therapy for basal cell carcinoma. *B,* Débridement of entire wound—including skin, orbicularis oris, and mucosa—with medial and lateral undermining. *C,* Direct closure with alignment of white roll and vermilion wet line.

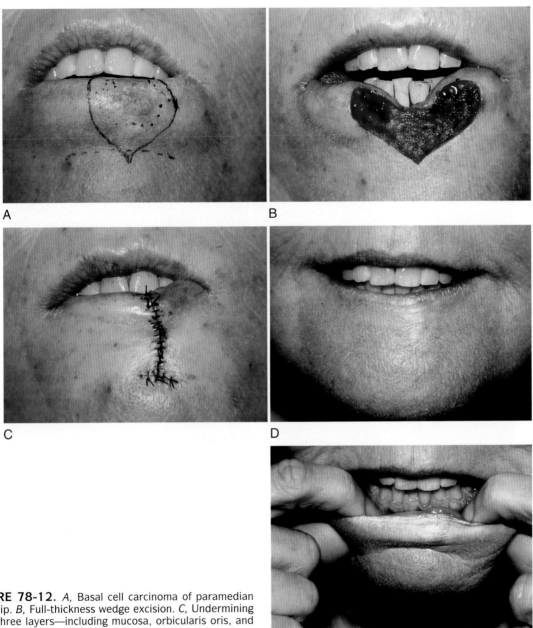

FIGURE 78-12. *A,* Basal cell carcinoma of paramedian lower lip. *B,* Full-thickness wedge excision. *C,* Undermining of all three layers—including mucosa, orbicularis oris, and skin—and direct closure. *D* and *E,* Final result after direct closure reconstruction.

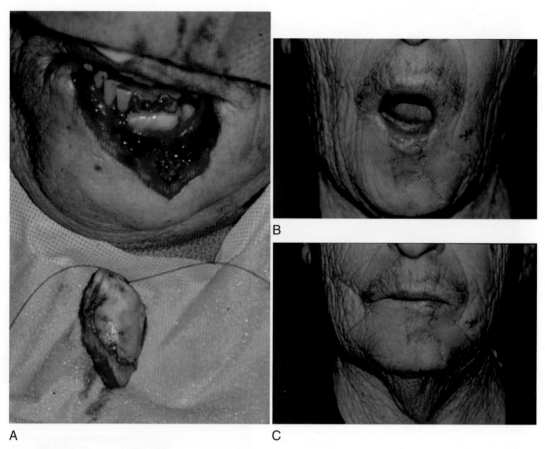

FIGURE 78-13. *A,* Wide excision of squamous cell carcinoma of left lower lip, including skin, orbicularis oris, and mucosa. *B* and *C,* Result with reconstruction by wide lateral undermining of skin, muscle, and mucosa.

FIGURE 78-14. *A,* Paracentral upper lip defect after Mohs therapy for basal cell carcinoma, with loss of skin and partial orbicularis oris in hair-bearing area. *B,* Débridement of entire wound with full-thickness large wedge excision of all three layers of skin, orbicularis oris, and mucosa. *C,* Paramedian defect after débridement, with adjacent undermining of all three layers. *D,* Direct closure with alignment of hair-bearing philtrum column and vermilion. *E* to *G,* Mature postoperative wound with imperceptible deformity.

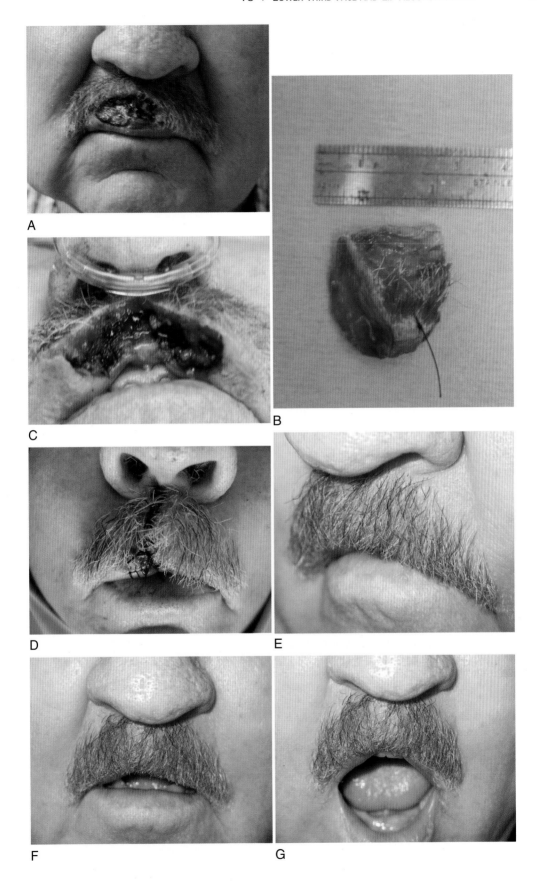

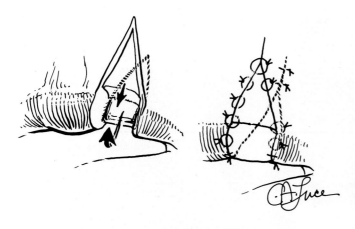

FIGURE 78-15. Wedge excision closure with inside and outside V-Y advancement flaps. (From Zide BM: Deformities of the lips and cheeks. In McCarthy JG, ed: Plastic Surgery. Philadelphia, WB Saunders, 1990:2009.)

advancement for alignment of skin and vermilion (Fig. 78-15).[13,14] This method requires the simultaneous advancement of a mucosal-vermilion flap to cover lost vermilion.

FLAP RECONSTRUCTION

For lip defects greater than 30% of horizontal dimension, the use of adjacent tissue for reconstruction is mandatory. A V-shaped wedge excision may be combined with a rectangular advancement flap from the labial mental area.[15] This technique was later modified by Owens[16] to reconstruct the entire lower lip. Again, mucosal advancement flaps are used for vermilion.

In 1974, Johanson et al[17] described a technique that allowed reconstruction of up to two thirds of the lower lip by a "staircase" technique. Usually, two to four steps are needed to allow closure, but the disadvantage of this technique is that the scars are noticeable, and the lip may appear to be tight (Fig. 78-16). In 1954, Schuchardt[18] described a modification of the W or barrel-shaped excision, which is extended around the labial mental fold to the submental region. On occasion, a triangle-shaped excision from the submental region is necessary to correct for the advancement; again, this may result in a tight lip (Fig. 78-17).

An opposing lip flap, or Abbe[19,20] flap, is used to reconstruct both upper and lower lip defects. Typically, however, it is used when defects of the upper lip, usually in the central portion, need to be reconstructed from the lower lip (Fig. 78-18). An opposing flap from the lower lip is carried on its arterialized pedicle (the labial artery) to the upper lip. This flap is ideal for reconstruction in men as the lower lip provides hair-bearing tissue for continuity (Fig. 78-19). For lower lip defects, the upper lip in the area lateral to the philtrum is suitable for transfer to the lower lip. The central philtral area is not suitable for transfer because of its aesthetic irreplaceability. The Abbe flap can subsequently be divided 7 to 10 days later, after the flap receives adjacent blood supply from its inset into the upper lip.

For a lip flap transposition, the patient obviously must be cooperative because constant motion of the mouth and lips will compromise the reconstruction. The patient must maintain upper and lower lip approximation for the time the flap is attached to both lips. On occasion, Ivy loops for mandibulomaxillary fixation on a temporary basis have allowed the flap to heal in its new position without the constant motion of an uncooperative mouth. The labial artery runs very superficial to the oral mucosal border of the vermilion. For this reason, a small pedicle can be designed

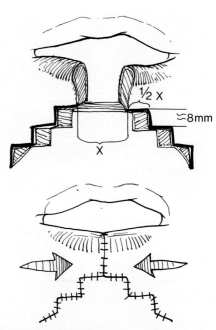

FIGURE 78-16. The staircase or stepladder method introduced by Johanson et al[17] in 1974 may be used for both central and lateral defects. Although function and sensation may be preserved, the incisions are usually obvious. (From Zide BM: Deformities of the lips and cheeks. In McCarthy JG, ed: Plastic Surgery. Philadelphia, WB Saunders, 1990:2009.)

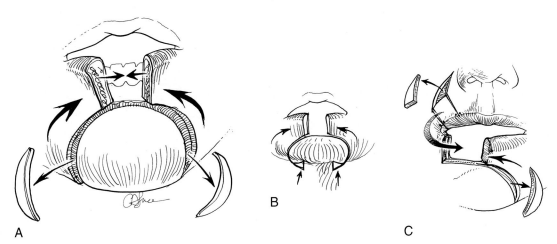

FIGURE 78-17. *A* and *B,* The Schuchardt procedure rotates and advances the cheek and lip to provide closure. The skinfolds are removed as crescents *(A)* or submental triangles *(B). C,* An example of unilateral Schuchardt procedure combined with an Abbe-type flap. (From Zide BM: Deformities of the lips and cheeks. In McCarthy JG, ed: Plastic Surgery. Philadelphia, WB Saunders, 1990:2009.)

both for comfort and for ease of division and insetting 7 to 10 days after the transposition.

A modification of the Abbe flap described by Stein[21] and subsequently popularized by Wexler and Dingman[22] involves the excision of two upper lip flaps on either side of the philtrum that are transposed to fill a large, central lower lip defect (Fig. 78-20). This flap, like the Abbe flap, is subsequently divided, and the vermilion is restored. The switch flap has even been described as a free composite graft from time to time, but better fullness, more pliable tissue, and a more predictable result will be achieved if it is used and designed as a vascularized flap. The donor areas are closed primarily, and its scar is usually insignificant. Secondary procedures may be necessary to correct any vermilion discrepancies at the flap inset site. It has been reported that the muscle portion of the Abbe flap becomes innervated by appositional nerve ingrowth called neurotization.[23] Even if neurotization

does not occur, the living muscle acts as a link of the broken chain reconstituting the competency of the oral stoma.

The Estlander flap[24] is a transposition flap from the upper lip used to repair defects of the lateral lower lip (Fig. 78-21). Obviously, a secondary procedure is usually needed to reconstruct the obliterated commissure. A modification of the Estlander flap is a reverse Abbe flap, which has the advantage of maintaining the commissure by transposing the flap just medial to the commissure.

The Gillies[4] fan flap is an extension of the Estlander flap. It combines a rotation around the commissure with additional tissue from the nasolabial fold. This allows partial continuity of the oral sphincter, which may undergo reinnervation (Figs. 78-22 to 78-25).

Karapandzic[25] and later Jabaley et al[26] modified the Gillies fan flap in an attempt to leave the

Text continued on p. 820

FIGURE 78-18. *A,* Central upper lip full-thickness defect, with design of shield-shaped flap (Abbe flap) from lower lip based on inferior labial artery. *B,* Transposition of central Abbe flap, with donor site inferior edge descending to labial mental sulcus. *C,* Maturation of wound—end result. (From Lesavoy MA: Lip deformities and their reconstruction. In Lesavoy MA, ed: Reconstruction of the Head and Neck. Baltimore, Williams & Wilkins, 1981:95.)

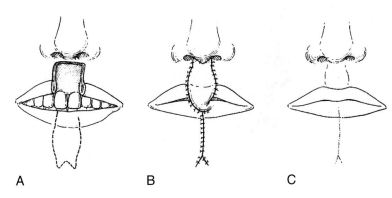

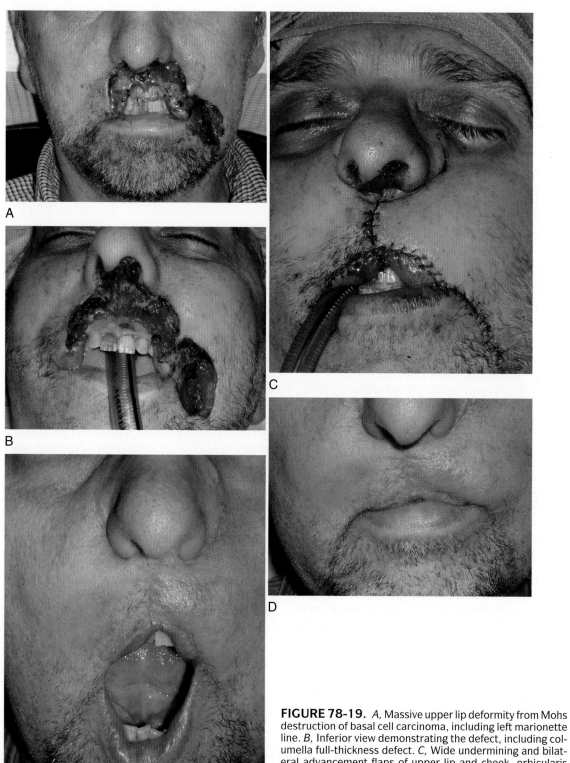

FIGURE 78-19. *A,* Massive upper lip deformity from Mohs destruction of basal cell carcinoma, including left marionette line. *B,* Inferior view demonstrating the defect, including columella full-thickness defect. *C,* Wide undermining and bilateral advancement flaps of upper lip and cheek, orbicularis oris, upper lip mucosa and sulcus, and free vermilion and direct closure of left marionette line. *D,* Maturing scars after primary advancement flap closures. *E,* Demonstration of microstomia and lack of philtral columns, philtral dimple, and upper lip tubercle.

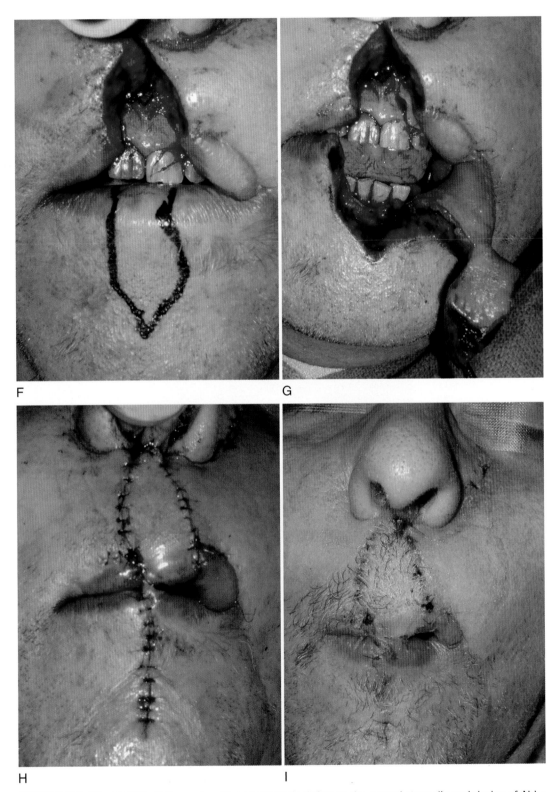

FIGURE 78-19, cont'd. *F,* Reconstruction of anatomic defect at the central upper lip and design of Abbe flap from lower lip to be based on the left lower labial artery. *G,* Elevation of full-thickness Abbe flap based on left inferior labial artery. *H,* Inset of Abbe flap to upper lip with 180-degree transposition. *I,* Wound healing of Abbe flap inset.   *Continued*

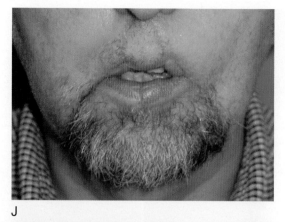

J

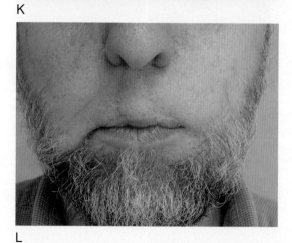

K

L

FIGURE 78-19, cont'd. *J,* Maturation of Abbe flap in upper lip position with good philtral columns and tubercle and imperceptible donor site scar of lower lip. *K,* Functional correction of microstomia. *L,* Final result of upper lip reconstruction with Abbe flap transposition and direct closure of left marionette line.

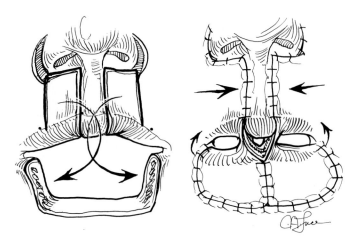

FIGURE 78-20. The double Abbe flap developed by Wexler and Dingman[22] may be used to close 75% central defects of the lower lip. (From Zide BM: Deformities of the lips and cheeks. In McCarthy JG, ed: Plastic Surgery. Philadelphia, WB Saunders, 1990:2009.)

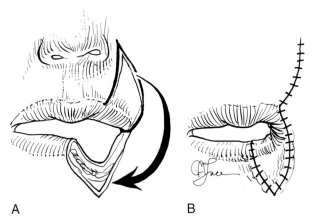

A   B

FIGURE 78-21. A and B, The Estlander flap. Although this flap provides closure for lower lip defects, it produces a rounded commissure that may require secondary revision. (From Zide BM: Deformities of the lips and cheeks. In McCarthy JG, ed: Plastic Surgery. Philadelphia, WB Saunders, 1990:2009.)

FIGURE 78-22. A to C, Fan flap reconstruction for upper lip defects, including skin, orbicularis oris, and mucosa. (Modified from Gillies HD, Millard DR Jr: Principles and Art of Plastic Surgery. Boston, Little, Brown, 1957.)

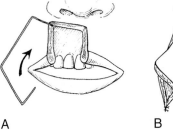

A

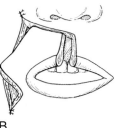

B

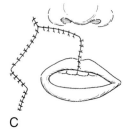

C

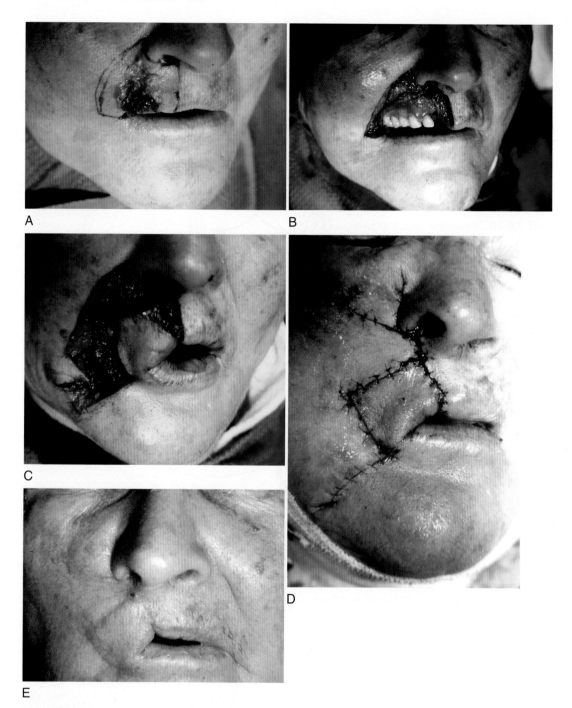

FIGURE 78-23. *A,* Squamous cell carcinoma of right upper lip; markings with 1-cm margin for histopathologic examination. *B,* Defect of right upper lip encompassing approximately 40% of horizontal and vertical defect, including commissure. *C,* Transposition of fan flap. *D,* Closure of multiple donor advancements. *E,* Resultant healed, immature reconstruction requiring future correction of microstomia.

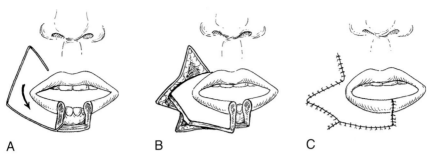

FIGURE 78-24. *A to C,* Fan flap reconstruction for full-thickness lower lip defects. (Modified from Gillies HD, Millard DR Jr: Principles and Art of Plastic Surgery. Boston, Little, Brown, 1957.)

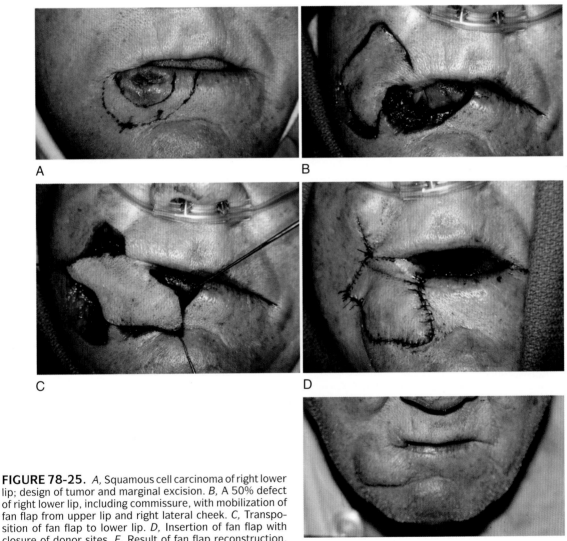

FIGURE 78-25. *A,* Squamous cell carcinoma of right lower lip; design of tumor and marginal excision. *B,* A 50% defect of right lower lip, including commissure, with mobilization of fan flap from upper lip and right lateral cheek. *C,* Transposition of fan flap to lower lip. *D,* Insertion of fan flap with closure of donor sites. *E,* Result of fan flap reconstruction, with some flap contraction and "pincushioning."

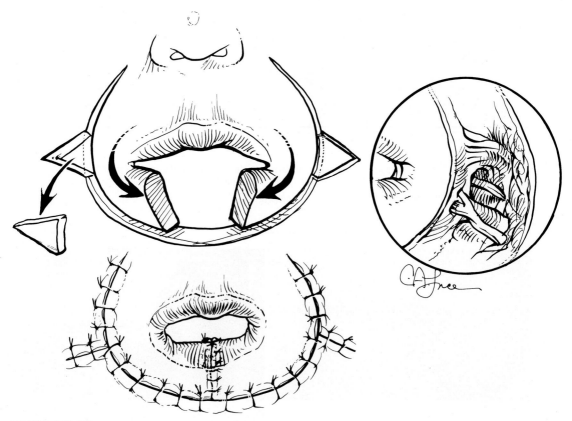

FIGURE 78-26. The Karapandzic technique produces a functioning sphincter and may be used bilaterally. Central defects of up to 80% may be reconstructed. (From Zide BM: Deformities of the lips and cheeks. In McCarthy JG, ed: Plastic Surgery. Philadelphia, WB Saunders, 1990:2009.)

neurovascular supply intact. Tissue from the naso-labial fold, including the lower fold, is rotated medially and provides the proper muscle orientation. This flap can be designed as a unilateral or bilateral flap (Fig. 78-26). This flap works best for central defects of the lower lip, and its main disadvantage, microstomia, often requires a secondary commissuroplasty.

COMMISSURE RECONSTRUCTION

The reconstruction of a normal commissure is frequently mandated after electrical burns of the mouth, in neoplastic extirpation, and in secondary staged revisions of lip flaps.

Electrical burns of the lip commissure are frequently observed in children between the ages of 1 and 4 years (Fig. 78-27). Most of these children bite the free end of a "live electrical extension cord," and because the oral commissures are usually moist, they subsequently have decreased resistance to the electrical current. For that reason, the damage is fairly localized to the commissures of the lip.

Early treatment of lip commissure electrical burns is still debatable.[27] Some think that immediate excision of the damaged tissue and direct closure should ensue. However, in general, most plastic surgeons believe that conservative therapy with topical antibiotics and "tincture of time" will allow the eschars to separate and the wound to demarcate.[27] Secondary healing will then occur and result in a deformity that can later be reconstructed. These patients may need to be hospitalized as excessive bleeding from the labial artery may be observed 24 to 48 hours after injury to the commissure. Bleeding at this site can be distressing, and even dangerous, if the child is at home under the care of his or her parents and not trained medical personnel.

In reconstructing the vermilion at the commissure, one must remember the principles that the upper lip, cosmetically, is more important and that sharing of the vermilion of the lower lip gives the most pleasing results. Spacial and anatomic relationships are important structures of a normal commissure. This is analogous to ear reconstruction, when a well-constructed ear in an incorrect position is not pleasing (Fig. 78-28).

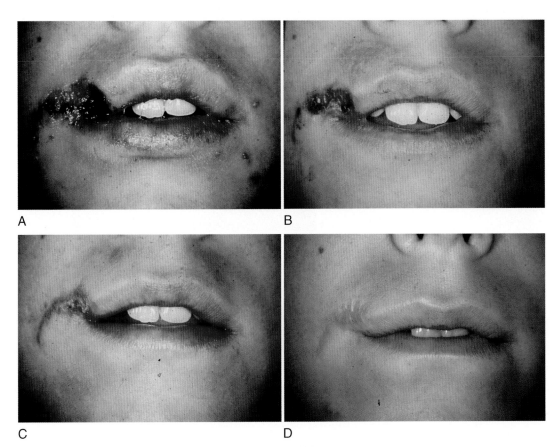

A

B

C

D

FIGURE 78-27. *A,* Traumatic avulsion of right commissure. *B,* Débridement and conservative treatment with dressing changes. *C,* Contraction and secondary closure of wound. *D,* Final result with only secondary closure and no flap reconstruction.

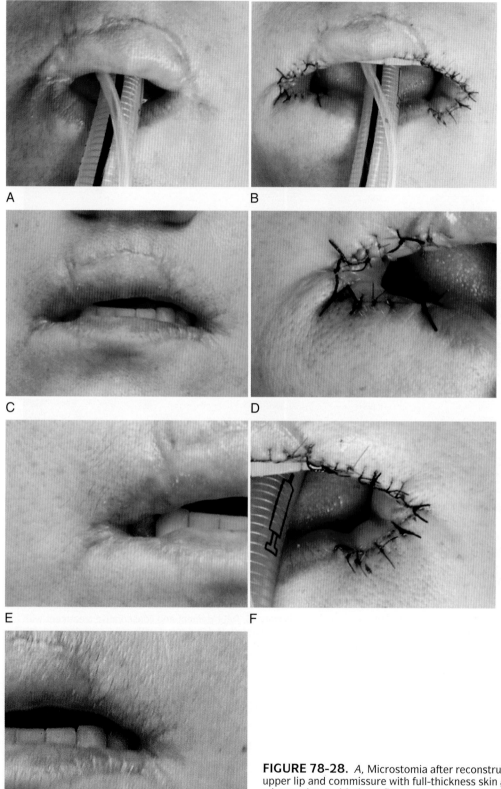

FIGURE 78-28. *A*, Microstomia after reconstruction of entire upper lip and commissure with full-thickness skin graft. *B*, Commissuroplasty with three-flap mucosal advancements. *C*, Healed commissure reconstruction. *D*, Right commissuroplasty. *E*, Healed right commissure. *F*, Left commissuroplasty. *G*, Healed left commissure.

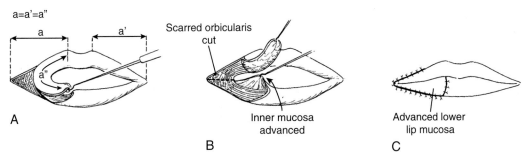

FIGURE 78-29. *A,* Commissure flap design, measurements of the normal from the height of the Cupid's bow on the nonaffected side to the commissure. The defect measurement is transposed along the vermilion mucosa to the lower lip on the affected sided. *B,* Elevation of vermilion mucosal flap and incision of cicatricial commissure. *C,* Insertion of upper lip commissuroplasty flap with advancement of lower lip mucosa for closure of donor site. (From Lesavoy MA: Lip deformities and their reconstruction. In Lesavoy MA, ed: Reconstruction of the Head and Neck. Baltimore, Williams & Wilkins, 1981:95.)

Careful measurement and knowledge of the "normal" are most important so that reconstruction of the commissure is placed symmetrically to the opposite normal commissure. One determines the most lateral aspect of the neocommissure, which usually lies at an imaginary vertical line dropped from the midportion of the pupil. One must also determine the point on this vertical line at which the commissure should lie in a horizontal plane (Fig. 78-29). This can be determined on the normal side by measuring the distance from the lower eyelid to the normal commissure. The distance should then be measured from the normal commissure to the height of the normal Cupid's bow, and this distance is transposed from the ipsilateral Cupid's bow height to the distance of the vermilion of the lower lip that corresponds. This vermilion flap is then raised from the lower lip, based on the ipsilateral upper lip vermilion; the scar and orbicularis are incised to the predetermined point, and the vermilion is inset for reconstruction of the upper lip half of the commissure. The donor site on the lower lip can then be reconstructed by advancement of the adjacent lower lip buccal mucosa. This technique seems to offer advantages of upper lip camouflage and maintains continuity of the upper lip vermilion. It also eliminates the need for three flaps that draw at the angle of the mouth and subsequently tend to contract (Fig. 78-30).[3]

RECONSTRUCTION OF TOTAL UPPER AND LOWER LIP DEFECTS

For massive deformities of the lower lip, bilateral lower lip and cheek advancements can be accomplished as described by Bernard.[28] This type of reconstruction can be satisfactory in some patients; however, when competency of the lower lip is needed to prevent drooling, this operation sometimes falls short. Webster et al[29] added several technical refinements to the procedure in 1960. In their modification, a tumor is excised as a quadrilateral segment. Buccal mucosal membrane flaps are used to provide vermilion. The Webster modification allows the design of a sensate, aesthetic, and functional reconstructive result with a competent and innervated oral stoma (Fig. 78-31).

In major defects of the upper or lower lip as a result of trauma, vigorous and sharp débridement must be carried out and all devitalized tissue must be discarded. Raw bone ends can be covered and saved for later reconstruction by closing oral mucosa to overlying skin. After an appropriate period, swelling and edema will subside and future plans for reconstruction can be decided. In these types of devastating presentations, the airway is of greatest importance at the initial injury, and tracheostomy is almost immediately imperative. Although it is not within the scope of this chapter to discuss bone reconstruction of the mandible or maxilla, one should keep in mind that stabilization or reconstruction of these structures is essential for an optimal aesthetic and functional outcome (Fig. 78-32).

In massive trauma, distant flaps are often needed. For reconstruction of an entire mouth, it is wise to plan not only flap coverage but also camouflage. In this vein, a temporal frontal scalp flap can be used (Fig. 78-33). A misdirected shotgun blast frequently will destroy entire anterior portions of the face, and patients such as these can illustrate graphically the essence of reconstructive surgery (Fig. 78-34). Concern must be directed toward identification of the defect, and reconstruction of the entire upper lip must be planned. Not only is bone stabilization and reconstruction imperative, but also the timing of this procedure must coincide with soft tissue addition.

For reconstruction of the upper lip, a delayed temporal frontal scalp flap based on the anterior branch

Text continued on p. 831

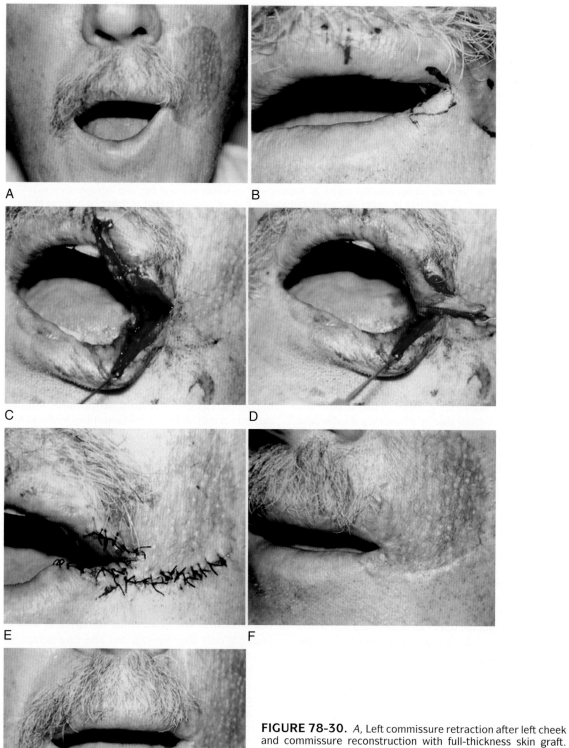

FIGURE 78-30. *A,* Left commissure retraction after left cheek and commissure reconstruction with full-thickness skin graft. *B,* Design of lower lip commissure vermilion mucosal flap for commissuroplasty. *C,* Mobilization and elevation of vermilion mucosal flap and incision of commissure scar. *D,* Transposition of vermilion mucosal flap. *E,* Inset of vermilion mucosal flap for upper lip, commissure, and advancement of lower lip mucosa for closure of donor site. *F* and *G,* Final result of vermilion mucosal commissuroplasty.

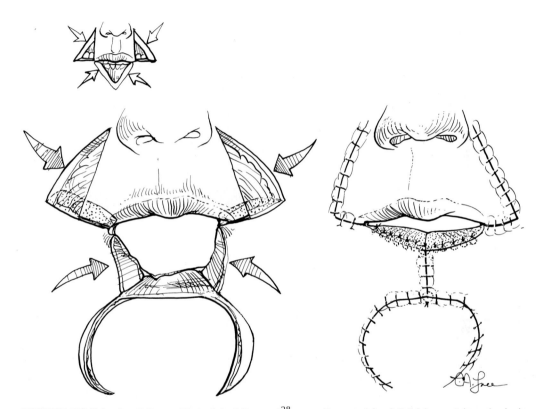

FIGURE 78-31. *Small figure:* The original Bernard[28] operation used for full-thickness triangular incisions. *Large figures:* The Webster[29] modification provided major technical advances. Mucosal flaps *(stippled)* were used for vermilion reconstruction. The nasolabial excisions became partial thickness. Schuchardt[18] flaps facilitated cheek advancement. (From Zide BM: Deformities of the lips and cheeks. In McCarthy JG, ed: Plastic Surgery. Philadelphia, WB Saunders, 1990:2009.)

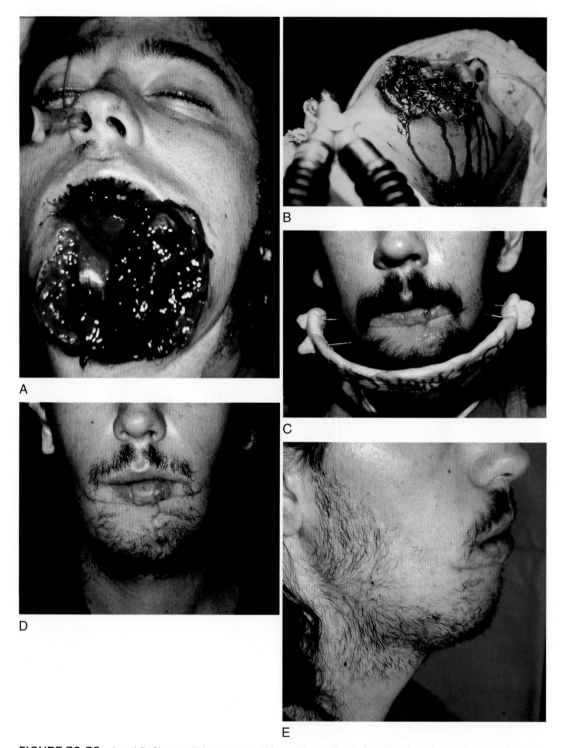

FIGURE 78-32. *A* and *B*, Shotgun injury to mandible and lower lip. *C*, Stabilization of mandibular defect with external fixator. *D* and *E*, Final result after bone graft into mandible and lower lip reconstruction.

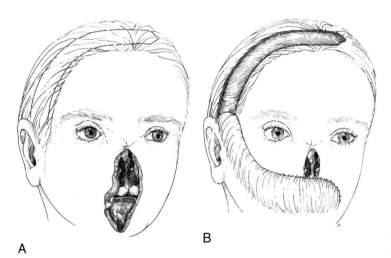

FIGURE 78-33. *A* and *B,* Temporal frontal scalp flap for total upper lip reconstruction. (From Lesavoy MA: Lip deformities and their reconstruction. In Lesavoy MA, ed: Reconstruction of the Head and Neck. Baltimore, Williams & Wilkins, 1981:95.)

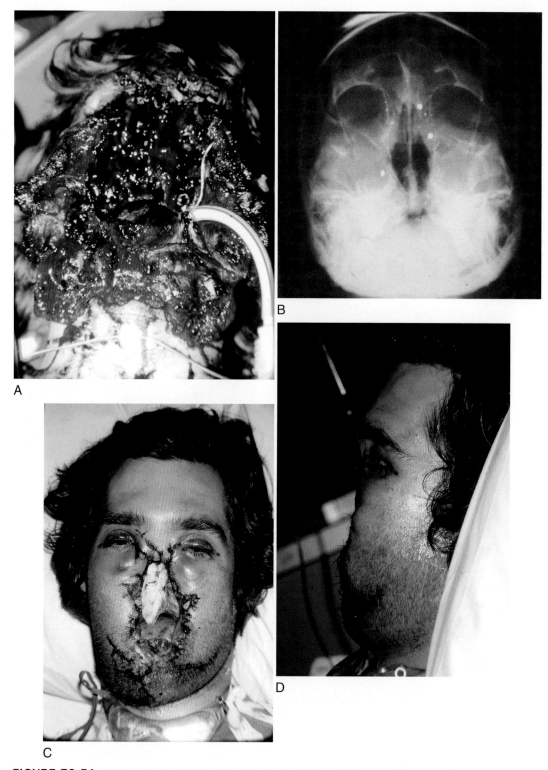

FIGURE 78-34. *A,* Massive facial deformity after shotgun injury. *B,* Bone evidence showing destruction of maxilla and mandible. *C,* Débridement and advancement of soft tissue. *D,* Lateral view.

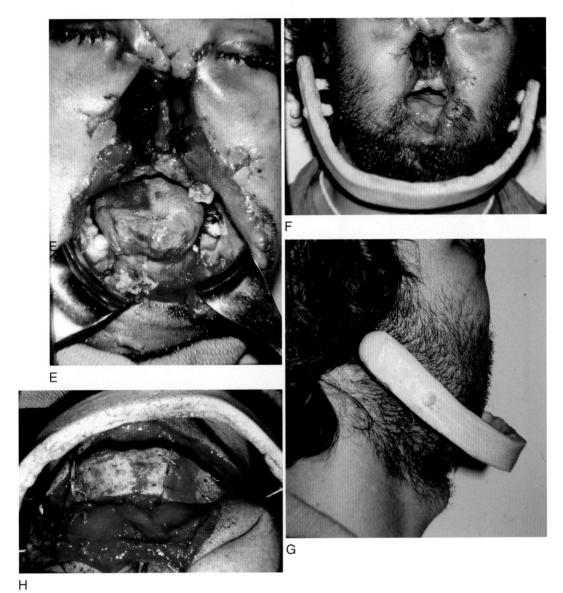

FIGURE 78-34, cont'd. *E,* Intraoral view with absent nose, septum, maxilla, hard palate, central mandible, and anterior tongue. *F* and *G,* Bone stabilization of mandible with external fixator.   *Continued*

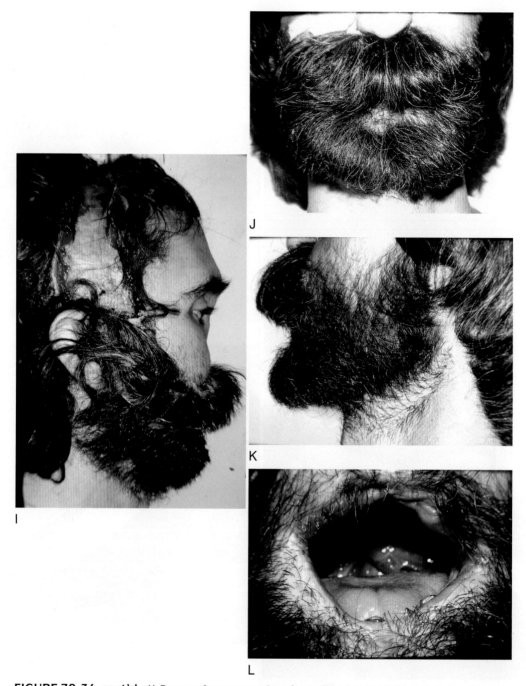

FIGURE 78-34, cont'd. *H,* Bone graft reconstruction of mandible. *I,* Lateral view of hair-bearing scalp flap of upper lip reconstruction with donor site skin grafting. *J* and *K,* Result of hair-bearing upper lip reconstruction and mandibular bone reconstruction. *L,* Upper and lower lip reconstruction before dentures.

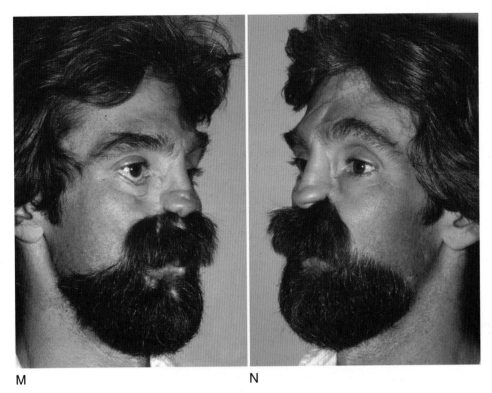

M   N

FIGURE 78-34, cont'd. *M* and *N,* Final result—facial reconstruction.

of the superficial temporary artery can be elevated and lined with a split-thickness skin graft. Once the flap has been transposed into the upper lip position, the skin graft can be discarded if good flap coverage can be maintained for lining by turnover adjacent mucosal book flaps. A maxillary prosthetic obturator is important for maintenance of these lip flaps to prevent contraction. Three weeks after the inset, division and return of the temporal pedicle can be accomplished. In this way, an upper lip can be reconstructed in the male patient to allow good soft tissue augmentation and hairy camouflage of this area (Fig. 78-34*M*). Obviously, this is not appropriate in the female patient.

CHEEK RECONSTRUCTION

Anatomy

The cheeks can be divided into zones, namely, a suborbital, a preauricular, and a buccal mandibular area (Fig. 78-35). Reconstruction of a defect in any of these areas is, obviously, dependent on its horizontal size and depth.

Reconstruction

Depending on the laxity of adjacent skin, some full-thickness skin defects can be closed primarily with

adequate adjacent undermining (Fig. 78-36). Obviously, the lines and creases of the face must be maintained and used to their optimal advantage (Fig. 78-37). Intermittently, Z-plasties or even W-plasties can be used to release scars inappropriately positioned

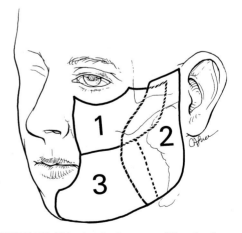

FIGURE 78-35. Aesthetic zones of the cheek: zone I, suborbital; zone 2, preauricular; and zone 3, buccomandibular. The zones may overlap considerably. Zone 3 may require lining as well as cover. (From Zide BM: Deformities of the lips and cheeks. In McCarthy JG, ed: Plastic Surgery. Philadelphia, WB Saunders, 1990:2009.)

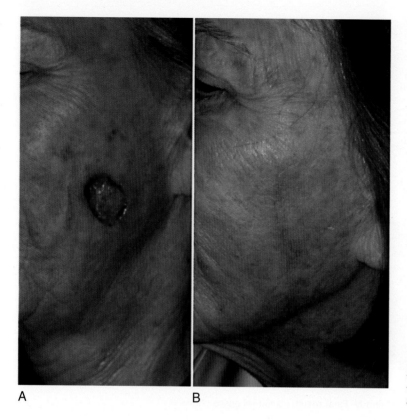

A   B

FIGURE 78-36. *A* and *B,* Full-thickness skin defect after Mohs therapy for basal cell carcinoma with advancement and direct closure.

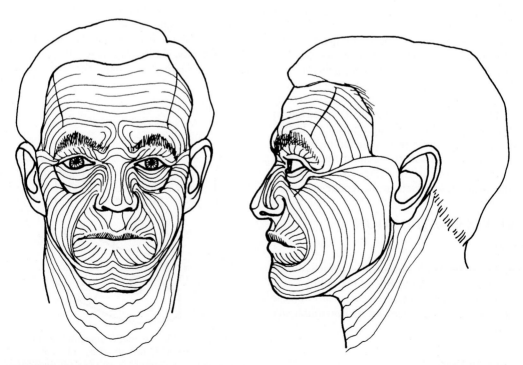

FIGURE 78-37. Facial wrinkle lines. (From Mullin WR: Surgery of the forehead and cheek regions. In Lesavoy MA, ed: Reconstruction of the Head and Neck. Baltimore, Williams & Wilkins, 1981:29.)

opposite the underlying muscle directional pull (see Chapter 12).

Secondarily, if direct closure cannot be obtained, a split- or full-thickness skin graft is the next reconstructive option to consider. An advantage is that rapid wound closure can be obtained, but this can be at the expense of a relatively poor aesthetic endpoint.

Tumor resection or trauma may leave minor or large defects in the cheeks and lower face in both adult and pediatric patients. Debulking or correction of massive defects may require multiple, staged procedures with the use of local or distant flaps. Lymphangioma or "cystic hygroma" was first described by Wernher[30] in a monograph published in 1843. A cystic lymphatic anomaly can be diagnosed in utero by ultrasonography as early as 12 weeks of gestation.[31] The characteristic progression of a lymphatic malformation is enlargement commensurate with a child's growth. Determination of a lesion's growth pattern is a critical step in an accurate diagnosis. Lymphatic anomalies are not neoplastic in term of invasion of tissue, but there is often massive and complex involvement of adjacent normal tissue. Resection of these lesions often requires multiple, staged procedures for debulking and secondary cosmesis (Fig. 78-38).

For other defects resulting from tumor resection or traumatic injury that cannot be closed primarily, local flaps such as rhomboid flaps (Limberg or Dufourmentel flaps) (Figs. 78-39 and 78-40),[32-34] V-Y or local transposition flaps,[35,36] and posteriorly based or anteriorly based cervicofacial advancement flaps[37] (Fig. 78-41) can be used effectively to reconstruct complex defects (Figs. 78-42 and 78-43).

In addition to local flaps, tissue expanders may be used to increase the amount of skin soft tissue volume available for reconstruction, with the advantage of color match (if local tissue is expanded) as well as skin and tissue of similar texture and quality.[38] Numerous studies have confirmed improved vascularity of expanded tissue, affording more reliability when it is based on smaller random or axial patterns.[39-41] Expanded tissue may be used for primary defect closure, for donor defect closure, or as a full-thickness skin graft. The incidence of complications of tissue expansion in head and neck reconstruction continues to make the use of these devices somewhat controversial; however, the benefits may outweigh the risks in specific patients with massive, complex defects. The procedure of tissue expansion is well tolerated in adults and children and in patients requiring serial expansion and reconstruction (Fig. 78-44).

For large zone 3 defects, it may be necessary to use regional flaps such as deltopectoral flaps (Fig. 78-45),[42] cervicohumeral flaps (Fig. 78-46),[43] pectoralis major flaps (Figs. 78-47 and 78-48),[44] trapezius flaps (Fig. 78-49),[45,46] latissimus flaps, and free flaps for optimal reconstruction. Careful preoperative planning for elevation of these flaps is essential. When planning a reconstruction for a cheek defect, one must be concerned with the depth of the wound. If the full-thickness defect encroaches onto the oral mucosa or the maxillary sinus, various lining flaps are paramount in the reconstructive plan. Various techniques to provide lining include primary closure when possible, forehead flap transposition,[47] turnover book flaps (see Fig. 78-42),[48] folded skin flaps,[49] musculocutaneous flaps transposed from distant areas, and ultimately free flaps. Coleman, Nahai, and Mathes[50] presented and advocated the use of the platysma flap for cheek lining (Fig. 78-50). The pectoralis major musculocutaneous flap based on the dominant thoracoacromial pedicle has a standard arc of rotation that will provide coverage up to the level of the inferior orbital rim (Fig. 78-51; see Fig. 78-45).

In some unique situations, such as subcutaneous paucity of tissue as seen in Romberg disease or residual contour defects from cicatricial retraction, subcutaneous filling with dermal grafts, dermal fat grafts,[51-53] or free fat injections[54,55] may be used for defect correction (Fig. 78-52; see Fig. 78-38L). The etiology of progressive hemifacial atrophy, or Romberg disease, is unknown. Not only may it involve the subcutaneous tissue and skin, but it may also include the muscles and osteocartilaginous framework. Treatment for the atrophy is, in general, recommended after progression of the disease ceases. However, well-vascularized tissue flaps may maintain volume even in the progressive stage of the disease. Regarding free flap reconstruction, the parascapular flap, omental flap, groin flap, and various muscle flaps, such as the latissimus dorsi, the serratus anterior, and the gracilis, are excellent choices (Figs. 78-53 and 78-54).[56-63]

Reconstruction for acquired defects secondary to aging or cosmetic surgery may be required. For example, witch's chin deformity, a term originally coined by Gonzalez-Ulloa[64] in 1972 to describe ptosis of the premental soft tissues, a prominent submental crease, and, often, a loss of bone projection, has a number of procedures that have been described for its correction.[65-68] These procedures take into account tightening of the soft tissues of the chin but do not address any bone reconstruction. The witch's chin deformity results from laxity and gravitational movement, producing ptosis of the soft tissue and musculature of the chin at the mentum. Repair by use of the anteriorly based, de-epithelialized, triangular flaps—buried posteriorly in a subcutaneous pocket—can easily correct this witch's chin deformity without sacrifice of tissue (Figs. 78-55 to 78-58).[69]

Text continued on p. 857

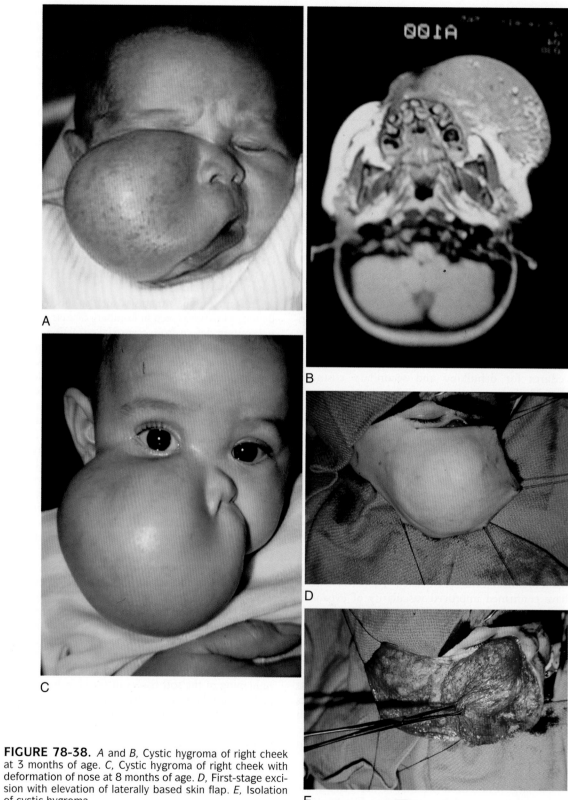

FIGURE 78-38. *A* and *B,* Cystic hygroma of right cheek at 3 months of age. *C,* Cystic hygroma of right cheek with deformation of nose at 8 months of age. *D,* First-stage excision with elevation of laterally based skin flap. *E,* Isolation of cystic hygroma.

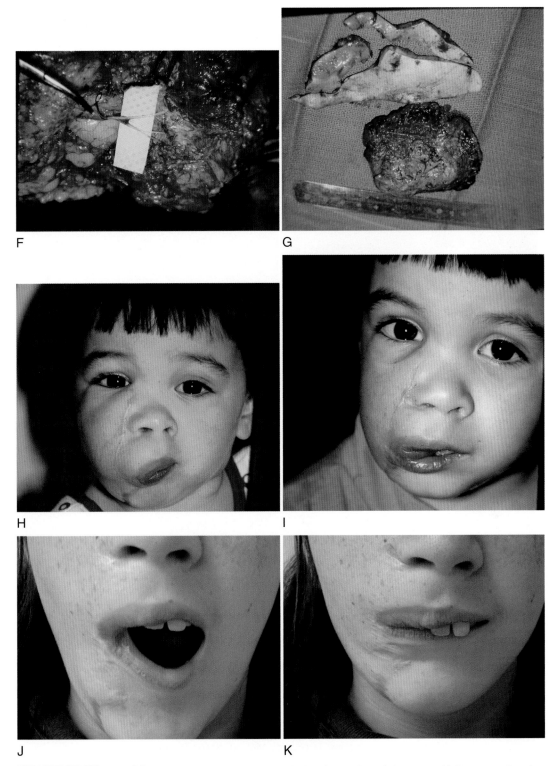

FIGURE 78-38, cont'd. *F,* Isolation of facial nerves. *G,* Specimen of cystic hygroma. *H,* Postoperative view at the age of 3 years. *I,* Age 4 years, after re-excision. *J* and *K,* Age 14 years.   *Continued*

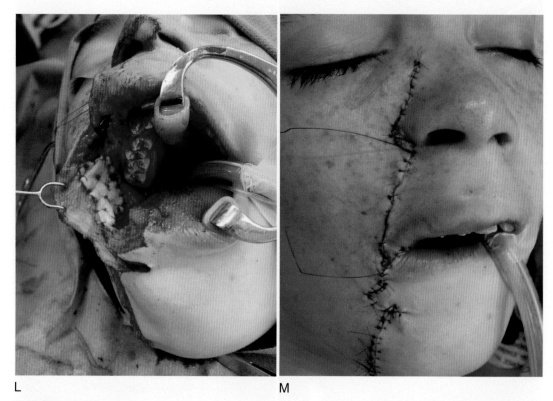

L   M

FIGURE 78-38, cont'd. *L,* Release of right buccal mucosal contraction with full-thickness skin graft. *M,* Intraoperative closure.

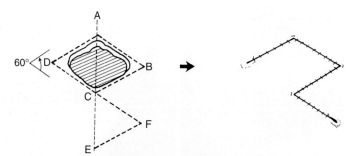

FIGURE 78-39. The Limberg[32] flap designed for use in a rhomboidal defect with a small angle of about 60 degrees. A-C is extended to E and D-C is extended to F so that C-F = A-B and E-F = C-B. Mobility of the local area is a must. (From Mullin WR: Surgery of the forehead and cheek regions. In Lesavoy MA, ed: Reconstruction of the Head and Neck. Baltimore, Williams & Wilkins, 1981:29.)

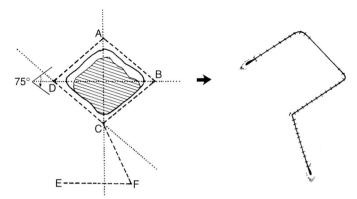

FIGURE 78-40. The Dufourmentel flap is used for rhomboidal defects with small angles of about 75 degrees. A-C and D-C are extended, and the resulting angle is bisected so that C-F = A-B and E-F = C-B. E-F is horizontal to D-B. As in the Limberg flap, local mobility is a must. (From Mullin WR: Surgery of the forehead and cheek regions. In Lesavoy MA, ed: Reconstruction of the Head and Neck. Baltimore, Williams & Wilkins, 1981:29.)

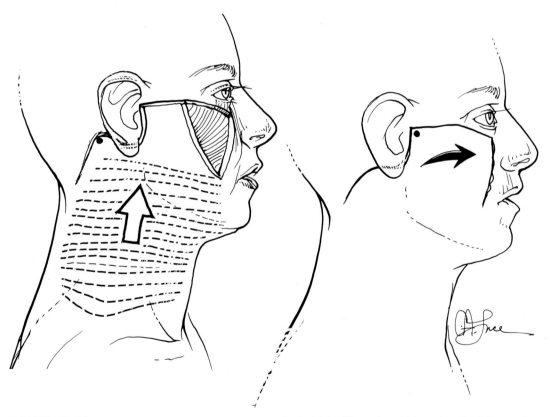

FIGURE 78-41. An anteriorly and inferiorly based cervicofacial flap[37] may be widely undermined for rotation and advancement to close the lateral aspect of the suborbital region. (From Zide BM: Deformities of the lips and cheeks. In McCarthy JG, ed: Plastic Surgery. Philadelphia, WB Saunders, 1990:2009.)

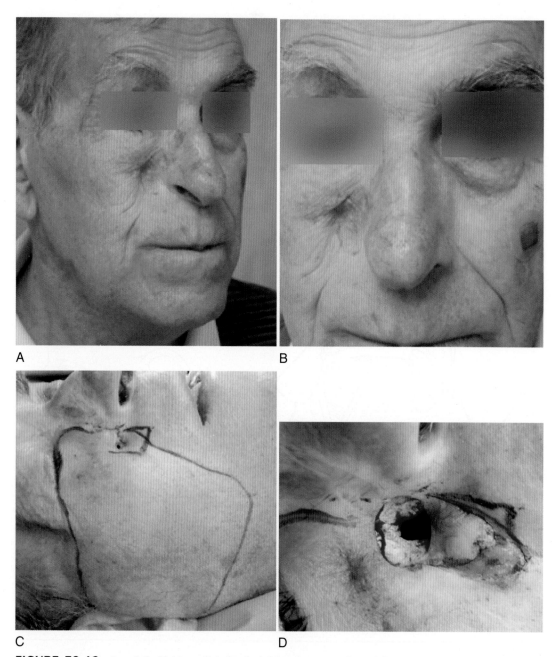

FIGURE 78-42. *A* and *B,* Right medial cheek defect after resection of maxillary sinus-cutaneous fistula. *C,* Design of posteriorly based cheek flap advancement and superiorly based turnover flap for closure of maxillary sinus–cutaneous fistula. *D,* Preparation of superiorly based turnover book flap.

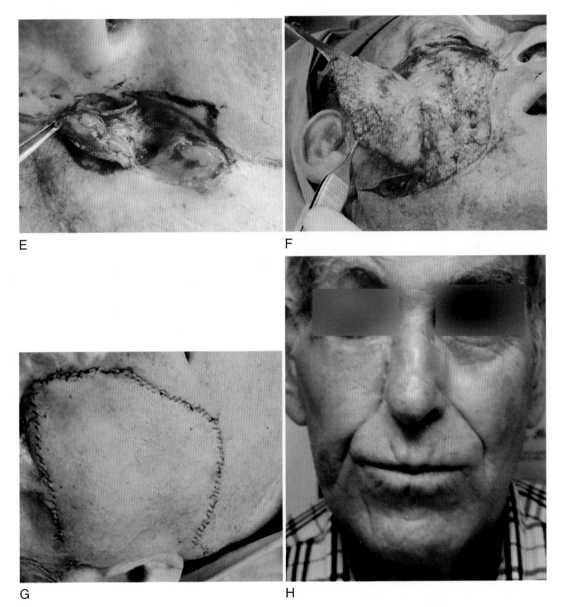

FIGURE 78-42, cont'd. *E,* Transposition of turnover book flap for cutaneous lining of maxillary sinus-cutaneous fistula. *F,* Elevation of posteriorly based cheek advancement flap. *G,* Inset of cheek advancement flap. *H,* Final result with two-flap closure.

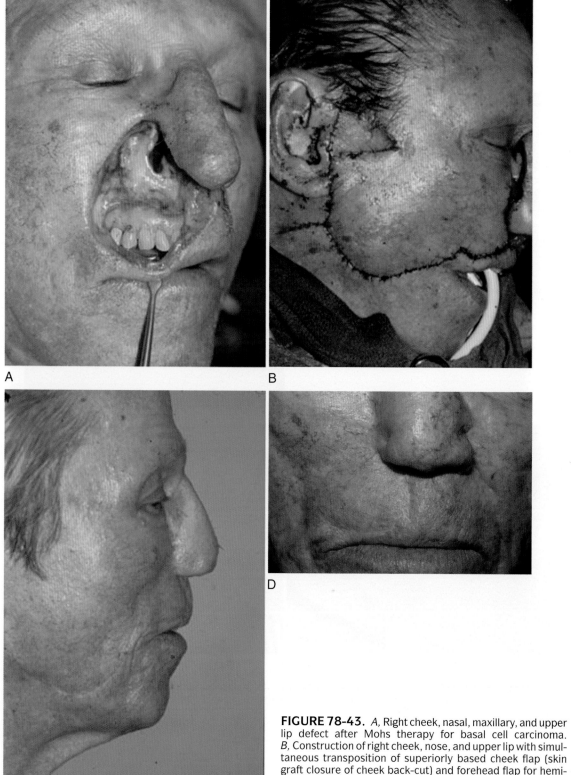

FIGURE 78-43. *A,* Right cheek, nasal, maxillary, and upper lip defect after Mohs therapy for basal cell carcinoma. *B,* Construction of right cheek, nose, and upper lip with simultaneous transposition of superiorly based cheek flap (skin graft closure of cheek back-cut) and forehead flap for heminasal reconstruction. *C* and *D,* Final result of right cheek, upper lip, and nasal reconstruction.

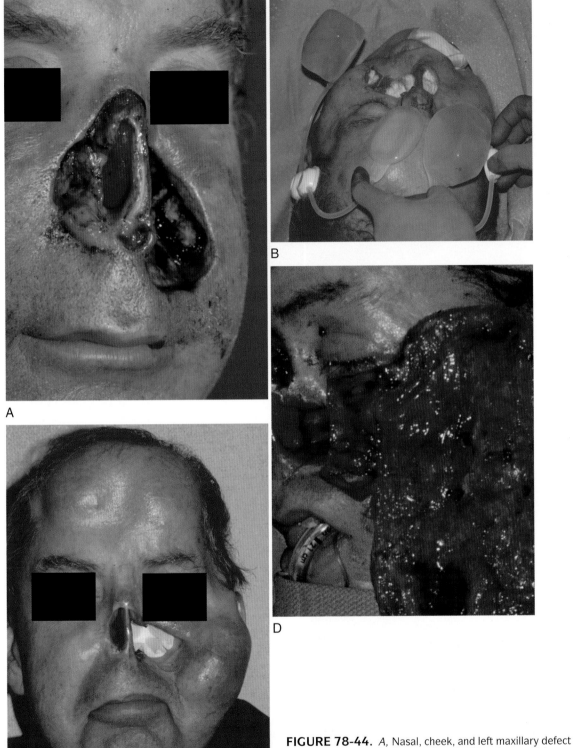

FIGURE 78-44. *A,* Nasal, cheek, and left maxillary defect after Mohs therapy for invasive basal cell carcinoma. *B,* Insertion of two tissue expanders in forehead for nasal reconstruction and one tissue expander in left cheek for cheek reconstruction. *C,* Postoperative view with tissue expanders in place. *D,* Cutaneous lining of maxillary sinus with turnover book flaps. *Continued*

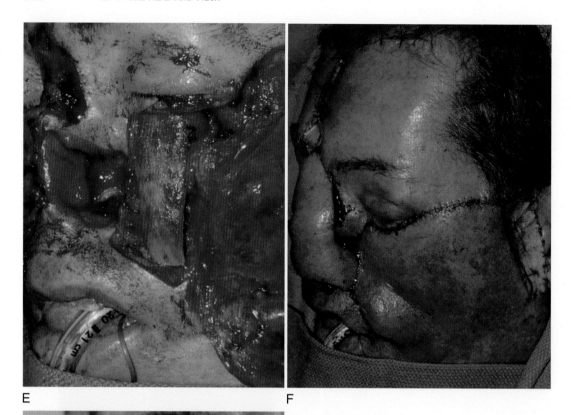

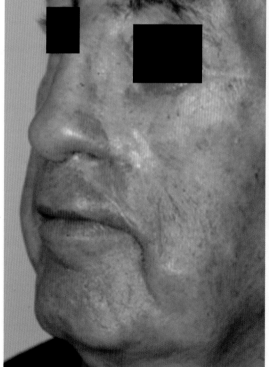

FIGURE 78-44, cont'd. *E,* Osseous rib graft (superficial to cutaneous lining flap of maxillary sinus) for bone stabilization of maxilla. *F,* Inferiorly based cheek transposition flap for maxillary bone graft coverage and simultaneous forehead flap for nasal reconstruction. *G,* Reconstruction of left maxillary sinus lining, bony maxilla, cheek, nose, and left upper lip. Forehead flap—nasal reconstruction.

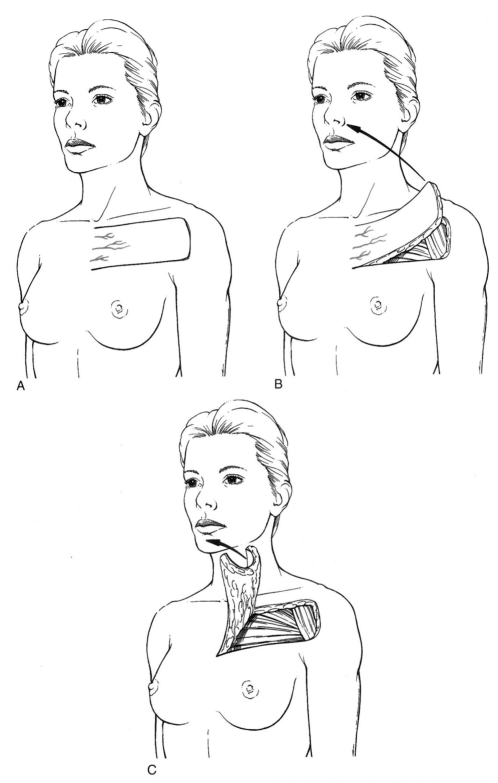

FIGURE 78-45. Deltopectoral flap: arc of rotation. *A,* Standard flap design. *B,* Arc to lower neck. *C,* Tubed flap arc to lower oral cavity. (From Mathes SJ, Nahai F: Reconstructive Surgery: Principles, Anatomy, and Technique. New York, Churchill Livingstone, 1997:417.)

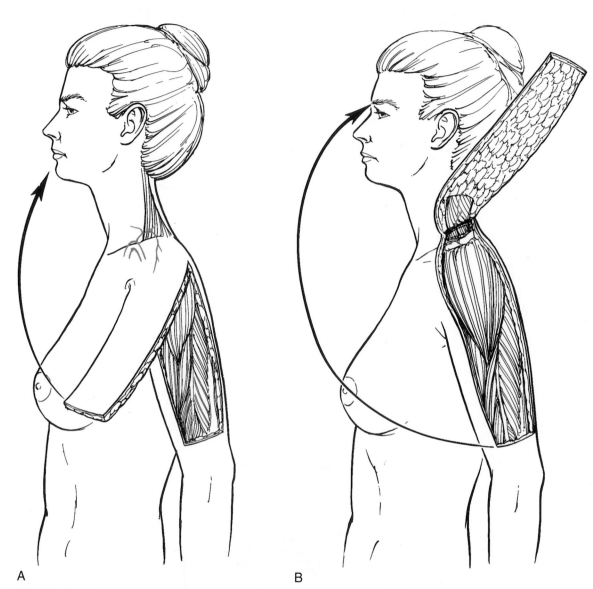

A   B

FIGURE 78-46. Extended lateral (cervicohumeral) flap: arc of rotation. With elevation of the fasciocutaneous extension of the superior trapezius flap territory from the upper lateral arm, the point of rotation is located at the acromioclavicular joint at the lateral base of the neck. The flap will reach the middle and inferior thirds of the face, ear, and oral cavity. *A,* Arc to neck and inferior face (anterior trapezius fibers to acromioclavicular joint intact). *B,* Arc to neck and superior face (superior trapezius fibers of insertion elevated with flap). (From Mathes SJ, Nahai F: Reconstructive Surgery: Principles, Anatomy, and Technique. New York, Churchill Livingstone, 1997:661.)

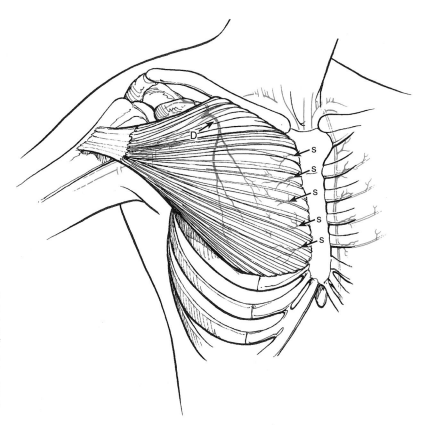

FIGURE 78-47. Pectoralis major flap. Dominant pedicle: pectoral branch of thoracoacromial artery (D). Secondary pedicle: perforating branches of internal mammary artery (s). (From Mathes SJ, Nahai F: Reconstructive Surgery: Principles, Anatomy and Technique. New York, Churchill Livingstone, 1997: 442.)

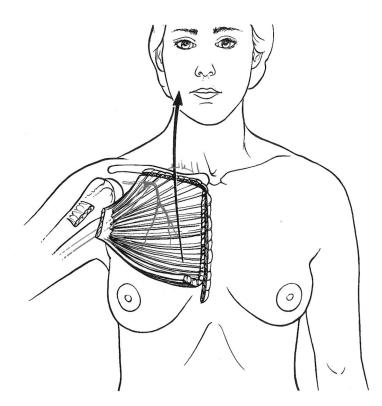

FIGURE 78-48. Pectoralis major flap: arc of rotation of standard flap to middle third of the face. Based on the single dominant thoracoacromial pedicle, the muscle will provide coverage for the head and neck up to the level of the inferior orbital rim. Division of the muscle either at its insertion or through the anterior axillary fold will allow further flap rotation and increase the arc of rotation by as much as 3 to 5 cm. (From Mathes SJ, Nahai F: Reconstructive Surgery: Principles, Anatomy, and Technique. New York: Churchill Livingstone, 1997:448.)

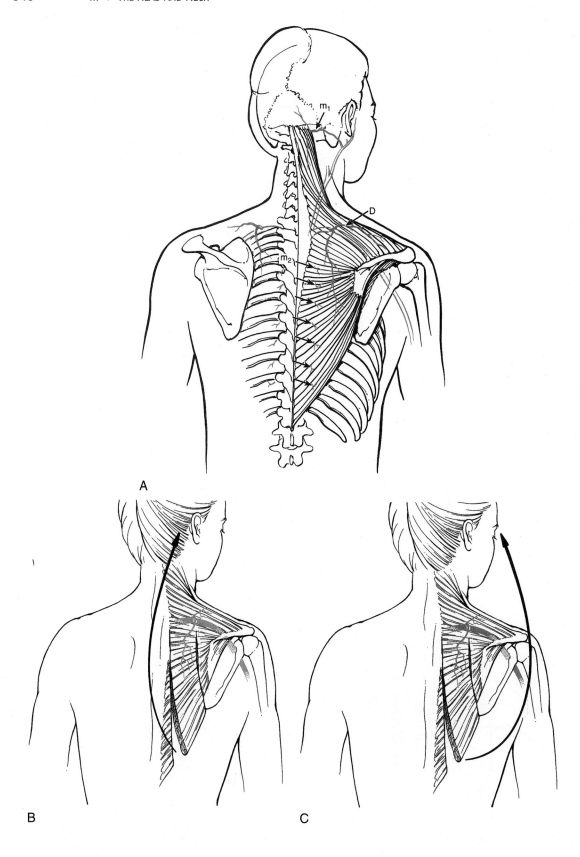

A

B   C

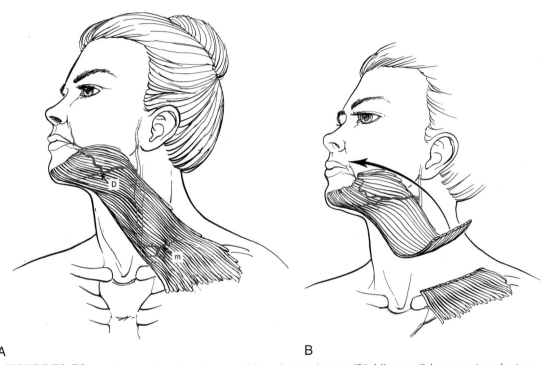

A   B

FIGURE 78-50. *A,* Platysma flap. Dominant pedicle: submental artery (D). Minor pedicle: suprasternal artery (m). *B,* Platysma flap arc of rotation, standard flap. Based on the dominant pedicle, the entire muscle may be elevated as a flap with a rotation point at the level of the mandible. It will reach midline neck defects, the chin, and even the upper lip. It will also reach the intraoral cavity from the central buccal sulcus to the anterior tonsillar pillar. (From Mathes SJ, Nahai F: Reconstructive Surgery: Principles, Anatomy, and Technique. New York, Churchill Livingstone, 1997:326, 327.)

FIGURE 78-49. *A,* Vertical trapezius musculocutaneous flap. Dominant pedicle: transverse cervical artery (D). Minor pedicles: branch of occipital artery (m$_1$); perforating intercostal arteries (m$_2$; see arrows). *B,* Posterior arc of rotation of vertical standard flap. With a rotation point at the posterior base of the neck, the muscle will reach the posterior skull, cervical and thoracic vertebral column, midface, and neck. With release of the superior muscle fibers, the point of rotation will be in the posterior midneck. The flap will now reach the anterior neck, scalp, and face. *C,* Posterior arc of vertical standard flap to anterior neck and face. (From Mathes SJ, Nahai F: Reconstructive Surgery: Principles, Anatomy and Technique. New York, Churchill Livingstone, 1997:658.)

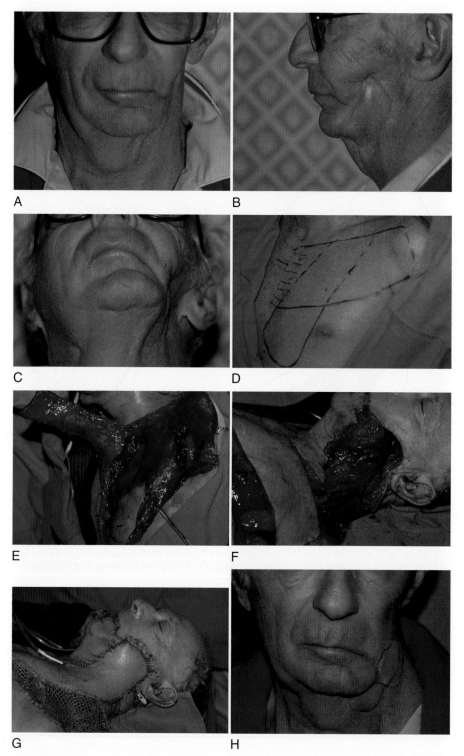

FIGURE 78-51. *A* to *C,* Left mandible and cheek deformity after hemimandibulectomy, irradiation, and salivary fistula. *D,* Design of left deltopectoral flap for cover and pectoralis major musculocutaneous flap for lining. *E,* Elevation of left deltopectoral flap and mobilization of left pectoralis major musculocutaneous flap based on thoracoacromial pedicle. *F,* Transposition of pectoralis major musculocutaneous flap for closure of salivary fistula and lining of oral cavity. *G,* Myocutaneous coverage of pectoralis major muscle flap with deltopectoral flap transposition. *H,* Final result.

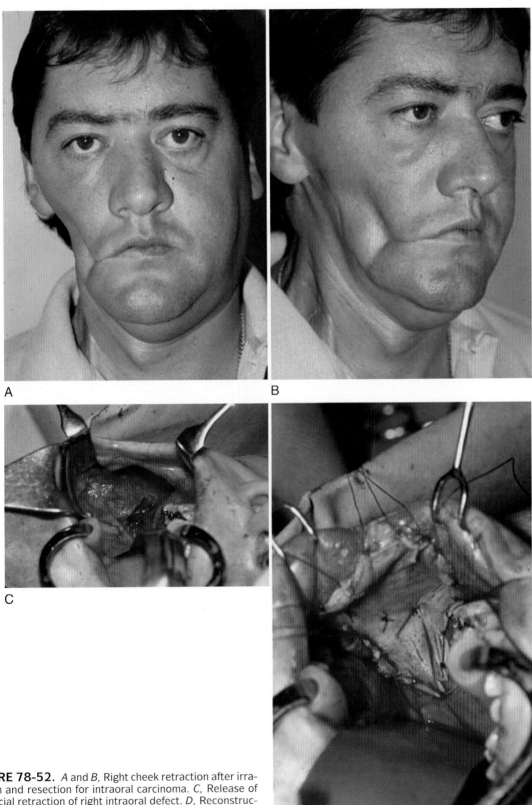

FIGURE 78-52. *A* and *B*, Right cheek retraction after irradiation and resection for intraoral carcinoma. *C*, Release of cicatricial retraction of right intraoral defect. *D*, Reconstruction of intraoral defect with full-thickness skin graft.

Continued

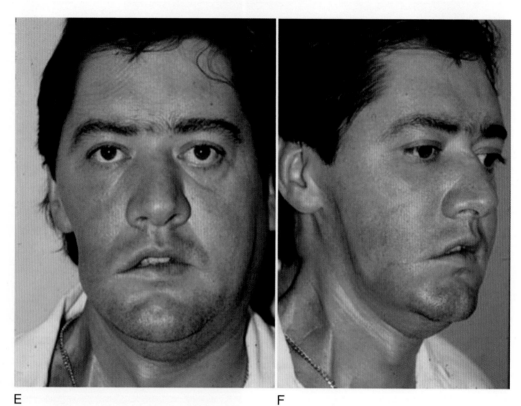

E   F

FIGURE 78-52, cont'd. *E* and *F,* Excellent contour after reconstruction.

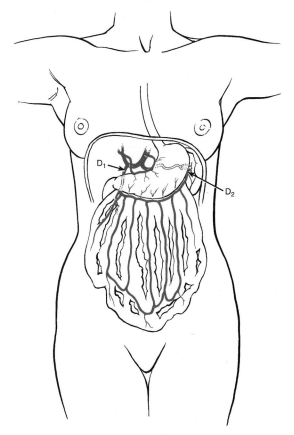

FIGURE 78-53. Omental flap. Dominant pedicles: right gastroepiploic artery and vein (D_1); left gastroepiploic artery and vein (D_2). (From Mathes SJ, Nahai F: Reconstructive Surgery: Principles, Anatomy, and Technique. New York, Churchill Livingstone, 1997:1142.)

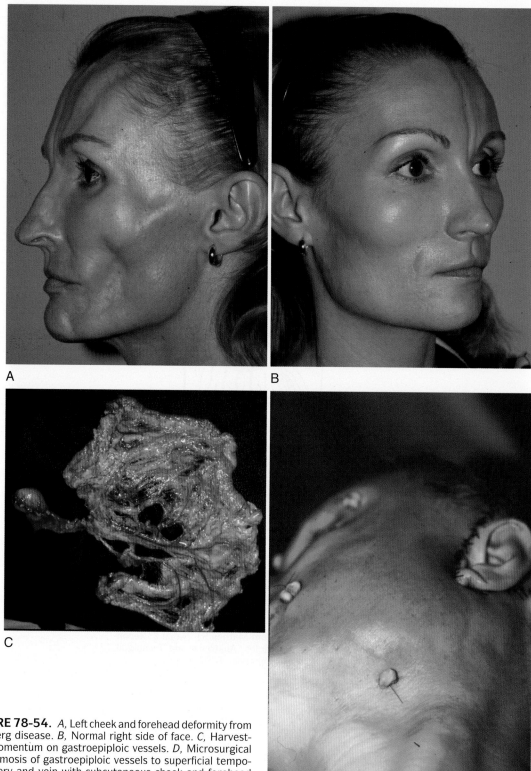

FIGURE 78-54. *A,* Left cheek and forehead deformity from Romberg disease. *B,* Normal right side of face. *C,* Harvesting of omentum on gastroepiploic vessels. *D,* Microsurgical anastomosis of gastroepiploic vessels to superficial temporal artery and vein with subcutaneous cheek and forehead undermining and bolster stabilization of omentum.

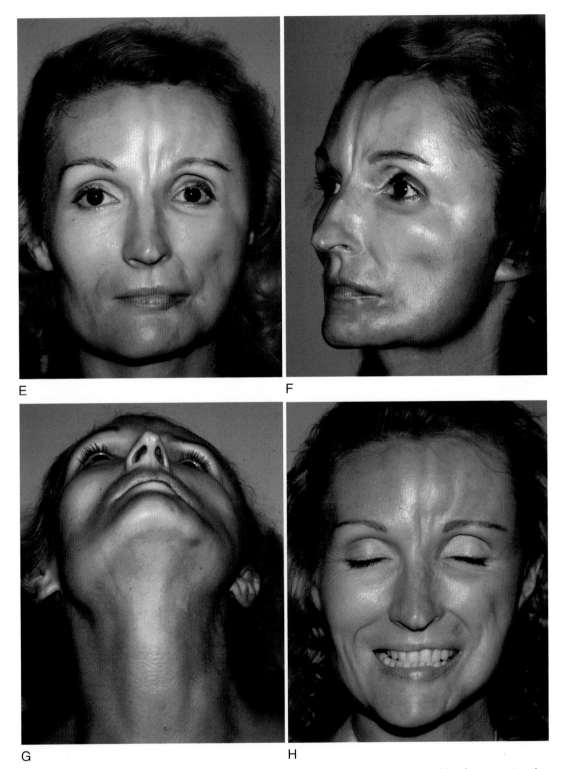

FIGURE 78-54, cont'd. *E to G,* Final result after omentum microsurgical transposition for reconstruction of Romberg disease. *H,* Good animation status after reconstruction.

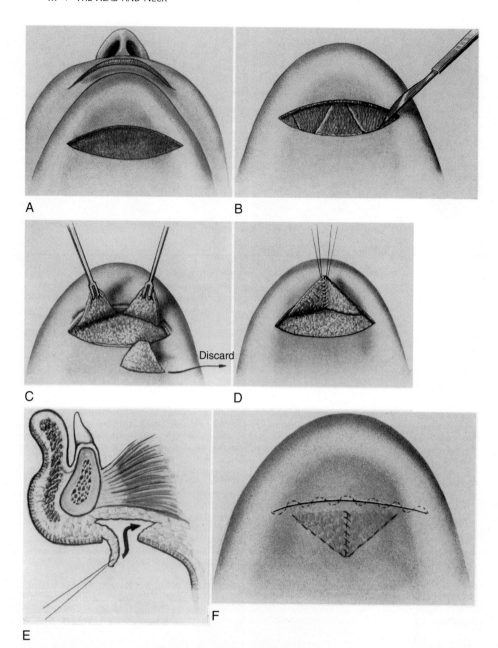

A

B

C

Discard

D

E

F

FIGURE 78-55. *A,* An ellipse with the submental fold as its long axis is de-epithelialized. *B,* Two divergent anteriorly based triangular flaps are formed in the de-epithelialized skin. *C,* The medial intervening triangle of skin is excised. *D,* The converging flaps are sutured together. *E,* The skin posterior to the ellipse is undermined to the hyoid bone. *F,* The flaps are inset, and the posterior skin edge is advanced and sutured to the anterior edge of the ellipse. (From Lesavoy ML, Creasman C, Schwartz RJ: A technique for correcting witch's chin deformity. Plast Reconstr Surg 1996;97:842.)

FIGURE 78-56. *A,* Preoperative view of patient with witch's chin deformity. *B,* Postoperative view of witch's chin correction. *C,* Diagram of intraoperative submental crease, triangular flaps. *D,* De-epithelialization of anteriorly based triangular flaps. *E* and *F,* Elevation of anteriorly based triangular flaps. *G,* Medial approximation of anteriorly based flaps. *H,* Final closure. (*A* and *B* from Lesavoy ML, Creasman C, Schwartz RJ: A technique for correcting witch's chin deformity. Plast Reconstr Surg 1996;97:842.)

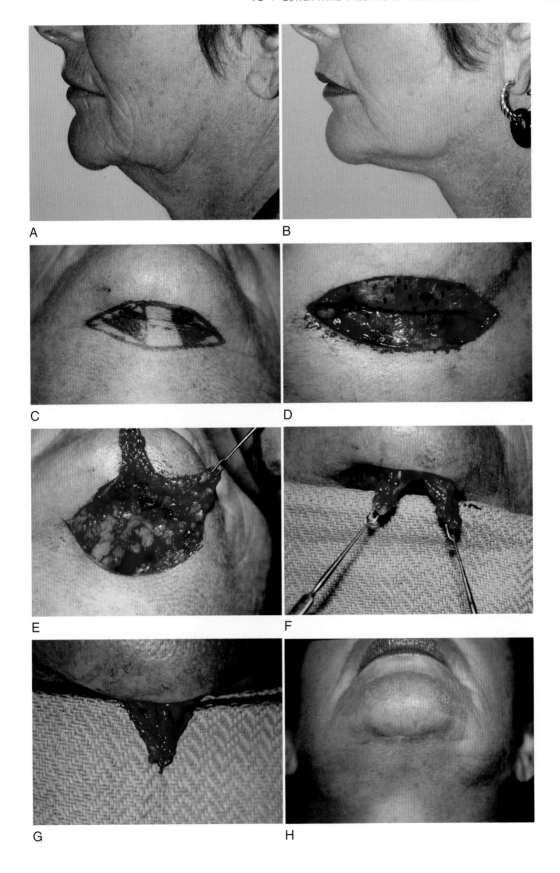

A

B

C

D

E

F

G

H

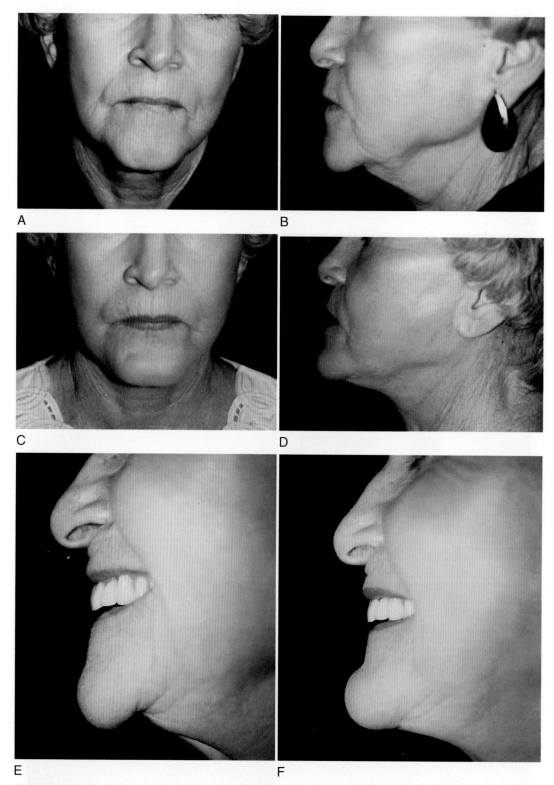

A   B

C   D

E   F

FIGURE 78-57. *A, C,* and *E,* Preoperative views of patient with witch's chin deformity. *B, D,* and *F,* Post-operative views after correction of witch's chin deformity.

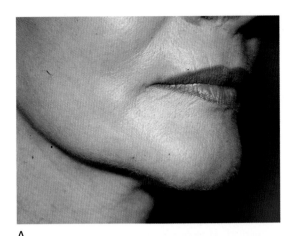

A

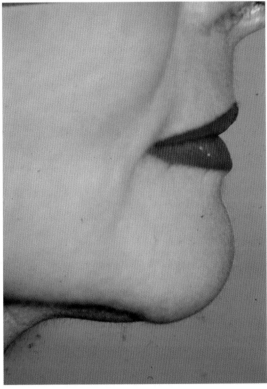

B

FIGURE 78-58. *A*, Preoperative view of patient with witch's chin deformity. *B*, Postoperative view of correction of witch's chin deformity.

REFERENCES

1. Constantinidis J, Federspiel P, Iro H: Functional and aesthetic objectives in the lip reconstruction. Facial Plast Surg 1999;15:337.
2. Mazzola RF, Lupo G: Evolving concepts in lip reconstruction. Clin Plast Surg 1984;11:583.
3. Lesavoy MA: Lip deformities and their reconstruction. In Lesavoy MA, ed: Reconstruction of the Head and Neck. Baltimore, Williams & Wilkins, 1981:95.
4. Gillies HD, Millard DR Jr: Principles and Art of Plastic Surgery. Boston, Little, Brown, 1957.
5. Kawamoto HK: Correction of major defects of the vermilion with a cross-lip vermilion flap. Plast Reconstr Surg 1979;64:315.
6. Wilson JSP, Walker EP: Reconstruction of the lower lip. Head Neck Surg 1981;4:29.
7. Bakamjian V: The use of tongue flaps in lower lip reconstruction. Br J Plast Surg 1964;17:76.
8. Bretteville-Jensen G: Reconstruction of the lower lip after central excisions. Br J Plast Surg 1973;26:247.
9. Stranc MF, Robertson GA: Steeple flap reconstruction of the lower lip. Ann Plast Surg 1983;10:4.
10. Rayner CR, Arscott GD: A new method of resurfacing the lip. Br J Plast Surg 1987;40:454.
11. Louis A: Memoire sur l'operation du bec de lievre, ou l'on etabli le premier principe de l'art de reunir les plaies. Mem Acad Roy Chir 1768;4:385.
12. Webster JP: Crescentic peri-alar cheek excision for upper lip flap advancement with a short history of upper lip repair. Plast Reconstr Surg 1955;16:434.
13. Spira M, Stal S: V-Y advancement of a subcutaneous pedicle in vermilion lip reconstruction. Plast Reconstr Surg 1983;72:562.
14. Davidson TM, Bartlow GA, Bone RC: Surgical excisions from and reconstructions of the oral lips. J Dermatol Surg Oncol 1980;6:133.
15. Andrews EB: Repair of lower lip defects by the Hagedorn rectangular flap method. Plast Reconstr Surg 1964;34:27.
16. Owens N: Simplified method of rotating skin and mucous membrane flaps for complete reconstruction of the lower lip. Surgery 1944;5:196.
17. Johanson B, Aspelund E, Breine U, Holmstrom H: Surgical treatment of non-traumatic lower lip lesions with special reference to the step technique. Scand J Plast Reconstr Surg 1974;8:232.
18. Schuchardt K: Operationen im Gesicht und im kieferbereich Operationen an den Lippen. In Bier A, Braun H, Kümmel H, eds: Chirurgische Operationslehre. Leipzig, JA Barth, 1954.
19. Abbe RA: A new plastic operation for the relief of deformity due to double harelip. Med Rec 1898;53:477.
20. Abbe R: A new plastic operation for the relief of deformity due to double harelip. The classic reprint. Plast Reconstr Surg 1968;42:481.
21. Stein SAW: Laebedannelse (Cheiloplastik) udfort paa en ny methode. Hospitalsmeddelelson (Copenh) 1848;1:212.
22. Wexler MR, Dingman RO: Reconstruction of the lower lip. Chir Plast (Berl) 1975;3:23.
23. Smith JW: The anatomical and physiologic acclimatization of tissue transplanted by the lip switch technique. Plast Reconstr Surg 1960;26:40.
24. Estlander JA: Eine Methode aus der einen Lippe Substanzverluste der anderen zu ersetzen [A method of reconstructing loss of substance in one lip from the other lip]. Arch Klin Chir 1872;14:622. Classic reprint; translated from the German by Dr. Borje Sundell. Plast Reconstr Surg 1968;42:360.
25. Karapandzic M: Reconstruction of lip defects by local arterial flaps. Br J Plast Surg 1974;27:93.
26. Jabaley ME, Clement RL, Orcutt TW: Myocutaneous flaps in lip reconstruction. Applications of the Karapandzic principle. Plast Reconstr Surg 1977;59:680.
27. Canady JW, Thompson SA, Bardach J: Oral commissure burns in children. Plast Reconstr Surg 1996;97:738, discussion 745, 746-755.
28. Bernard C: Cancer de la levre inferieure opere par un procede nouveau. Bull Mem Soc Chir Paris 1853;3:357.
29. Webster RC, Coffey RJ, Kelleher RE: Total and partial reconstruction of the lower lip with innervated muscle bearing flaps. Plast Reconstr Surg 1960;25:360.
30. Wernher A: Die angeborenen Kysten-Hygrome und die ihnen verwandten Geschwulste in anatomischer, diagnosticher und therapeutischer Beziehung. Giessen, GF Heyer, Vater, 1843.

31. Garden AS, Benzie RJ, Miskin M, Gardner HA: Fetal cystic hygroma colli: antenatal diagnosis, significance, and management. Am J Obstet Gynecol 1986;154:221.

32. Limberg AA: Mathematical Principles of Local Plastic Procedures on the Surface of the Human Body. Leningrad, Medgis, 1946.

33. Lister GD, Gibson T: Closure of rhomboid skin defects: the flaps of Limberg and Dufourmentel. Br J Plast Surg 1972;25:300.

34. Jeris W, Salyer K, Busquets M, Atkins R: Further application of Limberg and Dufourmentel flaps. Plast Reconstr Surg 1975;58:196.

35. Mustardé JC: Repair and Reconstruction in the Orbital Region. Edinburgh, Churchill Livingstone, 1980.

36. Jackson IT: Local Flaps in Head and Neck Reconstruction. St. Louis, CV Mosby, 1985.

37. Juri J, Juri C: Advancement and rotation of a large cervicofacial flap for cheek repairs. Plast Reconstr Surg 1979;64:692.

38. Argenta LC, Watanabe MJ, Grabb WC: The use of tissue expansion in head and neck reconstruction. Ann Plast Surg 1983;11:31.

39. Spence R: Experience with novel uses of tissue expanders in burn reconstruction of the face and neck. Ann Plast Surg 1992;28:453.

40. Cherry GW, Austad ED, Pasky K, et al: Increased survival and vascularity of random pattern skin flaps elevated in controlled, expanded skin. Plast Reconstr Surg 1983;72:680.

41. Baker SR, Swanson NA: Clinical applications of tissue expansion in head and neck surgery. Laryngoscope 1990;100:313.

42. Bakamjian VY: A two-stage method of pharyngoesophageal reconstruction with a primary pectoral skin flap. Plast Reconstr Surg 1965;36:173.

43. Mathes SJ, Vasconez LO: The cervicohumeral flap. Plast Reconstr Surg 1978;61:7.

44. Ariyan S: The pectoralis major myocutaneous flap, a versatile flap for reconstruction in the head and neck. Plast Reconstr Surg 1979;63:73.

45. Panje W, Cutting C: Trapezius osteomyocutaneous island flap for reconstruction of the anterior floor of the mouth and mandible. Head Neck Surg 1980;3:66.

46. Baek SM, Biller HF, Krespi YP, Lawson W: The lower trapezius island myocutaneous flap. Ann Plast Surg 1980;5:108.

47. McGregor IA, Reid WH: Simultaneous temporal and deltopectoral flaps for full-thickness defects of the cheek. Plast Reconstr Surg 1970;45:326.

48. Chongchet V: Subcutaneous pedicle flaps for reconstruction of the lining of the lip and cheek. Br J Plast Surg 1977;30:38.

49. Sharzer LA, Kalisman M, Silver CE, Strauch B: The parasternal paddle: a modification of the pectoralis major myocutaneous flap. Plast Reconstr Surg 1981;67:753.

50. Coleman JJ, Nahai F, Mathes SJ: The platysma musculocutaneous flap: experience with 24 cases. Plast Reconstr Surg 1983;72:315.

51. Yano H, Tanaka K, Murakami R, et al: Microsurgical dermal fat retransfer for progressive hemifacial atrophy. J Reconstr Microsurg 2005;21:15.

52. Leaf N, Zarem HA: Correction of contour defects of the face with dermal and dermal-fat grafts. Arch Surg 1972;105:715.

53. Williams HB, Crepeau RJ: Free dermal fat flaps to the face. Ann Plast Surg 1979;3:1.

54. Moscona R, Ullman Y, Har-Shai Y, Hirshowitz B: Free-fat injections for the correction of hemifacial atrophy. Plast Reconstr Surg 1989;84:501, discussion 508.

55. Chajchir A, Benzaquen I: Fat-grafting injection for soft-tissue augmentation. Plast Reconstr Surg 1989;84:921, discussion 935.

56. Longaker MT, Siebert JW: Microvascular free-flap correction of severe hemifacial atrophy. Plast Reconstr Surg 1995;96:800.

57. Upton J, Albin RE, Mulliken JB, Murray JE: The use of scapular and parascapular flaps for cheek reconstruction. Plast Reconstr Surg 1992;90:959.

58. Tweed AE, Manktelow RT, Zuker RM: Facial contour reconstruction with free flaps. Ann Plast Surg 1984;12:313.

59. Jurkiewicz MJ, Nahai F: The omentum: its use as a free vascularized graft for reconstruction of the head and neck. Ann Surg 1982;195:756.

60. Harashina T, Fujino T: Reconstruction in Romberg's disease with free groin flap. Ann Plast Surg 1981;7:289.

61. Dunkley MP, Stevenson JH: Experience with the free "inverted" groin flap in facial soft tissue contouring; a report on 6 flaps. Br J Plast Surg 1990;43:154.

62. Jones NF: The contribution of microsurgical reconstruction to craniofacial surgery. World J Surg 1989;13:454.

63. Mordick TG 2nd, Larossa D, Whitaker L: Soft-tissue reconstruction of the face: a comparison of dermal-fat grafting and vascularized tissue transfer. Ann Plast Surg 1992;29:390.

64. Gonzalez-Ulloa M: Ptosis of the chin: the witch's chin. Plast Reconstr Surg 1972;50:54.

65. Feldman JJ: The ptotic (witch's) chin deformity: an excisional approach. Plast Reconstr Surg 1992;90:207.

66. Field LM: Correction by a flap of suprahyoid fat of a witch's chin caused by a submental retracting scar. J Dermatol Surg Oncol 1981;7:719.

67. Burke LO: Correction of the deep submental crease by dermafat "roll flap." Presented at the fifteenth annual meeting of the American Society for Aesthetic Plastic Surgery, Las Vegas, April 22, 1982.

68. Peterson RA: Correction of the senile chin by derma-fat flaps, chin implant, and platysma plication. Presented at the fifteenth annual meeting of the American Society for Aesthetic Plastic Surgery, Las Vegas, April 22, 1982.

69. Lesavoy ML, Creasman C, Schwartz RJ: A technique for correcting witch's chin deformity. Plast Reconstr Surg 1996;97:842.

✦

Midface Reconstruction

Kɪʏᴏɴᴏʀɪ Hᴀʀɪɪ, MD ✦ Hɪʀᴏᴛᴀᴋᴀ Aꜱᴀᴛᴏ, MD, PhD
✦ Aᴋɪʜɪᴋᴏ Tᴀᴋᴜꜱʜɪᴍᴀ, MD, PhD

ANATOMIC STRUCTURES OF THE MIDFACE
    Specific Organs
    Soft Tissues
    Bones
    Vessels and Nerves
MORBIDITY AND ETIOLOGY
PREOPERATIVE EVALUATION
    Type I Defect
    Type II Defect

Type III Defect
Type IV Defect
Type V Defect
OPERATIVE MANAGEMENT
    Skin and Soft Tissue Defects
    Skeletal Defects
    Muscle Defects

The midface includes the cheek, maxilla, palate, orbit, and nose. The face presents a human's identity to others. In addition, functions such as respiration, mastication, deglutition, and speech are greatly influenced by midface morbidity. The goal of midface reconstruction, therefore, is to minimize functional as well as aesthetic defects. However, in general, less attention has been paid to reconstruction of the midface than of other areas of the head and neck, especially in cancer treatments.[1,2] Because three-dimensional reconstruction of the skin, bone, and mucosa complex is required, technical difficulties may interfere with adequate midface reconstruction. Reconstructive options, however, have been greatly expanded with the introduction of various procedures during the last few decades, including microvascular free tissue transfers.[3,4]

ANATOMIC STRUCTURES OF THE MIDFACE

The midface represents the central portion of the face and includes a wide area of soft tissues and musculature supported mainly by the maxillary and zygomatic bony scaffolds. It extends to the orbit and the anterior skull base. Sagging or downward deviation of the ocular globe caused by an inadequate or absent orbital floor frequently leads to diplopia and eye pain as well as facial disfigurement.[5] A watertight seal between the nasoethmoidal and intracranial spaces is a prerequisite in defects of the anterior skull base to minimize life-threatening infections. Three-dimensional structures of the midface consist of various elements, such

as skin and subcutaneous tissues, muscles, bones, and oronasal mucosal lining, which makes reconstruction complex and difficult. It is made more difficult by the need for optional aesthetic reconstruction as well as functional restoration.

Specific Organs

Eyes are an important focal point in the midface and serve as the primary antenna of the central nervous system. Maxillary and zygomatic bones support the orbital bones and their contents. Impairment of the orbital bones as well as of the extraocular muscles may cause dislocation of the globes, frequently resulting in diplopia and eye pain. Enophthalmos and hypophthalmos caused by orbital bone deficiencies also lead to severe functional morbidity as well as an asymmetric appearance (Fig. 79-1).

The nose acts as both a respiratory and olfactory organ. It serves as the primary airway in the upper respiratory system, filtering inspired air and providing warmth and humidification. Inability to breathe through the nose causes discomfort, chronic oral drying, and olfactory dysfunction.[5] The functional roles of the paranasal sinuses are still controversial, but they apparently reduce the weight of the facial skeleton and head and also protect the brain from anterior impact. Their function is not critical, but the sinus spaces are important to maintain the volume of the anterior face. In addition to respiratory and olfactory functions, the nose itself is aesthetically important because of its central location in the face. It often presents a significant challenge to a reconstructive surgeon.

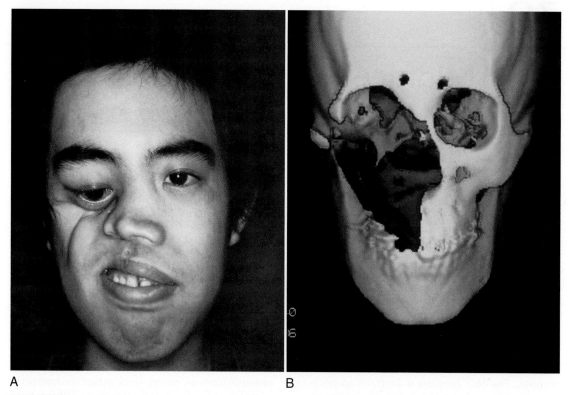

FIGURE 79-1. *A,* Severe depression deformity of the cheek and downward dislocation of the eye after resection of a right maxillary carcinoma including a large part of the maxillary bone. The patient complained of diplopia and eye pain. *B,* A three-dimensional computed tomography scan of the same patient is shown.

Soft Tissues

Facial skin has unique characteristics including rich sebaceous glands, color, texture, and flexibility. The aesthetic facial units first mentioned by Gonzalez-Ulloa et al[6] need to be considered in reconstruction of the midface. Skin in such widely differing areas as the cheek, nose, lips, and orbital regions must be matched according to the criteria mentioned. The lips are defined from the cheek by the nasolabial sulcus running from the nasal ala to the angle of the mouth. Relaxed skin tension lines or wrinkle lines are also important landmarks to note for minimizing incisional scars on the face.[7]

Facial subcutaneous fat consists of small and dense fat particles and tends to accumulate in the buccal region. The buccal fat pad is deeply in the cheek between the masseter and buccinator muscles, forming the wall of the cheek with the buccinator muscle.

Posteriorly in the cheek, the masseter muscle covers the vertical ramus of the mandible. The parotid gland, the largest salivary gland, is located subcutaneously in the posterior cheek, forming a flattened and three-sided pyramid. The superficial surface of the parotid gland is covered by a dense parotid fascia, partly connected to the superficial musculoaponeurotic system,

blending caudally with the platysma fascia and anteriorly to masseter muscle fascia.[8] Clinically, the parotid gland is separated into two portions by the facial nerves. The superficial and large portion anteriorly covers the posteroinferior portion of the masseter muscle. Posteriorly, it covers the ramus and temporomandibular joint of the mandible. It also extends cephalically to the zygoma while it tapers caudally and overlaps the posterior belly of the digastric muscles. The deep and relatively small portion of the parotid gland is mostly located beneath the mandibular ramus. The function of the subcutaneously underlying mimetic musculature innervated by the facial nerves is extremely important. The mimetic muscles allow humans to communicate emotionally with others through various expressions. Treatment of a paralyzed face, therefore, has been a great challenge for reconstructive plastic surgeons.[9]

Bones

The skeletal framework of the midface consists of thicker segments of pillar bones, the so-called buttresses, which form the major support system of the face.[10,11] As Coleman[12] emphasized, the buttresses of the midface are vertically and horizontally oriented and form a three-dimensional skeletal support, preventing soft tissue collapse inward and downward (Fig. 79-2). The paired maxillary and zygomatic bones, palatine bones, orbital bones, and nasofrontal bones serve as the buttresses. Of these, the three vertical buttresses of the maxilla—the nasofrontal, zygomatic, and pterygomaxillary—maintain the midfacial projection and vertical height. The lower horizontal buttress, chiefly consisting of the palatal bone and maxillary alveolus, provides a normal occlusal plane to the mandible. It also keeps facial width and proportion in close connection with the vertical buttresses. The upper horizontal buttress, consisting of the infraorbital rim and zygomatic arch, supports the eyes and forms the zygomatic prominence, aesthetically important in manifesting a three-dimensional form of the face. Between these buttresses, thin membranous bones intervene to separate cavities and are lined with oronasal mucosa.

Vessels and Nerves

The blood supply to the midface is primarily from branches of the external carotid artery. The facial artery, accompanied by the anterior facial vein, is the only significant cutaneous blood supply of the cheek. However, many close anastomoses with other arteries also serve the midface (e.g., infraorbital, buccal, transverse facial arteries). Sacrifice of the facial artery itself, therefore, leaves no impairment of blood supply to the midface. The deeper blood supply is derived from the branches of the internal maxillary artery, a branch of the external carotid artery, as well as from communicating branches of the external carotid artery. Abundant blood supply from many arteries frequently makes hemostasis difficult in patients with severe trauma.

There are two major nervous systems in the midface, the trigeminal and facial nerves. The sensory nerves originating from the sensory branches of the trigeminal nerve contribute to sensory innervation to the face; the motor branches of the trigeminal nerve innervate the muscles of mastication, such as the temporal, masseter, and pterygoid muscles. The facial nerve chiefly supplies the motor branches to the mimetic muscles.

Finally, lymph drainage of the midface gathers primarily into the parotid and submaxillary lymph nodes and flows to the cervical lymphatic system.

MORBIDITY AND ETIOLOGY

Congenital anomalies, trauma, tumor resection, degenerative diseases, or diseases with an unknown etiology can cause midfacial morbidity. A hemifacial microsomia, although uncommon, typically presents as underdevelopment of the cheek including the mandible, maxilla, and soft tissues. It is sometimes

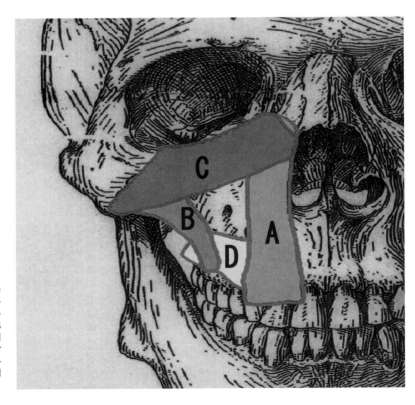

FIGURE 79-2. Schema of the maxillary buttresses: A, nasomaxillary buttress; B, zygomatic buttress; C, upper horizontal buttress mainly consisting of the infraorbital rim and zygomatic arch; D, lower horizontal buttress mainly consisting of the palatine bone and alveolus.

accompanied by facial paralysis because of loss of the mimetic muscles (Fig. 79-3). Severe facial clefts may also require soft tissue reconstruction as well as skeletal rearrangement with a craniofacial procedure. Devastating trauma, such as a gunshot wound or industrial accident, often leads to deficiencies in soft tissues and supportive bones. Deep burns frequently leave thick, wide scars that are best reconstructed with skin grafts.

Defects and morbidity after resection of tumors, however, represent the majority of patients requiring midface reconstruction. For example, radical orbital-nasal-maxillary resection for maxillary carcinoma results in massive and complex defects of the orbital content, maxillary and zygomatic bones, palate, mucosal lining of the oronasal cavity, and sometimes soft tissues of the face. Exposure of the brain through an anterior skull base defect should be immediately sealed from the upper aerodigestive tract to prevent a life-threatening infection (Fig. 79-4). An adequate dental prosthesis may also be required for normal mastication and facial appearance to be regained.

In addition to malignant tumors, extensive resection of a large vascular malformation, such as arteriovenous malformation or lymphangioma, may leave skin, soft tissue, and bone defects (Fig. 79-5). Facial paralysis may become a problem when a wide and deep vascular malformation of the cheek is resected. Parotid tumors, particularly if they are malignant, frequently also result in facial paralysis as well as a soft tissue depression after resection.

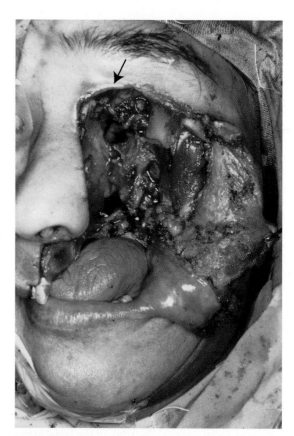

FIGURE 79-4. A large cheek defect with exposure of the brain through a defect of the anterior skull base *(arrow).* Immediate sealing of the brain from the aerodigestive tract is required to prevent a life-threatening infection.

Irradiation, preoperatively or postoperatively, may also cause some sequelae, such as bone necrosis, chronic radiation ulcers, and contractures. Surgery and adjuvant radiotherapy for soft tissue sarcoma or retinoblastoma in children frequently result in underdevelopment of the cheek and the mandible. Such degenerative diseases as progressive hemifacial atrophy (Romberg disease), lipodystrophy, and localized morphea also cause a severe depression of the cheek, leading to significant cosmetic defects.

PREOPERATIVE EVALUATION

It is important preoperatively to evaluate the type of defect present and the anatomic location. The patient and the patient's requirements should also be carefully assessed. A complete understanding of the functional and aesthetic relationship of the normal midfacial units is also indispensable. For example, the goal of surgical therapy for maxillary cancers is total extirpation of the tumor with cure of the patient. However, resection of the maxillary bone, paranasal sinus, palate, zygoma, and possibly orbit results in

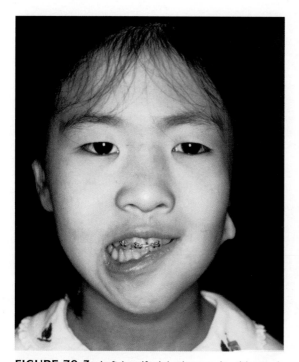

FIGURE 79-3. Left hemifacial microsomia with paralysis of the lower face.

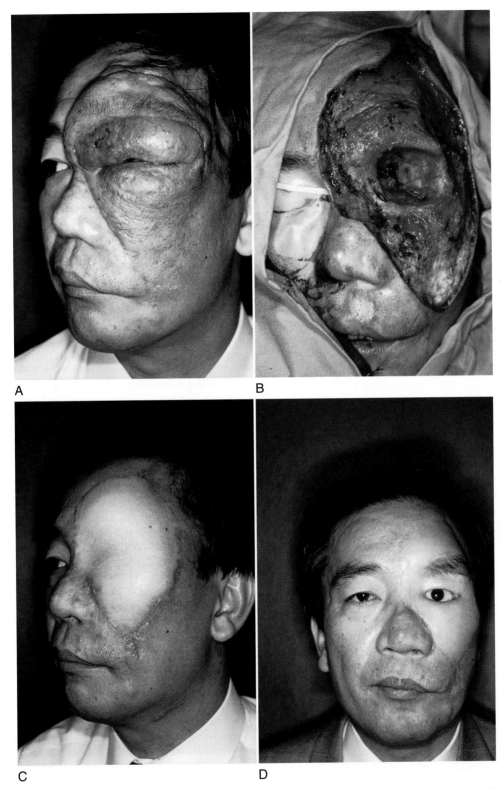

FIGURE 79-5. A 44-year-old man with a severe arteriovenous malformation of the left upper cheek including the eye. *A,* Preoperative view. *B,* Soft tissue defects after extensive resection including the eye. *C,* Immediate coverage with a free latissimus dorsi flap, 4 months postoperatively. *D,* Final result, 2 years postoperatively, after eye socket and eyebrow reconstruction.

significant functional and aesthetic defects and severe morbidity (Fig. 79-6).[13]

A reconstruction algorithm should be regulated by the type of patient, the size of the defect, the anatomic location of the defect, and the structures involved. Wells and Luce[13] proposed a classification of midfacial defects after resection of maxillary malignancies into five unique types according to the size of the skin defect, the extent of the loss of maxillary buttress, the size of the palatal defect, and the loss of orbital support. In the following sections, these types of midfacial defects are listed and categorized in accordance with the size and depth of the defect, location, and structures involved.

Type I Defect

A type I defect includes the cutaneous and superficial subcutaneous tissues. The underlying bony framework and deep structures are mostly intact. No penetrating defects to the aerodigestive cavities are noted. Surgery for burn scar, traumatic scar, and various nevi for which laser treatment is ineffective frequently results in a type I defect. When a skin defect cannot be closed directly, various standard reconstructive modalities for skin

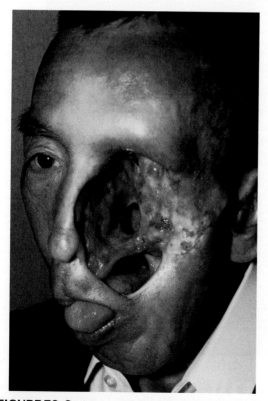

FIGURE 79-6. A full-thickness defect of the cheek after extensive resection of an advanced maxillary cancer and radiation treatment.

replacement are required. A simple skin graft or local flap reconstruction is the preferred choice.[14] Tissue expansion can provide a sufficient local skin flap with good color and texture from the surrounding region to close a relatively large defect, although some authors have reported a high complication rate.[15]

Type II Defect

Deeper soft tissue defects, sometimes including the mimetic and masticatory muscles, require greater bulk to restore facial contour. These are classified as type II defects and are frequently caused by progressive hemifacial atrophy (Romberg disease), lipodystrophy, localized morphea, severe hemifacial microsomia, and ablative surgery for extended malignant tumors of the parotid gland. Facial skin and intraoral mucosa are intact or minimally involved.

A de-epithelialized free skin flap or omental free flap is the ideal reconstructive option for augmentation of missing soft tissues for type II defects (Fig. 79-7).[16,17] A galea-temporoparietal fascia or temporal muscle flap can also augment a depressed orbital region and upper cheek with a simple technique when the defect is limited (Fig. 79-8).[18,19] A conventional pedicle flap from a distant area would be a choice only when local tissues cannot be employed or no vessels are available for free vascularized tissue transfers. A free autogenous fat or dermal fat graft is indicated when a defect is relatively small and has a well-vascularized bed.

When loss of the mimetic muscles results in facial paralysis (which greatly distresses patients because of facial asymmetry as well as dysfunction), a neurovascularized free muscle or musculocutaneous flap can often provide a good result (Fig. 79-9).[20,21]

Type III Defect

A full-thickness defect of the cheek predominantly results from resection of advanced malignant neoplasms. Simultaneous reconstruction of a through-and-through defect of both internal lining and external coverage requires a difficult and complex reconstructive procedure.[22-24] Pedicled or free musculocutaneous flaps, such as the pectoralis major, trapezius, latissimus dorsi, or rectus abdominis flap, can form two or more separated skin paddles on the muscle pedicle. This can then be safely folded to provide flaps for simultaneous coverage of both the internal lining and external skin defect of the cheek (Fig. 79-10).[25-29] In most situations, free musculocutaneous flaps are the most versatile choice because of their reliable vascularity. However, free fasciocutaneous flaps, such as the radial forearm flap, may also serve as a folded flap.[30,31]

Reconstruction of a total or subtotal nasal defect is also a challenging procedure because the nose is located

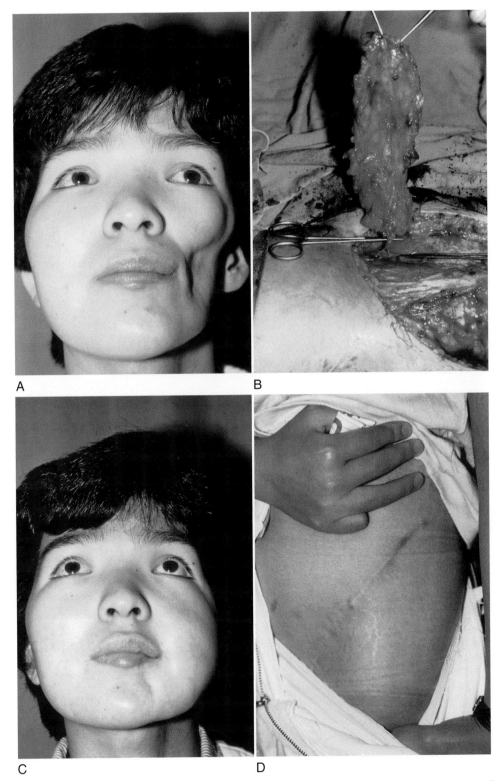

FIGURE 79-7. A 20-year-old woman with severe progressive hemifacial atrophy (Romberg disease). *A,* Preoperative view. *B,* Elevation of a de-epithelialized groin flap, which was transferred to augment the depressed cheek. *C,* Two years postoperatively. *D,* A scar directly closing the donor defect is well accepted by the young woman. (From Hirabayashi S, Harii K, et al: A review of free de-epithelialized skin flap transfer for patients with progressive hemifacial atrophy. J Jpn Soc Plast Reconstr Surg 1987;7:260.)

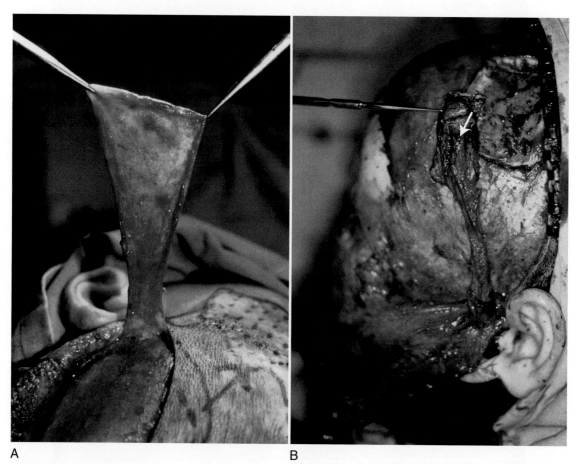

A   B

FIGURE 79-8. *A,* Elevated galea-temporoparietal flap. *B,* A vascularized calvarial bone segment *(arrow)* elevated with a temporoparietal flap.

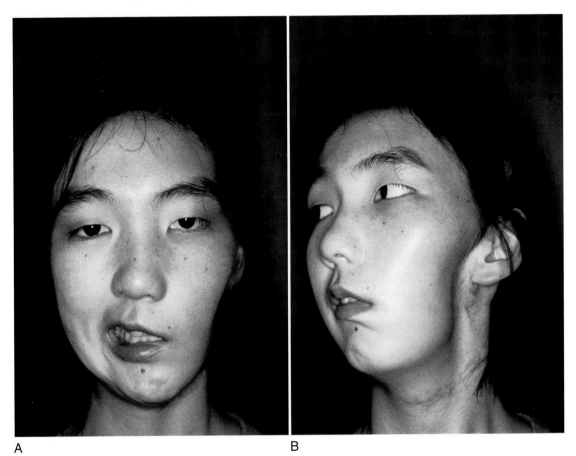

FIGURE 79-9. *A* and *B,* The patient with facial paralysis and cheek depression after extensive parotidectomy including the facial nerve is a good candidate for a neurovascular free muscle or musculocutaneous flap.

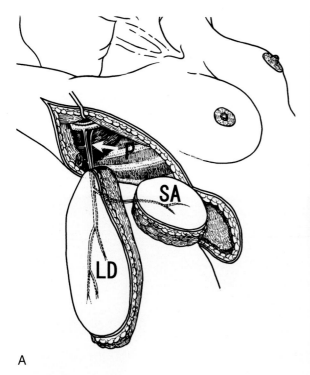

A

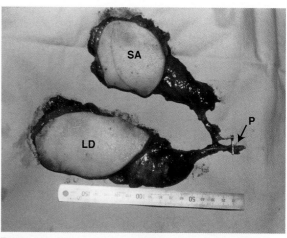

B

FIGURE 79-10. A double musculocutaneous flap with the latissimus dorsi and serratus anterior muscles, nourished by a common pedicle of the thoracodorsal-subscapular vessels, is available for closure of full-thickness cheek defects. *A,* Schema of flaps. *B,* Isolated flaps. LD, latissimus dorsi flap; SA, serratus anterior flap; P, thoracodorsal-subscapular vessel pedicle.

in the center of the face and therefore requires a good aesthetic result.[32] A forehead flap is the best reconstructive option for the nose because of its good color and texture match and proper skin thickness. An expanded forehead flap can provide a sufficient amount of tissue for reconstruction of the total nose.[33,34] A free flap may be an alternative if forehead skin is not available or the patient refuses the use of forehead skin because of its conspicuous donor scar (Fig. 79-11). The free flaps currently used, however, are either a poor color and texture match or of an unfit thickness. Development of a new flap or prefabricated flap would be required to achieve a better result.[35]

Type IV Defect

Type IV defects include deformities to bony structures or bony frameworks (buttresses) of the maxilla and zygoma leading to significant aesthetic deformities of the cheek as well as serious functional morbidity of the eye and dentition. Trauma, severe congenital facial cleft, and tumor ablation may cause this type of defect. Although a large defect of the anterior maxillary wall may cause a depression deformity of the cheek from collapse of the subcutaneous soft tissues into the paranasal sinus, loss of the multiplanar buttresses causes severe deformities of the orbit, cheek, and alveolus.[36,37] Type IV defects are further divided into two subtypes, IVA and IVB.

TYPE IVA DEFECT

Partial loss of the maxilla with loss of the palate and alveolar ridge is a type IVA defect. The nasomaxillary and zygomaticomaxillary buttresses and floor of the orbit including Lockwood ligament are intact. In maxillary cancer cases, this type of bone defect is usually associated with loss of the internal mucosal lining, which permits use of a free skin graft and allows the use of a denture prosthesis. The prosthesis also serves as a palatal obturator and assists in maintaining midfacial projection.

TYPE IVB DEFECT

A type IVB defect indicates a more extensive loss of the maxillary bone including the nasomaxillary and zygomaticomaxillary buttresses, palate, and floor of the orbit. Total maxillectomy for maxillary cancer frequently leads to this type of defect. Devastating trauma, such as a gunshot wound, also causes an extensive defect of the maxilla; however, this type of defect occurs in far fewer patients than do those defects resulting from resection of maxillary cancer. Reconstruction of the bony constitution, especially the upper horizontal buttress and orbital floor, is required for maintenance of facial contour and prevention of dislocation of the globe (Fig. 79-12). When soft tissue lining is complete, an autogenous free bone graft or costal cartilage graft may safely replace the

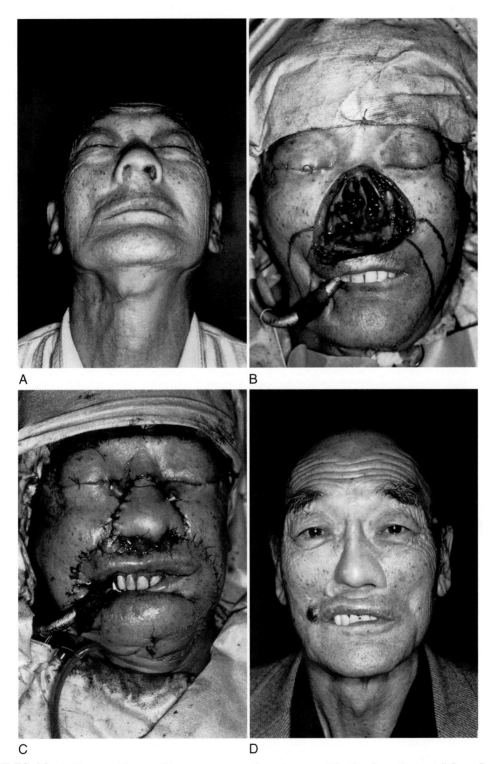

FIGURE 79-11. A 69-year-old man with a squamous cell carcinoma originating from the nostril floor. Despite an innocuous external appearance, the tumor was invasive to a wide area of the nose. *A,* Preoperative view. *B,* Extensive nasal defect after wide resection of the tumor required immediate reconstruction for nasal function and appearance. *C,* Because the defect was too extensive in this particular case, a free radial forearm flap was employed instead of a standard forehead flap. The lining was made by bilateral nasolabial flaps. An iliac bone strut was also used to support the nasal height. *D,* Good appearance obtained 6 months postoperatively. (From Takushima A, Asato H, Harii K: Reconstructive rhinoplasty for large nose defects. Jpn J Plast Reconstr Surg 2003;46:881.)

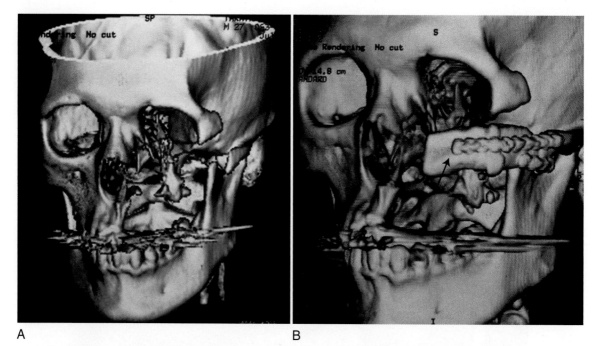

A   B

FIGURE 79-12. *A,* Three-dimensional computed tomographic image of an extensive loss of the upper part of the maxillary bone after resection of a sarcoma in a 27-year-old man. *B,* Three-dimensional computed tomographic image, 6 months postoperatively, after reconstruction of the upper horizontal buttress by a free scapular osteocutaneous flap to correct the downward dislocation of the eye. Arrow indicates a well-surviving scapular bone segment placed into the bone defect of the upper maxillary buttress.

buttresses.[38] A vascularized calvarial bone graft pedicled by the temporoparietal fascia is especially useful for reconstruction of infraorbital and zygomatic regions of the midface.[39-41] However, its size is limited, and difficulty in fabrication may be a problem. In contrast, a free vascularized bone graft or osteocutaneous flap offers a more reliable bone replacement option for extensive bone defects, although the surgical technique is more complex.[42,43]

Reconstruction of the alveolar ridge is also important to affix dentures. Osseointegration has now been popularized in restorative dentistry to stabilize prostheses,[44,45] but it frequently requires an adequate bony support or platform using vascularized bone grafts.[46,47]

Type V Defect

A total maxillectomy with palatectomy for maxillary cancer or devastating injury to the midface may frequently result in massive defects, or a type V defect, combining the maxillary bony framework, mucosal lining, and cutaneous coverage. Reconstruction is challenging for these defects because the complex maxillary framework or buttresses should be replaced by a suitable support; extensive soft tissue replacement may also be required. In most instances, free flaps are the

best reconstructive option because they provide various types of composite tissues in addition to adequate vascularity in a single-stage operation (Fig. 79-13). Of the free flaps currently used, the free scapular osteocutaneous flap and fibular osteocutaneous flap are preferred. These flaps provide a well-vascularized bony support as well as skin flaps for covering skin or mucosal defects. Dual transfer of the osteocutaneous flap and radial forearm flap is also useful for reconstruction of complex defects including maxillary bone, mucosal lining, and skin.

FIGURE 79-13. A 57-year-old man with a large low-grade adenocarcinoma originating from the bilateral maxillary sinuses. *A,* Preoperative view. *B,* Extensive defects of the lower part of the bilateral maxillary bones including oral mucosa and cheek skin. *C,* For immediate closure of these extensive defects, double free flaps including the latissimus dorsi flap (LD) and serratus anterior flap with a rib segment of 10 cm (SA) were harvested and transferred with anastomoses between the facial vessels and thoracodorsal vessels (P). The rib segment was fixed to the bilateral zygomatic arches with miniplates and K-wire. *D* and *E,* Postoperative view and computed tomographic image (arrow indicates the grafted rib segment) 6 months later.

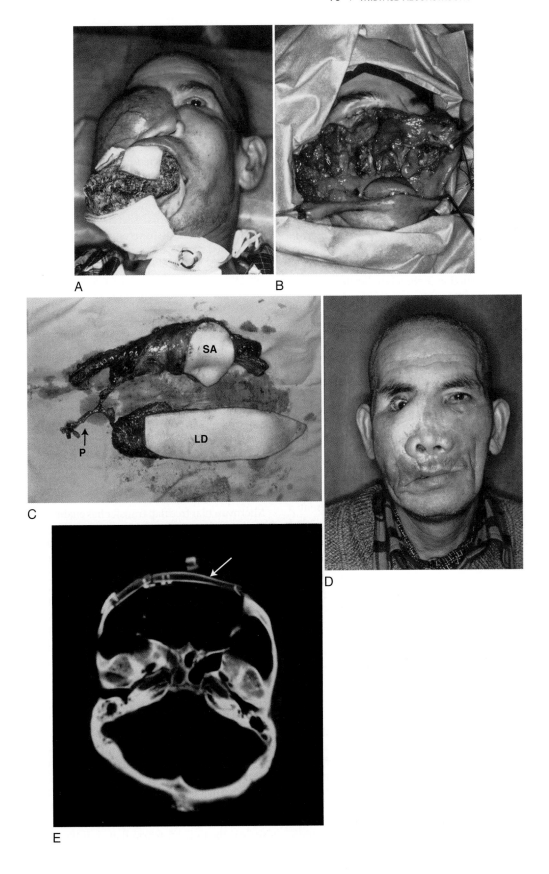

OPERATIVE MANAGEMENT
Skin and Soft Tissue Defects

SKIN GRAFT

A free skin graft is the most simple and traditional surgical treatment option when a defect is limited to the skin or superficial cutaneous layer (type I defect, such as postexcisional defect of scar tissue after a burn injury or trauma). The regional aesthetic units should be considered to obtain inconspicuous scar margins of skin grafts.[6] Full-thickness skin grafts usually produce better cosmetic results than do split-thickness skin grafts. The skin graft, however, cannot usually provide skin of an analogous color or texture, and the aesthetic result is frequently poor (with the possible exception of resurfacing eyelids with a postauricular skin graft). Recruitment of free skin grafts in midface reconstruction is therefore limited from an aesthetic standpoint.

LOCAL FLAP AND SOFT TISSUE EXPANSION

A good functional and aesthetic result requires reconstruction to replace missing tissue with similar tissue. Local flaps, such as rhomboid flaps or subcutaneous flaps, can migrate skin with similar color and texture to the missing skin.[48] They produce a good aesthetic result for closure of relatively small but deeper defects. However, secondary scarring after the use of local flaps should always be considered. A flap developed in the forehead can safely provide skin of good-quality color and texture for reconstruction of the nose and midface, but resulting scars in the forehead may present a problem.[22] An expanded forehead flap can provide a sufficient soft tissue flap with minimal donor site scars for reconstruction of a total defect of the nose (Fig. 79-14). A malar flap or cervicofacial fasciocutaneous flap[49,50] is another option for closure of relatively large and full-thickness defects of the cheek. Soft tissue expansion can greatly extend the application of local flaps for large defects in the head and neck.[15,51] An expanded cervicofacial flap can be especially useful for extending the flap to the high cephalad level of the cheek and the lower eyelid (Fig. 79-15).[52] For larger defects, distant or free flaps may be required.

DISTANT FLAP

Before introduction of the musculocutaneous flap, the deltopectoral flap developed by Bakamjian[53] was the preferred procedure for head and neck reconstruction. Staged procedures and limited reach of the pedicle, however, make this reconstruction difficult and lengthy, and it has now been primarily replaced with musculocutaneous flaps such as the pectoralis major, latissimus dorsi, and trapezius.[54] Of these, the pectoralis major musculocutaneous flap developed by Ariyan[55] is one of the preferred musculocutaneous flaps for head and neck reconstruction. The pectoralis major musculocutaneous flap can be extended up to the cheek and infraorbital regions, although vascularity of a skin paddle developed from the distal portion of the pectoralis major muscle may sometimes be unstable. The donor site scar and resulting disfigurement, however, may be a problem for some patients.

The latissimus dorsi muscle has a long vascular pedicle, and its pedicled musculocutaneous flap can reach the zygomaticotemporal region.[56] Vascularity of a large skin island developed on the muscle is highly reliable when the flap includes one or more musculocutaneous perforators. Several skin paddles can be designed on the latissimus dorsi muscle and employed as a folded flap to close a full-thickness defect of the oral and pharyngeal regions. The main drawback of the latissimus dorsi musculocutaneous flap for head and neck reconstruction is the difficulty in positioning the patient for simultaneous resection and flap dissection. This frequently requires a change in the patient's position during surgery and lengthens the operation time.

Other pedicled musculocutaneous flaps, such as the trapezius and sternomastoid flaps, may also be employed for repair of cheek and midface defects. However, because of freedom of flap design and the ability to transfer various types of tissues, the microvascular free flap is generally more versatile than the pedicled flap in head and neck reconstruction.

MICROVASCULAR FREE FLAPS

Microvascular free flap transfer has enabled the development of many new fields of reconstructive surgery in the head and neck. Free skin flaps, such as the groin and deltopectoral flaps, were first employed for resurfacing cutaneous defects of the face and neck[57] or for augmentation of depressed areas of the face as a de-epithelialized flap.[58] A sufficient amount of soft tissue required in the recipient site can be transferred in a one-stage operation. Selection of adequate donor tissue matching the recipient defect provides the best reconstructive option.

Midface reconstruction, however, has been greatly advanced by clinical introduction of various reliable microvascular free flaps, such as free musculocutaneous and fasciocutaneous flaps, in the 1980s. Free musculocutaneous flaps, such as the latissimus dorsi and rectus abdominis flaps, provide a thick soft tissue flap suitable for repair of large or deep midfacial and cheek skin defects. These musculocutaneous flaps can be folded and used to reconstruct a full-thickness cheek defect (Figs. 79-16 and 79-17).[25,28,29] When a skin defect is relatively small and thin, free fasciocutaneous flaps, such as the radial forearm flap, dorsalis pedis flap, or

Text continued on p. 877

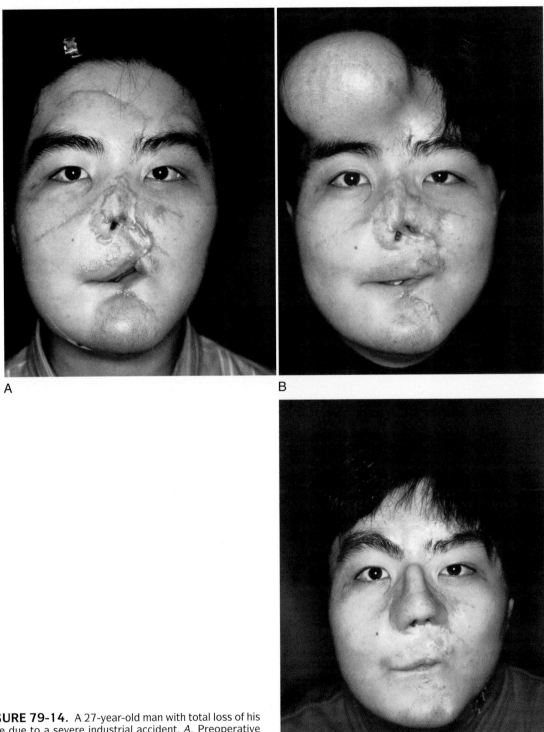

FIGURE 79-14. A 27-year-old man with total loss of his nose due to a severe industrial accident. *A*, Preoperative view. *B*, Expanded forehead flap used for nasal reconstruction. *C*, The reconstructed nose shows good appearance with good color and texture matching to the face 1$\frac{1}{2}$ years later. The donor site scar is also acceptable.

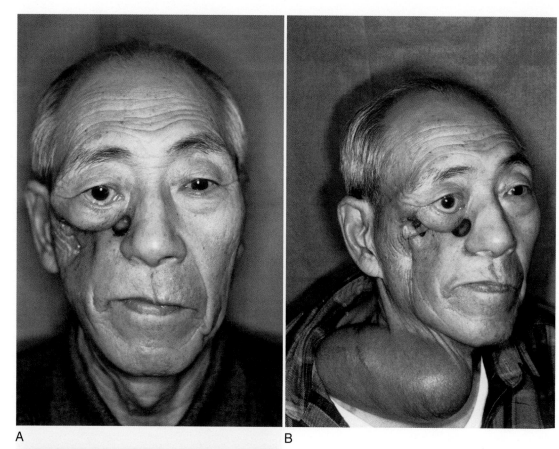

A

B

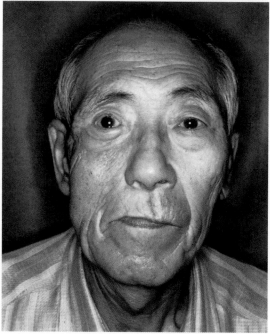

C

FIGURE 79-15. A 72-year-old man had a wide fistula and downward dislocation of the left eye 3 years after treatment of a maxillary cancer. *A*, Preoperative view. *B*, Neck skin fully expanded with a 410-mL expander inserted into the lower neck region in the first-stage operation. *C*, Four months after the first-stage operation, a subscapular osteocutaneous flap was transferred to reconstruct the upper horizontal buttress of the maxillary bone and defect of the mucosal lining. Simultaneously, a cervicofacial flap with the expanded neck skin was used to resurface the cheek skin defect. Good aesthetic appearance was obtained 1 year postoperatively. (From Mochizuki Y, Ueda K, et al: Microsurgical treatment assisted by a tissue expansion procedure for repairing a postoperative deformity due to maxillary cancer. J Jpn Soc Reconstr Microsurg 2001;14:24-31. Courtesy of Professor Kazuki Ueda.)

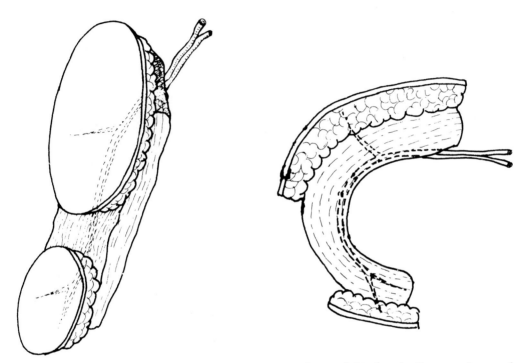

FIGURE 79-16. Schema of a folded free musculocutaneous flap available for simultaneous closure of a full-thickness cheek defect.

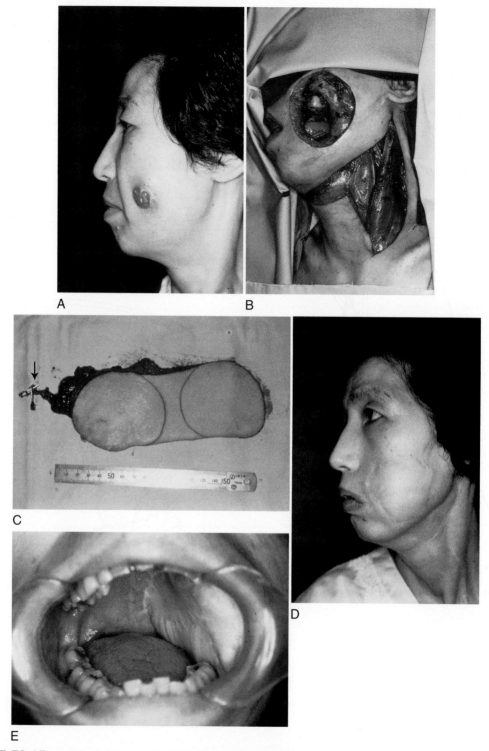

FIGURE 79-17. A 55-year-old woman with squamous cell carcinoma originating from the left buccal mucosa and invading the cheek skin. *A,* Preoperative view. *B,* A full-thickness cheek defect after extensive resection of the tumor and modified neck dissection. *C,* An isolated rectus abdominis flap is going to be folded (arrow shows the pedicle inferior epigastric vessels). *D* and *E,* Five years postoperatively, good closure of both external surface and internal lining is achieved in a single operation. (From Nakatsuka T, Harii K, Yamada A, et al: Versatility of a free inferior rectus abdominis flap for head and neck reconstruction: analysis of 200 cases. Plast Reconstr Surg 1994;93:762-769.)

anterolateral thigh flap, offer excellent reconstructive options.

Skeletal Defects

When a maxillary defect is small and has good soft tissue coverage, an autogenous free bone or costal cartilage graft can survive. Bioinactive or biocompatible alloplastic materials, such as titanium mesh and hydroxyapatite, may be advocated when poor local tissue factors such as irradiation and scar do not exist. In contrast, a vascularized bone graft or osteocutaneous flap can reliably provide various types of vascularized bone segments with or without cutaneous flaps for osseous reconstruction of maxillary defects. These flaps can recruit the missing buttresses of the maxilla so that facial contour can be maintained aesthetically. The free scapular osteocutaneous flap is among the most preferred donor flaps because it can simultaneously provide a well-vascularized segment of the lateral border and inferior angle of the scapula as well as skin.[42] Great freedom in spatial orientation of skin and bone segments enables the surgeon to achieve a three-dimensional reconstruction of a complex defect of the maxilla and midface (Fig. 79-18). A relatively thin scapular bone segment may also be an option for reconstruction of a maxillary bone defect. A long stalk of the circumflex-subscapular vessel pedicle can be anastomosed to the external carotid branches, but an interpositional vessel graft or flow-through flap should be used when the recipient vessels are beyond the length of the flap's vascular stalk.[59] The authors recommend employing a radial forearm flap as a flow-through flap in patients with severe midfacial deformities after treatment of maxillary cancer for which several types of tissue flaps including vascularized bone segments are required. In most instances, a scapular osteocutaneous flap is attached to the distal stump of the radial vessels when a maxillary buttress needs to be reconstructed (Fig. 79-19).

The angular branch of the thoracodorsal vessels can also nourish the inferolateral segment of the scapula[60] and be transferred with a latissimus dorsi flap for reconstruction of type V defects. A combination scapular flap, latissimus dorsi flap, and serratus anterior flap, sometimes including ribs, is available for reconstruction of multiple defects in the midface.[61,62]

Muscle Defects

Irreversible or long-standing facial paralysis due to permanent damage to the facial nerve, resection of the mimetic muscles, or congenital deficiency is one of the most challenging problems in midfacial and cheek reconstruction. Microneurovascular free transplantation of various skeletal muscles has now been popularized and is a well-established procedure, often yielding natural or nearly natural cheek movement on smiling.[63-66] For a successful result to be obtained with this procedure, selection of an adequate motor nerve in the cheek is extremely important. In some patients who have undergone tumor resection including the facial nerves and mimetic muscles, a residual branch of the facial nerve may be available for reinnervation of a transplanted muscle. Because suitable facial nerve branches are frequently unavailable in the paralyzed cheek, a two-stage method combining a cross-facial nerve graft and muscle graft has long been championed and promises a good result with a natural or nearly natural smile.[64,65] However, this procedure requires a staged operation and a lengthy waiting period before contraction of a transplanted muscle is obtained. Sequelae such as hypoesthesia and paresthesia in the lateral foot after harvesting of a sural nerve segment for a cross-

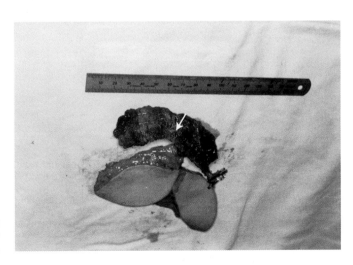

FIGURE 79-18. A scapular osteocutaneous flap with two separated skin paddles (arrow shows a vascularized scapular bone segment).

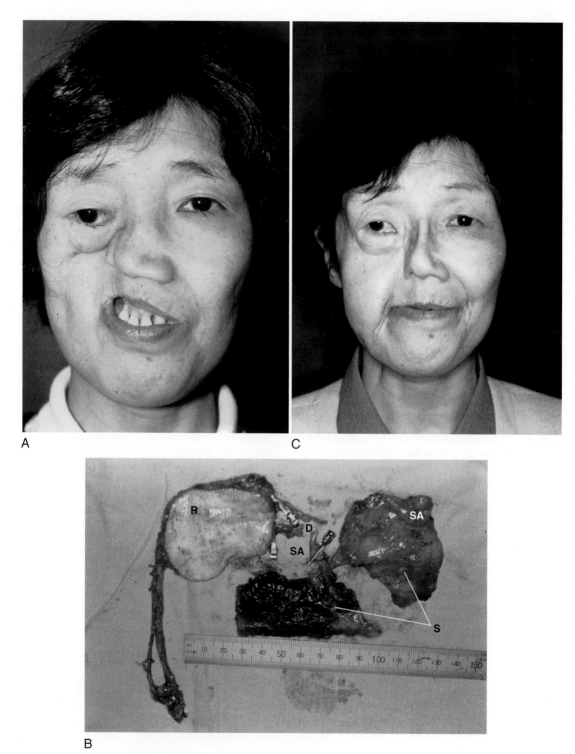

FIGURE 79-19. A severe cheek deformity in a 45-year-old woman after treatment of a right maxillary carcinoma. *A,* Preoperative view. *B,* A sequentially linked radial forearm flap (R) with a scapular osteocutaneous flap (S) is shown. The radial forearm flap was used to reconstruct the oral mucosal defect, and the scapular osteocutaneous flap was used to reconstruct the upper horizontal buttress of the maxilla and augment the depressed cheek. The radial vessels of the forearm flap were anastomosed to the facial vessels; the circumflex scapular vessels (SA) nourishing the scapular flap were anastomosed to the distal end of the radial vessels (D). *C,* Good facial appearance is obtained 8 years postoperatively.

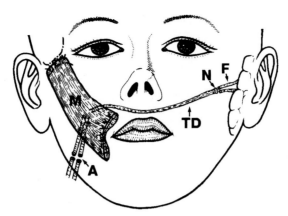

FIGURE 79-20. Schema of the one-stage reconstruction of a paralyzed face with a latissimus dorsi muscle segment in which the thoracodorsal motor nerve is crossed through the upper lip and sutured to the contralateral facial nerve branches. M, latissimus dorsi muscle; A, site of vascular anastomosis; N, site of nerve suture; TD, thoracodorsal nerve; F, intact facial nerve in the nonparalyzed cheek. (From Harii K, Asato H, Yoshimura K, et al: One-stage transfer of the latissimus dorsi muscle for reanimation of a paralyzed face: a new alternative. Plast Reconstr Surg 1998;102:942.)

face nerve graft may also occur and cannot be disregarded.

To overcome the drawbacks of the two-stage method, a one-stage method has been developed with use of the latissimus dorsi muscle segment.[21] The thoracodorsal nerve is directly crossed through the upper lip and sutured to the contralateral nonparalyzed facial nerve branches (Fig. 79-20).[21] Through a preauricular face lift incision on the paralyzed cheek, the cheek skin is widely undermined to develop a subcutaneous pocket to accept a subsequent muscle graft. Through an additional small incision in the submandibular region, the facial artery and vein (respectively) are exposed as the recipient vessels. During preparation of the recipient cheek, a segment of the latissimus dorsi muscle (an average of about 3 cm wide and 8 cm long), with its neurovascular pedicle, is harvested by another operative team. The thoracodorsal nerve should be dissected proximally to its origin from the posterior cord of the brachial plexus to obtain sufficient length (≥13 cm). This provides enough length to reach the contralateral facial nerve branches exposed through a small incision, less than 2 cm long, at the anterior margin of the parotid gland. The isolated muscle segment is then transferred to the recipient cheek and fixed between the zygoma and the nasolabial region under proper tension. The neurovascular anastomoses are then carried out under an operating microscope. Reinnervation of the transferred latissimus dorsi muscle is established at a mean of 7 to 8 months postoperatively (Fig. 79-21).

SUMMARY

Reconstruction of the midface is a challenging and difficult task for reconstructive plastic surgeons. Many defects are composite, involving many layers of skin, subcutaneous soft tissues, maxillary scaffolds, and mucosa. Aesthetic as well as functional results are important because morbidity seriously influences a patient's quality of life. Development of microvascular tissue transfer now offers various reconstructive options and has greatly improved the results of midface reconstruction. Multidimensional approaches, including conventional surgical and prosthetic procedures, however, should be considered in accordance with the individual patient and specific defect.

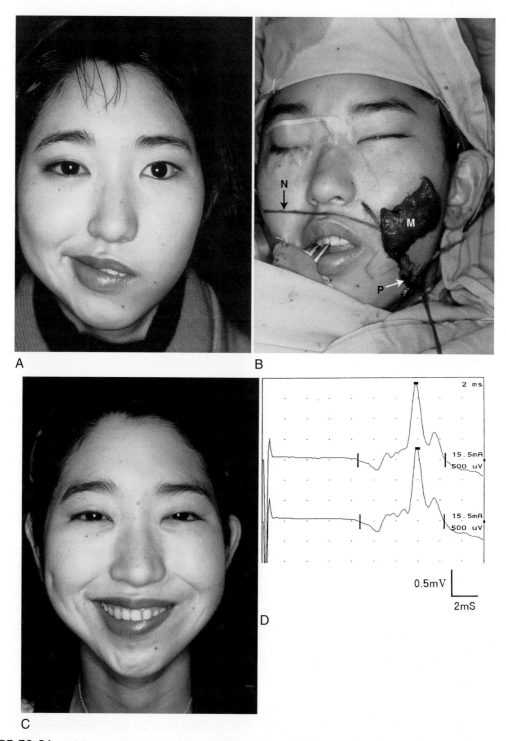

FIGURE 79-21. A 22-year-old woman with severe incomplete left facial paralysis after parotidectomy more than 10 years earlier. *A,* Preoperative view on smiling. *B,* Smile reconstruction as accomplished with a one-stage transfer of the latissimus dorsi muscle segment. The transferred latissimus dorsi muscle is shown. M, muscle; N, thoracodorsal nerve crossing the upper lip to the contralateral cheek; P, thoracodorsal vessels anastomosing to the recipient facial vessels. *C* and *D,* At 3½ years postoperatively, a natural smile is obtained with high evoked potentials from the transferred muscle on stimulation of the contralateral facial nerve. (From Harii K, Asato H, Yoshimura K, et al: One-stage transfer of the latissimus dorsi muscle for reanimation of a paralyzed face: a new alternative. Plast Reconstr Surg 1998;102:945.)

REFERENCES

1. Foster RD, Anthony JP, Singer MI, et al: Microsurgical reconstruction of the midface. Arch Surg 1996;131:960-966.
2. McCarthy JG, Kawamoto H, Grayson BH, et al: Surgery of the jaws. In McCarthy JG, ed: Plastic Surgery, vol 2. Philadelphia, WB Saunders, 1990:1456.
3. Harii K: Microvascular Tissue Transfer. New York, Igaku-Shoin, 1983.
4. Soutar DS, ed: Microvascular Surgery and Free Tissue Transfer. London, Edward Arnold, 1993.
5. Tatum SA: Concepts in midface reconstruction. Otolaryngol Clin North Am 1997;30:563-592.
6. Gonzalez-Ulloa M, Castillo A, Stevens E, et al: Preliminary study of the total restoration of the facial skin. Plast Reconstr Surg 1954;13:151-161.
7. Borges AF: Relaxed skin tension lines (RSTL) versus other skin lines. Plast Reconstr Surg 1984;73:144-150.
8. Mitz V, Peyronie M: The superficial musculo-aponeurotic system (SMAS) in the parotid and cheek area. Plast Reconstr Surg 1976;58:80-88.
9. Bunnel S: Surgical repair of the facial nerve. Arch Otolaryngol 1937;25:235-259.
10. Manson PN, Hoopes JE, Su CT: Structural pillars of the facial skeleton: an approach to the management of Le Fort fractures. Plast Reconstr Surg 1980;66:54-61.
11. Gruss JS, Mackinnon SE: Complex maxillary fractures: role of buttress reconstruction and immediate bone grafts. Plast Reconstr Surg 1986;78:9-22.
12. Coleman JJ III: Microvascular approach to function and appearance of large orbital maxillary defects. Am J Surg 1989;158:337-341.
13. Wells MD, Luce EA: Reconstruction of midfacial defects after surgical resection of malignancies. Clin Plast Surg 1995;22:79-89.
14. Stark RB, Kaplan JM: Rotation flaps, neck to cheek. Plast Reconstr Surg 1972;50:230-233.
15. Antonyshyn O, Gruss JS, Zuker R, Mackinnon SE: Tissue expansion in head and neck reconstruction. Plast Reconstr Surg 1988;82:58-68.
16. Jurkiewickz MJ, Nahai F: The use of free revascularized grafts in the amelioration of hemifacial atrophy. Plast Reconstr Surg 1985;76:44-54.
17. Harii K: Clinical application of free omental flap transfer. Clin Plast Surg 1978;5:273-281.
18. Holmes AD, Marshall KA: Uses of temporalis muscle flap in blanking out orbits. Plast Reconstr Surg 1979;63:337-343.
19. Avelar JM, Psillakis JM: The use of galea flaps in craniofacial deformities. Ann Plast Surg 1981;6:464-469.
20. Harii K: Microneurovascular free muscle transplantation. In Rubin LR, ed: The Paralyzed Face. St. Louis, Mosby–Year Book, 1991:178-200.
21. Harii K, Asato H, Yoshimura K, et al: One-stage transfer of the latissimus dorsi muscle for reanimation of a paralyzed face: a new alternative. Plast Reconstr Surg 1998;102:941-951.
22. McGregor IA, Reid WH: The use of the temporal flap in the primary repair of full-thickness defects of the cheek. Plast Reconstr Surg 1966;38:1-9.
23. Bunkis J, Mulliken JB, Upton J, Murray JE: The evolution of techniques for reconstruction of full-thickness cheek defects. Plast Reconstr Surg 1982;70:319-327.
24. Harii K, Ono I, Ebihara S: Closure of total cheek defects with two combined myocutaneous free flaps. Arch Otolaryngol 1982;108:303-307.
25. Fujino T, Maruyama Y, Inuyama M: Double-folded free myocutaneous flap to cover a total cheek defect. J Maxillofac Surg 1981;9:96-100.
26. Bhathena HM, Kavarana NM: The folded, bipaddled pectoralis major composite flap in oral cancer reconstruction. Br J Plast Surg 1989;42:441-446.
27. Guillamondegui OM, Campbell BH: The folded trapezius flap for through-and-through cheek defects. Otolaryngol Head Neck Surg 1987;97:24-27.
28. Pribaz JJ, Morris DJ, Mulliken JB: Three-dimensional folded free-flap reconstruction of complex facial defects using intraoperative modeling. Plast Reconstr Surg 1994;93:285-293.
29. Nakatsuka T, Harii K, Yamada A, et al: Versatility of a free inferior rectus abdominis flap for head and neck reconstruction: analysis of 200 cases. Plast Reconstr Surg 1994;93:762-769.
30. Savant DN, Patel SG, Deshmukh SP, et al: Folded free radial forearm flap for reconstruction of full-thickness defects of the cheek. Head Neck 1995;17:293-296.
31. Duffy FJ, Gan BS, Israeli D, et al: Use of bilateral folded radial forearm free flaps for reconstruction of a midface gunshot wound. J Reconstr Microsurg 1998;14:89-96.
32. Burget GC: Aesthetic restoration of the nose. Clin Plast Surg 1995;12:463-480.
33. Adamson JE: Nasal reconstruction with the expanded forehead flap. Plast Reconstr Surg 1988;81:13-20.
34. Bolton LL, Chandrasekhar B, Gottlieb ME: Forehead expansion and total nasal reconstruction. Ann Plast Surg 1988;21:210-216.
35. Shaw WW: Microvascular reconstruction of the nose. Clin Plast Surg 1981;8:471-480.
36. Coleman JJ III: Osseous reconstruction of the midface and orbits. Clin Plast Surg 1994;21:113-124.
37. Yamamoto Y, Minakawa H, Kawashima K, et al: Role of buttress reconstruction in zygomaticomaxillary skeletal defects. Plast Reconstr Surg 1998;101:943-950.
38. Wolfe SA: Autogenous bone grafts versus alloplastic material in maxillofacial surgery. Clin Plast Surg 1982;9:539-540.
39. McCarthy JG, Zide BM: The spectrum of calvarial bone grafting: introduction of the vascularized calvarial bone flap. Plast Reconstr Surg 1984;74:10-18.
40. Rose EH, Norris MS: The versatile temporoparietal fascial flap: adaptability to a variety of composite defects. Plast Reconstr Surg 1990;85:224-232.
41. Ilankovan V, Jackson IT: Experience in the use of calvarial bone grafts in orbital reconstruction. Br J Oral Maxillofac Surg 1992;30:92-96.
42. Swartz WM, Banis JC, Newton ED, et al: The osteocutaneous scapular flap for mandibular and maxillary reconstruction. Plast Reconstr Surg 1986;77:530-545.
43. Nakayama B, Matsuura H, Hasegawa Y, et al: New reconstruction for total maxillectomy defect with a fibula osteocutaneous free flap. Br J Plast Surg 1994;47:247-249.
44. Albrektsson T: A multicenter report on osseointegrated oral implants. J Prosthet Dent 1986;60:75-84.
45. Parel SM, Tjellstrom A: The United States and Swedish experience with osseointegration and facial prostheses. Int J Oral Maxillofac Implants 1991;6:75-79.
46. Anthony JP, Foster RD, Sharma AB, et al: Reconstruction of a complex midfacial defect with the folded fibular free flap and osseointegrated implants. Ann Plast Surg 1996;37:204-210.
47. Reece GP, Lemon JC, Jacob RF, et al: Total midface reconstruction after radical tumor resection: a case report and overview of the problem. Ann Plast Surg 1996;36:551-557.
48. Brobyn TJ, Cramer LM, Hulnick SJ, Kodsi MS: Facial resurfacing with the Limberg flap. Clin Plast Surg 1976;3:481-494.
49. Juri J, Juri C: Advancement and rotation of a large cervico-facial flap for cheek repairs. Plast Reconstr Surg 1979;64:692-696.
50. Cook TA, Israel JM, Wang TD, et al: Cervical rotation flaps for midface resurfacing. Arch Otolaryngol Head Neck Surg 1991;117:77-82.
51. Azzolini A, Riberti C, Cavalca D: Skin expansion in head and neck reconstructive surgery. Plast Reconstr Surg 1992;90:799-807.

52. Kawashima T, Yamada A, Ueda K, et al: Tissue expansion in facial reconstruction. Plast Reconstr Surg 1994;94:944-950.

53. Bakamjian VY, Poole M: Maxillo-facial and palatal reconstructions with the deltopectoral flap. Br J Plast Surg 1977;30:17-37.

54. Mathes SJ, Nahai F: Clinical Applications for Muscle and Musculocutaneous Flaps. St. Louis, CV Mosby, 1982.

55. Ariyan S: Pectoralis major, sternomastoid, and other musculocutaneous flaps for head and neck reconstruction. Clin Plast Surg 1980;7:89-109.

56. Barton FE, Spicer TE, Byrd HS: Head and neck reconstruction with the latissimus dorsi myocutaneous flap: anatomic observations and report of 60 cases. Plast Reconstr Surg 1983;71:199-204.

57. Harii K, Ohmori K, Torii S, Sekiguchi J: Microvascular free skin flap transfer. Clin Plast Surg 1978;5:239-263.

58. Shintomi Y, Ohura T, Honda K, Iida K: The reconstruction of progressive facial hemiatrophy by free vascularized dermis fat flaps. Br J Plast Surg 1981;34:398-409.

59. Wells MD, Luce EA, Edwards AL, et al: Sequentially linked free flaps in head and neck reconstruction. Clin Plast Surg 1994;21:59-67.

60. Seneviratne S, Duong C, Taylor GI: The angular branch of the thoracodorsal artery and its blood supply to the inferior angle of the scapula: an anatomical study. Plast Reconstr Surg 1999;104:85-88.

61. Harii K: Myocutaneous flaps—clinical applications and refinements. Ann Plast Surg 1980;4:440-456.

62. Maruyama Y, Urita Y, Onishi K: Rib–latissimus dorsi osteomyocutaneous flap in reconstruction of a mandibular defect. Br J Plast Surg 1985;38:234-237.

63. Harii K, Ohmori K, Torii S: Free gracilis muscle transplantation, with microneurovascular anastomoses for the treatment of facial paralysis. A preliminary report. Plast Reconstr Surg 1976;57:133-143.

64. Harii K: Refined microneurovascular free muscle transplantation for reanimation of paralyzed face. Microsurgery 1988;9:169-176.

65. O'Brien BM, Pederson WC, Khazanchi RK, et al: Results of management of facial palsy with microvascular free-muscle transfer. Plast Reconstr Surg 1990;86:12-22.

66. Terzis JK, Noah ME: Analysis of 100 cases of free-muscle transplantation for facial paralysis. Plast Reconstr Surg 1997;99:1905-1921.

Facial Paralysis

Ronald M. Zuker, MD, FRCSC, FACS ✦ Ralph T. Manktelow, MD, FRCSC
✦ Gazi Hussain, MBBS, FRCSA

THE CLINICAL PROBLEM

CLASSIFICATION AND ETIOLOGY

ANATOMY
    Facial Nerves
    Facial Muscles

ASSESSMENT OF THE PATIENT

TREATMENT PLANNING

NONSURGICAL MANAGEMENT

SURGICAL MANAGEMENT
    Brow
    Upper Eyelid

    Lower Eyelid
    Nasal Airway
    Upper Lip and Cheek (Smile Reconstruction)
    Lower Lip

ASSOCIATED SUBSPECIALTY MANAGEMENT

GENETIC IMPLICATIONS OF CONGENITAL FACIAL
PARALYSIS

AREAS OF FURTHER RESEARCH AND
DEVELOPMENT

Facial paralysis is a devastating condition with profound functional, aesthetic, and psychosocial consequences. It affects both young and old and may be congenital or acquired. Unfortunately, despite decades of effort and significant advances, there remains a need for the development of additional procedures for the multitude of problems associated with a paralyzed face.

THE CLINICAL PROBLEM

Paralysis of the facial muscles leads to many adverse consequences for the patient. Function of the muscles vital for the protection of the eye, maintenance of the nasal airway, oral continence, and clear speech may be lost. These muscles support the face at rest and enable an individual to wink, pucker the lips, and express emotions of surprise, joy, anger, and sorrow (Figs. 80-1 and 80-2).

Brow ptosis is more commonly a problem in the older patient. The weight of the forehead tissue may cause sagging of the eyebrow inferiorly over the superior orbital margin, which causes an asymmetric shape and obstructs the upward gaze. This may be complicated by overactivity of the contralateral frontalis muscle, which increases the discrepancy between eyebrow height. At rest, the depressed eyebrow gives the impression of unhappiness or excessive seriousness. With animation, the asymmetry of the brows and wrinkling of the forehead are accentuated.

The orbicularis oculi muscle is crucial for the protection of the eye. It enables eyelid closure and provides a physical barrier against wind and foreign matter. Repetitive blinking is also important for control of the even spread of tear film in a lateral to medial direction to prevent drying of the cornea. The tear film passes into the inferior fornix and migrates along the lower lid margin into the inferior and superior puncta. The effective drainage of tears is also dependent on a functioning orbicularis oculi muscle; its action on the lacrimal sac establishes a pump-like effect that facilitates the efficient clearance of tears.

When the eyelids are open, the palpebral aperture has the shape of an asymmetric ellipse. The distance between the upper and lower eyelid is 9 to 11 mm at its widest point. In the neutral gaze position, the upper eyelid covers 2 to 3 mm of the superior corneal limbus; the lower eyelid lies at the level of the inferior corneal limbus. Thus, there is normally no scleral show.

With eye closure, the majority of movement occurs in the upper eyelid while the lower lid remains relatively static. However, with squinting or smiling, there is up to 2 mm of upward movement in the lower eyelid. The main functions of the inferior orbicularis oculi are the maintenance of lid margin contact with the globe and assistance with tear drainage.

Patients with facial paralysis are troubled by significant discomfort in the eye because of corneal exposure and desiccation. This drying frequently

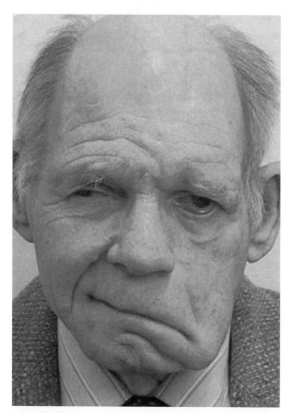

FIGURE 80-1. Facial paralysis produces marked asymmetry at rest between the paralyzed side and the nonparalyzed side. The asymmetry is particularly severe in the older patient.

produces a reflex tear flow. Excessive tears poorly managed by the paralyzed eyelids result in overflow. Therefore, patients with dry eyes often present with excessive tearing. This tearing problem can be distressing and is exacerbated by the downward inclination of the face (e.g., during reading).

The appearance of the paralyzed eye is also of concern to the patient. The eye has a widened palpebral aperture and is unable to convey expression. Thus, when the patient smiles, the paralyzed eyelids remain open instead of slightly closing. With the passage of time, the lower eyelid develops an ectropion, causing the inferior lacrimal punctum to pull away from the eye. An ectropion further exacerbates tearing and increases the risk of excessive corneal exposure.

The other major concern for patients with facial paralysis is the inability to control their lips. This affects the patient's ability to speak, eat, and drink properly. For example, many patients with facial paralysis have difficulty producing *b* and *p* sounds. Buccinator paralysis leads to problems in control of food boluses. Food tends to pocket in the buccal sulcus of the paralyzed portion of the face; therefore, many patients chew only

on the contralateral side. Patients frequently bite the cheek while chewing. This type of paralysis also severely affects normal facial expressions. The main complaint heard from patients is their inability to smile. This should not be regarded as an aesthetic issue. It is a functional disability because it directly impairs communication. Paralysis of the orbicularis oris results in drooling and difficulty in controlling the mouth (e.g., drinking from a glass).

The emotional effects of facial paralysis cannot be underestimated. The unilaterally paralyzed face presents obvious asymmetry at rest, exacerbated with an attempt to smile (see Fig. 80-2). As a result, these patients avoid situations in which they are required to smile. They become characterized as serious and unhappy, and their psychosocial functioning is frequently poor. A patient with bilateral facial paralysis has a severe disability because his or her face cannot convey emotion. To make matters worse, the patient is frequently treated as mentally disabled rather than physically disabled.

CLASSIFICATION AND ETIOLOGY

Facial paralysis can take many forms. It can be classified anatomically and as congenital or acquired, and it can be broken down further into unilateral or bilateral categories. In addition, the degree of muscle involvement varies from total to partial paralysis. More than 50% of the patients with facial paralysis suffer from Bell palsy and often recover fully.

Congenital facial paralysis is present at birth. This is the most common form of facial paralysis seen in a pediatric setting. It may be isolated with involvement of the facial nerve and its musculature only, or it may be part of a congenital syndrome. Three types of isolated congenital facial paralysis can be identified. The first and most common is the panfacial form; all components of the facial nerve are affected. The second most common form affects only the mandibular branch of the facial nerve; here, the clinical effects are restricted to lack of lower lip depression. The third form involves the buccal branches of the facial nerve, and consequent muscle weakness may lead to elevation of the commissure and upper lip. All three forms are variable in that they may be complete or incomplete.

It is estimated that facial paralysis occurs in 2.0% of live births.[1] In the majority of patients, it is believed to be the result of intrauterine pressure on the developing fetus from the sacral prominence. The facial nerve is superficial and easily compressed. This leads to the panfacial type and buccal branch variety of congenital facial paralysis. It is believed, however, that the mandibular branch component and syndromic forms of facial paralysis may have a different etiology. In the authors' experience, the cause of unilateral facial paralysis was congenital in two thirds of the patients

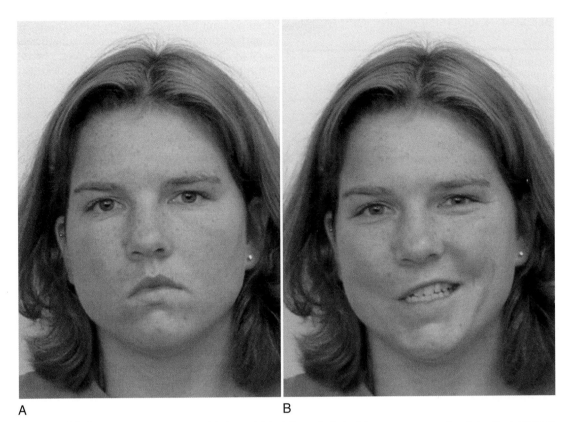

FIGURE 80-2. *A,* At rest, the right-sided partial facial paralysis in this young woman is minimally evident as seen by a slight deviation of the mouth to her left and a slightly wider palpebral aperture in her right eye. *B,* With smiling, the asymmetry becomes more apparent.

encountered and acquired in one third of the patients. Acquired facial paralysis resulted from intracranial tumors in 50% of the patients; the other 50% of the patients acquired facial paralysis from extracranial trauma. The majority of traumas were related to surgical procedures, most commonly cystic hygroma excision. In infants, the nerve is superficial at birth and can easily be traumatized through external compression or surgical misadventure. In contrast, the cause of facial paralysis for the majority of adults is acquired, from either intracranial lesions or inflammatory processes, such as Bell palsy.

Congenital facial paralysis may be syndromic. In other words, it may be associated with other anomalies. The most common unilateral syndromic condition associated with facial paralysis is hemifacial microsomia. All tissues of the face can be affected to a variable degree, including the facial nerve musculature. The most common bilateral congenital facial paralysis is a result of Möbius syndrome. The functional effects of congenital facial paralysis tend to gradually worsen as the influence of gravity and aging prevail.

Bilateral facial paralysis may be the result of bilateral intracranial tumors or bilateral skull base trauma, but it is usually found to be the congenital bilateral facial paralysis of Möbius syndrome. Various cranial nerves accompany the seventh nerve's involvement, specifically the sixth, ninth, tenth, and twelfth. Möbius syndrome is also associated with trunk and limb anomalies in about one third of the patients, the most common being talipes equinovarus and a variety of hand anomalies, including Poland syndrome. The cranial nerve involvement is usually bilateral and severe but often incomplete. There is frequently some residual function in the lower component of the face (the cervical and mandibular branch regions). The incidence of Möbius syndrome is estimated to be about 1 in 200,000 live births.

Acquired facial paralysis may also be unilateral or bilateral through local disruption of the nerve at various locations. Damage to the nerve may be intracranial in the nucleus or the peripheral nerve, extracranial in the peripheral nerve, or the result of damage to the muscle itself. Intracranial and extracranial neoplasms, Bell palsy, and trauma are the most common causes seen in the adult setting. Although recovery is the rule in Bell palsy, at least 10% of patients are left with some degree of paralysis that may be severe. Bilateral acquired facial paralysis is usually the result of skull

TABLE 80-1 ✦ CLASSIFICATION OF FACIAL PARALYSIS

Extracranial
  Traumatic
    Facial lacerations
    Blunt forces
    Penetrating wounds
    Mandible fractures
    Iatrogenic injuries
    Newborn paralysis
  Neoplastic
    Parotid tumors
    Tumors of the external canal and middle ear
    Facial nerve neurinomas
    Metastatic lesions
  Congenital absence of facial musculature
Intratemporal
  Traumatic
    Fractures of petrous pyramid
    Penetrating injuries
    Iatrogenic injuries
  Neoplastic
    Glomus tumors
    Cholesteatoma
    Facial neurinomas
    Hemangiomas
    Meningiomas
    Acoustic neurinomas
    Squamous cell carcinomas
    Rhabdomyosarcoma
    Arachnoidal cysts
    Metastatic
  Infectious
    Herpes zoster oticus
    Acute otitis media
    Chronic otitis media
    Malignant otitis externa
  Idiopathic
    Bell palsy
    Melkersson-Rosenthal syndrome
  Congenital: osteopetroses
Intracranial
  Iatrogenic injury
  Neoplastic
  Congenital
    Absence of motor units
  Syndromic
    Hemifacial microsomia (unilateral)
    Möbius syndrome (bilateral)

base fractures, intracranial lesions usually in the brainstem, or intracranial surgery.

Throughout all of these areas, however, facial paralysis constitutes a spectrum of involvement. It may be complete or incomplete to varying degrees, obvious in some patients, and subtle in others (Table 80-1).

ANATOMY

Facial Nerves

The extratemporal portion of the seventh cranial nerve begins at the stylomastoid foramen. It is in a deep position below the earlobe but becomes more superficial before it passes between the superficial and deep portions of the parotid gland. As it enters the parotid gland, the facial nerve usually divides into two main trunks. These two trunks then further divide within the substance of the gland. In a series of anatomic dissections, Davis[2] demonstrated several branching patterns of the facial nerve. Traditionally, it is taught that this results in five divisions of the facial nerve: frontotemporal, zygomatic, buccal, marginal mandibular, and cervical. In practice, however, there is no distinct separation between the zygomatic and buccal branches either in their location or in the muscles they innervate. In reference to the nerves that supply the midface, it is preferable to use the term zygomaticobuccal branches.

At their exit from the parotid gland, the facial nerve branches lie approximately 10 mm from the skin surface[3]; however, they become progressively more superficial from there. This is particularly true in the temporal gland. It is 5 cm distal to the parotid gland and may be only a few millimeters deep to the surface.

On leaving the parotid, the facial nerve may have 8 to 15 branches making up the five divisions. Distally, there is further arborization and interconnection of these branches (Fig. 80-3). The net effect is a great deal

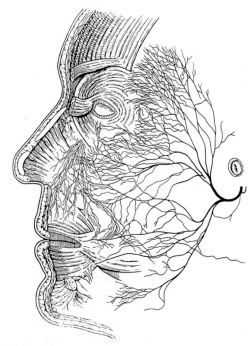

FIGURE 80-3. A typical pattern of facial nerve branching. The main branch is divided into two components, each of which then branches in a random manner to all parts of the face. The extensive distal arborization and interconnections are apparent. (From May M: Anatomy for the clinician. In May M, Shaitken BM, eds: The Facial Nerve. New York, Thieme, 2000:43.)

of functional overlap between the branches. For example, a single zygomaticobuccal branch may supply innervation to the orbicularis oculi as well as to the orbicularis oris.

The temporal division consists of three or four branches[4] that run obliquely along the undersurface of the temporoparietal fascia after crossing the zygomatic arch in a location 3 to 5 cm from the lateral orbital margin. The lower branches run along the undersurface of the superior portion of the orbicularis oculi for 3 to 4 mm before entering the muscle to innervate it.[5] According to Ishikawa,[4] the upper two branches enter the frontalis muscle at the level of the supraorbital ridge and are usually located up to 3 cm above the lateral canthus. The nerves usually lie approximately 1.6 cm inferior to the frontal branch of the superficial temporal artery. Because there is relatively little adipose tissue at the lateral border of the frontalis, those nerves are virtually subcutaneous and susceptible to injury.

The zygomaticobuccal division consists of five to eight branches with significant overlap of muscle innervation such that one or more branches may be divided without causing weakness. These nerves supply innervation to the lip elevators as well as to the lower orbicularis oculi, orbicularis oris, and buccinator. Functional facial nerve mapping and cross-facial nerve grafting require the precise identification and stimulation of these zygomaticobuccal branches to isolate the exact branches responsible for smiling. These nerves lie deep near the parotid-masseteric fascia in the same plane as the parotid duct. There are sometimes connections between the lower branches and the marginal mandibular division.

The marginal mandibular division consists of one to three branches[6] whose course begins up to 2 cm below the ramus of the mandible and arcs upward to cross the mandible halfway between the angle and mental protuberance. It has been well documented[4,5,7] that these branches lie on the deep surface of the platysma and cross superficially to the facial vessels approximately 3.5 cm from the parotid edge. Nelson and Gingrass[7] described separate branches to the depressor anguli oris, depressor labii inferioris, and mentalis and a variable superior ramus supplying the upper platysma and lower orbicularis oris.

The cervical division consists of one branch that leaves the parotid well below the angle of the mandible and runs on the deep surface of the platysma, which it innervates by entering the muscle at the junction of its cranial and middle thirds. This point of entry is 2 to 3 cm caudal to the platysma muscle branch of the facial vessel.[8]

Facial Muscles

Facial musculature consists of 17 paired muscles and one unpaired sphincter muscle, the orbicularis oris

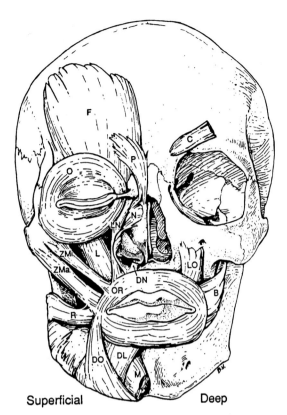

Superficial   **Deep**

F-Frontalis
P-Procerus
O-Orbicularis oculi
OR-Orbicularis oris
N-Nasalis
LN-Levator labii superioris alaeque nasi
L-Levator labii superioris
ZMi-Zygomaticus minor
ZMa-Zygomaticus major
R-Risorius
DO-Depressor anguli oris
DL-Depressor labii inferioris
M-Mentalis
DN-Depressor nasi

C-Corrugator supercilii
B-Buccinator
LO-Levator anguli oris

FIGURE 80-4. The muscles of facial expression are present in two layers. The buccinator, depressor labii inferioris, levator anguli oris, and corrugator are in the deeper layer.

(Fig. 80-4). The subtle movements that convey facial expression require coordination between all of these muscles.

The major muscles affecting the forehead and eyelids are the frontalis, corrugator, and orbicularis oculi. There are two groups of muscles controlling the movement of the lips. The lip retractors include the levator labii superioris, levator anguli oris, zygomaticus major and minor for the upper lip, and depressor labii inferioris and depressor anguli oris for the lower lip. The antagonist to these lip-retracting muscles is the orbicularis oris, which is responsible for oral continence and some expressive movements of the lips.

Freilinger et al[5] have demonstrated that the mimetic muscles are arranged in four layers. The depressor anguli oris, part of the zygomaticus minor, and the orbicularis oculi are the most superficial, whereas the buccinator, mentalis, and levator anguli oris make up the deepest layer. Except for the three deep muscles, all other facial muscles receive innervation from nerves entering their deep surfaces.

The muscles that are clinically important or most often require surgical management in patients with facial paralysis are the frontalis, orbicularis oculi, zygomaticus major, levator labii superioris, orbicularis oris, and depressor labii inferioris.

The frontalis muscle is a bilateral broad sheet-like muscle 5 to 6 cm in width and 1 mm thick.[6] The muscle takes origin from the galea aponeurotica at various levels near the coronal suture and inserts onto the superciliary ridge of the frontal bone and into fibers of the orbicularis oculi, procerus, and corrugator supercilii. It is firmly adherent to the skin through multiple fibrous septa but glides over the underlying periosteum. The two muscles fuse in the midline caudally; however, this is often a fibrous junction. Not only is the frontalis essential to elevate the brow, but also its tone at rest keeps the brow from descending. This tone is lost in the patient with facial paralysis, which allows the brow to fall and potentially obscure upward gaze.

The orbicularis oculi muscle acts as a sphincter to close the eyelids. Upper eyelid opening is performed by the levator palpebrae superioris muscle innervated by the third cranial nerve and the Müller muscle, which is a smooth fiber muscle innervated by the sympathetic nervous system. The orbicularis oculi muscle is one continuous muscle but has three subdivisions: pretarsal, covering the tarsal plate; preseptal, overlying the orbital septum; and orbital, forming a ring over the orbital margin. The pretarsal and preseptal portions function together when a patient blinks, whereas the orbital portion is recruited during forceful eye closure and to lower the eyebrows. According to Jelks, the preseptal portion of the orbicularis oculi is under voluntary control, whereas the pretarsal provides reflex movement.

The pretarsal orbicularis oculi overlies the tarsal plate of the upper and lower eyelids. The tarsal plates are thin, elongated plates of connective tissue that support the eyelids. The superior tarsal plate is 8 to 10 mm in vertical height at its center but tapers medially and laterally, whereas the inferior tarsal plate is 3.8 to 4.5 mm in vertical height. The skin overlying the pretarsal orbicularis is the thinnest in the body and is adherent to the muscle over the tarsal plate. The skin is more lax and mobile over the preseptal and orbital regions. The eyelid skin also becomes thicker over the orbital part of the muscle. The preseptal orbicularis provides support to the orbital septa and is more mobile except at the medial and lateral canthi, where the muscle is firmly attached to the skin. The orbital portion of the orbicularis oculi extends in a wide circular fashion around the orbit. It originates medially from the superomedial orbital margin, the maxillary process of the frontal bone, the medial canthal tendon, the frontal process of the maxilla, and the inferomedial margin of the orbit. In the upper eyelid, the fibers sweep upward into the forehead and cover the frontalis and corrugator supercilii muscles; the fibers continue laterally to be superficial to the temporalis fascia.[9,10] Because this muscle is one of the superficial group of mimetic muscles,[3] in the lower eyelid the orbital portion lies over the origins of the zygomaticus major, levator labii superioris, levator labii superioris alaeque nasi, and part of the origin of the masseter muscle. There are multiple motor nerve branches that supply the upper and lower portions of the orbicularis oculi, and these enter the muscle just medial to its lateral edge.

Freilinger[5] has extensively studied the three major lip elevators, zygomaticus major, levator labii superioris, and levator anguli oris, and provided data on their length, width, and thickness (Table 80-2).

The zygomaticus major takes origin from the lower lateral portion of the body of the zygoma; the orbicularis oculi and zygomaticus minor cover its upper part. Its course is along a line roughly from the helical root of the ear to the commissure of the mouth, where it leads into the modiolus. The modiolus is the point of common attachment at which the fibers of the zygomaticus major and minor, orbicularis oris,

TABLE 80-2 ◆ DIMENSIONS OF THE LEVATORS OF THE UPPER LIP

Muscle	Length (mm)	Width (mm)	Thickness (mm)
Zygomaticus major	70	8	2
Levator labii superioris	34	25	1.8
Levator anguli oris	38	14	1.7

From Freilinger G, Gruber H, Happak W, Pechmann U: Surgical anatomy of the mimic muscle system and the facial nerve: importance for reconstructive and aesthetic surgery. Plast Reconstr Surg 1987;80:686.

buccinator, risorius, levator anguli oris, and depressor anguli oris come together. Deep fibers of the zygomaticus major are angled upward from the modiolus to fuse with the levator anguli oris, whereas caudal fibers continue into the depressor anguli oris. The main nerve to the zygomaticus major enters the deep surface of the upper third of the muscle.

The levator labii superioris originates along the lower portion of the orbital margin above the infraorbital foramen. The muscle courses inferiorly, partially inserting into the nasolabial crease. The lateral fibers pass inferiorly into the orbicularis oris, and the deepest fibers form part of the modiolus. The nerve to this muscle reaches it by first passing underneath the zygomaticus major muscle to supply the levator labii superioris on its deep surface.

The levator anguli oris is the third lip elevator. It takes origin from the maxilla below the infraorbital foramen and inserts into the modiolus. Because this muscle belongs to the deepest layer, it is innervated on its superficial surface by the same branch that supplies innervation to the buccinator.

Three muscles along with the zygomaticus minor serve to elevate the lip. The zygomaticus muscles move the commissure at an angle of approximately 45 degrees, the levator anguli oris elevates the commissure vertically and medially, and the levator labii superioris elevates the lip vertically and laterally to expose the upper teeth.

The orbicularis oris is a complex muscle that functions as far more than a sphincter of the mouth; it serves to pucker and purse the lips. It makes up the bulk of the lip, as skin overlies it superficially and mucous membrane is attached on its deep surface. In the lower lip, the fibers sweep around to attach into the opposite modiolus and form concentrated bands of muscle. In the upper lip, however, these fibers decussate in the midline to insert into the opposite philtral column. In fact, the philtral dimple is formed by the decussation of these fibers. Philtral columns are formed by the insertion of the orbicularis, and a portion of the levator labii superioris, into the skin.[11] The levator labii superioris fibers reach the philtral columns by coursing above the surface of the orbicularis oris to insert into the lower philtral columns and vermilion border as far medially as the peak of Cupid's bow. Anatomically and functionally, the orbicularis oris muscle consists of two parts, superficial and deep. The deep layers of the muscle encircle the orifice of the mouth and function as a constrictor. The superficial component also brings the lips together, but its fibers can contract independently to provide expression.[12] The protrusion of the vermilion is caused by the most superficial fibers of the superficial component, which are reflected anteriorly to insert into the skin of the vermilion border. This roll of muscle is known as the pars marginalis and

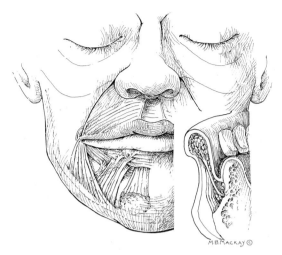

FIGURE 80-5. The depressor anguli oris can be seen in the corner of the mouth. Muscle contraction pulls the corner of the mouth down as in the expression of sadness. The depressor labii inferioris goes into the orbicularis oris of the midlateral portion of the lower lip and pulls the lip down. The muscle's function is apparent in an open-mouth smile showing the lower teeth. The mental nerve lies on the deep surface of the depressor labii inferioris.

gives the orbicularis a J shape when it is viewed in cross section.

The lower lip depressors consist of the depressor labii inferioris, also known as the quadratus labii inferioris, and the depressor anguli oris, also known as the triangularis (Fig. 80-5). The platysma may be considered a weak depressor of the lower lip through its insertion into the other lower lip depressors and the modiolus. The mentalis, however, is not a lip depressor. Its indirect action on the lip is to elevate it.[9] The mentalis arises from the anterior mandible at the level of and below the incisor roots, and its fibers are directed downward to insert into the skin of the chin at the soft tissue prominence. With contraction, the lower lip is pulled firmly against the teeth and the skin of the chin is wrinkled. The depressor labii inferioris arises from the lateral surface of the mandible, which is inferior and lateral to the mental foramen. It runs medially and superiorly to insert into the lower border of the orbicularis oris and its surface. Through fibrous septa, it attaches to the vermilion and the skin of the middle third of one side of the lip.[10] Its action is to draw the lower lip downward and laterally and to evert the vermilion (e.g., as in showing the lower teeth). The depressor anguli oris arises from the mandible laterally and is superficial to the depressor labii inferioris. The medial fibers insert directly into the skin at the labiomandibular crease; the remainder blend into the modiolus.[13] It depresses the angle of the mouth (e.g., in frowning).

ASSESSMENT OF THE PATIENT

Facial nerve paralysis does not result in the same sequelae in all patients, and facial nerve palsy is not in itself a diagnosis. A thorough history and examination will reveal the presence of a complete or partial seventh nerve paralysis and, if the paralysis is partial, the specific muscles affected and the extent of the paralysis. Has there been any return of function? Is this improvement continuing or has it reached a plateau? The history must include any eye symptoms, such as dryness, excessive tearing, incomplete closure, discomfort when the patient is outdoors, and use of artificial tears. The patient should be questioned about the nasal airway, oral continence, speech, and level of psychosocial functioning and social interactions.

The patient's concerns and expectations must be sought. For some, attaining a symmetric appearance at rest is more important than achieving a smile. In comparison to the younger patient, the older patient is more likely to be worried about brow ptosis, ectropion, and drooping of the cheek.

The level of injury to the nerve, if it is not known, can be assessed clinically. Injury to the nerve within the bony canal may result in loss of ipsilateral taste appreciation, hyperacusis, and facial weakness because the chorda tympani and nerve to the stapedius may be injured at this level. Injury to the seventh cranial nerve near the geniculate ganglion will also result in decreased secretory function of the nose, mouth, and lacrimal gland.

Examination of the face begins with the brow. Its position at rest and with movement must be noted. The superior visual field may be diminished by the ptotic brow.

The eye must be thoroughly assessed. Visual acuity in each eye should be documented. The height of the palpebral aperture should be measured and compared with the nonparalyzed side. The degree of lagophthalmos and the presence of a Bell reflex will indicate the risk of corneal exposure. The lower eyelid position should be measured. Tone in the lower eyelid can be assessed by the use of the snap test. This is done by gently pulling the eyelid away from the globe and releasing it. The eyelid normally snaps back against the globe; however, this fails to occur in the patient with poor lid tone. The position of the inferior canalicular punctum should be assessed. Is it applied to the globe or is it rolled away and exposed? In addition, the patient should be examined for corneal ulceration.

The nasal airway is examined next. Forced inspiration may reveal a collapsed nostril due to a loss of muscle tone in the dilator naris and drooping of the cheek. An intranasal examination should also be done.

Examination of the mouth and surrounding structures documents the amount of philtral deviation, the presence or absence of a nasolabial fold, the amount of commissure depression and deviation, the degree to which the upper lip droops, and the presence of vermilion inversion. With animation, the amount of bilateral commissure movement is recorded; it is also noted how much of the upper incisors show when the patient is smiling. The patient's lower teeth are also examined with regard to how much they show when the patient is smiling. Speech should be assessed. An intraoral examination is performed to check dental hygiene and to look for evidence of cheek biting.

The presence of synkinesis, the simultaneous contraction of two or more groups of muscles that normally do not contract together,[14] should be documented. Synkinesis is thought to occur from a misdirected sprouting of axons. The most common types of synkinesis are eye closure with smiling,[15] brow wrinkling when the mouth is moved,[16] and mouth grimacing when the eyes are closed.

An assessment of the other cranial nerves, particularly the fifth, is also performed. Cranial nerve involvement may exacerbate the morbidity of facial nerve paralysis. These nerves should also be assessed as possible donor motor nerves.

TREATMENT PLANNING

Treatment must be individualized. However, in general, the aims of treatment are to protect the eye, to provide symmetry at rest, and then to provide movement. The ultimate goal is to restore involuntary, independent, and spontaneous facial expression. The goals of treatment for the eye are to maintain vision, to provide protection, to maintain function of the eyelids, to improve cosmesis, and to enable the eye to express emotion. The goals for the mouth are to correct asymmetry, to provide oral continence, to improve speech, and to provide a balanced symmetric smile that the patient will use in social settings. Clearly, the accomplishment of all these goals is difficult, and they cannot be achieved completely.

The patient must be counseled as to what are real and achievable expectations. It is clearly impossible to restore intricate movements to all facial muscles, and the patient who is appropriately informed is more likely to be satisfied with his or her outcome.

NONSURGICAL MANAGEMENT

Nonsurgical management of the patient with facial paralysis applies primarily to the eye and can frequently make the difference between a comfortable eye and a painful one. Nonsurgical maneuvers can protect the eye while surgery is being planned and are regularly used in concert with the surgical management of the eye. In some instances, surgery may be avoided. Nonsurgical management of the eye consists of

TABLE 80-3 ✦ NONSURGICAL MANEUVERS TO PROTECT THE EYE

Lid taping, particularly while sleeping
Soft contact lenses
Moisture chambers, which can be taped to the skin around the orbit
Modification of eyeglasses to provide a lateral shield
Forced blinking exercises in a patient with weak eye closure
Eye patches
Temporary tarsorrhaphy

protecting the eye and maintaining eye lubrication (Table 80-3).

Eye lubrication can be provided by a number of commercially available preparations. This includes clear watery drops containing either hydroxypropyl methylcellulose or polyvinyl alcohol along with other agents including preservatives. These drops function by adsorbing into the cornea and lubricating it. Although the duration of action will vary, most are retained on the surface of the eye between 45 and 120 minutes.[17] Thus, to be most effective, they should be instilled frequently during the day. Thicker ointments containing petrolatum, mineral oil, or lanolin alcohol are retained longer and can be used at night to protect and "seal" the eyelids during sleep. The patient who presents with excessive tearing may in fact have a dry eye and may benefit by the use of artificial tears. Corneal ulceration should be managed with prompt referral for ophthalmologic assessment.

In patients in whom there is incomplete facial nerve paralysis or recovering muscle activity after nerve injury, function may be improved with neuromuscular retraining supervised by an experienced therapist. This consists of various treatment modalities such as biofeedback, electromyography, and self-directed mirror exercises using slow, small, and symmetric movements.[18] Patients can often relearn some facial movements or strengthen movements that are weak.

SURGICAL MANAGEMENT

Deciding on a surgical procedure can initially seem daunting. There are a number to choose from, and selecting the most appropriate reconstruction may be confusing. It is important to listen to each patient carefully to identify which aspects of the paralysis are most troublesome and to treat each region of the face separately. The age of the patient, duration of the facial paralysis, condition of the facial musculature and soft tissues, and status of potential donor nerves and muscles will all influence treatment options. One must consider the patient's needs carefully and match the needs of the patient with the skill of the surgeon (Table 80-4).

Brow

There are at least three approaches to a brow lift: direct excision of the tissue above the brow (direct brow lift), open brow lift performed through a coronal incision, and endoscopic brow lift. Unilateral frontalis paralysis may cause a difference in brow heights of up to 12 mm. A direct brow lift is best able to correct such

TABLE 80-4 ✦ MOST COMMON SURGICAL OPTIONS FOR EACH REGION OF THE FACE

Brow

Direct brow lift (direct excision)
Coronal brow lift with static suspension
Endoscopic brow lift

Upper Eyelid (Lagophthalmos)

Gold weight
Temporalis transplantation
Spring
Tarsorrhaphy

Lower Eyelid (Ectropion)

Tendon sling
Lateral canthoplasty
Horizontal lid shortening
Temporalis transplantation
Cartilage graft

Nasal Airway

Static sling
Alar base elevation
Septoplasty

Commissure and Upper Lip

Microneurovascular muscle transplantation with use of ipsilateral seventh nerve, cross-facial nerve graft, or other cranial nerve for motor innervation
Temporalis transplantation with or without masseter transplantation
Static slings
Soft tissue balancing procedures (rhytidectomy, mucosal excision or advancement)

Lower Lip

Depressor labii inferioris resection
Muscle transplantation (digastric, platysma)
Wedge excision

a large discrepancy. Direct brow lift involves excision of a segment of skin and frontalis muscle just above and parallel to the eyebrow. If the incision is placed just along the first line of hair follicles, the resulting scar is usually less noticeable. Frontalis shortening by excision and repair provides a reliable correction, which minimally relaxes over time. However, overcorrection is still required. Slight overcorrection is particularly beneficial if the person's normal side of the forehead is quite active during facial expression. Branches of the supraorbital nerve should be identified and preserved because they lie deep to the muscle (Fig. 80-6).

Brow lift may be performed through a coronal incision with or without a fascial graft to suspend the brow from the temporalis fascia or medially on the frontal bone. Whereas the scar is concealed, this is a larger operation than a direct brow lift and may not achieve as adequate a lift.

The authors have had limited experience with endoscopically assisted brow lifts for facial paralysis. The amount of lift required in the patient with facial paralysis is usually more than can be achieved from a unilateral endoscopic brow lift. It is likely that with time, there will be gradual drooping. Therefore, the longevity of results in patients with facial paralysis has yet to be demonstrated with this procedure, especially when a large unilateral lift is required.

Weakening of the contralateral normal frontalis muscle by transection of the frontal nerve or resection of strips of muscle is occasionally useful to control wrinkle asymmetry.

Upper Eyelid

Several techniques are available for the management of lagophthalmos. These are all directed at overcoming the unopposed action of the levator palpebrae superioris. Because of its relative technical ease and reversibility, lid loading with gold prostheses is the most popular technique. The patient's eyelid configuration is important in determining whether the bulge of the gold weight will be visible when the eye is open. If the amount of exposed eyelid skin above the lashes is more than 5 mm when the eye is open, the gold weight is likely to be noticeable to the patient. If the distance is less than 5 mm, the gold weight will roll back and be covered by the supratarsal skinfold (Fig. 80-7).

Because of its inertness, 24-carat gold is used; allergic reactions are rare, but if they occur, platinum weights are also available. Prostheses are available in weights ranging from 0.8 to 1.8 g. Adequate improvement in eye closure can be obtained with a weight of 0.8 to 1.2 g, giving the patient a comfortable eye without weight-related problems.[19] The appropriate weight is selected by taping trial prostheses to the upper eyelid

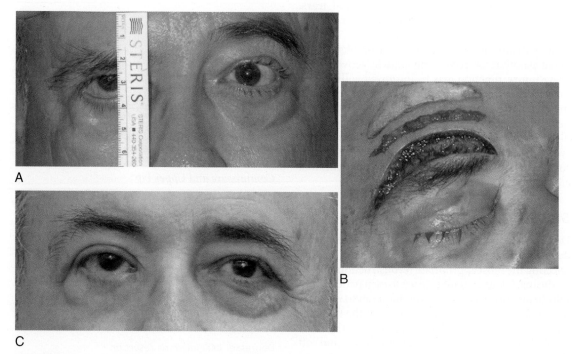

FIGURE 80-6. *A,* Assessment of the amount of brow depression on the paralyzed side compared with the normal eyebrow on the patient's left. *B,* Excision of skin and a strip of frontalis muscle to correct brow ptosis. *C,* Postoperative appearance.

prosthesis is fixed to the upper half of the tarsal plate by permanent sutures, which pass through the tarsal plate. Care should be taken not to interfere with the insertion of Müller muscle (Fig. 80-8). With proper placement, the prosthesis should be hidden in the upper eyelid skin crease when the eye is open. The closure produced by the gold weight is slow, and the patient must be instructed to consciously relax the levator muscle for 1 to 2 seconds to allow the eyelid to descend (Fig. 80-9). Complications include extrusion, excessive capsule formation causing a visible lump, and irritation of the eye by the weight. If these occur, the weight can easily be removed, replaced, or repositioned.

The authors have used the gold weight alone 27 times. The incidence of complications requiring removal of the weight was 2%, and 8% required revision of the weight. In 52% of the patients, good symptomatic improvement was obtained. Of these patients, 64% subsequently required lower lid support with a static sling. As a result, it has become much more common to recommend both a gold weight and a lower eyelid sling at the same operative sitting, which results in a 95% good improvement in symptoms.

An alternative procedure for eyelid closure is the palpebral spring described by Morel-Fatio, which consists of a wire loop with two arms.[20] One arm is sutured along the lid margin, and the other arm is fixed to the inner aspect of the lateral orbital rim. When the eye is open, the two arms are brought close to each other; when the eyelid is relaxed, the "memory" of the wire loop moves the arms apart, causing closure of the eyelid (Fig. 80-10).

The advantage of this procedure is that it is not dependent on gravity. However, problems with malpositioning of the spring, spring breakage or weakening, pseudoptosis due to excessive spring force, and

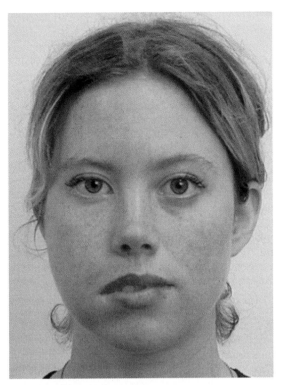

FIGURE 80-7. Right facial paralysis in a young woman with total paralysis of the orbicularis oculi showing ideal eyelid configuration that allows gold weight insertion without visibility.

over the tarsal plate with the patient awake. The lightest weight that will bring the upper eyelid within 2 to 4 mm of the lower lid and cover the cornea should be used. As long as the patient has an adequate Bell phenomenon, complete closure is not necessary. The

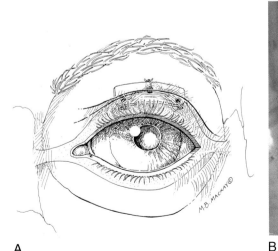

A

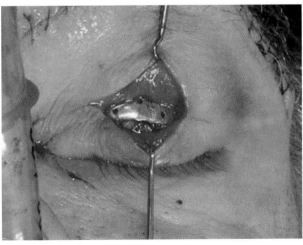

B

FIGURE 80-8. *A*, Placement of gold weight directly above the cornea on the upper half of the tarsal plate. *B*, Gold weight sutured in place with the knots turned away from the skin.

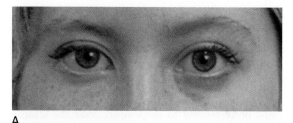

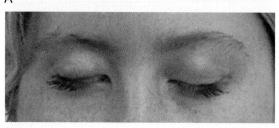

FIGURE 80-9. *A*, Postoperative appearance of the patient shown in Figure 80-7 after a gold weight is fixed to the right upper eyelid. *B*, Eye closure is shown after gold weight insertion.

skin erosion have prevented the widespread use of this procedure. It is certainly a more involved procedure than insertion of the gold weight, and results may be dependent on the surgeon's skill level.

For short-term use, there are implantable devices. These include magnetized rods inserted into the upper and lower eyelids and silicon bands sutured to the lateral and medial canthal ligaments.

Temporalis muscle transplantation has the advantage of using autogenous tissue, thereby avoiding the use of foreign materials. First described by Gillies,[21] this procedure has since been modified by several authors.[22] A 1.5-cm-wide flap of temporalis muscle

based inferiorly is raised along with the overlying temporalis fascia. Because both the blood supply and motor nerve innervation enter the muscle on its inferior deep surface, the flap remains functional. The fascia is then elevated off the muscle from its inferior surface, attached to the left, and usually reinforced with sutures to the muscle superiorly (Fig. 80-11). The flap is passed subcutaneously to the lateral canthus, where the fascial strips are tunneled along the upper and lower lid margins and sutured to the medial canthal ligament (Fig. 80-12). With activation of the muscle, the fascial strips are pulled tight, causing eyelid closure. This technique has the advantage of addressing both upper eyelid lagophthalmos and lower eyelid ectropion. Use of the temporalis transfer for only the upper eyelid and a static sling for the lower eyelid allows better muscle excursion and therefore better eyelid closure. It is preferable to use a 2-mm strip of tendon; fascia appears to stretch, resulting in loss of effective eyelid movement. The disadvantages of this transfer are that with muscle contraction, the lid aperture changes from an oval to a slit shape; there may be skin wrinkling over the lateral canthal region and an obvious muscle bulge over the lateral orbital margin. Movements of the eyelids during chewing may also be a disturbing feature for the patient. Nevertheless, this procedure usually provides an excellent static support, eye closure on command, and good lubrication of the eye through distribution of the tear film.

Microneurovascular muscle transplantation for orbicularis function is a relatively new procedure. Platysma transplantation procedures that involve revascularization with the superficial temporal artery and vein and reinnervation with a cross-facial nerve graft are tedious and complex and should be reserved for patients for whom simpler techniques are unsuccessful. Transplantation of the platysma

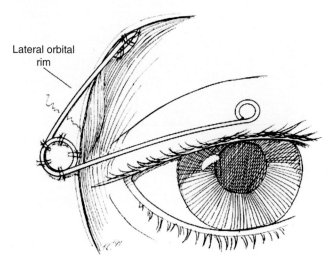

Lateral orbital rim

FIGURE 80-10. Palpebral spring in right upper eyelid. (From Levine RE: The enhanced palpebral spring. Operative Techniques Plast Reconstr Surg 1999;6:152.)

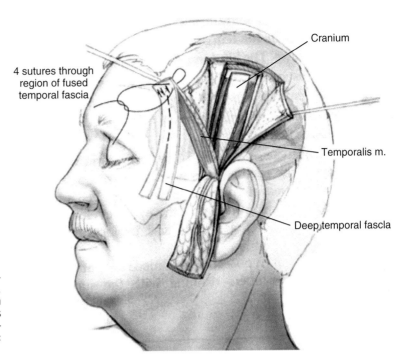

FIGURE 80-11. Elevation of temporalis muscle for transfer to eye. (From Salimbeni G: Eyelid animation in facial paralysis by temporalis muscle transfer. Operative Techniques Plast Reconstr Surg 1999;6: 159.)

may also produce some undesirable thickening of the eyelids.

Historically, lateral tarsorrhaphy has been one of the mainstay treatments for paralyzed eyelids. The McLaughlin lateral tarsorrhaphy[23] may provide a reasonably acceptable cosmetic result. However, horizontal lid length is decreased, which detracts from the aesthetic appeal and obstructs lateral vision. This procedure consists of resection of a segment of lateral skin, cilia, and orbicularis from the lower lid and a matching segment of conjunctiva and tarsus from the upper lid. The two raw surfaces are sutured together, preserving the upper eyelashes. At present, the main indication for lateral tarsorrhaphy is for the patient with an anesthetic cornea, severe corneal exposure, or failure of aesthetically more acceptable techniques.

Lower Eyelid

The orbicularis oculi muscle, through its attachment to the canthal ligaments, holds the lower eyelid firmly against the globe and with contraction is able to raise the lid 2 to 3 mm. Ordinarily, the eyelid margin rests at the level of the limbus of the eye. With paralysis of the orbicularis, tone in the muscle is lost. Gravity causes the lower eyelid to stretch and sag, resulting in scleral show. Over time, the lid and inferior canalicular punctum roll away from the globe, resulting in an ectropion (Fig. 80-13). Therefore, management is directed at resuspending the lid and reapposing the punctum to the globe.

Pronounced ectropion with lid eversion and more than 2 to 3 mm of scleral show is usually associated

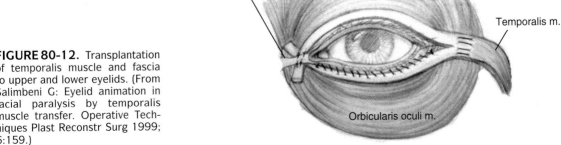

FIGURE 80-12. Transplantation of temporalis muscle and fascia to upper and lower eyelids. (From Salimbeni G: Eyelid animation in facial paralysis by temporalis muscle transfer. Operative Techniques Plast Reconstr Surg 1999; 6:159.)

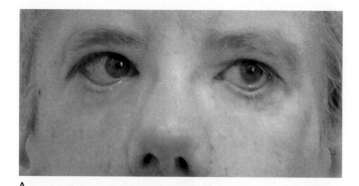

A

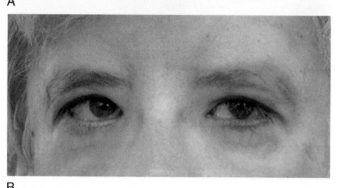

B

FIGURE 80-13. *A,* Marked bilateral ectropion in lower eyelids in a 52-year-old woman with Möbius syndrome. *B,* Postoperative appearance after tendon sling insertion to lower eyelids.

with symptoms of dryness and aesthetic concerns. This situation requires support of the entire length of the eyelid. This is best achieved with a static sling passed 1.5 to 2 mm inferior to the gray line of the eyelid and fixed both medially and laterally (Fig. 80-14).[24] Tendon provides longer lasting support with less stretching than the fascia lata. A 1.5-mm-wide strip of tendon is sutured to the lateral orbital margin in the region above the zygomaticofrontal suture and tunneled subcutaneously along the lid anterior to the tarsal plate. Proper placement is crucial; too low of a position will exacerbate the ectropion. In the elderly patient with particularly lax tissues, too superficial or high placement may result in an entropion. The sling is then passed around the anterior limb of the medial canthal ligament and sutured to itself. Subcutaneous tunneling of the tendon graft is facilitated by the use of a curved Keith needle. This procedure provides good support to the lower lid. It does not deform the eyelid, it is not apparent to an observer, and the effect appears to last well. If the sling is placed too loosely, it may be tightened at the lateral orbital margin.

Lateral examination of the eye and eyelid will determine its vector.[25] A negative vector occurs when the globe is anterior to the lid margin and the lid margin is anterior to the cheek prominence. In patients with a relatively proptotic eye, the lower eyelid sling will correct ectropion, but it may not decrease scleral show. In patients with a positive vector, in which the globe

is posterior to the lid margin and the lid margin is posterior to the cheek prominence, the sling will be effective. However, lateral fixation of the tendon graft may need to be through a drill hole, 2 to 3 mm posterior to the lateral orbital margin, because fixation to the frontal periosteum may lift the lateral eyelid away from the globe. The authors have used the lower lid sling on 25 occasions, and in combination with a gold weight to the upper lid, it results in a 95% improvement in symptoms (see Fig. 80-13*B*). Two patients have had complications from the lower lid sling procedure, which required the sling to be tightened. One patient required revision because the sling exacerbated the ectropion, and one required epilation of some lower eyelashes because of entropion.

Milder eyelid problems consisting of lower lid laxity and minimal scleral show may be treated with lateral canthoplasty. Jelks[26] has described various techniques of canthoplasty, such as the tarsal strip, dermal pennant, and inferior retinacular lateral canthoplasty. The canthal ligament must be reapproximated to the position of Whitnall tubercle, which is situated not only above the horizontal midpupillary line but also 2 to 3 mm posterior to the lateral orbital margin.

Horizontal lid shortening may be required to deal with redundant and stretched lower eyelid tissue. The Kuhnt-Szymanowski procedure can be modified not only to excise a wedge of tarsus and conjunctiva but also to resuspend the lateral canthus. This procedure

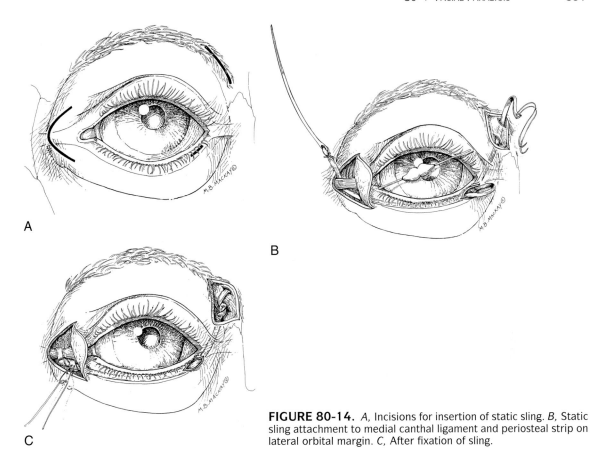

FIGURE 80-14. *A,* Incisions for insertion of static sling. *B,* Static sling attachment to medial canthal ligament and periosteal strip on lateral orbital margin. *C,* After fixation of sling.

tends to distort and expose the caruncle and does not provide a lasting correction.

Cartilage grafts to prop up the tarsal plate have also been used. By augmentation of the middle lamella and suturing of the cartilage to the inferior orbital margin, there will be less of a tendency for the lower eyelid to migrate inferiorly. However, results may be poor because the cartilage tends to rotate into a more horizontal position rather than a vertical one, producing a visible bulge and minimal eyelid support.

In patients with isolated medial ectropion that includes punctal eversion, the lower lid can be repositioned against the globe by direct excision of a tarsoconjunctival ellipse. This causes a vertical shortening of the inner aspect of the lower lid and helps reposition the punctum against the globe. Medial canthoplasty will also support the punctum.

Nasal Airway

Paralysis of the nasalis and levator alaeque nasi combined with drooping and medial deviation of the paralyzed cheek leads to support loss of the nostril, collapse of the ala, and reduction of airflow. Nasal septal deviation, which occurs in patients with congenital facial paralysis, may further accentuate any breathing difficulties. In the patient who complains of significant symptoms, the correction of the airway collapse is best accomplished by the elevation and lateral support of the alar base with a sling of tendon and by upper lip and cheek elevation procedures. Septoplasty may be indicated to provide an improvement in airway patency.

Upper Lip and Cheek (Smile Reconstruction)

The majority of patients with facial paralysis who present for reconstruction do so for either correction of an asymmetric face at rest or reconstruction of a smile. However, significant functional problems are associated with paralysis of the oral musculature, including drooling and speech difficulties. The flaccid lip and cheek can also lead to difficulties with chewing food, cheek biting, and pocketing of food in the buccal sulcus due to paralysis of the buccinator. However, the main emphasis of surgery is usually centered on reconstruction of a smile.

The surgeon and patient must have clearly defined goals. For the patient who solely requests symmetry at rest, static techniques such as slings and soft tissue procedures can produce this. For the patient who is willing to apply conscious effort and desires static correction as well as the ability to achieve a smile, regional muscle transplantations of the temporalis or masseter can provide excellent results. Free muscle transplantations innervated by cranial nerves other than those in the face can also provide satisfying results for the patient. However, the only techniques currently available to restore both voluntary and involuntary facial movements plus symmetry at rest require the use of the seventh nerve. This nerve is most easily used when it is combined with a free functioning muscle transplantation. The surgeon must have the skills to undertake this complex procedure.

FREE MUSCLE TRANSPLANTATION

It is not possible to restore complete symmetry of all movements because of the complexity of muscle interaction and the number of facial muscles involved. There are 18 separate muscles of facial expression, and of these, 5 are elevators of the upper lip and 2 are depressors of of the lower lip. A transplanted muscle can only be expected to produce one function and movement in one direction.

If the facial nerve is used to reinnervate the transplanted muscle, a smile and laughter will be spontaneous. When other nerves are used (e.g., the fifth, eleventh, or twelfth), teeth clenching or other movements are required to activate the smile. With time, the smile movement will often become less of a conscious effort and more spontaneous.

The patient's suitability for free muscle transplantation and reinnervation must be carefully assessed. This includes an assessment of the patient's ability to undergo a substantial operative procedure with general anesthesia as well as an evaluation of comorbidities that may affect the functioning of microneurovascular muscle transplantation. The patient should also be counseled with regard to the time that it could take to achieve full movement, which is usually around 18 months. It is generally recognized that reinnervation does not often occur in older individuals. However, it is difficult to determine which patient should be classified as "old" because muscle reinnervation can occur at any age. However, it is the authors' practice to be reluctant to perform functioning muscle transplantations on patients who are older than 60 years.

Smile Analysis

Preoperative planning is crucial. It is recognized that the unopposed smile on the normal side in unilateral facial paralysis will be an exaggerated expression of the same movement after reconstruction of the paralyzed side. Therefore, careful analysis of the patient's smile on the nonparalyzed side will instruct the surgeon in establishing a symmetric smile. As Paletz and Manktelow[27] have shown, individuals have various types of smiles. It is important to assess the direction of movement of the commissure and upper lip. How vertical is the movement? What is the strength of the smile and where around the mouth is the force most strongly focused? What is the relative amount of movement of the upper lip compared with the commissure and what is the position of the nasolabial fold with smiling? Is there a labial mental fold? Once these features have been determined, an estimate of the muscle's size, point of origin, tension, direction of movement, and placement can be planned (Fig. 80-15).

Technique Options

One-stage procedures for smile reconstruction with free muscle transplantations would seem to be the most appealing approach; however, for numerous reasons, they may not necessarily provide the best results (see Table 80-4). If the ipsilateral facial nerve trunk is available, it would seem to be an ideal source of reinnervation for a muscle flap. However, the exact branches to the lip elevators may be difficult to determine. If incorrect innervation is used, muscle contraction may take place only when the patient performs some facial movement other than smiling, such as closing the eyes or puckering the lips.

Single-stage muscle flaps with innervation from the contralateral facial nerve have been reported. This technique requires the use of a muscle with a long nerve segment, such as the latissimus dorsi or rectus abdominis.[28] However, even the gracilis[29] has been used. The nerve is tunneled across the lip and coapted to the facial nerve branches on the opposite side of the face. The advantages here are that the patient undergoes only one operation and there is only one site of coaptation for regenerating axons to cross. There does not appear to be any significant denervation atrophy of the muscle while it awaits reinnervation. However, although the muscle may function with facial movement, it may not contract when the patient smiles. This is because the facial nerve branches that are used are close to the mouth and are usually found through a nasolabial incision on the unaffected side. This approach does not allow thorough facial nerve mapping to be performed; thus, the most appropriate nerve branches may not be recruited. Also, this approach does not allow an assessment of what remaining branches have been left intact.

When there is neither an ipsilateral nor a contralateral facial nerve available to act as a donor, as in Möbius syndrome or other causes of bilateral facial paralysis, another cranial nerve must be used to reinnervate a muscle flap. This procedure can be performed in one stage, and it is our practice to use the nerve to the masseter muscle.[29] Zuker et al have shown that in children, this provides a symmetric smile with

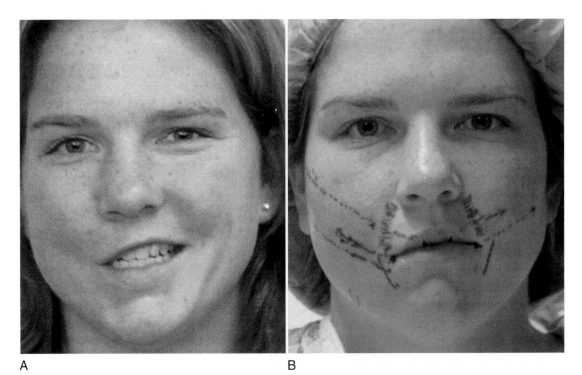

A   B

FIGURE 80-15. *A,* Patient shown smiling. Note direction of movement of the commissure and the mid-upper lip on the normal left side, location of the fold in the nasolabial area, and shape of the upper and lower lip. *B,* The nasolabial folds and directions of movement have been marked on the normal left side and copied on the paralyzed side. The desired position of the muscle is outlined by two dotted lines across the cheek.

excellent muscle excursion. These patients may never achieve involuntary movement or a truly spontaneous smile. However, in many children and in 50% of the adults, there would appear to be some cortical "rewiring" such that these people are able to activate a smile without performing a biting motion and without conscious effort.

In treatment of patients with unilateral facial paralysis, it is preferable to perform a two-stage reconstruction consisting of facial nerve mapping and cross-facial nerve grafting followed by a microneurovascular muscle transplantation.

AUTHORS' PREFERRED METHOD: TWO-STAGE MICRONEUROVASCULAR TRANSPLANTATION

Cross-Facial Nerve Graft. The first stage of this procedure involves a dissection of the facial nerve on the unaffected side through a preauricular incision with a submandibular extension (Fig. 80-16). The zygomaticobuccal nerve branches medial to the parotid gland are meticulously identified and individually stimulated with a micro-bipolar electrical probe attached to a stimulator source that allows variable voltage and frequency control (Fig. 80-17). Disposable stimulators used to identify the presence of motor nerves do not provide reliable controlled tetanic muscle contraction that will allow muscle palpation

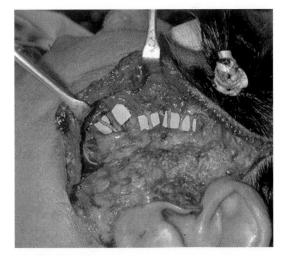

FIGURE 80-16. The cross-facial nerve graft is inserted through a preauricular incision. The parotid gland can be seen immediately in front of the left ear, and branches of the facial nerve supplying the muscles of the mouth and eye are seen superficial to the background material.

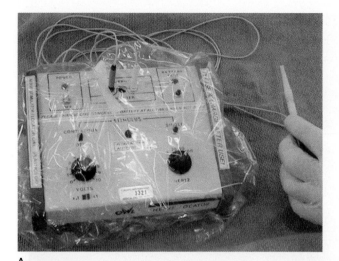

A

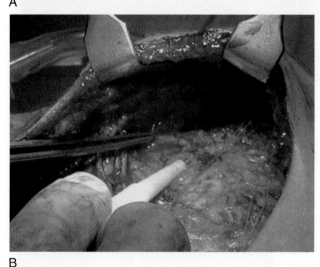

B

FIGURE 80-17. *A*, A portable electrical stimulator with variable voltage and frequency control is put in a sterile plastic bag placed close to the operating site so that the surgeon can adjust the voltage as needed. *B*, Bipolar electrical probe establishes an electrical current between the electrodes and a localized stimulus to a small area of tissue.

and clear visual identification of which muscle is being stimulated. Facial nerve mapping clearly identifies which nerve fibers stimulate the orbicularis oris and oculi muscles as well as the lip retractors. When stimulated, the facial nerve branches that produce a smile and no other movement are selected (Fig. 80-18). It is sometimes difficult to find "smile" branches that do not contain some orbicularis oculi function. There are usually between two and four nerve branches that activate the zygomaticus and levator labii superioris. This allows one or two branches to be used for the nerve graft coaptation while function of the normal facial muscles is preserved (Fig. 80-19).

The sural nerve is the usual donor nerve. This is harvested with the use of a nerve stripper (Fig. 80-20). The advantage of the stripper is that the patient is left with only two scars, one above the heel and the other below the popliteal fossa. Stripping of the nerve does not appear to affect its function as a graft.[30]

The proximal ends of the donor facial nerve branches are sutured to the distal end of the nerve graft such that regenerating axons will travel in a distal to proximal direction down the graft. The sural nerve is often split longitudinally and half is used. This modification was done for a number of reasons. Most surgeons agree that the amount of excursion gained in a muscle innervated by a traditional cross-facial nerve graft is usually less than desired. The reasons for this are likely to be related to decreasing nerve regeneration in the longer nerve graft, only partial regeneration of the graft's nerve fibers due to inadequate fiber input of regenerating nerve fibers, and the need for two nerve coaptations. Because there is usually a size mismatch between the large cross-sectional area of the sural graft and the small donor facial nerve branches, splitting provides a better end-to-end match. Splitting requires an interfascicular dissection under the operating microscope. It is usually technically

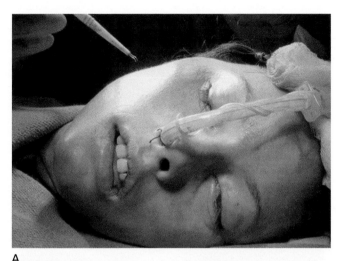

A

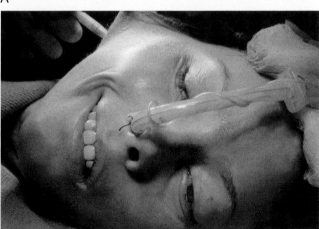

B

FIGURE 80-18. *A,* Patient with left facial paralysis under anesthesia. Facial nerve branches are prepared for functional nerve mapping of her right facial nerve. *B,* Stimulation of a branch of the facial nerve to the zygomaticus major, an ideal branch for coaptation to a cross-facial nerve graft.

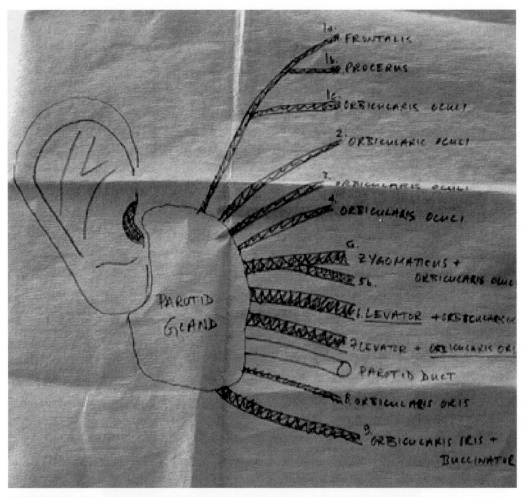

FIGURE 80-19. A functional nerve map is made of the branches of the facial nerve supplying the eye and mouth. The map identifies the muscles that contract when each branch is stimulated.

possible to perform an interfascicular split on a 10-cm length of sural nerve graft, whereas it is often not possible on a long graft because of nerve fiber crossovers between fascicles (Fig. 80-21). In the past, a 25-cm nerve was used for the nerve graft and passed subcutaneously across the face to the opposite pre-tragal area. After a period of 12 months, the second stage was performed. The current practice is to use a short nerve graft, approximately 10 cm in length, and to bank the free end in the upper buccal sulcus. This should provide an innervated graft that is better. In addition, the waiting period between the first and second stages is reduced with use of a short cross-facial nerve graft from 12 months to around 6 months. Patients who have had short nerve grafts achieve stronger muscle contraction than was previously

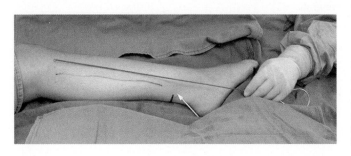

FIGURE 80-20. A nerve stripper is used for removal of the sural nerve. The arrow points to the incision for the insertion of the stripper. The stripper is brought out through a small posterior incision below the popliteal fossa. The sural nerve is seen lying on the calf under the stripper.

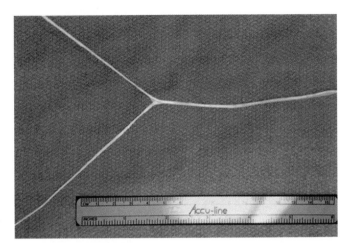

FIGURE 80-21. With use of the operating microscope, a sural nerve can usually be split longitudinally. Although interfascicular branching is present to a limited extent, it is usually possible to split a 10- to 15-cm length of sural nerve graft without division of crossover fascicles.

obtained with traditional long cross-facial nerve grafts (Table 80-5).

Gracilis Muscle Transplantation. Many muscles are available for functioning muscle transplantation for lower facial reconstruction (Table 80-6). The muscle should be transplantable by vascular anastomoses and have a suitable motor nerve for nerve coaptation to the face. Initially, surgeons attempted to find a muscle that was exactly the right size for the face. However, a more suitable approach is to pare down a muscle to the desired size before transplantation.[31] This concept allows the surgeon to use many different muscles and to customize the muscle to fit the functional requirements of the face. For example, a lightly structured face with only a partial paralysis will require a small piece of muscle. A large face with a strong movement of the mouth to the normal side and a total paralysis will require a large piece of muscle.

The gracilis muscle is suitable for facial paralysis reconstruction. The neurovascular pedicle is reliable and relatively easy to prepare. A segment of muscle can be cut to any desired size based on the neurovascular pedicle. This allows the surgeon to customize the muscle to the patient's facial requirements. There is no functional loss in the leg. Because the scar is in the medial aspect of the thigh, it is reasonably well hidden. However, the scar usually does spread. The thigh is far enough removed from the face that a simultaneous preparation of the muscle and the face is easily accomplished. The gracilis is the preferred muscle for transplantation because the anatomy is well known and the technique of preparing it for transplantation well described (Figs. 80-22 to 80-24).[32]

The muscle is usually split longitudinally and the anterior portion of the muscle is used. The amount of muscle that is taken varies from 30% to 70% of the cross section of the muscle, depending on the muscle size and needs of the face. The muscle can usually be split longitudinally without concern; however, on occasion, the vascular pedicle enters in the middle of the muscle on the deep surface. In this situation, it may be necessary to remove a portion of the anterior part of the muscle as well as the posterior to pare down the width of the muscle. After facial measurements are taken, a piece of muscle with a little extra length is removed. The end of the muscle that is to be inserted into the face is oversewn with mattress sutures, placing

TABLE 80-5 ✦ OPTIONS FOR MICRONEUROVASCULAR MUSCLE TRANSPLANTATION

One-stage	Muscle innervated by ipsilateral facial nerve (if available)
	Muscle with long nerve segment innervated by contralateral seventh nerve branches
	Muscle innervated by masseter, hypoglossal, or accessory nerve
Two-stage	Cross-facial nerve graft followed by the muscle transplantation

TABLE 80-6 ✦ MUSCLES AVAILABLE FOR MICRONEUROVASCULAR TRANSPLANTATION

Gracilis
Pectoralis minor
Rectus abdominis
Latissimus dorsi
Extensor carpi radialis brevis
Serratus anterior
Rectus femoris
Abductor hallucis

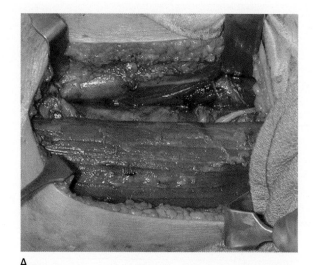

A

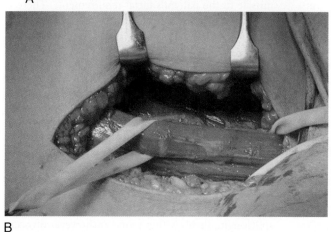

B

FIGURE 80-22. *A,* Preparation of gracilis muscle in right thigh. The motor nerve is seen in the right upper corner of the dissection adjacent to the vascular pedicle. *B,* A longitudinal split of the anterior half of the gracilis muscle.

one more than the number of sutures inserted about the lips.

Attaching the muscle to the mouth is a critical part of the procedure (Fig. 80-25). It is usually inserted into the fibers of the paralyzed orbicularis oris above and below the commissure and along the upper lip (Fig. 80-26A and B). Preoperative smile analysis determines the points of insertion. The preoperative smile analysis is also crucial for determining the origin of the muscle, which may be attached to the zygomatic body, arch, temporal fascia, or preauricular fascia. Intraoperative traction on the orbicularis oris while the movement of the mouth is observed will verify the correct placement of the sutures. The correct tension is difficult to determine because the mechanical tension within the muscle, the degree of tone that the muscle develops, and the gravitational and muscle forces within the face will influence the eventual position (Fig. 80-26C).

The vascular pedicle is usually anastomosed to the facial vessels; however, the facial vein may occasion-

ally be absent. There is invariably a large transverse facial vein that may be used instead. The superficial temporal vessels may also be used. The gracilis is positioned so that its hilum is close to the mouth and the motor nerve can be tunneled into the upper lip. The upper buccal sulcus incision is reopened, and the free end of the nerve graft is identified and coapted to the gracilis muscle motor nerve.

Movement does not usually occur until 6 months or more have elapsed, and maximal movement is usually gained by 18 months. At this stage, an assessment is made of the resting tension in the muscle and its excursion with smiling. It is not uncommon for the patient to require a third procedure to adjust the muscle (i.e., either tightening or loosening), and this can be combined with other touch-up procedures such as debulking or an adjustment of the insertion of origin.

With this procedure, patients usually gain around 50% as much movement on the paralyzed side as on

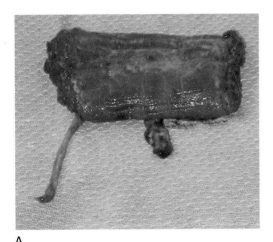

A

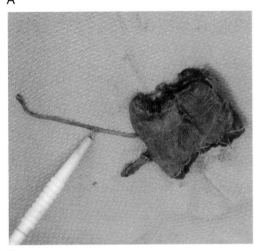

B

FIGURE 80-23. *A,* After removal of the segment of gracilis muscle, the motor nerve can be seen to the lower left and the pedicle inferiorly. The right-hand side demonstrates the distal end of the muscle, which has been oversewn with multiple mattress sutures. *B,* The marked muscle shortening is shown that is possible in the gracilis muscle with motor stimulation.

courses downward and anteriorly from the superoposterior border of the masseter in an oblique fashion. The nerve is always on the undersurface of the masseter muscle and enters this surface of the muscle belly approximately 2 cm below the zygomatic arch. The nerve courses through the muscle, giving off a variety of branches. Thus, the nerve can be traced distally, divided, and reflected proximally and superiorly to be in a position suitable for neural coaptation. The muscle transplant procedure is done much the same as described in the section on unilateral facial paralysis.

The origin and the insertion are the same, as is the revascularization process. The motor nerve to the transplanted muscle (segmental gracilis) is coapted to the motor nerve of the masseter. There is a remarkable similarity in size, and excellent reinnervation can be achieved. In fact, for patients with Möbius syndrome, the oral commissure movement accomplished by a gracilis transplant innervated by the masseter motor nerve comes within 2 mm of normal movement. There is approximately 15 mm of movement normally achieved at the oral commissure. With gracilis muscle transplantation innervated by the motor nerve to the

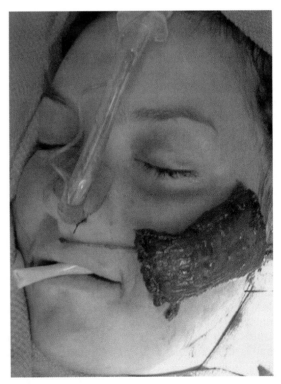

FIGURE 80-24. The muscle has been removed and placed on the face to demonstrate its approximate position. The muscle's motor nerve is placed across the cheek in the position for coaptation to the cross-facial nerve graft in the upper buccal sulcus.

the nonparalyzed side. This provides them with an excellent resting position and a pleasing smile that is totally spontaneous.

MUSCLE TRANSPLANTATION IN THE ABSENCE OF SEVENTH NERVE INPUT. The concept of muscle transplantation in the absence of seventh nerve input can be applied to bilateral facial paralysis and Möbius syndrome. An effective motor nerve must be used to power the muscle. The use of the twelfth nerve and eleventh nerve has been described, but preference is now given to the motor nerve to the masseter. This is a branch of the trigeminal (fifth nerve) and as such is almost always normal in patients who have bilateral facial paralysis, including Möbius syndrome. The nerve

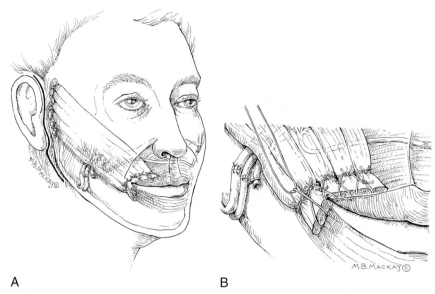

A   B

FIGURE 80-25. *A,* The muscle is placed in the face by vascular anastomosis to the facial artery and the vein. Nerve coaptation to the cross-facial nerve graft is accomplished. The muscle is attached about the mouth and to the preauricular and superficial temporal fascia. *B,* Insertion into the paralyzed orbicularis oris is accomplished with figure-of-eight sutures placed through the orbicularis oris and behind the mattress sutures at the end of the muscle. This ensures strong muscle fixation to the mouth, which should prevent dehiscence.

masseter, the average recovery of function is 13 mm.[29] The benefit of the cross-facial nerve graft, of course, is that it provides for spontaneity of activity, whereas the motor nerve to masseter does not and requires conscious activity. With a muscle that is innervated with a cross-facial nerve graft, the patient develops spontaneous expression because the muscle is controlled by the facial nerve on the normal side. However, when the masseter motor nerve is used, the smile movement must be learned as part of a conscious effort, although many patients may be able to smile without conscious effort and without needing to close the jaw. Patients with Möbius syndrome have each side revised separately with the procedures placed at least 2 months apart. Innervation of the segmental gracilis muscle transplant by the motor nerve to masseter is now the preferred reconstruction. It has proved to be extremely effective in helping improve lower lip incompetence and drooling as well as speech irregularities, especially those requiring bilabial sound production. Most important, however, it is effective in providing the patient with an acceptable level of smile animation that is not possible with other techniques (Figs. 80-27 and 80-28).

REGIONAL MUSCLE TRANSPLANTATION

Patients who are not suitable candidates for free muscle transplantation may be candidates for regional muscle transplantation. These techniques, which have been in use for many decades, involve the transplantation of either the temporalis or masseter muscle or both. Because these muscles are innervated by the trigeminal nerve to activate a smile, the patient must clench the teeth.

The retrograde temporalis muscle transplantation, as first described by Gillies,[21] involves detaching the origin of the muscle from the temporal fossa and turning it over the zygomatic arch to extend to the oral commissure. Frequently, a fascial graft is required to achieve the necessary length to reach the mouth. This leaves a significant hollowing in the temporal region that can be filled with an implant. Baker and Conley[33] recommend leaving the anterior portion of the temporalis behind to partially camouflage the temporal hollowing. Another aesthetic disadvantage of the temporalis transplantation is the bulge of muscle present where it passes over the arch of the zygoma. To avoid these complications, McLaughlin[23] described an antegrade temporalis transplantation. Through an intraoral, scalp, or nasolabial incision, the temporalis muscle is detached from the coronoid process of the mandible and brought forward. Fascial grafts are used to reach the angle of the mouth.

The temporalis provides excellent static positioning as well as voluntary activity. It is capable of producing an oblique lift to the mouth. There is, however, no control of the direction of movement.

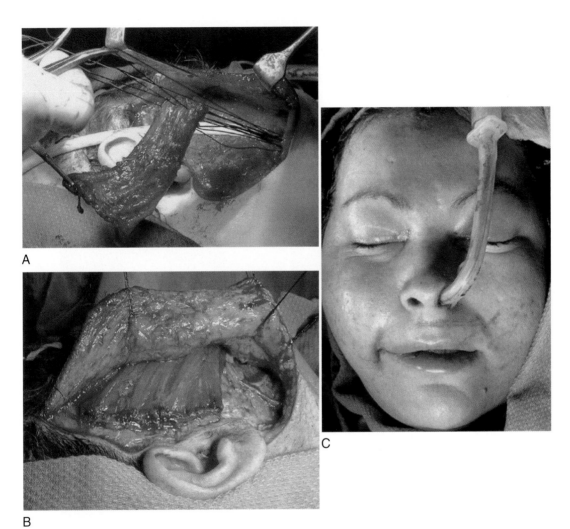

FIGURE 80-26. *A,* Traction of the sutures that are placed in the orbicularis muscle allows assessment of the expected shape of the smile. They are then placed through the muscle to fix it to the mouth. *B,* The muscle has been attached into the superficial temporal, parotid, and preauricular fascia. *C,* The muscle has been inserted on the patient's right side and sutured to the paralyzed orbicularis oris, showing slight overcorrection with good placement of the nasolabial and labiomental folds.

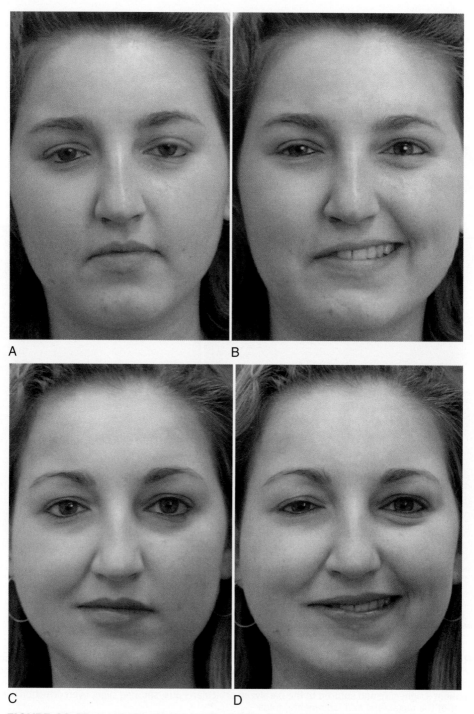

A   B

C   D

FIGURE 80-27. *A,* Preoperative view of a patient with partial right facial paralysis at rest. *B,* On smiling, she has only 1 to 2 mm of movement at the right commissure. *C,* After cross-facial nerve grafting and microneurovascular muscle transplantation, she is nicely balanced at rest. *D,* On smiling, she has a spontaneous movement of the right side of her mouth and a nearly symmetric nasolabial fold and upper lip.

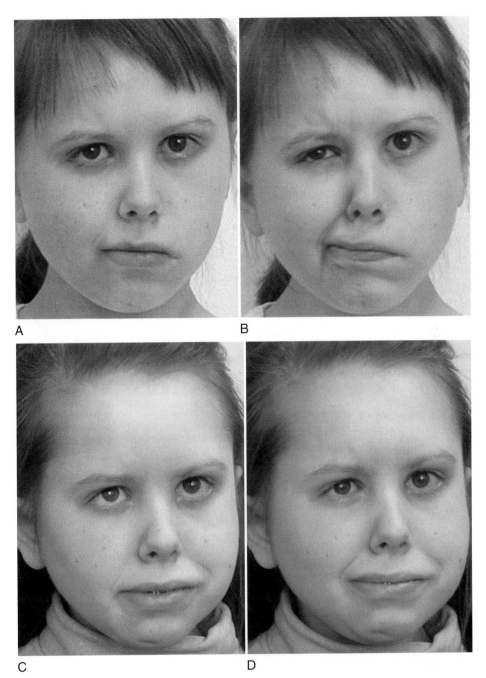

FIGURE 80-28. *A,* Preoperative view of a patient with complete left and partial right facial paralysis secondary to a brainstem tumor. *B,* On smiling, there is some zygomaticus and levator function. *C,* After microneurovascular muscle transplantation innervated with the masseter motor nerve, there is improved position at rest. *D,* Patient shown smiling.

The masseter muscle transplantation as described by Baker and Conley[33] involves transplanting the entire muscle or the anterior portion from its insertion on the mandible and inserting it around the mouth. Rubin[34] recommends separating the most anterior half of the muscle only and transposing it to the upper and lower lip. During the splitting dissection, the surgeon must be cautious not to injure the masseteric nerve, which enters the muscle on the deep surface superior to its midpoint.

Good static control of the mouth can be achieved with the masseter transplantation; however, it lacks sufficient force and excursion to produce a full smile, and the movement produced is too horizontal for most faces. Patients frequently have a hollow over the angle of the mandible.

Rubin[34] has advocated transplanting the temporalis and masseter muscles together (Fig. 80-29). The temporalis provides motion to the upper lip and nasolabial fold; the masseter provides support to the corner of the mouth and lower lip.

STATIC SLINGS

Static slings are used to achieve symmetry at rest without providing animation. They can be used alone or as an adjunct to dynamic procedures to provide immediate support. The goal is to produce a facial position equal to or slightly overcorrected from the resting position on the normal side. The slings can be made of fascia (tensor fascia lata), tendon, or prosthetic material such as Gore-Tex. In our experience, Gore-Tex produces an undesirable inflammatory reaction. When fascia lata is taken from the thigh, it is preferable to repair the donor defect or an uncomfortable and unsightly muscle hernia may develop. The authors' preference, however, is to use tendon (palmaris longus, plantaris, or extensor digitorum longus) (Fig. 80-30).

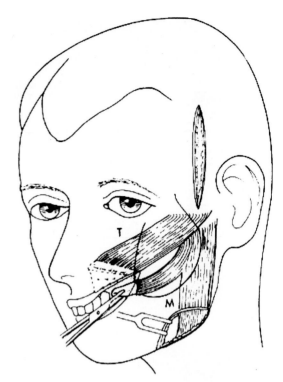

FIGURE 80-29. Transplantation of both the temporalis and a portion of the masseter muscle to the periorbital region. (From Rubin LE: Reanimation of the paralyzed face using the contiguous facial muscle technique. Operative Techniques Plast Reconstr Surg 1999;6:167.)

Tendon can easily be harvested and woven through tissues. Curved, pointed forceps are useful for inserting the tendon through the tissues of the oral commissure and upper lip and the temporalis and zygomatic fascia. Exposure can be through a nasolabial combined with a preauricular approach or a preauricular approach alone.

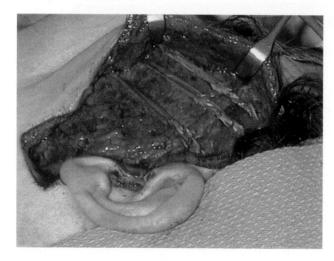

FIGURE 80-30. Static slings of plantaris tendon in place to support the mouth and cheek.

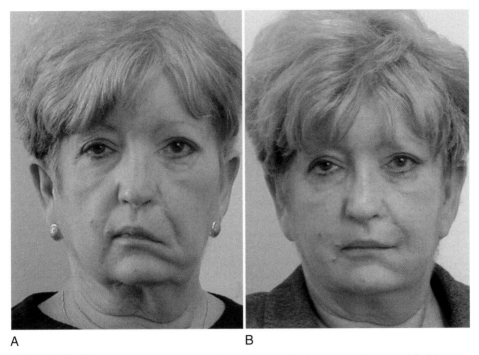

A   B

FIGURE 80-31. *A,* Preoperative view of an elderly patient at rest with marked facial asymmetry. Previous surgery elsewhere had placed a visible scar in the left nasolabial area. *B,* Improvement in facial symmetry after insertion of static slings to the mouth.

When tension is applied to the grafts, the force should be distributed evenly around the mouth with a little overcorrection. This is done to compensate for the difference in facial tone when the patient is awake and for postoperative stretching. The graft is then attached to the temporal fascia or to the zygoma, depending on the desired direction of pull. Multiple grafts should be inserted, usually three, to provide an even lift to the corner of the mouth and upper lip (Fig. 80-31). It is important to position the sling properly to achieve the correct elevation with regard to the upper lip and corner of the mouth. It is possible to insert the static sling too tightly, particularly in the upper lip, which establishes a corridor through which air and liquid can escape.

SOFT TISSUE REBALANCING

Soft tissue procedures are a useful adjunct to both dynamic and static management. These procedures involve suspension and repositioning of the lax structures. This will include rhytidectomy with or without plication or suspension of the superficial musculoaponeurotic system; midface subperiosteal lifts may also be beneficial. Procedures on the nasolabial fold usually do not help define this important structure. Asymmetry of the upper lips may be corrected by mucosal excisions. These procedures, which may be minor, will often be of great benefit to patients.

Lower Lip

The lower lip deformity caused by marginal mandibular nerve palsy may be part of a generalized facial paralysis or may occur in isolation as a congenital defect or secondary to trauma or surgery. It is a particular risk during rhytidectomy or parotid and upper neck surgery. The marginal mandibular nerve consists of one to three branches and supplies the depressor labii inferioris, depressor anguli oris, mentalis, and portions of the lower lip orbicularis oris. The orbicularis oris also receives innervation from buccal branches and the contralateral marginal mandibular nerves. The muscle function that is missed most by the patient is that of the depressor labii inferioris. Paralysis of this muscle results in the inability to depress, lateralize, and evert the lower lip. In the normal resting position, the deformity is not usually noticeable as the lips are closed and the depressors are relaxed. However, when the patient is talking, the paralyzed side stays in an elevated position, whereas the nonparalyzed side is able to move inferiorly and away from the teeth. The deformity is most accentuated when the patient attempts a full smile, showing his or her teeth.

Problems with speech and eating may occur, but most patients are concerned primarily with the asymmetric appearance of the lower lip during speech and smiling. The inability to express rage and sorrow, which require a symmetric lower lip depression, is also of concern.

Many techniques have been described for the correction of marginal mandibular nerve palsy, including operating on the affected side to try to animate it or operating on the unaffected side to minimize its function. Puckett et al[35] described a technique of excising a wedge of skin and muscle but preserving orbicularis oris on the unaffected side. Glenn and Goode[36] described a full-thickness wedge resection of the paralyzed side of the lower lip. Edgerton[37] described transplantation of the anterior belly of the digastric muscle. The insertion of the digastric muscle to the mandible on the paralyzed side is divided and attached to a fascia lata graft that is then secured to the mucocutaneous border of the involved lip. Conley[38] modified this technique by leaving the mandibular insertion intact but divided the tendon between anterior and posterior bellies, rotated the muscle, and reattached the tendon to the lateral aspect of the lower lip. As branches of the nerve to mylohyoid innervate the anterior belly of the digastric, activation of the muscle requires a movement other than smiling. This is difficult to coordinate for most patients, and the result is that the digastric transplantation tends to act more as a passive restraint on the lower lip rather than as an active depressor. Terzis[8] has further modified the digastric transplantation by combining it with a cross-facial nerve graft coapted to a marginal mandibular nerve branch on the unaffected side, thereby allowing the possibility of spontaneous activation with smiling.

In patients in whom the facial paralysis is less than 24 months in duration and there is evidence of remaining depressor muscle after needle electromyography, Terzis recommends a mini hypoglossal nerve transplantation to the cervicofacial branch of the facial nerve. This involves division of the cervicofacial branch proximally and coaptation of the distal stump to a partially transected (20% to 30%) hypoglossal nerve. In patients with long-standing paralysis with a functional ipsilateral platysma muscle (i.e., an intact cervical division of the facial nerve), Terzis suggests transplantation of the platysma muscle to the lower lip.

The approach to depressor muscle paralysis has been to achieve symmetry both at rest and with expression by performing a selective myectomy of the depressor labii inferioris of the nonparalyzed side. This was first reported by Curtin[39] in 1960 and later by Rubin,[34] although details of their techniques are not provided. The depressor resection can be performed as an outpatient procedure under local anesthetic and can be preceded by an injection of either long-acting local anesthetic or botulinum toxin into the depressor labii inferioris. This injection allows the patient a chance to decide whether to proceed with the muscle resection based on the loss of function of the depressor. As a result of this operation, the shape of the smile is altered on the normal side, and the lower lip is now symmetric with the opposite side (Fig. 80-32).

The depressor labii inferioris is marked preoperatively by asking the patient to show the teeth and palpating over the lower lip. The muscle can be felt as a band passing from the lateral aspect of the lower lip inferiorly and laterally to the chin. Through an intraoral buccal sulcus incision, the muscle is identified; it is partly hidden by the orbicularis oris, whose fibers must be elevated to reveal the more vertically and obliquely oriented fibers of the depressor labii inferioris, which measures approximately 1 cm in width. Care must be taken to preserve the branches of the mental nerve during the dissection (see Fig. 80-5). Once the muscle has been identified, the central portion of the muscle belly is resected. Simple myotomy will not produce long-standing results, whereas results from myectomy have been permanent.

The authors have performed depressor labii inferioris resections on 27 patients, and these were reviewed with a follow-up questionnaire.[40] Of these patients, 77% stated that their lower lip was more symmetric with smiling; half of these patients thought that their smile had changed from being significantly asymmetric to completely symmetric. Before the muscle resection, 53% of the patients were concerned about lower lip asymmetry in expressing other emotions, such as sorrow or anger. After the muscle resection, 80% of the patients now thought that having a symmetric lower lip in expressing other emotions was more acceptable. Speech was unchanged in 73% of the patients and improved in 27% after depressor labii inferioris resection. Some authors have suggested that depressor muscle resection will result in a deterioration of oral continence. However, in our series, 89% of the patients stated that oral continence was either unchanged or improved. Three patients reported a slight increase in drooling after depressor labii inferioris resection.

ASSOCIATED SUBSPECIALTY MANAGEMENT

Facial paralysis crosses many subspecialty lines. Limited eye closure, tear transport, and ectropion dictate the involvement of ophthalmologists as well as oculoplastic surgeons. Intranasal airflow may be limited and symptomatic, necessitating involvement of nasal surgeons often with otolaryngology background. Otolaryngologists may also be consulted for associated hearing loss, stapedial malfunction, or other components involving the middle ear. In certain patients, brainstem involvement may cause difficulty in dealing with oral secretions, aspiration, and swallowing. This may

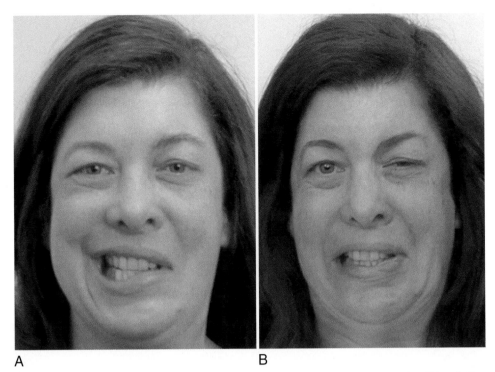

FIGURE 80-32. Patient showing a "full dental" smile before depressor resection *(A)* and after depressor resection *(B)*, with marked improvement in symmetry of the lower lip.

occur congenitally, such as in patients with Möbius syndrome, or it may be acquired, such as in patients with intracranial tumors. These situations may require the involvement of otolaryngologists.

There are other functional issues that may need to be addressed by subspecialists. For example, feeding may be a problem for infant or adult patients. Feeding experts from occupational therapy may be helpful in providing techniques for mechanical assistance. After surgical intervention, occupational therapy is also helpful in assisting with an exercise program to improve muscle excursion and symmetry of smile. Speech is often affected by facial paralysis. Speech therapy can help improve articulation errors and provide appropriate lip placement.

The psychosocial aspects of facial paralysis are enormous. Surgeons tend to focus on the physical, but it is extremely important to keep the entire patient in mind. A battery of psychosocial support personnel should be available to work with the surgeon for the overall benefit of the patient. This team should include social workers, clinical psychologists, developmental psychologists, and psychiatrists. It is important to sort out the various needs of the patient—not just from a physical standpoint but also from a psychosocial standpoint. Only then can true success in surgical management be achieved.

GENETIC IMPLICATIONS OF CONGENITAL FACIAL PARALYSIS

A majority of patients with congenital facial paralysis have unilateral and isolated involvement. It is believed to be the result of a compression of the fetal face that limits facial nerve development. Consequently, there are no genetic implications. Parents have no predisposition for additional children with facial paralysis, nor does the patient have any greater increased likelihood of facial paralysis than that of the general population. The same can be said for patients with unilateral syndrome, which occurs with hemifacial microsomia, for example. This is thought to be acquired at an early stage of fetal development because of environmental factors. Thus, again, there are no genetic implications. The same is not true, however, for all patients with Möbius syndrome. Although most are thought to be sporadic, there has been a surge of interest in the genetics of the condition.[41] There have been pedigrees described indicating that certain forms of Möbius syndrome are inherited by an autosomal dominant gene with variable expressivity (Fig. 80-33).

Incomplete penetration is also thought to account for the inconsistency of involvement. Certain chromosomes have also been identified in specific patients,[42] and a reciprocal translocation between the

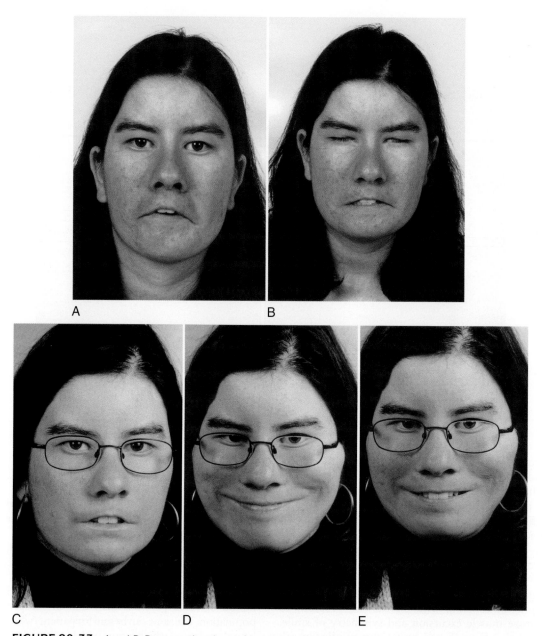

FIGURE 80-33. *A* and *B*, Preoperative views of a patient with Möbius syndrome at rest and with maximum animation. *C*, Postoperative view of a patient after muscle transplantation to the lower face at rest. *D*, Patient with closed-mouth smile. *E*, Patient smiling and showing teeth.

long arm of chromosome 13 and the short arm of chromosome 1 has been described.[43] A great deal of interest has been stimulated relative to the genetic aspects of Möbius syndrome and its relationship to other behavioral conditions. Research is under way in these areas and will undoubtedly shed light on inheritance features as well as the etiologic factors involved in Möbius syndrome.

AREAS OF FURTHER RESEARCH AND DEVELOPMENT

Although significant progress has been made in the management of facial paralysis, much is yet to be done. Acceptable commissure movement can be achieved, but upper lip elevation is far more difficult. The short distance of the muscle involved and the challenging access have proved difficult to overcome. However, new techniques are emerging, and work in this area continues.

Across any nerve repair, there is considerable loss of axonal continuity. Improved nerve coaptation techniques with the use of neurotrophic factors will undoubtedly be instrumental in providing further improvement. From a physical standpoint, does the length of the nerve graft affect recovery? Does its vascular nature or the technique of harvest result in alteration of function? Laboratory research in these areas is ongoing and could again provide some level of improvement in recovery. The placement, anchorage, and direction of movement of the muscle transplant are critical to success. Improvements have been made in these areas, but asymmetry continues to be a challenge. Further attention needs to be drawn to the direction of the smile and the positioning of the muscle relative to the oral commissure and nasolabial crease.

Fundamental to progress in any field is an assessment tool that is reliable, universally acceptable, and as simple as possible to use. In facial paralysis, it is necessary to measure muscle excursion, direction of movement, volume symmetries, and contour irregularities to assess the results of repair and reconstruction. For comparison of results from center to center, a common tool is needed. Also, to assess results from a psychosocial standpoint, a reliable common instrument of evaluation is needed if meaningful conclusions are to be drawn. Progress has been made on the physical measurement and the psychosocial profile tools,[44] and there is hope that these will be universally accepted and applied in the future.

In addition to these technical issues, concepts need to evolve with respect to new areas of development. Eye expression is an area that has not as yet been addressed. Also, thus far, oral movement has been directed at commissure and upper lip elevation. Orbicularis oris function or reconstruction of the depressors has not been addressed. Finally, there is not as yet an effective method of managing synkinesis. This is an extremely disturbing phenomenon with psychosocial and functional implications. We are just beginning to see how Botox injection techniques can be effective in other areas of muscle overactivity, and perhaps some level of synkinesis control will evolve with this technique. Much is yet to be done for the patient with facial paralysis, and further research and development in this area will continue to yield improvements.

REFERENCES

1. Falco NA, Eriksson E: Facial nerve palsy in the newborn: incidence and outcome. Plast Reconstr Surg 1990;85:1.

2. Davis RA, Anson BJ, Budinger JM, Kurth LR: Surgical anatomy of the facial nerve and parotid gland based upon a study of 350 cervico-facial halves. Surg Gynecol Obstet 1956;102:385.

3. Rudolph R: Depth of the facial nerve in facelift dissection. Plast Reconstr Surg 1990;85:537.

4. Ishikawa Y: An anatomical study of the distribution of the temporal branch of the facial nerve. J Craniomaxillofac Surg 1990;18:287.

5. Freilinger G, Gruber H, Happak W, Pechmann U: Surgical anatomy of the mimic muscle system and the facial nerve: importance for reconstructive and aesthetic surgery. Plast Reconstr Surg 1987;80:686.

6. Baker DC, Conley J: Avoiding facial nerve injuries in rhytidectomy: anatomical variations and pitfalls. Plast Reconstr Surg 1979;64:781.

7. Nelson DW, Gingrass RP: Anatomy of the mandibular branches of the facial nerve. Plast Reconstr Surg 1979;64:479.

8. Terzis JK, Kalantarian B: Microsurgical strategies in 74 patients for restoration of dynamic depressor muscle mechanism: a neglected target in facial reanimation. Plast Reconstr Surg 2000;105:1917.

9. Zide BM, McCarthy J: The mentalis muscle: an essential component of chin and lower lip position. Plast Reconstr Surg 1989;83:413.

10. Rubin L, ed: The Paralyzed Face. St. Louis, Mosby-Year Book, 1991.

11. Latham RA, Deaton TG: The structural basis of the philtrum and the contour of the vermilion border: a study of the musculature of the upper lip. J Anat 1976;121:151.

12. Fára M: The musculature of cleft lip and palate. In McCarthy JG, ed: Plastic Surgery. Philadelphia, WB Saunders, 1990:2598.

13. Pessa JP, Garza PA, Love VM, et al: The anatomy of the labiomandibular fold. Plast Reconstr Surg 1998;101:482.

14. May M: Microanatomy and pathophysiology of the facial nerve. In May M, ed: The Facial Nerve. New York, Thieme, 1986:63.

15. Guerrissi JO: Selective myectomy for post paretic facial synkinesis. Plast Reconstr Surg 1991;87:459.

16. Neely JG: Computerized quantitative dynamic analysis of facial motion in the paralyzed and synkinetic face. Am J Otol 1992;13:97.

17. Tears Naturale II [product information]. Alcon Canada, Inc., 2001.

18. Diels HJ: Neuromuscular retraining for facial paralysis. Otolaryngol Clin North Am 1997;30:727.

19. Manktelow RT: Use of the gold weight for lagophthalmos. Operative Techniques Plast Reconstr Surg 1999;6:157.

20. Levine RE: The enhanced palpebral spring. Operative Techniques Plast Reconstr Surg 1999;6:152.

21. Gillies H: Experiences with fascia lata grafts in the operative treatment of facial paralysis. Proceedings of the Royal Society of Medicine, London, England, August 1934. London, England, John Bale, Sons, and Danielsson, 1935.

22. Salimbeni G: Eyelid reanimation in facial paralysis by temporalis muscle transfer. Operative Techniques Plast Reconstr Surg 1999;6:159.

23. McLaughlin CR: Surgical support in permanent facial paralysis. Plast Reconstr Surg 1953;11:302.

24. Carraway JH, Manktelow RT: Static sling reconstruction of the lower eyelid. Operative Techniques Plast Reconstr Surg 1999;6:163.

25. Jelks GW, Jelks EB: Preoperative evaluation of the blepharoplasty patient. Clin Plast Surg 1993;20:213.

26. Jelks GW, Glat PM, Jelks EB, et al: Evolution of the lateral canthoplasty: techniques and indications. Plast Reconstr Surg 1997;100:1396.

27. Paletz JL, Manktelow RT, Chaban R: The shape of a normal smile: implications for facial paralysis reconstruction. Plast Reconstr Surg 1993;93:784.

28. Koshima I, Tsuda K, Hamanaka T, Moriguchi T: One-stage recon-struction of established paralysis using a rectus abdominis muscle transfer. Plast Reconstr Surg 1997;99:234.
29. Zuker RM, Goldberg CS, Manktelow RT: Facial animation in children with Moebius syndrome after segmental gracilis muscle transplant. Plast Reconstr Surg 2000;106:1.
30. Koller R, Frey M, Rab M, et al: Histological examination of graft donor nerves harvested by the stripping technique. Eur J Plast Surg 1995;18:24.
31. Manktelow RT, Zuker RM: Muscle transplantation by fascicu-lar territory. Plast Reconstr Surg 1984;73:751.
32. Manktelow RT: Microvascular Reconstruction. Anatomy, Appli-cations, and Surgical Technique. New York, Springer-Verlag, 1986.
33. Baker DC, Conley J: Regional muscle transposition for rehabilitation of the paralyzed face. Clin Plast Surg 1979;6: 317.
34. Rubin L: Re-animation of total unilateral facial paralysis by the contiguous facial muscle technique. In Rubin L, ed: The Paralyzed Face. St. Louis, Mosby-Year Book, 1991:156.
35. Puckett CL, Neale HW, Pickerell KL: Dynamic correction of unilateral paralysis of the lower lip. Plast Reconstr Surg 1975;55:397.
36. Glenn MG, Goode RL: Surgical treatment of the marginal mandibular lip deformity. Otolaryngol Head Neck Surg 1987;97:462.
37. Edgerton MT: Surgical correction of facial paralysis: a plea for better reconstruction. Ann Surg 1967;165:985.
38. Conley J, Baker DC, Selfe RW: Paralysis of the mandibular branch of the facial nerve. Plast Reconstr Surg 1982;70:569.
39. Curtin JW, Greely PW, Gleason M, Braver D: Supplementary procedures for the improvement of facial nerve paralysis. Plast Reconstr Surg 1960;26:73.
40. Presented at the Canadian Society of Plastic Surgery meeting, Jasper, Canada. June 2001.
41. Kremer H, Kuyt LP, van den Helm B, et al: Localization of a gene for Möbius syndrome to chromosome 3q by linkage analy-sis in a Dutch family. Hum Mol Genet 1996;5:1367.
42. Slee JJ, Smart RD, Viljoen DL: Deletion of chromosome 13 in Möbius syndrome. J Med Genet 1991;28:413.
43. Ziter FA, Wiser WC, Robinson A: Three generation pedigree of a Möbius syndrome variant with chromosome translocation. Arch Neurol 1977;34:437.
44. Jugenburg M, Hubley P, Yandell H, et al: Self-esteem in children with facial paralysis: a review of measures. Can J Plast Surg 2001;9:143.

✦ Oral Cavity Reconstruction

JOANNE J. LENERT, MD ✦ GREGORY R. D. EVANS, MD

THE PROBLEM

SCOPE AND COMPLEXITY
   Statistics
   Risk Factors
   Genetics
   Nutrition
   Concurrent Medical Problems
   Social Issues
   Rehabilitation
   Surveillance

THE ORAL CAVITY
   Anatomy
   Function

TREATMENT OF ORAL CAVITY DEFECTS
   Preoperative Evaluation
   Treatment Goals
   Site-Specific Treatment Goals

ALGORITHM FOR SURGICAL TREATMENT

SPECIFIC SURGICAL TECHNIQUES
   Primary Closure and Secondary Healing

   Skin Grafts
   Local and Regional Flaps
   Musculocutaneous Flaps
   Free Flaps

INTRAOPERATIVE AND POSTOPERATIVE CARE

COMPLICATIONS
   Flap Loss
   Hematoma
   Neck Flap Necrosis
   Infection
   Fistula
   Donor Site Complications
   Need for Revision

OUTCOMES
   Surgical
   Functional
   Oncologic
   Quality of Life

UNSOLVED PROBLEMS

THE PROBLEM

The oral cavity is the inlet to the aerodigestive tract. Its contents perform an array of functions viewed as second nature by the average human. These functions include speech, mastication, deglutition, maintenance of oral and oronasal competence, salivation, and early digestion. Oral cavity reconstruction aims to restore form and function to a complex configuration of tissues. Just as reanimation of the paralyzed face can never truly recreate the intricate movements of the normal facial musculature, so present reconstructive techniques cannot restore full function to the oral cavity after radical resection. Nonetheless, the application of certain basic principles allows the reconstructive surgeon to achieve wound closure and to optimize form and function in the patient with a large intraoral defect.

The focus of this chapter is oncologic reconstruction of the oral cavity. In general, the principles discussed are easily applied to the reconstruction of traumatic and other nononcologic defects.

SCOPE AND COMPLEXITY

Statistics

Most patients requiring major reconstruction of the oral cavity carry a diagnosis of malignant neoplasia (Fig. 81-1). By far, the most common malignant tumor of the oral cavity is squamous cell carcinoma (86%).[1] Other primary tumors of the oral cavity are verrucous carcinoma, sarcoma, melanoma, and lymphoma; minor salivary gland tumors include adenocarcinoma, mucoepidermoid carcinoma, and adenoid cystic carcinoma. Metastatic tumors are also seen, most commonly from lung, kidney, breast, and skin.[2]

Worldwide, cancers of the mouth and oropharynx account for about 363,000 new cases and 200,000 deaths annually. The age-standardized incidence rates (cases per 100,000 population per year) are similar in developed and developing countries: 13.5 versus 11.5 for men and 3.0 versus 5.1 for women.[3]

Oral cavity and pharynx together represent the seventh leading site of new cancer in men in the United States (3% of all cancer cases).[4] Although this site is

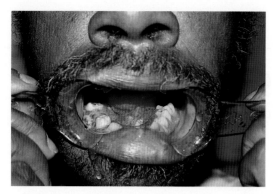

FIGURE 81-1. T4 squamous cell carcinoma of the floor of mouth with mandibular invasion.

not yet among the top 10 cancer sites in women, the incidence of oral cancer in women continues to increase as the number of female smokers rises.[5] Of all head and neck cancer sites, oral cavity cancer (not including pharynx) makes up about 14%, second only to larynx (21%).[1] On the basis of earlier data, an estimated 19,400 new cases of oral cavity cancer were expected to occur in the United States in the year 2003, including 7100 tumors of the tongue, 9200 tumors of the mouth, and 3100 tumors arising in other locations in the oral cavity.[4]

The 5-year relative cancer survival rate (adjusted for normal life expectancy) for cancers of the oral cavity and pharynx is about 54% (United States, 1989-1996), a number that has been fairly constant since the mid-1970s. The survival rates for patients with head and neck squamous cell carcinoma follow a general pattern: the more posterior and inferior the site, the worse the prognosis. Thus, the inclusion of pharyngeal cancers in these statistics skews the numbers somewhat in a negative direction. The age-adjusted death rates (deaths per 100,000 population per year) from oral cavity and pharynx cancers are 3.2 for men and 1.1 for women. Looking at oral cavity tumors alone, 5200 deaths were expected to occur in the United States in the year 2003, 1700 from tongue cancers, 1900 from mouth cancers, and 1600 from other oral cavity cancers.[4]

Risk Factors

Tobacco use is the major risk factor for the development of squamous cell carcinoma of the oral cavity throughout the world. Alcohol use has an independent carcinogenic effect and potentiates the effects of tobacco use.[6] Thus, excessive use of both tobacco and alcohol results in a synergistic 15-fold increase in the risk of oral cancer compared with abstinence from both. Geographic differences in the type of tobacco habit (smoking versus chewing) are reflected in large differences in the relative frequencies of tumor location.

Where tobacco chewing predominates, most oral and pharyngeal cancers are found in the oral cavity. In contrast, in locations where smoking is more common, tumor incidence is split more evenly between oral cavity and pharynx.[3]

Other proposed risk factors for oral cancer include poor oral hygiene, mechanical irritation from teeth or dentures, betel nut use, heredity, syphilis, and viruses.[5] The oncogenic potential of viruses is an area of current research. The human papillomavirus is associated with a large fraction of verrucous carcinomas and may well play a central etiologic role in their formation. Cancers of the tonsil and cancers of the tongue are also strongly correlated with human papillomaviruses on the basis of molecular epidemiologic data. The carcinogenic effect of human papillomavirus probably relates, at least in part, to the degradation of the tumor suppressor protein p53 in human papillomavirus–infected cells.[7]

Genetics

Although tobacco use and alcohol use account for a large majority of oral cavity cancers in the United States, only a minority of individuals exposed to tobacco and alcohol develop head and neck cancer. It is clear that host-specific factors must also influence the risk for development of cancer. In fact, heritable differences in susceptibility to environmental insults have been identified at almost every stage of carcinogenesis. For example, many tobacco carcinogens require metabolic activation before exerting their carcinogenic effect. Interindividual variation in activation or detoxification will cause differences in carcinogen concentration, which will manifest as differences in susceptibility.

DNA repair capability is also relevant for upper aerodigestive tract cancers. Assays have been developed to measure mutagen sensitivity, revealing a spectrum of DNA repair capability within the general population. Mutagen sensitivity appears to be an independent risk factor for cancer development, after controlling for the effects of alcohol and tobacco use. Ideally, the measurement of susceptibility markers by this and similar assays will enable the identification of high-risk population subgroups that can be targeted for intensive preventive strategies.[8]

Nutrition

Malnutrition, iron deficiency, and avitaminosis, particularly riboflavin deficiency, appear to increase the risk of carcinoma of the oral cavity. Perhaps more important, pain, poor dietary habits, alcohol abuse, and tumor burden may result in nutritional deficiency and weight loss in the patient with oral cavity cancer. Immune suppression and impaired wound healing may result, compromising reconstructive efforts and depressing the host response to malignant disease. Side effects from surgery and adjuvant therapy may have a negative impact on dietary intake, resulting in further weight and protein loss.[5] The treating physician must be mindful of the need to evaluate nutritional status and to provide perioperative nutritional support to these high-risk patients. The severely malnourished patient should receive preoperative nutritional replacement in an effort to decrease operative morbidity and mortality.[9]

Concurrent Medical Problems

Due to the association of oral cavity cancer with smoking and alcohol abuse, as well as the elderly nature of the affected population, concurrent medical problems are common. A good review of systems, and additional work-up as indicated, should be performed to identify chronic obstructive pulmonary disease and coronary artery disease in every patient. Liver disease should be considered in heavy drinkers. Consultation with internal medicine is often advisable to optimize medical status and to minimize operative morbidity and mortality. The surgical plan will occasionally change if the operative risks are high.

Social Issues

Cancer of the head and neck disproportionately affects the elderly and individuals in lower income brackets. In addition, the number of head and neck mucosal cancers is disproportionately greater among African Americans than among whites, and the incidence appears to be increasing in this minority group. Not only is head and neck cancer more prevalent among African Americans, it is more lethal. The 5-year cancer survival rate for oral cavity and pharynx cancer is 59% for whites compared with 35% for blacks (United States, 1992-1998).[4] This may simply reflect a more advanced stage at presentation, which may be tied to economic disadvantage and limited access to resources. Alternatively, racial differences may result from as yet unidentified environmental and biologic factors.

Rehabilitation

Treatment of the patient with oral cavity cancer does not end when the wound is healed. Present treatments continue to result in high rates of poor functional outcome. Most reconstructions become temporarily swollen and stiff regardless of their ultimate characteristics. Oral function may take months to be recovered, and this period is exacerbated and lengthened by postoperative radiotherapy.

The combination of the loss of tongue function and xerostomia leaves many patients with poor speech and severe dysphagia. These alterations in function may have a profound impact on the patient physically and socially. Speech impairment may cause the patient to change employment or to withdraw from social interaction. Difficulty managing oral secretions may render the patient an "oral cripple" who will not eat or even appear in public. Dysphagia and aspiration can result in nutritional compromise and even life-threatening infection. Early and continued involvement of the speech therapist and dietitian helps optimize the patient's post-treatment quality of life. The importance of rehabilitation cannot be overemphasized.

Surveillance

During the past 20 to 30 years, marginal if any improvement in overall survival has occurred for patients with both early and locally advanced squamous cell carcinoma of the head and neck. Despite successful primary therapy, the majority of patients with advanced local and regional disease will die of local recurrence, distant metastasis, or second primary tumor. Although patients with early-stage disease can be treated effectively with single-modality local therapy (surgery or radiotherapy), these patients have a 4% to 7% annual risk for development of a second primary tumor. A new primary cancer remains the principal cancer-related cause of death for patients with early-stage disease.[10] Both recurrent tumors and second primaries may be eminently treatable. Thus, close surveillance for a lifetime is indicated in patients with both early- and late-stage disease.

THE ORAL CAVITY
Anatomy

The lips form the anterior border of the oral cavity. The posterior border is delineated by an imaginary vertical plane joining the junction of the hard and soft palates with the circumvallate papillae of the tongue (Fig. 81-2). The bony support of the oral cavity comes from the maxilla superiorly and the mobile mandible inferiorly. The oral cavity is lined by a moist mucous membrane that is continuous with the skin at the vermilion border of the lips. The oral mucosa is composed of stratified squamous epithelial cells overlying a vascular fibrous connective tissue, the lamina propria, which provides structural support for the mucosa. In areas where extensibility is required (e.g., the buccal mucosa), a submucosa composed of loose fatty connective tissue is present. Elsewhere (e.g., the hard palate or gingivae), the submucosa is absent and the mucous membrane is attached directly to the underlying bone or muscle. Regional variations reflect different functional requirements at different sites.

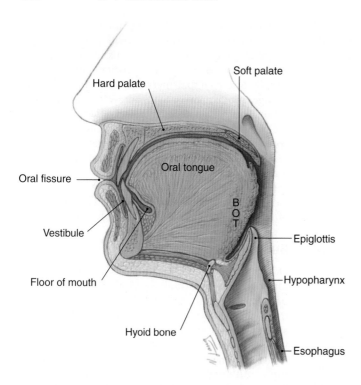

FIGURE 81-2. The oral cavity (median section). The oral cavity is highlighted in gold and the oropharynx in pink. BOT, base of tongue.

The oral cavity consists of an outer smaller part, the vestibule, and an inner larger part, the oral cavity proper (see Fig. 81-2). The vestibule is a slit-like space bounded externally by the lips and cheeks and internally by the gums and teeth. It communicates with the outside world through the oral fissure. It is limited above and below by the reflection of the mucous membrane from the lips and cheeks to the gums. Stensen duct, carrying secretions from the parotid gland, empties into the oral cavity through a small papilla in the buccal mucosa opposite the second upper molar tooth. Tumors originating in the oral vestibule commonly involve the labial or buccal sulcus, the buccal mucosa along the cheek, or the alveolar or gingival mucosa.

The teeth are arranged in rows on the maxillary and mandibular alveolar arches and form a boundary that separates the vestibule and the oral cavity proper (see Fig. 81-2). On either side of each arch, alveolar mucosa covers the alveolar bone and fuses with the gingival mucosa, which forms a free edge around the mucosal margins of the crowns of the teeth. The integrity of the lining of the mouth is maintained by the close attachment of the epithelium of the gingival mucosa to the surfaces of the teeth. The gingivae of the vestibule and the oral cavity proper become continuous in the interdental spaces. The mucosa behind the mandibular third molar, extending upward along the inner surface of the ascending ramus of the mandible, makes up the retromolar trigone (Fig. 81-3). It is continuous above with the maxillary tuberosity.

The oral cavity proper contains the lingual gingival and alveolar mucosa, the floor of mouth, the oral tongue, and the hard palate (see Figs. 81-2 and 81-3). The tongue is a muscular organ composed of interlacing bundles of striated muscle. The intrinsic muscles of the tongue alter its shape. The extrinsic muscles of the tongue (genioglossus, hyoglossus, styloglossus, and palatoglossus) originate outside the tongue and insert into it, acting mainly to alter its position. The entire tongue receives its primary blood supply from the lingual branches of the external carotid arteries. The facial and ascending pharyngeal arteries give additional branches to the lingual root that communicate anteriorly with the lingual arteries.

The oral tongue, or anterior two thirds of the tongue, lies free in the oral cavity (Fig. 81-4). The median sulcus and underlying lingual septum divide the tongue longitudinally in the midline. A V-shaped groove, the sulcus terminalis, separates the oral tongue from the base of tongue. Just posterior to the apex of the sulcus terminalis is the foramen cecum, a pit-like depression representing the caudal remnant of the thyroglossal duct. Anterior to the sulcus terminalis are the circumvallate papillae. The papillae possess taste buds and also receive saliva through the ducts of minor salivary glands in the area. The dorsum of the tongue is lined with a specialized mucosa designed for mastication and taste. The roughness of this mucosa results from multiple and varied papillae along its surface. The tongue's ventral surface, in contrast, is smooth and without

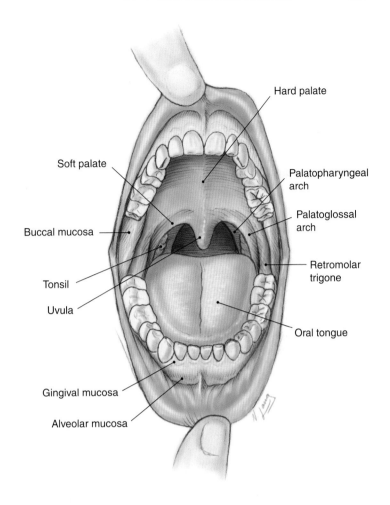

FIGURE 81-3. The oral cavity (intra-oral view).

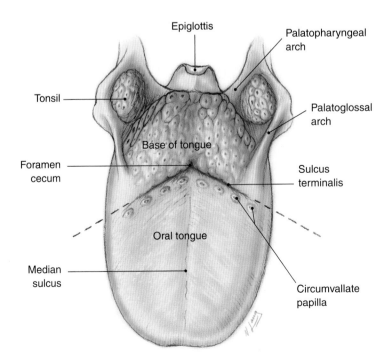

FIGURE 81-4. The tongue.

surface papillae. In the midline, a fold of mucous membrane, the frenulum, loosely connects the ventral surface of the oral tongue to the floor of mouth.

The posterior third of the tongue, or base of tongue, is considered part of the oropharynx, not the oral cavity (see Figs. 81-2 and 81-4). The base of tongue is fixed to the hyoid bone. Its embryologic development differs from that of the oral tongue, as does the structure of its covering membrane. Its mucous membrane has no papillae. Underlying nodules of lymphoid tissue, the lingual tonsils, give its dorsal surface a cobblestone appearance.

The floor of mouth is a horseshoe-shaped area formed by reflections of mucous membrane from the mandibular alveolus to the ventral surface of the tongue (Fig. 81-5). Its posterior limit is the anterior tonsillar pillar. Minor salivary glands are visible as small submucosal bulges on either side of the frenulum. The paired sublingual glands are seen as larger bulges emerging from under the tongue more posteriorly. Each sublingual gland has multiple excretory ducts, most of which open separately into the floor of mouth along an elevation of mucous membrane called the sublingual fold. Others join with the ipsilateral submandibular duct (Wharton duct), and the ducts exit together at the sublingual papilla that sits adjacent to the lingual frenulum near its base.[11, 12]

The hard palate forms the roof of the oral cavity (see Figs. 81-2 and 81-3). Anterolaterally, it blends with the alveolar and gingival mucosae. Posteriorly, it is continuous with the soft palate. The bony plate of the hard palate is composed of the palatine process of the maxilla and the horizontal process of the palatine bone, each fused in the midline with its counterpart from the opposite side. A specialized mucoperiosteum covers the bone.

The soft palate, like the base of tongue, is considered part of the oropharynx (see Figs. 81-2 and 81-3). A muscular structure encased in mucous membrane, it has a free posterior border and hangs suspended between the oropharynx and the nasopharynx.

Extending laterally and downward from each side of the soft palate are two curved folds of mucous membrane. The anterior fold contains the palatoglossus muscle and hence is named the palatoglossal arch. It joins the soft palate with the lateral tongue at the junction of the oral and oropharyngeal portions. The posterior fold, the palatopharyngeal arch, contains the palatopharyngeus muscle. It runs laterally and posteriorly from the uvula to the lateral wall of the oropharynx. The palatoglossal and palatopharyngeal arches are also called the anterior and posterior tonsillar pillars, respectively, and together they compose the isthmus of the fauces.

The oral cavity communicates with the oropharynx through an aperture created by the anterior tonsillar pillars, the soft palate, and the surface of the base of tongue. The anterior and posterior tonsillar pillars, as well as the palatine tonsil sitting in the fossa between them (see Figs. 81-2 and 81-3), are considered part of the oropharynx.[12, 13]

Tumors originating in the oral cavity proper may arise in the oral tongue, the floor of mouth, the hard palate, or the alveolar or gingival mucosa. Tumors do not generally observe the anatomic boundaries defined before. Thus, tumors of the base of tongue may invade the oral tongue, and tumors of the retromolar trigone may extend onto the soft palate. As demonstrated in the clinical cases shown later in this chapter, reconstruction of the oral cavity often requires simultaneous reconstruction of adjacent involved non–oral cavity structures.

Function

The primary functions of the oral cavity are mastication, deglutition, and speech. Each is reviewed.

MASTICATION

Normally, solid food is chewed and mixed with saliva to form a soft bolus during mastication. Voluntary

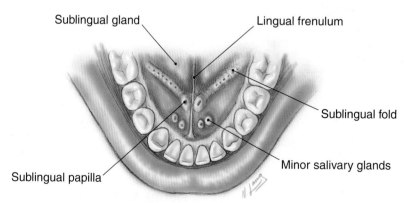

Sublingual gland

Lingual frenulum

Sublingual fold

Minor salivary glands

Sublingual papilla

FIGURE 81-5. The floor of mouth.

rotary motion at the temporomandibular joint allows the mandibular and maxillary teeth to move relative to each other, permitting chewing and grinding. The tongue assists during mastication by moving food to the grinding surfaces of the teeth. It then pulls the food into a semicohesive bolus for transport into the pharynx.

DEGLUTITION

Deglutition, or swallowing, is a complex process by which the bolus moves from the mouth through the pharynx and esophagus. Swallowing is traditionally described in three stages.

The first stage of swallowing is voluntary. During this stage, the tongue lifts and propels the bolus posteriorly through the oral cavity. The tip of the tongue is pressed against the hard palate by the intrinsic muscles of the tongue. Movement spreads backward rapidly, pushing the bolus from behind the tip of the tongue to the posterior part of the mouth. The hyoid bone is lifted and pulled forward. The posterior tongue rises and the palatoglossal arches move together, pushing the bolus through the oropharyngeal isthmus into the oropharynx.

The second stage of swallowing is involuntary and rapid, triggered by sensory receptors as the bolus passes into the oropharynx. Movements of the palatopharyngeal arches, the pharynx, and the soft palate combine to isolate the oropharynx from the nasopharynx, preventing the bolus from passing upward. As the bolus passes through the oropharynx, the larynx and pharynx are elevated, drawn upward with the hyoid bone. Movements of various pharyngeal and laryngeal muscles act to protect the airway as successive contractions of the superior and middle pharyngeal constrictors propel the bolus over the epiglottis and into the hypopharynx. The third and final stage is effected by the inferior constrictor, which forces the bolus into the esophagus.

SPEECH

Speech is a highly complex function brought about by an intricate assembly of structures. The larynx is specifically designed for phonation. Variations in the opening between the vocal folds alter the pitch of sounds produced by the passage of air through the folds. Sounds emanating from the larynx are translated into intelligible speech by articulatory and resonating structures in the pharynx, nose, and mouth. Although several articulators are used during the production of speech, the tongue is the most important. The tongue is active during the production of all vowels and is essential for the production of many consonants. Consonants are associated with particular anatomic sites, for example, labials (p and b), dentals (t and d), and nasals (m and n). At each site, a partial obstruction or con-striction of the vocal tract produces noise, which is superimposed on or interrupts the flow of laryngeal tones. Subtle position changes in the larynx, pharynx, palate, tongue, and circumoral muscles, rendered with speed and dexterity, bring about the fluctuations of sound that define human speech.[12, 14]

TREATMENT OF ORAL CAVITY DEFECTS

Preoperative Evaluation

When faced with a head and neck patient, the reconstructive surgeon's best approach is to return to the basics of evaluation. A complete history and physical examination are performed. In choosing a reconstructive technique, it is vital to know the patient's general medical status. Although free flaps may be unavoidable for certain defects, a quicker alternative, such as a pectoralis flap, may be a satisfactory choice in a patient with severe medical problems. An abnormal vascular history or finding may obviate certain reconstructive options. For example, a history of carotid disease or a bruit on examination may make free tissue transplantation a less desirable choice because of underlying vascular disease. Receptor vessel selection favors anastomosis to an external carotid branch rather than to the main artery, avoiding risk of carotid embolism or thrombosis.

A tumor history is obtained, with attention to details that affect the extent of resection. Lip numbness in a patient with a floor of mouth tumor, for example, suggests that the inferior alveolar nerve may be involved and that mandibular resection may be required. The tumor is inspected and palpated, and nodal status is assessed. Knowledge of previous surgery and radiation therapy in the area of the tumor is imperative, and old operative notes are studied when they are available. Imaging studies are reviewed.

Potential donor sites are examined, and factors that will prevent the use of a specific flap are noted. For example, previous abdominal surgery or morbid obesity may argue against the use of the rectus abdominis flap. An abnormal Allen test result will preclude the use of the radial forearm flap (unless arterial reconstruction is planned). Alternative free flap donor sites are identified, and the availability of the pectoralis flap is assessed. The potential risks of reconstruction are discussed with the patient, as is the likelihood of postoperative speech and swallowing dysfunction. In many cases, the method of reconstruction is not chosen until the extirpative defect is visualized and the plan is conveyed to the patient. Nevertheless, the patient can be evaluated and prepared for the most likely alternatives.

Communication with the head and neck surgeon is vital in predicting the defect and hence planning the reconstruction. If neck dissection is planned, plastic surgery input in planning the incision may be advisable. Information about the likelihood of postoperative irradiation may affect the choice of reconstructive technique. Preoperative involvement of dentistry and prosthodontics may simplify intraoperative decision-making. Prefabrication of dental or palatal splints, when indicated, will help optimize postoperative function. Early involvement in care of the patient by speech therapy and social service may help allay the perioperative and postoperative concerns of the patient and the patient's family.

Treatment Goals

The first goal of reconstruction is to permit complete removal of the tumor. Reconstructive concerns should not compromise the ablative procedure, although the reconstructive options should be considered in the overall surgical plan. Conversely, the ability to reconstruct should not be the ultimate factor in determining resectability. The advent of free tissue transplantation has certainly made larger resections possible because tissue availability is usually not a concern. However, successful transplantation of tissue does not always translate into restoration of form and function. The extirpative surgeon must weigh the benefits of larger and larger resections, including the potential for cure or palliation, against the morbidity and functional sequelae of such procedures.

Second, the reconstruction must achieve wound closure. Ideally, primary wound healing is achieved in a single stage without fistulas or other complications that may delay adjuvant therapy. Thus, immediate reconstruction has become routine, and reliability of the reconstruction is key. Patients often have advanced disease, indicating either a limited survival or the need for adjuvant therapy. Despite poor prognosis, excellent palliation is afforded the patient when primary wound healing is achieved. In contrast, a failed reconstruction wastes potential "quality" time and may prevent optimal treatment, most often by delaying radiation therapy. Reconstructive failure also prolongs hospitalization and increases cost.

Third, the reconstructive technique should not add to the patient's morbidity. The donor defect and complications at the donor site must be minimized.

Fourth, the reconstruction should aim to restore function. Restoration of speech and swallowing is critical to ensure a satisfactory quality of life. In a general sense, restoration of function is best accomplished by returning uninvolved structures to their normal anatomic position, by allowing mobile structures to move as they would have moved, and by replacing missing structures with tissue of similar surface area and volume.

Finally, the reconstruction should aim to restore a normal appearance, maintaining cosmesis at both the recipient and donor sites.

Site-Specific Treatment Goals

TONGUE

In a broad sense, oral function is determined ultimately by tongue function. Structural alterations of the tongue, along with changes in sensibility and motion, will result in poor control of the food bolus and a distorted swallow reflex with aspiration. Speech will similarly be affected in a negative way by the loss of precisely coordinated tongue movements.

The extent of resection dictates functional outcome in non-reconstructed patients after partial glossectomy. Resections that preserve innervation to the residual tongue and tongue mobility will result in the best function postoperatively. If sensibility is preserved, primary closure of the defect may optimize functional outcome as long as there is no tethering. Most defects that involve less than 10% to 20% of the tongue can be closed primarily without any significant difficulty in speech and swallowing. However, if primary closure distorts the anatomy or results in significant tension at the suture line, a different reconstructive option should be chosen. In the absence of communication with the neck, small defects that cannot be closed without tension are sometimes best left to heal by secondary intention.[15]

For larger defects that cannot be closed primarily, the quality of the reconstruction will determine the degree of speech and swallowing impairment in many patients. After partial glossectomy, the goals of reconstruction are to preserve mobility of the residual tongue segment and to restore shape and volume. The restoration of sensation to a flap remains of theoretical but unproven benefit. If 30% or more of the native tongue remains after resection, a thin, pliable flap such as the radial forearm is desirable to preserve tongue mobility without adding excessive bulk. Preservation of even a small tongue remnant may improve swallowing and speech as long as the remaining portion of the tongue is able to contact the palate.

In contrast, reconstruction after total or nearly total glossectomy requires replacement of a large tissue volume and elimination of dead space. The reconstruction must provide bulk, so that the neotongue can act as an obturator to prevent aspiration. The rectus abdominis musculocutaneous flap is often a good choice for this defect. In heavy patients, the rectus flap may provide too much bulk. In this situation, the surgeon can excise the skin paddle and use muscle and fascia alone to close the defect. The exposed intraoral flap may then be skin grafted or, alternatively, allowed to remucosalize spontaneously. Surprisingly good speech and swallowing can often be achieved if the surgeon makes the effort during the reconstruction to make the tongue as large as possible. This may involve folding the flap or placing darts at the edge of the skin paddle to augment the volume.

Reconstructed glossectomy patients must learn mechanisms to position the neotongue for optimal speech and swallowing. Some patients are unable to achieve contact between the tongue or neotongue and the palate after reconstruction. This results in speech problems and a tendency for food to collect in the palatal arch during swallowing. Palatal augmentation with a prosthesis may improve speech and swallowing in these patients.

FLOOR OF MOUTH

The goals after floor of mouth excision are similar to those after partial glossectomy. In fact, the two defects often occur simultaneously in the same patient. Preservation of tongue mobility is of paramount importance. Small nonirradiated defects may be allowed to heal secondarily or may be resurfaced with skin grafts, even when periosteum or bone is exposed. In cases of previous or planned radiation, for large defects, or when a significant amount of bone is exposed, flap closure is preferable. The flap must be thin and supple. In most circumstances, the free radial forearm is the flap of choice because of its characteristics, reliability, and low donor site morbidity. When anterior segmental mandibulectomy is performed during resection of a floor of mouth tumor, an osteocutaneous flap is required for reconstruction. In most cases, the flap of choice is the free fibula (see Chapter 82).

During reconstruction, an effort should be made to maintain the lingual vestibule, and sufficient height should be restored to the floor of mouth so that saliva and food particles do not pool there. For this reason, when a floor of mouth resection includes resection of the mylohyoid complex, the defect is best managed by the use of a flap because a skin graft will produce a significant depression under the tongue.[16] The gingivobuccal sulcus must also be maintained. Failure to do so will lead to drooling and oral incompetence. Portions of the flap may be anchored to the underlying bone to achieve this result. Late sulcus reconstruction with local tissue rearrangement and skin grafting is difficult because of tissue scarring and contracture, especially if the patient has been irradiated.

BUCCAL MUCOSA

The buccal mucosa is specialized to provide extensibility of the cheek tissues during mandibular excursion. Inadequate replacement of buccal tissue may interfere with mouth opening and denture wear. Small superficial defects can be closed primarily or allowed to heal by secondary intention. Larger defects may be amenable to closure with skin or mucosal grafts or mucosal rotation flaps, but these techniques are limited by the loss of excursion brought about by tissue loss and wound contraction. When necessary, thin pliable flaps, such as the platysma flap or radial forearm free flap, are used to replace missing mucosa. Excess bulk in this region should be avoided because the patient will tend to bite the flap during mastication.

A high percentage of patients with cancer of the buccal mucosa present in late stages. Invasion of the underlying cheek musculature and the cheek skin may occur. As the cancer enlarges, it may grow posteriorly to invade the pterygoid muscles; inferiorly into the mandible; or superiorly into the upper alveolar ridge, palate, or maxillary sinus. Through-and-through defects of the cheek may require two flaps (a lining flap plus an external flap), a folded or double-paddle flap, or a flap and graft. The primary goals in reconstruction of these complex defects are to replace missing lining and skin, to close the orocutaneous fistula, and to prevent trismus.[17, 18]

LOWER AND UPPER ALVEOLAR RIDGE

Tumors of the lower gingiva frequently involve bone and require at least partial mandibular resection. When marginal mandibulectomy is performed for a small cancer, there may be adequate mucosa remaining for direct closure over the bone. In the nonirradiated patient, the transected raw surface of the mandible will usually accept a skin graft when primary closure is not possible or compromises function.[17, 18]

After extensive marginal mandibulectomy, reinforcement of the remaining mandibular rim with a low-profile reconstruction plate is recommended, especially when postoperative radiotherapy is planned. Before or after radiotherapy, the reconstruction must achieve wound closure and must cover the residual bone (and plate, if present) with well-vascularized soft tissue, preserving the sulcus. A radial forearm free flap is often a good choice. In contrast, an osteocutaneous flap is the preferred reconstruction if segmental mandibulectomy is required (see Chapter 82).

Small, superficial cancers of the maxillary alveolar ridge can be excised and left to heal by secondary intention. Larger cancers may require alveolectomy or maxillectomy.[18]

PALATE

The palate divides the upper airway into oral and nasal parts, allows intelligible speech, and aids in deglutition. Tumors of the hard palate are rare, and minor salivary gland tumors represent a high percentage of tumors diagnosed. Defects resulting from resection of small superficial lesions of the hard palate or upper alveolus may be skin grafted or left open to heal secondarily.

Bone involvement by tumor may require alveolectomy or partial or total maxillectomy. With resection of palatal bone, a palatal obturator is required. When full-thickness resection of the hard palate is anticipated, preoperative dental evaluation should include the fabrication of an immediate obturator when possible. The use of such a prosthesis provides for improved comfort of the patient and hygiene in the early postoperative period and helps prevent collapse of the adjacent soft tissues.[17] In the rare patient, residual structures will be inadequate for stabilization of the prosthesis. Osseointegrated implants may provide stabilization in some cases. Alternatively, an osteocutaneous flap can be used to reconstruct the hard palate or to provide a platform for osseointegrated implants.

The soft palate is often secondarily involved with tumor by direct extension of an oral cavity cancer. Large soft palate defects are, in general, best rehabilitated prosthetically. In long-term follow-up, flaps tend to "sag" into the oral cavity over time, and the need for revision is common. Flaps are generally ineffective in restoring velopharyngeal closure in this highly dynamic region. The adjacent lateral and posterior pharyngeal wall should be reconstructed surgically. The cut edges of the oral and nasal lining of the soft palate margin are then sutured to each other to achieve wound closure. An immediate surgical obturator is not used unless the entire soft palate has been removed. A delayed surgical prosthesis, followed by a definitive obturator, is recommended for patients with less extensive defects of the posterior or lateral borders of the soft palate. Ideally, this appliance interacts with the normally functioning velopharyngeal complex on the opposite side to help restore speech and swallowing. In practice, defects of the soft palate are difficult to manage because the goal of restoring oronasal separation in an active manner is often impossible to achieve.[19, 20]

In summary, the use of prostheses, combined with the judicious use of fasciocutaneous, myocutaneous, or osteocutaneous flaps, will best achieve the goals of palatal reconstruction: to restore oronasal competence and to preserve swallowing and speech.

RETROMOLAR TRIGONE

Small retromolar trigone lesions are treated by excision, often accompanied by marginal mandibulectomy of the ascending ramus to obtain clear margins. Primary closure or skin grafting may be adequate. However, retromolar trigone carcinomas are often diagnosed late and frequently extend to adjoining regions including the mandible, pterygopalatine muscles, cheek, tonsil, floor of mouth, soft palate, and tongue.[17] Resection of an aggressive retromolar trigone tumor often results in a large composite defect that includes significant intraoral lining and the ipsilateral

hemimandible. The goals of reconstruction include replacement of missing lining, restoration of contour, and prevention of mandibular drift.

The best reconstruction for a posterior mandibular defect is controversial, but there is some consensus that bony reconstruction of the mandible is not required.[16–18, 21] If the bony resection involves only the ramus and part of the body on one side, a reasonably good reconstruction can be achieved with a soft tissue flap, such as a rectus abdominis free flap. The bulk of the flap fills the space left by the resected jaw, restoring contour. The skin paddle replaces missing oral lining, restoring function by preventing contractures that might otherwise tether the tongue and mandible. Mandibular drift will occur but is minimized by postoperative physical therapy.

In fact, mandibular drift results from the disinsertion of the pterygoid muscles from the mandible during the resection and is not completely prevented by bone replacement. Inadequate replacement of the soft tissue loss can exacerbate the drift by worsening the forces of scar contracture. Many patients are poor candidates for bony reconstruction because of medical problems, unfavorable tumor prognosis, or advanced age. Donor site morbidity and operative time are both considerably reduced in these difficult cases when reconstruction is performed with soft tissue alone.

In contrast, resection of the anterior arch of the mandible results in significant functional deficit and major aesthetic deformity. If the mandibular defect extends anteriorly beyond the symphysis, bony reconstruction is required. It is also reasonable to consider bony reconstruction of a posterior defect in a young patient with a good prognosis, as long as oral lining is adequately replaced.

ALGORITHM FOR SURGICAL TREATMENT

In most cases, the patient is admitted on a same-day surgery basis. The patient is brought to the operating room and placed in a supine position on the operating table. Sequential compression devices are applied routinely, and broad-spectrum antibiotics covering oral flora are administered. General anesthesia is induced. A Foley catheter (preferably with a temperature probe) is inserted, and appropriate monitoring is established. An arterial line is routine. If a radial forearm flap is planned, the donor site must be protected from arterial and venous punctures.

The reconstructive surgeon should be present at the start to ensure that appropriate positioning and preparation of the patient are carried out. A shoulder roll is placed to extend the neck. The head and neck team may perform examination under anesthesia and tracheotomy at this time. The patient is then positioned and prepared for surgery. An effort is made to prepare potential flap donor sites at this time, but this is not always possible. If use of a skin or vein graft is anticipated, the donor site may be prepared as well. Ideally, the patient is double grounded so that cautery is available at the recipient and donor sites simultaneously.

The extirpation is begun. A lip-splitting incision or mandibulotomy may be needed to provide adequate exposure for both resection and reconstruction. The tumor is removed with frozen section control of the margins. Once the nature of the defect is determined, the reconstructive team can begin to harvest the flap, as long as the donor site is far enough from the head and neck region to avoid interfering with the extirpative effort. In complex cases, it may be best to delay flap design until tumor resection (with appropriate margin control) is complete. This ensures proper flap selection and adequate flap size and shape. If free tissue transplantation is planned, it is best to evaluate the recipient vessels before raising the flap when possible.

The defect is examined. Remaining anatomic structures are identified. Portions of the defect where primary closure can be achieved or where a prosthesis is preferable to autogenous reconstruction are identified. The defect is measured, and the tissue requirements (bulk, lining, or both) are identified. When the defect is complex, design and partial insetting of an Esmarch template may be useful.

Once the requirements of the wound are known, the reconstructive technique is chosen. The flap is designed and elevated. The recipient vessels are prepared, and vein grafts are harvested if required. An arteriovenous loop can be created before flap harvest to minimize ischemia time. All other preparatory work at the recipient site should be performed before division of the flap vessels. This may include primary closure of amenable areas, mobilization of mucoperiosteum for insetting, and burring down of sharp corners at osteotomy sites.

The flap is rotated into position or harvested and brought to the recipient site. When a free flap is used, it is advisable to perform at least some of the insetting before the anastomoses are performed to allow accurate placement of sutures in the absence of bleeding and flap edema. Insetting is done with vertical or horizontal mattress sutures or tightly spaced interrupted sutures of 3–0 Vicryl, attempting to secure a "watertight" closure.

The microvascular anastomoses are performed to large high-flow vessels when possible. End-to-side anastomoses to the external carotid artery and internal jugular vein are preferred when these vessels are available. When the recipient vessels have been irradiated, dissection must proceed with care, manipulation must be limited, and blood flow through the vessels must be assessed before the anastomoses are performed. In patients with known or suspected atherosclerotic disease of the carotid artery, manipulation of the carotid must be minimized. In this situation, anastomosis to a branch of the external carotid artery rather than to the main vessel is preferred to minimize the risk of embolic stroke.

After microanastomosis, insetting is completed. Drains are placed as indicated. A site for external Doppler monitoring is identified and marked with a suture on the flap skin paddle if possible (Fig. 81-6A). Otherwise, an internal Doppler probe is placed (Fig. 81-6B), preferably on the flap vein. The neck incision is closed in layers. A feeding tube for postoperative alimentation is placed through the nose into the stomach unless a gastrostomy tube is already present. The donor site is then closed over drains or skin grafted, dressed, and splinted as indicated.

During surgery and in the early postoperative period, the patient is kept warm and well hydrated, and the use of vasoconstricting agents and diuretics is avoided. Anticoagulants are not used routinely after free flap transplantation but may be given at the surgeon's discretion. Postoperatively, the flap is monitored closely. After free flap transplantation, the flap color, capillary refill, and arterial and venous Doppler signals are checked every hour for at least 48 hours after surgery, then on a tapering schedule through postoperative day 5. Congestion, pallor, or loss of Doppler signal necessitates emergency re-exploration of the flap.

SPECIFIC SURGICAL TECHNIQUES

Primary Closure and Secondary Healing

Primary closure is often possible for small defects of the lateral tongue or buccal mucosa, where direct approximation will not cause tethering of the tongue or interference with mandibular excursion. Small defects of the buccal mucosa, buccal sulcus, floor of mouth, or hard palate may be left open or packed with Xeroform to allow healing by secondary intention.

Skin Grafts

Split-thickness skin grafts can be used to close superficial defects of the alveolus, the palate, or the dorsum or lateral edge of the tongue (Fig. 81-7). In these locations, contraction of the graft is unlikely to cause a functional problem. Grafts are often preferred for resurfacing the alveolus, where the mobility of a flap skin paddle can interfere with dental rehabilitation. The tendency for grafts to contract in extensible areas such as the floor of mouth or buccal surface makes

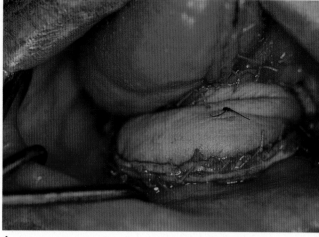

A

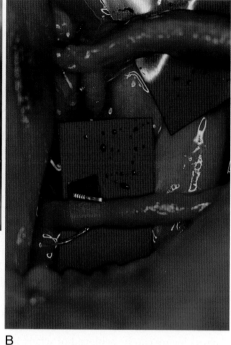

B

FIGURE 81-6. Free flaps are monitored with an external Doppler probe *(A)* at a specified site (note suture) or with an implantable Doppler probe *(B)*.

them less useful in these areas unless the defect is small. Increased risk of partial or total graft loss due to scarring and radiation change also limits the usefulness of skin grafts in the oral cavity.

Immobilization of intraoral grafts remains challenging. Special splints can be fabricated and sutured in place, or multiple quilting sutures can be placed to hold the graft in position.[22]

Local and Regional Flaps

A litany of local and regional flaps has been used for oral cavity reconstruction. Tongue flaps[23, 24] were frequently used to close small oral defects in the past but have fallen into disfavor because of the tethering and functional disturbance that result. Nasolabial,[25] forehead,[26, 27] and temporalis muscle[28] flaps, once used extensively, are rarely indicated now that free tissue transplantation is available. The facial artery musculomucosal flap[29] has proved useful for small defects of the hard palate, alveolus, tonsillar fossa, and floor of mouth but has found limited application.

The deltopectoral flap[30] is an axial-pattern cutaneous flap based medially on the second, third, and fourth anterior perforating branches of the internal mammary arteries. The flap extends laterally over the deltoid muscle, and additional flap length may be obtained by delaying the flap. The deltopectoral flap revolutionized head and neck reconstruction, but the flap has fallen into disfavor because of its poor reliability

without surgical delay.[31] It is used only rarely, when other flaps have failed or are not available.

Musculocutaneous Flaps

Several musculocutaneous flaps have been described for head and neck reconstruction. A superiorly based sternocleidomastoid muscle flap is occasionally useful to augment mandibular coverage. The sternocleidomastoid musculocutaneous flap,[32, 33] in contrast, is unreliable and rarely used. Lateral and inferior trapezius musculocutaneous flaps have been employed for intraoral reconstruction.[34–36] The lateral flap has poor flap reliability and leaves an unacceptable functional deficit at the donor site. The inferior flap design is reliable unless its pedicle has been divided at the neck base during the neck dissection. However, intraoperative positioning difficulties limit the usefulness of the trapezius for this indication. Use of the latissimus dorsi musculocutaneous flap is also well described.[37–40] The flap is safe and reliable, but the patient must be repositioned for access to the donor site. In addition, extensive dissection is required before the latissimus will match the anterior reach of the pectoralis major flap. The latissimus flap has been used in salvage situations when free tissue transplantation cannot be performed and the pectoralis flap has failed or is unavailable.

The pectoralis major musculocutaneous flap is still widely used, and the platysma flap has a more limited role in the reconstruction of specific defects.

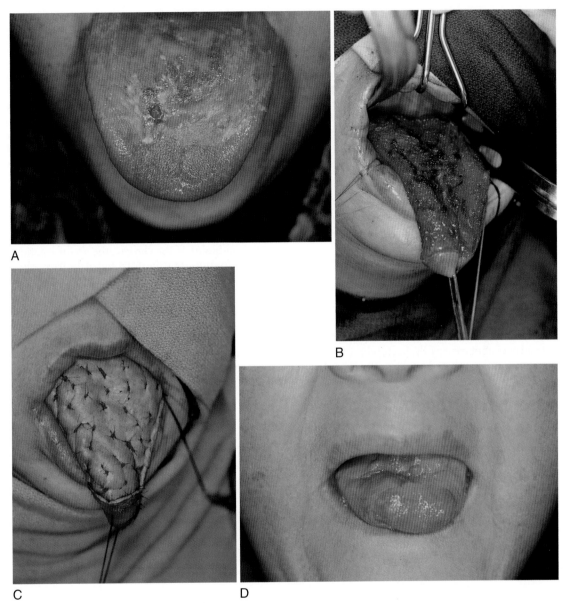

FIGURE 81-7. Tongue reconstruction with a split-thickness skin graft. *A,* Long-standing leukoplakia and biopsy-proven dysplasia of the tongue. *B,* Defect after mucosal resection of dorsal and partial ventral surfaces of tongue. *C,* Split-thickness skin graft sutured in place with multiple quilting sutures. *D,* Result 10 weeks after surgery. (From Butler CE: "Tongue sandwich" bolster for skin graft immobilization. Head Neck 2002;24:706-707. Reprinted by permission of John Wiley & Sons, Inc.)

These flaps are discussed in further detail in the following sections.

PECTORALIS MAJOR FLAP

First described for head and neck reconstruction by Ariyan in 1979,[41] the pectoralis major musculocutaneous flap provided adequate quantities of skin to resurface large intraoral defects and proved more reliable than earlier techniques, including the deltopectoral flap. It quickly became the workhorse of head and neck reconstruction. Relegated to a secondary role by the advent of microvascular free tissue transplantation, it nonetheless remains an extremely useful flap for oral cavity reconstruction.

The pectoralis major musculocutaneous flap is used most often when recipient vessels are not available or when a patient is considered too sick to tolerate free tissue transplantation. It is best used to reconstruct defects requiring tissue bulk, such as total glossectomy and composite posterior mandible defects. The flap also plays an extremely important role in salvage reconstruction.

The pectoralis major muscle flap is sometimes used to provide external cover, alone or in conjunction with free tissue transplantation to the oral cavity. Although the flap has been shown to reach above the zygoma in some patients, it is reliable only for coverage of the neck and lower face. The pectoralis muscle flap is occasionally used to bolster a primary mucosal repair or to close a small intraoral defect.

Anatomy

The pectoralis major muscle is a large, fan-shaped muscle arising from the medial half of the clavicle, the sternum, and the upper seven costal cartilages. It inserts into the crest of the greater tubercle of the humerus and acts as a medial rotator and adductor of the humerus. It is innervated by the lateral and medial pectoral nerves.[42]

The muscle receives its primary blood supply from the thoracoacromial artery and a secondary blood supply from segmental parasternal perforators arising medially from the internal mammary artery. For most head and neck applications, the pectoralis major musculocutaneous flap is based on the pectoral branch of the thoracoacromial artery. The thoracoacromial artery leaves the subclavian artery at about the midpoint of the clavicle, and the pectoral branch heads inferolaterally at a right angle to the clavicle. It courses between the pectoralis major and minor muscles, then enters the undersurface of the pectoralis major. The vessel then runs inferomedially with the lateral pectoral nerve along a line drawn from the tip of the shoulder to the xiphoid process (Fig. 81-8).[43] Laterally, there are rich anastomoses between the lateral thoracic artery and the pectoral branch of the thoracoacromial artery.[42]

Flap Design

Once the surgical defect is defined, the cutaneous portion of the flap is designed. With the pivot point at the midpoint of the clavicle, the arc of rotation is checked to ensure that the distal end of the flap as drawn will reach the farthest edge of the defect.

The reliability of the paddle (skin island) is optimized by including the skin overlying the vascular axis of the flap, particularly that in the vicinity of the nipple-areolar complex. To minimize the donor defect in women, the skin paddle may be designed medially along the sternum with an extension into the inframammary

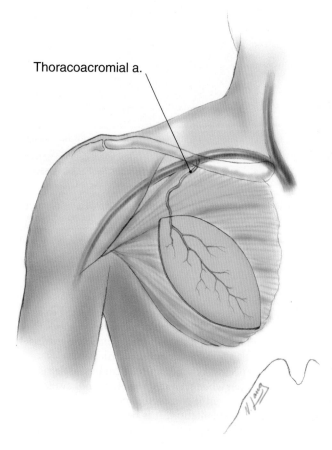

Thoracoacromial a.

FIGURE 81-8. The pectoralis major musculocutaneous flap. The thoracoacromial vessels join the subclavian vessels at about the middle third of the clavicle. They turn to travel along an axis drawn from the shoulder to the xiphoid process, running inferomedially on the deep surface of the pectoralis major muscle. A skin paddle is outlined along the vascular axis.

fold. This design is less reliable, however, and some authors prefer to avoid the use of the musculocutaneous flap in women.[44]

An extended pectoralis flap may be designed, with the skin paddle extending below the inferior border of the pectoralis muscle.[45] In this case, a large portion of the paddle must still lie over the muscle, and the flap should include the anterior rectus sheath deep to the inferior skin extension. The extended flap is not reliable in its distal portion, particularly in smokers and in patients with thick subcutaneous tissue.

If desired, the deltopectoral flap can be designed and partially elevated within the design of the pectoralis flap. This technique surgically delays the deltopectoral flap and preserves it for later use if needed.[42]

For small intraoral defects, a muscle flap can be used for intraoral lining. The muscle may be skin grafted or allowed to remucosalize. Significant contracture may occur with the use of muscle-only flaps, and thus this technique is not recommended for large defects.

Flap Dissection

The edges of the paddle are incised, beveling outward, until the muscle is reached. The adjacent skin is elevated off the muscle in all directions to better define the anatomy and to mobilize the chest skin for later primary closure. The lateral edge of the pectoralis major muscle is identified, and the plane between the major and minor muscles is developed. The pectoralis major is divided distally and medially, with care taken to control the parasternal perforators. When an extended pectoralis flap has been designed, the anterior rectus fascia underlying the skin paddle must be harvested with the flap. The muscle is lifted in a cephalad direction, and the vascular pedicle is identified on its deep surface. With the pedicle in view, the muscle is divided laterally. An attempt is made to preserve the lateral border of the muscle in situ for aesthetic reasons. Ideally, the muscle portion of the flap is narrowed dramatically as the dissection proceeds to decrease the bulk of the flap.

The pedicle dissection is facilitated by an incision from the superior corner of the skin paddle to the midclavicular region or, alternatively, by an incision parallel to the clavicle. As the clavicle is approached, the flap can be developed as an island flap, attached only by its vascular pedicle (Fig. 81-9). It may be helpful to leave some adventitial tissue intact around the pedicle to help prevent traction injury when the flap is transplanted. For longer reach of the flap, a segment of clavicle can be removed and replaced, allowing the pedicle to pass under the clavicle (Fig. 81-10).

The flap is rotated into position and inset into the mouth. It is advisable to suspend the flap from a nonmobile structure to lessen the tension on the suture line and to offset the unavoidable downward pull on the flap.

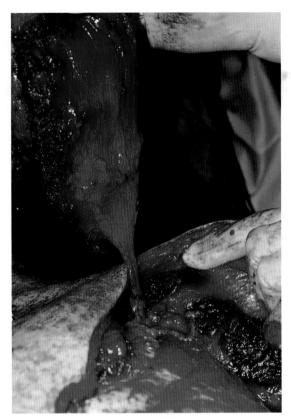

FIGURE 81-9. The pectoralis major musculocutaneous flap. The flap can be dissected as a true island flap. (Courtesy of Dr. Howard Langstein.)

In oral cavity reconstruction, the pectoralis donor site is generally small enough to be closed primarily over drains. Otherwise, a split-thickness skin graft is applied to the chest wall. If the nipple is harvested with the skin paddle, it can be excised and reapplied to the chest wall as a free graft.

Advantages and Disadvantages

The advantages of the pectoralis major flap are its straightforward design, ease of dissection, and relative reliability. The flap can be dissected with the patient supine, and microsurgical expertise is not required. The muscle portion of the flap is large enough to cover and protect the carotid artery in those patients undergoing radical neck dissection. Although excess bulk can be a disadvantage, the pectoralis major flap is specifically selected when bulk is beneficial, such as after subtotal or total glossectomy when the larynx is spared. The indications for this flap may increase in the very thin male patient when it becomes a rational alternative to the fasciocutaneous free flaps. The pectoralis flap is indispensable in salvage situations when free flap reconstruction has failed or resulted in significant complications.

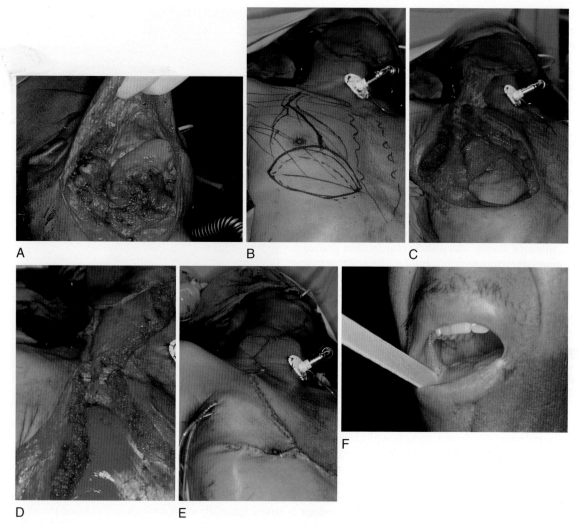

FIGURE 81-10. Reconstruction with a pectoralis major musculocutaneous flap. *A,* Defect of right hemimandible, floor of mouth, buccal mucosa, and retromolar trigone after resection of third-time recurrent osteosarcoma of the mandible. The mandible had previously been reconstructed with an iliac crest free flap. *B,* Design of the pectoralis major musculocutaneous flap. The skin paddle extends beyond the distal end of the pectoralis muscle. A portion of the anterior rectus fascia is taken in continuity with the pectoralis muscle. *C,* Flap raised. *D,* Flap rotated into defect. An incision has been made joining the chest and oral cavity wounds, and a segment of clavicle has been removed. *E,* Immediate postoperative result. A split-thickness skin graft has been placed over the muscle in the neck. *F,* Well-healed flap 4 months after surgery. (Courtesy of Dr. Howard Langstein.)

Although the muscle portion of the pectoralis flap is reliable, the skin paddle is not. As a result, wound healing problems and orocutaneous fistulas are more common after pectoralis flap reconstruction of the oral cavity than after free flap reconstruction.[44, 46] For this reason, some would argue that free flap reconstruction is preferable to pectoralis flap reconstruction even in patients with serious medical problems, who are likely to tolerate complications poorly. Other disadvantages include a limited arc of rotation and bulkiness, which tends to resolve with time if the nerves to the transplanted muscle are severed. However,

contractures occur frequently, and late revisions are not uncommon.[46]

PLATYSMA FLAP

The platysma flap is especially useful for resurfacing the buccal sulcus and buccal mucosa, where thin pliable tissue is desired.[47] For this application, the lower cervical skin is carried on the superiorly based platysma muscle and turned inward to replace the missing oral mucosa (Fig. 81-11).

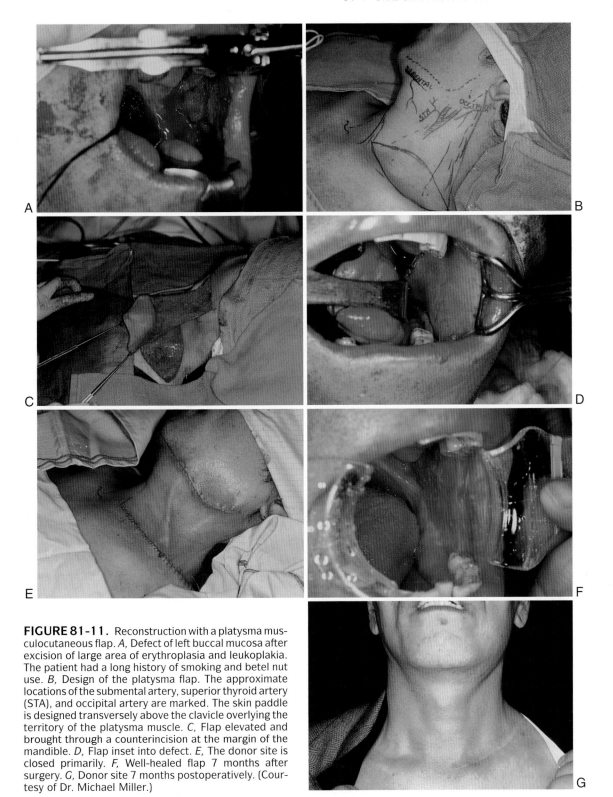

FIGURE 81-11. Reconstruction with a platysma musculocutaneous flap. *A,* Defect of left buccal mucosa after excision of large area of erythroplasia and leukoplakia. The patient had a long history of smoking and betel nut use. *B,* Design of the platysma flap. The approximate locations of the submental artery, superior thyroid artery (STA), and occipital artery are marked. The skin paddle is designed transversely above the clavicle overlying the territory of the platysma muscle. *C,* Flap elevated and brought through a counterincision at the margin of the mandible. *D,* Flap inset into defect. *E,* The donor site is closed primarily. *F,* Well-healed flap 7 months after surgery. *G,* Donor site 7 months postoperatively. (Courtesy of Dr. Michael Miller.)

Anatomy

The platysma is a thin subcutaneous sheet-like muscle that extends from the lower face across the mandible, neck, and clavicles to the level of the first or second ribs. The muscle extends laterally toward each acromion. A generous arterial system traverses the platysma on its way to the skin of the neck. Blood supply comes superiorly from the facial artery, inferiorly from the transverse cervical artery, medially from the thyroid arteries, and laterally from the occipital and postauricular arteries.[48] A random anastomosing network connects these vessels as the dermal-subdermal plexus. In contrast to the multiaxial arterial supply, the venous drainage is vertically oriented through the external jugular vein and other superficial veins of the neck.[49, 50]

The platysma musculocutaneous flap will generally survive if the arterial blood supply from at least one region is preserved.[48] When the flap is used for intraoral reconstruction, the submental branch of the facial artery typically provides the flap's arterial supply. The submental artery branches from the facial artery just before it turns to cross the inferior border of the mandible at the anterior edge of the masseter muscle. Owing to numerous anastomoses with ipsilateral and contralateral lingual, inferior labial, and superior thyroid arteries, the submental artery will vascularize the flap even if the ipsilateral facial artery has been ligated.[48, 50]

The platysma muscle receives innervation from the cervical branch of the facial nerve, which enters its deep surface superolaterally between the angle of the mandible and the sternocleidomastoid muscle. Meticulous dissection on the deep surface of the muscle allows preservation of these branches when the superior arc of rotation is used.[48, 51]

Flap Design

The patient can demonstrate the anatomy of the platysma preoperatively by voluntarily activating the muscle. The skin island may be designed at any site over the muscle. It is usually designed over the inferior portion of the platysma muscle immediately above the clavicle. Design as a horizontal ellipse allows primary closure of the donor defect.

Flap Dissection

A short transverse counterincision is made about 2 cm below the mandible, through skin and subcutaneous tissue but not platysma. The skin paddle is then incised to the level of the platysma muscle. Superiorly, a skin flap is elevated off the platysma to the level of the upper incision. Inferiorly, the platysma is divided and then separated from the deep structures in a caudad to cephalad direction. The fascia of the sternocleidomastoid muscle is included with the flap as much as

possible. This prevents inadvertent damage to the circulation of the thin platysma muscle and may incorporate some additional fascial circulation. If possible, the cutaneous branch of the superior thyroid artery is preserved to augment inflow to the flap. A major superficial vein of the neck (usually the external jugular) is included with the flap to facilitate venous drainage. During the dissection, the marginal mandibular branch of the facial nerve is identified and avoided. On completion of the dissection, the flap is rotated into the defect so that the skin paddle replaces the absent mucosa.[48]

Advantages and Disadvantages

The proximity of the platysma flap to the oral cavity makes it especially useful for resurfacing the buccal sulcus and buccal mucosa. The pliability and thinness of the platysma musculocutaneous flap permit draping over the mandible and allow mucosal replacement without excessive bulk. The donor area is generally hairless. The donor site can usually be closed primarily, leaving a satisfactory scar, and the sacrifice of the platysma muscle results in minimal contour deformity in the neck.[50, 51]

The primary disadvantage of the flap is the relative unreliability of the skin paddle, which can result in partial flap loss, dehiscence, wound healing delay, and fistula formation.[51, 52] Preoperative radiation makes use of the platysma flap hazardous, and although many successful outcomes with radiated platysma flaps have been reported in the literature,[50, 52] it is preferable to use a free flap in irradiated patients. Prior neck incisions that have separated the skin, the muscle, or both from the blood supply prevent the use of this flap. After flap dissection, sensation is diminished over the neck and upper anterior chest skin because of interruption of the transverse cervical and supraclavicular nerves. Necrosis of the neck skin flap with healing delay, dehiscence, and exposure of vital structures may occur.[52]

An intact facial artery is not crucial for survival of the flap. However, the connection between the submental artery and the facial artery must be preserved. The superior and inferior labial arteries appear to be the most important anastomotic vessels. For this reason, lip-splitting incisions are a contraindication to the use of the platysma flap if the facial artery has been ligated.[50]

Free Flaps

Microvascular surgery has revolutionized the management of carcinoma of the head and neck. Because of the high reliability of free tissue transplantation, immediate single-stage reconstruction is now possible for almost all patients. The variety of flaps available allows an excellent match of the reconstruction to the defect. Reliable immediate reconstruction yields superior functional and aesthetic results, reduces morbidity, and maximizes quality of life in patients who may have a reduced life expectancy. The introduction of well-vascularized tissue into a scarred or irradiated wound bed dramatically increases the chances that primary wound healing will be achieved.

For these reasons, microvascular techniques have become firmly established in the field of head and neck reconstruction. Obviously, free flaps demand microsurgical expertise, patient management skills, and proper anesthetic technique to make them reliable. Appropriate instrumentation and a postoperative care unit staffed with experienced personnel are also required.[53]

Although a variety of free flaps are available for repair of any given intraoral defect, every microsurgeon has a few favorite flaps used frequently because of their reliability in his or her hands. These flaps include the radial forearm and rectus abdominis free flaps. One of these two flaps will be suitable for almost any intraoral defect not requiring bone. Both flaps are described in the following sections.

An occasional patient will be a poor candidate for both the radial forearm flap and the rectus flap. It is therefore useful to have one or two second-line flaps that are used only in selected patients. The lateral thigh flap serves this purpose and is also described. The parascapular flap, latissimus flap, lateral arm flap, and others may also be used, depending on the defect and the preferences and experience of the surgeon.

It is preferable to repair all defects with a single flap whenever possible to minimize operating time and complexity. On occasion, a second free flap is required to provide sufficient tissue to repair a large or complex defect. When a second flap is necessary, it is preferable to perform separate end-to-end anastomoses to the cervical great vessels rather than to connect the flaps in sequence.

RADIAL FOREARM FLAP

The radial forearm flap is a versatile fasciocutaneous flap from the volar wrist that provides thin viable skin useful in a variety of reconstructive situations. Invented in China,[54,55] the flap was first used for intraoral reconstruction by Soutar et al.[56] Clinical experience has since proved the radial forearm flap to be an excellent choice for oral lining restoration when bulk is not required.

Anatomy

The brachial artery typically divides into the radial and ulnar arteries about 1 cm below the antecubital fossa. The radial artery runs longitudinally along the volar aspect of the forearm, passing between the brachioradialis and pronator teres muscles, then between the brachioradialis and flexor carpi radialis tendons in the lower two thirds of its course. As it travels, it gives off branches that pass along the anterolateral intermuscular septum between the flexor carpi radialis and brachioradialis. These septocutaneous perforators branch to the skin, subcutaneous tissue, muscle, and bone, forming a rich vascular network in the subcutaneous layer. The artery becomes progressively more superficial and is covered only by skin and fascia at the wrist. As it crosses the wrist, the radial artery branches and joins with the deep branch of the ulnar artery to form the deep palmar arch.[57]

Three separate venous systems, two superficial and one deep, provide drainage for the flap. These systems are the cephalic vein, the basilic vein, and the venae comitantes that travel with the radial artery. The superficial and deep systems are equally capable of draining the forearm flap. The venae comitantes may be used for flap transplantation, but they are occasionally quite small. Consequently, it is advisable to elevate the cephalic or basilic vein with the flap in case the venae comitantes are inadequate.[58]

Sensory innervation of the flap is provided by the medial and lateral antebrachial cutaneous nerves of the forearm. If a sensate flap is desired, one of these branches can be harvested with the flap and sutured to the lingual nerve or to a cutaneous nerve in the neck. The lateral antebrachial cutaneous nerve passes deep to the cephalic vein at the elbow and descends along the radial border of the forearm to the wrist. It innervates the skin over the lateral half of the volar surface of the forearm. The medial antebrachial cutaneous nerve pierces the deep fascia with the basilic vein at about midforearm level and divides into anterior and posterior branches. The anterior branch supplies the skin over the medial half of the volar surface of the arm. Division of the lateral or medial antebrachial cutaneous branches is often required during flap dissection, even if the flap is not neurotized. Therefore, all patients should be advised of the potential for sensory loss. After nerve division, the cut end of the nerve should be buried in muscle to minimize the risk of painful neuroma.

The radial sensory nerve travels from below the fascia to the subcutaneous plane, emerging between the tendons of the extensor carpi radialis longus and the brachioradialis at about the juncture of the distal and middle thirds of the forearm. The nerve may exit anywhere from the midportion of the forearm to a few centimeters proximal to the radial styloid. The radial sensory nerve lies superficial to the radial artery and arborizes after reaching its superficial location. It must be preserved during dissection of the radial forearm flap.[58]

Flap Design

Patency of the ulnar artery and deep palmar arch must be confirmed preoperatively with an Allen test. If the

Allen test result is borderline, the presence of a Doppler signal in the radial palmar arch and digital arteries during manual compression of the radial artery is reassuring. If the vascular anatomy of the hand is uncertain, Doppler flow studies or arteriography should be performed before this flap is raised. Absence of collateral circulation precludes the use of the radial forearm flap or at least necessitates vascular reconstruction. Invasive studies are rarely performed, and it is preferable to choose an alternative flap when adequate collateral circulation is in doubt.[58]

The radial forearm flap is remarkably robust. The fasciocutaneous branches of the distal part of the radial artery will generally support a large territory, including the skin of almost the entire forearm as well as the distal third of the upper arm. The shape, size, and location of the flap may be designed freely on this large territory (Fig. 81-12).

The nondominant arm is chosen as the donor site unless there is a contraindication to its use, such as previous surgery or lack of a patent palmar arch. The chosen arm is marked in clinic at the preoperative visit to prevent inadvertent venous or arterial puncture before flap harvest. Simultaneous harvest and tumor extirpation may be performed. This is often logistically difficult, however, and the harvest of the radial

forearm flap frequently must await completion of the resection. In addition, the exact size of the defect will not be known until after the extirpation is completed, and unexpected bone resection may alter the choice of flap.

In the operating room, the landmarks for flap design are drawn. A line drawn from a point 1 cm below the center of the antecubital fossa to the tubercle of the scaphoid corresponds to the surface anatomy of the radial artery and the anterolateral intermuscular septum.[57] The flap is designed along this axis, adjusting for recipient site requirements and for factors such as hairlessness. The cephalic or basilic vein is also marked. If a long pedicle is desired, the flap is designed distally on the forearm. If pedicle length is not an issue, the flap is moved proximally, with the distal edge of the flap 2 to 5 cm proximal to the wrist crease. This offers thicker flap skin for reconstruction and less potential for exposure of the flexor tendons after flap harvest.[58]

Flap Dissection

The flap is dissected under tourniquet control. The arm is exsanguinated with an Esmarch bandage or simply by elevation. The upper arm tourniquet is inflated. The distal incision is made, and the flexor

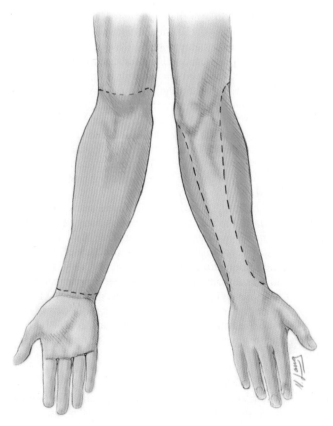

FIGURE 81-12. Territory of the radial forearm flap.

tendons, radial artery, venae comitantes, and brachioradialis tendon are identified (Figs. 81-13 and 81-14). If the cephalic or basilic vein is to be harvested with the flap, it is isolated distally, ligated, and dissected with the flap. The ulnar incision is made through skin, subcutaneous tissue, and deep fascia. Suturing the antebrachial fascia to the skin may help prevent shearing. The ulnar aspect of the flap is elevated in the subfascial plane, dissecting toward the radial artery. The deep fascia encircling the palmaris longus tendon must be divided to preserve the tendon on the forearm. During the dissection, care is taken to preserve the paratenon on the flexor tendons to facilitate skin graft take. The flap is dissected from distal to proximal, tracing the exposed radial vascular bundle and taking care not to damage the fasciocutaneous branches emerging from the intermuscular septum.

The radial side of the flap is then raised toward the radial artery, preserving the cephalic vein with the flap if desired. The superficial branch of the radial nerve must be identified and preserved. If the nerve is injured, neurorrhaphy is required. The brachioradialis muscle is retracted laterally, and the radial vascular bundle is dissected along its radial side from the wrist proximally. The selected superficial vein is dissected proximally to the required length.

The distal end of the radial vascular bundle is then divided and ligated. (Alternatively, this can be done earlier in the dissection.) The flap is elevated in a distal to proximal direction on its radial artery pedicle with the venae comitantes and the chosen superficial vein intact. The lateral or medial antebrachial cutaneous nerve may be included for neurotization of the flap. The forearm incision may be extended as far as the bifurcation of the brachial artery, depending on the pedicle length required. The vessel diameter increases as the antecubital fossa is approached, facilitating the microvascular anastomoses. If desired, the cephalic vein may be followed to its junction with the venae comitantes, so that one venous anastomosis will

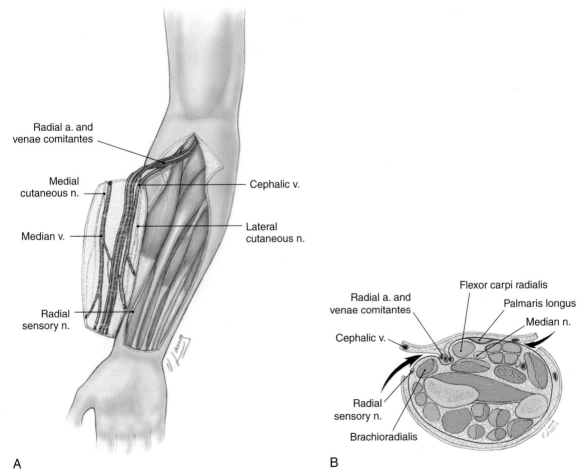

A   B

FIGURE 81-13. The radial forearm flap. *A*, Dissection of the flap (see text for details). *B*, Cross section of the distal forearm just above the wrist crease.

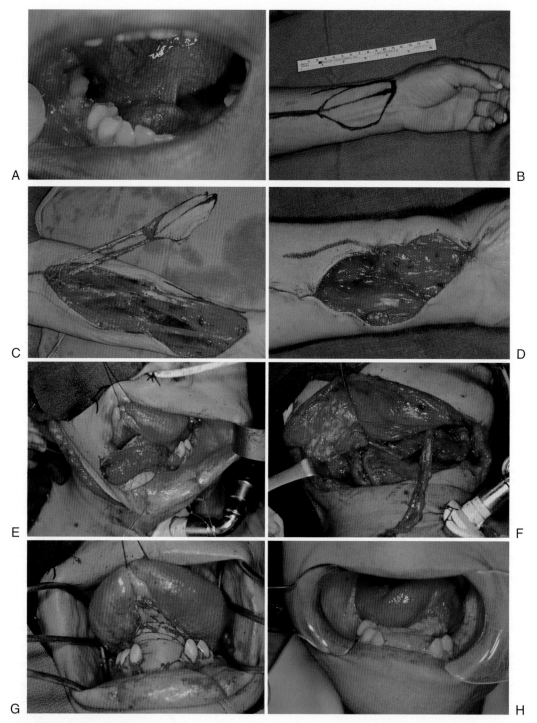

FIGURE 81-14. Reconstruction of the floor of mouth with a free radial forearm flap. *A,* Squamous cell carcinoma of floor of mouth. *B,* Design of the radial forearm flap. *C,* Flap raised. *D,* Donor site defect after partial primary closure. Note the radial sensory nerve in the wound. *E,* Defect of the floor of mouth and ventral tongue, with flap ready for inset. *F,* Flap vessels tunneled through floor of mouth defect into neck wound, ready for anastomosis. The radial artery and cephalic vein were anastomosed end-to-side to the external carotid artery and the internal jugular vein, respectively. *G,* Flap inset. A split-thickness skin graft resurfaces the ventral tongue. *H,* Well-healed flap and graft 1 month after surgery. (Courtesy of Dr. Charles Butler.)

drain both the superficial and deep venous systems of the flap.

After dissection, the tourniquet is released and the vascularity of the hand is assessed. Reconstruction of the radial artery with an interposition vein graft is usually not required. However, if flow to the radial side of the hand through the palmar arch is insufficient, the radial artery is reconstructed with any available forearm vein. If a need for reconstruction is anticipated, the flap is elevated nearly completely before the radial artery is divided. This allows continued blood flow through the artery during dissection, minimizing the ischemia time of the hand. The radial artery is then divided distally, the flap is elevated with the radial artery pedicle, and the radial artery is reconstructed.[58]

After preparation of the recipient vessels, the flap is harvested and transplanted as detailed previously (see "Algorithm for Surgical Treatment"). Three-dimensional defects are closed easily with this flap because the flap can be rotated on itself for insetting.

Closure of the forearm donor site proceeds simultaneously with flap insetting. Primary closure of part or all of the wound is performed when possible. An unmeshed full- or split-thickness skin graft is placed over the remaining open wound. Meticulous hemostasis is essential for successful skin graft take. The paratenon must be intact, and every effort to advance muscle over the tendons should be made before skin grafting. Rotational flaps may be necessary to obtain adequate coverage of the vein graft after arterial reconstruction. The radial sensory nerve also requires muscle or skin coverage to decrease the risk of exposure and neuroma formation.[59]

Dressings and a volar splint are applied with the hand in the position of function. The wrist and hand are immobilized for 5 days, at which time the dressing is removed, the graft is examined, and active and passive motion is begun.[58]

Advantages and Disadvantages

Advantages of the radial forearm flap include the superficial and constant anatomy of the radial artery, the large caliber of the artery (2 to 4 mm at the elbow), and the extensive length of the pedicle. All of these factors facilitate flap dissection and microsurgical transplantation and help account for the reliability of the flap (see Fig. 81-14).[57]

The flap provides thin tissue that is well vascularized over a large territory, making it extremely malleable. Three-dimensional defects are easily filled, and the flap can be rotated on itself for insetting. Portions of the skin may be de-epithelialized to facilitate closure of complex wounds. In addition, the potential for creating a sensate flap exists.

Disadvantages of the radial forearm flap are primarily related to its donor site morbidity. Only narrow or purely fascial flaps have donor sites that can be closed primarily. Skin grafting is generally required, and problems with poor graft take, delayed wound healing, and tendon exposure are common. A persistent deformity in a prominent and visible location is the rule. Anesthesia and dysesthesias over the radial dorsum of the hand may result from dissection of the radial sensory nerve. Several authors[60–62] recommend suprafascial elevation of the radial forearm flap. Suprafascial harvest may decrease the incidence of partial graft loss, tendon exposure, wrist stiffness, and diminished grip strength without increasing the incidence of flap failure.

RECTUS ABDOMINIS FLAP

The rectus abdominis musculocutaneous flap is useful in the reconstruction of total or subtotal glossectomy defects, hemimandibulectomy defects, and complex intraoral defects. This well-vascularized flap provides bulk, decreases dead space, and conforms around exposed vital structures.[63] On occasion, the musculocutaneous flap may provide too much bulk. In this instance, the skin paddle can be excised and muscle and fascia alone used for closure of the defect. The exposed intraoral tissue may then be skin grafted or, alternatively, allowed to remucosalize. In rare situations, the rectus muscle can be used to wrap an anterior mandibular reconstruction plate when mandibular reconstruction with vascularized bone is not an option.[64]

Anatomy

The rectus abdominis is a long, flat muscle that originates from the pubic symphysis and crest and inserts into the fifth, sixth, and seventh costal cartilages. The function of the muscle is to flex the vertebral column. A fascial sheath encloses the rectus muscle, except below the arcuate line where a posterior fascial cover is absent. At least three tendinous insertions are consistently present. The average muscle length, width, and thickness are 30, 6, and 0.6 cm, respectively,[65] but wide variations among patients exist.

A dual, interconnecting blood supply perfuses the muscle. The deep superior epigastric vessels reach the muscle lateral to the xiphoid and run along its posterior surface for a short distance before entering the substance of the muscle. The major blood supply, however, is by the deep inferior epigastric artery, which originates from the external iliac artery immediately above the inguinal ligament. The artery and its venae comitantes travel medially, then pass anterior to the arcuate line and turn superiorly to run along the anterior surface of the posterior rectus sheath. The artery usually divides into lateral and medial branches below the level of the umbilicus. From each branch, a vertical row of cutaneous perforators pierces the muscle to supply the overlying skin. The largest perforators are usually in the medial row, just below the umbilicus. There are no significant perforators inferior to the arcuate line. The lateral and medial branches pass upward through the muscle to communicate with the superior epigastric system above the level of the umbilicus.

The rectus abdominis free flap is based on the deep inferior epigastric vessels. If it is harvested at its takeoff from the iliac artery, the average arterial diameter is 2.7 mm, and the pedicle length ranges from 7 to 15 cm. The artery runs with two venae comitantes, which occasionally join before their junction with the external iliac vein. The average vein diameter is 3.0 mm.[65] The innervation of the rectus abdominis muscle comes from the ventral rami of the lower six or seven segmental thoracic spinal nerves. The ability to transfer the rectus abdominis muscle for functional recovery is limited by this segmental innervation.[63]

To maximize blood supply to the flap, the flap is harvested with both rows of perforators. This is done by taking the full width of the rectus muscle with the flap, as described later, or by preserving small strips of muscle medial and lateral to both rows. Alternatively, the flap may be raised on either the lateral or medial branch alone, leaving the other branch and its attached muscle intact. A final option is to perform a deep inferior epigastric perforator flap, dissecting the perforators from within the muscle and leaving the entire muscle in situ.

Previous abdominal surgery may preclude the use of the free rectus flap. Upper abdominal surgery does not disrupt the inferior epigastric pedicle, and flap transplantation can usually proceed. Lower abdominal surgery, however, may result in injury to the inferior epigastric vascular system. If the patient has lower abdominal scars, the vessels should be explored to assess the status of the pedicle before complete flap elevation.[63]

Flap Design

The skin island (paddle) of the rectus abdominis musculocutaneous flap may be oriented in a vertical, oblique, or transverse direction. For head and neck reconstruction, a vertical rectus abdominis musculocutaneous flap is used in most cases (Fig. 81-15). An attempt is made to capture the periumbilical perforators in the paddle design. Placement of the medial edge of the skin ellipse in the midline will guarantee capture of at least the medial row of perforators. On occasion, the muscle is wider than anticipated or is displaced laterally because of a wide diastasis. It is easy to miss the lateral row of perforators in the flap design in these situations. Assessment of the laxity of the abdominal wall will help the surgeon estimate the maximum flap width that can be taken without compromising primary closure.

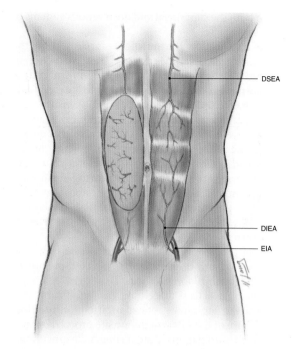

FIGURE 81-15. The vertical rectus abdominis musculocutaneous flap. The deep inferior epigastric artery (DIEA) arises from the external iliac artery (EIA) and anastomoses with the deep superior epigastric artery (DSEA) above the umbilicus. The skin paddle is shown overlying the right rectus abdominis muscle, capturing blood supply from the lateral and medial rows of perforators.

Because of the distance of the donor site from the head and neck, flap harvest can proceed during tumor extirpation. If the ultimate size of the defect is unknown, the flap is designed as large as possible (based on skin laxity) and subsequently tailored to fit the defect. Thoughtful orientation of the cutaneous paddle relative to the inferior epigastric pedicle will allow maximal flap reach. The muscle should not be relied on for restoration of missing tissue bulk because atrophy will occur. Rather, the skin and fat of the skin paddle should provide the bulk required.

Flap Dissection

The skin paddle is incised down to deep fascia, beveling outward to capture as many perforators as possible. The flap is elevated off the fascia from lateral to medial until the lateral perforators are seen entering the skin paddle from the underlying rectus muscle. A similar dissection is performed medially, and the medial row of perforators is identified. Next, the anterior rectus sheath is opened just lateral to the lateral row. The fascial incision is extended inferiorly to facilitate dissection of the deep inferior epigastric vessels.

The muscle is mobilized from its sheath laterally and the pedicle is identified. Once it is clear that the pedicle is suitable for free tissue transplantation, the fascial incision is extended to circumscribe all the perforators to the flap. The muscle is freed from the anterior sheath. Special care is required at the tendinous inscriptions to ensure that the pedicle, which may run superficially under the inscription, is not injured. The superior aspect of the muscle, above the level of the skin paddle, is divided with electrocautery. If needed for the reconstruction, additional muscle may be harvested superiorly. The superior epigastric vessels are ligated.

At this point, a few sutures placed between the skin and the harvested rectus fascia or muscle will help prevent shear injury to the perforators during the remaining dissection and flap transplantation. The muscle is elevated from the posterior sheath. Intercostal nerves and vessels are divided between clips or ties as they are encountered laterally. Vascular branches in the loose areolar tissue between the rectus muscle and the posterior sheath are similarly ligated (or cauterized if small) and divided.

Dissection continues from superior to inferior until the muscle is completely freed from its sheath. The muscle is divided inferiorly below the point of pedicle entry, with care taken to protect the pedicle. The deep inferior epigastric vessels are dissected to their respective junctions with the external iliac artery and vein to maximize pedicle length.

The recipient site is prepared, and the flap is harvested. The flap is inset, and the microanastomoses are performed. After the microanastomoses are complete, the abdominal fascia is closed carefully, making sure to include both layers of the anterior rectus sheath in the closure. Synthetic mesh is used to reinforce the closure only if necessary. The abdominal skin and subcutaneous tissue are mobilized and closed in layers over drains.

Advantages and Disadvantages

The rectus abdominis flap is extremely useful for reconstruction of complex defects of the oral cavity and pharynx. The vascular pedicle of the rectus flap is large, constant, reliable, and long. Flap dissection is technically easy, and flap failure is uncommon. Abundant tissue is available, and the skin paddle is versatile. The size and shape of the paddle can be varied to suit any number of recipient site requirements, and the good blood supply enables thinning, de-epithelializing, or folding of the flap as needed. The richly vascularized flap provides excellent coverage and protection of exposed vital structures or prostheses, enhances wound healing, and tolerates radiation well. Importantly, the supine position for flap harvest is favorable for most head and neck defects, and the donor site is easily hidden by clothing.[66]

The rectus abdominis is an excellent choice for the total glossectomy defect in which a large volume of tissue has been resected (Fig. 81-16). Replacing the missing tissue with this bulky flap helps decrease the risk of aspiration. The flap can be shaped into a dome by de-epithelializing triangular darts along the edges of the skin paddle. An effort is made to maximize the intraoral volume of the flap, allowing it to fill the oral cavity as completely as possible while still allowing mouth closure. The excess volume is needed to compensate for the muscle atrophy that will occur during the first 6 months after surgery.[66]

The flap can be folded on itself to provide continuous closure of complex intraoral defects that extend into the pharynx and beyond (Fig. 81-17). The skin paddle can be used for lining replacement, skin replacement, or both (Figs. 81-18 and 81-19). In obese patients, the rectus muscle or muscle and fascia may be harvested without skin for tongue or oral cavity reconstruction. Significant contraction of the lining surface should be expected, however, when a skin paddle is not used. Another way to decrease the bulk of the flap is to use a deep inferior epigastric artery perforator flap.

Another common indication for the rectus abdominis musculocutaneous flap is the posterior mandibular defect (see Figs. 81-17 and 81-18). Most of the functional morbidity in patients with posterior mandibular composite defects is due not to the bone deficiency but to the associated loss of soft tissue lining. A reasonably good reconstruction of a posterior mandibular defect can be achieved with soft tissue alone by use of a rectus abdominis free flap. The bulk of the flap restores contour and helps minimize lateral drift of the jaw. The skin paddle replaces absent intraoral lining and helps restore function. Provided the remaining mandible is in good position, both function and appearance can be almost normal. Soft tissue reconstruction has the advantages of relatively low donor site morbidity, short operative times, and high success rates. However, if the mandibular defect is segmental and the original condyle has been preserved, a bony reconstruction is usually indicated.[21, 66]

The chief disadvantage of the rectus flap is the donor defect. Weakness of the abdominal wall as well as abdominal bulge or hernia can result from harvest of the rectus muscle and its anterior sheath. In addition, the flap is bulky in obese patients, and it may require considerable thinning secondarily with use for intraoral reconstruction.[66] Sensory neurotization of the skin paddle is difficult to achieve because of the muscle's multisegmental innervation.

LATERAL THIGH FLAP

Although a wide variety of options are available for reconstruction of the oral cavity, a radial forearm or rectus abdominis free flap is usually the best choice

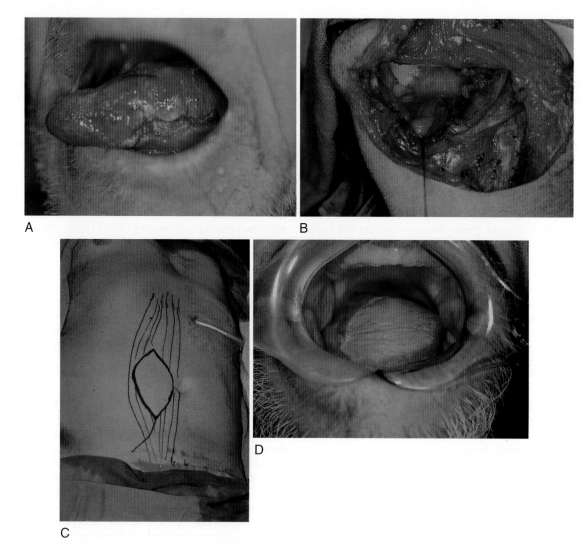

FIGURE 81-16. Tongue reconstruction with a free vertical rectus abdominis musculocutaneous flap. *A,* Deeply infiltrative squamous cell carcinoma of the tongue. At surgery, the tumor extended into the suprahyoid musculature and the submandibular space, with direct invasion of the sublingual and submandibular glands. *B,* Subtotal glossectomy defect includes most of the floor of mouth. A remnant of tongue remains at the posterior aspect of the defect on the right (held by suture). A left modified neck dissection has been performed. *C,* Design of the vertical rectus abdominis musculocutaneous flap. Anastomoses were performed end-to-side to the external carotid artery and internal jugular vein. *D,* Well-healed flap 2 months after surgery. (Courtesy of Dr. Charles Butler.)

when medium to large defects are encountered. These techniques have high success rates, acceptable donor site morbidity, and lower complication rates than comparable regional flaps. They can generally achieve the reconstructive goals in one stage. With the radial forearm and the rectus abdominis free flaps, the reconstructive surgeon can repair almost any soft tissue oral defect that might be encountered. On occasion, however, these flaps are not available. Therefore, it is helpful to have an additional flap or two in one's armamentarium for reconstruction of the difficult head and neck defect. The lateral thigh flap fits into this category of "backup" flap.

The lateral thigh flap is a fasciocutaneous flap based on the third perforator of the profunda femoris artery. Baek[67] first described the flap in 1983, and Hayden[68,69] and Miller[70] later elucidated its use for head and neck reconstruction. The lateral thigh flap can provide thin pliable tissue suitable for replacing the lining of the oral cavity.

Anatomy

The profunda femoris artery branches from the common femoral artery and descends along the medial side of the femur, terminating in connections with the upper muscle branches of the popliteal artery. The first major branches of the profunda femoris are the medial

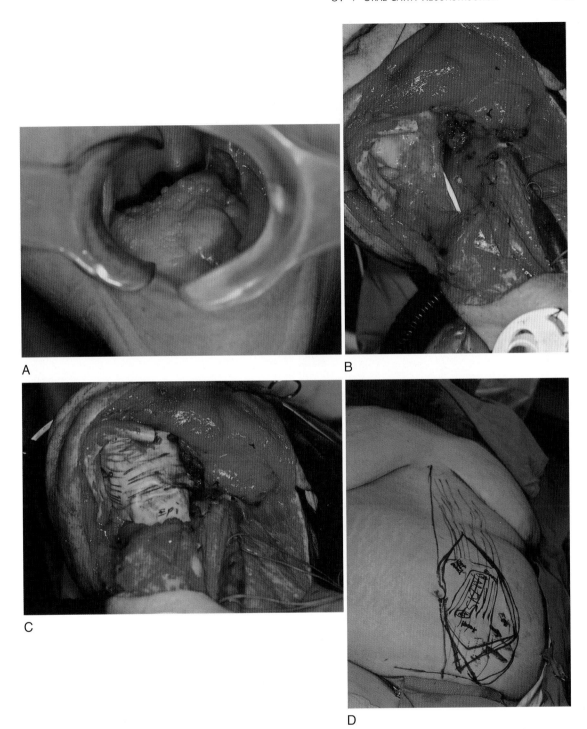

FIGURE 81-17. Reconstruction of complex intraoral defect with free vertical rectus abdominis musculocutaneous flap. *A,* Recurrent squamous cell carcinoma of the tongue base and left tonsillar pillar after multiple excisions, chemotherapy, and radiation therapy. *B,* Defect includes the entire tongue and floor of mouth, the left posterior mandible, the left soft palate, and portions of the oropharynx and nasopharynx. Left modified neck dissection has been performed, with preservation of the internal jugular vein but sacrifice of the external carotid artery. *C,* An Esmarch template is prepared and inset into the defect. *D,* The template is sterilized and transplanted to the abdomen to assist in vertical rectus abdominis musculocutaneous flap design.   *Continued*

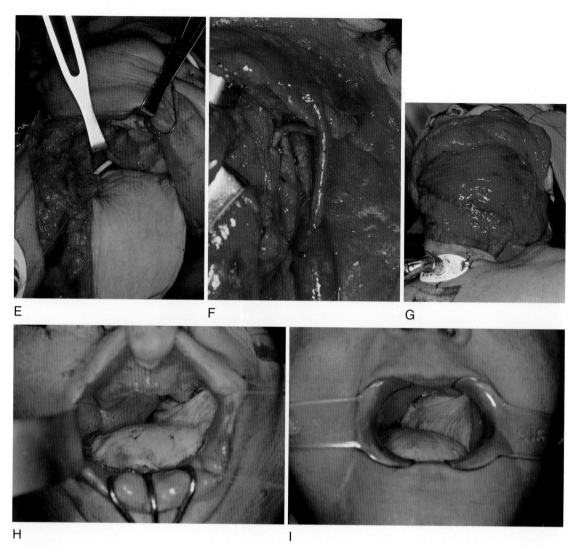

FIGURE 81-17, cont'd. *E,* The flap is inset along the posterior pharynx, inferiorly to the level of the epiglottis (note suture), and along the superior gingivobuccal sulcus before the microvascular anastomoses are performed. *F,* The deep inferior epigastric artery is anastomosed end-to-end to the stump of the superior thyroid artery. The external carotid artery stump is oversewn. The vein is anastomosed end-to-side to the internal jugular vein. Intraoral insetting is then completed. *G,* Revascularized rectus muscle in position before closure. *H,* Immediate postoperative appearance of skin paddle. *I,* Well-healed flap 4 weeks after surgery. (From Butler CE, Lewin JS: Reconstruction of large composite oromandibulomaxillary defects with free vertical rectus abdominis myocutaneous flaps. Plast reconstr Surg 2004;113(2):499-507.)

and lateral circumflex femoral arteries. More distally, four perforating arteries pass through the attachment of the adductor magnus muscle along the linea aspera of the femur to supply the tissues of the lateral thigh (Fig. 81-20). These perforators terminate in the plexus of the superficial fascia and supply the overlying skin. Each artery is accompanied by paired venae comitantes.[70]

The principal artery to the lateral thigh skin is the third perforating artery, although the fourth perforator is the dominant vessel in a small minority of patients.[69] The caliber of the third perforating artery ranges from 1.5 to 2.5 mm, and the caliber of the venae

comitantes is similar. The length of the pedicle (from the origin to the level of the superficial fascia) ranges from 4.5 to 9.0 cm.[70] Injection studies have demonstrated that the potential territory of the third perforator includes nearly the entire lateral thigh.

Flap Design

The surface landmarks are identified with the patient in the supine position with a lift under the buttock, the knee slightly flexed, and the hip internally rotated. The intermuscular septum is identified between the vastus lateralis anteriorly and the biceps femoris posteriorly. This is easy to visualize in thin

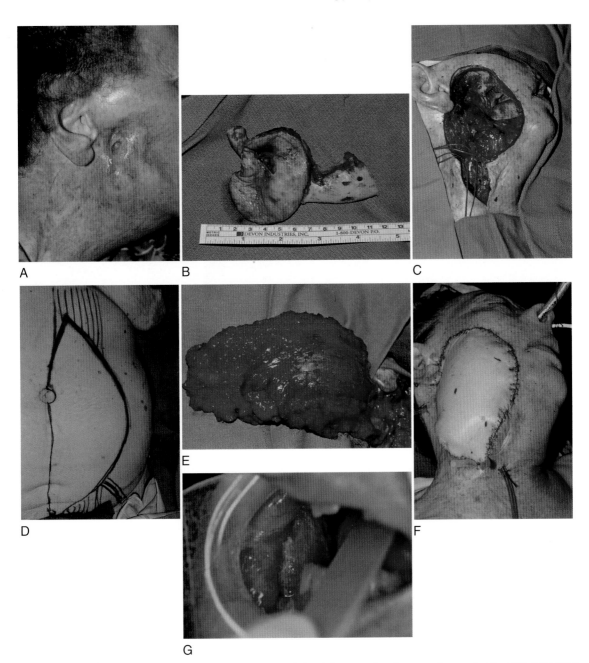

FIGURE 81-18. Combination of free vertical rectus abdominis musculocutaneous flap and skin graft for reconstruction of complex facial defect with intraoral component. *A*, Osteoradionecrosis of the mandible 5 years after parotidectomy and radiation therapy for salivary duct carcinoma. The patient is without evidence of recurrent disease. *B*, Resection specimen included posterior mandible and facial skin as well as buccal mucosa. *C*, Defect after extirpation. Note intraoral mucosal defect. *D*, Design of vertical rectus abdominis musculocutaneous flap. *E*, Revascularized vertical rectus abdominis musculocutaneous flap with split-thickness skin graft sutured to muscle surface. The grafted portion of the flap was inset into the mucosal defect by use of a parachute suture technique. *F*, Flap inset. *G*, Healing graft 3 weeks after surgery. (From Butler CE: Skin grafts used in combination with free flaps for intraoral oncological reconstruction. Ann Plast Surg 2001;47:294-298.)

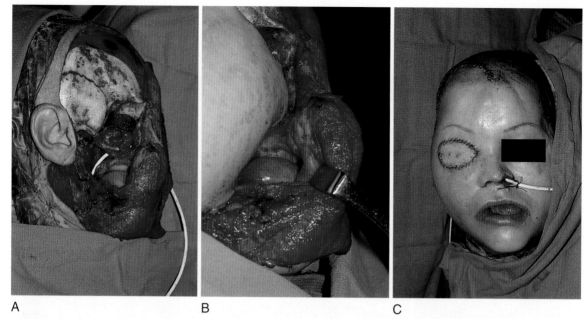

A   B   C

FIGURE 81-19. Free transverse rectus abdominis musculocutaneous flap alone for reconstruction of complex facial defect with intraoral component. *A,* Defect after resection of recurrent sarcoma of temporal region. Note intraoral and orbital components. *B,* Initial inset of skin paddle of free transverse rectus abdominis musculocutaneous flap into the intraoral defect. A separate region of the skin paddle is inset into the orbital exenteration defect. The remainder of the paddle is de-epithelialized or debulked. *C,* Immediate postoperative result. (Courtesy of Dr. David Chang.)

patients, especially after muscle relaxation. In heavier patients, the landmarks for the septum are the posterior aspect of the lateral condyle of the femur and the posterior aspect of greater trochanter (Fig. 81-21). The cutaneous branch of the third perforating branch of the profunda femoris is located on this line about midway between the greater trochanter and the lateral condyle. Its location can be confirmed by Doppler examination.[67, 69, 70]

The flap is designed on the posterolateral aspect of the thigh, incorporating the identified third perforator in the design. A longitudinal elliptical design facilitates primary closure of the donor site. Large flaps can be harvested without any peripheral necrosis, but these are rarely necessary for oral cavity reconstruction. The thickness of the tissue can be estimated by pinching the skin. The thinnest tissue lies anteriorly, over the area of the vastus lateralis muscle, and the flap is usually designed to include this area.[70]

Flap Dissection

A knee bolster and a heel cushion are used to position the leg. The anterior incision is made, and the flap is elevated in the relatively avascular plane between the superficial fascia and the fascia lata. The third perforator usually becomes visible on the undersurface of the flap near the intermuscular groove. The perforator courses most often through the substance of the short head of the biceps femoris muscle, exiting posterior to the intermuscular groove. The perforator only rarely passes through the intermuscular septum with no intramuscular component.[70] Thus, an intramuscular dissection is required (Fig. 81-22). The pedicle is dissected from within the substance of the short head of the biceps muscle by dividing the overlying fibers. Branches to the muscle are ligated and divided, unless the muscle is to be included in a composite flap. A large branch supplying the short head of the biceps femoris muscle is commonly seen about 3 cm beneath the superficial fascia. Inclusion of the muscle allows the skin and muscle to be inset somewhat independently but significantly shortens the pedicle length.

An assistant standing opposite the surgeon retracts upward and anteriorly to help the surgeon visualize the pedicle as it exits the fascial hiatus at the linea aspera. Careful control of various muscle branches from the pedicle near the hiatus is required. The linea aspera is split lengthwise, and the pedicle is followed to the point where it disappears behind the linea aspera and joins the main trunk of the profunda femoris artery. It will eventually be ligated and divided at this level. Once the vascular pedicle is dissected, the posterior part of the flap is raised until the entire flap is isolated on its vascular pedicle.[67, 69, 70]

For head and neck applications, the donor site can often be closed primarily. Wide undermining is

The donor site morbidity is significantly less than that of the radial forearm flap, especially when large flaps are required. In many cases, the donor defect can be closed primarily. The scar is easily hidden, and there is no functional deficit related to flap harvest. When there is a volume deficit at the recipient site, thicker portions of thigh skin or the muscle may be harvested with the skin flap to fill dead space or to restore contour. The donor site is distant from the head and neck, and harvest does not require repositioning of the patient. As a result, simultaneous resection and flap harvest are possible. The lateral femoral cutaneous nerve can be harvested with the flap, giving sensory potential to the transplanted skin.

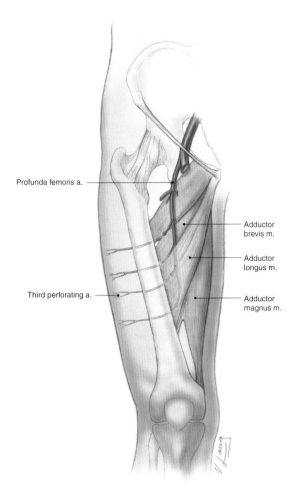

FIGURE 81-20. Anatomy of the perforating system of the profunda femoris artery. The profunda femoris artery passes deep to the adductor longus muscle medial to the femur. The third perforating branch of the profunda femoris artery passes behind the linea aspera of the femur below the lower border of the adductor brevis muscle. It then penetrates the fibers of the adductor magnus muscle (see also Fig. 81-23) to reach the lateral thigh.

performed, and suction drainage is applied routinely. If primary closure is not possible, a split-thickness skin graft is applied. Graft take in this location is often patchy. For this reason, some authors advocate a relaxing incision in the medial thigh, allowing primary closure over the intermuscular septum laterally. A skin graft is then applied medially, directly on the medial thigh musculature.[69]

Advantages and Disadvantages

The lateral thigh free flap is a useful alternative in head and neck reconstruction (Fig. 81-23), particularly when the radial forearm flap is not available. It provides one of the largest surface areas of any skin flap available.

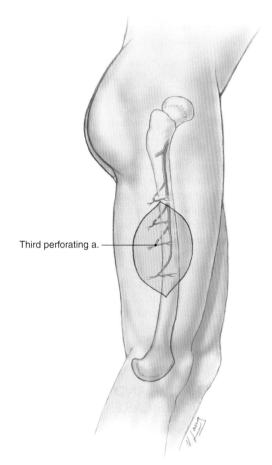

FIGURE 81-21. Design of the lateral thigh flap. A line is drawn from the greater trochanter to the lateral condyle of the femur. This line corresponds to the lateral intermuscular septum and is the axis of the flap. The third perforating branch of the profunda femoris artery is marked at the midpoint of this line.

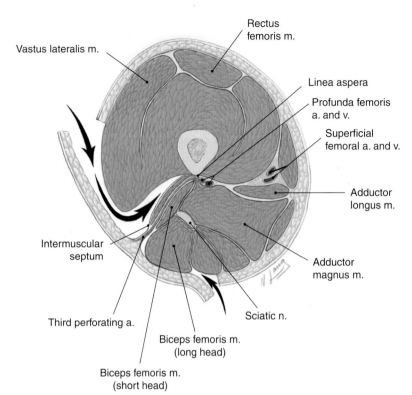

Rectus
femoris m.

Vastus lateralis m.

Linea aspera

Profunda femoris
a. and v.

Superficial
femoral a. and v.

Adductor
longus m.

Intermuscular
septum

Adductor
magnus m.

Third perforating a.

Sciatic n.

Biceps femoris m.
(long head)

Biceps femoris m.
(short head)

FIGURE 81-22. Dissection of the lateral thigh flap at the level of the third perforating artery. The course of the vessel is through the short head of the biceps femoris muscle in most patients. Therefore, an intramuscular dissection is usually required.

The chief disadvantages of the lateral thigh flap relate to its vascular pedicle, which is shorter, smaller, and more variable than that of other commonly used flaps. Anastomoses are often best performed end-to-end to branches of the external carotid artery and internal jugular vein; therefore, the presence of suitable recipient vessels should be confirmed before flap harvest. There is considerable variation among patients in the thickness of the subcutaneous tissue and the amount of hair present. The flap may not be a good choice in obese patients when a thin pliable flap is required. The donor site is occasionally hairy in men. If postoperative radiotherapy is required, however, this feature becomes only a relative contraindication because irradiation permanently depilates the skin of the transplanted flap. Seromas at the donor site are common even when suction drainage is used.[69, 70]

INTRAOPERATIVE AND POSTOPERATIVE CARE

During and after flap reconstruction, the patient is kept warm and well hydrated. The use of vasoconstricting agents is avoided. The patient is transferred to intensive care and ventilated through the tracheotomy overnight, after which weaning from the ventilator is begun. Diuretics are avoided in the first few days after surgery unless there is a clear indication for diuresis. Intravenous antibiotics are continued for several days.

Urine output is monitored closely as an indicator of volume status.

In patients undergoing free flap transplantation, postoperative flap monitoring is performed with a hand-held Doppler device at a site on the skin paddle marked intraoperatively with a Prolene suture. Alternatively, the free flap is monitored with an implantable Doppler device placed on the flap vein. Monitoring is performed on an hourly basis for 48 to 72 hours and then on a tapering schedule through postoperative day 5. Loss of the Doppler signal or visible flap congestion or pallor demands re-exploration. Monitoring by trained and experienced personnel is essential if thrombosis is to be recognized early enough to salvage the flap.

Anticoagulation is not used routinely after free flap transplantation. Certainly, aspirin, dextran, or heparin can be administered at the surgeon's discretion. In the event of vessel thrombosis requiring revascularization, systemic anticoagulation with intravenous heparin is used for 5 days.

Feeding through a nasogastric feeding tube placed at surgery is begun once bowel function has returned. Oral hygiene can be improved with neomycin power sprays or Peridex mouth rinses starting a few days after surgery. Oral feeding is delayed for 7 to 10 days, depending on the location of the reconstruction and the patient's surgical and adjuvant therapy history. A modified barium swallow examination is performed

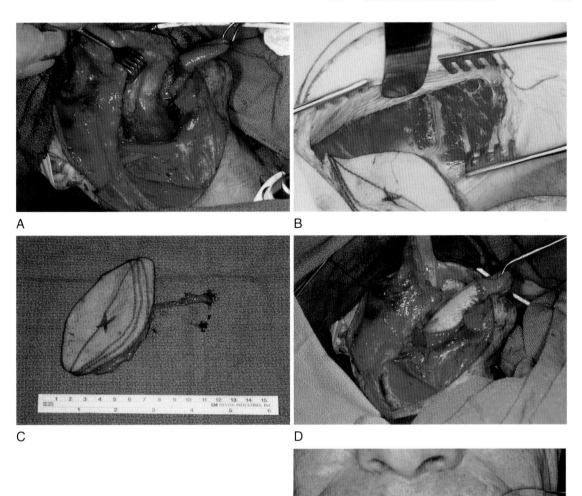

FIGURE 81-23. Intraoral reconstruction with a free lateral thigh flap. *A,* Defect after re-excision of an inadequately excised leiomyosarcoma involving the right tongue and palatoglossal fold. Right hemiglossectomy was performed after mandibular osteotomy with mandibular swing for access. The tip of the tongue has been preserved. *B,* Free lateral thigh flap partially dissected. The vastus lateralis is retracted anteriorly. The intramuscular dissection through the short head of the biceps muscle is in progress. *C,* The harvested flap. *D,* The flap is partially inset. *E,* Well-healed flap and excellent tongue mobility 2 months after surgery. (Courtesy of Dr. Michael Miller.)

before the initiation of feeding. This study may identify a leak at the repair but is done primarily to assess swallowing function and degree of aspiration.

Drains are removed from the neck when drainage is less than 15 mL per day and from the flap donor site when drainage is less than 30 mL per day. If an implantable Doppler device is used, the wire is brought through the neck incision or through a separate incision and carefully secured to the skin. Wires are maintained until 2 to 3 weeks after surgery, at which time gentle traction on the wire will cause it to detach from the vascular sheath, allowing removal.

COMPLICATIONS

Flap Loss

Partial flap loss is seen with both pedicled and free flaps but is more common after pedicled flap reconstruction. Management of partial flap loss depends on the degree of loss. Minor flap loss can generally be left to heal secondarily. More significant flap loss may require surgical intervention, ranging from débridement alone to skin graft or a second flap.

Total flap loss is usually seen after microsurgical failure of a free flap. The rates of flap failure are low (see "Outcomes"), and early total reconstructive loss may be reversible. Many flaps that fail do so because of poor management of the patient, poor operative design, or poor microsurgical technique. The patient needs to be kept warm, sedated, pain free, and well hydrated in the postoperative period. If flap viability is in question, surgical exploration is required. The salvage rate is highly dependent on the speed of recognition of the problem. Prompt re-exploration may result in salvage of the flap after either arterial or venous thrombosis, although flaps generally tolerate ischemia better than congestion. If flow is re-established, steroids may be helpful in minimizing flap edema, and anticoagulation is indicated. If salvage attempts are unsuccessful, the flap must be discarded and another reconstruction performed.

In this situation, a second free flap is not necessarily contraindicated. Second free flaps play an important role in salvaging head and neck reconstructions in selected patients. Despite an earlier failure, the majority of second free flaps are successful, even when the same recipient vessels are used.[71,72] Salvage with a pedicled flap, usually the pectoralis major, is indicated when the adequacy of the recipient vessels is poor or in question, when the patient is medically unstable, and, in some instances, when the reason for loss of the first flap is poorly understood. When major flap loss has resulted in fistulization and infection, it is usually best to temporize by establishing a controlled fistula rather than to try to achieve primary wound healing in a compromised wound bed.

Hematoma

Large hematomas at the recipient site require re-exploration, evacuation of clot, and control of bleeding. Hematomas are easily confused with and sometimes caused by venous congestion of a free flap. Conversely, compression of a free flap pedicle by an expanding hematoma can result in microvascular occlusion and flap loss. Therefore, the pedicle should be examined at the time of re-exploration to ensure that there is no active bleeding at the anastomoses and that flow through the flap is preserved.

Neck Flap Necrosis

Necrosis of the edge of the neck skin flap is not uncommon. This complication is usually of no consequence, and the area of tissue loss will heal quickly by secondary intention. When large portions of the skin flap are lost, exposure of vital structures including the great vessels and vascular microanastomoses may occur. Anastomotic thrombosis and carotid blowout may result. Return to the operating room, débridement, and flap coverage of the vessels, usually with a pectoralis major muscle flap, are indicated to avoid these disastrous complications.

Infection

Wound infection usually presents as erythema and drainage from the neck incision. These findings may represent a localized abscess or may be the first sign of fistulization. Antibiotics and local wound care with daily packing are indicated.

Fistula

In many cases, the presence of a fistula is obvious because the communication between the oral cavity and the skin can be visualized. A wound infection characterized by copious amounts of drainage long after the wound is opened and antibiotics are begun may well represent a fistula even if an orocutaneous connection cannot be identified. Patients with these findings should be given a presumptive diagnosis of fistula and treated as such. The patient is allowed nothing by mouth and treated with local wound care until drainage decreases and partial healing is evident. Contrast studies or the "grape juice test" may confirm the presence of a fistula when the diagnosis is in question.

Donor Site Complications

Potential donor site complications include hematoma, seroma, infection, dehiscence, wound healing delay, partial or total skin graft loss, tendon exposure (after radial forearm flap), hernia or abdominal bulge (after rectus abdominis flap), and contour deformity. It is important to minimize these complications to avoid delay in adjuvant therapy.

Need for Revision

Not infrequently, surgical revision is required to optimize functional and aesthetic outcomes in the patient with head and neck cancer. Alveoloplasty, flap debulking, release of contractures, and scar revision are relatively simple interventions that may significantly improve outcome. Release of a tethered tongue and correction of late deformities in the oral cavity may require skin grafting or even free flap reconstruction. The radial forearm flap is particularly useful for this purpose and does not add excessive intraoral bulk. In general, revisions should be delayed until the edema has fully resolved, usually at least 3 months. After radiation therapy, longer delay is often advisable. Revision after radiotherapy should be approached with caution because the wound healing capacity has been permanently altered in the irradiated area.

OUTCOMES

Outcome assessment of oral cavity reconstruction is multifaceted. Surgical outcome is reflected in flap loss, complication, and revision rates as well as in donor site morbidity statistics. Functional and aesthetic outcomes are more difficult to quantitate. Oncologic outcomes continue to be suboptimal. As cancer treatment improves, however, the demands on the reconstructive surgeon will only increase.

Surgical

There is no doubt that the addition of microvascular free tissue transplantation to the reconstructive armamentarium has greatly improved our ability to achieve reliable, effective, and safe single-stage reconstruction. Watkinson and Breach[73] reported a flap success rate of 95% with no mortality in 77 cases of head and neck free flap reconstruction. Urken et al[74] quoted an overall success rate of 93.5% in 200 cases of free flap reconstruction. Schusterman et al[75] cited a similar overall flap success rate (94%) and a complication rate of 36% in 308 free flaps for head and neck reconstruction. Studies have shown that free flaps compare favorably with the best available pedicled flap, the pectoralis major musculocutaneous flap. Kroll et al[46] compared the rectus abdominis free flap with the pectoralis musculocutaneous flap for head and neck reconstruction and found fewer complications and a lower incidence of flap loss in the free flap group. A study by Schusterman and Horndeski[76] demonstrated no increased incidence of postoperative medical complications in patients undergoing free flap reconstruction, despite longer operative times compared with the control (non–free flap) group.

Functional

The assessment of oral cavity reconstruction results has moved beyond measurements of flap loss and complication rates. The focus has shifted from achieving primary mucosal healing to improving functional results. As stated eloquently by Boyd, "The more we anticipate (and produce) primary healing and a reasonable appearance following radical ablative surgery, the more we are inclined to shift our magnifying lens to areas once considered of secondary importance. The quality of dental rehabilitation, the articulation of speech, the ease of swallowing, and the maintenance of normal intraoral sensation have come to reflect our abilities as reconstructive surgeons no less than anastomotic patency rates, bony union, the absence of complications, and the shortening of hospital stay."[77]

Ultimately, a combination of the nature of the resection and the type of flap reconstruction determines intraoral function. Despite early hopes that free flap reconstruction would solve the problem of restoring function, it has become clear that immobile and insensate flaps cannot replace the dynamic and complex functions of the human tongue in swallowing and speech.[78] Several modifications of the free tissue design and inset have been proposed to help optimize intraoral function and are discussed. These modifications include neurotization of the flap, alteration of the shape of the flap, and transfer of mucus-producing flaps.

MOTOR NEUROTIZATION

Attempts have been made to restore function by use of innervated muscle and musculocutaneous flaps powered by the hypoglossal nerve. Haughey[79] used innervated free and pedicled latissimus dorsi flaps for tongue reconstruction, orienting the muscle fibers perpendicular to the long axis of the skin component in an attempt to provide a contractile muscle sling that would raise the new tongue toward the palate for speech and swallowing.

Unfortunately, a single reinnervated muscle cannot duplicate the complex intrinsic musculature of the tongue. Voluntary neotongue motion can be elicited, but the result is a bunching up of the tongue with no useful function for food transport or articulation.[80] However, reinnervation of a transplanted muscle does provide maintenance of muscle bulk. If atrophy of the flap will result in inadequate bulk of the reconstructed tongue, innervation of the muscle may be considered.[16] In general, atrophy is not a concern with musculocutaneous flaps because the cutaneous portion of the flap maintains the desired bulk. In general, pure muscle flaps are not reinnervated because a palatal prosthesis will assist with palatal contact if neotongue bulk is deficient.

SENSORY NEUROTIZATION

Intact intraoral sensation facilitates the presentation of ingested material to the teeth for chewing and to the tongue for swallowing. Normal sensation prevents the pooling of saliva and resultant drooling. Evidence also links intraoral sensation to the quality of speech.[77] When sensory feedback is removed, the highly coordinated functions of chewing and swallowing are grossly impaired. Effective sweeping of the floor of the mouth by the tongue is lost, and oral hygiene deteriorates. Loss of the afferent sensory arm of the swallow reflex may result in dysphagia and aspiration.[81]

Some spontaneous sensory recovery in noninnervated flaps has been reported.[82, 83] Hermanson et al,[84] however, found no evidence of light touch or pain sensation in any noninnervated free flap to the lower extremity. In 1977, David[85] was the first to report the use of a sensory innervated flap (a pedicled deltopectoral flap) for intraoral reconstruction. The use of sensory innervated free flaps to the head and neck soon followed.[86, 87]

In 1990, Urken et al[88] were the first to publish a report on the use of the neurotized radial forearm free flap for oral cavity reconstruction. The cutaneous nerves of the forearm were anastomosed to the great auricular nerve, and as a result, sensory feedback was not appropriate for the defect. Hayden[81] reported results of suturing the lateral antebrachial cutaneous nerve of transplanted radial forearm flaps to the stumps of glossopharyngeal and lingual nerves within oral and pharyngeal resections. He demonstrated temperature differentiation and two-point discrimination in innervated flaps and hypothesized that careful choice of the recipient nerve resulted in return of sensation appropriate to the defect.

Boyd et al[77] used sophisticated testing to show that innervated flaps were superior to noninnervated flaps in every sensory modality tested, including pain, temperature, and two-point discrimination. The innervated flaps had sensation of the same order as that of the normal tongue and better than that of the contralateral unoperated forearm. In contrast, noninnervated free radial forearm flaps and pedicled pectoralis flaps had nondetectable two-point discrimination. Boyd conceded that his measurements of intraoral function were rather abstract, but he reported his impression that patients developed useful sensation that helped them talk, maintain oral continence, chew, and swallow. Subjective testing on the ability to sense food in the mouth supported this belief but could not readily be subjected to statistical analysis.

FLAP GEOMETRY

In the past, reconstruction after total glossectomy focused on resurfacing the intraoral defect with a skin flap or graft to prevent scar contracture and distortion of the intraoral structures. This created a dead space in the oral cavity that allowed pooling of saliva and food. Speech was poor, and patients ate by tilting their heads back and allowing gravity to pull the bolus into the pharynx.

Salibian et al[80] demonstrated with cineradiography that glossectomy patients reconstructed with free groin flaps push food from the mouth into the oropharynx by closing the jaw and pressing the flap against the palate. The food is then squeezed from the oropharynx into the hypopharynx by constrictor muscle contractions while the flap is kept in contact with the palate. These observations led Salibian to recommend shaping the flap into a cylinder so that it touches the hard and soft palate and completely obliterates the oral cavity when the jaw is closed.

Other authors have also advised shaping the flap to improve neotongue function. Kroll and Baldwin[66] recommended de-epithelializing triangular darts along the edges of the rectus flap skin paddle during insetting, letting the flap fill the oral cavity as completely as possible while still allowing mouth closure. Similarly, Kiyokawa et al[89] attempted to maximize tissue volume by orienting the rectus abdominis musculocutaneous flap in a "money pouch" configuration. The excess volume generated by these geometric adaptations compensates for postoperative muscle atrophy and may help maintain the neotongue-palatal contact necessary for optimal swallowing function.

MUCOSAL FLAPS

Xerostomia can be a disabling problem for the irradiated patient with head and neck cancer. In efforts to prevent or treat xerostomia, several authors have recommended the use of mucosal flaps in reconstruction. Hayden[81] described the use of a gastric or jejunal visceral flap in patients with recurrent disease or a second primary when a large defect in the oral cavity or oropharynx is expected. He believes that the added benefit of mucus production allows treatment of dry mouth in the process of treatment of the cancer. Jones et al[90] argued that free gastric transplantation exposes the patient to the risk of altered gastric motility as well as peptic ulceration of the flap. In addition, the limited diameter of the jejunum makes its use for larger defects a problem. Jones described free colon transplantation for resurfacing of the oral cavity. The donor tissue is abundant and capable of resurfacing large convoluted surfaces with thin, supple, mucus-secreting tissue that allows unimpaired tongue mobility, swallowing, speech, and denture wear, thus enabling a "functional" reconstruction.

It is intuitive that improved intraoral sensation, advantageous geometry, and mucus production will have a positive impact on intraoral function. Unfortunately, a direct relationship between postoperative function and these flap modifications cannot be assumed. Numerous other factors, such as the extent of resection and exposure to radiation therapy, affect the recovery of swallowing and speech. Evaluation of the true functional advantage of these modifications awaits the outcome of prospective blinded studies. Matched populations of patients with similar defects and reconstructions must be assessed by objective measurement of accepted parameters of functional outcome before the true value of these techniques is known.[81]

Oncologic

Early-stage squamous cell carcinoma of the oral cavity is often curable with surgery or radiotherapy. Unfortunately, the majority of patients present with advanced disease. Despite advances in combined-modality treatment, including wider resections enabled by better reconstructive techniques, the oncologic outcomes for these patients have not dramatically improved. Furthermore, patients cured of their initial early-stage head and neck cancers remain at high risk for development of a second primary tumor.

Spurred by discoveries in molecular biology, investigators are currently studying numerous modalities in the search for better ways to control and potentially to cure advanced local, regional, and metastatic disease. Multiple chemotherapeutic agents have been administered, singly and in combination, for adjuvant and neoadjuvant therapy.[91] Molecular radiosensitizers have been delivered in attempts to achieve larger differentials between the responses of tumors and normal tissues to radiation. Antibody-based therapy and gene therapy have been given in attempts to reverse tumorigenesis by blocking pathways that lead to tumor cell proliferation. Agents designed to inhibit tumor angiogenesis, invasion, and metastasis are under investigation.

Efforts to improve survival rates for patients "cured" of head and neck cancer have focused on prevention of new malignant tumors, the most important cause of mortality in patients with early-stage disease.[8,92] The high incidence of field cancerization, in which large areas of multicentric superficial premalignant and malignant change exist, makes prevention difficult. This "condemned mucosa" is extremely difficult to treat by conventional therapies because of the diffuse nature of the disease and the difficulty in defining the extent of the condition. One approach is chemoprevention,[92] the use of chemical agents to reverse, halt, or delay carcinogenesis. Another is photodynamic therapy,[93, 94] whereby a photosensitizing drug selectively localizes in tumors and leads to preferential tumor necrosis when the tissue is exposed to laser-generated light. Multiple studies demonstrate the effectiveness of photodynamic therapy for early superficial cancers of the mucosa of the upper aerodigestive tract. The technique allows relatively large affected areas to be treated with preservation of normal tissue and can be repeated as often as necessary. Further controlled studies will help elucidate the role of chemoprevention and photodynamic therapy in the treatment and prevention of head and neck cancer.

As better cancer treatments are identified, the requirements for reconstruction will change. The defects may be bigger, smaller, or nonexistent. The impact of radiotherapy, chemotherapy, and as yet unidentified modalities on the patient and the tissues will affect reconstructive choices. Reconstructions may even become carriers of anticancer therapy. As oncologic outcomes improve, the expectations of patients, now living long and full lives, will rise, and the importance of achieving functional and aesthetic reconstructions will only increase.

Quality of Life

Ultimately, the assessment of outcome of cancer treatment lies not with the health care provider but with the patient. More and more, investigators are considering the patient's quality of life in outcome assessment. Quality of life is a term used to describe the nontraditional outcome measures of functional status and psychosocial well-being. Quality of life is multidimensional and complex, and tools designed to measure it reflect the patient's view of the effectiveness of therapy.[95, 96]

Cancer-related disability, particularly in the head and neck region, affects all aspects of a patient's life. From a general health standpoint, the disease is chronic and often terminal. General health surveys, such as the Medical Outcomes Studies Short-Form 36 (SF-36)[97] and the Functional Assessment of Cancer Therapy (FACT) Scale,[98] measure conditions such as pain perception, energy level, feelings of nausea, depression, and ability to interact with others. A composite score is generated, and treatment efficacy is analyzed as it relates to physical, emotional, functional, and social well-being.

Disease-specific multiple-domain instruments have also been developed. In the patient with head and neck cancer, treatment may result in reduced ability to perform important activities of daily living and may involve gross disfigurement and secondary self-image problems. Methods such as the University of Washington Quality of Life Scale,[99] the FACT Head and Neck Subscale,[100] and the Performance Status Scale for Head and Neck Cancer[100] are designed to determine specific functional limitations resulting from the disease process. These scales attempt to measure the impact of speech and swallowing difficulties on the patient's ability to eat and communicate as well as the levels of physical and emotional discomfort resulting from treatment.

Evaluation of treatment outcomes by standard clinical trial endpoints can only be enhanced by the inclusion of quality of life assessment. The results of quality of life studies will add to our understanding of the impact of treatment, including reconstruction, and will help us refine our treatment choices to better serve our patients.

UNSOLVED PROBLEMS

Restoration of form, function, and quality of life after radical resection of the oral cavity remains an elusive goal. As improvements in reconstructive surgery happen, the expectations of patients and physicians alike adjust upward. We must see the flaws in our present reconstructive methods, and we must demand ever better results. Advances in the field of oncology may eventually come to pass that will change and possibly even eradicate the role of the reconstructive surgeon in the treatment of head and neck cancer. In the meantime, we must strive for better ways to restore oral function, and we must find better ways to measure function and quality of life so that we can demonstrate the value of our methods. We must look to tissue engineering to develop functional tissue constructs that will bypass the need for donor sites (and donor site morbidity) while yielding superior results. Finally, we must investigate ways in which the reconstructive method itself will contribute to the oncologic management of the patient.

REFERENCES

1. Hoffman HT, Karnell LH, Funk GF, et al: The National Cancer Data Base Report on Cancer of the Head and Neck. Arch Otolaryngol Head Neck Surg 1998;124:951.
2. Cawson RA, Binnie WH, Speight PM, et al: Metastases in the jaws and soft tissues. In Cawson RA, Binnie WH, Speight P, et al, eds: Lucas's Pathology of Tumors of the Oral Tissues, 5th ed. London, Churchill Livingstone, 1998:425.
3. Parkin DM, Pisani P, Ferlay J: Global cancer statistics. CA Cancer J Clin 1999;49:33.
4. Jemal A, Murray T, Samuels A, et al: Cancer Statistics, 2003. CA Cancer J Clin 2003;53:5.
5. Blair EA, Callender DL: Head and neck cancer. The Problem. Clin Plast Surg 1994;21:1.
6. Decker J, Goldstein JC: Risk factors in head and neck cancer. N Engl J Med 1982;306:1151.
7. Steinberg BM, DiLorenzo TP: A possible role for human papillomaviruses in head and neck cancer. Cancer Metastasis Rev 1996;15:91.
8. Spitz MR: Risk factors and genetic susceptibility. In Hong WK, Weber RS, eds: Head and Neck Cancer: Basic and Clinical Aspects. Boston, Kluwer Academic, 1995:73.
9. Bumpous JM, Snyderman CH: Nutritional considerations in patients with cancer of the head and neck. In Myers EN, Suen JY, eds: Cancer of the Head and Neck, 3rd ed. Philadelphia, WB Saunders, 1996:105.
10. Lippman SM, Clayman GL, Huber MH, et al: Biology and reversal of aerodigestive tract carcinogenesis. In Hong WK, Weber RS, eds: Head and Neck Cancer: Basic and Clinical Aspects. Boston, Kluwer Academic, 1995:89.
11. Hiatt JL, Gartner LP: The oral cavity, palate, and pharynx. In Hiatt JL, Gartner LP: Textbook of Head and Neck Anatomy, 2nd ed. Baltimore, Williams & Wilkins, 1987:31.
12. Williams PL, Warwick R: Splanchnology. In Williams PL, Warwick R: Gray's Anatomy, 36th British ed. Philadelphia, WB Saunders, 1980:1227.
13. Hiatt JL, Gartner LP: Palate, pharynx, and larynx. In Hiatt JL, Gartner LP: Textbook of Head and Neck Anatomy, 2nd ed. Baltimore, Williams & Wilkins, 1987:245.
14. Casper JK, Colton RH: Characteristics of alaryngeal and glossectomy speech. In Casper JK, Colton RH: Clinical Manual for Laryngectomy and Head/Neck Cancer Rehabilitation, 2nd ed. San Diego, Singular Publishing Group, 1998:157.
15. Reece GP, Kroll SS, Miller MJ, et al: Functional results after oropharyngeal reconstruction: a different perspective. Arch Otolaryngol Head Neck Surg 1999;125:474.
16. Panje WR: Immediate reconstruction of the oral cavity. In Thawley SE, Panje WR, eds: Comprehensive Management of Head and Neck Tumors, vol I. Philadelphia, WB Saunders, 1987:563.
17. Shah JP, Shemen LJ, Strong EW: Buccal mucosa, alveolus, retromolar trigone, floor of mouth, hard palate, and tongue tumors. In Thawley SE, Panje WR, eds: Comprehensive Management of Head and Neck Tumors, vol I. Philadelphia, WB Saunders, 1987:551.
18. Alvi A, Myers EN, Johnson JT: Cancer of the oral cavity. In Myers EN, Suen JY, eds: Cancer of the Head and Neck, 3rd ed. Philadelphia, WB Saunders, 1996:321.
19. Evans JH, Wright RF: Prosthetic rehabilitation. In Close LG, Larson DL, Shah JP, eds: Essentials of Head and Neck Oncology. New York, Thieme, 1998:356.
20. Davis BK, Roumanas ED, Nishimura RD: Prosthetic-surgical collaborations in the rehabilitation of patients with head and neck defects. Otolaryngol Clin North Am 1997;30:631.
21. Kroll SS, Robb GL, Miller MJ, et al: Reconstruction of posterior mandibular defects with soft tissue using the rectus abdominis free flap. Br J Plast Surg 1998;51:503.
22. Schramm VL, Myers EN: Skin grafts in oral cavity reconstruction. Arch Otolaryngol 1980;106:528.
23. Chambers RG, Jaques LD, Mahoney WD: Tongue flaps for intraoral reconstruction. Am J Surg 1969;118:783.
24. Druck NS, Lurton J: Repair of anterior floor of mouth defects: the island pedicle tongue flap. Laryngoscope 1978;88:1372.
25. Cohen IK, Edgerton MT: Transbuccal flaps for reconstruction of the floor of mouth. Plast Reconstr Surg 1971;48:8.
26. McGregor IA: Temporal flap in intraoral repair: its use in repairing the post-excisional defect. Br J Plast Surg 1963;16:318.
27. Lewis MB, Remensnyder JP: Forehead flap for reconstruction after ablative surgery for oral and oropharyngeal malignancy. Plast Reconstr Surg 1978;62:59.
28. Bradley P, Brockbank J: The temporalis muscle flap in oral reconstruction. J Maxillofac Surg 1981;9:139.
29. Pribaz J, Stephens W, Crespo L, et al: A new intraoral flap: facial artery musculomucosal (FAMM) flap. Plast Reconstr Surg 1992;90:421.
30. Bakamjian VY: A two-stage method for pharyngoesophageal reconstruction with a primary pectoral skin flap. Plast Reconstr Surg 1965;36:173.
31. Park JS, Sako K, Marchetta FC: Reconstructive experience with the medially based deltopectoral flap. Am J Surg 1974;128:548.
32. Ariyan S: One stage reconstruction for defects of the mouth using a sternomastoid myocutaneous flap. Plast Reconstr Surg 1979;63:618.
33. Parkash S, Ramakrishnan K, Ananthakrishnan N: Sternomastoid based island flap for lining after resection of oral carcinomas. Br J Plast Surg 1980;33:115.
34. Mathes SJ, Vasconez LO: The cervicohumeral flap. Plast Reconstr Surg 1978;61:7.
35. McCraw JB, Magee WP, Kalwaic H: Uses of the trapezius and sternomastoid myocutaneous flaps in head and neck reconstruction. Plast Reconstr Surg 1979;63:49.
36. Demergasso F, Piazza MV: Trapezius myocutaneous flap in reconstructive surgery for head and neck cancer: an original technique. Am J Surg 1979;138:533.
37. Quillen CG, Shearin JC Jr, Georgiade NG: Use of the latissimus dorsi myocutaneous island flap for reconstruction in the head and neck area. Plast Reconstr Surg 1978;62:113.
38. Barton FE Jr, Spicer TE, Byrd HS: Head and neck reconstruction with the latissimus dorsi myocutaneous flap: anatomic observations and report of 60 cases. Plast Reconstr Surg 1983;71:199.
39. Sabatier RE, Bakamjian VY: Transaxillary latissimus dorsi flap reconstruction in head and neck cancer. Limitations and refinements in 56 cases. Am J Surg 1985;150:427.
40. Davis JP, Nield DV, Garth RJ, et al: The latissimus dorsi flap in head and neck reconstructive surgery: a review of 121 procedures. Clin Otolaryngol 1992;17:487.
41. Ariyan S: The pectoralis major myocutaneous flap. A versatile flap for reconstruction in the head and neck. Plast Reconstr Surg 1979;63:73.
42. Stringer SP: Flaps and grafts for reconstruction. In Million RR, Cassisi NJ, eds: Management of Head and Neck Cancer: A Multidisciplinary Approach, 2nd ed. Philadelphia, JB Lippincott, 1994:157.
43. Ariyan S: Further experiences with the pectoralis major myocutaneous flap for the immediate repair of defects from excisions of head and neck cancer. Plast Reconstr Surg 1979;64:605.

44. Kroll SS, Goepfert H, Jones M, et al: Analysis of complications in 168 pectoralis major myocutaneous flaps used for head and neck reconstruction. Ann Plast Surg 1990;25:93.

45. Magee WP Jr, Gilbert DA, McInnis WD: Extended muscle and musculocutaneous flaps. Clin Plast Surg 1980;7:57.

46. Kroll SS, Reece GP, Miller MJ, et al: Comparison of the rectus abdominis free flap with the pectoralis major myocutaneous flap for reconstructions in the head and neck. Am J Surg 1992;164:615.

47. Futrell JW, Johns ME, Edgerton MT, et al: Platysma myocutaneous flap for intraoral reconstruction. Am J Surg 1978;136:504.

48. Hurwitz DJ, Rabson JA, Futrell JW: The anatomic basis for the platysma skin flap. Plast Reconstr Surg 1983;72:302.

49. Futrell JW, Rabson JA: Discussion of: Coleman JJ 3rd, Jurkiewicz MJ, Nahai F, et al: The platysma musculocutaneous flap: experience with 24 cases. Plast Reconstr Surg 1983;72:322.

50. McGuirt WF, Matthews BL, Brody JA, et al: Platysma myocutaneous flap: caveats reexamined. Laryngoscope 1991;101:1238.

51. Coleman JJ 3rd, Jurkiewicz MJ, Nahai F, et al: The platysma musculocutaneous flap: experience with 24 cases. Plast Reconstr Surg 1983;72:315.

52. Ruark DS, McClairen WC Jr, Schlehaider UK, et al: Head and neck reconstruction using the platysma myocutaneous flap. Am J Surg 1993;165:713.

53. Batchelor A: The oral cavity. In Soutar DS, Tiwari R, eds: Excision and Reconstruction in Head and Neck Cancer. Edinburgh, Churchill Livingstone, 1994:119.

54. Song R, Gao Y, Song Y, et al: The forearm flap. Clin Plast Surg 1982;9:21.

55. Yang G, Chen B, Gao Y: Forearm free skin flap transplantation. Nat Med J China 1981;61:139.

56. Soutar DS, Scheker LR, Tanner NS, et al: The radial forearm flap: a versatile method for intra-oral reconstruction. Br J Plast Surg 1983;36:1.

57. Strauch B, Yu H: Forearm region. In Strauch B, Yu H: Atlas of Microvascular Surgery: Anatomy and Operative Approaches. New York, Thieme, 1993:44.

58. Evans GR, Kroll SS: Intraoral soft tissue reconstruction. In Schusterman MA, ed: Microsurgical Reconstruction of the Cancer Patient. Philadelphia, Lippincott-Raven, 1997:13.

59. Evans GR, Schusterman MA, Kroll SS, et al: The radial forearm free flap for head and neck reconstruction: a review. Am J Surg 1994;168:446.

60. Webster HR, Robinson DW: The radial forearm flap without fascia and other refinements. Eur J Plast Surg 1995;18:11.

61. Chang SC, Miller G, Halbert CF, et al: Limiting donor site morbidity by suprafascial dissection of the radial forearm flap. Microsurgery 1996;17:136.

62. Lutz BS, Wei FC, Chang SC, et al: Donor site morbidity after suprafascial elevation of the radial forearm flap: a prospective study in 95 consecutive cases. Plast Reconstr Surg 1999;103:132.

63. Evans GR: The rectus abdominis flap. In Evans GR, ed: Operative Plastic Surgery. New York, McGraw-Hill, 2000:362.

64. Wenig BL, Keller AJ: Microvascular free-tissue transplantation with rigid internal fixation for reconstruction of the mandible following tumor resection. Otolaryngol Clin North Am 1987;20:621.

65. Strauch B, Yu H: Abdominal wall and cavity. In Strauch B, Yu H: Atlas of Microvascular Surgery: Anatomy and Operative Approaches. New York, Thieme, 1993:448.

66. Kroll SS, Baldwin BJ: Head and neck reconstruction with the rectus abdominis free flap. Clin Plast Surg 1994;21:97.

67. Baek SM: Two new cutaneous free flaps: the medial and lateral thigh flaps. Plast Reconstr Surg 1983;71:354.

68. Hayden RE: Lateral cutaneous thigh flap. In Baker SR, ed: Microvascular Reconstruction of the Head and Neck. New York, Churchill Livingstone, 1989:211.

69. Hayden RE: Lateral thigh flap. Otolaryngol Clin North Am 1994;27:1171.

70. Miller MJ, Reece GP, Marchi M, et al: Lateral thigh free flap in head and neck reconstruction. Plast Reconstr Surg 1995;96:334.

71. Amin AA, Baldwin BJ, Gurlek A, et al: Second free flaps in head and neck reconstruction. J Reconstr Microsurg 1998;14:365.

72. Kroll SS, Schusterman MA, Reece GP, et al: Timing of pedicle thrombosis and flap loss after free-tissue transfer. Plast Reconstr Surg 1996;98:1230.

73. Watkinson JC, Breach NM: Free flaps in head and neck reconstructive surgery: a review of 77 cases. Clin Otolaryngol 1991;16:350.

74. Urken ML, Weinberg H, Buchbinder D, et al: Microvascular free flaps in head and neck reconstruction. Report of 200 cases and review of complications. Arch Otolaryngol Head Neck Surg 1994;120:633.

75. Schusterman MA, Miller MJ, Reece GP, et al: A single center's experience with 308 free flaps for repair of head and neck cancer defects. Plast Reconstr Surg 1994;93:472.

76. Schusterman MA, Horndeski G: Analysis of the morbidity associated with immediate microvascular reconstruction in head and neck cancer patients. Head Neck 1991;13:51.

77. Boyd B, Mulholland S, Gullane P, et al: Reinnervated lateral antebrachial cutaneous neurosome flaps in oral reconstruction: are we making sense? Plast Reconstr Surg 1994;93:1350.

78. Marks SC: Surgical management of head and neck cancer. Hematol Oncol Clin North Am 1999;13:655.

79. Haughey BH: Tongue reconstruction: concepts and practice. Laryngoscope 1993;103:1132.

80. Salibian AH, Allison GR, Rappaport I, et al: Total and subtotal glossectomy: function after microvascular reconstruction. Plast Reconstr Surg 1990;85:513.

81. Hayden RE: Free flap transfer for restoration of sensation and lubrication to the reconstructed oral cavity and pharynx. Otolaryngol Clin North Am 1994;27:1185.

82. Hoppenreijs TJ, Freihofer HP, Brouns JJ, et al: Sensibility and cutaneous reinnervation of pectoralis major myocutaneous island flaps. A preliminary clinical report. J Craniomaxillofac Surg 1990;18:237.

83. Shindo ML, Sinha UK, Rice DH: Sensory recovery in noninnervated free flaps for head and neck reconstruction. Laryngoscope 1995;105:1290.

84. Hermanson A, Dalsgaard CJ, Arnander C, et al: Sensibility and cutaneous reinnervation in free flaps. Plast Reconstr Surg 1987;79:422.

85. David DJ: Use of an innervated deltopectoral flap for intraoral reconstruction. Plast Reconstr Surg 1977;60:377.

86. Franklin JD, Withers EH, Madden JJ, et al: Use of the free dorsalis pedis flap in head and neck repairs. Plast Reconstr Surg 1979;63:195.

87. Matloub HS, Larson DL, Kuhn JC, et al: Lateral arm free flap in oral cavity reconstruction: a functional evaluation. Head Neck 1989;11:205.

88. Urken ML, Weinberg H, Vickery C, et al: The neurofasciocutaneous radial forearm flap in head and neck reconstruction: a preliminary report. Laryngoscope 1990;100:161.

89. Kiyokawa K, Tai Y, Inoue Y, et al: Functional reconstruction of swallowing and articulation after total glossectomy without laryngectomy: money pouch–like reconstruction method using rectus abdominis myocutaneous flap. Plast Reconstr Surg 1999;104:2015.

90. Jones TR, Lee G, Emami B, et al: Free colon transfer for resurfacing large oral cavity defects. Plast Reconstr Surg 1995;96:1092.

91. Khattab J, Urba SG: Chemotherapy in head and neck cancer. Hematol Oncol Clin North Am 1999;13:753.

92. Papadimitrakopoulou VA: Carcinogenesis of head and neck cancer and the role of chemoprevention in its reversal. Curr Opin Oncol 2000;12:240.

93. Gluckman JL, Portugal LG: Photodynamic therapy for cancer of the head and neck. In Hong WK, Weber RS, eds: Head and Neck Cancer: Basic and Clinical Aspects. Boston, Kluwer Academic, 1995:159.

94. Biel MA: Photodynamic therapy and the treatment of head and neck neoplasia. Laryngoscope 1998;108:1259.
95. Deleyiannis FW, Weymuller EA: Quality of life in patients with head and neck cancer. In Myers EN, Suen JY, eds: Cancer of the Head and Neck, 3rd ed. Philadelphia, WB Saunders, 1996:904.
96. Terrell JE: Quality of life assessment in head and neck cancer patients. Hematol Oncol Clin North Am 1999;13:849.
97. Ware JE: SF-36 Health Survey: Manual and Interpretation Guide. Boston, The Health Institute, 1993.
98. Cella DF, Tulsky DS, Gray G, et al: The Functional Assessment of Cancer Therapy scale: development and validation of the general measure. J Clin Oncol 1993;11:570.
99. Hassan SJ, Weymuller EA: Assessment of quality of life in head and neck cancer patients. Head Neck 1993;15:485.
100. List MA, D'Antonio L, Cella DF, et al: The Performance Status Scale for Head and Neck Cancer Patients and the Functional Assessment of Cancer Therapy—Head and Neck Scale. A study of utility and validity. Cancer 1996;77:2294.

♦

Mandible Reconstruction

DAVID A. HIDALGO, MD ♦ JOSEPH J. DISA, MD

HISTORICAL REVIEW

ETIOLOGY OF MANDIBLE DEFECTS

CLASSIFICATION OF MANDIBLE DEFECTS

NONVASCULARIZED METHODS OF MANDIBLE
RECONSTRUCTION
    Nonvascularized Bone Grafts
    Prosthetic Plates and Regional Soft Tissue Flaps

REGIONAL OSTEOMUSCULOCUTANEOUS FLAPS

FREE FLAP MANDIBLE RECONSTRUCTION
    Donor Site Development and Evolution
    Flap Selection
    Donor Site Morbidity
    Graft Fixation Methods

PREOPERATIVE PREPARATION
    Systemic Risk Factor Screening
    Donor Site Studies
    Mandible Template Fabrication

OPERATIVE APPROACH TO FREE FLAP
RECONSTRUCTION
    Recipient Site Preparation
    Graft Shaping and Insetting
    Microvascular Considerations
    Postoperative Care

SPECIAL PROBLEMS
    Secondary Reconstruction
    Radiation and Reconstruction
    Pediatric Mandible Reconstruction

DENTAL RECONSTRUCTION
    Soft Tissue Procedures
    Osseointegrated Implants

FUNCTIONAL OUTCOME

HISTORICAL REVIEW

One of the most challenging problems faced by the reconstructive surgeon is the reconstruction of mandibular defects. Attempts at reconstruction of the mandible date to the late 1800s, when Martin[1] used a prosthetic appliance to replace a missing segment of mandible in 1889. Eight years later, Partsch[2] was able to restore the continuity of the mandible with a metal band. During the next 2 decades, various materials, such as silver wire, hard rubber, and ivory, were used to bridge gaps within the mandible.

The major advances in mandibular reconstruction occurred during the extensive clinical experience obtained from treatment of traumatic facial injuries in World Wars I and II. In addition, increasing experience during the 20th century with surgical treatment of tumors involving the mandible led to the development of modern-day mandibular reconstruction.

The first major advance in mandible reconstruction resulted from the development of bone grafting techniques for jaw defects. Initially, rib and tibia were used as a source of bone graft. However, Lindemann[3] in 1916 and Klapp[4] in 1917 recognized the superiority of cancellous bone. On the basis of

these observations, iliac bone became the preferred graft material.

In 1931, Ivy[5] recorded his results with immediate iliac bone grafting for a mandible defect; this graft is recorded to have remained intact and to have functioned well 38 years later. The superiority of iliac crest as a bone graft donor site is due to the presence of cancellous bone, as opposed to cortical bone grafts, which are merely acellular and a poor source of osteocytes. In addition, cancellous bone, particularly when it is fragmented, has a significant surface contact with the surrounding soft tissue, is much more cellular, and is rapidly revascularized.

During World War I, fixation of the bone graft was accomplished by rigid external support. Subsequently, during World War II, internal stabilization became favored. Converse[6] described use of a fenestrated metal tray to reconstruct the body of the mandible destroyed by a gunshot wound. The tray was made of fenestrated tantalum and was filled with fragmented bone graft. In a second stage, the tray was removed, and further iliac bone grafting was done to reinforce the reconstructed mandible. During the next 40 years, multiple combinations of prosthetic material and bone grafts were used to reconstruct the mandible. Boyne[7,8] described the use of a chromium-cobalt alloy crib to support cancellous bone grafts and to act as an internal splint. He subsequently described a titanium tray for the same purpose. Swanson,[9] in 1983, used a wire-reinforced silicone tray, but this was abandoned because of a high failure rate. Mandible reconstruction with use of titanium mesh trays and cancellous bone grafts after tumor resection was reported by Boyne and Zarem[10] in 1976 with an 88% success rate.

Leake and Rappoport[11] in 1972, Schwartz[12] in 1984, and Albert et al[13] in 1986 described the Dacron-urethane prosthesis as an alternative to metallic prosthesis. These authors described a success rate of more than 88% in developing solid functional mandibles. Despite a small number of successful reports of use of bone grafts for mandible reconstruction, failure of the reconstruction remained a problem. Nonvascularized bone grafts have a poor tolerance to infection, particularly when they are used to reconstruct defects after cancer surgery by an intraoral approach. In the setting of preoperative or postoperative irradiation, bone grafts generally do not revascularize and subsequently resorb. Although the addition of prosthetic trays provides better fixation for the bone graft while tissue ingrowth in neovascularization takes place, the failure rate of these devices remains high secondary to wound contamination from saliva and ultimate hardware exposure.

There are multiple reports of sterilization of a resected autogenous segment of mandible by freeze-drying techniques or irradiation. The theory is that the replaced, biologically inert mandible would serve as a scaffold for new bone growth. Despite encouraging preliminary reports, long-term results have been uniformly unsuccessful, and this procedure has been abandoned.[14-16]

Kellman and Gullane[17] have reported AO stainless steel plate reconstruction of mandibular defects for oropharyngeal malignant disease. The authors noted a 17% exposure rate in lateral mandibular reconstructions and a 48% exposure rate for anterior arch reconstruction. In an effort to improve the results of alloplastic mandibular replacement, Raveh[18,19] designed the titanium-coated hollow screw and reconstruction plate system (THORP). This system makes use of hollow screws so that new bone is actually incorporated into the prosthesis. Although the author reports an 85% success rate, the incidence of plate fracture and exposure remains high, especially in the setting of radiotherapy. In general, alloplasts in mandibular resections are advantageous as temporary spacing devices before definitive reconstruction with vascularized bone.

In the late 1980s, musculocutaneous flaps were introduced for head and neck reconstruction. Some of these flaps required an underlying bone segment based on the periosteal blood supply from the muscle.

Of note, pectoralis major flaps with associated rib, sternocleidomastoid with clavicle, trapezius with scapula, and temporalis muscle with parietal bone from the skull were used for mandibular reconstruction with marginal success.[20-23] These techniques largely suffered from the poor quality of local bone available for transfer, the unreliable blood supply to the bone segments, and a nonideal bone–soft tissue orientation. This resulted in less than ideal function and aesthetics.

At present, the "gold standard" for mandibular reconstruction is through the use of vascularized bone grafts transferred by microvascular technique. Reconstruction of a segmental defect of the mandible with vascularized bone allows primary healing, delivers well-vascularized tissue that is able to withstand adjuvant radiotherapy, and allows dental rehabilitation with osseointegrated implants. These factors result in optimal function and aesthetics, thus affecting the overall quality of life of patients requiring mandibular reconstruction.

Vascularized bone grafts were first reported in the late 1980s. The iliac crest became widely used, and a variety of other flaps, including the dorsalis pedis flap with the second metatarsal bone, the groin flap with the iliac crest, and the osteocutaneous scapula flap, were described.[24-27] The next echelon of osteocutaneous flaps for mandible reconstruction included the radial forearm and the fibula free flaps.[28,29] In the current era of microsurgery, vascularized bone transfer has become the technique of choice for mandible reconstruction with success rates of more than 96% and optimal functional and aesthetic outcome.

ETIOLOGY OF MANDIBLE DEFECTS

Segmental defects in the mandible can result from benign and malignant tumors as well as from trauma. Although trauma, such as that sustained after a motor vehicle accident, can contribute to segmental loss of mandible, it is more common for penetrating trauma, such as a high-velocity gunshot wound or a shotgun wound, to result in this problem. In this circumstance, immediate reconstruction with either a vascularized or a nonvascularized mandible substitute is rarely if ever performed primarily. Typically, the extent of soft tissue devascularization needs to be established before a definitive mandible reconstruction is performed. Multiple débridement procedures, fixation of remaining mandibular segments, and stabilization of a soft tissue injury are necessary before definitive reconstruction to minimize complications related to or loss of the reconstructed mandible.[30]

Reconstruction after resection of benign tumor, such as ameloblastoma and other odontogenic benign tumors, can be performed with either a vascularized or nonvascularized bone, depending on the location and size of the defect. Malignant tumors in the mandible often require adjuvant radiation therapy as part of the overall treatment plan. These tumors require a wider margin of resection and often involve soft tissue resection along with the bone.[31] Composite resection of the mandible for malignant disease typically includes resection of the associated soft tissues. Ideal reconstruction includes the use of vascularized bone and soft tissue to replace missing bone and lining. This technique will expedite healing and the subsequent use of adjuvant radiation therapy. Even though nonvascularized and prosthetic methods of mandible reconstruction can be considered for small, lateral segmental mandibular defects, the use of vascularized bone leads to the most rapid recovery and the best long-term results. The selection of donor site, the use of single or multiple flaps, and the method of reconstruction ultimately rest on experience with the various techniques, the amount of bone reconstruction required, and the amount of intraoral and extraoral soft tissue that needs to be replaced. The need for adjuvant radiation therapy or the desire for postoperative osseointegrated dental implants will affect the selection.

CLASSIFICATION OF MANDIBLE DEFECTS

There have been several classification schemes that categorize mandible defects. Some only classify the bone defect,[32] whereas another is more comprehensive by including a classification of the associated soft tissue defect.[33] The latter is complex because separate subcategorization of the soft tissue defect into tongue, mucosa, external skin, and neurologic components is proposed. The number of specific defects that can be described by this system is myriad. Although comprehensive, it may not ultimately prove practical to use for comparison of methods of reconstruction and their outcomes.

Defects of the mandible can be broadly grouped into anterior and lateral types on the basis of the predominant component of the defect. The simple system of Jewer et al[32] describes the various subtypes of anterior and lateral defects in a manner easy to visualize (Fig. 82-1). Lateral defects are given the designation L when the condyle is not included and H when it is. Central defects that include both canine teeth are termed C. Either single letters or a combination of letters can describe all defects. A defect that extends from the angle of the mandible across the midline as far as the opposite canine is termed an LC defect, for example. An angle-to-angle defect is termed LCL, and a complete hemimandible defect is H. Multiple possibilities can be described with this system. The extent of the bone loss alone does not correlate with functional or aesthetic results because almost any type or

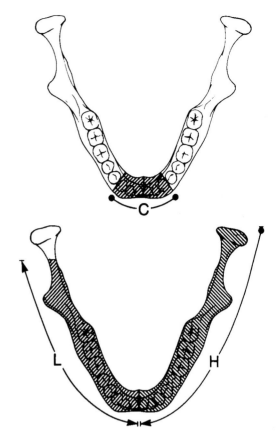

FIGURE 82-1. HCL classification system. This is based on reconstructive considerations rather than on classic anatomic landmarks. C represents the central segment of the mandible containing the canines and the incisor teeth. For C to be included in the designation, the whole segment must be present. L represents a lateral segment of any length that does not include the condyle. H is the same as L except that it includes the condyle. Letters are combined to describe various possibilities: LC, HC, LCL, and HCL. To this bone defect, the letters m, s, or ms can be added to signify an additional requirement for mucosa, skin, or both, respectively. (From Boyd J: Use of reconstruction plates in conjunction with soft-tissue free flaps for oromandibular reconstruction. Clin Plast Surg 1994; 21:72.)

length of bone defect can be reconstructed with great precision by current techniques.

The extent of soft tissue involvement is probably best categorized from a practical point of view as none (bone only), intraoral component, external component (skin), or combined intraoral and external defect. This has previously been described in conjunction with the HCL concept, and the authors proposed adding the letters o for bone only, m for mucosa, s for skin, and ms for combined soft tissue defects.[34] The functional and aesthetic results correlate most closely with the degree of soft tissue loss. Bone-only defects typically achieve excellent results, and combined mucosal and skin defects usually yield poor results. Defects with intraoral soft tissue loss usually achieve results in between, depending on the amount of soft tissue loss involved.

NONVASCULARIZED METHODS OF MANDIBLE RECONSTRUCTION
Nonvascularized Bone Grafts

The refinement of microsurgical technique combined with the availability of microsurgeons has led to the increased availability of vascularized bone reconstruction for mandible defects. As a result, nonvascularized methods of bone reconstruction are less popular. Any method of nonvascularized bone reconstruction relies on the surrounding soft tissue bed and adjacent mandibular ends to revascularize the graft. Angiogenesis into the bone graft will not occur in the absence of adequate blood supply in the surrounding tissues. Thus, pathologic conditions such as previous irradiation, extensive scar tissue from contamination, infection, prior surgery or trauma, and lack of soft tissue covering over the graft result in environments that are unfavorable to nonvascularized bone grafting.[35]

Indications for nonvascularized reconstruction are small defects, including the ramus or the body of the mandible; bone-only defects not requiring soft tissue reconstruction; defects resulting from resection of benign tumors; and defects resulting from treatment of mandibular fracture nonunions. Large defects and anterior defects are best treated with vascularized bone grafts.[36-38] Reconstruction of the mandible with nonvascularized bone grafts requires the use of autogenous bone and a method of graft fixation to the remaining native mandible. Cortical-cancellous iliac crest or rib is typically used for mandible reconstruction. The most popular method of stabilizing the autograft is with large titanium (or other metal composition) reconstruction plates, typically more than 2 mm in thickness. Rigid fixation is accomplished by use of AO principles, which recommend three or four screws on each side of the native mandible to rigidly fix the plate in place. Bone grafts are then fixed to the plate with similar screws.[39,40] Methods of grafting include block-type cortical-cancellous grafts; freeze-dried mandibular allografts, which are hollowed out and packed with particulate cancellous marrow; and cortical bone, such as rim or inner table ilium, in combination with densely packed particulate cancellous marrow.[35]

Another method of fixation of nonvascularized bone graft uses alloplastic trays. Titanium mesh trays packed with particulate cancellous marrow have been used successfully since 1976.[41] This method has resulted in a success rate of up to 88% in nonirradiated patients. However, graft failure approximates 50% in the setting of radiation therapy. The advantage of a titanium plate is its rigidity, reducing the need for mandibular immobilization. However, the ideal containment method for particulate cancellous marrow is one that ensures ideal mandibular shape, is biocompatible, and is resorbed after the graft heals. Freeze-dried allogeneic grafts of mandible or ilium are useful to meet these requirements. The grafts can be shaped into the desired size, fashioned into a porous tray to allow ingrowth of new bone, and densely packed with particulate cancellous marrow.[42]

Hyperbaric oxygen therapy in conjunction with nonvascularized bone grafts has been successful in the setting of irradiated recipient sites. Marx and colleagues have developed a protocol that uses preoperative and postoperative hyperbaric oxygen to improve the vascular bed in previously irradiated tissue.[43] The protocol involves the use of 20 sessions of hyperbaric oxygen at either 2.4 atmospheres of absolute pressure for 90 minutes or 2 atmospheres of pressure for 121 minutes per session before mandible reconstruction. This is then followed by 10 supplemental sessions after reconstruction. At 6 months, the patient is evaluated for possible revisional surgery, and if this is necessary, the patient will again undergo presurgical and postsurgical hyperbaric oxygen treatments.[44]

Indications for this technique in an era when vascularized mandibular reconstruction is readily available are questionable. Although success with this technique is demonstrated, there are clearly limitations, including accessibility to hyperbaric oxygen chambers, potential for aggravating active malignant disease, and specific medical contraindications (optic neuritis and immunosuppression). In addition, in the setting of inadequate soft tissue, a regional myocutaneous flap may be necessary to provide coverage of the graft. A well-planned vascularized bone transfer can accomplish all of these goals without the need for hyperbaric oxygen and provide the optimal mandible reconstruction.

Prosthetic Plates and Regional Soft Tissue Flaps

Classification of mandibular defects as previously described in this chapter is critical in selecting a plate method of mandibular reconstruction. By use of the HCL system of mandibular classification as described by Boyd, in which C represents the central segment of the mandible containing the canines and incisor teeth, L represents a lateral segment of any length of mandible excluding the condyle, and H is the same as L but includes the condyle,[34] mandibular defects can be based on reconstructive difficulty rather than on anatomic landmarks. A prospective evaluation of patients undergoing plate and flap reconstruction of mandible defects showed an overall failure rate requiring plate removal of 20%. Careful analysis demonstrated a failure rate of 35% for the central segment, whereas it was only 5% for a lateral defect (H or C).[45] Given the success of free tissue transplantation for mandibular reconstruction, plate and soft tissue flap should be limited to lateral or posterior defects in patients who are not otherwise candidates for vascularized mandibular reconstruction.

Several good options for plate reconstruction of the mandible exist. Traditional AO reconstruction plates are readily available. These were initially made of stainless steel but are now more commonly made of composite metals such as titanium or Vitallium. Plate thicknesses greater than 2.5 mm are typically used for this purpose. Three or four screws on either side of the native mandible are necessary for rigid fixation.[39] Another option includes the use of titanium hollow screw reconstructive plates (THORP). The hollow screws used in this system allow ingrowth of bone to lock each screw in place permanently. With use of the THORP system, rigidity does not rely on compression of the plate against the mandible, but rather each screw head is fixed to the plate by means of expansion bolts.[46] Titanium locking plates, in which the receptive holes in the plates are threaded to allow double-threaded screws to attach the plate to the bone and the screw to the plate, have most recently been introduced. These plates potentially represent an advance over the THORP system.

There are several principles in regard to shaping of the reconstruction plate. In the setting of immediate reconstruction when the tumor has not violated the outer cortex of the mandible, the plate should be shaped against the native mandible before resection. If possible, drill holes placed in the native mandible on either side of the segment to be resected will allow accurate fixation of the plate to maintain the exact shape of the remaining mandible. The plate is aligned along the lower border of the mandible to maintain facial height, to avoid tooth roots, and to keep it away from the oral mucosa. If the plate is used in the setting of delayed reconstruction or in situations in which tumor or trauma has violated the native shape of the mandible, the plate can be fashioned by use of a prefabricated template as described later.

When there is not adequate soft tissue to cover the reconstruction plate, it should be covered by a soft tissue flap. Boyd and colleagues have popularized the use of radial forearm free tissue transplantation in conjunction with the reconstruction plate. For lateral or posterior segment reconstruction, Boyd reports a 96% success rate.[47] The advantages of this technique include an excellent aesthetic and functional result with minimal donor site disability when it is used for specific indications, including lateral and posterior low-volume defects in debilitated elderly patients and those patients with poor prognoses. The major recognized weakness in this system is the tendency toward plate fracture, plate loosening, or plate exposure through the skin. When a free tissue transplantation is not available or not desirable, other regional soft tissue flaps can be used to cover the plate, such as a pectoralis major musculocutaneous flap, trapezius musculocutaneous flap, or latissimus musculocutaneous flap. All of these methods of reconstruction avoid the need for free tissue transfer; however, the flaps suffer from excessive bulk, limitations in arc of rotation, disturbances in shoulder function, and lack of reliability of the skin island, particularly when a random segment of skin attached to muscle is necessary. Several modifications of the pectoralis major flap have been made to deal with these problems: vertically oriented parasternal skin island, which tends to be less bulky than traditional skin islands; two-stage procedure with prefabrication of a skin-grafted muscle that is subsequently transferred; extension of the skin island to include the rectus fascia for more cephalad defects; and resection of the medial portion of the clavicle to add length to the flap.[48-50]

Although it is technically simple to harvest, the latissimus dorsi musculocutaneous flap is limited in head and neck reconstruction for several reasons. The skin island is unreliable because it is designed over the distal aspect of the muscle, which is necessary for transfer to the head and neck region. Most authors agree that it is safer to transplant the latissimus dorsi flap as a free flap. The pedicle can be compressed or twisted as it is tunneled between the pectoralis major and minor muscles, which may lead to flap compromise.[51]

The trapezius musculocutaneous flap can be used to cover the reconstruction plate as well. The skin island is designed over the acromioclavicular joint, and the flap is carried on the transverse cervical artery. The skin island designed over the proximal muscle segment is based on the superficial (ascending) branch of the transverse cervical artery; the deep (descending) neurovascular branch is divided so the flap can reach the oropharynx. Advantages of this flap include its proximity to the operative field and the thin, pliable skin of the proximal deltoid area. Disadvantages include the variable origin of the superficial branch of the artery and an undependable venous drainage system. Previous neck dissection or irradiation may make this donor site unusable.[52-54]

Another regional flap described in mandible reconstruction is the sternocleidomastoid flap. This flap is most reliable when it is based on the occipital artery. At least partial flap loss has been described in up to 50% of patients when this flap is used. The advantages of the sternocleidomastoid flap include ease of elevation and location within the head and neck region. The disadvantages of this flap include the loss of protection of the great vessels, the contraindication to use in the setting of a clinically positive neck on the ipsilateral side, the contour deformity, and the unreliable skin island.[55]

The platysma musculocutaneous flap has also been described for oromandibular coverage. Experience with this flap is limited. The thinness and pliability of the muscle skin paddle make it ideal for reconstruction in the oral cavity with negligible functional impairment. However, in the setting of previous irradiation to the neck, this flap is unreliable. Skin loss has been described in up to 30% of patients, thus limiting its utility.[56]

REGIONAL OSTEOMUSCULOCUTANEOUS FLAPS

Reconstruction of the mandible gradually evolved from free bone grafts to tubed osteocutaneous skin flaps, then to osteomusculocutaneous flaps, then most recently to free flaps. Tubed osteocutaneous flaps using the medial portion of the clavicle were developed to improve the viability of free bone grafts. This technique tubed a skin flap around a segment of clavicle and transferred it to the mandibular defect in stages. Bone viability with this technique as measured by tetracycline uptake was demonstrated to be superior to that seen with free bone grafts.[57] These flaps were used with some success clinically, although disadvantages included shoulder instability problems, the need for staged procedures, and a limited amount of bone.

Osteomusculocutaneous flaps based on a sternomastoid, pectoralis major, or trapezius muscle carrier were next described.[21,22,58-61] The advantages were single-stage transfer and insetting based on the muscle carrier and improved bone vascularity. Although one study demonstrated improved bone survival with use of sternum instead of rib attached to a pectoralis pedicle, a portion of the fifth or sixth rib has been a more popular clinical option when the pectoralis muscle is selected as a carrier.[62] The trapezius muscle can be used to transfer a portion of the spine of the scapula measuring as much as 10 to 14 cm in length. Advantages of pedicled osteomusculocutaneous flaps are marginal and few compared with currently available free flap alternatives: a contiguous donor site, possibly less operating time, and no requirement for microvascular anastomoses.

Pectoralis and trapezius flaps are the best remaining choices today, but both are rarely indicated. Disadvantages include the limited amount of bone that can be included with the muscle carrier, poor vascularity of the bone segment due to its tenuous vascular supply at the end of the flap, limited insetting flexibility imposed by muscle tethering, unwanted soft tissue bulk due to the muscle pedicle, absence of a reliable skin component, and potential for increased morbidity at the surgical site due to a contiguous donor

site. The proposed advantage of avoiding a microvascular anastomosis by selecting a local flap does not offset the many disadvantages enumerated. It also overlooks the many advantages of free tissue transplantation, including the ability to provide not only the required tissue types in adequate amounts but also tissue having ideal characteristics to satisfy the specific defect requirements.

Pedicled osteomusculocutaneous flaps have a limited role in mandible reconstruction today. The trapezius flap with scapula may be used for short lateral mandible defects when microvascular capability either is not available or has failed in one or more previous attempts. It has been successfully used to reconstruct longer bone defects, but this is not recommended given the superiority of free flap alternatives.[63] The pectoralis flap with rib could be used in similar circumstances for a limited anterior mandible defect (Fig. 82-2).[64]

FREE FLAP MANDIBLE RECONSTRUCTION

Donor Site Development and Evolution

The first attempts to reconstruct segmental mandible defects with vascularized bone used either rib flaps or groin flaps with attached ilium.[65-68] Rib grafts were harvested with an anterior blood supply from the internal mammary vessels, by a posterolateral approach using the intercostal arteries, or in a more complicated posterior dissection that included the nutrient artery to the bone together with the intercostal arteries.[69,70] It became evident that periosteal circulation alone was sufficient to maintain bone viability and that the anterior approach was the most favorable because the patient could be positioned supine. Obtaining greater length of the internal mammary vessels can lengthen the pedicle, but this increases the chest wall defect. An alternative approach of harvesting either serratus anterior muscle or latissimus dorsi muscle with rib based on the thoracodorsal vessels has also been reported but not widely used.[71,72] Use of the rib provides adequate bone length, but the dissection with all approaches is tedious; chest tube drainage is usually required postoperatively, and segmental osteotomy of the rib to simulate mandible shape compromises graft blood supply. Moreover, the bone is thin and would not likely support osseointegrated implants. Although inclusion of a skin island with the rib has been described, it never became popular.[73] Proximity of the chest to the head and neck area and the potential for compromised pulmonary function postoperatively due to pain are other unfavorable characteristics leading to the adoption of other donor sites. Use of the groin flap with attached ilium presents difficulties owing to the short vascular pedicle of the flap and the marginal

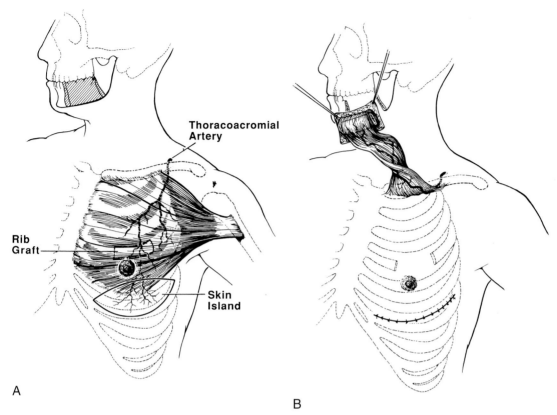

FIGURE 82-2. Pectoralis major osteomusculocutaneous flap. *A*, Design of the flap. Note the rib and skin island components and the thoracoacromial pedicle. *B*, Transfer of the flap. (From McCarthy JG, Kawamoto H, Grayson BH, et al: Surgery of the jaws. In McCarthy JG, ed: Plastic Surgery. Philadelphia, WB Saunders, 1990:1188.)

blood supply to the bone. Both the rib and the groin flap donor sites are no longer appropriate choices for clinical use.

Another early donor site developed for free flap reconstruction of the mandible is the second metatarsal and toe.[74-76] The bone component can be raised with a thin, pliable skin island and the dorsalis pedis vessels. This development was an improvement over the rib in that flap dissection is easier, the vascular pedicle is of large diameter and abundant length, the donor site is distant from the head and neck area, and the skin island is reliable, large, and thin. The aesthetic compromise of the foot is considerable because of the requirement for skin graft closure and the narrowing of the foot from second ray deletion. In addition, the bone stock is not uniform in thickness, and the articulation of the toe joints may or may not be ideally located for optimal application at the recipient site. These limitations and the subsequent development of better donor sites have relegated the second metatarsal to a minor role in mandible reconstruction.

Use of the ilium based on the deep circumflex iliac artery represented the first major advance in free flap mandible reconstruction. It remains the workhorse flap today in many centers. Taylor[24,77] was the first to

recognize the superiority of the deep circumflex iliac artery in providing robust blood supply to the bone compared with previous attempts to use the superficial circumflex iliac artery by the groin flap. This vessel is a branch of the external iliac artery just proximal to the inguinal ligament. It courses toward the anterior superior iliac spine and bifurcates into an ascending branch that supplies the overlying skin and a continuation of the main vessel along the inner aspect of the ilium.[78] The blood supply is not truly segmental as it is in the case of the fibula, and long segments of harvested bone have less blood supply at the distal end of the graft. However, this has not proved to constitute a significant limitation clinically.

This donor site offers bone of maximum thickness and height and is second only to the fibula in the amount of usable length, with as much as 14 to 16 cm available (Fig. 82-3). It accommodates osseointegrated implants easily. The ilium has an intrinsic shape that contains within it a replica of a hemimandible oriented upside-down. The anterior superior iliac spine represents the angle of the mandible, and the iliac crest represents the body. The portion of bone between the anterior superior iliac spine and the anterior inferior iliac spine represents the ramus. The curve of the bone

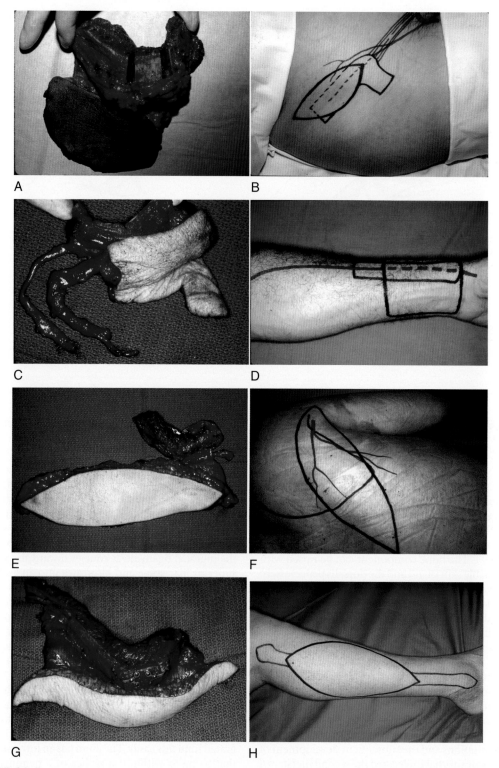

FIGURE 82-3. Free flap donor sites. *A,* Ilium. Tall, thick bone stock and the adjacent skin island are shown. *B,* The ilium donor site. The inguinal ligament and course of the deep circumflex iliac artery are shown. *C,* Radius. The pedicle is long and of large diameter, the skin is thin and pliable, and the bone is thin. *D,* The radius donor site. *E,* Scapula. The bone and large skin island are shown independent of one another, with the pedicle seen projecting to the right in between. *F,* The scapula donor site. *G,* Fibula. The pedicle is shown in the upper left, the long anterior-type defect graft in the middle with portions of the flexor hallucis longus muscle visible on either side, and the skin island below. *H,* The fibula donor site is shown with a large skin island that will need skin graft closure.

makes the ipsilateral hip the proper choice for reconstructing a lateral mandible defect. The design can also be reversed with respect to the portion that represents the ramus and body, but this provides less overall graft length.[79] Whereas this similarity in bone shape between the mandible and ilium is convenient, the ilium graft does not precisely duplicate the mandible shape. Other donor site choices can actually produce more accurate mandible shapes by means of carefully planned osteotomies. Anterior defects can be reconstructed by use of a multiply osteotomized segment of the iliac crest portion of the bone.

The skin island overlying the ilium tends to be bulky and not very mobile. This makes it difficult to position intraorally. Moreover, the blood supply is often tenuous given that the primary supply arises from the superficial circumflex iliac artery. It is not practical to isolate the superficial circumflex iliac artery for anastomosis in addition to the deep circumflex iliac artery, although this has been reported.[80] Some authors have proposed either using a second free flap taken from the radial forearm for the skin component or harvesting a portion of the internal oblique muscle to use as intraoral lining.[81,82] Use of a second flap provides the ideal combination of tissue (ample bone and thin skin) but obviously complicates the procedure by having two separate donor site wounds and two sets of anastomoses to perform. Use of the internal oblique muscle can provide reliable tissue for intraoral mucosal replacement, but this practice enlarges the donor site defect considerably, complicates the dissection, and can contribute to abdominal wall laxity problems. Despite these limitations, the ilium remains a popular choice for mandible reconstruction.[81,83,84]

The radial forearm donor site was first developed as a skin free flap before use as an osteocutaneous free flap for mandible reconstruction.[85] The thin, pliable, mostly hairless nature of the forearm skin was recognized as an ideal replacement material for oral mucosa.[86,87] Up to 10 cm of split radius can be included with the overlying skin for mandible reconstruction. The amount of bone length available is limited to the portion lying between the insertions of the pronator teres muscle proximally and the brachioradialis muscle distally.[88] The thickness of the bone is limited to one cortex because at least 60% of its circumference must remain intact to prevent postoperative fracture, the worst donor site complication that can occur with this site. The flap can also include the palmaris longus muscle and tendon, although there is rarely a need for this tissue. The skin portion of the flap can also be innervated because it contains the anterior branches of the medial and lateral antebrachial cutaneous nerves.

The forearm flap is based on the radial artery, its venae comitantes, and the cephalic vein. The artery can be followed proximally between the brachioradialis and flexor carpi radialis muscles to obtain a long pedicle (see Fig. 82-3). Several small branches of the artery supply the bone in a random fashion. When the cephalic vein is used with the artery, the pedicle vessels have a relatively large diameter that facilitates performance of the microvascular anastomoses. The radial artery does not need to be reconstructed. A normal Allen test result is a prerequisite for use of this donor site.

The donor site must be closed with a skin graft. It is therefore important to leave the paratenon intact over the flexor carpi radialis and any other tendons that may be exposed during the course of flap dissection.

The outstanding qualities of this donor site include its location, which allows a two-team approach to resection and reconstruction; its ideal skin island; its long pedicle of large-diameter vessels; and its ease of dissection. Its disadvantages include the poor quality and limited length of the bone it provides, its lack of substantial soft tissue bulk when this quality is needed, its requirement for skin graft closure of the donor site, and the generally poor appearance of the donor site. Despite these limitations, this donor site has been used successfully to reconstruct composite defects of the mandible.[89]

The scapula donor site was first described as a skin free flap based on the cutaneous branches of the circumflex scapular artery.[90-92] The circumflex scapular artery is a branch of the subscapular artery that approaches the lateral border of the scapula and supplies the periosteum of the bone and adjacent muscles. Its cutaneous branch traverses the triangular space bounded by the teres major, teres minor, and long head of the triceps to supply the overlying skin.[93] The cutaneous branch divides into transverse and descending branches that allow the skin island design to be oriented in either direction. The lateral border of the scapula including its tip can be harvested as a free flap together with a skin island that can measure as long as 30 cm (see Fig. 82-3). The maximum length of bone that can be obtained ranges from 10 to 14 cm.[94] Although the bone tends to be thin, it is able to accommodate osseointegrated implants. The bone does not have a segmental blood supply, so the distal portions of the bone have marginal blood supply when multiple osteotomies are performed in a long graft.

An advantage of this donor site is that there is great flexibility in insetting of the skin island because it is not attached directly to the bone. Moreover, it is possible to design two separate skin islands or to harvest the bone with both a skin island and a muscle flap if the thoracodorsal artery is included in the pedicle. This enables the latissimus dorsi muscle either with or without skin to be included with the flap. No other donor site offers as much associated soft tissue in one flap or greater insetting flexibility of the soft tissue component. The primary disadvantage of this donor site is its location on the back. Use of this donor site for mandible reconstruction requires changing the patient's position several times and does not allow a simultaneous two-team approach to resection and reconstruction. The posterior donor site location has greatly limited its popularity. A less important disadvantage is that the skin island is thick compared with other alternatives, such as the forearm skin.

The fibula was first recognized as a vascularized bone graft donor site for long bone reconstruction in 1975.[95] It was found to be ideally suited to replace segmental defects of the radius, ulna, humerus, and femur as a "double-barrel" graft.[96-100] It was subsequently adapted to mandibular reconstruction when it was demonstrated that the bone could be safely osteotomized multiple times to simulate the subtle nuances of mandible shape.[101]

The fibula has up to 25 cm of useful length, enough to reconstruct any mandible defect. It has a consistent shape throughout its length, which makes it the ideal bone stock for duplicating mandible shape.[102] It has a robust segmental blood supply by the large-diameter peroneal artery that parallels the course of the bone and can allow it to function as a flow-through flap to supply a second free flap in tandem. This segmental blood supply allows the bone to be osteotomized as many times as necessary to reproduce mandible shape accurately. The osteotomized segments can be as short as 1 cm and survive completely. The fibula has adequate dimensions to support the use of osseointegrated implants.[103]

The bone can be harvested to include the flexor hallucis longus muscle. This muscle can be sacrificed without significant functional deficit at the donor site. It is conveniently located on the graft to fill in the submental soft tissue defect that typically accompanies mandible resection. Another advantage of this donor site is its distant location from the head and neck area. Although flap dissection was originally described from a posterior approach, the lateral approach is more popular and allows a simultaneous two-team approach to resection and reconstruction.[104]

The fibula can be harvested with a skin island based on a septocutaneous blood supply (see Fig. 82-3).[105,106] Initial reports were somewhat skeptical about the reliability of the skin vascularity, but subsequent investigation and experience demonstrated that the skin island is reliable in more than 90% of patients.[107] It has become established that the skin island blood supply is most reliable when the skin island is designed over the distal half of the leg because most of the septocutaneous vessels reach the skin in this area.[108] Whereas it was previously reported that inclusion of a significant cuff of muscle was important to ensure adequate blood supply to the skin, later reports confirmed the general perception that the skin island can be harvested with a reliable blood supply based on the septocutaneous supply alone.[109,110] Rarely, when vascularity is in doubt, it is possible to preserve the musculocutaneous branches until adequate septocutaneous supply is confirmed. The musculocutaneous perforators require intramuscular dissection and may prove to arise from the anterior tibial vessels and not the peroneal vessels. This can complicate the graft revascularization process.[111] This problem occurs only when the septum appears to be completely devoid of vessels or when the skin island is designed proximally on the leg. The former situation is unusual and the latter can be avoided. Harvesting a longer segment of bone and preserving maximum septum length even after shortening of the bone can contribute to the maximum preservation of septocutaneous blood supply.[112] In any event, large skin islands can be reliably harvested with the fibula, although those wider than 6 cm typically require skin graft closure of the donor site. More recent developments in skin island technology include restoration of sensation by neural anastomosis of the lateral sural cutaneous nerve contained within the skin island and separation of the skin island into two independent parts for improved insetting flexibility.[113,114] Although the skin island of the fibula is thicker than that of the forearm, it works well for both mucosal and external skin replacement.

The fibula has great flexibility in terms of design. The ipsilateral leg is usually chosen for a lateral mandible defect. The angle of the mandible is positioned where the peroneal artery enters the bone. This maximizes pedicle length. Anterior reconstructions have the design shifted farther down the bone to effectively lengthen the pedicle. When the contralateral neck vessels will be used for anastomosis, the contralateral leg is chosen. In this case, the design is shifted to the most distal part of the bone to lengthen the pedicle maximally (Fig. 82-4).

There are few disadvantages of the fibula donor site. Skin island viability problems are rare. Patients who have peroneal artery–dominant legs are not candidates for use of the fibula.

Flap Selection

Each of the donor sites described has characteristics that render it more or less useful in flap selection to address specific problems in mandible reconstruction (Table 82-1). The outstanding qualities of the fibula donor site make it the first choice for the majority of mandible defects, particularly the anterior type. Other donor sites are far less commonly indicated. However, there are specific instances when an alternative choice may be superior (Table 82-2).[115,116] A large posterior intraoral soft tissue defect that includes the lateral pharyngeal wall, the tonsillar pillars, and portions of the soft palate in conjunction with a short defect of the

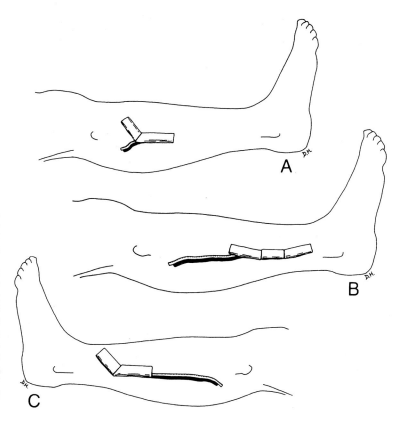

FIGURE 82-4. *A*, The bone design for a right hemimandible graft is shown drawn on the right leg. Note that the angle of the mandible graft is positioned at the point where the pedicle approximates the fibula. *B*, The bone design for an anterior graft requiring only partial right body replacement is shown drawn on the right leg. Note that the graft is shifted distally to increase pedicle length. *C*, The bone design for a right hemimandible graft, in which the left-side neck vessels will be used, is shown drawn on the left leg. (From Hidalgo DA: Free flap mandibular reconstruction. Clin Plast Surg 1994;21:25.)

TABLE 82-1 ✦ COMPARISON OF FREE FLAP DONOR SITES FOR MANDIBLE RECONSTRUCTION*

Donor Site	Tissue Characteristics			Donor Site Characteristics	
	Bone	*Skin*	*Pedicle*	*Location*	*Morbidity*
Fibula	A	C	B	A	A
Ilium	B	D	D	B	C
Scapula	C	B	C	D	B
Radius	D	A	A	C	D

*Flaps are rated best to worst, A to D.
Revised from Cordeiro PG, Hidalgo DA: Conceptual considerations in mandibular reconstructions. Clin Plast Surg 1995;22:61.

TABLE 82-2 ✦ ALGORITHM FOR FLAP SELECTION

	Tissue Defect Type		
	Bone Only	*Bone + Skin or Mucosa*	*Bone + Skin + Mucosa*
First choice	Fibula	Fibula	Fibula + skin free flap*
Second choice	Ilium	Radial forearm†	Scapula

*Either radial forearm fasciocutaneous or rectus abdominis myocutaneous flap.
†Only for lateral defect with small bone component.

ramus and adjacent body is an ideal situation for selection of the radius donor site. The thin pliable skin island is optimal for resurfacing an area such as this. The small amount of unicortical bone available still permits restoration of bone continuity with a single osteotomy. There is no concern for the adequacy of thin radius bone to accept osseointegrated implants because they are rarely necessary in the region of the molar teeth posteriorly.[117] The radius donor site should not be used for anterior reconstruction because of the paucity of both bone and soft tissue bulk it provides. Patients with anterior defects reconstructed with the radius often appear tissue deficient postoperatively, having a hollow submental contour due to soft tissue deficiency and a poorly supported lower lip due to inadequate bone thickness.

The scapula is a reasonable choice when the soft tissue component of the defect is massive and the bone defect, even if it is substantial, is mostly of secondary concern because of the scope of the wound closure problem itself. The abundant size of the skin island available with this flap permits closure of complex soft tissue defects that possess both intraoral and skin components. The massive nature of these defects usually includes partial loss of facial nerve function, and these patients have an obvious skin patch visible. These limiting aesthetic issues and the generally poor prognosis associated with massive defects usually obviate any concern about the thickness and sometimes bulky nature of the back skin. The scapula is the best choice for a lateral bone defect with a mucosal replacement requirement *and* a sternomastoid defect associated with a concomitant radical neck dissection. The latissimus dorsi muscle can be harvested on a common pedicle with the scapula flap in this situation and used to replace the sternomastoid muscle. Neck contour is thereby restored. This application is rare in occurrence.

The ilium is not indicated for anterior defects because it possesses no clear advantage compared with other choices. It is a secondary choice for lateral defects. Its fixed shape, nonsegmental blood supply, problematic skin island, and donor site morbidity potential are important restrictive factors. The ilium constitutes a reasonable choice in the rare case in which the fibula is not available as an option.

There are occasions when two free flaps used simultaneously provide the best solution. This occurs in the case of massive defects in which there is substantial loss of bone and a large volume of soft tissue including both skin and intraoral mucosa. Whereas the scapula donor site alone can solve many of these problems, the bone quality and location of this donor site make it less appealing than the alternative of using two separate flaps that have ideal tissue characteristics and donor site location. The fibula is most often combined with the radial forearm fasciocutaneous flap for this application. The fibula provides the ideal bone

stock, and the skin island from the forearm provides the best quality skin including the potential for sensory reinnervation. The distant donor site location for each makes simultaneous flap harvest by two teams convenient. This is also important to minimize the increased operative time required for a double flap approach. Either the fibula or forearm skin can be used internally or externally in these cases, depending on the specific defect. The rectus abdominis musculocutaneous flap can be used together with the fibula when there is a particularly large volume soft tissue defect. Other combinations of flaps have been reported, including fibula–rectus femoris, fibula–tensor fascia lata, iliac crest–radial forearm, and iliac crest–tensor fascia lata.[118]

Separate neck recipient vessels for each flap can be used, or one flap with flow-through characteristics (fibula, radial forearm) can provide recipient vessels for the second flap. "Piggyback" technique increases the possibility of loss of both flaps but may prove necessary when there is a paucity of suitable ipsilateral or contralateral recipient vessels in the neck because of previous surgery, irradiation, or both. A skin island on the second flap provides a convenient means of monitoring both flaps.[119]

Donor Site Morbidity

Donor site morbidity in free flap reconstruction has the potential for accurate study because the donor site is remote from the primary wound. An early study of 300 consecutive patients showed an overall morbidity rate of 20%, with secondary procedures required in 7.7% and major complications occurring in 2.3%.[120] Some of the recommendations by the authors to reduce morbidity included avoidance of excessive tension during closure, careful retraction of adjacent structures, obtaining complete hemostasis, and closure of the wound immediately after pedicle division.

Additional studies of morbidity have focused on specific donor sites. Most attention has been focused on the fibula, one of the most popular donor sites used for mandible reconstruction. Acute morbidity associated with this donor site is low and includes incomplete skin graft (large skin islands), infection (usually skin-grafted patients), hematoma, and discomfort with early ambulation. The most significant morbidity occurs in patients requiring skin graft closure because of harvest of a large skin island. As many as half experience delayed healing of the donor site, although this delay seldom results in the need for additional surgery.[121]

Long-term morbidity of the fibula donor site has been well studied. A decrease in ankle flexion and extension up to 29% has been demonstrated, consistent with the muscles affected by harvest of the fibula. Ankle inversion and eversion were shown to be affected in one study but not in another.[122,123] Strength is measurably decreased in the donor leg, and disturbances in gait with abnormal load transmission have also been demonstrated.[124] Despite measurable findings, these studies have also reported that the clinical impact of decreased ankle function is minimal.

Although significant long-term symptoms are unusual with the fibula donor site, as many as one of three patients may experience minor symptoms. These include mild discomfort and edema usually associated with prolonged standing or extensive ambulation, hypesthesia in the distribution of either the superficial or deep peroneal nerve, and mild ankle instability. The majority of patients experience loss of hallux flexion, but this too appears to be of little practical concern.

The radius donor site has the potential for significant morbidity if fracture should occur. The incidence of postoperative fracture was reported to be as high as 15% in one study.[125] Management of this complication often requires open reduction with internal fixation and an iliac bone graft. Some fractures can be managed with cast immobilization alone. Use of a keel-shaped (beveled) osteotomy technique appears to reduce the likelihood of fracture.[126,127] However, one study demonstrated only a 5% benefit to use of this technique, and bone strength and resistance to torque loads were reduced more than 70% by removal of as little as one quarter of the bone depth.[128] Avoidance of fracture is largely dependent on careful longitudinal osteotomy of the bone such that adequate structural rigidity remains, use of a different donor site in elderly women with decreased bone density, and adequate postoperative immobilization. Compromised range of motion of the wrist can occur after fracture.

Soft tissue problems with the radius donor site include incomplete skin graft take, numbness in the radial nerve distribution, and poor aesthetics.[89] Minor tendon exposure can occur in as many as one third of patients. The site of tendon exposure almost always heals uneventfully without the need for secondary surgery. The issue of poor aesthetics is due to the exposed location of the distal volar forearm and the requirement of a skin graft to achieve wound closure. Whereas there have been suggestions to shift the design of the skin island more to the ulnar aspect of the forearm or to use tissue expanders for removal of the skin graft secondarily, neither option is practical or completely effective in improving aesthetics.[129]

Morbidity associated with the scapula donor site includes wide scars that may hypertrophy, seromas, and decreased shoulder range of motion. Poor scars are largely unavoidable owing to the nature of back skin and because large skin islands place the wound under a considerable amount of tension. Avoidance of seromas requires that drains be left in for as long as 3 weeks. Compromised range of motion of the shoulder can occur when the maximum amount of scapula border is harvested. This possibility is even greater if the latissimus dorsi muscle is included as a second flap (with contiguous blood supply); this option is useful to reconstruct a sternomastoid muscle defect resulting from a concomitant radical neck dissection. Compromised range of motion can be minimized with a program of postoperative physical therapy.[94]

The ilium donor site is associated with contour deformities when large portions of bone have been harvested, although it is possible to minimize this problem by harvesting only the inner cortex of the bone. There are also problems with delayed ambulation due to pain, long-term gait disturbance, possible damage to the lateral femoral cutaneous nerve or femoral nerve itself, and, rarely, hernia formation.[130] Delayed ambulation in frail, elderly patients due to pain can lead to systemic complications such as pneumonia and pulmonary embolism. Attenuation of the lateral abdominal wall can also occur, causing a significant bulge without hernia formation. The potential for abdominal wall problems increases when portions of the internal oblique muscle are included with the flap.[82] Avoidance of abdominal wall structural problems requires meticulous closure of the donor site by experienced personnel. Prosthetic mesh may be required to provide adequate strength to the closure.

Other donor sites are rarely used. Donor site morbidity with use of vascularized rib has not been well documented. There is the potential for compromised pulmonary function postoperatively due to splinting and possibly a post-thoracotomy type pain syndrome. Donor site morbidity with the metatarsal has been cited as low, but no report has studied postoperative gait in detail. Distal sensory deficits can be expected.

Graft Fixation Methods

Before the advent of free flap mandible reconstruction, patients were commonly restored secondarily. Biphase external fixators were popular in these patients and were placed at the time of resection by the ablative surgeon. These fixators consisted of at least two threaded bars screwed into the mandible on each side of the segment planned for resection. Their opposite ends pierced the skin and were attached to a bar connecting the two sides. The resection was then performed with this bar in place. The bar was replaced with an acrylic substitute at the conclusion of the procedure. This method of fixation, although crude, served to stabilize the floating segments in a relatively normal anatomic position (Fig. 82-5). This technique was intended to prevent collapse of the lower face due to wound contraction forces and presumably to facilitate a later reconstructive effort. These devices today are largely obsolete given that most mandible

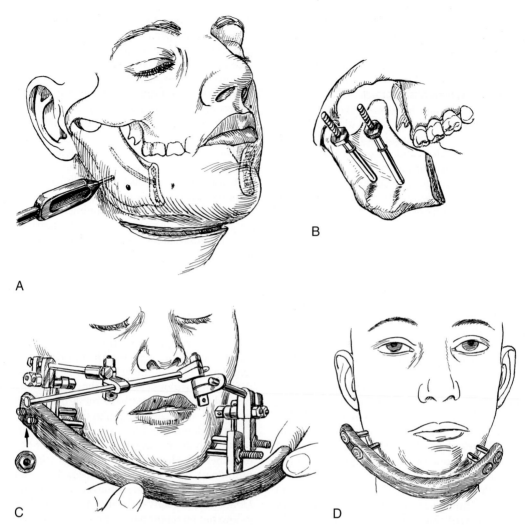

FIGURE 82-5. The biphase external fixation appliance. *A*, Drill holes are made percutaneously. *B*, The bone screws are threaded into position. *C*, An acrylic bar is fashioned to replace the temporary connecting bar hardware. *D*, The completed external fixation in place. (From McCarthy JG, Kawamoto H, Grayson BH, et al: Surgery of the jaws. In McCarthy JG, ed: Plastic Surgery. Philadelphia, WB Saunders, 1990:1188.)

reconstructions are performed as a primary procedure.

Early fixation of multiply osteotomized free flaps for mandible reconstruction used interosseous wires. This method was effective even though establishment of adequate resistance to torsional stress across multiple osteotomies could be a problem. The method was tedious and lacked precision. Kirschner wires were sometimes used as an adjunct to interosseous wire fixation.

Today, fixation hardware includes both reconstruction plates and miniplates. These two types of hardware involve different approaches to the graft shaping process. Reconstruction plates of either the AO or titanium hollow screw (THORP) type are first shaped to the mandible before resection.[131,132] The

specimen is then removed, and the shaped plate is used as a template to shape the bone graft. The bone graft is osteotomized, and the individual segments are fixed to the plate. The ends of the reconstruction plate are longer than the graft to allow fixation to the native mandible on each end. Miniplates, in contrast, are used to span a single osteotomy and allow the graft shaping process to continue sequentially from one segment to the next. Miniplate hardware is simplified by relying on only a few different plate shapes and by using self-tapping screws of various lengths (Fig. 82-6).

Both methods provide adequate rigidity, although reconstruction plates add unnecessary bulk to the outer surface of the bone graft that is particularly noticeable in anterior reconstructions. Reconstruction plates may also prove more difficult to remove later if

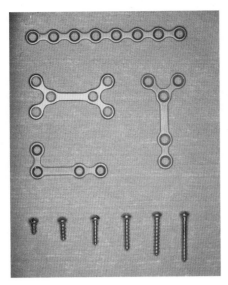

FIGURE 82-6. Miniplate fixation systems are simple. Only a few plate styles and screw sizes are required. (From Hidalgo D: Refinements in mandible reconstruction. Operative Techniques Plast Reconstr Surg 1996;3:257.)

necessary either to eliminate infection or in preparation for dental reconstruction. Reconstruction plates achieved a bone union rate of 95% and miniplates 99%.[133,134] It is clear that mandible fixation does not require compression for normal healing to occur.

Complications due to fixation are surprisingly rare given the nature of the oral wound environment and the length of time the wound is open during surgery. Potential problems include infection, which may result in either hardware exposure or possibly the development of an orocutaneous fistula. Hardware that becomes exposed intraorally or involved in infection is not removed until clinical union of the bone is demonstrated. It may take 6 weeks or more until the plates can be removed without adversely affecting stability. The development of osteomyelitis is very rare in the absence of radiation therapy. Nonunion and plate fractures are other unusual complications that may require additional surgery.

Portions of hardware placed for fixation must often be removed before the placement of osseointegrated implants. This usually requires only removal of screws that traverse the sites proposed for implant placement. This is performed as a minor secondary procedure after the graft demonstrates clinical union. On occasion, hardware may exhibit impending extrusion of the skin along the inferior border of the mandible when miniplates are used. The miniplates can be removed when it is convenient given the low propensity for infection in this setting.

Intermaxillary fixation plays an important adjunctive role in mandible reconstruction. Patients with lateral defects are placed into fixation before graft insetting so that preoperative occlusion is preserved. This practice also decreases errors in graft shaping and thereby contributes to improved aesthetic results. Intermaxillary fixation is not usually helpful in the case of anterior reconstructions because there are usually few teeth available on the lateral segments to allow use of the technique. Intermaxillary fixation is typically released after insetting is complete, although arch bars are usually left in place postoperatively. Patients who have a condyle graft are usually maintained in intermaxillary fixation for at least 1 week postoperatively. This allows the condyle graft to become stabilized in the glenoid fossa.

PREOPERATIVE PREPARATION
Systemic Risk Factor Screening

Preoperative preparation of the patient undergoing mandible resection is based on a multidisciplinary team approach. It includes head and neck surgeons, reconstructive surgeons, radiation oncologists, pathologists, maxillofacial prosthodontists, speech and occupational therapists, internists, psychologists, and social workers.[135] Preparation begins with the history and physical examination to define the extent of disease, to identify other relevant medical problems, to assess nutritional status, to study donor sites, and to evaluate the recipient site for potential vascular problems. It continues with biopsy, panendoscopy, and radiologic studies that include computed tomographic or magnetic resonance scans, chest radiography, and Panorex study. The scans precisely define the anatomic boundaries of local disease as well as assess regional lymph node status. They serve as an important guide for planning surgical resection. Other essential steps in preoperative preparation include screening studies to detect underlying cardiopulmonary and liver disease, dental consultation, and specific studies of the donor site when indicated.

Dental consultation before surgery is important for optimal planning of dental reconstruction. It allows impressions and models to be made and enables the dentist or oral surgeon to anticipate an intraoperative request to provide intermaxillary fixation during the reconstructive procedure. Dental rehabilitation may entail one or more operative procedures after successful mandibular reconstruction; this includes selective removal of fixation hardware and placement of osseointegrated implants.

Cardiopulmonary disease, overt or subclinical, is the leading cause of serious perioperative morbidity in patients undergoing mandible reconstruction. A cardiac stress test and pulmonary function studies should be strongly considered for any patient older than 45 years and are mandatory for patients with preexisting cardiopulmonary disease. Whereas results of these studies rarely constitute an absolute contraindication to surgery for a serious oncologic condition, they can contribute to optimal intraoperative and postoperative management when significant problems are identified and quantified beforehand.

Most mandible reconstruction procedures are limited in their invasiveness to more superficial portions of the body. They are less disturbing from a physiologic point of view compared with general surgical procedures that involve major body cavities, for example. As such, the primary risks to patients undergoing mandible reconstruction are prolonged anesthesia and, to a lesser degree, blood loss. Fluid shifts are usually not major and are generally easy to monitor and correct.

Donor Site Studies

Donor site studies are rarely needed and are donor site specific. The scapula donor site does not need preoperative study. The forearm donor site usually requires only an Allen test to establish the adequacy of collateral circulation. The deep circumflex iliac artery of the ilium donor site does not require angiography. The fibula donor site does not require angiography if pedal pulses are normal and there are no stigmata of peripheral vascular disease evident.[136] There is one congenital anomaly that must be ruled out if pulses are abnormal in either a healthy young patient or an older patient without other evidence of peripheral vascular disease. This is the rare condition in which the peroneal artery is dominant and both the anterior and posterior tibial arteries are more vestigial structures. Harvest of the fibula in a peroneal artery–dominant patient can result in distal ischemia. Angiography should be performed when this condition is suspected. Awareness of this condition will either suggest use of a different donor site or require a plan to reconstruct the peroneal artery with a vein graft.

Mandible Template Fabrication

Mandible templates are useful devices for assisting in accurate graft shaping while the graft is left attached at the donor site, a practice that minimizes graft ischemia time during the procedure.[107] Although the surgical specimen provides key information for the graft shaping process, templates provide an accurate model of the bone in a single dimension and facilitate the graft shaping process. A lateral cephalogram, for example, provides a replica of the lateral view of the mandible. Either the radiograph itself can be cut out and sterilized or the pattern can be traced on a thin piece of acrylic plastic, which is then cut out and used as a more durable template. A transverse cut from a computed tomographic or magnetic resonance

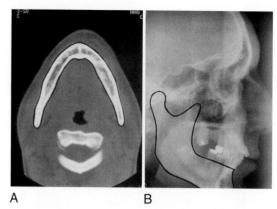

FIGURE 82-7. Mandible templates. *A,* A computed tomographic scan section below the tooth roots and magnified to 1:1 ratio is the basis for fabrication of a template in the transverse plane. *B,* A lateral cephalogram is used to fabricate a lateral template. Templates can be made out of either thin acrylic plastic or x-ray film on the basis of these studies. These templates are useful for both anterior and lateral reconstructions. (From Hidalgo D: Refinements in mandible reconstruction. Operative Techniques Plast Reconstr Surg 1996;3:257.)

imaging scan of the mandible taken below the tooth root level and reproduced at 1:1 scale allows fabrication of a template showing the curve of the inferior border of the mandible (Fig. 82-7). The lateral and inferior view templates are used together to assist in the graft shaping process described later.

OPERATIVE APPROACH TO FREE FLAP RECONSTRUCTION
Recipient Site Preparation

Preparation of the recipient site for free tissue transfer begins after the mandibulectomy has been performed. Ideally, the vessels in the ipsilateral neck are used as recipient vessels. When this is not possible because of previous resection or when prior surgery, irradiation, or severe peripheral vascular disease renders them unusable, the contralateral neck vessels are used. When it is present, the internal jugular vein is prepared by circumferentially dissecting it to allow vascular control for an end-to-side anastomosis with the flap vessels. If preserved, branches of the internal jugular veins, such as the common facial vein, can be used in an end-to-end fashion for the microvascular anastomosis. The external jugular vein can also be used and anastomosed end-to-end with the flap vein when it is available. The external jugular vein is ideally left attached to the lower neck skin flap to prevent injury during neck dissection. Branches of the external carotid artery are typically used to provide inflow to the free flap. The superior thyroid artery is the first major branch of the external carotid artery. This vessel, along with the facial artery and lingual artery, is easily exposed. The facial artery is commonly divided distally during neck dissection, and a more proximal segment can be used as a recipient vessel. Division of the digastric muscle at its midpoint with preservation of the underlying hypoglossal nerve will expose the facial and lingual arteries. These vessels typically loop under the hypoglossal nerve, which runs from the skull base between the internal and external carotid artery. Depending on the local anatomy, the facial artery can be left looping under the hypoglossal nerve or dissected free and brought over the top of it. Ideally, two recipient arteries and two recipient veins are identified before the free flap is rendered ischemic to ensure adequate inflow and venous drainage at the free flap while simultaneously minimizing ischemia time. End-to-side anastomosis between the flap artery and the external carotid artery is also a viable alternative to an end-to-end anastomosis with one of the branches of the external carotid artery.

Preparation of two arterial inflow sites will obviate the need to dissect an additional recipient site artery while the flap is ischemic; preparation of two venous recipient sites will allow anastomosis of multiple veins to drain the flap. With proper preoperative planning and flap design, the need for vein grafts is rare.[115,137]

Either subsequent to or before recipient vessel preparation, the recipient bed is prepared for insetting before division of the flap pedicle in transfer of the shaped graft to the head. This occurs by partially closing the deepest aspect of the oral wound while exposure to this area is ideal. The ends of the native mandible are prepared by exposing enough bone to allow room for plate fixation. If necessary, the mandibular ends can be step cut with removal of one or more teeth to improve the gingival closure. If the oral cavity is not adequately closed, contamination of the fixation hardware will occur, and this may lead to an orocutaneous fistula. In the setting of adequate lower dentition, after segmental mandibular resection, maxillomandibular fixation with arch bars and elastic bands is performed before insetting of the graft. This maneuver allows the neomandible to be fixated with the native mandible in its appropriate anatomic location, thus maintaining optimal occlusion after reconstruction.[102]

Graft Shaping and Insetting

Mandible defects are grouped into two types for graft shaping purposes: anterior and lateral. Anterior defects include the bone segment between the canine teeth and usually a portion of the adjacent mandible body on one or both sides. Lateral defects include a variable portion of the ramus and body and may extend as far as the symphysis in the case of a hemimandible defect. Many defects have elements of both types, but one predominates for purposes of graft shaping.

The bone of all commonly used donor sites can be safely transected completely at each planned osteotomy site. "Greenstick" fractures do not have a role in mandible reconstruction. Osteotomies must be done with care for all graft types because circulation to the most distal bone segments is maintained by soft tissue attachments alone. These soft tissue attachments are tenuous in the case of the radius, scapula, and ilium. The fibula has an excellent blood supply throughout the length of the graft because the peroneal artery parallels the course of the bone.

Graft shaping is aided greatly in primary cases by having the surgical specimen available for measurement and study of the nuances of its shape. Most osteotomy sites require angulation in more than one plane to reproduce a precisely shaped substitute for the resected portion of the mandible.[102] A "no-touch" method of handling the specimen is mandatory.

The lateral template assists in accurate reproduction of the angle formed between the ramus and body. It also assists in determination of the correct length of the ramus and body segments of the graft in conjunction with measurements taken directly from the surgical specimen. The inferior template helps determine the proper curve of the body segment in a lateral graft and the correct splay angle that the body segments make with the anterior segment in the case of an anterior graft.

The most important goal in graft shaping is accurate reproduction of the contour of the inferior aspect of the mandible.[107] Graft height is less important given that most donor sites have bone of adequate dimension to support the placement of osseointegrated implants. These implants form the foundation for dental prostheses that are able to compensate for any deficiency in graft height.

ANTERIOR GRAFTS

Anterior grafts consist of a central segment attached to a lateral segment on each side. This design type minimizes the number of osteotomies necessary to reproduce the curve of the anterior mandible accurately. There is in fact no advantage to a graft design that has an osteotomy corresponding in location to the mandible symphysis. The small amount of projection lost by having an anterior segment that spans the midline is of no clinical significance. The anterior segment usually measures 2 cm in length.

The first step in graft shaping is proper location of the anterior segment along the length of the donor site bone. Its position is determined by pedicle considerations. The pedicle must comfortably reach the region of the angle of the mandible when the graft is finished and inset. The graft design is therefore shifted

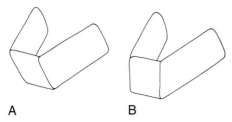

FIGURE 82-8. The anterior graft central segment should *not* be oriented in the same plane as the body segments during graft fabrication *(A)*. It should be oriented instead in a vertical plane to allow proper placement of osseointegrated implants later *(B)*.

along the length of the bone to the appropriate location that yields adequate pedicle length. The fibula has the most versatility in this regard compared with other donor sites.

The osteotomy performed on each end of the anterior segment must be angled correctly in two planes because the body segments diverge away in both a backward and upward direction from the anterior segment. Correct determination of these two angles will keep the anterior face of the anterior segment parallel to a coronal plane, a necessary requirement for proper orientation of osseointegrated implants placed at a later date (Fig. 82-8). The osteotomies at each end of the anterior segment must be identical in both planes. Lack of osteotomy symmetry can result in asymmetric divergence of the body segments backward, a twist to the mandible, or both. Both the lateral and inferior templates assist in determining the proper angles of the osteotomies.

Graft segments are fixed with miniplates placed in perpendicular planes at each osteotomy site for maximum rigidity. Plates are placed on the anterior

surface of the anterior segment to first fix the angle between this segment and each of the body segments. The contour of the inferior surface is then checked with the template for accuracy. A plate is then placed along the inferior border of the anterior segment spanning both osteotomies (Fig. 82-9*A*).

Measurements taken from the surgical specimen help ensure accuracy (Fig. 82-9*B*). The measurement between the ends of the body segments on the specimen reflects the angle of divergence of the body segments. This must be accurately reproduced in the graft (Fig. 82-9*B*, measurement D). The graft ends are purposely left long as it is shaped at the donor site. Osteotomy of the body segments to determine their final length (Fig. 82-9*B*, measurements B and C) is done during insetting. The angle of the resection osteotomy on each end of the specimen is observed for reference during insetting.

Insetting of anterior grafts is often more challenging than insetting of lateral grafts because the remaining mandible is a less stable platform to work with compared with the typical lateral defect, in which the remaining native mandible can be secured in place with intermaxillary fixation (Fig. 82-10). There is commonly a lack of adequate dentition on the lateral mandibular segments to permit the use of intermaxillary fixation. The nonstabilized lateral segments can contribute to insetting errors because they can move freely in many directions. The only stable landmarks for reference are often the midline and the curve of the maxillary arch. Possible anterior graft insetting errors include prognathism, retrognathia, excessive lower facial height or inadequate lower facial height, and twisting or canting of the mandible when it is viewed from the front. Insetting is often partly intuitive, and experience therefore plays an important role in determining the accuracy of insetting. The inferior

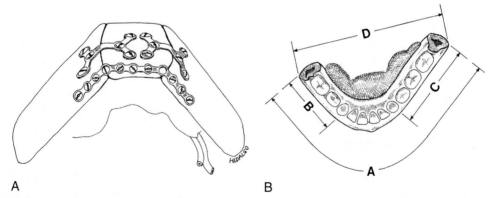

FIGURE 82-9. *A,* The anterior graft shows the central segment fixed to body segments with two plates spanning each osteotomy for maximum stability against torsional stress. *B,* Anterior defect grafts typically have different body segment lengths B and C. Measurement D is determined by both the splay angle of the body segments away from the central segment and the individual body segment lengths. This important reference should not be overlooked during graft fabrication.

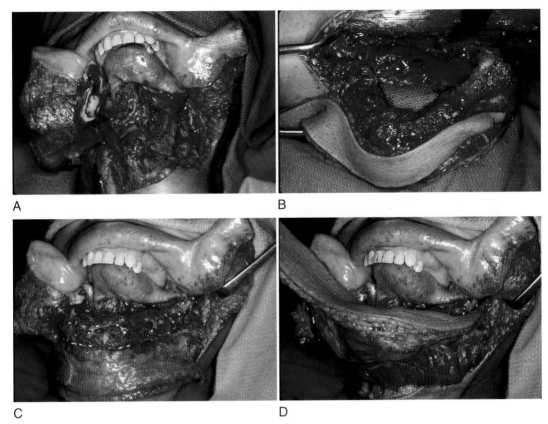

A   B

C   D

FIGURE 82-10. A typical anterior defect. *A,* Reflected skin flaps reveal extent of resection. The ends of the lateral mandible segments are seen. Note absence of the anterior floor of mouth and submental musculature. *B,* A fibula graft with a long narrow skin island is shown. The graft has been shaped and fixed with miniplates while still attached to the leg. *C,* The bone portion of the graft has been inset. The skin island hangs at its inferior edge. *D,* The skin island is being inset to replace the anterior floor of the mouth before final wound closure. Note the flexor hallucis longus muscle that will be used to fill in the submental dead space.

template is a key adjunct in this process. Miniplates are placed across the body osteotomies and also along the inferior border of the mandible to complete the insetting process (Fig. 82-11).

LATERAL GRAFTS

Lateral grafts are planned along the length of the donor site bone in such a way that pedicle length is maximized when the graft is complete. This plan uses the same principle advocated for anterior graft design. The fibula donor site has the greatest versatility in planning graft location along its length. The ipsilateral leg is selected for lateral or hemimandibular defects in the typical case in which the ipsilateral neck vessels are available for microvascular anastomoses. However, the opposite leg is selected in the unusual circumstance in which adequate ipsilateral neck vessels are not present. The graft design is shifted distally to allow lengthening of the pedicle to reach the opposite side of the neck. The body segment is located proximal to the ramus segment on the fibula (which will be angled anteriorly) so that the associated flap soft tissues will come to lie in the submental area, as they do in the more common case when the ipsilateral leg is selected. The forearm donor site has no limitations in this regard. The scapula and ilium are less versatile choices when the opposite-side neck vessels are required for microvascular anastomoses; vein grafts may be required when either of these two donor sites is selected.

The first step in shaping the lateral graft is to locate the site of the angle of the mandible on the donor site bone. The lateral template is used to help determine the angle of the two osteotomies needed to form the correct angle between the ramus and body segments of the graft. Bisecting its angle marks the template. The template is then aligned with the graft along its ramus component and then along its body component, marking the bone in reference to the mark on the template each time. This method defines a wedge-shaped piece of bone that, when it is removed,

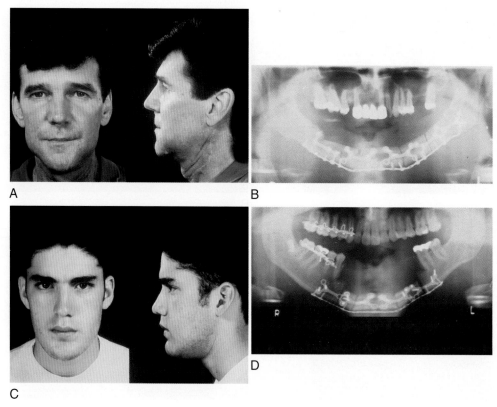

FIGURE 82-11. *A,* Postoperative views of an anterior reconstruction. *B,* Postoperative Panorex. *C,* Postoperative views of an anterior reconstruction. *D,* Postoperative Panorex. (From Hidalgo DA: Free flap mandibular reconstruction. Clin Plast Surg 1994;21:25.)

establishes the correct angle on the graft (Fig. 82-12). The specimen is checked to note the small angle at which the ramus diverges away from the body in a coronal plane. This is duplicated on the graft as the angle is formed. A miniplate is placed on the lateral surface of the graft, and a second straight plate is placed along the inferior border of the graft (Fig. 82-13).

The ramus defect is typically partial length. Its extent is measured on the specimen and precisely duplicated on the graft. When resection is planned high on the ramus, it is usually best to disarticulate the mandible specimen because fixation of a graft with a long ramus component is technically difficult when only a short condyle-containing segment remains in situ. Several

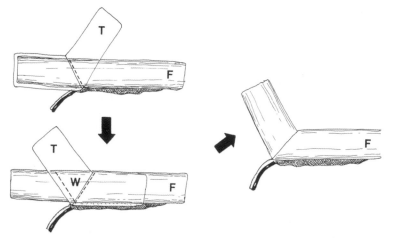

FIGURE 82-12. Template-guided osteotomy design. A plastic template (T) for lateral graft fabrication is positioned parallel to the fibula, and the angle of the template is marked on the bone *(top)*. The template is then rotated so that its other end is now parallel to the bone, and the angle is again marked. This determines the wedge (W) of bone necessary to remove for the angle of the mandible to be reproduced with precision *(bottom)*. The wedge is then removed, and the graft ends are folded together *(right)*.

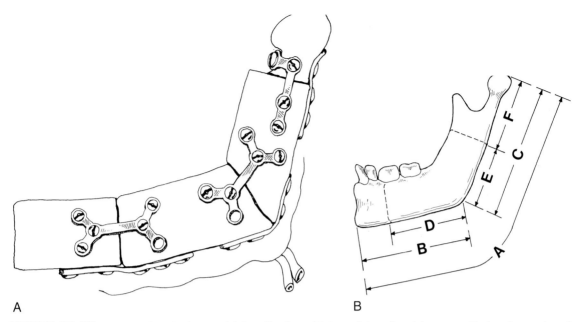

FIGURE 82-13. *A,* Lateral graft shows miniplate fixation with two plates placed in perpendicular planes at each osteotomy site. *B,* Lateral defect graft measurements D and E must be accurate to restore overall lengths B and C to normal.

options then exist for management of the condyle defect. The graft ramus can be left short as one alternative, leaving a gap where the condyle used to be. A second option is to duplicate the total length of the ramus including the condyle. The end of the graft is rounded to approximate the shape of the condyle. Aesthetic and functional results with use of these two methods have not been well studied. Prosthetic condyles are available as another option. However, they are not patient specific in design, and their long-term compatibility with the soft tissues of the glenoid fossa is unknown. Perhaps the best option is to transplant the native condyle as a nonvascularized graft onto the proximal end of the mandible graft. This method allows accurate restoration of posterior facial height and preserves tandem temporomandibular joint function. The condyle segment should contain a small portion of the ramus to facilitate fixation to the graft with miniplates (Fig. 82-14). The total posterior height of the mandible (see Fig. 82-13B, measurement C) is measured on the specimen before harvesting of the condyle. The correct total length of the ramus with the condyle graft must match the original measurement.

The transplanted condyle has been demonstrated to survive intact for at least 10 years in some patients and to degrade with time in others.[138] However, despite these differences, use of the condyle as a nonvascularized graft has not resulted in pain, temporomandibular joint syndrome symptoms, infection, ankylosis, or trismus.[134]

The condyle segment can be considered for use only if it can be established to be free of disease. Analysis of bone scrapings is neither practical nor of proven reliability. If any doubt exists as to the proximal extent of disease, the condyle segment should not be harvested from the specimen for use.

The body segment of a lateral graft usually requires an osteotomy to establish the proper curve. The inferior template helps determine the best site of the osteotomy as well as the correct angle. The body osteotomy must sometimes be angled in two planes at the osteotomy site. The lateral template provides useful information in this regard by showing whether the body segment is straight or angulated either slightly upward or downward on the lateral view. Miniplates are placed along the external surface of the graft and along its inferior border to stabilize the osteotomy (see Fig. 82-13A). The end of the body segment is purposely left long. The final osteotomy that determines overall graft length is best made during the insetting process.

Insetting of the lateral graft is greatly assisted by first stabilizing the remaining native mandible with intermaxillary fixation. This ensures maintenance of preoperative occlusion and facilitates accurate determination of overall graft length.

The most important spatial relationship to establish with precision in insetting of the lateral graft, assuming an accurate graft shape to begin with, is the angle of the mandible in three dimensions. The angle

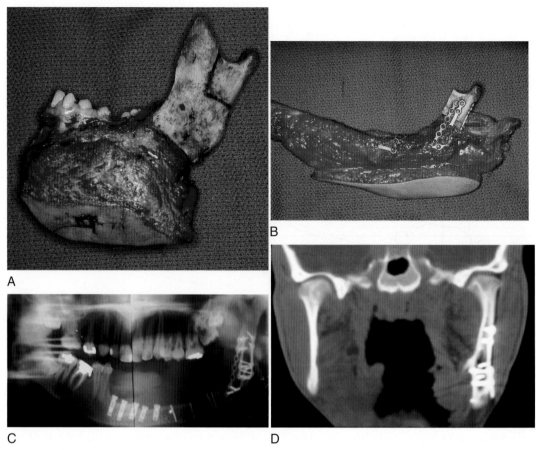

FIGURE 82-14. Condyle transplantation. *A,* Surgical specimen showing a tumor of the mandible body with adjacent soft tissue including skin. The condyle segment is shown marked for resection. *B,* The condyle graft is shown mounted to the fibula free flap that has just been separated from the donor site. *C,* Panorex study at 3 years shows condyle graft appearing intact. *D,* Computed tomographic scan at 3 years confirms complete survival of condyle graft.

must be located an equivalent distance from the midline in a sagittal plane compared with the opposite (normal) side, otherwise the facial contour will have either a bowed out or collapsed appearance, depending on the nature of the error. The angle must also be located in the same transverse plane as the normal side or the facial contour will be uneven from the front view, with one side being either lower or higher than the other.[139] Errors in the transverse plane are largely avoided by accurate graft shaping that establishes an equivalent posterior height of the mandible on both sides. Insetting with intermaxillary fixation in place aids in determining the correct overall graft length. This helps avoid an error in locating the angle of the mandible either too far anteriorly or posteriorly in relation to the opposite side.

The condyle end of the graft, if it is present, is inset into the glenoid fossa first. It is not necessary to attempt to close the joint capsule because the exposure is difficult and the benefit unproven. Miniplates are placed along the external surface and inferior border of the ramus end of the graft to fix it to the condyle segment when it has been left in situ.

The final step in the insetting process is the osteotomy and fixation of the anterior end of the graft. The curved transverse plane template is helpful in determining the precise location and angle of the osteotomy on the graft. The graft is then fixed in place with miniplates along its anterior and inferior surfaces. This completes the insetting process (Figs. 82-15 to 82-17).

Microvascular Considerations

The microvascular anastomosis is performed after bone insetting is complete. What is available and what is convenient to use guide selection of the appropriate recipient vessels. As indicated before, the superior thyroid artery, facial artery, lingual artery, or external carotid artery can be used. One or two venous anastomoses

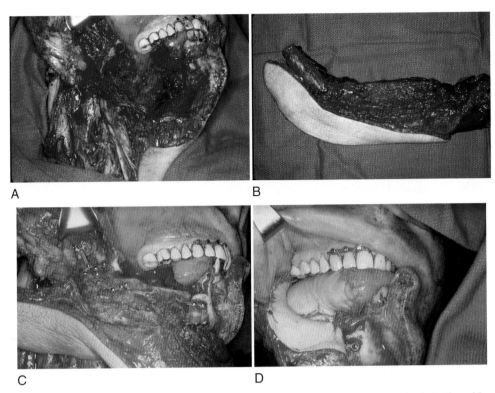

FIGURE 82-15. A typical lateral defect. *A,* The bone defect extends from the parasymphysis to the midramus. The soft tissue defect includes the lateral floor of the mouth and a portion of the tongue. *B,* The fibula graft is shown shaped, fixed, and divided from the donor site. *C,* The bone has been inset, and the skin island hangs from its inferior border. *D,* The skin island has been folded on itself to reconstruct the tongue and the lateral floor of the mouth.

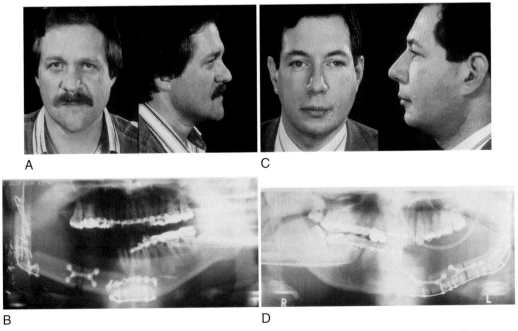

FIGURE 82-16. *A,* Postoperative views of a lateral reconstruction. This was a bone-only defect. *B,* Postoperative Panorex. *C,* Postoperative views of a lateral reconstruction. There was an intraoral skin island and condyle graft. *D,* Postoperative Panorex.

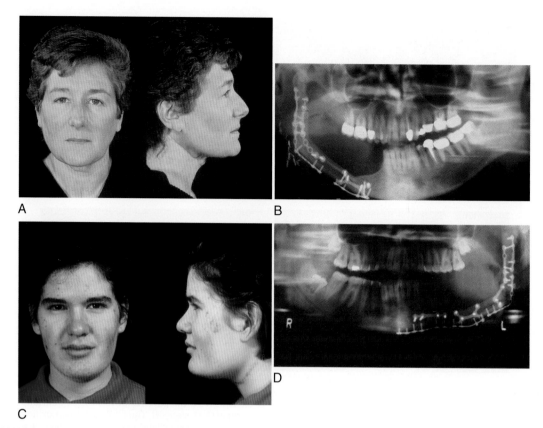

FIGURE 82-17. *A,* Postoperative views of a lateral reconstruction. There was a small intraoral skin island. (From Hidalgo D: Refinements in mandible reconstruction. Operative Techniques Plast Reconstr Surg 1996;3:257.) *B,* Postoperative Panorex. (From Cordeiro PG, Hidalgo DA: Conceptual considerations in mandibular reconstructions. Clin Plast Surg 1995;22:61.) *C,* Postoperative views of a lateral reconstruction. There was a small intraoral skin island. *D,* Postoperative Panorex.

are performed to a branch of the internal jugular vein, to the internal jugular vein itself, or to the external jugular vein.

The microvascular anastomosis is accomplished by use of the operating microscope, and the largest available recipient vessels are used. In the setting of end-to-end anastomoses, a double approximating microvascular clamp is used to position the donor and recipient vessels. Vessel ends are trimmed, dilated, and flushed with heparinized saline solution. In the setting of an end-to-side anastomosis, side-biting vascular clamps or angled vascular clamps are used to control the recipient vessels. Anastomoses are accomplished with 9-0 nylon suture in the continuous suture technique. This technique places two sutures 180 degrees apart on the vessels. One suture is used continuously on the back wall of the vessel and then tied to the tail of the opposite suture. The second suture is used on the anterior wall of the vessel and tied to the tail of the opposite suture.[140] After both the arterial and venous anastomoses are accomplished, clamps are removed, confirming adequate inflow and venous drainage

from the flap. Before the operative microscope is removed, the head of the patient is turned from side to side and flexed to ensure that kinking or twisting of the vascular pedicle, which could potentially compromise the flap in the postoperative period, does not occur.

Postoperative Care

Ten minutes before the division of the free flap, patients are given 3000 units of heparin. Anticoagulation is not routinely used postoperatively. The exception to this is patients with the development of intraoperative thrombosis prompting revision of the artery or vein. Work at our institution has demonstrated that the routine postoperative use of low-molecular-weight dextran results in a significantly higher incidence of postoperative systemic (pulmonary and cardiac) complications with no change in overall flap outcome.[141]

The skin island for replacement of the intraoral lining or external skin is used to monitor the flap when it is present. Color, capillary refill, and Doppler ultrasonography are used to monitor free flap viability. If a skin island is not included with the bone flap, arterial patency is monitored with a Doppler device. Routine conventional monitoring techniques have resulted in a 99.5% free flap survival rate in more than 700 free flaps performed in our institution.[142] Free flaps are monitored on an hourly basis after surgery, every 2 hours for the next 48 hours, and every 4 hours for the next 48 hours. During the postoperative period, prophylactic systemic antibiotics and conventional analgesics are used.

Maxillomandibular fixation placed intraoperatively is released after 5 days if the condyle has not been reconstructed and after 7 to 10 days if a condylar reconstruction has been performed. Exercises to increase incisal opening of the mandible are initiated. Temporary tracheostomy is performed routinely during segmental mandibulectomy and reconstruction. During the postoperative period, the tracheostomy is gradually downsized and removed at approximately 7 to 10 days. Approximately 5 days postoperatively, twice-daily oral hygiene with aerosolized saline-bicarbonate solution is performed. When the integrity of the oral closure is ensured, usually after 7 to 10 days, liquids are started. The diet is gradually progressed to a soft diet; foods requiring the greatest masticatory effort are not permitted until after 6 weeks.

In the setting of a fibula donor site, a posterior splint is used to immobilize the lower extremity. The patient is out of bed to a chair with the leg elevated within 48 hours. The posterior splint is taken down at 5 days postoperatively. In the absence of a skin graft to the donor site, ambulation is encouraged, initially with the use of a walker. Full weight bearing on the donor extremity is allowed. If a skin graft is necessary, ambulation is delayed for 10 to 14 days postoperatively. Bone healing is followed by conventional panoramic radiographic (Panorex) studies at approximately 3 months and periodically thereafter. Bone scans are not routinely obtained.[102]

SPECIAL PROBLEMS
Secondary Reconstruction

Secondary reconstruction poses an even greater challenge than primary reconstruction does. The extent of soft tissue and bone loss is not precisely known and tends to be underestimated as a result of wound contraction forces. Facial distortion is not prevented by the use of external fixators, previously popular devices that are rarely used today. Examination of operative and pathology reports usually adds little useful information to guide the task of secondary reconstruction. Patients previously treated with radiation therapy pose additional problems. It is more difficult to dissect fibrotic areas, and there is a higher incidence of wound healing problems and infection. Fortunately, most mandible reconstructions today are performed as primary procedures. There is little indication to delay reconstruction given the techniques currently available.

Template fabrication based on radiologic studies is also useful in secondary reconstruction. Templates modeled on the normal side can be used to assist in reconstruction of a lateral defect on the opposite side. Computed tomographic scans obtained before the original resection are often available and can be used to fabricate a template of the inferior border of the mandible for reconstruction of anterior defects. The goals in secondary reconstruction, as in primary reconstruction, are to reproduce the shape of the inferior border of the mandible accurately and to inset the graft so that the maxillary and mandibular arches are properly aligned. Careful design of vascularized bone will result in the restoration of facial symmetry and set the stage for successful dental reconstruction later.

Soft tissue contraction and radiation-induced fibrosis may prevent the skin envelope from expanding adequately to accommodate insertion of a vascularized graft of the appropriate dimensions. It may therefore be necessary to include a skin island externally to allow wound closure without excessive tension. This can serve as a convenient means of monitoring the flap. It may be possible to improve aesthetics later by excising the skin island after healing is complete and all swelling has resolved.

One advantage of delayed reconstruction is that it is possible to stay out of the oral cavity in some patients. This limits the scope of the wound and reduces the potential for postoperative infection and fistula, particularly in patients who have been irradiated. Although it is often unnecessary to recreate a through-and-through wound for lateral defects, secondary reconstruction of anterior defects usually does require interposition of a skin island to restore adequate dimension to the anterior floor of the mouth.

Secondary reconstruction may require several staged procedures when the defect is large. Some patients may require more than one free flap for adequate restoration of the missing tissue (Fig. 82-18). Other patients may require local flaps for reconstruction of the lip if the oral aperture is severely contracted.

Secondary mandible reconstruction in the presence of a radical neck dissection poses additional considerations. Recipient vessel availability and whether the radical neck defect itself will be reconstructed determine flap selection. For example, use of the scapular flap including the latissimus dorsi muscle can reconstruct the mandible and sternomastoid muscle defect simultaneously, although such a procedure is challenging technically. Flap design is also influenced by a need to use the contralateral neck as a source of

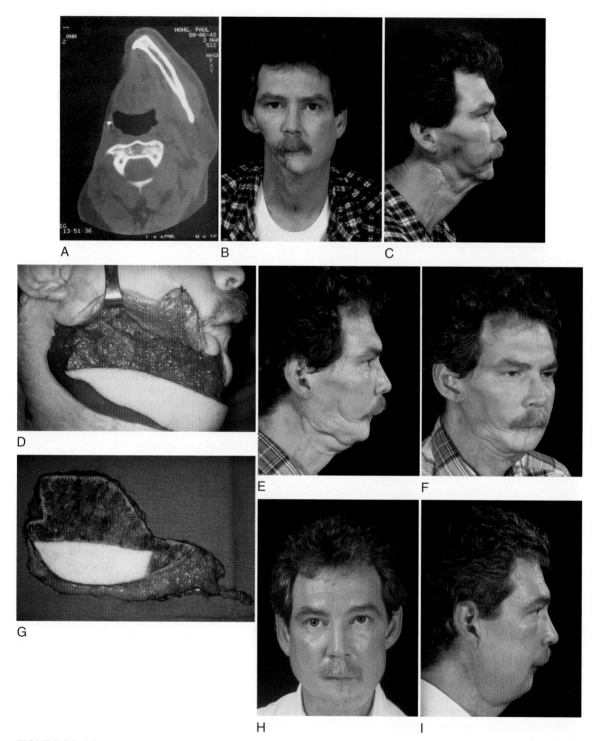

FIGURE 82-18. Secondary reconstruction of an extensive bone and soft tissue defect. *A,* The computed tomographic scan indicates the extent of tissue loss. *B* and *C,* Preoperative views. *D,* The fibula free flap is shown in place. A skin island was used to compensate for contracted soft tissue and to allow primary wound closure. *E* and *F,* Postoperative views after the first procedure. *G,* A partially de-epithelialized scapula free flap is then used in a second procedure to fill in the remaining soft tissue deficit. *H* and *I,* Postoperative views of the patient 10 years later.

recipient vessels. When the fibula is selected to reconstruct a lateral defect in this setting, the contralateral leg is chosen. The design of the flap is shifted distally on the bone to lengthen the pedicle adequately to reach the opposite side of the neck. It is best to avoid vein grafts to lengthen the pedicle of a flap. This goal can almost always be achieved with proper flap selection and design.

The aesthetic improvement for the patient undergoing secondary reconstruction of the mandible is often dramatic. However, the aesthetic results of primary reconstruction are usually superior and constitute one of the main reasons that primary reconstruction is preferred.

Radiation and Reconstruction

Mandible reconstruction in the setting of prior radiation therapy is problematic. Conventional nonvascularized bone grafts in the setting of prior irradiation have a high failure rate.[65] The reason for this failure rate is the effect of ionizing radiation on the region of the mandible. In concert with tumor control, ionizing radiation also has acute and chronic effects on the soft tissue and bone in the area of the mandible.[143,144] The chronic effects of irradiation include skin atrophy, edema, changes in pigment, cholangiectasis, xeroderma, and increased susceptibility to breakdown after minor breakdown with poor healing.[145] On histologic examination, obliterative endarteritis, decreased number of blood vessels, decreased cellularity, and increased accumulation of soluble collagen are responsible for poor diffusion of oxygen in irradiated tissues.[146] This unfavorable environment to wound healing results in difficulty for mandibular reconstruction. The use of vascularized tissue is necessary to combat this problem.

Early approaches involved the use of vascularized pedicled flaps or wrapping of local muscle and musculocutaneous flaps around nonvascularized bone grafts. The survival of free nonvascularized bone grafts in irradiated areas that are wrapped by muscle flaps has been demonstrated in the animal model.[147] This technique has been demonstrated clinically with use of the sternocleidomastoid and clavicle combination, trapezius and scapular spine combination, and pectoralis major with anterior fifth rib combination for mandible reconstruction in the setting of prior irradiation. Owing to problems with the sternocleidomastoid-clavicle combination in the setting of a neck dissection, the pectoralis major with anterior fifth rib is preferred for mandible reconstruction using pedicled flaps.[148] The trapezius-scapular flap is also useful in this setting, although the short arc of rotation limits its use to defects involving the horizontal ramus. An additional technique described for reconstruction of the irradiated mandible with a local pedicled

musculo-osseous flap is that of the lateral pectoral composite flap. This flap differs from previously described pectoralis major-rib flaps in that the majority of the pectoralis major is preserved, thus preserving function of the shoulder.[64]

The utility of free tissue transplantation to provide a living bone graft in the setting of irradiation was demonstrated initially in a dog model. This research demonstrated that regular fracture repair between the host bone and the revascularized bone graft was possible and required a considerably shorter healing time than in the setting of a conventional free bone graft. The authors proposed that the vascularized graft carried its own blood supply and could actively participate in the repair process.[149] Early clinical use of microvascular flaps after composite resection and irradiation for recurrent oral cancer was demonstrated by Rosen et al[76,150] in Canada. In their initial report, 14 patients underwent microsurgical free flap procedures for reconstruction after composite resection of radiation-recurrent oral cancer. Their initial approach used metatarsal bone and associated soft tissue based on the dorsalis pedis vessels. Subsequently, they expanded this approach to include vascularized iliac crest grafts. The overall survival with this technique was 93%.

Free tissue transplantation is currently the mainstay of therapy in the setting of prior irradiation and mandible reconstruction. The advantages of this technique include not only the availability of the ideal bone stock but also the ability to transplant composite tissues containing well-vascularized muscle and skin to bring in new blood supply to an already compromised area. This method maximizes wound healing as well as providing optimum function and aesthetics for the patient.

A special subset of reconstruction after radiation involves osteoradionecrosis. Osteoradionecrosis is a severe complication after radiation therapy for head and neck cancer. The problem involves not only the mandible but also the associated soft tissues. Therefore, for treatment to be effective, all tissues involved must be managed appropriately.[151]

The reported incidence of osteoradionecrosis of the mandible ranges from 0.8% to 37.0%.[152] Osteoradionecrosis can present as prolonged bone exposure that does not heal for more than 3 to 6 months or a pathologic fracture with intact mucosa. This condition is suggested to be secondary to radiation-induced obliteration of the inferior alveolar artery and radiation fibrosis of the mandibular periosteum.[153] The site of necrosis in osteoradionecrotic mandibles is typically the buccal cortex. Mandibular bone marrow is often replaced by dense, fibrous, poorly vascularized tissue with associated occlusion of the inferior alveolar artery and its branches. Collateral circulation is further diminished by surgical ligation of branches of the external carotid artery. In general, the most vulnerable portion of the mandible is the premolar, molar, and retromolar buccal cortex. This area has a lack of muscle attachments and a dependence on the inferior alveolar artery for blood supply.[154]

Risk factors for the development of osteoradionecrosis include older patients with a history of tobacco and ethanol abuse, radiation therapy of more than 65 Gy (particularly more than 70 to 75 Gy), adjunctive use of radioactive implants to boost tumoricidal doses, advanced or recurrent tumors, bone involvement by tumor, and poor intraoral hygiene.[155,156] The incidence of osteoradionecrosis is higher in dentulous patients than in edentulous patients. This incidence is particularly associated with postirradiation dental extraction.[157]

Osteoradionecrosis is best managed by prevention. Effective measures taken before irradiation include completion of all restorative or periodontal treatment with an opportunity for wound healing for 2 to 3 weeks. Severely diseased teeth require extraction; remaining teeth should be managed with meticulous oral hygiene, fluoride treatments, dietary supplementation, and antifungal or antibiotic agents as needed. After the completion of radiation therapy, close dental follow-up is mandatory.[151] As noted, postirradiation dental extraction is definitively associated with the development of osteoradionecrosis. As a result, Marx et al[158] recommend pre-extraction hyperbaric oxygen therapy consisting of 20 preoperative treatments at 2.4 atmospheres.

Management of osteoradionecrosis centers on adequate surgical débridement and wound closure. Attempts to use hyperbaric oxygen alone in the management of this condition are generally unsuccessful, although some patients do heal. At this time, hyperbaric oxygen is considered an adjunct to aggressive management of the osteonecrotic bone.[43,146] Failure to control osteoradionecrosis is generally thought to be secondary to inadequate débridement, which results in a failure to recognize the absolute extent of the disease process. Restoration of mandibular continuity is generally performed with vascularized bone flaps.

With the exception of the Marx protocol,[43,146] bone grafts are generally unsuccessful. The Marx protocol describes at least 20 preoperative hyperbaric oxygen treatments at 2.4 atmospheres to induce neoangiogenesis. After several weeks, cadaveric mandible is burred out and filled with cancellous bone from the patient and placed through an extraoral incision. An additional 20 to 40 hyperbaric oxygen treatments are then given. The advantages of this include decreased donor site morbidity, good contour of the mandible, and possibility for dental rehabilitation, and the procedure does not require microvascular skills. The disadvantages include the need to delay reconstruction to complete hyperbaric oxygen treatments, expense

and time involved with the treatments, and long time for healing as the graft heals by creeping substitution.

Vascularized flaps such as the fibula free flap provide bone with its own inherent blood supply in soft tissue replacement as needed. Because microvascular techniques are widely available, this method of reconstruction after irradiation or after osteoradionecrosis is preferred.

Pediatric Mandible Reconstruction

Disease causing segmental mandible defects in the pediatric population is uncommon. Enucleation and curettage usually manage problems such as odontogenic cysts. Odontogenic tumors such as ameloblastoma may require segmental resection, but the bone gap is often short and may be amenable to nonvascularized bone graft reconstruction. More severe problems are caused by nonodontogenic tumors, such as osteogenic sarcoma, chondrosarcoma, Ewing sarcoma, and fibrosarcoma, although these entities are rare.[159] The principles for reconstruction of significant segmental defects of the mandible are the same as in the adult population.

Use of the fibula in pediatric mandible reconstruction does not appear to impair growth of the leg. It is not generally necessary or of proven benefit to try to place the growth center of the transplanted fibula-mandible near the condyle. Inclusion of the proximal fibula growth center is technically possible to achieve this position but may interfere with knee stability.

Very young patients with advanced tumors may be best reconstructed initially with a reconstruction plate and soft tissue free flap. Definitive secondary reconstruction with an osseous free flap can be undertaken later when mandible growth is complete and survival ensured.

Intermaxillary fixation is often not possible or practical in the pediatric population as an adjunct to facilitate graft insetting. Insetting is therefore a more intuitive process in terms of re-establishment of facial symmetry and proper maxillary and mandibular arch alignment.

DENTAL RECONSTRUCTION
Soft Tissue Procedures

The best functional and aesthetic results after mandible reconstruction occur with the use of vascularized bone. For these results to be optimized, postoperative oral and dental rehabilitation is critical. In the multidisciplinary approach to head and neck cancer management, maxillofacial prosthodontics specializes in the rehabilitation of cancer patients, including facial defects.[160]

Evaluation of the patient for oral rehabilitation after oromandibular reconstruction includes assessment of incisal opening and occlusion; function of the temporomandibular joints; depth of the vestibule between the tongue, mandible, and cheeks; and thickness and character of the supporting tissue covering the reconstructed mandible. Adequate incisal opening is necessary for mastication and for dental rehabilitation. Maintenance of proper occlusion during the initial reconstruction will help optimize overall functional results. Whether the dental rehabilitation will be a permanent fixed prosthesis such as an osseointegrated dental implant or a removable prosthesis anchored to remaining teeth, adequate vestibular depth is necessary so that the prosthesis will sit properly and function optimally.

Two procedures are routinely used to correct the problems of vestibular depth: a vestibuloplasty with split-thickness skin graft and the placement of osseointegrated dental implants. The skin island associated with an osseous free flap, such as fibula or iliac crest, is often much thicker than the native mucosa over the mandible. This results in a blunting of the anterior or lateral vestibule, providing a difficult platform for a removable dental prosthesis. With soft tissue from the radial forearm flap, the thin and pliable nature of the skin tends to make this less of a problem. Vestibuloplasty can be performed to apply a layer of thin skin over the reconstructed mandible to allow prosthesis placement. The reconstructed alveolar ridge can be palpated through the skin island of the free flap. Dissection can be carried down to the osseous free flap without incising the periosteum, thus exposing the bone. This dissection will leave a suitable base for acceptance of the split-thickness skin graft. Dissection can be carried down along the lingual and buccal sulcus of the free flap to establish a vestibule that is 1 to 1.5 cm in depth.[161,162]

The split-thickness skin graft is harvested in the usual fashion, at a thickness of 0.015 to 0.018 inch. Ideally, a premade acrylic resin surgical stent is used to fix the skin graft in place. Circummandibular wires or interdental wires in a dentate patient are used to hold the stent in place, and this is then left for 3 to 5 days. Once the stent is removed, any excess skin is trimmed and the stent is revised as necessary. The stent continues to be worn as an internal prosthesis until adequate skin graft healing is obtained.[163]

Osseointegrated Implants

An alternative to deepening the vestibule to allow prosthetic rehabilitation of dentition is placement of dental implants. This method places permanent fixtures in the neomandible, which will then support the prosthesis. Adequate bone stock is mandatory for proper seating and integration of dental implants. In a comparative study of neomandibular bone thickness, it was determined that safe osseointegration of dental implants requires a bone height of 10 mm or more and a bone width of 5.75 mm or more. A comparison of multiple measurements of the iliac crest, scapula, fibula, and radius donor site revealed that the iliac crest and fibula had bone dimensions that are consistently adequate for implant placement; the radius has the highest number of bone segments inadequate for implant placement.[164]

After adequate bone stock has been established, the next factor for consideration is whether the bone has been irradiated. Controversy exists as to whether dental implants are possible in the setting of irradiated bone. Most authors believe that irradiation is a relative contraindication to the placement of osseointegrated dental implants; however, the decision depends on how much of the mandible is irradiated. Research is currently under way to determine whether hyperbaric oxygen as a pretreatment in irradiated bone will improve implant success.[165,166]

Osseointegrated dental implant placement typically requires a two-stage procedure. In the first stage, the reconstructed alveolar ridge is exposed by an incision made down to the bone over the crest of the ridge. The skin island and the underlying periosteum are dissected away from the bone until the bone is exposed. The bone is then flattened with a burr, and a small notch made with the burr marks the position for the implant. Drill holes are made in the bone for implant placement. Ideally, 5 mm is placed between implants. Implants should be placed in the superior and inferior cortex of the grafted bone but not through the inferior cortex of the bone. The flaps are closed primarily over the implants, and the implants are allowed to integrate for 3 months before they are used to support and retain a prosthesis (Figs. 82-19 and 82-20).[163]

Three basic types of prosthesis can provide function and aesthetics for mandibular reconstruction. These include removable prosthesis, fixed prosthesis, and a combination of removable and fixed prosthesis. Removable prostheses are retained to acceptable teeth or dental implants and can be removed by the patient. Fixed prostheses are fixed to remaining teeth or implants and cannot be removed by the patient or a dentist. These require careful and thorough oral hygiene. The combination fixed-removable prosthesis can be removed only by the dentist for evaluation of the implants and remaining dentition. Again, oral hygiene needs to be systematic and intense. Without adequate and proper oral hygiene and maintenance, prostheses and implants often fail. Ultimately, oral hygiene is easier for the patient when the prostheses are removable.[160,167,168]

Optimum functional and aesthetic dental restoration can be expected in 90% or more of

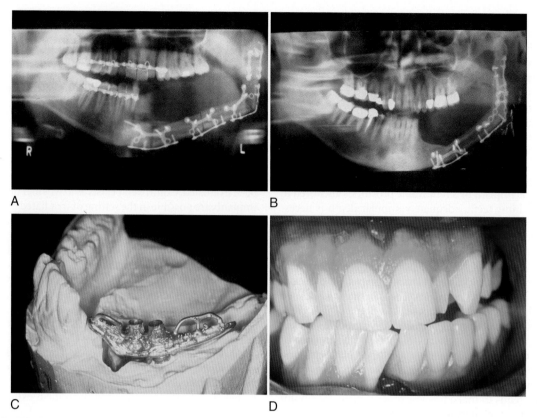

FIGURE 82-19. Dental rehabilitation after free flap reconstruction of a lateral defect. *A,* Postoperative Panorex taken before partial miniplate removal. *B,* Osseointegrated implants are shown in place. *C,* The prosthesis "super-structure" is fabricated on a dental model. *D,* The completed prosthesis is shown mounted to the implants.

nonirradiated patients receiving osseointegrated dental implants.[103,169] Whereas most implants are placed in a delayed fashion, there are reports of primary insertion of dental implants at the time of mandible reconstruction. Opponents of this procedure state that implant placement may not be ideal to restore good occlusion when implants are placed primarily. In addition, there is the risk of placing implants in the newly revascularized bone, which could potentially compromise the endosteal circulation of the bone flap, thus limiting osseointegration and ultimately contributing to implant failure. However, it has been demonstrated that in patients who are in good general and oral conditions with benign disease and thus do not require postoperative radiation therapy, primary insertion of dental implants can be successfully accomplished.[170] The obvious advantage of this procedure is complete oral rehabilitation in a shorter time as noted; however, selection of patients is imperative in this setting.

FUNCTIONAL OUTCOME

The functional outcome of mandible reconstruction is evaluated by long-term functional outcome, aesthetic appearance, and bone retention. Bone height and bone mass have been evaluated after fibula free flap mandible reconstruction. With a mean follow-up of more than 2.5 years and up to 10 years, it has been shown that fibula free flaps maintain their bone height, which is a reflection of bone mass, in more than 90% of patients irrespective of previous irradiation, the placement of osseointegrated dental implants, and the anterior or lateral position of the reconstruction.[171]

The long-term functional outcome of free flap mandible reconstruction examines speech, diet, and overall aesthetics. In an evaluation of 151 consecutive patients during a 10-year period, 36% of patients returned to normal speech, 27% returned to nearly normal speech, 28% were intelligible, and only 9% were unintelligible. The best speech results were generally seen in patients with hemimandibular and lateral reconstructions; the worst results were in central reconstructions.[116] The overall quality of speech could largely be attributed to the amount of intraoral soft tissue resected. As the mandibulectomy specimen extends to include intraoral soft tissue such as anterior and lateral floor of mouth and, in particular, the tongue, the speech results worsen. The skin island from

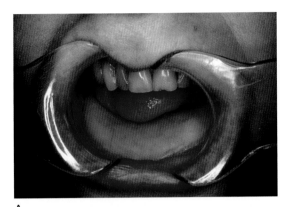

A

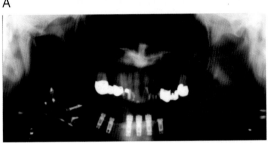

B

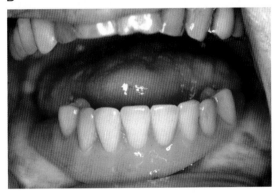

C

FIGURE 82-20. Dental rehabilitation after free flap reconstruction of an anterior defect. *A,* A well-healed fibula skin island is shown replacing the anterior floor of the mouth. *B,* Panorex shows six osseointegrated implants in place after a previous procedure removed graft fixation hardware in the area. Three of the implants are shown with extension collars in place. *C,* The completed prosthesis is shown mounted to the implants.

the fibula free flap is not as mobile as the normal intra-oral soft tissues. Therefore, when it is necessary to reconstruct missing tongue with skin island from the fibula, some tethering can be expected with a reduction in the overall quality of speech.

When the same group of patients was examined for functional results in terms of returning to unrestricted diet, it was found that 45% of patients are able to return to an unrestricted diet after mandible reconstruction, whereas 45% eat a soft diet; 5% of patients return to a liquid diet, whereas only 5% require tube feeding to sustain nutrition.[116] The same limitations in central or anterior reconstruction were found in terms of diet evaluation as with speech. The majority of patients returning to an unrestricted diet had either hemimandibular or lateral reconstructions; the majority of the anterior reconstruction patients returned to a soft diet.[116]

Finally, aesthetic evaluation can be expected to yield 32% of patients with an excellent aesthetic result, 27% with a good result, 27% with a fair result, and 14% with a poor result. Hemimandibular and lateral reconstructions can be expected to reveal the best aesthetic results; anterior reconstructions and, in particular, those patients requiring placement of external skin by either the fibula skin island or a second free flap demonstrated less quality in the aesthetic result. The poor result of this reconstruction is due to the cutaneous texture and color mismatch that is inevitable after a soft tissue flap is used to reconstruct a composite defect that includes external facial skin.[116]

REFERENCES

1. Martin C: De lymphadenopathy prosthese immediate, appliquee a lymphadenopathy resection des maxillaires: rhino-plastie sur appareil prothetique permanent; restauration de lymphadenopathy face, levres, nez, langue, voute et voile du palais. Paris, Masson et Cie, 1889.
2. Partsch: Prosthesis of lower jaw after resection. Arch Klin Chir 1897;55:746.
3. Lindemann A: Bruhn's Ergebnisse aus dem Düsseldorfer Lazarett, Behandlungen der Kieferschussverletzungen. Wiesbaden, 1916:243.
4. Klapp R, Schroeder H: Die Unterkieferschussbruche. Berlin, Hermann Meusser, 1917.
5. Ivy RH: Extensive loss of substance of mandible due to removal of sarcoma, replaced by bone graft from crest of ilium. Int J Orthod 1921;7:483.
6. Converse JM: Early and late treatment of gunshot wounds of the jaw in French battle casualties in North Africa and Italy. J Oral Surg 1945;3:112.
7. Boyne PJ: Restoration of osseous defects in maxillofacial casualties. J Am Dent Assoc 1969;78:767.
8. Boyne PJ: Implants and transplants. Review of recent research in the area of oral surgery. J Am Dent Assoc 1973;87:1074.
9. Swanson LT, Habal MB, Leake DL, Murray JE: Compound silicone-bone implants for mandibular reconstruction: development and application. Plast Reconstr Surg 1973;51: 402.
10. Boyne PJ, Zarem H: Osseous reconstruction of the resected mandible. Am J Surg 1976;132:49.
11. Leake DL, Rappoport M: Mandibular reconstruction: bone induction in an alloplastic tray. Surgery 1972;72:332.
12. Schwartz HC: Mandibular reconstruction using the Dacron-urethane prosthesis and autogenic cancellous bone: review of 32 cases. Plast Reconstr Surg 1984;73:387.
13. Albert TW, Smith JD, Everts EC, Cook TA: Dacron mesh tray and cancellous bone in reconstruction of mandibular defects. Arch Otolaryngol Head Neck Surg 1986;112:53.
14. Cummings CW, Leipzig B: Replacement of tumor-involved mandible by cryosurgically devitalized autograft. Human experience. Arch Otolaryngol 1980;106:252.

15. Leipzig B, Cummings CW: The current status of mandibular reconstruction using autogenous frozen mandibular grafts. Head Neck Surg 1984;6:992.

16. Hamaker RC, Singer MI: Irradiated mandibular autografts update. Arch Otolaryngol Head Neck Surg 1986;112:277.

17. Kellman RM, Gullane PJ: Use of the AO mandibular reconstruction plate for bridging of mandibular defects. Otolaryngol Clin North Am 1987;20:519.

18. Raveh J, Stich H, Sutter F, Greiner R: Use of titanium-coated hollow screw and reconstruction system in bridging of lower jaw defects. J Oral Maxillofac Surg 1984;42:281.

19. Raveh J, Sutter F, Hellem S: Surgical procedures for reconstruction of the lower jaw using the titanium-coated hollow-screw reconstruction plate system: bridging of defects. Otolaryngol Clin North Am 1987;20:535.

20. Ketchum LD, Masters FW, Robinson DW: Mandibular reconstruction using a composite island rib flap. Plast Reconstr Surg 1974;53:471.

21. Siemssen SO, Kirkby B, O'Connor TP: Immediate reconstruction of a resected segment of the lower jaw, using a compound flap of clavicle and sternocleidomastoid muscle. Plast Reconstr Surg 1978;61:724.

22. Bell MS, Baron PT: The rib-pectoralis major osteomyocutaneous flap. Ann Plast Surg 1981;6:347.

23. Panje WR, Cutting C: Trapezius osteomyocutaneous island flap for reconstruction of the anterior floor of mouth and mandible. Head Neck Surg 1980;3:66.

24. Taylor GI, Townsend P, Corlett R: Superiority of the deep circumflex iliac vessels as the supply for free groin flaps. Clinical work, Plast Reconstr Surg 1979;64:745.

25. Silverberg B, Banis JC Jr, Acland RD: Mandibular reconstruction with microvascular bone transfer. Series of 10 patients. Am J Surg 1985;150:440.

26. Coleman JJ, Sultan MR: The bipedicle osteocutaneous scapula flap: a new subscapular system free flap. Plast Reconstr Surg 1991;87:682.

27. O'Brien BM, Morrison WA, MacLeod AM, Dooley BJ: Microvascular osteocutaneous transfer using the groin flap and iliac crest, the dorsalis pedis flaps and second metatarsal. Br J Plast Surg 1979;32:188.

28. Soutar DS, Widdowson WP: Immediate reconstruction of the mandible using a vascularized segment of radius. Head Neck Surg 1986;8:232.

29. Hidalgo DA: Fibula free flap: a new method of mandible reconstruction. Plast Reconstr Surg 1989;84:71.

30. Thorne CH: Gunshot wounds to the face. Clin Plast Surg 1992;19:233.

31. Patel SG, Shah JP: Tumors of the oropharynx. In Shah JP, ed: Cancer of the Head and Neck. Hamilton, Ontario, BC Decker, 2001:127.

32. Jewer DD, Boyd JB, Manktelow RT, et al: Orofacial and mandibular reconstruction with the iliac crest free flap: a review of 60 cases and a new method of classification. Plast Reconstr Surg 1989;84:391.

33. Urken M, Weinberg H, Vickery C, et al: Oromandibular reconstruction using microvascular composite free flaps. Arch Otolaryngol Head Neck Surg 1991;117:733.

34. Boyd JB, Gullane PJ, Rostein LE, et al: Classification of mandibular defects. Plast Reconstr Surg 1993;92:1266.

35. Eppley BL: Nonvascularized methods of mandible reconstruction. Operative Techniques Plast Reconstr Surg 1996;3:226.

36. Duncan MJ, Manktelow RT, Zuker RM, et al: Mandibular reconstruction in the radiated patient: the role of osteocutaneous free tissue transfer. Plast Reconstr Surg 1985;76:829.

37. Coleman JJ, Wooden WA: Mandibular reconstruction with composite microvascular tissue transfer. Am J Surg 1990;160:390.

38. Markowitz B, Taleisnick A, Calcaterra T, et al: Achieving mandibular continuity with vascularized bone flaps: a comparison of primary and secondary reconstruction. J Oral Maxillofac Surg 1994;52:114.

39. Kim MR, Donoff RB: Critical analysis of mandibular reconstruction using AO reconstruction plates. J Oral Maxillofac Surg 1992;50:1152.

40. Schusterman MA, Reese GP, Krol SS, et al: Use of AO plate for immediate mandibular reconstruction in cancer patients. Plast Reconstr Surg 1991;88:588.

41. Boyne PJ, Zarem H: Osseous reconstruction of the resected mandible. Am J Surg 1976;49:132.

42. Carlson ER, Marks RE: Mandibular reconstruction with particulate bone cancellous marrow grafts: factors resulting in predictable reconstruction of the mandible. In Worthington P, Evans JR, eds: Controversies in Oral and Maxillofacial Surgery. Philadelphia, WB Saunders, 1994:288-300.

43. Marx RE, Ames JR: The use of hyperbaric oxygen therapy in bony reconstruction of the irradiated and tissue-deficient patient. J Oral Surg 1982;40:412.

44. Marx RE: Mandibular reconstruction. J Oral Maxillofac Surg 1993;51:466.

45. Boyd JB, Mulholland RS, Davidson J, et al: The free flap and plate in oromandibular reconstruction: long term review and indications. Plast Reconstr Surg 1995;95:1018.

46. Raveh J, Stich H, Sutter F, et al: Use of titanium coated hollow screw and reconstruction system in bridging of lower jaw defects. J Oral Maxillofac Surg 1984;42:281.

47. Boyd JB: Use of reconstruction plates in conjunction with soft tissue free flaps for oromandibular reconstruction. Clin Plast Surg 1994;21:69.

48. Murakamy Y, Sato S, Akira T, et al: Esophageal reconstruction with a skin grafted pectoralis major muscle flap. Arch Otolaryngol Head Neck Surg 1982;108:719.

49. Malloy PJ: Reconstruction of intermediate sized mucosal defects with pectoralis major myofascial flap. J Otolaryngol 1989;19:32.

50. Lee KY, Lore JM Jr: Two modifications of pectoralis major myocutaneous flaps. Laryngoscope 1986;96:363.

51. Davis JP: The latissimus dorsi flap in head and neck reconstructive surgery: a review of 121 procedures. Clin Otolaryngol 1992;17:47.

52. Demergasso F, Piazza MV: Trapezius myocutaneous flap in reconstructive surgery for head and neck cancer: an original technique. Am J Surg 1979;138:533.

53. Bertotti JA: Trapezius musculocutaneous island flap in the repair of major head and neck cancer. Plast Reconstr Surg 1980;65:16.

54. Mathes SJ, Nahai F: Muscle flap transposition with function preservation: technical and clinical considerations. Plast Reconstr Surg 1980;66:242.

55. Larson DL, Goepfert H: Limitations of the sternocleidomastoid musculocutaneous flap in head and neck cancer reconstruction. Plast Reconstr Surg 1982;70:328.

56. Coleman JJ III, Nahai F, Mathes SJ: Platysmal musculocutaneous flap: clinical and anatomic considerations in head and neck reconstruction. Am J Surg 1982;144:477.

57. Snyder C, Bateman J, Davis C, et al: Mandibulo-facial restoration with live osteocutaneous flaps. Plast Reconstr Surg 1970;45:14.

58. Cuono C, Ariyan S: Immediate reconstruction of a composite mandibular defect with a regional osteomusculocutaneous flap. Plast Reconstr Surg 1980;65:477.

59. Dufresne C, Cutting C, Valauri F, et al: Reconstruction of mandibular and floor of mouth defects using the trapezius osteomyocutaneous flap. Plast Reconstr Surg 1987;79:687.

60. Guillamondegui O, Larson D: The lateral trapezius musculocutaneous flap: its use in head and neck reconstruction. Plast Reconstr Surg 1981;67:143.

61. Panje W: Mandible reconstruction with the trapezius osteo-musculocutaneous flap. Arch Otolaryngol 1985;111:223.

62. Robertson G: A comparison between sternum and rib in osteomyocutaneous reconstruction of major mandibular defects. Ann Plast Surg 1986;17:421.

63. Gregor R, Davidge-Pitts K: Trapezius osteomyocutaneous flap for mandibular reconstruction. Arch Otolaryngol 1985; 111:198.

64. Little JW, McCulloch DT, Lyons JR: The lateral pectoral composite flap in one-stage reconstruction of the irradiated mandible. Plast Reconstr Surg 1983;71:326.

65. Daniel RK: Mandibular reconstruction with free tissue transfers. Ann Plast Surg 1978;1:346.

66. Serafin D, Villarreal-Rios A, Georgiade N: A rib-containing free flap to reconstruct mandibular defects. Br J Plast Surg 1977;30:263.

67. Harashina T, Nakajima H, Imai T: Reconstruction of mandibular defects with revascularized free rib grafts. Plast Reconstr Surg 1978;62:514.

68. McKee D: Microvascular bone transplantation. Clin Plast Surg 1978;5:283.

69. Thoma A, Heddle S, Archibald S, et al: The free vascularized anterior rib graft. Plast Reconstr Surg 1988;82:291.

70. Serafin D, Riefkohl R, Thomas I, et al: Vascularized rib-periosteal and osteocutaneous reconstruction of the maxilla and mandible: an assessment. Plast Reconstr Surg 1980;66:718.

71. Richards M, Poole M, Godfrey A: The serratus anterior/rib composite flap in mandibular reconstruction. Br J Plast Surg 1985;38:466.

72. Schmidt D, Robson M: One-stage composite reconstruction using latissimus myoosteocutaneous free flap. Am J Surg 1982;144:470.

73. Ariyan S, Finseth F: The anterior chest approach for obtaining free osteocutaneous rib grafts. Plast Reconstr Surg 1978;62:676.

74. Bell M, Barron P: A new method of oral reconstruction using a free composite foot flap. Ann Plast Surg 1980;5:281.

75. MacLeod A, Robinson D: Reconstruction of defects involving the mandible and floor of mouth by free osteo-cutaneous flaps derived from the foot. Br J Plast Surg 1982;35:239.

76. Rosen IB, Bell MS, Barron PT, et al: Use of microvascular flaps including free osseocutaneous flaps and reconstruction after composite resection for radiation-recurrent oral cancer. Am J Surg 1979;138:544.

77. Taylor G, Townsend P, Corlett R: Superiority of the deep circumflex iliac vessels as the supply for free groin flaps: experimental work. Plast Reconstr Surg 1979;64:595.

78. Hidalgo D: Deep circumflex iliac artery free flaps. In Shaw W, Hidalgo D: Microsurgery in Trauma. Mount Kisco, NY, Futura, 1987:327.

79. Taylor G: Reconstruction of the mandible with free composite iliac bone grafts. Ann Plast Surg 1982;9:362.

80. Salibian A, Rappaport I, Allison G: Functional oromandibular reconstruction with the microvascular composite groin flap. Plast Reconstr Surg 1985;76:819.

81. Boyd B: The place of the iliac crest in vascularized oromandibular reconstruction. Microsurgery 1994;15:250.

82. Urken M, Weinberg H, Vickery C, et al: The internal oblique–iliac crest free flap in composite defects of the oral cavity involving bone, skin and mucosa. Laryngoscope 1991;101:257.

83. David D, Tan E, Katsaros J, et al: Mandibular reconstruction with vascularized iliac crest: a 10 year experience. Plast Reconstr Surg 1988;82:792.

84. Shpitzer T, Neligan P, Gullane P, et al: The free iliac crest and fibula flaps in vascularized oromandibular reconstruction: comparison and long-term evaluation. Head Neck 1999;21:639.

85. Yang G, Gao YG, Chan BC, et al: Forearm free skin transplantation. Nat Med J China 1981;61:139.

86. Soutar D, McGregor I: The radial forearm flap in intraoral reconstruction: the experience of 60 consecutive cases. Plast Reconstr Surg 1986;78:1.

87. Soutar D, Scheker L, Tanner N, et al: The radial forearm flap: a versatile method for intraoral reconstruction. Br J Plast Surg 1983;36:1.

88. Hidalgo D: Forearm free flaps. In Shaw W, Hidalgo D: Microsurgery in Trauma. Mount Kisco, NY, Futura, 1987:283.

89. Swanson E, Boyd B, Manktelow R: The radial forearm flap: reconstructive applications and donor-site defects in 35 consecutive patients. Plast Reconstr Surg 1990;85:258.

90. dos Santos L: The vascular anatomy and dissection of the free scapular flap. Plast Reconstr Surg 1984;73:599.

91. Gilbert A, Teot L: The free scapular flap. Plast Reconstr Surg 1982;69:601.

92. Nassif T, Vidal L, Bovet J, et al: The parascapular flap: a new cutaneous microsurgical free flap. Plast Reconstr Surg 1982;69:591.

93. Hidalgo D: Scapular free flaps. In Shaw W, Hidalgo D: Microsurgery in Trauma. Mount Kisco, NY, Futura, 1987:257.

94. Swartz W, Banis J, Newton E, et al: The osteocutaneous scapular flap for mandibular and maxillary reconstruction. Plast Reconstr Surg 1986;77:530.

95. Taylor G, Miller G, Ham F: The free vascularized bone graft. Plast Reconstr Surg 1975;55:533.

96. Hurst L, Mirza M, Spellman W: Vascularized fibular graft for infected loss of the ulna: case report. J Hand Surg 1982;7:498.

97. Jones N, Swartz W, Mears D: The double-barrel free vascularized fibular bone graft. Plast Reconstr Surg 1988;81:378.

98. Pho R: Malignant giant cell tumor of the distal end of the radius treated by free vascularized fibular transplant. J Bone Joint Surg Am 1981;63:877.

99. Taylor G: Microvascular free bone transfer: a clinical technique. Orthop Clin North Am 1977;8:425.

100. Weiland A, Kleinert H, Kutz J, et al: Free vascularized bone grafts in surgery of the upper extremity. J Hand Surg 1979;4:129.

101. Hidalgo D: Fibula free flap: a new method of mandible reconstruction. Plast Reconstr Surg 1989;84:71.

102. Hidalgo DA: Free flap mandibular reconstruction. Clin Plast Surg 1994;21:25.

103. Zlotolow IM, Huryn JM, Piro JD, et al: Osseointegrated implants and functional prosthetic rehabilitation in microvascular free flap reconstructed mandibles. Am J Surg 1992;165:677.

104. Gilbert A: Vascularized transfer of the fibular shaft. Int J Microsurg 1979;1:100.

105. Carriquiry C, Costa A, Vasconez L: An anatomic study of the septocutaneous vessels of the leg. Plast Reconstr Surg 1985;76:354.

106. Yoshimura M, Shimada T, Hosakawa M: The vasculature of the peroneal tissue transfer. Plast Reconstr Surg 1990;85:917.

107. Hidalgo D: Aesthetic improvements in free-flap mandible reconstruction. Plast Reconstr Surg 1991;88:574.

108. Jones N, Monstrey S, Gambier B: Reliability of the fibular osteocutaneous flap for mandibular reconstruction: anatomical and surgical confirmation. Plast Reconstr Surg 1996;97:707.

109. Schusterman M, Reece G, Miller M, Harris S: The osteocutaneous free fibula flap: is the skin paddle reliable? Plast Reconstr Surg 1992;90:787.

110. Wei F, Chen H, Chuang C, et al: Fibular osteoseptocutaneous flap: anatomic study and clinical application. Plast Reconstr Surg 1986;78:191.

111. Winters H, Jongh G: Reliability of the proximal skin paddle of the osteocutaneous free fibula flap: a prospective clinical study. Plast Reconstr Surg 1999;103:846.

112. Anthony J, Ritter E, Young D, Singer M: Enhancing fibula free flap skin island reliability and versatility for mandibular reconstruction. Ann Plast Surg 1993;31:106.

113. Wei F, Chuang S, Yim K: The sensate fibula osteoseptocutaneous flap: a preliminary report. Br J Plast Surg 1994;4:544.

114. Yang K, Leung J, Chen J: Double-paddle peroneal tissue transfer of oromandibular reconstruction. Plast Reconstr Surg 2000;106:47.

115. Hidalgo DA, Disa JJ, Cordeiro PG, et al: A review of 716 consecutive free flaps for oncologic surgical defects: refinement in donor site selection and technique. Plast Reconstr Surg 1998;102:722.

116. Cordeiro PG, Disa JJ, Hidalgo DA, et al: Reconstruction of the mandible with osseous free flaps: a 10 year experience with 150 consecutive patients. Plast Reconstr Surg 1999;104:1314.

117. Zenn M, Hidalgo D, Cordeiro P, et al: Current role of the radial forearm free flap in mandibular reconstruction. Plast Reconstr Surg 1997;99:1012.

118. Wei F, Demirkan F, Chen H, et al: Double free flaps in reconstruction of extensive composite mandibular defects in head and neck cancer. Plast Reconstr Surg 1999;103:39.

119. Wells M, Luce E, Edwards A: Sequentially linked free flaps in head and neck reconstruction. Clin Plast Surg 1994;21:59.

120. Colen S, Shaw W, McCarthy J: Review of the morbidity of 300 free-flap donor sites. Plast Reconstr Surg 1986;77:948.

121. Hidalgo D, Rekow A: A review of 60 consecutive fibula free flap mandible reconstructions. Plast Reconstr Surg 1995;96:585.

122. Anthony J, Rawnsley J, Benhaim P, et al: Donor leg morbidity and function after fibula free flap mandible reconstruction. Plast Reconstr Surg 1995;96:46.

123. Lee E, Goh J, Helm R, et al: Donor site morbidity following resection of the fibula. J Bone Joint Surg Br 1990;72:129.

124. Youdas J, Wood M, Cahalan T, Chao EY: A quantitative analysis of donor site morbidity after vascularized fibula transfer. J Orthop Res 1988;6:621.

125. Thoma A, Khadaroo R, Grigenas O, et al: Oromandibular reconstruction with the radial-forearm osteocutaneous flap: experience with 60 consecutive cases. Plast Reconstr Surg 1999; 104:368.

126. Bardsley A, Soutar D, Elliot D, et al: Reducing morbidity in the radial forearm flap donor site. Plast Reconstr Surg 1990;86:287.

127. Weinzweig N, Jones N, Shestak K, et al: Oromandibular reconstruction using a keel-shaped modification of the radial forearm osteocutaneous flap. Ann Plast Surg 1994;33:359.

128. Meland N, Maki S, Chao E, et al: The radial forearm flap: a biomechanical study of donor-site morbidity utilizing sheep tibia. Plast Reconstr Surg 1992;90:763.

129. Hallock G: Refinement of the radial forearm flap donor site using skin expansion. Plast Reconstr Surg 1988;81:21.

130. Boyd B, Rosen I, Rotstein L, et al: The iliac crest and the radial forearm flap in vascularized oromandibular reconstruction. Am J Surg 1990;159:301.

131. Schusterman M, Reece G, Kroll S, et al: Use of the AO plate for immediate mandibular reconstruction in cancer patients. Plast Reconstr Surg 1991;88:588.

132. Vuillemin T, Raveh J, Sutter F: Mandibular reconstruction with the titanium hollow screw reconstruction plate (THORP) system: evaluation of 62 cases. Plast Reconstr Surg 1988;82:804.

133. Boyd J, Mulholland R: Fixation of the vascularized bone graft in mandibular reconstruction. Plast Reconstr Surg 1991;91:274.

134. Hidalgo D: Titanium miniplate fixation in free flap mandible reconstruction. Ann Plast Surg 1989;6:498.

135. Markowitz B, Calcaterra T: Preoperative assessment and surgical planning for patients undergoing immediate composite reconstruction of oromandibular defects. Clin Plast Surg 1994;21:9.

136. Disa J, Cordeiro P: The current role of preoperative arteriography in fibula free flaps. Plast Reconstr Surg 1998;102:1083.

137. Anthony JP, Foster RD: Mandibular reconstruction with the fibula osteocutaneous free flap. Operative Techniques Plast Reconstr Surg 1996;3:233.

138. Hidalgo D, Pusic AL: Free flap mandibular reconstruction: a 10-year follow-up study. Plast Reconstr Surg 2002;110:438.

139. Hidalgo D: Refinements in mandible reconstruction. Operative Techniques Plast Reconstr Surg 1996;3:257.

140. Cordeiro PG, Santamaria E: Experience with the continuous suture microvascular anastomosis in 200 consecutive free flaps. Ann Plast Surg 1998;40:1.

141. Singh BH, Kraus DH, Sharon Z, et al: Impact of perioperative fluid management on the development of complications and outcome of microvascular free tissue transfer. Plast Reconstr Surg; in press.

142. Disa JJ, Cordeiro PG, Hidalgo DA: Efficacy of conventional monitoring techniques in free tissue transfer: an eleven-year experience in 750 consecutive cases. Plast Reconstr Surg 1999;104:97.

143. Baker DG: The radiobiological basis for tissue reaction in the oral cavity following therapeutic x-irradiation. Arch Otolaryngol 1982;108:21.

144. Rubin P, Casarett GW: Clinical radiation pathology as applied to curative radiotherapy. Cancer 1968;22:767.

145. Miller SH, Rudolph R: Healing in the irradiated wound. Clin Plast Surg 1990;17:503.

146. Marx RE: Osteoradionecrosis: a new concept of its pathology. J Oral Maxillofac Surg 1983;41:283.

147. Lukash FN, Zingaro EA, Salig J: The survival of free nonvascularized bone grafts in irradiated areas by wrapping in muscle flaps. Plast Reconstr Surg 1984;74:783.

148. Pearlman NW, Albin RE, O'Donnell RS: Mandibular reconstruction in irradiated patients utilizing myosseous-cutaneous flaps. Am J Surg 1983;346:474.

149. Ostrup LT, Fredrickson JM: Reconstruction of mandibular defects after radiation using a free, living bone graft transferred by microvascular anastomosis. Plast Reconstr Surg 1975;55:563.

150. Rosen IB, Manktelow RT, Zucker RM, et al: Application of microvascular free osteocutaneous flaps in the management of postradiation recurrent oral cancer. Am J Surg 1985;150:474.

151. Sanger JR, Matloub HD, Yousif NJ, et al: Management of osteoradionecrosis of the mandible. Clin Plast Surg 1993;20:517.

152. Coffin F: The incidence and management of osteoradionecrosis of the jaws following head and neck radiotherapy. Br J Radiol 1983;56:851.

153. Bras J, de Jonge HK, Van Merkesteyn JP: Osteoradionecrosis of the mandible: pathogenesis. Am J Otolaryngol 1990;11:244.

154. Parint J: Detailed roentgenologic examination of the blood supply in the jaws and teeth by applying radioopaque solution. Oral Surg Oral Med Oral Pathol 1949;2:20.

155. Beumer J, Harrison RH, Sanders B, et al: Osteoradionecrosis: predisposing factors and outcome of therapy. Head Neck Surg 1984;6:19.

156. Kluth EV, Jain PR, Stuchell RN, et al: A study of factors contributing to the development of osteoradionecrosis of the jaws. J Prosthet Dent 1988;59:194.

157. Marciani RD, Ownby HE: Osteoradionecrosis of the jaws. J Oral Maxillofac Surg 1986;44:218.

158. Marx RE, Johnson RP, Klein SN: Prevention of osteoradionecrosis: a randomized prospective clinical trial of hyperbaric oxygen versus penicillin. J Am Dent Assoc 1985;111:49.

159. Havlik R: Reconstruction of the pediatric mandible. Operative Techniques Plast Reconstr Surg 1996;3:272.

160. Martin JW, Lemon JC, King GE: Maxillofacial restoration after tumor ablation. Clin Plast Surg 1994;21:37.

161. Anderson JO, Benson D, Waite DE: Intraoral skin grafts, an aid to alveolar ridge extension. J Oral Surg 1969;27:427.

162. Kruger GO: Ridge extension: review of indications and techniques. J Oral Surg 1958;16:191.

163. Martin JW, Lemon JC, Schusterman MA: Oral and dental rehabilitation after mandible reconstruction. Operative Techniques Plast Reconstr Surg 1996;3:264.

164. Frodel JL Jr, Funk GF, Capper DT, et al: Osseointegrated implants: a comparative study of bone thickness in four vascularized bone flaps. Plast Reconstr Surg 1993;92:449.

165. Schweiger JW: Titanium implants in irradiated dog mandibles. J Prosthet Dent 1989;62:201.

166. Gosta G, Tjellstrom A, Albrektsson T: Postimplantation irradiation for head and neck cancer treatment. Int J Oral Maxillofac Implants 1993;8:401.

167. Des Jardins RP: Tissue-integrated prosthesis for edentulous patients with normal and abnormal jaw relationships. J Prosthet Dent 1988;59:180.

168. Davidoff SR, Steinberg MA, Halperin AS: The implant-supported overdenture: a practical plan–prosthetic design. Compend Contin Educ Dent 1993;14:724.

169. Gurlek A, Miller MJ, Jacob RF, et al: Functional results of dental restoration with osseointegrated implants after mandible reconstruction. Plast Reconstr Surg 1998;101:650.

170. Chang YM, Santamaria E, Wei FC: Primary insertion of osseointegrated dental implants into fibula osseoseptocutaneous free flap for mandible reconstruction. Plast Reconstr Surg 1998;102:680.

171. Disa JJ, Winters RM, Hidalgo DA: Long term evaluation of bone mass in free fibula flap mandible reconstruction. Am J Surg 1997;174:503.

Hypopharyngeal and Esophageal Reconstruction

JOHN J. COLEMAN III, MD ✦ AMARDIP S. BHULLER, MD

REASONS FOR RECONSTRUCTION

HISTORY OF RECONSTRUCTION
    Pedicled Alimentary Grafts
    Microvascular Transplantation

AIMS IN RECONSTRUCTION

PATIENT FACTORS IN PROCEDURE CHOICE

SURGICAL TECHNIQUES
    Jejunal Free Flap
    Radial Forearm Fasciocutaneous Flap
    Pectoralis Major Musculocutaneous Flap
    Deltopectoral Flap
    Gastric Pull-up
    Colon Interposition
    Other Methods: Lateral Thigh, Ulnar Forearm, and
        Gastroepiploic

Ancient documents allude to attempts at repair of defects caused by trauma and disease. From the oldest surgical and medical texts of Egypt, such as the Edwin Smith papyrus (circa 3000 to 2500 BC), to the Indian *Sushruta* (600 BC), surgeons practiced reconstruction of the nose, ear, and scalp. After the Dark Ages, ancient knowledge again resurfaced through various schools and translations of Arabic texts. In 1430, Branca developed a method of restoring form to the nose by use of skin flaps based on the arms.[1] Reliance on skin flaps from either local tissues or distant, however, characterized reconstruction for the next 500 years until the advent of the musculocutaneous concept and the era of microsurgery. Until the 1970s, multiple-stage skin flaps with high failure rates made surgery on the pharynx perhaps more dangerous than the natural history of the disease afflicting it.

The loss of speech and transnasal breathing and the disruption of the alimentary canal that impairs swallowing are physically and psychologically devastating for patients undergoing resection of the pharynx, larynx, and cervical esophagus. Re-establishment of gastrointestinal tract continuity and relatively normal oral alimentation are the main goals of reconstruction of the hypopharynx and cervical esophagus. When laryngectomy accompanies the pharyngeal resection, it is desirable to include the facilitation of alaryngeal speech (which usually means establishing a patulous or widely patent passage between the oral cavity and the remaining esophagus). The ideal reconstructive method is a single-stage procedure with low morbidity and mortality that provides for rapid restoration

of function with brief hospitalization. Such techniques must preserve the direct route of the airway, rapidly restore deglutition, and facilitate voice rehabilitation. Donor site morbidity must be low, and optimally the method imports tissue of like character to the resected pharyngoesophagus (i.e., lined by epithelium) from outside the field of surgical dissection and adjuvant radiotherapy.

REASONS FOR RECONSTRUCTION

The majority of defects of the cervical esophagus and hypopharynx are made in the treatment of malignant disease. The malignant neoplasm most commonly treated is squamous cell carcinoma of the respiratory epithelium lining, the larynx, and the pharynx. Although laryngeal preservation has been achieved with combined chemotherapy and radiotherapy in some patients under protocol,[1] the standard therapy for advanced squamous cell carcinoma of the larynx and pharynx is resection with a margin of normal tissue with or without neck dissection (depending on the stage at presentation) followed by postoperative adjuvant radiotherapy. The natural history of glottic carcinoma is one of slow growth with lymph node metastases relatively uncommon. Thus, T1, T2, and sometimes T3 N0 glottic carcinomas may be treated with radiotherapy alone with surgery reserved for salvage of treatment failure. Squamous cell carcinomas of the supraglottic larynx and all sites in the pharynx are not, however, constrained anatomically, as is laryngeal carcinoma; they are characterized by early local invasion outward from their epicenter and early nodal metastases frequently bilaterally. Although T1 N0 lesions or an occasional T2 N0 lesion may be treated with radiotherapy, most of the supraglottic and pharyngeal lesions require en bloc resection and neck dissection with adjuvant radiotherapy. Because of the frequency of submucosal spread and axillary and lymphatic metastases to the mediastinum, not laterally to the neck, cervical esophageal squamous cell carcinoma may require total esophagectomy and mediastinal dissection as well as adjuvant radiotherapy.[2] Definitive radiotherapy for laryngeal tumors is usually 5500 to 7000 cGy to the central neck without lateral fields. For postoperative adjuvant radiotherapy, 5000 to 6000 cGy is administered to the primary site and one or both sides of the neck.

The pharynx is a compact, mobile space capable of expanding and contracting, with structures whose synergy controls the vegetative functions of alimentation and respiration as well as the corollary functions of swallowing and speech. The surgical oncologic principle of removing the tumor with a margin of 2 cm of normal tissue frequently results in complete removal of the larynx and pharynx, leaving a circumferential defect extending from the base of the tongue anteriorly around to the posterior pharynx. If the distal extent of the defect is at or above the thoracic inlet, reconstruction can be accomplished totally within the neck. Release of the sternocleidomastoid from the sternum and medial clavicle or resection of the manubrium and mobilization of the subclavian vessels will expose the esophagus to the arch of the aorta. If subtotal resection of the pharynx is performed for laryngeal or pharyngeal lesions, a strip of mucosa and muscle may be left along the prevertebral fascia. Because unopposed action of the longitudinally transected constrictor muscle occurs immediately beneath the mucosa, this tissue bunches on the prevertebral fascia and may seem thin and inadequate for use in the reconstruction. Careful stretching to both sides and repositioning of the mucosa and muscle on the prevertebral fascia with resorbable stitches will demonstrate its true extent and determine whether it should be preserved for use in reconstruction or discarded.

Preservation of the larynx after resection of pharyngeal cancer is sometimes possible, particularly when a tumor presents in the base of the tongue, tonsillar pillar, or posterior pharynx. In these patients, reconstruction must aim to facilitate normal function of the larynx, not impairing its motion, and to provide sensation to the area surrounding the larynx so that the airway will not be presented with such substances as saliva or food without sensory warning. Another common cause for reconstruction of the hypopharynx and cervical esophagus is stenosis and stricture, usually after surgery or radiotherapy. Primary closure of the pharynges-laryngectomy defect has resulted in

a 15% to 45% fistula rate.[2] In those patients developing fistulas, the subsequent stenosis rate reaches 80%.[2] Adequate oral alimentation is an important quality of life concern for patients who often present with late-stage disease and are at high risk for recurrent disease and death. Prevention of the fistula and subsequent stenosis is therefore paramount. Stenosis may also result from technical flaws, particularly with the distal esophageal suture line of the pharyngeal reconstruction. When stenosis and subsequent dysphagia do present in a hypopharyngeal reconstruction either early or late, it is important to rule out recurrent tumors by endoscopy and biopsy. This is not an uncommon phenomenon. Congenital abnormalities, such as a wide cleft of the palate, may require the introduction of soft tissue to adequately separate the oropharynx and nasal cavity. Microvascular transplantation of the radial forearm or scapula flap is an excellent choice in patients when local tissue is inadequate. Tracheoesophageal fistula is a rare cause but may require cervical esophageal or total esophageal reconstruction. Pediatric tumors such as rhabdomyosarcoma are usually treated with chemotherapy and radiotherapy without surgery, but the subsequent retardation of growth and stricture at the site of the tumor necrosis may require reconstruction early in life.

Reconstruction for trauma to the hypopharynx and cervical esophagus is relatively uncommon. Small perforations from ingested objects (pins, fish bones) rarely cause significant deformity and can usually be repaired primarily or allowed to fistulize and heal secondarily. Penetrating wounds from gunshots are larger and are likely to be fatal because of proximity of the carotid artery and jugular vein laterally and the spinal cord posteriorly. On occasion, unrecognized iatrogenic injury to the esophagus during thyroidectomy or other cervical operations or overzealous resection of mucosa during the treatment of Zenker diverticulum (Fig. 83-1) may result in stenosis requiring surgical intervention and subsequent reconstruction. Unfortunately, such iatrogenic injuries are often compounded by transection of the recurrent laryngeal, external laryngeal, or vagus nerve, causing further disturbance to the important synergy of motion and sensation in the laryngopharynx. Such injuries may present as a postoperative abscess from a leak, and only after resolution of the infection does the fistula or stenosis become apparent (Fig. 83-2).

Ingestion of caustic substances such as alkali (lye, cleaning fluid) and acids may cause extensive damage to the oral cavity, pharynx, and cervical esophagus. Most patients are toddlers, although there is a second peak of incidence in the 20- to 30-year age group, for which attempted suicide or psychosis is the more common etiology. Depending on the concentration and volume of the substances ingested and the duration of the contact, there is damage to the oral cavity structures,

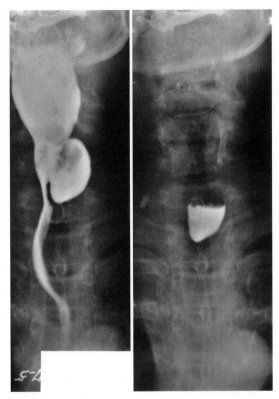

FIGURE 83-1. Zenker diverticulum caused by hypertension of the cricopharyngeus muscle with subsequent weakening of the muscle above and outpouching of mucosa. Treatment is by cricopharyngeus myotomy with or without resection of the diverticulum and closure.

the pharynx, the larynx, the cervical and thoracic esophagus, and the stomach. Coagulation of mucosal proteins results in full-thickness burn and perforation at any site. Contracture and epithelialization of the surface injury as well as deeper burns to the submucosa and muscle result in stenosis of the alimentary tube and synechiae of the walls of the pharynx and esophagus or a portion of the pharynx and tongue. To delineate the extent of injury, endoscopy, manometric studies of the esophagus, and computed tomography or magnetic resonance imaging are useful. If the proximal alimentary canal is heavily scarred, retrograde endoscopy through the gastrostomy and gastroesophageal junction is occasionally necessary to determine if there is any useful esophagus left or if total esophagectomy is indicated. Replacement of scarred, contracted tissue with epithelium-lined supple vascularized tissue is optimal. Because caustic ingestion may also result in immobility of the oral tongue with scarring of the floor of the mouth, velopharyngeal insufficiency caused by shortening of the soft palate and uvula and fixation to the pharyngeal wall, supraglottic stenosis caused by synechia of the epiglottis and

lateral and posterior pharyngeal wall, and esophageal stricture of varying length, the reconstruction plan must address all of these anatomic defects and functional disorders.

HISTORY OF RECONSTRUCTION

Billroth[3] reported the first laryngectomies. Reconstruction of the esophagus was not attempted until the late 19th century, and the proliferation of techniques during the next 100 years attests to the difficulty of the problem.[4] The easiest and simplest technique involved applying a split-thickness skin graft over a tubular or conical stent; this was rarely applicable in resections of any magnitude because of the high incidence of poor graft survival and stricture formation and reports of death caused by erosion of permanently implanted rigid stents into the great vessels and mediastinum. Wookey,[5] in 1942, reported cervical esophageal reconstruction with a laterally based rectangular neck flap of skin and platysma. In this method, the flap is raised when the laryngopharyngectomy is performed, and then suture of the cephalad margin to the base of the tongue and of the caudal margin to the esophagus in a tube establishes a lateral cervical sinus by suturing it to the fascia; this is later closed by mobilizing adjacent skin and grafting the donor neck several weeks after the resection. Wookey's method was an adaptation of the antethoracic skin tube reported by Bircher[6] in 1894 for the treatment of lye stricture. Unfortunately, this procedure had clear limitations, particularly the inadequacy of cervical skin supply resulting in difficulty in tubing of the skin. Furthermore, previous and subsequent radiotherapy decreased the likelihood of the successful reconstruction. Multiple descriptions of random flaps prepared by delay and tubing and ultimately waltzed to the neck for subsequent reconstruction characterized the next 50 years. Because of their multiple stages requiring prolonged hospitalization and the risk of complication and failure at each stage, they were infrequently attempted. If surgery was at all part of the therapy, the development of a permanent "controlled" cervical fistula was preferred.

Bakamjian[7] pushed the boundaries of head and neck surgery forward with the introduction of the deltopectoral flap in 1965. His method revolutionized reconstruction by reintroducing the concepts of arterial flap design advocated by Esser.[8] The deltopectoral flap is an axial-pattern flap based on perforators from the internal mammary artery lying just lateral to the sternum in the first through fourth intercostal spaces. This large flap, which could be rotated to the neck either tubed or untubed, allowed immediate reconstruction without the need to consider length-to-width ratios of prior flap design. In the second stage of the procedure, the base of the flap is divided and inset

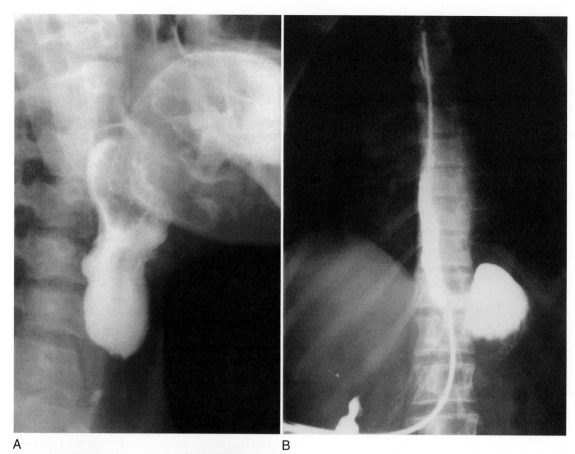

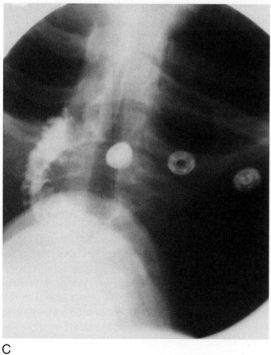

FIGURE 83-2. *A,* Complete obstruction of pharyngo-esophagus as a complication of partial transection of the esophagus during thyroidectomy. The level of the fistula with subsequent complete stenosis was below the vocal cords. *B,* Retrograde examination of the esophagus through the gastrostomy shows normal anatomy of the distal esophagus. *C,* Jejunal autograft resulted in re-establishment of alimentary continuity and swallowing without aspiration despite unilateral cord palsy secondary to recurrent laryngeal nerve injury at the time of thyroidectomy.

into the esophageal remnant, completely closing the defect. By performance of a delay procedure over the shoulder or axially down the arm, the length of the flap can be extended beyond the anterior axillary fold. Although difficulties with the flap were numerous and at least two stages were required to complete the reconstruction, it was markedly superior to the other methods then available and soon became the standard method of pharyngeal and indeed all head and neck reconstruction. In the 1970s, Ariyan[9] advocated the use of the pectoralis major flap to close oral and pharyngeal defects. Blood supply to the skin paddle is derived from perforators through the pectoralis major muscle from the subjacent thoracoacromial vessels. It is then transposed to the neck to close the pharyngeal defect. The skin island may be used as a patch or tube to establish the channel for alimentation in esophageal replacement. Limitations of the flap include the bulkiness and weight of the flap in most Americans, which increases the risk of dehiscence at the proximal anastomosis to the pharynx or base of tongue. Furthermore, the most distal end of the flap has a relatively sparse and random-pattern blood supply that may favor ischemic necrosis, particularly in the highly contaminated environment of the oropharynx. This was, however, a major breakthrough because reconstruction could be completed in one stage, improving the quality of life for patients and decreasing morbidity in these frequently malnourished and immunodeficient patients who have undergone multiple procedures. The pectoralis major musculocutaneous flap soon supplanted the deltopectoral flap for head and neck reconstruction with particular usefulness in patients with partial resections of the circumference of the pharynx and esophagus.

Pedicled Alimentary Grafts

Biondi proposed replacement of the esophagus with stomach brought into the chest through the diaphragmatic hiatus.[10] It was 40 years later, however, in 1933 when Oshawa[11] first described successful resection of the thoracic esophagus and immediate esophagogastrostomy. Sweet[12] verified that after ligation of the left gastroepiploic and short gastric vessels, the stomach remained totally viable and could be brought through the mediastinum to the level of the arch of the aorta. Brewer[13] performed a successful reconstruction of the cervical and thoracic esophagus with a subpharyngeal esophagogastrostomy in 1948. In 1907, Roux[14] attempted total antethoracic esophagoplasty by bringing the jejunum with its mesentery through the anterior mediastinum. Herzen, as described in Yudin,[15] reported a modified Roux method and subsequently performed the first successful procedure on a patient who had a stricture due to ingestion of lye. Yudin,[15] with several modifications of Herzen's operation,

described a series of 80 patients in 1944, most of whom suffered from caustic strictures. Because of the tethering effect of the small bowel mesentery, the distal bowel often failed to survive; the procedure was subsequently abandoned in favor of either esophagogastrostomy or right or left colon interposition. Kelling[16] in 1911 described replacement of the esophagus with the transverse colon. Vulliet,[17] to avoid the potential danger of mediastinitis should the operation fail, placed the left colon in a subcutaneous position in continuity with a tube of skin constructed to perform the proximal esophageal replacement.

In 1950, Orsini and Toupet[18] resurrected the use of colon interposition. Preference was given to the right colon and a transverse colon in the isoperistaltic position until 1954, when Goligher and Robin[19] reported a successful colon anastomosis to the pharynx in the antiperistaltic position. Baronofsky[20] subsequently confirmed the feasibility and utility of using the left and transverse colon in the antiperistaltic position because of the superior reliability of the vascular pedicle to these segments through the marginal artery.

Microvascular Transplantation

Because the diameter of the jejunum closely approximates that of the esophagus, Longmire[21] devised a procedure in which the jejunum was isolated on its mesenteric blood supply, implanted in a skin tube, and transplanted to the anterior chest to serve as an artificial esophagus. This procedure was the first recorded attempt to transfer a segment of bowel deprived of its native mesenteric blood supply to a different anatomic location. In 1947, following the concepts of Carrel,[22] Longmire described the modification of the Roux technique for antethoracic esophageal reconstruction designed to overcome the 22% incidence of distal necrosis of the segment of jejunum described with the Roux-Herzen procedure. Longmire, using a vascular clamp, temporarily occluded the first set of mesenteric vessels to the transposed bowel segment at the root of the mesentery. The second and third sets of vessels were divided at the mesenteric border, preserving the arcuate vessels. The loop was then advanced to the root of the neck in a subcutaneous tunnel. Two costal cartilages were resected at the left sternal border and the internal mammary vessels isolated. With use of binocular loupe magnification, anastomosis of the vessels supplying the distal mesenteric arcade to the internal mammary vessel was performed with 5-0 silk suture, setting the precedent for free transplantation of a portion of the alimentary tract for reconstruction of the cervical esophagus.

In 1959, Seidenberg[23] reported a technique of revascularizing the jejunal segment in the neck of dogs. The venous anastomosis was performed by use of a tantalum ring prosthesis; the arterial anastomosis was established by running continuous suture of 7-0 silk. Following this, a clinical procedure was performed but the patient died of a cerebrovascular accident on the seventh postoperative day. At autopsy, the vascular anastomoses to the jejunal segment were both noted to be patent. This led other surgeons to pursue free vascularized flaps. In 1961, Roberts[24] reported successful replacement of a cervical esophagus by revascularized free jejunal autograft in two patients. Also in 1961, Heibert[25] revascularized a free graft of gastric antrum in the neck to re-establish continuity of the cervical esophagus. Reports of successful jejunal transplantation by Nakayama[26] and Jurkiewicz[27] soon followed. Widespread acceptance of microvascular transplantation of free flaps, however, had to await the technological refinement of surgical instruments and suture material necessary to complete these procedures successfully. In the late 1970s and early 1980s, the renewed interest in the vascular supply to the muscle and skin that arose from the elucidation of the musculocutaneous concept led to the description of a number of fasciocutaneous flaps that were useful in pharyngeal and cervical esophageal reconstruction. Despite the relatively low incidence of abdominal complications in several large series of jejunal free autografts,[28,29] it was considered desirable to avoid laparotomy during these extensive head and neck procedures. The most important of the fasciocutaneous flaps is the free radial forearm flap, which was described by Yang[30] in 1981 and further refined by Harii.[31] After the initial report by Hayden,[32] Baek[33] reported a series of lateral thigh flaps for hypopharyngeal and cervical esophageal reconstruction. Numerous other flaps have been described for pharyngeal reconstruction, including free dorsalis pedis,[34] free ulnar,[35] free gastro-omental,[36] free ileocolic,[37] free tensor fasciae latae,[38] free rectus abdominis,[39] free lateral arm and free scapula,[40] and free peritoneal.[41] The free ulnar flap first described by Lovie[42] in 1984 appears to demonstrate a success rate comparable to that of the others described. Elective free tissue transplantation for pharyngeal reconstruction can now be accomplished with a success rate exceeding 90%, which greatly surpasses that of pedicled flaps.

AIMS IN RECONSTRUCTION

Advances in reconstructive technique have allowed surgeons to restore alimentary function in the head and neck even when the most radical local and locoregional resections have been performed. Clearly, the dominating tenet of surgical oncology remains resection of the primary tumor with a clear margin (usually around 2 cm) and removal of the real or potential lymphatic metastases. This along with adjuvant radiotherapy or chemotherapy is the critical step in providing the patient's highest priority, survival. The

reconstructive surgeon (should he or she be someone other than the extirpative surgeon) will help facilitate survival by providing a method that ensures a closed, healed wound. Furthermore, by analyzing the elements of the surgical defect, such as dimension, associated resection of the oral cavity structures or bone, previous or subsequent radiotherapy, and others, the reconstructive surgeon will be able to choose a technique that will return the patient to reasonable function and appearance, the two main parameters of quality of life, and do so in a time commensurate with the natural history of advanced squamous cell carcinoma of the pharynx. Clearly, this is best accomplished by a single-stage procedure. Only by having numerous procedures available for the specific needs of each patient will this successful approach be possible.

PATIENT FACTORS IN PROCEDURE CHOICE

In choosing the reconstructive procedure for a patient, the amount of esophagus resected, whether the defect is circumferential or partial, and whether the defect extends into the thorax or abdomen should significantly influence the reconstructive surgeon. Laryngectomy is usually a part of radical resection of lesions of the pharynx; therefore, the functional presence of the larynx is often not a consideration. However, when the larynx is left intact in a trauma patient or the occasional tumor resection, the status of its innervation (both motor and sensory) is critical. Potential sensate flaps, such as the radial forearm or lateral arm, are more useful in these patients than is the jejunum, whose secretory nature may cause problems with aspiration (Fig. 83-3).

Body habitus and preexisting comorbidities such as obesity, which make the use of thoracic musculocutaneous flaps less desirable, must also be considered. Renal failure treated with hemodialysis precludes the use of a radial forearm flap for reconstruction because this would waste a valuable access site for an arteriovenous fistula. Although it is certainly not a contraindication to visceral transfer, a history of intra-abdominal surgery with possible adhesions or other structural changes may limit certain techniques, such as colon interposition. Hepatic insufficiency with ascites is a major risk factor for bowel resection, however, and should suggest the use of another technique.

Although arteriosclerosis is a common systemic disorder in patients with pharyngeal carcinoma, it is rare to find occlusive disease in the neck so severe as to prevent microvascular anastomosis. The presence of a palpable facial artery at the mandibular notch is usually sufficient evidence of adequate arterial flow, but Doppler ultrasonography or rarely arteriography may be useful in preoperative evaluation. A more

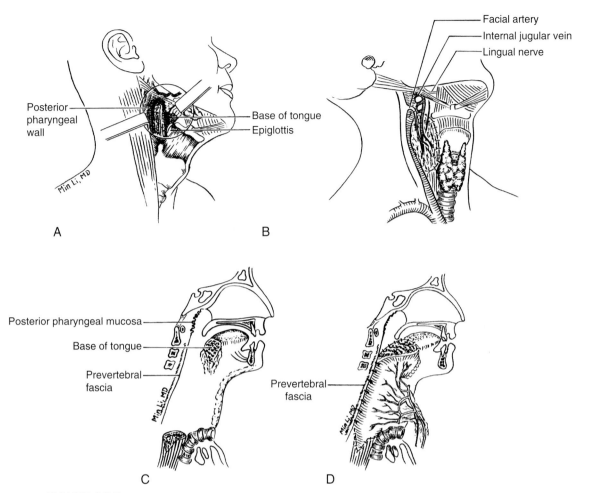

FIGURE 83-3. *A,* Partial pharyngectomy at or above the level of the larynx may form a defect of a size and complexity that requires flap closure. Function of the remaining larynx must be facilitated, which requires a flap of small dimensions and light weight. Because of its secretory mucosa, the jejunum is an inappropriate choice at this level. Whenever it is consistent with oncologic demands of the resection, superior laryngeal nerve function should be preserved. The posterolateral defect reveals the proximity of the epiglottis to the base of the tongue. Whatever reconstruction is used must allow the larynx to elevate to the level of the base of the tongue and epiglottis to effect closure of the respiratory tube during swallowing for prevention of aspiration. The facial or occipital artery can be dissected free above or below the posterior belly of the digastric muscle as a recipient vessel. The external jugular, internal jugular, or branch thereof serves as a recipient vein. *B,* A lightweight fasciocutaneous flap such as the radial forearm or the lateral arm flap is an excellent choice for reconstruction. Sensory neurotization of the flap by end-to-side anastomosis of a cutaneous sensory nerve to the lingual nerve may provide some protective sensation to the area closed by the flap. End-to-side venous anastomosis of the cephalic vein or venae comitantes to the internal jugular vein provides excellent venous outflow. *C,* Total laryngopharyngectomy is frequently required for tumors of the hypopharynx, particularly the piriform sinus, and for recurrence of laryngeal cancer after radiotherapy. The airway is re-established by permanent tracheostomy. The defect in the alimentary tube usually extends from the base of tongue and posterior pharyngeal wall to the inlet of the thoracic esophagus, resulting in a space bordered posteriorly by the prevertebral fascia and anteriorly by the skin of the neck. *D,* In the circumferential defect caused by the total laryngopharyngectomy, a jejunal free autograft is an excellent method of reconstruction; a tubular conduit is constructed from the base of the tongue and oropharyngeal mucosa to the hypopharynx or cervical or thoracic esophagus.

common problem is the lack of venous outflow secondary to previous neck dissection. Again, Doppler ultrasonography will provide a useful roadmap in such secondary resections and reconstructions. Multiple series of head and neck reconstruction have demonstrated that previous adjuvant or even curative radiotherapy is not a factor in the success of reconstruction by free tissue transplantation. The presence of pulsatile flow in a branch of the external carotid or subclavian at the time of neck exploration is satisfactory for continuation of the transplantation.

SURGICAL TECHNIQUES

To address the various problems of pharyngoesophageal reconstruction, the total reconstructive armamentarium available to the modern plastic surgeon should be considered. With all reconstructive techniques of the hypopharynx and cervical esophagus, the size and location of the defect are the dominant factors in determining the most appropriate technique. In patients with defects that extend inferiorly along the esophagus into the chest, techniques that use free tissue transplantation are more difficult, and gastric pull-up or colon interposition may present options more suitable. These procedures keep the anastomotic suture line out of the chest and may avoid the devastating complication of mediastinitis should there be an anastomotic leak or fistula at one of the suture lines. For defects that do not extend into the chest, the radial forearm flap and jejunal free flap are appropriate and frequently used; but fasciocutaneous flaps (such as the lateral thigh flap,[32] the free ulnar forearm flap,[35] and the lateral arm flap[40]) and viscera free transfer (such as the colon[37] and gastroepiploic[36] autograft) have been successfully described in small series. When there are no suitable vessels for microsurgical anastomosis because of previous surgery or irradiation, a pedicle flap may be required. In these instances, the pectoralis major flap is the preferred choice. Despite several small series demonstrating its successful use,[43-45] the pectoralis major flap has significant limitations, and a number of large series have shown a high complication rate, making it markedly inferior to free tissue transplantation.[46-48]

Preservation of cervical arteries and veins for safe microvascular anastomosis is of paramount importance in free tissue transplantation for reconstruction of the hypopharynx and cervical esophagus after pharyngolaryngectomy. Because most patients undergo pharyngolaryngectomy for squamous cell carcinoma of the hypopharynx and cervical esophagus, they may require simultaneous neck dissection, either unilateral or bilateral. It is therefore important that the surgeon save a proximal recipient vein as long as it does not compromise the therapeutic resection. Preservation of one jugular vein will facilitate end-to-

side anastomosis. When this is not possible, the cephalic vein can be transposed in situ as a graft, or a branch of the subclavian vein such as the transverse cervical can be used for venous anastomosis. Because of its location low in the neck, the transverse cervical artery is frequently spared in neck dissection and may not receive a full dose of adjuvant or therapeutic radiation. By division of its ascending branches as it courses laterally deep in the posterior triangle, it is mobilized with adequate length and caliber for microvascular anastomosis. To avoid anastomotic thrombosis due to accumulation of secretions from anastomotic leak, some surgeons recommend that the donor and recipient vessels be located high in the neck away from the dependent area. The position of the donor and flap vessels in the neck in the flexed, extended, and neutral positions is critical to the success of free tissue transplantation and reconstruction of the pharynx. Excessive pedicle length that results in kinking of the vessels on neck movement may result in thrombosis and graft necrosis. Similarly, inadequate length or poor positioning may result in anastomotic disruption or thrombosis. Because the pharyngoesophagus is a midline structure and the desired reconstructive goal is a simple conduit, a direct straight-line positioning of the reconstructive graft in the center of the neck is optimal in most patients. Redundancy and curving of the reconstructive segment may impair subsequent food bolus transit.

Jejunal Free Flap

The jejunum offers several advantages in its use as a free flap for hypopharyngeal and cervical esophageal reconstruction. The location of its donor site at a distance from the resection site allows two teams to work simultaneously. The appropriate selection and dissection of the vascular arcade will allow segments of bowel from 6 to 25 cm to be harvested, thus satisfying virtually any defect in the neck or upper mediastinum. When it is elevated appropriately, it has a homogeneous blood supply, and its lumen is similar in diameter to that of the cervical esophagus. Because it is a tubular structure, it serves as an excellent conduit for replacement of circumferential defects, particularly when the larynx has been removed. When laryngeal preservation has been accomplished, however, it should be used with caution unless the defect is below the level of the cricopharynges because of the risk of aspiration of its copious secretions. Several series have noted inferior esophageal or transesophageal speech with the jejunum, suggesting that the mucous secretions and uncoordinated contraction may impair the flow of air through the reconstructive segment.[49,50] Contraindications to the use of the jejunum are ascites and chronic inflammatory diseases of the bowel. Multiple previous laparotomies may make access difficult and potential donor tissue inadequate.

Because of the magnitude of combined resection and reconstruction, preoperative planning and preparation of the patient are critical. If there is dysphagia secondary to obstructing tumor, enteral feeding is implemented to approximate positive nitrogen balance, and adequate hemoglobin level is restored by transfusion if necessary. Similarly, pulmonary hygiene and preparation are important if aspiration or chronic obstructive pulmonary disease is present. In the operating room, a two-team approach will facilitate timely and efficient completion of the operation. As with any free tissue transplantation, hydration, maintenance of normothermia, and avoidance of systemic administration of vasoconstrictors are important elements of success. While the extirpative team works on the neck, the reconstructive team proceeds with the abdominal part of the operation. The abdomen is opened, and the ligament of Treitz is identified. A segment of jejunum with satisfactory jejunal vessels and arcade is identified at the site that will facilitate the formation of a tube jejunostomy just distal to the enteric anastomosis that results from the resection. The diameter of the jejunal vessel should be 2 to 4 mm for optimal microvascular anastomosis. Evaluation of the anatomic extent of the arcade is facilitated by transillumination of the mesentery. The length of jejunum required for cervical reconstruction will depend on the size of the defect after oncologic clearance has been achieved with confirmed clear margins. The wedge of supporting mesentery is divided by use of nonabsorbable ligatures. Because of the fragility of the veins, meticulous technique is required to prevent a mesenteric hematoma. Vessel loops are passed around the single artery and vein of the superior mesenteric arcade supplying the jejunal segment. The bowel is isolated, and a suture is used to mark the proximal or distal end of the bowel to ensure isoperistaltic placement. It is then divided between clamps, wrapped in a moistened laparotomy bed, and left perfusing in situ. A sutured or stapled anastomosis of the bowel proximal and distal to the segment is performed, the patency of the lumen is checked, and the mesentery is reapproximated (Fig. 83-4). The segment of bowel to be used for reconstruction is inspected for viability through its entire length, and any questionable bowel is resected along the mesenteric border (Fig. 83-5). Not until the oncologic portion of the procedure is completed and the vessels in the neck have been prepared for microvascular anastomosis is the bowel harvested by dividing the jejunal vessels. Before closure of the abdomen, a feeding jejunostomy distal to the bowel anastomosis is completed. After completion of the procedure in the neck, the defect is measured and suitable vessels are identified and prepared. The arterial inflow is provided by branches of the external

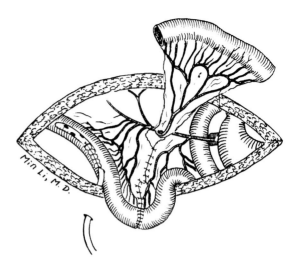

FIGURE 83-4. In harvesting of jejunum, the enteroenterostomies and closure of the mesentery should be performed with the autograft segment perfused in situ until the neck is completely prepared for transplantation.

carotid artery or by the transverse cervical artery selected to match the size of the donor and recipient vessels and to lie in the most favorable geometric configuration. If lumen size discrepancy is greater than 1.5:1, end-to-side anastomosis is recommended. Careful planning and adequate dissection of the vessels will usually obviate the need for a vein graft because this is thought to have a negative impact on graft survival. If necessary because of extensive inflammation, scarring, or arteriosclerosis, vessels in the contralateral neck or, as a last resort, the ipsilateral common carotid artery may be used. Once it is selected, the suitable artery is freed from surrounding tissue, and a soft noncalcified segment is chosen as the site of anastomosis. The superior thyroid artery, facial artery, and transverse cervical vessels are excellent choices. Because of the midline position of the reconstructed pharyngeal segment and the proximity of the internal jugular and carotid vessels, it is important to position the donor and recipient vessels so they lie in a comfortable geometric configuration that will prevent kinking of the vessels or accordion folding of the mesentery on neck movement and still allow the jejunal segment its straight pathway rather than curving in a bowed fashion.

After the vessels are occluded by microsurgical clamps and the final position of the anastomosis is determined, the blood flow is evaluated by loosening the clamp and observing for pulsatile flow. The clamp is then reapplied on the particular vein chosen in the same anatomic vicinity (external jugular vein, posterior facial vein, or internal jugular vein). When the internal jugular vein is chosen, vessel loops above and below the site chosen for anastomosis can be used to occlude the vein and to elevate it into a field where

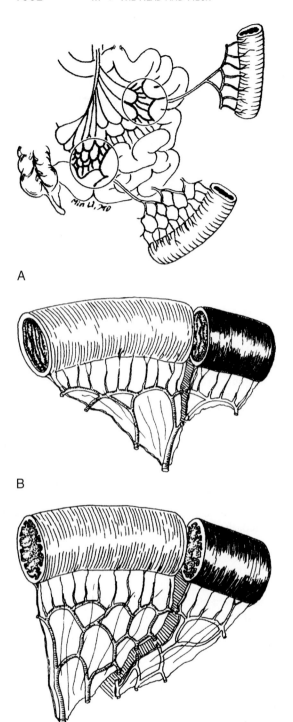

A

B

C

FIGURE 83-5. The number of arcades between the main mesenteric vessel and the bowel segment *(A)* is fewer in the proximal small bowel (jejunum) *(B)* than in the distal small bowel (ileum) *(C)*, making it easier to predict the relationship between the nutrient vessel and the bowel.

anastomosis will be facilitated. Veins that are in juxtaposition to the tracheostomy should not be used to avoid possible thrombosis from adjacent inflammation. Selection and preparation of the appropriate vessels are mandatory before harvesting of the free autograft to allow a shorter ischemic interval. After the viability of the jejunal segment has been confirmed on its native pedicle, the supplying vessels are divided and ligated; the jejunum is brought up to the head and neck and positioned in an isoperistaltic position. The most difficult visceral anastomosis (usually the proximal) is performed first when visibility is best, followed by microvascular anastomosis and finally the second (usually distal) visceral anastomosis. Adequate visualization for proper suture placement is critical to prevent fistula, particularly when the proximal anastomosis is high in the oropharynx or nasopharynx. To facilitate this, a mandibulotomy may be necessary. In the event of size discrepancy in the oral cavity or oropharynx, the proximal bowel can be opened along the antimesenteric border and tailored to fit the defect from the tongue to the posterior pharynx if necessary (Fig. 83-6). After completion of the proximal

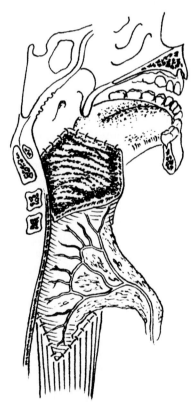

FIGURE 83-6. Splitting the jejunum along its antimesenteric border will increase the diameter of the lumen somewhat, accommodate defects of various shapes, and decrease the likelihood of circumferential scarring and subsequent stenosis. Insetting a portion of the flap in a V shape at the esophageal anastomosis will decrease the risk of stenosis.

pharyngojejunal anastomosis by either one-layer or two-layer technique with absorbable sutures, the vessels are positioned to avoid torsion and the flap is positioned in the midline. The deeper of the vessels undergoes an anastomosis first followed by the more superficial with 9-0 or 8-0 monofilament suture. If arteriosclerotic plaque is discovered during the anastomosis, it is critical to avoid dissection of the atheroma or formation of an intimal flap. In these patients, it is important that the needle be passed toward the plaque to fix it to the media and the adventitia rather than pushing it away. When the microvascular clamps are removed, perfusion of the jejunum will result in return of its normal color with pulsation of the vessels along the bowel, bleeding of the cut edges, peristalsis, and excessive mucous secretion. The length of the jejunal segment must be adjusted so it lies in a direct line of appropriate length to avoid redundancy with its subsequent dysphagia. The distal jejunal anastomosis is similarly performed with interrupted 3-0 absorbable suture. Triangular interdigitation of the jejunum into the esophagus may prevent stricture at the distal anastomosis (Fig. 83-7). Before closure of the overlying skin flap, the neck is moved through a full range of passive motion to ensure that there is no twisting or

torsion of the vessels or of the segment that would compromise blood flow. To maintain the vessels and the bowel segment in a satisfactory position, tacking sutures from the bowel or mesentery to the prevertebral fascia may be placed. If appropriate, the mesentery of the jejunum may be used to cover the previously irradiated carotid vessels. Monitoring can be performed by exteriorization of a small vascularized segment of jejunum or by leaving a small segment of the incision open for direct observation. Although many methods of invasive monitoring are described, external application of Doppler ultrasonography is preferred. Hourly monitoring is used for 48 to 72 hours. If there are no complications, a barium swallow study is performed at 7 to 10 days to evaluate patency and integrity of the visceral anastomoses (Fig. 83-8). If no leak is demonstrated, a liquid or soft diet is started. If a fistula develops, however, most will heal by secondary intention without surgery and can be managed on an outpatient basis with the patient allowed nothing by mouth. Radiation therapy is started at 4 to 6 weeks if indicated, and the jejunostomy tube is left to supplement nutrition during radiation therapy if necessary. Even in the presence of a fistula, radiation therapy should commence within 6 weeks to promote

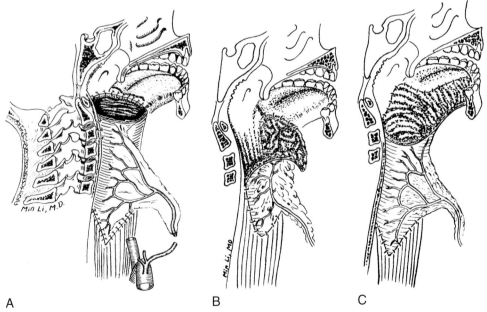

A   B   C

FIGURE 83-7. *A,* Reconstruction of a circumferential defect of the pharynx with a tube of jejunum. Careful suturing of the graft in one or two layers to the base of the tongue and the distal pharyngoesophagus is critical. Suture of the serosa of the jejunal graft to the prevertebral fascia will help mitigate the effects of gravity on the proximal suture line, particularly because uncoordinated muscle movement of the jejunum will occur on restoration of blood flow and may place traction on the proximal suture line. The transverse cervical vessels are excellent recipient vessels because the course of the mesenteric vessels places them lateral in the neck. *B,* When the defect after resection has an irregular border or is not completely circumferential, the jejunum may be divided along the antimesenteric border to make a patch for the reconstruction. *C,* Defects that include part of the oral cavity can be reconstructed with the jejunum, which is customized as necessary by dividing along the antimesenteric border and either keeping or discarding part of the jejunum to design a fillet and tube flap.

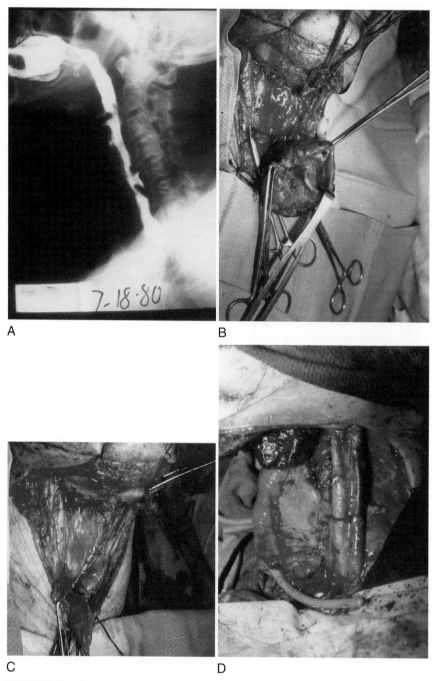

A

B

C

D

FIGURE 83-8. *A*, Radiologic appearance of squamous cell carcinoma of the cervical esophagus after failure of radiotherapy as the primary treatment. *B* and *C*, Defect after laryngopharyngectomy extends from the base of the tongue to the esophagus at the thoracic inlet. *D*, Segment of jejunum revascularized by end-to-end anastomosis to the superior thyroid artery and end-to-side anastomosis to the internal jugular vein.

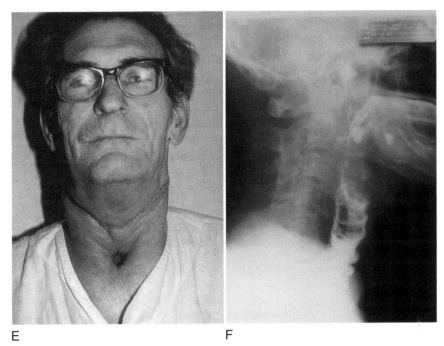

E   F

FIGURE 83-8, cont'd. *E* and *F*, Primary healing occurred. Barium swallow examination at 10 days demonstrates intact conduit between oral cavity and thoracic esophagus.

optimal oncologic outcomes. More than 50% of fistulas present at the beginning of radiation therapy will heal without surgery during or after irradiation.[51]

Radial Forearm Fasciocutaneous Flap

The radial forearm flap is a fasciocutaneous flap based on septocutaneous branches from the radial artery. It is a useful method for reconstruction of the hypopharynx and cervical esophagus in carefully selected patients who have undergone total laryngopharyngectomy or particularly in those with the larynx intact after partial resection. Its reliable homogeneous vascularity, ease of elevation, potential for sensory innervation, and long pedicle length with a large vessel diameter of approximately 2 to 4 mm make it attractive for microsurgical technique. The thin skin of the forearm with its pliability is amenable to the three-dimensional shaping necessary to reconstruct the posterior pharynx and tonsillar area. Because a very small flap can be designed, partial defects of the pharynx with the larynx intact may be reconstructed. Because the goal for esophageal speech is to facilitate the passage of air through a simple conduit, the flaccid noncontractile radial forearm is perhaps superior to the jejunum in restoring speech.

For defects proximal to the intact larynx or partial larynx, the nonsecretory nature of the forearm skin makes the radial forearm or other fasciocutaneous flaps superior to the jejunum for pharyngeal reconstruction.

The radial forearm fasciocutaneous free flap's blood supply relies on the radial artery, its venae comitantes, and the cutaneous veins of the forearm, most important of which is the cephalic vein (Fig. 83-9). Because the radial artery in the majority of patients is the dominant vessel to the deep palmar arch, supplying the princeps pollicis and the radialis indicis arteries, and interruption of flow may cause injury to the thumb and index finger, it is mandatory before a radial forearm free flap to determine that there is a patent anastomosis between the radial and ulnar arteries at the level of the deep palmar arch. Assessment of flow across the palmar arch is conventionally determined by performing an Allen test of patency of the ulnar and radial arteries and the completeness of patency of the palmar arch. Ultrasonic Doppler study and other techniques may be helpful when there is uncertainty about flow. A particular advantage of the radial forearm flap is the degree of freedom with which it can be designed to fit defects of variable size and shape encountered in attempting pharyngoesophageal reconstruction. Most of the volar surface of the arm can be included in the flap if its design is centered on the vessels and its various skin territories are connected to the central pedicle by subcutaneous and septocutaneous branches. To facilitate dissection during harvest, the arm may be exsanguinated with an elastic bandage and a tourniquet above the elbow inflated to

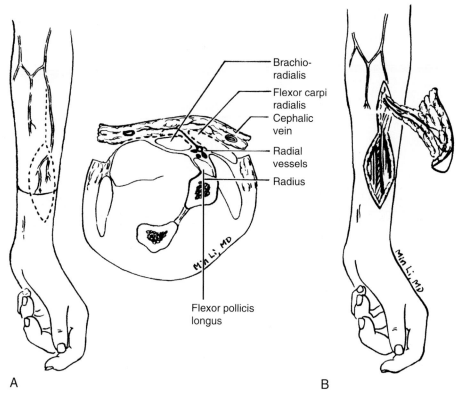

FIGURE 83-9. *A,* The radial forearm free flap is a fasciocutaneous flap supplied by septocutaneous branches of the radial artery and its venae comitantes that travel between the vessels and the skin between the brachioradialis muscle and flexor carpi radialis muscle. Most of the skin of the forearm can be centered on the vessels to raise the flap. The cephalic vein as well as the venae comitantes can be used for venous outflow. *B,* The radial forearm flap is a versatile tool for pharynx reconstruction. A patch of skin can be used for partial defects, or a circumferential defect can be reconstructed by tubing the flap to itself. The donor site is closed primarily or by split-thickness skin grafting.

100 mm Hg above the patient's baseline systolic pressure. This technique has been described in most reports of the radial forearm flap; the authors prefer simply to obtain hemostasis as the procedure is performed because release of the tourniquet may result in bleeding into the septum between the pedicle and the skin and subsequent edema of the flap. Design of the flap to contain the cephalic or another large cutaneous vein makes the microvascular anastomosis easier because the venae comitantes (although these can be dissected beyond the antecubital plexus to a larger caliber) are frequently small. The radial vessels are easily identified in the proximal forearm between the brachioradialis and flexor carpi radialis muscles. The dissection of the flap may proceed from the ulnar or radial side, raising the fascia off the brachioradialis and flexor carpi radialis, leaving them attached to the intramuscular septum. Beneath the vessels lie the radius and the flexor pollicis longus muscle. The fascia should be raised off this to prevent windows in the septocutaneous connections. After isolation of the flap on the radial vessels, they are divided distally and the flap is raised; the proximal pedicle is prepared for microvascular anastomosis,

and the flap is left in situ to be perfused until the recipient site is prepared for flap transplantation. If there is a complete pharyngeal defect, the flap may be tubed on the arm to decrease the ischemic time after transfer. Inset of the flap in the neck is done with precautions similar to those taken in jejunal free autograft; each stitch is placed carefully under full visualization. The length of the pedicle is useful if the internal jugular vein is not available for end-to-side anastomosis. The external jugular or transverse cervical vessels are particularly appropriate choices in such situations. The flap can be positioned so that the vessels are at either the cephalad or caudad margin to facilitate anastomosis. Interrupted absorbable stitches are used to perform the visceral anastomoses. If the margin of the flap is de-epithelialized, a second-layer closure may be performed along the suture lines by approximating the subcutaneous tissue of the radial forearm free flap over the first layer of suture, particularly along the proximal suture line. Triangular interdigitation of the radial forearm flap into the distal esophagus is helpful in preventing stricture. Injection of saline through the nasopharynx into the reconstructed area under pressure is useful to determine whether the flap is watertight.

In patients in whom the larynx is still intact, the lateral and medial antebrachial cutaneous nerves may be anastomosed to the greater auricular or lingual nerve in an attempt to provide protective sensation. Tracheoesophageal puncture may be performed either at the time of surgery or as a secondary procedure. Monitoring is performed by transcutaneous Doppler ultrasonography on the radial artery or direct visualization of an exteriorized portion of the flap or of the luminal surface with endoscopy. If the external suture line is intact at 10 days without evidence of fistula or infection, a barium swallow study is obtained to demonstrate patency and watertight seal. If there is no evidence of fistula, the feeding tube is removed and the patient begins a liquid diet. The donor site is reconstructed with a split-thickness sheet skin graft held in place with a pressure dressing, and the hand is splinted in the neutral position for 7 to 14 days to prevent graft shear over the flexor muscles of the arm (Fig. 83-10).

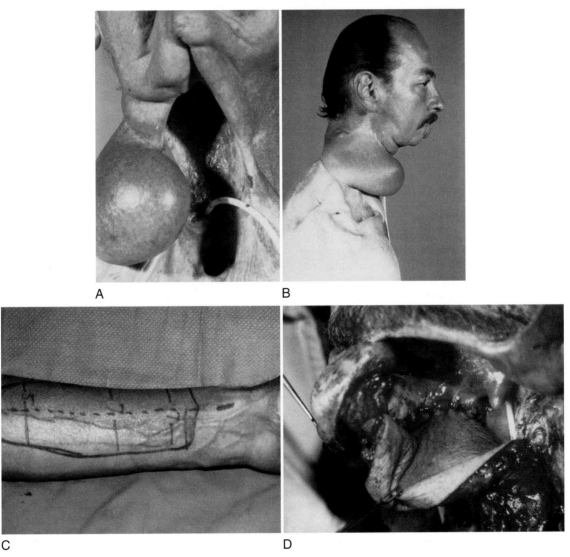

FIGURE 83-10. *A* and *B,* Patient who had previously undergone total glossectomy and laryngopharyngectomy with neck dissection for persistent squamous cell carcinoma of the base of the tongue after failure of radiation therapy. Multiple attempts at reconstruction with thoracic musculocutaneous flaps had failed, leaving a large oropharyngocutaneous fistula with the remnant of a trapezius musculocutaneous flap adjacent to it. *C* and *D,* A large radial forearm free flap was designed to provide a substitute for the missing oral and pharyngeal mucosa. The homogeneous blood supply at the flap and its light weight made it less likely than the bulky thoracic musculocutaneous flaps to pull away from the tenuous, irradiated residual mucosa of the oral cavity and pharynx. The microvascular anastomosis was performed between the radial vessels and the transverse cervical vessels. *Continued*

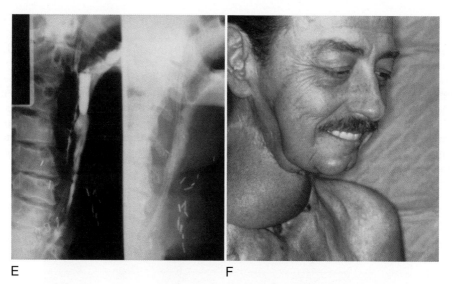

E   F

FIGURE 83-10, cont'd. *E* and *F,* The reconstruction healed primarily, restoring alimentary continuity. The patient was able to maintain weight adequately by peroral feedings.

Pectoralis Major Musculocutaneous Flap

Described in the mid-1970s and popularized in the early 1980s, the pectoralis major musculocutaneous flap was an important addition to the techniques available for hypopharyngeal and cervical reconstruction. Free tissue transplantation has superseded it to a great degree, however. In the unusual situation in which no vessels are available for microvascular anastomosis or in selected instances, the flap may be transposed from the thorax based on its main axial blood supply, the thoracoacromial vessels. If the skin island is designed below the fourth intercostal space, the deltopectoral flap based on the internal mammary perforators may be harvested from the ipsilateral chest wall (Fig. 83-11). The advantages of the pectoralis major musculocutaneous flap are its ease of harvest, absence of requirement for microvascular anastomosis, low donor site morbidity, and ample supply of well-vascularized muscle to cover the exposed carotid and jugular vessels. There are, however, several major disadvantages of the pectoralis major flap. The random blood supply of its distal end and the flap's excessive bulk in most Americans make it difficult to be tubed, and the considerable weight may increase tension on the proximal anastomosis, leading to fistula formation and subsequent stricture at the base of the tongue. Tracheoesophageal speech, although possible, is somewhat less likely to be achieved as the heavy flap tends to collapse on itself, narrowing the lumen and interfering with the flow of air through it to the mouth. Several

authors have described modifications of this technique, such as thinning or use of the muscle alone to circumvent some of these problems.[44,45,52]

In partial defects of the pharynx, the skin island is sutured to the remaining mucosa with one or two layers of interrupted stitches of absorbable suture. Passage of the suture through the prevertebral fascia as well as the mucosa will help prevent fistula caused by traction of the heavy flap on the suture line. This is particularly useful at the lateral extents of the cephalad base of the tongue suture line. Although it is somewhat more difficult with the bulky skin over the pectoralis muscle, some form of splaying or interdigitation of the flap into the distal esophageal segment is appropriate. When the pharyngeal defect is circumferential or complete, the skin island may be tubed, although this may be difficult because of its bulk and may result in a narrow lumen or fistula because of the long axial flap-to-flap suture line. Fabian[44] described a method of reconstruction of circumferential defects in which the posterior wall of the neopharynx is reconstructed with a split-thickness skin graft sutured to the prevertebral fascia. The remaining 270 degrees of lumen is reconstructed with the pectoralis flap sutured to the base of the tongue and esophagus at its cephalad and caudad margins and to the margin of the split-thickness skin graft and the prevertebral fascia at the lateral margins, thus forming a 360-degree reconstruction (Fig. 83-12).

The morbidity to the upper extremity and shoulder from loss of function with the pectoralis major musculocutaneous flap may be significant in patients

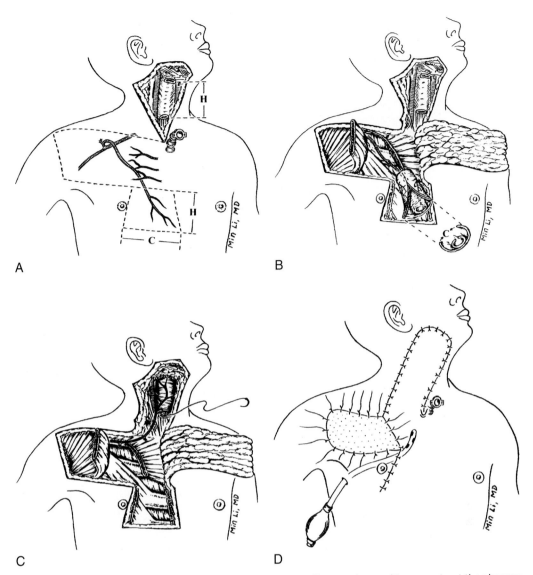

FIGURE 83-11. *A,* The pectoralis major musculocutaneous flap may be used to reconstruct the pharynx as either a patch or a tube. In planning the procedure, it is wise to design the flap so that if there is a fistula or some other subsequent requirement for tissue, the deltopectoral flap may be used. Flap design should allow raising of the pectoralis flap, which is based on the thoracoacromial vessels, leaving the perforators from the internal mammary vessels intact to supply the deltopectoral flap. This should be done whether the deltopectoral flap is elevated or not. H, length of defect and length of flap; C, circumference of defect and width of flap. *B,* The pedicle for the pectoralis flap is made up of the thoracoacromial vessels; if appropriate, it may be skeletonized to just proximal to the skin island. Muscle must be included beneath the skin island to transport perforators to the skin island. The bulk of the flap makes tubing of the flap somewhat difficult, but if this is done, the lumen should be constructed to match both the proximal and distal lumen size. The deltopectoral flap is reflected back to its perforator blood supply to facilitate fashioning of the tubed flap. *C,* Careful anastomosis of the skin of the flap to the mucosa proximal and distal is performed with interrupted 2-0 absorbable sutures. Fixation of the pectoralis flap to the prevertebral fascia will mitigate the effects of gravity on the bulky flap. *D,* When there is a cutaneous defect in the neck as well as the oropharyngeal defect, the deltopectoral flap can be transposed to cover most of the neck. The donor defect in the chest is minimized by advancing skin flaps from the inferior and lateral chest and the upper abdomen and skin grafting the residual defect.

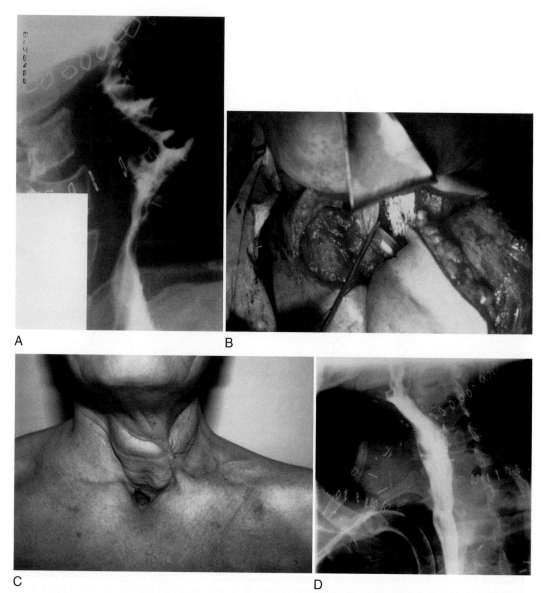

FIGURE 83-12. *A,* Patient with recurrent carcinoma of the cervical esophagus after failure of radiation therapy. Reconstruction with jejunal free autograft was unsuccessful. Necrotic jejunum was débrided. *B,* Because of the heavily irradiated neck with previous dissection and failure of the jejunum, a pectoralis major musculocutaneous flap was used for the salvage procedure. The lateral margins of the skin island were inset into the prevertebral fascia on both sides. The proximal margin of the skin flap is inset into the base of the tongue and oropharyngeal mucosa, and the distal margin is inset into the cervical esophagus in a 270-degree arc, constructing the anterior and lateral walls of the nasopharynx. The posterior wall is made by suturing the mucosa of the nasopharynx and cervical esophagus to the prevertebral fascia and covering the intervening prevertebral fascia with a split-thickness skin graft. *C* and *D,* Healed neck wound at 1 month after complete closure. Barium swallow examination showed intact reconstruction.

who have undergone previous or synchronous neck dissection.[45,52] Numerous series comparing complications and functional results have noted problems with the thoracic musculocutaneous flaps, especially compared with free tissue transplantation.[47,48]

Deltopectoral Flap

From 1965 when it was described by Bakamjian[7] until the late 1970s with the advent of the thoracic musculocutaneous flaps, the deltopectoral flap was the primary resource for pharyngeal reconstruction. Its axial blood supply is obtained from the perforating branches of the internal mammary vessels near the sternal margin; the skin and fascia overlying the cephalad chest wall may be raised from the midaxillary line to the blood supply 1 to 2 cm lateral to the sternal border. Further extension over the deltoid or down the arm may be designed but requires a delay procedure. This usually pliable skin and fascia may be tubed on itself and inset to the cephalad margin of a circumferential defect or inset to the margins of a partial defect. The proximal end of the flap is left open as a controlled fistula. After the flap has parasitized its blood supply from the inset margins (usually 14 to 21 days), the proximal blood supply of the flap on the chest wall is divided and the distal end inset to the esophageal margin, closing the controlled fistula. Thus, in two or three stages, the neopharynx is reconstructed.

Although an enormous improvement over the random thoracic skin flaps or multiple-stage waltzed flaps available before 1965, the deltopectoral flap has significant limitations. Despite its axial pattern, the most distal portion of the flap usually has a random blood supply, making it vulnerable to infection from the contaminated bacterial environment of the oropharynx. The twists and turns necessary to form a tubular conduit place its blood supply at some jeopardy when it is used for a circumferential reconstruction. Finally, the necessity of neovascularization from a surgically impaired or perhaps an irradiated environment makes ultimate success questionable. Because of these problems and the availability of more reliable single-stage methods, the deltopectoral flap is primarily an adjunct to other methods of pharynx reconstruction. It is particularly useful for replacing the skin of the neck when it is involved in the resection or has been severely damaged by previous radiotherapy. As mentioned earlier, this flap can be preserved in raising the pectoralis major musculocutaneous flap as a possible lifeboat, or it can be raised in combination with it by locating the skin island of the pectoralis major flap lower than the fourth intercostal space.

Gastric Pull-up

Total replacement of the esophagus is required when lesions of the hypopharynx or cervical esophagus extend directly into the thoracic esophagus or in patients with the skip lesions that sometimes characterize squamous cell carcinomas arising in the cervical esophagus. Unlike pharyngeal squamous cell carcinoma, which usually spreads laterally to the larynx or neck, cervical esophageal squamous cell carcinoma frequently spreads axially into the mediastinal lymph nodes or thoracic esophagus, requiring total esophagectomy for extirpation. Gastric pull-up allows a single-stage reconstruction of the entire esophagus with the advantage of a single anastomotic suture line out of the mediastinum.

The right gastric and right gastroepiploic vessels are the usual blood supply to the mobilized stomach for the gastric pull-up. The left gastric, the short gastrics, and the origin of the left gastroepiploic vessels are divided to allow mobilization of the stomach superiorly on the right gastric vessels after a Kocher maneuver has been performed. The stomach is passed through the hiatus of the diaphragm, and blunt manual dissection of the posterior mediastinum from above and below forms a passageway for delivery to the neck by traction on the cardia or remaining esophagus. Particular care is necessary in dissection behind the membranous trachea because perforation of this thin wall of the intrathoracic portion may result in tracheoesophageal fistula. When the proximal stomach has reached the neck, it is further mobilized to provide adequate length for two-layer pharyngogastric anastomosis, which is preferably performed end-to-side to the fundus (Fig. 83-13). Tacking sutures from the gastric serosa to the prevertebral fascia in the neck may mitigate traction forces somewhat and decrease the likelihood of an anastomotic leak. Vagotomy and pyloromyotomy or pyloroplasty are performed to aid with gastric emptying. Barium swallow examination is performed at 10 days, depending on the clinical picture. The stomach has a generous blood supply even based on these two vessels and is thus relatively radioresistant should adjuvant radiotherapy be required. The direct route through the mediastinum and the relatively large caliber of the lumen form a good conduit for swallowing. Disadvantages of the gastric pull-up include the increased perioperative morbidity and mortality secondary to transgression of both the abdominal and thoracic cavities. Mortality rates of 10% to 20% have been reported. Problems attendant on other forms of gastric surgery, such as dumping syndrome, massive gastric reflux and regurgitation, and dysphagia, may also occur in gastric pull-up. When a high pharyngogastric anastomosis is required, cephalad mobilization of the

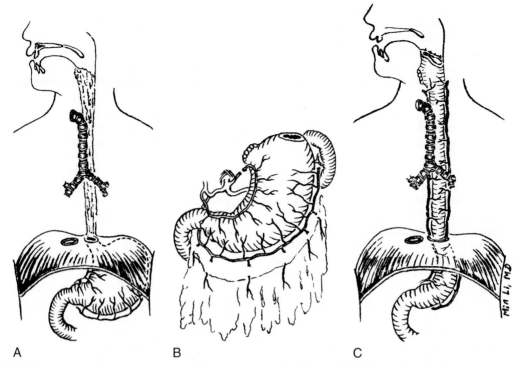

A   B   C

FIGURE 83-13. *A,* Tumors of the cervical esophagus or hypopharynx with significant distal extension or submucosal spread may require laryngopharyngectomy with total esophagectomy for adequate tumor clearance. *B,* Division of the short gastric vessels, the left gastric, and the left gastroepiploic and division of the omentum from the gastroepiploic will allow the stomach to be mobilized cephalad through the diaphragm. The blood supply to the stomach is from the right gastric and right gastroepiploic vessels. *C,* The stomach is passed through the posterior mediastinum behind the trachea and ordinarily will reach the pharynx. The gastroesophageal junction is closed and end-to-side anastomosis performed between the pharynx and the stomach tube. A pyloroplasty is necessary because the vagus nerves are divided in the gastric pull-up.

stomach may lead to increased tension on the anastomosis and ischemia of the distal end. Edema in the relatively narrow confines of the posterior mediastinum may result in distal ischemia. Despite these potential problems, gastric pull-up is an excellent method of total esophageal and pharyngeal reconstruction when oncologic considerations suggest its use.

Colon Interposition

Colon interposition based on the right, left, or middle colic vessels has been used for pharyngoesophageal reconstruction when total esophagectomy has been performed and when there has been previous gastric surgery or some other limitation to the use of the stomach. The ideal method of transposition is through the posterior mediastinum, but substernal and even subcutaneous routes have been described.[53] After several arcades are divided, the colon is brought by one of these routes to the neck. The distal anastomosis is performed to the fundus of the stomach and the proximal to the remaining pharyngoesophagus. The colon is reconstituted by colocolostomy or ileo-

colostomy as appropriate. Microvascular anastomosis of the most distal arcade has been described to improve viability of that segment farthest from the mesenteric blood supply.

Because of the somewhat tenuous blood supply of the colon segment (particularly in the elderly), the necessity for three viscera anastomoses, and the risk of total failure in the mediastinum, this method has been used less frequently in recent years.

Other Methods: Lateral Thigh, Ulnar Forearm, and Gastroepiploic

First described in 1984 for reconstruction of a cervical esophagus and hypopharynx and subsequently championed by Hayden,[32] the lateral thigh flap is a fasciocutaneous flap with a potentially larger surface area than the radial forearm flap. The lateral thigh flap, free of the excess bulk associated with musculocutaneous flaps, is relatively thin and pliable with a long vascular pedicle (usually about 8 to 12 cm) arising from the profunda femoris artery; vessel diameters are in the range of 3 mm. If it is harvested with the lateral femoral cutaneous nerve, the cutaneous island may be sensory innervated, providing potential benefit in swallowing or laryngeal protection. The donor site can usually be closed primarily; because of this flap's location in the leg, its use facilitates a two-team approach when extirpation and reconstruction are performed synchronously. The flap comprises the skin of the posterolateral thigh and underlying subcutaneous tissue. The long axis of the flap is placed over the intramuscular septum between the long head of the biceps femoris and the vastus lateralis muscles. The blood supply arises from the perforators of the profunda femoris, particularly the third of four perforators that travel deep to the adductor longus muscle and along the medial aspect of the femur before piercing a small amount of the margin of the adductor magnus and entering the subcutaneous tissue midway between the greater trochanter and the lateral femoral condyle. Skin islands up to 27 × 14 cm have been described,[33] and pedicle length may be increased by de-epithelialization of portions of the proximal flap. Venous drainage is through the venae comitantes of the perforators.

Although the lateral thigh flap has been described to be a reliable flap with considerable versatility,[32,33] the difficulty in dissecting the pedicle off the linea aspera of the femur and intramuscular septum has limited its popularity somewhat. Virtually every other fasciocutaneous flap has been described in small series as a useful tool in reconstruction of the pharynx.[30-35,38,40] The scapula flap[40] and lateral arm flap[33] as well as the free ulnar flap have had particular advocacy. Li[35] published 6 years' experience with the free ulnar forearm flap initially described by Lovie,[42] stating that its advantages include less conspicuous donor defect and provision of an ample amount of hairless skin. As with the radial forearm free flap, it is critical that an Allen test be performed to demonstrate the patency of the palmar arch and adequacy of supply by the radial vessels. A skin island up to 9 × 22 cm can be developed by placing the axis of the flap over the ulnar artery and vein. Similar to the radial forearm flap, the fascia is dissected off the flexor digitorum superficialis and profundus muscle and the flexor carpi ulnaris muscle, and the branches to these muscles are electrocoagulated within the muscles so that they are not injured in the intramuscular septum where they connect with the skin island. The basilic vein may be included as a venous outflow unit. Care must be taken not to injure the ulnar nerve in dissection of the flap. The donor defect is treated similarly to that of the radial forearm free flap by application of an unmeshed split-thickness skin graft.

In some patients, history of previous surgery and irradiation, oncologic dictates of the surgical resection, or some other reason may necessitate a segment of tissue to reconstruct the pharynx but no adjacent recipient vessels for microvascular anastomosis. In such instances, the gastroepiploic flap is an excellent choice.

A portion of the greater curvature of the stomach is harvested and vascularized by the gastroepiploic vessels. It can be used either as a patch or tubed for complete circumferential defects. By placing the segment of stomach fairly proximal on the greater curvature and by dissecting the gastroepiploic vessels off the greater curvature and following them back to their origin, a long vascular pedicle of large vessel diameter is obtained. This facilitates both reconstruction of the central pharyngeal defect and microvascular anastomosis at a distant cervical, thoracic, or axillary site (Figs. 83-14 and 83-15).

SUMMARY

Reconstruction of the pharynx and cervical esophagus has progressed dramatically in the last 20 years. With the proliferation of the techniques attendant on the development of microvascular surgery, there are numerous choices available for primary restoration or for secondary reconstruction necessary for recurrent disease or complications of primary surgery. Choice of a superior method from analysis of the literature is difficult, however, because of the relative rarity of the disease, the number of methods available, and the limited number of reports that measure restoration of function in addition to flap success and complications as endpoints. Clearly, the main risks of pharyngeal surgery (i.e., death, technique failure, fistula stenosis, and dysphagia) must be carefully considered. Furthermore, the local environment, particularly the presence of previous chemotherapy, radiotherapy, or surgery, is a critical factor. The recent increase in larynx-sparing protocols using chemoradiotherapy with surgery as salvage makes this an even more cogent consideration. Surkin's overview[48] in 1984 and Schechter's analysis[54] in 1987 both advocated the use of gastric pull-up as the optimal method of reconstructing the pharyngoesophagus. Schusterman,[55] however, in his 1990 series showed a much lower complication rate and higher ultimate success rate with jejunal free autograft. Graft failure was found to be 6% for the free jejunal autograft versus 13% for the gastric pull-up. Fistula occurred in 16% of patients reconstructed with jejunum and in 20% of patients with gastric pull-up. Like other authors, Schusterman noted a high rate of spontaneous resolution of fistula in the jejunum (75% as opposed to only 7% with the stomach), suggesting that the pharyngogastric anastomotic dehiscence is a function of ischemia rather than of mere technical error.

Although both methods had comparable success rates in swallowing (88% jejunum and 87% stomach), patients undergoing free jejunal autograft left the hospital earlier (10.6 versus 16 days) and resumed oral alimentation earlier (22.3 versus 29 days).[55] Carlson,[56] in his review of 20 years of experience of

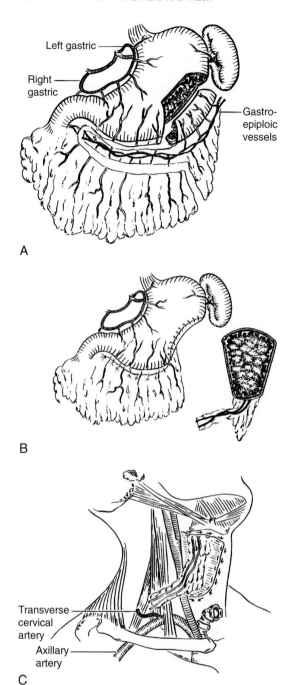

Left gastric

Right gastric

Gastro-epiploic vessels

A

B

Transverse cervical artery

Axillary artery

C

FIGURE 83-14. *A,* A segment of the greater curvature of the stomach vascularized by the gastroepiploic vessels can be harvested. This segment can be tubed or used as a patch; it is particularly useful when previous irradiation or surgery in the neck limits the choice of recipient vessels and a long vascular pedicle is desirable to reach the axilla or chest. *B,* The donor site on the greater curvature of the stomach is closed primarily in two layers or by stapling. *C,* The long pedicle allows reconstruction of the pharyngeal defect in the neck by microvascular anastomosis at a more distant site unaffected by previous surgery, irradiation, or a complication thereof.

reconstruction of the hypopharynx and cervical esophagus at the M.D. Anderson Cancer Center, demonstrated that the jejunal free autograft was superior to colon, stomach, deltopectoral flap, and musculocutaneous flap with respect to length of hospitalization, initiation of oral intake, and healing without fistula. He also noted that gastric pull-up and jejunal free autograft were equivalent and both superior to other techniques in avoidance of partial or total necrosis and functional success of the graft. Carlson concluded that because of its lower morbidity, the free jejunal autograft is the appropriate first choice when the defect is confined to the pharynx and cervical esophagus. Comparing the free jejunal autograft with the pectoralis major muscle during 10 years of pharyngoesophageal reconstruction, Coleman[46] in 1989 found that for both primary reconstruction (those done at the time of tumor resection) and secondary reconstruction (those done for complications such as fistulas, stenosis, and flap failure), the jejunal free autograft performed more reliably than the pectoralis major flap. In a series of 93 patients reconstructed with jejunal free autografts and 24 with pectoralis major musculocutaneous flaps, there was an initial success rate of 42% with pectoralis major versus 83% with the jejunum in primary reconstruction. Fistula appeared in 58% of patients with a pectoralis flap and in 24% of patients with the jejunum, requiring salvage surgery in 86% versus 29%. In secondary reconstruction, there was a 25% initial success rate for the pectoralis versus 56% for the jejunum, with 75% and 43% fistulas.[51] Subsequent comparisons by Shah[47] have shown similar experience.

In contrast to several negative American series, Lau[43] from Hong Kong reported good results when the pectoralis major was used as a patch for partial reconstruction of the pharynx and adequate results for resolution of circumferential defects. He reported 0% mortality, 97% graft success, 8.5% leak rate with 40% overall complications, and 97% swallowing success. This may be due to the flap's being less bulky in his population of patients. Experiencing a high fistula rate with early repair, Fabian[44] suggested that the circumferential defect be partitioned and that the anterior 270 degrees be repaired by the pectoralis major musculocutaneous flap; the posterior pharyngeal wall, the remaining portion of the circumferential defect, is covered by a split-thickness skin graft (see Fig. 83-12). The inset of the weighty pectoralis skin paddle into the prevertebral fascia presumably mitigates some of the effects of gravity. Using this method, he demonstrated a 95% graft success rate, a 3.3% fistula rate, and a 93% functional success in a series of 30 patients. Other authors have suggested modifications such as thinning of the pectoralis major flaps to improve results.[52]

There have been few comparisons of the radial forearm flap with the free jejunal autograft. Harii et al[57] published a 10-year experience of reconstruction

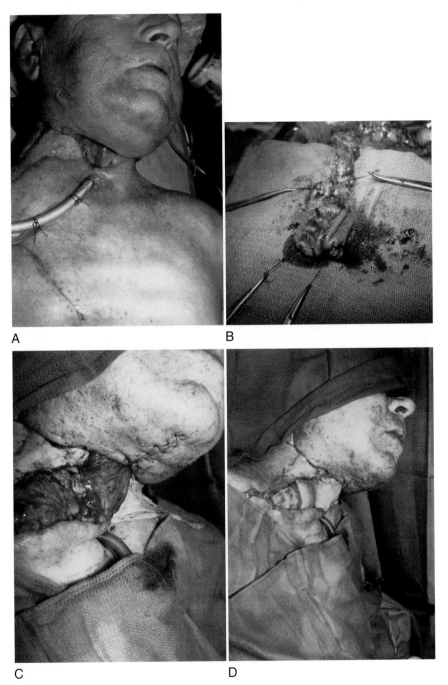

FIGURE 83-15. *A,* Patient with large pharyngocutaneous fistula after catastrophic failure of primary closure for laryngopharyngectomy and bilateral neck dissection after radiation failure for T3 N2 M2 squamous cell carcinoma of the larynx. The irradiated, exposed carotid artery is covered by a pectoralis major musculocutaneous flap that was used unsuccessfully to close the fistula. *B,* Because of the heavy irradiation, complex surgery, infection, and fistula, it was desirable to obtain recipient vessels outside the neck. A segment of the greater curvature of the stomach supplied by the gastroepiploic artery and vein was harvested. The long pedicle allowed microvascular end-to-side anastomosis to the axillary vessels. The omentum harvested with the flap covered the ipsilateral irradiated neck. The greater curvature of the stomach was closed primarily. *C* and *D,* The serosa of the stomach and the omentum were covered with split-thickness skin graft.   *Continued*

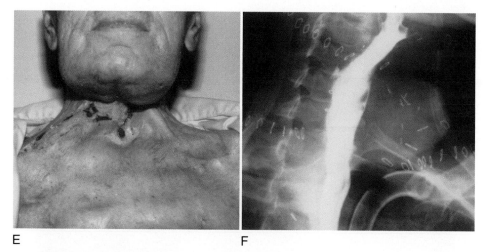

E   F

FIGURE 83-15, cont'd. *E* and *F,* The reconstruction healed primarily, restoring alimentary continuity, and the patient was able to eat by mouth and to swallow.

of the pharyngoesophagus, demonstrating 93% microvascular success rate with 0% mortality with the free jejunal flap and 100% microvascular success rate with 2.5% mortality with a free radial flap. Significantly more fistulas occurred in the forearm group (15 of 39 [39%]) than in the jejunal group (3 of 70 [4%]) and also significantly more strictures (13 of 33 [40%] as opposed to 6 of 64 [9%]). They concluded that the free jejunal flap should be used as the first choice but that in elderly high-risk patients, the radial forearm flap had the clear advantage of avoiding celiotomy. Su and Chiang[58] have addressed the problem of increased fistula and stricture rate by suggesting the use of a prefabricated forearm flap with the lateral anastomosis performed on the forearm to prevent the development of fistula.

Fasciocutaneous flaps such as the scapula, lateral arm, medial arm, and others appear to share the relatively high success rate of the radial forearm free flap (Fig. 83-16). With the lateral thigh flap, Hayden[32] demonstrated 97% swallowing success and microvascular flap survival with an 11% leak rate. Li[35] reported 95% flap survival with 15% fistula rate and 90% swallowing success rate with the free ulnar forearm flap; two of two patients in his series succeeded in obtaining esophageal speech.

Reported mortality rates have varied widely with technique, perhaps to some degree a function of the time of the report and improvements in perioperative care as well as in technique. Comparison studies published by Surkin[48] and Schechter[54] revealed a mortality rate of 5% to 16% for hypopharyngeal and cervical reconstruction. Perioperative mortality ranged from 0% to 6% with the pectoralis major musculocutaneous flap,[43,45,48,54] from 5% to 18% with gastric transposition,[43,48,56,59] and from 0% to 17% with the

free jejunal flap.[46,51,57,60-65] With only a small series of 18 patients, Biel[61] reported a mortality of 17% in 1987. Meta-analysis of large series of jejunal free autograft reveals a mortality of 3.5% in those series published after 1992 (475 patients).[28,56,57,60,62] The perioperative mortality rate for pharyngoesophageal reconstruction when the radial forearm flap is used ranges from 0% to 11%,[3,57,66-70] with meta-analysis revealing 3 deaths in 121 patients (2.6%).

Perioperative morbidity for patients undergoing reconstruction of the pharyngoesophagus ranges from

---

FIGURE 83-16. *A,* Resected tumor and ipsilateral neck dissection in an obese, diabetic, 54-year-old patient with a 50-pack a year smoking history who presented with a T3 N0 squamous cell carcinoma of the piriform sinus. Optimal oncologic treatment of this patient would include laryngopharyngectomy, ipsilateral radical neck dissection, and postoperative adjuvant radiotherapy in the range of 5000 to 6000 cGy to the primary site and each side of the neck. *B* and *C,* Design of lateral arm flap chosen to reconstruct anterior wall defect. The flap is raised in situ on the arm. *D,* Inset of lateral arm flap. Because of the proximity of the external carotid and internal or external jugular veins to the lateral wall of the pharynx reconstruction, the relatively short pedicle of the lateral arm flap is adequate. The position of the feeding tube shows that the defect could have been closed primarily, but the numerous risk factors for poor wound healing in this patient (obesity, diabetes, tobacco use, need for surgery and radiotherapy) suggest that interposition of well-vascularized soft tissue might decrease the risk of pharyngocutaneous fistula, delayed wound healing, and subsequent stenosis and dysphagia. *E* and *F,* After reconstruction, the wound healed primarily. The patient underwent adjuvant radiotherapy followed by a tracheoesophageal puncture for speech rehabilitation.

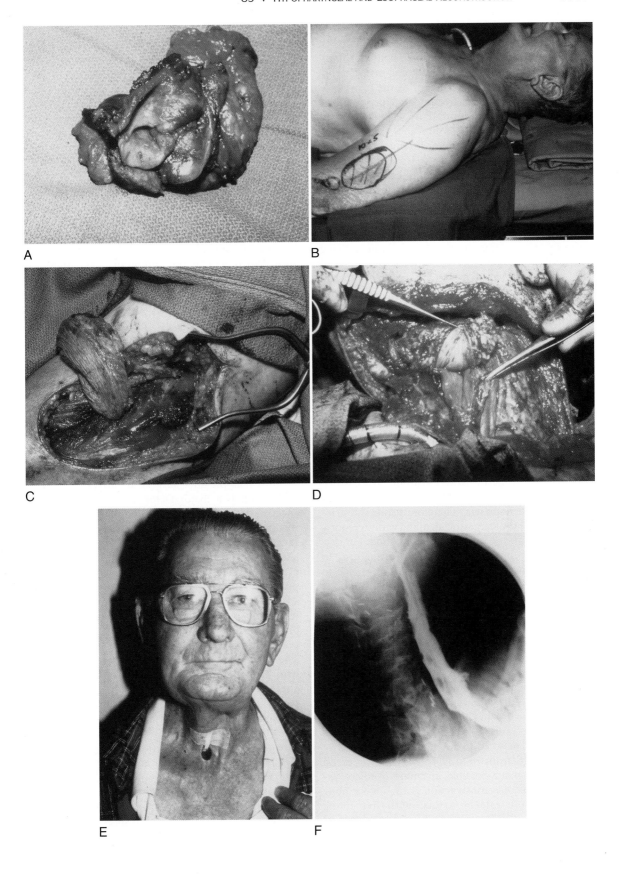

56% to 67% with the deltopectoral flap[48,71] and from 27% to 71% with pectoralis major musculocutaneous flaps.[43-45,48,72] A 32% to 52% perioperative morbidity rate is reported for patients undergoing gastric transposition.[43,48,71,72] In reconstruction of the pharyngoesophagus with the jejunal free autograft, perioperative morbidity has been reported in 4% to 6.4% of patients.[28,29,60-62] Shangold[63] found an average abdominal complication rate of 5.8% among 555 patients, consistent with that of smaller series. The variability in complication rates can probably be attributed to inclusion of infectious complications such as pneumonia and urinary tract infections in some series.[60] Thiele,[28] in the largest individual series to date, showed a 14.5% overall complication rate with the jejunum in 201 patients. A complication rate ranging from 50% to 55% has been reported with the use of the radial forearm flap for pharyngoesophageal reconstruction.[31,57,66,68]

In the subset of elderly patients with generally poor health, atherosclerosis, history of substance abuse, or previous surgery and radiotherapy who undergo procedures on the contaminated upper aerodigestive tract, the expectation for complications is certainly high. The predominant specific complications of pharyngoesophageal reconstruction are flap loss, fistula, and stenosis with subsequent dysphagia. It is difficult to obtain a clear understanding of the magnitude of these problems, particularly fistula, because clear differentiation of radiologic leak and clinical intracutaneous fistula is seldom made. There is, however, a clear relationship between the development of a fistula, radiologic or otherwise, and the subsequent problem of stenosis and dysphagia.. Therefore, fistula and stricture rates are intimately associated, and various reports demonstrate a wide range for each method. For deltopectoral flap, unplanned fistula rates are high, up to 58%, with subsequent stricture ranging from 23% to 100% incidence.[48,56,71] Similarly high rates of fistula (3% to 60%) and stricture (3% to 30%) are found with use of the pectoralis major musculocutaneous flaps.[43,46,48,54,72] Fistula after gastric transposition ranges from 2.5% to 31%[70]; two series (Cahow[59] in 1994 and Hartley[73] in 1999) reported 3.3% and 2.5%. Stenosis and stricture rates varied from 0% to 17%.[43,48,56,59,71-73]

With jejunal free autograft, fistula rates varied between 0% and 38%; subsequent stricture rates varied between 0% and 22%.[28,57,60,62,63] With fasciocutaneous flaps (radial forearm free flap), fistula rates were reported between 18% and 50%, and later stricture rates ranged from 0% to 39%.[31,52,57,66,67,69,74,75] Several series suggest that a possible advantage of microvascular methods of reconstruction is the higher nonsurgical closure rate of fistulas with free tissue transplantation, citing up to 66% success with local wound care.[51] The homogeneous blood supply and relatively light weight of the jejunum, gastroepiploic, and

fasciocutaneous flaps may facilitate this ability to heal without surgery (Fig. 83-17).

An important outcome of reconstruction of the pharyngoesophagus and a major determinant of good quality of life is successful peroral alimentation adequate to maintain weight and positive nitrogen balance. Again, numerous methods have shown variable success in achieving this outcome. Successful swallowing was obtained in 50% of patients with deltopectoral flaps in 79 to 90 days,[48,71] in 41% to 95% of patients with the pectoralis major flap in 9 to 70 days,[43,44,48,72] and in 83% to 100% of patients with the gastric transposition in 6 to 16 days.[43,48,59,71,72] Shektman[45] noted that patients undergoing surgery and adjuvant postoperative radiotherapy demonstrated significant delay in resumption of swallowing and full peroral alimentation. When jejunal free autografts were used for reconstruction, peroral alimentation was successful in 82% to 98% of patients in 8 to 16 days[46,55,56,61,64]; two large series of 402 and 450 patients demonstrated success rates of 82% and 90%, respectively.[28,57,60,62,63] An 89% to 100% graft success rate has been reported for patients who undergo a radial forearm free flap for pharyngoesophageal reconstruction; a large meta-analysis (121 patients) demonstrated 98% success, with 75% to 92% of patients resuming peroral alimentation between 7 and 29 days.[31,57,58,66,68,69]

The loss of speech has an enormously detrimental effect on quality of life. In treatment of a disease that frequently shortens the duration of life, it is important that the reconstructive surgeon restore speech as soon as possible after surgery. Clearly, the patient's motivation is a major factor in the resumption of speech after laryngectomy. Recognizing and providing treatment options for other problems such as mental depression and social isolation are critical to a successful outcome. An important study by Schechter et al[54] analyzed speech after reconstruction of the pharyngoesophagus by a numeric rating scale of 0 to 4 (0, no communication skills; 1, communication with electronic speech aids only; 2, single words or phrases or an electronic aid; 3, neoesophageal speech, but with poor volume; and 4, excellent neoesophageal speech). The average functional score for speech of patients who had undergone reconstruction of the pharyngoesophagus was as follows: deltopectoral flap, 1.4; pectoralis major musculocutaneous flap, 1.5; gastric transposition, 2.2; and free jejunal transposition, 0.9. They theorized that the negative intrathoracic pressure on the mediastinal portion of the gastric pouch facilitated the passage of air and thus production of alaryngeal speech. Tracheoesophageal puncture or the formation of a permanent fistula between the tracheostomy and the reconstructed neopharynx was developed to improve alaryngeal speech (Fig. 83-18). Medina[50] analyzed tracheoesophageal speech in 10 patients who had undergone pharyngoesophageal

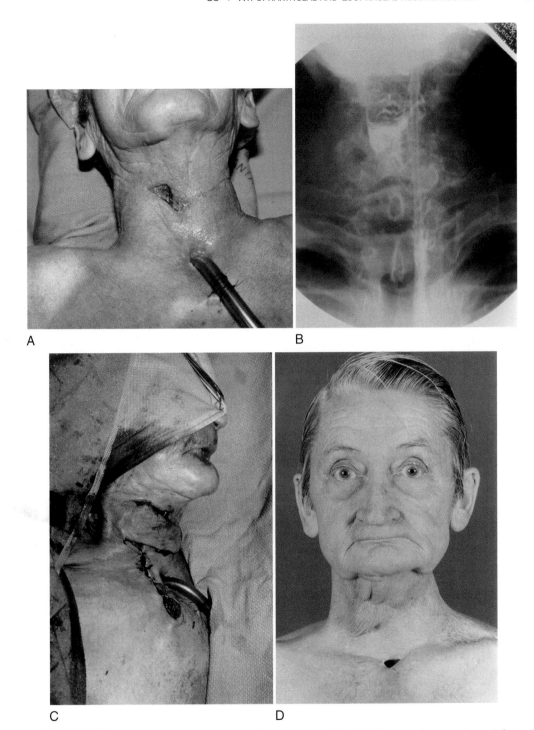

FIGURE 83-17. *A,* Fistula presenting 7 days after reconstruction of the laryngopharyngectomy defect in a patient who had previously been irradiated for squamous cell carcinoma of the larynx. The fistula may have been caused by replacement of a nasogastric tube. *B,* Barium swallow study demonstrates the fistula at the distal end of a jejunal free flap. *C,* Sternocleidomastoid flap design for closure. *D,* Single-layer closure of the fistula with a sternocleidomastoid flap was successful, probably because of well-vascularized tissue at the distal visceral anastomosis.

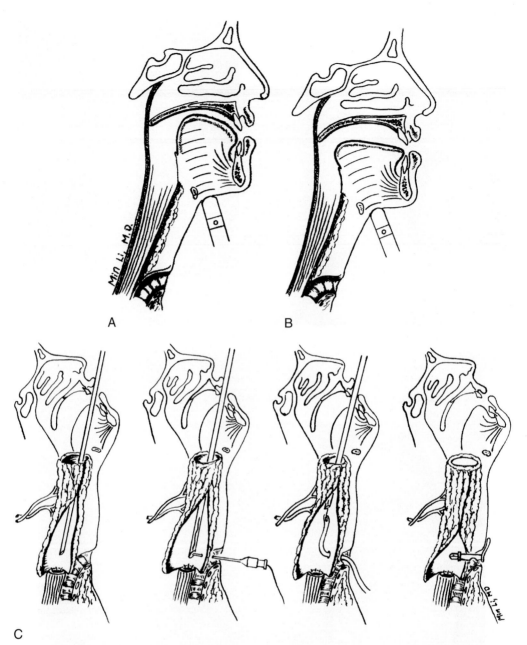

FIGURE 83-18. Various forms of alaryngeal speech possible with pharynx reconstruction. *A* and *B,* With the electrolarynx, the normal movements of the tongue, palate, teeth, and remaining pharynx modulate the vibratory signal produced by the instrument placed on the neck against the ventral tongue. *C,* Tracheoesophageal puncture with subsequent valve placement is the most successful method for the production of alaryngeal speech irrespective of the method of pharynx reconstruction. The puncture may be performed at the time of pharynx reconstruction or later. A bronchoscope visualizes the site of puncture and is used to retrieve a wire or piece of strong suture that directs a catheter through the cephalad portion of the tracheostome into the lumen of the pharyngoesophagus or reconstruction. This catheter is secured in place until a fistula is mature or an immediate prosthesis is inserted. When a fasciocutaneous flap or jejunal segment is used for reconstruction, it should be placed in such a position that the blood supply and the suture line will not lie adjacent to the puncture site.

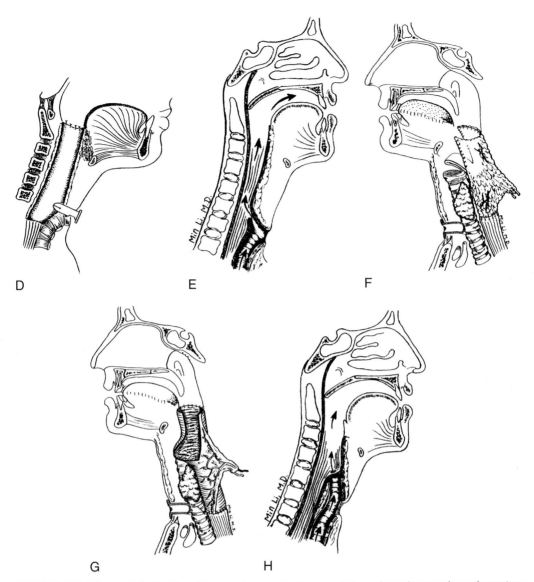

D   E   F

G   H

FIGURE 83-18, cont'd. *D,* Blom-Singer voice prosthesis placed through tracheoesophageal puncture into jejunal segment. *E,* Alaryngeal speech is produced by the modulation of air by the intact oropharyngeal structures. The flow of air is from the lungs and outside atmosphere through the fistula and into the pharynx and oral cavity. *F* and *G,* Various attempts at neoglottis reconstruction involve use of the jejunal reconstruction or fasciocutaneous flap. A side tracheostomy is made, leaving the cut end of the trachea in situ. This cut end of the trachea is then covered with a portion of the flap used, such as jejunum serosal surface *(F)* or segment of radial forearm flap *(G).* A small fenestration is made large enough to let air pass from the lungs into the pharynx but not so large as to allow aspiration of oropharyngeal contents. *H,* The route of the air that is modulated for speech is from the lungs and tracheostome through the fenestration and into the mouth.

reconstruction by cervical flaps, musculocutaneous flaps, gastric transposition, colon interposition, and jejunal free autograft combined with a pectoralis flap. He found no difference in result related to type of reconstruction. He did, however, note that the pitch or fundamental frequency and the loudness of patients undergoing laryngopharyngectomy and subsequent reconstruction were considerably diminished from those of patients undergoing laryngectomy and primary closure, and the overall quality of voice was perceived as less sharp and less clear, with less sustained volume. Maniglia,[49] in an assessment of five patients undergoing tracheogastric puncture after gastric pull-up, found similar inferior results, with lower pitch and a wet quality and slower rate of speech compared with patients undergoing primary closure.

Analysis of quality of speech after reconstruction with the jejunum has demonstrated problems with maintaining volume and projection and poor fluency because of a coarse, gravelly voice. The conjecture is that the somewhat random contractility of the jejunal segment interferes with airflow and the accumulated secretions result in a liquid, poorly intelligible articulation. Furthermore, the contractility and collapse of the segment do not provide a good vibratory surface. These problems have not been seen as frequently in patients reconstructed with the radial forearm fasciocutaneous flap. A number of series have demonstrated improved speech with radial forearm fasciocutaneous flaps and immediate or delayed tracheoesophageal puncture.[76,77] It appears that reconstruction with the radial forearm or other fasciocutaneous flaps allows variation of loud and soft speech, intelligibility, range of frequency, and other parameters of speech comparable to those seen in patients who do not require flap reconstruction after laryngectomy. With overall success rates ranging from 50% to 85%,[66,75] this is the most successful method of reconstruction for this rehabilitation issue.

REFERENCES

1. Mackay GJ, et al: Plastic and reconstructive surgery. In Sabiston DC, ed: Textbook of Surgery, 15th ed. Philadelphia, WB Saunders, 1996:1298-1329.
2. McConnel FM, Duck SW, Hester TR: Hypopharyngeal stenosis. Laryngoscope 1984;94:1162.
3. Schwartz AW: Dr. Theodor Billroth and the first laryngectomy. Ann Plast Surg 1978;1:513.
4. Edgerton MT: One stage reconstruction of the cervical esophagus and trachea. Surgery 1952;31:239.
5. Wookey H: The surgical treatment of cancer of the pharynx and upper esophagus. Surg Gynecol Obstet 1942;75:499.
6. Bircher E: Ein Beitrag zur plastischen Bildung eines neuen Oesophagus. Zentralbl Chir 1907;34:1479.
7. Bakamjian VY: A two-stage method for pharyngoesophageal reconstruction with a primary pectoral skin flap. Plast Reconstr Surg 1965;36:173.
8. Haeseker B: Dr. J.F.S. Esser and his influence on the development of plastic and reconstructive surgery [doctoral thesis]. Rotterdam, Netherlands, Erasmus University, 1983.
9. Ariyan S, Cuono CB: Myocutaneous flap in head and neck reconstruction. Head Neck Surg 1980;2:32.
10. Carlson GW, Coleman JJ, Jurkiewicz MJ: Reconstruction of the hypopharynx and cervical esophagus. Curr Probl Surg 1993;30:427.
11. Oshawa T: The surgery of the esophagus. Jpn J Surg 1933;10:604.
12. Sweet RH: Carcinoma of the mid-thoracic esophagus: its treatment by radical resection and high intrathoracic esophagogastric anastomosis. Ann Surg 1946;124:653.
13. Brewer LA III: One stage resection of carcinoma of the cervical esophagus with subpharyngeal esophagogastrostomy. Ann Surg 1949;130:9.
14. Roux C: L'oesophago-jejuno-gastrostomose, nouvelle operation pour retrecissement infranchissable de l'oesophage. Sem Med 1907;27:37.
15. Yudin SS: The surgical construction of 80 cases of artificial esophagus. Surg Gynecol Obstet 1944;78:561.
16. Kelling G: Oesophagoplastik mit Hilfe des Querkolon. Zentralbl Chir 1911;38:1209.
17. Vulliet H: De l'oesophagoplastie et des diverse modifications. Sem Med 1911;31:529.
18. Orsini P, Toupet A: Use of descending colon and left tail of transverse colon for esophagoplasty. Presse Med 1950;58:804.
19. Goligher JC, Robin IG: Use of left colon for reconstruction of pharynx and esophagus after pharyngectomy. Br J Surg 1954;42:283.
20. Baronofsky ID, Edelman S, Kreel I, et al: Surgical techniques. 1. The use of the left colon for esophageal replacement. J Mt Sinai Hosp 1960;27:88.
21. Longmire WP Jr: A modification of the Roux technique for antethoracic esophageal reconstruction. Surgery 1947;22:94.
22. Carrel A: Results of the transplantation of blood vessels, organs and limbs. JAMA 1908;51:1667.
23. Seidenberg B, Rosenak SS, Hurwitt ES, Som ML: Immediate reconstruction of the cervical esophagus by a revascularized isolated jejunal segment. Ann Surg 1959;149:162.
24. Roberts RE, Douglass FM: Replacement of the cervical esophagus and hypopharynx by a revascularized free jejunal segment. N Engl J Med 1961;264:342.
25. Heibert CA, Cummings GO: Successful replacement of the cervical esophagus by transplantation and revascularization of a free graft of gastric antrum. Ann Surg 1961;154:103.
26. Nakayama K, Yamamoto K, Tamiya T, et al: Experience with free autografts of the bowel with a new venous anastomosis apparatus. Surgery 1964;55:796.
27. Jurkiewicz MJ: Vascularized intestinal graft for reconstruction of the cervical esophagus and pharynx. Plast Reconstr Surg 1965;36:509.
28. Thiele DR, Robinson DW, Thiele DE: Free jejunal interposition reconstruction after pharyngolaryngectomy. Head Neck 1995;17:83.
29. Coleman JJ, Searles JM, Hester TR, et al: Ten years experience with the free jejunal autograft. Am J Surg 1987;154:389.
30. Yang G, Chen B, Gao Y, et al: Forearm free skin flap transplantation. Natl Med J China 1981;61:13.
31. Harii K, Ebihara S, Ono I, et al: Pharyngoesophageal reconstruction using a fabricated forearm free flap. Plast Reconstr Surg 1985;75:46.
32. Hayden R, Deschler D: Lateral thigh free flap for head and neck reconstruction. Laryngoscope 1999;109:1490.
33. Ha B, Baek C: Head and neck reconstruction using lateral thigh free flap: flap design. Microsurgery 1999;19:157.
34. Zuker RM, Manktelow RT, Palmer JA, Rosen IB: Head and neck reconstruction following resection of carcinoma using microvascular free flaps. Surgery 1980;88:461.
35. Li KK, Saliban AH, Allison GR, et al: Pharyngoesophageal reconstruction with the ulnar forearm flap. Arch Otolaryngol Head Neck Surg 1998;124:1146.
36. Guedon CE, Marmuse JP, Gehanno P, Barry B: Use of gastroomental free flaps in major neck defects. Am J Surg 1994;168:491.
37. Sartoris A, Succo G, Mioli P: Reconstruction of the pharynx and cervical esophagus using ileocolic free autograph. Am J Surg 1999;178:316.
38. Endo T, Nakayama Y: Pharyngoesophageal reconstruction: a clinical comparison between free tensor fasciae latae and radial forearm flaps. J Reconstr Microsurg 1997;13:93.
39. Nakatsuka T, Harii K, Asato H: Reconstruction of the cervical esophagus with a free inferior rectus abdominis flap. J Reconstr Microsurg 1999;15:509.
40. Ninkovic M, Harpf, Gunkel A, et al: One stage reconstruction of defects in the hypopharyngeal region with free flaps. Scand J Plast Reconstr Surg Hand Surg 1999;33:21.
41. Saito H, Kimura Y, Gota T: Free perineal skin flap for oropharyngeal reconstruction. Scand J Plast Reconstr Surg Hand Surg 1999;33:41.
42. Lovie MJ, Duncan GM, Glasson DW: The ulnar artery free flap. Br J Plast Surg 1984;37:486.

43. Lau WF, Lam KH, Wei WL: Reconstruction of hypopharyngeal defects in cancer surgery: do we have a choice? Am J Surg 1987;154:374.

44. Fabian RL: Pectoralis major myocutaneous flap reconstruction of the laryngopharynx and cervical esophagus. Laryngoscope 1988;98:1227.

45. Shektman A, Silver C, Strauch BA: A re-evaluation of hypopharyngeal reconstruction: pedicled flaps versus microvascular free flaps. Plast Reconstr Surg 1997;100:1691.

46. Coleman JJ: Reconstruction of the pharynx after resection for cancer: a comparison of methods. Ann Surg 1989;209:554.

47. Shah JP, Haribhakti V, Loree TR, Sutaria P: Complications of the pectoralis major myocutaneous flap in head and neck reconstruction. Am J Surg 1990;160:352.

48. Surkin MI, Lawson E, Biller HF: Analysis of the methods of pharyngoesophageal reconstruction. Head Neck Surg 1984;6:95.

49. Maniglia AJ, Leder SB, Goodwin WJ, et al: Tracheogastric puncture for vocal rehabilitation following total pharyngolaryngoesophagectomy. Head Neck 1989;11:52.

50. Medina JE, Nance A, Burns L: Voice restoration after total laryngopharyngectomy and cervical esophagectomy using the duckbill prosthesis. Am J Surg 1987;154:407.

51. Coleman JJ, Tan KC, Searles JM, et al: Jejunal free autograft: analysis of complications and their resolution. Plast Reconstr Surg 1989;84:589.

52. Shindo M, Constantino P, Friedman C: The pectoralis major myofascial flap for intraoral and pharyngeal reconstruction. Arch Otolaryngol Head Neck Surg 1992;118:707.

53. Silver CE: Surgery for Cancer of Larynx and Related Structures. New York, Churchill Livingstone, 1981.

54. Schechter GL, Baker JW, Gilbert DA: Functional evaluation of pharyngoesophageal reconstruction techniques. Arch Otolaryngol Head Neck Surg 1987;113:40.

55. Schusterman MA, Shestak K, deVries EJ, et al: Reconstruction of the cervical esophagus: free jejunal transfer versus gastric pull-up. Plast Reconstr Surg 1990;85:16.

56. Carlson GW, Schusterman MA, Guillamondegui OM: Total reconstruction of the hypopharynx and cervical esophagus: a twenty-year experience. Ann Plast Surg 1992;29:408.

57. Nakatsuka T, Harii K, Asato H: Comparative evaluation in pharyngo-esophageal reconstruction: radial forearm flap compared with jejunal flap. A 10-year experience. Scand J Plast Reconstr Surg Hand Surg 1998;32:307.

58. Su SY, Chiang YC: The fabricated radial forearm flap in pharyngolaryngeal surgery: saliva leakage and its prevention. Br J Plast Surg 1995;48:212.

59. Cahow CE, Sasaki CT: Gastric pull-up reconstruction for pharyngolaryngoesophagectomy. Arch Surg 1994;129:429.

60. Julieron M, Germain MA, Schwaab GR: Reconstruction with free jejunal autograft after circumferential pharyngolaryngectomy: eighty-three cases. Ann Otol Rhinol Laryngol 1998;107:581.

61. Biel MA, Maisel RE: Free jejunal autograft reconstruction of the pharyngoesophagus: review of a ten-year experience. Otolaryngol Head Neck Surg 1987;97:369.

62. Reece GP, Schusterman MA, Miller MJ: Morbidity and functional outcome of free jejunal transfer reconstruction for circumferential defects of the pharynx and cervical esophagus. Plast Reconstr Surg 1995;96:1307.

63. Shangold LM, Urken ML, Lawson W: Jejunal transplantation for pharyngoesophageal reconstruction. Otolaryngol Clin North Am 1991;24:1321.

64. Coleman JJ, Searles JM, Hester TR, et al: Ten years experience with the free jejunal autograft. Am J Surg 1987;154:389.

65. Bradford CR, Esclamado RM, Carroll WR, Sullivan MJ: Analysis of recurrence, complications and functional results with the free jejunal flap. Head Neck Surg 1994;16:149.

66. Anthony JP, Singer M, Deschler D: Long term functional results after pharyngoesophageal reconstruction with the radial forearm free flap. Am J Surg 1994;168:441.

67. Takato T, Harii K, Ebihara S: Oral and pharyngeal reconstruction using the free forearm flap. Arch Otolaryngol Head Neck Surg 1987;113:873.

68. Akin I, Torkut A, Ustunsoy E: Results of reconstruction with free forearm flap following laryngopharyngoesophageal resection. J Laryngol Otol 1997;3:48.

69. Cho BC, Kim M, Lee JH, et al: Pharyngoesophageal reconstruction with a tubed free radial forearm flap. J Reconstr Microsurg 1998;14:535.

70. Sullivan M, Talamonti M, Sithanandam K, et al: Results for reconstruction of the pharyngoesophagus. Surgery 1999;126:666.

71. Frederickson JM, Wagenfeld DJH, Denick JH, Pearson G: Gastric pull-up versus deltopectoral flap for reconstruction of the cervical esophagus. Arch Otolaryngol 1981;107:713.

72. Lam KH, Ho CM, Lau WF, et al: Immediate reconstruction of pharyngoesophageal defects. Arch Otolaryngol Head Neck Surg 1989;115:608.

73. Hartley BE, Bottrill ID, Howard DJ: A third decade's experience with the gastric pull-up operation for hypopharyngeal carcinoma: changing patterns of use. J Laryngol Otol 1999;113:241.

74. Kato H, Watanabe H, Iizuka T, et al: Primary esophageal reconstruction after resection of the cancer in the hypopharynx or cervical esophagus: comparison of free forearm skin tube flap, free jejunal transplantation and pull-through esophagectomy. Jpn J Clin Oncol 1987;17:255.

75. Stark B, Nathanson A: The free radial forearm flap: a reliable method for reconstruction of the laryngohypopharynx. Acta Otolaryngol 1998;118:419.

76. Deschler DG, Doherty ET, Reed CG: Tracheoesophageal voice following tubed free radial forearm flap reconstruction of the neopharynx. Ann Otol Rhinol Laryngol 1994;103:929.

77. Wenig BL, Keller AJ, Levy J: Voice restoration after laryngopharyngoesophagectomy. Otolaryngol Head Neck Surg 1989;10:11.

◆

Neck Reconstruction

Delora L. Mount, MD ◆ Stephen J. Mathes, MD

PEDIATRIC NECK PATHOLOGY AND
RECONSTRUCTION
    Surgical Anatomy and Embryology
    Skin and Subcutaneous Disorders
    Muscle Defects
    Vascular Anomalies
ACQUIRED NECK ANOMALIES
    Hypertrophic Neck Scar
    Cutaneous Malignant Neoplasms
    Oropharyngeal and Laryngeal Malignant Neoplasms

NECK RECONSTRUCTION
    Skin and Soft Tissue Replacement
    Local and Regional Fasciocutaneous Flaps
    Distant Fasciocutaneous Flaps
    Muscle and Musculocutaneous Flaps
    Omental and Jejunal Flaps
    Reconstruction of Specific Defects

Successful reconstruction of the neck must include a combined focus on function and form specific to the unique qualities of the neck structures. The neck functions to flex, extend, and rotate the head with easy range of motion. The normal neck skin and subcutaneous structures have soft and pliable texture, thin quality, and continuity with muscles of facial expression. The relatively superficial position of critical, vital structures (i.e., the carotid and jugular vascular systems and the respiratory and pharyngoesophageal conduits) requires immediate stable coverage.

An overview of embryology as it pertains to congenital neck problems is presented to explain the etiology of congenital anomalies encountered in the neck. Adult neck pathologic conditions with special emphasis on postextirpation oncologic reconstruction is discussed as it relates to reconstructive requirements within the neck.

The neck is a vital structure of aesthetic importance, with great emphasis on the quality, texture, and draping of the skin at the cervicomental angle, and is a focus of intervention in facial rejuvenation. This chapter focuses on pediatric and adult neck reconstruction with the goal of achievement of the optimal form and function when congenital or acquired deformity requires reconstruction.

PEDIATRIC NECK PATHOLOGY AND RECONSTRUCTION

Surgical Anatomy and Embryology

BRANCHIAL ARCH DERIVATIVES

Head and neck structures begin formation in the fourth week of embryonal gestation.[1] Guided by neural crest influence, the branchial apparatus, primarily the branchial arches and grooves, develops into the majority of the neck structures. Treatment and optimal timing of treatment of congenital neck abnormalities must be based on clear understanding of the embryologic anatomy and pathogenesis in this area, with particular emphasis on anatomic relationships of the various deformities with vital neck structures (i.e., the carotid arterial system). In the neck and lower head region, several anomalies occur when normal embryogenesis goes awry. Pharyngeal pouches and branchial arches constitute major structural precursors of neck structures.

Derivatives of the first branchial arch (mandibular arch) include the mandible and portions of the auricle.[2] Cartilaginous portions of the first arch branchial grooves form the auricular structures and the mandible; malformations and incomplete regression of structures result in preauricular tags, sinuses, and cysts (Fig. 84-1). Preauricular pits and tags are usually superficial in nature and are found in a triangular area of skin anterior to the ear.[2] They may discharge inspissated material or may, if blocked, develop acute cystic enlargement and pain. Treatment consists of careful local resection, including deep excision of any rudimentary cartilaginous stalk, or coring out of the epithelialized track.

Mandibular fusion to the cervical spine or sternum, which occurs with Klippel-Feil syndrome, constitutes a postnatal airway emergency. Other first arch syndromes include Treacher Collins syndrome and Pierre Robin sequence, which are reviewed elsewhere (see Chapter 90).

Second arch derivatives include stapes, hyoid bone, and muscles of facial expression. Failure of closure of

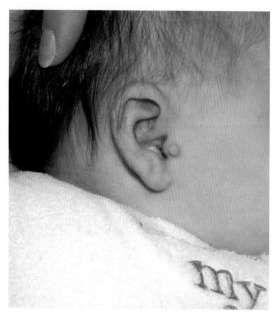

FIGURE 84-1. Lateral view of first arch remnant. The patient presented with incomplete regression of structures that form the cartilaginous portions of the first arch branchial grooves, which will become the auricular structures and the mandible.

the second branchial groove results in epithelialized sinuses that are typically located near the anterior border of the sternocleidomastoid muscle (Fig. 84-2A). They may discharge entrapped cellular material or develop acute cystic enlargement and pain if they become blocked or acutely infected. Frequently bilateral, these sinuses track deeply (Fig. 84-2B) and extend cephalad between the bifurcation of the internal and external carotid arteries. Distally, the track ends as an opening into the tonsil bed (Fig. 84-3). Obviously, careful dissection is paramount to uncomplicated resec-

tion of this type of cyst or sinus track. Recurrence is rare if the track is completely resected.

The third arch gives rise to the lower portion of the hyoid bone and stylopharyngeus muscles. Third arch abnormalities in the neck are unusual.

Cartilage from the fourth and sixth arches develops into laryngeal cartilages. The pharyngeal pouches of the fourth arch become the superior parathyroid glands. Abnormalities in the laryngeal cartilages may result in laryngeal clefts or webs. Congenital abnormalities of the third and fourth derivatives are present in DiGeorge syndrome, which consists of thymic and parathyroid absence.

AERODIGESTIVE EMBRYOLOGY

The trachea develops by a growing membranous partition by the tracheoesophageal septum across the endothelial tube at approximately 3 to 4 weeks of gestational age. Separation of the two tubes, trachea and esophagus, occurs from a caudal to cephalad direction.[1] When the dividing septum does not completely fuse or the separation is incomplete, persistent communication or tracheoesophageal fistula results. Tracheoesophageal fistula occurs in 1 in 4000 live births and is associated with early feeding abnormalities, aspiration pneumonia, and respiratory distress. Additional congenital anomalies including cardiac, gastrointestinal, and neurologic anomalies must be investigated in the patient with congenital tracheoesophageal fistula. All congenital tracheoesophageal fistulas are associated with some degree of esophageal atresia; the most common type is proximal esophageal atresia with distal tracheoesophageal fistula, accounting for 85% to 90% of all patients.[3] Early diagnosis is made by presence of fetal polyhydramnios, postnatal feeding difficulties with immediate vomiting, aspiration, choking, and possibly cyanosis. The diagnosis is confirmed clinically by inability to pass an orogastric

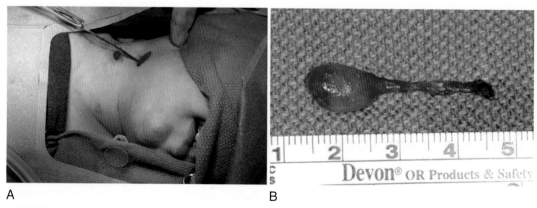

A   B

FIGURE 84-2. Failure of closure of the second branchial groove results in epithelialized sinuses that are typically located near the anterior border of the sternocleidomastoid muscle. *A,* Intraoperative view of branchial cyst. *B,* Intraoperative view of branchial cyst with track.

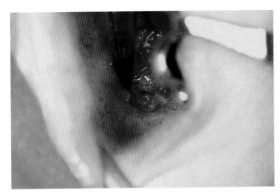

FIGURE 84-3. Tonsil bed branchial sinus. A branchial sinus track may end as an opening into the tonsil bed.

tube and radiographically with administration of contrast material.

Once accurate diagnosis is confirmed, surgical repair is required. Reconstruction requires anatomic separation of the trachea and esophagus and establishment of continuity of the esophageal tube. Most repairs are made as single-stage repairs, although multistage repairs may be necessary for the ill or premature infant. The trachea is closed through a thoracotomy and cervical approach with single- or double-layered repairs. Primary repair of the esophageal ends may require a myotomy,[4] extensive cephalad dissection, and a supportive buttress of the repair by interposition of muscle or soft tissue. Stricture, anastomotic leak, and recurrent tracheoesophageal fistula are potential complications of repair.[5]

Skin and Subcutaneous Disorders

CONGENITAL NECK WEB (PTERYGIUM COLLI)

Congenital neck web (pterygium colli) (Fig. 84-4) is most frequently associated with Turner syndrome, although it may be found also in other genetic abnormalities, such as trisomies 13, 18, and 21 (Down syndrome.) The incidence is 1 in 3000.[6,7] Turner syndrome is characterized by female phenotype, streak ovaries, web neck, and cubitus valgus.[8] Evidence suggests that the web is a remnant of regression of a posterior triangle cystic hygroma.[9] Hairline in the posterior web is significantly inferiorly displaced, and the soft tissue web extends from the mastoid-cranial base to the acromion-clavicular area.[7] Although functional limitations in neck range of motion are infrequent, aesthetic stigma of the web are important. Resection of excessive skin and platysma with layered closure of platysma and skin in lateral Z-plasty[10,11] or curvilinear and butterfly type of excisions[12-14] reduces risk of straight-line closure cicatricial contractures and anterior scars. Carefully planned excision with Z-plasty

closure or butterfly excision (Fig. 84-5) has been associated with minimal scar band and aesthetically appropriate scar and hairline placement. Typically, correction should occur before the child starts school.

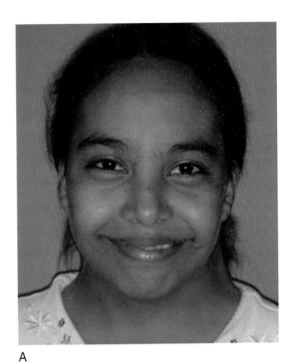

A

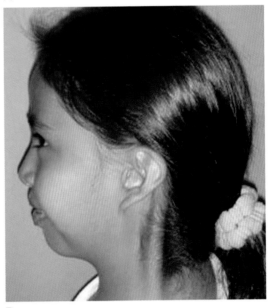

B

FIGURE 84-4. Congenital neck web (pterygium colli). Congenital neck web is most frequently associated with Turner syndrome, although it may be found also in other genetic abnormalities, such as trisomies 13, 18, and 21 (Down syndrome). *A*, Anterior view. *B*, Lateral view.
Continued

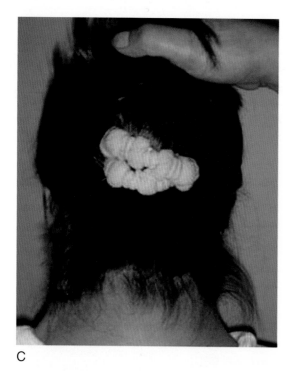

C

FIGURE 84-4, cont'd. *C,* Posterior view.

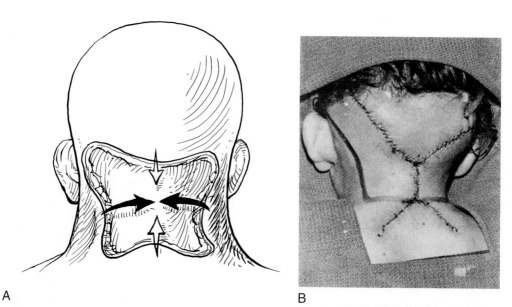

A

B

FIGURE 84-5. Butterfly correction of webbed neck in Turner syndrome. *A,* Redundant skin excised. *B,* Flaps sutured together at the midline. (From Shearin JC Jr, DeFranzo AJ: Butterfly correction of webbed-neck deformity in Turner's syndrome. Plast Reconstr Surg 1980;66:129.)

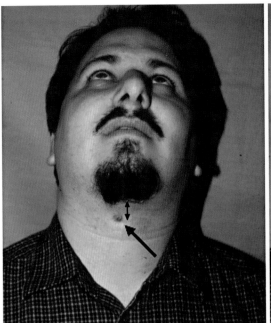

A

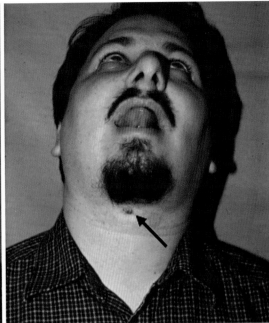

B

THYROGLOSSAL DUCT CYST

In contrast to the laterally based cysts that occur with retained pharyngeal sinus and branchial apparatus abnormalities, thyroglossal duct remnants and cysts occur in the midline. Thyroglossal duct cysts typically present with a midline palpable mass below the hyoid, with intermittent swelling, erythema, or infection (20%).[15] Diagnosis is usually based on clinical findings and imaging, including movement of the cyst with tongue protrusion, which demonstrates a soft tissue track extending from the midline infrahyoid anterior neck cephalad to the base of the tongue (Fig. 84-6A and B), best visualized with computed tomography or ultrasonography. Anatomically, the cyst and duct extend from below the hyoid and pass through the hyoid, ending at the foramen cecum as an opening at the base of the tongue. Ectopic thyroid tissue is noted as lingual thyroid in 8% of patients.[16] Treatment is cautious excision of the complete track with hyoid resection (Fig. 84-6C).[16-18] When a patient presents with active infection, many think that incision and drainage are unnecessary and increase the complication rate of later excision. Treatment is with conservative measures and antibiotics initially, followed by excision in a quiescent state (Fig. 84-7). Recurrence rates for thyroglossal duct cysts are 10%.[15]

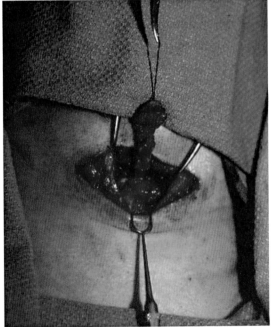

C

FIGURE 84-6. Thyroglossal duct cyst. Persistence of the thyroglossal duct may result in cysts or fistulas. *A* and *B*, Clinical presentation typically consists of a mass that may be visualized by having the patient extend the tongue. *C*, Intraoperative photograph of thyroglossal duct cyst. Extirpation includes the cyst, the body of the hyoid bone, and the track of the cyst or fistula.

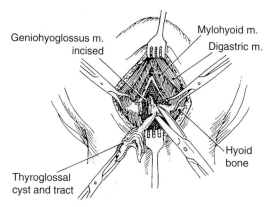

Geniohyoglossus m.
incised

Mylohyoid m.

Digastric m.

Hyoid
bone

Thyroglossal
cyst and tract

FIGURE 84-7. Dissection of the thyroglossal duct and cyst. (From Hoffman WV, Baker D: Pediatric tumors of the head and neck. In McCarthy JG, ed: Plastic Surgery. Philadelphia, WB Saunders, 1990:3175.)

CYSTIC HYGROMA

The incidence of cervical lymphangioma (cystic hygroma) in infants is 1.2 to 2.8 per 1000 births.[9] The neck is the most common site of lymphangioma occurrence, and the majority present as a painless mass in early infancy (Fig. 84-8).[9,19,20] Large cervical lymphangiomas may involve the tongue, pharynx, or floor of mouth and result in severe deformity and aerodigestive obstruction. In a large study, 74 consecutive patients were identified; 62% presented with cervical involvement, 9% of whom presented with symptoms of airway obstruction, and two required tracheostomy.[19] In fetuses diagnosed prenatally with large airway-obstructing cervical lymphangioma, planned cesarean section is often indicated with the surgical team standing by for establishment of an emergency surgical airway.

Cervical lymphangioma may be microcystic or macrocystic, and involvement in specific regions of the neck worsens outcome. Lesions in the posterior triangle have good response to treatment with low recurrence and complication rates for both surgical and nonsurgical treatments.[19,21] Suprahyoid neck lesions have the worst prognosis with high recurrence, incomplete treatment response, and higher incidence of concomitant airway obstruction.[21]

Treatments fall into two categories, surgical and sclerosant. Although spontaneous resolution may occur, it is infrequent.[22] Surgical therapy with debulking or complete resection has significant complications, including facial nerve injury (12% to 33%) and recurrence (10% to 37%).[9,21] Sclerotherapy has demonstrated encouraging results. In Japan, OK-432 (lyophilized and modified group A *Streptococcus pyogenes*) has been used as a sclerosant, presumably by inducing low-grade

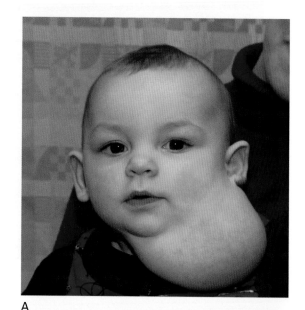

A

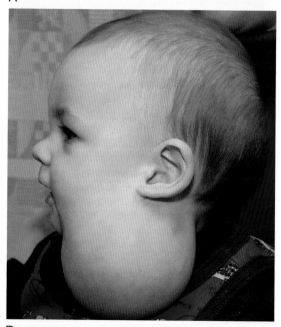

B

FIGURE 84-8. Cystic hygroma. *A,* Preoperative anterior view of toddler presenting with large cervical lymphangioma (cystic hygroma). *B,* Preoperative lateral view.

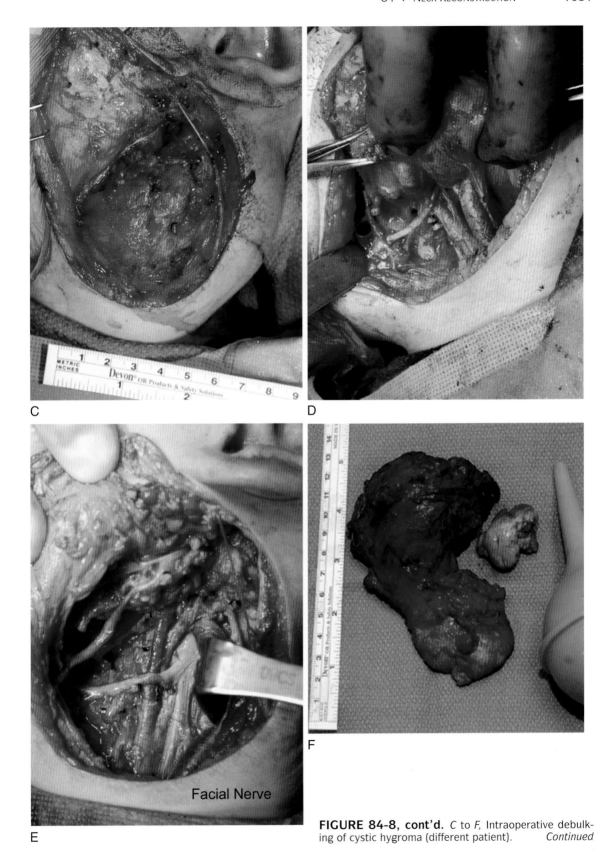

C

D

E

Facial Nerve

F

FIGURE 84-8, cont'd. *C* to *F,* Intraoperative debulking of cystic hygroma (different patient). *Continued*

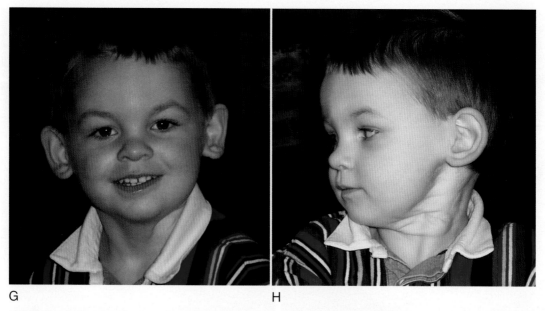

G   H

FIGURE 84-8, cont'd. *G,* Postoperative anterior view after debulking. *H,* Postoperative lateral view. A subsequent surgery is planned for correction of skin laxity.

inflammation and subsequent endothelial scar and contracture.[23] Side effects include fever, rash, and, in some patients, the need for multiple injections.[24] Current controlled trials are ongoing in the United States.[25] Bleomycin has also been used as a sclerosant for cervical lymphangioma. In one study, 88% achieved either complete resolution or more than 50% reduction in size when intralesional bleomycin was administered in a dosage of 0.3 to 0.6 mg/kg.[21] Unfortunately, however, sclerosant therapy is effective only in macrocystic disease.[26]

Muscle Defects

TORTICOLLIS

Torticollis occurs when the sternocleidomastoid muscle becomes spastic and sometimes fibrotic, inhibiting normal neck range of motion and producing a persistent head tilt (Fig. 84-9A). It can be secondary to intramuscular or intracapsular hematoma resulting from birth trauma or secondary to severe muscle spasm.[27,28] In the developing infant, a tilted head from untreated torticollis may cause inaccurate visual field discrimination and development of canted visual fields. In patients with extreme defects, compensatory strabismus may occur. In this instance, a child with complete treatment of sternocleidomastoid muscle imbalance may continue head tilt to comply with

patterned visual field development. Long-standing unresolved torticollis may result in positional plagiocephaly with secondary facial distortion and malocclusion (Fig. 84-9B).[29,30]

Torticollis may also occur from trauma or a spastic condition in later childhood or adulthood. Treatment of torticollis includes therapeutic release with range-of-motion exercises and, in late stages or resistant defects, botulinum toxin injection (in adults) and surgical release. Success varies with pathogenesis, age at presentation, and length of time of deformity. Current indications for treatment vary by severity and timing of onset. For a newborn with torticollis, manual muscle release and stretch through physical therapy and caregivers are often the only needed treatment. Physical and occupational therapy modalities of stretching and range-of-motion exercises are successful in 97% of patients.[31] In the subgroup of individuals with incomplete response to conservative treatment, sternocleidomastoid muscle transection, which can be safely performed endoscopically, is associated with successful resolution of head tilt and low morbidity.[32-36] Cordlike sternocleidomastoid bands and more than 30 degrees of rotational deformity are associated with higher failure rates with conservative therapy.[31]

In adults, botulinum toxin injection therapy has been used for several years for temporary muscle spasm blockade in treatment of spasmodic torticollis. In spastic individuals, when more permanent treatment is needed, a selective peripheral sternocleidomastoid muscle denervation procedure offers a safe surgical alternative. Selective denervation of the sternocleidomastoid muscle is associated with correction of head position in 77%, rare relapse, and low complication rate.[37] In addition to these surgical modalities, in the patient whose treatment has failed, open or endoscopic myofascial release by surgical transection may be required.

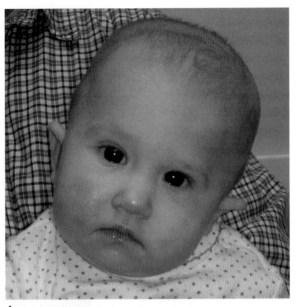

A

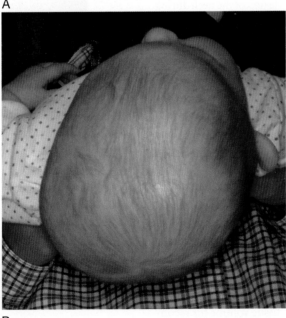

B

FIGURE 84-9. Torticollis. *A,* Torticollis occurs when the sternocleidomastoid muscle becomes spastic and sometimes fibrotic, inhibiting normal neck range of motion and producing a persistent head tilt. *B,* Long-standing unresolved torticollis may result in positional plagiocephaly with secondary facial distortion and malocclusion.

Vascular Anomalies

Vascular anomalies are discussed in detail in Chapter 106.

ACQUIRED NECK ANOMALIES

Hypertrophic Neck Scar

The neck structures are susceptible to unfavorable scar outcomes. The most difficult challenge of neck scarring is the severe burn scar. Progressive hypertrophic contracture of a burn scar leads to loss of range of motion of the neck and progressive functional inability, with secondary growth distortion of bone and soft tissues.[38] Prevention of neck burn scar contracture is most important in avoiding this unfavorable outcome. Second- and third-degree burns that require healing by secondary intention or excision and grafting are associated with high scar contracture rates.[39-42] Grafting with split-thickness grafts should be avoided because of risk of late progressive contracture. Full-thickness grafts are associated with lower rates of late contracture. Neck supports, specialized pressure garments, and aggressive physical therapy are indicated at the early healing phase to prevent onset of hypertrophic scar development. Risk of contracture is accentuated with noncompliant patients and debilitated patients. Controversy exists in the optimal prevention strategy for hypertrophic neck burn scars. Options include neck brace to prevent flexion of the neck during healing, customized pressure garments, topical treatment with hydrocolloids or silicone gel sheeting, massage, and intracicatrix steroid injections.[38,43-52] Prevention of unfavorable scarring with each of these modalities is dependent on the patient's compliance.

Once an individual develops an established hypertrophic neck burn scar, treatment indications include limitation of range of motion, unfavorable aesthetic appearance, and traction on the mandible. Long-standing limited burn scars may impair normal mandibular growth as well as produce cervical spine abnormalities.[38,53,54] Operative treatment options include resection and full-thickness grafting, W-plasty (Fig. 84-10) and Z-plasty for localized scar bands, and tissue expansion with local advancement or rotation flaps.

Tissue expansion is an effective method for replacement of scarred or inadequate adjacent tissue for primary closure of neck wounds (Fig. 84-11). Expansion results in increased soft tissue volume for reconstruction, with advantages of color match (if local tissue is expanded) and similar texture and quality.[55] Numerous studies have confirmed improved vascularity of expanded tissue, affording more reliability when it is based on smaller random or axial patterns.[56-58] During

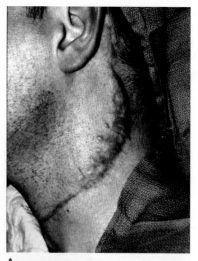

A

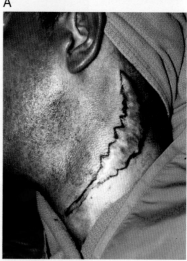

B

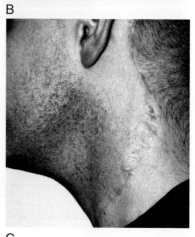

C

FIGURE 84-10. *A,* Patient presenting with large keloid scar on left lateral neck. *B,* Intraoperative design of W-plasty for scar revision. *C,* Postoperative view at 9 months.

expansion, the epidermis increases in thickness, demonstrated by increased mitotic activity, while the dermis progressively thins.[59-61] The procedure can be adapted to regional flap selection, for assurance of primary donor site defect closure, with use of immediately adjacent tissue for flap closure or use of the expanded skin as a full-thickness graft.[56,62] Placed in a subplatysmal plane in the neck, tissue expansion is well tolerated and produces excellent results in color and texture match without risk of vascular or airway compression.[56,58,63,64] The incidence of complications of tissue expansion in the neck is variable but notably higher than in other areas, such as trunk or scalp.[64,65] One study cited a complication rate of 69% in neck tissue expansion, with implant exposure and buckling most common.[64] However, despite the higher complication rate, the authors noted that reconstruction was accomplished satisfactorily in the majority of patients. The procedure of tissue expansion is well tolerated in adults and children and in patients requiring serial expansion and reconstruction.[66]

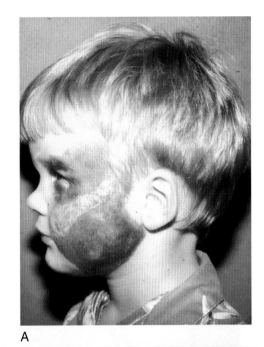

A

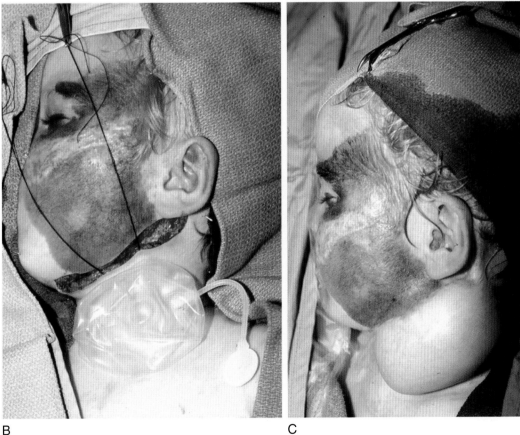

B   C

FIGURE 84-11. Neck expansion for superior neck and lateral face reconstruction. *A,* Lateral view of giant hairy nevus involving face and superior neck. *B,* Normal neck skin is elevated superficial to platysma for insertion of tissue expander. Note expander ready for insertion. *C,* Anterior view of expansion process completed at 3 months.   *Continued*

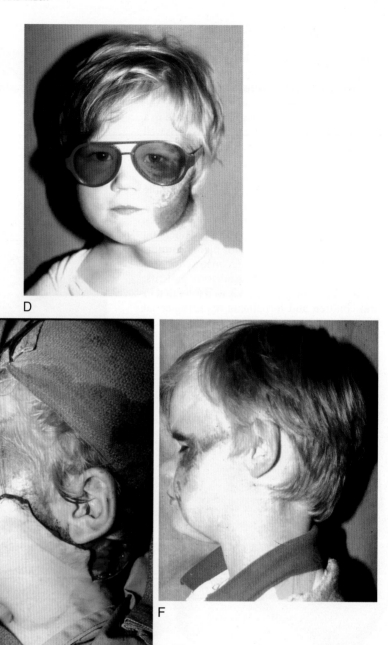

D

E

F

FIGURE 84-11, cont'd. *D* and *E,* Intraoperative view of expanded flap advanced to zygomatic arch, allowing resection of neck and lower and middle thirds of lateral face giant hairy nevus. *F,* Lateral view. Expanded inferior neck flap has provided stable coverage of neck and inferior two thirds of lateral face.

Cutaneous Malignant Neoplasms

Primary basal cell cancers are less common on the neck than on the face, probably secondary to the shading effect of the projected face and mandible. Effective treatment options include excision, cauterization, and cryotherapy (see Chapters 113 and 116). Squamous cell cancer of the neck is most frequently metastatic from the oropharynx or face. Melanoma can prima-rily arise in the neck region both cutaneously and mucosally, although it is much less common than primary cutaneous melanoma of the facial region. Options for treatment of primary skin malignant neo-plasms of the neck are the same as those for other areas of the body and include wide local excision, sentinel lymph node sampling for regional metastases, and in-continuity neck dissection when sentinel nodes are positive (Fig. 84-12).

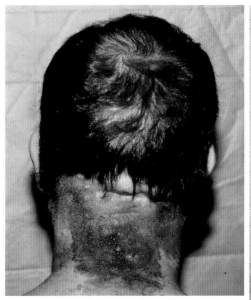

A

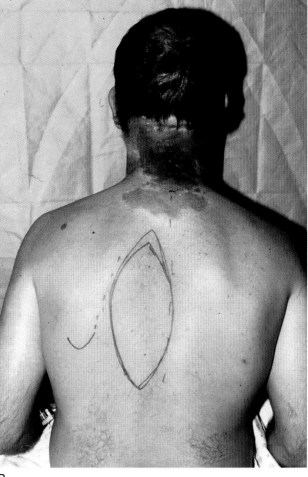

B

FIGURE 84-12. Malignant melanoma within posterior neck giant hairy nevus. *A,* Posterior view of giant hairy nevus of neck with invasive melanoma within inferior aspect of nevus based on biopsy. *B,* Posterior view of design of skin island for vertical trapezius musculocutaneous flap for immediate reconstruction of melanoma resection.

Continued

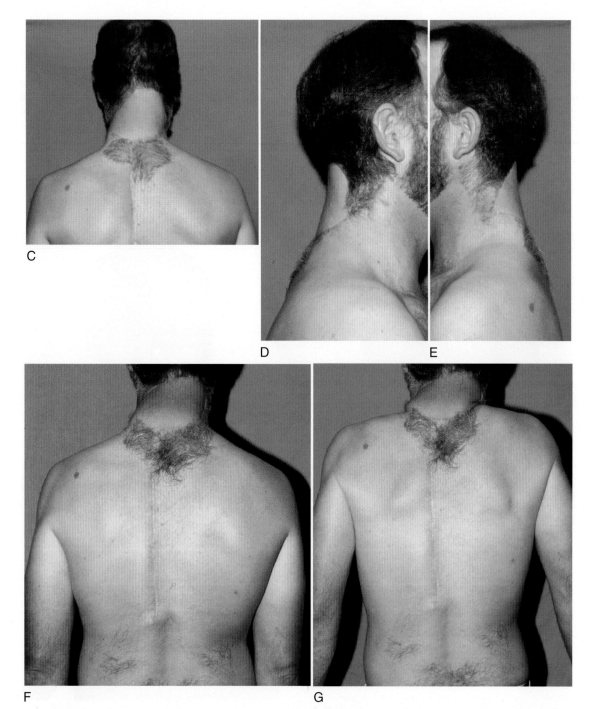

FIGURE 84-12, cont'd. *C,* Postoperative posterior view 6 months after melanoma resection and inset of vertical trapezius musculocutaneous flap. *D,* Right lateral view. Note that muscle with skin island provides natural contour to area of posterior neck dissection. *E,* Left lateral view. *F,* Posterior view: superior fibers of trapezius left intact. Note that with the shoulder at rest, there is no shoulder droop at the donor site. *G,* Posterior view of patient raising shoulders actively demonstrates trapezius function preservation.

Oropharyngeal and Laryngeal Malignant Neoplasms

By far, the most common malignant neoplasms affecting the neck are metastatic. One cannot treat lower face, mandibular, floor of mouth, and pharyngeal lesions without consideration of the impact on neck structures. Surgical removal of cervical lymph nodes is required for advanced stage oropharyngeal and laryngeal malignant disease, and irradiation is frequently required to reduce risk of local and regional recurrence. Extirpation by radical and modified radical neck dissection before and after extirpative radiation therapy significantly affects the neck structures. Wound healing, skin quality and pliability, cervicomental angle, and functional mobility are all negatively affected by radiation therapy and surgical extirpation. Besides the negative impact on neck aesthetic appearance, these treatments can also lead to wound breakdown and subsequent exposure of critical underlying structures and chronic fistulous communication to those structures.

Numerous successful reconstructive techniques have been described to address the post-extirpative neck.

NECK RECONSTRUCTION

Skin and Soft Tissue Replacement

In the nonirradiated neck, replacement of fine neck skin and subcutaneous tissue for cutaneous substitution and volume repletion can be performed by local tissue rearrangement with use of local flaps, such as rhomboid.[67] With local rotational flaps, Z-plasty,[68,69] or V-Y advancements, adjacent neck skin is used for repair, providing equal skin thickness and excellent color match. Limbs of an appropriately placed Z-plasty should emphasize a horizontal final suture line, and vertical orientation should be avoided because of high risk of scar band contracture. Emphasis on contour and selection of incisions is paramount. Transverse incisions with platysma and skin closures are optimal. Vertical incisions and T incisions are associated with high risk for scar contracture and unfavorable cervicomental angle aesthetic appearance. Skin grafts are seldom used as a single source of reconstruction and are primarily used to cover deeper buried muscle or omental flaps or after burn reconstruction.

Local and Regional Fasciocutaneous Flaps

Regional rotation flaps can be elevated satisfactorily and reliably based on angiosomal vascular territories and defined pedicles.[70,71] Large territories can be expanded and delayed as well as supercharged to increase reliable coverage of the neck.

LATERAL CERVICAL SKIN FLAPS

The lateral cervical skin flaps can be based superiorly, anteriorly, or posteriorly to be advanced or rotated into the defect. Delay is recommended for these random-pattern flaps if they are designed for greater than 2:1 length-to-width flap ratio (Fig. 84-13).[72]

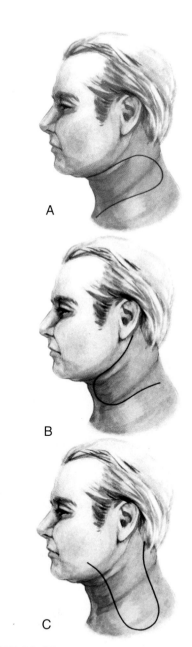

FIGURE 84-13. Lateral cervical skin flaps, which generally include the platysma muscle, can be based anteriorly *(A)*, posteriorly *(B)*, or superiorly *(C)*. (From Schuller D: Cervical skin flaps in head and neck reconstruction. Am J Otolaryngol 1981;2:62.)

PEDICLED OCCIPITAL ARTERY FLAP

Cervical coverage can be designed by pedicled fascio-cutaneous flap from an occipital donor site. The pedicled occipital artery flap is raised on reliable occipital artery positioned on the posterior aspect of the sternocleidomastoid and splenius capitis muscles. The artery, a derivative of the external carotid system, traverses the deep cervical fascia and enters the scalp at a point between the middle and medial third of the superior nuchal line.[71,73-75] The occipital flap can be designed as an inferior-based 15-cm-wide vertically oriented flap and will reliably rotate to the midline of the anterior neck. First, the occipital vessels are confirmed with Doppler study to ensure patency. The flap is designed with a 15-cm base extending cephalad to the most anterior hair-bearing scalp. The flap is elevated along the subgaleal plane to just below the level of the occipital protuberance. The mobilized flap is then rotated 90 degrees, below the ear, to be inset into the neck. The resultant rotational dog-ear can be treated with Burow triangle excision or secondarily with minor office revision. The occipital scalp donor site is grafted. Alterations in flap design may include a superior-based design, also termed nape of neck flap, in which the occipital artery is preserved at the level of the occipital protuberance and the skin flap is designed along skin and subcutaneous tissue overlying the lateral border of the trapezius (Fig. 84-14). In the superiorly based flap, the postauricular artery is also included in the flap design. Again, the donor site is grafted.[72]

SUBMENTAL ARTERY ISLAND FLAP

The submental artery island flap is based on the submental artery branch of the facial artery.[76] The flap uses skin and subcutaneous tissue and fascia in the submental area, with a reliable vascular pedicle of 8 cm (Fig. 84-15).[76,77] In addition to rotation for coverage of lower face and preauricular defects, it can be rotated to cover inferior neck and lateral neck defects.[77-79] A skin paddle of 4 to 10 cm can be raised as a standard flap,[80] with the possibility of 14×7 cm in an extremely lax neck.[81] The design of the flap is made with the patient in neck extension. The skin portion of the paddle is marked anterior in the submental area 1 to 2 cm posterior to the mandibular border. The skin paddle is elevated with dissection in the subplatysmal plane starting on the contralateral side from the pedicle. With continued dissection of the submental artery to the level of the anterior belly of the digastric muscle, the muscle is released and the flap is dissected to the level of the facial vessels. If longer reach is needed, additional dissection of the facial artery can facilitate length. Care must be taken to avoid traction or injury to the marginal mandibular nerve. The donor site is closed primarily in most instances, with skin grafting as an alternative. This flap has been reported to have successful use in a previously irradiated field, although authors caution that closure of the donor defect is compromised.[82] This flap has also been described for reconstruction of the cervical esophagus[80,81] and can be used for free microsurgical transfer.[77]

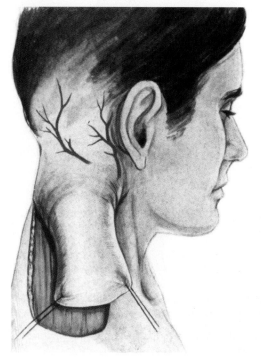

FIGURE 84-14. The nape of neck flap includes tissue that usually has not been included in radiation therapy ports and has a donor site that can readily be concealed by clothing. (From Schuller D: Cervical skin flaps in head and neck reconstruction. Am J Otolaryngol 1981;2:62.)

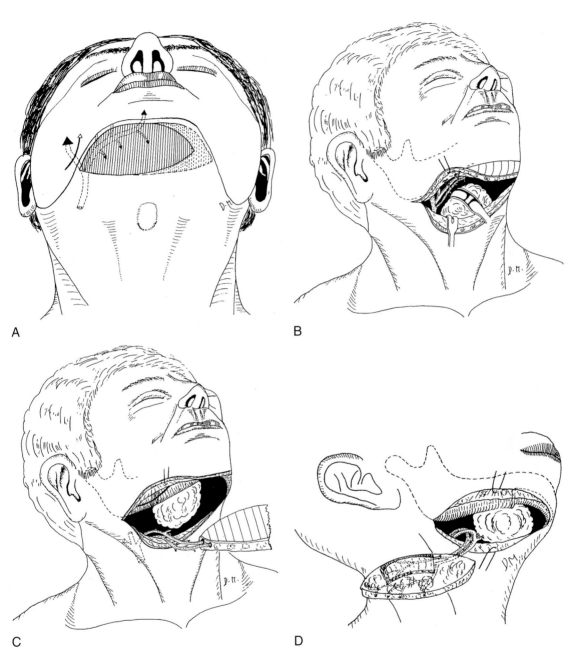

A

B

C

D

FIGURE 84-15. The submental artery island flap. *A,* Outlining of the flap. *B,* Undermining of the flap close to the submental gland. *C,* Raising of the flap from distal to proximal. *D,* Compound osteocutaneous flap. (From Martin D, Pascal JF, Baudet J, et al: The submental island flap: a new donor site. Plast Reconstr Surg 1993;92:867.)

DORSAL SCAPULAR ISLAND FLAP

Fasciocutaneous flaps based on the dorsal scapular artery (direct branch of subclavian artery or from trunk of transverse cervical artery)[70,83,84] provide thin and extensive tissue area for coverage of neck defects. In anatomic studies, the flap raised on this vessel (15 to 16 cm) can be rotated to the anterior neck, head, and upper chest wall (Fig. 84-16). Flaps can be used as large as 20 cm × 20 cm with standard harvest and 30 cm × 26 cm with pre-expanded delay.[85] Successful transfer of this flap requires the lower trapezius muscle (below the level of the spine of the scapula) to be included.[86] A complication of inset of this flap is venous insufficiency, which can be improved by flap delay with transection of the draining intercostal veins before transfer. Venous congestion can also be minimized by microsurgical supercharge of the venous system to recipient vessels in the neck.[85] Donor sites are closed by primary closure in most instances or by skin grafting. This flap is useful for both anterolateral and posterior neck defects.

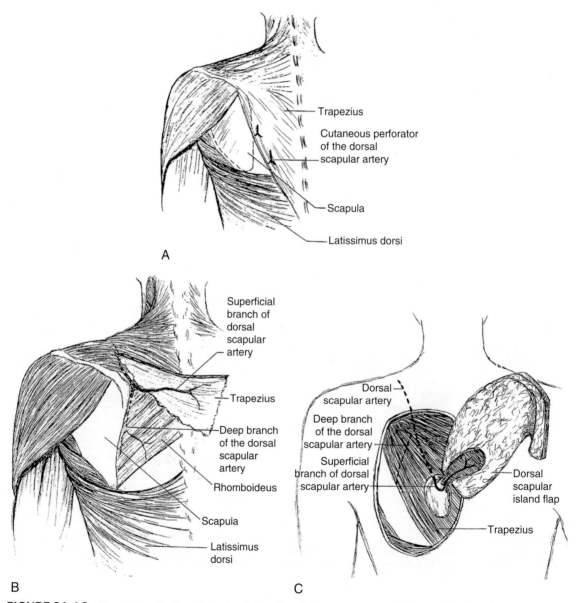

FIGURE 84-16. Dorsal scapular flap. *A*, Anatomic location of the cutaneous perforators of the dorsal scapular artery. *B*, Anatomy of the dorsal scapular artery. *C*, Illustration of the anatomy of the dorsal scapular island flap. (From Angrigiani C, Grilli D, Karanas YL, et al: The dorsal scapular island flap: an alternative for head, neck, and chest reconstruction. Plast Reconstr Surg 2003;111:67.)

DELTOPECTORAL FLAP

The deltopectoral flap was first described by Bakamjian in 1965.[87] The flap was developed at a time in history of increased resectional capability for head and neck tumors and advances in treatment with radiation therapy. The need for reconstructive tissue options outside the irradiated and resected fields drove innovation in flap design before widespread use of free tissue transfer techniques. Early experience with the technique did uncover shortcomings of the flap for uses in pharynx, face, and neck reconstruction,[87-89] but with modifications of the flap design and the delay principle, the deltopectoral flap remains a useful reconstructive flap in massive neck defects today.

Landmarks for elevation of the deltopectoral flap include the sternal edge, infraclavicular line, deltopectoral groove, and nipple (Figs. 84-17 and 84-18). The flap is designed diagonally upward across the upper chest and shoulder. The base lies over the second, third, and fourth costal cartilages; the upper border follows the infraclavicular line beyond the deltopectoral groove onto the anterior shoulder. A delayed flap can be extended safely to the tip of the shoulder. The lower border runs parallel to the upper border and usually lies a few centimeters above the position of the undisplaced nipple. The pedicle is designed by use of the perforating branches of the internal mammary artery located within 3 to 4 cm of the midsternal line. For transposition to the head and neck, skeletonization of the perforating vessels should be avoided. The patient is placed in the supine position. The ipsilateral arm may be abducted or adducted according to the surgeon's preference.[90]

Incisions are made through the skin and subcutaneous tissues down to the underlying pectoralis and deltoid muscle. The fascia overlying the muscle is included with the flap. The distal extent of the standard flap is just beyond the deltopectoral groove. However, with a delay, the flap can be safely extended to the tip of the shoulder.

Flap elevation proceeds from distal to proximal. The distal end is incised through skin and subcutaneous tissues down to and including the fascia over the deltoid. The dissection then proceeds rapidly through a relatively bloodless plane across the deltoid, across the deltopectoral groove, and onto the pectoralis major. The axially oriented vessels can sometimes be seen within 5 to 6 cm of the midline just above the fascia. The dissection is continued until the perforators are seen emerging through the pectoralis major muscle.

The delayed flap is outlined beyond the deltopectoral groove and onto the anterior border of the shoulder almost to the tip. That portion of the flap extending beyond the deltopectoral groove is then elevated and resutured into the donor site. A Silastic sheet or tissue expander may be placed beneath the area of flap delay.

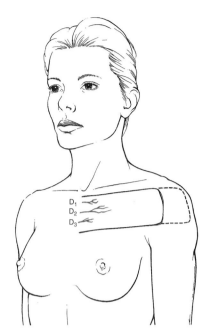

FIGURE 84-17. Deltopectoral flap. Dominant pedicles: perforating branches of internal mammary artery (D_1, D_2, D_3). (From Mathes SJ, Nahai F: Reconstructive Surgery: Principles, Anatomy, and Technique. New York, Churchill Livingstone, 1997:413.)

For staged reconstruction of the esophagus with a tubed deltopectoral flap, the flap is tubed with the cutaneous surface directed inside to provide lining for the neoesophagus. The upper border of the tubed flap is then approximated to the esophagus; the lower border remains open as a temporary controlled salivary fistula (Fig. 84-18C). At the second stage (usually 2 to 3 weeks later), the attached base of the deltopectoral flap is divided, the tubing is completed, and the distal esophageal anastomosis is completed.

The flap is inset according to the reconstructive requirements. For intraoral reconstruction, the tubed flap is approximated to the mucosa and muscle edges of the extirpative defect. The reconstruction is then completed at a second stage, when the tube is divided and the proximal divided portions of the flap are definitively inset. The second stage is usually performed 2 to 3 weeks after the initial reconstruction. In the meantime, the tubed deltopectoral flap serves as a controlled salivary fistula.

For the deltopectoral flap, preliminary expansion may enlarge the flap area and minimize the donor defect. With or without expansion, skin grafting is usually required for the donor area. In 10% of the flaps extending in length over the deltoid muscle (extended flap design with primary elevation), some necrosis is seen. This distal flap loss is avoided and the flap significantly lengthened by a primary delay procedure.[90]

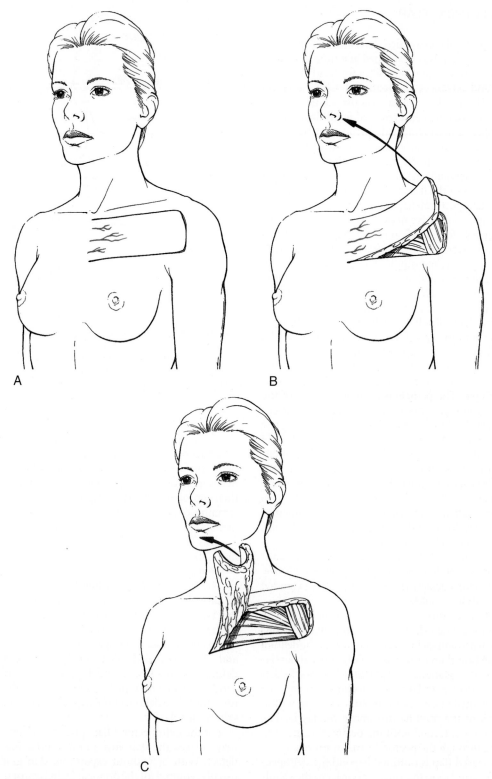

FIGURE 84-18. Deltopectoral flap arc of rotation. *A,* Standard flap design. *B,* Arc to lower neck. *C,* Tubed flap arc to lower oral cavity. (From Mathes SJ, Nahai F: Reconstructive Surgery: Principles, Anatomy, and Technique. New York, Churchill Livingstone, 1997:417.)

Distant Fasciocutaneous Flaps

Distant fasciocutaneous flaps are commonly selected for complex coverage of neck defects. Fasciocutaneous flaps provide reliable, versatile, thin flaps for microsurgical free tissue transplantation to multiple areas of the neck. Versatility of the flaps allows formation of tubes for reconstruction of pharyngeal and cervical esophageal conduits and folding for single-flap coverage of multiple areas. The highly concentrated vascular territories of the neck allow a great selection of recipient vessels for microvascular anastomosis.[91] The thin nature provides durability but less bulk than with muscle flaps, thereby improving contour as well as function.[92] Although any fasciocutaneous flap with a defined vascular pedicle greater than 1 to 2 mm can be used for microvascular composite tissue transplantation, this section discusses the three most commonly used fasciocutaneous microvascular transfers.

RADIAL FOREARM FLAP

Radial free forearm microvascular transplantation uses the thin surface of the ventral forearm skin for reconstruction of multiple neck defects. The flap is raised on the radial artery and paired venae comitantes or cephalic vein[93] (Fig. 84-19) and can be transferred as a sensory flap if the radial sensory branch is included.[94-96] The flap can be harvested at dimensions of 10 to 12 cm by 15 to 20 cm without delay. The thin and pliable nature of the forearm skin makes it particularly suitable for cutaneous reconstruction. In large series reports of reconstructions of the hypopharynx and upper esophagus, the radial free forearm microvascular transfer has been demonstrated to be a highly successful surgical transfer. Controversy exists in regard to the optimal reconstruction for circumferential segmental defects of the esophagus and lower pharynx reconstruction, although tubed radial free forearm microsurgical transplantation has been shown to be reliable and functional.[97] Others advocate free jejunal transplantation for circumferential pharyngoesophageal defects (see "Jejunal Flap").[98-102]

LATERAL THIGH FLAP

The anterolateral thigh flap is a thin, versatile fasciocutaneous or adipofascial perforator flap based on septal perforators from the lateral circumflex femoral vessel.[103-107] The flap may be harvested for sizes of 25×18 cm.[108] The septal perforators are mapped by Doppler study to distinct points on the overlying skin.[109] The flap (skin and subcutaneous tissue) is on average 7 mm thick, which compares favorably with the radial forearm (2 mm) and inferior epigastric territory (13 mm) (Fig. 84-20).[110] The flap can be safely thinned to 3 or 4 mm, with preservation of a small rim of fat at the level of the perforator vessels.[110-112] Advocates of this flap recommend that it not exceed 9 cm of skin paddle around the perforator, as further distance is unreliable.[113] This flap is transferred by microsurgical anastomosis of the lateral circumflex femoral pedicle (see Chapter 83 for description of technique). It is useful for extensive cutaneous tissue loss of the neck[114] and also has been successfully folded and tubed for reconstruction of circumferential pharyngoesophageal defects.[115] The anterolateral thigh donor defect is often grafted, although pre-expansion may allow primary donor defect closure.[116,117]

LATERAL ARM FLAP

The lateral arm flap was first described for microvascular composite tissue transplantation in 1982, when reliable lateral arm vessels were discovered to supply a large cutaneous territory. This territory supplied by the posterior radial collateral artery branch of the profunda brachii led to design on the posterolateral aspect of the upper arm extending from the deltoid insertion to the lateral epicondyle (Fig. 84-21).[118] Further studies on vascular territories reveal that the territories supplied by the posterior radial collateral artery extend well past the lateral condyle onto the radial aspect of the forearm.[119]

Elevation of this flap begins with an incision at the periphery of the skin island (Fig. 84-21); the fascia is exposed over the lateral head of the triceps muscle pos-

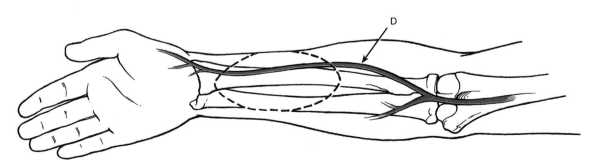

FIGURE 84-19. Radial arm flap. Dominant pedicle: radial artery (D). (From Mathes SJ, Nahai F: Reconstructive Surgery: Principles, Anatomy, and Technique. New York, Churchill Livingstone, 1997:776.)

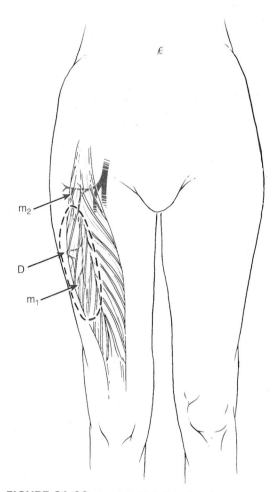

FIGURE 84-20. Lateral thigh flap. Dominant pedicle: septocutaneous branches of descending branch of lateral circumflex femoral artery (D). Minor pedicles: musculocutaneous branches of descending branch of lateral circumflex femoral artery (m_1); musculocutaneous branches of transverse branch of lateral circumflex femoral artery (m_2). (From Mathes SJ, Nahai F: Reconstructive Surgery: Principles, Anatomy, and Technique. New York, Churchill Livingstone, 1997:1164.)

teriorly and the brachialis and brachioradialis muscles anteriorly. The fascia is incised at the posterior and anterior limits of the flap and the posterior fascia is elevated, exposing the lateral head of the triceps muscle. Dissection proceeds anteriorly until the lateral intermuscular septum is reached. The fasciocutaneous perforating vessels may be visualized superficial to the deep fascia coursing from the intermuscular septum through the fascia.

An incision is made into the anterior fascia over the brachialis and radialis muscle. The fascia is elevated in a posterior direction until the anterior edge of the lateral intermuscular septum is reached. The distal fascia is incised to the level of the periosteum of the humerus, and the fascia anteriorly and posteriorly and inter-

muscular septum are elevated superiorly to the level of the deltoid insertion. At the distal end of the skin island, the fascial incision will expose the posterior antebrachial cutaneous nerve. This nerve is generally divided or may be left intact and separated from the vascular pedicle later if sensory nerve preservation is planned. Preservation of the nerve will increase the complexity of proximal flap dissection and is generally not necessary.

In the middle third of the upper arm, the muscle fibers of origin from the lateral head of the triceps muscle are incised, exposing the posterior radial collateral artery and associated venae comitantes as the intermuscular septum with overlying fascia and skin island is elevated.

In the proximal dissection of the flap, the lateral fibers of the triceps muscle are divided adjacent to their humeral attachments for vascular pedicle exposure. The radial nerve is visualized anterior to the posterior radial collateral artery and associated venae comitantes. It is carefully retracted to avoid injury during proximal pedicle dissection. At the level of the deltoid insertion, the bifurcation of the profunda brachii artery into the posterior radial collateral and the middle collateral artery is exposed. Flap elevation is completed when the flap is ready for transposition as an island flap or as a microvascular transplant based on the posterior radial collateral artery and associated venae comitantes.

Advantages of the flap include a reliable pedicle, ease of harvest with two concurrent operating teams, primary closure of donor site, and possibility of restoration of sensation to the transferred flap reconstruction.[120-123] Disadvantages of the flap include the relatively narrow width,[118] compared with other flaps, and short vascular pedicle often requiring vein grafts.[121]

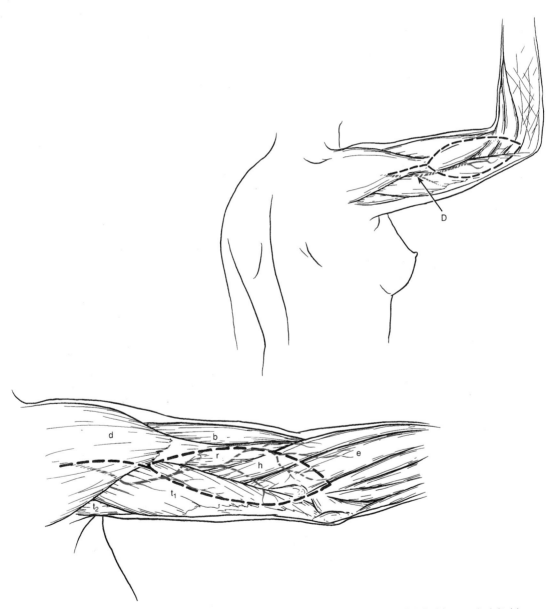

FIGURE 84-21. Lateral arm flap. Dominant pedicle: radial collateral artery (D). b, biceps; d, deltoid; e, extensor carpi radialis longus; h, brachioradialis; r, brachialis; t_1, lateral head of triceps; t_2, long head of triceps. (From Mathes SJ, Nahai F: Reconstructive Surgery: Principles, Anatomy, and Technique. New York, Churchill Livingstone, 1997:730.)

Muscle and Musculocutaneous Flaps

PLATYSMA FLAP

The platysma flap (Fig. 84-22) can be designed as a muscle or musculocutaneous flap based on the submental artery (branch of the facial artery) or inferiorly based suprasternal artery (branch of the suprascapular artery).[124] The flap will reach for coverage of the lower face,[125] intraoral reconstruction,[126,127] and anterior neck, and it is especially useful in stable coverage of tracheostomy sites (Fig. 84-23). Multiple modifications including bilateral flap elevation,[128,129] transverse orientation,[130] and innervated flaps[131] have improved the versatility of this flap. Major complications are infrequent, but minor complications, particularly partial loss of the skin island, occur frequently.[132] Its use is limited in the irradiated neck or extensive neck dissection without harming the flap or remaining neck skin closure.[127] In addition to proximally based and distally based pedicled flap elevation, the flap can be designed for microvascular transplantation, using the dominant blood supply, although its use as a free flap is rare.[90]

For the platysma flap, the anterior and posterior borders of the muscle are marked. The mandible represents the upper extent and the clavicle the lower extent of the muscle. The upper pedicle is located at the level of the mandibular notch deep to the muscle, and the inferior pedicle is located just behind the clavicle at the lateral border of the muscle. The skin island for the standard flap is located over the distal third of the muscle just above the clavicle. For the distally based flap, the island is placed over the central part of the muscle. The patient is positioned supine with the head turned to the opposite side. The muscle is exposed through parallel incisions over its origin and insertion or through the incisions around the skin island for the musculocutaneous flaps.[90]

When the standard flap is elevated, the muscle is easily identified under the skin. After the skin borders of the cutaneous island are incised, the superficial surface of the platysma muscle is identified and the midneck skin elevated from the muscle to the level of the larynx. A second transverse incision is made 3 cm below the mandible to complete exposure of the superior half of the platysma. The muscle fibers of origin are divided at the level of the clavicle, and the muscle with the overlying skin island is elevated superiorly. The external jugular vein and anterior jugular veins are included within the flap. The fascia overlying the sternocleidomastoid is also included with the flap. Segmental pedicles at the level of the midpoint of the flap are divided, and the flap is then elevated toward the mandible. The dominant pedicle is visualized deep to the surface of the muscle. This is a very thin muscle and dissection has to be performed sharply, with care taken not to injure the thin muscle fibers. For intraoral reconstruction, it is best to take the flap over the mandible because tunneling under the mandible may result in kinking of the vascular pedicle. In addition, the marginal mandibular branch of the facial nerve is deep to the platysma close to its insertion. This branch should be identified and preserved during flap elevation. The muscle and skin island are sutured into the defect. In most instances, the donor site is closed directly (Fig. 84-23A).[90]

For the distally based flap, the dissection proceeds in the opposite direction (Fig. 84-23B). The skin island is isolated, and the muscle is transected at the junction of its upper and middle thirds and dissected inferiorly. Release of the entire insertion of the muscle and mobilization of the facial artery will increase the arc of rotation (Fig. 84-24).

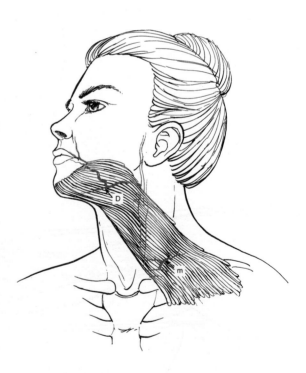

FIGURE 84-22. Platysma flap. Dominant pedicle: submental artery (D). Minor pedicle: suprasternal artery (m). (From Mathes SJ, Nahai F: Reconstructive Surgery: Principles, Anatomy, and Technique. New York, Churchill Livingstone, 1997:323.)

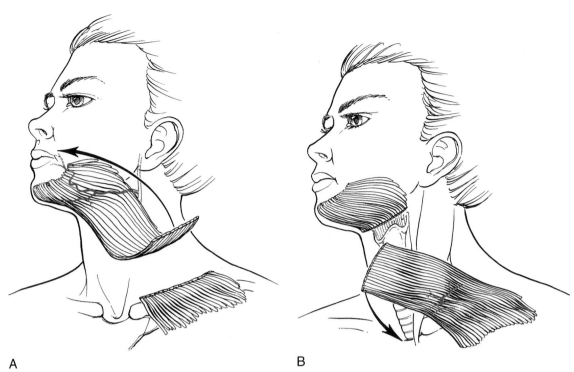

A   B

FIGURE 84-23. Platysma flap arc of rotation. *A,* Standard flap. Based on the dominant pedicle, the entire muscle may be elevated as a flap with a rotation point at the level of the mandible. It will reach midline neck defects, the chin, and even the upper lip. It will also reach the intraoral cavity from the central buccal sulcus to the anterior tonsillar pillar. *B,* Distally based flap. A small distal flap based on the inferior minor pedicle may be elevated for coverage of tracheostomy and other lower anterior neck defects. (From Mathes SJ, Nahai F: Reconstructive Surgery: Principles, Anatomy, and Technique. New York, Churchill Livingstone, 1997:326, 327.)

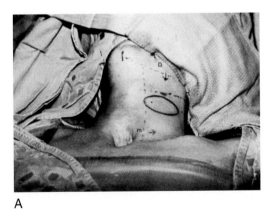

A

FIGURE 84-24. Platysma musculocutaneous flap. *A,* Adult singer noted unstable skin at site of long-term tracheostomy defect. Design of platysma musculocutaneous flap based on inferior minor pedicle (branch of facial artery) is demonstrated. D is site of entry of dominant pedicle (branch of facial artery); m is site of entry of minor pedicle (branch of transverse cervical artery).   *Continued*

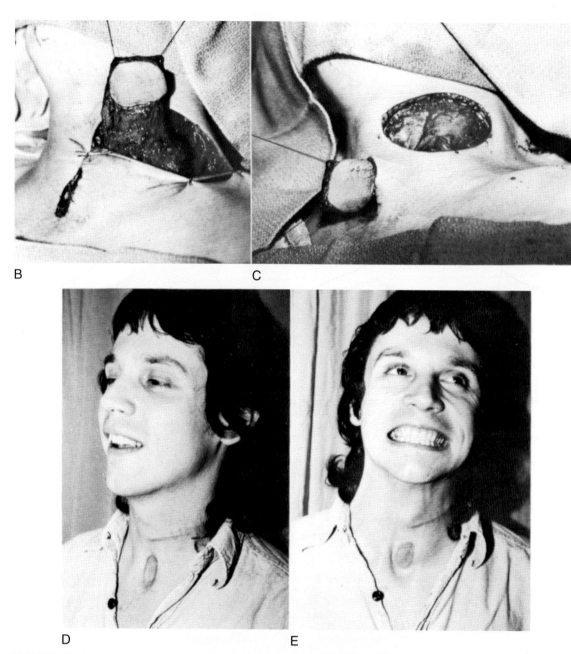

B   C

D   E

FIGURE 84-24, cont'd. *B,* Inferiorly based platysma musculocutaneous flap. Note design of skin island beneath left mandible. *C,* Platysma musculocutaneous flap tunneled beneath intact anterior neck skin to tracheostomy defect. *D,* Platysma muscle used for coverage of long-term tracheostomy defect. *E,* Absence of platysma contractions in left side of neck after transposition as flap to midline. (From Mathes SJ, Nahai F: Clinical Atlas of Muscle and Musculocutaneous Flaps. St. Louis, Mosby, 1979:186,187.)

STERNOCLEIDOMASTOID FLAP

The sternocleidomastoid flap can also be designed as a muscle or musculocutaneous flap. With a dominant pedicle (occipital artery) and multiple minor pedicles, the flap is versatile and reliable in transfer (Fig. 84-25). The flap is useful proximally or distally based and provides coverage of anterior and posterior neck defects in addition to the oral cavity (Fig. 84-

26).[83,90,127,133] The flap is associated with a high complication rate (30%) in one critique[134] and has limited application in head and neck reconstruction, especially when alternatives are available.[90]

The proximally based flap is primarily selected for oral cavity or distal third facial defects. The distally based flap is selected for anterior inferior neck defects. The skin island for a distally based sternocleidomas-

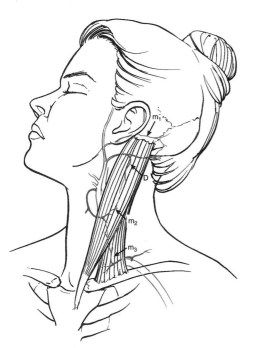

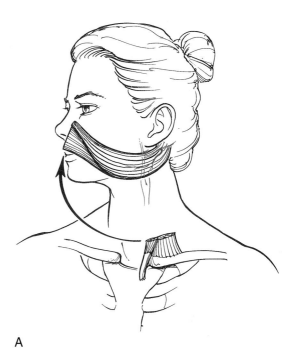

A

FIGURE 84-25. Sternocleidomastoid flap. Dominant pedicle: branch of occipital artery (D). Minor pedicles: branch of posterior auricular artery (m_1); branch of superior thyroid artery (m_2); branch of suprascapular artery (m_3). (From Mathes SJ, Nahai F: Reconstructive Surgery: Principles, Anatomy, and Technique. New York, Churchill Livingstone, 1997:356.)

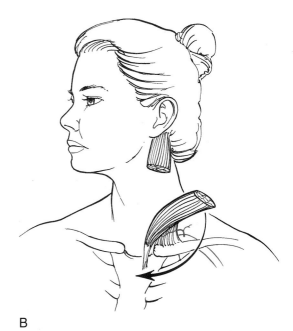

B

FIGURE 84-26. Sternocleidomastoid flap. *A,* Superior arc of rotation at the level of the carotid bifurcation. The lower two thirds of the muscle may be transposed for anterior neck and lower face coverage. *B,* Arc of rotation of distally based flap. Based on its distal vascular pedicles (branches of suprascapular artery and vein), the flap may be transposed for middle and lower neck coverage. (From Mathes SJ, Nahai F: Reconstructive Surgery: Principles, Anatomy, and Technique. New York, Churchill Livingstone, 1997:359, 360.)

toid flap is marked over the upper proximal muscle close to its insertion. The distal pedicle is deep to the lower third of the muscle. The patient is positioned supine with the head turned to the opposite side. The skin island is isolated, and the muscle is exposed through a parallel transverse neck incision or through a vertical incision directly over the muscle. The distally based flap is based on the branches of the suprascapular artery and vein. The muscle is outlined by drawing a line from the mastoid to the manubrium. The incision is made along that line and the muscle identified. The muscle is then divided at about midway along its length. The muscle is mobilized from above downward toward the distal vascular pedicle. The elevated flap is transposed into the defect. It is tunneled under the mandible for intraoral reconstruction.[90]

The eleventh cranial nerve has a close relationship to the muscle (passing through it at the junction of the upper and middle thirds). Injury to the nerve will denervate the trapezius. The internal jugular vein is close to the muscle and its origin, and one should use caution in this area. The great auricular nerve is closely related to the anterosuperior border of the muscle and should be preserved.[90]

PECTORALIS MAJOR FLAP

The pectoralis major flap is based on the thoracoacromial vessels and can be harvested as a muscle or myocutaneous flap (Fig. 84-27). As a type V muscle flap, the primary dominant arterial supply is the thoracoacromial artery with multiple segmental pedicles from intercostal perforators arising from the internal mammary system. These minor pedicles are divided in harvest of the flap. However, additional extension of the associated skin paddle can be achieved by inclusion of the upper abdominal fascia and overlying skin.[135-138] The flap will rotate to reach the floor of mouth, anterior neck, and lower neck pretracheal region (Fig. 84-28). There is a wide variation in complication rates with this flap (8% to 63%)[139-143]; however, reports show a low incidence of major complications, such as total flap loss. The flap and the thoracoacromial vessels are spared during radiation therapy for advanced head and neck tumors[140] and can expediently be harvested for single-stage reconstruction in the debilitated patient.

When the pectoralis major flap is used in head and neck reconstruction, once the skin island is isolated and the overlying skin separated from the muscle, the muscle is divided distally and mobilized proximally toward the clavicle and the dominant pedicle. This portion of the dissection is facilitated by the use of a lighted mammary retractor. It is not necessary to elevate the entire muscle. A wide central strip of muscle will contain a sufficient number of vessels to vascularize the muscle and the skin island. The vascular pedicle is visualized on the deep surface of the muscle and included with the flap. The dissection is completed up to the clavicle. The flap is then pulled through the clavicular incision.[90]

For reconstruction of the cervical esophagus, a tubed pectoralis musculocutaneous flap is available. A large skin island is designed on the pectoralis, and the muscle and skin are elevated. The flap is tubed so that the skin surface is on the inside, representing the lumen of the neoesophagus. The flap is then sutured into the esophageal defect; a skin graft is required for coverage of the outer muscular surface of the tubed flap (Fig. 84-29).

For head and neck reconstruction, the muscle or musculocutaneous pectoralis major flap is rotated 180 degrees if a skin island is designed for face coverage or turned over the clavicle for intraoral coverage. In general, the flap is passed over the clavicle and beneath the neck skin to reach intraoral or facial defects. The flap may also pass deep to the clavicle to reach the head and neck region. The muscle as well as the skin island is sutured into the defect.

The donor defect is usually closed directly for small skin islands. Larger skin islands require a skin graft or a secondary flap to close the donor area.[90]

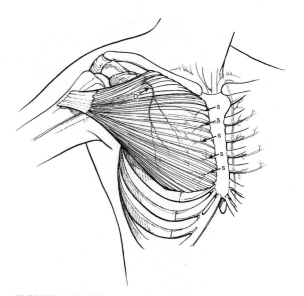

FIGURE 84-27. Pectoralis major flap. Dominant pedicle: pectoral branch of thoracoacromial artery (D). Secondary pedicle: perforating branches of internal mammary artery (s). (From Mathes SJ, Nahai F: Reconstructive Surgery: Principles, Anatomy, and Technique. New York, Churchill Livingstone, 1997:442.)

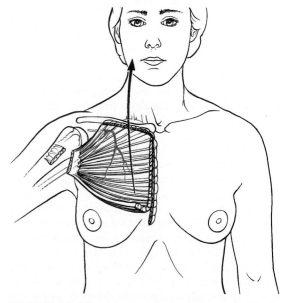

FIGURE 84-28. Pectoralis major flap: arc of rotation of standard flap. Based on the single dominant thoracoacromial pedicle, the muscle will provide coverage for the head and neck up to the level of the inferior orbital rim. Division of the muscle either at its insertion or through the anterior axillary fold will allow further flap rotation and increase the arc of rotation by as much as 3 to 5 cm. (From Mathes SJ, Nahai F: Reconstructive Surgery: Principles, Anatomy, and Technique. New York, Churchill Livingstone, 1997:448.)

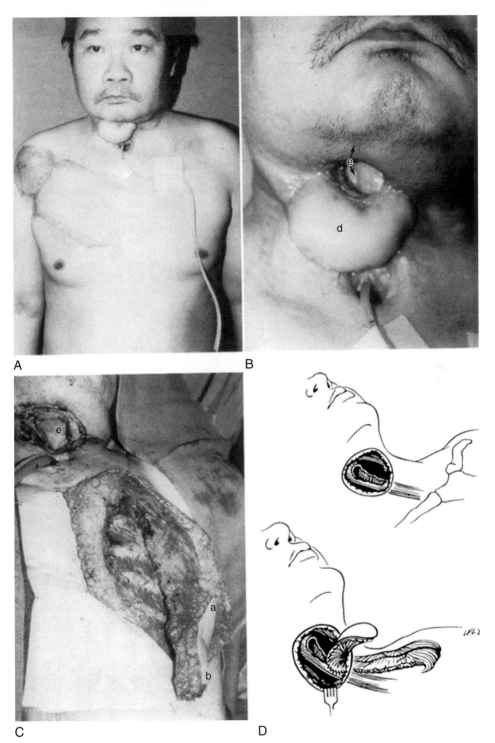

FIGURE 84-29. Pectoralis major musculocutaneous flap for reconstruction of a pharyngoesophageal fistula in a patient presenting with radiation necrosis and failed deltopectoral flap. *A,* Preoperative view. The patient had recurrent squamous cell carcinoma of the larynx after primary radiation therapy, which necessitated laryngectomy. Complications secondary to poor wound healing resulted in right-sided carotid rupture and necrosis of the anterior cervical esophageal wall. *B,* The deltopectoral flap failed to provide stable coverage. d, site of deltopectoral flap inset; e, anterior wall defect of the pharynx-cervical esophagus extending to the site of the tracheostomy. *C,* Deltopectoral flap excised; pharyngeal-cervical esophageal defect (e) débrided. The left pectoralis major musculocutaneous flap is elevated with a distal vertical skin island. a, superior aspect of skin island; b, inferior aspect. *D,* After flap transposition to the neck, the skin island is inset in the defect with the superior edge of the skin island sutured to the esophagus at the level of the trachea; the inferior portion is placed into the superior aspect of the pharyngeal defect.
Continued

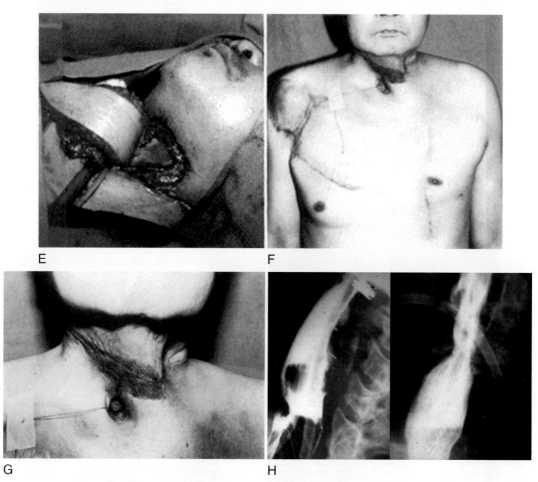

FIGURE 84-29, cont'd. *E,* Skin island tailored to fit defect in interior cervical esophagus. *F,* One month after reconstructive surgery, the patient demonstrated normal pharyngeal-esophageal continuity. *G,* Close-up view demonstrates stable coverage provided by skin grafts on the exposed deep surface of the pectoralis major muscle. *H,* Radiograph of barium swallow examination demonstrates restoration of pharyngeal-esophageal continuity with intact anterior wall at the site of the pharyngeal-esophageal reconstruction with the pectoralis major skin island. (From Mathes S: The pectoralis major flap. In Stark RB, ed: Plastic Surgery of the Head and Neck. New York, Churchill Livingstone, 1985:949.)

TRAPEZIUS FLAP

The trapezius muscle receives reliable vascularity through the dominant transverse cervical artery and vein and minor pedicle contribution through the dorsal scapular vessels and intercostal vessels (Fig. 84-30).[90] The rich vascularity allows the flap to be superiorly based (on the transverse cervical vessels) for high head and neck reconstructive needs and inferiorly based for trunk, axillary, or upper back reconstruction. The standard muscle flap design can also be extended to include a distal fasciocutaneous extension, that is, the cervicohumeral flap (Fig. 84-31). The extension allows a reliable and versatile cutaneous component for reconstruction of floor of mouth and cervical esophagus-pharynx as well as face and scalp coverage.[142,144-150]

For the vertical trapezius flap, an incision is made between the posterior base of the neck and the cephalad margin of the skin island. The incision is then made on the lateral edge of the planned skin island. The superficial surface of the trapezius muscle is identified above and lateral to the skin island over the scapula. The muscle is identified at the edge of the skin island, and the deep surface of the middle and lower thirds of the muscle is separated from the chest wall and rhomboid muscles. The medial skin island is incised, and the fibers of origin of the muscle from the vertebral column are divided to the level of the superior scapula. Above the scapula, the muscle is divided from its fibers of origin on the vertebral column and laterally toward the acromioclavicular joint as required for an adequate arc of rotation to the head and neck region. With division of fibers of origin from the thoracic vertebra to the C7-Tl spinous process and with release of fibers of insertion from the scapula, the flap has an adequate arc of rotation to reach the posterior skull, neck, and lateral lower third of the face (Figs. 84-32 and 84-33).[90]

The muscle with its skin island is generally passed through a tunnel superficial to the superior trapezius muscle fibers and beneath neck skin to reach posterior skull or lower facial defects. If the tunnel appears to constrict the flap base, the skin over the tunnel may be incised and the skin island incorporated into the closure or a skin graft used to cover the exposed muscle. If the anterior neck has severe scarring (i.e., prior radical neck dissection with adjuvant radiation therapy), the flap may require inset into the facial defect with the muscle base of the flap external to the neck skin. The exposed muscle is skin grafted or wrapped in moist gauze pending muscle division and completion of the flap inset in 3 to 6 weeks. The flap is rotated during its transposition to the anterior head and neck so that the skin island will be inset in either the oral cavity or the external cutaneous defect as required (Fig. 84-34).

For the extended lateral or cervicohumeral trapezius flap, the incision is made around the skin flap border centered over the acromioclavicular joint with the flap extending to the inferior aspect of the upper arm. Incision extends through the deep fascia, exposing the junction of the lateral head of the triceps and the long head of the biceps muscles at the anterior flap edge and the long head of the triceps muscle at the posterior flap edge beneath the distal flap. In the proximal flap, the superficial surface of the deltoid muscle is visualized at the flap edges.

The flap is elevated at the subfascial level to the base of the flap at the acromioclavicular joint. During flap elevation inferior to the deltoid insertion, the posterior septum is incised to elevate the deep fascia with the flap. Fasciocutaneous branches of the radial collateral artery and musculocutaneous perforating

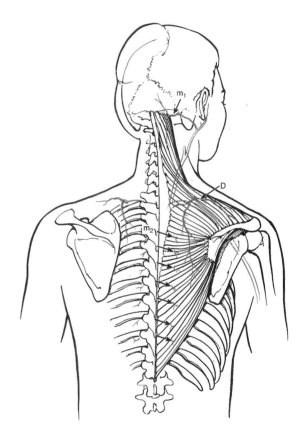

FIGURE 84-30. Vertical trapezius musculocutaneous flap. Dominant pedicle: transverse cervical artery (D). Minor pedicles: branch of occipital artery (m_1); perforating intercostal arteries (m_2; see arrows). (From Mathes SJ, Nahai F: Reconstructive Surgery: Principles, Anatomy, and Technique. New York, Churchill Livingstone, 1997: 652.)

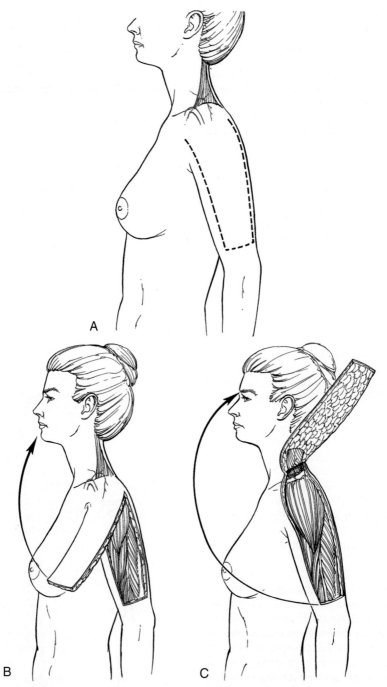

A

B

C

FIGURE 84-31. Extended lateral (cervicohumeral) flap. With elevation of the fasciocutaneous extension of the superior trapezius flap territory from the upper lateral arm, the point of rotation is located at the acromioclavicular joint at the lateral base of the neck. The flap will reach the middle and inferior thirds of the face, ear, and oral cavity. *A,* Flap design is based on the ascending branch of the transverse cervical artery. *B,* Arc to neck and inferior face (anterior trapezius fibers to acromioclavicular joint intact). *C,* Arc to neck and superior face (superior trapezius fibers of insertion elevated with flap). (From Mathes SJ, Nahai F: Reconstructive Surgery: Principles, Anatomy, and Technique. New York, Churchill Livingstone, 1997:657, 661.)

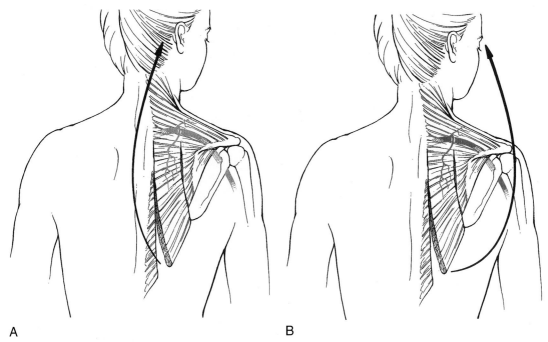

A   B

FIGURE 84-32. Vertical trapezius musculocutaneous flap. *A,* Posterior arc of rotation of vertical standard flap. With a rotation point at the posterior base of the neck, the muscle will reach the posterior skull, cervical and thoracic vertebral column, midface, and neck. With release of the superior muscle fibers, the point of rotation will be in the posterior midneck. The flap will now reach the anterior neck, scalp, and face. *B,* Posterior arc of vertical standard flap to anterior neck and face. (From Mathes SJ, Nahai F: Reconstructive Surgery: Principles, Anatomy, and Technique. New York, Churchill Livingstone, 1997:658, 659.)

vessels from the posterior humeral circumflex artery are divided during flap elevation. The flap point of rotation is generally at the level of the acromioclavicular joint. At the level of the acromioclavicular joint, it is possible to elevate the deep fascia at the lateral third of the clavicle and to release trapezius muscle fibers of insertion to the clavicle. Dissection deep to the anterior superior trapezius is continued until the anterior branch of the transverse cervical artery is reached. Care is taken to preserve both the vascular connections to the muscle and direct cutaneous branches of the transverse cervical artery. The flap arc of rotation can be increased by this maneuver, but this is generally not required if adequate flap length is included in the lateral upper arm.

The flap is rotated 120 to 180 degrees in an anterior arc to reach the head and neck region. The flap is tubed at its base and will require delayed flap base division and inset. Passage of the flap through a neck tunnel is not recommended to avoid constriction of the flap base.

The muscle is inset with the skin island located externally for cutaneous defects or internally for mucosal coverage. After radical neck dissection in conjunction with oral cavity extirpative surgery, the vertical trapezius muscle will provide carotid artery coverage and the distally located skin island will provide oral mucosal replacement.

For the vertical trapezius flap, direct donor site closure is recommended because a noticeable contour deformity will result if skin grafts are placed on the exposed rhomboid muscles. Furthermore, scapular motion during the early postoperative course is difficult to prevent and can result in skin graft disruption. After direct closure of the donor site, shoulder anterior rotation or abduction must be avoided to prevent disruption of the closure site. Direct donor site closure leaves a minimal donor site deformity. Furthermore, because the continuity of the superior muscle fibers is usually preserved, shoulder droop or weakness is avoided (see Fig. 84-12). The intact rhomboid and serratus muscles preserve the position and function of the scapula.

In the extended lateral cervicohumeral flap, skin edges at the flap borders are advanced for partial donor site closure. The remaining exposed muscle will require skin grafts. At second-stage flap inset, the flap base is returned to the donor site.

Text continued on p. 1062

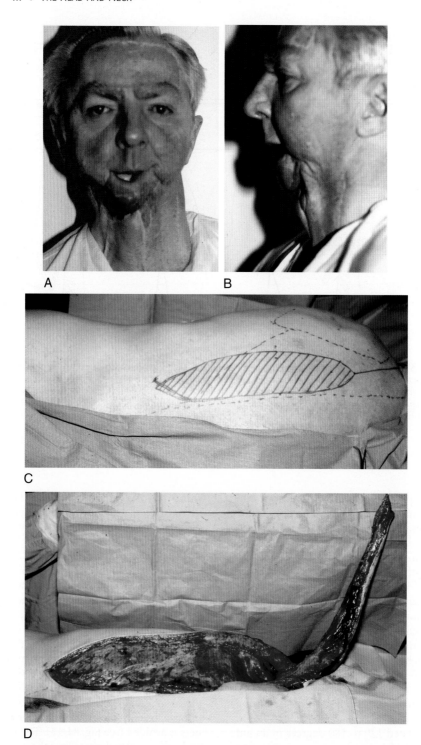

FIGURE 84-33. Vertical trapezius musculocutaneous flap. *A,* Anterior view. The patient presented with orocutaneous fistulas after resection and irradiation of floor of mouth cancer. *B,* Lateral view. Note lack of soft tissue at site of oral cutaneous fistulas. *C,* Intraoperative lateral decubitus view: design of skin island for vertical trapezius musculocutaneous flap. *D,* Intraoperative view. The flap is elevated and ready for transposition to anterior neck defect.

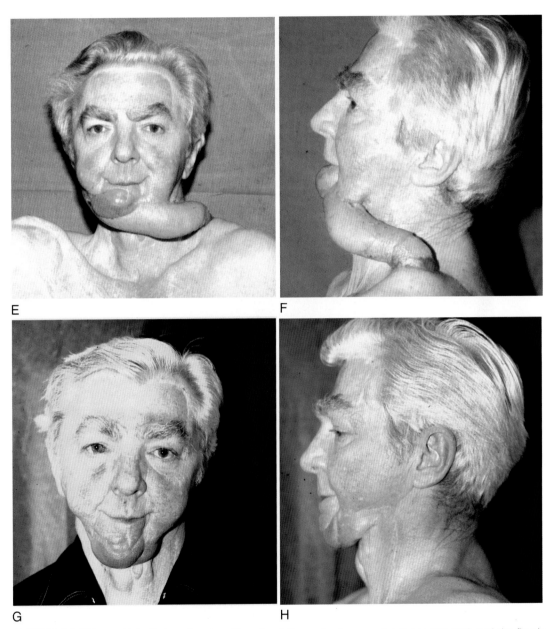

E

F

G

H

FIGURE 84-33, cont'd. *E,* Anterior view. The site of the oral cutaneous fistulas is resected, and the flap is inset with two layers—trapezius muscle (inferior fibers) and skin island. *F,* Lateral view. Base of flap is covered with skin grafts. *G,* Anterior view. Base of flap is divided and the flap inset. *H,* Lateral view. Note well-healed flap with closure of oral cutaneous fistulas.

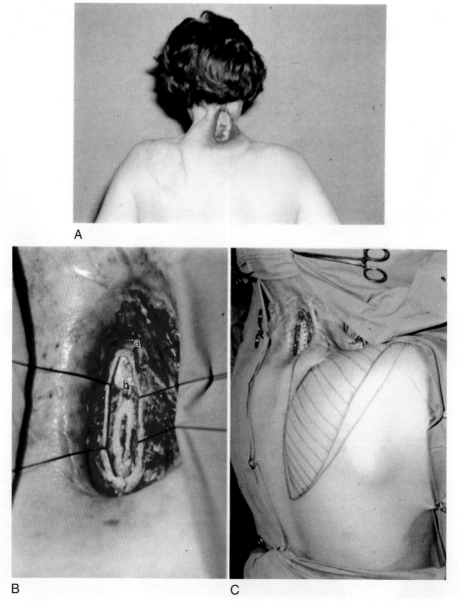

FIGURE 84-34. Posterior trapezius musculocutaneous flap. *A,* Defect is secondary to osteoradionecrosis of cervical vertebral column. Local random flaps from left shoulder have failed to provide stable coverage. *B,* Resection of nonviable tissue includes arachnoid. Note the underlying radiation necrosis of posterior commissure of cervical cord. a, arachnoid; b, posterior commissure of cervical cord. *C,* Fascia lata graft used to restore arachnoid continuity; design of posterior trapezius musculocutaneous flap.

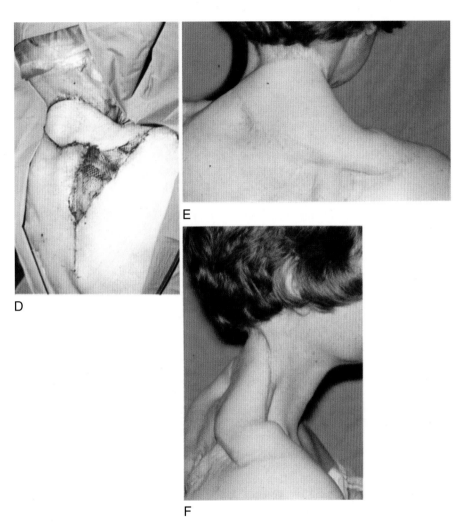

FIGURE 84-34, cont'd. *D,* Posterior trapezius musculocutaneous flap inset into posterior neck defect. Muscle provides coverage of fascia lata graft. The donor defect is skin grafted. *E,* Postoperative posterior view at 3 years demonstrates stable coverage for osteoradionecrosis of cervical vertebral column. *F,* Lateral view demonstrates flap inset. Preservation of anterior fibers of trapezius muscle provides function and avoids shoulder droop. (From Mathes SJ, Nahai F: Clinical Applications for Muscle and Musculocutaneous Flaps. St. Louis, CV Mosby, 1982. Cases similar to *A* and *C* are shown in Mathes SJ, Vasconez LO: Head, neck, and truncal reconstruction with the musculocutaneous flap: anatomical and clinical considerations. Transactions of the VII International Congress of Plastic and Reconstructive Surgery, Rio de Janeiro, 1979. São Paulo, Brazil, Cartgraf, 1980:178-182.)

One should keep in mind that if the patient has undergone a radical neck dissection or has severe inferior neck scarring from radiation therapy, the anterior ascending and posterior descending branches of the transverse cervical artery may be divided or injured. Therefore, preoperative selective arteriography is required to confirm patency of the transverse artery before its use as a flap in reconstructive surgery. When the trapezius muscle is denervated but the transverse cervical vessel remains intact, the vertical trapezius musculocutaneous flap may be used. However, flap elevation is difficult because of the thin, atrophic characteristics of the muscle fibers. The middle fibers of the trapezius muscle are carefully identified lateral to the skin island before separation of the muscle flap from the underlying rhomboid muscles. The flap base of the extended lateral (cervicohumeral) flap should be centered on the acromioclavicular joint to include both direct cutaneous and musculocutaneous branches of the ascending branch of the transverse cervical artery and associated veins. Because second-stage flap base division and inset are required, the vertical trapezius musculocutaneous flap design is preferable to obtain adequate arc of rotation, coverage, and donor site closure.[90]

LATISSIMUS DORSI FLAP

The latissimus dorsi flap is an extremely versatile flap for neck reconstruction (Fig. 84-35). It has a reliable and consistently large and anatomically predictable long vascular pedicle. The muscle itself is wide and relatively flat and thin. Its proximity to the neck makes it suitable for flap transposition (Fig. 84-36) in addition to the possibility of microvascular flap transplantation. It is a large muscle with a primary vascular pedicle (thoracodorsal) and multiple segmental vessels (intercostal branches and lumbar branches). Taken as a musculocutaneous flap, the cutaneous portion can be divided for internal pharyngeal wall reconstruction and additional outer skin paddle coverage as necessary. Disadvantages include the need for modified decubitus position for harvest and high risk of seroma formation postoperatively.[151] A survey of patients undergoing this procedure also noted subjective shoulder weakness, shoulder discomfort, and dissatisfaction with scar.[152] Current work is being done to develop techniques of muscle-sparing harvest and harvest of the skin portion as a perforator flap to reduce postoperative morbidity.[153]

The dominant vascular pedicle of the latissimus dorsi flap, the thoracodorsal artery and vein, is located in the posterior axilla and enters the lateral deep surface of the muscle approximately 15 cm below its insertion in the humerus. The minor segmental pedicles enter the muscle in two rows in the posterior trunk between the posterior ribs and paraspinous muscle.[90]

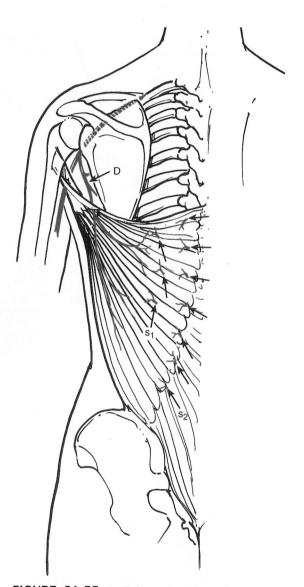

FIGURE 84-35. Latissimus dorsi musculocutaneous flap. Dominant pedicle: thoracodorsal artery (D). Secondary segmental pedicles: lateral row, branches of posterior intercostal artery and vein (s_1); medial row, branches of lumbar artery and vein (s_2). (From Mathes SJ, Nahai F: Reconstructive Surgery: Principles, Anatomy, and Technique. New York, Churchill Livingstone, 1997:566.)

The patient is placed in a lateral decubitus or prone position for flap elevation. The ipsilateral upper extremity is prepared and draped in the operative field to allow shoulder abduction during flap dissection. A beanbag or axillary roll with padding is placed on the opposite axilla to protect the dependent shoulder in the decubitus position. Similarly, protective padding is placed between the legs and feet. If flap transposition to the head, neck, or anterior thorax is planned, the beanbag is recommended. The bag is deflated and repositioned after flap elevation and donor site closure; the patient is then turned supine for completion of flap inset, often without repreparation and redraping, for breast reconstruction.

Incision around the skin island is made with a bevel away from the skin island, or a direct cutaneous linear incision is made overlying the surface of the muscle. Elevation of skin and subcutaneous tissue extends from the superficial surface of the muscle over the limits of the planned muscle dissection (generally to the posterior midline, the tip of the scapula, and 5 to 7 cm superior to the posterior superior iliac spine). This dissection to expose the superficial surface of the muscle includes elevation of skin in the posterior axilla to expose the muscle fibers of insertion.

The superior fibers of the muscle at the tip of the scapula and junction of the posterior superior latissimus muscle with the inferior trapezius muscle fibers are identified. The superior medial fibers of origin are divided, and the latissimus muscle is separated from the underlying scapula superficial to the fibers of insertion of the serratus anterior muscle. The remaining fibers of origin are divided from the vertebral column, the latissimus fibers of origin are separated from the paraspinous muscle fascia, and the lumbosacral fascia is divided to the level of the posterior axillary line.

The entire muscle is elevated toward the axilla. The minor vascular pedicles from the lumbar and posterior intercostal arteries are readily identified and divided as the flap is elevated toward its insertion. Congenital adhesions between the latissimus and serratus anterior muscles are divided to the level of the crossing branch from the thoracodorsal artery to the serratus anterior muscle. Superior elevation of the muscle exposes its deep surface in the posterior axilla. The thoracodorsal artery and vein are identified at the point of entrance into muscle. Congenital adhesions between the posterior superior latissimus and adjacent teres major muscle are then divided.

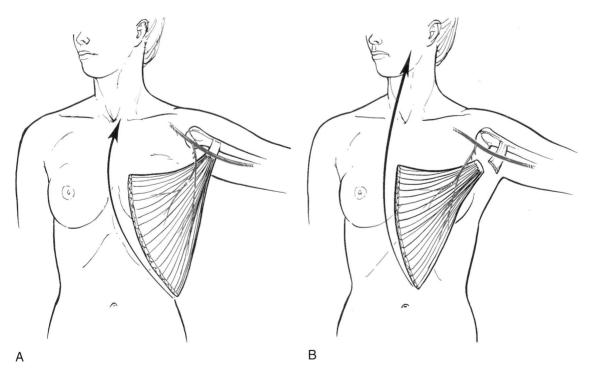

A   B

FIGURE 84-36. Latissimus dorsi musculocutaneous flap: anterior arc of rotation of standard flap. *A,* Arc to anterior thorax with insertion intact. *B,* Arc after release of muscle insertion. (From Mathes SJ, Nahai F: Reconstructive Surgery: Principles, Anatomy, and Technique. New York, Churchill Livingstone, 1997:574.)

The muscle reaches the superior abdomen and anterior chest wall through a subcutaneous tunnel superficial to the serratus anterior muscle. The latissimus muscle will reach the head and neck region through a tunnel between the chest wall and the pectoralis major fibers of insertion with the muscle coursing superficial to the lateral clavicle. The flap may also course superficial to the pectoralis major muscle (Fig. 84-37), although this position results in a reduced arc of rotation. In the face and neck, the muscle is inset with the skin island externally for midface defects or internally for the oral cavity (see Fig. 84-36). For the pharynx and esophagus, the muscle is inset with the skin island internally and partially or completely tubed as required for the esophagus. A double skin island may also be used, one island for pharyngeal or esophageal lining and a second island for face or neck coverage. Direct donor site closure is recommended because the use of skin grafts results in severe contour defects on the posterior chest wall. A skin island with a width of 5 to 7 cm will generally permit closure without excessive skin tension. Wider islands will

close directly in selected patients (Figs. 84-38 and 84-39).[90]

Omental and Jejunal Flaps

OMENTAL FLAP

The omentum is a unique tissue of the body, highly vascular and laden with bacteria-killing macrophages.[154] Because of its thin, pliable texture and vascular qualities, it serves an important role in flap selection for neck reconstruction. Intra-abdominally, it serves as a barrier and initial responder to local inflammation and infection. These functional capabilities of the omentum to provide vascular-rich, infection-resistant, pliable tissue make it extremely useful in contaminated and irradiated wounds.[154-157] The omental flap can also be modified to include a tube of gastric tissue along the greater curvature of the stomach to successfully provide both pharynx or esophageal replacement with the omental flap.[158]

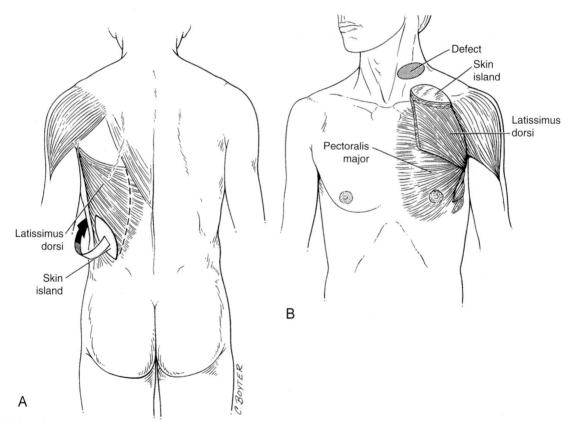

FIGURE 84-37. *A,* Latissimus dorsi skin island for head and neck reconstruction. *B,* Transposition of latissimus dorsi into neck over pectoralis major muscle. (From Mathes SJ, Nahai F: Clinical Applications for Muscle and Musculocutaneous Flaps. St. Louis, CV Mosby, 1982:208, 209.)

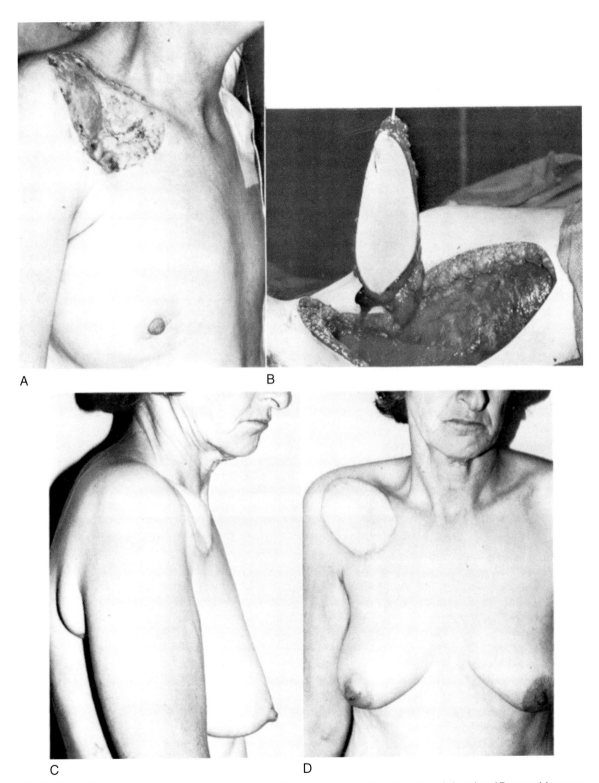

FIGURE 84-38. Latissimus dorsi musculocutaneous flap for coverage of lower neck and chest in a 45-year-old woman after chemosurgical excision of basal cell carcinoma over right clavicle. *A,* Right clavicle is exposed. *B,* The musculocutaneous flap is elevated and the pedicle is dissected. The flap is tunneled deep to the pectoralis major into the neck. *C* and *D,* Stable coverage of lower neck and chest defect is provided by latissimus dorsi musculocutaneous flap. (From Mathes SJ, Nahai F: Clinical Applications for Muscle and Musculocutaneous Flaps. St. Louis, CV Mosby, 1982:188.)

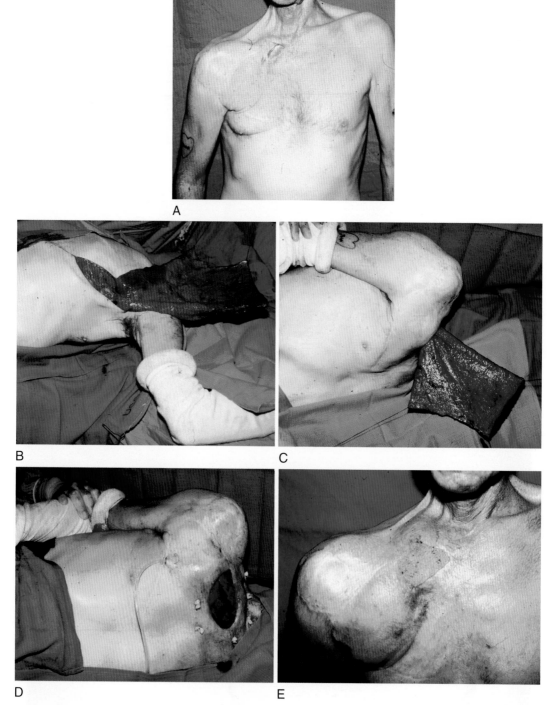

FIGURE 84-39. Latissimus dorsi musculocutaneous flap for coverage of lower neck and chest defect secondary to radiation. *A,* Exposed wound in lower neck and chest. *B,* Elevation of latissimus dorsi musculocutaneous flap. *C* and *D,* The flap is tunneled to the anterior chest and placed over the pectoralis major for coverage of the lower neck/chest wound. Wound coverage was completed with skin grafting. *E,* Patient is shown postoperatively with stable wound coverage.

The vascular pedicle for the omental flap includes the right gastroepiploic artery located within the anterior two layers of the omentum; it courses along the greater curvature of the stomach to communicate with the left gastroepiploic artery (Fig. 84-40). This pedicle rises from the gastroduodenal artery at the lower border of the pylorus of the stomach. The adjacent right gastroepiploic vein is a tributary of the superior mesenteric vein. The left gastroepiploic artery is located within the anterior two layers of the omentum and courses along the greater curvature of the stomach and joins the right gastroepiploic artery to complete a vascular arch between the two pedicles of the greater omentum. The left gastroepiploic artery arises from the splenic artery or its terminal branches at the level of the tail of the pancreas. The associated gastroepiploic vein is a tributary of the splenic vein.[90]

On entering of the peritoneal cavity through either a midline or transverse subcostal incision, the omentum is gently released from any pelvic or peritoneal adhesions and reflected over the stomach onto the region of the liver (Fig. 84-41A). This maneuver exposes the attachments of the paired posterior layers of the omentum with the transverse colon (Fig. 84-41B). The posterior omentum is released from its attachments to the colon along its antimesenteric border. Care is taken to avoid injury to the transverse mesocolon and its middle colic artery and vein.

The omentum is now returned to the inferior abdominal cavity to expose its anterior paired layer attachments to the greater curvature of the stomach. The short vascular branches extending from the gastroepiploic arch to the gastric wall along the greater curvature are divided immediately adjacent to the gastric wall to preserve a cuff of omentum with the gastroepiploic arch (Fig. 84-41C). A decision is now made about the location of the flap base on either the left or right gastroepiploic vessels. If the omentum is to be based on the right gastroepiploic artery and vein, then the left gastroepiploic artery and vein are ligated immediately distal to their junction with the splenic artery and vein adjacent to the pancreaticosplenic and gastrosplenic ligaments. The omentum is mobilized to within 3 cm of the gastric pylorus, at which point standard flap elevation is completed (Fig. 84-41D). For microvascular transplantation, the gastroepiploic artery and vein are dissected to the posterior pylorus as required for pedicle length.

If the omentum is to be based on the left gastroepiploic artery and vein, then the right gastroepiploic artery and vein are divided and ligated along the greater curvature of the stomach immediately proximal to the pylorus. The greater omentum is mobilized

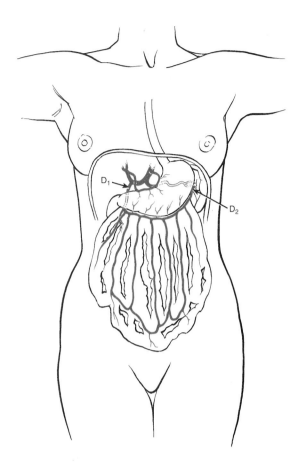

FIGURE 84-40. Omental flap. Dominant pedicles: right gastroepiploic artery and vein (D_1); left gastroepiploic artery and vein (D_2). (From Mathes SJ, Nahai F: Reconstructive Surgery: Principles, Anatomy, and Technique. New York, Churchill Livingstone, 1997:1142.)

from the greater curvature of the stomach to a point 5 to 7 cm proximal to the gastrosplenic ligament, where standard flap elevation is completed. A tunnel is required either over the costal margin or through the diaphragm to reach a neck defect. The tunnel for the omentum must be of adequate size to avoid flap compression. A tunnel size that is too large may result in a hernia defect (Fig. 84-42).

The omental flap will cover defects in the anterior neck. In general, the pectoralis muscle flap is selected, but the omental flap provides less bulk and is especially useful for coverage of the brachial plexus after neurolysis (Fig. 84-43). When regional flaps are unavailable, the omentum is an excellent option for neck coverage.

Text continued on p. 1072

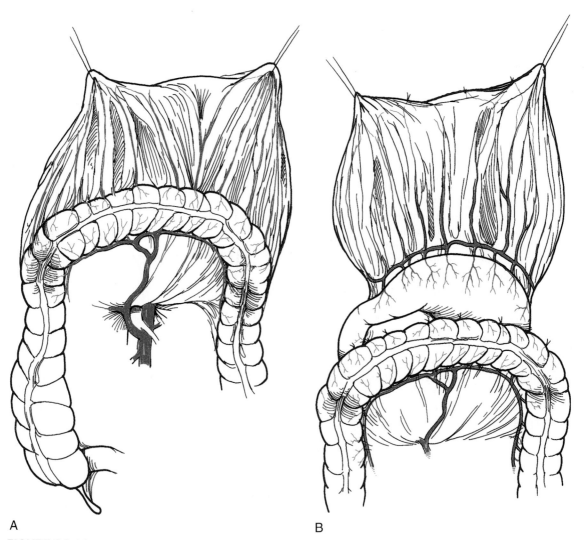

A

B

FIGURE 84-41. Omental flap elevation technique. *A,* Flap design (based on right gastroepiploic pedicle). *B,* Release of colon adhesions.

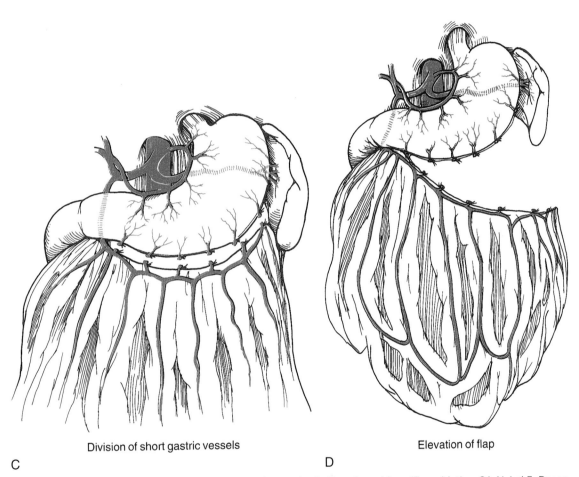

Division of short gastric vessels   Elevation of flap

C   D

FIGURE 84-41, cont'd. *C,* Division of short gastric vessels. *D,* Elevation of flap. (From Mathes SJ, Nahai F: Reconstructive Surgery: Principles, Anatomy, and Technique. New York, Churchill Livingstone, 1997:1150, 1151.)

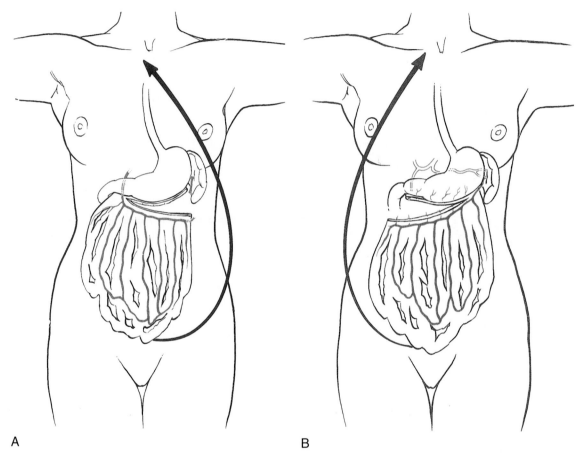

A   B

FIGURE 84-42. Omental flap: arc of rotation of standard flap. *A,* Arc to chest and mediastinum (right gastroepi-ploic-based flap). *B,* Arc to chest and mediastinum (left gastroepiploic-based flap). (From Mathes SJ, Nahai F: Reconstructive Surgery: Principles, Anatomy, and Technique. New York, Churchill Livingstone, 1997:1144, 1145.)

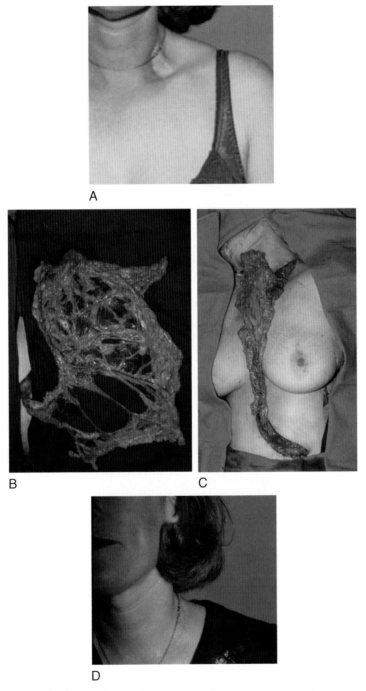

FIGURE 84-43. Omental flap for anterior neck coverage. *A,* Anterior view. The patient has undergone multiple procedures for thoracic outlet syndrome with resultant scar compression of the brachial plexus. *B,* Intraoperative view of omental flap based on right gastroepiploic artery and vein. *C,* Intraoperative view of arc of rotation of omental flap to anterior neck (omental flap will be passed through tunnel superficial to sternum). *D,* Postoperative anterior view at 6 months of flap inset after brachial plexus neurolysis.

JEJUNAL FLAP

The free jejunal microvascular transplantation has been used for many years for pharyngoesophageal reconstruction. The method represents the tissue most similar to native pharynx, with presence of intestinal smooth muscle wall, capability for peristalsis, and native mucosal lining. Inclusion of a contiguous segment of attached mesentery provides additional bulk and reliable buttress or coverage of the anastomosis and exposed great vessels. The technique is associated with much greater success and less morbidity, including fistula, than are nonintestinal origin, keratinized epithelial musculocutaneous flaps.[159] Free tissue jejunal autograft is an excellent method for pharyngeal reconstruction.[98,160] Recently, the tubed radial forearm flap is selected for pharyngeal reconstruction because the wall is more rigid, making it more suitable with the use of new valves (see "Radial Forearm Flap").

The pedicle for the jejunal flap is located within the mesentery (Fig. 84-44). The patient is placed in the supine position. Two teams work simultaneously; one team prepares the neck recipient site while the abdominal team harvests the jejunum. An upper midline incision is made, and the abdominal cavity is entered. The ligament of Treitz is identified, and a suitable segment with a single vascular arcade is selected within the first 30 to 60 cm of jejunum. The extent of bowel resection is then marked (Fig. 84-45A). A suture is often used to mark the bowel so that it can be oriented in the neck in an isoperistaltic position. With the bowel marked, the mesentery is incised from the bowel margin toward the center to expose the vascular pedicle (Fig. 84-45B). The mesentery is completely divided on each side, and usually the jejunal artery is dissected free from the surrounding tissues under loupe magnification and separated from the accompanying vein. The thin-walled jejunal veins make careful dissection in this area essential. After identification and isolation of this vascular pedicle, the bowel is divided proximally and distally. This maneuver isolates the loop of jejunum on its vascular pedicle (Fig. 84-45C). The continuity of the remaining bowel is then re-established with either staples or sutures (Fig. 84-45D). The mesentery is repaired, and the loop of jejunum is now ready for transplantation to the neck. Final vessel division is delayed until the recipient vessels in the neck are prepared. After harvest of the jejunum, the proximal portion of the jejunal pedicle is ligated, and the vessels are cut. The bowel is then transferred to the neck and placed in position, and the pedicle length is adjusted. The proximal and distal bowel anastomoses are performed before the microsurgical anastomosis. The abdominal defect is closed (Fig. 84-46).

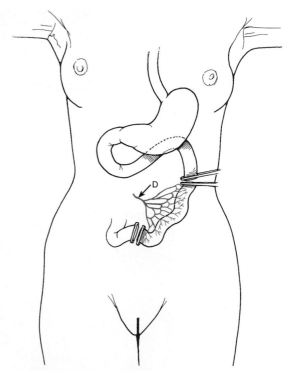

FIGURE 84-44. Jejunal flap. Dominant pedicle: jejunal artery and accompanying vein (D). (From Mathes SJ, Nahai F: Reconstructive Surgery: Principles, Anatomy, and Technique. New York, Churchill Livingstone, 1997:1128.)

Reconstruction of Specific Defects

CAROTID BLOWOUT

Earlier detection and improved diagnostic imaging modalities have resulted in treatment of head and neck cancer at an earlier stage. These advances contribute to the decline in number of patients presenting with large tumors and advanced disease. Improved treatments including radiation therapy and chemotherapy have reduced the incidence of local complications after extirpative surgery. Radical neck dissection necessitating sternocleidomastoid, jugular vein, and accessory cranial nerve XI resection has been replaced by modified radical dissection and limited neck dissection, preserving these vital structures. However, in patients with neck dissection and an irradiated field, complications such as aerodigestive-cutaneous fistulas, tracheoesophageal fistulas, and carotid blowout may require urgent surgical therapy.

Carotid blowout is a devastating sequela of neck extirpative surgery. The incidence of rupture after head and neck operations is 3% to 4%.[161,162] Risk factors associated with carotid rupture include heavily irradiated and chronically irradiated soft tissue and orocutaneous or pharyngocutaneous fistula.[163,164] Carotid rupture is associated with a high incidence of death

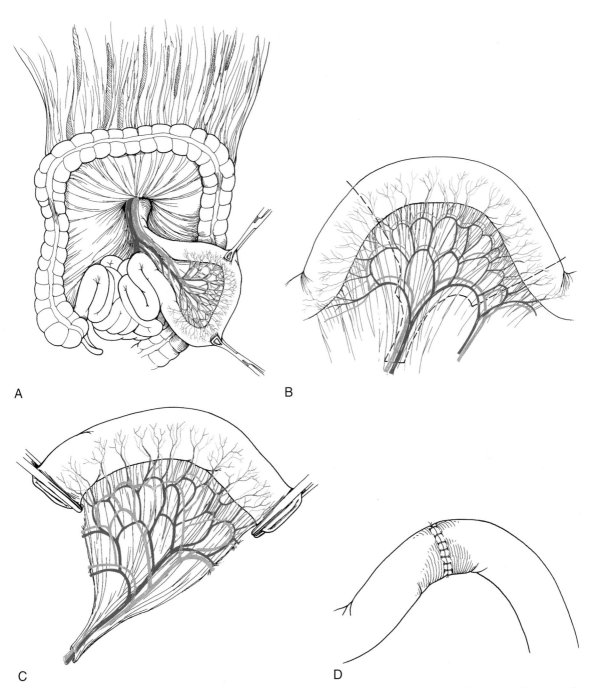

A

B

C

D

FIGURE 84-45. Jejunal flap elevation technique. *A,* Identification of proximal jejunum. *B,* Exposure of mesenteric pedicle. *C,* Jejunal flap design. *D,* Enteroenterostomy to re-establish bowel continuity. (From Mathes SJ, Nahai F: Reconstructive Surgery: Principles, Anatomy, and Technique. New York, Churchill Livingstone, 1997:1132, 1133.)

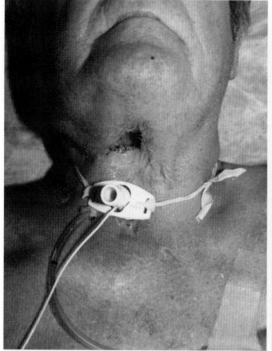

A

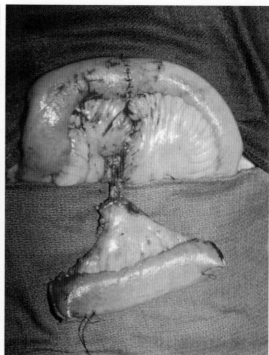

B

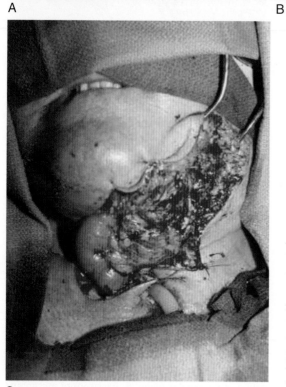

C

FIGURE 84-46. Jejunum for esophageal reconstruction. *A,* Anterior view of patient after resection of advanced laryngeal cancer. Note the submental region, pharynx, and right inferior neck-remaining cervical esophagus. *B,* Intraoperative view of segment of jejunum isolated on pedicle: branches of superior mesenteric artery and vein. Jejunojejunostomy is completed to restore jejunal continuity. Note that the extramesentery is part of transplant to be used for neck coverage. *C,* Intraoperative view. Jejunum is inserted into defect, providing alimentary continuity between the pharynx and the cervical esophagus. The extramesentery is used to provide vascularized coverage of the left lateral neck. The microanastomosis is between the jejunum's mesenteric vessels and the facial artery and vein in the left side of the neck.

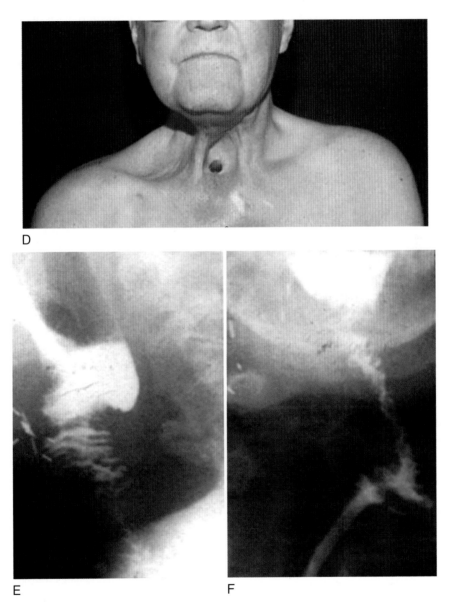

FIGURE 84-46, cont'd. *D,* Anterior view of patient 6 months after esophageal reconstruction. Note that skin grafts were placed directly on the mesenteric flap and have provided stable coverage. *E* and *F,* Radiographs of barium swallow examination confirm restoration of pharyngeal-esophageal continuity.

CAROTID RUPTURE

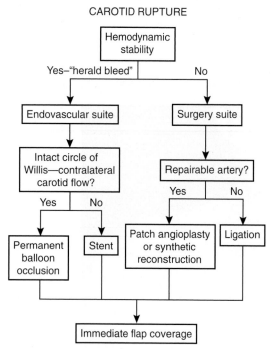

FIGURE 84-47. Algorithm for management of carotid rupture.

$(46\%)^{163}$ and neurologic morbidity (60%).[165] When carotid blowout occurs, urgent management to prevent exsanguination is required. Early carotid occlusion by ligation or endovascular balloon occlusion is sometimes required, although total occlusion is associated with 15% to 20% massive cerebral ischemia.[166] Coleman[163] advocates identification of patients at high risk and early treatment of risk factors, particularly poor wound healing, carotid artery exposure, and fistulas. Once rupture has occurred, because of skin necrosis, radiation effect, and lack of viable local tissue options, distant flap coverage concomitant with arterial treatment is generally required. After emergency vascular repair or ligation, options for muscle flap coverage include pectoralis major muscle or musculocutaneous flap, latissimus dorsi musculocutaneous flap, and trapezius musculocutaneous flap (if the trapezius muscle flap is selected, selective angiography is required to determine whether the transverse cervical artery is intact when the patient has undergone a neck dissection) (see Fig. 84-31).

Since 1995, additional techniques for emergent treatment of carotid rupture have been developed with use of endovascular techniques of balloon occlusion, selective embolization of carotid pseudoaneurysms, and endovascular stent placement.[166,167] Obviously, after control of hemorrhage with these techniques, adequate stable vessel coverage must still be obtained (Fig. 84-47).

EXPOSED CERVICAL SPINAL CORD AND OSTEOMYELITIS OF CERVICAL VERTEBRAE

Exposed cervical spine and posterior neck defects occur with complicated spinal fusions and diskectomies and are higher with the posterior surgical approach. Primary cervical osteomyelitis is uncommon, usually related to poor wound healing and exposure after posterior approach neck surgery. Exposure of the cervical spine dura, nerve roots, or proximal brachial plexus is associated with complicated wound infections and post-extirpative exposure. Treatment requires stable coverage of the defect, possibly into a deep cavity for protection of neural function (see Fig. 84-34).

REFERENCES

1. Moore KL: The Developing Human: Clinically Oriented Embryology. Philadelphia, WB Saunders, 1988.
2. Skandalakis J, Gray S: Embryology for Surgeons: The Embryological Basis for the Treatment of Congenital Anomalies. Baltimore, Williams & Wilkins, 1994.
3. Rowe M, O'Neill J Jr, Grosfeld E, et al: Essentials of Pediatric Surgery. St. Louis, Mosby, 1995.
4. Haight C, Towsley HA: Congenital atresia of the esophagus with tracheoesophageal fistula, extrapleural ligation of fistula and end-to-end anastomosis of esophageal segments. Surg Gynecol Obstet 1943;76:672.
5. Louhimo I, Lindahl H: Esophageal atresia: primary results of 500 consecutive treated patients. J Pediatr Surg 1983;18:217.
6. Vaughan VC, McKay RC: Endocrine system. In Nelson WE, McKay RJ, Vaughn VC, eds: Nelson's Textbook of Pediatrics, 10th ed. Philadelphia, WB Saunders, 1975.
7. Rossillon D, De May A, Lejour M: Pterygium colli: surgical treatment. Br J Plast Surg 1989;42:178.
8. Turner J: A syndrome of infantilism, congenital webbed neck and cubitus valgus. Endocrinology 1938;23:566.
9. Filston HC: Hemangiomas, cystic hygromas and teratomas of the head and neck. Semin Pediatr Surg 1994;3:147.
10. Cronin TD: Deformities of the cervical region. In Converse JM, ed: Reconstructive Plastic Surgery. Philadelphia, WB Saunders, 1964:1643.
11. McGregor IA: Fundamental Techniques of Plastic Surgery, 6th ed. New York, Churchill Livingstone, 1976.
12. Menick FF, Furnas DW, Achauer BM: Lateral cervical advancement flaps for the correction of webbed-neck deformity. Plast Reconstr Surg 1984;73:223.
13. Shearin JC Jr, DeFranzo AJ: Butterfly correction of webbed-neck deformity in Turner's syndrome. Plast Reconstr Surg 1980;66:129.
14. Agris J, Dingman RO, Varon J: Correction of webbed neck defects. Ann Plast Surg 1983;11:299.
15. Ostlie DJ, Burjonrappa SC, Snyder CL, et al: Thyroglossal duct infections and surgical outcomes. J Pediatr Surg 2004;39:396.
16. Telander RL, Deane SA: Thyroglossal and branchial cleft cysts and sinuses. Surg Clin North Am 1977;57:779.
17. Sistrunk W: Techniques of removal of cysts and sinuses of the thyroglossal duct. Surg Gynecol Obstet 1928;46:109.
18. Guarisco J: Congenital head and neck masses in infants and children. Ear Nose Throat J 1991;70:75.
19. Kennedy T, Whitaker M, Pellitteri P, et al: Cystic hygroma/lymphangioma: a rational approach to management. Laryngoscope 2001;111:1929.
20. Hancock BJ, St.-Vil D, Luks FL, et al: Complications of lymphangiomas in children. J Pediatr Surg 1992;27:220.

21. Orford J, Barker A, Thonell S, et al: Bleomycin therapy for cystic hygroma. J Pediatr Surg 1995;30:1282.

22. Ravitch M, Rush B: Cystic hygroma. In Ashcraft K, Holder TM, eds: Pediatric Surgery. Philadelphia, WB Saunders, 1993.

23. Ogita S, Tsuto T, Nakamura K, et al: OK-432 therapy for lymphangioma in children: why and how does it work? J Pediatr Surg 1996;31:477.

24. Ng J: Letter to the editor. J Pediatr Surg 1996;31:1463.

25. Greinwald JH, Burke DK, Sato Y, et al: Treatment of lymphangiomas in children: an update of Picibanil (OK-432) sclerotherapy. Otolaryngol Head Neck Surg 1999;121:381.

26. McMurray J: Personal communication, 2004.

27. Wolfort FG, Kanter MA, Miller LB: Torticollis. Plast Reconstr Surg 1989;84:682.

28. Davids JR, Wenger DR, Mubarak SJ: Congenital muscular torticollis: sequela of intrauterine or perinatal compartment syndrome. J Pediatr Orthop 1993;13:141.

29. Minamitani K, Inoue A, Okuno T: Results of surgical treatment of muscular torticollis for patients greater than 6 years of age. J Pediatr Orthop 1990;10:754.

30. Tse P, Cheng J, Chow Y, et al: Surgery for neglected congenital torticollis Acta Orthop Scand 1987;58:270.

31. Cheng JC, Au AW: Infantile torticollis; a review of 624 cases. J Pediatr Orthop 1994;14:802.

32. Armstrong D, Pickrell K, Fetter B, et al: Torticollis: an analysis of 271 cases. Plast Reconstr Surg 1965;35:14.

33. Burstein FD: Long-term experience with endoscopic surgical treatment for congenital muscular torticollis in infants and children: a review of 85 cases. Plast Reconstr Surg 2004;114:491.

34. Burstein FD, Cohen SR: Endoscopic surgical treatment for congenital muscular torticollis. Plast Reconstr Surg 1998;101:20.

35. Ling CM: The influence of age on the results of open sternomastoid tenotomy in muscular torticollis. Clin Orthop 1976;116:142.

36. Ferguson JW: Surgical correction of the facial deformities secondary to untreated muscular torticollis. J Craniomaxillofac Surg 1993;21:137.

37. Cohen-Gadol AA, Ahlskog JE, Matsumoto JY, et al: Selective peripheral denervation for the treatment of intractable spasmodic torticollis: experience with 168 patients at the Mayo Clinic. J Neurosurg 2003;98:1247.

38. Fricke NB, Omnell ML, Dutcher KA, et al: Skeletal and dental disturbances in children after facial burns and pressure garment use: a 4-year follow-up. J Burn Care Rehabil 1999;20:239.

39. Jonsson CE, Dalsgaard CJ: Early excision and skin grafting of selected burns of the face and neck. Plast Reconstr Surg 1991;88:83.

40. Cole JK, Engrav LH, Heimbach DM, et al: Early excision and grafting of face and neck burns in patients over 20 years. Plast Reconstr Surg 2002;109:1266.

41. Iwuagwu FC, Wilson D, Bailie F: The use of skin grafts in postburn contracture release: a 10-year review. Plast Reconstr Surg 1999;103:1198.

42. Kraemer MD, Jones T, Deitch EA: Burn contractures: incidence, predisposing factors, and results of surgical therapy. J Burn Care Rehabil 1988;9:261.

43. So K, Umraw N, Scott J, et al: Effects of enhanced patient education on compliance with silicone gel sheeting and burn scar outcome: a randomized prospective study. J Burn Care Rehab 2003;24:411, discussion 410.

44. Roques C: Massage applied to scars. Wound Repair Regen 2002;10:126.

45. Musgrave MA, Umraw N, Fish JS, et al: The effect of silicone gel sheets on perfusion of hypertrophic burn scars. J Burn Care Rehabil 2002;23:208.

46. Mustoe TA, Cooter RD, Gold MH, et al, International Advisory Panel on Scar Management: International clinical recommendations on scar management. Plast Reconstr Surg 2002;110:560.

47. Staley MJ, Richard RL: Use of pressure to treat hypertrophic burn scars. Adv Wound Care 1997;10:44.

48. Ward RS: Pressure therapy for the control of hypertrophic scar formation after burn injury: a history and review. J Burn Care Rehabil 1991;12:257.

49. Linares HA: From wound to scar. Burns 1996;22:339.

50. Rayner K: The use of pressure therapy to treat hypertrophic scarring. J Wound Care 2000;9:151.

51. Johnson J, Greenspan B, Gorga D, et al: Compliance with pressure garment use in burn rehabilitation. J Burn Care Rehabil 1994;15:180.

52. Chang P, Laubenthal KN, Lewis RW II, et al: Prospective, randomized study of the efficacy of pressure garment therapy in patients with burns. J Burn Care Rehabil 1995;16:473.

53. Uzunismail A, Iccen D: Long-term effect of postburn neck contractures on mandibular growth. Plast Reconstr Surg 1997;99:918.

54. Katsaros J, David DJ, Griffin PA, Moore MH: Facial dysmorphology in the neglected paediatric head and neck burn. Br J Plast Surg 1990;43:232.

55. Argenta LC, Watanabe MJ, Grabb WC: The use of tissue expansion in head and neck reconstruction. Ann Plast Surg 1983;11:31.

56. Spence R: Experience with novel uses of tissue expanders in burn reconstruction of the face and neck. Ann Plast Surg 1992;28:453.

57. Cherry GW, Austad ED, Pasky K, et al: Increased survival and vascularity of random pattern skin flaps elevated in controlled, expanded skin. Plast Reconstr Surg 1983;72:680.

58. Baker SR, Swanson NA: Clinical applications of tissue expansion in head and neck surgery. Laryngoscope 1990;100:313.

59. MacLennan SE, Corcoran J, Neale HW: Tissue expansion in head and neck burn reconstruction. Clin Plast Surg 2000;27:121.

60. LoGiudice J, Gosain AK: Pediatric tissue expansion: indications and complications. J Craniofac Surg 2003;14:866.

61. Takei T, Mills I, Katsuyuki A, et al: Molecular basis for tissue expansion: clinical implications for the surgeon. Plast Reconstr Surg 1998;101:247.

62. Bauer BS, Vicari F, Richard ME, et al: Expanded full-thickness skin grafts in children: case selection, planning, and management. Plast Reconstr Surg 1993;92:59.

63. Karacaoglan N, Uysal A: Reconstruction of postburn scar contracture of the neck by expanded skin flaps. Burns 1994;20:547.

64. Antonyshyn O, Gruss JS, Zuker R, Mackinnon SE: Tissue expansion in head and neck reconstruction. Plast Reconstr Surg 1988;82:58.

65. Manders EK, Schenden MJ, Furrey JA, et al: Soft-tissue expansion: concepts and complications. Plast Reconstr Surg 1984;74:493.

66. Hudson DA, Lazarus D, Silfen R: The use of serial tissue expansion in pediatric plastic surgery. Ann Plast Surg 2000;45:589.

67. Ertas NM, Bozdogan N, Erbas O, et al: The use of subcutaneous pedicle rhomboid flap in the treatment of postburn scar contractures. Ann Plast Surg 2004;53:235.

68. Daw JL Jr, Patel PK: Double-opposing Z-plasty for correction of midline cervical web. J Craniofac Surg 2003;14:774.

69. Hikade KR, Bitar GJ, Edgerton MT, Morgan RF: Modified Z-plasty repair of webbed neck deformity seen in Turner and Klippel-Feil syndrome. Cleft Palate Craniofac J 2002;39:261.

70. Taylor GI, Palmer JH: The vascular territories (angiosomes) of the body: experimental study and clinical applications. Br J Plast Surg 1987;40:113.

71. Ogawa R, Hyakusoku H, Murakami M, Gao JH: Clinical and basic research on occipito-cervico-dorsal flaps: including a study of the anatomical territories of dorsal trunk vessels. Plast Reconstr Surg 2004;113:1923.

72. Schuller D: Cervical skin flaps in head and neck reconstruction. Am J Otolaryngol 1981;2:62.

73. Floyd DC, Ali FS, Ilyas S, Brough MD: The pedicled occipital artery scalp flap for salvage surgery of the neck. Br J Plast Surg 2003;56:471.

74. Matloub JS, Yousif JN, Ye A, Sanger JR: The occipital artery flap for transfer of hair-bearing tissue. Ann Plast Surg 1992;29:491.

75. Tolhurst D, Carstens M, Greco R, Hurwitz D: The surgical anatomy of the scalp. Plast Reconstr Surg 1991;87:603.

76. Faltaous AA, Yetman RJ: The submental artery flap: an anatomic study. Plast Reconstr Surg 1996;97:56.

77. Martin D, Pascal JF, Baudet J, et al: The submental island flap: a new donor site. Anatomy and clinical applications as a free or pedicled flap. Plast Reconstr Surg 1993;92:867.

78. Curran AJ, Neligan P, Gullane PJ: Submental artery island flap. Laryngoscope 1997;107:1545.

79. Sterne GD, Januszkiewicz JS, Hall PN, Bardsley AF: The submental island flap. Br J Plast Surg 1996;49:85.

80. Vural E, Suen JY: The submental island flap in head and neck reconstruction. Head Neck 2000;22:572.

81. Janssen DA, Thimsen DA: The extended submental island lip flap: an alternative for esophageal repair. Plast Reconstr Surg 1998;102:835.

82. Wu Y, Tang P, Qi Y, Xu A: Submental island flap for head and neck reconstruction: a review of 20 cases. Asian J Surg 1998; 21:247.

83. McCraw J, Dibbell D, Carraway J: Clinical definition of independent myocutaneous vascular territories. Plast Reconstr Surg 1977;60:341.

84. Netterville J, Woo D: The lower trapezius flap; vascular anatomy and surgical technique. Arch Otolaryngol Head Neck Surg 1991;117:73.

85. Angrigiani C, Grilli D, Karanas YL, et al: The dorsal scapular island flap: an alternative for head, neck, and chest reconstruction. Plast Reconstr Surg 2003;111:67.

86. Tan KC, Tan BK: Extended lower trapezius island myocutaneous flap: a fasciomyocutaneous flap based on the dorsal scapular artery. Plast Reconstr Surg 2000;105:1758.

87. Bakamjian VY: A two-stage method for pharyngoesophageal reconstruction with a primary pectoral skin flap. Plast Reconstr Surg 1965;36:173.

88. Bunkis J, Mulliken JB, Upton J, Murray JE: The evolution of techniques for reconstruction of full-thickness cheek defects. Plast Reconstr Surg 1982;70:319.

89. Mazzola RF, Sambataro G, Oldini C: Our experience with pharyngoesophageal reconstruction. Ann Plast Surg 1979; 2:219.

90. Mathes SJ, Nahai F: Reconstructive Surgery: Principles, Anatomy, and Technique. New York, QMP/Churchill Livingstone, 1997.

91. Eckardt A, Fokas K: Microsurgical reconstruction in the head and neck region: an 18-year experience with 500 consecutive cases. J Craniomaxillofac Surg 2003;31:197.

92. Berger A, Bargmann HJ: Aesthetic aspects in reconstructive microsurgery. Aesthetic Plast Surg 1989;13:115.

93. Ichinose A, Tahara S, Yokoo S, et al: Fail-safe drainage procedure in free radial forearm flap transfer. J Reconstr Microsurg 2003;19:371.

94. Chicarilli ZN, Ariyan S, Cuono CB: Free radial forearm flap versatility for the head and neck and lower extremity. J Reconstr Microsurg 1986;2:221.

95. Dubner S, Heller KS: Reinnervated radial forearm free flaps in head and neck reconstruction. J Reconstr Microsurg 1992;8:467, discussion 469.

96. Weinzweig N, Davies BW: Foot and ankle reconstruction using the radial forearm flap: a review of 25 cases. Plast Reconstr Surg 1998;102:1999.

97. Anthony JP, Singer MI, Mathes SJ: Pharyngoesophageal reconstruction using the tubed free radial forearm flap. Clin Plast Surg 1994;21:137.

98. Carlson GW, Temple JR, Codner MA: Reconstruction of the pharynx and overlying soft tissue by a partitioned free jejunal flap. Plast Reconstr Surg 1996;97:460.

99. Disa JJ, Pusic AL, Hidalgo DA, Cordeiro PG: Microvascular reconstruction of the hypopharynx: defect classification, treatment algorithm, and functional outcome based on 165 consecutive cases. Plast Reconstr Surg 2003;111:652, discussion 661.

100. Shestak KC, Myers EN, Ramasastry SS, et al: Microvascular free tissue transfer for reconstruction of head and neck cancer defects. Oncology (Huntingt) 1992;6:101, discussion 110, 115, 121.

101. Gurtner G, Evans G: Advances in head and neck reconstruction. Plast Reconstr Surg 2000;106:672.

102. Colen SR, Baker DC, Shaw WW: Microvascular flap reconstruction of the head and neck. An overview. Clin Plast Surg 1983;10:73.

103. Song YG, Chen GZ, Song YL: The free thigh flap: a new free flap concept based on the septocutaneous artery. Plast Reconstr Surg 1984;37:149.

104. Lin DT, Coppit GL, Burkey BB: Use of the anterolateral thigh flap for reconstruction of the head and neck. Curr Opin Otolaryngol Head Neck Surg 2004;12:300.

105. Makitie AA, Beasley NJ, Neligan PC, et al: Head and neck reconstruction with anterolateral thigh flap. Otolaryngol Head Neck Surg 2003;129:547.

106. Hsieh CH, Yang CC, Kuo YR, et al: Free anterolateral thigh adipofascial perforator flap. Plast Reconstr Surg 2003;112:976.

107. Chen HC, Tang YB: Anterolateral thigh flap: an ideal soft tissue flap. Clin Plast Surg 2003;30:383.

108. Koshima I, Fukuda H, Yamamoto H, et al: Free anterolateral thigh flaps for reconstruction of head and neck defects. Plast Reconstr Surg 1993;92:421.

109. Tsukino A, Kurachi K, Inamiya T, Tanigaki T: Preoperative color Doppler assessment in planning of anterolateral thigh flaps. Plast Reconstr Surg 2004;113:241.

110. Nakayama B, Hyodo I, Hasegawa Y, et al: Role of the anterolateral thigh flap in head and neck reconstruction: advantages of moderate skin and subcutaneous thickness. J Reconstr Microsurg 2002;18:141.

111. Chana JS, Wei FC: A review of the advantages of the anterolateral thigh flap in head and neck reconstruction. Br J Plast Surg 2004;57:603.

112. Ozkan O, Coskunfirat OK, Ozgentas HE: An ideal and versatile material for soft-tissue coverage: experiences with most modifications of the anterolateral thigh flap. J Reconstr Microsurg 2004;20:377.

113. Kimura N, Satoh K, Hasumi T, Ostuka T: Clinical application of the free thin anterolateral thigh flap in 31 consecutive patients. Plast Reconstr Surg 2001;108:1193.

114. Koshima I, Nanba Y, Tsutsui T, et al: Free perforator flap for the treatment of defects after resection of huge arteriovenous malformations in the head and neck regions. Ann Plast Surg 2003;51:194.

115. Koshima I, Yamamoto H, Moriguchi T, Yozo O: Extended anterior thigh flaps for repair of massive cervical defects involving pharyngoesophagus and skin: an introduction to the "mosaic" flap principle. Ann Plast Surg 1994;32:321.

116. Hallock GG: The preexpanded anterolateral thigh free flap. Ann Plast Surg 2004;53:170.

117. Tsai FC: A new method: perforator-based tissue expansion for a preexpanded free cutaneous perforator flap. Burns 2003; 29:845.

118. Katsaros J, Schusterman M, Beppu M, et al: The lateral upper arm flap: anatomy and clinical applications. Ann Plast Surg 1984;12:489.

119. Kuek LB, Chuan TL: The extended lateral arm flap: a new modification. J Reconstr Microsurg 1991;7:167.

120. Ninkovic M, Harpf C, Schwabegger AH, et al: The lateral arm flap. Clin Plast Surg 2001;28:367.

121. Nahabedian MY, Deune EG, Manson PN: Utility of the lateral arm flap in head and neck reconstruction. Ann Plast Surg 2001;46:501.

122. Civantos FJ Jr, Burkey B, Lu FL, Armstrong W: Lateral arm microvascular flap in head and neck reconstruction. Arch Otolaryngol Head Neck Surg 1997;123:830.

123. Sullivan MJ, Carroll WR, Kuriloff DB: Lateral arm free flap in head and neck reconstruction. Arch Otolaryngol Head Neck Surg 1992;118:1095.

124. Hurwitz DJ, Rabson JA., Futrell JW: The anatomic basis for the platysma skin flap. Plast Reconstr Surg 1983;72:302.

125. Coleman JJ III, Jurkiewicz MJ, Nahai F, Mathes SJ: The platysma musculocutaneous flap. Plast Reconstr Surg 1983;72:315.

126. Futrell JW, Johns ME, Edgerton MT, et al: Platysma myocutaneous flap for intraoral reconstruction. Am J Surg 1978; 136:504.

127. Posnick JC, McCraw JB: Useful arterialized flaps for head and neck reconstruction. Ann Plast Surg 1987;19:359.

128. Zimman OA: Reconstruction of the neck with two rotation-advancement platysma myocutaneous flaps. Plast Reconstr Surg 1999;103:1712.

129. Zimman OA, Sokolowicz DG: Secondary pharyngeal reconstruction after pharyngolaryngectomy using two platysma myocutaneous flaps. Eur J Plast Surg 1989;12:237.

130. Ariyan S: The transverse platysma myocutaneous flap for head and neck reconstruction: an update. Plast Reconstr Surg 2003;111:378.

131. Fine NA, Pribaz JJ, Orgill DP: Use of the innervated platysma flap in facial reanimation. Ann Plast Surg 1995;34:326.

132. Coleman JJ III, Nahai F, Mathes SJ: Platysma musculocutaneous flap: clinical and anatomic considerations in head and neck reconstruction. Am J Surg 1982;144:477.

133. Ariyan S: The sternocleidomastoid myocutaneous flap. Laryngoscope 1980;90:676.

134. Larson DL, Goepfert H: Limitations of the sternocleidomastoid musculocutaneous flap in head and neck cancer reconstruction. Plast Reconstr Surg 1982;70:328.

135. Russell R, Feller A, Elliott LF, et al: The extended pectoralis major myocutaneous flap: uses and indications. Plast Reconstr Surg 1991;88:814.

136. Ariyan S: Further experiences with the pectoralis major myocutaneous flap for the immediate repair of defects from excision of head and neck cancers. Plast Reconstr Surg 1979;64:605.

137. Ariyan S: The pectoralis major myocutaneous flap. Plast Reconstr Surg 1979;63:73.

138. Magee WP, McCraw JB, Horton CE, McInnis W: Pectoralis "paddle" myocutaneous flaps: the workhorse of head and neck reconstruction. Am J Surg 1980;140:507.

139. Kroll SS, Reece GP, Miller MJ, Schusterman MA: Comparison of the rectus abdominis free flap with the pectoralis major myocutaneous flap for reconstructions in the head and neck. Am J Surg 1992;164:615.

140. Kroll SS, Goepfert J, Jones M, et al: Analysis of complications in 168 pectoralis major myocutaneous flaps used for head and neck reconstruction. Ann Plast Surg 1990;25:93.

141. Huang RD, Silver SM, Hussain A, et al: Pectoralis major myocutaneous flap: analysis of complications in a VA population. Head Neck 1992;14:102.

142. Baek SM, Lawson W, Biller HF: An analysis of 133 pectoralis major myocutaneous flaps. Plast Reconstr Surg 1982;69: 460.

143. Liu R, Gullane P, Brown D, Irish J: Pectoralis major myocutaneous pedicled flap in head and neck reconstruction: retrospective review of indications and results in 244 consecutive cases at the Toronto General Hospital. J Otolaryngol 2001;30:34.

144. Rosen HM: The extended trapezius musculocutaneous flap for cranio-orbital facial reconstruction. Plast Reconstr Surg 1985;75:318.

145. Demergasso F, Piazza MV: Trapezius myocutaneous flap in the reconstructive surgery for head and neck cancer. Am J Surg 1979;138:533.

146. Mathes SJ, Stevenson TR: Reconstruction of posterior neck and skull with vertical trapezius musculocutaneous flap. Am J Surg 1988;156:248.

147. Mathes SJ, Nahai F: Clinical Atlas of Muscle and Musculocutaneous Flaps. St. Louis, Mosby, 1979.

148. Panje W: Myocutaneous trapezius flap. Head Neck Surg 1980;2:206.

149. Papadopoulos O, Tsakoniatis N, Georgiou P, Christopoulos A: Head and neck soft-tissue reconstruction using the vertical trapezius musculocutaneous flap. Ann Plast Surg 1999;42: 457.

150. Ugurlu K, Ozcelik D, Huthut I, et al: Extended vertical trapezius myocutaneous flap in head and neck reconstruction as a salvage procedure. Plast Reconstr Surg 2004;114:339.

151. Rios JL, Pollock T, Adams WP Jr: Progressive tension sutures to prevent seroma formation after latissimus dorsi harvest. Plast Reconstr Surg 2003;112:1779.

152. Adams WP, Lipschitz AH, Ansari M, et al: Functional donor site morbidity following latissimus dorsi muscle flap transfer. Ann Plast Surg 2004;53:6.

153. Schwabegger A, Harpf C, Rainer C: Muscle-sparing latissimus dorsi myocutaneous flap with maintenance of muscle innervation, function and aesthetic appearance of the donor site. Plast Reconstr Surg 2003;111:1407.

154. Jurkiewicz MJ, Nahai F: The omentum: its use as a free vascularized graft for reconstruction of the head and neck. Ann Surg 1982;195:756.

155. Arnold PG, Irons GB: The greater omentum: extensions in transposition and free transfer. Plast Reconstr Surg 1981; 67:169.

156. Freeman JL, Brondbo K, Osborne M, et al: Greater omentum used for carotid cover after pharyngolaryngoesophagectomy and gastric "pull-up" or colonic "swing." Arch Otolaryngol 1982;108:685.

157. Losken A, Carlson GW, Culbertson JH, et al: Omental free flap reconstruction in complex head and neck deformities. Head Neck 2002;24:326.

158. Mixter RC, Rao VK, Katsaros J, et al: Simultaneous reconstruction of cervical soft tissue and esophagus with a gastro-omental free flap. Plast Reconstr Surg 1990;86:905.

159. Coleman JJ 3rd: Reconstruction of the pharynx after resection for cancer. A comparison of methods. Ann Surg 1989; 209:554, discussion 561.

160. Nahai F, Stahl RS, Hester TR, Clairmont AA: Advanced applications of revascularized free jejunal flaps for difficult wounds of the head and neck. Plast Reconstr Surg 1984; 74:778.

161. Heller KS, Strong EW: Carotid arterial hemorrhage after radical head and neck surgery. Am J Surg 1979;138:607.

162. Morrissey DD, Andersen PE, Nesbit GM, et al: Endovascular management of hemorrhage in patients with head and neck cancer. Arch Otolaryngol Head Neck Surg 1997;123:15.

163. Coleman JJ 3rd: Treatment of the ruptured or exposed carotid artery: a rational approach. South Med J 1985; 78:262.

164. Thawley SE: Complications of combined radiation therapy and surgery for carcinoma of the larynx and inferior hypopharynx. Laryngoscope 1981;91:677.
165. Chaloupka JC, Putman CM, Citardi MJ, et al: Endovascular therapy for the carotid blowout syndrome in head and neck surgical patients: diagnostic and managerial considerations. Am J Neuroradiol 1996;17:843.
166. Lesley WS, Chaloupka JC, Weigele JB, et al: Preliminary experience with endovascular reconstruction for the management of carotid blowout syndrome. AJNR Am J Neuroradiol 2003;24:975.
167. Warren FM, Cohen JI, Nesbit GM, et al: Management of carotid "blowout" with endovascular stent grafts. Laryngoscope 2002;112:428.

◆ Index

Note: **Boldface** *roman numerals indicate volume. Page numbers followed by f refer to figures; page numbers followed by t refer to tables.*

A

Abbe flap
  for cleft lip, **IV**:346, 348f, 349f
  for upper eyelid reconstruction, **V**:364-365, 366f
  for upper lip reconstruction, **III**:812-813, 813f-818f, **V**:381-383, 382f
Abbe-McIndoe procedure, **VI**:1282-1285, 1282f-1285f
ABBI system, **VI**:640-641
Abdomen. *See also* Abdominal wall.
  aesthetic proportions of, **VI**:119, 120f, 126, 362, 363f
  gunshot injury to, **I**:926, 926f, 1006, 1007f
  liposuction for, **VI**:96, 97, 110, 115, 227-230, 227f, 229f-230f, 278-279
Abdominal compartment syndrome, **I**:818, 1006
Abdominal wall. *See also* Abdominoplasty.
  acquired defects of, **I**:1006, 1007f, **VI**:1179, 1193. *See also* Abdominal wall reconstruction.
  after TRAM flap breast reconstruction, **VI**:843, 847, 859, 862, 865, 994-995
  anatomy of, **VI**:88-92, 90f, 91f, 1175-1179, 1176f, 1177f
  anterior-anterolateral, **VI**:1175-1178, 1176f, 1177f
  blood supply of, **VI**:371, 371f
  congenital defects of, **VI**:93
  contour deformity of, **VI**:120
  embryology of, **VI**:87-88, 89f
  fat accumulation in, **VI**:92-93, 92f, 93f
  layers of, **VI**:89
  lymphatic drainage of, **VI**:91
  muscles of, **VI**:89-91, 90f
  nerves of, **VI**:91-92, 1178
  pathology of, **VI**:92-93, 92f, 93f
  pinch test for, **VI**:122-123, 123f
  post-bariatric surgery, **VI**:120
  posterior-posterolateral, **VI**:1178-1179
  postpartum deformity of, **VI**:120
  tissue expansion in, **I**:563
  trauma-related defects of, **I**:1006, 1007f, **VI**:1179, 1193
  tumors of, **VI**:93
  vascular anatomy of, **VI**:91, 91f, 1178
Abdominal wall reconstruction, **I**:1006, 1007f, **VI**:1175-1194
  aesthetic considerations in, **VI**:1181
  algorithm for, **VI**:1192-1193
  anatomy for, **VI**:1175-1179, 1176f, 1177f
  anterior rectus abdominis fasciocutaneous flap for, **VI**:1185

Abdominal wall reconstruction
  (Continued)
  anterolateral thigh flap for, **VI**:1187-1191, 1190f
  bilateral rectus abdominis-internal oblique musculocutaneous flaps for, **I**:985, 989f
  care after, **VI**:1192
  cicatricial adhesion and, **VI**:1181
  closure techniques for, **VI**:1181-1183, 1181t, 1182f
  external oblique flap for, **I**:446-447, 447t, **VI**:1187, 1187f
  fascial grafts for, **I**:585, 586f, **VI**:1183-1184
  flaps for, **I**:446-448, 447f, 447t, **VI**:1181t, 1185-1192
    distant, **I**:447-448, **VI**:1187-1192, 1188f-1190f
    local, **I**:446-447, **VI**:1185-1187, 1186f, 1187f
  functional, **VI**:1180-1181
  gracilis flap for, **VI**:1192
  iliolumbar flap for, **VI**:1185
  infection and, **VI**:1180
  latissimus dorsi flap for, **I**:447, 447t, 448f, **VI**:1191-1192
  layered closure technique for, **VI**:1183
  local flaps for, **VI**:1185-1187, 1186f, 1187f
  mesh repair for, **I**:985, 988f, 1006, 1007f, **VI**:1184
  microvascular tissue transplantation for, **I**:448, **VI**:1187-1192, 1189f-1190f
  patient evaluation for, **VI**:1192-1193
  patient preparation for, **VI**:1193
  pedicled tensor fascia lata flap for, **VI**:1188, 1188f
  polyglactin 910 mesh for, **VI**:1184
  polyglycolic acid mesh for, **VI**:1184
  polypropylene mesh for, **VI**:1184
  polytetrafluoroethylene patch for, **VI**:1184
  prosthetic materials for, **VI**:1184-1185, 1185f
  rectus abdominis flap for, **I**:446-447, 447t, **VI**:1185, 1186f
  rectus femoris flap for, **I**:447-448, 450f, **VI**:1191
  relaxing incision technique for, **VI**:1182-1183, 1182f
  results of, **VI**:1192, 1192t
  sensory function and, **VI**:1181
  skin grafts for, **I**:985, 986f, **VI**:1183
  static, **VI**:1180

Abdominal wall reconstruction
  (Continued)
  tensor fascia lata flap for, **I**:380-381, 380f-381f, 447, 447t, 449f, 585, 586f, 985, 987f, **VI**:1188-1191, 1188f-1190f
  timing of, **VI**:1179, 1179t
  tissue expansion for, **VI**:1183
  zones for, **I**:446, 447f, 447t
Abdominoplasty, **VI**:87-116, 119-202
  adipose excess after, **VI**:376
  aesthetic considerations in, **VI**:126, 126f, 362, 363f
  anatomic considerations in, **VI**:124-126, 125f, 126f
  anesthesia for, **VI**:114-115
  arterial supply in, **VI**:125-126, 126f
  Baroudi, **VI**:146-153
    closure in, **VI**:152, 153f
    dressings in, **VI**:152
    excess skin resection in, **VI**:148-149, 149f
    fascial plication in, **VI**:148, 148f
    incision for, **VI**:147-148
    markings for, **VI**:146-147, 146f
    sutures in, **VI**:152
    umbilicoplasty in, **VI**:149-152, 150f
    umbilicus in, **VI**:147, 147f
  bony framework in, **VI**:122
  care after, **VI**:115, 145-146
  cigarette smoking and, **VI**:174-175, 364, 371
  classification of, **VI**:126-134, 127t, 130f-135f
  complications of, **VI**:115-116, 174-180, 362-378, 365f-378f. *See also* Abdominoplasty, secondary.
    prevention of, **VI**:378-379
  compression garments after, **VI**:115, 115f
  contraindications to, **VI**:116
  dietary supplements and, **VI**:175
  dog-ears after, **VI**:363, 365f, 366f
  edema after, **VI**:375-376
  embolism after, **VI**:115
  endoscopic, **I**:1047, **VI**:110, 165, 167
  enterocutaneous fistula after, **VI**:115-116
  fascial management in, **VI**:108-110, 109f-113f
  fascial plication in, **VI**:137, 139f, 139t, 140
  fat excision in, **VI**:140
  flap contour deficiency after, **VI**:375-376
  flap undermining in, **VI**:137, 138f
  goals of, **VI**:122
  hemorrhage and, **VI**:178-179, 372, 379
  hernia after, **VI**:377, 378

i

Abdominoplasty *(Continued)*
  historical perspective on, VI:87, 88f, 119-120, 121f
  in diastasis recti, VI:92-93, 94f, 95f, 110
  in hernia repair, VI:110, 111f-113f
  in weight-loss patient, VI:167-171, 169f, 170f
  incision for, VI:134-136, 134f-136f, 140, 142f
  indications for, VI:122
  informed consent for, VI:124
  ischemia and, VI:178
  lateral tension, Color Plate VI:125-3, VI:154-155, 154f-156f, 259, 260-262, 261f-263f
    indications for, VI:261
    markings for, VI:154, 154f
    technique of, VI:261-262, 264f, 371, 371f
  laxity after, VI:376-377, 377f, 378f
  lipectomy with, VI:101, 101f, 171-172, 172f, 173f, 376
  liposuction with, VI:96, 97, 98f, 101, 110, 115, 140, 141f
  male, VI:104, 104f-105f
  markings for, VI:140
  medical malpractice suits and, I:144
  mini-, VI:96, 96f, 158-165, 158f-164f
    Baroudi, VI:158, 160f
    extended, VI:158-159, 161f-164f
  modern, VI:97-101, 98f-100f
  modified, VI:96, 96f, 109f
  monsplasty with, VI:174
  muscle plication in, VI:376-377, 378f
  musculofascial deformity classification in, VI:137, 139f, 139t, 140
  musculofascial system evaluation in, VI:123-124, 125, 125f
  nerve injury after, VI:180, 181f, 372, 375
  obesity and, VI:175, 175t
  panniculectomy in, VI:101-104, 102f-104f
  patient classification for, VI:93, 94f, 95f
  patient evaluation for, VI:122-124, 123f
  patient position for, VI:140
  patient selection for, VI:122
  physical examination for, VI:122-124, 123f
  pinch test in, VI:122-123, 123f
  preexisting scars and, VI:114, 114f, 116
  preoperative preparation for, VI:140, 142
  rectus diastasis after, VI:377
  respiratory complications of, VI:378
  reverse, VI:113, 113f, 165, 165f-167f
  rib resection in, VI:113
  scar after, VI:179-181, 180f, 182f-189f, 372, 378
  scar tissue and, VI:114, 114f, 116
  secondary, VI:114, 180-189, 361-379
    adipose excess and, VI:376
    edema and, VI:375-376
    flap contour deficiency and, VI:375-376
    hematoma and, VI:372, 379
    nerve injury and, VI:372, 375
    rectus diastasis and, VI:377
    residual contour irregularity and, VI:181, 185f-187f
    scar and, VI:372, 378
    seroma and, VI:372, 379
    skin laxity and, VI:376-377, 377f, 378f

Abdominoplasty *(Continued)*
    skin loss and, VI:364, 371-372, 371f, 373f-374f
    skin redundancy and, VI:362-364, 363f-368f
    skin wrinkling and, VI:364, 369f-370f
    step-off deformity and, VI:376
    stretch marks and, VI:364
    umbilical deformity and, VI:181, 188-189, 188f, 189f
    umbilical ischemia and, VI:377, 379
    umbilicus eccentricity and, VI:377-379, 378f
    umbilicus malposition and, VI:378-379
    weight gain and, VI:376
  seroma after, VI:179, 185f, 372, 379
  skin examination for, VI:122-123, 123f
  skin excision for, VI:136-137, 136f, 137f
  skin incision for, VI:134-136, 134f-136f
  skin loss after, VI:364, 371-372, 371f, 373f-374f
  skin redundancy after, VI:362-364, 363f-368f
  skin wrinkling after, VI:364, 369f-370f
  standard, VI:97, 97f
    vs. lateral tension abdominoplasty, VI:260
  step-off deformity after, VI:376
  stretch marks after, VI:364
  subcutaneous fat in, VI:123
  technique of, VI:93-103, 98f-101f, 140, 142-145, 142f-145f
    Baroudi, VI:146-153, 146f-150f, 153f
    fascial management in, VI:108-110, 109f-113f
    in type I patient, VI:93, 94f, 96
    in type II patient, VI:93, 94f, 96, 96f
    in type III patient, VI:93, 95f, 96, 96f
    in type IV patient, VI:93, 95f, 97, 97f
    lateral tension, Color Plate VI:125-3, VI:154-155, 154f-156f, 259, 260-262, 261f-263f
    panniculectomy in, VI:101-104, 102f-104f
    umbilicoplasty in, VI:105-108, 106f-108f, 149-152, 150f, 172-174
  thromboembolism and, VI:175-178, 177t, 178f, 362, 378
  tissue necrosis and, VI:178, 178f, 179f
  type 0, VI:127t, 128f
  type 1, VI:127t, 129f
  type 2, VI:127t, 130f
  type 3, VI:127t, 131f
  type 4, VI:127t, 131f
  type 5, VI:127t, 132f
  type 6, VI:127t, 133f
  umbilical ischemia after, VI:377, 379
  umbilicoplasty in, VI:105-108, 106f-108f, 149-152, 150f, 172-174
  umbilicus circumscription in, VI:142, 142f
  umbilicus eccentricity after, VI:377-378, 378f
  umbilicus position in, VI:126, 126f, 136, 136f, 137f, 172-174
  weight gain after, VI:376
  without undermining, VI:155, 157, 157f
  wound complications in, VI:115, 178, 179f, 379
Abductor digiti minimi, VI:1406f, 1407, VII:32

Abductor digiti minimi flap, for foot reconstruction, I:462, 464
Abductor digiti minimi transfer, for low median nerve palsy, VIII:466
Abductor digiti quinti minimi transfer, for thumb opposition, VIII:342, 342f
Abductor hallucis, VI:1405, 1406f
Abductor hallucis-abductor digiti minimi flap, for foot reconstruction, VI:1419
Abductor hallucis flap, for foot reconstruction, I:462
Abductor pollicis brevis, VII:32
Abductor pollicis longus, VII:403
ABO blood group, in transplantation, I:271, 273
Abrasion
  facial, III:11, 12f
  traumatic tattoos with, III:12, 12f
Abrasion chondroplasty, for wrist, VII:134
Abscess
  after breast reduction, VI:578
  hand, VII:771, 777, 779-780, 779f, 780f
  peritonsillar, V:2
  retropharyngeal, V:2
Absorptive dressings, I:884-885, 885t
Abuse
  by health care providers, I:136-138
  child
    facial injury in, III:399-400, 399f
    hand burns in, VII:588, 590f
    radiologic evaluation of, III:399-400, 399f
  drug. *See also* Alcohol use.
    by surgeon, I:112
    in patient evaluation, I:85
    intra-arterial injection injury with, VII:807
Accessory abductor pollicis longus tendon transfer, for index finger abduction, VIII:479
Accessory meningeal artery, IV:81
Acclimatization, cold injury and, VII:649
Acetabular fossa, pressure sores of, VI:1347, 1347t, 1348f, 1349f
Acetaminophen, I:183
Acetazolamide, in acute mountain sickness prevention, I:861
Acetic acid injury, to hand, VII:654
Acetylcholinesterase, in prenatal diagnosis, I:1073
Acheiria, VIII:56-60
Achilles tendon
  débridement of, I:875-876, 875f-880f
  release of, I:866, 868f
  rupture of, I:1010, 1012, 1015f
Acinic cell carcinoma, of salivary glands, V:84-85
Acne, I:258, II:388, 390f
Acne cosmetica, after laser resurfacing, II:370-371
Acne keloidalis nuchae, I:944, 944f
Acne rosacea, V:254, 254f
Acquired immunodeficiency syndrome (AIDS)
  informed consent and, I:131
  Kaposi sarcoma and, V:299-300, 300f
  salivary gland lymphoma and, V:87
  skin cancer and, V:275, 397
  wound healing and, I:940-941, 941f

Acrocephalosyndactyly. *See* Apert syndrome.

Acrochordon, V:261

Acrofacial dysostosis (Nager syndrome), IV:101, 422, 423f, VIII:30, 30f, 62, 63f

Acromegaly, radiography in, VII:63, 64f

Acrospiroma, VII:960

Acrosyndactyly, VIII:146-147, 197f, 201-202, 201f, 202f. *See also* Constriction ring syndrome.
  classification of, VIII:146, 147f, 177-178
  treatment of, VIII:178-180, 178f, 179f

Acrylic, for facial skeletal augmentation, II:408

Acticoat, I:884t

Actinic cheilitis, V:446

Actinic keratoses, Color Plate V:113-1, V:266-268, 267f, 278, 278f, 279f, 393, 394f, 446, VII:960
  chemotherapeutic agents in, Color Plate V:116-2, V:278, 403-405, 404t
  of auricle, III:689
  pigmented, V:278, 279f

Acupuncture, in complex regional pain syndrome/reflex sympathetic dystrophy, VII:855

Adactyly, VIII:56-60

ADAM sequence, VIII:187

Adams-Oliver syndrome, V:41, VIII:187, 188f

Adapalene, II:395

Adductor canal syndrome, VII:876t

Adductor hallucis, VI:1408, 1408f

Adductor pollicis, VII:32
  in cleft hand, VIII:84, 93, 141f

Adenocarcinoma
  of nasal cavity, V:111
  of salivary glands, V:85-86, 86f

Adenoid cystic carcinoma
  of infratemporal fossa, V:145-148, 146f
  of lacrimal gland, V:115
  of nasal cavity, V:111
  of orbit, V:127, 134f
  of salivary glands, V:83-84, 86f

Adenoid hypertrophy, III:768

Adenoma, of salivary glands, V:76-77, 78f-80f

Adenomatoid odontogenic tumor, V:97, 200

Adenosine, in ischemic preconditioning, I:495

Adhesion cheiloplasty, IV:182-184, 183f-187f
  definitive, IV:184, 186f, 187f
  indications for, IV:183
  lateral lip incisions for, IV:183-184, 184f
  markings for, IV:183
  mucosal C flap for, IV:183, 183f
  mucosal closure for, IV:184, 186f
  muscle closure for, IV:184, 186f
  skin closure for, IV:184, 186f
  turbinate flap for, IV:184, 184f, 185f

Adhesives
  for facial prostheses, I:771-772, 771f
  in peripheral nerve repair, I:733

Adolescence, I:80-81, 80t

Adrenal gland, etomidate effects on, I:175

Advertising, ethics of, I:123

Aerodigestive system, vascular territories of, Color Plate I:15-13, I:343-344, 343f, 343t

Aesthetic surgery, II:31-45
  anesthesia consultation for, II:41
  limitations of, II:39
  patient approach in, II:33, 36-44
    anesthesia consultation and, II:41
    cautions in, II:38
    consent forms and, II:40-41, 42f, 43f
    consultation and, II:36-39, 37f
    goal determinations in, II:38-39
    initial contact and, II:33, 36
    photography and, II:39
    postoperative visits and, II:42-43
    three interview rule and, II:38
  payment for, II:40, 41f
  peer review consent form in, II:40-41, 42f
  photographic consent form in, II:40-41, 42f
  photography in, II:39
  psychological effects of, II:39
  scheduling of, II:39-41, 40f
  societal interest in, II:31-33, 32f, 33f, 34-35t, 36t
  staff for, II:42
  surgical consent form in, II:41, 43f
  unsatisfactory, II:43-44

Affirmative duty, I:140

Afipia felis infection (cat-scratch disease), VII:763-764

Age
  bone repair and, I:659
  cold injury and, VII:648
  distraction osteogenesis and, I:668-669
  microvascular surgery and, I:525
  rhinoplasty and, I:76

Aging
  body image and, I:68-69
  cartilage, I:623
  eyebrow, I:48-50, 49f, 220
  eyelid, II:128
  facial, II:171-174, 173f, 174f, 177, 178f, 215, 216t, 253-256, 254f, 255f, 340-341, 341f
  nasojugal groove, II:152
  neck, II:179-181, 180f, 181f, 297, 299-300, 301f, 302f
  pelvic tilt and, VI:259, 260f
  skin, II:340-341, 341f, 386-388, 387f, 388f

Air bag injury, III:455-456, VII:656

Airway
  after secondary rhinoplasty, II:793
  carbon dioxide laser fire in, I:202
  in craniofacial cleft, IV:416, 422
  in maxillary fracture, III:249
  in pediatric facial trauma, III:395, 397-398, 397f
  obstruction of
    after bilateral cleft lip repair, IV:238
    after rhinoplasty, II:559-560, 560f, 566, 768, 785, 788, 789
    congenital, I:1121-1122, 1121f
    in craniosynostoses, IV:476, 497
    in Nager syndrome, IV:422, 423f
    in Robin sequence, IV:512, 513, 514t
    in toxic epidermal necrolysis, I:797
    in Treacher Collins syndrome, IV:507
    mandibular distraction for, IV:422, 423f

Airway *(Continued)*
  preoperative evaluation of, I:168, 168f, 168t

Airway (artificial)
  mask, laryngeal, I:176, 177f
  nasopharyngeal, in craniofacial clefts, IV:416, 422
  oropharyngeal, cuffed, I:176
  tracheal, I:176-177
    in children, III:395, 397-398, 397f

Ajo, VI:176t

Alar cartilage
  anatomy of, III:188-189, 189f
  collapse of, after rhinoplasty, II:512
  flaring of, correction of, II:457-458, 458f, 785, 787f
  in unilateral cheiloplasty, IV:198-199
  malposition of, after rhinoplasty, II:535-536, 535f, 536f, 785, 786f
  reconstruction of, II:586, 588, 588f, 589f, 600, 605, 606f-612f
  reduction deformity of, after rhinoplasty, II:567, 567f
  resection of, in closed rhinoplasty, II:540, 542f, 545, 547
  retraction of, after open rhinoplasty, II:512

Albinism, oculocutaneous, V:399-400

Albright syndrome, fibrous dysplasia in, V:99, 101f

Alcohol use
  by surgeon, I:112
  cold injury and, I:857, VII:648
  head and neck cancer and, V:159
  in patient evaluation, I:85
  microvascular surgery and, I:525
  oral cavity cancer and, III:918

Alendronate sodium, in complex regional pain syndrome/reflex sympathetic dystrophy, VII:860

Alexithymia, VII:842-843

Alfentanil, I:181-182

Alkaline phosphatase, I:648, 649t

Alkyl mercuric agent injury, to hand, VII:654

Allen test, VII:35-36, 35f-36f, 45, 46f-47f, 797-798, 799f

Allergy, to local anesthetics, I:190

AlloDerm, I:313, 571, 574-576, 893, 1018, 1087t, 1088
  in burn treatment, I:824t, 827, VII:613
  indications for, I:574, 574f
  outcomes with, I:575-576
  uses of, I:574-575, 574f, 576f

AlloGro, I:1101t

AlloMatrix, I:1101t

Alloplastic materials, I:745-766. *See also* Implant(s).
  absorbable, I:746, 746t, 761, 761t
  advantages of, I:746, 746t
  applications of, I:746, 746t
  ceramic, I:693t, 696-700, 752-756, 753f-755f, 754t
  classes of, I:747
  corrosion of, I:751
  criteria for, I:746, 747t
  ductility of, I:750
  elasticity of, I:748-749, 749f
  fatigue of, I:750
  fracture stress of, I:750

Alloplastic materials (Continued)
  hardness of, I:750
  historical perspective on, I:745-746
  host response to, I:754t, 761-762, 762t
  impact tests for, I:750
  mechanical properties of, I:748-750,
    749f, 750t
  metal, I:751-752, 752t
  plasticity of, I:750
  polymer, I:756-760, 756f, 758f, 759f
  regulatory approval of, I:746-748
  safety testing of, I:748-751
  standards for, I:748-751
  strains on, I:748-750, 749f
  stresses on, I:748-750, 749f
  toughness of, I:749-750
  wear of, I:750-751
Aloe vera, in frostbite, I:860, 860t,
  VII:652
Alopecia. See Hair, scalp, loss of.
Alpha-fetoprotein, in prenatal diagnosis,
  I:1073
Alpha-hydroxy acids, II:397-399, 400f
Alpha particles, I:836
Alprostadil, VI:1234
Altitude sickness, I:861
Altruism, I:101
Alumina implants, I:755-756
Alveolar artery, IV:78f, 79
Alveolar bone, III:230, IV:71, 71f, V:163
  cleft. See Cleft alveolus.
  deficiency of, recombinant bone
    morphogenetic proteins in, I:662-
    663
  fracture of, III:245. See also Maxillary
    fracture.
    in children, III:405-409, 406f-408f
  tumors of, III:925. See also Oral cavity
    reconstruction.
Alveolar bone grafting
  in cleft alveolus, IV:263-266, 265f
  orthodontic treatment with, IV:286,
    288f, 289, 289f
  preparation for, IV:286, 287f
  quad helix expander in, IV:286, 287f
Alveolar molding. See also Nasoalveolar
  molding.
  in cleft lip, IV:177-178, 177f, 178f, 180-
    181
Alveolar nerve, IV:82
  neuroma of, VII:944
Alveolar soft part sarcoma, V:14
Ameloblastic fibro-odontoma, of
  mandible, V:98, 200
Ameloblastic fibroma, of mandible, V:97-
  98, 199-200
Ameloblastic fibrosarcoma, of mandible,
  V:99
Ameloblastoma
  of mandible, V:95, 95f, 197-199, 198f
  of maxilla, V:95, 96f-97f
American Board of Plastic Surgery, I:30,
  30f
American Medical Association, Principles
  of Medical Ethics of, I:113, 114t
American Society of Anesthesiologists,
  physical status classification of, I:170,
  171t
American Society of Plastic Surgeons,
  Code of Ethics of, I:113-122, 115t

Amitriptyline, in complex regional pain
  syndrome/reflex sympathetic
  dystrophy, VII:858-859
Amlodipine, in complex regional pain
  syndrome/reflex sympathetic
  dystrophy, VII:857
Amniocentesis, I:1073
  in twin-twin transfusion syndrome,
    I:1130
Amnion tubes, in peripheral nerve repair,
  I:735
Amniotic bands, I:54, 55f, 1130-1131,
  IV:414, 415f, VIII:190. See also
  Constriction ring syndrome.
Amperage, VII:598
Amputation
  arm
    congenital, VIII:51-61, 580, 584. See
      also Arm, transverse deficiency
      of; Phocomelia.
    therapeutic, VIII:584
      brachial plexus injury and,
        VIII:580
    traumatic, VIII:584
  auricle, III:34-36, 35f, 670, 672-677. See
    also Auricle, replantation of.
  finger. See Finger(s), amputation of.
  fingertip, VII:158-167, 159f-166f, 180-
    182
  foot
    Chopart, VI:1430
    in diabetes mellitus, VI:1443-1444,
      1448-1449
    Lisfranc, VI:1427, 1430, 1432f
  hand
    congenital, VIII:56-61, 58f, 60f, 584-
      587, 585f, 586f. See also
      Constriction ring syndrome.
    prostheses for, VIII:592, 598f, 599f,
      600, 600f, 601f
      body-powered, VIII:573-577, 574t,
        575f-579f
      in children, VIII:584-587, 585f,
        586f
    therapeutic, VIII:584
    traumatic, VIII:584
  in frostbite, I:860, 861f
  nasal, III:30
  prostheses for, I:781-788, VIII:573-580,
    583-606. See also Prostheses, upper
    extremity.
  thumb. See Thumb(s), amputation of.
  vs. reconstruction, VI:1367, VII:318-319
Amyotrophic lateral sclerosis, vs. nerve
  entrapment syndromes, VII:881
Anal sphincter reconstruction,
  vascularized muscle graft in, I:615
Analgesia. See also Anesthesia.
  epidural, I:195-196
  nonopioid, I:183-184
  opioid, I:171, 181-182, 181t
  opioid agonist-antagonist, I:182-183
Anastrozole, in breast cancer, VI:672
Anatomy. See also Vascular anatomy;
  Vascular territories and at specific
  structures.
  historical perspective on, I:13-18, 14f-
    23f
Ancrod, VI:1445
Anemia, Fanconi, V:401

Anencephaly, I:1128
Anergy, I:279
Anesthesia, I:167-204. See also Analgesia.
  ADA physical status classification for,
    I:170, 171t
  airway devices for, I:175-177, 177f
  airway evaluation for, I:168, 168f, 168t
  cardiovascular system evaluation for,
    I:168
  central nervous system evaluation for,
    I:169-170
  dental system evaluation for, I:168, 168f,
    168t
  endocrine system evaluation for, I:170
  gastrointestinal system evaluation for,
    I:169
  general, I:171-189, 172t
    bispectral index during, I:189
    cerebral function monitoring during,
      I:189
    complications of, I:200-202
    cuffed oropharyngeal airway with,
      I:176
    definition of, I:171
    face mask for, I:175-176
    fluid management and, I:184-186,
      186f
    goals of, I:171-172
    induction agents for, I:172-175, 172t
    intravenous adjuvants with, I:179-
      181, 179t
    laryngeal mask airway with, I:176,
      177f
    maintenance agents for, I:177-179
    muscle relaxants with, I:179-181, 179t
    neuromuscular blockade monitoring
      during, I:189
    opioid analgesics with, I:181-182,
      181t
    patient position and, I:187-189, 188f
    postanesthesia care unit for, I:199-
      202, 200t, 201t
    recovery from, I:199-202, 200t, 201t
    temperature regulation and, I:186-
      187
    tracheal intubation with, I:176-177
  historical perspective on, I:28
  in microvascular surgery, I:526
  local, I:192-194, 193f-199f. See also
    Nerve block(s).
  medication history and, I:170
  monitored care for, I:196-198
  office-based, I:198-199
  oral cavity evaluation for, I:168, 168f,
    168t
  preoperative evaluation for, I:167-171,
    168f, 168t, 169t, 171f, 171t, II:41
  preoperative medications and, I:170-
    171, 171f
  recovery after, I:199-202
  regional, I:189-196, 190t. See also Nerve
    block(s).
  reproductive system evaluation for, I:170
  respiratory system evaluation for, I:168-
    169
  surgical history and, I:170
  topical, in facial trauma, III:8
  upper extremity, VII:87-106, 112-113,
    113f
    adjuncts to, VII:94-97, 96t

Anesthesia *(Continued)*
  agents for, VII:92-94, 93t
  anatomy for, VII:91-92, 92f
  axillary blockade for, VII:101-102,
    101f
  clinical scenarios for, VII:105-106
  continuous catheter techniques for,
    VII:102
  cost of, VII:89
  digital nerve blocks for, VII:105
  efficiency of, VII:89
  elbow blocks for, VII:103-104, 104f
  in finger fracture, VII:425
  in hand surgery, VII:112-113, 113f
  infraclavicular block for, VII:100,
    100f
  interscalene block for, VII:97-99, 98f
  intravenous, VII:102-103
  isolated peripheral nerve blocks for,
    VII:103-105
  long-term outcomes and, VII:89
  median nerve block for, VII:103, 104-
    105, 104f, 105f
  multimodal analgesia and, VII:88
  needles for, VII:97, 98f
  patient preparation for, VII:89-91,
    90f
  preemptive analgesia and, VII:87-88
  radial nerve block for, VII:103, 104,
    104f
  recovery after, VII:89
  supraclavicular block for, VII:99-100,
    99f
  suprascapular block for, VII:100-101
  ulnar nerve block for, VII:103-104,
    104f, 105
  wrist blocks for, VII:104-105
Aneurysm, upper extremity, VII:813-814
Aneurysmal bone cyst
  of hand, VII:988
  of mandible, V:103, 195-196
Angelman syndrome, I:53
Angina, Ludwig, III:770, V:2
Angioblastoma
  giant cell, VIII:378, 379f
  of Nakagawa, V:36-37
Angiofibroma, nasopharyngeal, juvenile,
  V:11
Angiogenesis, VIII:370
Angiography
  before microvascular surgery, I:525
  in arteriovenous malformation, V:52,
    53f, VIII:398-399
  in foot, VI:1415
  in frostbite, VII:649
  in muscle transfer, VIII:493
  in pediatric trauma, VIII:428-429
  in upper extremity ischemia, VII:802
  in vascular thoracic outlet syndrome,
    VII:813, 813f
  in vasospastic disease, VII:816
  in venous malformation, VIII:383-384,
    387f
  of hand and wrist, VII:80, 82, 83f, 84f,
    649
  of hemangioma, VIII:373
Angioma, tufted, V:36-37
Angiosarcoma
  of mandible, V:107
  of upper extremity, VIII:378

Angiosome, I:332-334. *See also* Vascular
    territories.
  clinical implications of, I:333-334
  comparative anatomy of, I:330-332,
    332f, 333f
Animal bites
  facial, III:2-3, 3f, 30, 31f, 402, 402f, 403f
  hand, VII:762-764, 765f, 766t
  nasal, III:30, 31f
Ankle. *See also* Foot (feet).
  bones of, VI:1410, 1413f
  liposuction for, VI:232, 235, 235f, 236f,
    288
  reconstruction of, VI:1419, 1421f-1423f
Ankle block, I:194, 199f
Ankle/brachial index, I:964, VI:1412
Ankylosis, in temporomandibular joint
    dysfunction, III:543
Anonychia, VII:171, 185, 188, 188f
Anorexia nervosa, I:84-85, 84t
Anosmia, IV:461
Anterior thigh flap, for pressure sore
    treatment, VI:1347, 1349, 1349f, 1350f
Anterolateral compartment syndrome,
    VII:876f
Anterolateral thigh flap
  for abdominal wall reconstruction,
    VI:1187-1191, 1187f-1190f
  for neck reconstruction, III:1045, 1046f
Anthelix composite graft, in columella
    defect, II:586-589, 587f-589f
Anthropometry, facial, II:1-16. *See also*
    Cephalometry.
  chin in, II:5t, 15, 15f-18f
  eyebrows in, II:4t, 8, 10f
  eyes in, II:4t, 5t, 8, 10f, 11f
  facial heights in, II:2, 4-5t, 6-7, 6f-8f, 6t
  forehead in, II:4t, 5t, 7-8, 9f
  four-section canon in, II:6-7, 7f
  history of, II:2
  in skeletal augmentation, II:405, 406f
  lips in, II:4t, 5t, 13, 13f-15f
  neoclassical canons of, II:2, 3t
  nose in, II:4t, 5t, 8, 11-13, 11f
  soft tissue landmarks in, II:3f, 3t
  subnasale to gnathion height in, II:7, 8f
  teeth in, II:4t, 13, 13f-15f
  three-section canon in, II:6, 7f
  two-section canon in, II:6, 6f
Anthropometry, history of, II:2
Anti-interleukin-2, I:274t, 277-278
Antibiotics
  equipment coating with, I:763
  in breast augmentation, VI:28, 325-326
  in breast reduction, VI:557
  in chemical hand injury, VII:655
  in Fournier disease, VI:1253
  in genital lymphedema, VI:1255
  in hand implant patient, VII:762
  in hand infection, VII:766-767t, 777
  in head and neck procedures, V:186
  in irradiated tissue, I:841, 1055, 1055t
  in lymphatic malformation, V:43-44
  in pressure sore treatment, VI:1351
  in problem wounds, I:912-913t, 950,
    954-955, 956f
  topical, I:883-884, 884t
    for wound healing, I:224-225
    in hand surgery, VII:121
    with laser facial resurfacing, II:345

Antibody screening, for transplantation,
    I:274
Anticoagulation, microvascular surgery
    and, I:521-522, 525-526
Anticonvulsants, in complex regional pain
    syndrome/reflex sympathetic
    dystrophy, VII:857-858
Antidepressants
  in breast pain, VI:355
  in complex regional pain
    syndrome/reflex sympathetic
    dystrophy, VII:858-859
Antidotes, for chemical injury, VII:655t,
    656
Antiemetics, I:171, 202
Antigens
  in graft rejection, I:272-273
  in transplantation, I:270-271
Antilymphocyte globulin, I:274t, 277
Antithymocyte globulin, I:274t
Anxiety, in patient evaluation, I:82-84, 83t
Anxiolytics, preoperative, I:170-171, 171f
Apatitic calcium phosphate bone cement,
    I:694t, 702
Apert syndrome, III:778, IV:92, 93t, 99,
    VIII:20, 21t. *See also* Craniosynostosis
    (craniosynostoses), syndromic.
  classification of, VIII:170, 171f, 171t
  clinical presentation of, VIII:144-145,
    144f, 145f, 146t
  clinodactyly in, VIII:298, 298f
  genetic analysis in, I:58, 60-61, 61f-63f
  symphalangism in, VIII:265-266, 266f
  syndactyly in, IV:99, VIII:145-146, 145f,
    146t, 363-365, 363f
    treatment of, VIII:170-175
      first web space release in, VIII:172
      interdigital web space release in,
        VIII:172, 173f
      outcomes of, VIII:173, 175, 176f
      principles of, VIII:170, 172t
      secondary revision in, VIII:172-
        173, 174f, 175f
Aphallia, VI:1218, 1220f
Aplasia cutis congenita, III:610-611
  wound healing and, I:944
Apligraf, I:313-314, 893, 896f, 1087t, 1088-
    1089
  in epidermolysis bullosa, I:805, 806f
  in wound healing, I:1018-1019
Apnea, sleep, III:784-794. *See also* Sleep
    apnea.
Apnea index, III:775
Apocrine glands, I:298-299
Apoptosis
  in toxic epidermal necrolysis, I:795
  ischemic preconditioning and, I:495-496
  of osteocytes, I:646
Apprenticeship, I:35
Aquacel Ag, I:884t
Aquaphor, after laser resurfacing, II:370
Arbitration clause, of contract, I:136
Arcuate line, VI:1177-1178
Arcus marginalis, incision and release of,
    II:232, 234, 234f, 804, 804f
Areola, VI:791, 792f. *See also* Nipple(s).
  reconstruction of, I:302, VI:812-814,
    812t. *See also* Nipple
    reconstruction.
    dermal fat flap for, VI:796, 797f-799f

Areola (Continued)
management after, VI:814
skin grafts for, VI:813-814
tattooing in, Color Plate VI:139-1,
VI:814, 814f-816f
residual, after breast reduction, VI:1075-
1076, 1076f
L-Arginine, in ischemia-reperfusion injury,
I:494
Arglase, I:884t
Arm(s). See also Forearm; Hand(s);
Shoulder; Upper extremity.
amputation of
congenital, VIII:51-61. See also
Arm(s), transverse deficiency of;
Phocomelia.
therapeutic, VIII:584
brachial plexus injury and,
VIII:580
as flap carrier, I:367, 370f
desmoid tumors of, VII:954-955, 954f
fullness of, VI:291-313, 292f, 292t, 293f
breast reduction and, VI:292, 293f
classification of, VI:293, 293t
complications of, VI:292t, 312
etiology of, VI:291-293, 292t
evaluation of, VI:293-296, 293t, 294f,
294t
measurements for, VI:294, 294f
muscle tone and, VI:294
photography for, VI:295-296, 295f
pinch test for, VI:294, 296, 296f
skin tone and, VI:294
treatment of, VI:296-313
in group 1 patients, VI:296-300,
296f-303f
in group 2 patients, VI:300-308,
304f-308f
in groups 3 and 4 patients, VI:308-
312, 309f-313f
laser resurfacing of, II:367
liposuction for, VI:216-221, 218f-222f
lymphedematous, VI:292, 312, VII:995-
1004. See also Lymphedema, upper
extremity.
mangling injury to, VII:317-348
débridement for, VII:320
evaluation of, VII:318
provisional revascularization for,
VII:320-321
reconstruction for, VII:319-320
innervated gracilis transfer for,
VII:335, 338, 343f
latissimus dorsi flap in, VII:324,
325f, 326f
musculotendinous, VII:322
nerve injury in, VII:322
rectus abdominis flap in, VII:324-
326
soft tissue, VII:322-324
vascular, VII:321-322
skeletal stabilization for, VII:321
muscle transfer in, VIII:489-506
alternatives to, VIII:494
anatomy for, VIII:490-492, 490f,
491f
complications of, VIII:504
expectations for, VIII:494-495
extremity assessment for, VIII:493-
494

Arm(s) (Continued)
for anterior deltoid reconstruction,
VIII:502-503, 502f, 503f, 504,
506
for biceps reconstruction, VIII:501-
502, 502f, 504, 505f
for finger extension, VIII:500-501,
501f
for flexor aspect of forearm, VIII:497-
500, 498f, 499f, 504, 505f
for triceps reconstruction, VIII:502
gracilis for, VII:335, 338, 343f,
VIII:490-492, 490f, 491f, 494f,
496-497
historical perspective on, VIII:489-490
latissimus dorsi for, I:390, 400f-402f,
405, VIII:492
management after, VIII:503-504
muscle selection for, VIII:495-496
patient selection for, VIII:495
physiology of, VIII:492, 493f, 494f
preoperative planning for, VIII:495,
496f
recipient site for, VIII:495, 496f
skin coverage for, VIII:495-496
prosthetic, I:1149-1150, 1149f-1152f. See
also Prostheses, upper extremity.
body-powered, I:1149-1150, 1151f,
1154-1155
customization of, I:1150, 1152f
for congenital amputation, VIII:54-
56, 55f, 580
future trends in, I:1154-1155
limitations of, I:1154
materials for, I:1154
passive, I:1149-1150, 1150f
selection of, I:1150, 1153-1154, 1153f,
1154f
radial (preaxial) deficiency of, VIII:61-
80. See also Radial (preaxial)
deficiency.
transverse deficiency of, VIII:51-61
at forearm level, VIII:54-56, 55f
at upper arm level, VIII:51
incidence of, VIII:40t
intercalated, VIII:51-54. See also
Phocomelia.
ulnar deficiency of, VIII:101-110. See
also Ulnar deficiency.
Arnica, VI:175
Arnold nerve, III:4
Aromatase inhibitors, in breast cancer,
VI:672
Arrhinencephaly, IV:21, 383, 384f
Arrhinia, III:763, 764, 765f, IV:404, 407,
408f
Arrhythmias
in hypothermia, I:858
ketamine effects on, I:174
Arterial insufficiency, VI:1473-1484. See
also Lower extremity, arterial
insufficiency of.
wound healing and, I:219, 902-906,
904f, 963-964, 965f-966f
Arterial pressure, in upper extremity
ischemia, VII:798
Arterial stenosis, VII:796, 796f
Arteriectomy, in vasospastic disease,
VII:817
Arteriovenous fistula, of hand, VII:807

Arteriovenous malformation, III:775, V:6-
7, 51-54, VIII:397-407, 397t, 398f-
408f
angiography in, VIII:398-399
classification of, VIII:397-398, 397t
clinical features of, V:51, 52f, 52t,
VIII:397
embolization in, VIII:401, 401f-404f
in Parkes Weber syndrome, V:60
magnetic resonance imaging in,
VIII:398, 399f
management of, V:52-54, 53f-55f
pathogenesis of, V:51
pathophysiology of, VIII:397
radiologic features of, V:51-52
sclerotherapy in, VIII:399, 401
surgery in, VIII:401, 404-407, 404f-
408f
treatment of, VIII:399-407, 400f
type A, VIII:397, 398f, 400f
type B, VIII:397, 398f-401f, 403f, 404f
type C, VIII:398, 398f, 400f, 402f, 405f-
408f
ultrasonography in, VIII:398
vs. hand infection, VII:769
wound healing and, I:945, 946f
Arteritis, of upper extremity, VII:814-815,
814f
Artery(ies). See also Vascular anatomy;
Vascular territories.
arcades of, I:348, 348f, 349f
connective tissue relation of, I:344-345
historical studies of, I:15, 16f-17f, 18,
21f-23f
nerve relation to, I:345-347, 346f
origin of, I:350
radiation of, I:345
size of, I:347-348, 347f
tissue-engineered, Color Plate I:37-2,
I:1089-1091, 1090f, 1092f
Arthritis. See also Osteoarthritis.
in temporomandibular joint
dysfunction, III:541, 541f
septic, of hand, VII:782-784, 784f, 788-
789
Arthrodesis
in carpometacarpal joint osteoarthritis,
VII:722, 724
in Dupuytren disease, VII:752
in finger reconstruction, VII:216
in musicians' hands, VII:702
in proximal interphalangeal joint
osteoarthritis, VII:717, 718f
in radial (preaxial) deficiency, VIII:69
Arthrogryposis, hand in, VIII:147, 148f
Arthroplasty
in carpometacarpal joint osteoarthritis,
VII:720, 721f, 722f
in finger reconstruction, VII:215-216
in musicians' hands, VII:702
in proximal interphalangeal joint
osteoarthritis, VII:713-717, 714f-
716f, 718t
Arthroscopy
in temporomandibular joint
dysfunction, III:542-543
of wrist, VII:125-137. See also Wrist,
arthroscopy of.
Arthrotomy, in temporomandibular joint
dysfunction, III:543

Arytenoepiglottoplasty, III:768
Asian patient
  blepharoplasty in, II:107-108, 107t
  face lift in, II:248
Asphyxiating thoracic dystrophy, VI:484-
    485, 484f, 485f
Aspiration
  foreign body, in children, III:769-770
  in pediatric facial trauma, III:398
  with laryngeal mask airway, I:176
Aspiration pneumonitis, I:169
Aspirin
  in flap optimization, I:499t, 500
  in microvascular surgery, I:522
Asthma
  gastroesophageal reflux and, III:771
  preoperative evaluation of, I:169
  propofol anesthesia and, I:174
Atenolol, before neck lift, II:321
Athetoid-like movement, ketamine-related,
    I:175
Atracurium, I:180, 180t
Atrial fibrillation, in hypothermia, I:858
Auditory canal, stenosis of, III:34, 677-679,
    679f
Auricle
  acquired deformities of, III:669-670,
      672-695
    after face lift, II:732-736, 733f-735f
    of helical rim, III:681, 684f-686f, 685,
        VI:386-388, 387f
    of lobe, III:687, 689, 692f-695f
    of lower third, III:687
    of middle third, III:686-687, 688f-
        692f
    of upper third, III:685-686
    partial, III:681, 682f-684f
    reconstruction for, III:679-695
      composite grafts in, III:680, 683f,
          684f
      contralateral conchal cartilage graft
          in, III:680
      fascial flap in, III:680
      for helical rim loss, III:681, 684f-
          686f, 685, VI:386-388, 387f
      for lobe deformities, III:687, 689,
          692f-695f
      for lower third defects, III:687
      for middle third defects, III:686-
          687, 688f-692f
      for upper third defects, III:685-686
      historical perspective on, III:633-
          634
      ipsilateral conchal cartilage graft in,
          III:680, 682f
      prostheses for, III:680
      revolving door flap for, V:386-388,
          387f
      skin covering in, III:680
      tunnel procedure in, III:686-687,
          688f-692f
    trauma-related, III:30-36, 32f, 35f,
        679
    with tissue loss, III:679-680
    without tissue loss, III:677-679,
        679f
  actinic keratosis of, III:689
  amputation of, III:34-36, 35f, 670, 672-
      677. See also Auricle, replantation
      of.

Auricle (Continued)
    with narrow pedicle, III:34-35
    with wide pedicle, III:34, 35f
  anatomy of, III:31-32, 634-635, 635f
  anterior chonchal defect of, V:388
  burns of, III:33
  carcinoma of, III:689, 695
    petrous extension of, V:148-149
  cartilage graft from, I:624, 625, 625f,
      626f
    in alar reconstruction, II:600, 605,
        607f, 610f, 611f
  cauliflower, III:677
  composite graft from, for nasal
      reconstruction, II:586-589, 587f-
      589f, V:349
  congenital deformities of, III:633-669.
      See also Microtia.
    classification of, III:638, 638t
    diagnosis of, III:638
    drugs and, III:638
    etiology of, III:637-638
    facial abnormalities with, III:638, 639f
    genetic factors in, III:637-638
    in craniofacial microsomia, III:638,
        639f, IV:122, 124f, 125t, 546
    in Treacher Collins syndrome, IV:506-
        507, 509-510
    incidence of, III:637
    ischemia in, III:638
    middle ear abnormalities with, III:638
    rubella and, III:638
    urogenital abnormalities with,
        III:638-639
  constricted, III:662-663, 664f-668f
  cryptotic, III:663, 665, 669f
  degloving injury to, V:388
  embryology of, III:635-636, 637f,
      IV:115-117, 116f
  field blocks for, III:9-10, 11f
  hemangioma of, V:32
  hematoma of, III:32-33, 32f, 677
  irregular contour of, III:677
  keloids of, III:14-15, 15f
  laceration of, III:33
  nerve supply of, III:635, 635f
  prominent, III:665, 667, 669, 670f-672f
    antihelical fold restoration in, III:667,
        671f
    cartilage remodeling in, III:667, 669,
        671f, 672f
    conchal alteration in, III:667, 670f
    lateral cartilage alteration in, III:669,
        673f
  regional anesthesia of, I:191
  replantation of, III:670, 672-677
    cartilage fenestration for, III:673,
        676f, 677f
    composite graft for, III:672, 674f, 675f
    dermabrasion for, III:673, 676f
    fascial flap for, III:676
    microsurgical, III:36, 676-677
    postauricular skin removal for,
        III:673, 676f, 677f
    skin graft for, III:676
    with pedicle attachment, III:672, 674f
    with preserved cartilage, III:674
  sebaceous cysts of, III:689
  skin loss from, III:679
  suppurative chondritis of, III:33-34

Auricle (Continued)
  tissue expansion for, I:557
  trauma to, III:30-36, 32f, 35f. See also
      Auricle, acquired deformities of.
    anatomy for, III:31-32
    examination of, III:32, 32f
    surgical treatment of, III:32-36, 35f
      anesthesia for, III:32
  tumors of, III:689, 695
    petrous extension of, V:148-149
Auricular nerve block, in facial trauma,
    III:9-10
Auriculotemporal nerve block, in facial
    trauma, III:10-11, 11f
Authoritarianism, I:98t, 99-100
Automated Endoscope System for Optimal
    Positioning, I:1155
Automobile accidents, injury prevention
    and, III:455-456
Autonomy, I:101t, 102-104
Avascular necrosis
  condylar process fracture and, III:174,
      177
  Dupuytren disease fasciectomy and,
      VII:750-751, 751f
  in temporomandibular joint
      dysfunction, III:543-544
  mandibular fracture and, III:182
  orthognathic surgery and, II:685
Axilla
  burn-related contracture of, VII:630-
      633, 631f, 634f
  lymphatic malformations of, V:42, 43f,
      46, 46f
Axillary artery, in brachial plexus injury,
    VII:526
Axillary lymph nodes
  dissection of, VI:664-665, 664f
  sentinel biopsy of, VI:661-664, 662f
Axillary nerve block, I:193, 195f, VII:101-
    102, 101f
Axillary nerve entrapment, VII:909
Axon, VII:472, 474-475, 474f
  regeneration of, VII:477-481, 478f
  transport in, VII:476-477
Axonotmesis, I:725-726, 726f, VII:483-485,
    483t, 484f
Azathioprine, I:275t, 276

B
B-K mole syndrome, V:309-310
Bacille Calmette-Guérin (BCG), I:1056-
    1057
Bacitracin, I:884t
Back
  complex wounds of, reconstruction for,
      VI:442, 446-455
    after orthopedic manipulation,
        VI:450, 453f-455f
    clinical considerations in, VI:446
    for myelomeningocele, VI:434, 447-
        448, 448f-450f
    for radiation defects, VI:448, 450,
        451f, 452f
    in chronic osteomyelitis, VI:450
    omental flap for, VI:446-447, 447f
    pathophysiologic considerations in,
        VI:442, 446
  liposuction for, VI:227-230, 228f, 250,
      250f, 280-281, 280f

Back *(Continued)*
  lower, reconstruction of, VI:442, 445f, 446f
  Marjolin ulcer of, VI:446-447, 447f
  middle, reconstruction of, VI:441-442, 444f
  radiation injury to, latissimus dorsi flap reconstruction for, VI:448, 450, 451f, 452f
  reconstruction of, VI:441-450
    for complex wounds, VI:442, 446-450, 448f-455f
    for noncomplex wounds, VI:441-442, 443f-447f
    gluteal flap for, VI:442, 445f
    latissimus dorsi flap for, VI:441-442, 444f, 448, 450, 451f, 452f
    omental flap for, VI:446-447, 447f
    transverse flap for, VI:442, 446f
    trapezius flap for, VI:441, 443f
  tumor resection on, I:983
  upper, reconstruction of, VI:441, 442f, 443f
  wound healing on, I:983
Baclofen, in complex regional pain syndrome/reflex sympathetic dystrophy, VII:860
Bacon, Sir Francis, I:18, 18f
Baculum, VI:1311, 1311f
Balanitis xerotica obliterans, VI:1253-1254, 1273
Baldness, II:690-691. *See also* Hair, scalp, loss of; Hair restoration.
Baller-Gerold syndrome, III:778
Balloon digits, in constriction ring syndrome, VIII:202-203, 203f
Band-aid disease, I:945
Bannayan-Riley-Ruvalcaba syndrome, V:54-55, VIII:411-412
Barbiturates, for general anesthesia, I:172-173, 172t
Bariatric surgery, abdominoplasty after, VI:120. *See also* Abdominoplasty.
Baroudi abdominoplasty, VI:146-153
  closure in, VI:152
  dressings in, VI:152
  excess skin resection in, VI:148-149, 149f
  fascial plication in, VI:148, 148f
  incision for, VI:147
  markings for, VI:146-147, 146f
  sutures in, VI:152
  umbilicoplasty in, VI:149-152, 150f
  umbilicus in, VI:147, 147f
Basal cell carcinoma, V:282-290, 391-448
  biopsy of, V:403
  brachytherapy in, V:436
  chemical exposure and, V:275-276
  chemoprevention of, Color Plate V:116-2, V:277, 403-405, 404t
  chemotherapeutic agents in, V:286t, 288, 403-404, 404t
  chronic wounds and, V:275
  clinical features of, V:283
  diagnosis of, V:401-403, 401f, 402f
  dietary fat and, V:278
  epidemiology of, V:394
  etiology of, V:274-276, 274t, 282, 393
  follow-up for, V:436-437
  genetic features of, V:398-399, 398t

Basal cell carcinoma *(Continued)*
  histopathology of, Color Plate V:113-5, V:282-283, 283t, 401-403, 401f, 402f
  historical perspective on, V:391-393
  immune factors in, V:275
  in AIDS, V:397
  in atomic bomb survivors, V:396
  incidence of, V:273, 394, 395-396, 395t
  infiltrating, V:402
  metastatic, V:283, 435, 446-447
  mimics of, V:402-403
  morpheaform (sclerosing), Color Plate V:113-8, V:283, 285f, 402
  nevoid, V:290, 290f, 398, 398t, 399t
  nevus sebaceus of Jadassohn and, V:281-282, 281f, 282f
  nodular, Color Plates V:113-5 and V:113-6, V:283, 284f, 285f, 402, 402f
  of cheek, III:833, 840f-842f, V:346, 346f, 376f, 377f
  of forehead, V:348, 349f
  of glabella, V:355f
  of lower eyelid, V:367f-368f
  of medial canthus, V:353f, 373f-375f
  of nasal tip, V:349, 354f, 356f, 358f, 362f
  of nose, V:352f
  of paranasal area, V:380f
  of perionychium, VII:201, 201f
  of scalp, III:611-612, 612, V:346, 347f, 348, 348f
  of upper extremity, VII:961
  of upper eyelid, V:365f, 367f-368f
  organ transplantation and, V:396
  p53 gene in, Color Plate V:116-1, V:393
  photodynamic therapy in, V:286t, 406, 407f
  pigmented, Color Plate V:113-7, V:283, 285f
  porokeratosis and, V:282
  prevention of, Color Plate V:116-2, V:276-278, 277, 277t, 393-394, 403-405, 404t
  radiation therapy and, V:274-275, 435
  recurrence of, V:287-288, 287t, 289f, 414t, 415t, 416t, 419t, 435
  risk factors for, V:394-396, 395t
  shave biopsy in, V:408, 410, 410f
  superficial, V:283, 401, 401f
  treatment of, V:285-290, 286t, 287t, 406-437, 408t, 409t, 417f-418f, 419t
    algorithm for, V:417f-418f
    care after, V:436-437
    chemotherapeutic agents in, V:286t, 288, 403-404, 404t
    cryosurgery in, V:286t, 290, 408t, 409t, 411-413, 411f, 412f
    curettage and electrodesiccation in, V:285, 286t, 409t, 410-411
    5-fluorouracil in, V:286t, 288, 403-404
    frozen vs. permanent sections in, V:425
    full-thickness excision in, V:409t, 413-416, 414t, 415t, 416t, 425-426, 425f, 426f
    micrographic surgery in, V:286t, 288, 408t, 409t, 426-432. *See also* Mohs micrographic surgery.

Basal cell carcinoma *(Continued)*
  pathology processing in, V:414-416, 425-426, 425f, 426f
  photodynamic therapy in, V:286t, 406, 407f
  radiation therapy in, V:286t, 288, 408t, 419t, 432-437, 433f, 434t
  shave excision in, V:408, 409t, 410, 410f
  tumor margins in, V:414-416, 425-426, 425f, 426f
  ultraviolet radiation and, V:274, 274t
  vs. melanoma, V:310, 312f
  xeroderma pigmentosum and, V:279-280
Basal cell nevus syndrome, V:290, 290f
Basic fibroblast growth factor, in hemangioma, V:20
Basiliximab, I:274t
Bassoonist, hand disorders in, VII:695
Battered child syndrome, III:399-400, 399f, VII:588, 590f
Bazex syndrome, V:398
Bcl-2, I:496
Beads, antibiotic-impregnated, I:955, 956f, 977
Beauty, II:44-45, 44f
Beckwith-Wiedemann syndrome, macroglossia in, III:767-768, 767f
Bell flap, for nipple reconstruction, VI:807, 810f
Bell palsy, I:613-614, 614f, III:749f
Bell phenomenon, II:93
Belt lipectomy, VI:171-172, 172f, 173f
Beneficence, I:101-102, 101t
Bennelli round block technique, for breast reduction, VI:570-571, 572f
Bennett fracture, VII:434-436, 435f
  reversed, VII:436
Benzocaine, I:190t
Best practices, in evidence-based decision-making, I:46-47
Beta-hydroxy acids, II:399
Beta particles, I:836
Betel nut, head and neck cancer and, V:159
Biceps femoris flap, for lower extremity reconstruction, VI:1372
Biceps reconstruction
  gracilis transfer for, VII:338, 343f, VIII:501-502, 502f, 504, 505f
  latissimus dorsi flap for, I:400f-402f, 405
Biceps tendon transfer, for obstetric brachial plexus palsy, VII:557, 560f
Biceps to triceps transfer, for elbow extension, in tetraplegic patient, VIII:517-518, 519f
Bier block, I:192, 193f
Biesenberger technique, for breast reduction, VI:540, 542f
Biglycan, I:649t, 650
Biobrane, I:313, 893, 1087t
  in burn treatment, I:824t, 825
  in toxic epidermal necrolysis, I:797-798, 798f
Biofeedback therapy, in complex regional pain syndrome/reflex sympathetic dystrophy, VII:855
Bioglass, I:755

Biopsy
    breast, Color Plates VI:138-1 and 138-2,
        VI:638-642, 640f, 641t
        after augmentation, VI:355-356
    in bone tumor, VII:980-981
    in complex regional pain
        syndrome/reflex sympathetic
        dystrophy, VII:831
    in head and neck mass, V:167, 227-228
    in melanoma, V:311-313, 312t, 313f-
        315f, 324-325, 325f
    in salivary gland tumors, V:72-73, 72f
    nerve, in muscle transfer, VIII:494
    sentinel node, I:1062, VI:654, 661-664,
        662f
    skin, V:252, 263
Birth
    brachial plexus injury with, VII:539-
        562. See also Brachial plexus injury,
        obstetric.
    facial trauma with, III:398
Bispectral index, I:189
Bisphosphonates, in complex regional pain
    syndrome/reflex sympathetic
    dystrophy, VII:859-860
Bites
    dog, III:2-3, 3f, 30, 31f, 402, 402f, 403f
    facial, III:2-3, 3f, 30, 31f, 402, 402f, 403f
    hand, VII:47, 762-764, 765f, 766t, 768,
        768f
    in child abuse, III:399
    nasal, III:30, 31f
    snake, I:931-932, 934f, 935f, 1016-1017
    spider, I:931-932, 933f, 934f, 1017,
        VII:768, 768f
Black widow spider bite, I:931-932, 933f,
    934f, 1017
Bladder
    epidural block effects on, I:194-195
    exstrophy of, VI:1207-1208, 1208f, 1210f
    spinal block effects on, I:194-195
Blair, Vilray P., I:29
Blastocyst, IV:2
Bleeding. See also Hematoma;
    Hemorrhage.
    in hemangioma, V:28
    in Klippel-Trénaunary syndrome, V:60
    in maxillary fracture, III:238, 247, 249
    in nasal fracture, III:206
    in zygoma fracture, III:227
    with craniofacial cleft management,
        IV:461
    with palatoplasty, IV:263
Bleomycin, in lymphatic malformations,
    V:45
Blepharitis, in epidermolysis bullosa, I:805
Blepharoplasty, II:127-129, 130f-132f
    historical perspective on, I:33
    lower lid, II:111-121, 112f, 127-129,
        130f-132f
        anatomic analysis in, II:824-825, 824f,
            826f
        canthopexy in, II:115-123, 124-125,
            805. See also Canthopexy.
        complications of, II:823-824, 824t,
            825t, 826t. See also
            Blepharoplasty, lower lid,
            secondary.
        evaluation of, II:152
        excessive fat removal with, II:813

Blepharoplasty (Continued)
        fat grafting in, II:129, 150, 152-153,
            154f-156f
        laser resurfacing and, II:359-360,
            360f
        malar pad liposuction with, II:149-
            150, 151f
        patient selection for, II:128-129
        secondary, II:805-807, 805f-807f, 817-
            821, 817t, 819f-821f, 835-855
            anatomic analysis in, II:824-825,
                824f, 826f, 835, 835f, 836f,
                836t, 837t
            chemosis after, II:854, 855f
            complications of, II:851, 853f-855f,
                854-855
            corneal protection for, II:825, 827f
            dermal-orbicular pennant lateral
                canthoplasty, II:847-851, 848f-
                852f
            distraction test in, II:839, 840f
            epiblepharon after, II:851, 854, 854f
            evaluation for, II:835-841, 835f-
                843f, 836t
            excessive fat removal and, II:813
            fat-related complications of, II:851,
                853f
            fat retention and, II:805
            free skin graft in, II:818
            granuloma after, II:854-855
            horizontal lid shortening in, II:839,
                841f, 850-851, 851f, 852f
            iatrogenic defects and, II:808t, 811-
                813, 811f, 811t, 812f
            inferior retinacular lateral
                canthoplasty in, II:842-846,
                843t, 845f, 846f
            lamellar retraction and, II:820-821,
                820f, 821f
            lateral canthoplasty in, II:841-851,
                843t, 844t
            lid eversion and, II:839-840, 842f,
                843f
            lid retraction and, II:811-812, 811f,
                811t, 812f
            lower lid posture and, II:814, 817-
                818
            malar excess after, II:851, 854f
            malar fat descent and, II:840-841
            medial canthal laxity and, II:837,
                839, 840f
            midface deficits and, II:805-807,
                806f, 807f
            midfacial screw fixation in, II:850-
                851, 852f
            midlamellar retraction and, II:836,
                837f
            pentagonal wedge resection in,
                II:841
            shortened horizontal aperture and,
                II:812-813
            snap test in, II:839, 840f
            soft tissue to bone distance and,
                II:837, 840f
            subconjunctival hemorrhage after,
                II:854, 855f
            tarsal strip lateral canthoplasty in,
                II:843t, 846-847, 846f, 847f
            tarsal strip procedure in, II:850-
                851, 851f, 852f

Blepharoplasty (Continued)
            tarsoligamentous integrity and,
                II:837, 839, 840f, 841f
            tear trough implant in, II:806-807,
                807f
            transposition myocutaneous graft
                in, II:818-820, 819f
            vector relationships in, II:836-837,
                838f, 839f
            shortened horizontal aperture with,
                II:812-813
        skin excision, II:112-115, 113f-115f
        transconjunctival, II:122-124, 124f
    medical malpractice suits in, I:144
    secondary, II:801-807, 802t, 823-855. See
        also at Blepharoplasty, lower lid;
        Blepharoplasty, upper lid.
    upper lid, II:99-111, 127-129, 130f-132f
        anatomic analysis in, II:824-825, 824f,
            826f
        anchor (invagination), II:100-106,
            101t, 102f-105f
            Asian suture technique in, II:105
            asymmetry after, II:106, 110
            care after, II:106
            complications of, II:106
            edema after, II:106
            exophthalmos and, II:96
            infection after, II:106
            levator aponeurosis shortening
                with, II:106, 107f
            pseudoepicanthal folds after, II:106
            retrobulbar hemorrhage after,
                II:106
            webbing after, II:106
        asymmetry after, II:129, 803-804
        brow drop after, II:88, 88f
        brow position in, II:95-96
        brow ptosis and, II:102f, 104f, 109-
            111, 128, 801-802
        complications of, II:74, 823-824, 824t,
            825t. See also Blepharoplasty,
            upper lid, secondary.
        excessive skin excision in, II:99, 99f,
            751-753, 752f
        eyebrow lift and, II:224
        eyelid malposition in, II:751-753,
            752f-754f
        fat overexcision with, II:753, 754f
        free fat graft in, II:811
        globe prominence after, II:804
        in Asian patients, II:107-108, 107t
        laser resurfacing and, II:360, 360f
        lateral canthal tightening procedures
            after, II:239, 242, 242f
        levator aponeurosis sectioning with,
            II:810, 811f
        patient selection for, II:128-129
        results of, II:49f, 51f, 52f
        retraction after, II:803-804
        scarring with, II:810-811
        secondary, II:801-804, 802t, 815-817,
            815t, 816f, 817f, 827-835
            anatomic analysis in, II:824-825,
                824f, 826f
            corneal protection for, II:825, 827f
            evaluation for, II:827-829, 827t,
                828f
            exaggerated interbrow frown and,
                II:802-803

Blepharoplasty *(Continued)*
  excessive fat removal and, II:810, 810f
  excessive skin removal and, II:807-808, 808f
  Fansanella-Servat procedure in, II:831, 832f
  fat herniation and, II:814
  fat transposition in, II:810, 810f
  frontal lift in, II:804
  globe prominence and, II:804
  iatrogenic defects and, II:807-811, 807t
  inadequate fat reduction and, II:803
  lateral eyelid retraction and, II:808-810, 809f
  levator aponeurosis repositioning/fat grafting in, II:815-817, 817f
  levator lengthening in, II:809-810, 809f
  lid asymmetry and, II:803-804
  lid fold definition and, II:808, 809f
  lid retraction and, II:803, 804, 831, 833f, 834f, 835
  Müller muscle hematoma and, II:810
  orbital fat and, II:803
  orbital rim prominence and, II:804, 804f
  photo face and, II:802
  poor blink reflex and, II:808
  progressive degenerative changes and, II:813-814, 813t
  ptosis and, II:802, 810-811, 811f, 813, 827t, 828f, 829-831, 829f
  recurrent glabellar lines and, II:813-814
  recurrent transverse lines and, II:814
  sequelae of, II:237, 239-242, 240f-242f
  skin excision, II:99-100
Blindness
  in frontobasilar region fracture, III:335-338
  in maxillary fracture, III:252
  in orbital fracture, III:327
  with craniofacial cleft management, IV:459
Blink, postblepharoplasty impairment of, II:808
Blix curve, VII:26, 26f
Blood gases, in Robin sequence, IV:513
Blood group antigens, in transplantation, I:271, 273
Blood-nerve barrier, I:720, 722f, VII:475-476
Blood pressure
  opioid effects on, I:181
  propofol effects on, I:174
Blood transfusion, I:185-186
  in breast reduction, VI:557
Blood vessels. *See also* Vascular anatomy; Vascular territories.
  in tissue expansion, I:541-542, 542f, 543f
Blue nevus, V:264-265, 264f, 308-309
Blue rubber bleb nevus syndrome, V:47, 48f, VIII:389, 390f

Body contouring
  abdominal, VI:87-116, 119-202. *See also* Abdominoplasty.
  face and neck, II:184-211, 283-295, 297-336. *See also* Face lift; Neck lift.
  large-volume, VI:241-254. *See also* Liposuction, large-volume.
  lower body, Color Plates VI:125-1 and 125-2, VI:260, 268-271, 270f, 271f
  transverse flank-thigh-buttock, Color Plate VI:125-4, VI:262-265, 265f, 266f
  trunk and thigh, VI:257-271. *See also* Thigh lift; Trunk lift.
  upper extremity, VI:291-313. *See also* Arm(s), fullness of; Liposuction, upper extremity.
Body dysmorphic disorder, I:85-86, 85t, II:39, 514, 565-566
Body image, I:67-69, II:39
  aging and, I:68-69
  behavior and, I:68
  emotional response and, I:68
  in adolescence, I:68
  in childhood, I:68
  plastic surgery effects on, I:69
Body lift. *See also* Thigh lift; Trunk lift.
  lateral tension abdominoplasty for, Color Plate VI:125-3, VI:259, 260-262, 261f-264f
  lower body, Color Plates VI:125-1 and 125-2, VI:260, 268-271, 270f, 271f
  transverse flank-thigh-buttock, Color Plate VI:125-4, VI:262-265, 265f, 266f
Body mass index, VI:174-175, 175t
Bolus dressing, for skin grafts, I:308, 308f
Bone(s), I:639-650. *See also specific bones.*
  alkaline phosphatase in, I:648, 649t
  artificial, for nipple projection, VI:810t, 811
  biglycan in, I:649t, 650
  biopsy of, VII:980-981
  calcium phosphate of, I:640
  cancellous, I:640, 642f
  cortical, I:639-640, 640f
  débridement of, I:876, 878-879, 879f
  distraction osteogenesis of, I:667-671.
    See also Distraction osteogenesis.
  endochondral, I:639
  extracellular matrix of, I:648-650, 649t
  fracture of. *See* Fracture(s).
  in tissue expansion, I:541
  mechanical loading of, I:645-646
  membranous, I:639
  nerve implantation into, in neuroma treatment, VII:941-943
  osteoblasts of, I:641t, 642-645, 642f, 643f
  osteocalcin in, I:648, 649t, 650
  osteoclasts of, I:641t, 646-648, 647f
  osteocytes of, I:641t, 645-646, 645f
  osteonectin in, I:648, 649t
  osteopontin in, I:648, 649t
  proteoglycans in, I:649t, 650
  radiation effects on, I:841-842, 844f, 845f. *See also* Osteoradionecrosis.
  remodeling of, I:645-646
  resorption of, I:646
  ruffled border formation in, I:646
  sealing zone formation in, I:646

Bone(s) *(Continued)*
  sialoprotein in, I:648, 649t, 650
  transplantation of, I:280-281
  tumors of. *See specific sites and tumors.*
  type I collagen of, I:648, 649t
  Wolfe's law of, I:645-646
Bone cyst
  aneurysmal, V:103, 195-196, VII:988
  of mandible, V:103, 196-197
Bone-derived hydroxyapatite ceramics, I:693t, 696-697
Bone flap, I:387, 390, 390f, 390t, 391f-399f, 421
  fasciocutaneous flap with, I:390
  fibula for, I:390, 390t, 393f-395f
  iliac crest for, I:390, 390t, 395f-396f
  in fracture treatment, VI:1396-1399, 1398f
  radius for, I:390, 390t
  rib for, I:390, 391f, 392f
  scapula for, I:390, 390t, 397f-399f
Bone graft, I:671-680
  after tumor resection, VII:982-983
  allogeneic (allograft), I:281, 691-695
    corticocancellous, I:693t, 695
    demineralized, I:695
    disease transmission with, I:691-692
    formulations of, I:692, 693t
    history of, I:691
    immune response to, I:692
    incorporation of, I:692
    morselized, I:692, 693t, 695
    preservation of, I:691
    processing of, I:691
    rejection of, I:692
  alveolar
    in cleft alveolus, IV:263-266, 265f
    orthodontic treatment with, IV:286, 288f, 289, 289f
    preparation for, IV:286, 287f
    quad helix expander in, IV:286, 287f
  autologous (autograft), I:280, 671-672, 673-675t
    calvaria for, I:675t, 688-691, 689f-691f
    embryonic origin of, I:676-677, 677f
    fibroblast growth factor-2 for, I:678
    fibula for, I:674t, 686-688, 687f
    fixation of, I:672, 676
    greater trochanter for, I:673t, 684-685
    history of, I:671
    ilium for, I:673t, 680-684
      in adults, I:681-682, 681f-683f
      in children, I:682-684
      vascularized, I:684, 684f
    mechanical stress on, I:672
    metatarsus for, I:675t, 688
    olecranon for, I:673t, 684-685
    orientation of, I:677
    periosteum in, I:677
    recipient bed for, I:677-679
    recombinant bone morphogenetic proteins in, I:662-663
    revascularization of, I:678-679
    rib for, I:673t, 685-686, 686f, 687f
      vascularized, I:685-686
    scapula for, I:674t, 688
    sources of, I:673-675t, 680-691, 681f-684f, 686f, 687f, 689f-691f

Bone graft *(Continued)*
tibia for, I:673t, 680, 681f
vascularized, I:679-680, 684-686, 684f
calcium phosphate substitutes for, I:693-694t, 696-702, 1100, 1101t
calcium sulfate substitutes for, I:693t, 695-696, 1100, 1101t
in cleft alveolus, IV:181-182, 263-266, 265f
in craniofacial cleft, IV:431-433, 432f-435f
in craniofacial microsomia, IV:533, 534f-537f
in facial surgery, III:564
in finger reconstruction, VII:213-214
in metacarpal hypoplasia, VIII:59
in Treacher Collins syndrome, IV:431-432, 432f, 433f, 507-509, 508f
in unilateral cleft lip, IV:181
in upper extremity reconstruction, VII:321, 335, 342f
methyl methacrylate substitute for, I:702-703
substitutes for, I:693-694t, 695-703, 1100, 1101t
tissue-engineered, I:1100-1101, 1102t, 1103f
xenogeneic, I:695
Bone lining cells, I:644
Bone marrow, autologous, recombinant bone morphogenetic proteins with, I:663
Bone morphogenetic proteins, I:656t, 659-663, 660t
in bone repair, I:656t, 659-663, 660t
isoforms of, I:661
recombinant, I:662-663
signal transduction in, I:661
Bone scan
in complex regional pain syndrome/reflex sympathetic dystrophy, VII:845-846
in frostbite, VII:650
Bone substitutes, I:693-694t, 695-703
calcium phosphate, I:693t, 696-702, 1100, 1101t
calcium sulfate, I:693t, 695-696, 1100, 1101t
BoneSource, I:694t, 700-701
Borderline personality, I:72-73
Botryoid odontogenic cyst, V:191
Botulinum toxin
after obstetric brachial plexus repair, VII:549
complications of, II:69-70
for eyebrow lift, II:68-70, 68t, 69f, 232
for forehead rhytids, II:67-68, 68t
for torticollis, III:1032-1033
with laser facial resurfacing, II:345
Boutonnière deformity, VII:663, 664f
burns and, VII:625-627, 626f
infection and, VII:788-789
repair of, VII:416-417, 416f
Bowen disease, Color Plate V:113-4, V:266, 267f, 280-281, 280f, 437t, 442-443
Boxer fracture, VII:426-427, 427f
Boyes superficialis tendon transfer, for radial nerve palsy, VIII:458-459, 461

Brachial artery
anatomy of, VII:34-37, 792
catheterization of, thrombosis with, VII:806
embolism of, VII:807-808, 809f
pressure in, VI:1412
Brachial plexitis (Parsonage-Turner syndrome), VII:881
Brachial plexus. *See also* Brachial plexus injury; Thoracic outlet syndrome.
anatomy of, VII:515-516, 522-523, 522f, 523t
inflammation of, VII:881
variant anatomy of, VII:522-523
Brachial plexus block, I:192-193, 194f
catheter-delivered, VII:98f, 102
Brachial plexus injury. *See also* Thoracic outlet syndrome.
adult, VII:516-535
chart for, VII:524, 524f
Chuang triangle in, VII:528-529, 529f
classification of, VII:517f, 517t
degree of, VII:523-524
early exploration of, VII:523-524
electrodiagnosis of, VII:526
evaluation of, VII:524-526, 524f
four-root avulsion in, VII:532
Horner syndrome with, VII:525-526
infraclavicular, VII:520-522, 521f, 521t, 535
motor examination in, VII:525
pain with, VII:525
pathophysiology of, VII:523-524
patient history in, VII:524-525
postganglionic, VII:517t, 518, 519f, 535
preclavicular, VII:517t, 518, 520, 520f, 535
preganglionic, VII:516-518, 517t, 532-534, 533f, 534f
prosthesis for, VIII:580
radiography of, VII:526
retroclavicular, VII:517t, 518, 520, 520f, 535
sensory examination in, VII:525
single-root avulsion in, VII:535
supraclavicular, VII:516, 520-521, 521t
three-root avulsion in, VII:532
Tinel sign in, VII:525
total root avulsion in, VII:532, 533f, 534f
treatment of, Color Plate I:25-2, I:736-737, 737t, VII:526-535
delayed repair in, VII:527-528
electrodiagnosis in, VII:529
end-to-side neurorrhaphy in, VII:532
for infraclavicular injury, VII:535
for postganglionic injury, VII:535
for preclavicular injury, VII:535
for preganglionic injury, VII:532-535, 533f, 534f
for retroclavicular injury, VII:535
free muscle transplantation in, VII:532
functional sequelae of, VII:536
infraclavicular dissection in, VII:528-529, 529f
nerve grafting in, VII:530, 531f

Brachial plexus injury *(Continued)*
nerve transfer in, VII:530-532
neurolysis in, VII:530
neurorrhaphy in, VII:530
outcomes of, VII:536
rehabilitation after, VII:535-536
supraclavicular dissection in, VII:528
timing of, VII:523-524, 526-528
two-root avulsion in, VII:532-535
vascular injury with, VII:526
obstetric, VII:539-562
clinical presentation of, VII:540, 540f
computed tomographic myelography in, VII:542
differential diagnosis of, VII:542
elbow sequelae of, VII:557
electromyography in, VII:542
etiology of, VII:539
evaluation of, VII:540t, 541-542, 541t
forearm sequelae of, VII:557, 560f
growth effects and, VIII:444-445, 445f, 446
hand sequelae of, VII:557, 561f, 562
Horner syndrome in, VII:540, 540f
prosthesis for, VIII:580
recovery patterns in, VII:542
shoulder sequelae of, VII:549, 553-557, 554f-560f
treatment of, Color Plate I:25-2, I:736-737, 737t, VII:551-553
care after, VII:548-549, 548f
cross-innervation with, VII:549
goals of, VII:546-548, 547f
growth effects and, VIII:444-445, 445f, 446
incisions for, VII:543, 544f
indications for, VII:541, 542
intercostal nerve transfer in, VII:548
nerve transfer in, VII:548, 551f-552f
neurolysis in, VII:546
neuroma-in-continuity in, VII:543, 545f, 546
outcomes of, VII:540-541, 549, 550f-552f, 553f
patient position for, VII:543, 543f
phrenic nerve transfer in, VII:548
preparation for, VII:542-543
root avulsion in, VII:548
sural nerve graft in, VII:546-548, 547f
technique of, VII:543-546, 543f-545f, 546t
trumpet sign after, VII:549
ulnar nerve transfer in, VII:548
wrist sequelae of, VII:557, 561f, 562
Brachiocephalic shunt, steal syndrome with, VII:807, 808f
Brachioplasty, VI:291-292, 300, 306f, 307f, 308, 309f-311f, 312. *See also* Liposuction, upper extremity.
Brachioradialis, VII:24
nerve implantation into, VII:940-941, 943f, 944f
Brachioradialis transfer
for high median nerve palsy, VIII:469-470, 469f
for wrist extension, in tetraplegic patient, VIII:520-521, 521f

Brachycephaly, **IV:**137t, 149-154, 151f-
    155f, 469
Brachydactyly, **VIII:**21t, 41t
Brachytherapy, **I:**837, 837f, 838f
    in skin cancer, **V:**436
    wound healing and, **I:**983
Branchial arches
    anomalies of, **V:**3-4. *See also* Craniofacial
        microsomia.
    cyst of, **I:**945, **III:**1025-1026, 1026f, **V:**3
    embryology of, **III:**1025-1027, 1026f,
        1027f, **IV:**4, 5f
Brand's tendon transfer, for MCP joint
        flexion and interphalangeal extension,
        VIII:476-478, 476f, 477f
Brava system, **VI:**46
BRCA genes, **VI:**631, 657
Breast(s). *See also* Areola; Nipple(s).
    absence of, congenital, **VI:**522
    anatomy of, **VI:**510, 511f, 550-551
    asymmetry of, **I:**562
        after breast augmentation, **VI:**340-
            342, 341f
        after breast reconstruction, **VI:**1092,
            1092t, 1160-1163, 1161t, 1162t,
            1163f
        after breast reduction, **VI:**580, 1070
    augmentation of. *See* Breast augmentation.
    biopsy of, Color Plates **VI:**138-1 and
        138-2, **VI:**638-642, 640f, 641t
        after augmentation, **VI:**355-356
    blood supply of, Color Plates **VI:**137-1
        to 137-3, **VI:**551, 606-607, 606f
    boxy deformity of, after breast
        reduction, **VI:**580
    cancer of. *See* Breast cancer.
    congenital anomalies of, **VI:**509-533. *See*
        also specific anomalies.
    constricted development of, **VI:**513,
        515f, 521f, 524f-526f. *See also*
        Breast(s), tuberous.
    core needle biopsy of, Color Plate
        VI:138-2, **VI:**639-642, 640f, 641t
    cystic mass of, cancer vs., **VI:**638
    development of, **VI:**551
    during menstrual cycle, **VI:**551
    ectopic, **VI:**512-513, 512f, 513f
    embryology of, **VI:**509-510, 550
    examination of, **VI:**552-553, 632
    excisional biopsy of, **VI:**641-642, 641t
    fat injection in, **I:**584
    fine-needle aspiration of, Color Plate
        VI:138-1, **VI:**639, 641t
    hypertrophy of, **VI:**551-553, 552t. *See*
        also Breast reduction.
        in adolescent, **VI:**577
        physiological effects of, **VI:**553-554
        psychological aspects of, **VI:**554, 577
    hypoplasia of, **I:**561-563, 564f. *See also*
        Poland syndrome.
    imaging of. *See* Mammography.
    infection of
        augmentation and, **VI:**27, 29, 329,
            346-348
        free TRAM flap and, **VI:**872
        reduction and, **VI:**578
        secondary reconstruction and,
            VI:1108, 1111, 1124, 1124t,
            1127-1130, 1128f, 1129f, 1131-
            1132t, 1133f, 1134t

Breast(s) *(Continued)*
    innervation of, **VI:**550-551
    juvenile papillomatosis of, **V:**16
    lift of. *See* Mastopexy.
    liposuction for, **VI:**224-227, 226f, 281-
        282, 283f
    magnetic resonance imaging of, **VI:**635,
        635f
    male. *See* Gynecomastia.
    mammography of. *See* Mammography.
    pain in
        after augmentation, **VI:**352-355
        after reduction, **VI:**578
    photography of, **I:**160, 164f
    physiology of, **VI:**551-552
    ptosis of, **VI:**47-49, 48f, 48t. *See also*
        Mastopexy.
        after augmentation, **VI:**345-346
        after secondary reconstruction,
            VI:1105, 1107, 1107f
    radial scar of, Color Plate **VI:**138-2,
        VI:641
    reconstruction of. *See* Breast
        reconstruction.
    reduction of. *See* Breast reduction.
    self-examination of, **VI:**632
    size of, **VI:**553, 554-556, 555f. *See also*
        Breast augmentation; Breast
        reduction.
    supernumerary, **VI:**512-513, 512f, 513f
    tuberous, **I:**562-563, **VI:**513-522
        classification of, **VI:**514, 516f, 516t
        clinical presentation of, **VI:**514
        etiology of, **VI:**513-514, 516f
        incidence of, **VI:**513
        pectus excavatum and, **VI:**463, 465f
        treatment of, **VI:**514, 516-527, 523t
            implant reconstruction in, **VI:**517,
                521f, 522, 522f, 523f-526f
            Maillard Z-plasty in, **VI:**517, 518f
            Puckett technique in, **VI:**517, 522,
                522f
            Ribeiro technique in, **VI:**517, 520f-
                521f
            superior pedicle mammaplasty in,
                VI:517, 519f
            tissue expansion in, **VI:**522, 523f-
                526f
    tubular, **VI:**513, 514f
    ultrasonography of, **VI:**633-635, 634t
    wrinkling of
        after augmentation, **VI:**337-340, 337f,
            338t
        after reconstruction, **VI:**1121, 1121t
Breast augmentation, **VI:**1-30, 35-46
    aesthetic planning for, **VI:**9, 9f
    anesthesia for, **I:**204
    antibiotics for, **VI:**28, 325-326
    asymmetry after, **VI:**340-342, 341f
        etiology of, **VI:**340
        frequency of, **VI:**340
        in nipples, **VI:**342
        treatment of, **VI:**340-342
    biopsy after, **VI:**355-356
    Brava system for, **VI:**46
    breast cancer after, **VI:**356
    candidates for, **VI:**35
    capsular contracture after, **VI:**26-29, 26t,
        321-329. *See also* Breast
        augmentation, secondary.

Breast augmentation *(Continued)*
    axillary capsule and, **VI:**327-328
    bacterial contamination and, **VI:**325-
        326
    calcification and, **VI:**327, 327f
    capsule retention and, **VI:**328
    capsule thickness and, **VI:**322
    capsulectomy for, **VI:**326-328, 327t
    capsulotomy for, **VI:**326
    classification of, **VI:**321, 322t
    corticosteroids and, **VI:**325
    development of, **VI:**322
    etiology of, **VI:**27
    explantation for, **VI:**328-329, 328t
    hematoma and, **VI:**329
    histology of, **VI:**322
    implant extrusion and, **VI:**348-349
    implant filler and, **VI:**323-324, 323t
    implant position and, **VI:**324-325,
        324t
    implant surface and, **VI:**323, 323t
    infection and, **VI:**27, 329
    myofibroblasts and, **VI:**322
    prevention of, **VI:**27-28, 329
    scarring and, **VI:**27
    subglandular position and, **VI:**324-
        325, 324t
    subpectoral position and, **VI:**324-325,
        324t
    timing of, **VI:**322-323
    treatment of, **VI:**28-29, 326-329, 327f,
        327t, 328t
    capsulotomy after, **VI:**28-29, 326
    care after, **VI:**26
    complications of, **VI:**29-30, 39, 45-46.
        See also Breast augmentation,
        secondary.
    corticosteroids in, **VI:**28
    dissection for, **VI:**21, 23, 38-39, 39f, 40f
    endoscopic, **I:**1046-1047, 1046f, 1047f
    ethics and, **I:**116
    evaluation for, **VI:**35
    goals of, **VI:**8, 9f, 9t
    hematoma after, **VI:**29, 350-351
    immunomodulators in, **VI:**28
    implants for, **VI:**1-7, 2f, 5f, 5t, 6f
        alternative filler, **VI:**4
        anatomic-shaped, **VI:**5-7, 6f, 12, 13f
        breast cancer diagnosis and, **VI:**635-
            637, 636f, 637f
        cohesive gel, **VI:**324
        deflation of, **VI:**30
        dimensions of, **VI:**10-11, 11f
        double-lumen, **VI:**3
        explantation of, **VI:**318-320. *See also*
            Breast augmentation, secondary.
            mastopexy after, **VI:**82, 84
        extrusion of, **VI:**348-349
        failure of, **VI:**329-337. *See also* Breast
            augmentation, secondary.
        infection and, **VI:**346-348
        insertion of, **VI:**39, 41f
        low-bleed, **VI:**324
        malposition of, **VI:**30, 342-345
            combination, **VI:**344-345
            etiology of, **VI:**342-343, 345
            frequency of, **VI:**342-343
            inferior, **VI:**344
            lateral, **VI:**344
            medial, **VI:**343

Breast augmentation *(Continued)*
   superior, VI:343
     treatment of, VI:343-345
   material of, VI:46
   placement of, VI:37-39, 38f-41f
   rippling of, VI:30
   rupture of, VI:30, 330-337
     etiology of, VI:330-333, 331f, 332f
   safety of, VI:7-8
   saline-filled, VI:2-3, 11, 12f
     fill volume for, VI:339-340
     overfilling of, VI:339-340
     palpability of, VI:337-340, 339t
     rippling of, VI:30
     rupture of, VI:336-337
     secondary augmentation after,
       VI:316-317
     skin wrinkling with, VI:337-340,
       337f, 338t
       etiology of, VI:337-338, 337f
       treatment of, VI:339-340
     underfilling of, VI:339-340
   selection of, VI:11-12, 12f, 318, 318t,
     352-353
   shape of, VI:46
   silicone gel, VI:1-2, 2f, 4-5, 5t, 6f, 11,
     26-27
     displacement of, VI:30
     rupture of, VI:30, 333-336, 334t
       diagnosis of, VI:335
       outcomes of, VI:336
       treatment of, VI:335-336
     safety of, VI:7-8
     secondary augmentation after,
       VI:315-316
   size change in, VI:351-352
   sizers for, VI:23, 23f, 25, 39, 40f
   textured, VI:3-4, 5f, 11, 27
   in male-to-female transformation,
     VI:1315
   incisions for, VI:19-23, 20t, 21f-23f, 36-
     37, 36f
   infection after, I:921, VI:29, 346-348
     etiology of, VI:347
     frequency of, VI:347-348
     treatment of, VI:348
   informed consent for, VI:8
   inframammary incision for, VI:20-23,
     20t, 21f-23f, 36, 36f
   medical malpractice suits in, I:143
   Mondor disease after, VI:30
   motion exercises after, VI:28
   nipple sensation after, VI:29-30
   nonoperative, VI:46
   pain after, VI:352-355
     drug treatment of, VI:355
     evaluation of, VI:353-354
     frequency of, VI:352-353, 354t
     nutritional treatment of, VI:354-355
     treatment of, VI:354-355
   patient assessment for, VI:9-10, 10f
   patient positioning for, I:188, VI:20
   periareolar incision for, VI:20t, 23-24,
     24f, 36-37, 36f
   pocket selection for, VI:12, 14t, 15f-18f,
     19t
   povidone-iodine for, VI:325-326
   psychological factors in, I:76-77
   ptosis after, VI:345-346
     etiology of, VI:345

Breast augmentation *(Continued)*
   frequency of, VI:345
     treatment of, VI:345-346
   results of, VI:39, 42f-45f
   safety of, VI:7-8
   secondary, VI:315-357
     bimanual examination for, VI:320
     breast asymmetry and, VI:340-342,
       341f
     breast cancer and, VI:356
     capsular contracture and, VI:321-329,
       322t, 323t, 324t, 327f, 327t, 328f
     capsulectomy for, VI:319-320
     explantation for, VI:318-320
     frequency of, VI:315-318, 316t
     hematoma and, VI:350-351
     implant extrusion and, VI:348-349
     implant failure and, VI:329-337, 331f,
       332f, 334t
     implant malposition and, VI:342-345
     implant palpability and, VI:337-340,
       339t
     implant-related infection and,
       VI:346-348
     implant size change and, VI:351-352
     mastalgia and, VI:352-355, 354t
     mastopexy in, VI:82, 84, 346
     planning for, VI:318, 318t
     prevention of, VI:356
     ptosis and, VI:345-346
     reimplantation for, VI:320-321
     seroma and, VI:350, 351
     skin wrinkling and, VI:337-340, 337f,
       338f
     technique of, VI:35-39, 36f-41f
   seroma after, VI:29, 350, 351
   subglandular pocket for, VI:12, 14t, 15f,
     16f, 19t, 37-38, 38f
   subpectoral pocket for, VI:12, 14t, 17f,
     18f, 19t, 38, 38f
   thrombophlebitis after, VI:30
   transaxillary incision for, VI:20t, 25, 36f,
     37, 37f
   transumbilical approach to, VI:20t, 25-
     26, 46
   wound closure for, VI:39, 41f
Breast cancer, VI:631-783
   aromatase inhibitors in, VI:672
   axillary lymph nodes in
     dissection of, VI:654, 664-665, 664f
     nerve injury with, VI:665
     sentinel biopsy of, VI:661-664, 662f
   BRCA genes in, VI:631, 657
   breast augmentation and, VI:355-356
   breast-conserving therapy in, VI:646-
     648, 646t, 648f
     in ductal in situ disease, VI:672-673,
       672t, 673t
   breast reduction and, VI:581, 611, 1080-
     1081
   chemotherapy in, VI:666-667, 667t, 670-
     671
   cystic mass vs., VI:638
   diagnosis of, VI:632-643
     BI-RADS classification in, VI:633,
       633t, 634f
     biopsy in, Color Plates VI:138-1 and
       138-2, VI:633, 638-642, 640f,
       641t
     breast examination in, VI:632

Breast cancer *(Continued)*
     breast implants and, VI:635-637, 637f,
       638f
     core needle biopsy in, Color Plate
       VI:138-2, VI:639-642, 640f, 641t
     delay of, VI:637-638, 637f
     ductal lavage in, Color Plate VI:138-3,
       VI:642-643
     excisional biopsy in, VI:641-642, 641t
     fine-needle aspiration in, Color Plate
       VI:38-1, VI:639, 641t
     image-guided core biopsy in, VI:639
     magnetic resonance imaging in,
       VI:635, 635f
     mammography in, VI:632-633, 633t.
       See also Mammography.
     needle-localized excisional biopsy in,
       VI:641t, 642
     nipple aspiration in, Color Plate
       VI:138-3, VI:642-643
     open excisional biopsy in, VI:642
     ultrasonography in, VI:633-635, 634t
   ductal in situ, VI:672-673, 672t, 673t
   endocrine therapy in, VI:671-672
   HER-2/neu receptor in, VI:671
   hormone receptors in, VI:671
   in children, V:16
   in contralateral breast, VI:657
   in situ, VI:672-673, 672t, 673t
   incidence of, VI:631
   inflammatory, VI:773, 776, 779f-780f
   lobular in situ, VI:673
   lumpectomy in, VI:647-648, 648f
     axillary lymph node dissection with,
       VI:665
     breast reduction after, VI:620, 622,
       622f
     radiation therapy after, VI:667-668
   management of, VI:665-673
     endocrine therapy in, VI:671-672
     in in situ cancer, VI:672-673, 672t,
       673t
     neoadjuvant chemotherapy in,
       VI:666-667, 667t
     neoadjuvant radiation therapy in,
       VI:666
     postoperative adjuvant chemotherapy
       in, VI:670-671
     postoperative radiation therapy in,
       VI:667-670, 668t, 669t, 670t
     surgical, VI:643, 646-665, 646t. *See*
       also Breast reconstruction.
       lumpectomy in, VI:647-648, 648f
       lymph node dissection in, VI:664-
        665, 664f
       mastectomy in, VI:648-661. *See also*
        Mastectomy.
       nipple-areola complex in, VI:661
       quadrantectomy in, VI:648
       sentinel node biopsy in, VI:661-
        664, 662f
   mastectomy in, VI:648-661. *See also*
     Mastectomy.
   metastatic, VI:666
   micrometastases in, VI:663, 670-671
   nipple-areola complex in, VI:661
   node-negative, VI:671
   palpable, VI:633
   prophylactic mastectomy and, VI:657-
     659, 657t, 658f-659f

Breast cancer *(Continued)*
  psychological factors in, I:78-79
  quadrantectomy in, VI:648
  radiation therapy in, I:839, 839f, 840f,
      VI:666, 667-670, 668t, 669t, 670t
    complications of, I:910-911, 911f, 967,
        972f-973f
  raloxifene in, VI:671
  recurrence of
    after lumpectomy, VI:667, 668
    chest wall reconstruction in, VI:415f
    in ductal in situ disease, VI:672, 672t
    in node-negative disease, VI:671
    skin-sparing mastectomy and,
        VI:654-657, 656t
    subcutaneous mastectomy and,
        VI:651-652
  risk factors for, VI:631, 632t
  segmental resection (quadrantectomy)
      in, VI:648
  sentinel lymph node biopsy in, VI:654,
      661-664, 662f
  staging of, VI:643, 644-645t, 646t
  survival in, VI:646t
  tamoxifen in, VI:671
  trastuzumab in, VI:671
Breast-conserving therapy, in cancer,
    VI:646-648, 646t, 648f, 672-673, 672t,
    673t
Breast-feeding
  breast reduction and, VI:580-581, 611,
      625
  cleft palate and, IV:254
Breast implants
  explantation of, VI:82, 84, 318-320, 328-
      329, 328f, 1147-1150, 1148f-1149f,
      1149t
  for augmentation, VI:1-7, 2f, 5f, 5t, 6f.
      See also Breast augmentation,
      implants for.
  for reconstruction, VI:897-922, 923-932,
      966-970, 969f, 970f. *See also at*
      Expander-implant breast
      reconstruction.
  in pectus excavatum, VI:463, 465f, 470-
      471, 472f
  in Poland syndrome, VI:493, 495f
Breast lift. *See* Mastopexy.
Breast reconstruction, I:557-561, VI:673-
    783. *See also* Nipple reconstruction.
  after implant explantation, VI:84, 988f
  chest wall irradiation and, I:561
  complications of. *See* Breast
      reconstruction, secondary.
  contralateral breast in, VI:691, 695f, 782,
      922, 1024, 1027f
  deep circumflex iliac artery (Rubens)
      flap for, VI:764t, 1053-1055
    patient position for, VI:1055f
    selection of, VI:1063
    surgical technique for, VI:771, 771f,
        772f, 1059-1060, 1059f, 1061f,
        1062f
  deep inferior epigastric artery perforator
      flap for, VI:686, 762, 764t, 1040-
      1044
    anatomy of, VI:1040-1041
    bilateral, VI:1042
    complications of, VI:765t, 1044
    defect closure for, VI:1042, 1044

Breast reconstruction *(Continued)*
    surface markings for, VI:1040, 1041f
    surgical technique for, VI:765-766,
        766f, 1002, 1004f, 1007f, 1008,
        1011, 1011f, 1012f, 1020, 1020f,
        1040t, 1041-1042
    unilateral, VI:1042, 1042f, 1043f
    vascular anatomy of, VI:1040-1041,
        1041f
  delayed
    expander-implant. *See* Expander-
        implant breast reconstruction.
    implant-only, VI:679, 679t, 680, 681f
    latissimus dorsi flap for, VI:1023-
        1037. *See also at* Latissimus dorsi
        flap.
    microvascular. *See* Breast
        reconstruction, microvascular
        composite tissue transplantation
        (free flap) for.
    TRAM flap for, VI:973-997, 1001-
        1020. *See also at* Transverse
        rectus abdominis myocutaneous
        (TRAM) flap.
  expander-implant. *See* Expander-
      implant breast reconstruction.
  goals of, VI:674, 674t
  historical perspective on, I:33
  immediate, I:560-561, 560f, VI:674,
      675
    expander-implant in, VI:875-970. *See
        also* Expander-implant breast
        reconstruction.
    implant-only, VI:679, 679t, 680
    latissimus dorsi flap for, VI:819-832.
        See also at Latissimus dorsi flap.
    microvascular. *See* Breast
        reconstruction, microvascular
        composite tissue transplantation
        (free flap) for.
    transverse rectus abdominis
        myocutaneous flap for, VI:835-
        847, 849-872. *See also at*
        Transverse rectus abdominis
        myocutaneous (TRAM) flap.
  implant-only, VI:679, 679t, 680, 681f
  implants for. *See also* Expander-implant
      breast reconstruction.
    cancer diagnosis and, VI:635-637,
        636f, 637f, 678-679
    complications of. *See* Breast
        reconstruction, secondary.
    connective tissue disorders and,
        VI:679
    in latissimus dorsi flap procedure,
        VI:696, 701f-704f, 823f, 824f,
        827f, 830, 1034, 1035f, 1036
    in TRAM flap procedure, VI:738,
        742f-743f, 952, 955f-959f, 956
    magnetic resonance imaging of,
        VI:635, 636f, 637
    mammography of, VI:636-637, 637f
    placement of, I:558-559, 559f
    safety of, VI:677-679
    ultrasonography of, VI:637
  in acquired hypoplastic deformities,
      I:561-563, 564f
  in breast asymmetry, I:562
  in complex defect, VI:773-780, 774f,
      775f, 776t, 777f-780f

Breast reconstruction *(Continued)*
  in inflammatory breast cancer, VI:773,
      776, 779f-780f
  in obese patient, I:525
  in Poland syndrome, I:563, 564f, VI:432,
      434, 493, 495f, 506, 509, VIII:142-
      143
  in tuberous breast, I:562-563
  inferior gluteal artery perforator flap
      for, VI:764t, 769-771, 769t, 952,
      953f
  lateral transverse thigh flap for,
      VI:1055f, 1056f-1057f, 1057-1058,
      1058f, 1063
  latissimus dorsi flap for, VI:686, 688f,
      690-711, 690t, 691f-695f, 697f-
      711f. *See also* Latissimus dorsi
      flap.
  microvascular composite tissue
      transplantation (free flap) for,
      I:440, VI:686, 690, 761-772, 762f,
      1039-1050, 1049t, 1053-1065
    advantages of, VI:1039-1040
    contraindications to, VI:763
    deep circumflex iliac artery (Rubens
        flap), VI:764t, 1053-1055
      patient position for, VI:1055f
      selection of, VI:1063
      surgical technique for, VI:771, 771f,
          772f, 1059-1060, 1059f, 1061f,
          1062f
    deep inferior epigastric artery, VI:686,
        762, 764t, 1040-1044
      anatomy of, VI:1040-1041
      bilateral, VI:1042
      complications of, VI:765t, 1044
      defect closure for, VI:1042, 1044
      surface markings for, VI:1040,
          1041f
      surgical technique for, VI:765-766,
          766f, 1002, 1004f, 1007f, 1008,
          1011, 1011f, 1012f, 1020,
          1020f, 1040t, 1041-1042
      unilateral, VI:1042, 1042f, 1043f
      vascular anatomy of, VI:1040-1041,
          1041f
    disadvantages of, VI:1040
    flap selection for, VI:762, 763-765,
        764t
    indications for, VI:762-763, 763t
    inferior gluteal artery, VI:764t, 769t,
        770-771, 952, 953f
    lateral transverse thigh, VI:1055f,
        1056f-1057f, 1057-1058, 1058f,
        1063
    nomenclature for, VI:1040
    receptor vessels for, VI:1047-1049,
        1048t
    results with, VI:1049, 1049f, 1050f
    superficial inferior epigastric artery,
        VI:764t, 766, 768-769, 768f
    superior gluteal artery, VI:764t, 1044-
        1047, 1045t, 1060, 1062, 1063f,
        1064f
      anatomy of, VI:1044-1045
      complications of, VI:1047
      defect closure for, VI:1047
      donor scar with, VI:1046f
      surface markings for, VI:1044-
          1045, 1044f-1046f

Breast reconstruction (*Continued*)
    surgical technique for, VI:769-770,
      769t, 1047, 1048f, 1049f
    vascular anatomy of, VI:1045-1047
    TRAM flap for, I:433, VI:713, 718,
      720, 762, 764t, 765-766, 765t,
      767f. *See also* Transverse rectus
      abdominis myocutaneous
      (TRAM) flap.
  muscle flap for, I:559-560
  patient consultation for, VI:781-783
  psychological factors in, I:78-79
  radiation therapy and, VI:668-670, 668t,
    669t, 670t, 782
  referral for, VI:673-674
  secondary, VI:1083-1170
    axillary fullness and, VI:1138f, 1141
    chemotherapy and, VI:1168, 1170
    envelope deformity and, VI:1093-1111
      evaluation of, VI:1090, 1090t
      excess ptosis in, VI:1105, 1107,
        1107f, 1108t
      flap loss in, VI:1101-1105, 1102f,
        1102t, 1103f, 1104f, 1105t,
        1106t
      infection in, VI:1108, 1111
      mastectomy skin loss in, VI:1093-
        1101, 1093f-1095f, 1095t,
        1096f-1098f, 1099-1100t,
        1101t
      skin deficiency in, VI:1108, 1108f,
        1109f, 1110f
    epigastric fullness and, VI:1147
    evaluation for, VI:1090-1092, 1090t,
      1091t, 1092t
    expander-implants for, VI:1084-1086,
      1085t
    flaps for, VI:1086
    implant explantation and, VI:1147-
      1150, 1148f-1149f, 1149t
    incidence of, VI:1088-1090, 1089t
    indications for, VI:1087-1088, 1087t,
      1088t
    inframammary line problems and,
      VI:1091, 1092t, 1150-1151,
      1150t, 1153-1156, 1153f-1156f
    lumpectomy and radiation-related
      defects and, VI:1142-1147,
      1142f-1146f
    mound deformity and, VI:1111-1150
      capsular contracture in, VI:1111-
        1120, 1111t, 1112f, 1112t,
        1113t, 1114t, 1115t, 1116t,
        1117f-1120f
      contour defects in, VI:1137-1147,
        1137f, 1137t, 1138f-1140f,
        1142f-1146f
      evaluation of, VI:1090-1091, 1091t
      fat necrosis in, VI:1134-1135,
        1136t, 1137t
      implant extrusion in, VI:1121-1122
      implant failure in, VI:1122-1124,
        1122t, 1123t, 1125f-1128f
      implant palpability in, VI:1121,
        1121t
      implant-related infection in,
        VI:1124, 1124t, 1127-1130,
        1128f, 1129f, 1131-1132t,
        1133f, 1134t
      skin wrinkling in, VI:1121, 1121t

Breast reconstruction (*Continued*)
    nipple-areola problems and, VI:1092,
      1164-1167, 1165t
    position deformity and, VI:1150-
      1156, 1150t, 1152f-1156f
      evaluation of, VI:1091, 1092t
    radiation therapy and, VI:1167-1168,
      1169f-1170f
    reconstruction outcomes and,
      VI:1086-1087
    scar problems and, VI:1157-1160,
      1157t, 1158f-1160f
      evaluation of, VI:1091-1092, 1092t
    symmetry problems and, VI:1160-
      1163, 1161t, 1162t, 1163f
      evaluation of, VI:1092, 1092t
  superficial inferior epigastric artery
    fasciocutaneous flap for, VI:764t,
    766, 768-769, 768f
  superior gluteal artery perforator flap
    for, VI:764t, 769-770, 769t, 1044-
    1047, 1045t, 1060, 1062, 1063f,
    1064f
    anatomy of, VI:1044-1045
    complications of, VI:1047
    defect closure for, VI:1047
    donor scar with, VI:1046f
    surface markings for, VI:1044-1045,
      1044f-1046f
    surgical technique for, VI:769-770,
      769t, 1047, 1048f, 1049f
    vascular anatomy of, VI:1045-1047
  symmetry in, VI:675
  technique selection for, VI:674-675,
    675f, 676f
  timing of, VI:781-782
  tissue expansion for, I:557-558, 561,
    VI:674-675, 676-677, 677f. *See also*
    Expander-implant breast
    reconstruction.
  transverse rectus abdominis
    myocutaneous (TRAM) flap for,
    VI:686, 689f, 712-761. *See also*
    Transverse rectus abdominis
    myocutaneous (TRAM) flap.
  tubed pedicle flap for, VI:686, 687f
Breast reduction, VI:539-581. *See also*
  Nipple reconstruction.
  abscess after, VI:578
  after radiation therapy, VI:575
  antibiotics for, VI:557
  asymmetry after, VI:580
  Bennelli round block technique for,
    VI:570-571, 572f
  Biesenberger technique of, VI:540, 542f
  blood flow after, VI:579
  blood transfusion for, VI:557
  boxy deformity after, VI:580
  breast cancer and, VI:581, 611, 1080-
    1081
  breast-feeding and, VI:580-581, 611, 625
  breast pain after, VI:578
  breast size for, VI:554-556, 555f
  cellulitis after, VI:578
  central mound technique for, VI:540,
    547f, 563
  complications of, VI:578-581, 611
  definition of, VI:539
  dermal-lipoglandular flap for, VI:603,
    604f

Breast reduction (*Continued*)
  dog-ears and, VI:581, 1068, 1071f
  drains for, VI:557
  epinephrine infiltration for, VI:557
  fat necrosis after, VI:578-579
  fibrocystic disease after, VI:1081
  goals of, VI:601
  Goes technique for, VI:571, 573f
  Hall-Findlay technique for, VI:564,
    567f
  hematoma after, VI:578
  Hester technique for, VI:540, 547f, 563
  historical perspective on, VI:539-550,
    540f-549f, 550t
  horizontal bipedicle technique for,
    VI:543f, 561
  horizontal scar technique for, VI:570
  hospitalization for, VI:557-558
  in adolescent, VI:577
  inadequate, VI:580
  inadequate mastopexy effect after,
    VI:581
  indications for, VI:553-554, 553t, 607-
    608
  infection after, VI:578
  inferior pedicle technique for, VI:559-
    560, 561f, 562f, 601-629, 602f, 616f-
    617f, 619f
    after lumpectomy and radiation,
      VI:620, 622, 622f
    breast cancer risk and, VI:611
    breast circulation and, Color Plates
      VI:137-1 to 137-3, VI:605f, 606-
      607, 607f
    breast-feeding and, VI:611, 625
    complications of, VI:611, 622, 624t,
      625
    de-epithelialization in, VI:615, 616f
    historical perspective on, VI:601, 603,
      603f-605f
    in gigantomastia, VI:608-609, 608f,
      621f, 626f-629f
    in large macromastia, VI:609-610,
      609f
    in moderate macromastia, VI:610,
      610f
    intraoperative positioning in, VI:615
    keyhole design in, VI:603, 605f
    markings for, VI:612-615, 613f-614f
    nipple-areola circulation check in,
      Color Plate VI:132-4, VI:618,
      620
    nipple-areola malposition after,
      VI:622, 623f, 624f
    nipple-areola necrosis after, VI:625
    nipple-areola positioning in, VI:612-
      615, 613f-614f, 617f, 618, 619f
    nipple-areola sensation after, VI:611,
      625
    patient age and, VI:610-611
    pedicle elevation in, VI:615-618, 616f-
      617f
    physical examination before, VI:611
    preoperative preparation in, VI:612-
      615, 613f-614f
    results of, VI:625, 626f-629f
    scars after, VI:611-612
    sutures for, VI:617f, 618
    tobacco use and, VI:611
    vs. vertical reduction, VI:612t

Breast reduction *(Continued)*
  Wise pattern resection in, VI:601-603, 602f
  with nipple-areolar grafts, VI:620, 621f
  intramammary scarring after, VI:580
  L-shaped scar technique for, VI:570, 570f, 571f
  lactation after, VI:1077-1078
  Lassus-Legour technique for, VI:563-568, 564f-566f, 568f, 569f
  lateral pedicle technique for, VI:561, 563
  liposuction for, VI:556, 558, 559f
  lower pole amputation for, VI:574, 575f-577f
  major, VI:556
  mammography after, VI:558, 1080
  Marchac short-scar technique for, VI:568-570, 569f
  massive, VI:556
  McKissock technique for, VI:540, 543f, 561
  medial pedicle technique for, VI:563
  medical malpractice suits in, I:143-144
  menopause after, VI:1078, 1079f
  nipple graft for, VI:574, 575f-577f
  nipple hypopigmentation in, VI:556
  nipple location for, VI:556
  nipple loss after, VI:579
  nipple numbness after, VI:579
  overresection with, VI:580
  pain after, VI:578
  Passot nipple transposition in, VI:539, 540f
  patient age and, VI:610-611
  patient position for, I:188
  patient selection for, VI:608-612, 608f, 609f, 610f
  periareolar techniques for, VI:570-574, 572f, 573f
  physical examination before, VI:611
  Pitanguy technique for, VI:540, 544f-546f, 561
  pregnancy after, VI:1077-1078
  psychological factors in, I:77
  quality of life after, VI:577-578
  recurrent hypertrophy after, VI:580, 1077-1078, 1078f-1080f
  results of, VI:547f, 577-578, 593-597, 594f-597f, 625, 626f-629f
  scars and, VI:580, 1068, 1069f, 1070f
  Schwarzmann technique of, VI:539-540, 541f
  secondary, VI:574, 580, 622, 1067-1081
    asymmetry and, VI:1070
    breast cancer after, VI:1080-1081
    complications of, VI:1081
    dog-ears and, VI:1068, 1071f
    epidermal cyst and, VI:1077
    fat necrosis and, VI:1068, 1070
    fibrocystic disease and, VI:1081
    high nipple and, VI:1074-1075, 1075f
    irregular pigmentation and, VI:1076
    liposuction in, VI:1078
    mammography after, VI:1080
    medicolegal considerations in, VI:1068
    nipple-areola contour irregularity and, VI:1076-1077
    nipple convergence and, VI:1075

Breast reduction *(Continued)*
    nipple divergence and, VI:1075, 1076f
    nipple necrosis and, VI:1072, 1074, 1074f
    overreduction and, VI:1070, 1072, 1072f
    patient-physician relationship in, VI:1067-1068
    postmenopausal, VI:1078, 1079f
    pregnancy and, VI:1077-1078, 1080f
    ptosis and, VI:1079-1080
    regrowth and, VI:1077-1078, 1078f, 1079f
    residual areola and, VI:1075-1076, 1076f
    scars and, VI:1068, 1069f, 1070f
    surgical technique of, VI:1078, 1080f
    underreduction and, VI:1069f, 1072, 1073f
    wound dehiscence and, Color Plate VI:149-1, VI:1070, 1071f
  seroma after, VI:578
  short-scar techniques for, VI:563-574, 563t, 564f-573f
  skin necrosis after, VI:578
  small-to-moderate, VI:556
  SPAIR technique for, VI:571, 573f
  Strombeck technique for, VI:540, 543f, 561
  superior pedicle technique for, VI:544f-546f, 561
  superomedial pedicle technique of, VI:540, 548f, 549f
  technique selection for, VI:554-555, 554t
  tobacco use and, VI:611
  upper arm fullness and, VI:292, 293f
  vertical bipedicle technique for, VI:543f, 561, 603, 603f
  vertical scar technique for, VI:563-564, 564f-567f, 585-599, 611-612
    breast shape after, VI:598
    closure for, VI:589, 591f, 592f
    complications of, VI:597-598
    de-epithelialization for, VI:587-588, 588f
    dissection for, VI:588-589, 588f-590f
    excess scarring with, VI:597-598
    excision markings for, VI:586-587, 587f
    incisions for, VI:588-589, 588f-590f
    mammostat for, VI:587-588, 588f
    markings for, VI:586-587, 586f, 587f
    modifications of, VI:592-593, 593f
    nipple position for, VI:586, 586f, 598
    patient selection for, VI:585-586
    results of, VI:593-597, 594f-597f
    SPAIR modification of, VI:592-593
    vs. inferior pedicle technique, VI:611-612, 612t
  weight gain after, VI:1077, 1078f
  Wise-pattern procedure for, VI:540, 546f, 558-559, 560f, 601-603, 602f
Breathing, periodic, III:775
Bretylium tosylate, in complex regional pain syndrome/reflex sympathetic dystrophy, VII:854-855
British Association of Plastic Surgeons Council, I:13f
Bromelain, VI:175, 177t

Bronchopleural fistula, VI:428-431, 429t, 430f
Brown recluse spider bite, I:931-932, 933f, 934f, 1017
  vs. hand infection, VII:768, 768f
Browpexy, II:64. *See also* Eyebrow lift.
Buccal fat
  anatomy of, II:170, 171f
  overexcision of, II:738-740, 739f
Buccal mucosa, V:163, 163f
  reconstruction of, III:925. *See also* Oral cavity reconstruction.
  verrucous carcinoma of, V:162
Buccal sulcus incision, for facial surgery, III:564
Buccinator, IV:59f, 73f
Buerger disease, VI:1475, VII:814-815, 814f
Bulimia nervosa, I:84-85, 85t
Bunnell transfer, for low median nerve palsy, VIII:465-466, 466f, 467f
Bupivacaine, I:190-191, 190t
  for facial anesthesia, III:7-8, 7t
Burkhalter transfer, for low median nerve palsy, VIII:463-464, 463f-465f
Burkitt lymphoma, of mandible, V:107, 212
Burns, I:811-832
  after breast reconstruction, VI:832
  anesthesia and, I:203
  burn center referral for, I:815, 815t
  compartment syndrome with, I:818, VII:591, 600-601
  complications of, I:203, 828-830
  contracture with
    in axilla, VII:630-633, 631f, 634f
    in elbow, VII:633, 635
    in hand, VII:616-624, 618f-620f, 622f, 623f
    in shoulder, VII:630-633, 631f, 634f
  degree of, I:816, 816f, 816t, 817-818, 817f
  depth of, I:816, 816f, 816t, 817-818, 817f
  electrical, I:831. *See also* Hand burns, electrical.
  epidemiology of, I:813-815, 813f-815f
  first degree, I:816, 816f, 816t
  gastrointestinal ulcers with, I:829
  heterotopic ossification with, I:829-830, VII:635-636
  hypertrophic scar after, I:830-831, 830f
  in child abuse, III:399
  infection with, I:828-829
  Marjolin ulcer after, I:916, 917f, III:612, V:275, 276f, 437-439, 437f, 437t, VI:446-447, 447f, VII:614
  of axilla, VII:630-633, 631f
  of ear, III:33
  of elbow, VII:633-636, 634f, 635-636
  of face, III:45-75. *See also* Facial burns.
  of hand, VII:605-642. *See also* Hand burns.
  of scalp, I:1004-1006, 1005f-1060f, III:611
  of shoulder, VII:630-633, 631f, 634f
  pathophysiology of, I:815-821, 816f, 816t
  prognosis for, I:813-814
  psychological factors in, I:78

Burns *(Continued)*
  radiation. *See* Radiation injury.
  second degree, I:816, 816f, 816t, 817, 817f
  skin cancer and, V:275
  smoke inhalation with, I:831-832, 832f
  tar, I:831
  third degree, I:816, 816f, 816t, 817-818, 817f
  total body surface area in, I:813-814, 814f, 815f
  treatment of, I:821-828
    AlloDerm in, I:824t, 827
    Biobrane in, I:824t, 825
    biologic dressings in, I:823-825, 824f, 824t, VII:592
    colloid administration in, I:820, 820t
    complications of, I:828-830
    crystalloid administration in, I:820-821, 820t
    cultured epidermal autograft in, I:818, 825, 826f
    débridement in, I:822-823, 1000
    dermal replacement materials in, I:824t, 825-827, 827f
    escharotomy in, I:818, 818f, 1000
    fluid resuscitation in, I:203, 818-821, 819f, 820t
    historical perspective on, I:811-813, 812t
    Integra in, I:824t, 826-827, 827f
    isolation for, I:829
    nutrition in, I:821, 821t, 1004
    ointments in, I:822
    pain control in, I:828
    reconstruction after, I:830-831, 830f
    rehabilitation in, I:827-828
    skin graft in, I:818, 822, 823-827, 824f, 824t, 826f, 827f
    split-thickness skin graft in, I:824f, 824t, 825, 826f
    surgical, I:822-823
    topical dressings in, I:822
    TransCyte in, I:824t, 825
    wound care in, I:821-827, 824f, 824t, 826f, 827f
  wound healing and, I:930-931, 930f, 931f, 1000, 1004-1006, 1005f-1006f
Buschke-Löwenstein tumors, V:446
Busulfan, limb deformity and, VIII:61-62
Butorphanol, I:182-183
Buttocks
  hemangioma of, V:28f
  lift for, Color Plate VI:125-4, VI:262-265, 265f, 266f
  liposuction of, VI:230, 230f, 231f

C

Caffeine, in obstructive sleep apnea, III:776
Calcaneal nerve, neuroma of, VII:919-920, 945
Calcaneus, pressure sores of, VI:1347, 1347t
Calcification, vs. hand infection, VII:767-768
Calcifying epithelial odontogenic tumor, V:199
Calcitonin, in complex regional pain syndrome/reflex sympathetic dystrophy, VII:859-860

Calcitonin gene-related peptide, in complex regional pain syndrome/reflex sympathetic dystrophy, VII:838-839
Calcium alginate, I:225t, 884-885, 885t
Calcium carbonate, for hydrofluoric acid burn, VII:656
Calcium channel blockers, in complex regional pain syndrome/reflex sympathetic dystrophy, VII:856-857
Calcium gluconate, for hydrofluoric acid burn, VII:656
Calcium phosphate bone substitutes, I:693t, 696-700, 1000, 1001t
  in vivo properties of, I:697-700
Calcium phosphate cements, I:694t, 700-702
Calcium phosphate implants, I:753-756, 754f, 755f
Calcium sulfate bone substitutes, I:693t, 695-696, 1000, 1001t
Calcium sulfate implants, I:755
Calculi, of salivary glands, V:75, 75f, 76f
Calf, liposuction for, VI:232, 234f-236f, 235, 288
Calvarial bone graft, I:675t, 688-691, 689f
  for cranioplasty, III:549, 554f, 555, 555f-557f
  for rhinoplasty, II:552-553, 553f
  in pediatric head injury, III:442, 444, 445f
  vascularized (temporoparietal flap), I:688-691, 690f, 691f
CAM walker boot, VI:1443
Camitz transfer, for low median nerve palsy, VIII:466, 467f, 468f
Camptodactyly, VIII:280, 286-294
  anatomy of, VIII:288, 289f, 290f
  clinical presentation of, VIII:288-289
  differential diagnosis of, VIII:289, 292
  incidence of, VIII:40t, 41t, 286-287
  outcomes of, VIII:293-294
  pathogenesis of, VIII:287-288, 288f-290f
  radiology of, VIII:289, 291f, 292
  syndromic associations of, VIII:287, 287f
  treatment of, VIII:292-293, 293f, 564-565
Canaliculus, trauma to, III:25-26, 26f
Cancer, I:1053-1064. *See also specific cancers.*
  aggressiveness of, I:1057-1058
  atomic bomb and, I:843, 847f
  barriers to, I:1058
  breast. *See* Breast cancer.
  classification of, I:1060-1061
  clinical evaluation of, I:1060-1061
  doubling time of, I:1057-1058
  histologic classification of, I:1060-1061
  in burn scar, VII:614
  morphologic classification of, I:1060
  pathobiology of, I:1057-1060
    cellular differentiation in, I:1057
    critical mass in, I:1057-1058
    radiation-induced, I:842-844, 845t, 846f, 847f
  recurrence of, I:1058-1059, 1059f
  spread of, I:1061-1062, 1062f
  submicroscopic tumor levels in, I:1058-1060

Cancer *(Continued)*
  surgery for, I:1054, 1061-1063, 1062f
    recurrence and, I:1058-1059, 1059f
    tumor margins and, I:1058-1060, 1058f
  thickness of, I:1061
  TNM classification of, I:1060
  treatment of, I:1061-1063, 1062f
    chemotherapy in, I:1055-1056, 1063
    history of, I:1053-1057
    immunotherapy in, I:1056-1057
    photoradiation in, I:1063-1064, 1064t
    radiation therapy in, I:1054-1055, 1055f, 1055t, 1063-1064
      nerve repair after, I:738
    surgery in, I:1054, 1061-1063, 1062f
  upper extremity ischemia in, VII:815
  wound healing and, I:916-918, 916f-918f, 981, 983, 984f
Candidiasis, V:401
  after laser resurfacing, II:371, 371f
Cannula
  for liposuction, VI:194-196, 195f, 209, 238
  nasal, I:175
Canthal tendon, lateral, II:81, 81f
Cantharides, hand injury from, VII:654
Canthopexy, III:738
  corono-, II:124-125, 125f
  lateral, II:111-112, 112f, 115-122, 239, 242, 242f
    exophthalmos and, II:96
    in secondary lower lid repair, II:818-819, 819f, 821, 821f
    into bone, II:118-122, 120f-123f
    into periosteum, II:115-118, 116f, 117f, 119f
    transnasal, III:745, 748f-751f
  medial
    in orbital hypertelorism, IV:372, 373f, 375-376
    transnasal, III:743-745, 743t, 744f-747f
Canthoplasty, lateral
  dermal-orbicular pennant, II:847-851, 848f-852f
  in lower lid laxity, III:896
  in secondary blepharoplasty, II:841-851, 843t, 844t
  inferior retinacular, II:842-846, 843t, 845f, 846f
  tarsal strip, II:843t, 846-847, 846f, 847f
Canthus
  lateral
    cat-like appearance of, II:236
    in eyebrow lift, II:221
  medial
    dystopia of, with craniofacial cleft management, IV:461
    reconstruction of, forehead flap for, V:369, 373f-375f
    webs of, after facial burn excision and grafting, III:60, 61f-62f
Cantrell, pentalogy of, VI:483-484
Capases, in apoptosis, I:496
Capillaries, I:317, 319f
  in tissue expansion, I:541-542, 542f, 543f
  malformations of. *See* Capillary malformations.
Capillaroscopy, in hand ischemia, VII:797

Capillary-arteriovenous malformation (Parkes Weber syndrome), V:60, 60f, VIII:309, 312t, 412-413, 413t

Capillary blood velocity, in complex regional pain syndrome/reflex sympathetic dystrophy, VII:846

Capillary-lymphatic-venous malformation (Klippel-Trénaunay syndrome), V:56-60, 58f, 59f, VIII:408-409, 409f, 410f, 413t
  bleeding in, V:60
  imaging of, V:57-58, 59f
  macrodactyly in, VIII:309, 311f, 316-317
  management of, V:58, 60
  overgrowth in, V:58

Capillary malformations, V:37-41, VIII:380, 381f
  clinical presentation of, V:37-39, 37f, 38f
  cosmetic creams in, V:39-40, 39f
  in Klippel-Trénaunay syndrome, V:56-60, 58f, 59f, VIII:408-409, 409f, 410f, 413t
  in Parkes Weber syndrome, V:60, 60f, VIII:309, 312t, 412-413, 413t
  in Sturge-Weber syndrome, V:39, 39f, VIII:380
  laser therapy for, V:40, 40f
  management of, V:39-40, 39f, 40f
  operative management of, V:40, 40f
  pathogenesis of, V:37
  radiological features of, V:39

Capillary refill test, VII:45-46, 46f-47f

Capitohamate ligament, VII:456f

Capitotrapezoid ligament, VII:456f

Capsaicin, in complex regional pain syndrome/reflex sympathetic dystrophy, VII:857

Capsulectomy, in secondary breast augmentation, VI:319-320

Capsulitis, in temporomandibular joint dysfunction, III:537

Capsulopalpebral fascia, II:85

Capsulotomy, after breast augmentation, VI:28-29, 326

Carbamazepine, in complex regional pain syndrome/reflex sympathetic dystrophy, VII:858

Carbon dioxide/Er:YAG laser, for facial resurfacing, II:351-355, 353f-355f

Carbon dioxide laser
  airway fire hazard of, I:202
  anesthesia for, I:202
  eye protection with, I:202
  for facial resurfacing, II:70, 70f, 347, 350, 351f
  for neck resurfacing, II:366, 366f
  hazards of, I:202

Carbonated calcium phosphate cement, I:694t, 701-702

Cardiomyocytes, after infarction, I:612

Cardiomyoplasty, I:615

Cardiopulmonary bypass, fetal, I:1125

Carotid artery, II:85, 85f, IV:78f, 81
  injury to, with mandibular fracture treatment, III:181
  occlusion of, in fetal sheep, IV:114
  rupture of, III:1072, 1076, 1076f

Carotid-cavernous sinus fistula, in frontobasilar region fractures, III:335

Carpal bones, VII:17-18, 17f, 20. See also Hand(s).
  ballottement tests for, VII:54
  fracture of, VII:464-467, 465f, 466f
    in children, VIII:423-424
  greater arc of, VII:19, 20f
  instability of, VII:134-135, 467-468, 467f, 468f
  lesser arc of, VII:19, 20f
  ligaments of, VII:20-21
  motion of, VII:20-21

Carpal coalition, VIII:272

Carpal hand, VIII:56-60

Carpal instability, VII:134-135, 467-468, 467f, 468f

Carpal tunnel syndrome, I:45, VII:876t, 885-889
  coexisting compressions in, VII:885
  failed decompression in, VII:885-889, 886f-888f
  in musician, VII:702-703
  internal neurolysis in, VII:884
  motor branch of median nerve in, VII:885, 888
  postoperative management in, VII:884-885, VIII:562-563
  vs. cubital tunnel syndrome, VII:894-895
  vs. reflex sympathetic dystrophy/chronic regional pain syndrome, VII:849-850, 852

Carpectomy, VII:133

Carpenter syndrome, III:778, IV:100. See also Craniosynostosis (craniosynostoses), syndromic.

Carpometacarpal joint
  finger
    dislocation of, VII:434, 435f
    fracture-dislocation/subluxation of, VII:434-436
    osteoarthritis of, VII:57f, 719-724
      abductor pollicis longus tenoplasty for, Color Plate VII:191-1, VII:720-722, 723f
      arthrodesis for, VII:722, 724
      Silastic arthroplasty for, VII:720, 721f, 722f
  thumb, VII:17, 17f, 23
    dislocation of, VII:433-434
    fracture-dislocation/subluxation of, VII:434-436, 435f

Cartilage, I:621-634
  age-related changes in, I:623
  anatomy of, Color Plate I:23-2, I:622, 623t
  elastic, Color Plate I:23-1, I:621
  flexibility of, I:623-624, 623f, 624f
  for nipple projection, VI:809, 810t, 811
  function of, I:622-623
  healing of, I:628-629
  hyaline, Color Plate I:23-1, I:621
  injury to, I:628-629
  neocartilage interaction with, I:628-629, 629f
  perichondrium of, I:623-624, 624f
  tissue-engineered, Color Plate I:37-3, I:1097-1099, 1098f, 1099t
  tumor of, in children, V:12
  types of, I:622, 623t

Cartilage graft, I:281, 621-634
  allogeneic (allograft), I:281, 626-627, 628
  autologous (autograft), I:281
  bioengineering for, I:622, 627, 629-633, 629f
  cells for, I:630
  collagen for, I:631
  fibrin for, I:631-632
  hyaluronan for, I:631
  hydrogels for, I:631
  perichondrial simulation for, Color Plate I:23-4, I:633, 634f
  polyglycolic acid scaffold for, I:632, 632f, 633
  poly(ethylene oxide) scaffold for, I:632-633
  polytetrafluoroethylene for, Color Plate I:23-3, I:633, 634f
  scaffolds for, I:630-633
  sodium alginate for, I:631
  cryopreservation for, I:627-628
  disease transmission with, I:628
  donor site for, I:622, 624-626, 625f, 626f
  freeze-drying for, I:628
  from ear, I:624, 625, 625f, 626f
  from nasal septum, I:624, 625f, 626, II:459, 459t
  from rib, I:623, 623f, 624-625, 625f
  in alar reconstruction, II:600, 605, 606f-612f
  in nasal lining skin graft, II:618, 623f-625f
  in rhinoplasty, II:458-461
    from ear, II:459-460, 459t, 460f
    from rib, II:459-461, 459t, 460f, 461f
    from septum, II:459, 459t
  indications for, I:621
  perichondrium for, I:626
  periosteum for, I:626
  preservation techniques for, I:627-628
  refrigeration for, I:627
  xenogeneic (xenograft), I:281, 626-627, 628

Cartilaginous auditory tube, IV:58f

Case-control study design, I:38, 40f

Case reports, I:38-39

Case series, I:38-39

Casuistry, I:105-106

Cat-scratch disease, VII:763-764

Categorical imperative, I:99

Catheter
  antibiotic-coated, I:763
  epidural, in pain management, I:195-196

Cauliflower ear, III:677

Causalgia, VII:826, 835, 851-852. See also Complex regional pain syndrome/reflex sympathetic dystrophy.

Cavernous nerve repair, Color Plate I:25-3, I:737-738

Cbfa1, IV:9

CD18 monoclonal antibody, in experimental neutrophil-mediated reperfusion injury, I:491-492, 492f, 493f, 496

CD11b/CD18, in neutrophil-endothelial adhesion, I:489-490, 490f

Celecoxib, I:183-184

Cell adhesion molecules, in nerve regeneration, VII:480

Cellist, hand disorders in, VII:694, 698f
Cellulite, VI:92, 282
Cellulitis. *See also* Infection.
  after breast reduction, VI:578
  after free TRAM flap, VI:872
  assessment of, I:864, 865f
  lymphatic malformations and, V:44, 45f,
    VIII:393
Celsus, I:27
Cemental dysplasia, periapical, V:98
Cementifying fibroma, V:98
Cemento-osseous dysplasia, V:202, 204
Cementoblastoma, V:98, 202
Central giant cell granuloma, V:102-103,
  208-209
Central mound technique, for breast
  reduction, VI:540, 547f, 563
Central nervous system. *See also* Peripheral
    nerve(s).
  bispectral index of, I:189
  congenital anomalies of. *See*
    Encephalocele;
    Meningoencephalocele.
  hypersensitive state of, VII:87-88, 88f
  injury to, VI:1317, 1318t. *See also*
    Pressure sore(s); Spastic hand;
    Tetraplegia.
  monitoring of, during anesthesia, I:189
  preoperative evaluation of, I:169-170
Centrofacial flattening procedure, in
    Treacher Collins syndrome, IV:509,
    509f
Cephalometry, II:15, 18-28, 19f, 20t, 21t.
    See also Anthropometry.
  chin in, II:26, 28f
  cranial base in, II:23
  facial height in, II:26
  in craniofacial microsomia, IV:129-131,
    129f, 130f
  landmarks for, II:19f, 20t
  mandible in, II:24, 26, 26f, 27f
  maxilla in, II:23, 24f
  orbits in, II:23, 23f
  reference planes for, II:20f, 21t
  soft tissues in, II:19, 26-27
  step 1 (tracing), II:19, 21, 21f
  step 2 (regions), II:23-27, 23f-28f
  teeth in, II:23-24, 25f
  worksheet for, II:22t
Cephalopolysyndactyly, VIII:21t, 22
Ceramic implants, I:693t, 696-700, 752-
    756, 753f-755f, 754t
Cerberus protein, IV:2
Cerebral blood flow
  in hypothermia, I:858
  propofol effects on, I:174
Cerebral edema, high-altitude, I:861
Cerebral ischemia, with craniofacial cleft
    management, IV:459
Cerebrospinal fluid leak
  after closed rhinoplasty, II:564
  fistula and, I:924, 924f, IV:459
  in frontobasilar region fracture, III:334-
    335
  in maxillary fracture, III:239, 251-252
  in nasoethmoidal-orbital fracture,
    III:313-314, 314f, 315, 330
  in pediatric facial trauma, III:455
  with craniofacial cleft management,
    IV:459

Cerebrum, anomalies of, in craniofacial
    microsomia, IV:122
Cervical spine
  injury to. *See also* Spastic hand;
    Tetraplegia.
    facial fracture and, III:83-85, 84f
  osteomyelitis of, neck reconstruction in,
    III:1076
Cervicofacial fascia, II:297, 299, 300f, 301-
    302, 303f
Cervicofacial flap
  for cheek reconstruction, III:833, 837f-
    840f
  for midface reconstruction, III:872, 874f
Cervicofacial hike procedure, II:234, 236f
Cervicohumeral flap, for cheek
    reconstruction, III:833, 844f
CHAOS (congenital high airway
    obstruction syndrome), I:1121-1122,
    1121f
Charcot neuroarthropathy, VI:1444-1445.
    See also Diabetes mellitus, foot
    reconstruction in.
CHARGE syndrome, choanal atresia in,
    III:763-764
Checkrein ligaments, VII:22, 664-665, 667f
Cheek(s). *See also* Cheek reconstruction.
  aesthetic zones of, III:831, 831f
  anatomy of, III:26, 831, 831f
  basal cell carcinoma of, III:833, 840f-
    842f
  blood supply of, III:26
  cervicofacial hike for, II:234, 236f
  giant hairy nevus of, I:551, 554f
  hemangioma of, V:28f, 32
  innervation of, III:26
  superficial lift of, II:244, 245f-248f
  trauma to, III:26-27, 27f, 28f
  wrinkle lines of, III:831-833, 832f
Cheek flap, for lower eyelid reconstruction,
    V:360, 364f, 368f, 369, 370f
Cheek lift, II:244, 245f-248f
Cheek reconstruction, III:831-857, V:369,
    375-381, 376f-380f
  advancement flap for, V:375-376, 378f-
    380f, 381
  anatomy for, III:831-833, 832f
  cervicofacial flap for, III:833, 837f-840f
  cervicohumeral flap for, III:833, 844f
  deltopectoral flap for, III:833, 843f, 848f
  direct closure in, III:831, 832f
  Dufourmentel flap for, III:833, 837f
  finger flap for, V:381
  in basal cell carcinoma, III:833, 840f-
    842f
  in cystic hygroma, III:833, 834f-836f
  in intraoral carcinoma, III:833, 849f-
    850f
  in Romberg disease, III:833, 852f-853f,
    865f
  in witch's chin deformity, III:833, 854f-
    857f
  island flap for, V:381
  Limberg flap for, III:833, 836f
  Mustardé rotation flap for, I:551, 553,
    554f
  omental flap for, III:833, 851f, 852f-853f
  pectoralis major flap for, III:833, 845f,
    848f
  platysma flap for, III:833, 847f

Cheek reconstruction *(Continued)*
  rhomboid flap for, V:346, 346f
  rotation flap for, V:369, 375, 376f, 377f
  skin graft for, III:833, 849f-850f
  tissue expansion for, III:833, 841f-842f,
    V:388, 388f
  transposition flap for, V:376, 381
  trapezius flap for, III:833, 846f
Cheilitis, actinic, V:446
Cheiloplasty. *See also at* Cleft lip, unilateral;
    Lip reconstruction.
  adhesion, IV:182-184, 183f-187f
  Mohler's, IV:200-202, 200f-203f
  rotation-advancement, IV:186, 188-195,
    188f-196f, 202, 204f, 205f
Chemical injury
  intravenous, I:932, 935f, 936, 936f, 1012,
    1016, 1016f
  of hand, VII:653-656, 653t, 655t
Chemical peels, facial, II:70, 258-259, 343-
    344, 343t, 379-380, 379t, 380f
Chemical sympathectomy, in frostbite,
    VII:652
Chemosis, with periorbital reconstruction,
    III:745
Chemotherapy, I:1055-1056
  adjuvant, I:1063
  extravasation of, I:932, 935f, 936, 936f,
    1012, 1016, 1016f
  hair loss and, II:691
  in actinic keratoses, Color Plate V:116-2,
    V:404-405, 404t
  in breast cancer, VI:666-667, 667t, 670-
    671, 1168, 1170
  in melanoma, I:983
  in skin cancer, V:286t, 288, 403-406,
    404t
  wound healing and, I:221, 911, 937
Cherry, George, I:32
Cherubism, V:12, 101-102, 101f, 102f, 209
Chest wall
  anatomy of, VI:411-413, 412f
  congenital anomalies of, VI:431-434,
    433f, 457-533. *See also specific*
    anomalies and at Chest wall
    reconstruction.
    mammary, VI:509-533. *See also at*
      Breast(s).
    thoracic, VI:457-509. *See also at*
      Rib(s); Sternum; Thorax.
  osteoradionecrosis of, I:910-911, 911f,
    967, 972f-973f
Chest wall reconstruction, I:441, 445f, 446,
    985, 990, 991f, VI:411-438
  anatomy for, VI:411-413, 412f
  evaluation for, VI:413
  historical perspective on, VI:411
  in cleft sternum, VI:431, 479-482, 481f,
    482f, 483t
  in ectopia cordis, VI:482-483, 483f
  in Jeune syndrome, VI:484-485, 484f,
    485f
  in pectus carinatum, VI:432, 477-478,
    479f, 480f
  in pectus excavatum, VI:431-432, 458-
    477. *See also* Pectus excavatum.
  in pentalogy of Cantrell, VI:483-484
  in Poland syndrome, VI:432, 434, 490-
    493, 492f, 494f, 495f. *See also*
    Poland syndrome.

Chest wall reconstruction *(Continued)*
  in posterior midline chest wall defects,
    VI:434-436, 435f-438f
  in sternal infection, VI:425-427, 425t,
    427f, 428f
  in sternal tumors, VI:427
  indications for, VI:413, 424t
  latissimus dorsi flap for, I:441, 446,
    VI:414-417, 414f, 415f, 420f-421f
  metallic bars in, VI:432
  methyl methacrylate glue in, VI:414
  omental flap for, Color Plate VI:132-2,
    I:446, 990, 991f, VI:417, 424, 427,
    428f, 435-438, 437f, 438f
  outcomes of, VI:424-425
  pectoralis major flap for, I:441, 445f,
    990, VI:414, 416, 416f-419f, 426-
    427f
  polypropylene mesh in, VI:414
  polytetrafluoroethylene mesh in, VI:414,
    415f
  Ravitch procedure for, VI:432, 433f
  rectus abdominis flap for, I:446, VI:417
  serratus anterior flap for, Color Plate
    VI:132-1, I:446, VI:417, 422f, 423f
  silicone implants for, VI:432
  thoracoepigastric flap for, I:990
  trapezius flap for, I:990
Chilblain, I:858
Child abuse
  facial injury in, III:399-400, 399f
  hand burns in, VII:588, 590f
  radiologic evaluation of, III:399-400,
    399f
Children. *See also specific congenital
    anomalies and syndromes.*
  acute life-threatening events in, III:771
  alveolar soft part sarcoma in, V:14
  arrhinia in, III:763, 764, 765f
  arteriovenous malformation in, III:775,
    V:6-7, 51-54, 52f-54f, VIII:397-407,
    397t, 398f-408f. *See also*
    Arteriovenous malformation.
  branchial arch disorders in, I:945,
    IIII:1025-1027, 1026f, 1027f, V:3-4
  breast cancer in, V:16
  breast papillomatosis in, V:16
  burns in, VII:587-588, 589f
  capillary malformations in, V:37-41,
    37f-40f. *See also* Capillary
    malformations.
  cartilage tumors in, V:12
  choanal atresia in, III:763-764
  chondrosarcoma in, V:15
  congenital anomalies in
    amputation, VIII:185-211. *See also*
      Constriction ring syndrome.
    craniofacial, IV:15-41. *See also*
      Craniofacial cleft(s); Craniofacial
      syndromes; Craniosynostosis
      (craniosynostoses).
    digit duplication, VIII:215-261. *See
      also* Polydactyly.
    digit growth, VIII:265-317, 323-365.
      See also at Finger(s); Thumb(s).
    digit separation, VIII:139-180. *See
      also* Syndactyly.
    upper extremity, VIII:25-49, 51-131,
      580, 584. *See also at* Arm(s);
      Hand(s).

Children *(Continued)*
  vascular, V:19-61, VIII:369-413, 370t.
    See also Capillary
    malformations; Hemangioma;
    Vascular malformations; Venous
    malformations.
  cranial growth in, III:382f, 383f, 388,
    388f
  craniopharyngioma in, III:767
  cutaneous adnexal tumors in, V:12-13,
    13f
  cutis marmorata telangiectasia
    congenita in, V:40-41, 41f
  dermoid cysts in, III:765, V:4, 4f, 5f
  digital fibrous tumors in, V:11
  epiglottitis in, III:770
  Ewing sarcoma in, V:15, 107, 212,
    VII:991
  facial growth in, III:382-388, 382f-386f,
    383t, 388f
  facial trauma in, III:381-456, 770. *See
    also* Facial fracture(s), pediatric;
    Facial trauma, pediatric.
  fibromatosis colli in, V:10-11
  fibrosarcoma in, V:14
  fibrous dysplasia in, V:12, 12f
  fingernail injury in, VIII:426
  fingertip injury in, VIII:426, 427f
  forearm fracture in, VIII:420-423, 422f
  foreign body aspiration in, III:769-770
  fracture in, VIII:420-424, 422f
  gastroesophageal reflux disease in,
    III:771
  glioma in, III:765
  glottic webs in, III:769
  hemangioma in, III:772-774, 773f, V:20-
    34. *See also* Hemangioma.
  hemangiopericytoma in, V:14-15
  kaposiform hemangioendothelioma in,
    V:35-36, 36f
  lacrimal duct cyst in, III:765
  laryngomalacia in, III:768-769
  leiomyosarcoma in, V:15
  lipomatosis in, V:9-10
  liposarcoma in, V:15
  Ludwig angina in, III:770, V:2
  lymphadenopathy in, V:2
  lymphatic malformations in, V:7-8, 8f,
    42-47, 43f-46f
  lymphoma in, III:771-772
  malignant mesenchymoma in, V:15
  nasoethmoid meningoencephalocele in,
    III:765, 765f
  nasopharyngeal angiofibroma in, V:11
  nasopharyngeal carcinoma in, V:16
  nasopharyngeal hamartoma in, III:766
  nasopharyngeal obstruction in, III:763-
    767, 764f-766f
  nasopharyngeal teratoma in, III:766,
    766f
  neck reconstruction in. *See* Neck
    reconstruction, pediatric.
  neuroblastoma in, V:13, 119
  neurofibroma in, V:8-9, 9f, 10f
  nose in, III:388, 389f, 390-391
  odontogenic tumors in, V:11, 11f
  osteoblastoma in, V:11-12
  osteogenic tumors in, V:11-12
  osteoid osteoma in, V:11-12
  osteosarcoma in, V:15

Children *(Continued)*
  paranasal sinuses of, III:386f, 387-388,
    388f
  peripheral nerve injury in, VIII:427-428
  pharyngotonsillitis in, III:770
  pilomatrixoma of, V:12-13, 13f
  piriform aperture stenosis in, III:763
  pyogenic granuloma in, V:3, 3f, 34-35,
    35f
  respiratory papillomatosis in, III:770
  retinoblastoma in, V:15
  retropharyngeal abscess in, V:2
  rhabdomyosarcoma in, III:772, V:13-14,
    14f, 114, 114f, 115, 118, 127, 129f,
    VII:973
  salivary gland tumors in, V:15-16
  sternal wound infection in, I:981
  subglottic hemangioma in, III:768
  subglottic stenosis in, III:769
  synovial sarcoma in, V:14
  tendon injury in, VII:378-379, 378f,
    VIII:28-29, 28f, 424-426, 580-582
  teratoma in, V:5-6
  thyroglossal duct remnants in, V:4
  thyroid cancer in, V:16
  tissue expansion in, I:546-547
  tuberculosis in, V:2
  tufted angioma in, V:36-37
  tumors in, V:1-16
    benign, V:2-13. *See also specific benign
      tumors.*
    diagnosis of, V:1-2
    etiology of, V:1
    malignant, V:13-16, 14f. *See also
      specific malignant tumors.*
  radiation-induced, V:149, 152f-153f
  turbinate hypertrophy in, III:765
  upper extremity trauma in, VIII:417-
    429. *See also at* Hand(s); Hand
    reconstruction.
    emergency care in, VIII:417-418, 418t
  vascular anomalies in, III:774-775, V:19-
    61, VIII:369-413, 370t. *See also*
    Capillary malformations;
    Hemangioma; Vascular
    malformations; Venous
    malformations.
  vascular injury in, VIII:428-429
  venous malformations in, V:6, 8f, 47-51.
    See also Venous malformations.
  vocal cord paralysis in, III:769
Chimeric flaps, in microvascular surgery,
  I:526-527, 527f
Chin
  aesthetic analysis of, II:5t, 15, 15f-18f,
    26, 28f
  augmentation of, II:414, 418-419, 418f-
    420f
    implant design for, II:414, 418, 418f
    implant failure after, III:599, 600f
    implant position for, II:418, 419f
    implant selection for, II:418
    technique for, II:418-419, 420f
  cephalometric analysis of, II:26, 28f
  reconstruction of, III:599, 600f-602f
    after radiation injury, III:599, 601f-
      602f
    iliac osteocutaneous flap for, III:599,
      603f-604f
    in craniofacial cleft, IV:444-446, 445f

Chin (Continued)
    in craniofacial microsomia, IV:533, 538f, 539f, 550, 551f, 552f
    in obstructive sleep apnea, III:790-791, 792f
    microsurgical, III:599, 603f-604f
    witch's deformity of, III:833, 854f-857f
2-Chloroprocaine, I:190t
Choanal atresia, III:763-764, IV:422, 422f
Choke arteries, I:319f, 324, 326f
Cholesterol, defects in, IV:12
Choline acetyltransferase, after reinnervation, I:608
Chondritis, suppurative, of ear, III:33-34
Chondrocytes, in tissue engineering, Color Plate I:37-3, I:1097-1099, 1098f, 1099t
Chondroma
    mandibular, V:207
    periosteal, VII:984, 985f
Chondromalacia, of wrist, VII:134
Chondrosarcoma
    in children, V:15
    in Maffucci syndrome, V:56
    of hand, VII:988, 989f
    of mandible, V:106-107, 108f-109f, 211-212
    radiation-related, V:149, 152f-153f
Chopart amputation, VI:1430
Chordee, VI:1208, 1210-1212, 1211f, 1212f
Chorionic villus sampling, I:1073-1074
Chromatolysis, VII:478-479, 478f
Chromic acid injury, of hand, VII:653-654
Chromosome analysis, I:54-55, 56f
Chronic obstructive pulmonary disease, propofol anesthesia and, I:174
Chronic regional pain syndrome. See Complex regional pain syndrome/reflex sympathetic dystrophy.
Chronic venous insufficiency, VI:1464-1473. See also Lower extremity, chronic venous insufficiency of.
Chuang triangle, in brachial plexus injury, VII:528-529, 529f
Chylothorax, congenital, I:1125
Cigarette smoking
    abdominoplasty and, VI:175, 364, 371
    breast reconstruction and, I:905, VI:995-996
    breast reduction and, VI:611
    cessation of, I:168-169, VII:802
    head and neck cancer and, V:159
    microvascular surgery and, I:525
    oral cavity cancer and, III:918
    replantation surgery and, VII:567
    skin cancer and, V:394
Ciliary neurotrophic factor, VII:480
Cimetidine, preoperative, I:171
Cinefluoroscopy, in velopharyngeal dysfunction, IV:317, 317f
Circulation. See also Vascular anatomy; Vascular territories.
    historical studies of, I:15-18, 15f-18f
Circumcision, necrosis after, VI:1217-1218, 1219f
Circumferential torsoplasty, VI:171-172, 172f, 173f
Cisatracurium, I:180t, 181
Civatte, poikiloderma of, II:388, 390f
Clagett procedure, VI:430-431

Clarinetist, hand disorders in, VII:695
Clasped thumb, VIII:282-286, 283f-286f
    classification of, VIII:283
    clinical presentation of, VIII:282-283, 284f
    differential diagnosis of, VIII:283, 285f
    outcomes of, VIII:286
    treatment of, VIII:283, 285f, 286f, 564
Claw hand, VIII:471-473, 472f, 473f
Clear cell hidradenoma, V:259
Clear cell odontogenic tumor, V:199
Cleft, craniofacial. See Craniofacial cleft(s).
Cleft alveolus, IV:50, 50f, 51, 169f, 181-182
    bone grafting in, IV:181-182, 263-266, 265f
        donor site for, IV:264-265
        rationale for, IV:263
        technique of, IV:265-266, 265f
        timing of, IV:263-264
    classification of, IV:82-87, 85f, 85t
    external taping for, IV:177-178, 177f, 178f
    gingivoperiosteoplasty for, IV:181-182
    Grayson method molding for, IV:178-179, 179f
    Liou method molding for, IV:178, 179f
    periosteoplasty in, IV:181
Cleft hand, VIII:80, 82-101, 82t, 350-353, 351f, 352f
    adductor pollicis muscle in, VIII:84, 93, 141f
    angiography in, VIII:84, 87f-88f
    associated malformations of, VIII:84
    atypical, VIII:110-131, 353-355, 353f, 354f. See also Symbrachydactyly.
    classification of, VIII:80, 82, 82t, 83f
    cleft depth in, VIII:83f, 84, 85f
    clinical presentation of, VIII:84-92, 85f-92f
    flexion contractures in, VIII:84, 90f, 96
    genetics of, VIII:84
    incidence of, VIII:82
    pathogenesis of, VIII:82-84
    single-digit, VIII:84, 87f-89f, 98, 98t
    thumb duplication in, VIII:86f, 98
    treatment of, VIII:92-98, 93t
        adductor pollicis in, VIII:93
        aesthetics of, VIII:92, 92f
        digital flexion contracture in, VIII:96
        first web space in, VIII:97-98, 97f
        foot treatment and, VIII:101
        in monodactylic hand, VIII:98, 98t
        incisions for, VIII:93, 94f, 95f
        index ray in, VIII:93
        indications for, VIII:92
        intermetacarpal ligament reconstruction in, VIII:93, 96f
        metacarpal osteotomy in, VIII:93
        outcomes of, VIII:98, 100f, 101
        thumb in, VIII:98, 99f
Cleft lip, IV:45-53, 250-251. See also Cleft palate.
    AlloDerm augmentation in, I:575
    alveolus and, IV:50, 50f, 51. See also Cleft alveolus.
    bilateral, IV:217-244
        anatomy of, IV:217-220, 218f, 219f
        cleft palate and, IV:50-51, 51f
        complete, IV:50-51, 51f
        incomplete, IV:49-50, 50f, 220, 220f

Cleft lip (Continued)
        orthodontics in, IV:277-280, 279f-282f. See also Cleft lip, orthodontics in.
        repair of, IV:220-244
            Abbe flap for, IV:346, 347f, 348f
            airway obstruction after, IV:238, 240
            banked forked flap for, Color Plate IV:94-1, IV:229-231, 229f-232f
            bleeding after, IV:240
            breast-feeding after, IV:238
            care after, IV:238
            cartilage-based, IV:231-238, 233f-243f
            complications of, IV:238, 240, 242-244
            Cupid's bow deformity and, IV:346
            flap loss after, IV:242
            infection after, IV:242
            lateral vestibular web correction for, IV:233-234
            lip construction in, Color Plate IV:94-1, IV:226-227, 227f, 229f
            lower lateral cartilage repositioning for, IV:231-238, 233f-243f
            medial crura footplate repositioning in, IV:237-238, 243f
            nasoalveolar molding in, IV:236, 239f-241f
            one-stage, IV:234-236, 234f-238f
            prolabial unwinding flap in, IV:235
            without nasoalveolar molding, IV:236-237, 242f
            midface growth deficiency after, IV:242
            nasoalveolar molding in, IV:278, 281f-282f, 341, 342f
            premaxilla malposition after, IV:242
            projecting premaxilla in, IV:220-225, 221f-226f
                 elastic traction for, IV:221, 222f
                 gingivoperiosteoplasty for, IV:225, 226f
                 lip adhesion for, IV:221
                 lip repair alone for, IV:221, 221f
                 nasoalveolar molding for, IV:222-225, 223f, 224f
                 pin-retained appliance for, IV:221-222, 222f
            scarring after, IV:242, 348-349
            skin-based, Color Plate IV:94-1, IV:229-231, 229f-232f
            sulcus abnormalities after, IV:346-347
            vermilion deficiency after, IV:346, 346f, 347f
        secondary deformity with, IV:339-351. See also Cleft lip, secondary deformity with.
    blood supply in, IV:52
    classification of, IV:46-47, 48f
    constriction ring syndrome and, VIII:187, 187f
    definition of, IV:45, 46f
    embryology of, IV:6-8, 7f, 45-46, 46f-47f

Cleft lip *(Continued)*
  fetal intervention for, I:1129
  in Van der Woude syndrome, IV:102-
    103
  median, IV:23, 24f
  minimal, IV:48, 48f
  morphologic varieties of, IV:47-51, 48f-
    51f
  muscle anatomy in, IV:52
  nasal deformity with, II:557, 558f, IV:51,
    51f, 52
  orthodontics in, IV:271-307
    anterior crossbite in, IV:282-283,
      284f, 285f
    distraction procedures and, IV:293,
      296-308, 297f-307f
    in infancy, IV:271-280, 274f-282f
    permanent dentition and, IV:290,
      292f, 293-308, 293f-295f
    posterior crossbite in, IV:282, 283f
    protrusive premaxilla and, IV:290,
      291f, 292f
    transitional dentition and, IV:283,
      285f, 286-290, 286f-289f
  osseous morphology in, IV:51
  pathologic anatomy of, IV:51-52
  prenatal diagnosis of, Color Plate I:36-6,
    IV:165-166
    magnetic resonance imaging in,
      I:1070, 1071f
    neonatal outcome and, I:1071-1072
    ultrasonography in, I:1069, 1070f
  secondary deformity with, IV:339-351
    Cupid's bow abnormalities as, IV:346
    evaluation of, IV:339-340, 340f
    intervention for, IV:341-351, 342f-
      351f
      in lip length abnormalities, IV:349-
        350, 350f
      in lip width abnormalities, IV:350-
        351, 351f
      in orbicularis abnormalities,
        IV:347-348, 349f
      in scar, IV:348-349
      in sulcus abnormalities, IV:346-347
      in vermilion abnormalities, IV:342-
        346, 343f-348f
      normal anatomy and, IV:341
      timing of, IV:340
    long lip as, IV:349-350, 350f
    orbicularis muscle deformities as,
      IV:347-348, 349f
    prevention of, IV:341, 342f
    scars as, IV:348-349
    short lip as, IV:349
    sulcus abnormalities as, IV:346-347
    tight lip as, IV:350
    vermilion deficiency as, IV:343-346,
      344f-348f
    vermilion malalignment as, IV:342-
      343, 342f-344f
    wide lip as, IV:350-351, 351f
  soft tissue morphology in, IV:51-53
  unilateral, IV:165-211
    alveolar molding for, IV:177-178,
      177f, 178f, 180-181
    cheiloplasty for, IV:173-177, 176f
      adhesion, IV:182-184, 183f-187f.
        See also Adhesion cheiloplasty.
      adjustments at, IV:199-200

Cleft lip *(Continued)*
      aesthetic assessment after, IV:207
      alar base in, IV:198
      alar cartilage in, IV:198-199
      care after, IV:205-206
      complications of, IV:206-208
      correction of, IV:208-210
      Cupid's bow peaking after, IV:208
      function after, IV:206-207
      historical perspective on, IV:173,
        174f-175f
      horizontal lip length in, IV:200
      infrasill depression after, IV:210
      lateral lip deficiency after, IV:209
      lateral orbicularis peripheralis
        muscle in, IV:199
      lip border in, IV:200
      long lateral lip after, IV:208
      lower lateral cartilage correction
        after, IV:209
      medial orbicularis peripheralis
        muscle in, IV:199
      Mohler's technique of, IV:200-202,
        200f-203f. *See also* Mohler's
        cheiloplasty.
      nasal molding after, IV:205-206,
        206f
      nasal repair with, IV:195, 197-199,
        197f, 198f
      nostril floor in, IV:200
      orbicularis oris muscle in, IV:199
      palatoplasty and, IV:210
      patient satisfaction with, IV:207-
        208
      plans for, IV:175, 176f
      principles of, IV:184-185
      rhinoplasty after, IV:210
      rotation-advancement, IV:186,
        188-195, 188f-196f, 202, 204f,
        205f. *See also* Rotation-
        advancement cheiloplasty.
      short lateral lip after, IV:208
      Tennison, IV:204-205, 341-342,
        342f
      treatment after, IV:175-177, 176f
      treatment before, IV:173, 176f
      turned-out alar base after, IV:209
      two-stage, IV:182-184, 183f-187f
      vermilion deficiency after, IV:208,
        209f
      vertical lip length in, IV:199-200
      vestibular webbing after, IV:209
      wide nostril after, IV:209
    classification of, IV:167, 167f-169f
    codes for, IV:167, 167f
    columella evaluation in, IV:173
    complete, IV:49, 49f
      cleft palate and, IV:50, 50f
      embryology of, IV:6, 7f
    Cupid's bow measurements in,
      IV:170-171, 172f
    dental plate for, IV:177f, 178, 178f,
      180
    genetics of, IV:166-167
    gingivoperiosteoplasty for, IV:181-
      182, 210-211
    Grayson nasoalveolar molding for,
      IV:178-179, 180f
    incidence of, IV:166, 166t
    incomplete, IV:48-49, 49f

Cleft lip *(Continued)*
    lateral lip measurements in, IV:171-
      173, 172f
    Liou nasoalveolar molding for,
      IV:178, 179f
    lip measurements in, IV:170-171, 172f
    maxilla molding for, IV:180-181
    nasoalveolar molding for, IV:178-179,
      179f, 180f, 181, 273-277, 275f-
      278f
    nostril floor skin evaluation in, IV:173
    orthodontics in. *See also* Cleft lip,
      orthodontics in.
    in infancy, IV:273-277, 274f-278f
    pathology of, IV:167-169, 168f-170f
    periosteoplasty for, IV:181
    philtral column identification in,
      IV:171, 172f
    prenatal diagnosis of, IV:165-166
    presurgical nasoalveolar molding for,
      IV:177-181, 177f-180f
    primary bone grafting for, IV:181
    secondary deformity with, IV:339-
      351. *See also* Cleft lip, secondary
      deformity with.
    three-dimensional measurements of,
      IV:169-170, 171f
    vermilion deficiency in, IV:172f, 173,
      343-345, 344f, 345f
Cleft nose, III:764, IV:51, 52, 354, 356-362
  after Tennison cheiloplasty, IV:341-342,
    342f
  anatomy of, IV:354, 356f
  evaluation of, IV:339-340
  repair of, IV:354, 356-360, 357f-360f
    nasoalveolar molding for, IV:360-361,
      360f, 361f
    open vs. closed, IV:361-362
    timing of, IV:340, 354, 356
  with orbital hypertelorism, IV:376, 377f
Cleft palate, IV:55-67, 249-266. *See also*
  Cleft lip.
  anatomy of, IV:76, 77f
    muscular, IV:72-76, 73f-75f, 77f
    neural, IV:81-82
    osseous, IV:70-71, 70f, 71f
    surface, IV:69-70
    vascular, IV:76-81, 78f-80f
  bilateral, IV:250, 250f, 251
  classification of, IV:55-57, 56f, 56t, 57t,
    82-88, 250-253, 250f
    American Association for Cleft Palate
      Rehabilitation, IV:16f, 83
    Davis and Ritchie, IV:55, 56t
    Kernahan and Strack, IV:83, 83t
    LAHSHAL, IV:56-57, 57f, 85, 87t, 88f
    Pruzansky, IV:82-83
    Spina, IV:83
    striped Y, IV:55, 56f, 57f, 57t, 83, 85,
      86f, 87f
    symbolic, IV:83, 85, 86f, 87f
    Veau's, IV:55, 56f, 82, 82f
    Villar-Sancho, IV:83, 85f, 85t
  complete, IV:250, 250f
  constriction ring syndrome and,
    VIII:187, 187f
  cranial base anomalies with, IV:71
  embryology of, IV:6, 8
  eustachian tube function and, IV:255-
    256

Cleft palate (Continued)
  feeding and, IV:254-255
  fetal intervention for, I:1129
  growth retardation and, IV:253-254
  historical perspective on, IV:249-250
  in Van der Woude syndrome, IV:102-103
  incomplete, IV:250, 250f, 251-253, 252f
  levator palatini muscle in, IV:251, 252f
  maxillary growth and, IV:256-257, 262
  orthodontics in
    distraction procedures and, IV:293, 296-308, 296f-307f
    permanent dentition and, IV:290, 292f, 293-308, 293f-295f
    transitional dentition and, IV:283, 285f, 286-290, 286f-289f
  palatoplasty for, IV:253-262. See also Palatoplasty.
  prenatal diagnosis of, I:1069, 1070t, 1071-1072
  secondary deformity with, IV:351-354
    evaluation of, IV:339-340
    fistula as, IV:352-354, 353f, 355f
  speech and, IV:255, 255f, 256
  submucous, IV:253, 317-318
  swallowing and, IV:254-255
  syndromic associations of, IV:257
  unilateral, IV:250, 250f, 251
  velopharyngeal insufficiency and, III:777
  with cleft lip and alveolus, IV:250-251
Cleft sternum, VI:479-482, 481f, 482f, 483t
  clinical presentation of, VI:480-481, 481f
  etiology of, VI:479
  hemangioma and, V:26f
  incidence of, VI:479
  treatment of, VI:481-482, 482f, 483t
  vascular malformation and, VI:481
Cleidocranial dysplasia, in mice, IV:9
Cleland ligament, VII:16, 17f, 731, 731f
Clenched fist syndrome, vs. reflex sympathetic dystrophy/chronic regional pain syndrome, VII:848
Clicking, with condylar process fracture, III:515
Clinodactyly, VIII:294-298, 295f-298f
  delta phalanx and, VIII:294-295, 295f
  incidence of, VIII:39
  Kirner, VIII:295-296
  outcomes of, VIII:297-298
  treatment of, VIII:296-297, 296f-298f
Clitoroplasty, in male-to-female transformation, Color Plates VI:156-8 and 156-9, VI:1314-1315
Clivus, tumor of, V:149, 150f-152f
Clomiphene citrate, ear deformity and, III:638
Clonal deletion, I:278-279
Clonazepam, in complex regional pain syndrome/reflex sympathetic dystrophy, VII:858
Clonidine
  in complex regional pain syndrome/reflex sympathetic dystrophy, VII:856
  preoperative, I:171
Clostridial myonecrosis, of hand, VII:782
Cloverleaf skull deformity, IV:476-477

Clubfoot, in constriction ring syndrome, VIII:192, 194f
Clubhand. See Radial (preaxial) deficiency; Ulnar deficiency.
Coagulation, in venous malformations, V:49
Coblation, facial, II:378-379
Cobweb syndrome, VIII:190
Cocaine
  for facial anesthesia, III:7-8, 7t
  nasal reconstruction and, III:573
  topical, I:190t, 191
Cohort study, I:37-38, 38f, 44, 47
Cold injury, I:855-861, VII:647-653. See also Frostbite.
  acclimatization and, VII:649
  age and, VII:648
  alcohol use and, I:857, VII:648
  environmental moisture and, VII:648-649
  environmental temperature and, VII:648
  immobilization and, I:857
  medical disease and, I:857
  mental illness and, VII:648
  overexertion and, I:857
  paralysis and, I:857
  peripheral vascular disease and, VII:648
  risk factors for, I:857, 857t
  sensitization to, I:857
  vasoconstriction and, I:857
  vasodilatation and, I:857
Cold therapy, in hand therapy, VIII:571
Collaboration, I:24-25
Collagen
  for bioengineered cartilage, I:631
  in Dupuytren disease, VII:735
  in wound healing, I:212-213, 214-215, 214f
  of bone, I:648, 649t
  of dermis, I:296
  of tendon, I:592, 593f
Collagen conduit, for nerve repair, VII:500
Collagen injection
  in lower third face lift, II:282-283
  in wrinkle treatment, II:258
Collagen vascular disease
  breast reconstruction and, VI:979
  lower extremity, VI:1475-1476, 1477f
Collagenases, in wound healing, I:214, 225-226
Collagraft, I:1101t
Colloid administration, in burn treatment, I:820, 820t
Coloboma
  lower eyelid, IV:427, 427f, 428f, 506, 506f
  upper eyelid, V:364-365, 366f
Colon cancer, I:1059, 1059f
Colonic flap, I:379, 379t
  for esophageal reconstruction, III:997, 1012
Color duplex imaging, in upper extremity ischemia, VII:800
Commissural ligaments, of thumb, VII:732, 732f
Commissure, labial
  in craniofacial microsomia, IV:541, 542f-543f
  reconstruction of, III:820-823, 821f-823f, V:385

Common interosseous artery, VII:792
Common plantar digital nerve, neuroma of, VII:922-923, 923f
Communication, physician
  as expert witness, I:128-130
  for informed consent, I:148-149
Comparative genomic hybridization, in prenatal diagnosis, I:1074
Compartment syndrome
  abdominal, I:818, 1006
  burns and, I:818, VII:591, 600-601
  lower extremity, I:339, VII:876t
  of foot, VI:1415, 1417, 1418f
Complement
  in graft rejection, I:272
  in wound healing, I:209-210
Complex regional pain syndrome/reflex sympathetic dystrophy, III:363-365, 363-364t, VII:823-866, 934, 935f
  alexithymia in, VII:842-843
  biopsy in, VII:831
  bone scan in, VII:845-846
  calcitonin gene-related peptide in, VII:838-839
  capillary blood velocity in, VII:846
  central mechanisms in, VII:844-845
  classification of, VII:825-826, 825t
  clinical manifestations of, VII:830-836, 831f, 832f, 832t, 833t, 836f
  definition of, VII:824-825
  diagnosis of, VII:825-826, 825t, 845-847
  differential diagnosis of, VII:847-850, 848f, 849f
  E-phase theory of, VII:840
  edema in, VII:831, 832f
  electromyography in, VII:846
  etiology of, VII:839-845, 841f, 842t
  functional assessment in, VII:847
  galvanic skin conduction in, VII:846
  historical perspective on, VII:826-828
  incidence of, VII:828
  inflammation in, VII:837-839
  internuncial pool theory of, VII:840
  magnetic resonance imaging in, VII:846
  myofascial dysfunction in, VII:833-835, 848
  nerve conduction tests in, VII:846
  nerve injury and, VII:826-827, 835
  neurokinin A in, VII:838-839
  neuropeptides in, VII:837-839
  neurotransmitters in, VII:827, 837-838
  opioid pain control system in, VII:843
  pain in, VII:824-825, 830-831, 831f
  pathophysiology of, VII:836-839
  precipitating events in, VII:829-830
  prevention of, VII:862
  prognosis for, VII:828-829, 862-863
  psychophysiologic mechanisms of, VII:840-843, 841f, 842t
  radiography in, VII:845
  recurrence of, VII:865
  shoulder-hand syndrome in, VII:835-836, 836f
  stage I in, VII:832, 832f, 832t
  stage II in, VII:832t, 833, 833f
  stage III in, VII:832t, 833, 833f
  substance P in, VII:837-839
  Sudeck atrophy in, VII:827, 836, 836f
  sweat response in, VII:846
  sympathetic block in, VII:847

Complex regional pain syndrome/reflex sympathetic dystrophy *(Continued)*
sympathetic nervous system in, VII:827-828, 839
terms for, VII:824, 824t, 825, 827
thermography in, VII:846
trauma-based classification of, VII:826
treatment of, VII:850-864
acupuncture in, VII:855
alendronate sodium in, VII:860
anti-inflammatory medications in, VII:857
antianxiety agents in, VII:859
anticonvulsants in, VII:857-858
antidepressants in, VII:858-859
baclofen in, VII:860
biofeedback therapy in, VII:855
bisphosphonates in, VII:859-860
calcitonin in, VII:859-860
calcium channel blockers in, VII:856-857
capsaicin in, VII:837-838, 857
carbamazepine in, VII:858
clonazepam in, VII:858
clonidine in, VII:856
corticosteroids in, VII:857
dimethyl sulfoxide in, VII:857
electrical stimulation in, VII:852-853, 855
gabapentin in, VII:858
hand therapy in, VII:860-861, VIII:563
individualization of, VII:863
intravenous infusion in, VII:854-855
litigation and, VII:863, 864-866
mannitol in, VII:857
medical, VII:855-860
mexiletine in, VII:860
nerve block in, VII:853-854
nifedipine in, VII:856-857
objective results of, VII:863
opioids in, VII:859
phenoxybenzamine in, VII:856
phentolamine in, VII:856
phenytoin in, VII:858
physician attitude and, VII:830, 863, 864
placebo effect in, VII:843
prazosin in, VII:856
principles of, VII:862-864
propranolol in, VII:856
psychotherapy in, VII:861-862
sleep aids in, VII:859
stellate ganglion block in, VII:853-854
subclavian vein decompression in, VII:852
surgical, VII:851-852, 863-864
sympathectomy in, VII:851-852
sympatholytics in, VII:855-857
tiagabine in, VII:858
tramadol in, VII:860
transcutaneous electrical nerve stimulation in, VII:855
valproic acid in, VII:858
trigger points in, VII:833-835
type I, VII:835
type II, VII:835
vs. carpal tunnel syndrome, VII:849-850
vs. central pain syndromes, VII:831
vs. connective tissue disorders, VII:847

Complex regional pain syndrome/reflex sympathetic dystrophy *(Continued)*
vs. conversion disorder, VII:848
vs. factitious wounding, VII:848, 848f
vs. malingering, VII:847-848
vs. myofascial dysfunction, VII:848
vs. psychiatric disorders, VII:847-848, 848f
vs. Volkmann ischemic contracture, VII:848-849, 849f
Composite tissue transplantation. *See* Microvascular surgery.
Compound A, I:179
Compound nevus, V:308, 308f
Compression therapy, in venous insufficiency, I:964
Computed tomographic myelography, in obstetric brachial plexus palsy, VII:542
Computed tomography
in arteriovenous malformation, V:51-52
in condylar process fracture, III:516, 516f
in congenital hand anomalies, VIII:38
in craniofacial microsomia, IV:131-132, 131f
in facial fracture repair, III:467, 468f
in frontoethmoidal meningoencephalocele, IV:409f
in head and neck cancer, V:228
in Kienböck disease, VII:68
in maxillary fracture, III:239
in nasal fracture, III:196-197, 199f
in nasoethmoidal-orbital fracture, III:314-315
in orbital fracture, III:275-276
in orbital hypertelorism, IV:366-367, 368f
in pectus excavatum, VI:459, 460f, 462f
in pediatric facial trauma, III:392, 393f, 395, 395t, 397f
in peripheral nerve injury, I:729, 730f
in salivary gland tumors, V:73
in sternal infection, VI:426
in temporomandibular joint dysfunction, III:542, 543
in wrist injury, VII:458
in zygoma fracture, III:214, 215f
of craniofacial clefts, IV:401, 402f
of hand and wrist, VII:66, 68, 68f
Computer-assisted surgery
in cranioplasty, III:547, 548f, 556, 557f
in craniosynostosis, IV:490
in rhinoplasty, II:437, 439f, 770, 772
Conduction, of heat, I:855-856, 856f
Condylar process fracture, III:511-532, 512t. *See also* Mandibular fracture.
anatomy of, III:512-515, 512f-514f
classification of, III:171f-174f, 512-513, 512f
clicking with, III:515
clinical examination of, III:515
computed tomography of, III:516, 516f
crepitation with, III:515
diagnosis of, III:515-517, 516f, 517f
dislocation with, III:514, 514f
displacement with, III:513-514, 513f, 514f
etiology of, III:511
evaluation of, III:512

Condylar process fracture *(Continued)*
facial asymmetry with, III:515
facial nerve and, III:514-515
in children, III:412, 414-421, 414f-416f, 419f-420f
lateral override with, III:513, 513f
lower lip anesthesia with, III:515
malocclusion with, III:515
medial override with, III:513, 513f
pain with, III:515
panoramic tomography of, III:516-517, 517f
standard radiography of, III:517
temporomandibular joint dysfunction and, III:539-541, 540f
treatment of, III:517-529
closed, III:517-519, 518t
vs. open reduction, III:175, 177-179
endoscopic, III:174f, 472-485, 519-529
age and, III:520
bailout strategy for, III:529
check trocar placement for, III:524
comminution and, III:477, 520-521, 520f
computed tomography before, III:473, 479f, 481f, 483f
concomitant illness and, III:521-522
confirmed reduction for, III:528f, 529, 529f
contraindications to, III:473, 519t
dislocated condylar head and, III:521
displacement and, III:477, 485
edentulousness and, III:485
extraoral, III:477
fracture location and, III:477, 520, 520f
fracture reduction for, III:524-525, 526-527, 526f-528f
growth and, III:485
ideal patient for, III:521f, 522
indications for, III:473
intraoral approach for, III:522-523, 523f-525f
management after, III:529, 530f
maxillomandibular fixation and, III:485
operative portals for, III:473, 474f-475f
panoramic tomography after, III:529, 530f
patient preference and, III:522
proximal fragment displacement and, III:521
rationale for, III:519
results of, III:477, 478f-484f, 528f, 529, 530f, 531, 531f
rigid fixation application for, III:517f, 525-526
submandibular approach for, III:523-524
surgical positioning for, III:522, 522f
technique of, III:473-477, 474f-476f, 522-529, 522f-529f
with condylar head malpositioning, III:477

Condylar process fracture (Continued)
  goals of, III:517
  nonsurgical, III:517-519, 518t
  open, III:170-181, 172f-174f, 176f,
    517-519, 518t
    avascular necrosis and, III:174, 177
    Risdon incision for, III:175, 176f
    vs. closed reduction, III:175, 177-
    179
Condylion, II:19f, 20t
Connective tissue, vascular tissue relation
    to, I:344-345
Connective tissue disorders
  breast implants and, VI:679
  upper extremity ischemia in, VII:815
  vs. reflex sympathetic dystrophy/chronic
    regional pain syndrome, VII:847
Conscious sedation, I:196-198
Consent. See Informed consent.
Constriction ring syndrome, VIII:146-147,
    147f, 185-211
  acrosyndactyly in, VIII:146-147, 197f,
    201-202, 201f, 202f
    classification of, VIII:146, 147f, 177-
    178
  flexed digits in, VIII:208-209
  floppy index finger in, VIII:208, 209f
  sinuses in, VIII:203, 204f
  two-fingered, VIII:205, 207, 207f,
    208f
  associated malformations in, VIII:186-
    189, 187f, 187t, 188f
  autoamputation in, VIII:191f, 192
  balloon digits in, VIII:202-203, 203f
  classification of, VIII:146, 147f, 177-178,
    185
  clinical presentation of, VIII:190, 192-
    196, 192f-195f
  depth of, VIII:188-189, 189f, 190f
  differential diagnosis of, VIII:189, 196,
    196t
  double digit in, VIII:203-205, 204f
  extrinsic theory of, VIII:190, 191f
  fingernails in, VIII:195, 195f, 210
  flexed digits in, VIII:208-209
  floppy index finger in, VIII:208, 209f
  growth and, VIII:210f, 211
  hypoplastic nails in, VIII:210
  in twins, VIII:186, 186f
  incidence of, VIII:40t, 186
  intrauterine trauma and, VIII:190
  intrinsic theory of, VIII:189-190
  lower limb, VIII:200f, 203, 203f
  of thumb, VIII:203, 205, 355-360, 356f-
    359f
  pathogenesis of, VIII:189-190, 191f
  pointed amputation stumps in, VIII:210
  short double digit in, VIII:203, 204f, 205
  short thumb in, VIII:203, 205
  side-by-side short digits in, VIII:207-
    208
  sinuses in, VIII:203, 204f
  soft tissue asymmetries in, VIII:209-210,
    209f
  swelling in, VIII:190f, 195-196, 197f,
    202-203, 203f
  terminology of, VIII:185, 186t
  treatment of, VIII:178-180, 178f, 179f,
    196-211
    complications of, VIII:209f, 210-211

Constriction ring syndrome (Continued)
    digital lengthening in, VIII:205, 205f,
    206f
    digital transposition in, VIII:205,
    207f
    fetal, VIII:196, 197f
    principles of, VIII:196, 198
    technique of, VIII:198-200, 199f, 200f
    timing of, VIII:196
    toe transfer in, VIII:179, 179f, 357f,
    359-360, 359f
    Z-plasty in, VIII:198, 199f, 200f
    two-fingered hand in, VIII:205, 207,
    207f, 208f
  vs. Adams-Oliver syndrome, VIII:187,
    188f
Contact dermatitis, after laser resurfacing,
    II:370
Contact lenses, periorbital surgery and,
    II:89-90, 91
Contract, I:134-136
Contraction, in wound healing, I:213-214,
    213f
Contracture
  burn scar
    in elbow, VII:633, 635
    in hand, VII:616-624, 618f-620f, 622f,
    623f
    in shoulder, VII:630-633, 631f, 634f
  Dupuytren, VII:668-669, 669f, 671, 736,
    737f. See also Dupuytren disease.
  in musician, VII:696-697, 697f, 701
  of fingers, VII:659-672. See also
    Finger(s), contractures of.
  vs. wound contraction, I:213-214
Convection, heat loss with, I:856, 856f
Converse, John Marquis, I:2-4, 3f
Conversion disorder, vs. reflex sympathetic
    dystrophy/chronic regional pain
    syndrome, VII:848
CoolTouch, II:376, 377f
Cooper, Astley, I:28
Copper-based antiaging preparation,
    II:401
Cor pulmonale, obstructive sleep apnea
    and, III:786, 786f
Coralline hydroxyapatite implants, I:693t,
    696, 754, 755f
Core-binding factor α1, in osteoblast
    differentiation, I:644
Core body temperature, in hypothermia,
    I:858
Core needle biopsy, in breast cancer, Color
    Plate VI:138-2, VI:639-642, 640f,
    641t
Cornea
  evaluation of, II:93
    protective shields for, in blepharoplasty,
    II:825, 827f
Corneal abrasion, with laser resurfacing,
    II:375
Coronal brow lift, II:60-61, 61f, 62f
Coronal incision, for facial surgery,
    III:563-564, 564f
Coronary artery bypass graft, sternal
    wound infection after, I:915, 915f,
    977, 980-981, 980f
Coronary artery disease, preoperative
    evaluation of, I:168
Coronocanthopexy, II:124-125, 125f

Coronoid process
  hypertrophy of, III:539
  in zygomatic arch fracture, III:209-210,
    210f, 211f
Coronoplasty, in female-to-male
    transformation, VI:1310
Corrosive agent injury, to hand, VII:653t,
    654, 656
Corrugator superciliaris, II:81-82, 82f
  in brow mobility, II:55, 56f
  nerve ablation in, II:223
  transection of, II:223
Corticosteroids
  in breast augmentation, VI:28
  in complex regional pain
    syndrome/reflex sympathetic
    dystrophy, VII:857
  in Dupuytren disease, VII:740
  in flap optimization, I:499t, 500
  in hemangioma, V:6, 29-30, 29f,
    VIII:375
  in immunosuppression, I:275-276, 275t
  in kaposiform hemangioendothelioma,
    V:36
  in toxic epidermal necrolysis, I:798
  in trigger finger, VII:685
  wound healing and, I:221
Cortisol, etomidate effects on, I:175
Corundum implant, I:756
Corynebacterium parvum, I:1056
Cosmetics, in capillary malformations,
    V:39-40, 39f
Cost-effectiveness analysis, in evidence-
    based decision-making, I:44-45
Costochondral graft, in craniofacial cleft
    management, IV:430, 430f, 431f
Counterreaction, I:70
Countertransference, I:70-71
Covermark, V:39-40
Cowden syndrome, V:55
Cranial base
  cephalometric analysis of, II:23
  in cleft palate, IV:71
Cranial nerve abnormalities, in
    craniofacial microsomia, IV:122-124
Cranial sutures
  absence of. See Craniosynostosis
    (craniosynostoses).
  embryology of, IV:11
Cranial vault remodeling
  in craniofacial microsomia, IV:541
  in craniosynostoses, IV:502-504
Craniofacial cleft(s), IV:15-41. See also
    Cleft lip; Cleft palate.
  AACPR classification of, IV:20, 20t
  amniotic bands and, IV:414, 414f, 415f
  classification of, IV:20-22, 20t, 21t, 22f,
    381-385, 382t, 383t, 384f
  computed tomography of, IV:401, 402f
  environmental factors in, IV:413
  epidemiology of, IV:15
  etiology of, IV:15-16, 411-413, 412f
  eyelid deficiency in, IV:426-428, 427f,
    428f
  fusion failure theory of, IV:18
  genetics of, IV:411-413, 412f
  in craniofacial microsomia, IV:541,
    542f-543f
  Karfik classification of, IV:20, 21t, 381-
    382, 382t

Craniofacial cleft(s) (Continued)
   management of, IV:414-461
      airway in, IV:416, 422
      alveolar bone grafting in, IV:432, 434f
      anosmia with, IV:461
      anterior maxilla graft in, IV:432
      Australian Craniofacial Unit
         protocols for, IV:416, 417-419t
      blindness with, IV:459
      blood loss with, IV:461
      bone distraction in, IV:430-431, 446
      bone grafting in, IV:431-433, 432f-
         435f
      canthal dystopia with, IV:461
      cerebral ischemia with, IV:459
      cerebrospinal fistula with, IV:459
      cleft closure in, IV:422, 424-426, 424f-
         426f
      complications of, IV:458-459, 461
      costochondral graft in, IV:430, 430f,
         431f
      diplopia with, IV:461
      dural damage with, IV:458-459
      enophthalmos with, IV:461
      epilepsy with, IV:459
      epiphora with, IV:461
      eyelid reconstruction in, IV:426-428,
         427f, 428f
      facial bipartition osteotomy in,
         IV:439, 439f
      fronto-orbital osteotomy in, IV:435,
         436f
      genioplasty in, IV:444-446, 445f
      gliosis with, IV:459
      hydrocephalus with, IV:459
      intracranial hematoma with, IV:459
      inverted L ramus osteotomy in,
         IV:444, 444f
      keratitis with, IV:461
      Le Fort I osteotomy in, IV:439, 441,
         441f
      Le Fort II osteotomy in, IV:439, 440f
      Le Fort III osteotomy in, IV:439, 439f
      mandibular osteotomy in, IV:441,
         443-444, 443f, 444f
      midface osteotomy in, IV:439-446,
         439f-445f
      nasal bone grafting in, IV:433, 434f,
         435f
      nasopharyngeal intubation in, IV:416,
         422
      neurosurgical complications of,
         IV:458-459
      orbital expansion in, IV:429-430, 429f
      orbital osteotomy in, IV:435-439,
         436f-439f
      orthodontics in, IV:431
      osseointegration in, IV:446, 448f
      osteotomy in, IV:433, 435-446
      partial orbital osteotomy in, IV:435-
         436, 437f
      principles of, IV:414-416, 416f
      results of, IV:446, 449f-453f, 454,
         454f-457f, 458, 458f-460f
      sagittal split ramus osteotomy in,
         IV:441, 443, 443f
      segmental maxillary osteotomy in,
         IV:441, 442f
      total orbital osteotomy in, IV:436,
         438f

Craniofacial cleft(s) (Continued)
      vascularized tissue transfer in, IV:446,
         447f
      vertical subsigmoid ramus osteotomy
         in, IV:443-444, 444f
      zygoma graft in, IV:432
   midline agenesis in, IV:404, 406f, 407, 408f
   number 0 (median), IV:2-3, 21, 22f, 23,
      24f, 385, 387f
   number 1 (paramedian facial), IV:21,
      22f, 23, 25f, 385, 387, 388f
   number 2 (paramedian facial), IV:21,
      22f, 23, 25, 26f, 387, 389, 389f
   number 3 (oro-naso-ocular), IV:21, 22f,
      25-26, 27f, 389-390, 390f, 417t
      management of, IV:417t, 425f, 427-428
   number 4 (oro-ocular), IV:21, 22f, 26,
      28f, 29, 391, 391f, 417t
      management of, IV:417t, 424-426,
         425f, 426f, 427-428, 454, 457f
   number 5 (oro-ocular), IV:21, 22f, 29-
      30, 29f, 392, 392f, 417t
      management of, IV:417t, 424, 425f,
         427-428, 454, 457f
   number 6, 7, 8 combination, IV:33-35,
      34f-35f. See also Treacher Collins
      syndrome.
   number 6 (zygomatic-maxillary), IV:22f,
      30, 31f, 392-393, 393f, 407t, 418t
   number 7 (temporozygomatic), IV:22f,
      30, 32f, 393-394, 394f, 418t, 419t
      closure of, IV:422, 424f
   number 8 (frontozygomatic), IV:22f, 33,
      33f, 394-395, 395f, 396f, 418t
   number 9 (upper lateral orbital), IV:22f,
      35, 35f, 394-395, 396f, 419t
      management of, IV:419t, 446, 452f
   number 10 (upper central orbital),
      IV:22f, 35-36, 36f, 395, 397, 397f,
      402f, 419t
      management of, IV:419t, 446, 451f
   number 11 (upper medial orbital),
      IV:22f, 37, 37f, 397, 398f
   number 12, IV:37, 38f, 397-398, 398f
   number 12 (paramedian cranial), IV:22f
   number 13 (paramedian cranial),
      IV:22f, 37, 39f, 399, 399f
   number 14 (midline cranial), IV:22f, 38-
      39, 40f-41f, 399-400, 400f
   number 30 (lower jaw), IV:39
   pathogenesis of, IV:19-20, 413-414
      fusion failure theory of, IV:18
      neuromeric theory of, IV:18-19, 19f
   radiation exposure and, IV:413
   stapedial artery loss and, IV:20
   teratogens in, IV:413
   Tessier classification of, IV:21-22, 22f,
      385, 386f, 400-401
   van der Meulen classification of, IV:20-
      21, 21t, 382, 383f
   vs. normal morphogenesis, IV:16-19, 17f
Craniofacial complex, embryology of,
   IV:1-12
   branchial structures in, IV:4, 5f
   defects in, IV:11-12
   early patterning in, IV:2, 3f
   facial primordia in, IV:4, 6-8, 6f, 7f
   neural crest in, IV:2, 3-4, 3f
   palatal fusion in, IV:8
   skeletal development in, IV:8-11, 10f

Craniofacial microsomia, III:777, IV:101-
   102, 113-132, 385, 401, 403f-406f,
   404, 407t
   bilateral, IV:126, 126f
   cephalometric analysis in, IV:129-131,
      130f
   cerebral anomalies in, IV:122
   classification of, IV:126-129, 127f, 128t,
      132t
      OMENS, IV:128-129, 132t
      phenotypic, IV:127-128
      Pruzansky, IV:521, 522f
      SAT (alphanumeric), IV:128, 128t,
         401, 403f-405f, 407t
      surgical-anatomic, IV:128, 129f
   computed tomography in, IV:131-132,
      131f
   cranial nerve abnormalities in, IV:122-
      124
   diagnostic criteria for, IV:126
   differential diagnosis of, IV:126
   distraction osteogenesis in, III:780-783,
      780f-783f, IV:523-525, 524f-532f
   ear malformations in, III:638, 639f,
      IV:122, 124f, 125t, 546
   electromyography in, IV:124
   embryology of, IV:11, 115-117, 116f
   etiopathogenesis of, IV:113-115, 114f
   extracraniofacial anomalies in, IV:125,
      125t
   facial growth in, IV:125-126
   genetic theory of, IV:114-115
   grading system for, IV:127, 127f
   growth studies in, IV:550-551, 553
   lateral pterygoid muscle impairment in,
      IV:120-122
   macrostomia in, IV:81t, 124-125, 124f
   mandibular deformity in, IV:117-120,
      118f-120f, 125t
   mastoid process deformity in, IV:120
   morphology of, IV:401, 404f-406f, 407t
   muscle function in, IV:120-122
   natural history of, IV:125-126
   nervous system abnormalities in,
      IV:122-124
   OMENS classification of, IV:128-129,
      132t
   omental fat flap in, I:579, 580f
   orbital deformity in, IV:120, 122f
   pathology of, IV:117-126, 118f-121f,
      123f, 124f, 125t
   phenotypic classification of, IV:127-128
   Pruzansky classification in, IV:521, 522f
   reconstruction for, IV:101-102, 418t,
      421f, 521-553
      absent ramus and condyle in, IV:533
      algorithm for, IV:549-550
      auricular reconstruction in, IV:546
      bone grafts in, IV:533, 534f-537f
      commissuroplasty in, IV:541, 542f-
         543f
      cranial vault remodeling in, IV:541
      evaluation for, IV:521, 522f
      fronto-orbital advancement in, IV:541
      gastrostomy in, IV:523
      genioplasty in, IV:533, 538f, 539f, 550,
         551f, 552f
      historical perspective on, IV:522-523
      in adolescent, IV:550
      in adult, IV:550

Craniofacial microsomia (Continued)
in child, IV:549-550
in infant, IV:549
in neonate, IV:549
intraocclusal splints in, IV:540
Le Fort I osteotomy in, IV:533, 538f-540f, 540
mandibular distraction in, IV:523-525, 524f-532f
maxillomandibular distraction in, IV:525, 532f, 533
maxillomandibular orthognathic surgery in, IV:533, 538f-540f, 540-541
microvascular free flap in, IV:541, 544f, 545f
occlusion management in, IV:546-549, 547f, 548f
ramus osteotomies in, IV:540-541, 541f
results of, IV:454, 455f, 456f
tracheostomy in, IV:523
SAT (alphanumeric) classification of, IV:128, 128t, 401, 403f-405f, 407t
skeletal pathology of, IV:117-120, 118f-121f
skin deficiency in, IV:124-125, 124f
soft tissue pathology of, IV:120-125, 123f, 124f, 125t
surgical-anatomic classification of, IV:128, 129f
teratogen theory of, IV:113-114, 114f
transgenic mouse model of, IV:114-115
twin studies of, IV:115
unilateral, IV:126
zygoma deformity in, IV:120
Craniofacial syndromes, IV:91-110. See also Craniofacial cleft(s); Craniosynostosis (craniosynostoses) and specific syndromes.
airway obstruction in, III:776-784
craniofacial growth in, IV:95-96, 97f
cultural practices and, IV:91-92
diagnosis of, IV:96
etiology of, IV:92-93
genetic factors in, IV:92-93, 93f, 93t
historical perspective on, IV:91-92
management team for, IV:96, 98
molecular biology of, IV:92-93
psychological factors in, I:79-80
surgery in, IV:103-106
indications for, IV:103-104
outcomes of, IV:104-105, 105t
rigid internal fixation in, IV:105-106
timing of, IV:104, 104t
types of, IV:93-95
Craniofrontonasal syndrome, IV:107, 414, 414f. See also Frontonasal malformation.
Craniopharyngioma, nasopharyngeal, III:767
Cranioplasty, III:547-561
calvarial bone for, III:549, 554f, 555, 555f-557f
inner table harvest of, III:549, 555, 556f, 557f
outer table harvest of, III:549, 554f, 555f
computer-aided, III:547, 548f, 556, 557f
hydroxyapatite for, III:555-556

Cranioplasty (Continued)
in female-to-male transformation, VI:1315
latissimus dorsi muscle flap for, III:557
mesh-only technique for, III:549, 551f-552f
methyl methacrylate for, III:548-549, 550f-552f
microvascular composite tissue transplantation for, III:556-561, 558f-560f
omental free tissue transfer for, III:557-561, 558f-560f
patient position for, III:548
porous polyethylene for, III:555, 557f, 561, 561f
rectus abdominis flap for, III:557
screw stabilization for, III:549, 552f
sleeve molding technique for, III:549, 550f
split rib for, III:549, 553f
temporal hollowing and, III:561, 561f
timing of, III:548
Craniosynostosis (craniosynostoses)
genetic analysis in, I:58, 60-61, 61f-63f
nonsyndromic, IV:98-99, 135-162, 137t, 138f-140f, 495
coronal
bilateral, IV:137t, 149-154, 150f-155f, 469
unilateral, IV:137t, 145-149, 145f-148f, 150f-155f, 469, 471-472, 472f-474f
epidemiology of, IV:98, 98t
evaluation of, IV:138-140, 138f-140f, 138t
follow-up for, IV:140, 140f
functional issues in, IV:466
genetic factors in, IV:135-136
growth and, IV:95-96, 97f
intracranial pressure in, IV:103
lambdoid, IV:159-162, 160f-162f
metopic, IV:137t, 154-158, 156f-160f, 472-474, 475f, 476f
multiple, IV:98, 162
reconstruction for, IV:103-106, 138-162
calvariectomy defect site in, IV:139-140, 140f
fixation system in, IV:105-106
historical perspective on, IV:136
in bilateral coronal synostosis (brachycephaly), IV:149-154, 150f-155f, 469, 471-472, 472f-474f
in lambdoid synostosis, IV:159-162, 160f-162f
in metopic synostosis (trigonocephaly), IV:137t, 154-158, 156f-160f, 472-474, 475f, 476f
in sagittal synostosis (scaphocephaly), IV:137t, 140-145, 141f-144f, 466-469, 468f, 470f, 471f
in turribrachycephaly, IV:477, 502-504, 503f
in unilateral coronal synostosis (plagiocephaly), IV:145-149, 145f-148f, 469, 471-472, 472f-474f

Craniosynostosis (craniosynostoses) (Continued)
indications for, IV:103-104
intracranial pressure and, IV:103, 136
outcomes of, IV:136-137
resorbable suture materials in, IV:106
timing of, IV:136, 138-139, 139f
sagittal, IV:137t, 140-145, 141f-144f, 466-469, 468f, 470f, 471f
syndromic, IV:91-100. See also specific syndromes.
airway obstruction in, IV:497
definition of, IV:94
dental evaluation in, IV:497
diagnosis of, IV:96
dysmorphology of, IV:495, 496f
epidemiology of, IV:98, 98t
etiology of, IV:92-93, 93f, 93t, 94
evaluation of, IV:475-476, 497
gene therapy in, IV:490
growth and, IV:95-96, 466
historical perspectives on, IV:91-92
intracranial pressure in, IV:103, 496-497
monitoring of, IV:497
neurocognitive development in, IV:465-466
neurologic evaluation in, IV:497
ophthalmoscopic examination in, IV:497
prenatal diagnosis of, IV:94-95
reconstruction for, IV:103-106, 474-491, 495-517. See also Robin sequence; Treacher Collins syndrome.
algorithm for, IV:490, 490t
Bandeau osteotomy in, IV:499-500, 499f
computer-assisted, IV:490
cranial vault remodeling in, IV:502-504, 503f
distraction osteogenesis in, IV:485-486
evaluation for, IV:497
facial bipartition procedure in, IV:501, 502f
fixation system in, IV:105-106
fronto-orbital advancement in, IV:498-500, 498f-500f
functional considerations in, IV:496-497
historical perspective on, IV:136, 465
in cloverleaf skull deformity, IV:476-477
in Robin sequence, IV:511-515. See also Robin sequence.
in Treacher Collins syndrome, IV:504-511. See also Treacher Collins syndrome.
indications for, IV:103-104, 497-498
intracranial pressure and, IV:103
intracranial volume and, IV:465-466
Le Fort II osteotomy in, IV:482, 485, 485f, 486f
Le Fort III osteotomy in, IV:500-501, 500f

Craniosynostosis (craniosynostoses)
    (Continued)
        midface procedures in, IV:477-485,
            478f-489f, 500-501, 500f-502f
        minimally invasive procedures for,
            IV:487
        monobloc advancement in, IV:485,
            488f, 489f, 501, 501f
        monobloc distraction in, IV:485,
            488f
        monobloc osteotomy in, IV:485,
            487f
        orthognathic procedures in,
            IV:501-502
        outcomes of, IV:104-105, 105t
        posterior-then-anterior vault
            remodeling in, IV:504
        resorbable suture materials in,
            IV:106
        results of, IV:491
        staged approach to, IV:498-502,
            498f-502f
        subcranial Le Fort III osteotomy in,
            IV:477-482, 478f-483f
        Le Fort I advancement osteotomy
            with, IV:482, 484f
        timing of, IV:104, 104t
        total cranial vault remodeling in,
            IV:502-504, 503f
    single-suture, IV:98
    sutural manipulation in, IV:490
Cranium
    acquired defects of, III:564-565, 566f-
        573f
    anatomy of, III:547
    congenital defects of, IV:15-41. See also
        Craniofacial cleft(s); Craniofacial
        syndromes; Craniosynostosis
        (craniosynostoses).
    embryology of, IV:8-11, 10f
    postnatal growth of, III:382f, 383f, 388,
        388f
    reconstruction of. See Cranioplasty.
Creativity, I:1-2
Cremasteric muscle, VI:91
Creosote, skin cancer and, V:275-276
Crepitus
    in condylar process fracture, III:515
    in de Quervain syndrome, VII:678
Crimes, I:136-138
Critical arterial stenosis, VII:796, 796f
Cross-finger flap, VII:164-166, 164f, 165f
Crossmatching, for transplantation, I:274
Crouzon syndrome, III:777-778, IV:92, 99-
    100. See also Craniosynostosis
    (craniosynostoses), syndromic.
    genetic analysis in, I:58, 60-61, 61f-63f
Crow's feet, II:242, 243f
Cryogen spray, II:378
Cryosurgery, in skin cancer, V:286t, 290,
    409t, 411-413, 411f
Cryotherapy, in hand therapy, VIII:571
Cryptorchidism, VI:1245-1246, 1245f, 1261
Cryptotia, III:663, 665, 669f
Cubital tunnel syndrome, VII:876t, 894-912
    diagnosis of, VII:894-895, 896f-897f
    in musician, VII:703
    nonoperative treatment of, VII:895
    surgical management of, VII:895, 897-
        902, 897f-900f, 901t

Cubital tunnel syndrome (Continued)
        anatomy-related failure of, VII:895,
            897t
    complications of, VII:901-902
    historical perspective on, VII:895
    medial antebrachial cutaneous nerve
        neuroma after, VII:901-902
    meta-analysis of, VII:898, 901, 901t
    musculofascial lengthening technique
        in, VII:898f-900f
    postoperative care in, VII:901, 901t,
        VIII:562-563
    pressure measurements after, VII:895,
        897f
Cuffed oropharyngeal airway, I:176
Cultured epidermal autograft, in burn
    treatment, I:818, 825, 826f
Cumulative trauma disorder, VII:688-689
    ergonomic consultation for, VII:690
    etiology of, VII:688-689
    metabolic changes in, VII:689
    nerve compression in, VII:689
    prevention of, VII:689-690
    psychosocial factors in, VII:689, 691
    repetition in, VII:688
    treatment of, VII:690-691
Cupid's bow, after cleft lip repair, IV:346
Curettage and electrodesiccation, in skin
    cancer, V:285, 286t, 409, 410-411
Curling's ulcers, I:829
Cutaneous nerves, I:327-329, 328f, 345-
    347, 346f
Cutaneous perforators, I:297, 322-324,
    325f, 326f, 336f, 351, 353f, 354f
    connective tissue relation of, I:344
    direct, Color Plate I:15-1, I:323-324
    Doppler mapping of, I:355
    indirect, I:323
    of face, I:340-341, 340f, 341f
    of forearm, Color Plate I:15-4, I:334
    size of, I:347-348, 347f
Cutaneous veins, I:324-326, 326f
Cutis marmorata telangiectasia congenita,
    V:40-41, 41f, VIII:378, 380, 380f
Cyanosis, choanal atresia and, III:764
Cyclopamine, teratogenicity of, IV:12
Cyclophosphamide, in toxic epidermal
    necrolysis, I:799
Cyclosporine, I:275t, 276
Cylindroma, Color Plate V:112-3, V:83-84,
    86f, 259-260, 259f
Cyst(s)
    bone, aneurysmal, V:103, 195-197,
        VII:988
    botryoid, V:191
    branchial arch, I:945, III:1025-1026,
        1026f, V:3
    breast, VI:638
    dentigerous, V:93, 95, 191-192, 192f
    dermoid, III:765, IV:107-108, 108f, V:4,
        4f, 5f
    epidermal, V:255, 255f
    eruption, V:192
    fat injection and, I:584
    fissural, V:94
    ganglion, VII:70, 136, 196-198, 198f,
        199f, VIII:563
    gingival, V:92-93, 191
    glandular, V:193
    globulomaxillary, V:94

Cyst(s) (Continued)
    Gorlin, V:93, 193-194
    inclusion, in constriction ring
        syndrome, VIII:203, 204f
    keratin (milia), V:255-256
    laryngeal, III:769
    mandibular, V:92-95, 94f, 103, 189, 190t,
        191-197, 192f, 194f, 195f
    nasopalatine, V:94
    nonodontogenic, V:195, 196f
    odontogenic, V:92-95, 94f, 190t, 191-
        195, 192f, 194f
    of perionychium, VII:188, 191, 200
    palatal, V:94
    paradental, V:94, 195
    periodontal, V:93, 94, 191
    pilar, V:255
    radicular, V:93-94, 194-195
    residual, V:94
    sebaceous, of auricle, III:689
    thyroglossal duct, III:767, 1029, 1029f,
        1030f
Cystic adenomatoid malformation, I:1124-
    1125
Cystic hygroma
    cheek reconstruction in, III:833, 834f-
        836f
    neck reconstruction in, III:1030-1032,
        1030f-1032f
Cytokines
    in bone repair, I:655-658, 656-657t
    in nerve regeneration, VII:480
    in toxic epidermal necrolysis, I:795

D

Da Vinci Surgical System, I:1155-1157,
    1156f, 1157f
Daclizumab, I:274t
Dacryocystitis, in maxillary fracture,
    III:251
Dacryocystorhinostomy, III:328, 743, 743f
Dakin solution, in burn treatment, I:822
Danazol, in breast pain, VI:355
Dandy-Walker syndrome, I:1128-1129,
    V:26f
Database analysis, in evidence-based
    decision-making, I:42-44, 43t
De Quervain syndrome, VII:54, 676-680
    clinical presentation of, VII:676-677
    cortisone injection in, VII:679-680, 679f
    crepitus in, VII:678
    differential diagnosis of, VII:677-678
    Finkelstein maneuver in, VII:678, 678t
    in musician, VII:702
    nonoperative treatment of, VII:679-680,
        679f
    pain in, VII:678
    patient history in, VII:677
    physical examination in, VII:677-678,
        678f
    radiography in, VII:678-679
    treatment of, VII:679-680, 679f,
        VIII:559-560, 560f
    vs. radial sensory nerve entrapment,
        VII:904
DEB test, VIII:62
Débridement, I:300, 863-883
    biologic agents for, I:873
    gauze dressing for, I:873
    in bronchopleural fistula, VI:429

Débridement *(Continued)*
in burn treatment, I:822-823
in diabetic ulcers, I:981
in facial trauma, III:11
in frostbite, I:860, 860t, VII:652
in necrotizing soft-tissue infection,
I:976-977
in osteomyelitis, I:977
in sternal infection, I:980, VI:426
in traumatic tattoo, III:12
in upper extremity mangling injury,
VII:320
infection assessment and, I:879-880
maggots for, I:873
nonsurgical tools for, I:873
of acute wound, I:880-881
of chronic wound, I:882-883
of infected wound, I:881-882, 881f, 882f
operative, I:955-958
after radiation therapy, I:958
flap coverage after, I:962-963, 962f, 963f
instruments for, I:958, 958t, 959f-962f
reconstruction after, I:958, 962-963,
962f, 963f
revascularization and, I:957-958
serial, I:956-957
tissue viability criteria in, I:957-958
pharmacologic, I:955
techniques of, I:866-868, 870f
for bone, I:876, 878-879, 879f
for fascia, I:875
for muscle, I:875
for skin, I:873-875, 874f
for subcutaneous tissue, I:875
for tendon, I:875-876, 875f-878f
tools for, I:870-872, 870f-872f
Wood's lamp examination for, I:956, 957f
wound assessment for, I:864-866, 865f-
868f
Decision analysis, in evidence-based
decision-making, I:44-45
Decubitus ulcers. *See* Pressure sores.
Deep circumflex iliac artery composite
flap, I:390, 395f-396f
Deep circumflex iliac artery (Rubens) flap,
VI:764t, 1053-1055
patient position for, VI:1055f
selection of, VI:1063
surgical technique for, VI:771, 771f,
772f, 1059-1060, 1059f, 1061f,
1062f
Deep facial fascia, II:162f, 165-167, 167f
Deep inferior epigastric artery perforator
flap, VI:686, 762, 764t, 1040-1044
anatomy of, VI:1040-1041, 1041f
bilateral, VI:1042
complications of, VI:765t, 1044
defect closure for, VI:1042, 1044
surface markings for, VI:1040, 1041f
surgical technique for, VI:765-766, 766f,
1002, 1004f, 1007f, 1008, 1011,
1011f, 1012f, 1020, 1020f, 1040t,
1041-1042
unilateral, VI:1042, 1042f, 1043f
Deep venous thrombosis, VI:175-178,
177t, 178f
after abdominoplasty, VI:362
after free TRAM flap, VI:872
liposuction and, VI:237-238
microvascular surgery and, I:525-526

Defense mechanisms, I:69-70
Deformation, I:53-54
Degloving injury
to auricle, V:388
to nose, III:30
Deglutition, III:923
Delay procedure, in flap optimization,
I:357-358, 357f, 358f, 367-371, 369f-
371f, 494, 499t, 500
Delta phalanx, VIII:294-295, 295f
Deltoid flap, I:405-407, 405f-407f
Deltoid reconstruction, VIII:502-503, 502f,
503f, 504, 506
Deltoid to triceps transfer, for elbow
extension, in tetraplegic patient,
VIII:512-517, 513f-515f, 517f
Deltopectoral flap
for esophageal reconstruction, III:1011
for facial reconstruction, I:381, 382f-
386f, III:833, 843f, 848f
for head and neck reconstruction,
III:1043, 1044f, V:223, 224f, 226t
Demander personality, I:74
Dendritic cells, in graft rejection, I:272
Denervation, I:607
Denial, I:69
Dental implants
after mandibular reconstruction,
III:984-986, 986f, 987f
osseointegrated, I:524, 524f
recombinant bone morphogenetic
proteins with, I:662-663
Dental plate, in cleft lip, IV:177f, 178, 178f,
180
Dental splint, in maxillary fracture, III:257,
257f
Dentigerous cyst, V:93, 95, 191-192, 192f
Dentition. *See* Tooth (teeth).
Deontology, I:98-99, 98t
Deoxyribonucleic acid (DNA), analysis of,
IV:94-95
Dependent personality, I:72, 73
Depigmentation, with carbon dioxide laser
resurfacing, II:70, 70f
Depression, in patient evaluation, I:82,
83t
Depressor anguli oris, III:889
Depressor labii inferioris, III:889, 889f
resection of, in lower lip paralysis,
III:912, 913f
Depressor supercilaris, II:55, 56f
Dermablend, V:39-40
Dermabrasion, facial, II:343, 343t
Dermagraft, I:893, 1087t, 1088
Dermagraft-TC, I:313
Dermal-epidermal junction, I:296
Dermal fat flap, for nipple reconstruction,
VI:796, 797f-799f
Dermal graft, I:569-576. *See also* Skin graft.
allograft, I:571, 574-576
indications for, I:574, 574f
outcomes of, I:575-576
sources of, I:571, 574, 574f
uses of, I:574-575, 574f, 576f
autogenous, I:570-571
harvesting of, I:570-571, 570f, 571f
indications for, I:570
outcomes of, I:571, 572f, 573f
sutures for, I:571
historical perspective on, I:569-570

Dermal-lipoglandular flap, for breast
reduction, VI:603, 604f
Dermal-orbicular pennant lateral
canthoplasty, II:847-851, 848f-852f
Dermatitis
contact, after laser resurfacing, II:370
pustular, VII:784-785
radiation, I:843
Dermatofibroma, Color Plate V:112-4,
V:260-261, 260f, 399, VII:952, 952f
Dermatofibrosarcoma protuberans, V:298-
299, 299f
Dermatoheliosis, II:387
Dermatolipectomy, suprapubic, VI:408, 409f
Dermis, I:294f, 296. *See also* Skin.
in tissue expansion, I:541
Dermis-fat graft, I:301f, 578-579, 579f
Dermofasciectomy, in Dupuytren disease,
VII:748-750, 749f, 750f
Dermoid cyst, III:765, V:4, 4f, 5f
Desepiphysiodesis, posttraumatic,
VIII:446, 447f
Desflurane, I:178-179, 178t
Desiccant agent injury, to hand, VII:653t,
654, 656
Desmoid
abdominal, VI:93
upper extremity, VII:954-955, 954f
Desmoplastic fibroma, V:103, 206-207
Dextran
in flap optimization, I:499t, 500
in microvascular surgery, I:522
Diabetes mellitus
amputation in, VI:1448-1449
common peroneal nerve compression
in, VII:912
Dupuytren disease in, VII:738
foot reconstruction in, VI:1443-1450
amputation alternatives for, VI:1448-
1449
outcomes of, VI:1449-1450
preoperative evaluation for, VI:1446
vacuum-assisted closure device in,
VI:1449
wound management for, VI:1446-
1448, 1447f, 1448f
gangrene in, VII:782
hemorheologic abnormalities in,
VI:1445-1446, 1445f, 1450
neuropathy in, VI:1444-1445, 1450,
VII:923-924
preoperative evaluation of, I:170
tarsal tunnel release in, VI:1448, 1448f
ulcers in, I:981, 982f
wound healing in, I:219-220, 942-943,
943f
Diabetic neuropathy, VI:1444-1445, 1450,
VII:923-924
Dialysis, steal syndrome with, VII:807, 808f
Diaphragm
agenesis of, VI:434
anatomy of, VI:413
Diaphragmatic hernia, congenital, I:1122-
1124, 1123f
Diastasis recti, VI:92-93, 94f, 95f, 110
Diazepam
in complex regional pain
syndrome/reflex sympathetic
dystrophy, VII:859
preoperative, I:171f

Diclofenac, I:183-184
  in skin cancer, V:404t, 406
Diepoxybutane test, in Fanconi anemia,
    VIII:325
Diet
  breast pain and, VI:354-355
  large-volume liposuction and, VI:242
  skin cancer and, V:278
Dietary supplements, abdominoplasty and,
    VI:175
Dieting, medications for, I:170
Difficult patient, I:73-75
Digastric muscles, after face lift, II:740-
    741, 741f
DiGeorge syndrome, IV:102
Digit. See Finger(s); Thumb(s).
Digital arteries, VII:37, 794-795, 795f
  in finger reconstruction, VII:221, 221f
  of nail unit, VII:171-172
  thrombosis of, VII:810
Digital nerve block, VII:105
Digital nerve repair, I:735, VII:508
Diltiazem, in complex regional pain
    syndrome/reflex sympathetic
    dystrophy, VII:857
Dimethyl sulfoxide (DMSO)
  hand injury from, VII:654
  in complex regional pain
    syndrome/reflex sympathetic
    dystrophy, VII:857
Dimple sign, VII:54
Diplegia, spastic, interferon-alfa and, V:30-
    31
Diplopia
  in orbital fracture, III:275, 277t, 281,
    284-285, 284f, 286, 325-326
  in zygoma fracture, III:210-212, 211f,
    213, 227-228, 228f
  with craniofacial cleft management,
    IV:461
Diprosopus, IV:407
Disomy, uniparental, I:53
Disruption, I:53-54
Dissatisfied patient, I:87, 87t
Distant learning, I:1142
Distortion, I:69
Distraction osteogenesis, I:667-671, 667f,
    III:778-784
  age-related factors in, I:668-669
  blood supply in, I:669
  device stability for, I:670-671
  fractionated protocols for, I:670
  histology of, I:668, 669f
  history of, I:667-668
  in cleft lip and palate, IV:293, 296, 303-
    308, 304f-308f
  in constriction ring syndrome, VIII:205,
    205f, 206f
  in craniofacial cleft, IV:430-431, 446
  in craniofacial microsomia, III:780-783,
    780f-783f, IV:523-533, 524f-532f,
    546, 548f
  in craniosynostosis, IV:485-486
  in hand reconstruction, VII:628, 629
  in micrognathia, III:776-778, 776f, 778f,
    780-783, 780f-783f
  in obstructive sleep apnea, III:778-780
  in radial (preaxial) deficiency, VIII:70f,
    73, 74f, 75
  in Robin sequence, III:781, IV:515

Distraction osteogenesis (Continued)
  in thumb reconstruction, VII:291-292,
    628-629
  latency period for, I:669-670
  metacarpal, VIII:57-59, 58f
  midface, III:783-784
  rate of, I:670
  stages of, I:668, 669f
  timing of, I:669-670
Diuretics, in altitude sickness, I:861
Diverticulum, Zenker, III:994, 995f
Dizziness, postoperative, I:202
DMSO (dimethyl sulfoxide)
  hand injury from, VII:654
  in complex regional pain
    syndrome/reflex sympathetic
    dystrophy, VII:857
Dobutamine, microvascular surgery and,
    I:521
Dog
  bites by, III:2-3, 3f, 30, 31f, 402, 402f,
    403f
  vascular territories in, I:330-332, 333f
Dog-ears
  after abdominoplasty, VI:363, 365f, 366f
  after breast reduction, VI:581, 1068,
    1071f
Dopamine, microvascular surgery and,
    I:521
Doppler imaging
  in foot, VI:1412, 1414, 1414f
  in upper extremity ischemia, VII:800
  of flap, I:497t, 498-499
Dorsal arteries, of hand, VII:37
Dorsal intercarpal ligament, VII:455, 455f
Dorsal radiocarpal ligament, VII:455, 455f
Dorsal retinaculum, zone VII extensor
    tendon injury under, VII:418-420,
    419f
Dorsal reversed homodigital flap, for finger
    reconstruction, VII:228, 231, 232f
Dorsal scapular island flap, for neck
    reconstruction, III:1042, 1042f
Dorsalis pedis artery, VI:1404-1405, 1404f,
    1409, 1411f, 1412f
Double crush syndrome, VII:878-879,
    880f, 903-904
Double opposing tab flap, for nipple
    reconstruction, VI:807, 811f
Double opposing Z-plasty technique, in
    palatoplasty, IV:259-261, 261f
Down syndrome, macroglossia in, III:768
Dreams, ketamine-induced, I:175
Dressings
  absorptive, I:884-885, 885t
  after laser facial resurfacing, II:363-364
  biologic, I:823-825, 824f, 824t
  bolus, I:308, 308f
  film, I:224, 225t
  Flexzan, II:364
  foam, I:224, 225t, 884-885, 885t
  for Benelli mastopexy, VI:54
  for burns, I:822, 823-825, 824f, 824t,
    VII:592
  for closed rhinoplasty, II:550, 551f
  for fingertip, VII:156-157
  for fractures, VI:1390
  for hand surgery, VII:121-122
  for hemangioma, V:28
  for lower extremity, I:224, VI:1469

Dressings (Continued)
  for pressure sores, VI:1350-1351
  for skin grafts, I:307-309, 308f
  for syndactyly, VIII:166-167
  gauze, I:224, 225t, 873
  hydrocolloid, I:224, 225t
  hydrogel, I:224, 225t
  in Dupuytren disease, VII:746, 747f
  in lower extremity edema, I:224
  silicone, I:224, 225t, 227
  subatmospheric pressure, I:224, 225t
  wound, Color Plate I:32-1, I:224, 225t,
    873, 883-886, 885f
Drowsiness, postoperative, I:202
Drug abuse
  by surgeon, I:112
  in patient evaluation, I:85
  intra-arterial injection injury with,
    VII:807
Duck, vascular territories in, I:330-332,
    333f
Ductal lavage, in breast cancer, Color Plate
    VI:138-3, VI:642-643
Dufourmentel flap, for cheek
    reconstruction, III:833, 837f
Duplication
  craniofacial, IV:407, 409f, 419t
  digital, VIII:215-261. See also
    Polydactyly.
  maxillary, IV:407, 409f
Dupuytren, Guillaume, I:27, VII:729
Dupuytren disease, VII:729-754, 954
  adult digital fibroma and, VII:954
  age and, VII:739
  alcoholism and, VII:738
  amputation in, VII:752
  assessment of, VII:739-740, 740f
  bilaterality of, VII:739
  biomechanical pathology in, VII:734
  clinical presentation of, VII:735-740,
    735f-738f
  collagen type III in, VII:735
  contractures in, VII:668-669, 669f, 670f,
    671, 736, 737f, VIII:561
    in musician, VII:696-697, 697f, 701
  dermofasciectomy in, VII:748-750, 749f,
    750f
  differential diagnosis of, VII:736-738,
    737f, 738f
  enzymatic fasciotomy in, VII:740-741
  epidemiology of, VII:739
  family incidence of, VII:739
  fasciectomy in, VII:742, 743-751
    central slip tenodesis test in, VII:745
    checkrein release in, VII:745, 746f
    closure after, VII:745-746, 746f
    complications of, VII:750-751, 751f
    dressing for, VII:746, 747f
    dynamic splinting after, VII:746
    hand positioning for, VII:743, 743f
    incisions for, VII:743-745, 743f
    infection after, VII:751
    neurovascular injury with, VII:750-
      751, 751f
    open palm technique for, VII:747, 747f
    reflex sympathetic dystrophy after,
      VII:751
    skin graft in, VII:748-750, 749f, 750f
    skin necrosis after, VII:750-751, 751f
    wound dehiscence after, VII:751, 751f

Facial fracture(s) *(Continued)*
panoramic view in, III:106, 108f, 109f
posteroanterior mandibular view in, III:103, 105f
profile view in, III:96, 97f
reverse Waters position in, III:92, 94f
semiaxial (superoinferior) closed projection in, III:92, 95f
submentovertex position in, III:97, 102f
superoinferior anterior occlusal view in, III:97, 100f
superoinferior central occlusal view in, III:97, 99f
temporomandibular joint views in, III:103, 105-106
Titterington position in, III:92, 95f
verticosubmental position in, III:97, 102f
Waters position for, III:90, 92f
visual acuity in, III:86-87, 87f
endoscopic management of, III:463-507
contraindications to, III:472
development of, III:469-471
evolution of, III:469, 507
in condylar neck, III:472-485
in frontal sinus, III:492, 501f-504f, 503-504
in internal orbit, III:504-507, 505f-507f
in mandibular symphysis, III:485-491, 487f-490f
in zygomatic arch, III:491-492, 494f-503f
indications for, III:472
instrumentation for, III:471, 471f
skill acquisition for, III:471-472
frontobasilar, III:330-344. *See also* Frontobasilar region fracture.
Glasgow Coma Scale in, III:81, 83, 83t
gunshot-related, III:344, 350-361. *See also* Face, gunshot wounds to.
head injury with, III:81, 83, 83t
hemorrhage in, III:79-81, 80f-82f
management of, III:110-145
airway in, III:78-79, 79t
arterial ligation in, III:81
computed tomography in, III:467, 468f
coronal incision for, III:111, 111f
dental fixation in, III:118, 120-128
acrylic splints in, III:127, 129f
anatomy for, III:118, 120-122, 120f-122f
arch bar method wiring in, III:123-126, 124f-127f
Eyelet method wiring in, III:122-123, 123f
Gilmer method wiring in, III:122, 122f
intermaxillary fixation screw in, III:128, 130f
monomaxillary vs. bimaxillary, III:128
orthodontic bands in, III:127, 128f
wiring techniques in, III:122-128, 122f-127f
embolization in, III:81

Facial fracture(s) *(Continued)*
endoscopic, III:463-507. *See also* Facial fracture(s), endoscopic management of.
fracture stabilization in, III:128, 131-145
appliances for, III:128, 131-138, 132f-139f
bone grafts for, III:138-145, 140f-143f, 144t
historical perspective on, III:464-465
incision for, III:111-118, 111f
blepharoplasty, III:111-114, 111-114f, 115t, 116f
coronal, III:111, 111f
extraoral, III:111f, 116, 118, 119f, 120f
intraoral, III:111f, 114-116, 116f-118f
sequelae of, III:466-467
minimally invasive, III:469-472
nasal packing in, III:79-81, 80f, 81f
planning for, III:467, 468f
residual skeletal malreduction with, III:465-466, 466f
soft tissue malpositioning with, III:466
timing in, III:85
undesirable outcomes of, III:465-467, 466f
mandibular, III:145-187. *See also* Mandibular fracture.
maxillary, III:229-264. *See also* Maxillary fracture.
mechanism of injury of, III:77-78
nasal, III:187-208. *See also* Nasal fracture.
nasoethmoidal-orbital, III:305, 307-330. *See also* Nasoethmoidal-orbital fracture.
open repair of, III:463, 464f
orbital, III:264-305. *See also* Orbital fracture.
pain after, III:361-366, 363-364t
pediatric, III:402-454, 770
abuse-related, III:399-400, 399f
alveolar, III:405-409, 406f-408f
birth-related, III:398
complications of, III:454-455
condylar, III:412, 414-421, 414f-416f, 419f-420f
ethmoid, III:434-438, 435f-438f
etiology of, III:402, 404
evaluation of, III:456t
frontal bone, III:438-444, 440f-445f
incidence of, III:404-405, 404t, 405t, 407f
Le Fort, III:448-453, 448t, 449f-451f
malocclusion and, III:411-412
mandibular, III:409-411, 410f-413f
Panorex exam in, III:395, 396f
maxillary, III:448-453, 448t, 449f-451f
midfacial, III:421-424, 421f-424f, 448-453, 448t, 449f-451f
nasal, III:432-434, 433f
nasoethmoidal-orbital, III:393f-394f, 434-438, 435f-438f
orbital, III:424-432, 425f-428f, 429t, 430f-431f, 434-438, 435f-438f

Facial fracture(s) *(Continued)*
plate translocation in, III:454
prevention of, III:457-456
resorbable fixation in, III:454
rigid fixation in, III:453-454
subcondylar, III:770
supraorbital, III:445-448, 445f-448f
zygomatic, III:397f, 424-432, 425f-426f
zygoma, III:208-229, 424-432. *See also* Zygoma, fracture of.
Facial nerve
anatomy of, II:167-169, 168f, 169f, III:4-5, 4f
at forehead, II:57-58, 58f
in face lift, II:256-257, 257f, 302-304, 305f
in facial paralysis, III:886-887, 886f
in periorbital surgery, II:86, 86f
in salivary gland tumors, V:69, 71f
cervical division of, III:886f, 887
frontal division of, II:83
in craniofacial microsomia, IV:123, 124
injury to, III:27, 361-366, 883-915. *See also* Facial paralysis.
in children, III:401
in liposuction, VI:220
neck lift and, II:332-334, 335f
nerve blocks in, III:365-366
neurolysis in, III:366
rhytidectomy and, II:206, 207f
subperiosteal midface lift and, II:236
treatment of, III:365-366
mandibular division of, III:886f, 887
repair of, I:737, 737t
temporal division of, II:58, 59f, 82, III:886f, 887
zygomaticobuccal division of, III:886f, 887
Facial nerve block, I:191-192, 192f
Facial paralysis, III:883-915
acquired, III:181, 884-885
anatomy for, III:886-889, 886f, 887f, 888t, 889f
asymmetry in, III:883, 884f, 885f
bilateral, III:885-886
brow ptosis in, III:883
classification of, III:884-886, 886t
congenital, III:884-885, 913-914, 913f
ectropion with, III:884, 895-897, 896f, 897f
emotional effects of, III:884
eye in, III:883-884, 890, 891
fascial graft for, I:585
feeding in, III:913
lagophthalmos in, III:748, 749f, 891t, 892-895, 893f-895f
mouth assessment in, III:890
patient assessment in, III:890
psychosocial aspects of, III:913
smile impairment with, III:884, 885f
smile restoration in, III:877, 879, 879f, 880f
speech impairment with, III:884
synkinesis in, III:890
tearing with, III:883-884
treatment of, III:890-915
brow lift in, III:891-892, 891t
contralateral facial nerve in, III:898, 899-903, 899f-902f

Facial paralysis *(Continued)*
future directions in, III:914-915
lower eyelid in, III:895-897, 896f, 897f
lower lip in, III:911-912, 913f
masseter muscle nerve in, III:898-899, 905-906
masseter muscle transplantation in, III:910, 910f
nasal airway in, III:897
neuromuscular retraining in, III:891
nonsurgical, III:890-891, 891t
nonvascularized muscle graft in, I:612
planning for, III:890
smile reconstruction in, III:897-911. *See also* Smile reconstruction.
subspecialty, III:912-913
sural nerve in, III:900, 902f
surgical, III:891-912, 891t
temporalis muscle transplantation in, III:906, 910, 910f
upper eyelid in, III:748, 749f, 891t, 892-895, 893f-895f
tumor-related, III:885
unilateral, III:885
Facial prostheses, I:770-781
acrylic buttons for, I:772, 772f
adhesives for, I:771-772, 771f
anatomic fitting of, I:772-773, 772f
color for, Color Plate I:27-3, I:776
for ear, I:776-778, 776f, 777f
for eye, I:772f, 780-781
for nose, Color Plate I:27-4, I:778, 778f, 779f
for orbit, I:778-780, 779f, 780f
impressions for, I:774-775, 775f
materials for, I:775-776, 775f
osseointegration of, Color Plate I:27-2, I:773-774, 773f, 774f
retention of, Color Plate I:27-1, I:771-773, 771f, 772f
titanium, Color Plate I:27-2, I:773-774, 773f, 774f
Facial reconstruction. *See also* Cheek reconstruction; Chin, reconstruction of; Forehead reconstruction; Nasal reconstruction; Neck reconstruction.
deltopectoral flap for, I:381, 382f-386f, III:833, 843f, 848f
pectoralis major flap for, I:423, 423f-427f, III:833, 845f, 848f
bone (rib) with, I:390, 391f, 392f
skeletal augmentation for, II:405-425. *See also* Facial skeleton, augmentation of.
tissue expansion in, I:551, 553, 554f, 555f
trapezius flap for, I:423, 428f-430f, III:833, 846f
Facial resurfacing, II:339-380, 385-401
chemical peels for, II:343-344, 343t, 379-380, 379t, 380f
coblation for, II:378-379
dermabrasion for, II:343, 343t
future trends in, II:379-380, 379t, 380f
laser, II:339-380
acne cosmetica after, II:370-371
anesthesia for, II:346
antibiotics in, II:345, 365
Aquaphor after, II:365, 370
botulinum toxin with, II:345

Facial resurfacing *(Continued)*
brow lift with, II:358-359, 360f
candidates for, II:341, 341t
care after, II:361, 363-365
clinical evaluation for, II:340-344, 341f, 341t
CO_2, II:70, 70f, 347, 350, 351f
complications of, II:368-376, 371f, 372f, 374f, 375f, 756
contact dermatitis after, II:370
contraindications to, II:342-343, 342t
CoolTouch, II:376, 377f
corneal abrasion with, II:375
creams after, II:365
cryogen spray with, II:378
delayed healing with, II:342, 374-375
demarcation lines with, II:344
dilated pores with, II:376
diode, II:377-378
dual-mode Er:YAG (Sciton Contour), II:356, 357f
ectropion with, II:375
edema with, II:368
Er:YAG, II:347, 350-351, 352f, 378
hyperpigmentation with, II:345
erythema with, II:369-370
exudate with, II:368-369
eyebrow lift and, II:232, 233f
eyelid, II:258-259
eyelid surgery with, II:359-360, 360f
face lift with, II:360-361, 362f, 363f
Flexzan dressing after, II:364
fluence and, II:346-347
FotoFacial, II:376-377, 378f
full-face vs. regional, II:344
globe puncture with, II:375
healing after, II:361, 363
herpes simplex virus infection and, II:342, 345, 346f
historical perspective on, II:339-340
hydroquinone with, II:345
hyperpigmentation with, II:342, 345, 372-373
hypopigmentation with, II:373-374, 374f
indications for, II:341-342
infection after, II:371-372, 371f
isotretinoin and, II:342
lower lid laxity and, II:342-343
milia after, II:370-371
Nd:YAG, II:376, 377f
nonablative, II:376-380, 377f, 378f
open vs. closed dressings for, II:363-364
OxyMist after, II:365
periorbital, II:258-259, 359-360, 360f
petechiae with, II:376
physical principles of, II:346-347, 347f
preparation for, II:344-346
pulse duration and, II:346
pulsed dye, II:377
re-epithelialization after, II:361, 364
recommendations for, II:356, 358
rhytidectomy with, II:360-361
safety precautions for, II:349, 349t
scleral show with, II:375
sequential CO_2/Er:YAG, II:351-353, 353f, 354f
simultaneous CO_2/Er:YAG (Derma-K), II:353-355, 355f

Facial resurfacing *(Continued)*
skin sensitivity after, II:370
skin thickness and, II:348t
SkinLaser, II:377-378
synechia with, II:375, 375f
tissue interactions with, II:348-349, 348f
tooth cracks with, II:375-376
topical agents after, II:364-365
toxic shock syndrome after, II:372
variable-pulsed erbium (CO_3), II:356, 358f
wavelength and, II:346, 347f
yeast infection after, II:371, 371f
pharmacologic, II:385-401
copper-based preparations for, II:401
furfuryladenine for, II:401
historical perspective on, II:386
hydroxy acids for, II:385-386, 397-400, 400f
patient selection for, II:388, 390
topical retinoids for, II:385, 390-397, 391t. *See also* Retinoids.
vitamin C for, II:400-401
vitamin E for, II:401
procedure selection for, II:343-345, 343t
Facial skeleton
acquired deformities of, III:563-604. *See also* Facial fracture(s).
access incisions for, III:563-564
bone grafts for, III:564
coronal incisions for, III:563-564, 564f
in chin, III:599, 600f-604f
in cranium, III:564-565, 566f-573f
in irradiated orbit, III:582
in mandible, III:594, 598f-599f
in maxilla, III:582, 593f-597f, 594
in nasoethmoid fracture, III:580, 581f
in nose, III:565, 573, 574f-579f
in orbitozygomatic fracture, III:580, 582, 583f-592f
in post-traumatic enophthalmos, III:580, 582, 583f-592f
intraoral incisions for, III:564
lower eyelid incisions for, III:564
skeletal augmentation in, II:405-425. *See also* Facial skeleton, augmentation of.
soft tissue coverage for, III:564
augmentation of, II:405-425
acrylic for, II:408
alloplastic materials for, II:407-408, 407f
anesthesia for, II:408-409
anthropometric measurements for, II:405, 406f
for soft tissue depressions, II:423, 425, 425f
implant for, II:407-408, 407f
immobilization of, II:408
positioning of, II:408
shape of, II:408
of chin, II:414, 418-419, 418f-420f
of forehead, II:409, 409f, 410, 410f
of infraorbital rim, II:412, 416f-417f
of lower third, II:414, 418-423, 418f-424f
of malar midface, II:410-411, 411f-413f

Facial skeleton *(Continued)*
of mandible, II:414, 418-423, 418f-424f
of mandibular ramus, II:419, 421-423, 421f-424f
of middle third, II:410-414, 411f-417f
of paranasal midface, II:412, 414f, 415f
of supraorbital rim, II:409, 410, 410f
of upper third, II:409-410, 409f, 410f
physical examination for, II:405
planning for, II:405-406, 406f
polyethylene for, II:407f, 408
polysiloxane (silicone) for, II:407
polytetrafluoroethylene (Gore-Tex) for, II:407-408
cephalometric analysis of, II:15, 18-28, 19f, 20t, 21t. *See also* Facial analysis, cephalometric.
congenital disorders of. *See* Craniofacial cleft(s); Craniofacial syndromes.
Facial trauma
bone, III:77-367, 563-604. *See also* Facial fracture(s) *and fractures at specific structures.*
nerve, III:883-915. *See also* Facial paralysis.
pain after, III:361-366, 363-364t
pediatric, III:381-456. *See also* Facial fracture(s), pediatric.
abuse-related, III:399-400, 399f
aspiration in, III:398
birth-related, III:398
computed tomography in, III:392, 393f, 395, 395t, 397f
CSF rhinorrhea with, III:455
dental injury in, III:405-409, 406f-408f
dog bites and, III:402, 402f, 403f
emergency treatment of, III:395, 397-398, 397f
endotracheal tube in, III:395, 397-398, 397f
etiology of, III:381-382
evaluation of, III:391-392
facial nerve injury in, III:401
healing of, III:400-401
hematoma in, III:399, 400, 401-402
hemorrhage in, III:397-398
in infant, III:398-399
lacerations in, III:400, 401
nasal packing in, III:397-398
Panorex exam in, III:395, 396f
radiologic evaluation of, III:392-395, 393f-394f, 395t, 396f, 397f
scarring after, III:400-401, 401f
soft tissue injury in, III:400-402, 401f
tracheal stenosis in, III:398
soft tissue, III:1-39
anatomy in, III:3-5, 4f, 5f
assaults and, III:2
bites and, III:2-3, 3f
clinical examination of, III:5-6
collisions and, III:1-2
débridement in, III:4
etiology of, III:1-3, 2f, 3f
evaluation of, III:3-6, 4f, 5f
falls and, III:1
in children, III:400-402, 401f
incidence of, III:1-3, 2f, 3f

Facial trauma *(Continued)*
innervation in, III:4-5, 4f
Langer's lines in, III:3
nasal examination in, III:6
ocular examination in, III:6
oral cavity examination in, III:6
road accidents and, III:2
sports injury and, III:2
treatment of, III:6-38
anesthesia in, III:6-11, 7t, 8f-11f
auricular nerve block for, III:9-10
auriculotemporal nerve block for, III:10-11, 11f
epinephrine for, III:6-7, 7t
infraorbital nerve block for, III:8-9, 9f
local infiltration for, III:7-8
mental nerve block for, III:9, 10f
nerve blocks for, III:8-11, 8f-11f
ophthalmic nerve block for, III:8, 8f
ring block for, III:10-11, 11f
sodium bicarbonate buffering in, III:7
topical anesthetics for, III:8
débridement in, III:11
for abrasions, III:11, 12f
for avulsions, III:14
for cheek injury, III:26-27, 27f, 28f
for ear injury, III:30-36, 32f, 35f
for eyebrow injury, III:17, 20-23, 21f-23f
for eyelid injury, III:23-26, 23f-26f
for lacerations, III:13-14, 13f, 14f
for mouth injury, III:36-38, 38f
for nasal injury, III:27-30, 31f
for scalp and forehead injury, III:15-17, 18f-20f
for traumatic tattoo, III:12-13, 12f
irrigation in, III:11, 12f
keloids and, III:14-15, 15f
vascular perfusion in, III:3-4
wound healing and, I:1006-1008, 1008f
Factitial disorders, I:944
vs. hand infection, VII:768
vs. reflex sympathetic dystrophy/chronic regional pain syndrome, VII:848, 848f
Falls
by children, III:400
by infant, III:398-409
Famotidine, preoperative, I:171
Fan flap, for lip reconstruction, III:813, 817f-819f, V:383
Fanconi anemia, V:401, VIII:31, 325
Fansanella-Servat procedure, II:831, 832f
Fascial débridement, I:875, 976
Fascial flaps, I:374-377, 375f, 376f, 377t, 417, 586-588, 587f. *See also* Flap(s) *and at specific flaps and procedures.*
advantages of, I:417
arc of rotation of, I:375, 375f
disadvantages of, I:417
outcomes of, I:586-588, 587f
section of, I:421
type A, I:376-377, 376f, 377t, 390
type B, I:376-377, 376f, 377t, 390
type C, I:376f, 377, 377t
Fascicle, VII:474-475, 474f

Fasciectomy, in Dupuytren disease, VII:742, 743-751. *See also* Dupuytren disease, fasciectomy in.
Fasciitis
necrotizing, I:911, 914, 914f, 974, 976-977
abdominal, VI:93
of hand, VII:781-782, 782f, 783f
nodular, VII:952-953
Fasciocutaneous flaps, I:358-359, 374-377, 376f, 377t, 378f, 417. *See also* Flap(s) *and at specific flaps and procedures.*
advantages of, I:417
arc of rotation of, I:375, 376f
disadvantages of, I:417
free, I:412-413, 414f
reverse transposition, I:409-411, 411f, 412f
section of, I:421
type A, I:376-377, 376f, 377t, 378f, 390
type B, I:376f, 377, 377t, 378f, 390, 410, 412f
type C, I:376f, 377, 377t, 378f
with vascularized bone, I:390, 390t, 393f
Fasciotomy
in Dupuytren disease, VII:741-742
in hand burns, VII:592, 600-601
needle, VII:742
open, VII:741-742
subcutaneous, VII:741
Fasting, preoperative, I:169
Fat
buccal, II:170, 171f
overexcision of, II:738-740, 739f
injection of. *See* Fat injection.
malar. *See* Malar fat pads.
orbital, III:271-272, 272f
postblepharoplasty, II:803, 810, 810f, 814
suction removal of. *See* Liposuction.
tissue-engineered, I:1095-1096
Fat embolism, with liposuction, VI:238
Fat graft, I:576-579
dermis-fat, I:301f, 578-579, 579f
free, I:578, 580f
historical perspective on, I:576-578, 577f
Fat injection, I:579-584
cyst formation with, I:584
fat harvest for, I:580, 582, 582f
in face lift, II:249-250, 250f
in facial atrophy, II:751, 752f
indications for, I:579-580
mammary, I:584
middle cerebral artery embolism with, I:583-584
outcomes of, I:582-584
penile, I:584
pseudocyst formation with, I:584
technique of, I:582, 583f, 584f
Fat necrosis
after breast reduction, VI:578-579, 1068, 1070
after TRAM flap breast reconstruction, VI:865, 994
Feeding, cleft palate and, IV:254-255
Feet. *See* Foot (feet).
Felon, VII:772, 772f, 777, 778f
Feminist ethics, I:106-107
Femoral cutaneous nerve, lateral, entrapment of, VII:909-910, 911f

Femoral nerve block, I:193-194, 198f
Fentanyl, I:181-182
Ferguson-Smith syndrome, V:400, 441
Fetal surgery, I:1072, 1117-1131
  fetoscope in, I:1118-1119
  historical perspective on, I:1117
  in amniotic band syndrome, I:1130-1131
  in cardiac disorders, I:1125-1126
  in cleft lip and palate, I:1129
  in cystic adenomatoid malformation, I:1124-1125
  in diaphragmatic hernia, I:1122-1124, 1123f
  in hemangioma, I:1122
  in high airway obstruction syndrome, I:1121, 1121f
  in hydronephrosis, I:1126-1127, 1126t
  in hydrothorax, I:1125
  in intracranial anomalies, I:1128-1129
  in myelomeningocele, I:1128
  in neck disorders, I:1121-1122, 1121f, 1122t
  in neurologic disorders, I:1128-1129
  in sacrococcygeal teratoma, I:1127-1128
  in thoracic disorders, I:1122-1125, 1123f
  in twin-twin transfusion syndrome, I:1129-1130
  in vascular malformations, I:1122
  incision for, I:1118, 1119f
  maternal care during, I:1119
  minimally invasive techniques for, I:1118-1119
  monitoring during, I:1119-1120, 1120f
  placental vessel catheterization in, I:1120, 1120f
  preterm labor and, I:1120-1121
  selection for, I:1118, 1118t
  standard techniques for, I:1118, 1119f
  ultrasonography in, I:1118, 1120
Fetus
  evaluation of, I:1067-1076. See also Prenatal diagnosis.
  renal function in, I:1126-1127, 1126t
  surgery on. See Fetal surgery.
  wound healing in, Color Plate I:11-1, I:217-218, 217f
FGFR1 gene, VIII:20
FGFR2 gene, IV:11, 92, 93t, VIII:20
FGFR3 gene, IV:92, 93t
Fibonacci sequence, VII:401-402
Fibrin, for bioengineered cartilage, I:631-632
Fibro-odontoma, ameloblastic, V:98, 200
Fibroblast
  in fetal wound healing, I:217-218
  in keloids, I:222
  in wound healing, I:210f, 211-213, 211f
Fibroblast growth factors
  in bone repair, I:657t, 658, 660t, 665-666
  in wound healing, I:212t, 216, 226, 1018
  receptors for, mutations in, I:58, 60-61, 61f-63f
Fibrocartilage, Color Plate I:23-1, I:621
Fibrolipoma, VII:958
Fibroma
  ameloblastic, V:97-98, 199-200
  cementifying, V:98, 204
  chondromyxoid, V:207
  desmoplastic, V:103, 206-207

Fibroma (Continued)
  infantile, of digits, VII:953-954, 953f
  odontogenic, V:98, 201-202
  ossifying, V:206, 208f
  tendon sheath, VII:953, 953f
Fibromatoses
  juvenile, V:10-11
  upper extremity, VII:954-955, 954f
Fibromatosis colli, V:10-11
Fibromyalgia, double crush syndrome in, VII:903-904
Fibronectin, in wound healing, I:212
Fibrosarcoma
  ameloblastic, V:99
  in children, V:14
  of head and neck, V:118-119
  of mandible, V:99, 107, 213
Fibrous dysplasia
  in children, V:12, 12f
  of frontal bone, III:565, 571f-572f
  of mandible, V:99-101, 100f, 101f, 206, 207f
  of orbit, V:127, 130f-131f, 144
Fibrous tumors, V:11, VII:952-956, 952f-955f
Fibula
  for bone graft, I:674t, 686-688, 687f
  transfer of, for upper extremity reconstruction, VII:335, 342f
Fibula flap, for mandible reconstruction, I:390, 390t, 393-395f, III:964f, 966, 967f, 968-969
Fibular tunnel syndrome, VII:876t
Field cancerization, V:160
Filariasis, I:907, 909f, VI:1457, 1457f
Film dressings, I:224, 225t
Finasteride, in hair restoration, II:693-694, III:626, 628
Fine-needle aspiration. See also Biopsy.
  in breast cancer, Color Plate VI:138-1, VI:639, 641t
  of head and neck mass, V:167
  of salivary gland tumors, V:72-73, 72f
Finger(s). See also Fingertip; Hand(s); Thumb(s).
  amputation of
    congenital, VIII:56-61. See also Constriction ring syndrome.
     bone graft in, VIII:59
     metacarpal distraction lengthening in, VIII:57-59, 58f
     metacarpal transposition in, VIII:57
     nubbin excision in, VIII:56
     phalangeal transfer in, VIII:57
     prostheses in, VIII:56
     toe transfer in, VIII:59-60, 60f
     web deepening in, VIII:57
    difficult cases of, VIII:603-604, 603f-606f
    prostheses for, VIII:589-592, 590f-597f, 600, 602f, 603
    therapeutic, VII:207-212, 208t, 209t
     burns and, VII:627-630, 629f
     distal phalangeal, VII:210-211, 211f, 212, 223f-225f
     impairment with, VII:208, 210f
     in central polydactyly, VIII:243
     levels of, VII:208, 210

Finger(s) (Continued)
    middle phalangeal, VII:210-211, 222, 226f
    postoperative care of, VIII:566-567
    proximal phalangeal, VII:212, 212f, 222, 226f, 227f
    ray, VII:211-212, 212f
    traumatic. See also Finger(s), injury to; Finger reconstruction.
     burn-related, VII:627-630, 629f
     in musician, VII:701
     replantation for. See Finger replantation.
  anatomy of, VII:731-732, 731f, VIII:287-288, 288f, 545f
  arteries of, VII:221, 221f
  bone tumors of, VII:979-991, 980f
    benign, VII:983-988, 984f-987f
    biopsy in, VII:980-981
    imaging of, VII:980, 980f
    malignant, VII:988-991, 989f, 990f
    resection of, VII:981-982, 982t
     reconstruction after, VII:982-983
    staging of, VII:981
  boutonnière deformity of, VII:663, 664f
    burns and, VII:625-627, 626f
    infection and, VII:788-789
    repair of, VII:416-417, 416f
  burn scar contracture of, VII:616-624, 617t, 618f-620f, 622f, 624f
  carpometacarpal joint of
    dislocation of, VII:434, 435f
    fracture-dislocation of, VII:434-436, 435f
    osteoarthritis of, VII:57f, 719-724
     abductor pollicis longus tenoplasty for, Color Plate VII:191-1, VII:720-722, 723f
     arthrodesis for, VII:722, 724
     Silastic arthroplasty for, VII:720, 721f, 722f
  Cleland ligaments of, VII:731, 731f
  constriction ring syndrome of, VIII:139-165. See also Constriction ring syndrome.
  contractures of, VII:659-672
    biomechanics of, VII:665, 667f
    burn scar and, VII:616-624, 617t, 618f-620f, 622f, 624f
    cartilage necrosis and, VII:672
    checkreins in, VII:664-665, 667f, 669
    chondral fracture and, VII:661
    collateral ligament changes in, VII:663-665, 665f-667f
    complications of, VII:671-672
    Dupuytren, VII:668-669, 669f, 671, 736, 737f, VIII:561. See also Dupuytren disease.
    in musician, VII:696-697, 697f, 701
    extension, VII:660-661, 661f, 669-671, 671f
    extrinsic tightness test in, VII:662, 663f
    flexion, VII:659, 660f, 668-669, 669f, 670f, 671-672
    hyperextension and, VII:671-672
    intrinsic tightness test in, VII:662, 663f
    neurovascular ischemia with, VII:672

Finger(s) *(Continued)*
  nonoperative treatment of, VII:665-
       668, 667f, 668f
  operative treatment of, VII:668-671,
       669f-671f
  pathophysiology of, VII:665, 667f
  relapse of, VII:671, 672
  seesaw effect in, VII:661-663, 662f-
       664f
  splinting for, VII:665-668, 667f, 668f
  treatment of, VII:665-672, 667f-671f
  volar plate in, VII:660, 663-665, 665f-
       667f
  deformities of, VIII:277-317. *See also*
       specific deformities.
  differential diagnosis of, VIII:280
  terminology for, VIII:280
  dermatofibroma of, VII:952, 952f
  deviation of, VIII:294-298, 295f-298f.
       See also Clinodactyly.
  dislocation of
     at carpometacarpal joint, VII:434,
          435f
     at distal interphalangeal joint,
          VII:448-449, 448f
     at metacarpophalangeal joint,
          VII:439-440, 440f
     at proximal interphalangeal joint,
          VII:441-445, 442f-444f
  duplication of, VIII:215-261. *See also*
       Polydactyly.
  embryology of, VIII:277-280
  extension restoration of, tendon transfer
       for, VIII:483
  extensor tendons of, VII:401-420. *See*
       also Extensor tendon(s).
  extrinsic extensors of, VII:24-25
  extrinsic flexors of, VII:26-29
  fascial anatomy of, VII:731-732, 731f
  fibrous tumors of, V:11
  flexion deformity of, VIII:286-294. *See*
       also Camptodactyly.
  flexion-extension arc of, VII:402-403,
       402f
  flexion restoration of, tendon transfer
       for, VIII:483, 486
  flexor tendons of, VII:351-394. *See also*
       Flexor tendon(s).
  focal dystonia of, in musician, VII:703-
       704
  foreign body in, VII:57, 58f
  fracture-dislocation of
     at carpometacarpal joint, VII:434-
          436, 435f
     at distal interphalangeal joint,
          VII:449-450, 450f
     at metacarpophalangeal joint, VII:441
     at proximal interphalangeal joint,
          VII:445-448, 445f-447f
     postoperative care of, VIII:561-562
  fracture of, VII:423-451. *See also* Finger
       reconstruction.
  anesthesia for, VII:425
  complex, VII:213-214, 214f, 214t
  distal phalangeal, VII:432-433, 433f,
       VIII:561-562
  early active motion for, VII:424-425
  evaluation of, VII:423-424, 424t
  in children, VIII:424-426
  in musicians, VII:701

Finger(s) *(Continued)*
  internal fixation for, VII:139-150,
       143t, 321
  90-90 wiring for, VII:145, 147f
  bone compression and, VII:140-
       141, 141f
  bridge plate for, VII:147, 150f
  compression plate in, VII:147, 148f
  general principles of, VII:140-142
  indications for, VII:139-140, 140f,
       140t
  Kirschner wires for, VII:141, 143t
  lag screw principle for, VII:142-
       143, 144f, 145f
  mini-condylar plate for, VII:147,
       149f
  movement and, VII:142, 142f
  philosophy of, VII:147, 150
  plate applications for, VII:143t,
       145, 148f, 149f, 150
  rules for, VII:147, 149f
  screws for, VII:142, 142f, 143f, 143t,
       1695t
  soft tissue handling and, VII:142
  tension band principle for, VII:143,
       145, 146f, 147f
  timing of, VII:141
  malunion or nonunion of, VII:429
  metacarpal, VII:425-429, 426f-429f
  postoperative care of, VIII:562
  metacarpophalangeal joint, VII:215-
       216
  middle phalangeal, VII:430, 432, 432f
  perionychium deformity in, VII:180,
       181f
  phalangeal, VII:429-433, 430f-432f
  postoperative care of, VIII:561-562
  proximal phalangeal, VII:429-430,
       430f, 431f, VIII:562
     in children, VIII:424
  reconstruction for, VII:212-218. *See*
       also Finger reconstruction.
  simple, VII:213, 213t
  splint for, VII:425, 425f
  tetanus prophylaxis for, VII:424, 424t
  treatment principles for, VII:424-425,
       425f
  frostbite of, VII:647-653. *See also*
       Frostbite.
  functional capacity of, VII:401-403, 402f
  furuncle of, VII:771
  ganglion of, VII:70, 196-198, 198f, 199f
  giant cell tumor of, VII:70, 71f, 698f,
       955-956, 955f
  gigantism of, VIII:298-317. *See also*
       Macrodactyly.
  Grayson ligaments of, VII:731, 731f
  hemangioma of, VII:70, 76f
  hemorrhage in, VII:68, 69t
  herpetic whitlow of, VII:766t, 768, 784
  imaging of, VII:55-84
  angiography in, VII:80, 82, 83f, 84f
  computed tomography in, VII:66, 68,
       68f
  magnetic resonance angiography in,
       VII:79-80, 80f, 81f
  magnetic resonance imaging in,
       VII:69-79, 69t, 70t, 71f-78f, 79t
  plain film radiography in, VII:55-65,
       56f-65f

Finger(s) *(Continued)*
  radionuclide imaging in, VII:65-66, 67f
  tomography in, VII:65, 66f
  ultrasonography in, VII:68-69
  in obstetric brachial plexus palsy,
       VII:557, 561f, 562
  index, abduction of, tendon transfer for,
       VIII:479
  infantile fibroma of, VII:953-954, 953f
  infection of, VII:759-789, 770, 771f. *See*
       also Hand infection; Perionychium,
       infection of.
  apical space, VII:771
  post-traumatic, VII:46-47, 48f
  pulp space, VII:772, 772f, 777, 778f
  injury to, VII:207-208, 208t, 209t. *See*
       also Finger(s), amputation of;
       Finger(s), fracture of; Finger
       reconstruction; Finger
       replantation.
  Allen test in, VII:45, 46f-47f
  amputation after, VII:318-319
  bite, VII:47
  bone evaluation in, VII:47-48
  capillary refill test in, VII:45
  Doppler ultrasonography in, VII:45
  evaluation of, VII:45-50, 46f-47f, 318
     Allen test in, VII:45, 46f-47f
     bone and joint assessment in,
          VII:47-48
     capillary refill in, VII:45
     circulation assessment in, VII:45-
          46, 46f-47f
     infection assessment in, VII:46-47,
          48f
     muscle-tendon assessment in,
          VII:48-49, 49f, 50f
     patient history for, VII:45
     sensation assessment in, VII:49
     skin assessment in, VIII:46-47
  flexor tendon sheath infection with,
       VII:47, 48f
  infections after, VII:46-47, 48f
  ischemic. *See* Hand(s), ischemic
       injury to.
  joint evaluation in, VII:47-48
  muscle-tendon evaluation in, VII:48-
       49, 49f, 50f
  occult fracture with, VII:48
  patient history in, VII:45
  reconstruction for, VII:317-348. *See*
       also Finger reconstruction.
  skin examination in, VII:46-47
  suppurative tenosynovitis with,
       VII:46-47
  interphalangeal joints of. *See*
       Interphalangeal joints.
  melanoma of, V:326, 331f
  metacarpophalangeal joints of. *See*
       Metacarpophalangeal joints.
  motion of, VII:21-22, 21f
  muscles of, VII:32-34, 33f
     anatomy of, VIII:287-288, 288f, 545f
     in camptodactyly, VIII:288, 289f, 290f
  nerves of, VII:37-41, 38f-40f
  osteoarthritis of, VII:57f, 707-724, 708f-
       709f, 719f
     abductor pollicis longus tenoplasty
          for, Color Plate VII:191-1,
          VII:720-722, 723f

Finger(s) *(Continued)*
arthrodesis for, VII:717, 718f, 722, 724
arthroplasty for, VII:713-717, 714f-716f, 718t
diagnosis of, VII:710-711
Herbert screw for, VII:711-712, 712f, 713f
indications for, VII:711
postoperative care in, VIII:563-564
Silastic arthroplasty for, VII:720, 721f, 722f
overgrowth of, VIII:298-317. *See also* Macrodactyly.
prosthetic, I:782, 782f, 786, VIII:589-592, 590f-597f
pyogenic granuloma of, VII:956
radioulnar deviation of, VIII:294-298. *See also* Clinodactyly.
reconstruction of, VII:212-247. *See also* Finger reconstruction.
rheumatoid arthritis of, postoperative care in, VIII:563, 564f, 565f
ring avulsion injury of, VII:567, 569f
skin sensitivity of, VII:218, 220f
small, ulnar deviation of, tendon transfer for, VIII:478
splinting of, VIII:567-568, 568t, 569f, 569t, 570f
in camptodactyly, VIII:292
swan-neck deformity of, VII:403, 405f, 413-414, 414f, 663, 664f
treatment of, VIII:548t, 550-551
symphalangism of, VIII:265-269, 266f-268f
synovial sheath of, VII:29, 32
transverse retinacular ligaments of, VII:731-732
trigger, VII:684-686, 684f, 686f, VIII:280-282, 560, 561f
in musician, VII:702
ulceration of, in Raynaud disease, I:905-906, 906f
vincula of, VII:29, 31f
web spaces of
burn scar contracture of, VII:617, 617t, 618f-620f, 620-624, 622f, 624f
in cleft hand, VIII:97-98, 97f
infection of, VII:772, 777, 779, 779f
release of, VIII:159-161, 160f-162f, 335f, 339-340
in Apert syndrome, VIII:172, 173f
webbing of. *See* Syndactyly.
Finger bank, VII:218
Finger flap
cross-, VII:164-166, 164f, 165f
for cheek reconstruction, V:381
for finger reconstruction, VII:220-237. *See also* Finger reconstruction, flaps for.
Finger reconstruction, VII:212-247. *See also* Thumb reconstruction.
arthrodesis in, VII:216
arthroplasty in, VII:215-216
bone grafts in, VII:213-214
débridement in, VII:212-213, 213t
DIP joint transfer in, VII:216, 218, 218f, 219f
dorsal reversed homodigital flap for, VII:228, 231, 232f

Finger reconstruction *(Continued)*
finger bank parts for, VII:218
flaps for, VII:220-237, 220t, 221f, 222t
distal phalanx, VII:210, 211f, 220t, 222, 223f-225f
dorsal digital, VII:220t, 228, 231-237, 232f-239f
lateral first-toe, VII:237, 241f, 242
palmar digital, VII:220t, 222, 226f-231f, 228
partial first-toe, VII:242, 242f
second-toe, VII:237, 240f, 242-244, 243f
toe, VII:237, 239t, 240-242, 240f-242f
gracilis muscle transfer for, VIII:500-501, 501f
homodigital advancement flap for, VII:220t, 222, 223f, 226f, 227f
homodigital reverse-flow flap for, VII:220t, 222, 224f, 225f
in complex fracture, VII:213-214, 214f, 214t
in joint fracture, VII:214-218, 215f-219f
in proximal interphalangeal joint fracture, VII:214-218, 215f-219f
in simple fracture, VII:213, 213t
island flap for, VII:166-167, 220-247, 220t
perforator island metacarpal flap for, VII:237, 239f
reverse-flow palmar metacarpal flap for, VII:228, 228f
reverse-flow second metacarpal flap for, VII:231, 235f, 236f
reverse-flow thenar flap (Miami flap) for, VII:228, 229f, 230f-231f
reversed first dorsal metacarpal artery flap for, VII:231, 233f, 234f
reversed ulnar parametacarpal flap for, VII:231, 237, 238f
second-toe flaps for, VII:237, 240f, 242-244, 243f
skin coverage in, VII:218, 220, 220f
toe transfer for, VII:216, 217f, 338, 344f-345f, 345, 346f, 348
multiple, VII:244-247, 244f-247f
Finger replantation, VII:565-584
after ring avulsion injury, VII:567, 569f
arterial repair in, VII:574-575
care after, VII:576
centers for, VII:565-566
cost of, VII:580
failure of, VII:577-578, 577f, 580
fasciotomy in, VII:574
for multiple injured digits, VII:567, 570, 570f-571f
historical perspective on, VII:565
in children, VIII:440, 444, 444f
incisions in, VII:573, 574f
indications for, VII:566-567, 567f
initial care for, VII:566
leech therapy after, VII:577, 577f
monitoring after, VII:576, 577f
neurorrhaphy in, VII:575
osteosynthesis in, VII:574
outcome of, VII:578-581, 579t, 580t
patient preparation for, VII:571
patient's satisfaction with, VII:580
physical therapy after, VII:577-578
range of motion after, VII:579-580

Finger replantation *(Continued)*
sensory function after, VII:578-579
tendon repair in, VII:575-576
thrombosis after, VII:576, 577f
transportation for, VII:566
vein repair in, VII:576
vs. revascularization, VII:578
Fingernails. *See* Perionychium.
Fingertip, VII:153-167
amputation of, VII:158-167, 159f-166f, 180-181
anatomy of, VII:153-154, 154f
cold intolerance of, VII:156
dressings for, VII:156-157
glomus tumor of, VII:957-958, 957f
injury to, VII:155-167
classification of, VII:155, 155f
composite grafts for, VII:158
cross-finger flap for, VII:164-166, 165f, 166f
healing by secondary intention for, VII:156-157
Hueston rotation advancement flap for, VII:162
in children, VIII:426, 427f
in musicians' hands, VII:699, 701
island flaps for, VII:166-167
Kutler lateral V-Y flap for, VII:159-160, 159f
linear (amputation) closure for, VII:157
local flaps for, VII:158-167, 159f-161f, 163f-166f
Moberg volar advancement flap for, VII:161-162, 161f
perionychium reconstruction in, VII:180-182
reconstruction strategies for, VII:154-156
skin grafts for, VII:157-158
thenar flap for, VII:162-163, 163f, 164f
volar V-Y flap for, VII:160-161, 160f
innervation of, VII:154
melanoma of, V:326, 330f
pyogenic granuloma of, VII:956
Finkelstein maneuver, in de Quervain syndrome, VII:678, 678t
First dorsal metacarpal artery flap, reversed, for finger reconstruction, VII:231, 233f, 234f
First web space
deficiency of, VIII:339-340
in cleft hand, VIII:97-98, 97f
release of, VIII:159-161, 160f-162f, 335f, 339-340
in Apert syndrome, VIII:172, 173f
Fissural cyst, of mandible, V:94
Fistula, I:922-924, 922t
after hypospadias repair, VI:1272, 1272f
bronchopleural, VI:428-431, 429t, 430f
carotid-cavernous sinus, III:335
cerebrospinal fluid, I:924, 924f
with craniofacial cleft management, IV:459
enterocutaneous, I:923, 923f, 993-995, 994f
esophageal reconstruction and, III:1018, 1019f
gastrointestinal, I:922t, 923, 923f

Fistula *(Continued)*
  genitourinary, I:922t, 923-924
  in frontobasilar region fractures, III:335
  in zygoma fracture, III:227, 229
  intestinal, I:923
  maxillary sinus-cutaneous, III:833, 838f-839f
  oral-antral, III:227, 229
  orocutaneous, I:967
  palatal, IV:263, 264f, 352-354, 353f, 355f
  pancreatic, I:923
  pharyngocutaneous, I:922-923, 967
  pharyngoesophageal, I:923, 923f, 967, 970f-971f
  pulmonary, I:922, 922t, 923
  rectovaginal, I:924
  tracheocutaneous, I:922
  tracheoesophageal, congenital, III:1026-1027
  wound healing and, I:922-924, 922t, 923f, 924f, 967, 970f-971f
Flank, liposuction for, VI:250, 250f
Flank-thigh-buttock lift, Color Plate VI:125-4, VI:262-265, 265f, 266f
Flap(s), I:365-473, 483-501. *See also specific flaps and procedures.*
  abdominal visceral, I:379, 379t
  advancement, I:369f
  antibiotic use and, I:472
  anticoagulation and, I:472
  arc of rotation of, I:368f, 369f, 372, 373f, 417-418, 418f, 419f
  arm carrier for, I:367, 370f
  axial, I:371-372, 372f, 484, 484f
  bipedicle, I:367, 369f
  blood flow of, I:483-484
    elevation and, I:485-486
    monitoring of, I:496-499, 497t
    regulation of, I:484-486, 485t
  bone, I:387, 390, 390f, 390t, 391f-399f, 421
  classification of, I:367-379, 368f-374f, 374t, 375t, 375f, 376f, 377t, 378f, 379t
  colonic, I:379, 379t
  color of, I:496-497
  combination, I:407-408, 408f
  complications of, I:472-473
  composite, I:359-361, 360f, 361f, 412, 413f
  definition of, I:483-484
  delayed transfer of, I:367-371, 369f-371f
    physiology of, I:368, 371
  design of, I:471
  donor site complications and, I:415-416, 473
  Doppler monitoring of, I:497t, 498-499
  errors and, I:473
  failure of, I:415, 486-488, 487f
  fascial, I:374-377, 375f, 376f. *See also* Fascial flaps.
  fasciocutaneous, I:358-359, 374-377, 376f, 377t, 378f. *See also* Fasciocutaneous flaps.
  fluorescein monitoring of, I:497, 497t
  for breast reconstruction, I:433-440, 434f-440f. *See also* Breast reconstruction.
  for facial reconstruction, V:345-390. *See also* Facial flap(s).

Flap(s) *(Continued)*
  for foot reconstruction, I:454, 462-464. *See also* Foot reconstruction.
  for head and neck reconstruction, I:421-430. *See also* Head and neck reconstruction.
  for lower extremity reconstruction, I:454, 455f-461f. *See also* Lower extremity reconstruction.
  for mediastinal reconstruction, I:440-441, 442f-444f
  free (microvascular composite tissue transplantation), I:412-413, 414f, 523-533. *See also* Microvascular surgery.
  hematoma of, I:488
  historical perspective on, I:15, 18, 19f, 22f, 365-367, 366t
  inadequate design of, I:473
  inadequate preparation for, I:473
  ischemia of, I:486-488, 487f, 495-496
  ischemic preconditioning and, I:494-495, 495t, 499t, 500
  jejunal, I:379, 379t
  loss of, I:415, 473
  monitoring of, I:472, 496-499, 497t
  muscle, I:372-374, 373f, 374t, 375t. *See also* Muscle flaps.
  musculocutaneous, I:359, 360f, 373f, 417
    skin territory of, I:418, 420
  omental, I:379, 379t
  patient positioning for, I:471-472
  perforator, I:355-358, 377, 379. *See also* Microvascular surgery.
    axes of, I:355-356, 356f
    dimensions of, I:356-358, 357f, 358f
    necrosis of, I:357
    nomenclature for, I:479
    surgical delay for, I:357-358, 357f, 358f
  pH monitoring of, I:497t, 498
  photoplethysmography of, I:497t, 498
  prefabrication of, I:409
  prelamination of, I:408-409
  preoperative evaluation for, I:467-468, 471
  random-pattern, I:367, 368f, 370f, 484, 484f
  reperfusion injury to, I:486-494, 487f, 489f
    experimental models of, I:491-494, 492f, 493f
    free radicals in, I:491
    integrin-Ig-like ligand adhesion in, I:489-490, 489f
    neutrophil-endothelial adhesion in, I:488-489, 490f
    nitric oxide inhibition of, I:493-494
    platelet-activating factor in, I:491
    selectin-carbohydrate adhesion in, I:490
  reverse-flow, I:409-411, 411f, 412f
  rotation, I:367, 369f
  safety of, I:473
  segmental, I:384, 386, 386f
  selection of, I:413, 415-421, 415f, 418f, 419f
    donor site considerations in, I:415-416
    errors in, I:473

Flap(s) *(Continued)*
  functional considerations in, I:416-417
  obesity and, I:471
  preoperative considerations in, I:467-468, 471
  recipient site considerations in, I:416
  reconstructive ladder in, I:413, 415, 415f
  reconstructive triangle in, I:415, 415f
  reliability considerations in, I:471
  safety considerations in, I:415
  skeletal reconstruction and, I:416
  tobacco use and, I:471
  weight-bearing and, I:416
  sensory, I:405-407, 405f-407f
  septocutaneous, I:358-359, 526-527, 527f
  spectroscopy of, I:497t, 498
  splitting of, I:384, 386, 386f
  supercharging of, I:413, VI:720
  temperature monitoring of, I:497, 497t
  tissue expansion for, I:380-384, 380f-386f, 416. *See also* Tissue expansion.
  tissue mobility and, I:345
  transcutaneous oxygen tension of, I:497-498, 497t
  tubed pedicle, I:367, 370f
  V-Y advancement, I:367, 369f
  vascular anatomy of, I:367, 367f-369f, 371-372, 372f, 373f. *See also* Vascular territories.
    bone, I:317-361, 390, 390t
    fasciocutaneous, I:358-359, 374-377, 376f, 378f
    muscle, I:359, 360f, 372-374, 374f
  venous, I:412, 413f
  venous occlusion in, I:486-487
  viability of, I:486-488, 487f
    aspirin and, I:499t, 500
    delay procedure and, I:494, 499t, 500
    dextran and, I:499t, 500
    heat shock and, I:495
    heparin and, I:499t, 500-501
    hypothermia and, I:499t, 500
    ischemic preconditioning and, I:494-495, 495t, 499t, 500
    leeches and, I:499t, 501
    monitoring of, I:496-499, 497t
    monophosphoryl lipid A and, I:495
    neovascularization and, I:496
    optimization of, I:499-501, 499t
    steroids and, I:499t, 500
Flexion strap, for finger contracture, VII:667f, 668
Flexner, Abraham, I:12
Flexor carpi radialis, VII:34
Flexor carpi radialis tendon transfer, for radial nerve palsy, VIII:456t, 458, 461f
Flexor carpi ulnaris tendon transfer
  for obstetric brachial plexus palsy, VII:561f, 562
  for radial nerve palsy, VIII:456-458, 456t, 457f-460f
Flexor digiti minimi brevis, VI:1408, 1408f, VII:32
Flexor digitorum brevis, VI:1406f, 1407
Flexor digitorum brevis flap, for foot reconstruction, I:462, 462f, 463f

Flexor digitorum profundus, VII:27, 28, 29
assessment of, VII:48, 49f
function of, VII:31-32
isolated rupture of (Jersey finger),
VII:379, 380f
Flexor digitorum superficialis, VII:26-27,
48, 49f
Flexor digitorum superficialis tendon,
I:599
Flexor digitorum superficialis tendon
transfer
for low median nerve palsy, VIII:465-
466, 466f, 467f
for radial nerve palsy, VIII:458-459, 461
for thumb flexion-adduction, VIII:479
for thumb flexion restoration, VIII:483,
485f
for thumb opposition, VIII:342-343
Flexor hallucis brevis, VI:1405, 1406f,
1408, 1408f
Flexor pollicis brevis, VII:32
Flexor pollicis longus, VII:27
Flexor pollicis longus tendon transfer
for high median nerve palsy, VIII:469-
470
for key pinch restoration, VIII:522, 524-
527, 525f-527f
Flexor pollicis longus tendon transfer, for
high median nerve palsy, VIII:470f
Flexor superficialis finger, VII:382
Flexor tendon(s), VII:351-394
anatomy of, VII:29-32, 30f, 31f, 352-356,
354f
biomechanics of, VII:353-355, 355f,
358-362
collagen of, VII:353
endotenon of, VII:353, 354f
epitenon of, VII:353, 354f
evaluation of, VII:48-49, 48f
force generation and, VII:360-361, 361t
healing of, VII:357-358
histology of, VII:353
infection of, VII:47
injury to, VII:48-49, 49f, 50f, 351-394
clinical assessment of, VII:363-365,
363f-365f
computed tomography of, VII:364
fibroblastic response to, VII:357
healing response to, VII:357-358
historical perspective on, VII:352
imaging of, VII:363-365
in children, VII:378-379, 378f,
VIII:28-29, 28f, 424-426
inflammatory response to, VII:357
MRI of, VII:364-365
partial laceration in, VII:379-381
pharmacologic treatment of, VII:358
remodeling response to, VII:357
repair for, VII:365-372. See also Flexor
tendon reconstruction.
biomechanics in, VII:358-360
complications of, VII:377
core sutures for, VII:359, 369-370,
370f
Dran-Houser early motion
protocol in, VII:374, 375f
early controlled active flexion in,
VII:374-377
early motion protocols in, VII:372-
377, 373f-375f

Flexor tendon(s) (Continued)
epitenon suture in, VII:360, 370-
371, 371f
force generation and, VII:360-361
gapping and, VII:359
grasping loops for, VII:360
historical perspective on, VII:352
in children, VII:378-379, 378f,
VIII:425-426
in isolated FDP rupture, VII:379,
380f
in partial lacerations, VII:379-381
in zone I injury, VII:366-372, 367f-
371f
in zone III injury, VII:372
in zone IV injury, VII:372
in zone V injury, VII:372
incisions for, VII:366, 367f
Indiana early controlled active
flexion in, VII:376
Kleinert early motion protocol in,
VII:374
knot placement in, VII:359
locking loops in, VII:360
outcomes of, VII:377-378, 378f
preoperative preparations for,
VII:366
principles of, VII:352, 365-366
rehabilitation after, VII:372-377,
373f-375f
Silfverskiöld and May's early
controlled active flexion in,
VII:376
strength in, VII:359, 360, 361-362,
361t, 362f, 362t
suture techniques in, VII:359, 361-
362, 361t, 362f, 362t, 369-371,
370f, 371f
tendon sheath repair in, VII:371-
372
timing of, VII:365
unassisted early active motion in,
VII:376
work of flexion and, VII:358-359
ultrasonography of, VII:364
zone I, VII:48-49, 49f, 366-372, 367f-
371f
zone III, VII:48-49, 49f, 372
zone IV, VII:48-49, 49f, 372
zone V, VII:48-49, 49f, 372
nutrition of, VII:356
physiology of, VII:356-358, 357f
postoperative care in, VIII:566
pulley system of, VII:353-355, 355f, 358
reconstruction of, VII:381-394. See also
Flexor tendon reconstruction.
tenosynovitis of, VII:684-686, 684f, 686f
vascular system of, VII:356, 357f
zones of, VII:355-356, 356f
Flexor tendon reconstruction, VII:381-394
active tendon implants for, VII:382
complications of, VII:392-393
contraindications to, VII:382-383
first stage of, VII:390-391, 391f
flexor sheath in, I:596, 596f
graft healing and, VII:383-384
imaging for, VII:383, 383f
incisions for, VII:386
indications for, VII:381-382, 381t
motors for, VII:387, 389

Flexor tendon reconstruction (Continued)
pulleys for, VII:386-387, 386f-388f
results of, VII:393-394, 394t
second stage of, VII:391-392, 391f, 392f
single-stage, VII:382
suture techniques in, VII:390
tendon graft for, VII:384-386, 385f
extensor digitorum longus for,
VII:385
flexor digitorum superficialis for,
VII:385-386
healing of, VII:383-384
length of, VII:389-390, 389f
palmaris longus for, VII:384
plantaris for, VII:384-385, 385f
tip to palm, VII:389, 389f
tip to wrist, VII:389, 389f
vascularized, VII:386
third stage of, VII:392, 393f
timing of, VII:383
two-stage, VII:382
vascularized tendon grafts for, VII:386
Fluids
in burn injury, I:203, 818-821, 819f,
820t
in toxic epidermal necrolysis, I:797
maintenance formulas for, I:185-186
management of, I:184-186, 186f
preoperative intake of, I:169
Fluorescein monitoring, of flaps, I:497,
497t
Fluorescent in situ hybridization, I:54-55,
56f
in prenatal diagnosis, I:1074, 1075f
5-Fluorouracil
in actinic keratoses, Color Plate V:116-2,
V:404-405, 404t
in basal cell carcinoma, V:286t, 288, 403-
404
Flutist, hand disorders in, VII:694f, 695-
696
Foam dressings, I:224, 225t, 884-885, 885t
Focal dystonia, in musicians' hands,
VII:703-704
Fontanels, embryology of, IV:11
Food, preoperative restrictions on, I:169
Foot (feet). See also Foot reconstruction.
amputation of, VI:1425-1426, 1427,
1429f, 1430, 1432f, 1441, 1443
anatomy of, VI:1403-1411, 1404f-1414f
arterial anatomy of, VI:1404-1405, 1404f
bones of, VI:1410-1411, 1413f
cleft hand surgery and, VIII:101
clinical evaluation of, VI:1411-1417
angiography in, VI:1415
ankle/brachial indices in, VI:1412
compartment pressures in, VI:1415
Doppler flow studies in, VI:1412,
1414, 1414f
duplex imaging in, VI:1414
gait analysis in, VI:1415, 1416f
plain films in, VI:1415, 1417
sensory assessment in, VI:1415
tissue perfusion studies in, VI:1414-
1415
toe pressures in, VI:1412
compartment release in, VI:1417, 1418f
compartment syndrome of, VI:1415,
1417, 1418f
compartments of, VI:1405, 1406f

Foot (feet) (Continued)
diabetic, VI:1443-1450. See also Diabetes mellitus, foot reconstruction in.
dorsal soft tissue of, VI:1403-1405, 1404f
in capillary-lymphatic-venous malformation, V:58, 58f
isosulfan blue dye evaluation of, VI:1417
Ledderhose disease in, VII:737, 738f
L'Nard splint for, VI:1443
melanoma of, V:327, 332f
muscles of, VI:1405-1410, 1405f-1409f
neuroma of, VII:933, 933f, 945
osteomyelitis of, VI:1415, 1417, 1440, 1440f, 1443
plantar soft tissue of, VI:1405-1410, 1405f-1413f
fourth layer of, VI:1409-1410, 1409f-1413f
second layer of, VI:1407-1408, 1407f
superficial layer of, VI:1405-1407, 1406f
third layer of, VI:1408, 1408f
pulses in, VI:1411-1412
tarsal tunnel syndrome in, VII:917-922
ulcers of, I:866, 868f, 943, 943f, 981, 982f
vascular evaluation of, VI:1411-1415
venous malformations of, V:48f
weight on, VI:1411

Foot reconstruction, I:454, 462-464, 462f-464f, VI:1403-1450
abductor digiti minimi flap for, I:462, 464
abductor hallucis-abductor digiti minimi muscle flap for, VI:1419
abductor hallucis flap for, I:462
ankle, VI:1419, 1421f-1423f
antibiotics after, VI:1443
CAM walker boot after, VI:1443
care after, VI:1443
deltoid flap for, I:405-407, 405f-407f
dorsal, VI:1419, 1420f
extensor digitorum brevis muscle flap for, VI:1419, 1421f
flexor digitorum brevis flap for, I:462, 462f, 463f
forefoot amputation in, VI:1425-1426, 1429f
heel pad flaps for, VI:1435, 1437f, 1438f
hindfoot amputation in, VI:1441, 1443
in diabetes, VI:1443-1450, 1447f, 1448f. See also Diabetes mellitus, foot reconstruction in.
intrinsic muscle flaps for, VI:1431-1435, 1433f, 1434f
lateral supramalleolar flap for, VI:1419, 1423f
L'Nard splint after, VI:1443
medial plantar artery flap for, VI:1435, 1436f
microvascular surgery for, I:464, 464f, VI:1427, 1432f, 1436, 1440-1441, 1440f-1442f
midfoot amputation in, VI:1427, 1430, 1432f
neurovascular island flap for, VI:1424-1425, 1426-1427, 1426f, 1430f
plantar
forefoot, VI:1419, 1424-1426, 1425f-1428f
hindfoot, VI:1430-1443, 1433f, 1434f, 1436f-1442f

Foot reconstruction (Continued)
midfoot, VI:1426-1427, 1431f, 1432f
sensory flap for, I:406f-407f
reinnervation in, VI:1450
retrograde lateral plantar artery flap for, I:462
sensory flap for, I:406f-407f
suprafascial flaps for, VI:1425, 1427
sural artery flap for, VI:1435-1436, 1439f
sural neurocutaneous flap for, VI:1419, 1422f
toe fillet flap for, VI:1424, 1425f
V-Y flaps for, VI:1425, 1427, 1427f, 1428f, 1431f

Forced duction test, in orbital fracture, III:288, 288f

Forearm. See also Arm(s); Upper extremity.
cutaneous perforators of, Color Plate I:15-4, I:334
flexor aspect reconstruction of, muscle transfer for, VIII:497-500, 498f, 499f, 504, 505f
hemangioma of, VII:70, 73f
rotation of, in obstetric brachial plexus palsy, VII:557, 560f
ulnar deficiency at, VIII:103, 105f, 106f, 107, 110, 110f
vascular territories of, I:334-337
clinical implications of, I:336-337
donor site morbidity and, I:336-337
free flap donor sites and, I:337
of bones, I:335-336
of muscles, Color Plates I:15-5 to 15-7, I:335, 336-337
of skin, Color Plate I:15-4, I:334
Volkmann ischemic contracture and, I:337

Forearm flaps. See Radial forearm flap; Ulnar forearm flap.

Forefoot
amputation of, VI:1425-1426, 1429f
reconstruction of, VI:1419, 1424-1426, 1425f-1428f

Forehead. See also Forehead reconstruction.
aesthetic analysis of, II:4t, 5t, 7-8, 9f, III:609, 609f
anatomy of, II:81-83, 82f, 83f, III:699-701, 700f-703f
anterior region of, III:699, 700f
arterial supply of, III:700-701, 701f
augmentation of, II:409, 409f, 410, 410f
defects of, III:702-703
eyebrows of, II:47-74, III:699-700, 700f. See also Eyebrow(s).
facial nerve of, II:57-58, 58f
frontalis of, III:700, 700f
glabellar lines of, postblepharoplasty recurrence of, II:813-814
glabellar region of, III:699, 700f
hemangioma of, V:32
innervation of, III:701, 702f
laceration of, III:13, 13f
loose areolar layer of, III:700, 700f
pericranium of, III:700, 700f
pretemporal regions of, III:699, 700f
reconstruction of, III:613, 699-773, 704-705t. See also Forehead reconstruction.

Forehead (Continued)
reduction of, in male-to-female transformation, VI:1315
redundant skin of, II:50
rhytids of, II:48-50, 49f, 67-68, 68t
skin of, III:700, 700f
subcutaneous layer of, III:700, 700f
subunits of, III:699-700, 700f
tissue layers of, III:700, 700f
transverse lines of, postblepharoplasty recurrence of, II:814
unrejuvenated, II:749-751, 750f

Forehead flap
for head and neck reconstruction, V:223, 225f
for medial canthus reconstruction, V:369, 373f-375f
for midface reconstruction, III:872, 873f
for nasal reconstruction, II:581-584, 582f, 583f, V:349, 353f, 355f, 360, 361f, 362f
for upper eyelid reconstruction, V:367f, 369, 371f-372f

Forehead reconstruction, III:699-773, 704-705t
bilobed flap for, III:708
closure by secondary intention in, III:703, 704t
crane principle in, III:706, 707f
direct wound edge approximation in, III:703, 704t
distant flaps for, III:705t, 716-717, 717f-722f
eyebrows in, III:723, 727f, 728-730, 728t
flap prefabrication in, III:705t
four-flap scalp flap for, III:716, 718f, 720f
full-thickness skin grafting in, III:706t, 708
local flaps in, III:705t, 708-712, 709f-712f
microvascular composite tissue transplantation in, III:705t, 717, 723, 725f-726f, 727t
rhomboid flap for, III:708, 710f, 712f
secondary, II:720-721, 723f
Shutter flap for, III:708, 711f
skin grafting in, III:703, 704t, 706-708, 706t, 707f
temporoparietal flap for, I:371-372, 372f
three-flap scalp flap for, III:716, 717f
tissue expansion in, I:551, III:705t, 713-716, 713f-716f, V:348, 350f
vertical pedicled trapezius musculocutaneous flap for, III:716-717, 719f, 722f
Worthen flap for, III:708, 709f

Foreign body
airway, III:769-770
finger, VII:57, 58f
vs. hand infection, VII:768, 769f

Formaldehyde, squamous cell carcinoma and, V:276

Formic acid injury, to hand, VII:654

FotoFacial, II:376-377, 378f

Four-flap technique
for forehead reconstruction, III:716, 718f, 720f
for scalp reconstruction, III:613, 615f

Fournier disease, VI:1250-1253

Fracture(s), VI:1383-1399. *See also* at
  specific sites.
  Bennett, VII:434-436, 435f
  bone repair in, I:650-659
    age-related factors in, I:659
    angiogenesis in, I:654-658, 656-657t
    blood supply in, I:653-658, 654f, 655f,
      656-657t
    bone morphogenetic proteins in,
      I:656t, 659-663, 660t
    compression plating in, I:651, 651f
    cytokines in, I:655-658, 656-657t
    fibroblast growth factor-2 in, I:657t,
      658, 660t, 665-666
    fibrous union in, I:652
    immobilization in, I:658-659
    inflammatory phase of, I:652, 653f
    periosteum in, I:652
    platelet-derived growth factor in,
      I:657t, 660t, 666-667
    primary, I:650-652, 650f
    remodeling phase of, I:652, 653f
    reparative phase of, I:652, 653f
    secondary, I:650f, 652, 653f
    transforming growth factor-β in,
      I:656t, 660t, 663-665
    vascular endothelial growth factor in,
      I:655, 657t, 658
  boxer, VII:426-427, 427f
  carpal bone, VII:464-467, 465f, 466f
    in children, VIII:423-424
  distal radius, VII:460-463, 461f, 462f
    arthroscopy-assisted fixation of,
      VII:136
    in children, VIII:420-423
  distal tibial, I:1008, 1010, 1011f-1014f
  facial, III:77-367. *See also* Facial
    fracture(s) *and specific fractures.*
  finger, VII:423-451. *See also* Finger
    reconstruction.
    anesthesia for, VII:425
    complex, VII:213-214, 214f, 214t
    early active motion for, VII:424-425
    evaluation of, VII:423-424, 424t
    in children, VIII:424
    malunion or nonunion of, VII:429
    metacarpal, VII:425-429, 426f-429f
    perionychium deformity in, VII:180,
      181f
    phalangeal, VII:429-433, 430f-432f
    simple, VII:213, 213t
    splint for, VII:425, 425f
    tetanus prophylaxis for, VII:424,
      424t
    treatment principles for, VII:424-425,
      425f
  hand, VII:423-451. *See also* Finger(s),
    fracture of.
    fixation of, VII:321
    in children, VIII:424, 425f
    in musician, VII:701
  infection with, VI:1385-1387, 1387f
  lunate, in children, VIII:424
  mandibular, III:145-187. *See also*
    Condylar process fracture;
    Mandibular fracture.
  maxillary, III:229-255, 582, 593f-594f.
    See also Maxillary fracture.
  naso-orbital-ethmoid, III:580, 581f
  open, VI:1383-1385, 1384t

Fracture(s) *(Continued)*
  orbital, III:264-305. *See also* Orbital
    fracture.
  orbitozygomatic, III:580
  pediatric, VIII:420-424, 422f
    evaluation of, III:391-392
    facial, III:402-454. *See also* Facial
      fracture(s), pediatric.
    radiologic evaluation of, III:392-395,
      393f-394f, 395t, 396f, 397f
  radius, VII:460-463, 461f, 462f
    in children, VIII:420-423, 422f
  rib, in children, III:400
  Salter classification of, VIII:424, 425f
  scaphoid, VII:464-465, 464f, 465f
    arthroscopy-assisted fixation of,
      VII:136-137
    computed tomography in, VII:68
    in children, VIII:423-424
  skull
    in children, III:438-444, 439t, 440f
    in infant, III:398-399
    pseudogrowth of, III:440, 442, 443f
  treatment of, VI:1384f, 1388-1399
    amputation in, VI:1387-1388
    antibiotic beads in, VI:1390, 1391f
    débridement in, VI:1388-1390,
      1389f
    fixation in, VI:1393, 1394f
    hyperbaric oxygen in, VI:1390-1391
    nutrition in, VI:1391-1392
    reconstruction in, VI:1392-1399,
      1394f, 1398f
      bone graft in, VI:1395-1396
      dead space management in,
        VI:1393-1395
      free vascularized bone flaps in,
        VI:1397-1399, 1398f
      Ilizarov technique in, VI:1395
      pedicle bone flaps in, VI:1396-
        1397
    vacuum-assisted closure in,
      VI:1392
    wound dressing in, VI:1390
  triquetrum, VII:466-467
    in children, VIII:424
  ulnar, in children, VIII:420-423, 422f
  wound healing impairment and, I:1008-
    1010, 1009f-1014f
Fracture-dislocation
  at carpometacarpal joint, VII:434-436,
    435f
  at distal interphalangeal joint, VII:449-
    450, 450f
  at metacarpophalangeal joint, VII:441
  at proximal interphalangeal joint,
    VII:445-448, 445f-447f
Franceschetti-Zwahlen-Klein syndrome.
  See Treacher Collins syndrome.
Frankfort horizontal, II:3f, 3t, 20f, 21t
Fraud, I:136-138
Freckles, V:261, 261f
Free radicals
  in ischemia, I:487-488, 487f, VII:117
  in neutrophil-endothelial adhesion,
    I:491
Freeman-Sheldon syndrome, VIII:147,
  148f
Frey syndrome, V:87-88, 88f
Froment sign, VII:50, 52f

Frontal bone, III:547
  anatomy of, III:331, 333f
  encephalocele of, IV:376, 377f
  fibrous dysplasia of, III:565, 571f-572f
  fracture of (Le Fort IV), III:330-333,
    333f, 338-339, 338f, 339f. *See also*
    Frontobasilar region fracture.
    clinical manifestations of, III:333-337
    in children, III:438-444, 440f-445f
    reconstruction for, III:565, 569f-570f
  gunshot injury to, III:565, 567f-568f
  pediatric, fracture of, III:438-444, 440f-
    445f
  strength of, III:332-333, 333f
Frontal hairline brow lift, II:62, 62f, 63f
Frontal sinus
  anatomy of, III:309, 339
  fracture of, III:339-344, 340f, 438-440
    diagnosis of, III:339-341
    infection and, III:340
    mucocele and, III:341
    treatment of, III:341-344, 342f-350f
      cranialization in, III:341-342, 343f
      cranioplasty in, III:344, 344f-350f
      endoscopic, III:342, 344, 492, 501f-
        504f, 503-504
      galeal flaps in, III:342, 343f
      hydroxyapatite cement in, III:344,
        346f
      methyl methacrylate in, III:344,
        347f-349f
      titanium mesh in, III:344, 350f
  mucocele of, III:341
  obliteration of, III:565, 566f
Frontalis
  anatomy of, II:52-53, 53f, 81, 82f, 83f,
    III:607, 608f, 888
  dynamics of, II:87-88, 87f
Fronto-orbital advancement, in
  craniofacial microsomia, IV:541
Fronto-orbital osteotomy, IV:435, 436f
Frontobasilar region fracture, III:330-344
  anatomy for, III:331-332, 332f
  carotid-cavernous sinus fistula in,
    III:335
  classification of, III:332-333
  clinical manifestations of, III:333-337
  cranial nerve injury in, III:334
  CSF rhinorrhea in, III:334-335
  frontal lobe injury in, III:334
  globe displacement in, III:335
  meningitis in, III:335
  optic nerve injury in, III:335-338
  orbital apex syndrome in, III:335, 336f
  orbital emphysema in, III:335
  pneumocephalus in, III:335
  superior orbital fissure syndrome in,
    III:335
  visual loss in, III:335-338
Frontoethmoidal meningoencephalocele
  classification of, IV:383, 385
  computed tomography in, IV:409f
  management of, IV:416, 419t, 431, 454,
    458, 459f, 460f
  morphology of, IV:407, 409, 409f, 410f,
    411, 411f
    naso-orbital, IV:411, 411f
    nasoethmoidal, IV:407, 410f
    nasofrontal, IV:408, 410f
  pathogenesis of, IV:414

Frontonasal malformation, IV:106-110, 107f
  dermoid in, IV:107-108, 108f
  encephalocele in, IV:108-109, 108f
  glioma in, IV:108, 108f
  hypertelorism in, IV:109-110, 109f
Frostbite, I:858-860, VII:647-653
  acclimatization and, VII:649
  age and, VII:648
  alcohol use and, VII:648
  aloe vera in, VII:652
  angiography in, VII:649
  blisters with, I:859, 859f, 860
  chemical sympathectomy in, VII:652
  débridement in, VII:652
  degrees of, I:859, 859f
  environmental factors in, VII:648-649
  environmental moisture and, VII:648-649
  environmental temperature and, VII:648
  eschar incision in, VII:652, 653f
  eschar with, I:859, 859f
  evaluation of, VII:649-651, 649t, 650f
  host factors in, VII:648
  late sequelae of, VII:652-653
  low-molecular-weight dextran in, VII:652
  magnetic resonance imaging in, VII:650-651
  mental illness and, VII:648
  neurologic effects of, VII:648
  pathophysiology of, I:859, 859f, VII:647-648, 648f
  pentoxifylline in, VII:652
  peripheral vascular disease and, VII:648
  physical therapy for, VII:652, 653f
  predisposing factors in, VII:648-649
  prehospital care for, VII:651
  radiography in, VII:649, 650f
  recombinant tissue plasminogen activator in, VII:652
  sympathectomy in, VII:652
  symptoms of, I:860
  thermography in, VII:649, 650f
  treatment of, I:860, 860t, 861f, VII:651-652, 651f, 652t
  triple-phase bone scan in, VII:650
  wind chill index and, I:856
Functional transfers
  in tetraplegia, VIII:507-540. See also Tetraplegia, upper extremity function restoration in.
  muscle, I:390, 400f-404f, 405, VIII:489-506. See also Arm(s), muscle transfer in.
  nerve, VII:503-505, 504f, 530-532, 548, 551f-552f
  tendon, VIII:453-486. See also Hand reconstruction, tendon transfer in.
  toe. See Toe transfer.
Funduscopy, II:93
Fungal infection
  of hand, VII:766t, 785, 785f
  of perionychium, VII:194, 196
Furfuryladenine, II:401
Furstenberg test, III:766
Furuncle, of hand, VII:771

G
Gabapentin
  in breast pain, VI:355
  in complex regional pain syndrome/reflex sympathetic dystrophy, VII:857-858
Gait analysis, VI:1415, 1416f
Galea aponeurotica, II:82, 82f, III:607, 608f
Galeal flap
  for frontal sinus fracture treatment, III:342, 343f
  for scalp reconstruction, III:617, 617f
Galen, I:13-14, 14f
Galvanic skin conduction, in complex regional pain syndrome/reflex sympathetic dystrophy, VII:846
Gamma particles, I:836
Ganglion
  in musicians' hands, VII:702
  interphalangeal, VII:196-198, 198f, 199f
  magnetic resonance imaging of, VII:70
  of wrist, VII:136, 702
  postoperative care of, VIII:563
Ganglionectomy, arthroscopic, VII:136
Gangrene
  abdominal, VI:93
  Fournier, I:911
  gas, I:914
  Meleney, I:911
  of hand, VII:782
  synergistic, I:911, 914f, 1004f
Garlic, VI:176t, 177t
Gastric bypass surgery
  abdominoplasty after, VI:167-172
    care after, VI:170-171
    markings for, VI:168
    preoperative evaluation for, VI:168
    preparation for, VI:168
    technique of, VI:168-170, 169f, 170f
  suprapubic dermolipectomy after, VI:408, 409f
Gastric pull-up, for esophageal reconstruction, III:1011-1012, 1012f
Gastrocnemius, arterial supply of, Color Plates I:15-10 and 15-11, I:338
Gastrocnemius flap, for lower extremity reconstruction, I:454, 455f, 456f, VI:1374, 1375f
Gastroepiploic flap, for esophageal reconstruction, III:1013, 1014f-1016f
Gastroesophageal reflux, III:771
Gastrointestinal system
  opioid effects on, I:181
  preoperative evaluation of, I:169
  venous malformations of, V:47, 48, 48f, 50-51
Gastroschisis, VI:93
  wound healing and, I:945, 947, 948f
Gastrostomy, in craniofacial microsomia, IV:523
Gastrulation, IV:2
Gauze dressing, I:224, 225t, 873
Gender dysphoria syndrome, VI:1306
Gender identity disorder, VI:1305-1316
  anatomic considerations in, VI:1307-1308, 1307t
  embryologic considerations in, VI:1307-1308, 1307t
  female-to-male surgery for, VI:1308-1312

Gender identity disorder *(Continued)*
    coronoplasty in, VI:1310
    hysterectomy in, VI:1311-1312
    mastectomy in, VI:1308
    penile stiffening techniques in, VI:1311, 1311f
    phalloplasty in, Color Plate VI:156-2, VI:1308-1310, 1310f
    scrotoplasty in, VI:1310-1311
    vaginectomy in, VI:1311-1312
  historical perspective on, VI:1305-1306
  hormone therapy for, VI:1307
  incidence of, VI:1306
  male-to-female surgery for, Color Plates VI:156-3 to 156-9, VI:1312-1316
    augmentation mammaplasty in, VI:1315
    clitoroplasty in, Color Plates VI:156-8 and 156-9, VI:1314-1315
      graft or local flap for, VI:1314-1315
      pedicled dorsal glans for, VI:1315, 1315f
    facial skeleton feminization in, VI:1315
    mentoplasty in, VI:1315
    reduction thyroid chondroplasty in, VI:1315
    rhinoplasty in, VI:1315
    rib resection in, VI:1316
    vaginoplasty in, Color Plates VI:156-3 to 156-7, VI:1312-1314
      local flaps for, VI:1312
      penile inversion for, Color Plate VI:156-5, VI:1312
      rectosigmoid technique for, VI:1313-1314, 1313f, 1314f
      skin graft for, VI:1312
    voice alteration procedures in, VI:1316
  medical management of, VI:1306-1307
  trial cross-living in, VI:1307
Gene linkage study, IV:94
Gene therapy
  in craniosynostosis, IV:490
  in peripheral nerve repair, I:738-739
  in wound healing, I:226
Genetics, I:51-65. *See also specific disorders.*
  chromosomal analysis in, I:54-55, 56f
  ethical aspects of, I:64-65
  imprinting in, I:53
  Mendelian, I:51-52, 52f, 53f
  microarray analysis in, I:58, 60f
  mitochondrial, I:53
  non-Mendelian, I:52-53
  Northern blot in, I:55-56
  nucleic acid analysis in, I:55
  polymerase chain reaction in, I:56, 58, 59f
  prenatal diagnosis in, I:1067-1076. *See also* Prenatal diagnosis.
  Southern blot in, I:55-56, 57f
  uniparental disomy in, I:53
Genicular artery, Color Plates I:15-9 and 15-10, I:338
Genioplasty. *See also* Chin.
  after implant failure, III:599, 600f
  after radiation injury, III:599, 601f-602f
  iliac osteocutaneous free flap for, III:599, 603f-604f
  in craniofacial cleft, IV:444-446, 445f

Genioplasty *(Continued)*
  in craniofacial microsomia, IV:533, 538f, 539f, 550, 551f, 552f
  in obstructive sleep apnea, III:790-791, 792f
  microsurgical, III:599, 603f-604f
Genitalia
  change in. *See* Gender identity disorder.
  female
    cosmetic surgery for, VI:404-408, 406f-408f
    reconstruction of, VI:1281-1289, 1295-1304. *See also* Vaginal reconstruction.
  male, VI:1197-1256. *See also* Penis; Scrotum; Testis (testes).
    acquired defects of, VI:1218, 1221, 1224f
    anatomy of, VI:1198-1201, 1199f
    blood supply to, VI:1201-1204, 1201f-1205f
    congenital defects of, VI:1207-1218
    cosmetic surgery for, VI:389-404. *See also at* Penis.
    embryology of, VI:1198, 1199f
    lymphatic supply to, VI:1206
    nerve supply to, VI:1205-1206, 1206f
    reconstruction of, VI:1221, 1223-1247. *See also* Penile reconstruction.
Genitofemoral nerve injury, in abdominoplasty, VI:375
Gentamicin, topical, I:884t
Ger, Ralph, I:32
Giant cell angioblastoma, VIII:378, 379f
Giant cell granuloma, central, V:102-103, 208-209
Giant cell tumor
  of hand, VII:70, 71f, 698f, 702, 955-956, 955f, 987-988, 987f
  of metacarpal head, VII:987, 987f
  of perionychium, VII:200
  of tendon sheath, VII:955-956, 955f
  of wrist, VII:70, 74f
Giant nevus
  of face, I:551, 554f
  of scalp, III:612
Gibbs ringing artifact, I:1071f
Gigantism, digital. *See* Macrodactyly.
Gigantomastia, VI:552-553, 574, 575f-577f, 608-609, 608f, 621f, 626f-629f. *See also* Breast reduction.
Gillies, Sir Harold Delf, I:12, 12f, 28-29, 29f
Gillies fan flap, III:813, 817f-819f, V:383
Gingival cyst, V:92-93, 191
Gingival plexus, IV:80f
Gingivoperiosteoplasty, IV:181-182, 210-211, 225, 226f
Ginkgo biloba, I:170, VI:176t
Ginseng, VI:176t
Glabella, II:3f, 3t, 19f, 20t
Glabellar flap, for nasal reconstruction, V:349, 357f
Glabellar lines, postblepharoplasty recurrence of, II:813-814
Glandular cyst, of mandible, V:193
Glasgow Coma Scale
  in facial fracture, III:81, 83, 83t
  in pediatric head injury, III:438, 439t

Glass implants, I:753f, 755
GLI3 gene, VIII:22
Glioma
  nasal, III:765, IV:108, 108f
  optic nerve, V:115
Gliosis, with craniofacial cleft management, IV:459
Globe. *See also* Eye(s); Orbit.
  anatomy of, III:271-272, 271f
  displacement of, in frontobasilar region fractures, III:335
  evaluation of, II:93
  in blepharoplasty, II:96, 804
  in craniosynostosis, IV:476
  in orbital fracture, III:288, 289f, 326-328
  in zygoma fracture, III:210-212, 211f, 227-228, 228f
  postblepharoplasty prominence of, II:804
  puncture of, with laser resurfacing, II:375
  rupture of, in orbital fracture, III:288, 289f
Globulomaxillary cyst, V:94
Glomangioma, V:47
Glomus tumor, VII:198, 200, 957-958, 957f, VIII:377
Glossectomy, V:236
Glossopharyngeus, IV:73f
Glossotomy, V:234, 234f
Glottis
  cancer of, V:241-246, 241f, 244f-247f, 244t, 245t
  in gastroesophageal reflux disease, III:771
  webs of, III:769
Glucose, serum, tissue perfusion and, VI:1445, 1445f
Gluteal thigh flap, for pressure sores, VI:1323f, 1324t, 1325, 1327, 1331f, 1332f, 1338, 1343f
Gluteus maximus, for anal sphincter reconstruction, I:615
Gluteus maximus flap
  for back reconstruction, VI:442, 445f
  for groin and perineal reconstruction, I:452, 454
  for lower extremity reconstruction, VI:1369-1370, 1370f
  for pelvic reconstruction, I:403f-404f
  for pressure sores, I:464-465, 467f-470f, VI:1324-1325, 1324t, 1328f-1330f, 1334, 1337f-1339f, 1338
  segmental, I:384, 386f, 387f
Gnathion, II:3f, 3t, 19f, 20t
Goes technique, for breast reduction, VI:571, 573f
Gold implants, I:745, 752
Gold weights, in lagophthalmos, III:748, 749f, 892-893, 893f, 894f
Goldenhar syndrome (oculoauriculovertebral sequence), III:777, IV:113, 422, 424f. *See also* Craniofacial microsomia.
Gonadal sex, VI:1198
Gonion, II:19f, 20t
Good Samaritan service, I:132
Gore-Tex, I:756, 756f
Gorlin cyst, V:93, 193-194

Gorlin syndrome (nevoid basal cell carcinoma syndrome), III:611-612, V:93, 290, 290f, 398, 398t, 399t
  genetic analysis in, I:62-64, 64f
  midfacial reconstruction in, I:385f-386f
Gout
  of proximal interphalangeal joint, VII:77f
  vs. hand infection, VII:764, 767, 767f
  wound healing and, I:943
Gracilis
  anatomy of, VIII:490-492, 490f, 491f
  harvest of, VIII:496-497
  physiology of, VIII:492, 494f
Gracilis flap
  for abdominal wall reconstruction, VI:1192
  for lower extremity reconstruction, VI:1372-1373, 1372f
  for perineal reconstruction, I:451, 451f
  for pressure sores, I:465, 465f, 466f, VI:1324t, 1327, 1333-1334, 1333f, 1335f
  for vaginal reconstruction, VI:1285-1286, 1286f, 1287f, 1301, 1302f, 1303f
Gracilis transfer
  complications of, VIII:504
  for biceps reconstruction, VII:338, 343f, VIII:501-502, 502f, 504, 505f
  for deltoid reconstruction, VIII:502-503, 502f, 503f, 504, 506
  for facial paralysis, I:613-614, 614f, III:903-906, 904f, 905f, 908f, 909f
  for finger extension, VIII:500-501, 501f
  for flexor aspect of forearm, VIII:497-500, 498f-500f, 504, 505
  for upper extremity reconstruction, VII:335, 343f, VIII:490-492, 490f, 491f, 494f, 496-497
  harvest of, VIII:496-497
  management after, VIII:503-504
Graft(s)
  bone, I:671-680. *See also* Bone graft.
  cartilage, I:621-634. *See also* Cartilage graft.
  dermal, I:569-576. *See also* Dermal graft; Skin graft.
  fascial, I:584-588, 586f, 587f
  fat, I:576-579, 577f-578f
  muscle, I:610-616, 614f. *See also* Muscle graft.
  nerve, VII:495-503. *See also* Nerve graft.
  skin, I:293-314. *See also* Skin graft.
  tendon, I:598-599, 599f. *See also* Tendon graft.
Grafton DMB gel, I:1101t
Granulation tissue, in wound healing, I:213
Granulocytes, in graft rejection, I:271
Granuloma
  giant cell, of mandible, V:102-103, 208-209
  pyogenic, I:945, V:310, 312f
    in children, V:3, 3f, 34-35, 35f
    of finger, VII:956
    of perionychium, VII:200
    of upper extremity, VII:956-957, VIII:376, 377f
  vs. hand infection, VII:767, 768f

Granuloma annulare, vs. hand infection, VII:769

Grasp
cylinder, VII:254, 255f
development of, VIII:41-42, 43f-44f
key pinch, VII:254, 255f, VIII:521, 522f. *See also* Key pinch.
restoration of. *See at* Tetraplegia, upper extremity function restoration in.

Gray (Gy), I:836

Grayson ligament, VII:731, 731f

Grayson nasoalveolar molding, IV:178-179, 180f

Great auricular nerve
anatomy of, II:171, 172f, 189
injury to, II:205-206, 206f

Greater palatine neurovascular bundle, in palatoplasty, IV:258

Greig syndrome, VIII:21t, 22

Groin, reconstruction of, I:448, 451-454, 452f, 453f

Groin flap
for lower extremity reconstruction, VI:1374, 1376, 1376f
for mandible reconstruction, III:962-963

Growth
brachial plexus injury and, VIII:444-445, 445f, 446
cleft lip and, IV:242
cleft palate and, IV:253-254, 256-257, 262
condylar process fracture and, III:485
constriction ring syndrome and, VIII:210f, 211
cranial, III:382f, 383f, 388, 388f
craniosynostosis and, IV:466
facial
in craniofacial microsomia, IV:125-126
in craniofacial syndromes, IV:95-96
postnatal, III:382-388, 382f-386f, 383t, 388f
mandibular, III:382f-386f, 388-390, 390f
after facial burn treatment, III:69-70
in craniofacial microsomia, IV:550-551, 553
midface, III:390-391, 453-454
nasal, III:388, 389f, 390-391
pediatric hand reconstruction and, VIII:439-448. *See also* Hand reconstruction, pediatric.
upper extremity prosthesis and, VIII:54-56, 55f, 580
vascular territories effects of, I:347-348, 347f

Growth factors
in fetal wound healing, I:218
in tissue expansion, I:542, 544f
in wound healing, I:212t, 215-217, 226, 888-890, 1017-1018
neurotrophic, I:723, 723f

Growth plate
injury to, VIII:440-444, 440f-444f
transplantation of, VIII:446

Guanethidine, in complex regional pain syndrome/reflex sympathetic dystrophy, VII:855

Guedel airway with cuff, I:176

Guitarist, hand disorders in, VII:694-695, 695f

Gunpowder tattoo, III:12-13

Gunshot injury
abdominal, I:926, 926f, 1006, 1007f
facial, I:1006-1008, 1008f, III:344, 350-361, 823, 826f, 828f-831f. *See also* Face, gunshot wounds to.
upper extremity, I:1008, 1009f

Guyon canal
anatomy of, VII:41
trauma to, VII:894

Guyon canal syndrome, VII:876t, 893-894, 894f

Gynecomastia, VI:527-533
acquired, VI:527, 527t, 528t
classification of, VI:528-529, 528t
clinical presentation of, VI:528-529
drug-induced, VI:527, 528t
etiology of, VI:527, 527t
grade I, VI:528t, 529-531, 530f, 531f
grade II, VI:528t, 532f, 533
grade III, VI:528t, 533-534, 533f
histology of, VI:528
incidence of, VI:527
liposuction for, VI:221, 223-224, 223f-225f, 281-282, 283f
nonoperative treatment of, VI:529
operative treatment of, VI:529-532, 530f-533f
skin cancer and, VI:529
testicular cancer and, VI:528-529

H

Hair
growth of, I:297, II:691, 693, 693f, III:625
scalp. *See also* Hair restoration.
anatomy of, II:688-690, 688f, 689f
density of, II:690
exit angle of, II:690
growth cycles of, II:691, 693, 693f, III:625
loss of, II:690-691. *See also* Hair restoration.
after brow lift, II:72-73, 74f
burn-related, III:611
chemical-related, III:611
cicatricial, III:610, 610t
classification of, II:691, 692f
in women, III:4-5, 626
infection-related, III:611
male pattern, II:690-691, 692f, III:625-626, 627f
radiation-related, III:611
with face lift, II:721-722, 724f
shape of, II:690
terminal, II:690
types of, II:690
vellus, II:690

Hair follicles, I:294f, 297, 298f
in skin grafts, I:312
occlusion of, after laser resurfacing, II:370

Hair restoration, II:687-713
anesthesia for, II:708-709, 709f
artificial hair for, II:712-713
automated, II:713
bouquet formation with, II:712, 712f
cloning for, II:713

Hair restoration *(Continued)*
complications of, II:709-712, 709f-712f
cornrow appearance after, II:710-712, 711f, 712f
donor-site scarring after, II:710, 710f
expanded hair-bearing flaps for, II:697, 698f
finasteride for, II:693-694
follicular units for, II:694, 695f, 696f
frontal-temporal recession and, II:688-689, 689f
hair grafts for, II:694, 695f, 696f, III:628-629, 628f
hairline design in, II:703-704, 703f-705f
in eyebrow reconstruction, III:23, 23f, 728, 728f, 729-730, 729f, 731f
instrumentation for, II:704-706
ischemia-related complications of, II:691
medical treatment for, II:693-694, III:626, 628
minoxidil for, II:693-694
patient evaluation for, II:699, 702-704, 702f-705f
scalp flaps for, II:694-697, 696f, III:630
scalp reduction for, II:697, 699, 700f, 701f, III:629, 629f
session number for, II:707-708, 708f
technique of, II:704-707, 706f, 707f
temporal alley after, II:712, 712f
tissue expansion for, I:551, III:629-630

Hairline
after face lift, II:716-721, 717f-723f
frontal-temporal recession of, II:688-689, 689f
in auricular reconstruction, III:656, 658, 660f
in eyebrow lift, II:221-222, 222f
natural, II:688-690, 689f

Hall-Findlay technique, for breast reduction, VI:564, 567f

Haller index, VI:459, 460f

Halo nevus, Color Plate V:114-2, V:265, 265f, 311, 314f

Halothane, I:177-178, 178t

Hamartoma, nasopharyngeal, III:766

Hamulus, IV:74f

Hand(s). *See also* Finger(s); Thumb(s); Wrist.
abscess of, VII:771, 777, 779-780, 779f, 780f
acute suppurative arthritis of, VII:772
air bag injury to, VII:656
Allen test of, VII:35-36, 35f-36f, 45, 46f-47f, 797-798, 799f
amputation of
congenital, VIII:56-61, 58f, 60f, 584-587, 585f, 586f. *See also* Constriction ring syndrome.
prostheses for, VIII:592, 598f, 599f, 600, 600f, 601f
body-powered, VIII:573-577, 574t, 575f-579f
in children, VIII:584-587, 585f, 586f
therapeutic, VIII:584
vs. reconstruction, VII:318-319
anatomic center of, VII:18-19, 18f
anatomy of, VII:13-41, 729-733, 730f
arterial, VII:34-37, 35f-36f, 792-796, 793f-795f

Hand(s) *(Continued)*

    cutaneous, **VII**:14-15, 14f, 15f

    fascial, **VII**:16, 16f, 17f, 729-731, 730f

    muscle, **VII**:24-34, 26f-28f, 30f-32f

    nerve, **VII**:37-41, 38f-40f

    osseous, **VII**:16-19, 17f

    vascular, **VII**:34-37, 35f-36f, 221, 221f, 792-797, 793f-796f

  aneurysmal bone cyst of, **VII**:988

  angiography of, **VII**:80, 82, 83f, 84f, 649

  arterial arches of, **VII**:792-794, 793f, 794f

  arthritis of, postoperative care in, **VIII**:563, 564f, 565f

  basal cell carcinoma of, **VII**:961

  bite injury to, **VII**:47, 762-764, 765f, 766t, 768, 768f

  blood supply of, **VII**:34-37, 35f-36f, 221, 221f, 792-797, 793f-796f

  bone tumors of, **VII**:979-991

    benign, **VII**:983-991, 984f-987f

    biopsy of, **VII**:980-981

    evaluation of, **VII**:979-981, 980f

    malignant, **VII**:988-991, 989f, 990f

    reconstruction after, **VII**:982-983

    resection of, **VII**:981-982, 982t

    staging of, **VII**:981, 981f

  bones of, **VII**:16-19, 17f

    evaluation of, **VII**:47-48

  burns of, **VII**:587-602, 605-642. *See also* Hand burns.

  bursae of, **VII**:47, 48f

  carpal, **VIII**:56-60

  central deficiency of, **VIII**:80, 82-101. *See also* Cleft hand.

  chemical injury to, **VII**:653-656, 653t, 655t, 768

  chondroma of, **VII**:984, 985f

  chondrosarcoma of, **VII**:988, 989f

  chronic, **VII**:823-866. *See also* Complex regional pain syndrome/reflex sympathetic dystrophy.

    evaluation of, **VII**:49-54, 51f-53f

    joint testing in, **VII**:50, 52f

    muscle testing in, **VII**:50, 52f, 53

    nerve testing in, **VII**:50, 51f, 53, 53f

    provocative maneuvers in, **VII**:53-54

    sudomotor function in, **VII**:50

  circulatory testing in, **VII**:35-36, 35f-36f, 45, 46f-47f, 797-798, 799f

  cleft. *See* Cleft hand.

  cold injury to. *See* Frostbite.

  complex regional pain syndrome/reflex sympathetic dystrophy of, **VII**:823-866. *See also* Complex regional pain syndrome/reflex sympathetic dystrophy.

  computed tomography of, **VII**:66-68, 68f

  congenital anomalies of, **VIII**:20-21, 21t, 25-49. *See also specific anomalies.*

    amputation, **VIII**:185-211. *See also* Constriction ring syndrome.

    angiography in, **VIII**:38-39

    classification of, **VIII**:31-36, 32-35t, 36f, 37f

    computed tomography in, **VIII**:38

    deformation sequence in, **VIII**:28, 28f, 29f

Hand(s) *(Continued)*

    disruption sequence in, **VIII**:28, 28f, 29f

    dysharmonic maturation in, **VIII**:38

    evaluation of, **VIII**:27, 40-42, 42f

    functional evaluation in, **VIII**:41-42, 43f-44f

    growth-related changes in, **VIII**:48-49, 48f

    hand dominance in, **VIII**:42

    heterogeneity of, **VIII**:29

    historical perspective on, **VIII**:25, 26f, 31

    incidence of, **VIII**:39-40, 40t, 41t

    longitudinal, **VIII**:61-131. *See also* Cleft hand; Symbrachydactyly.

    magnetic resonance imaging in, **VIII**:38

    malformation association in, **VIII**:28-29

    malformation sequence in, **VIII**:28, 28f, 29f

    nonspecificity of, **VIII**:29

    ossification center evaluation in, **VIII**:37-38

    prehension evaluation in, **VIII**:41-42, 43f-44f

    prosthesis for, **VIII**:564. *See also* Hand(s), prosthetic.

    radiology in, **VIII**:36-39, 36-40, 37f

    secondary deformity with, **VIII**:47, 47f

    skeletal maturation evaluation in, **VIII**:36-38

    syndromic, **VIII**:30-31, 30f, 39-40

    terminology for, **VIII**:27-30, 28f, 29f

    transverse, **VIII**:56-61, 58f, 60f

    treatment of, **VIII**:45-49, 47f, 48f

      timing of, **VIII**:42, 45-46, 45f, 46f, 48-49

    variance in, **VIII**:29

  constriction ring syndrome of, **VIII**:185-211. *See also* Constriction ring syndrome.

  contagious pustular dermatitis of, **VII**:784-785

  contracture of, **VII**:659-672. *See also* Finger(s), contractures of; Hand(s), stiff.

    burn-related, **VII**:616-624, 617t, 618f-620f, 622f, 624f

    in Dupuytren disease, **VII**:668-669, 669f, 670f, 671, 696-697, 697f, 701, 736, 737f, **VIII**:561

  cumulative trauma disorder of, **VII**:688-691

    etiology of, **VII**:688-689

    prevention of, **VII**:689-690

    treatment of, **VII**:690-691

  de Quervain syndrome of, **VII**:54, 675f, 676-680, 676f, 676t, 679f

  dermatofibroma of, **VII**:952, 952f

  desmoid of, **VII**:954-955

  digital arteries of, **VII**:794-795, 795f

  dominance of, **VIII**:42

  Dupuytren disease of, **VII**:668-669, 669f, 671, 729-754, 736, 737f. *See also* Dupuytren disease.

    in musician, **VII**:696-697, 697f, 701

Hand(s) *(Continued)*

  dysmorphology of, **VIII**:27-30, 28f. *See also* Hand(s), congenital anomalies of.

  electrical injury to, **VII**:590, 591f, 598-602, 636-638, 638f-642f

  enchondroma of, **VII**:63, 65f, 980, 980f, 984, 984f

  epidermolysis bullosa of, **VIII**:431-437, 432f, 434f-437f

  epithelioid sarcoma of, **VII**:970-972, 971f

  evaluation of, **VII**:45-50, 46f-47f, 318

    Allen test in, **VII**:35-36, 35f-36f, 45, 46f-47f, 797-798, 799f

    angiography in, **VII**:80, 82, 83f, 84f

    bone and joint assessment in, **VII**:47-48

    capillary refill in, **VII**:45

    circulation assessment in, **VII**:45-46, 46f-47f

    computed tomography in, **VII**:66-68, 68f

    infection assessment in, **VII**:46-47, 48f

    magnetic resonance imaging in, **VII**:69-80, 69t, 70t, 71f-78f

    muscle-tendon assessment in, **VII**:48-49, 49f, 50f

    patient history for, **VII**:45

    plain film radiography in, **VII**:55-65, 56f-65f

    radionuclide imaging in, **VII**:65-66, 67f

    sensation assessment in, **VII**:49

    skin assessment in, **VII**:46-47

    tomography in, **VII**:65, 66f

    ultrasonography in, **VII**:68-69

  Ewing sarcoma of, **VII**:991

  extension contracture of, **VII**:660-661, 661f

  extensor tendons of, **VII**:401-420. *See also* Extensor tendon(s).

  extrinsic extensors of, **VII**:24-25

  fascia of, **VII**:16, 16f, 17f, 729-731, 730f

  fibrolipoma of, **VII**:958

  fibroma of, **VII**:953-954, 953f

  first web space of

    deficiency of, **VIII**:339-340

    in cleft hand, **VIII**:97-98, 97f

    release of, **VIII**:159-161, 160f-162f, 172, 335f, 339-340

  five-fingered, **VIII**:360, 361f, 362f

  flexor tendons of, **VII**:351-394. *See also* Flexor tendon(s).

  fracture of, **VII**:423-451. *See also* Finger(s), fracture of.

    in children, **VIII**:424, 425f

  furuncle of, **VII**:771

  giant cell tumor of, **VII**:955-956, 955f, 987-988, 987f

  glomus tumor of, **VII**:957-958, 957f

  growth of, **VIII**:48, 48f

    pediatric hand reconstruction and, **VIII**:439-446, 440f-445f

  hypoplasia of, **VIII**:147-148. *See also* Syndactyly.

  in Apert syndrome, **VIII**:144-146, 144f, 145f, 146t, 170-175, 171t, 172t, 173f-176f

Hand(s) *(Continued)*
  in arthrogryposis, VIII:147, 148f
  in Freeman-Sheldon syndrome,
    VIII:147, 148f
  in Poland syndrome, VIII:141-144, 142f,
    143f, 144t, 175, 177, 177f
  in tetraplegia, VIII:507-540. *See also*
    Tetraplegia, upper extremity
    function restoration in.
  infection of, VII:759-789. *See also* Hand
    infection.
  injury to, VII:804-807, 805f, 805t
    air bag, VII:656
    bite, VII:47, 762-764, 765f, 766t, 768,
      768f
    burn, VII:605-642. *See also* Hand
      burns.
    chemical, VII:653-656, 653t, 655t, 768
    closed, VII:804, 805f
    cold. *See* Frostbite.
    cumulative, VII:688-691
    electrical, VII:590, 591f, 598-602, 636-
      638, 638f-642f
    evaluation of, VII:45-49, 46f-50f. *See*
      also Hand(s), evaluation of.
    iatrogenic, VII:806-807
    ischemic, VII:791-819. *See also*
      Hand(s), ischemic injury to.
    mangling, VII:317-348. *See also* Hand
      reconstruction.
    open, VII:804
    pediatric, VIII:418-420
      débridement in, VIII:418-419, 420f
      emergency care in, VIII:417-418
      evaluation of, VIII:418, 419f
      reconstruction in, VIII:419-420,
        420f, 439-448. *See also* Hand
        reconstruction, pediatric.
    treatment of, VII:805-807. *See also*
      Hand reconstruction.
  intersection syndrome of, VII:680-681,
    681f
  ischemic injury to, VII:791-819
    acquired arteriovenous fistula and,
      VII:807, 808f
    aneurysm and, VII:813-814
    arterial reconstruction in, VII:806
    arteritis and, VII:814-815, 814f
    definition of, VII:791-792
    digital artery thrombosis and, VII:810
    embolism and, VII:807-808, 809f
    evaluation of, VII:797-802
      Allen test in, VII:797-798, 799f
      capillaroscopy in, VII:797
      color duplex imaging in, VII:800
      contrast arteriography in, VII:802,
        803f
      digital temperature in, VII:798
      Doppler study in, VII:798, 799f
      laser Doppler perfusion imaging in,
        VII:800
      magnetic resonance angiography
        in, VII:802
      noninvasive vascular testing in,
        VII:798, 800
      office examination in, VII:797-798
      patient history in, VII:797
      physical examination in, VII:797-798
      plethysmography in, VII:800, 800f,
        801f

Hand(s) *(Continued)*
    radionuclide imaging in, VII:800
    segmental arterial pressure in,
      VII:798
    ultrasonography in, VII:798, 800
    in Buerger disease, VII:814-815, 814f
    in connective tissue disorders, VII:815
    in neonate, VII:815
    in neoplastic disease, VII:815
    in sepsis, VII:815
    in vasospastic disease, VII:815-819,
      817f-819f
    incidence of, VII:791-792
    medical management in, VII:802
    mycotic aneurysm and, VII:814
    nonsurgical management in, VII:802,
      804
    radial artery aneurysm and, VII:814
    radial artery thrombosis and, VII:810
    thoracic outlet syndrome surgery and,
      VII:810-813, 813f
    thrombolytic therapy in, VII:802, 804
    tourniquet-related, VII:115-118
    traumatic, VII:804-807, 805f, 805t
      closed, VII:804, 805f
      iatrogenic, VII:806-807
      open, VII:804
      signs of, VII:805t
      treatment of, VII:805-807
    ulnar artery aneurysm and, VII:813-
      814
    ulnar artery thrombosis and, VII:808-
      810, 810f-812f
    with arterial cannulation, VII:806
    with arterial harvest, VII:807
    with drug injection, VII:807
  joint axes of, VII:14-15, 15f
  joints of, VII:16-24, 17f, 19f
    motion of, VII:21-22, 21f
  Kaplan's cardinal line of, VII:14, 14f
  keratoacanthoma of, VII:962, 962f
  keratoses of, VII:960
  laser resurfacing of, II:367
  lipoma of, VII:70, 958
  longitudinal deficiency of, VIII:61-131
    central, VIII:80, 82-101. *See also* Cleft
      hand.
    classification of, VIII:61
    radial (preaxial), VIII:61-80. *See also*
      Radial (preaxial) deficiency.
    ulnar, VIII:101-110. *See also* Ulnar
      deficiency.
  longitudinal fascial fibers of, VII:730,
    730f
  magnetic resonance imaging of, VII:69-
    80, 69t, 70t, 71f-78f
  malignant fibrous histiocytoma of,
    VII:970, 972
  mangled, VII:317-348. *See also* Hand
    reconstruction.
  median nerve of, VII:38, 39f, 41
  melanoma of, V:326-327, 331f, VII:965-
    969, 965f, 966t, 968t
  metastatic disease of, VII:991
  microarterial system of, VII:795-796
  mirror, VIII:17, 19, 19f, 21t, 249-254. *See*
    also Mirror hand.
  multiple enchondromatosis of, VII:984-
    985
  muscles of, VII:24-34

Hand(s) *(Continued)*
    assessment of, VII:48-50, 49f, 50f
    extensor, VII:24-25
    flexor, VII:26-29, 27f, 28f
    intrinsic, VII:32-34, 33f
    pronator, VII:25-26
    retinacular system of, VII:29-32, 30f,
      31f
    supinator, VII:25-26
  musicians', VII:693-704. *See also*
    Musicians' hands.
  necrotizing fasciitis of, VII:781-782,
    782f, 783f, 789
  neural fibrolipoma of, VII:958
  neurilemoma of, VII:958-959
  neurofibroma of, VII:70, 72f, 958-959
  nevi of, VII:959
  nodular fasciitis of, VII:952-953
  ossification centers of, VII:26, 27f
  osteoarthritis of, VII:57f, 707-725
    diagnosis of, VII:709
    epidemiology of, VII:707, 709
    etiology of, VII:707
    macrodactyly and, VIII:303, 304f
    postoperative care in, VIII:563-564
    treatment of, VII:710-725
      conservative, VII:710
      endoprostheses for, VII:710
      in carpometacarpal joint of first
        ray, VII:719-724, 721f-723f
      in distal interphalangeal joints,
        VII:710-712, 712f, 713f
      in metacarpophalangeal joint,
        VII:717-719, 718t, 719f
      in proximal interphalangeal joints,
        VII:713-717, 714f-716f, 718f
      in thumb, VII:724, 724f, 725f
      indications for, VII:709-710
  osteoblastoma of, VII:986
  osteochondroma of, VII:985, 985f, 986f
  osteogenic sarcoma of, VII:988, 990,
    990f
  osteoid osteoma of, VII:985-986, 986f
  osteomyelitis of, VII:65f, 784, 789
  palmar fascia of, VII:16, 16f, 729-731,
    730f
  paronychia of, VII:771, 777, 778f
  plain film radiography of, VII:55-65,
    56f-65f
    in acromegaly, VII:63, 64f
    in Hurler syndrome, VII:63, 64f
    specialized views for, VII:61-65, 63f,
      64f
    views for, VII:55-57, 56f-58f
  point tenderness in, VII:48
  prosthetic, I:782, 782f, 787, VIII:601
    active, I:782-785, 783f-785f
    aesthetic, VIII:586f, 588f, 592, 598f,
      599f, 600, 600f, 601f
    battery-powered, I:783-785, 785f,
      VIII:577-578, 579f, 580f
    body-powered, VIII:573-577, 574t,
      575f-579f
    complete, I:787
    fitting of, VIII:580
    in symbrachydactyly, VIII:130f, 131
    myoelectric, I:783-785, 785f
    partial, I:787
    passive, I:785-786
    shoulder-powered, I:783, 784f

Hand(s) *(Continued)*
  telemetry system for, I:788
  wrist-powered, I:783-784
  provocative testing of, VII:53-54
  pyogenic granuloma of, VII:956
  radial nerve of, VII:38, 38f
  radionuclide imaging of, VII:65-66, 67f
  reflex sympathetic dystrophy of,
      VII:823-866. *See also* Complex
      regional pain syndrome/reflex
      sympathetic dystrophy.
  replantation of, I:284-285, VII:565-584,
      568f, 572f, 573f. *See also* Hand
      replantation.
  retinacular system of, VII:29-32, 30f, 31f
  rhabdomyosarcoma of, VII:973
  sarcoma of, VII:968-970
  sensation testing in, VII:49
  septic arthritis of, VII:782-784, 784f,
      788-789
  skin of, VII:14
    evaluation of, VII:46-47, 48f
    in finger reconstruction, VII:218,
        218t, 220, 220f. *See also* Finger
        reconstruction, flaps for.
    preoperative preparation of, VII:114-
        115
    sudomotor function testing of, VII:50
  spastic, VIII:543-553
    assessment of, VIII:544-547, 546f,
        546t
    etiology of, VIII:543-544, 544f
    treatment of, VIII:547-553, 548t
  splinting of, VIII:567-568, 568t, 569f,
      569t, 570f
  squamous cell carcinoma of, VII:962-
      964, 963f
  stiff, VII:659-672
    collateral ligament changes and,
        VII:663-665, 665f-667f
    complications of, VII:671-672
    extension contracture and, VII:660-
        661, 661f
    flexion contracture and, VII:659, 660f
    nonoperative treatment of, VII:665-
        668, 667f, 668f
    operative treatment of, VII:668-671,
        669f-671f
      complications of, VII:671-672
    pathophysiology of, VII:665, 667f
    seesaw effect and, VII:661-663, 662f-
        664f
    treatment of, VII:665-672, 667f-671f
    volar plate changes and, VII:663-665,
        665f-667f
  subcutaneous tissue of, VII:14
  surgery on. *See* Hand reconstruction;
      Hand replantation; Hand surgery.
  sweat gland tumors of, VII:960, 961f,
      964-965
  synovial cell sarcoma of, VII:70, 75f,
      972-973
  synovial sheaths of, VII:29, 32, 47
  tendinitis of, VII:54
    in musician, VII:702
    therapy for, VIII:559-561, 559f-561f
  tendons of, VII:29-32, 30f, 31f. *See also*
      Extensor tendon(s); Flexor
      tendon(s).
    evaluation of, VII:48-49, 49f

Hand(s) *(Continued)*
  tenosynovitis of, VII:675-688
    extensor tendon, VII:675-684, 676f.
        See also De Quervain syndrome.
    fifth dorsal compartment, VII:676f,
        683
    first dorsal compartment, VII:676-
        680, 676f. *See also* De Quervain
        syndrome.
    flexor tendon, VII:684-686, 684f, 686f
    fourth dorsal compartment, VII:676f,
        682-683
    pyogenic, VII:773, 773f, 774f, 788
      treatment of, VII:780-781, 781f
    second dorsal compartment, VII:676f,
        680-681, 681f
    sixth dorsal compartment, VII:676f,
        683-684
    third dorsal compartment, VII:676f,
        681-682, 682f
  tomography of, VII:65, 66f
  transplantation of, I:77-78, 284-285. *See
      also* Hand replantation.
  transverse deficiency of
    at carpal level, VIII:56-60
    at metacarpal level, VIII:56-60, 58f,
        60f
    at phalangeal level, VIII:60-61
  transverse fascial fibers of, VII:730-731,
      730f
  tumors of
    bone, VII:979-991, 984f-987f, 989f,
        990f
    fibrous, VII:952-956, 953f-955f
    malignant, VII:960-973, 962f, 963f,
        965f, 966t, 971f
    pigmented, VII:959-960
    soft tissue, VII:949-973, 950t
    sweat gland, VII:960, 960f, 964-965
    vascular, VII:956-958, 957f
  two- and three-digit, VIII:147-148, 148f,
      168, 169f
  two-point discrimination in, VII:49
  ulnar deficiency of, VIII:101-110, 104f,
      109f. *See also* Ulnar deficiency.
  ulnar nerve of, VII:38-39, 40f, 41
  ultrasonography of, VII:68-69
  vascular anatomy of, VII:34-37, 35f-36f,
      221, 221f, 792-797, 793f-796f
  veins of, VII:37
  vertical fascial fibers of, VII:730f, 731
  viral infection of, VII:768, 784-785
  web spaces of
    burn scar contracture of, VII:617,
        617t, 618f-620f, 620-624, 622f,
        624f
    in cleft hand, VIII:97-98, 97f
    infection of, VII:772, 777, 779, 779f
    release of, VIII:159-161, 160f-162f,
        335f, 339-340
      in Apert syndrome, VIII:172, 173f
Hand burns, VII:587-602, 605-642
  blisters with, VII:592
  chemical, VII:653-656, 653t, 655t
  classification of, VII:605, 606t
  compartment syndrome with, VII:591,
      600-601
  conservative treatment of, VII:607
  cooling for, VII:590
  early excision in, VII:605-607

Hand burns *(Continued)*
  electrical, VII:590, 591f, 598-602, 636-
      638, 638f-642f
    alternating current in, VII:599
    clinical features of, VII:600
    compartment syndrome with,
        VII:600-601
    cutaneous, VII:600
    direct current in, VII:599
    epidemiology of, VII:598
    immediate management of, VII:637
    muscle, VII:600
    pathophysiology of, VII:599-600, 636-
        637
    staged reconstruction after, VII:637-
        638, 638f-641f
    tissue destruction with, VII:599-600
    treatment of, VII:600-602
      fasciotomy in, VII:600-601
      grafting in, VII:602
      immediate, VII:637
      splinting in, VII:601
      staged reconstruction in, VII:637-
          638, 638f-641f
      wound care in, VII:601
      wound coverage in, VII:602
    types of, VII:600
  flames and, VII:588
  grease fires and, VII:588, 590f
  heterotopic ossification with, VII:635-
      636
  hot tar and, VII:590
  in child abuse, VII:588, 590f
  in toddler, VII:587-588, 589f
  inflammation with, VII:606
  joint deformities with, VII:624-627,
      624t, 625f, 626f
  nonoperative treatment of, VII:607
  patterns of, VII:587-590, 589f, 590f
  postoperative care of, VIII:566
  pressure therapy in, VII:615
  reconstruction for, VII:613-630, 642f
    AlloDerm in, VII:613
    amputations in, VII:627-630, 629f
    distal interphalangeal joint
        deformities and, VII:627
    distraction lengthening in, VII:628,
        629
    dorsal contracture and, VII:617
    full-thickness vs. split-thickness skin
        grafts in, VII:607, 609
    grade IV contracture and, VII:617, 618f
    historical perspective on, VII:605-610
    hypertrophic scars and, VII:614-616
    immobilization in, VII:609-610, 616
    Integra in, VII:611-613, 612f
    joint deformities and, VII:624-627,
        624t, 625f, 626f
    metacarpophalangeal joint
        deformities and, VII:624, 624t,
        625f
    mobilization in, VII:609-610
    osteoplastic thumb reconstruction in,
        VII:630
    outcomes of, VII:605, 606t
    phalangization in, VII:628
    pollicization in, VII:628, 629f
    proximal interphalangeal joint
        deformities and, VII:625-627,
        626f

Hand burns *(Continued)*
scar contracture and, VII:616-624, 617t, 618f-620f, 622f, 624f
skin grafts in, VII:592-597, 593f-597f, 607-609, 608f, 617, 619f, 620f
skin substitutes in, VII:610-613, 610t, 611f, 612f
splinting in, VII:609-610
toe to thumb transfer in, VII:630
unstable scars and, VII:614
volar contracture and, VII:617
web space contracture and, VII:617, 620-624, 622f, 623f
scalding, VII:588, 590f
scarring with, VII:592, 616-624, 617t, 618f-620f
silicone gel therapy in, VII:615
treatment of, VII:587-602, VIII:565-566. *See also* Hand burns, reconstruction for.
biologic dressings in, VII:592
digit grafts in, VII:597
escharotomy in, VII:591-592
exposed bone in, VII:597-598
fasciotomy in, VII:592
for dorsal surface, VII:592-595, 593f-595f
for entire hand, VII:597, 597f
for fourth-degree burns, VII:597
for palmar surface, VII:595-597, 595f, 596f
gauze wrapping in, VII:593, 595, 596
Goulian knife in, VII:593, 593f
graft attachment in, VII:593, 594f, 595f
graft harvest for, VII:593, 594f, 595-596, 595f
grafting techniques in, VII:592-597, 593f-597f
hyperpigmentation with, VII:596
immediate, VII:590-592
Kirschner wires in, VII:597
philosophy of, VII:587, 588f
results of, VII:587, 588f
topical agents in, VII:592
tourniquet in, VII:592-593
wound management in, VII:592
Hand-heart syndrome, VIII:21t
Hand infection, VII:759-789
after fracture fixation, VII:760
anatomy of, VII:770-775, 771f-775f
apical space, VII:771
bites and, VII:762-764, 765f
boutonnière deformity after, VII:788-789
bursal, VII:773, 773f, 781
catheter-related, VII:762
clostridial, VII:782
complications of, VII:788-789
deep, VII:772-775, 773f-776f
deep palmar space, VII:773-775, 774f, 775f, 779-780, 780f
differential diagnosis of, VII:764, 767-770, 767f-770f
dorsal subaponeurotic space, VII:774f, 775, 780
drug abuse and, VII:760, 761f
etiology of, VII:759
examination of, VII:775-776
fungal, VII:766t, 785, 785f

Hand infection *(Continued)*
gangrenous, VII:782
gonococcal, VII:761-762
Gram stain for, VII:776
historical perspective on, VII:759
hypothenar space, VII:779-780
imaging of, VII:776, 776f
in diabetic patient, VII:760-761, 761f, 782
in HIV patient, VII:761
incidence of, VII:759-762
intermediate-depth, VII:771-772, 772f
joint, VII:782-784, 784f
laboratory tests in, VII:776
midpalmar space, VII:779, 780f
motion loss after, VII:788
mycobacterial, VII:774f, 785-788, 786f, 787f
necrotizing, VII:766t, 781-782, 782f, 783f, 789
Nocardia, VII:788
organisms in, VII:762-764, 763f, 764f
osteomyelitic, VII:784
palmar space, VII:773-775, 774f, 775f, 779-780, 780f
Parona space, VII:780
pathogenesis of, VII:759
patient history in, VII:775
postmastectomy, VII:762
postoperative, VII:120-121, 760
pulp space, VII:772, 772f, 777, 778f
radial bursa, VII:773, 773f, 781
septic, VII:782-784, 784f
Staphylococcus aureus in, VII:762, 763f, 764f
superficial, VII:771
thenar space, VII:779, 780f
toxic shock syndrome with, VII:762
treatment of, VII:766-767t, 775-777
antibiotics for, VII:766-767t, 777
drainage for, VII:777
principles of, VII:776-777
ulnar bursa, VII:773, 773f, 781
viral, VII:768, 784-785
vs. arteriovenous malformation, VII:769
vs. brown recluse spider bite, VII:768, 768f
vs. calcification, VII:767-768
vs. chemotherapeutic infiltration injury, VII:768
vs. factitious illness, VII:768
vs. foreign body, VII:768, 769f
vs. gout, VII:764, 767, 767f
vs. granuloma annulare, VII:769
vs. herpetic whitlow, VII:768
vs. metastatic lesions, VII:768-769, 769f
vs. pseudogout, VII:769
vs. pyoderma gangrenosum, VII:768
vs. pyogenic granuloma, VII:767, 768f
vs. rheumatoid arthritis, VII:769-770, 770f
vs. sarcoidosis, VII:770
vs. silicone synovitis, VII:769
web space, VII:772, 777, 779, 779f
Hand reconstruction, VII:317-348
after burns, VII:613-630, 642f. *See also* Hand burns, reconstruction for.
arterial anastomoses for, VII:323-324
arteriography in, VII:323
consent for, VII:320

Hand reconstruction *(Continued)*
débridement in, VII:320
delayed, VII:319
early, VII:319-320
free fibula transfer in, VII:335, 342f
innervated gracilis transfer in, VII:335, 338, 343f
joint problems in, VII:338, 345
lateral arm flap for, VII:328, 330, 330f-333f
latissimus dorsi flap for, VII:324, 325f, 326f, VIII:492
musculotendinous reconstruction in, VII:322
nerve grafting in, VII:322
pediatric, VIII:439-448
growth anomaly prevention in, VIII:446
growth anomaly treatment in, VIII:446, 447f, 448f
growth plate injury and, VIII:440-444, 440f-444f
negative growth effects in, VIII:440-446, 440f-445f
paralysis and, VIII:444-445, 445f
poor planning of, VIII:445-446
positive growth effects in, VIII:439-440
postirrigation culture before, VII:320
postoperative management in, VII:323
provisional revascularization in, VII:320-321
radial forearm flap for, VII:327-328, 329f
rectus abdominis flap for, VII:324-326, 327f
scapular flap for, VII:330, 333, 334f, 335f
serratus anterior flap for, VII:326, 328f
skeletal stabilization in, VII:321
soft tissue flaps in, VII:322-335, 325f-345f
planning of, VII:323-324
temporoparietal fascia flap for, VII:333, 335, 336f-341f
tendon transfer in, VIII:453-486
bone healing and, VIII:454
direction of, VIII:455
donor muscle-tendon for, VIII:454-455
for clawing, VIII:472-473, 473f
for combined nerve injury, VIII:481-482
for flexion-adduction of thumb, VIII:478-479
for high median-high ulnar nerve palsy, VIII:482
for high median nerve palsy, VIII:466, 469-470, 469f, 470f
for high ulnar nerve palsy, VIII:479, 481
for index finger abduction, VIII:479
for low median nerve palsy, VIII:462-466, 463f-468f
for low ulnar nerve palsy, VIII:471-472, 472f, 475-476, 476f
for MCP joint flexion, VIII:473-475, 474f
for MCP joint flexion and interphalangeal extension, VIII:475-477, 475f-478f

Hand reconstruction (*Continued*)
for median-low ulnar nerve palsy, VIII:481-482
for posttraumatic reconstruction, VIII:483-486, 484f, 485f
for radial nerve palsy, VIII:455-462, 456f, 456t, 457f-461f
for ulnar deviation of small finger, VIII:478
general principles of, VIII:454-455, 454t
in leprosy, VIII:470, 471t
postoperative care of, VIII:567
soft tissue healing and, VIII:454
techniques for, VIII:455
timing of, VIII:455
timing of, VII:319-320
toe transfer in, VII:338, 344f-345f, 345, 346f, 348
vascular reconstruction in, VII:321-322
vs. amputation, VII:318-319
Hand replantation, VII:565-584, 568f, 572f, 573f
arterial repair in, VII:574-575
care after, VII:576
centers for, VII:565-566
cold preservation for, VII:566
contraindications to, VII:567
failure of, VII:577-578, 577f
fasciotomy in, VII:574
historical perspective on, VII:565
indications for, VII:566-567
initial care for, VII:566
leech therapy after, VII:577, 577f
monitoring after, VII:576, 577f
neurorrhaphy in, VII:575
osteosynthesis in, VII:574
outcome of, VII:581
patient preparation for, VII:571
physical therapy after, VII:577-578
reperfusion injury and, VII:571
T shunt in, VII:571, 573f
tendon repair in, VII:575-576
thrombosis after, VII:576, 577f
transportation for, VII:566
vein repair in, VII:576
Hand-Schüller-Christian disease, V:103-104, 209
Hand surgery, VII:3-10, 109-122. *See also* Hand burns, reconstruction for; Hand reconstruction; Hand replantation.
anesthesia for, VII:87-106, 112-113, 113f. *See also* Anesthesia, upper extremity.
antibiotic ointment for, VII:121
antiseptic for, VII:115
care after, VII:122. *See also* Hand therapy.
current research in, VII:9-10
diagnosis for, VII:109-110, 110f, 111f
dressings for, VII:121-122
elevation after, VII:122
goals of, VII:112
hair removal for, VII:115
handwashing for, VII:114-115
historical origins of, VII:3-4, 4f
instruments for, VII:118, 119t
irrigation for, VII:121
microsurgical innovations in, VII:8

Hand surgery (*Continued*)
modern contributions to, VII:6-7
nerve grafting in, VII:9
operating room organization for, VII:113-114
patient position for, VII:113-114
planning for, VII:112-113, 113f
post-tourniquet syndrome with, VII:117-118
post-World War II contributions to, VII:7-8
principles of, VII:5-6, 5f, 6f, 112
reconstructive choices in, VII:112
skin preparation for, VII:114-115
splints for, VII:121-122
suture materials for, VII:118-120
tables for, VII:114
tissue equilibrium and, VII:112
tourniquet for, VII:115-118, 116f, 118f
muscle effects of, VII:116-117
nerve effects of, VII:117
vs. nonoperative management, VII:110-112
war-related contributions to, VII:6-7
wound infection after, VII:120-121
Hand therapy, VIII:557-572
cold therapy in, VIII:571
educational component of, VIII:568-570
electrical stimulation therapy in, VIII:572
evaluation for, VIII:557-558, 558t
for amputations, VIII:566-567
for arthritis, VIII:563-564, 564f, 565f
for burns, VIII:565-566
for camptodactyly, VIII:564-565
for carpal tunnel syndrome, VIII:562-563
for Colles' fracture, VIII:562
for congenital deformities, VIII:564-565
for congenital limb deficiency, VIII:564
for cubital tunnel syndrome, VIII:562-563
for de Quervain tenosynovitis, VIII:559-560, 560f
for distal phalanx fractures, VIII:561-562
for Dupuytren contracture, VIII:561
for extensor tendon repairs, VIII:566, 567f
for flexor tendon repairs, VIII:566
for fractures, VIII:561-562
for ganglion cyst, VIII:563
for lateral epicondylitis, VIII:558, 559f
for mallet finger, VIII:566, 567f
for medial epicondylitis, VIII:558
for metacarpal fractures, VIII:562
for nerve compression injuries, VIII:562-563
for osteoarthritis, VIII:563-564
for proximal phalanx fractures-dislocations, VIII:562
for radial clubhand, VIII:565
for radial tunnel syndrome, VIII:562-563
for rheumatoid arthritis, VIII:563, 564f, 565f
for tendon injuries, VIII:566
for tendon transfers, VIII:567
for tendonitis, VIII:558-561, 559f-561f
for thumb-in-palm, VIII:564

Hand therapy (*Continued*)
for trigger finger, VIII:560, 561f
for wrist flexor-extensor tendinitis, VIII:560-561
heat therapy in, VIII:571
in complex regional pain syndrome/reflex sympathetic dystrophy, VII:860-861, VIII:563
iontophoresis in, VIII:572
splinting in, VIII:567-568, 568t, 569f, 569t, 570f
transcutaneous electrical nerve stimulation in, VIII:572
ultrasound in, VIII:571-572
Handedness, VIII:42
Hard tissue replacement compound, I:703
Harvey, William, I:15, 15f, 16f-18f, 18
Hatchet flap, for eyebrow reconstruction, V:348-349, 351f
Hateful patient, I:73-75
Head and neck. *See also* Head and neck cancer; Head and neck reconstruction.
anatomy of, V:218-220, 218f, 219f
arteriovenous malformation of, III:775
biopsy of, V:167, 227-228
desmoplastic melanoma of, V:119-120, 120f
fetal, surgery on, I:1121-1122, 1121f, 1122t
fibrosarcoma of, V:118-119
hemangioma of, III:772-774, 773f
hemangiopericytoma of, V:119
injury to. *See* Head injury.
leiomyosarcoma of, V:119
liposarcoma of, V:119
malignant fibrous histiocytoma of, V:119
mass in, V:167
neuroblastoma of, V:119
neurofibrosarcoma of, V:119
neuroma of, VII:944
rhabdomyosarcoma of, V:115, 118
soft tissue sarcoma of, V:115, 118-120, 120f
synovial cell sarcoma of, V:119
unknown primary cancer in, V:249
vascular malformations of, III:774-775
vascular territories of, I:339-344
of anterior neck muscles, Color Plate I:15-13, I:343-344, 343t
of internal nose, Color Plate I:15-13, I:343
of lateral muscles, Color Plate I:15-13, I:342-343
of muscles, I:341-343, 342t, 343t
of muscles of facial expression, Color Plate I:15-12, I:340f, 341-342
of muscles of mastication, Color Plate I:15-12, I:342
of ocular muscles, I:342
of palate, I:343-344
of posterior neck muscles, Color Plate I:15-13, I:342
of salivary glands, I:344
of skin, Color Plate I:15-12, I:340-341, 340f, 341f
of superficial musculoaponeurotic system, Color Plate I:15-12, I:340-341, 340f, 341f
of thyroid gland, I:344
of tongue, I:343, 343f

Head and neck cancer, V:159-180, 217-250.
  See also Laryngeal cancer; Lip(s),
  cancer of; Oral cavity, cancer of;
  Oropharyngeal cancer.
  anatomy for, V:218-220, 218f, 219f
  biopsy in, V:167, 227-228
  cervical lymphatics in, V:160-161, 219-
    220, 219f, 221
  clinical manifestations of, V:226-227
  computed tomography in, V:228
  endoscopy in, V:227, 228
  epidemiology of, V:159-160
  evaluation of, V:167-169, 168f, 226-228
  field cancerization in, V:220, 249
  functional radical dissection of, V:472-
    473, 472f, 473f
  hematogenous spread of, V:467
  histology of, V:220
  hypopharyngeal, V:236-237
  laboratory evaluation in, V:228
  laryngeal, V:237-246. *See also* Laryngeal
    cancer.
  lymphatic spread of, V:160-161, 162f,
    219-220, 219f, 221
  metastatic, V:166-167, 166f, 465-473
    biopsy in, V:467-468
    cervical lymphatics in, V:160-161,
      466-467, 466f
    computed tomography in, V:468
    distant sites of, V:467
    evaluation of, V:467-468
    fine-needle aspiration biopsy in,
      V:468
    magnetic resonance imaging in, V:468
    sentinel node biopsy in, V:468
    treatment of, V:466-473
      functional radical dissection in,
        V:472-473, 472f, 473f
      lymph node status and, V:466-467
      radical neck dissection in, V:469-
        473, 469f-473f
    unknown primary in, V:466
  nasopharyngeal, V:246-247
  oropharyngeal, V:229-236. *See also*
    Oropharyngeal cancer.
  pain in, V:226
  paranasal sinus, V:247-249, 248f
  physical examination in, V:227
  premalignant lesions in, V:160
  psychological factors in, I:79
  radical dissection of, V:469-473, 469f-
    473f
  radiology in, V:169
  recurrence of, V:184-185
  risk factors for, V:220
  second primary in, V:249
  spread of, V:160-162, 220, 466-467, 466f
  staging of, V:167-169, 168f
  surgical anatomy for, V:163-166, 163f-
    165f
  treatment of, V:169-179, 171f-177f, 217-
    218
    airway complications of, V:249
    complications of, V:249
    guidelines for, V:220-221
    outcomes of, V:185-186
    photoradiation (photodynamic
      therapy) in, I:1063-1064, 1064t
    radiation therapy in, mandibular
      osteonecrosis after, III:983-984

Head and neck cancer *(Continued)*
    resection in, V:220-221
      reconstruction after, V:221-226,
        222f-225f, 226t. *See also* Head
        and neck reconstruction.
    second primary after, V:249
    wound healing and, I:981, 983
Head and neck reconstruction, V:185, 221-
  226, 222f-225f, 226t
    deltopectoral flap for, III:1043, 1044f,
      V:223, 224f, 226t
    dorsal scapular island flap for, III:1042,
      1042f
    forehead flap for, V:223, 225f
    jejunal flap for, III:1072, 1072f-1075f,
      V:226, 226t
    lateral arm flap for, III:1045-1047
    lateral cervical skin flaps for, III:1039,
      1039f
    lateral thigh flap for, III:1045, 1046f
    latissimus dorsi flap for, I:423, 429f-
      432f, 430, III:1062-1064, 1062f-
      1066f, V:222, 223f, 226t
    microvascular tissue transplantation for,
      I:430, 431f-432f, V:225-226, 226t
    nasolabial flap for, V:223, 224f, 226t
    omental flap for, III:1064, 1067-1071,
      1067f-1071f
    pectoralis flap for, I:423, 423f-427f,
      III:1052-1054, 1052f-1054f, V:221-
      222, 222f, 226t
    pedicled occipital artery flap for,
      III:1039f, 1040, 1040f
    platysma flap for, I:422, 422f, III:1048,
      1048f-1050f
    radial forearm flap for, III:1045, 1045f,
      V:226, 226t
    rectus abdominis flap for, V:226, 226t
    sternocleidomastoid flap for, I:421,
      III:1050-1051, 1051f
    submental artery island flap for,
      III:1040, 1040f
    temporalis flap for, I:421, V:223-225
    temporoparietal flap for, I:371-372,
      372f, V:223
    tissue expansion in, I:547-548, 551, 553,
      554f, 555f
    trapezius flap for, I:423, 428-430f,
      III:1055-1062, 1055f-1061f, V:222-
      223, 223f, 226t
Head injury
  in facial fracture, III:81, 83, 83t
  pediatric, III:400, 438-444
    calvarial bone graft in, III:442, 444, 445f
    evaluation of, III:438, 439f
    Glasgow coma scale in, III:438, 439t
    wound healing and, I:1006-1008, 1008f
Headache
  after dural puncture, I:194
  postoperative, I:202
Healos, I:1101t
Health Care Quality Improvement Act
    (1986), I:133
Health-related quality of life, I:41-42, 42f, 42t
Hearing
  in cleft palate, IV:255-256
  in craniofacial microsomia, IV:122, 123
  in head and neck cancer, V:226-227
  in Treacher Collins syndrome, IV:506-
    507, 509-510

Heart
  ectopic thoracic placement of, VI:482-
    483, 483f
  etomidate effects on, I:175
  in pectus excavatum, VI:461
  ketamine effects of, I:174
  local anesthetic effects on, I:189-190
  myoblast cell grafting into, I:612
  opioid effects on, I:181
  preoperative evaluation of, I:168, 169t
  rapacuronium effects on, I:180
  succinylcholine effects on, I:179
  transplantation of, cutaneous basal cell
    carcinoma and, V:396
Heart block, fetal, I:1125, 1126
Heart failure
  cardiomyoplasty in, I:615
  hemangioma and, V:29
Heat, body, loss of, I:855-856, 856f, 857,
    857t. *See also* Frostbite; Hypother-
    mia.
Heat shock, in flap optimization, I:495
Heat therapy, in hand therapy, VIII:571
Hedgehog pathway, I:62, 64f
Hedonism, I:98
Heel pad flaps, for foot reconstruction,
    VI:1435, 1437f, 1438f
Heel pain syndrome, VII:876t
Heggers-Robson protocol, in frostbite,
    VII:651, 652t
Help-rejecting personality, I:74
Hemangioendothelioma, VIII:378, 379f
  kaposiform, V:35-36, 36f, VIII:376-377,
    378f
Hemangioma, V:6, 7f, 20-34, VII:956-957,
    VIII:370-376, 371t, 372f-375f, 956-
    957
  angiography of, VIII:373
  bleeding from, V:28
  cardiovascular complications of, V:29
  cervicofacial, III:772-774, 773f
  cleft sternum and, VI:481
  clinical features of, V:21-25, 22f-25f,
    VIII:371, 371t
  congenital, V:24, 25f, VIII:371, 373f
  corticosteroid therapy for, V:29,
    VIII:375
  differential diagnosis of, V:25, 26f,
    VIII:373-374
  distribution of, V:22
  dressings for, V:28
  embolization in, V:31, VIII:376
  familial, V:21
  fetal, I:1122
  genetic factors in, V:21
  hand, VII:70, 76f
  incidence of, VIII:370
  interferon alfa for, V:30-31, VIII:375-
    376
  involuted phase of, V:20f, 21, 22-23, 23f,
    34, 35f
  involuting phase of, V:20f, 21, 22, 23f,
    32-34, 33f, VIII:370, 371, 372f
  laser therapy in, V:31, 31f
  life cycle of, V:20-21, 20f
  lumbosacral, V:26, 26f
  magnetic resonance imaging of, V:27,
    27f, VIII:373, 374f
  management of, V:27-34, VIII:374-376
    corticosteroids in, V:29-30, 29f,
      VIII:375

Hemangioma *(Continued)*
embolization in, V:31, VIII:376
interferon-alfa in, V:30-31, 30f, VIII:375-376
laser therapy in, V:31, 31f
medical therapy for, VIII:375-376
observation in, V:27
operative, V:31-34, 32f-35f, VIII:376
topical, V:28
multiple, V:22, 22f, 24-25
natural history of, VIII:370
noninvoluting, VIII:371
of buttocks, V:28f
of cheek, V:28f, 32
of ear, V:32
of extremities, V:28f
of eyelid, V:32
of face, III:772-774, 773f, V:28f-30f, 31, 31f, 33f
of fingers, VII:70, 76f
of forearm, VII:70, 73f
of forehead, V:32
of head and neck, III:772-774, 773f, V:34
of labia majora, VI:1292f
of lip, V:32, 33f, 35f, 379f
of liver, V:24-25, 29
of mandible, V:104, 210
of nasal tip, V:361f
of nose, V:34, 34f
of salivary gland, V:78-79, 81f
of scalp, V:32f
pathogenesis of, V:20-21, 20f
proliferating phase of, V:20-21, 20f, 22, 32, 32f, VIII:371, 372f
radionuclide imaging of, VIII:373
shunting in, V:25
social response to, V:27
structural anomalies with, V:25-26, 26f
subglottic, III:768, V:28-29, 31
telangiectatic, V:41
ulceration of, V:28, 28f, VIII:374, 375f
ultrasonography of, V:26-27, VIII:371, 373
viral infection and, V:21
vs. vascular malformation, V:19-20, 25, 26f
wound healing and, I:945
Hemangiomatosis, VIII:371
Hemangiopericytoma, VIII:377-378
in children, V:14-15, VIII:377-378
of head and neck, V:119
of orbit, V:115, 118f
Hematoma
flap, I:488
in child abuse, III:399, 400
in hand and wrist, VII:68, 69t
in nasal fracture, III:196, 204, 206-208, 207f
in nasoethmoidal-orbital fracture, III:325, 328
in pediatric facial trauma, III:399, 400, 401-402, 433-434
in zygoma fracture, III:209, 210f, 214
of ear, III:32-33, 32f, 677
of nasal septum, III:29-30, 196, 204, 206-208, 207f, 433-434
subungual, VII:175, 177
with abdominoplasty, VI:372, 379
with body lift, VI:271

Hematoma *(Continued)*
with breast augmentation, VI:29, 350-351
with breast reduction, VI:578
with brow lift, II:72
with craniofacial cleft management, IV:459
with facial liposuction, VI:213
with free TRAM flap, VI:872
with neck lift, II:320-323, 332
with neck liposuction, VI:220
with pressure sore treatment, VI:1351
with rhytidectomy, II:204-205, 205f
Hemiarrhinia, III:764
Hemidesmosomes, I:296
Hemiexophthalmos, II:93, 96-97
Hemifacial atrophy, IV:555-568
correction of, IV:556-561, 557f
care after, IV:560-561
donor site for, IV:561, 568f
fat injection for, IV:556
inframammary extended circumflex scapular flap for, IV:556-560, 559f, 560f
parascapular flap for, IV:559-560, 560f, 562f-565f, 568f
revisions after, IV:561, 562f-567f
silicone injection for, IV:556
superficial inferior epigastric flap for, IV:556, 557f, 566f-567f
timing of, IV:556
in connective tissue disorders, IV:555-556
in Romberg disease, III:833, 852f-853f, 865f, IV:555
Hemifacial microsomia. *See* Craniofacial microsomia.
Hemihypertrophy, macrodactyly and, VIII:308, 309f, 316
Hemilaryngectomy, V:243-244, 243f, 244f, 244t
Hemiplegia, spastic, VIII:543-544, 544f
Hemodialysis, wound healing and, I:943-944
Hemorrhage
abdominoplasty and, VI:178-179
after closed rhinoplasty, II:561-562
after mandibular fracture treatment, III:181
after orthognathic surgery, II:684-685
after secondary rhinoplasty, II:797
in hand and wrist, VII:68, 69t
in Kasabach-Merritt phenomenon, V:36
in lymphatic vascular malformation, III:775
in pediatric facial trauma, III:397-398
retrobulbar, after blepharoplasty, II:106
Hemostasis, in wound healing, I:209, 210f
Heparin
in flap optimization, I:499t, 500-501
in microvascular surgery, I:521-522
Hepatitis C, informed consent and, I:131
HER-2/neu receptor, VI:671
Herbal medicine, I:170, VI:175, 176t, 177t
Herbert screw, in osteoarthritis, VII:711-712, 712f, 713f
Hering's law, II:831, 834f, 835
HERMES system, I:1155

Hernia, VI:91
after abdominal surgery, I:985, 986f, 987f, 989f
after abdominoplasty, VI:377, 378
after free TRAM flap, VI:872
diaphragmatic, I:1122-1124, 1123f
epigastric, VI:92-93
periumbilical, VI:93
Herpes simplex virus infection, laser facial resurfacing and, II:342, 345, 346f
Herpetic whitlow, VII:194, 196f, 784
vs. hand infection, VII:768
Hester technique, for breast reduction, VI:540, 547f, 563
Heterotopic ossification, burn-related, I:829-830, VII:635-636
Hidradenitis suppurativa, wound healing and, I:940, 941f
Hidradenoma, clear cell, V:259
High airway obstruction syndrome, I:1121-1122, 1121f
Hindfoot reconstruction, VI:1430-1443, 1433f, 1434f, 1436f-1442f
Hip, liposuction for, VI:227-230, 227f, 229f-230f, 250, 250f, 280-281, 280f, 281f
Histiocytosis X, V:103-104
Histrionic personality, I:72
HLA typing, in transplantation, I:270-271, 273-274
Holoprosencephaly, IV:2-3, 22f, 23, 24f, 385, 387. *See also* Craniofacial cleft(s).
classification of, IV:21
Sonic hedgehog gene in, I:64, IV:3
Holt-Oram syndrome, VIII:21t, 275-276, 276f
hypoplastic thumb in, VIII:326
radial defects in, VIII:62
Homodigital advancement flap, for finger reconstruction, VII:220t, 222, 223f, 226f, 227f
Homodigital reverse-flow flap, for finger reconstruction, VII:220t, 222, 224f, 225f
Horner syndrome, VII:525-526, 540, 540f
Hospital privileges, peer review of, I:133-134
Hot packs, in hand therapy, VIII:571
House intrinsic tenodesis, in tetraplegia, VIII:531-532, 533f-534f
Hubbard tank, in hypothermia, I:858
Hueston rotation advancement flap, for fingertip reconstruction, VII:162
Hugh Johnson sign, VII:735
Human bite, hand infection from, VII:762-764, 765f, 766t
β-Human chorionic gonadotropin, in prenatal diagnosis, I:1073
Human immunodeficiency virus (HIV) infection
informed consent and, I:131
Kaposi sarcoma and, V:299-300, 300f
salivary gland lymphoma and, V:87
skin cancer and, V:275
wound healing and, I:940-941, 941f
Human papillomavirus (HPV) infection, III:770
skin cancer and, V:291, 292t

Humerus
  fracture of, arterial injury with, VII:804, 805f
  osteosarcoma of, VII:990, 990f
  rotational osteotomy of, VII:557, 558f
Hung span procedure, for scaphocephaly, IV:469, 470f, 471f
Hurler syndrome, VII:63, 64f
Hutchinson freckle, V:311, 313f
Hyaluronan, for bioengineered cartilage graft, I:631
Hyaluronic acid
  in tendon healing, I:595
  in wound healing, I:212
  injection of, for lower third face lift, II:283
Hyaluronic acid conduit, for nerve repair, VII:500
Hydralazine, before neck lift, II:322
Hydranencephaly, I:1128
Hydrocarbons, skin cancer and, V:275-276
Hydrocephalus
  fetal intervention for, I:1128-1129
  in craniosynostoses, IV:103, 476, 496-497
  in Crouzon syndrome, IV:100
  with craniofacial cleft management, IV:459
Hydrochloric acid injury, VII:654, 656
Hydrocolloid dressings, I:224, 225t
Hydrofluoric acid injury, VII:654, 656
  specific antidote for, VII:656
Hydrogel
  for cartilage graft, I:631
  in tissue engineering, I:1093-1095, 1095f, 1095t
Hydrogel dressing, I:224, 225t
Hydrogen peroxide, in flap ischemia, I:487-488, 487f
Hydronephrosis, congenital, I:1126-1127, 1126t
Hydrops fetalis
  cystic adenomatoid malformation and, I:1124, 1125
  pericardial teratoma and, I:1126
Hydroquinone, with laser facial resurfacing, II:345
Hydrothorax, congenital, I:1125
Hydroxy acids, II:397-400, 400f
  misconceptions about, II:400
  side effects of, II:399
Hydroxyapatite, for cranioplasty, III:555-556
Hydroxyapatite implants, I:693t, 696-700, 754, 755f
  bone-derived, I:693t, 696-697
  coralline, I:693t, 696, 754, 755f
  in vivo properties of, I:697-700
  laboratory-produced, I:693t, 697
  ocular, I:781
  sintered, I:755
Hydroxyl radical, in flap ischemia, I:487-488, 487f
Hygroma, cystic
  cheek reconstruction in, III:833, 834f-836f
  neck reconstruction in, III:1030-1032, 1030f-1032f
Hyoid suspension, in obstructive sleep apnea, III:790-791, 792f

Hyperbaric oxygen, I:952-954, 954f
  in Fournier disease, VI:1253
  in ischemic wounds, I:492
  in mandible reconstruction, III:960
  in smoke inhalation, I:832
  in wound healing, I:893, 895-897
Hypernasality, in velopharyngeal dysfunction, IV:313
Hyperostosis, macrodactyly and, VIII:307-308, 307f, 316
Hyperpigmentation
  after hand burn treatment, VII:596
  after laser resurfacing, II:342, 345, 372-373, 372f
  after liposuction, VI:239
  of skin graft, I:311
Hypersensitivity reactions, to implant, I:764
Hypertelorism, IV:107f, 109-110, 109f, 365-379, 366f
  computed tomography in, IV:366-367, 368f
  pathology of, IV:366, 366f, 367f
  reconstruction for, IV:417t, 420f
    bipartition procedure in, IV:372, 374, 375f
    combined craniofacial osteotomy in, IV:367, 369-372, 369f-374f
    longitudinal studies of, IV:376, 378f
    medial canthopexy in, IV:372, 373f, 375-376
    nasal reconstruction in, IV:376, 377f
    planning for, IV:366-367, 367f-369f
    results of, IV:446, 449f, 450f, 454, 458f
    soft tissue cleft coverage in, IV:376, 377f
    subcranial osteotomy in, IV:374
    U-shaped osteotomy in, IV:374-375, 376f
Hypertension
  intracranial, in craniosynostosis, IV:475
  postoperative, I:200-201
  preoperative evaluation of, I:168
Hyperthermia, malignant, I:179, 187
Hyperthyroidism, exophthalmos with, III:752, 753f, 754f
Hypoglossal nerve transplantation, in lower lip paralysis, III:912
Hyponasality, in velopharyngeal dysfunction, IV:313
Hyponychium, VII:172f
  defects of, VII:192, 193f
Hypopharyngeal reconstruction, III:993-1022
  colon interposition for, III:1012
  complications of, III:1016, 1018-1021, 1019f-1021f
  deltopectoral flap for, III:1011
  fasciocutaneous flaps for, III:998, 999f, 1016, 1017f
  fistula with, III:1018, 1019f
  gastric pull-up for, III:1011-1012, 1012f
  gastroepiploic flap for, III:1013, 1014f-1016f
  goals of, III:998
  historical perspective on, III:995, 997-998
  indications for, III:993-995
  jejunal flap for, III:1000-1005, 1001f-1005f, 1014

Hypopharyngeal reconstruction (Continued)
  lateral arm flap for, III:1016, 1017f
  lateral thigh flap for, III:1012-1013
  mortality with, III:1016
  patient factors in, III:998, 1000
  pectoralis major flap for, III:1008-1011, 1009f, 1010f
  radial forearm flap for, III:1005-1007, 1006f-1008f, 1014, 1016
  results of, III:1013-1014, 1016-1022, 1017f, 1019f-1021f
  speech after, III:1018, 1020f-1021f, 1022
  ulnar forearm flap for, III:1013
Hypopharynx
  anatomy of, V:218-219. See also Hypopharyngeal reconstruction.
  cancer of, V:236-237
Hypopigmentation, after laser resurfacing, II:373-374, 374f
Hypopnea, III:775
Hypospadias, VI:1259-1277, 1260f
  anatomy of, VI:1261
  chordee and, VI:1260-1261
  classification of, VI:1260
  cryptorchidism and, VI:1261
  distal, VI:1259, 1260f, 1262-1267
    flip-flap procedure in, VI:1267, 1269f
    glans reapproximation procedures in, VI:1263-1265, 1264f-1267f, 1274, 1276f
    meatoplasty and glansplasty procedure in, VI:1265, 1268f, 1274
    tubularized incised plate repair in, VI:1265, 1267, 1268f, 1274-1275, 1275t, 1276f
    urinary diversion in, VI:1271-1272, 1272f
  embryology of, VI:1261
  etiology of, VI:1259
  flat glans and, VI:1275, 1277f
  incidence of, VI:1259
  megameatus and, VI:1277, 1277f
  mild, VI:1259, 1260f
  proximal, VI:1259, 1260f, 1267, 1269-1271
    inner preputial island flap in, VI:1271, 1271f, 1275
    two-stage glans-splitting Bracka technique in, VI:1267, 1269-1271, 1269f, 1270f, 1276f
  surgical repair of, VI:1262-1271, 1264f-1271f
    algorithm for, VI:1275-1277, 1276f
    fistula after, VI:1272, 1272f
    flat glans and, VI:1275, 1277f
    lichen sclerosus et atrophicus after, VI:1273
    meatal problems after, VI:1272-1273, 1273f
    megameatus and, VI:1277, 1277f
    outcomes of, VI:1274
    skin problems after, VI:1273
    stricture after, VI:1273
Hypothenar muscles, VII:32
Hypothermia, I:858. See also Frostbite.
  anesthetic-induced, I:187
  in flap optimization, I:499t, 500
Hypovolemia, I:185

Hypoxia
in craniosynostoses, IV:497
in Robin sequence, IV:513
Hysterectomy, in female-to-male
transformation, VI:1311-1312
Hysterical paralysis, vs. reflex sympathetic
dystrophy/chronic regional pain
syndrome, VII:848

I

Ibuprofen, I:183-184
in frostbite, I:860, 860t
Ice massage, in hand therapy, VIII:571
Ice packs, in hand therapy, VIII:571
Iliohypogastric nerve, VI:92, 1178
injury to, in abdominoplasty, VI:375
Ilioinguinal nerve, VI:92, 1178
injury to, in abdominoplasty, VI:375
Iliolumbar flap, for abdominal wall
reconstruction, VI:1185
Ilium flap, I:390, 390t, 395f-396f
for chin reconstruction, III:599, 603f-
604f
for mandible reconstruction, III:963-
965, 964f, 968, 969
Ilium graft, I:673t, 680-684
in adults, I:681-682, 681f-683f
in children, I:682-684
Iloprost, in flap salvage, I:488
Imiquimod, in skin cancer, V:404t, 406
Immersion foot, I:858-859
Immersion tank protocol, in hypothermia,
I:858
IMMIX extenders, I:1101t
Immobilization
cold injury and, I:857
in bone repair, I:658-659
in extensor tendon repair, VII:410-412
in hand burn reconstruction, VII:609-
610, 616
Immune globulin, intravenous, in toxic
epidermal necrolysis, I:799
Immune system, I:270-279. See also at
Transplantation.
B lymphocytes in, I:271-272
blood group antigens in, I:271
complement in, I:272
dendritic cells in, I:272
granulocytes in, I:271
immunoglobulins in, I:272
in head and neck cancer, V:159-160
in skin cancer, V:275
macrophages in, I:271
major histocompatibility complex in,
I:270-271
minor histocompatibility antigens in,
I:271
natural killer cells in, I:271
rejection cascade in, I:271-273
skin-specific antigens in, I:271
T lymphocytes in, I:272-273
Immunodeficiency. See also Human
immunodeficiency virus (HIV)
infection.
skin cancer and, V:397
Immunoglobulins, in graft rejection,
I:272
Immunologic tolerance, I:278-279, 285
Immunomodulators, in breast
augmentation, VI:28

Immunosuppression
cancer and, V:275, 291
for transplantation, I:274-278, 274t,
275t, 285. See also Transplantation,
immunosuppression for.
wound healing and, I:941-942
Immunotherapy, I:1056-1057
Implant(s). See also Alloplastic materials.
alumina, I:755-756
antibiotic-coated, I:763
breast
explantation of, VI:82, 84, 318-320,
328-329, 328f, 1147-1150, 1148f-
1149f, 1149t
for augmentation, VI:1-7, 2f, 5f, 5t, 6f.
See also Breast augmentation,
implants for.
for reconstruction, VI:897-922, 923-
932, 966-970, 969f, 970f. See also
at Expander-implant breast
reconstruction.
in pectus excavatum, VI:463, 465f,
470-471, 472f
in Poland syndrome, VI:493, 495f
calcium phosphate, I:753-756, 754f, 755f
calcium sulfate, I:755
carcinogenicity of, I:763-764, 764t
ceramic, I:693t, 696-700, 752-756, 753f-
755f, 754t
complications of, I:761-764, 762t
corundum, I:756
dental
after mandibular reconstruction,
III:984-986, 986f, 987f
osseointegrated, I:524, 524f
recombinant bone morphogenetic
proteins with, I:662-663
economics of, I:765
elastomer, I:758-760
exposure of, I:764
extrusion of, I:764
failure of, I:764
glass, I:755
gold, I:745, 752
historical perspective on, I:745-746
hydroxyapatite, I:693t, 696-700, 754,
755f, 781
hypersensitivity reactions to, I:764
in chest reconstruction, VI:432
in mastopexy, VI:81-82, 83f
in pectus excavatum, VI:463, 464f, 465f,
470-471, 472f
in Poland syndrome, VI:490-493, 492f,
494f, 495f
infection with, I:762-763
mechanical properties of, I:748-750,
749f, 750t
metal, I:751-752, 752t
nickel-titanium alloy, I:752
nipple, VI:809
platinum, I:752
polymer, I:756-760, 756f, 758f, 759f
polyolefin, I:757-758, 758f, 759f
polyethylene terephthalate, I:757
prominence of, I:764
removal of, I:764-765
silver, I:752
stainless steel, I:751-752, 752t
surgical placement of, I:751, 751t
tantalum, I:752

Implant(s) (Continued)
thermoplastic, I:756-758, 756f, 758f,
759f
thermoset, I:760
titanium, I:752, 752t
toxicity of, I:763
tricalcium phosphate, I:755
with tissue expansion, I:543-544
Implied consent, I:132, 146-147
Impotence. See Erectile dysfunction.
Impressions, for facial prostheses, I:774-
775, 775f
Imprinting, I:53
Incision inferius, II:19f, 20t
Incision superius, II:19f, 20t
Incisive foramen, IV:70-71, 70f
Inclusion cyst, in constriction ring
syndrome, VIII:203, 204f
Indian hedgehog growth factor, in
osteoblast differentiation, I:644-645
Infant. See also Children and specific
congenital anomalies and disorders.
birth-related facial trauma in, III:398
brachial plexus injury in, VII:539-562.
See also Brachial plexus injury,
obstetric.
digital fibroma in, VII:953-954, 953f
facial trauma in, III:398-399. See also
Facial trauma, pediatric.
fall-related injury in, III:398-399
melanotic neuroectodermal tumor in,
III:772
physical abuse of, III:399-400
thrombosis in, VII:808, 815
trigger thumb in, VII:687-688
Infection
blepharoplasty and, II:106
breast
augmentation and, VI:27, 29, 329,
346-348
free TRAM flap and, VI:872
reduction and, VI:578
secondary reconstruction and,
VI:1108, 1111, 1124, 1124t,
1127-1130, 1128f, 1129f, 1131-
1132t, 1133f, 1134t
burns and, I:828-829
closed rhinoplasty and, II:563
finger, VII:770, 771, 771f, 772, 772f, 777,
778f
hand, VII:759-789. See also Hand
infection.
hypothermia and, I:187
implant-related, I:762-763
laser resurfacing and, II:371-372, 371f
liposuction and, VI:236-237
lymphatic malformation and, V:44, 45f,
VIII:393
mandibular fracture and, III:181-182
maxillary fracture and, III:249, 251
neck lift and, II:332
oral cavity reconstruction and, III:950
orthognathic surgery and, II:685
perionychium, VII:192-196, 195f, 196f
pressure sore, VI:1322, 1351
radiation therapy and, I:840f, 841, 842f,
843f, 1054-1055, 1055f, 1055t
rhytidectomy and, II:210, 211f
scalp, III:611
secondary rhinoplasty and, II:793, 797

Infection (Continued)
skin graft, I:312
sternal, VI:425-426, 425t, 427f
tissue expansion and, I:565-566
wound, I:220, 911-918, 912-913t, 914f, 915f, 916t. See also Wound(s), management of; Wound(s), problem.
anaerobic, I:913t, 914
antibiotics for, I:912-913t
bone, I:914-915, 915f, 977, 978f, 979f
culture for, I:882
débridement and, I:881-882, 881f
gram-negative, I:912-913t
gram-positive, I:912t
hydrogen peroxide for, I:882, 882f
necrotizing, I:911, 914, 914f, 974, 976-977
soft tissue, I:911, 914, 914f, 974, 976-977
spinal, I:981
spread of, I:879-880
sternal, I:914-915, 915f, 977, 979f, 980-981, 980f
Inferior gluteal artery perforator flap, VI:764t, 769t, 770-771, 952, 953f
Inferior gluteus maximus flap, for pressure sore treatment, VI:1324-1325, 1324t, 1328f-1330f
Inferior retinacular lateral canthoplasty, II:842-846, 843t, 845f, 846f
Inflammation. See also Infection.
in complex regional pain syndrome/reflex sympathetic dystrophy, VII:837-839
in fetal wound healing, I:218
in wound healing, I:209-211, 210f, 211f, 212t
Informed consent, I:103-104, 146-148, 148t
capacity for, I:103-104
communication approaches to, I:148-149
confidentiality and, I:104
conflicts of interest and, I:131-132
documentation of, I:148
elements of, I:147-148, 148t
for abdominoplasty, VI:124
for breast augmentation, VI:8
for large-volume liposuction, VI:244
historical perspective on, I:105-106
in medical malpractice suits, I:131-132
information for, I:103
Informed refusal, I:146
Infraclavicular block, VII:100, 100f
Inframammary extended circumflex scapular flap, for hemifacial atrophy, IV:556-560, 559f, 560f
Infraorbital artery, IV:78f, 79
Infraorbital hollowness, arcus marginalis release for, II:232, 234, 234f
Infraorbital nerve, IV:81-82
decompression of, III:366
injury to
in nasoethmoidal-orbital fracture, III:329-330
in orbital fracture, III:290
in zygoma fracture, III:212, 212f, 213, 229
pain with, III:361
neuroma of, VII:944

Infraorbital nerve block, I:191-192, 192f, III:8-9, 9f
Infratemporal fossa, tumors of, V:144-148, 146f-148f
Infratrochlear nerve, II:55-56
Ingrown fingernail, VII:204
Inheritance. See also Genetics.
autosomal, I:51-52, 52f
Mendelian, I:51-52, 52f, 53f
mitochondrial, I:53
non-Mendelian, I:52-53
sex-linked, I:52, 53f
Insulin-like growth factor 1, in wound healing, I:212t, 216
Insurance Portability Act, I:136
Integra, I:313, 893, 1087t, 1088, 1088f
in burn treatment, I:824t, 826-827, 827f, VII:611-613, 612f
in scar revision, I:260f, 263
in wound healing, I:1018
Integrins, in wound healing, I:212
Intellectualization, I:70
Interbrow frown, postoperative, II:802-803
Intercanthal axis tilt, II:78
Intercarpal ligament, VII:455, 455f
Intercellular adhesion molecule 1, I:490, 490f
Intercostal nerves, VI:1178
Interferon, in skin cancer, V:404t, 405-406
Interferon-alfa
in hemangioma, III:774, V:30-31, 30f, VIII:375-376
in kaposiform hemangioendothelioma, V:36
Interleukin-6, in nerve regeneration, VII:480
Intermaxillary elastics, during mandibular distraction, IV:546, 548f
Intermetacarpal ligaments, VII:22
Internal oblique muscle, VI:1177
Internet, I:1140-1142. See also Telemedicine.
Interorbital space, III:309
Interosseous muscles, VII:22, 32, 33f
evaluation of, VII:32-34, 33f, 50, 52f
plantar, VI:1409, 1409f
Interosseous nerve
anterior, entrapment of, VII:876t, 889-892, 890f-893f
posterior, entrapment of, VII:876t, 904, 906, 906f
Interosseous recurrent artery, Color Plate I:15-6, I:335
Interphalangeal joints. See also Finger(s).
contractures of. See Finger(s), contractures of.
distal
axis of rotation of, VII:22
degrees of freedom of, VII:22
dislocation/subluxation of, VII:448-449
dorsal, VII:448, 448f
lateral, VII:449
volar, VII:448-449
extension of, VII:403, 406-408, 406f, 407-408, 407f
tendon transfers for, VIII:475-477, 475f-477f
fracture-dislocation/subluxation of, VII:449-450

Interphalangeal joints (Continued)
dorsal, VII:449
volar, VII:449-450, 450f
fusion of, VIII:265-269, 266f-268f
motion of, VII:21-22, 21f
osteoarthritis of, VII:707, 708f-709f, 710-712
diagnosis of, VII:710-711
Herbert screw for, VII:711-712, 712f, 713f
indications for, VII:711
passive flexion of, VII:403, 407f
transfer of, in PIP joint reconstruction, VII:216, 218, 218f, 219f
proximal
axis of rotation of, VII:22
congenital contracture of. See Camptodactyly.
degrees of freedom of, VII:22
dislocation/subluxation of, VII:441-445, 442f
dorsal, VII:442-444, 442f, 443f
lateral, VII:444-445
volar, VII:444, 444f
extension of, VII:403, 406-408, 406f, 407f
tendon transfers for, VIII:475-477, 475f-477f
fracture-dislocation/subluxation of, VII:445-448
dorsal, VII:445-446, 445f, 446f
K-wire for, VII:447-448, 447f
splinting for, VII:447
volar, VII:446-447
fracture of, VII:216f
arthrodesis in, VII:216
arthroplasty in, VII:215-216
DIP joint transfer in, VII:216, 218, 218f, 219f
external fixation in, VII:215, 215f
open reduction and internal fixation for, VII:447-448, 447f
splint for, VII:447
toe joint transfer in, VII:216, 216f
fusion of, VIII:265-269, 266f-268f
gouty tophus of, VII:77f
motion of, VII:21-22, 21f
osteoarthritis of, VII:713-717
arthrodesis (plate and screws) for, VII:717, 718f
arthroplasty (Silastic implant) for, VII:713-717, 714f-716f, 718t
reconstruction of, VII:338, 345. See also Finger reconstruction.
Interscalene nerve block, I:192, 194f, VII:97-99, 98f
Intersection syndrome, VII:680-681, 681f
Intracavernosal injection therapy, VI:1234
Intracranial pressure
in craniosynostoses, IV:103, 476, 496-497
in Crouzon syndrome, IV:100
ketamine effects on, I:175
Intradermal nevus, V:308, 308f
Intranasal lining flaps, II:577-579, 578f, 579t, 613, 617f, 618, 619f-621f, 626f-629f
Intraoral splint, IV:303, 304f

Intrathoracic defects, VI:427-431, 429t, 430f

Intravelar veloplasty, IV:261, 262f

Intrinsic muscle flaps, for foot reconstruction, VI:1431-1435, 1433f, 1434f

Intubation
  nasopharyngeal, in Treacher Collins syndrome, IV:416, 422
  tracheal, I:176-177
    of children, III:395, 397-398, 397f

Inverted L ramus osteotomy, IV:444, 444f

Iodoflex, topical, I:884t

Iodosorb, topical, I:884t

Iontophoresis, in hand therapy, VIII:572

Iowa classification, of radial (thumb) polydactyly, VIII:216, 216f

Irrigation
  in chemical injury, VII:654-655
  in facial trauma, III:11, 12f
  of wound, I:950, 951f

Ischemia, I:608-609
  flap, I:486-488, 487f. *See also* Necrosis, flap.
  hand, VII:791-819. *See also* Hand(s), ischemic injury to.
  in abdominoplasty, VI:178
  no-reflow phenomenon and, I:608-609

Ischemic preconditioning, in flap optimization, I:494-495, 495t, 499t, 500

Ischium, pressure sores of, I:999t, 1000, 1001f, 1004f, VI:1324-1334, 1324t, 1326f-1333f, 1335f

Isoflurane, I:178, 178t

Isolation, for burn patient, I:829

Isotretinoin, V:277, 405
  ear deformity and, III:638
  laser resurfacing and, II:342

J

Jackson-Weiss syndrome, III:778, IV:93t, 100. *See also* Craniosynostosis (craniosynostoses), syndromic.
  genetic analysis in, I:58, 60-61, 61f-63f

Jacobson nerve, III:4

Jadassohn, nevus sebaceus of, V:257, 281-282, 281f, 282f, 399

Jaffe-Lichtenstein syndrome, V:206

James Barrett Brown Award, I:23-24, 24t

Jaw. *See* Mandible; Orthognathic surgery.

Jejunal flap, I:379, 379t
  for esophageal reconstruction, III:997-998, 1000-1005, 1001f-1005f, 1014
  for head and neck reconstruction, III:1072, 1072f-1075f, V:226, 226t

Jersey finger, VII:379, 380f

Jervine, teratogenicity of, IV:12

Jeune syndrome, VI:484-485, 484f, 485f

Joint jack, for finger contracture, VII:666-667, 667f

Joule's law, VII:598-599

Jowls
  after face lift, II:744-745, 745f
  sagging of, II:281-282

Junctional nevus, V:308, 308f

Juncturae tendinum, VII:405, 407f

Justice, I:101t, 104-105, 122-123

K

Kant, Immanuel, I:98-99

Kaplan's cardinal line, VII:14, 14f

Kaposi sarcoma, V:299-300, 300f

Kaposiform hemangioendothelioma, V:35-36, 36f, VIII:376-377, 378f

Karapandzic flap, for lip reconstruction, III:813, 820, 820f, V:383, 384f

Karyotype, I:54, 56f

Kasabach-Merritt syndrome, III:773-774, 773f, V:35-36, 36f, VII:956

Kava, VI:176t

Kazanjian, Varastad H., I:29

Keloids, I:222, 227t, III:14-15, 15f
  hypertrophic, I:938, 939f
  treatment of, I:228-230, 229f

Keratin cysts (milia), V:255-256

Keratinocyst, odontogenic, V:93, 94f, 192-193, 194f

Keratinocytes, I:295
  in keloids, I:222
  in toxic epidermal necrolysis, I:795
  in wound healing, I:214
  tissue-engineered, I:1087-1088, 1087t

Keratitis
  postblepharoplasty, II:808
  with craniofacial cleft management, IV:461

Keratitis, ichthyosis, and deafness (KID) syndrome, V:401

Keratoacanthoma, V:268-269, 269f, 280, 280f, 437t, 439-442
  clinical features of, V:439-440, 439f, 440t
  epidemiology of, V:439
  etiology of, V:439
  Ferguson-Smith, V:441
  giant, V:440-441
  Grzybowski-type, V:441
  histology of, V:440, 441f
  incidence of, V:439
  Muir-Torre, V:441
  of hand, VII:962, 962f
  of perionychium, VII:200
  subungual, V:441, VII:200
  treatment of, V:441-442

Keratosis
  actinic, V:266-268, 267f
  lichenoid, V:446
  seborrheic, V:253-254, 254f, 310, 312f
  upper extremity, VII:960

Ketamine, I:172t, 174-175, 184

Ketorolac, I:183-184

Key pinch, VII:254, 255f, VIII:521, 522f
  development of, VIII:41-42, 43f-44f
  restoration of, VIII:521-527, 523f, 525f-528f
    brachioradialis to FPL transfer for, VIII:527-529, 528f, 529f
    Brand-Moberg pollicis longus tenodesis for, VIII:508-509, 508f, 522, 524-527, 525f-527f
    flexor pollicis longus tenodesis for, VIII:522, 524-527, 525f-528f
    functional neuromuscular stimulation for, VIII:536, 538, 539f
    in IC group 1 and 2, VIII:521-527, 523f, 525f-527f
    in IC group 2 and 3, VIII:527-529, 528f, 529f

Key pinch *(Continued)*
    results of, VIII:482, 540
    split FPL to EPL interphalangeal stabilization for, VIII:522, 523f
    winch procedure for, VIII:518, 520, 520f

Kidneys
  compound A effects on, I:179
  fetal, I:1126-1127, 1126t

Kienböck disease, VII:66f, 68

Kirner deformity, VIII:295-296

Kite flap, for finger reconstruction, VII:231, 233f, 234f

Kleeblattschädel, IV:476-477

Kleinman-Reagan shear test, VII:458

Klippel-Trénaunay syndrome, V:56-60, 58f, 59f, VIII:408-409, 409f, 410f, 413t
  macrodactyly in, VIII:309, 311f, 316-317

Knee
  anastomoses around, I:339
  liposuction for, VI:288, 288f
  prosthetic, infection with, I:919, 922f, 996, 996f-997f

Knuckle-Jack splint, VII:667f, 668

Knuckle pads, VII:736-737, 737f

Krukenberg procedure, VIII:54

Kuhnt-Szymanowski procedure, III:896-897

Kutler lateral V-Y flap, for fingertip reconstruction, VII:159-160, 159f

Kuttner tumor, V:3

Kutz elevator, VII:177, 177f

L

Labetalol, before neck lift, II:321-322

Labia majora
  fat injections for, VI:408
  hemangioma of, VI:1292f

Labia minora
  anatomy of, VI:404-405
  dehiscence of, VI:408, 408f
  hypertrophy of, VI:1290f, 1291f
  reduction of, VI:404-405, 406f, 407-408, 407f, 1289-1292

Labial artery, IV:78f, 80f

Labial cleft. *See* Cleft lip.

Labiomental groove (fold), II:13, 14f

Labioplasty, VI:404-405, 406f, 407-408, 407f, 1289-1292, 1290f-1292f

Labyrinth, embryology of, IV:115-117, 116f

Laceration
  ear, III:33
  facial, III:13-14, 13f, 14f
    in children, III:400, 401
  in child abuse, III:399
  nasal, III:30
  with brow lift, II:72, 73f

Lacrimal duct
  cyst of, III:765
  injury to, with closed rhinoplasty, II:564

Lacrimal gland
  ptosis of, II:128
  tumors of, V:115

Lacrimal sac, groove for, III:269

Lacrimal system
  examination of, in orbital fracture, III:273
  injury to, in nasoethmoidal-orbital fracture, III:328
  obstruction of, in maxillary fracture, III:251

Lagophthalmos, III:892-895, 893f-895f
   after brow lift, II:71
   gold weight for, III:748, 749f, 892-893,
      893f, 894f
   lateral tarsorrhaphy for, III:895
   palpebral spring in, III:893-894, 894f
   platysma transplantation for, III:894-
      895
   temporalis muscle transplantation for,
      III:894, 895f
Lambdoid craniosynostosis, IV:159-162,
   160f-162f
Lamellar graft, in secondary lower lid
   repair, II:820-821, 820f, 821f
Lamina densa, I:296
Lamina lucida, I:296
Laminin, in nerve regeneration, VII:480
Langerhans cell, I:295
Langerhans cell disease, V:209
Langer's lines, III:3
Large cohort studies, in evidence-based
   decision-making, I:44
Large-volume liposuction, VI:241-254. See
   also Liposuction, large-volume.
Laryngeal cancer, V:237-246
   anatomy for, V:237-238, 237f
   staging of, V:238
   treatment of, V:238-246
      at glottis, V:241-246, 241f, 244f-247f,
         244t, 245t
      at supraglottis, V:239-241, 240f-242f,
         240t
      neck reconstruction in, III:1039
Laryngeal cleft, III:769
Laryngeal mask airway, I:176, 177f
Laryngectomy
   glottic, V:243-246, 244f-247f
   supracricoid, V:246, 247f
   supraglottic, V:240-241, 240f-242f
   total, V:244-246, 245f, 245t, 246f
Laryngomalacia, III:768-769
Laryngotracheobronchitis, III:768
Larynx
   anatomy of, V:218-219, 237-238, 237f
   arterial supply of, Color Plate I:15-13,
      I:343-344, 343t
   atresia of, I:1121-1122, 1121f
   cancer of. See Laryngeal cancer.
   cleft of, III:769
   cyst of, III:769
   lymphoma of, III:771-772
Laser Doppler, for flap monitoring, I:497t,
   498-499
Laser Doppler fluxmetry, in upper
   extremity ischemia, VII:800
Laser Doppler perfusion imaging, in upper
   extremity ischemia, VII:800
Laser resurfacing
   facial, II:339-380. See also Facial
      resurfacing.
   nonfacial, II:365-368, 366f
Laser therapy
   in capillary malformations, V:40, 40f
   in hairline management, III:656, 658,
      660f
   in hemangioma, V:31, 31f
   in lymphatic malformations, V:45
   in pediatric hemangioma, V:6
   in peripheral nerve repair, I:733
   in traumatic tattoo, III:12

Laser therapy (Continued)
   in twin-twin transfusion syndrome,
      I:1130
   in venous malformations, V:50
LASIK surgery, periorbital surgery and,
   II:90
Lassus-Legour technique, for breast
   reduction, VI:563-564, 564f-566f,
   567-568, 568f, 569f
Lateral arm flap
   for esophageal reconstruction, III:1016,
      1017f
   for neck reconstruction, III:1045-1047,
      1047f
   for upper limb reconstruction, VII:328,
      330, 330f-333f
Lateral cervical skin flaps, for neck
   reconstruction, III:1039, 1039f
Lateral femoral cutaneous nerve
   entrapment of, VII:909-910, 911f
   injury to, in abdominoplasty, VI:375
Lateral first-toe flap, for finger
   reconstruction, VII:237, 241f, 242
Lateral supramalleolar flap, for foot
   reconstruction, VI:1419, 1423f
Lateral sweep syndrome, II:237, 238f
Lateral tension abdominoplasty, Color
   Plate VI:125-3, VI:259, 260-262, 261f-
   264f
Lateral thigh flap
   for esophageal reconstruction, III:1012-
      1013
   for lower extremity reconstruction,
      VI:1377, 1377f
   for neck reconstruction, III:1045, 1046f
   for oral cavity reconstruction, III:941-
      942, 944-948, 948f, 949f
   transverse, for breast reconstruction,
      VI:1055f, 1056f-1057f, 1057-1058,
      1058f, 1063
Latissimus dorsi, anatomy of, VI:496f, 690,
   691f, 819-821, 820f
Latissimus dorsi flap, I:423, 428f
   arc of rotation of, I:418, 418f
   breast reconstruction with, I:433, 434f,
      435f, VI:686, 688f, 690-712, 690t
      after subcutaneous mastectomy,
         VI:652
      complications of, VI:704, 712, 831-
         832, 1036-1037
      contraindications to, VI:691t
      contralateral breast in, VI:691, 695f,
         1024, 1027f
      delayed, VI:1023-1037
         anatomy for, VI:1028-1030, 1029f
         blood supply for, VI:1029-1030,
            1029f
         complications of, VI:1036-1037
         contraindications to, VI:1024, 1028
         contralateral breast size and,
            VI:1024, 1027f
         donor site for, VI:693f-694f, 1030-
            1031, 1031f
         extended flap for, VI:1035-1036,
            1036f, 1037f
         flap elevation for, VI:1032-1034,
            1032f, 1033f
         flap placement for, VI:696, 701f-
            704f, 1033-1034, 1033f,
            1034f

Latissimus dorsi flap (Continued)
      flap thickness and, VI:1024, 1028f
      implant for, VI:696, 702f-704f,
         1034, 1035f, 1036
      marking for, VI:691, 693f-694f,
         695f, 1030-1031, 1031f
      mastectomy skin flap thickness
         and, VI:1024, 1028f
      patient positioning for, VI:1031-
         1032, 1031f
      prior radiation therapy and,
         VI:1024, 1026f, 1027f
      reconstruction site marking for,
         VI:691, 695f, 1031
      results of, VI:709f-711f
      skin island design for, VI:691, 693f-
         694f
   endoscopic harvest of, I:1039-1046,
      1040f
      after lumpectomy, I:1045-1046,
         1045f, 1046f
      after segmental mastectomy,
         I:1045-1046, 1045f, 1046f
      care after, I:1044
      complications of, I:1046
      dissection in, I:1042-1043, 1042f
      division in, I:1043, 1043f
      flap examination in, I:1041, 1041f
      implant pocket creation in, I:1043
      in partial mastectomy, I:1045-1046,
         1045f, 1046f
      patient positioning for, I:1041-
         1042, 1041f
      patient selection for, I:1040
      preoperative markings for, I:1040-
         1041, 1040f
      results of, I:1044, 1044f
      sutures in, I:1043, 1043f, 1044,
         1044f
   immediate, VI:819-832
      after breast augmentation, VI:826
      after mastopexy, VI:822, 826
      after prophylactic mastectomy,
         VI:826, 827f
      after radiation therapy, VI:822, 824f
      anatomy for, VI:819-821, 820f
      complications of, VI:831-832
      contraindications to, VI:826
      donor site complications after,
         VI:831
      expander for, VI:829-830, 831f
      flap elevation for, VI:828-829, 828f-
         830f
      flap insetting for, VI:705f, 829-830,
         831f
      flap molding for, VI:830, 831f
      flap necrosis after, VI:831
      for excessively thin skin, VI:822
      for partial mastectomy defects,
         VI:822, 825f
      for ptotic breasts, VI:826
      historical perspective on, VI:819
      implant for, VI:704, 705f, 823f,
         824f, 827f, 830
      indications for, VI:821-826, 821f-
         825f
      marking for, VI:690-691, 692f
      patient assessment for, VI:821
      planning for, VI:690-691, 692f,
         826-827, 827f, 828f

Latissimus dorsi flap *(Continued)*
    prosthesis migration after, VI:831-832
    results of, VI:706f, 707f, 708f, 821-822, 821f, 822f
    sensation after, VI:832
    seroma after, VI:831
    skin island design for, VI:691, 693f-694f
    skin necrosis after, VI:831
    thermal injury after, VI:832
    thoracodorsal nerve in, VI:830-831
  indications for, VI:691t
  technique of, VI:695-712, 697f-707f.
      See also Latissimus dorsi flap, breast reconstruction with, delayed; Latissimus dorsi flap, breast reconstruction with, immediate.
    dissection for, VI:696, 698f-701f
    donor site closure in, VI:696, 700f
    flap inset in, VI:696, 701f-704f, 704, 705f
    implant placement in, VI:696, 702f-704f, 704, 705f, 706f
    implant pocket in, VI:696, 701f-704f
    incisions for, VI:695-696, 697f
    patient position in, VI:695, 697f
    preoperative markings for, VI:690-695, 692f-695f
    results of, VI:706f-711f
    thoracodorsal artery in, VI:690, 691f
    thoracodorsal nerve in, VI:696
    vascular anatomy in, VI:690, 691f
  for abdominal wall reconstruction, I:447, 447t, 448f, VI:1191-1192
  for back reconstruction, VI:441-442, 444f, 448, 450, 451f, 452f
  for chest wall reconstruction, I:441, 446, VI:414-417, 414f, 415f, 420f-421f
  for cranioplasty, III:557
  for head and neck reconstruction, I:423, 429f-432f, 430, III:1062-1064, 1062f-1066f, V:222, 223f, 226t
  for lower extremity reconstruction, VI:1364, 1366f
  for mandible reconstruction, III:961
  for mediastinum reconstruction, I:441
  for scalp reconstruction, I:429f-432f, 430, III:620, 621f
  for smile reconstruction, III:877, 879, 879f, 880f
  for upper extremity reconstruction, I:400f-402f, 405, VII:324, 325f, 326f, VIII:492
  in Poland syndrome, VI:490, 491f, 493, 496f-500f, 501-506, 501f-505f
  segmental, I:384
Latrodectus bite, I:931-932, 933f, 934f, 1017
Le Fort I osteotomy
  in craniofacial cleft, IV:439, 441, 441f
  in craniofacial microsomia, IV:533, 538f-540f, 540
  in orthognathic surgery, II:660, 662, 662f
  Le Fort III with, IV:482, 484f

Le Fort II osteotomy
  in craniofacial cleft, IV:439, 440f
  in craniosynostosis, IV:482, 485, 485f, 486f
Le Fort III osteotomy
  in craniofacial cleft, IV:439, 439f
  subcranial, IV:477-482, 478f-481f
    Le Fort I advancement osteotomy with, IV:482, 484f
    midface advancement with bone graft with, IV:480-482, 481f-483f
    midface distraction devices with, IV:479-480, 479f, 480f
Leapfrog Group, I:43, 43t, 48
Ledderhose disease, VII:737, 738f
Leeches, I:499t, 501, VII:577, 577f
Leg. *See* Lower extremity.
Legal issues. *See also* Ethics; Medical malpractice; Professionalism.
  abuse and, I:136-138
  contracts and, I:134-136
  criminal offenses and, I:118-119
  expert witness testimony and, I:112-113
  fraud and, I:136-138
  in peer review, I:133-134
  informed consent and, I:103-104
Leiomyosarcoma
  in children, V:15
  of head and neck, V:119
Lentigo, V:261, 261f
Leprosy, tendon transfers in, VIII:470, 471t
Leriche sympathectomy, in vasospastic disease, VII:817
Leser-Trélat, sign of, V:254
Letrozole, in breast cancer, VI:672
Letterer-Siwe disease, V:104, 209
Leukemia, wound healing and, I:916, 918
Leukoplakia, Color Plate V:113-2, V:160, 268, 268f, 279, 445
Leukotriene B$_4$, in flap ischemia, I:488
Levator anguli oris, III:888t, 889
Levator aponeurosis
  blepharoplasty-related shortening of, II:106, 107f
  disinsertion of, acquired ptosis and, II:829-831, 830f-831f
  in secondary upper periorbital repair, II:815-817, 817f
  inadvertent sectioning of, II:810, 811f
  lengthening of, II:106, 107f
  plication of, in eyelid ptosis, II:134-135, 134f, 135f
  postblepharoplasty lengthening of, II:809-810, 809f
  reinsertion of, in eyelid ptosis, II:135-136, 136f-138f
Levator labii superioris, III:748, 750, 888t, 889
Levator palpebrae superioris, II:83, 84f, 133, 143-144, 143f, III:331-332, 750. *See also* Eyelid(s).
Levator scapulae transfer, for obstetric brachial plexus palsy, VII:557, 559f
Levator veli palatini
  anatomy of, IV:58f, 59f, 60-61, 60t, 61f, 72, 73f, 74f, 75, 75f, 312f, 351-352, 352f
  in cleft palate, IV:251, 252f, 261, 262f
  magnetic resonance imaging of, IV:65, 66f, 67f

Levobupivacaine, I:190t, 191
Liability. *See* Medical malpractice.
Lichen planus, V:160
Lichen sclerosus et atrophicus, VI:1253-1254, 1273
Lichenoid keratosis, V:446
Lid-switch flap, for upper eyelid reconstruction, V:364-365, 366f
Lidocaine, I:190, 190t
  for facial anesthesia, III:7-8, 7t
Life support protocols, in hypothermia, I:858
Lim1, IV:2
Limberg flap, for cheek reconstruction, III:833, 836f
Linburg-Comstock syndrome, VII:696
Linea alba, VI:91
Linea semicircularis, VI:91
Linea semilunaris, VI:91, 1178
Linguini sign, VI:636f, 637
Linton procedure, I:964
Liou nasoalveolar molding, IV:178, 179f
Lip(s). *See also* Lip lift; Lip reconstruction.
  cancer of, V:160-162, 161f, 445
    biopsy of, V:167
    epidemiology of, V:159-160
    evaluation of, V:167-169
    laboratory studies in, V:169
    metastases from, V:160-162, 162f, 166-167
    radiology of, V:169
    reconstruction after, V:185
    recurrence of, V:184-185
    TNM staging of, V:167-169
    treatment of, V:169-170, 170t, 171f-173f
      goals of, V:169-170
      outcomes of, V:185-186
      radiotherapy in, V:183-184
  cleft. *See* Cleft lip.
  commissure of
    in craniofacial microsomia, IV:541, 542f-543f
    reconstruction of, III:820-823, 821f-823f, V:385
  deformities of
    acquired, III:799-831. *See also* Lip reconstruction.
    congenital. *See* Cleft lip.
  functions of, III:801
  lower
    aesthetic analysis of, II:4t, 5t, 13, 13f-15f
    anatomy of, III:36, 799, 800f, IV:341, V:163
    anesthesia of, with condylar process fracture, III:515
    avulsion of, III:37
    blood supply to, III:799, 800f
    deformity of, after facial burn excision and grafting, III:66-69, 67f-68f
    depressors of, III:889, 889f
    dysesthesia of, with condylar process fracture, III:515
    function of, III:801
    hemangioma of, V:32
    in facial paralysis, III:911-912, 913f
    innervation of, III:799, 800f
    laceration of, III:37, 805-806, 806f-807f

Lip(s) *(Continued)*
  leukoplakia of, V:268, 395
  muscles of, III:799, 800f
  trauma to, III:37
  upper
    aesthetic analysis of, II:4t, 5t, 13, 13f-
      15f
    anatomy of, III:36, 799, 800f, IV:341,
      V:163
    avulsion of, III:37, 38f
    blood supply to, III:799, 800f
    defects of, direct closure for, V:381
    flat, after facial burn excision and
      grafting, III:62, 64f-65f, 66
    hemangioma of, V:32, 33f, 35f, 379f
    innervation of, III:799, 800f
    laceration of, III:37, 38f
    leukoplakia of, V:268, 395
    levators of, III:888-889, 888t
    long, after cleft lip repair, IV:349-350,
      350f
    muscles of, III:799, 800f
    short, after cleft lip repair, IV:349
    tight, after cleft lip repair, IV:350
    trauma to, III:37, 38f
    wide, after cleft lip repair, IV:350-351,
      351f
Lip augmentation, II:278-279, 749
  AlloDerm for, I:574, 574f
Lip lift, II:276-279, 276f-279f, 277t
  central, II:276-277, 276f, 277f
  corner, II:277-278, 278f, 279f
  supra-vermilion, II:277
Lip reconstruction, III:799-857. *See also at*
  Cleft lip.
  commissure in, III:820-823, 821f-823f,
    V:385
  lower
    after facial burn excision and grafting,
      III:66-69, 67f-68f
    anatomy for, III:799-801, 800f
    direct closure for, III:805-812, 806f-
      811f
    double Abbe flap for, III:813, 817f
    Estlander flap for, III:813, 817f
    fan flap for, V:383
    flaps for, V:383-385, 384f, 385f
    full-thickness skin graft for, III:801,
      803f, 804f
    in total defects, III:823, 825f, 826f
    Karapandzic flap for, III:813, 820,
      820f, V:383, 384f
    Schuchardt procedure in, III:812, 812f
    staircase flap for, III:812, 812f
    tongue flap for, V:383, 385, 385f
    Webster advancement technique for,
      V:385
    wedge excision in, III:806, 809, 810f
  upper
    Abbe flap for, III:812-813, 813f-816f,
      V:381-383, 382f
    after facial burn excision and grafting,
      III:62, 64f-65f, 66
    anatomy for, III:799-801, 800f
    direct closure in, III:805-812, 806f-
      811f, 807f
    fan flap for, III:813, 817f, 818f, V:383
    flaps for, V:381-383, 382f
    full-thickness skin graft in, III:801,
      802f

Lip reconstruction *(Continued)*
  in basal cell carcinoma, III:833, 840f
  in cleft lip. *See* Cleft lip.
  in total defect, III:823, 827f-831f
  perialar crescentic flap for, V:379f, 381
  temporal frontal scalp flap for,
    III:823, 827f
  wedge excision in, III:806, 811f
  vermilion reconstruction in, III:801,
    805, 805f, 806f
Lipectomy
  belt, VI:171-172, 172f
  with abdominoplasty, VI:101, 101f, 171-
    172, 172f, 173f, 376
Lipodermatosclerosis, of lower extremity,
  VI:1466
Lipoma, of hand, VII:70, 958
Lipomatosis, in children, V:9-10
Lipomatous macrodactyly, VIII:301, 303-
  304, 303f-305f
Liposarcoma
  in children, V:15
  of head and neck, V:119
Liposuction, I:361, VI:193-239
  abdominal, VI:227-230, 227f, 229f-230f,
    278-279
    with abdominoplasty, VI:96, 97, 98f,
      101, 110, 115, 140, 141f
  anesthesia for, I:202-203, VI:199-200,
    203-204
  ankle, VI:232, 235, 235f, 236f, 288
  arm, VI:216-221, 218f-222f, 249, 249f
  back, VI:227-230, 228f, 250, 250f, 280-
    281, 280f
  bleeding with, VI:203, 209, 235
  breast
    female, VI:224-227, 226f, 281-282,
      283f, 556, 558, 559f
    male, VI:221, 223-224, 223f-225f
  buttocks, VI:230, 230f, 231f
  calf, VI:232, 234f-236f, 235, 288
  cannulas for, VI:194-196, 195f, 209
    misdirection of, VI:238
  care after, VI:210, 212
  complex deformities after, VI:387
  complications of, VI:235-239
    cosmetic, VI:238-239
    medical, VI:235-238
  compression garments after, VI:210, 212
  contour irregularity after, VI:238-239,
    381
    overcorrection and, VI:383, 384f-386f
    prevention of, VI:387-388
    skin retraction and, VI:386-387
    types of, VI:382-387, 383f-386f
    undercorrection and, VI:382-383
  core body temperature for, VI:204
  deaths with, I:202-203
  deep venous thrombosis with, VI:237-
    238
  draping for, VI:205, 208
  dysesthesia after, VI:238
  endpoint evaluation for, VI:209-210,
    211f
  epinephrine-related mortality in, I:203
  face, Color Plates VI:123-4 and 123-5,
    VI:212-213, 213f-215f
  fat embolism with, VI:238
  flank, VI:250, 250f
  fluid imbalance with, VI:237

Liposuction *(Continued)*
  fluid replacement in, I:186, VI:200, 203,
    203f
  hematoma with, VI:235
  hip, VI:227-230, 227f, 229f-230f, 250,
    250f, 280-281, 280f, 281f
  hyperpigmentation after, VI:239
  in gynecomastia, VI:221, 223-224, 223f-
    225f
  in neck lift, II:319, 330f-331f, 334
  infection with, VI:236-237
  infiltrating cannulas for, VI:194, 194f
  instrumentation for, VI:193-197, 194f-
    197f
  knee, VI:288, 288f
  large-volume, Color Plate VI:124-1,
    VI:241-254, 245f-246f
    anesthesia for, VI:244, 247
    consultation for, VI:241-244
    contraindications to, VI:241
    definition of, VI:241
    drug discontinuation for, VI:242, 243-
      244t
    evacuation for, VI:251, 251f
    fluid management in, I:202-203,
      VI:247-248
    heat preservation during, VI:247
    hypothermia during, VI:247
    incisions for, VI:244
    infiltration for, VI:248
    informed consent for, VI:244
    lidocaine for, VI:248
    markings for, VI:244, 246f
    of arms, VI:249, 249f
    of back, VI:250, 250f
    of hip and flank, VI:250, 250f
    of thigh, VI:250-251, 250f
    patient examination for, Color Plate
      VI:124-2, VI:242
    patient history for, VI:242, 243-244t
    patient positioning for, VI:247, 247f,
      248
    patient selection for, VI:241
    photography for, VI:242
    planned stages for, VI:244
    results of, VI:252f-254f
    thrombosis prevention for, VI:247
    ultrasound-assisted, VI:248-251, 249f,
      249t, 250f, 251f
  left lateral decubitus position for,
    VI:208, 208f
  lidocaine for, VI:199-200, 200t, 203-204
    toxicity of, VI:237
  local anesthesia for, VI:199-200, 200t,
    203-204
  lower extremity, VI:231-235, 232f-236f,
    273-277, 282-288, 286f-288f
    care after, VI:289-290
    complications of, VI:274-275, 275t
    fat assessment for, VI:274
    infiltration for, VI:277
    marking for, VI:275-276, 276f
    patient selection for, VI:273-275,
      274f, 274t
    physical examination for, VI:273,
      274f
    pinch test in, VI:289
    planning for, VI:275
    power-assisted, VI:275
    principles of, VI:288-289

Liposuction *(Continued)*
ultrasound-assisted, VI:275
wetting solution for, VI:276-277, 277t
malar pad, II:149-150, 151f
medical malpractice suits in, I:145
neck, Color Plate VI:123-6, VI:213-216, 215f-217f
operative report form for, VI:204-205, 206f
patient evaluation for, VI:197-199, 198f-202f
physical examination for, VI:198-199, 199f-202f
pinch thickness after, VI:210, 211f
positioning for, VI:208-209, 208f-211f
povidone-iodine for, VI:205, 207f
power-assisted, VI:196, 196f
preparation for, VI:204-212
marking in, VI:204, 205f
prone position for, VI:208-209, 209f, 210f
pulmonary embolus with, VI:237-238
right lateral decubitus position for, VI:208
secondary, VI:381-388
complex deformities and, VI:387
overcorrection and, VI:383, 384f-386f
patient selection for, VI:382
physician-patient relationship in, VI:381-382
skin retraction after, VI:386-387
timing of, VI:387
undercorrection and, VI:382-383
seroma with, VI:235-236
skin irritations after, VI:239
skin laxity and, VI:199
skin necrosis with, VI:237
skin retraction after, VI:386-387
smoothness assessment after, VI:210
stem cells from, I:612, 613f
suction pumps for, VI:196-197
supine position for, VI:209, 211f
suprapubic, VI:408, 409f
technique of, Color Plate VI:123-2, VI:209
thigh, VI:231-232, 232f-234f, 250-251, 250f, 282-288, 284f. *See also* Thigh lift.
anterior, VI:285-288
care after, VI:289-290
circumferential, VI:285-288, 287f
lateral, VI:283, 286f
marking for, VI:276f
medial, VI:283, 285, 285f, 286f
trunk, VI:227-230, 227f-230f, 273-282, 280f, 281f, 283f. *See also* Trunk lift.
care after, VI:289-290
complications of, VI:274-275, 275t
fat assessment for, VI:274
gender-related variations in, VI:277-278, 278f-279f
infiltration for, VI:277
patient selection for, VI:273-275, 274f, 274t
physical examination for, VI:273, 274f
pinch test in, VI:289
planning for, VI:275
power-assisted, VI:275
principles of, VI:288-289
ultrasound-assisted, VI:275
wetting solution for, VI:276-277, 277t

Liposuction *(Continued)*
ultrasound-assisted, VI:196-197, 196f, 197f, 387
for lower extremity, VI:275
for trunk, VI:275
large-volume, VI:248-251, 249f, 249t, 250f, 251f
upper extremity, VI:291-313, 292f, 292t, 293f
complications of, VI:292t, 312
in group 1 patients, VI:296-300, 296f-303f
in group 2 patients, VI:300-308, 304f-308f
in groups 3 and 4 patients, VI:308-312, 309f-313f
in lymphedematous arm, VI:292, 312
measurements for, VI:294, 294f
muscle tone and, VI:294
patient evaluation for, VI:293-296, 293t, 294f, 294t
patient's weight and, VI:295
photography for, VI:295-296, 295f
pinch test for, VI:294, 296, 296f
skin tone and, VI:294
superwet solution for, VI:297, 297t
visceral perforation with, VI:238
visual assessment of, VI:210
volumes in, VI:210
warming blanket for, VI:204
weight gain after, VI:387
wetting infusion for, VI:194, 194f, 195f, 208
wound closure for, VI:210
Lisfranc amputation, VI:1427, 1430, 1432f
Lister's tubercle, EPL tendon rupture at, VII:418, 419f
Literature evaluation, I:37
Liver, hemangioma of, V:24-25, 29
Liver spots, V:261, 261f
Long lip, after cleft lip repair, IV:349-350, 350f
Loose bodies, at wrist, VII:131, 133
Loving cup ear, II:734-736, 735f
Low-molecular-weight dextran, in frostbite, VII:652
Lower body lift, Color Plates VI:125-1 and 125-2, VI:260, 268-269, 269f, 270f
complications of, VI:269-271
Lower extremity. *See also* Lower extremity reconstruction.
amputation of
in arterial insufficiency, VI:1479
vs. reconstruction, VI:1367
anatomy of, VI:1357, 1360-1362, 1360f-1363f
arterial insufficiency of, VI:1473-1484
amputation in, VI:1479
diagnosis of, VI:1473-1476, 1475f
differential diagnosis of, VI:1474-1476
evaluation of, VI:1476
free flaps for, VI:1480, 1483
limb salvage in, VI:1479
local flaps for, VI:1480
medical treatment for, VI:1476, 1483
revascularization for, VI:1479-1480
soft tissue procedures for, VI:1480
surgical treatment of, VI:1479-1483, 1481f-1482f

Lower extremity *(Continued)*
aspirin after, VI:1483
care after, VI:1483
heparin after, VI:1483
outcomes of, VI:1484
vascular-microvascular reconstruction for, VI:1480-1483, 1481f-1482f
vs. collagen vascular disease, VI:1475-1476, 1477f
vs. diabetic ulcers, VI:1475
vs. hematologic disease, VI:1476
vs. thromboangiitis obliterans, VI:1475
vs. vasculitis, VI:1476, 1478f
vs. venous disease, VI:1474
chronic venous insufficiency of, VI:1464-1473
air plethysmography in, VI:1467
ankle/brachial index in, VI:1467
antibiotics in, VI:1470
Apligraf in, VI:1472
classification of, VI:1468
compression therapy in, VI:1468-1469
Daflon in, VI:1470
débridement in, VI:1470
diagnosis of, VI:1466-1468, 1467f
diuretics in, VI:1469
fibrin cuff theory of, VI:1466
free tissue transfer in, VI:1472, 1473f, 1474f
granulocyte-macrophage colony-stimulating factor in, VI:1472-1473
growth factors in, VI:1472
ifetroban in, VI:1470
medical treatment of, VI:1468-1470
occlusive dressing in, VI:1469
pentoxifylline in, VI:1470
pharmacologic therapy in, VI:1469-1470
photoplethysmography in, VI:1467
skin grafts in, VI:1470-1471, 1471f
stanozolol in, VI:1470
surgical treatment of, VI:1470-1472, 1471f
ultrasonography in, VI:1467
white cell trapping in, VI:1466
collagen vascular disease of, VI:1475-1476, 1477f
compartment anatomy of, VI:1360-1361, 1362f
compartment syndromes of, I:339
compression dressing for, I:224
connective tissue framework of, I:339
cutaneous vessels of, I:339
diabetic ulcers of, VI:1475
edema of, I:224. *See also* Lymphedema, lower extremity.
in diabetes mellitus, I:219-220
innervation of, VI:1361-1362, 1363f
lipodermatosclerosis of, VI:1466
liposuction for, VI:273-277, 282-288, 286f-288f, 288t
care after, VI:289-290
complications of, VI:274-275, 275t
fat assessment for, VI:274
infiltration for, VI:277
marking for, VI:275-276, 276f

Lower extremity *(Continued)*
  patient selection for, VI:273-275,
      274f, 274t
  physical examination for, VI:273, 274f
  pinch test in, VI:289
  planning for, VI:275
  power-assisted, VI:275
  principles of, VI:288-289
  ultrasound-assisted, VI:275
  wetting solution for, VI:276-277, 277t
  lymphatic system of, Color Plates
      VI:161-1 to 161-4, VI:1455-1456.
      See also Lymphedema, lower
      extremity.
  lymphedema of, VI:1455-1464. *See also*
      Lymphedema, lower extremity.
  melanoma of, V:326-327, 331f, 332f
  metastatic disease of, VI:1476
  muscles of, vascular territories of, Color
      Plates I:15-9 to 15-11, I:338-339,
      338t
  neuroma of, VII:944-945
  nonhealing wounds of, I:219-220
  osteoradionecrosis of, I:974, 975f
  pyoderma gangrenosum of, VI:1467,
      1476
  replantation of, VI:1369
  sarcoma of, I:983
  skin of, vascular territories of, Color
      Plate I:15-8, I:337-338
  thromboangiitis obliterans of, VI:1475
  tissue expansion in, I:563-565
      failure of, I:920
  tumor ablation in, VI:1368-1369
  ulcers of
      arterial, I:903-904, 904f, 965f-966f
      carcinoma and, I:916, 916f
      diabetic, I:942-943, 943f, 981, 982f
      ischemic, I:903-904, 904f
      venous, I:906-907, 906f, 907f,
          VI:1464-1465, 1465f, 1467,
          1467f. *See also* Lower extremity,
          chronic venous insufficiency of.
  vascular anatomy of, VI:1357, 1360,
      1360f, 1361f
  vascular territories of, Color Plates I:15-
      8 to 15-11, I:337-339, 338t
  venous drainage of, VI:1465-1466
  wound healing in, I:965f-966f, 1008,
      1010, 1011f-1012f
Lower extremity reconstruction, I:454,
    455f-461f, VI:1355-1379. *See also* Foot
    reconstruction.
  after tumor ablation, VI:1368-1369
  anatomy for, VI:1357, 1360-1362, 1360f-
      1363f
  biceps femoris flap for, VI:1372
  compartment anatomy for, VI:1360-
      1361, 1362f
  fasciocutaneous flaps for, VI:1374, 1376-
      1379, 1376f-1379f
  flap failure in, VI:1367
  gastrocnemius flap for, I:454, 456f,
      VI:1374, 1375f
  gluteus maximus flap for, VI:1369-1370,
      1370f
  gracilis flap for, VI:1372-1373, 1372f
  groin flap for, VI:1374, 1376, 1376f
  historical perspective on, VI:1355-1356
  in osteomyelitis, VI:1367-1368, 1368f

Lower extremity reconstruction
    (Continued)
  in traumatic wounds, VI:1363-1367,
      1365f, 1366f
  lateral thigh flap for, VI:1377, 1377f
  latissimus flap for, VI:1364, 1366f
  medial thigh flap for, VI:1376-1377, 1377f
  microvascular tissue transplantation for,
      I:454
  musculocutaneous flaps for, VI:1369-
      1374, 1370f, 1371f
  neural anatomy for, VI:1361-1362, 1363f
  primary closure in, VI:1357, 1358f, 1359f
  principles of, VI:1356-1357
  reconstructive ladder in, VI:1357
  rectus femoris flap for, VI:1371-1372
  replantation for, VI:1369
  saphenous flap for, VI:1378, 1379f
  soft tissue coverage for, VI:1364, 1366f,
      1367
  soft tissue expansion for, VI:1362-1363
  soleus flap for, I:409-410, 411f, 454,
      457f-461f, VI:1373
  sural flap for, VI:1377-1378, 1378f
  tensor fascia lata flap for, VI:1370-1371,
      1371f
  vascular anatomy for, VI:1357, 1360,
      1360f, 1361f
  vs. amputation, VI:1367
Loxosceles bite, I:931-932, 933f, 934f, 1017
Ludwig angina, III:770, V:2
Lumbricals, VI:1407-1408, 1407f, VII:32
Lumpectomy, VI:647-648, 648f
  axillary lymph node dissection with,
      VI:665
  breast reduction after, VI:620, 622, 622f
  endoscopic latissimus dorsi breast
      reconstruction after, I:1045-1046,
      1045f, 1046f
  psychological factors in, I:79
  radiation therapy after, VI:667-668
Lunate bone, VII:19
  fracture of, in children, VIII:424
  in Kienböck disease, VII:66f, 68
Lungs
  burn-related infection of, I:829
  ketamine effects on, I:174-175
  metastatic disease of, V:162
Lunotriquetral instability, VII:134-135
Lunotriquetral ligament, VII:21, 456f
Lunula, VII:154, 154f, 172f
Lye injury, to hand, VII:654
Lymph
  accumulation of. *See* Lymphedema.
  daily flow of, I:907
Lymph nodes, axillary
  dissection of, VI:664-665, 664f
  sentinel biopsy of, I:1062, VI:654, 661-
      664, 662f
Lymphadenectomy
  in cancer, I:1061-1062, 1062f
  in head and neck cancer, V:179, 183,
      183f
  in melanoma, V:327, 329-330, 329t, 332-
      336, 333t, 334f-338f
Lymphadenopathy, in children, V:2
Lymphangioma
  cervical, III:1030, 1032
  of wrist, VII:80, 81f
  upper extremity, I:983, 984f

Lymphangioma circumscriptum, V:46-47
Lymphangiomatosis, VIII:392
Lymphangioplasty
  in lower extremity lymphedema, VI:1462
  in upper extremity lymphedema,
      VII:1002, 1002f
Lymphangiosarcoma, VI:1464
Lymphatic malformations, V:7-8, 8f, 42-47,
      VIII:389-397, 391f-396f
  axillary, V:42, 43f, 46, 46f
  cellulitis in, V:44, 45f
  cervical, V:42, 44f, 46
  clinical features of, V:42, 43f, VIII:390-
      392, 391f, 392f
  facial, V:42, 43f, 44f, 45-47, 46f
  fetal, I:1122, 1122t
  infection with, VIII:393
  magnetic resonance imaging in,
      VIII:392, 393f
  management of, V:43-47
      antibiotics in, V:43-44
      laser therapy in, V:45
      operative, V:45-47, 46f, VIII:394-397,
          394f-396f
      sclerotherapy in, V:44-45
  multifocal, V:42
  pathogenesis of, V:42, VIII:389-390
  radiologic features of, V:42-43, 44f
  resection of, V:45-47, VIII:394-397,
      394f-396f
  sclerotherapy in, VIII:394
  ultrasonography in, VIII:392
  wound healing and, I:945
Lymphatic system. *See also* Lymphatic
      malformations; Lymphedema.
  cervical
      anatomy of, V:219-220, 219f
      in head and neck cancer, V:160-161,
          162f, 179, 183
Lymphatic-venous anastomoses
  in lower extremity lymphedema,
      VI:1463-1464
  in upper extremity lymphedema,
      VII:1002-1004, 1003f, 1004f
Lymphedema
  genital, VI:1255-1256, 1464
  lower extremity, I:907-908, 908f, 909f,
      964, VI:1455-1464
      aplastic, VI:1457
      bridging flap techniques for, VI:1462-
          1463
      cancer treatment and, VI:1457, 1457f
      classification of, VI:1456-1457, 1456f
      compression for, VI:1460-1461, 1461f,
          1462f
      computed tomography in, VI:1460
      congenital, VI:1456-1457, 1456f
      contrast lymphography in, VI:1459
      diagnosis of, VI:1458-1460, 1458f,
          1459f
      dietary treatment of, VI:1461
      excisional surgery for, VI:1461
      hypoplastic, VI:1457
      indirect lymphangiography in,
          VI:1459
      liposuction for, VI:1461-1462
      lymphangioplasty for, VI:1462
      lymphangiosarcoma and, VI:1464
      lymphatic-venous anastomoses for,
          VI:1463-1464

Lymphedema *(Continued)*
  lymphoscintigraphy in, VI:1459
  magnetic resonance imaging in,
    VI:1459-1460
  medical treatment of, VI:1460-1461,
    1461f, 1462f
  natural history of, VI:1457-1458
  obstructive, VI:1457
  pharmacologic treatment of, VI:1461
  primary, VI:1456-1457, 1456f
  secondary, VI:1457, 1457f
  surgical treatment of, VI:1461-1464
  ultrasonography in, VI:1460
  vs. chronic venous insufficiency,
    VI:1458
  vs. lipidemia, VI:1458, 1459f
  upper extremity, I:964, VI:292, 312,
    VII:995-1004
    anatomy of, VII:996
    complications of, VII:1004
    definition of, VII:995-996
    diagnosis of, VII:996-998, 997f
    flow augmentation treatment in,
      VII:1001-1004, 1002f-1004f
    infection and, VII:999
    lymphangiography in, VII:997-998
    lymphatic-venous anastomoses in,
      VII:1002-1004, 1003f, 1004f
    lymphoscintigraphy in, VII:998
    medical treatment of, VII:998, 998f
    pathophysiology of, VII:996
    postmastectomy, VI:292, 312
    prevention of, VII:999t
    secondary, VII:995
    stockinette sling for, VII:998, 998f
    tissue ablation in, VII:1000-1001,
      1000f, 1001f
    Wick lymphangioplasty in, VII:1002,
      1002f
Lymphedema praecox, I:908f, VI:1456-
  1457, VII:995
Lymphedema tarda, VII:995
Lymphocyte
  B, I:271-272
  T, I:272-273, 278-279
Lymphocyte toxicity assay, in toxic
  epidermal necrolysis, I:795
Lymphoma
  mandibular, V:107, 213
  orbital, V:114
  pediatric, III:771-772
  salivary gland, V:86-87, 87f
  T-cell, cutaneous, V:300, 300f
Lymphoscintigraphy, in melanoma, V:320-
  324, 323f, 324f, 324t

M

Ma huang, I:170, VI:176t
McCarthy, Joseph G., I:4-5, 4f
Macrocephaly, cutis marmorata
  telangiectasia congenita and, V:41
Macrodactyly, VIII:298-317
  classification of, VIII:300
  definition of, VIII:298-300, 299f
  epiphysiodesis in, VIII:313, 446, 448f
  hemihypertrophy and, VIII:308, 309f,
    316
  hyperostosis and, VIII:307-308, 307f,
    316
  in Maffucci syndrome, VIII:309-310

Macrodactyly *(Continued)*
  in Proteus syndrome, VIII:308-309, 316
  lipomatous, VIII:301, 303-304, 303f-
    305f
  nerve decompression in, VIII:311, 313
  nerve excision in, VIII:314
  nerve territory-oriented, VIII:300-301,
    301f, 302f, 316
  neurofibromatosis and, VIII:304-307,
    306f, 316
  neurolysis in, VIII:314
  nonsyndromic, VIII:310, 313f
  outcomes of, VIII:315-317
  psychological concerns in, VIII:311
  skeletal reduction in, VIII:314-315, 315f
  soft tissue debulking in, VIII:313-314,
    314f
  vascular malformation and, VIII:309-
    310, 311f, 312f, 316-317
Macroglossia, III:767-768, 767f
Macromastia, VI:552-554, 552t, 607-608.
  See also Breast reduction.
  psychological effects of, VI:608
Macrophage
  in graft rejection, I:271
  in wound healing, I:210-211, 211f, 212t
Macrophage colony-stimulating factor, in
  osteoclast differentiation, I:647
Macrostomia, in craniofacial microsomia,
  IV:124-125, 124f
Mafenide acetate, I:822, 950
Maffucci syndrome, V:55-56, 57f, VII:984-
  985, VIII:410-411, 411f, 412f, 984-985
  macrodactyly in, VIII:309-310
Maggots, for débridement, I:873
Magnetic resonance angiography, of hand
  and wrist, VII:79-80, 80f, 81f
Magnetic resonance imaging, VII:69, 69t,
  70t
  before posterior pharyngeal flap, IV:324
  in arteriovenous malformation, V:51-52,
    53f, VIII:398, 399f
  in breast cancer, VI:635, 635f
  in breast implant rupture, VI:635, 636f
  in complex regional pain
    syndrome/reflex sympathetic
    dystrophy, VII:846
  in congenital hand anomalies, VIII:38
  in fetal diaphragmatic hernia, I:1123
  in ganglion cyst, VII:70
  in hand frostbite, VII:650-651
  in hemangioma, V:27, 27f, VIII:373,
    374f
  in ischemia, VII:802
  in lymphatic malformation, VIII:392,
    393f
  in peripheral nerve injury, I:729, 730f
  in prenatal diagnosis, I:1070, 1070f,
    1071f
  in salivary gland tumors, V:73-74, 73t
  in temporomandibular joint
    dysfunction, III:542
  in venous malformation, V:49, 49f,
    VIII:383, 384f
  in wrist injury, VII:458-459
  of breast implants, VI:635, 636f, 637
  of hand and wrist, VII:69-79, 69t, 70t,
    71f-78f, 79t
  of levator veli palatini muscle, IV:65,
    66f, 67f

Magnetic resonance imaging *(Continued)*
  of palate, IV:65, 66f, 67f
  of uvular muscle, IV:65, 66f
  water on, VII:69-70, 69t, 70t
Maillard Z-plasty, in tuberous breasts,
  VI:517, 518f
Major histocompatibility complex, in
  transplantation, I:270-271, 273-274
Malar bone. *See* Zygoma.
Malar crease, II:150
Malar eminence, II:92
Malar fat pads, II:253-254, 254f
  aging-related changes in, II:232, 234f,
    254-256, 255f, 259
  elevation of, II:234, 235f
  liposuction of, II:149-150, 151f
Malar hypoplasia, suborbital, II:96-97
Malar implant
  for face lift, II:269, 271
  postblepharoplasty, II:806-807, 807f
Malformation, I:53-54. *See also specific
  malformations and structures.*
Malignant fibrous histiocytoma
  of head and neck, V:119
  of mandible, V:107
  of upper extremity, VII:970, 972
Malignant hyperthermia, I:179, 187
Malignant mixed tumor, of salivary glands,
  V:86
Malingering, I:944, VII:847-848
Maliniac, Jacques, I:31
Mallet finger, VII:413, 432-433, 433f, 449-
  450, 450f
Malnutrition
  oral cavity cancer and, III:918-919
  pressure sores and, VI:1318
  salivary gland enlargement and, V:74
  wound healing and, I:220-221, 918-919,
    918f, 981
Malocclusion
  class I, II:649, 650f
  class II, II:649, 650f
  class III, II:649, 650f
  in condylar process fracture, III:515
  in mandibular fracture, III:185-186,
    187f
  in maxillary fracture, III:239, 240f, 252-
    253, 252f
  in panfacial fracture, III:257, 257f
  in pediatric facial fracture, III:411-412
  in zygoma fracture, III:213
  transverse dimension of, II:649, 650f
  vertical dimension of, II:649, 650f
Malpractice. *See* Medical malpractice.
Mammaplasty. *See* Breast augmentation;
  Breast reconstruction; Breast
  reduction; Mastopexy.
Mammography, VI:632-633, 633t, 634f
  after breast reduction, VI:558, 1080
  before breast reduction, VI:553
  misinterpretation of, VI:638
  screening, VI:633
    breast implant and, VI:635-637, 636f,
      637f
Mammotome system, VI:640
Mandible. *See also* Mandible
  reconstruction; Maxilla;
  Orthognathic surgery.
  adenomatoid odontogenic tumor of,
    V:97, 200

Mandible *(Continued)*
  ameloblastic fibro-odontoma of, V:98, 200
  ameloblastic fibroma of, V:97-98, 199-200
  ameloblastic fibrosarcoma of, V:99
  ameloblastoma of, V:95, 95f, 197-199, 198f
  anatomy of, III:146-150, 147f-149f, 150t, 151f, 535-537, 536f, 537f
  aneurysmal bone cyst of, V:103, 195-196
  angiosarcoma of, V:107
  augmentation of, II:414, 418-423, 418f-424f
  avascular necrosis of, III:182
  birth-related injury to, III:398
  bone cyst of, V:196-197
  botryoid odontogenic cyst of, V:191
  Burkitt lymphoma of, V:107, 212
  calcifying epithelial odontogenic tumor of, V:97, 199
  cementifying fibroma of, V:98, 204
  cemento-osseous dysplasia of, V:202, 204
  cementoblastoma of, V:98, 202
  central giant cell granuloma of, V:102-103, 208-209
  cephalometric analysis of, II:24, 26, 26f, 27f
  cherubism of, V:101-102, 102f, 209
  chondroma of, V:207
  chondromyxoid fibroma of, V:207
  chondrosarcoma of, V:106-107, 211-212
  clear cell odontogenic tumor of, V:199
  coronoid hyperplasia of, V:209-210
  cysts of, V:91-95, 94f, 189-197, 190t, 192f, 194f, 195f
  defects of. *See also* Mandible reconstruction.
    classification of, III:959-960, 959f
    etiology of, III:958-959
    exogenous transforming growth factor-β in, I:664
    in craniofacial microsomia, IV:117-120, 118f-120f, 125t
  dentigerous cyst of, V:93, 191-192, 192f
  desmoplastic fibroma of, V:103, 206-207
  ectomesenchymal odontogenic tumors of, V:98
  embryology of, IV:9, 10f, 11, 17, 17f
  eruption cyst of, V:192
  Ewing sarcoma of, V:107, 212
  exostoses of, V:205-206
  fibrosarcoma of, V:107, 213
  fibrous dysplasia of, V:101-102, 102f, 206, 207f
  focal osteoporotic bone marrow defect of, V:197
  fracture of, III:145-187. *See also* Mandibular fracture.
  gingival cyst of, V:92-93, 191
  glandular cyst of, V:193
  Gorlin cyst of, V:93, 193-194
  granular cell odontogenic fibroma of, V:202
  growth of
    after facial burn excision and grafting, III:69-70
    in craniofacial microsomia, IV:550-551, 553

Mandible *(Continued)*
  hemangioma of, V:104, 210
  histiocytosis X of, V:103-104
  in craniofacial microsomia, IV:117-120, 118f-120f, 125t
  in zygomatic arch fracture, III:209-210, 210f, 211f
  juxtacortical osteosarcoma of, V:211
  Langerhans cell disease of, V:209
  lateral periodontal cyst of, V:93, 94, 191
  lymphoma of, V:213
  malignant fibrous histiocytoma of, V:107
  median cyst of, V:94, 195, 196f
  mesenchymal chondrosarcoma of, V:211-212
  metastatic carcinoma of, V:213
  multiple myeloma of, V:212
  neurofibroma of, V:210
  neurogenic tumors of, V:210
  neuroma of, V:210
  non-Hodgkin lymphoma of, V:107
  nonodontogenic cysts of, V:195, 196f
  nonodontogenic tumors of, V:190t, 204-213
    benign, V:190t, 206-210, 207f, 208f
    malignant, V:190t, 210-213
  odontoameloblastoma of, V:98, 200
  odontogenic carcinoma of, V:98-99, 204
  odontogenic cysts of, V:92-95, 94f, 190t, 191-195, 192f, 194f
  odontogenic fibroma of, V:98, 201-202
  odontogenic keratocyst of, V:93, 94f, 192-193, 194f
  odontogenic myxoma of, V:98, 202, 203f
  odontogenic sarcoma of, V:204
  odontogenic tumors of
    benign, V:190t, 197-204, 198f, 201f, 202f
    malignant, V:190t, 204
  odontoma of, V:200-201, 201f
  ossifying fibroma of, V:206, 208f
  osteitis of, III:182
  osteoblastoma of, V:99, 205
  osteoid osteoma of, V:99, 205
  osteoma of, V:99, 205
  osteomyelitis of, III:182
  osteoradionecrosis of, I:918, 918f, 967, 968f-969f, III:983-984
  osteosarcoma of, V:104, 106, 106f, 210-211
  paradental cyst of, V:94, 195
  periapical cemental dysplasia of, V:98
  peripheral odontogenic fibroma of, V:202
  Pinborg tumor of, V:199
  plasma cell neoplasm of, V:212-213
  postnatal growth of, III:382f-386f, 388-390, 390f
  pseudocysts of, V:190t, 195-197
  radicular cyst of, V:93-94, 194-195
  recombinant bone morphogenetic proteins for, I:663
  resection of, III:594, 598f-599f, 958-959
  residual cyst of, V:94
  rotation of, after mandibular fracture treatment, III:186-187
  schwannoma of, V:210
  solitary plasmacytoma of, V:212-213

Mandible *(Continued)*
  squamous odontogenic tumor of, V:97, 199
  static bone cyst of, V:196-197
  symphysis fracture of, III:485-491, 487f-490f
  tumors of, V:91-109, 92t, 197-213. *See also specific tumors.*
    odontogenic, V:95-97, 95f, 190t, 197-204, 198f, 201f, 202f
    resection of, V:121-122, 226f, 235-236, 235t
  vascular lesions of, V:210
Mandible reconstruction, III:957-987, V:121-122
  after tumor resection, III:594, 598f-599f, 958-959
  biphase external fixators in, III:969-970, 970f
  cardiopulmonary disease evaluation before, III:971-972
  dental consultation in, III:971
  dental reconstruction and, III:984-986, 986f, 987f
  fibula flap for, I:390, 390t, 394f-395f, III:964f, 966, 967f, 968-969
  forearm flap for, III:964f, 965, 968
  free flap for, III:962-971, 972-981
    anastomoses for, III:978, 980
    anterior graft design and insetting for, III:973-975, 974f-976f
    care after, III:980-981
    donor site for, III:962-966, 964f, 967f, 972
    donor site morbidity with, III:968-969
    graft shaping for, III:973-978, 974f-980f
    lateral graft design and insetting for, III:975-978, 976f-980f
    recipient site preparation for, III:972-973
    selection of, III:966-968, 967t
  functional outcome after, III:975-976
  graft fixation methods in, III:969-971, 970f, 971f
  groin flap for, III:962-963
  historical perspective on, III:957-958
  hyperbaric oxygen in, III:960
  ilium flap for, III:963-965, 964f, 968, 969
  latissimus dorsi flap for, III:961
  mandible template fabrication for, III:972, 972f
  miniplate fixation systems in, III:970-971, 971f
  musculocutaneous flap for, III:961-962
  nonvascularized bone grafts in, III:960
  osteomusculocutaneous flaps in, III:962, 963f
  osteoradionecrosis and, III:983-984
  pediatric, III:984
  preparation for, III:971-972
  prosthetic plates in, III:960-962
  radiation and, III:983-984
  radius flap for, III:964f, 965, 968, 969
  rib flap for, III:962
  scapula flap for, I:390, 390t, 397f-399f, III:964f, 965-966, 968, 969
  second metatarsal flap for, III:963
  secondary, III:981-983, 982f

Mandible reconstruction (Continued)
soft tissue flaps in, III:961-962
sternocleidomastoid flap for, III:961-962
systemic risk factor screening before,
    III:971-972
trapezius flap for, III:961, 962
two flaps in, III:968
Mandible-splitting procedures, V:121
in oropharyngeal cancer, V:233-234,
    234f, 234t
Mandibular condyle, III:536-537, 537f
ankylosis of, III:418
dislocation of, III:418-421, 419f-420f,
    544
fracture of, III:511-532. See also
    Condylar process fracture.
growth of, III:417
hypoplasia of, III:539
osteochondroma of, III:539
postnatal growth of, III:389-390, 390f
reconstruction of, III:543, 544
restitutional remodeling of, III:417-418
rheumatoid arthritis of, III:541, 541f
Mandibular distraction
extraoral, IV:523, 524f
for airway obstruction, IV:422, 423f
growth after, IV:551, 553
in craniofacial cleft, IV:430-431, 446
in craniofacial microsomia, III:780-783,
    780f-783f, IV:523-525, 524f-532f,
    546, 548f
in micrognathia, III:780-783, 780f-783f
intermaxillary elastics during, IV:546,
    548f
intraoral, IV:523, 525f
transport, IV:525, 532f
vectors for, IV:525, 531f
Mandibular fracture, III:145-187. See also
    Maxillary fracture.
anatomy in, III:146-150, 147f-149f, 150t,
    151f
classification of, III:150, 152f, 153f
condylar, III:511-532. See also Condylar
    process fracture.
dental injury with, III:155, 156
diagnosis of, III:150, 152-154
    clinical examination in, III:150, 152-
        154, 153f
    computed tomography in, III:108f-
        110f, 154
    radiographic examination in,
        III:102f-108f, 154
in children, III:395, 396f, 409-411, 410f-
    413f
in infant, III:409-410
malunion of, III:185, 186f-188f
mechanism of injury in, III:145-146
nonunion of, III:182-185, 183f
Panorex exam in, III:395, 396f
symphysis, endoscopic management of,
    III:485-491, 487f-490f
complications of, III:490, 490f
computed tomography before, III:486
contraindications to, III:486
indications for, III:485-486
results of, III:486, 489f, 490
technique of, III:486, 487f, 488f, 490-
    491
treatment of, III:154-181
antibiotics in, III:154-155

Mandibular fracture (Continued)
avascular necrosis after, III:182
carotid artery injury in, III:181
closed reduction in, III:155, 155f, 156
complications of, III:181-187
dental fixation in, III:155
early complications of, III:181-182
external pin fixation in, III:180-181
facial nerve injury in, III:181
hemorrhage with, III:181
implant failure after, III:187
increased facial width after, III:186-
    187
infection after, III:181-182
intermaxillary fixation in, III:156
late complications of, III:182-187
malocclusion after, III:185-186
malunion after, III:185, 186f-188f
mandible rotation after, III:186-187
nonunion after, III:182-185, 183f
open reduction and internal fixation
    in, III:156-161, 158f
callus removal in, III:162, 163f
cooling irrigation in, III:162
facial nerve in, III:159
fixation devices for, III:161-164,
    163f-165f
for oblique fracture, III:164
in angle fracture, III:166, 169, 169f
in body fracture, III:116f, 117f, 166
in comminuted fracture, III:169f,
    178, 178f
in coronoid fracture, III:169-170,
    170f
in edentulous mandible, III:178-
    180, 179f
in parasymphysis fracture, III:139f,
    163f, 164, 166, 167f-168f
in subcondylar fracture, III:174,
    175
in symphysis fracture, III:164, 166,
    167f-168f
intraoral vs. extraoral approach to,
    III:116f, 119f, 157-159, 158f,
    159f
mental nerve injury in, III:162
miniplates in, III:159, 159f, 161f
occlusal pattern in, III:162-163,
    164f
plate-bending errors in, III:134f,
    164
plates for, III:134f-137f, 159-161,
    159f-162f, 163-164, 164f
screw failure in, III:162, 163f
screw-related errors in, III:164
soft tissue mobilization in, III:158,
    159f-161f
soft tissue removal in, III:162
sutures for, III:158
osteitis after, III:182
osteomyelitis after, III:182
protocol for, III:156-157f, 156-157t
temporomandibular joint ankylosis
    after, III:182
tooth reimplantation in, III:155
tooth root precautions in, III:187
Mandibular ligaments, II:169, 170f, 174f
Mandibular nerve, rhytidectomy-related
    injury to, II:206
Mandibular nerve palsy, III:911-912, 913f

Mandibular osteotomy, IV:441, 443-444,
    443f, 444f
Mandibular plane, II:20f, 21t
Mandibular ramus. See also Mandible;
    Mandibular condyle.
augmentation of, II:419, 421-423, 421f-
    424f
inverted L osteotomy of, IV:444, 444f
reconstruction of, in craniofacial
    microsomia, IV:533, 540-541,
    541f
sagittal split osteotomy of, IV:441, 443,
    443f
vertical subsigmoid osteotomy of,
    IV:443-444, 444f
Mandibular swing procedure, V:147-148,
    147f
Mandibulectomy, V:121-122, 226f, 235-
    236, 235t
Mandibulofacial dysostosis. See Treacher
    Collins syndrome.
Mandibulotomy, V:177, 178f, 179, 179f
Mangling injury, VII:317-348. See also
    Arm(s), mangling injury to; Finger
    reconstruction; Hand reconstruction;
    Thumb reconstruction; Upper
    extremity reconstruction.
débridement after, VII:320
evaluation of, VII:318
provisional revascularization after,
    VII:320-321
salvage vs. amputation management
    after, VII:318-319
skeletal stabilization after, VII:321
skin loss with, VII:322-323
Manipulative personality, I:74
Mannitol, in complex regional pain
    syndrome/reflex sympathetic
    dystrophy, VII:857
Marchac short-scar technique, for breast
    reduction, VI:568-570, 569f
Margin reflex distance, II:91
Marionette lines, II:276, 279
Marjolin ulcer, I:916, 917f, V:275, 276f,
    437-439, 437f, 437t
of back, VI:446-447, 447f
of hand, VII:614
of scalp, III:612
Masseter muscle transplantation, in facial
    paralysis, III:910, 910f
Masseteric cutaneous ligaments, II:174f
Mast cells
in ischemia-reperfusion injury, I:493
opioid effects on, I:181
Mastalgia, VI:353
augmentation and, VI:352-355
reduction and, VI:578
Mastectomy, I:1063, VI:648-661
breast reconstruction after. See Breast
    reconstruction.
breast reduction after, VI:620, 622, 622f
complex defect after, VI:773-780, 774f,
    775f, 776t, 777f-780f
    thoracoepigastric flap for, VI:773,
        776, 776t, 777f-780f
    TRAM flap for, VI:773, 775f, 776t
    vertical rectus abdominis flap for,
        VI:773, 774f
in gender identity disorder, VI:1308
lymphangiosarcoma after, VI:1464

Mastectomy *(Continued)*
lymphedema after, VI:292, 312. *See also* Lymphedema, upper extremity.
modified radical, VI:643, 646, 646t, 659-660, 660f
 axillary lymph node dissection with, VI:664-665, 664f
 nerve injury with, VI:665
nipple-areola complex in, VI:661, 791
prophylactic, I:44-45, VI:657-659, 657t, 658f-659f, 673
 nipple-areola complex in, VI:791
psychological factors in, I:78
radiation therapy after, VI:668, 978
radical, VI:643, 646t, 648-649, 660-661
scar from, breast reconstruction and, VI:977, 977f, 978f, 990-991, 991f
simple, VI:646t, 649
skin-sparing, VI:646t, 652-657, 653f-655f, 656t
 inadequate skin envelope and, VI:948-951, 948t, 949f-951f, 949t
 single-stage reconstruction and, VI:923-924, 924f, 925f
 TRAM flap reconstruction and, VI:976-977
subcutaneous, VI:650-652, 651f
total, VI:649, 650f, 650t, 652
Mastication, III:922-923
muscles of, III:535, 536f
 arterial supply of, Color Plates I:15-12 and 15-13, I:340f, 342, 342t
Mastoid process, in craniofacial microsomia, IV:120
Mastopexy, VI:47-86
after breast augmentation, VI:346
after implant explantation, VI:82, 84
anesthesia for, I:204
augmentation, VI:81-82, 83f
Benelli, VI:50-54, 51f-56f
 advantages of, VI:51
 areola fixation for, VI:53, 55f
 cerclage stitch for, VI:53, 55f
 disadvantages of, VI:50-51
 dissection for, VI:51, 51f, 52f
 dressing for, VI:54
 flap fixation for, VI:51, 53, 53f, 54f
 indications for, VI:50-51
 markings for, VI:51, 51f
 U suture for, VI:53-54, 56f
Chiari L-shaped scar technique for, VI:68-73
 advantages of, VI:68-69
 disadvantages of, VI:69
 dissection for, VI:71-73, 73f
 indications for, VI:68-69
 markings for, VI:69, 71, 71f, 72f
 results of, VI:73, 74f
complications of, VI:84-86
concentric, VI:50
cosmetic problems after, VI:85-86
disappointment after, VI:85-86
flap necrosis after, VI:85
Goes, VI:54-58, 56f-61f
 advantages of, VI:54-55
 disadvantages of, VI:55-56
 dissection for, VI:56, 57f
 fixation for, VI:56, 58f
 indications for, VI:54

Mastopexy *(Continued)*
 markings for, VI:56, 56f
 mixed mesh for, VI:56, 59f, 60f
 inverted T closure for, VI:77-78, 79f
 Lassus, VI:58, 60-62, 62f
 Lejour, VI:63-64, 64f, 65f
liposuction for, VI:78-81, 80f, 81f
nipple loss with, VI:84-85
nipple malposition after, VI:85
patient selection for, VI:49
periareolar techniques of, VI:49-58, 50f-61f
 Benelli, VI:50-54, 51f-56f
 Goes, VI:54-58, 56f-61f
scars after, VI:85
short horizontal scar technique for, VI:73-76, 75f-78f
vertical scar (short scar) techniques for, VI:58, 60-81
 Chiari, VI:68-73, 71f-74f
 Lassus, VI:58, 60-62, 62f
 Lejour, VI:63-64, 64f, 65f
 preferred variation on, VI:64, 66-68, 66f-70f, 83f
 short horizontal scar technique with, VI:73-76, 75f-78f
Matrix metalloproteinases
in actinic keratoses, V:278
in wound healing, I:214
Mattress, for pressure sore prevention, VI:1319
Maxilla. *See also* Mandible; Orthognathic surgery.
adenomatoid odontogenic tumor of, V:97
ameloblastic fibro-odontoma of, V:98
ameloblastic fibroma of, V:97-98
ameloblastic fibrosarcoma of, V:99
ameloblastoma of, V:95, 96f-97f
anatomy of, III:229-232, 230f, 231f, IV:70-71, 70f
aneurysmal bone cyst of, V:103
angiosarcoma of, V:107
body of, III:230, 230f
Burkitt lymphoma of, V:107
calcifying epithelial odontogenic tumor of, V:97
cementifying fibroma of, V:98
cementoblastoma of, V:98
central giant cell granuloma of, V:102-103
cephalometric analysis of, II:23, 24f
cherubism of, V:101-102, 102f
chondrosarcoma of, V:106-107
dentigerous cyst of, V:93
desmoplastic fibroma of, V:103
duplication of, IV:407, 409f
ectomesenchymal odontogenic tumors of, V:98
edentulous, fracture of, III:247, 249f-251f
embryology of, IV:9, 10f, 11, 17, 17f
Ewing sarcoma of, V:107
fibrosarcoma of, V:107
fibrous dysplasia of, V:99-102, 100f-102f
fracture of, III:229-255. *See also* Maxillary fracture.
frontal process of, III:230, 230f
globulomaxillary cyst of, V:94
Gorlin cyst of, V:93

Maxilla *(Continued)*
hemangioma of, V:104
histiocytosis X of, V:103-104
hypoplasia of, IV:404, 406f
in cleft palate, IV:256-257, 262
lateral periodontal cyst of, V:93, 94
malignant fibrous histiocytoma of, V:107
median palatal cyst of, V:94
muscles of, III:231-232
nerves of, III:230-231, 231f
non-Hodgkin lymphoma of, V:107
odontoameloblastoma of, V:98
odontogenic carcinoma of, V:98-99
odontogenic cyst of, V:92-95, 92t, 94f
odontogenic fibroma of, V:98
odontogenic myxoma of, V:98
odontoma of, V:98
osteoblastoma of, V:99
osteoid osteoma of, V:99
osteoma of, V:99
osteosarcoma of, V:104, 106
paradental cyst of, V:94
periapical cemental dysplasia of, V:98
postnatal growth of, III:388
radicular cyst of, V:93-94
reconstruction of, III:582, 594, 595f-597f
residual cyst of, V:94
squamous odontogenic tumor of, V:97
tumors of, III:582, V:91-109, 92t. *See also specific tumors.*
 resection of, III:582, 594, 595f-597f, V:122-123
zygomatic process of, III:230, 230f
Maxillary artery, IV:78f
Maxillary fracture, III:229-255, 582, 593f-594f
airway in, III:249
anterior, III:234f
bleeding with, III:238
blindness with, III:252
cerebrospinal fluid leak with, III:239, 251-252
classification of, III:232-238, 232t, 233f-236f
clinical examination of, III:238-239
complex (panfacial), III:255-264
 complications of, III:261-264
 definition of, III:256, 256f
 treatment of, III:256-264, 262f-263f
  dental splint in, III:257, 257f
  displacement after, III:263-264, 264f, 265f
  reconstruction order for, III:257-261, 259f, 261f
  soft tissue reconstruction in, III:260, 260f
complicated, III:235f
complications of, III:247, 249, 251-255, 252f
computed tomography in, III:239
diagnosis of, III:238-239
edema with, III:238
extraocular muscle injury in, III:255
hemorrhage with, III:247, 249
in children, III:448-453, 448t, 449f-451f
infection with, III:249, 251
lacrimal obstruction with, III:251
Le Fort I, III:232, 232t, 233f
 in children, III:448, 448t, 452

Maxillary fracture (*Continued*)
  Le Fort II, III:133f, 232, 232t, 248f-249f
    blindness in, III:252
    edentulous, III:249f-251f
    in children, III:421-422, 423f-424f,
      449, 452
    rhinorrhea in, III:251-252
  Le Fort III, III:232t, 233, 233f, 239, 240f
    blindness in, III:252
    edentulous, III:249f-251f
    in children, III:449, 452
    rhinorrhea in, III:251-252
  malocclusion in, III:239, 240f
  malunion of, III:253, 254f-255f
  maxillary mobility in, III:238, 239
  mechanisms of, III:231, 238
  muscle action in, III:231-232
  nasolacrimal duct injury in, III:255
  nonunion of, III:252, 253
  palpation in, III:239
  para-alveolar, III:234f
  parasagittal, III:234f
  posterolateral (tuberosity), III:235f
  radiography in, III:239
  sagittal, III:233-238, 234f, 236f-237f
  treatment of, III:239, 241-247
    anterior approach in, III:241
    canthal ligament in, III:241
    complications of, III:252-255, 252f
    craniofacial exposure in, III:244
    frontal zygomatic process in, III:242,
      244f
    in alveolar fracture, III:245
    in edentulous maxilla, III:247, 249f-
      251f
    in Le Fort fracture, III:245-246, 246f,
      248f-249f
    intermaxillary fixation in, III:245
    malunion after, III:253, 254f-255f
    occlusal deviation after, III:252-253,
      252f
    palate in, III:241-242, 243f, 244
    plate and screws in, III:242-243, 244
    reconstruction sequence in, III:241,
      242f, 243-244
    Rowe disimpaction forceps in,
      III:253, 254f-255f
    soft tissue in, III:241-242, 243f-244f
    zygomaticomaxillary suture in, III:239
Maxillary plane, II:20f, 21t
Maxillary sinus-cutaneous fistula, III:833,
    838f-839f
Maxillary sinuses, III:230, 231f
Maxillary swing procedure, V:149, 150f-
    152f
Maxillomandibular distraction, in
    craniofacial microsomia, IV:525, 532f,
    533
McCune-Albright syndrome, V:206
McGregor's patch, II:257
McKissock technique, for breast reduction,
    VI:540, 543f, 561
McMaster Health Index Questionnaire,
    I:42, 42t
Meatoplasty and glansplasty procedure,
    VI:1265, 1268f, 1274
Medial antebrachial cutaneous nerve,
    neuroma of, VII:901-902, 945
Medial plantar artery flap, for foot
    reconstruction, VI:1435, 1436f

Medial thigh flap, for lower extremity
    reconstruction, VI:1376-1377, 1377f
Medial thigh lift, VI:265-268, 267f, 268f
Median face syndrome. *See* Frontonasal
    malformation.
Median mandibular cyst, V:94, 195, 196f
Median nerve
  anatomy of, VII:38, 39f, 41, 472
  evaluation of, VII:50, 53, 53f
  fibrolipoma of, VII:958
  injury to. *See also* Median nerve palsy.
    repair of, I:736
      nerve transfer for, VII:504-505,
        504f
      outcomes of, VII:508-509
      postoperative course of, VII:506
      thumb in, VII:34
  laceration of, VII:39, 41
  neuroma of, VII:945
  neurotization of, in brachial plexus
    injury, VII:531-532
  radial artery association with, VII:889,
    890f
  tourniquet-related injury to, VII:117
Median nerve block, I:193, 196f, 197f
  at elbow, VII:103, 104f
  at wrist, VII:104-105, 105f
Median nerve palsy
  high
    high ulnar nerve palsy with, tendon
      transfer for, VIII:482
    tendon transfer for, VIII:466, 469-470
      brachioradialis for, VIII:469-470,
        469f
      flexor pollicis longus for, VIII:469-
        470, 470f
      indications for, VIII:466, 469
  low
    contracture prevention with, VIII:462
    low ulnar nerve palsy with, tendon
      transfer for, VIII:481-482
    tendon transfer for, VIII:462-466
      anatomic considerations in,
        VIII:462-463
      extensor indicis proprius for,
        VIII:463-464, 463f-465f
      outcomes of, VIII:463
      palmaris longus for, VIII:466, 467f,
        468f
      ring finger flexor digitorum
        superficialis for, VIII:465-466,
        466f, 467f
Mediastinum reconstruction, I:440-441,
    442f-444f
  latissimus dorsi flap for, I:441
  omental flap for, I:441
  pectoralis major flap for, I:440-441,
    442f-444f
Medical malpractice, I:127-133, 139-149
  affirmative duty and, I:140
  causation in, I:130
  consent-in-fact and, I:146-147
  cross-examination in, I:130
  defendant witness in, I:130
  definition of, I:139-140
  disclosure and, I:140
  expert witness in, I:128-130
  family disapproval and, I:142
  impeachment in, I:130
  implied consent and, I:132, 146-147

Medical malpractice (*Continued*)
  in abdominoplasty, I:144
  in blepharoplasty, I:144
  in breast augmentation, I:143
  in breast reduction, I:143-144
  in face lift, I:144
  in rhinoplasty, I:144
  in scarring, I:144
  in septoplasty, I:144
  in skin resurfacing, I:145
  in suction-assisted lipectomy, I:145
  informed consent and, I:131-132, 146-
    148, 148t
  insurance company duty and, I:128
  multiple surgeries and, I:142
  National Physicians Data Bank
    reporting of, I:128
  patient anger and, I:141, 141f
  patient demands and, I:142
  patient expectations and, I:141, 141f
  patient immaturity and, I:142
  patient indecision and, I:142
  patient motivation and, I:140, 141f
  patient refusal and, I:146
  patient secrecy and, I:142
  patient selection and, I:139
  personal counsel for, I:128
  personality conflicts and, I:142
  prevention of, I:139, 140-141
  prudent patient test and, I:146
  religion-based treatment refusal and,
    I:147
  risk management and, I:132-133
  speciality and, I:132
  standard of care and, I:139-140
  surgery-specific, I:142-146, 143f, 144f
  technology and, I:127
  testimony in, I:128-131
  type A personality and, I:132
  warranty and, I:140
Medications
  patient history of, I:170
  preoperative, I:170-171
MEDPOR implant, for lower eyelid
    retraction, II:136, 139-142, 141f-142f
Megalin gene, IV:12
Meibomian glands, carcinoma of, V:296-
    298, 297f
Meige disease, VI:1456-1457
Meissner corpuscles, in nerve injury,
    VII:482
Melanin, I:295
Melanocytes, I:295
Melanocytic (nevomelanocytic) nevus,
    V:261-263, 262f
  congenital, V:263-264
Melanoma, V:305-343, VII:965-969, 965f,
    968t
  ABCD of, V:311, 313f
  acral-lentiginous, V:315-316, 316f,
    VII:201-203, 201f
  amelanotic, V:318, 318f
  atypical nevus and, V:309
  B-K mole syndrome and, V:309-310
  biopsy of, V:311-313, 312t, 313f-315f
  Clark classification of, V:318-319, 318f
  classification of, V:313, 315-319
    clinical, V:315
    histologic, V:318-319, 318f
    morphologic, V:315-318, 316f, 317f

Melanoma (Continued)
  clinical evaluation of, V:311-313, 312t,
    313f-315f, 319-325, 320t
    computed tomography in, V:319-320,
      320f
    gallium scan in, V:320, 321f, 321t
    lymphatic mapping in, V:320-324,
      323f, 324f, 324t
    magnetic resonance imaging in,
      V:320, 322f
    positron emission tomography in,
      V:320, 323f
    sentinel lymph node biopsy in, V:324-
      325, 325f
  depigmentation of, Color Plate V:114-1,
    V:311, 314f
  desmoplastic, Color Plate V:114-3,
    V:119-120, 120f, 316-318, 317f,
    VII:968
  differential diagnosis of, V:310-313,
    312f, 313f
  formaldehyde and, V:276
  histology of, Color Plates V:114-1 and
    114-2, V:311, 318-319, 318f
  historical perspective on, V:305-307,
    306f, 307f, 307t
  incidence of, V:273
  lentigo maligna, V:315, 316f
  metastatic, I:916, 983
  multiple, V:311
  nodular, V:315, 316f
  of head and neck, III:1037, 1037f-1038f,
    V:119-120, 120f
  of nasal cavity, V:111
  of orbit, V:111, 112f, 115, 116f-117f
  of paranasal sinuses, V:111
  of perionychium, VII:201-203, 201f
  of scalp, III:612
  of upper extremity, VII:965-969, 965f,
    968t
  recurrence of, V:338-342, 339f-341f,
    342t, VII:968
  risk for, V:263, 264
  staging of, V:315, 319, 319f, VII:966-967,
    966t
  subungual, VII:201-203, 201f
  superficial spreading, V:315, 316f
  treatment of, V:325-329
    adjuvant therapies in, V:342-343
    axillary lymphadenectomy in, V:333,
      336, 336f
    cervical lymphadenectomy in, V:332,
      334f, 335f
    complications of, V:336, 338-342
    for extremities, V:326-327, 330f-332f
    for face, V:326, 328f-329f
    for feet, V:327, 332f
    for fingers, V:326, 331f
    for fingertips, V:326, 330f
    for hands, V:326-327, 331f
    for head and neck, V:326, 328f-329f
    for legs, V:326-327, 331f
    for trunk, V:327, 333f
    historical perspective on, V:306-307,
      307f, 307t
    inguinofemoral lymphadenectomy in,
      V:336, 337f, 338f
    lesion depth and, V:325
    lymphadenectomy in, V:327, 329-330,
      329t, 332-336, 333t, 334f-338f

Melanoma (Continued)
    monitoring after, V:336, 339t
    recurrence after, V:338-342, 339f-
      341f, 342t
    resection width in, V:326
    skin grafts in, V:326, 327f
Melanonychia striata, VII:196, 197f
Melanotic neuroectodermal tumor of
  infancy, III:772
Melasma, II:396-397, 398f
Meningeal artery, accessory, IV:81
Meningioma, V:127, 128f, 145
Meningitis
  in frontobasilar region fracture, III:335
  in nasoethmoidal-orbital fracture,
    III:330
Meningocele, in spinal root avulsion, I:729,
  730f
Meningoencephalocele, frontoethmoidal
  classification of, IV:383, 385
  computed tomography in, IV:409f
  management of, IV:416, 419t, 431, 454,
    458, 459f, 460f
  morphology of, IV:407, 409, 409f, 410f,
    411, 411f
  naso-orbital, IV:411, 411f
  nasoethmoidal, III:765, 765f, IV:407,
    410f
  nasofrontal, IV:408, 410f
  pathogenesis of, IV:414
Meningomyelocele, I:945
Mental nerve block, I:191-192, 192f, III:9,
  10f
Mental status, in hypothermia, I:858
Mentalis, III:889
Menton, II:19f, 20t
Mentoplasty, in male-to-female
  transformation, VI:1315
Meperidine, I:181-182
Mepivacaine, I:190t
  for facial anesthesia, III:7-8, 7t
Meralgia paresthetica, VII:876t, 910
Merkel cell, I:295-296
  in nerve injury, VII:482
Merkel cell carcinoma, V:295-296, 296f,
  437t, 443-445, 443f, 444f
Mesenchymoma, V:15
Mesoneurium, VII:475
Meta-analysis, in evidence-based decision-
  making, I:45, 46f
Metacarpal arteries, VII:37
Metacarpal bones, VII:17-18, 17f
  finger
    congenital remnants of, VIII:56-60
      bone grafting for, VIII:59
      lengthening of, VIII:57-59, 58f
      toe transfer for, VIII:59-60, 60f
      transposition of, VIII:57
      web deepening of, VIII:57
    contracture of, VII:736, 737f. See also
      Dupuytren disease.
    fracture of, VII:426-429, 427f-429f
      K-wires for, VII:428
      malrotation with, VII:427-428
      malunion or nonunion of, VII:429
      open reduction and internal
        fixation for, VII:428-429, 429f
    thumb, fracture of, VII:425-426, 426f
Metacarpal boss, in musicians' hands,
  VII:702

Metacarpal flap, for finger reconstruction,
  VII:228, 228f, 231, 235f, 236f, 239f
Metacarpal synostosis, VIII:268-269
  classification of, VIII:268, 269f
  clinical presentation of, VIII:268, 269f
  incidence of, VIII:268
  outcomes of, VIII:272
  treatment of, VIII:270-272, 271f, 273f-
    275f
Metacarpophalangeal joints
  finger
    arthrodesis in, VII:216
    arthroplasty in, VII:215-216
    burn-related contracture of, VII:624,
      624t, 625f
    congenital amputation at, VIII:56-60,
      60f
    dislocation of, VII:439-440, 440f
    dislocation/subluxation of, VII:439-
      440, 440f
    dorsal dislocation of, VII:439-440,
      440f
    first, VII:24
    flexion of, tendon transfers for,
      VIII:473-478, 474f-478f
    fracture-dislocation of, VII:441
    fracture-dislocation/subluxation of,
      VII:441
    fracture of, VII:215-216
    fusion of, VIII:265-269, 266f
    hyperextension of, VII:406-407,
      409f
    motion of, VII:21, 21f
    osteoarthritis of, VII:717-719, 719f
  thumb
    dislocation/subluxation of, VII:437-
      438, 437f-439f
    dorsal dislocation of, VII:438
    fracture-dislocation/subluxation of,
      VII:440-441, 441f
    osteoarthritis of, VII:724, 725f
Metal implants, I:751-752, 752t
Metallic bars, in chest reconstruction,
  VI:432
Metastases
  from basal cell carcinoma, V:283, 435,
    446-447
  from breast cancer, VI:663, 670-671
  from head and neck cancer, V:166-167,
    166f, 465-473. See also Head and
    neck cancer, metastatic.
  from melanoma, I:916, 983
  from oral cavity cancer, V:160-162, 162f,
    166-167, 167f
  from squamous cell carcinoma, V:160-
    162, 162f, 166-167, 291, 294-295,
    294f, 447-448
  hand, VII:991
    vs. infection, VII:768-769, 769f
  lower extremity, VII:1476
  mandibular, V:213
  nasal cavity, V:113
  orbital, V:115
  paranasal, V:113
  pulmonary, V:162
  salivary gland, V:87
Metatarsals, VI:1410-1411, 1413f
  for bone graft, I:675t, 688
Methohexital, I:172, 172t
8-Methoxypsoralen, V:276

Methyl methacrylate, I:702-703
  for chest wall reconstruction, VI:414
  for cranioplasty, III:548-549, 550f-552f
  for facial prostheses, I:775
Metoclopramide, preoperative, I:171
Metoidioplasty, in female-to-male
    transformation, VI:1308-1310, 1309f,
    1310f
Metopic craniosynostosis, IV:137t, 154-
    158, 156f-160f, 472-474, 475f, 476f
Mexiletine, in complex regional pain
    syndrome/reflex sympathetic
    dystrophy, VII:860
Miami flap, for finger reconstruction,
    VII:228, 229f, 230f-231f
Mibelli, porokeratosis of, V:401
Microarray analysis, I:58, 60f
Microcephaly, I:1128
Microelectrodes, in peripheral nerve
    repair, I:739
Micrognathia, III:763, 764f, 776-778, 776f,
    778f
  distraction osteogenesis in, III:780-783,
    780f-783f
Microophthalmia, reconstruction for,
    III:752, 761f, 762
Microsomia. See Craniofacial microsomia.
Microstomia, after facial burn excision and
    grafting, III:69, 70f-71f
Microtia, III:639-642
  associated deformities with, III:638-639,
    639t
  bilateral, III:660-662, 664f
  clinical characteristics of, III:639, 639t,
    640f, 641f
  drug-associated, III:638
  genetic factors in, III:637-638
  in utero factors in, III:638
  incidence of, III:637
  reconstruction for, III:633-669
    anatomy for, III:634-635, 635f
    anesthesia for, III:635, 635f
    bilateral, III:660-662, 664f
    care after, III:647, 649
    earlobe transposition in, III:649-650,
      650f, 651f
    first stage of, III:642, 643-649, 644f-
      649f
    fourth stage of, III:642, 650, 652f-
      654f
    framework fabrication for, III:645,
      645f-647f, 654f, 658, 661f
    historical perspective on, III:633-
      634
    framework implantation for, III:645-
      647, 648f-649f
    hairline management in, III:646, 648,
      660f
    historical perspective on, III:633-634
    middle ear in, III:635-637
    Nagata technique in, III:658, 661f
    patient activities after, III:649
    planning of, III:642-643, 643f
    preoperative consultation for,
      III:642
    results of, III:640f, 641f
    rib cartilage for, III:644-645, 644f
    second stage of, III:642, 649-650,
      650f, 651f
    secondary, III:660, 662f, 663f

Microtia (Continued)
    skin grafting for, III:642, 650-651,
      655f, 656, 656f-657f
    sulcus formation in, III:650-651, 655f,
      656, 656f-657f
    third stage of, III:642, 650-651, 655f,
      656, 656f-657f
    timing of, III:639, 641-642
    tragal construction in, III:650, 652f-
      654f
Microvascular surgery, I:412-413, 414f,
    507-533. See also Replantation.
  advantages of, I:523
  alcohol abuse and, I:525
  anastomosis in, I:516-523
    end-to-end, I:517-518, 517f, 518f
    end-to-side, I:518-519, 519f
    failure of, I:521-523
    patency of, I:521
    sequence of, I:516
    sleeve, I:518, 518f
    suturing technique for, I:516-517, 517f
    thrombosis of, I:521
  anastomotic devices for, I:512-513
  anesthesia for, I:526
  angiography before, I:525
  anticoagulative agents and, I:521-522
  arterial graft in, I:520
  aspirin and, I:522
  benefits of, I:508
  bipolar coagulator for, I:511-512
  blood flow factors in, I:520-521
  chimeric flaps in, I:526-527, 527f
  cigarette smoking and, I:525
  clamps for, I:511, 512f
  computed thermography monitoring in,
    I:531
  definition of, I:508
  dextran during, I:522
  disadvantages of, I:508-509, 523, 523f
  dissection techniques in, I:514
  donor site complications in, I:532, 532f
  donor tissue for, I:527-528, 528f, 528t,
    529f
  Doppler monitoring in, I:531
  during pregnancy, I:522
  endoscopic techniques in, I:526
  exposure for, I:514
  failure of, I:523, 523f, 531-532
  fibrin glue in, I:513
  forceps for, I:511, 511f
  heparin during, I:521-522
  historical perspective on, I:507-508
  in abdominal wall reconstruction, I:448,
    VI:1187-1192, 1189f-1190f
  in breast reconstruction, VI:686, 690,
    761-772, 1039-1050. See also Breast
    reconstruction, microvascular
    composite tissue transplantation
    (free flap) for.
  in children, I:525
  in chin reconstruction, III:599, 603f-
    604f
  in craniofacial microsomia, IV:541, 544f,
    545f
  in cranioplasty, III:556-561, 558f-560f
  in forehead reconstruction, III:705t,
    717, 723, 725f-726f, 727t
  in head and neck reconstruction, I:430,
    431f-432f, V:225-226, 226t

Microvascular surgery (Continued)
    in hindfoot reconstruction, I:464, 464f,
      VI:1436, 1440-1441, 1440f-1442f
    in lower extremity reconstruction, I:454,
      VI:1472, 1473f, 1474f, 1480-1483,
      1481f-1482f
    in mandible reconstruction, III:962-971,
      964f, 967f, 967t, 972-981, 974f-980f
    in midface reconstruction, III:872, 875f,
      876f, 877
    in midfoot reconstruction, VI:1427,
      1432f
    in nasal reconstruction, II:626, 629-647,
      630f-645f
    in older patients, I:525
    in oral cavity reconstruction, III:934-
      948, 936f-938f, 942f-946f, 948f
    in penile reconstruction, VI:1228, 1230-
      1245. See also Penile
      reconstruction, microsurgical.
    in pressure sore treatment, VI:1322
    in scalp reconstruction, III:620, 622f
    in smile reconstruction, III:898, 899-
      906, 899f-909f
    in thumb reconstruction, VII:258-269.
      See also Thumb reconstruction, toe
      transfer for.
    in transplantation, I:282-285
    in upper extremity reconstruction,
      VII:323-335, 325f-341f. See also at
      Upper extremity reconstruction.
    infection and, I:524
    innervated flap in, I:528-529
    instruments for, I:510-513, 511f, 512f
    irradiation effects in, I:525
    ischemia time in, I:521
    lasers and, I:513
    learning curve for, I:509
    magnifying loupes for, I:510
    microdialysis monitoring in, I:531
    microscopes for, I:509, 510f
    microsutures for, I:512, 512f
    monitoring in, I:530-531
    needle holders for, I:511
    obesity and, I:525
    patient evaluation for, I:524-525
    perforator flaps in, I:526-527, 527f
    photoplethysmography monitoring of,
      I:531
    planning for, I:513-514
    polytetrafluoroethylene graft in, I:520
    porcine graft in, I:520
    prefabrication in, I:529-530
    prelamination in, I:530
    recipient vessel selection in, I:514
    results of, I:531-532
    scissors for, I:511
    stapler for, I:513
    suturing technique in, I:516-517, 517f
    synthetic graft in, I:520
    team for, I:514
    thin flap in, I:529, 529f
    thromboprophylaxis in, I:525-526
    timing of, I:523-524
    training for, I:513
    ultrasonography monitoring in, I:530-
      531
    vascular complications of, I:531
    vasoactive agents and, I:521
    vasospasm in, I:515-516, 516f

Microvascular surgery *(Continued)*
  vein grafts in, I:519-520
  venous flaps in, I:530
  vessel preparation in, I:514-515, 515f
  vessel size discrepancy in, I:520, 520f
Midazolam, I:171f, 173f
Midcarpal clunk test, VII:458
Middle cerebral artery embolism, fat
    injection and, I:583-584
Midface, III:859-861, 861f. *See also* Face
    lift, midface; Midface reconstruction.
  aging of, II:232, 234f
  bones of, III:860-861, 861f
  defects of, III:861-862, 862f. *See also*
    Midface reconstruction.
    evaluation of, III:862, 864-871, 865f-
      871f
    postresection, III:859, 860f, 862, 864f
    type I, III:864
    type II, III:864, 865f-867f
    type III, III:864, 868, 868f, 869f
    type IV, III:868, 870, 870f
    type IVA, III:868
    type IVB, III:868, 870, 870f
    type V, III:870, 871f
  definition of, II:217
  distraction osteogenesis for, III:783-784
  fat injections into, II:249-250, 250f
  implants for, II:249
  nerves of, III:861
  postnatal growth of, III:390-391
    plate translocation and, III:454
    rigid fixation and, III:453-454
  postresection defect in, III:859, 860f,
    862, 864f
  sarcoma of, V:139
  soft tissues of, III:860
  tumors of, V:135-139, 136f-138f
  vessels of, III:861
Midface osteotomy, IV:439-446, 439f-445f
Midface reconstruction, III:859-881. *See
    also* Cheek reconstruction; Nasal
    reconstruction.
  cervicofacial flap for, III:872, 874f
  forehead flap for, III:872, 873f
  in arteriovenous malformation, III:863f
  in nose loss, III:873f
  in parotidectomy, III:867f, 880f
  in Romberg disease, III:833, 852f-853f,
    865f
  in tumor resection, III:869f, 870f, 871,
    871f, 874f, 876f, 878f
  microvascular free flaps for, III:872,
    875f, 876f, 877
  muscle defects in, III:877, 879, 879f, 880f
  musculocutaneous flaps for, III:872, 875f
  skeletal defects in, III:877, 877f, 878f
  skin graft in, III:872
  smile restoration in, III:877, 879, 879f,
    880f
  tissue expansion in, III:872, 874
Midfoot reconstruction, VI:1426-1427,
    1431f, 1432f
Midline agenesis, IV:404, 406f, 407, 408f
Milia, II:370, V:255-256
Milk lines, VI:512, 512f
Milton, Stuart, I:32
Mimetic muscles, II:162-165, 162f, 164f
  arterial supply of, Color Plates I:15-12
    and 15-13, I:340f, 341-342, 342t

Mini-abdominoplasty, VI:158-159, 158f-
    164f
  Baroudi, VI:158, 160f
  extended, VI:158-159, 161f-164f, 165
Minors, treatment of, I:147. *See also*
    Children; Informed consent.
Minoxidil, for hair restoration, II:693-694,
    III:626
Mirror hand, VIII:17, 19, 19f, 21t, 249-254
  clinical presentation of, VIII:250-251,
    251f-253f
  elbow in, VIII:251, 253f
  Entin's procedure in, VIII:253
  forearm in, VIII:251
  historical perspective on, VIII:249, 250f
  inheritance of, VIII:250
  pathogenesis of, VIII:250
  terminology for, VIII:249
  thumb in, VIII:253, 254f
  treatment of, VIII:251-254, 253f, 254f
  wrist in, VIII:251, 253
Mivacurium, I:179-180, 180t
Moberg-Brand flexor pollicis longus
    tenodesis, VIII:522, 524-527, 525f-
    527f
Moberg volar advancement flap, for
    fingertip reconstruction, VII:161-162,
    161f
Möbius syndrome, smile reconstruction in,
    III:905-906, 913-914, 913f
Mohler's cheiloplasty, IV:200-202, 200f-
    203f
  C flap for, IV:201, 201f
  closure for, IV:201-202, 202f
  incisions for, IV:200-201, 200f, 201f
  lateral incisions for, IV:201
  results of, IV:202, 203f
Mohs micrographic surgery, V:286t, 288,
    408t, 426-432
  advantages of, V:430
  disadvantages of, V:430-432, 431f, 431t,
    432f, 432t
  for penile cancer, VI:1255
  indications for, V:430, 430t
  on scalp, III:612
  technique of, V:427-430, 428f, 429f
Moisture, environmental, cold injury and,
    VII:648-649
Mole. *See* Nevus(i).
Molluscum contagiosum, V:252-253, 253f
Moment arm, of tendon, VII:28, 28f
Mondor disease, after breast
    augmentation, VI:30
Monitored anesthesia care, I:196-198
Monobloc osteotomy, IV:485, 487f-489f
  distraction with, IV:485, 488f
Monoclonal antibodies, in experimental
    neutrophil-mediated reperfusion
    injury, I:491-492, 492f, 493f
Monocytes, in wound healing, I:210, 211f
Monophosphoryl lipid A, in flap
    optimization, I:495
Monsplasty, VI:174
Morton neuroma, VII:876t, 922-923, 923f
Morula, IV:2
Motor retraining, after peripheral nerve
    injury, VII:507
Motor units, I:606-607
Mountain sickness, I:861
Mouth. *See* Oral cavity.

Movements
  etomidate-related, I:175
  ketamine-related, I:175
MSX2 gene, IV:11, 92, 93t
Mucocele
  of airway, III:767
  of frontal sinus, III:341
  of salivary glands, V:75
Mucoepidermoid carcinoma, of salivary
    glands, V:79, 82-83, 83f-85f
Muenke syndrome, I:58, 60-61, 61f-63f
Müller muscle, II:83-84, 84f, 143, 143f,
    144f
  hematoma of, II:810
  transection of, II:145f, 147
Multiple hereditary exostoses,
    osteochondroma in, VII:985, 985f
Multiple myeloma, of mandible, V:212
Munchausen syndrome, I:944
Munsell color system, for facial prostheses,
    Color Plate I:27-3, I:776
Mupirocin 2%, I:884t
Muriatic acid injury, to hand, VII:654
Muscle(s). *See also specific muscles.*
  after peripheral nerve repair, VII:506
  anatomy of, I:605-607, 606f
  atrophy of
    in nerve injury, VII:481-482
    rate of, I:607-608
  classification of, I:329-330, 329f-332f,
    329t, 605
  contraction of, I:606-607
  débridement of, I:875
  denervation of, I:607
  electrical stimulation of, I:615-616
  electromyography of, I:608, 609f
  experimental laceration of, I:609-610
  facial, arterial supply of, Color Plates
    I:15-12 and 15-13, I:340f, 341-343,
    342t
  fast fibers of, I:606-607, 608
  force of, VII:26, 26f
  forearm, vascular territories of, Color
    Plates I:15-4 to 15-7, I:335
  functional transfer of, I:390, 400f-404f,
    405, VIII:489-506. *See also* Arm(s),
    muscle transfer in.
  in tissue expansion, I:541, 541f
  injury response of, I:607-608
  ischemia of, I:608-609
  lower extremity, vascular territories of,
    Color Plates I:15-9 to 15-11, I:338-
    339, 338f
  motor units of, I:606-607
  myoblast (satellite cell) of, I:611-612
  myofibers of, I:605, 606f
  neck, arterial supply of, Color Plate I:15-
    13, I:340f, 342-343, 342t
  nerve implantation into, in neuroma
    treatment, VII:939-941, 940f-944f
  nerve supply of, I:328-330, 329f, 329t
  neurotization of, I:607
  opioid effects on, I:181
  physiology of, VIII:492, 493f, 494f
  plasticity of, I:608
  regeneration of, I:609-610
  reinnervation of, I:607-608
  resting tension of, I:607, 608
  shape of, VII:27-28
  slow fibers of, I:606, 608

Muscle(s) (Continued)
structure of, I:1096, VII:24-25
tenotomy effect on, I:608
tourniquet-related injury to, VII:116-117
type I, I:329-330, 329f, 329t, 330f, 347f
type II, I:329f, 329t, 330, 330f
type III, I:329f, 329t, 330, 331f
type IV, I:329f, 329t, 330, 332f
vascular anatomy of, I:325-330, 327f, 328f, 607
veins of, I:326-327, 327f, 354
Muscle conduit, for nerve repair, VII:500
Muscle dysmorphia, I:86
Muscle flaps, I:372-374, 373f, 374t, 375t, 417. See also Flap(s) and specific flaps and procedures.
advantages of, I:417
arc of rotation of, I:372, 373f, 410, 417-418, 418f, 419f
combination, I:407-408, 408f
disadvantages of, I:417
distally based, I:409, 409t, 410f
for abdominal wall reconstruction, I:446-447, 447f-450f, 447t. See also Abdominal wall reconstruction.
for breast reconstruction, I:430, 433-440, 434f-440f. See also Latissimus dorsi flap; Transverse rectus abdominis myocutaneous (TRAM) flap.
for chest reconstruction, I:441, 445f, 446. See also Chest wall reconstruction.
for facial reconstruction, V:345-390. See also Facial flap(s).
for foot reconstruction, I:454, 462-464, 462f-464f. See also Foot reconstruction.
for groin and perineum reconstruction, I:448, 451-454, 451f-453f
for head and neck reconstruction, I:421-430. See also Head and neck reconstruction.
for lower extremity reconstruction, I:454, 455f-461f. See also Lower extremity reconstruction.
for mediastinal reconstruction, I:440-441, 442f-444f
for pressure sores, I:464-467, 465f-470f. See also Pressure sores.
for upper extremity reconstruction, VII:323, 324-326, 325f-328f. See also Arm(s), mangling injury to.
functional, I:390, 400f-404f, 405
osseous, I:390, 391f, 392f, 421
prefabrication of, I:409
prelamination of, I:408-409
reverse-flow, I:409-411, 411f, 412f
segmental transfer of, I:384, 386, 386f-389f
selection of, I:413, 415-421, 415f, 418f, 419f
skin territory of, I:418, 420
splitting for, I:384, 386, 386f-389f
type I (one vascular pedicle), I:372, 374f, 374t
type II (dominant vascular pedicle and minor pedicle), I:372-373, 374f, 374t

Muscle flaps (Continued)
type III (two dominant pedicles), I:373, 374f, 375t
type IV (segmental vascular pedicles), I:373, 374f, 375t
type V (one dominant vascular pedicle and secondary segmental vascular pedicles), I:374, 374f, 375t
Muscle graft, I:610-616
nonvascularized, I:610-612
clinical applications of, I:612
experimental studies of, I:610-612, 611f
reinnervation of, I:607-608
vascularized, I:613-616
in anal reconstruction, I:615
in extremity reconstruction, I:614-615
in facial reanimation, I:613-614, 614f
in genitourinary reconstruction, I:615
Muscle relaxants, with anesthesia, I:179-181, 179t
Muscle transfer, I:390, 400f-404f, 405, VIII:489-506. See also Arm(s), muscle transfer in.
Musculocutaneous flaps, I:359, 360f, 417, 418, 420. See also Flap(s); Muscle flaps and specific flaps and procedures.
Musculus uvulae, IV:72, 74f, 75-76, 75f
Musicians' hands, VII:693-704
air playing for, VII:699
amputation injury in, VII:701
carpal tunnel syndrome in, VII:702-703
cubital tunnel syndrome in, VII:703
de Quervain tendinitis in, VII:702
Dupuytren contracture in, VII:701
electromyography for, VII:696
evaluation of, VII:694-696, 694f, 695f
fingertip injury in, VII:699, 701
focal dystonia in, VII:703-704
fracture in, VII:701
ganglion in, VII:702
instrument interface with, VII:694-696, 695f
metacarpal boss in, VII:702
nerve compression syndrome in, VII:702-703
nerve laceration in, VII:701
position of function of, VII:699
radial tunnel syndrome in, VII:703
surgical treatment of, VII:696-699
arthrodesis in, VII:702
incisions for, VII:697-699, 698f
indications for, VII:696-697, 697f, 697t
rehabilitation after, VII:699, 700f
results of, VII:704, 704t
videotaping of, VII:696
tendon injury in, VII:701
tumors in, VII:698f, 702
Mustard gas injury, to hand, VII:654
Mustardé rotation flap, I:551, 553, 554f
Mycobacterium infection, of hand, VII:785-788, 786f, 787f
Mycophenolate mofetil, for immunosuppression, I:275t, 276
Myectomy, digastric, II:741, 741f
Myelin, compression-related changes in, VII:877
Myelography, cervical, in brachial plexus injury, VII:519f, 526

Myelomeningocele
fetal surgery for, I:1128
reconstruction for, I:387f, VI:434, 447-448, 448f-450f
Myoblast
in regeneration, I:611-612
in tissue engineering, I:1096-1097, 1097f
Myocardial infarction, myocyte proliferation after, I:612
Myoclonus, etomidate-related, I:175
Myofascial dysfunction
in complex regional pain syndrome/reflex sympathetic dystrophy, VII:833-835, 848
temporomandibular, III:537
Myofibers, I:605, 606f
Myofibroblast
contraction of, VII:734
differentiation of, VII:734-735
in Dupuytren disease, VII:734-735
Myonecrosis, clostridial, VII:782
Myositis, necrotizing, I:977
Myotendinous junction, I:592-, 594
Myxoma, odontogenic, V:98, 202, 203f

N

Nagata technique, in auricular reconstruction, III:658, 661f
Nager syndrome (acrofacial dysostosis), IV:101, 422, 423f, VIII:30, 30f, 62, 63f
Nails. See Perionychium.
Nakagawa, angioblastoma of, V:36-37
Nalbuphine, I:182-183
Naproxen, I:183-184
Narcissistic personality, I:71-72
Nasal artery, IV:78f
Nasal cannula, I:175
Nasal cavity. See Nose.
Nasal fracture, III:187-208
bleeding with, III:206
classification of, III:191-196, 192f-195f
complications of, III:204, 206-208, 207f
contractures with, III:208
diagnosis of, III:196-197
bimanual examination in, III:196, 197f
computed tomography in, III:196-197, 199f
radiography in, III:196-197, 198f
facial swelling with, III:206
frontal impact, III:189-191, 190f, 192f-195f, 196
hematoma in, III:196, 204, 206-208, 207f
infection with, III:206, 208
lateral impact, III:189, 191, 192f-195f
malunion of, III:208
mechanisms of, III:189-191, 190f
misdiagnosis of, III:208
osteitis with, III:208
pediatric, III:432-434, 433f
septal subperichondrial fibrosis with, III:206, 208
sites of, III:189-191, 190f
synechiae with, III:208
treatment of, III:197-204
closed reduction in, III:197
percutaneous compression in, III:192f-193f, 201-204
open reduction in, III:197-201, 200f, 201f, 203
in compound fractures, III:204, 205f

Nasal molding, after cheiloplasty, IV:205-206, 206f

Nasal packing, in facial fracture, III:79-81, 80f, 81f

Nasal pit, III:765

Nasal reconstruction, II:573-643. *See also* Rhinoplasty.
  airway construction in, II:576
  alar cartilage reconstruction in, II:600, 605, 606f-612f
  alar margin defect in, II:586, 588, 588f, 589f
  anesthesia for, I:203
  bilobed flap for, II:590, 591f, 592f, V:349, 354f, 357f
  cartilage grafts for, II:600, 605, 606f-612f
    nasal lining skin grafts with, II:618, 623f-625f
  checklist for, II:577t
  cheek repair in, II:576-577
  columellar defects in, II:586, 586f
  composite ear graft for, II:586-589, 587f-589f, V:349
  contracture release in, II:575-576
  contralateral mucoperichondrial flap for, II:617f, 618, 619f
  deep defect, II:600, 605-622
    alar cartilage reconstruction in, II:605, 606f-612f
    cartilage graft in, II:618, 623f-625f
    composite, II:613, 613f-616f, 631, 641f-645f, 646
    full-thickness, II:605, 613-622, 613f-625f
    intranasal lining flaps in, II:613, 617f, 618, 619f-622f
    Menick nasal lining technique in, II:618, 626, 626f-629f
  design principles in, II:574-575, 575f
  eyebrow separation in, II:584-585
  facial landmarks in, II:600, 603f, 604f
  flaps for, II:575, V:349, 352-360, 352f-363f
  forehead flap for, II:581-584, 582f, 583f, V:349, 353f, 355f, 360, 361f, 362f
    blood supply for, II:582-583, 582f
    healing of, II:585-586
    lengthening of, II:583-584, 583f
    pattern design for, II:581-582
    size for, II:28, 582
    subunit principle for, II:597-599, 598f-599f
  full-thickness skin graft for
    for nasal lining, II:618, 623f-625f
    from forehead, II:590-595, 593f-596f
    from postauricular area, II:605, 613
    secondary, II:594
  glabellar flap for, V:349, 357f
  historical perspective on, I:19f, 27, 28f, II:573-574, 574f
  in composite defects, II:613, 613f-616f, 631, 641f-645f, 646
  intermediate flaying operation in, II:584, 584f, 585f
  intranasal lining flaps in, II:577-579, 578f, 579f, 613, 617f, 618, 619f-621f, 626f-629f
  island forehead flap for, V:349, 355f

Nasal reconstruction (*Continued*)
  large superficial defect, II:595, 597-600, 597f-599f, 601f-604f
  lateral advancement flap for, V:349, 352f
  malposition in, II:575
  Menick nasal lining technique in, II:618, 626, 626f-629f
  microvascular free tissue transfer for, II:626, 629-647
    airway preservation in, II:631, 638f-640f
    layer-by-layer stages for, II:631, 641f-645f, 646
    multiple graft paddles for, II:629, 631, 632f-637f
    nasal lining flap for, II:631, 638f-640f
    principles of, II:646
    septal pivot flap for, II:626, 629, 630f-631f
    staging of, II:646-647
  model for, II:574, 600, 646
  nasal lining for
    flaps in, II:577-579, 578f, 579t, 613, 617f, 618, 619f-621f, 626f-629f
    free microvascular flap in, II:626, 629-631, 630f-640f
    full-thickness skin graft in, II:618, 623f-625f
    Menick technique in, II:618, 626, 626f-629f
    triple-island radial forearm flap in, II:631, 638f-640f
  nasal platform in, II:575, 576f, 577
  nasolabial island flap for, II:599-600, 601f-604f
  nasolabial lining flap for, II:578f, 579
  nose-lip-cheek confluence in, II:600, 603f, 604f
  operative stage 1 in, II:577-584
    bone grafts in, II:579-580, 580t
    cartilage grafts in, II:579-580, 580t
    contralateral septal lining flap for, II:578f, 579
    forehead flaps in, II:581-584, 582f, 583f
      blood supply for, II:582-583, 582f
      length for, II:583-584, 583f
      lengthening of, II:583-584, 583f
      pattern design for, II:581-582
      size for, II:582
    nasal lining flaps in, II:577-579, 578f, 579t
    nasal margin lining flap in, II:579
    nasal site in, II:577
    nasal skin cover in, II:580-581, 581f, 581t
    nasolabial lining flap in, II:578f, 579
    skin thickness zones in, II:580-581, 581f, 581t
    turnover lining flap in, II:577, 578f, 579
  operative stage 2 in, II:584, 585f
  operative stage 3 in, II:584-585
  pedicled transverse neck flap for, V:360, 363f
  principles of, II:574-575, 575f, 595, 597-600, 597f-599f
    in composite defects, II:613, 613f-616f, 631, 641f-645f, 646
  Rintala flap for, V:349, 358f

Nasal reconstruction (*Continued*)
  rotation flap for, V:349, 356f
  scar excision in, II:575-576
  septal pivot flap for, II:626, 629, 630f-631f
  skin quality in, II:575
  skin thickness zones in, II:575, 575f, 580-581, 581f, 581t
  small superficial defect, II:586-594
    zone 1, II:586
    zone 2, II:590-594, 591f-596f
    zone 3, II:586-589, 587f-589f
  stages of, II:613, 613f-616f, 631, 641f-645f, 646-647
  subunit principle in, II:595, 597-600, 597f-599f
  three-dimensional patterns for, II:574-575
  timing of, II:585-586
  tissue expansion in, I:553, 556f
  tissue volume replacement in, II:577
  transposition flap for, V:349, 356f, 357f
  transverse pedicle flap for, V:349, 359f-360f
  triple-island radial forearm flap for, II:631, 638f-640f
  turnover lining flap for, II:577, 578f, 579
  upper lip repair in, II:576-577
  volume deficiency in, II:577

Nasal septum
  anatomy of, III:188-189, 189f
  deformity of
    after rhinoplasty, II:770
    birth-related, III:764
  examination of, II:526-527
  fracture of, III:190f, 191, 196f. *See also* Nasal fracture.
    hematoma in, III:204, 206-208, 207f
    treatment of, III:204, 206f
  graft from, I:624, 625f, 626
  hematoma of, III:29-30, 196, 204, 206-208, 207f
  in children, III:433-434
  in facial paralysis, III:897
  perforation of, with secondary rhinoplasty, II:797
  postnatal growth of, III:390-391
  postoperative collapse of, II:563, 563f
  subperichondrial fibrosis of, III:206, 208

Nasal spine, II:19f, 20t

Nasal tip, II:492, 494f, 520, 520f, 521f
  contour of, II:528-530, 529f, 530f
  deformity of, after facial burn excision and grafting, III:60-62, 63f
  inadequate projection of, after rhinoplasty, II:780, 781f-784f, 791
  overprojection of, after rhinoplasty, II:784-785
  pink
    after closed rhinoplasty, II:564
    after secondary rhinoplasty, II:797
  projection of, II:532, 534f, 535, 535f
  reconstruction of, V:349, 356f, 358f-363f

Nash, John, I:18

Nasion, II:3f, 3t, 19f, 20t

Nasoalveolar molding
  bilateral cleft lip repair with, IV:278, 281f-282f, 341, 342f
    lower lateral cartilage repositioning and, IV:236, 239f-241f

Nasoalveolar molding *(Continued)*
  projecting premaxilla and, IV:222-225, 223f, 224f
  cleft nose repair with, IV:360-361, 360f, 361f
  unilateral cleft lip repair with, IV:273-277, 275f-278f
    Grayson method for, IV:178-179, 180f
    Liou method for, IV:178, 179f
    passive method for, IV:181
Nasoethmoidal-orbital fracture, III:305, 307-330, 307f, 580, 581f
  anatomy of, III:308-310, 308f
  bilateral, III:314-315, 316f
  bimanual examination in, III:313, 314
  brain injury with, III:308, 310, 313, 315
  classification of, III:311-312
  clinical examination in, III:312-314, 313f
  complications of, III:324-330
  computed tomography in, III:314-315
  CSF rhinorrhea in, III:313-314, 314f, 315f, 330
  diagnosis of, III:312-315
  diplopia in, III:325-326
  facial appearance in, III:311
  globe injury in, III:326-328
  hematoma in, III:328
  hypertelorism in, III:311
  in children, III:393f-394f, 434-438, 435f-438f
  infraorbital nerve injury in, III:329-330
  intranasal examination in, III:313
  intraorbital hematoma in, III:328
  lacrimal system injury in, III:328
  lamina papyracea injury in, III:310
  mechanisms of, III:310-311, 311f
  meningitis in, III:330
  misdiagnosis of, III:208
  orbital fractures with, III:310, 318f
  pathology of, III:310-311
  pneumocephalus in, III:315
  ptosis in, III:328
  retrobulbar hematoma in, III:325
  telecanthus in, III:311
  treatment of, III:315, 320-324
    bone grafts in, III:322, 322f, 323f, 325
    canthal reattachment in, III:323-324
    complications of, III:324-330
    coronal incision for, III:322-323
    exposure for, III:315, 320-321, 320f-321f
    implant complications after, III:325
    lower eyelid incisions in, III:329
    medial orbital rim wires in, III:321-322, 323f
    open-sky technique in, III:319f
    transnasal wires in, III:321-322, 323f
    vertical midline nasal incision for, III:322
  type I, III:312, 315, 316f-317f
  type II, III:312, 315, 318f
  type III, III:312, 315, 319f
  type IV, III:312, 315
Nasoethmoidal-orbital region. *See* Ethmoid; Nasoethmoidal-orbital fracture; Orbit.
Nasofacial angle, II:474, 474f

Nasojugal groove, II:92. *See also* Malar fat pads.
  aging-related changes in, II:152
  anatomy of, II:152
Nasolabial angle, II:474-475, 475f
Nasolabial flap
  for head and neck reconstruction, V:223, 224f, 226t
  for nasal reconstruction, II:578f, 579, 599-600, 601f-604f
Nasolabial fold, II:279-280, 280f
  augmentation of, II:279
  excision of, II:279-280, 280f
Nasolacrimal duct injury, in maxillary fracture, III:255
Nasomaxillary complex, postnatal growth of, III:390-391
Nasopalatine artery, IV:78f
Nasopalatine duct cyst, V:94
Nasopharynx
  cancer of, V:246-247. *See also* Oropharyngeal cancer.
  in children, V:16
  congenital hamartoma of, III:766
  congenital obstructive disorders of, III:763-765, 764f, 765f
  endoscopy of, in velopharyngeal dysfunction, IV:315-317, 317f
  intubation of, in craniofacial clefts, IV:416, 422
  juvenile angiofibroma of, V:11
  mass of, III:765-767, 765f, 766f
  teratoma of, III:766, 766f
Natural killer cells, in graft rejection, I:271
Nausea, postoperative, I:201-202
  prevention of, I:184, 185t
Neck. *See also* Head and neck; Neck lift; Neck reconstruction.
  acne keloidalis of, I:944, 944f
  aging-related changes in, II:297, 299-300, 301f, 302f
  arterial supply of, Color Plates I:15-12 and 15-13, I:340, 340f, 341f, 342-343
  basal cell cancer of, III:1037
  chemical resurfacing of, II:368
  congenital web of (pterygium colli), III:1027, 1027f-1028f, 1028f
  contracture of, after facial burn excision and grafting, III:70-72, 72f
  dug-out deformity of, II:738, 738f
  embryology of, III:1025-1027, 1026f, 1027f
  hypertrophic scar of, III:1034-1035, 1034f
  laser resurfacing of, II:365-368, 366f
    CO_2, II:366, 366f
    Er:YAG, II:367
  liposuction of, Color Plate VI:123-6, VI:213-216, 215f-217f
    irregular contours from, III:334
  melanoma of, III:1037, 1037f-1038f
  neuroma of, VII:944
  platysma of, II:163, 176, 176f
    aging-related changes in, II:179-181, 180f, 181f, 298f, 299, 300f, 301f
  scar of
    skin graft resurfacing for, I:260-263, 261f-262f, 264f
    Z-plasty for, I:251, 254f

Neck *(Continued)*
  subcutaneous fat of, overexcision of, II:736-737, 736f, 737f
  subplatysmal fat of, overexcision of, II:738, 738f
  tissue expansion in, I:551, 553, 555f
  torticollis of, III:398, 1032-1033, 1033f, IV:98-99
  trauma to, wound healing and, I:1006-1008
  webs of
    after facial burn excision and grafting, III:73, 73f
    congenital (pterygium colli), III:1027, 1027f-1028f, 1028f
  wrinkled graft of, after facial burn excision and grafting, III:72, 73f
Neck flap
  for cheek reconstruction, V:375-376, 378f-380f, 381
  for nasal reconstruction, V:360, 363f
Neck lift, II:283-295, 297-336, 298f-299f. *See also* Face lift.
  anatomy for, II:300-304, 303f-305f
  atenolol before, II:321
  care after, II:319-320
  chin implants in, II:285, 287f
  complications of, II:320-323, 332-336, 335f
  composite technique of, II:309
  deep plane technique of, II:309
  direct, II:290, 293, 293f-295f
  facial nerve injury with, II:332-334, 335f
  hematoma after, II:320-323, 332
  hydralazine before, II:322
  in male, II:306
  incisions for, II:305-308
  infection after, II:332
  labetalol before, II:321-322
  lazy S-type postauricular incision for, II:306-308, 307f
  liposuction in, II:284-285, 286f, 287f, 334
    platysmaplasty with, II:285, 288f, 290f-292f
  modified, II:290
  nerve injury with, II:332-334, 335f
  nifedipine after, II:322
  pain after, II:320
  patient dissatisfaction with, II:334
  patient evaluation for, II:283-284, 284f
  patient selection for, II:304-305
  postauricular incision for, II:306-308, 307f
  preauricular incision for, II:305-306
  results of, II:298f-299f
  scar after, II:320
  skin flap technique of, II:308-309
  skin necrosis after, II:332
  Skoog technique of, II:309
  SMAS-platysmal rotation flap technique of, II:309-319, 311f-312f
    complications of, II:320-323, 332-336, 335f
    dissection for, II:312-315, 313f, 314f, 316f-318f
    flap mobilization for, II:315-316, 318f, 319f
    liposuction with, II:319, 330f-331f

Neck lift (Continued)
    results of, II:319, 324f-331f
    sutures for, II:316, 319, 319f-321f,
        323f
    vector diagram of, II:322f
Neck reconstruction, III:1025-1077. See
        also Head and neck reconstruction.
    deltopectoral flap for, III:1043, 1044f
    dorsal scapular island flap for, III:1042,
        1042f
    in carotid blowout, III:1072, 1076, 1076f
    in cervical osteomyelitis, III:1076
    in cutaneous neoplasms, III:1037,
        1037f-1038f
    in exposed cervical spinal cord, III:1076
    in hypertrophic neck scar, III:1034-
        1035, 1034f
    in laryngeal neoplasms, III:1039
    in oropharyngeal neoplasms, III:1039
    jejunal flap for, III:1072, 1072f-1075f
    lateral arm flap for, III:1045-1047
    lateral cervical skin flaps for, III:1039,
        1039f
    lateral thigh flap for, III:1045, 1046f
    latissimus dorsi flap for, III:1062-1064,
        1062f-1066f
    omental flap for, III:1064, 1067-1071,
        1067f-1071f
    pectoralis major flap for, III:1052-1054,
        1052f-1054f
    pediatric, III:1025-1033
        anatomy for, III:1025-1027, 1026f,
            1027f
        in cystic hygroma, III:1030-1032,
            1030f-1032f
        in pterygium colli, III:1027, 1027f-
            1028f, 1028f
        in thyroglossal duct cyst, III:1029,
            1029f, 1030f
        in torticollis, III:1032-1033, 1033f
    pedicled occipital artery flap for,
        III:1039f, 1040, 1040f
    platysma flap for, III:1048, 1048f-1050f
    radial forearm flap for, III:1045, 1045f
    sternocleidomastoid flap for, III:1050-
        1051, 1051f
    submental artery island flap for,
        III:1040, 1040f
    tissue expansion for, I:553, 555f,
        III:1034-1035, 1035f-1036f
    trapezius flap for, III:1055-1062, 1055f-
        1061f
Necrosis. See also Osteoradionecrosis.
    after circumcision, VI:1217-1218, 1219f
    avascular
        condylar process fracture and, III:174,
            177
        Dupuytren disease fasciectomy and,
            VII:750-751, 751f
        mandibular fracture and, III:182
        of temporomandibular joint, III:543-
            544
        orthognathic surgery and, II:685
    cartilage, finger contracture and,
        VII:672
    fat
        breast reduction and, VI:578-579,
            1068, 1070
        TRAM flap breast reconstruction and,
            VI:865, 994

Necrosis (Continued)
    flap, I:357
        breast reconstruction and, VI:831
        mastopexy and, VI:85
        open rhinoplasty and, II:510-511,
            511f
        oral cavity reconstruction and, III:950
        pressure sore treatment and, VI:1351
    nipple, after breast reduction, VI:1072,
        1074, 1074f
    skin
        body lift and, VI:270-271
        neck lift and, II:332
        of back, VI:448, 450, 451f, 452f
        rhytidectomy and, II:210
Necrotizing fasciitis, I:911, 914, 914f, 974,
        976-977
    abdominal, VI:93
    of hand, VII:781-782, 782f, 783f
Necrotizing sialometaplasia, V:75, 77f
Necrotizing soft tissue infection, I:911,
        914, 914f, 974, 976-977
Neomycin, topical, I:884t
Neonate. See Infant.
Neoumbilicoplasty, VI:188-189, 189f
Nerve. See Peripheral nerve(s).
Nerve block(s)
    ankle, I:194, 199f
    auricular, III:9-10
    auriculotemporal, III:10-11, 11f
    axillary, I:193, 195f, VII:101-102, 101f
    Bier, I:192, 193f
    brachial plexus, I:192-193, 194f, VII:98f,
        102
    central neuraxis blocks for, I:194-196
    digital, VII:105
    elbow, VII:103-104, 104f
    epidural, I:194-196
    extremity, I:192-194, 193f-199f
    facial, I:191-192, 192f
    femoral, I:193-194, 198f
    in complex regional pain
        syndrome/reflex sympathetic
        dystrophy, VII:853-854
    in facial trauma, III:7-8, 7t, 8-11, 8f-11f
    in post-traumatic pain, III:365
    infraclavicular, VII:100, 100f
    infraorbital, III:8-9, 9f
    interscalene, I:192, 194f, VII:97-99, 98f
    intravenous, I:192, 193f
    isolated, VII:103-105
    median nerve, I:193, 196f, 197f, VII:103,
        104-105, 104f, 105f
    mental, I:191-192, 192f, III:9, 10f
    monitoring of, I:189
    obturator, I:193-194, 198f
    ophthalmic, I:191-192, 192f, III:8, 8f
    radial nerve, I:193, 196f, 197f, VII:103,
        104, 104f
    sciatic, I:193
    spinal, I:194-196
    supraclavicular, I:193, VII:99-100, 99f
    suprascapular, VII:100-101, 101f
    ulnar nerve, VII:103-104, 104f, 105
    wrist, VII:104-105
Nerve chip, I:1155
Nerve conduction study, I:728t, 729,
        VII:486-487, 494
    after peripheral nerve repair, VII:506
    in brachial plexus injury, VII:526

Nerve conduction study (Continued)
    in complex regional pain
        syndrome/reflex sympathetic
        dystrophy, VII:846
Nerve entrapment syndromes, VII:875-
        924, 876t
    axillary nerve, VII:909
    brachial plexus, VII:906-909, 908f, 909f
    carpal tunnel, VII:882, 885-889
    common peroneal nerve, VII:910, 912,
        913f-915f
    conservative treatment of, VII:881-883
    cortisone injection in, VII:882
    cubital tunnel, VII:882, 882f
    deep peroneal nerve, VII:915-917, 916f
    diagnosis of, VII:878-881, 880f
    double crush, VII:878-879, 880f, 903-
        904
    electrodiagnostic studies in, VII:879-881
    electromyography in, VII:879-880
    gliding limitation in, VII:877-878
    grading of, VII:876-878, 877t, 878t
    in diabetes, VII:923-924
    lateral femoral cutaneous nerve,
        VII:909-910, 911f
    median nerve, VII:889-892
    myelin changes with, VII:877
    nerve conduction study in, VII:879-880
    neural degeneration with, VII:877-878,
        878t
    nonoperative treatment of, VII:881-883
    pathophysiology of, VII:876-878, 877t
    plantar digital nerve, VII:922-923, 923f
    posterior interosseous nerve, VII:904,
        906
    quantitative sensory testing in, VII:879-
        880
    radial sensory nerve, VII:902-904, 903f,
        905f
    radial tunnel, VII:904, 906, 906f
    staging of, VII:876-878, 877t
    superficial peroneal nerve, VII:912, 915
    surgical management of, VII:883-885
        decompression in, VII:883
        internal neurolysis in, VII:883-884
        mobilization in, VII:884-885
        neurolysis in, VII:883-884
        procedure codes for, VII:883
        technical considerations in, VII:883
    symptoms of, VII:875-876
    tarsal tunnel, VII:917-922, 918f-921f,
        922t
    tuning fork test in, VII:877
    two-point discrimination in, VII:877
    ulnar nerve, VII:893-902
    vibrometry in, VII:877
    vitamin B₆ in, VII:882
    vs. amyotrophic lateral sclerosis, VII:881
    vs. syrinx, VII:881
Nerve fibers, VII:472-475, 473f, 474f
Nerve gap, VII:495-505, 496f
    grafting for, VII:495-503, 498f
Nerve graft, I:733-734, 734f, 735f, VII:495-
        503, 498f. See also Peripheral nerve
        repair and reconstruction.
    after prostatectomy, I:737-738
    allogeneic (allograft), I:282, VII:500-
        503, 501f, 502f
    autologous (autograft), I:281-282
    donor nerve for, VII:497

Nerve graft (Continued)
  harvest of, VII:497-498, 498f
  in brachial plexus injury, I:736-737,
    VII:530, 531f
  in facial nerve injury, I:737, 737t
  in lower extremity, I:736
  in neuroma treatment, VII:937, 939
  in upper extremity, I:735-737, 737t,
    VII:322
  outcomes of, VII:509
  pedicled, VII:498-499
  radiation and, I:738
  rehabilitation after, I:738
  rosebud technique for, VII:494f, 497
  vascularized, VII:499
  vs. non-neural conduit, VII:499-500
Nerve territory-oriented macrodactyly,
    VIII:300-301, 301f, 302f, 316
Nerve transfer, VII:503-505, 504f
  criteria for, VII:503
  in brachial plexus injury, VII:530-532,
    548, 551f-552f
Neural crest, IV:2, 3-4, 3f, 9
Neural plate, IV:2, 3f
Neural tube, IV:2, 3f
  defects of, VI:434, 447-448, 448f-450f
    fetal surgery for, I:1128
  incomplete fusion of, IV:3
  prenatal evaluation of, Color Plate I:36-
    6
Neurapraxia, I:725, 726f, VII:483, 483t,
    484f
Neurilemoma, VII:958-959
Neuroblastoma, V:13, 119
Neurocranium, IV:9, 10f
Neurofibroma
  in children, V:8-9, 9f, 10f
  of hand, VII:70, 72f, 958-959
  of mandible, V:210
  orbital, V:139-144
    group 1, V:140
    group 2, V:140-142, 140f-141f
    group 3, V:142-144, 142f-143f
Neurofibromatosis
  macrodactyly and, VIII:304-307, 306f,
    316
  orbitopalpebral, III:565, 573f
Neurofibrosarcoma, of head and neck,
    V:119
Neurokinin A, in complex regional pain
    syndrome/reflex sympathetic
    dystrophy, VII:838-839
Neurolysis, I:732
  in brachial plexus injury, VII:530
  in macrodactyly, VIII:314
  in post-traumatic pain, III:366
Neuroma, VII:929-945
  anatomic sites of, VII:930t
  clinical presentation of, VII:930-931,
    933f
  diagnosis of, VII:933t
  formation of, VII:929-930, 932f
  Morton, VII:922-923, 923f
  of calcaneal nerve, VII:919-920
  of head and neck, VII:944
  of lower extremity, VII:933, 933f, 936,
    937f, 944-945
  of mandible, V:210
  of medial antebrachial cutaneous nerve,
    VII:901-902

Neuroma (Continued)
  of thorax, VII:943-944
  of upper extremity, VII:937, 938f, 940-
    941, 943f, 944f, 945
  of wrist, VII:940-941, 943f, 944f
  posterior interosseous nerve
    decompression and, VII:904, 906,
    906f
  reflex sympathetic dystrophy and,
    VII:934, 935f
  treatment of, VII:933t, 936-941
    distal target end organ reinnervation
      in, VII:936-939, 937f, 938f
    nerve into bone implantation in,
      VII:941-943
    nerve into muscle implantation in,
      VII:939-941, 940f-944f
    nonoperative, VII:936
    vs. collateral sprouting, VII:931-933, 934f
Neuroma-in-continuity, I:726, 726f,
    VII:483t, 484f, 485, 494, 495f
  in obstetric brachial plexus injury,
    VII:543, 545f, 546
Neuromuscular electrical stimulation, in
    hand therapy, VIII:572
Neuromuscular retraining, in facial
    paralysis, III:891
Neuropathy
  diabetic, VI:1444-1445. See also Diabetes
    mellitus, foot reconstruction in.
  entrapment, VII:875-924, 876t. See also
    Nerve entrapment syndromes.
  in frostbite, VII:652-653
Neurorrhaphy
  end-to-side, VII:505, 532
  in brachial plexus injury, VII:530, 532
Neurotmesis, I:726, 726f, VII:483t, 484f,
    485
Neurotransmitters
  axonal transport of, VII:476-477
  in complex regional pain
    syndrome/reflex sympathetic
    dystrophy, VII:827-828, 837-838
  in pain physiology, III:362-363
Neurotrophins, in nerve regeneration,
    VII:480
Neurotrophism, VII:480-481, 482f
Neurotropism, VII:480-481, 482f
Neurotube, in neuroma treatment,
    VII:936-937, 937f, 938f
Neurovascular territories, I:327-330, 328f,
    329f, 329t
Neutrophils
  in flap reperfusion injury, I:488-494,
    489f, 490f
  in wound healing, I:210, 211f
Nevoid basal cell carcinoma syndrome
    (Gorlin syndrome), III:611-612,
    V:194f, 290, 290f, 398, 398t, 399t
  genetic analysis in, I:62-64, 64f
  midfacial reconstruction in,
    deltopectoral flap for, I:385f-386f
Nevus(i)
  atypical, V:266, 266f, 309, 311f
  blue, V:47, 48f, 264-265, 264f, 308-309,
    VIII:389, 390f
  compound, V:308, 308f
  congenital, V:309, 309f, 310f
  dysplastic (atypical), V:266, 266f, 309,
    311f

Nevus(i) (Continued)
  epidermal, V:256-257
  giant, I:551, 554f
  halo, Color Plate V:114-2, V:265, 265f,
    311, 314f
  intradermal, V:308, 308f
  junctional, V:308, 308f
  melanocytic, V:261-263, 262f
    congenital, V:263-264
  of scalp, III:612
  spindle cell, V:265-266, 265f
  Spitz, V:265-266, 265f
  subungual, VII:196, 198f
  supraorbital, V:351f
  upper extremity, VII:959
  verrucous, V:257, 257f
Nevus sebaceus, Color Plate V:112-2,
    V:257-258, 257f
Nevus sebaceus of Jadassohn, III:611,
    V:257, 281-282, 281f, 282f, 399
Nickel-titanium alloy implant, I:752
Nicotine patch, in upper extremity
    ischemia, VII:802
Nifedipine
  after neck lift, II:322
  in complex regional pain
    syndrome/reflex sympathetic
    dystrophy, VII:856-857
Nikolsky sign, I:795
Nipple(s). See also Nipple reconstruction.
  anatomy of, VI:791, 792f
  artificial, VI:807, 809
  artificial bone implant for, VI:810t, 811
  aspiration of, in breast cancer, Color
    Plate VI:138-3, VI:642-643
  asymmetry of, after breast
    augmentation, VI:342
  autogenous tissue implant for, VI:809,
    810t, 811
  cancer of, VI:661
  costal cartilage implant for, VI:809, 810t,
    811
  hypopigmentation of, after breast
    reduction, VI:556
  implant for, VI:809, 810t, 811
  in breast augmentation, VI:342
  location of, for breast reduction, VI:556
  loss of
    after breast reduction, VI:579
    mastopexy-related, VI:84-85
  malposition of
    after breast reduction, VI:1074-1075,
      1075f, 1076f
    after mastopexy, VI:85
  necrosis of
    after breast reduction, VI:1072, 1074,
      1074f
    after reconstruction, VI:812, 813f
  numbness of, after breast reduction,
    VI:579
  reconstruction of, VI:862, 864f, 865
  sensation in, after breast augmentation,
    VI:29-30
  supernumerary, VI:510, 510t, 512f
Nipple-areola complex, VI:791, 792f. See
    also Areola; Nipple(s).
  fluorescein circulation check in, Color
    Plate VI:132-4, VI:618, 620
  free graft of, VI:620, 621f
  in mastectomy, VI:661

Nipple-areola complex *(Continued)*
    in subcutaneous mastectomy, VI:652
    malposition of, after breast reduction, VI:622, 623f, 624f
    necrosis of, after breast reduction, VI:625
    position of, in inferior pedicle breast reduction, VI:612-615, 613f-614f
    reconstruction of, VI:792-817. *See also* Areola, reconstruction of; Nipple reconstruction.
    sensation of, after breast reduction, VI:611, 625
    vascular anatomy of, Color Plate VI:137-2, VI:606-607, 607f
Nipple graft, for breast reduction, VI:574, 575f-577f, 620
Nipple reconstruction, I:302, VI:862, 864f, 865. *See also* Areola, reconstruction of.
    after TRAM flap breast reconstruction, VI:813, 815f, 985f, 986f, 993
    alloplastic materials in, VI:809
    artificial bone in, VI:810t, 811
    autogenous tissues in, VI:809, 810t, 811
    bell flap for, VI:807, 810f
    complications of, VI:812
    costal cartilage graft for, VI:809, 810t, 811
    dermal fat flap for, VI:796, 797f-799f
    double opposing tab flap for, VI:807, 811f
    ectoprosthesis in, VI:807, 809
    goals of, VI:792, 792t
    local flaps for, VI:794-811, 795t, 797f-805f, 808f-811f
        complications of, VI:812, 813f
    management after, VI:811
    necrosis after, VI:812, 813f
    nipple positioning for, VI:793, 794f
    nipple projection after, VI:812, 812f
    skate flap for, VI:796, 800f-806f, 807
    skin grafts for, I:302, VI:793-794, 794t
    star flap for, VI:807, 808f, 809f
    timing of, VI:792-793
Nitric acid injury, to hand, VII:654
Nitric oxide, in ischemia-reperfusion injury, I:493-494
Nitrofurazone, in burn treatment, I:822
Nitroglycerin, after fetal surgery, I:1120-1121
Nitrous oxide, I:179
No-reflow phenomenon, I:608-609
Nocardia infection, of hand, VII:788
Nodular fasciitis, VII:952-953
Nodules
    in Dupuytren disease, VII:735, 735f
    plantar (Ledderhose disease), VII:737, 738f
NOG gene, VIII:265
Non-Hodgkin lymphoma, V:107
Noncompete clause, I:135
Nonmaleficence, I:101t, 102
Nonsteroidal anti-inflammatory drugs (NSAIDs), I:183-184
    in temporomandibular joint dysfunction, III:542
    in tendon healing, I:595
Norian, I:694t, 701-702
Normothermia, I:186-187

Northern blot, I:55-56
Nose. *See also* at Nasal; Naso-; Rhinoplasty.
    abrasions of, III:29
    acne rosacea of, V:254, 254f
    acquired defects of, III:565, 573, 574f-579f
    adenocarcinoma of, V:111
    adenoid cystic carcinoma of, V:111
    aesthetic analysis of, II:4t, 5t, 8, 11-13, 11f
    agenesis of, III:763, 764, 765f
    airflow through, II:522-524, 523f
    AlloDerm graft in, I:575, 575f
    anatomy of, III:27-29, 187, 188-189, 189f, V:218, 219f
        functional, II:521-524, 521f-523f
        structural, II:519-520, 519f
    arterial supply of, Color Plates I:15-12 and 15-13, I:340-341, 341f, 343, 343t
    avulsion injury of, III:30, 31f
    base of, II:530, 531f, 532f
    bifid, IV:414, 414f
    birth-related injury to, III:398
    bite injury of, III:30, 31f
    blood supply of, III:28-29
    bridge of, II:530, 531f, 532f
    cartilage graft from, I:626
    cartilage of, III:188-189, 189f
    cleft. *See* Cleft nose.
    congenital piriform aperture stenosis of, III:763
    craniopharyngioma of, III:767
    degloving injury to, III:30
    dermoid cyst of, III:765, V:4, 5f
    embryology of, IV:17, 17f
    encephalocele of, III:766
    esthesioneuroblastoma of, V:111-112, 113f
    fracture of, III:187-208. *See also* Nasal fracture.
    glioma of, III:765
    in facial paralysis, III:897
    innervation of, III:28
    laceration of, III:30
    length of, II:475, 476f
    lengthening of, II:505-507, 506f-508f, III:573, 576f-579f
    lower cartilaginous vault of, II:520
    mass of, in children, III:765-767, 765f, 766f
    melanoma of, V:111
    meningoencephalocele of, III:765, 765f
    metastatic tumors of, V:113
    mid-dorsal notch of, II:560, 561f
    middle cartilaginous vault of, II:520
        collapse of (inverted V deformity), II:519, 520f
    nonepidermoid carcinoma of, V:111
    packing of, in pediatric facial trauma, III:397-398
    papilloma of, V:110-111
    paralysis of, III:897
    postnatal growth of, III:388, 389f, 390-391
    prosthetic, Color Plate I:27-4, I:778, 779f
    regional anesthesia of, I:191-192
    resection of, in midface tumors, V:135
    septum of. *See* Nasal septum.

Nose *(Continued)*
    short, lengthening of, II:505-507, 506f-508f
    skin thickness in, II:528, 528f, 529f
    squamous cell carcinoma of, V:111
    teratoma of, III:766, 766f, V:112-113
    tip of, II:492, 494f, 520, 520f, 521f
        contour of, II:528-530, 529f, 530f
        deformity of, after facial burn excision and grafting, III:60-62, 63f
        inadequate projection of, after rhinoplasty, II:780, 781f-784f, 791
        overprojection of, after rhinoplasty, II:784-785
        pink
            after closed rhinoplasty, II:564
            after secondary rhinoplasty, II:797
        projection of, II:532, 534f, 535, 535f
        reconstruction of, V:349, 356f, 358f-363f
        trauma to, III:27-30, 31f. *See also* Nasal fracture.
            anatomy for, III:27-29
            evaluation of, III:6, 29
            nonsurgical management of, III:29
            surgical management of, III:29-30
    tumors of, V:109-113, 110f
    turbinates of, II:524, 527
    upper cartilaginous vault of, II:519
    valves of, II:521, 522f, 526
    vascular anomalies of, V:25, 26f
Notochordal process, IV:2
Nucleic acid analysis, I:55
Nucleus ambiguus, IV:81
Nuland, Sherwin B., I:13
Nuss procedure, in pectus excavatum, VI:469-470, 469f, 470f, 475-477, 477t
Nutrition
    in burn treatment, I:821, 821t
    in toxic epidermal necrolysis, I:798-799

O

Obesity. *See also* Liposuction.
    abdominoplasty and, VI:175, 175t
    microvascular surgery and, I:525
    obstructive sleep apnea and, III:786, 786f
    TRAM flap breast reconstruction and, VI:977-978, 978f, 995
    wound healing and, I:221, 943
Oblique muscles, VI:89, 90f, 91, 1177
Oblique retinacular ligament
    in DIP extension, VII:407-408
    in PIP extension, VII:403, 406f, 407f
Oboeist, hand disorders in, VII:695
O'Brien, Bernard, I:32
Observational study design, I:37-39, 38f-40f
    case-control, I:38, 40f
    case reports, I:38-39
    case series, I:38-39
    cohort, I:37-38, 38f
Obsessive-compulsive personality, I:71-72
Obturator nerve block, I:193-194, 198f
Occipital artery, IV:78f
Occipital artery flap, for neck reconstruction, III:1039, 1039f, 1040
Occipitalis, III:607, 608f

Occlusal plane, II:20f, 21t
Occlusion. *See also* Malocclusion.
  in craniofacial microsomia, IV:546-549,
    547f, 548f
Oculoauriculofrontonasal syndrome,
  III:777
Oculoauriculovertebral sequence
  (Goldenhar syndrome), III:777,
  IV:113, 422, 424f. *See also* Craniofacial
  microsomia.
Odontoameloblastoma, V:98, 200
Odontogenic carcinoma, V:98-99, 204
Odontogenic cysts, V:92-95, 94f, 190t, 191-
  195, 192f, 194f
Odontogenic fibroma, V:98, 201-202
Odontogenic keratinocyst, V:93, 94f, 192-
  193, 194f
Odontogenic myxoma, V:98, 202, 203f
Odontogenic sarcoma, V:204
Odontogenic tumors
  benign, V:190t, 197-204, 198f, 201f, 202f
  malignant, V:190t, 204
Odontoma, V:98, 200-201, 201f
Ohm's law, VII:598-599
Ointments, in burn treatment, I:822
OK-432, in lymphatic malformations, V:45
OKT3, I:274t, 277
Olecranon, for bone graft, I:673t, 684-685
Oligodactyly, postaxial, VIII:21t
Oligohydramnios, constriction ring
  syndrome and, VIII:190
Ollier disease, VII:984-985
Omental flap, I:379, 379t, 579, 580f, 581f
  for back reconstruction, VI:446-447,
    447f
  for cheek reconstruction, I:580f, III:833,
    851f, 852f-853f
  for chest wall reconstruction, Color
    Plate VI:132-2, I:446, VI:417, 424,
    427, 428f, 435-438, 437f, 438f, 990,
    991f
  for cranioplasty, III:557-561, 558f-560f
  for mediastinum reconstruction, I:441,
    581f
  for neck reconstruction, III:1064, 1067-
    1071, 1067f-1071f
  for sternal wound, I:579, 581f
  in craniofacial microsomia, I:579, 580f
Omphalitis, VI:93
Omphalocele, VI:93
  wound healing and, I:945, 947f
Omphalomesenteric duct remnants, VI:93
Oncocytic carcinoma, of salivary glands,
  V:86
Oncocytoma, of salivary glands, V:77-78
Onychocryptosis, VII:204
Onycholysis, VII:185
Onychomycosis, VII:194, 196
OOPS (operation on placental support),
  I:1121, 1121f, 1122
Ophthalmic nerve block, I:191-192, 192f,
  III:8, 8f
Opioid(s), I:181-182, 181t
  in complex regional pain
    syndrome/reflex sympathetic
    dystrophy, VII:859
  preoperative, I:171
Opioid agonist-antagonists, I:182-183
Opponens digiti minimi, VII:32
Opponens pollicis brevis, VII:32

Optic canal, III:272-273, 273t
Optic foramen, III:269, 272-273, 332
Optic nerve
  anatomy of, III:332, 332f, 336-337
  decompression of, V:101, 101f
  glioma of, V:115
  injury to
    anterior, III:337
    in frontobasilar region fracture,
      III:335-338
    posterior, III:337
    treatment of, III:337-338
Oral-antral fistula, in zygoma fracture,
  III:227, 229
Oral cavity. *See also* Lip(s); Oral cavity
  reconstruction; Tongue.
  alveolar ridge of, V:163
  anatomy of, III:36, 919-922, 920f-922f,
    V:163-166, 163f, 164f, 218, 219f
  buccal mucosa of, V:163, 163f
  cancer of, III:917-919, 918f, V:160-162,
    161f. *See also* Oropharyngeal
    cancer.
    biopsy of, V:167
    epidemiology of, V:159-160
    evaluation of, V:167-169
    genetics of, III:918
    in African Americans, III:919
    laboratory studies in, V:169
    malnutrition and, III:918-919
    metastases from, V:160-162, 162f,
      166-167, 167f
    radiology of, V:169
    reconstruction after, V:185
    recurrence of, V:184-185
    rehabilitation after, III:919
    risk factors for, III:918
    surveillance for, III:919
    TNM staging of, V:167-169
    treatment of, V:169, 170, 170t, 174f-
      176f, 177-179
      composite resection with
        mandibulectomy in, V:177,
        179f
      goals of, V:169-170
      lymph node management in,
        V:179, 183-184, 183f
      mandibulotomy in, V:177, 178f
      outcomes of, V:185-186
      pull-through procedure in, V:177
      radiotherapy in, V:183-184
      transoral resection in, V:177, 177f,
        178f
  electrical burns of, III:75
  erythroplakia of, V:160
  evaluation of
    in facial trauma, III:6
    in head and neck cancer, III:923-924
    in temporomandibular joint
      dysfunction, III:542
  floor of, III:922, 922f, V:163f, 164
  functions of, III:922-923, V:166
  hard palate of, V:163f, 164
  leukoplakia of, V:160, 268, 268f, 279
  lichen planus of, V:160
  photography of, I:160, 163f
  premalignant lesions of, V:160
  preoperative evaluation of, I:168, 168f,
    168t
  retromolar trigone of, V:163f, 164

Oral cavity *(Continued)*
  roof of, III:921f, 922
  soft palate of, V:164f, 165
  squamous cell carcinoma of, V:160-162,
    161f
    metastases from, V:160-162, 162f,
      166-167, 167f
  trauma to, III:36-38, 38f
  verrucous carcinoma of, V:162
Oral cavity reconstruction, III:917-954. *See
  also* Lip reconstruction.
  after facial burn excision and grafting,
    III:69, 70f-71f
  algorithm for, III:926-927
  care after, III:949-949
  complications of, III:949-950
  donor site complications of, III:950
  Doppler monitoring for, III:927, 927f
  fistula after, III:950
  flap geometry and, III:952
  flap loss after, III:949-950
  flap necrosis after, III:950
  for alveolar ridges, III:925
  for buccal mucosa, III:925
  for floor of mouth, III:925
  for palate, III:925-926
  for retromolar trigone, III:926
  for tongue, III:924-925, 927-928, 929f,
    941, 942f-944f
  free flaps for, III:934-948, 936f-938f,
    942f-946f, 949f
  goals of, III:924
  hematoma after, III:950
  infection after, III:950
  lateral thigh flap for, III:941-942, 944-
    948, 949f
    advantages of, III:947-948
    anatomy of, III:942, 944
    design of, III:944, 946
    disadvantages of, III:947-948
    dissection of, III:946-947, 948f
  local and regional flaps for, III:928
  motor neurotization after, III:951
  oncologic outcomes after, III:952-953
  pectoralis major flap for, I:424f-425f,
    III:929-932
    advantages of, III:931-932
    anatomy of, III:930, 930f
    design of, III:930-931
    disadvantages of, III:931-932
    dissection of, III:931, 931f, 932f
  platysma flap for, III:932-934, 933f
    advantages of, III:934
    anatomy of, III:934
    design of, III:934
    disadvantages of, III:934
    dissection of, III:934
  preoperative evaluation for, III:923-924
  primary closure for, III:927
  quality of life after, III:953
  radial forearm flap for, III:935-939
    advantages of, III:939
    anatomy of, III:935
    design of, III:935-936, 936f
    disadvantages of, III:939
    dissection of, III:936-939, 937f, 938f
  rectus abdominis flap for, III:939-941,
    942f-946f
    advantages of, III:941
    anatomy of, III:939-940

Oral cavity reconstruction *(Continued)*
design of, III:940, 940f
disadvantages of, III:941
dissection of, III:940-941
results of, III:950-953
revision after, III:950
sensory neurotization after, III:951-952
site-specific, III:924-926
skin grafts for, III:927-928, 929f
xerostomia after, III:952
Orbicular arch redraping, for lower eyelid
ectropion, II:234, 235f
Orbicularis arch, redraping of, II:234, 235f
Orbicularis marginalis flap, for unilateral
cheiloplasty, IV:189, 190f
Orbicularis oculi, II:83, 84f, III:888. *See
also* Eyelid(s).
in brow mobility, II:54, 55f, 56f
inappropriate fat resection from, II:753,
755-756
innervation of, II:218
postblepharoplasty dysfunction of,
II:808
repair of, III:745, 748, 749t
Orbicularis oris, II:218, 220f, III:889. *See
also* Lip(s).
anatomy of, IV:52, 349f
deformities of. *See also* Cleft lip.
after cleft lip repair, IV:347-348, 349f
Orbicularis retaining ligament, II:217, 219f
Orbit. *See also* Eye(s); Globe; Periorbital
surgery.
adenoid cystic carcinoma of, V:127, 134f
anatomy of, II:80, 80f, III:266-273, 267f,
331-332, 332f
anterior, III:266, 267f
middle, III:266, 267f
posterior, III:266, 267f
blood supply to, II:85, 85f
cephalometric analysis of, II:23, 23f
congenital absence of, III:752, 761f, 762
contraction of, III:752, 762
dimensions of, III:267f
esthesioneuroblastoma of, V:111-112,
113f
exenteration of, III:752, 755f-760f
expansion of, in craniofacial cleft
management, IV:429-430, 429f
fat of, III:271-272, 271f
fibrous dysplasia of, V:127, 130f-131f,
144
floor of
anatomy of, III:266-267, 267f
fracture of, III:273, 282f-283f, 297,
299-300, 304. *See also*
Frontobasilar region fracture.
fracture of, III:264-305. *See also* Orbital
fracture.
hollow, after face lift, II:753, 754f, 755f
hypertelorism of, IV:365-379. *See also*
Hypertelorism.
in craniofacial microsomia, IV:120, 122f
irradiation-related defect of, III:582
lateral wall of, III:269, 270
fracture of, III:303-304, 303f, 327-328
lymphoma of, V:114
medial wall of, III:267-269, 268f-269f
fracture of, III:301-303, 302f
melanoma of, V:111, 112f, 115, 116f-
117f

Orbit *(Continued)*
meningioma of, V:127, 128f
metastatic tumors of, V:115
neurofibroma of, V:139-144
group 1, V:140
group 2, V:140-142, 140f-141f
group 3, V:142-144, 142f-143f
neurofibromatosis of, III:565, 573f
postblepharoplasty prominence of,
II:804, 804f
prosthetic, I:778-780, 779f, 780f
rhabdomyosarcoma of, V:114, 114f, 127,
129f
roof of, III:270
anatomy of, III:331-332, 332f
fracture of, III:304-305, 305f-307f,
330-344
clinical manifestations of, III:333-
337
mechanisms of, III:333
squamous cell carcinoma of, V:127,
132f-133f
tumors of, V:113-115, 114f
resection of, V:127-135, 127t, 128f-
133f
walls of, III:267-270, 268f-269f
fracture of, III:269, 270, 301-304,
302f, 303f, 327-328
reconstruction of
in children, III:432
Kawamoto technique (thin cranial
bone graft) in, III:432
Orbital apex syndrome, III:335, 336f
Orbital emphysema, in frontobasilar
region fracture, III:335
Orbital fat, III:271-272, 272f
postblepharoplasty, II:803, 810, 810f,
814
Orbital fissure, superior, III:269
Orbital fracture, III:264-305, 580. *See also*
Frontobasilar region fracture;
Nasoethmoidal-orbital fracture.
blow-in, III:274f, 275f, 281
blowout, III:276-281
classification of, III:288-290, 289f,
290f
computed tomography of, III:269,
270f
diagnosis of, III:286-288, 286f-288f
diplopia in, III:281, 284-285, 325-
326
double-hinged, III:276
enophthalmos in, III:278-281, 285,
286f
extraocular muscle injury in, III:284-
285, 284f, 286f
force transmission in, III:266-267,
267f
forced duction test in, III:288, 288f
globe injury in, III:326-328
globe position in, III:285
globe rupture in, III:288, 289f
impure, III:281, 294-295
in children, III:429, 431-432
intraorbital nerve in, III:290
mechanisms of, III:276-281, 276t,
277t, 278f, 282f-284f
nerve injury in, III:284-285, 290
oculorotatory movements in, III:288-
289, 289f

Orbital fracture *(Continued)*
ophthalmologic examination in,
III:273, 326-327
single-hinged, III:270f, 276
treatment of, III:290-300, 291t
alloplastic implants in, III:296-297,
297f-300f
bone grafts in, III:282f-283f, 295,
296f
diplopia after, III:326
endoscopic, III:292-294, 293f
indications for, III:291, 291t
nonsurgical, III:292
oral-antral fistula closure in,
III:297
orbital floor reconstruction in,
III:295
soft tissue closure in, III:294-295
subperiosteal dissection in, III:294-
295
timing of, III:291-292
volume changes with, III:281
white-eyed, III:290, 290f
with nasoethmoidal-orbital fracture,
III:318f
comminuted, III:300-301
computed tomography in, III:275-276
diagnosis of, III:273, 275-276, 275f
diplopia in, III:275, 277t, 284f
endoscopic treatment of, III:504-507,
505f-507f
contraindications to, III:504
indications for, III:504
results of, III:504-507, 507f
technique of, III:504, 505f, 506f
in children, III:393f-394f, 424-432, 425f-
428f, 429t, 430f-431f, 434-438,
435f-438f
in zygoma fracture, III:210-212, 211f,
212f, 304
inferior oblique muscle in, III:269, 270f,
271f
inferior rectus muscle in, III:269, 270f,
272f
linear, III:297, 299-300
of floor, III:273, 282f-283f, 297, 299-300,
304
of lateral wall, III:269, 270, 303-304,
303f, 327-328
of medial wall, III:301-303, 302f
of roof, III:304-305, 305f-307f, 330-344.
See also Frontobasilar region
fracture.
radiography in, III:275-276
in children, III:426-427, 427f
supraorbital, in children, III:445-448,
445f-448f
trap-door, in children, III:432
with nasoethmoidal-orbital fracture,
III:310
Orbital hypertelorism. *See* Hypertelorism.
Orbital osteotomy, IV:435-439, 436f-
439f
partial, IV:435-436, 437f
total, IV:436, 438f
Orbital rim, postoperative prominence of,
II:804, 804f
Orbital septum, II:83, 84f, 218, 220f,
III:272
Orbitale, II:3f, 3t, 19f, 20t

Orbitomalar septum, II:257, 258f
OrCel, I:893
Organ system failure, wound healing and, I:943-944
Organoids, tissue engineering of, I:1096-1097
Oropharyngeal airway, cuffed, I:176
Oropharyngeal cancer, V:229-236
  biopsy of, V:167
  epidemiology of, V:159-160
  evaluation of, V:167-169
  laboratory studies in, V:169
  neck reconstruction in, III:1039
  radiology of, V:169
  reconstruction after, V:185
  recurrence of, V:184-185
  squamous cell, V:160-162, 161f
    metastases from, V:160-162, 162f, 166-167
  staging of, V:167-169, 229
  treatment of, V:169-170, 179, 180f-182f, 229-235
    glossectomy in, V:236
    goals of, V:169-170
    lateral pharyngectomy in, V:231-233, 232f, 233f, 233t
    lymph node management in, V:179, 183-184, 183f
    mandible-splitting procedures in, V:233-234, 234f, 234t
    mandibulectomy in, V:226f, 235-236, 235t
    midline glossotomy in, V:234, 234f
    outcomes of, V:185-186
    radiotherapy in, V:183-184, 183t
    suprahyoid pharyngectomy in, V:230-231, 230f, 231f, 231t
  verrucous, V:162
Oropharynx. See also Oral cavity.
  anatomy of, V:164-166, 164f, 165f
  cancer of. See Oropharyngeal cancer.
  congenital anomalies of, III:767-768, 767f
  functions of, V:166
Orthodontics. See also Orthognathic surgery.
  cleft lip/palate
    anterior crossbite in, IV:282-283, 284f, 285f
    in infancy, IV:271-280, 274f-282f
    permanent dentition and, IV:290, 292f, 293-308, 293f-295f
    posterior crossbite in, IV:282, 283f
    protrusive premaxilla and, IV:290, 291f, 292f
    transitional dentition in, IV:283, 285f, 286-290, 286f-289f
  in craniofacial cleft, IV:431
  in craniofacial microsomia, IV:546-549, 547f, 548f
Orthognathic surgery, II:649-685
  avascular necrosis after, II:685
  complications of, II:684-685
  dental complications after, II:684
  double-jaw, II:660-662
  hemorrhage after, II:684-685
  historical perspective on, II:649-655, 651f-653f, 653t, 654f, 655f
  mandibular osteotomy in, II:649-651, 651f

Orthognathic surgery (Continued)
  maxillary osteotomy in, II:651-652, 652f
  symphyseal osteotomy in, II:652-653, 653f
  in class III malocclusion, II:658, 658f
  in cleft lip and palate, IV:293, 296-308, 297f-308f
  in craniofacial microsomia, IV:533, 538f-540f, 540-541
  in facial concavity and anterior divergence (class III deformity), II:666, 668-675, 669f-674f
  in facial convexity and posterior divergence (class II deformity), II:663-666, 664f-667f
  in vertical facial deficiency (short-face patient), II:658, 659f, 675, 681f-683f
  in vertical facial excess (long-face patient), II:662f, 675, 676f-680f
  infection after, II:685
  labiomental fold in, II:659
  Le Fort I osteotomy for, II:660, 662f
    prediction tracing for, II:660, 662f
    splint for, II:662
  mandibular advancement surgery for, II:663-666, 664f-667f
    prediction tracing for, II:660, 661f
  maxillary advancement surgery for, II:666, 668-675, 669f-674f
  model surgery for, II:661-662
  neurosensory loss after, II:684
  orthodontic considerations in, II:663
  planning for, II:655-662
    abbreviations for, II:653t
    cephalometric analysis for, II:653-655, 653t
    facial convexity/concavity in, II:656, 657f
    facial disproportion in, II:649f, 658-660, 659f
    facial divergence in, II:656, 656f
    facial morphology in, II:656-658, 656f, 657f
    historical perspective on, II:653-655, 654f, 655f
    prediction tracing in, II:660-661, 661f, 662f
    soft tissue evaluation in, II:656-658
  unfavorable results of, II:659-660
Osler, William, I:12-13
Osseointegration
  in craniofacial cleft management, IV:446, 449f
  of facial prosthesis, Color Plate I:27-2, I:773-774, 773f, 774f
  of prosthetic ear, I:777
Ossification, heterotopic, burn-related, I:829-830, VII:635-636
Osteitis
  after mandibular fracture treatment, III:182
  radiation, I:841, 844f
Osteoarthritis
  in temporomandibular joint dysfunction, III:541
  of hand, VII:707-725. See also Hand(s), osteoarthritis of.
Osteoarthrosis, in temporomandibular joint dysfunction, III:539, 540f

Osteoblastoma, V:11-12, 99, 205, VII:986
Osteoblasts, I:641t, 642-645, 642f, 643f
  differentiation of, I:643-645
  platelet-derived growth factor effects on, I:667
  transforming growth factor-β effects on, I:664
Osteocalcin, I:648, 649t, 650
Osteochondroma, VII:985, 985f, 986f
Osteoclast, I:641t, 646-648, 647f
Osteoclast differentiation factor, I:647-648
Osteoclastogenesis inhibitory factor, I:648
Osteocyte, I:641t, 645-646, 645f
Osteogenic protein 1, I:662, 663
Osteogenic sarcoma, VII:988, 990, 990f
Osteoma, V:99, 205
  osteoid, V:11-12, 99, 205, VII:985-986, 986f
Osteomyelitis, VI:1385-1387
  after mandibular fracture treatment, III:182
  classification of, VI:1386-1387, 1387f
  diagnosis of, VI:1386
  in diabetes mellitus, VI:1446
  of arm, VII:324-326, 327f
  of back, VI:450
  of foot, VI:1415, 1417, 1440, 1440f, 1443
  of hands, VII:65f, 784, 789
  of lower extremity, VI:1367-1368, 1368f
  of neck, III:1076
  of wrist, VII:78, 78f
  pressure sores and, VI:1320-1321
  squamous cell carcinoma and, V:275
  wound healing and, I:914-915, 915f, 977, 978f, 979f
Osteonectin, I:648, 649t
Osteopontin, I:648, 649t
Osteoporosis, Sudeck, VII:827, 836, 836f. See also Complex regional pain syndrome/reflex sympathetic dystrophy.
Osteoradionecrosis, I:841-842, 845f
  of chest wall, I:910-911, 911f, 967, 972f-973f
  of lower extremity, I:974, 975f
  of mandible, I:918, 918f, 967, 968f-969f
  of sacrum, VI:448, 450, 451f
  wound healing and, I:967, 968f-969f, 972f-973f, 974, 975f-976f
Osteosarcoma, V:104, 106, 106f, 210-211
  in children, V:15
  juxtacortical, V:211
OsteoSet, I:1101t
Osteotendinous junction, I:594
Osteotomy, IV:433, 435-446
  facial bipartition, IV:439, 439f
  fronto-orbital, IV:435, 436f
  in central polydactyly, VIII:243-244, 244f
  inverted ramus, IV:444, 444f
  Le Fort I, IV:439, 441, 441f. See also at Le Fort.
  Le Fort II, IV:439, 440f
  Le Fort III, IV:439, 439f
  mandibular, IV:441, 443-444, 443f, 444f
  midface, IV:439-446, 439f-445f
  orbital, IV:435-439, 436f-439f
  partial orbital, IV:435-436, 437f
  sagittal split ramus, IV:441, 443, 443f
  segmental maxillary, IV:441, 442f

Osteotomy (*Continued*)
  total orbital, IV:436, 438f
  vertical subsigmoid ramus, IV:443-444, 444f
Otitis media, cleft palate and, IV:256
Otohematoma, III:32-33, 32f, 677
Otx2, IV:2
Outcomes research, I:35-48
  best practices and, I:46-47
  case series and, I:47
  collaborative research and, I:47
  data simulation in, I:44-45
  database analysis in, I:42-44, 43t
  evidence in, I:36f, 36t, 37-45
    experimental study design and, I:37
    literature evaluation and, I:37
    observational study design and, I:37-39, 38f-40f
    study design and, I:37-39, 38f-40f
  expert opinion and, I:47
  health-related quality of life and, I:41-42, 42f, 42t
  high-volume centers and, I:48
  in head and neck cancer, V:185-186
  meta-analysis in, I:45, 46f
  patient-oriented, I:39-41, 40f, 41t
  patient preference and, I:41-42, 43f
  physician profiling and, I:47-48
  quality of life model for, I:45-46
  questionnaires and, I:47
  randomized trials and, I:47
Overexertion, cold injury and, I:857
Oxalic acid injury, to hand, VII:654, 656
Oxidizing agent injury, to hand, VII:653-654, 653t
Oxygen
  consumption of
    altitude sickness and, I:861
    hypothermia and, I:187
  face mask administration of, I:175-176
  hyperbaric, I:952-954, 954f
    in Fournier disease, VI:1253
    in ischemic wounds, I:492
    in mandible reconstruction, III:960
    in smoke inhalation, I:832
    in wound healing, I:893, 895-897
  nasal cannula administration of, I:175
  tissue, wound healing and, I:902, 904f, 944
Oxygen tension, transcutaneous, for flap monitoring, I:497-498, 497t

P

p53 gene, skin cancer and, Color Plate V:116-1, V:277, 393
Pacinian corpuscles, in nerve injury, VII:482
Padgett, Earl, I:31
Paget disease, Color Plate V:113-11, V:295, 295f
Pain. *See also* Complex regional pain syndrome/reflex sympathetic dystrophy; Nerve entrapment syndromes.
  after breast augmentation, VI:352-355
  after breast reduction, VI:578
  after neck lift, II:320
  after peripheral nerve repair, VII:505
  after TRAM flap breast reconstruction, VI:1014

Pain (*Continued*)
  epidural catheter for, I:195-196
  etomidate-related, I:175
  facial, III:361-366. *See also* Facial nerve, injury to.
  in burn treatment, I:828
  in de Quervain syndrome, VII:678
  in head and neck cancer, V:226
  in scars, I:239
  nerve blocks for, III:365, VII:853-854
  neurolysis for, III:366
  physiology of, III:362-363
  postmastectomy, VI:665
  postoperative, I:201
  propofol-related, I:174
  with brachial plexus injury, VII:525
  with condylar process fracture, III:515
  with infraorbital nerve injury, III:361
Palatal plane, II:20f, 21t
Palatal plexus, IV:80f
Palatal split sequence, in craniofacial clefts, IV:422
Palate. *See also* Palatoplasty.
  anatomy of, IV:57-67, 69-82, 351-352, 352f
    muscular, IV:57-64, 58f, 59f, 72-76, 73f-75f, 77f
    neural, IV:65, 81-82
    on magnetic resonance imaging, IV:65, 66f, 67f
    osseous, IV:57, 57f, 58f, 70-71, 70f, 71f
    vascular, Color Plate I:15-13, I:343-344, 343t, IV:64-65, 76-81, 78f-80f
  bones of, IV:57, 57f, 58f, 70-71, 70f, 71f
  cleft. *See* Cleft palate.
  cyst of, V:94
  embryology of, IV:6-8, 7f
  fistula of, IV:263, 264f, 352-354, 353f, 355f
  hard, III:921f, 922, V:163f, 164
  lengthening of, in velopharyngeal dysfunction, IV:332
  levator veli palatini muscle of, IV:58f, 59f, 60-61, 60t, 61f
  life-type prosthesis for, in velopharyngeal dysfunction, IV:332-333
  magnetic resonance imaging of, IV:65, 66f, 67f
  mucosa of, IV:69-70
  muscles of, IV:57-64, 58f, 59f, 72-76, 73f-75f, 77f
  nerves of, IV:65, 81-82
  palatoglossus muscle of, IV:58f, 59f, 60t, 63-64
  palatopharyngeus muscle of, IV:58f, 59f, 60t, 62-63, 63f
  Passavant ridge of, IV:69, 73f
  pharyngeal constrictor muscles of, IV:58f, 59f, 60t, 64, 64f
  reconstruction of, III:925-926. *See also* Oral cavity reconstruction; Palatoplasty.
  salpingopharyngeus muscle of, IV:58f, 59f, 60t, 62
  soft, III:921f, 922, V:164f, 165
  surface anatomy of, IV:69-70
  tensor veli palatini muscle of, IV:58f, 59f, 61-62, 62f
  uvular muscle of, IV:58f, 59f, 60t, 62, 63f
  vascular anatomy of, IV:76-81, 78f-80f

Palatine artery, IV:77, 78f, 79f, 80-81
Palatine bone, IV:70f, 71
Palatine nerve, IV:79f, 82
Palatine neurovascular bundle, in palatoplasty, IV:258
Palatoglossus, IV:58f, 59f, 60t, 63-64, 75, 79f, 312f
Palatopharyngeus, IV:58f, 59f, 60t, 62-63, 63f, 73f, 74f, 75, 79f, 312f
Palatoplasty, IV:253-262
  alveolar bone grafting with, IV:263-266, 265f
  bleeding with, IV:263
  double opposing Z-plasty technique of, IV:259-261, 261f
  fistula formation with, IV:263, 264f, 352-354, 353f, 355f
  greater palatine neurovascular bundle in, IV:258
  in Robin sequence, IV:251-253, 252f
  intravelar veloplasty with, IV:261, 262f
  outcomes of, IV:262-263
  patient preparation for, IV:257-258, 257f
  primary pharyngeal flap with, IV:262
  pushback (Veau-Wardill-Kilner) technique of, IV:258-259, 259f
  respiratory depression with, IV:263
  timing of, IV:256-257
  two-flap technique of, IV:259, 260f
  two-stage, IV:262
  vomer flaps with, IV:261-262
  von Langenbeck technique of, IV:258, 258f
Palatothyroideus, IV:74f
Palmar metacarpal flap, reverse-flow, for finger reconstruction, VII:228, 228f
Palmaris brevis, VII:32
Palmaris tendon, I:599
  transfer of, for low median nerve palsy, VIII:466, 467f, 468f
Palpebral arteries, II:85, 85f
Palpebral spring, in lagophthalmos, III:893-894, 894f
Palsy
  Bell, I:613-614, 614f, III:749f
  brachial plexus, VII:516-535, 539-562. *See also* Brachial plexus injury.
  Erb, VII:540, 540f, 550f
  mandibular nerve, III:911-912, 913f
  median nerve, VIII:462-470, 463f-468f
  radial nerve, VIII:455-462, 456t, 457-461f, 466
  ulnar nerve, VIII:471-472, 472f, 475-476, 476f, 479, 481-482
Pancuronium, I:180t
Panfacial fracture. *See* Maxillary fracture, complex (panfacial).
Panniculectomy, VI:101-104, 102f-104f, 137, 138f
Panoramic tomography, of condylar process fracture, III:516-517, 517f, 529, 530f
Panorex exam, in pediatric facial trauma, III:395, 396f
Papilledema, in craniosynostosis, IV:475
Papilloma, of nasal cavity, V:110-111
Papillomatosis, juvenile, V:16
Paradental cyst, V:94, 195
Paraffin, in hand therapy, VIII:571

Paralysis. *See also* Palsy; Tetraplegia.
 cold injury and, I:857
 hysterical, vs. reflex sympathetic
  dystrophy/chronic regional pain
  syndrome, VII:848
Paranasal sinuses. *See also specific sinuses.*
 adenocarcinoma of, V:111
 adenoid cystic carcinoma of, V:111
 metastatic tumors of, V:113
 papilloma of, V:110-111
 postnatal development of, III:386f, 387-
  388, 388f
 squamous cell carcinoma of, V:111
 teratoma of, V:112-113
 tumors of, V:109-113, 110f, 247-249, 248f
Paranoid personality, I:72
Parascapular flap, for hemifacial atrophy,
 IV:559-560, 560f, 562f-565f, 568f
Paratenon, I:591, 592f
Parkes Weber syndrome, V:60, 60f,
 VIII:309, 312f, 412-413, 413t
Paronychia, VII:771, 777, 778f
Parotid duct
 anatomy of, II:170, 171f
 trauma to, III:26-27, 27f, 28f
Parotid gland. *See also* Salivary glands.
 anatomy of, II:302, 304f, III:26, V:69, 70f
 arterial supply of, I:344
 innervation of, V:71f
Parotid-masseteric fascia, II:162f, 165
Parotidectomy, Frey syndrome and, V:87-
 88, 88f
Parsonage-Turner syndrome, VII:881
Passavant ridge, IV:69, 73f
Passot procedure, in breast reduction,
 VI:539, 540f
Pasteurella multocida infection, of hand,
 VII:763
patched gene, I:62-64, 64f
Patient history
 medication, I:170
 psychiatric, I:81-87, 82t, 83t, 84t, 85t
 surgical, I:170
Patient position, I:187-189, 188f. *See also at*
 specific procedures.
 lateral decubitus, I:188f, 189
 standard prone, I:188-189, 188f
Pectoralis major, absence of, in Poland
 syndrome, VI:432
Pectoralis major flap, I:423, 423f
 for cheek reconstruction, III:833, 845f,
  848f
 for chest wall reconstruction, I:441,
  445f, VI:414, 416, 416f-419f, 426-
  427, 427f, 990
 for esophageal reconstruction, I:426f-
  427f, III:1008-1011, 1009f, 1010f,
  1014
 for facial reconstruction, I:390, 391f,
  392f, 423, 423f-427f, III:833, 845f,
  848f
 for head and neck reconstruction, I:423,
  423f-427f, III:1052-1054, 1052f-
  1054f, V:221-222, 222f, 226t
 for mandible reconstruction, III:962,
  963f
 for mediastinum reconstruction, I:440-
  441, 442f-444f
 for oral cavity reconstruction, I:424f-
  425f, III:929-932, 930f-932f

Pectoralis major flap *(Continued)*
 for pharyngoesophageal fistula, I:426f-
  427f, 970f-971f
 segmental, I:384, 387, 388f, 389f
 vascularized bone with, I:390, 391f, 392f
Pectoralis transfer, in radial deficiency,
 VIII:75, 76f
Pectus carinatum, VI:432, 477-478, 479f,
 480f
Pectus excavatum, VI:431-432, 458-477
 aesthetic considerations in, VI:461
 cardiac function in, VI:461
 classification of, VI:461, 462f, 462t
 clinical presentation of, VI:459, 460f
 computed tomography in, VI:459, 460f,
  462f
 etiology of, VI:458
 evaluation of, VI:458, 459f
 Haller index in, VI:459, 460f
 incidence of, VI:458
 physiology of, VI:459-461, 461t
 psychological considerations in, VI:459,
  461
 respiration in, VI:460-461, 461t
 severity index in, VI:459, 460f
 treatment of, VI:461, 463-477, 477t
  bioabsorbable mesh in, VI:471, 475,
   475t
  complications of, VI:477, 477t
  custom implant in, VI:463, 464f, 470-
   471, 472f
  in mild defects, VI:463
  in severe defects, VI:463
  indications for, VI:461, 463
  minimally invasive, VI:469-470, 469f,
   470f, 475-477
  Nuss procedure in, VI:469-470, 469f,
   470f, 475-477, 477t
  plates and screws in, VI:475
  principles of, VI:463, 464f, 465f
  Ravitch procedure in, VI:463, 466f-
   468f, 469, 475, 476t, 477t
  resection and sternal fixation in,
   VI:471, 473-475, 473f, 474f, 475t
  results of, VI:475-477, 476t
  silicone implants in, VI:470-471,
   472f
  timing of, VI:461, 463
 tuberous breasts with, VI:463, 465f
 ventilatory mechanics in, VI:460
Peer review, I:133-134
Pelvic tilt, age-related, VI:259, 260f
Pelvis
 age-related tilt of, VI:259, 260f
 pressure sores of, VI:1347, 1349, 1349f
Pen-phen, I:170
Penile reconstruction
 after cancer surgery, VI:1255
 artificial erection for, VI:1218, 1221
 fasciocutaneous flaps for, VI:1226-1227
 flaps for, VI:1223, 1225f-1228f, 1226-
  1227
 in agenesis, VI:1218, 1220f
 in balanitis xerotica obliterans, VI:1253-
  1254, 1254f
 in buried penis, VI:1213, 1214f-1216f
 in chordee, VI:1208, 1210-1212, 1211f,
  1212f
 in epispadias, VI:1207-1208, 1208f
 in Fournier disease, VI:1250-1253

Penile reconstruction *(Continued)*
 in gender identity disorder, Color Plate
  VI:156-2, VI:1308-1310, 1310f,
  1311f
 in hypospadias of, VI:1259-1277. *See*
  also Hypospadias.
 in lipoid lymphogranuloma, VI:1256
 in lymphedema, VI:1255-1256
 in male pseudohermaphroditism,
  VI:1213
 in micropenis, VI:1213, 1216-1218,
  1217f, 1217t
 in penoscrotal transposition, VI:1218,
  1222f
 in Peyronie disease, VI:1248-1250,
  1251f, 1252f
 in skin cancer, VI:1254-1255
 in trauma-related injury, VI:1218, 1221,
  1224f
 in true pseudohermaphroditism, VI:1213
 meshed split-thickness graft
  urethroplasty in, VI:1246, 1246t,
  1247f-1249f
 microsurgical, VI:1228, 1230-1245
  aesthetic considerations in, VI:1242-
   1243
  donor site morbidity in, VI:1243,
   1244f
  for phallic construction, Color Plate
   VI:156-2, VI:1235-1245, 1236f-
   1238f, 1240f, 1241t, 1242f-1244f,
   1310, 1311f
  for replantation, VI:1228, 1230-1232,
   1230f-1233f
  for revascularization, VI:1232, 1234-
   1235
  forearm flap for, VI:1235-1237, 1236f,
   1238f, 1240f
  historical perspective on, VI:1235-
   1239, 1236f-1238f, 1239t
  in children, VI:1243-1245
  prostheses in, VI:1239, 1241, 1241t
  sensory preservation in, VI:1239
  technique of, VI:1235-1245, 1236f-
   1238f, 1240f, 1241t, 1242f-1244f
  testicular autotransplantation with,
   VI:1245-1246, 1245f
  urethral reconstruction in, VI:1239
 musculocutaneous flaps for, VI:1227,
  1229f
 principles of, VI:1246, 1246t, 1247f-
  1249f
 sequelae of, VI:1246, 1246t, 1247f-1249f
 Singapore flaps for, VI:1226-1227, 1229f
 skin grafts in, VI:1221, 1223, 1224f
 thigh flaps for, VI:1226-1227, 1229f
Penis, VI:389-404
 agenesis of, VI:1218, 1220f
 AlloDerm grafts for, VI:395
  complications of, VI:398, 399
 anatomy of, VI:390-391, 1261
 blood supply of, VI:1201-1204, 1201f-
  1205f
 Buck's fascia of, VI:1199, 1199f
 buried. *See* Penis, hidden.
 cancer of, VI:1254-1255
 chordee of, VI:1208, 1210-1212, 1211f,
  1212f, 1260-1261
 circumcision-related necrosis of,
  VI:1217-1218, 1219f

Penis (Continued)
circumference of, VI:389-390
Colles' fascia of, VI:1200, 1200f
construction of, in female-to-male transformation, VI:1308-1310, 1309f, 1310f
curvature of, VI:390, 1208, 1210-1212, 1211f, 1212f
dartos fascia of, VI:1199, 1199f
dermal fat grafts for, VI:394-395, 394f
complications of, VI:397-398, 398f, 399
embryology of, VI:1198, 1199f, 1261, 1263f
epispadic, VI:1207-1208
examination of, VI:390
fascia of, VI:1199-1200, 1199f, 1200f
fat injections of, I:584, VI:393
complications of, VI:396-397, 397f, 398f
Fournier disease of, VI:1250-1253
girth increase in, VI:393-395, 394f, 395f
complications of, VI:396-399, 397f, 398f
glans of, VI:1199
hidden, VI:401f, 402-403, 403f, 404f, 1213, 1214f-1216f
hypospadias of, VI:1259-1277. See also Hypospadias.
inversion of, in male-to-female transformation, Color Plate VI:156-5, VI:1312
length of, VI:389-390
lengthening of, VI:391-393, 391f, 392f
complications of, VI:395-396, 396f, 397f, 398-399
results of, VI:392-393, 393f
lipoid lymphogranuloma of, VI:1256
lymphatic supply of, VI:1206
lymphedema of, VI:1255-1256, 1464
measurement of, VI:389-390
micro-, VI:1213, 1216-1218, 1217f, 1217t
nerve supply of, VI:1205-1206, 1206f
Peyronie disease of, VI:1248-1250, 1251f, 1252f, VII:737
prosthetic, infection with, I:919, 921
protective withdrawal of, VI:1198-1199
reconstruction of. See Penile reconstruction.
replantation of, VI:1228, 1230-1232, 1230f-1233f
revascularization of, VI:1232, 1234-1235
Scarpa's fascia of, VI:1199, 1200f
scrotalization of, VI:396, 396f
skin cancer of, VI:1254-1255
skin of, VI:390-391
stretching devices for, VI:392-393, 393f
suspensory ligament of, VI:390
release of, VI:391-393, 391f-393f
trauma to, VI:1218, 1221, 1224f
tunical tissues of, VI:1199, 1199f
V-Y flap for, VI:391-393, 391f, 392f
reversal of, VI:398-399
venous system of, VI:1202-1203, 1204f, 1205f
Penoscrotal transposition, VI:1218, 1222f
Penoscrotal web, VI:399-402
Z-plasty for, VI:400f, 401-402
Pentalogy of Cantrell, VI:483-484

Pentoxifylline
in diabetes mellitus, VI:1445-1446
in frostbite, VII:652
Perforator flaps, I:355-358, 377, 379, 526-527, 527f. See also Microvascular surgery.
axes of, I:355-356, 356f
dimensions of, I:356-358, 357f, 358f
necrosis of, I:357
nomenclature for, I:479
surgical delay for, I:357-358, 357f, 358f
Perialar crescentic flap, for upper lip reconstruction, V:379f, 381
Periapical cemental dysplasia, V:98
Periarterial sympathectomy, in vasospastic disease, VII:817-818, 818f, 819f
Pericardiocentesis, fetal, I:1126
Perichondrium
for cartilage graft, I:626
simulation of, for bioengineered cartilage graft, Color Plate I:23-4, I:633, 634f
Pericranium, III:16, 607, 608f
Perilunate ligament instability, VII:467, 467f
Perineum
impaired wound healing of, I:967, 974f, 990, 992f, 993
reconstruction of, I:448, 451-454, 451f, 452f, 990, 992f, 993, 993f-994f
Periodic breathing, III:775
Periodontal cyst, V:93, 94
Periodontal plexus, IV:80f
Perionychium, VII:171-204
absence of, VII:171, 185, 188, 188f
amputation of, VII:180-182
anatomy of, VII:154, 154f, 171, 172f
basal cell carcinoma of, VII:201, 201f
cornified, VII:188, 189f, 190f
cysts of, VII:188, 191, 200
embryology of, VII:171
function of, VII:173
ganglion of, VII:196-188, 198f, 199f
giant cell tumors of, VII:200
glomus tumors of, VII:198, 200
growth of, VII:173
hematoma of, VII:175, 177
hooked, VII:191, 191f
in distal phalanx fracture, VII:180, 181f
in syndactyly, VIII:168
infection of, VII:192-196
bacterial, VII:194, 195f
epidemiology of, VII:192-193
fungal, VII:194, 196
viral, VII:194, 196f
inflammatory lesions of, VII:200
ingrown, VII:204
injury to, VII:173-192
assessment and management of, VII:175, 177-182, 177f-181f
epidemiology of, VII:173-175, 176f
in children, VIII:426
keratoacanthoma of, VII:200
Kutz elevator for, VII:177, 177f
laceration of, VII:177-178, 177f-181f
melanoma of, VII:201-203, 201f, 967-968
nerve supply of, VII:172-173
physiology of, VII:173, 173f-175f
pigmented lesions of, VII:196, 197f, 198f

Perionychium (Continued)
pincer deformity of, VII:202f, 203-204, 203f
prosthetic, VIII:589, 590f
reconstruction of, VII:182-192, 242, 242f
in anonychia, VII:185, 188, 188f
in cornified nail bed, VII:188, 189f, 190f
in eponychial deformities, VII:191-192, 192f
in fingertip amputations, VII:180-182
in hooked nail, VII:191, 191f
in hyponychial defects, VII:192, 193f
in nail spikes and cysts, VII:188, 191
in onycholysis, VII:185
in split nail, VII:182-185, 183f, 184f, 186f-187f
ridges of, VII:181f, 182
spikes of, VII:188, 191
split, VII:182-185, 183f, 184f, 186f-187f
squamous cell carcinoma of, VII:200-201, 200f
subungual hematoma of, VII:175, 177
transverse ridges of, VII:182
tumors of, VII:196-203
benign, VII:196-200, 197f-199f
malignant, VII:200-203, 200f-203f
vascularity of, VII:171-172
Periorbita, III:272
Periorbital fat, herniation of, II:218
Periorbital surgery, II:77-125. See also at Canthus; Eyebrow(s); Eyelid(s); and specific extraocular muscles and specific disorders.
aesthetic considerations in, II:77-80, 78f, 78t, 79f
anatomy for, II:80-86, 80f-86f
patient evaluation for, II:89-94
contact lens wear and, II:89-90
dry eyes and, II:90
exophthalmos and, II:90
external ocular examination in, II:91-92
extraocular muscle examination in, II:93
eyebrow examination in, II:91
eyelid examination in, II:91-92
four-finger lift in, II:89
globe examination in, II:93
lateral canthal tendon in, II:91-92, 92f
malar eminence in, II:92-93, 92f
observational examination in, II:89
ocular examination in, II:90-94
orbital examination in, II:92-93, 92f
patient history in, II:89-90, 90t
photoface reflex and, II:79-80, 79f, 88
photography in, II:94, 94t
pupils examination in, II:93
refractive surgery and, II:90
retinal examination in, II:93
Schirmer test in, II:93-94, 93f
tear film examination in, II:93-94, 93f
tear trough test in, II:92-93, 92f
visual acuity in, II:90-91
visual field examination in, II:90
planning for, II:94-97, 94t
brow position and, II:95
enophthalmos and, II:96

Periorbital surgery *(Continued)*
  exophthalmos and, II:96
  eyelid ptosis and, II:95-96
  hypoplastic supraorbital rim and, II:96
  lower eyelid tonicity and, II:95
  suborbital malar hypoplasia and,
    II:96-97
  supraorbital rim prominence and,
    II:96
  tear trough deformity and, II:97, 97f
secondary, II:801-822
  for failure to correct, II:801-807, 802t,
    804f, 805f-807f
  for iatrogenic defects, II:807-813,
    807t, 808f, 808t, 809f-812f
  for progressive degenerative changes,
    II:813-814, 813t
  techniques of, II:814-821, 816f, 817f,
    819f-821f
    for lower repair, II:817-821, 817t,
      819f-821f
    for upper repair, II:815-817, 815t,
      816f, 817f
Periosteoplasty, IV:181
Periosteum, I:639-640, 640f
  facial, II:162f, 166-167
  in bone graft, I:677
  in cartilage graft, I:626
  in primary bone repair, I:652
Peripheral nerve(s), I:719-739. *See also*
    specific nerves.
  anatomy of, VII:472-475, 473f, 474f
  artery relation to, I:327-329, 328f, 345-
    347, 346f
  awake stimulation of, VII:492, 494
  axoplasmic transport of, VII:476-477
  biopsy of, in muscle transfer, VIII:494
  blood-nerve barrier of, I:720, 722f,
    VII:475-476
  blood supply of, VII:475-476, 476f
  chromatolysis of, VII:478-479, 478f
  collateral sprouting of, VII:931-933,
    934f
  degeneration of, Color Plate I:25-1,
    I:723-724, 724f, VII:877-878, 878t,
    929-930, 932f
  embryology of, I:720
  entrapment of, VII:875-924. *See also*
    Nerve entrapment syndromes.
  epineurium of, I:721, 722f
  excursion of, VII:477
  fascicular patterns of, VII:475
  fibers of, VII:472-475, 473f, 474f
  gross anatomy of, VII:472, 473f
  growth factor effects on, I:723, 723f
  histologic staining of, VII:494
  injury to, I:723-724, 724f, VII:477-509,
    929-930, 932f. *See also* Nerve
    entrapment syndromes; Peripheral
    nerve repair and reconstruction.
    cellular response to, VII:477-481, 478f
    classification of, I:725-726, 726f,
      VII:482-486, 483t, 484f
    closed, VII:488, 489f
    compression with, VII:477
    computed tomography in, I:729, 730f
    degenerative change with, Color Plate
      I:25-1, I:723-724, 724f
    electrodiagnostic testing in, I:727-
      729, 728t, VII:486-488

Peripheral nerve(s) *(Continued)*
    electromyography in, I:727-728, 728t,
      VII:487
    electroneuronography in, I:728, 728t
    end-organ response to, VII:481-482
    evaluation of, I:726-727, 727t,
      VII:486-488, 487f
    fifth-degree (neurotmesis), I:726,
      726f, VII:483t, 484f, 485
    first-degree (neurapraxia), I:725, 726f,
      VII:483, 483t, 484f
    fourth-degree (neurotmesis), I:726,
      726f, VII:483t, 484f, 485
    imaging studies in, I:729, 730f
    in children, VIII:427-428
    in musician, VII:701, 702-703
    longitudinal patterns of, VII:485-486
    magnetic resonance imaging in, I:729,
      730f
    motor responses to, VII:481-482
    nerve conduction study in, I:728t,
      729, VII:486-487, 494
    open, VII:490, 490f
    patient history in, VII:486, 487f
    perceptual recovery after, I:724, 727,
      727t
    repair of. *See* Peripheral nerve repair
      and reconstruction.
    second-degree (axonotmesis), I:725,
      726f, VII:483, 483t, 484f
    sensory nerve action potentials in,
      VII:487
    sensory responses to, VII:482
    sixth-degree (neuroma-in-continuity),
      I:726, 726f, VII:483t, 484f, 485,
      494, 495f, 543, 545f, 546
    somatosensory evoked potentials in,
      I:728t, 729
    third-degree (axonotmesis), I:725-
      726, 726f, VII:483t, 484-485,
      484f
    tourniquet-related, VII:117
    two-point discrimination test in,
      I:727
    vibratory threshold testing in, I:727
    wallerian degenerative change with,
      I:723-724, 724f
  monofascicular, VII:472, 474f
  morphology of, I:720-723, 722f
  motor end plate of, I:723
  motor pathways of, VII:472, 473f
  myelination of, I:720
  neurotropism of, VII:480-481, 482f
  oligofascicular, VII:472, 474f
  perineurium of, I:720-721
  physiology of, I:720-723, 721f-723f,
    VII:475-477
  polyfascicular, VII:472, 474f
  regeneration of, I:724, 725f, VII:477-
    481, 478f, 482f
    Tinel sign in, I:727
  sensory pathways of, VII:472, 473f
  serial evaluation of, I:730
  sympathetic pathways of, VII:472, 473f
  tissue-engineered, I:1091-1093, 1093t,
    1094f
  topography of, I:721-723, 722f, VII:475
  tourniquet-related injury to, VII:117
  transfer of, I:282, VII:503-505, 504f
  vascularity of, I:723

Peripheral nerve repair and
    reconstruction, I:719-739, VII:490-
    505
  adhesives in, I:733
  after cancer-related radiation therapy,
    I:738
  after radical retropubic prostatectomy,
    Color Plate I:25-3, I:737-738
  algorithms for, VII:488-490, 489f, 490f
  amnion tubes in, I:735
  awake stimulation in, VII:492, 494
  biodegradable nerve conduit in, I:735
  blood flow assessment in, VII:491
  coaptation sutures for, I:731, 732f
  electrophysiologic monitoring after,
    VII:506
  end-to-side neurorrhaphy in, I:733,
    VII:505
  epineurial, I:731-732, 732f, VII:491-492,
    493f
  fascicular, I:731-732, 732f, VII:491-492,
    493f
  fascicular identification in, VII:492, 494
  gene therapy in, I:738-739
  histologic staining in, VII:494
  historical perspective on, I:719-720
  in brachial plexus injury, I:736-737
  in facial nerve injury, I:737, 737t
  in lower extremity, I:736
  in neuroma-in-continuity, VII:494, 495f
  in upper extremity, I:735-736, 737t
  intraoperative nerve conduction study
    in, VII:494
  lasers in, I:733
  management after, I:738, VII:505-507
  microelectrodes in, I:739
  microsurgical, VII:491-492, 493f
  motor retraining after, I:738, VII:507
  nerve allograft in, I:735, VII:500-503,
    501f, 502f
  nerve conduction study in, VII:494
  nerve gap in, VII:494-505, 496f
  nerve graft in, I:733-735, 734f, 734t,
    737t, VII:493f, 494-503, 498f, 501f,
    502f, 509. *See also* Nerve graft.
  nerve transfer in, VII:503-505, 504f
  neurolysis in, I:732
  non-neural conduits in, I:735, 738,
    VII:499-500
  outcomes of, I:735-738, 737t, VII:507-
    509, 507t
  pain management after, VII:505
  pedicled nerve graft in, VII:498-499
  postoperative compression and, VII:506
  primary, I:731, 732f
  principles of, I:731-733, 732f
  rehabilitation after, I:738
  sensory re-education after, VII:506-507
  silicone nerve conduit in, I:735
  splinting after, VII:505
  sutures for, I:731, 732f
  tension and, I:731, VII:491
  Tinel sign after, VII:506
  tissue engineering in, I:738-739
  vascularized nerve graft in, I:733-734,
    734t, VII:499
  vein grafts in, I:735
Peripheral vascular disease, cold injury
    and, VII:648
Peritoneum, VI:1175-1176

Peritonsillar abscess, V:2

Peroneal artery, Color Plates I:15-8 to 15-10, I:338

Peroneal nerve
common, compression of, VII:910, 912, 913f-915f
deep, compression of, VII:876t, 915-917, 916f
repair of, I:736
superficial, compression of, VII:912, 915

Peroneus brevis, arterial supply of, Color Plates I:15-9 and 15-11, I:338

Peroneus longus, arterial supply of, Color Plates I:15-9 and 15-11, I:338

Personality, I:69-70
borderline, I:72-73
demanding, I:74
dependent, I:72, 73
hateful, I:73
help-rejecting, I:74
histrionic, I:72
manipulative, I:74
narcissistic, I:71-72
obsessive-compulsive, I:71
of dissatisfied patient, I:87, 87t
paranoid, I:72
self-destructive, I:73-74
types of, I:71-73

Petechiae, with laser resurfacing, II:376

Petrosectomy, V:148-149

Petrous bone, carcinoma of, V:148-149

Peyronie disease, VI:1248-1250, 1251f, 1252f, VII:737

Pfeiffer syndrome, III:778, IV:92, 93t, 100, VIII:20, 21t, 363-365, 363f. See also Craniosynostosis (craniosynostoses), syndromic.
genetic analysis in, I:58, 60-61, 61f-63f

pH, for flap monitoring, I:497t, 498

Phalangealization, for thumb reconstruction, VII:295, 296, 298f, 299f, 628

Phalanges. See Finger(s); Thumb(s); Toe(s).

Phalloplasty. See Penile reconstruction.

Pharyngeal artery, IV:78f, 81

Pharyngeal bulb prosthesis, in velopharyngeal dysfunction, IV:332-333

Pharyngeal constrictor muscle, IV:312f
inferior, IV:58f, 59f
middle, IV:58f, 59f
superior, IV:58f, 59f, 60t, 64, 64f, 73f, 74f, 76, 79f

Pharyngeal flap, posterior, IV:318-324
complications of, IV:322, 324
historical perspective on, IV:318-319
magnetic resonance imaging before, IV:324
outcomes of, IV:319, 322, 323f, 333-334
technique of, IV:319, 320f-323f
with palatoplasty, IV:262

Pharyngeal plexus, IV:81

Pharyngeal walls, V:165

Pharyngectomy
lateral, V:231-233, 232f, 233f, 233t
suprahyoid, V:230-231, 230f, 231f, 231t

Pharyngoepiglotticus muscle, IV:58f

Pharyngoesophageal fistula, pectoralis major flap for, I:426f-427f

Pharyngoplasty, sphincter, IV:325-332
complications of, IV:331-332
historical perspective on, IV:325, 326f-328f
outcomes of, IV:325, 330-331, 333-334
technique of, IV:325, 329f

Pharyngoscopy, in obstructive sleep apnea, III:786, 786f

Pharyngotonsillitis, in children, III:770

Pharynx. See also at Hypopharyngeal; Pharyngeal.
cancer of. See Oropharyngeal cancer.
posterior wall augmentation in, in velopharyngeal dysfunction, IV:332

Phenols, hand injury from, VII:654

Phenotypic sex, VI:1198

Phenoxybenzamine, in complex regional pain syndrome/reflex sympathetic dystrophy, VII:856

Phentolamine, in complex regional pain syndrome/reflex sympathetic dystrophy, VII:856

Phenylephrine, microvascular surgery and, I:521

Phenytoin, in complex regional pain syndrome/reflex sympathetic dystrophy, VII:858

Phlebography, in upper extremity venous malformations, VIII:383

Phleboliths, in venous malformations, V:49, 49f

Phocomelia, VIII:51-54
clinical presentation of, VIII:51-53, 52f, 53f
prosthesis in, VIII:54
treatment of, VIII:53-54

Phosphorus, hand injury from, VII:654

Photo face reflex, II:79-80, 79f, 88, 802

Photocarcinogens, V:276

Photodynamic therapy, in cancer, I:1063-1064, 1064t, V:286t, 404t, 406, 407f

Photography, I:151-165, II:39, 94, 94t
aperture for, I:153
background for, I:159
body, I:160, 164f
breast, I:160, 164f
cameras for, I:151-153
consent for, I:164-165
depth of field in, I:153, 154f
digital, I:156-159, 165
extremity, I:160
f/stop for, I:153
facial, I:159, 161f, 162f
film for, I:156
flash, I:154-156, 155f
head angle in, I:159-160, 162f
historical perspective on, I:151
in large-volume liposuction, VI:242
in upper extremity body contouring, VI:295-296, 295f
intraoperative, I:159
intraoral, I:160, 163f
lenses for, I:151-153, 153f
lighting for, I:159
medicolegal aspects of, I:160, 164-165
photo face phenomenon and, II:79-80, 79f, 88, 802
resolution in, I:157-159, 158f
shutter speed for, I:153

Photography (Continued)
single-lens reflex camera for, I:152, 157
standardization of, I:159-160, 160f
zoom lenses for, I:152

Photoplethysmography, for flap monitoring, I:497t, 498

Physical therapy. See also Hand therapy.
after finger replantation, VII:577-578
in chemical hand injury, VII:655
in frostbite, VII:652, 653f

Physician-patient relationship, I:70-71

Physician profiling, I:47-48

Pi procedure, for scaphocephaly, IV:467-469, 468f

Pianist, hand disorders in, VII:694, 694f, 695, 704

Piano key sign, VII:54

Pierre Robin syndrome. See Robin sequence.

Pig, vascular territories in, I:330-332, 332f

Pigmentation
after laser resurfacing, II:372-374, 372f, 374f
after liposuction, VI:239

Pigmented tumors, VII:959-960

Pilar cysts, V:255

Pilomatrixoma, V:12-13, 13f, 258

Pincer nail, VII:202f, 203-204, 203f

Pinch. See Key pinch.

Pinch test
after liposuction, VI:289
in abdominoplasty, VI:122-123, 123f, 362, 363f
in lower extremity liposuction, VI:289
in upper extremity body contouring, VI:294, 296, 296f
of abdomen, VI:122-123, 123f

Pindborg tumor, V:97, 199

Pink tip, after rhinoplasty, II:564, 797

Piriform sinus, cancer of, V:236-237

Pisiform, VII:19

Pisohamate ligament, VII:454, 454f

Pitanguy technique, for breast reduction, VI:540, 544f-546f, 561

Pixy ear, II:734-736, 735f

Placenta
catheterization of, I:1120, 1120f
intraoperative oxygenation by, I:1121, 1121f, 1122

Plagiarism, I:115-116

Plagiocephaly, IV:137t, 145-149, 145f-148f, 150f-155f, 469, 471-472, 472f-474f
differential diagnosis of, IV:98

Plantar artery, VI:1409, 1410f-1413f

Plantar artery flap, for foot reconstruction, I:462

Plantar digital nerve, common, neuroma of, VII:922-923, 923f

Plantar flap, for foot reconstruction, VI:1425, 1427f, 1428f

Plantar muscles, VI:1405-1410, 1405f-1409f

Plantar nerves, VI:1410

Plantar ulcers, Achilles tendon release for, I:866, 868f

Plasmacytoma, solitary, V:212-213

Plasmapheresis, in toxic epidermal necrolysis, I:799

Plastic surgery. *See also* Aesthetic surgery.
  definition of, I:11-12
  ethics in, I:93-124. *See also* Ethics.
  evidence-based decision-making in,
      I:35-48. *See also* Evidence-based
      decision-making.
  historical perspective on, I:13-18, 27-34
  informed consent for, I:103-104, 146-
      148, 148t
  innovation in, I:1-2, 12-25, 30-34
    collaboration and, I:24-25
    observation in, I:12-18, 14f-23f
    profile for, I:18-19, 23-25, 24t
  joy of, I:25
  medical malpractice in, I:127-133, 139-
      149. *See also* Medical malpractice.
  outcomes research in, I:35-48. *See also*
      Outcomes research.
  professionalism in, I:100-101, 109-113.
      See also Professionalism.
Plastic Surgery, subject format of, I:5-12, 6-
    9t, 11t
Plastic Surgery (McCarthy), I:4-5
Platelet-activating factor, in neutrophil-
    endothelial adhesion, I:491
Platelet-derived growth factor
  in bone repair, I:657t, 660t, 666-667
  in wound healing, I:212t, 215, 1018
Platelet-endothelial cell adhesion molecule
    1, I:493
Platinum implants, I:752
Platysma, II:163, 176, 176f
  aging-related changes in, II:179-181,
      180f, 181f, 298f, 299, 300f, 301f
  support for, II:176, 176f, 302
  transplantation of, in lagophthalmos,
      III:894-895
Platysma bands, II:176, 176f, 179-181,
    180f-182f
  correction of, II:194, 196-201, 197f-201f
  residual, II:741-742, 742f, 743f
Platysma flap, I:422
  for cheek reconstruction, III:833, 847f
  for head and neck reconstruction, I:422,
      422f, III:1048, 1048f-1050f
  for mandible reconstruction, III:962
  for oral cavity reconstruction, III:932-
      934, 933f
Platysmaplasty, II:285, 288f, 290f-292f
Plethysmography, in upper extremity
    ischemia, VII:800, 800f, 801f
Pleural effusion, congenital, I:1125
Pleural space, Clagett procedure for,
    VI:430-431
PLUG (plug the lung until it grows), in
    fetal diaphragmatic hernia, I:1123,
    1123f
Pneumonitis, aspiration, I:169
Pogonion, II:3f, 3t, 19f, 20t
Poikiloderma congenitale, V:400
Poikiloderma of Civatte, II:388, 390f
Poland syndrome, VI:485-509, VIII:141-
    144
  breast reconstruction in, I:563, 564f,
      VI:432, 434, 493, 495f, 506, 509,
      VIII:142-143, 143f
  chest x-ray in, VI:488
  clinical presentation of, VI:486, 488,
      488f, VIII:141-144, 142f, 143f, 144t
  complex (severe), VI:489, 506, 507f-509f

Poland syndrome *(Continued)*
  digit length in, VI:489
  etiology of, VI:486
  evaluation of, VI:488-489
  historical perspective on, VI:485, 486f
  incidence of, VI:486
  mammography in, VI:488
  occupational restrictions in, VI:489
  simple form of, VI:489
  symbrachydactyly in, VIII:110-111
  symphalangism in, VIII:265-266, 266f
  syndactyly in, VI:488, VIII:141-144,
      142f, 143f, 144t, 175, 177
  treatment of, VI:489-508, VIII:175, 177,
      177f
    custom implants in, VI:490-493, 492f,
        494f, 495f
    functional muscle transfer in, VI:493,
        496f-500f, 501-506, 501f-505f
    indications for, VI:489
    latissimus dorsi flap in, VI:490, 491f,
        493, 496f-500f, 501-506, 501f-
        505f
    mesh prosthesis in, VI:490, 490f
    microvascular flap transplantation in,
        VI:493
    outcomes of, VIII:177
    split rib graft in, VI:490, 490f
    timing of, VI:489-490
    tissue expansion in, I:563, 564f
Pollex abductus, VIII:343
Poly-L-lactic acid, I:757
Polyamide, I:757
Polyarteritis nodosa, wound healing and,
    I:939
Polydactyly, VIII:215-261
  balanced, VIII:215-216
  central, VIII:215, 216f, 234-244, 234f
    amputation for, VIII:243
    associated anomalies with, VIII:235
    bone fusion for, VIII:243
    classification of, VIII:235, 237f
    clinical presentation of, VIII:235-238,
        238f-241f
    digital transpositions for, VIII:243
    incidence of, VIII:235
    inheritance of, VIII:235, 236f
    intrinsic muscles in, VIII:242-243
    osteotomy for, VIII:243-244, 244f
    tendon reconstruction for, VIII:243
    terminology for, VIII:234-235
    treatment of, VIII:238, 241-244, 241t,
        242f, 244f, 245f
  complications of, VIII:244
  fused bones in, VIII:243
  hidden, VIII:239f
  incidence of, VIII:39, 40t, 218, 218t, 235,
      245
  inheritance of, VIII:234f
  mirror hand, VIII:17, 19, 19f, 21t, 249-
      254
    clinical presentation of, VIII:250-251,
        251f-253f
    elbow in, VIII:251, 253f
    Entin's procedure in, VIII:253
    forearm in, VIII:251
    historical perspective on, VIII:249,
        250f
    inheritance of, VIII:250
    pathogenesis of, VIII:250

Polydactyly *(Continued)*
    terminology for, VIII:249
    thumb in, VIII:253, 254f
    treatment of, VIII:251-254, 253f, 254f
    wrist in, VIII:251, 253
  outcomes of, VIII:244, 245f
  postaxial, VIII:22, 215
  preaxial, VIII:21t, 215
  radial (thumb), VIII:215-229, 360-362
    at distal phalanx, VIII:218, 219f, 222-
        224, 223f-225f, 224t
    at metacarpal, VIII:221-222, 222f,
        223f
    at proximal phalanx, VIII:220-221,
        220f, 221f, 224-227, 225f-227f,
        227t
    classification of, VIII:216-218, 216f,
        217f, 229
    clinical presentation of, VIII:218-222,
        219f-223f, 229-230, 232-233
    etiology of, VIII:218
    German classification of, VIII:216,
        217f
    incidence of, VIII:218, 218t
    Iowa classification of, VIII:216, 216f
    special cases of, VIII:232-234, 232f,
        233f
    terminology for, VIII:215-216, 216f
    treatment of, VIII:222-229
      at distal phalanx, VIII:222-224,
          223f-225f, 224t
      at metacarpal, VIII:227-229, 228f,
          229t
      at proximal phalanx, VIII:224-227,
          225f-227f, 227t
      individualized, VIII:233, 233f
      with triphalangeal components,
          VIII:231, 231f
    with triphalangeal components,
        VIII:229-232, 230f, 231f
  syndactyly with, VIII:241-242, 244f
  ulnar, VIII:215, 216f, 245-249
    classification of, VIII:245-246, 246f
    clinical presentation of, VIII:246
    incidence of, VIII:245
    inheritance of, VIII:245
    syndromic associations of, VIII:245
    terminology for, VIII:245
    treatment of, VIII:246-249, 247f-249f
  unbalanced, VIII:215-216
Polyester conduit, for nerve repair, VII:500
Polyethylene, for facial skeletal
    augmentation, II:407f, 408
Polyethylene terephthalate (Dacron), I:757,
    1089
Polyglycolic acid, for bioengineered
    cartilage graft, I:632, 632f, 633
Polyglycolic conduit, for nerve repair,
    VII:500
Polyglycolide, I:757
Polyhydramnios, CHAOS and, I:1122
Polyhydroxy acids, II:399
Polyisoprene implants, I:760
Polymastia, VI:512-513, 512f, 513f
Polymer implants, I:756-760, 756f, 758f,
    759f
Polymer scaffolds, in tissue engineering,
    Color Plate I:37-1, I:1082-1083, 1083t
Polymerase chain reaction, I:56, 58, 59f
Polymethyl methacrylate, I:757

Polymyxin B, topical, I:884t
Polyolefin implants, I:757-758, 758f, 759f
Polyp, umbilical, VI:93
Polypropylene mesh, I:757-758
in chest wall reconstruction, VI:414
Poly(ethylene oxide) scaffold, for bioengineered cartilage graft, I:632-633
Polysomnography
in obstructive sleep apnea, III:776
in Robin sequence, IV:513
Polytetrafluoroethylene (e-PTFE, Gore-Tex), I:756, 756f, 1089
for bioengineered cartilage graft, Color Plate I:23-3, I:633, 634f
for chest wall reconstruction, VI:414, 415f
for facial skeletal augmentation, II:407-408
Polythelia, VI:510, 510t, 512f
Polyurethane
for facial prostheses, I:775, 775f
for implants, I:760
Popliteal artery, Color Plate I:15-8, I:338
Popliteus, arterial supply of, Color Plates I:15-10 and 15-11, I:338
Pores, dilated, with laser resurfacing, II:376
Porion, II:3f, 3t, 19f, 20t
Porocarcinoma, V:298, 298f
Porokeratosis, V:282, 401, 446
Poroma, V:258-259, 259f, VII:960
Porous polyethylene, for cranioplasty, III:555, 557f, 561, 561f
Port-wine stain, III:774, V:6
Post-tourniquet syndrome, VII:117-118
Postanesthesia care unit, I:199-200
bypassing of (fast-tracking), I:200, 201t
step-down (phase II) unit of, I:200, 200t
Postaxial polydactyly, VIII:22
Posterior midline chest wall defects, VI:434-436, 435f-438f
Postmastectomy pain syndrome, VI:665
Posture, aging-related changes in, VI:259, 260f
Potassium, serum, reperfusion injury and, VII:571
Potassium permanganate injury, to hand, VII:654
Povidone-iodine solution, in burn treatment, I:822
Prader-Willi syndrome, uniparental disomy in, I:53
Prazosin, in complex regional pain syndrome/reflex sympathetic dystrophy, VII:856
Preeclampsia, fetal CHAOS and, I:1122
Pregnancy
abdominoplasty after, VI:120. See also Abdominoplasty.
after TRAM flap breast reconstruction, VI:996
microvascular surgery during, I:522
Premaxilla, protrusive, IV:290, 291f, 292f
Prenatal diagnosis, I:1067-1076. See also Fetal surgery.
acetylcholinesterase in, I:1073
alpha-fetoprotein in, I:1073
amniocentesis in, I:1073
β-human chorionic gonadotropin in, I:1073

Prenatal diagnosis (Continued)
chorionic villus sampling in, I:1073-1074
comparative genomic hybridization in, I:1074
fluorescent in situ hybridization in, I:1074, 1075f
in cleft lip, Color Plate I:36-6, I:1069, 1070, 1070t, 1071-1072, 1071f, IV:165-166
in cleft palate, I:1069, 1070t, 1071-1072
in craniosynostoses, IV:94-95
magnetic resonance imaging in, I:1070, 1070f, 1071f
ultrasonography in, Color Plates I:36-1 to 36-6, I:1067-1072
Preosteoblast, I:644
Pressure-flow testing, in velopharyngeal dysfunction, IV:314-315, 314f-316f
Pressure sores, I:942, 942f, 999-1000, 999t, 1001f-1004f, VI:1317-1335
acetabular, VI:1347, 1347t, 1348f, 1349f
anatomic distribution of, VI:1318-1319, 1318t, 1321
calcaneus, VI:1347, 1347t
classification of, VI:1319, 1319t
defect analysis of, VI:1321-1322
depth of, VI:1321
etiology of, VI:1317-1318
evaluation of, VI:1320-1321
grading of, VI:1319, 1319t
infection of, VI:1322
ischial, I:465, 465f, 466f, 467, 470f, VI:1324-1334, 1324t, 1326f-1333f, 1335f
malignant degeneration of, VI:1351
malnutrition and, VI:1318
muscle spasm and, VI:1318
nonsurgical treatment of, VI:1321
osteomyelitis and, VI:1320-1321
pelvic, VI:1347, 1349, 1349f
prevention of, VI:1319, 1319t, 1320f, 1320t
sacral, I:465, 467, 467f-469f, VI:1335, 1336-1338, 1336f-1339f
site-specific pressure in, VI:1318
size of, VI:1321
spinal cord injury and, I:942, 942f
surgical history and, VI:1322, 1323f
treatment of, I:219, 464-467, VI:1321-1352
anterior thigh flap for, VI:1347, 1349, 1349f, 1350f
antibiotics for, VI:1351
complications of, VI:1351
drains for, VI:1351
dressings for, VI:1350-1351
flap necrosis after, VI:1351
flap selection for, VI:1324, 1324t
for acetabular fossa, VI:1347, 1347t, 1348f, 1349f
for calcaneus, VI:1347, 1347t
for ischium, VI:1324-1334, 1324t, 1326f-1333f, 1335f
for pelvis, VI:1347, 1349, 1349f
for sacrum, VI:1335, 1336-1338, 1336f-1339f
for trochanter, VI:1338, 1340-1346, 1340f-1346f

Pressure sores (Continued)
gluteal thigh flap for, VI:1323f, 1324t, 1325, 1327, 1331f, 1332f, 1338, 1343f
gluteus maximus flap for, I:464-465, 467f-470f, VI:1324t, 1334, 1337f-1339f, 1338
gracilis flap for, I:465, 465f, 466f, VI:1324t, 1327, 1333-1334, 1333f, 1335f
hematoma after, VI:1351
infection after, VI:1351
inferior gluteus maximus island flap for, VI:1324-1325, 1324t, 1328f-1330f
management after, VI:1349-1351
microvascular tissue transplantation in, VI:1322
mobilization after, VI:1351
outcomes of, VI:1351-1352
pedicled flaps in, VI:1322
positioning after, VI:1349-1350
preoperative planning for, VI:1322, 1324, 1324t
rectus abdominis flap for, VI:1324t, 1325, 1326f-1327f, 1338, 1344f
rectus femoris flap for, VI:1338, 1342f
rehabilitation after, VI:1351
sensory flap for, VI:1349, 1350t
seroma after, VI:1351
tensor fascia lata flap for, I:465, VI:1338, 1340f-1342f, 1345, 1345f
vastus lateralis flap for, VI:1345-1347, 1346f
wound separation after, VI:1351
trochanter, VI:1338, 1340-1346, 1340f-1346f
Pressure therapy, in burned hand, VII:615
Preterm labor, fetal surgery and, I:1120-1121
Prezygomatic space, II:217, 219f
Prilocaine, I:190t
for facial anesthesia, III:7-8, 7t
Pro Osteon, I:1101t
Procaine, I:190t
for facial anesthesia, III:7-8, 7t
Procerus, II:81, 82f
in brow mobility, II:54-55, 56f
Processed lipoaspirate cells, I:612, 613f
Professionalism, I:100-101, 109-113
Board certification and, I:110
chemical impairment and, I:112
competence and, I:109-110
disability and, I:110-111
discipline and, I:111-112
expert witness testimony and, I:112-113
peer review and, I:110-111
residency training and, I:110
training and, I:110
Progressive hemifacial atrophy (Romberg disease), III:833, 852f-853f, 865f, IV:555
Projection, I:69
Pronasale, II:3f, 3t
Pronator quadratus, VII:25
Pronator syndrome, VII:876t, 889-892, 890f-893f
Pronator teres, VII:25
Proplast, I:756-757

Propofol, I:172t, 173-174, 173f, 182f
Propranolol, in complex regional pain syndrome/reflex sympathetic dystrophy, VII:856
Prostacyclin, VII:797
in flap salvage, I:488
microvascular surgery and, I:521
Prostatectomy, cavernous nerve repair after, Color Plate I:25-3, I:737-738
Prostheses, I:769-788. *See also* Implant(s).
dental, III:984-986, 986f, 987f
facial, I:770-781. *See also* Facial prostheses.
thumb, I:786-787, VII:284-285
upper extremity, I:781-788, VIII:573-580, 574f. *See also* Hand(s), prosthetic.
active, I:782-785, 783f-785f
aesthetic, VIII:583-606
contraindications to, VIII:604
digital, VIII:589-592, 590f-597f
fingernail, VIII:589, 590f
for adolescents, VIII:587, 588f
for adults, VIII:587, 589
for children, VIII:584, 587, 587f
forearm, VIII:600
hand, VIII:586f, 588f, 592, 598f, 599f, 600, 600f, 601f. *See also* Hand(s), prosthetic.
in bilateral amputation, VIII:600, 602f, 603
in difficult cases, VIII:603-604, 603f-606f
in unilateral amputation, VIII:584-600, 587f, 588f, 590f-601f
long-term results with, VIII:604
psychological aspects of, VIII:604, 606
selection of, VIII:583-584, 585f, 586f
shoulder, VIII:600
body-powered, VIII:573-577, 574t, 575f-578f
digital, I:786, VIII:589-592, 590f-597f
elbow, VIII:577, 577f
externally powered, VIII:577-580, 579f, 580f
growth and, VIII:580
hybrid, VIII:580
in brachial plexus injury, VIII:580
in congenital arm amputee, VIII:54-56, 55f, 580
in phocomelia, VIII:54
in transverse deficiencies, VIII:54-56, 55f
objectives of, I:781-782, 782f
passive, I:785-786
shoulder, VIII:577, 578f, 600
telemetry systems for, I:788
thumb, I:786-787
transhumeral, VIII:577, 578f
types of, I:782-786, 783f-785f
Protein kinase C
in ischemic preconditioning, I:495
in tissue expansion, I:542
Proteoglycans, of bone, I:649t, 650
Proteus syndrome, V:55, 56f, VIII:409
macrodactyly in, VIII:308-309, 316
Protoplasmic poisons, hand injury from, VII:653t, 654

Proximal row carpectomy, VII:133
Pseudoaneurysm, of ulnar artery, VII:83f
Pseudocyst, fat injection and, I:584
Pseudoepicanthal fold, after blepharoplasty, II:106
Pseudogout, vs. hand infection, VII:769
Pseudohermaphroditism, female, VI:1212-1213
Pseudoptosis, II:91, 95, 110
Pseudosynovial sheath, for nerve repair, VII:500
Psoralen-ultraviolet A (PUVA) therapy, V:276
Psychiatric illness, I:81-87, 82t, 83t, 84t, 85t
cold injury and, VII:648
Psychological factors/reactions, I:67-88. *See also* Personality.
in adolescents, I:68, 80-81, 80t
in augmentation mammaplasty, I:76-77
in breast cancer, I:78-79
in burn treatment, I:78
in children, I:68, 79-81
in craniofacial anomalies, I:79-80
in facial surgery, I:75
in hand transplantation, I:77-78
in head and neck cancer, I:79
in patient selection, I:81-87, 82t, 83t, 84t, 85t
in reduction mammaplasty, I:77
in rhinoplasty, I:75-76
perioperative, I:70
Psychomimetic reactions, ketamine-induced, I:175
Psychotherapy, in complex regional pain syndrome/reflex sympathetic dystrophy, VII:861-862
PTEN gene, V:55
Pterygium, of eponychium, VII:185, 186f-187f
Pterygium colli, III:1027, 1027f-1028f, 1028f
Pterygoid muscle, IV:58f, 59f, 71, 71f
in craniofacial microsomia, IV:120-122
Pterygomandibular raphe, IV:59f
Ptosis
breast. *See* Breast(s), ptosis of.
eyebrow. *See* Eyebrow(s), ptosis of.
upper eyelid. *See* Eyelid(s), upper, ptosis of.
PU.1, in osteoclast differentiation, I:648
PubMed, I:1141
Puckett technique, in tuberous breasts, VI:517, 522, 522f
Pull-through procedure, in oral cavity cancer, V:177
Pulmonary edema
high-altitude, I:861
nitroglycerin-related, in pregnant patient, I:1121
Pulmonary embolism, VI:175-178, 177t, 178f
free TRAM flap and, VI:872
microvascular surgery and, I:525-526
with liposuction, VI:237-238
Punctum, closure of, II:94
Pupils, evaluation of, II:93
Pushback (Veau-Wardill-Kilner) technique, of palatoplasty, IV:258-259, 259f

Pyoderma gangrenosum, VI:1467, 1476
vs. hand infection, VII:768
wound healing and, I:940, 940f
Pyogenic granuloma, I:945, V:310, 312f
in children, V:3, 3f, 34-35, 35f
of finger, VII:956
of perionychium, VII:200
of upper extremity, VII:956-597, VIII:376, 377f
Pyramidalis, VI:91, 1177

Q

Quadrangular space syndrome, VII:876t
Quadrantectomy (segmental resection), in breast cancer, VI:648
Quadratus plantae muscles, VI:1407, 1407f
Quadrilateral space, axillary nerve compression in, VII:909
Quality of life, health-related, I:41-42, 42f, 42t
Questionnaires, I:40-41, 40f, 41t, 47
Qui tam prosecution, I:136, 137

R

Rabbit, vascular territories in, I:330-332, 333f
Rad, I:836
Radial artery, Color Plates I:15-4 and 15-5, I:335
anatomy of, VII:34, 792
aneurysm of, VII:803f, 814
catheterization of, thrombosis with, VII:806
dominance of, VII:796-797
harvest of, ischemia with, VII:807
in brachial plexus injury, VII:526
median nerve association with, VII:889, 890f
thrombosis of, VII:810
Radial (preaxial) deficiency, VIII:61-80
associated anomalies in, VIII:62-64, 62t, 63f
classification of, VIII:64-65, 64f, 66f
clinical presentation of, VIII:65, 67f, 68f
growth plate injury and, VIII:440, 441f-443f
incidence of, VIII:40t, 62
pathogenesis of, VIII:61-62
treatment of, VIII:65, 65t, 67-77, 565
arthrodesis in, VIII:69
centralization in, VIII:68f, 69-73, 70f-72f, 78-80, 79f
history of, VIII:69, 70f
technique of, VIII:69, 71f-72f, 73
complications of, VIII:78-80, 79f
distraction lengthening in, VIII:73, 74f, 75
elbow flexion in, VIII:75, 76f
microvascular transfer in, VIII:75, 78f
muscle transfer in, VIII:75, 76f
outcomes of, VIII:80, 81f
passive stretching in, VIII:68-69
preoperative distraction in, VIII:70f, 73, 75
radialization in, VIII:73, 74f
splinting in, VIII:69
tendon transfer in, VIII:75
timing of, VIII:67-68
ulnar lengthening in, VIII:75, 77f
ulnar straightening in, VIII:75

Radial (preaxial) deficiency (Continued)
  type I (short radius), VIII:64, 64f
  type II (hypoplastic radius), VIII:64, 64f
  type III (partial absence), VIII:64-65, 64f
  type IV (total absence), VIII:64f, 65, 66f, 79f, 80, 81f
Radial forearm flap, I:409, 410, 410f, 412f
  for esophageal reconstruction, III:1005-1007, 1006f-1008f, 1014, 1016
  for head and neck reconstruction, III:1045, 1045f, V:226, 226t
  for mandible reconstruction, III:964f, 965, 968
  for nasal reconstruction, II:631, 638f-640f
  for oral cavity reconstruction, III:935-939, 936f-938f
  for thumb reconstruction, VII:290, 290f-291f
  for upper extremity reconstruction, VII:327-328, 329f
Radial nerve. See also Radial nerve palsy.
  anatomy of, VII:38, 38f
  entrapment of, VII:34, 876t, 902-904, 903f, 905f
  evaluation of, VII:53, 53f
  repair of, I:736, VII:503
  tourniquet-related injury to, VII:117
Radial nerve block, I:193, 196f, 197f
  at elbow, VII:103, 104f
  at wrist, VII:104, 105f
Radial nerve palsy, VII:34, VIII:506f
  tendon transfer for, VIII:455-462, 456t
    abductor digiti minimi for, VIII:466
    extensor brevis pollicis for, VIII:466
    extensor digiti minimi for, VIII:466
    flexor carpi radialis for, VIII:456t, 458, 461f
    flexor carpi ulnaris for, VIII:456-458, 456t, 457f-460f
    flexor digitorum superficialis for, VIII:458-459, 461
    indications for, VIII:455-456
    outcomes of, VIII:462
Radial polydactyly, VIII:360-362
Radial recurrent artery, Color Plates I:15-4 and 15-5, I:335
Radial styloidectomy, VII:133
Radial tunnel syndrome, VII:703, 876t, VIII:562-563
Radiation, of heat, I:855, 856f
Radiation injury, I:835-852
  acute, I:839, 839f, 847-848, 848f, 849f
  carcinogenic, I:842-844, 844t, 846, 847t
  chronic, I:840-841, 840f
  historical perspective on, I:835-836
  infection in, I:839, 840f, 841, 842f, 843f
  late ulceration in, I:850-852, 851f
  mechanisms of, I:838
  sacral necrosis with, VI:448, 450, 451f
  salivary gland tumors and, V:71-72
  skin cancer and, V:274-275
  subacute, I:839-840, 840f
  systemic, I:838-839, 839t
  to bone, I:841-842, 844f, 845f. See also Osteoradionecrosis.
  to orbit, III:582
  to scalp, III:611
  to skin, I:839-841, 839f, 840f, V:274-275, VI:448, 450, 451f, 452f

Radiation injury (Continued)
  treatment of, I:845-852, 848f-851f
  with whole-body exposure, I:838-839, 839t
  wound healing and, I:844-845
Radiation sickness, I:839
Radiation therapy. See also Radiation injury.
  adjuvant, I:1063
  biologic effects of, I:838-845, 839f, 839t
  breast reconstruction and, VI:668-670, 668f, 669t, 670t, 782
    latissimus dorsi flap in, VI:822, 824f
    TRAM flap in, VI:978, 978f, 979f, 994, 996
  breast reduction after, VI:575
  carcinogenic effect of, I:842-844, 844t, 846, 847t
  energy sources for, I:836-838, 836t
  historical perspective on, I:835-836, 1054-1055
  in basal cell carcinoma, V:286t, 288
  in breast cancer, I:910-911, 911f, VI:666, 667-670, 668t, 669t, 670t, 978
  in Dupuytren disease, VII:740
  in giant cell tumor, VII:988
  in head and neck cancer, V:183-184, 183t
  in retinoblastoma, V:149, 152f-153f
  in skin cancer, V:409t, 423t, 432-436, 434t
  infection with, I:841, 842f, 843f, 1054-1055, 1055f, 1055t
  local biologic effects of, I:839-841, 839f, 840f
  lymphedema and, I:907
  mandible reconstruction and, III:983-984
  microvascular surgery and, I:525
  nerve repair after, I:738
  orbital, III:582
  surgery after, I:841, 842f, 843f, 849-850, 850f
  systemic biologic effects of, I:838-839, 839t. See also Radiation injury.
  wound healing and, I:220, 844-845
Radicular cyst, V:93-94, 194-195
Radiocarpal joint, VII:19
Radiocarpal ligament, VII:21, 455, 455f
Radiography, I:836. See also Computed tomography; Magnetic resonance imaging; Radionuclide imaging.
  in acromegaly, VII:63, 64f
  in battered child syndrome, III:399-400, 399f
  in brachial plexus injury, VII:526
  in complex regional pain syndrome/reflex sympathetic dystrophy, VII:845
  in condylar process fracture, III:517
  in de Quervain syndrome, VII:678-679
  in facial fracture, III:90-110. See also Facial fracture(s), diagnosis of, radiographic.
  in frostbite, VII:649, 650f
  in head and neck cancer, V:169
  in maxillary fracture, III:239
  in nasal fracture, III:196-197, 198f
  in orbital fracture, III:275-276, 426-427, 427f

Radiography (Continued)
  in radius fracture, VII:460, 461f
  in thumb amputation, VII:256
  in thumb reconstruction, VII:258, 259f
  in zygoma fracture, III:214
  of fingers, VII:55-65, 56f-65f
  of hand and wrist, VII:55-65, 56f-65f, 458, 460f. See also Wrist, plain film radiography of.
Radiolunate ligaments, VII:454, 454f
Radionuclide imaging
  in complex regional pain syndrome/reflex sympathetic dystrophy, VII:845-846
  in hemangioma, V:27, VIII:373
  in salivary gland tumor, V:74
  in upper extremity ischemia, VII:800
  of hand and wrist, VII:65-66, 67f
Radioscaphocapitate ligament, VII:454, 454f
Radioscaphoid impingement, VII:133
Radioulnar joint, distal
  computed tomography of, VII:66, 68
  evaluation of, VII:54
  injury to, VII:463-464, 463f
Radioulnar ligament, VII:454, 454f, 456
Radioulnar synostosis, VIII:272, 275-277
  clinical presentation of, VIII:275-276, 276f
  embryology of, VIII:275
  incidence of, VIII:272, 275
  outcomes of, VIII:276-277
  treatment of, VIII:276, 277f-279f
Radius
  fracture of, VII:460-463
    arthroscopy-assisted fixation of, VII:136
    classification of, VII:460
    evaluation of, VII:460, 461f
    in children, VIII:420-423, 422f
    nonoperative treatment of, VII:461
    operative treatment of, VII:461-463, 462f
    radiography in, VII:460, 461f
  osteochondroma of, VII:985, 986f
  osteosarcoma of, VII:990, 990f
  reconstruction of, after tumor resection, VII:983
  vascular territories of, I:335-336
Radius flap, I:390, 390t
  for mandible reconstruction, III:964f, 965, 968, 969
Radix, recession of, after rhinoplasty, II:773, 778f, 789
Raloxifene, in breast cancer, VI:671
Ranitidine, preoperative, I:171
Ranula, III:767
Rapacuronium, I:180, 180t
Rapamycin, I:277
Rationalization, I:70
Ravitch procedure, VI:432, 433f
  in pectus carinatum, VI:478, 479f
  in pectus excavatum, VI:463, 466f-468f, 469, 475, 476t, 477t
Raynaud syndrome, VII:815-819
  diagnosis of, VII:816
  digital blood flow in, VII:648
  in vascular thoracic outlet syndrome, VII:811-812
  Leriche sympathectomy in, VII:817

Raynaud syndrome (Continued)
periarterial sympathectomy in, VII:817-818, 818f, 819f
secondary, VII:816-817
sympathectomy in, VII:817-818, 817f-819f
RB gene, VII:988
Reagan-Linscheid test, VII:54
Receptor(s)
fibroblast growth factor, I:58, 60-61, 61f-63f
HER-2/neu, VI:671
hormone, VI:671
sensory, I:723
temperature, I:856
Reconstructive ladder, I:413, 415, 415f, 1148-1149, 1149f
Reconstructive Plastic Surgery (Converse), I:2-4
Reconstructive triangle, I:415, 415f
Rectus abdominis, VI:89, 90f, 1177
Rectus abdominis-external oblique flap, for breast reconstruction, Color Plate VI:143-2, VI:934, 935f-937f
Rectus abdominis flap
for abdominal wall reconstruction, I:446-447, 447t, VI:1185, 1187f
for breast reconstruction, I:433. See also Transverse rectus abdominis myocutaneous (TRAM) flap.
for chest wall reconstruction, I:446, VI:417
for complex post-mastectomy defect, VI:773, 774f
for cranioplasty, III:557
for groin and perineal reconstruction, I:451-452, 452f, 453f
for head and neck reconstruction, V:226, 226f
for oral cavity reconstruction, III:939-941, 940f, 942f-946f
for pressure sore treatment, VI:1324t, 1325, 1326f-1327f, 1338, 1344f
for upper extremity reconstruction, VII:324-326, 327f
for vaginal reconstruction, VI:1286-1289, 1287f, 1288f
Rectus abdominis-internal oblique flap, for abdominal wall reconstruction, I:985, 989f
Rectus femoris flap
for abdominal wall reconstruction, I:447-448, 450f, VI:1191
for groin and perineal reconstruction, I:451
for lower extremity reconstruction, VI:1371-1372
for pressure sore treatment, VI:1338, 1342f
Rectus myocutaneous flap, for vaginal reconstruction, VI:1299, 1301, 1301f, 1303
Rectus sheath, VI:1176, 1177f
Red nose, after rhinoplasty, II:564
Reducing agent injury, to hand, VII:653t, 654, 656
Reflex sympathetic dystrophy. See Complex regional pain syndrome/reflex sympathetic dystrophy.

Refractive surgery, periorbital surgery and, II:90
Refrigeration, for cartilage graft, I:627
Regression, I:69
Rehabilitation, upper extremity. See Hand therapy; Prostheses; Splint(s).
Reliability, of questionnaire, I:40-41, 40f
ReliefBand, I:202
Religion, treatment and, I:147
Remifentanil, I:181-182
Renal failure, wound healing and, I:943-944
Reperfusion injury, I:487-494, 487f, 489f, 608-609
experimental models of, I:491-494, 492f, 493f
free radicals in, I:491
integrin-Ig-like ligand adhesion in, I:489-490, 489f
neutrophil-endothelial adhesion in, I:488-489, 490f
nitric oxide inhibition of, I:493-494
platelet-activating factor in, I:491
selectin-carbohydrate adhesion in, I:490
Replantation
auricle, III:670, 672-677, 674f-677f
lower extremity, VI:1369
penile, VI:1228, 1230-1232, 1230f-1233f
scalp, III:17, 19f-20f, 620-625, 623f-624f
upper extremity. See Finger replantation; Hand replantation.
Replantation toxemia, I:609
Repression, I:69
Reproductive system, preoperative evaluation of, I:170
Residual cyst, of mandible, V:94
Resistance, electrical, VII:598
Respiration
heat loss with, I:855, 856f
in craniosynostoses, IV:497
in Jeune syndrome, VI:485
in pectus excavatum, VI:460-461, 461t
thorax in, VI:412-413, 412f
Respiratory system. See also Airway.
after palatoplasty, IV:263
desflurane effects on, I:178-179, 178t
enflurane effects on, I:178, 178t
etomidate effects on, I:175
halothane effects on, I:178, 178t
isoflurane effects on, I:178, 178t
ketamine effects on, I:174-175
obstruction of, III:763-794
adult, III:784-794. See also Sleep apnea.
pediatric, III:763-784
craniofacial anomalies in, III:776-784, 776f, 778f, 781f-783f
foreign body in, III:769-770
gastroesophageal reflux disease in, III:771
infection in, III:770
nasopharyngeal, III:763-767, 764f-766f
oropharyngeal, III:767-768, 767f
sleep apnea in, III:775-776
trauma in, III:770
vascular anomalies in, III:772-775, 773f
opioid effects on, I:181
preoperative evaluation of, I:168-169
sevoflurane effects on, I:179

Retin-A, in skin cancer, V:405
Retina, evaluation of, II:93
Retinaculum
orbital, II:80-81, 81f
wrist, VII:29-32, 30f, 31f, 418-420, 419f, 456
Retinoblastoma, V:15, 149, 152f-153f
Retinoids, II:390-397, V:277
dermal effects of, II:393-394, 393f, 394f
desquamation with, II:396, 396f, 397f
dyspigmentation resolution with, II:396-397, 398f
ear deformity and, III:638
effects of, II:391-394, 392f, 392t, 393f, 394f
epidermal effects of, II:392-393, 393f, 397, 398f
formulations of, II:395-401, 396f-399f
in skin cancer, V:404t, 405
irritation with, II:396
mechanism of action of, II:394-395
melasma resolution with, II:396-397, 398f
misconceptions about, II:396-397, 396f-399f
patient instruction guide for, II:391t
pharmacokinetics of, II:394-395
photosensitivity and, II:397
rosy glow with, II:392-393, 393f
teratogenicity of, II:397, IV:12
vehicles for, II:395, 396
Retinol, II:395-396
Retro-orbicularis oculi, inappropriate fat resection from, II:753, 755-756
Retrobulbar hemorrhage, after blepharoplasty, II:106
Retrograde lateral plantar artery flap, for foot reconstruction, I:462
Retromolar trigone, V:163f, 164
reconstruction of, V:926. See also Oral cavity reconstruction.
Retropharyngeal abscess, V:2
Reverse abdominoplasty, VI:165, 165f-167f
Reverse-flow flap, I:409-411, 411f, 412f
Reversed first dorsal metacarpal artery flap, for finger reconstruction, VII:231, 233f, 234f
Reversed ulnar parametacarpal flap, for finger reconstruction, VII:231, 237, 238f
Revolving door flap, for auricle reconstruction, V:386-388, 387f
Revue de Chirurgie Plastique, I:31
Rewarming
in frostbite, I:860, 860t, VII:651, 652t
in hypothermia, I:858
Rhabdomyosarcoma, III:772, V:13-14
of head and neck, V:13-14, 14f, 115, 118
of orbit, V:114, 114f, 127, 129f
of upper extremity, VII:973
Rheumatoid arthritis
in temporomandibular joint dysfunction, III:541, 541f
of hand, VII:63, 63f, 769-770, 770f, VIII:563, 564f, 565f
vs. infection, VII:769-770, 770f
wound healing in, I:937-938
Rhinitis
after closed rhinoplasty, II:563
after secondary rhinoplasty, II:797

Rhinophyma, V:254, 254f
Rhinoplasty, II:427-471. *See also* Nasal reconstruction.
  aesthetic analysis in, II:437-444, 439f-445f
    alar base width in, II:439, 441f
    alar-columellar relationship in, II:439-440, 441f, 442, 442f, 443f
    alar rims in, II:439, 441f
    bony base width in, II:438-439, 441f
    facial thirds in, II:437-438, 439f, 440f
    horizontal facial plane in, II:438, 440f
    ideal proportions in, II:437, 439f
    nasal base in, II:442, 444f
    nasal dorsum in, II:438, 440f, 443, 444f
    nasofrontal angle in, II:442-443, 444f
    tip projection in, II:443, 444f, 445f
    tip rotation in, II:444, 445f
  age-related psychological factors and, I:76
  body dysmorphic disorder and, II:565-566
  cleft nose, IV:354, 356-360, 357f-360f, 362
  closed, II:428-429, 517-569
    aesthetic examination for, II:527
    airway obstruction after, II:559-560, 560f, 566
    alar cartilage malposition and, II:535-536, 535f, 536f
    alar cartilage reduction deformity after, II:567, 567f
    anatomic variants and, II:531-536, 533f-538f
    anatomy and, II:518-520, 519f
    care after, II:550, 551f, 561-562
    cerebrospinal fluid rhinorrhea after, II:564
    circulatory complications of, II:563
    cleft nasal deformity and, II:557, 558f
    complications of, II:559-564, 559f-562f
    dressings for, II:550, 551f
    edema with, II:475, 478
    false assumptions of, II:524, 525f
    follow-up for, II:554-556, 555f
    global effects of, II:524, 525f
    graft problems after, II:561, 561f
    hemorrhage after, II:561-562
    in body dysmorphic disorder, II:565-566
    in donor site-depleted patient, II:557, 559
    inadequate tip projection and, II:532, 534f, 535, 535f
    infection after, II:563
    lacrimal duct injury after, II:564
    low dorsum and, II:531, 533f
    low radix and, II:531, 533f
    mid-dorsal notch after, II:560, 561f
    middle vault collapse after, II:560, 560f
    narrow middle vault and, II:531-532, 533f, 534f
    nasal deviation and, II:556
    nasal layers in, II:519, 519f
    nasal valve examination for, II:526
    overresected dorsum after, II:567, 567f

Rhinoplasty (*Continued*)
    patient complaints in, II:526
    patient dissatisfaction after, II:564-566
    patient history in, II:526
    patient interview for, II:524-526
    photographs before, II:527
    pink tip after, II:564
    planning for, II:524-536
      aesthetic examination in, II:527
      external examination in, II:527
      goal setting in, II:527
      intranasal examination in, II:526-527
      nasal base-bridge height balance and, II:530, 531f, 532f
      patient interview in, II:524-526
      photographs in, II:527
      preoperative patient-physician discussions in, II:527-528
      skin thickness and, II:528, 528f, 529f
      soft tissue parameters in, II:528-530
      tip lobular contour and, II:528-530, 529f, 530f
    posterior packs after, II:561-562
    red nose after, II:564
    revision after, II:527-528
    rhinitis after, II:563
    secondary, II:564-569
      after open rhinoplasty, II:567-568, 568f
      planning for, II:525
    septal collapse and, II:556-557, 557f, 563, 563f
    septal perforation with, II:562-563
    septum examination for, II:526-527
    skin thickness and, II:528, 528f, 529f
    soft tissue contraction after, II:518, 519f, 524
    supratip deformity with, II:518, 519f, 566f, 567
    technique of, II:536-554
      alar cartilage resection in, II:540, 542f, 545
      alar wedge resection in, II:547
      alloplastic augmentation in, II:553-554, 555f
      calvarial bone graft for, II:552-553, 553f
      columella graft in, II:548
      conchal cartilage graft in, II:552, 552f
      costal cartilage graft in, II:553, 554f
      dorsal resection in, II:539-540, 541f-542f
      dorsum graft in, II:543f-544f, 548
      lateral wall graft in, II:548
      maxillary augmentation in, II:554, 555f
      mid-dorsal notch and, II:539-540
      nasal spine-caudal septum in, II:540, 542f
      osteotomy in, II:547
      patient preparation in, II:537-538
      radix graft in, II:543f-544f, 548, 560f, 561, 562f
      segmental tip grafting in, II:549-550, 549f

Rhinoplasty (*Continued*)
      septal graft in, II:543f, 547-548
      septoplasty in, II:542f-543f, 545-546
      skeletonization in, II:538-539, 541f
      spreader graft in, II:544f, 548
      sutures for, II:481-482, 486f
      tip graft in, II:495, 544f-545f, 548-550, 549f, 561, 562f
      turbinectomy in, II:546-547
      upper lateral cartilages-shortening in, II:545
      wound closure in, II:547
    tip lobular contour and, II:528-530, 529f, 530f
    tissue equilibrium in, II:518-519
    turbinate examination for, II:527
    vs. open rhinoplasty, II:475-478, 477f, 530-531
  historical perspective on, I:33
  in adolescent, I:81
  in cheiloplasty patient, IV:210
  in male-to-female transformation, VI:1315
  medical malpractice suits in, I:144
  open, II:427-428, 428f, 428t, 473-514
    aesthetic analysis in, II:437-444, 439f-445f, 474-475, 474f-476f
    aesthetic outcomes of, II:470
    alar collapse after, II:512
    alar retraction after, II:512
    broad nasal base with, II:507, 509, 509f, 510f
    columellar scar after, II:511, 512f
    complications of, II:470, 470t, 510-513, 511f-513f
    contraindications to, II:475-478, 477f
    deformity after, II:510, 511f, 567-568, 568f
    early complications of, II:510, 511f
    edema with, II:475, 478
    examination for, II:430, 436-444, 436t
      computer imaging in, II:437, 439f
      photography in, II:436-437, 437f
    flap necrosis after, II:510-511, 511f
    for deviated nose with dorsal hump, II:464-467, 465f-466f
    for deviated nose with tip asymmetry, II:461-464, 462f-464f
    for short, wide nose with bulbous tip, II:467-470, 468f-469f
    functional outcomes of, II:470
    in the difficult patient, II:512
    indications for, II:475, 477f
    informed consent for, II:430, 431f-434f, 473
    nasal history for, II:430, 435f-436f
    nasofacial angle in, II:474, 474f
    nasolabial angle in, II:474-475, 475f
    outcomes of, II:470, 470t
    patient history for, II:430, 435f-436f
    short nose with, II:505-507, 506f-508f
    supratip deformity after, II:511-512, 513f
    technique of, II:444-461, 445t, 478-504
      alar contour graft in, II:455, 455f
      alar flaring correction in, II:457-458, 458f
      anesthesia for, II:445-446, 446f, 446t, 478, 478f

Rhinoplasty (Continued)
 cartilage grafts for, II:450-451, 451f, 458-461
  from ear, II:459-460, 459t, 460f
  from rib, II:459-461, 459t, 460f, 461f
  from septum, II:459, 459t
 caudal margin of lateral crus in, II:447, 448f
 cephalic trim in, II:451-452, 452f
 closure for, II:455-456, 456f, 504, 504f
 columellar-septal suture for, II:481, 482f-485f
 columellar strut in, II:452, 452f, 453f, 495, 497, 498f-500f
 combination tip graft in, II:455, 455f
 component nasal dorsum surgery in, II:447-450, 448f-450f
 depressor septi muscle translocation in, II:457, 457f
 dorsal hump reduction in, II:448-450, 449f, 450f
 dorsum grafting for, II:488-492, 490f-493f
 ear cartilage graft for, II:489-492, 490f-493f, 493-495
 final evaluation for, II:502, 504, 504f
 incisions for, II:475, 476f, 478-479
 inferior turbinoplasty in, II:451, 452f
 infralobular tip graft in, II:453-454, 454f
 intercrural suture in, II:453, 454f, 480, 481f
 interdomal suture in, II:453, 453f, 480, 481f
 irrigation after, II:455, 456f
 lateral crural mattress suture for, II:480-481, 482f
 lateral crus reconstruction for, II:497, 501f
 lateral osteotomy for, II:486, 488, 488f, 489f
 medial crural suture in, II:452-453, 453f
 medial osteotomy for, II:486, 488f
 nasal splints in, II:456, 456f
 nasal tip sutures in, II:452-453, 453f, 454f
 onlay tip graft in, II:454-455, 454f
 osteotomy for, II:482, 486, 487f, 488, 488f, 489f
 oxymetazoline-soaked pledgets for, II:446, 446f
 percutaneous osteotomy in, II:455
 septal reconstruction in, II:450-451, 451f
 septoplasty for, II:497, 502, 502f-504f
 skin envelope dissection in, II:447, 448f
 splint for, II:504, 504f
 spreader grafts in, II:450, 450f
 stair-step incision for, II:447, 447f, 475, 476f

Rhinoplasty (Continued)
 submucosal tunnel creation in, II:448, 448f
 sutures for, II:479-482, 479f-486f
 tandem graft for, II:489-492, 490f-493f
 taping in, II:456, 456f
 throat pack for, II:446
 tip graft in, II:453-455, 454f, 455f, 492-495, 493f-496f
 tip support graft for, II:493, 494f
 transdomal suture in, II:453, 454f, 479-480, 480f
 tip overprojection with, II:504-505, 505f
 video imaging for, II:474
 vs. closed rhinoplasty, II:475-478, 477f, 530-531
 psychological factors and, I:75-76
 secondary, II:765-799
  airway management after, II:793
  augmentation methods for, II:789-791, 790f
  care after, II:791, 793, 794f-796f
  complications of, II:793, 797
  compromised airflow and, II:768
  computer imaging for, II:770, 772
  dorsum deformity and, II:768-770, 769f, 771f
  evaluation for, II:766-767, 766t
  for alar cartilage malposition, II:785, 786f
  for columella asymmetry, II:785, 787f, 791
  for flaring alar bases, II:785, 787f
  for inadequate tip projection, II:780, 781f-784f, 791
  for low dorsum, II:773, 776f-779f, 780, 789, 790f
  for narrowed middle vault, II:780
  for overprojected tip, II:784-785
  for recessed radix, II:773, 778f, 789
  for secondary airway obstruction, II:785, 788, 789
  graft malposition after, II:797, 798f
  graft materials for, II:772-773, 774f, 791, 792f-793f
  hemorrhage after, II:797
  incisions in, II:478-479
  infection after, II:793, 797
  lateral wall support in, II:789, 791
  nose evaluation for, II:766-767, 766t
  open vs. closed, II:773, 775f
  patient disappointment after, II:797, 799
  patient reasons for, II:767-768
  pink tip after, II:797
  planning for, II:773
  rhinitis after, II:797
  septal deformity and, II:770
  septal perforation with, II:797
  skin deformity and, II:770
  steps of, II:788-789
  sutures in, II:481-482
  tip deformity and, II:770
  vs. primary rhinoplasty, II:788
 sexual identity–related psychological factors and, I:76

Rhinorrhea. See Cerebrospinal fluid leak.
Rhomboid flap, V:346-348
 for cheek reconstruction, V:346, 346f
 for scalp reconstruction, V:346-348, 346f-349f
Rhytidectomy. See Face lift.
Rhytids. See Wrinkles (rhytids).
Rib(s)
 anatomy of, VI:412-413, 412f
 bone graft from, I:673t, 685-686, 686f, 687f
 cartilage graft from, I:623, 623f, 624-625, 625f
  for auricular reconstruction, III:644-645, 644f-647f, 650-651, 656, 659f
 congenital anomalies of, VI:484-485, 484f, 485f
 fracture of, in children, III:400
 pectoralis major flap with, I:390, 391f, 392f
 resection of, in male-to-female transformation, VI:1316
 split, I:685, 686f
  for cranioplasty, I:685, 687f, III:549, 553f
Rib flap, I:390, 391f, 392f, III:962
Ribbon sign, in upper extremity injury, VII:321, 322
Ribeiro technique, in tuberous breasts, VI:517, 520f-521f
Rice bodies, VII:786, 786f
Ring block, in facial trauma, III:10-11, 11f
Rintala flap, for nasal reconstruction, V:349, 358f
Robin sequence, III:776-777, IV:93-94, 102, 251-253, 252f, 511-515
 airway obstruction in, IV:512, 513, 514t
 aspiration in, IV:512-513
 blood gases in, IV:513
 distraction osteogenesis in, III:781, IV:515
 dysmorphology of, IV:511-513
 etiology of, IV:511
 evaluation of, IV:513
 failure to thrive in, IV:512, 513
 management of, IV:513-515
  distraction osteogenesis in, IV:515, 781
  nasopharyngeal tube placement in, IV:513-514
  positioning in, IV:513
  surgery in, IV:514-515, 514t
  tongue-lip adhesion procedure in, IV:514-515, 516f
 mandibular growth in, IV:253
 mortality in, IV:513
 syndromic associations of, IV:511
Robotics, I:1147-1158
 for surgical assistance, I:1155-1157, 1156f-1158f
 future trends in, I:1154-1155
 historical perspective on, I:1147, 1148, 1148f
 indications for, I:1148-1149, 1149f
 prosthetic options in, I:1149-1150, 1150f-1152f
 selection of, I:1150, 1153-1154, 1153f, 1154f
 vs. replantation, I:1150, 1153-1154, 1154f

Rocuronium, I:180-181, 180t
Rofecoxib, I:183-184
Rolando fracture, of carpometacarpal joint, VII:436
Romberg disease, III:833, 852f-853f, 865f, IV:555. See also Hemifacial atrophy.
Rombo syndrome, V:398
Ropivacaine, I:190t, 191
    for facial anesthesia, III:7-8, 7t
Rotation-advancement cheiloplasty, IV:186, 188-195, 188f-196f
    alar-facial groove for, IV:194-195
    C flap for, IV:186, 188f, 189
    for incomplete cleft, IV:202, 204f, 205f
    inferior turbinate flap for, IV:189, 190f
    lateral lip incisions for, IV:189, 190f
    lip border closure for, IV:192, 194, 194f
    lip skin closure for, IV:194, 194f, 195f
    lower lateral cartilage fixation for, IV:194-195, 196f
    lower lateral cartilage release for, IV:189, 190f
    medial incisions for, IV:188, 188f
    muscle reconstruction for, IV:192, 193f
    nostril floor closure for, IV:194
    nostril floor reconstruction for, IV:190, 192, 193f
    orbicularis marginalis flap for, IV:189, 190f
    orbicularis peripheralis muscle closure for, IV:191, 193f
    orbicularis peripheralis muscle release for, IV:191, 191f
    overrotation in, IV:186, 189
    philtral column for, IV:195
    piriform mucosal deficiency correction for, IV:190, 192f
    rotation adequacy in, IV:186, 188f, 189f, 194, 196f
    vermilion triangular flap for, IV:189-190, 190f-192f
Rotation flap, I:367, 369f
    for cheek reconstruction, I:551, 553, 554f
    for nasal reconstruction, V:349, 356f
    for neck lift, II:309-319, 311f-314f, 316f-331f
    for unilateral cleft lip, IV:186, 188-195, 188f-196f
Rothmund-Thomson syndrome, V:400
Rubber implants, I:760
Rubens flap. See Deep circumflex iliac artery (Rubens) flap.
Rubenstein-Taybi syndrome, VIII:297f, 363-365, 363f, 364f
Runx2, IV:9

S

Sacrococcygeal teratoma, I:1127-1128, V:5-6
Sacrum
    osteoradionecrosis of, latissimus dorsi free flap for, VI:448, 450, 451f
    pressure sores of, I:999t, 1000, 1002f, 1030f, VI:1335, 1336-1338, 1336f-1339f
Saddle-nose deformity, III:573, 574f-575f
Saethre-Chotzen syndrome, III:778, IV:92, 93t, 100, VIII:21t. See also Craniosynostosis (craniosynostoses), syndromic.

Sagittal craniosynostosis, IV:137t, 140-145, 141f-144f, 466-469, 468f, 470f, 471f
Sagittal split ramus osteotomy, IV:441, 443, 443f
St. John's wort, I:170, VI:176t
Salivary glands. See also Parotid gland.
    acinic cell carcinoma of, V:84-85
    adenocarcinoma of, V:85-86, 86f
    adenoid cystic carcinoma of, V:83-84, 86f
    anatomy of, II:302, 304f, III:26, V:69-70, 70f
    arterial supply of, I:344
    hemangioma of, V:78-79, 81f
    inflammation of, V:74, 75f
    innervation of, V:71f
    lymphoma of, V:86-87, 87f
    malignant mixed tumor of, V:86
    malnutrition-related enlargement of, V:74
    metastatic tumors of, V:87
    monomorphic adenoma of, V:77, 80f
    mucocele of, V:75
    mucoepidermoid carcinoma of, V:79, 82-83, 83f-85f
    necrotizing metaplasia of, V:75, 77f
    oncocytic carcinoma of, V:86
    oncocytoma of, V:77-78
    pleomorphic adenoma of, V:76-77, 78f, 79f
    prominent, after face lift, II:739-740, 740f
    pseudocyst of, III:767
    squamous cell carcinoma of, V:86
    stenosis of, V:75, 76f
    stones in, V:75, 75f, 76f
    tumors of, V:70-88, 74t, 107, 109, 163
        benign, V:76-79, 78f-82f
        computed tomography of, V:73
        diagnosis of, V:72-74, 72f, 73t
        epidemiology of, V:70-72, 71t
        fine-needle aspiration of, V:72-73, 72f
        imaging of, V:73-74, 73t
        in children, V:15-16
        magnetic resonance imaging of, V:73-74, 73t
        malignant, V:79, 80t, 82-88, 82t, 83f-88f
        metastatic, V:87
        non-neoplastic, V:74-75, 74t, 75f-77f
        radiation exposure and, V:71-72
        radionuclide scan of, V:74
        sialography in, V:74
        ultrasonography of, V:74
    Warthin tumor of, V:77, 81f
Salpingopharyngeus, IV:58f, 59f, 60t, 62, 73f, 74f, 76, 312f
Samhita, I:27
Saphenous flap, for lower extremity reconstruction, VI:1378, 1379f
Saphenous nerve, neuroma of, VII:945
Sarcoidosis, vs. hand infection, VII:770
Sarcoma, VII:968-973, 971f
    biopsy of, VII:969
    epithelioid, VII:970, 971f
    evaluation of, VII:969
    Ewing, V:15, 107, 212, VII:991
    in children, V:13-15, 14f
    Kaposi, V:299-300, 300f
    midface, V:139

Sarcoma (Continued)
    odontogenic, V:204
    osteogenic
        of hand, VII:988, 990, 990f
        radiation-induced, I:843-844
    presentation of, VII:969
    soft tissue, V:13-15, 14f
    staging of, VII:969
    synovial
        in children, V:14
        of head and neck, V:119
        of upper extremity, VII:70, 75f, 972-973
    treatment of, VII:969-970
Sartorius flap, for groin and perineal reconstruction, I:451
SAT (alphanumeric) classification, of craniofacial microsomia, IV:128, 128t, 401, 403f, 404f, 405f, 407t
Satellite cell, in muscle regeneration, I:611-612
Scalp, III:607-630. See also Scalp reconstruction.
    anatomy of, III:15-16, 607-609, 608f-610f
    aplasia cutis congenita of, III:610-611
    arterial supply of, III:609, 610f
    basal cell carcinoma of, III:612
    burns of, I:1004-1006, 1005f-1006f, III:611
    cicatricial alopecia of, III:610, 610t
    dysplastic nevus of, III:612
    evaluation of, III:612-613
    giant nevus of, III:612
    hair of. See Hair, scalp.
    hemangioma of, V:32f
    infection of, III:611
    innervation of, III:16
    lacerations of, III:611
    layers of, III:607, 608f, VII:336f
    lymphatic network of, III:609
    Marjolin ulcer of, III:612
    melanoma of, III:612
    microsurgical replantation of, III:17, 19f-20f, 620-625, 623f-624f
    Mohs micrographic surgery on, III:612
    nerve supply of, III:609, 609f
    nevoid basal cell carcinoma of, III:611-612
    nevus sebaceus of Jadassohn of, III:611, V:281-282, 281f, 282f
    primary closure for, III:613
    radiation injury to, III:611
    reduction of, for male pattern baldness, III:629, 629f
    skin cancer of, III:611
    squamous cell carcinoma of, III:612
    trauma to, III:15-17, 18f-20f, 611
        anatomy in, III:15-16
        etiology of, III:15
        microsurgical replantation for, III:17, 19f-20f
        nonsurgical management of, III:16
        skin graft for, III:17
        surgical management of, III:16-17, 18f-20f
    tumors of, III:611-612
    vascular supply of, III:16
    venous drainage of, III:16
    venous supply of, III:609, 610f
    xeroderma pigmentosum of, III:612

Scalp flap
  for eyebrow reconstruction, III:728-729, 730f
  for forehead reconstruction, III:716, 717f, 718f, 720f
  for hair restoration, II:694-697, 696f, III:630
  for scalp reconstruction, III:613-618, 615f-618f, 620
  for upper lip reconstruction, III:823, 827f
Scalp reconstruction, I:548, III:613-630. See also Hair restoration.
  distant flaps for, III:619-620, 621f
  four-flap technique for, III:613, 615f
  galeal flap for, III:617, 617f
  in male pattern baldness, I:551
  latissimus dorsi flap for, I:429f-432f, 430, III:620, 621f
  local flaps for, III:613-618, 614f-618f
  microsurgical replantation for, III:17, 19f-20f, 620-625, 623f-624f
  microvascular composite tissue transplantation for, III:620, 622f
  pectoralis major flap for, III:620, 621f
  rhomboid flap for, V:346-348, 347f, 348f
  serial tissue expansion in, I:548, 550f, 552f
  split-thickness skin grafting for, III:613
  temporoparietal fascial flap for, III:617-618, 618f
  three-flap technique for, III:613, 616f
  tissue expansion in, I:548-551, 549f, 550f, 552f, III:618-619, 619f, V:388, 388f
  trapezius flap for, III:620
Scalp replantation, III:17, 19f-20f, 620-625, 623f-624f
Scaphocapitate ligament, VII:456f
Scaphocephaly, IV:137t, 140-145, 141f-144f, 466-469
  hung span procedure for, IV:469, 470f, 471f
  pi procedure for, IV:467-469, 468f
Scaphoid bone, VII:19
  blood supply to, VII:20
  evaluation of, VII:54
  fracture of, VII:48, 464-465, 464f, 465f
    arthroscopy-assisted fixation of, VII:136-137
    computed tomography in, VII:68
    in children, VIII:423-424
  tubercle of, VII:20, 20f
  Watson test of, VII:54
Scaphoid nonunion advanced collapse, VII:465-466, 465f, 466f
Scapholunate ligament, VII:21, 456f
  dissociation of, VII:467-468, 467f, 468f
Scaphotrapezium trapezoid ligament, VII:456f
Scapula, for bone graft, I:674t, 688
Scapula flap
  dorsal, for neck reconstruction, III:1042, 1042f
  for mandible reconstruction, I:390, 390f, 397f-399f, III:964f, 965-966, 968, 969
  for upper extremity reconstruction, VII:330, 333, 334f, 335f

Scar(s), I:221-222, 226-230, 239. See also Scar revision.
  aesthetic implications of, I:236
  after abdominoplasty, VI:179-181, 180f, 182f-189f
  after body lift, VI:271
  after breast reduction, VI:580
  after cleft lip repair, IV:242, 348-349
  after coronal brow lift, II:60-61, 61f, 62f
  after mastectomy, VI:977, 977f, 978f, 990-991, 991f
  after neck lift, II:320
  after upper extremity liposuction, VI:312
  assessment of, I:237-238, 237t, 238f, 238t
  burn-related, I:830-831, 830f
    in hand, VII:614-624, 616-624, 617t, 618f-620f, 622f, 623f
    malignant transformation in, VII:614
    unstable, in hand, VII:614
  camouflage of, I:258-259, 259f
  classification of, I:226, 227t
  crosshatched, with face lift, II:731-732, 732f
  definition of, I:235, 236t
  discoloration of, I:239
  facial
    face lift-related
      crosshatched, II:731-732, 732f
      misplacement of, II:722, 725f, 726f, 727-730, 727f-731f
      wide, II:730-731, 731f
    skin graft resurfacing for, I:263, 265f-266f
  formation of, I:214-215, 214f
  hypertrophic, I:221-222, 227t, 237, 938, 938f
    after face lift, II:730-731, 731f
    after facial burn excision and grafting, III:51-54, 52f-54f, 74, 75f
    after hand burns, VII:614-616
    after laser resurfacing, II:374-375
    after rhytidectomy, II:210
    donor-site, after facial burn excision and grafting, III:74, 75f
    neck, reconstruction in, III:1034-1035, 1034f
    pressure garment prevention of, VII:615
    treatment of, I:227-228, 229f
  medical malpractice suits for, I:144
  neck
    reconstruction for, III:1034-1035, 1034f
    skin graft resurfacing for, I:260-263, 261f-262f, 264f
    Z-plasty for, I:251, 254f
  pain in, I:239
  plastic surgery effects of, I:230
  prevention of, I:227, 228t
  revision of, I:235-266. See also Scar revision.
  squamous cell carcinoma in, V:437-439, 437f, 437t
  tensile strength of, I:215, 215f
  terminology for, I:236-237, 237t
  treatment of, I:227-230, 229f
  with skin graft, I:311

Scar revision, I:235-266
  after tracheostomy, I:255, 257f, 258, 258f
  anatomic landmark restoration in, I:244-245
  broken-line closure technique for, I:258-259, 259f, 260f
  care after, I:263
  conservative treatment before, I:242-243, 243t
  direct excision in, I:245
  evaluation for, I:239-240, 240t
  examination for, I:240
  fusiform, I:244, 245f
  in face, I:248, 249f-250f
  indications for, I:238-239
  informed consent for, I:240-241
  instruments for, I:243, 243f, 243t
  preoperative counseling for, I:241
  resurfacing for, I:259-263, 259f-262f
  serial excision in, I:245-248, 246f
  skin grafts for, I:259-263, 259f-262f
  staging of, I:242
  sutures for, I:243, 244f
  timing of, I:241-242
  tissue expansion in, I:245-248, 247f
  unsatisfactory result of, I:241
  W-plasty in, I:244, 245f
  wound plate in, I:244
  YV-plasty in, I:255-258, 255f-258f
  Z-plasty in, I:244, 245f, 248-254, 248t, 249f-254f
Schirmer test, II:93, 93f
Schwann cells, VII:472, 474
  cold storage of, VII:502
  in allograft, VII:501-502, 502f
  in nerve regeneration, VII:479-480
Schwannoma
  of mandible, V:210
  of upper extremity, VII:958-959
Schwarzmann technique, for breast reduction, VI:539-540, 541f
Sciatic nerve block, I:193
Sciatic nerve injury, I:736, VII:502-503
Scleral show, II:78
Scleroderma, IV:555-556, 562f-563f. See also Hemifacial atrophy.
  ulnar artery narrowing in, VII:84f
  wound healing in, I:937
Sclerotherapy
  in arteriovenous malformation, VIII:399, 401
  in lymphatic malformation, V:44-45, VIII:394
  in venous malformation, V:50, 50f, VIII:384-385, 386f
Scrotoplasty, in female-to-male transformation, VI:1309, 1310-1311
Scrotum
  construction of, in female-to-male transformation, VI:1309, 1310-1311
  lymphedema of, VI:1255-1256, 1464
  nerve supply of, VI:1206, 1206f
  reconstruction of, VI:1223
  reduction of, VI:403-404, 405f
Seal limb. See Phocomelia.
Seat belt injury, III:455
Sebaceous carcinoma, V:296-298, 297f
Sebaceous cyst, of auricle, III:689

Sebaceous glands, I:297-298
  hyperplasia of, V:256
  occlusion of, after laser resurfacing,
    II:370
Seborrheic keratosis, V:253-254, 254f, 310,
    312f
Sebum, I:297-298
Second metacarpal flap, reverse-flow, for
    finger reconstruction, VII:231, 235f,
    236f
Second metatarsal flap, for mandible
    reconstruction, III:963
Second-toe flap, for finger reconstruction,
    VII:237, 240f, 242-244, 243f
Second-toe transfer, for thumb
    reconstruction, VII:271-272, 273f,
    296-297, 298f
Sedation, conscious, I:196-198
Sedation-analgesia, I:196-198
Sedatives, preoperative, I:170-171, 171f
Segmental maxillary osteotomy, IV:441, 442f
Segmental resection (quadrantectomy), in
    breast cancer, VI:648
Seizures, propofol effects on, I:174
Selectins, I:490, 490f, 491
Selective serotonin reuptake inhibitors, in
    complex regional pain
    syndrome/reflex sympathetic
    dystrophy, VII:859
Self-destructive personality, I:73-74
Sella-nasion plane, II:20f, 21t
Semmes-Weinstein monofilament testing,
    I:865-866, 867f
Sensation, in hand, VII:50
Sensory flap
  for foot reconstruction, I:405-407, 405f-
    407f
  for pressure sore treatment, VI:1349,
    1350t
Sensory nerve action potentials, in
    peripheral nerve injury, VII:487
Sensory re-education, after peripheral
    nerve injury, VII:506-507
Sensory receptors, I:723
Sentinel node biopsy, I:1062, VI:654, 661-
    664, 662f
  false-negative, VI:663
  mastectomy and, VI:664
Sepsis
  in lymphatic malformation, V:44, 45f
  upper extremity ischemia in, VII:815
Septal pivot flap, for nasal reconstruction,
    II:626, 629, 630f-631f
Septic arthritis, of hand, VII:782-774, 784f
Septo-aponeurotic sling, II:84
Septocutaneous flap, I:526-527, 527f
Septum. See Nasal septum; Orbital septum.
Seroma
  after abdominoplasty, VI:179, 185f
  after body lift, VI:271
  after breast augmentation, VI:29, 350,
    351
  after breast reconstruction, VI:831
  after breast reduction, VI:578
  after liposuction, VI:235-236
  after pressure sore treatment, VI:1351
Serratus anterior flap
  for chest wall reconstruction, Color
    Plate VI:132-1, I:446, VI:417, 422f,
    423f

Serratus anterior flap (Continued)
  for upper extremity reconstruction,
    VII:326, 328f
  intrathoracic transposition of, VI:430
Serum imbibition, by skin graft, I:309-310
Sevoflurane, I:178t, 179
Sexual harassment, I:118
Shaken baby syndrome, III:400
Shave excision, in skin cancer, V:408, 409t,
    410, 410f
SHH gene, IV:3
Shh protein, IV:12
Shivering, I:856-857, 858
Short lip, after cleft lip repair, IV:349
Short-Watson sign, VII:736
Shoulder
  after obstetric brachial plexus palsy
    treatment, VII:549, 553-557, 554f-
    560f
  burns of, contracture with, VII:630-633,
    631f, 634f
  dislocation of, arterial injury with,
    VII:804
  prostheses for, VII:347f, VIII:600
  rotation contracture of
    humeral osteotomy for, VII:557, 558f
    soft-tissue release for, VII:553, 554f-
      557f
    trapezius and levator scapulae muscle
      transfer for, VII:557, 559f
  ulnar deficiency at, VIII:105f, 106f, 107
Shoulder-hand syndrome, VII:835-836,
    836f. See also Complex regional pain
    syndrome/reflex sympathetic
    dystrophy.
Sialadenitis, V:2-3, 74, 75f
Sialadenosis, V:74
Sialography, in salivary gland tumor, V:74
Sialolithiasis, V:75, 75f, 76f
Sialometaplasia, necrotizing, V:75, 77f
Sialoprotein, I:648, 649t, 650
Silicone
  conduit of, for nerve repair, I:735,
    VII:499
  dressings of, I:224, 225t, 227
  for breast prosthesis. See at Breast
    augmentation; Expander-implant
    breast reconstruction.
  for facial reconstruction, I:775-776,
    II:407
  gel formulation of, in burned hand
    treatment, VII:615
Silicone synovitis, vs. hand infection,
    VII:769
Silver implants, I:752
Silver nitrate, I:822, 950
Silver sulfadiazine, I:822, 884t, 950
Silverlon, I:884t
Singapore flap
  for penile reconstruction, VI:1226-1227,
    1229f
  for vaginal reconstruction, VI:1297,
    1298f, 1299f
Sinus
  in constriction ring syndrome, VIII:203,
    204f
  wound healing and, I:945
Sinuses. See Paranasal sinuses.
Sirolimus, I:275t
SiteSelect system, VI:641

SIX3 gene, IV:3
Sjögren's syndrome, VI:1475-1476, 1477f
Skate flap, for nipple reconstruction,
    VI:796, 800f-806f, 807
Skeletal traction, in Dupuytren disease,
    VII:751
Skin. See also Skin graft.
  acne-prone, II:388, 390f
  acne rosacea of, V:254, 254f
  actinic keratoses of, Color Plate V:113-1,
    V:266-268, 267f, 278, 278f, 393,
    394f, 446
    chemotherapeutic agents in, Color
      Plate V:116-2, V:278, 403-405,
      404t
    pigmented, V:278, 279f
  aging of, II:340-341, 341f
    sun exposure and, II:386-388, 387f,
      388f
    altered, II:387-388, 389f, 390f
  anatomy of, I:294-299, 294f
  apocrine glands of, I:298-299
  artificial
    in hand burn treatment, VII:610-613,
      610t, 611f, 612f
    in toxic epidermal necrolysis, I:797-
      798, 798f
    in wound healing, I:1018-1019
  basal cell carcinoma of, V:282-290, 391-
    448. See also Basal cell carcinoma.
  bioengineered replacements for, I:224,
    225t, 893
  biopsy of, V:252, 263
  biosynthetic, I:313-314
  blood supply to, I:296-297, 367, 367f,
    420
  Bowen disease of, Color Plate V:113-4,
    V:266, 267f, 280-281, 280f, 437t,
    442-443
  burns of, I:811-832. See also Burns.
  cancer of
    basal cell, V:391-448. See also Basal
      cell carcinoma.
    gynecomastia and, VI:529
    melanoma, V:305-343. See also
      Melanoma.
    premalignant lesions and, V:278-282,
      278f-282f
    sebaceous, V:296-298, 297f
    squamous cell, V:391-448. See also
      Squamous cell carcinoma.
  chemical sensitivity of, laser resurfacing
    and, II:370
  cold injury to, I:858-860, VII:647-653.
    See also Frostbite.
  color of, V:391-392, 392t
  cylindroma of, Color Plate V:112-2,
    V:259-260, 259f
  cysts of, V:255-256, 255f
  débridement of, I:873-875, 874f
  deficiency of, in craniofacial
    microsomia, IV:124-125, 124f
  dermal-epidermal junction of, I:294f,
    296
  dermatofibroma of, Color Plate V:112-4,
    V:260-261, 260f
  dermatofibrosarcoma protuberans of,
    V:298-299, 299f
  dermis of, I:294f, 296
  eccrine glands of, I:299

Skin *(Continued)*
eccrine poroma of, V:258-259, 259f
ephelides of, V:261, 261f
epidermal cyst of, V:255, 255f
epidermal nevus of, V:256-257
epidermis of, I:294-296, 294f
epidermodysplasia verruciformis of,
    V:281
epidermolysis bullosa of, I:800-806,
    VIII:431-437, 432f. *See also*
    Epidermolysis bullosa.
examination of, V:251-252
facial, II:161, 162f
    aging-related changes in, II:297, 299-
        300
    thickness of, II:348t
Fitzpatrick types of, V:391, 392t
freckles of, V:261, 261f
hair follicles of, I:297, 298f
hand, VII:14-15
    evaluation of, VII:46-47, 48f
    in finger reconstruction, VII:218,
        218t, 220, 220f. *See also* Finger
        reconstruction, flaps for.
hyperpigmentation of
    after hand burn treatment, VII:596
    after laser resurfacing, II:342, 345,
        372-373, 372f
    after liposuction, VI:239
hypertrophic scarring of. *See* Scar(s),
    hypertrophic.
hypopigmentation of, after laser
    resurfacing, II:373-374, 374f
Kaposi sarcoma of, V:299-300, 300f
keratoacanthoma of, V:268-269, 269f,
    280, 280f, 437t, 439-442, 439f, 440t,
    441f
laxity of, after abdominoplasty, VI:376-
    377, 377f, 378f
lentigo of, V:261, 261f
leukoplakia of, V:268, 268f, 279
loss of, after abdominoplasty, VI:364,
    371-372, 371f, 373f-374f
Marjolin ulcer of, I:916, 917f, III:612,
    V:275, 276f, 437-439, 437f, 437t,
    VI:446-447, 447f, VII:614
melanocytic nevus of, V:261-263, 262f
melanoma of, V:305-343. *See also*
    Melanoma.
Merkel cell carcinoma of, V:295-296,
    296f, 437t, 443-445, 443f, 444f
milia of, V:255-256
molluscum contagiosum of, V:252-253,
    253f
necrosis of
    after breast reconstruction, VI:831
    after breast reduction, VI:578
    after neck lift, II:332
    after rhytidectomy, II:210
    after TRAM flap breast
        reconstruction, VI:872, 994
    liposuction and, VI:237
nevus of, V:261-266. *See also* Nevus(i).
nevus sebaceus of, Color Plate V:112-2,
    V:257-258, 257f
nevus sebaceus of Jadassohn of, V:257,
    281-282, 281f, 282f, 399
Paget disease of, Color Plate V:113-11,
    V:295, 295f
perforator flaps of. *See* Perforator flaps.

Skin *(Continued)*
periorbital, assessment of, II:91
photoaging of, II:386-388, 386t, 387f,
    388f
phototypes of, V:274, 274t
pigmentation of
    after facial burn excision and grafting,
        III:70, 72f
    after hand burn treatment, VII:596
    after laser resurfacing, II:342, 345,
        373-374, 374f
    after liposuction, VI:239
pilar cyst of, V:255
pilomatricoma of, V:258
porokeratosis of, V:282
premalignant lesions of, V:278-282,
    278f-282f
pressure sores of, VI:1317-1332. *See also*
    Pressure sores.
radiation effects on, I:839-841, 839f,
    840f. *See also* Radiation injury.
redundancy of, after abdominoplasty,
    VI:362-364, 363f-368f
resurfacing of, II:339-380, 365-368, 366f.
    See also Facial resurfacing.
sebaceous carcinoma of, V:296-298, 297f
sebaceous glands of, I:297-298
sebaceous hyperplasia of, V:256
squamous cell carcinoma of, V:290-295,
    391-448. *See also* Squamous cell
    carcinoma.
substitutes for, I:312-314, 890, 892-893,
    894f
sun exposure of, II:386-388, 387f, 388f-
    390f
sunscreen for, V:276-277, 277t
sweat gland tumors of, V:258-261, 259f,
    260f
T-cell lymphoma of, V:300, 300f
tissue-engineered, I:1087-1089, 1087t,
    1088f
toxic epidermal necrolysis of, I:793-799.
    See also Toxic epidermal necrolysis.
transplantation of, I:279-280
trichoepithelioma of, V:260, 260f
tumors of. *See also specific tumors.*
    benign, V:251-269
    malignant, V:273-300. *See also* Basal
        cell carcinoma; Squamous cell
        carcinoma.
        epidemiology of, V:273-274
        etiology of, V:274-276, 393, 394f
        prevention of, V:276-278, 277t,
            393-394
    neck reconstruction in, III:1037,
        1038f-1039f
vascular anatomy of, I:367, 367f, 371,
    420
vascular anomalies of, V:19-61. *See also*
    Capillary malformations;
    Hemangioma; Vascular
    malformations; Venous
    malformations.
venous drainage of, Color Plate I:15-14,
    I:355
verruca vulgaris of, Color Plate V:112-1,
    V:252, 253f
verrucous nevus of, V:257, 257f
viral tumors of, Color Plate V:112-1,
    V:252-254, 253f

Skin *(Continued)*
wrinkling of. *See also* Wrinkles (rhytids).
    after abdominoplasty, VI:364, 369f-
        370f
    after breast augmentation, VI:337-
        340, 337f, 338t
    after breast reconstruction, VI:1121,
        1121f
xeroderma pigmentosum of, Color Plate
    V:113-2, V:279-280
Skin graft, I:293-314. *See also* Dermal graft
    *and at specific disorders and
    procedures.*
allogeneic (allograft), I:280, 313, 890,
    893
autologous (autograft), I:279-280
avulsed skin for, I:302
contraction of, I:311
contraindications to, I:300t
donor sites for, I:301-303, 301f
    for facial defects, I:302
    infection of, I:302
    treatment of, I:302
dressings for, I:307-309, 308f
failure of, I:312, 312t
for auricle replantation, III:676
for auricular reconstruction, III:642,
    650-651, 655f, 656, 656f-657f
for burns, I:818, 822, 823-827, 824f,
    824t, 826f, 827f. *See also at* Facial
    burns; Hand burns.
for cheek reconstruction, III:833, 849f-
    850f
for Dupuytren disease, VII:748-750,
    749f, 750f
for facial scars, I:263, 265f-266f
for fingertip reconstruction, VII:157-
    158
for forehead reconstruction, III:703,
    704f, 706-708, 706t, 707f
for lower extremity, VI:1470-1471, 1471f
for lower lid blepharoplasty, II:818
for midface reconstruction, III:872
for nail absence, VII:185, 188f
for nasal reconstruction, II:590-595,
    593f-596f, 594, 605, 613, 618, 623f-
    625f
for neck scar, I:260-263, 261f-262f, 264f
for nipple reconstruction, I:302, VI:793-
    794, 794t
for oral cavity reconstruction, III:927-
    928, 929f
for penile reconstruction, VI:1221, 1223,
    1224f
for scalp reconstruction, III:17, 613
for scar revision, I:259-263, 259f-262f
for tongue reconstruction, III:927-928,
    929f
for upper extremity injury, VII:322-323
for vaginoplasty, VI:1285, 1312
full-thickness, I:300-301
    donor sites for, I:301-302, 301f
    harvesting of, I:305
    preparation of, I:305-306
hair follicles in, I:312
harvesting of, I:303-305, 303f-306f
    dermatomes for, I:304, 305, 305f, 313f
    storage after, I:309
hematoma formation with, I:306-307
historical perspective on, I:293-294

Skin graft (Continued)
  hyperpigmentation of, I:311
  in children, I:302, 311
  in melanoma treatment, V:326, 327f
  in syndactyly treatment, VIII:166, 168
  indications for, I:300t
  infection of, I:312
  maturation of, I:311-312
  nerve growth in, I:311
  postoperative care for, I:307-309, 308f
  preparation of, I:305-307
  recipient wound preparation for, I:299-
    300
  revascularization of, I:310-311
  sensation in, I:311-312
  serum imbibition by, I:309-310
  shearing of, I:312
  split-thickness, I:300-301
    application of, I:306-307, 307f
    donor sites for, I:301, 301f
    harvesting of, I:303-305, 303f-305f
    meshing of, I:306, 306f
    preparation of, I:306
  stent compound in, I:309
  storage of, I:309
  survival of, I:309-312
  sweat gland function in, I:312
  thin, after facial burn excision and
    grafting, III:74, 74f
  tissue expansion for, I:547
  xenogeneic (xenograft), I:280, 313, 890,
    892-893, 894f
Skin grafts
  for abdominal wall reconstruction,
    I:985, 986f, VI:1183
  for areola reconstruction, VI:813-814
Skin pits, in Dupuytren disease, VII:735,
  735f
Skin slough, after face lift, II:746-748
Skin-specific antigens, in transplantation,
  I:271
Skin tags, V:261
SkinLaser, II:377-378
Skull. See also Cranio-; Cranium.
  fracture of
    pediatric, III:398-399, 438-444, 439t,
      440f-445f
    pseudogrowth of, III:440, 442, 443f
  osteomyelitis of, I:915, 915f, 978f
Skull base
  anatomy of, V:123-124, 124f
  anterior, tumors of, V:124-139
    malignant, V:127-139, 127t, 128f-
      133f, 136f-138f. See also Orbit,
      tumors of.
    nonmalignant, V:124-127, 125f-126f
    posterior, tumors of, V:139-149, 140f-
      143f, 146f-148f, 150f-152f
Sleep apnea, obstructive, III:784-794
  cor pulmonale and, III:786, 786f
  diagnosis of, III:784-787, 785f, 785t,
    786f
  obesity and, III:786, 786f
  pediatric, III:775-776
    distraction osteogenesis in, III:778-
      780
    gastroesophageal reflux and, III:771
  pharyngoscopy in, III:786, 786f
  tracheostomy in, III:786
  treatment of, III:787-794, 787t

Sleep apnea, obstructive (Continued)
    fascial tongue sling in, III:789-790,
      790f, 791f
    hyoid suspension in, III:790-791, 792f
    sliding window genioplasty in,
      III:790-791, 792f
    tongue advancement in, III:789-791,
      790f, 791f
    tracheostomy in, III:786, 791-794,
      793f, 794f
    uvulopalatopharyngoplasty in,
      III:787-789, 788f
  with craniofacial clefts, IV:422
Sliding window genioplasty, in obstructive
  sleep apnea, III:790-791, 792f
Sling procedure, for lower eyelid
  ectropion, II:147-149, 148f-149f
Small area variation, in evidence-based
  decision-making, I:43
Small-vessel disease, in diabetes mellitus,
  VI:1445-1446, 1445f. See also Diabetes
  mellitus, foot reconstruction in.
SMAS. See Superficial musculoaponeurotic
  system (SMAS).
SMAS roll-Vicryl mesh preparation,
  II:193-194, 193f-195f
Smile. See also Smile reconstruction.
  impairment of, III:884, 885f
Smile block, after face lift, II:748-749, 749f
Smile reconstruction, III:897-911
  free muscle transplantation for, III:898-
    906
    one-stage, III:877, 879, 879f, 880f,
      898-899
      planning for, III:898, 899f
    two-stage, III:899-906
      cross-facial nerve graft in, III:899-
        903, 899f-903f, 903t
      gracilis muscle in, III:903-905,
        904f-907f
      masseter motor nerve in, III:905-
        906, 908f, 909f
  regional muscle transplantation for,
    III:906, 910, 910f
  soft tissue rebalancing in, III:911
  static slings for, III:910-911, 910f
Smith-Lemli-Opitz syndrome, IV:12
Smoke inhalation, I:831-832, 832f
Snakebite, I:931-932, 934f, 935f, 1016-
  1017
SNRPN gene, I:53
Sodium alginate, for bioengineered
  cartilage graft, I:631
Sodium bicarbonate, for facial anesthetics,
  III:7
Sodium hypochlorite
  hand injury from, VII:654
  in burn treatment, I:822
Sodium nitroprusside, microvascular
  surgery and, I:521
Soleus, arterial supply of, Color Plates I:15-
  10 and 15-11, I:338
Soleus flap, for lower extremity
  reconstruction, I:409-410, 411f, 454,
  457f-461f, VI:1373
Somatization, I:70
Somatosensory evoked potentials
  in brachial plexus injury, VII:529
  in peripheral nerve injury, I:728t
Southern blot, I:55-56, 57f

SPAIR technique, for breast reduction,
  VI:571, 573f
Spanish fly, hand injury from, VII:654
Spasm. See also Vasospasm.
  muscle, pressure sores and, VI:1318,
    1319, 1320t
  sternocleidomastoid muscle (torticollis),
    III:398, 1032-1033, 1033f, IV:98-99
Spastic diplegia, interferon-alfa and, V:30-
  31
Spastic hand, VIII:543-553
  assessment of, VIII:544-547, 546f, 546t
  botulinum toxin in, VIII:547
  electrical stimulation in, VIII:547
  etiology of, VIII:543-544, 544f
  muscle tone assessment in, VIII:546
  nerve blocks in, VIII:547
  phenol in, VIII:547
  range of motion assessment in, VIII:546
  treatment of, VIII:547-553
    balance with, VIII:552-553
    complications of, VIII:552-553
    for finger swan-neck deformity,
      VIII:548t, 550-551
    for thumb-in-palm deformity,
      VIII:548t, 549-550
    for wrist flexion deformity, VIII:548-
      549, 548t
    goals of, VIII:547-548
    outcomes of, VIII:553
    principles of, VIII:548, 548t
    technique of, VIII:551-552
  wrist function assessment in, VIII:546,
    546t
Spasticity, VIII:543-544, 544f. See also
  Spastic hand.
Spectroscopy, for flap monitoring, I:497t,
  498
Speech, III:923
  after esophageal reconstruction,
    III:1018, 1020f-1021f, 1022
  cleft palate and, IV:255, 255f, 256
  facial paralysis and, III:884
  in velopharyngeal dysfunction, IV:313
Sphenoid bone, III:332, IV:71
Sphenopalatine artery, IV:77, 78f
Sphincter pharyngoplasty, IV:325-332
  complications of, IV:331-332
  historical perspective on, IV:325, 326f-
    328f
  outcomes of, IV:325, 330-331, 333-334
  technique of, IV:325, 329f
Spider bites, I:931-932, 933f, 934f, 1017
Spina bifida, closure for, I:945
Spinal accessory nerve injury,
  rhytidectomy and, II:206, 208f, 209f
Spinal block, I:194-196
Spinal cord
  cervical
    exposure of, neck reconstruction in,
      III:1076
    injury to, facial fracture and, III:84-85
  congenital anomalies of. See
    Myelomeningocele; Spina bifida.
  hypersensitive (wind-up) state of,
    VII:87-88, 88f
  injury to, VI:1317. See also Spastic hand;
    Tetraplegia.
    etiology of, VI:1317
    incidence of, VI:1317

Spinal cord *(Continued)*
life expectancy with, **VI:**1317, 1318t
pressure sores and, **VI:**1317-1352. *See also* Pressure sores.
prevalence of, **VI:**1317
wound healing and, **I:**942, 942f
Spinal surgery
latissimus dorsi flap reconstruction after, **VI:**450, 454f, 455f
wound infection after, **I:**981, 999
Spiradenoma, eccrine, **VII:**960, 961f
Spitz nevus, **V:**265-266, 265f
Splint(s)
after peripheral nerve repair, **VII:**505
counterforce, in tennis elbow, **VII:**904
dental, **III:**257, 257f
hand/finger, **VII:**121-122, **VIII:**567-568, 568t, 569f, 569t, 570f
in camptodactyly, **VIII:**292
in chemical hand injury, **VII:**655
in cryptotia, **III:**663, 669f
in Dupuytren disease, **VII:**746
in electrical hand injury, **VII:**601
in epidermolysis bullosa, **VIII:**436, 436f, 437f
in extensor tendon reconstruction, **VII:**411-412, 412f, 413f
in finger contracture, **VII:**665-668, 667f, 668f
in finger fracture, **VII:**425, 425f, 447
in hand burns, **VII:**601, 609-610
in hand surgery, **VII:**121-122
in peripheral nerve repair, **VII:**505
in radial (preaxial) deficiency, **VIII:**69
intraocclusal, **IV:**540
intraoral, **IV:**303, 304f
knuckle-jack, **VII:**667f, 668
L'Nard, **VI:**1443
nasal, **II:**456, 456f, 504, 504f
Split hand-split foot, **VIII:**21t
Split rib, **I:**685, 686f
for cranioplasty, **I:**685, 687f, **III:**549, 553f
Sporothrix infection, of hand, **VII:**785, 785f
Squamous cell carcinoma, **V:**290-305, 391-448
brachytherapy in, **V:**436
chemical exposure and, **V:**275-276
chemoprevention of, **V:**277, 403-405, 404t
chemotherapy in, **V:**403-406, 404t
chronic wounds and, **V:**275, 276f
clinical features of, Color Plate **V:**113-10, **V:**292, 293f
diagnosis of, **V:**403
dietary fat and, **V:**278
epidermodysplasia verruciformis and, **V:**281
epidermolysis bullosa and, **I:**800, 803f, 804-805
etiology of, **V:**274-276, 274t, 276f, 290-291, 391-392, 393
follow-up for, **V:**436-437
formaldehyde and, **V:**276
genetic features of, **V:**399-401, 400f
histopathology of, **V:**291-292
historical perspective on, **V:**391-393
human papillomavirus infection and, **V:**291, 292t
immune factors in, **V:**275
in AIDS, **V:**397

Squamous cell carcinoma *(Continued)*
in high-risk patient, **V:**424t
in scar, **V:**437-439, 437f, 437t
in situ (Bowen disease), Color Plate **V:**113-4, **V:**266, 267f, 280-281, 280f, 281f, 437t, 442-443
incidence of, **V:**273, 396-398, 397t
leukoplakia and, **V:**279
lower extremity ulcer and, **I:**916, 916f
lymphadenectomy in, **V:**294-295
lymphatic spread of, **V:**435, 447-448
metastatic, **V:**160-162, 162f, 166-167, 291, 294-295, 294f, 447-448
mortality from, **V:**397
of cheek, **V:**377f
of head and neck, **V:**160-162, 166-167, 166f
of lip, **V:**445
of lower eyelid, **V:**364f
of nasal cavity, **V:**111
of orbit, **V:**127, 132f-133f
of paranasal sinuses, **V:**111
of perionychium, **VII:**200-201, 200f
of salivary glands, **V:**86
of scalp, **III:**612
of upper extremity, **VII:**962-964, 963f
organ transplantation and, **V:**397
osteomyelitis and, **V:**275
photodynamic therapy in, **V:**406, 407f
porokeratosis and, **V:**282
premalignant lesions in, Color Plate **V:**113-1, **V:**278-280, 278f-280f
prevention of, **V:**276-278, 277t, 393-394
radiation therapy and, **V:**274-275, 434, 434f
radiation therapy in, **V:**409t, 423t, 432-436, 434t
recurrence of, **V:**292, 294f, 414t, 415t, 416t, 419t, 422t
risk factors for, **V:**395t
sinus tracks and, **V:**275
treatment of, **V:**292-294, 406-437, 408t, 420f-422f, 423t
algorithm for, **V:**420f-422f
chemotherapy in, **V:**403-406, 404t
cryosurgery in, **V:**408t, 409t, 411-413, 411f
curettage and electrodesiccation in, **V:**409t, 410-411
frozen vs. permanent sections in, **V:**425
full-thickness excision in, **V:**409t, 413-416, 414t, 415t, 416t, 425-426, 425f, 426f
micrographic surgery in, **V:**408t, 409t, 426-432. *See also* Mohs micrographic surgery.
pathology processing in, **V:**414-416, 425-426, 425f, 426f
photodynamic therapy in, **V:**406, 407f
radiation therapy in, **V:**408t, 409t, 423t, 432-437, 434t
shave excision in, **V:**408, 409t, 410, 410f
ultraviolet radiation and, **V:**274, 274t, 290-291
variants of, **V:**437-446, 437t
verrucous, **V:**294, 294f, 445-446, 445f
vs. keratoacanthoma, **V:**269, 280, 280f
well-differentiated, Color Plate **V:**113-9
xeroderma pigmentosum and, **V:**279-280
Squamous epitheliomas, self-healing, **V:**400

Squamous odontogenic tumor, **V:**97, 199
Stainless steel implants, **I:**751-752, 752t
Staircase flap, for lip reconstruction, **III:**812, 812f
Standard of care, **I:**139-140
Stapedial artery, in craniofacial cleft development, **IV:**20
Staphylococcus aureus infection
after rhytidectomy, **II:**210, 211f
in hand, **VII:**762, 763f, 764f
in irradiated skin, **I:**1054-1055, 1055f
in paronychium, **VII:**194
Star flap, for nipple reconstruction, **VI:**807, 808f, 809f
Static sling, in facial paralysis, **III:**896, 897f, 910-911, 910f, 911f
Stellate ganglion block, in complex regional pain syndrome/reflex sympathetic dystrophy, **VII:**853-854
Stem cells
from liposuctioned fat, **I:**612, 613f
in muscle regeneration, **I:**611-612
in tissue engineering, **I:**1084-1085, 1085f
in wound healing, **I:**1019
Stenosing tenosynovitis, of finger, **VIII:**560, 561f
Stenosis
arterial, **VII:**796, 796f
external auditory canal, **III:**677-679, 679f
piriform aperture, **III:**763
salivary gland, **V:**75, 76f
subglottic, **III:**769
tracheal, **III:**398
Stent compound, **I:**309
Stepladder sign, **VI:**637
Sternocleidomastoid flap
for head and neck reconstruction, **I:**421, **III:**1050-1051, 1051f
for mandible reconstruction, **III:**961-962
Sternocleidomastoid muscle
birth-related injury to, **III:**398
spasm of (torticollis), **III:**398, 1032-1033, 1033f, **IV:**98-99
Sternotomy, infection after, **VI:**425-426, 425t, 427f
Sternum, **VI:**457-482
anatomy of, **VI:**413
cleft, **VI:**479-482, 481f, 482f, 483t. *See also* Cleft sternum.
congenital cleft of, **VI:**431
embryology of, **VI:**457
infection of, **I:**914-915, 979f
after coronary artery bypass graft, **I:**915, 915f, 977, 980-981, 980f
after sternotomy, **VI:**425-426, 425t, 427f
pectus carinatum of, **VI:**477-478, 479f, 480f
pectus excavatum of, **VI:**458-477. *See also* Pectus excavatum.
radiation-induced sarcoma of, **VI:**416, 416f
wound in, omental flap for, **I:**579, 581f
Stevens-Johnson syndrome, **I:**794, 794t. *See also* Toxic epidermal necrolysis.
drugs in, **I:**794-795
epidemiology of, **I:**794-795
pathogenesis of, **I:**795
Stewart-Treves syndrome, **VI:**1464, **VII:**1004

Stickler syndrome, IV:102
Stiff hand, VII:659-672. *See also* Hand(s), stiff.
Stiles-Bunnell tendon transfer, VIII:475-476, 476f
Stimulan, I:1101t
Stomion, II:3f, 3t
Stones, of salivary glands, V:75, 75f, 76f
Streptokinase, in upper extremity ischemia, VII:802, 804
Stretch marks, after abdominoplasty, VI:364
Stroke volume, in pectus excavatum, VI:461
Strombeck technique, for breast reduction, VI:540, 543f, 561
Struthers, ligament of, VII:889, 889f
Study design, I:37-39, 38f-40f
    experimental, I:37
    observational, I:37-39, 38f-40f
Sturge-Weber syndrome, V:39, 39f, VIII:380
Styloglossus, IV:73f
Styloidectomy, radial, VII:133
Stylopharyngeus, IV:58f, 59f, 73f, 76
Subatmospheric pressure dressing, I:224, 225t
Subclavian artery, in brachial plexus injury, VII:526
Subclavian vein decompression, in complex regional pain syndrome/reflex sympathetic dystrophy, VII:852
Subgaleal fascia, III:607, 608, 608f
Subglottic stenosis, III:769
Sublabiale, II:3f, 3t
Sublimation, I:70
Sublingual gland, V:70, 70f. *See also* Salivary glands.
Submandibular gland, V:69-70, 70f. *See also* Salivary glands.
    arterial supply of, I:344
    prominent, after face lift, II:739-740, 740f
Submental artery island flap, for neck reconstruction, III:1040, 1040f
Subnasale, II:3f, 3t
Substance abuse
    by surgeon, I:112
    in patient evaluation, I:85
Substance P, in complex regional pain syndrome/reflex sympathetic dystrophy, VII:837-839
Succinylcholine, I:179, 179t
Sudden infant death syndrome, gastroesophageal reflux and, III:771
Sudeck atrophy, VII:827, 836, 836f. *See also* Complex regional pain syndrome/reflex sympathetic dystrophy.
Sufentanil, I:181-182
Sulcus abnormality, after cleft lip repair, IV:346-347
Sulfuric acid injury, to hand, VII:654, 656
Summary suspension, I:134
Sunlight
    actinic keratosis and, VII:960
    skin cancer and, V:274, 274t, 275, 290-291, 393
    skin exposure to, II:386-388, 387f, 388f-390f

Sunscreen, V:276-277, 277t
Supercharging, I:413, VI:720
Superficial cervicofacial fascia, II:297, 299, 300f, 301-302, 303f
Superficial fascial system, VI:259
Superficial inferior epigastric artery flap
    for breast reconstruction, VI:764t, 766, 768-769, 768f
    for hemifacial atrophy, IV:556, 557f, 566f-567f
Superficial musculoaponeurotic system (SMAS), II:162, 162f, 163-165, 164f, 165f, 175, 176-177
    arterial supply of, Color Plates I:15-12 and 15-13, I:340-341, 340f, 341f
    buttonholing of, II:748, 748f
    deep fasciae relationship to, II:166, 167f
    dissection of, II:175, 176-177, 201, 201f
    elevation of, II:181, 189-192, 190f-192f
    extended dissection of, II:189-192, 191f, 192f
    fixation of, II:192-194, 193f-196f, 201
    injury to, II:748, 748f
    redraping of, II:181, 184f
    wide dissection and, II:178-179
Superficial musculoaponeurotic system (SMAS)ectomy, II:175
Superficial musculoaponeurotic system (SMAS) flap, II:742-744, 743f, 744f, 745, 745f, 748, 748f
    high, II:744, 744f
    injury and, II:748, 748f
    low, II:742-744, 743f
Superficial musculoaponeurotic system (SMAS) graft, II:249, 249f
Superficial musculoaponeurotic system (SMAS)–platysmal rotation flap, II:309-319, 311f-312f
    complications of, II:320-323, 332-336, 335f
    dissection for, II:312-315, 313f, 314f, 316f-318f
    flap mobilization for, II:315-316, 318f, 319f
    liposuction with, II:319, 330f-331f
    results of, II:319, 324f-331f
    sutures for, II:316, 319, 319f-321f, 323f
    vector diagram of, II:322f
Superior gluteal artery perforator flap, VI:764t, 1044-1047, 1045t, 1060, 1062, 1063f, 1064f
    anatomy of, VI:1044-1045
    complications of, VI:1047
    defect closure for, VI:1047
    donor scar with, VI:1046f
    surface markings for, VI:1044-1045, 1044f-1046f
    surgical technique for, VI:769-770, 769t, 1047, 1048f, 1049f
    vascular anatomy of, VI:1045-1047
Superior oblique muscle, III:331-332
Superior orbital fissure syndrome, III:335, 336f
Superior pedicle mammaplasty, in tuberous breasts, VI:517, 519f
Superior transverse ligament of Whitnall, II:133
Supernumerary breasts, VI:512-513, 512f, 513f

Superoxide anion, in flap ischemia, I:487-488, 487f
Suppressor cells, in transplantation, I:279
Suprabrow excision, II:59-60, 60f
Supraclavicular block, I:193, VII:99-100, 99f
Supraglottis, cancer of, V:239-241, 240f-242f, 240t
Supramalleolar flap, for foot reconstruction, VI:1419, 1423f
Supraorbital artery, II:80
Supraorbital nerve, II:80
    anatomy of, II:56-57, 57f
    blockade of, I:191-192, 192f
    injury to, III:361
Supraorbital rim. *See also* Orbit.
    augmentation of, II:96, 409, 410, 410f
    fracture of, in children, III:445-448, 445f-448f
    hypoplasia of, II:96
    in blepharoplasty, II:96
    postoperative prominence of, II:804, 804f
Suprapubic fat, liposuction of, VI:408, 409f
Suprascapular block, VII:100-101, 101f
Supratrochlear nerve
    anatomy of, II:56, 57f
    injury to, III:361
Supratrochlear nerve block, I:191-192, 192f
Supraventricular tachyarrhythmias, fetal, I:1125-1126
Sural artery, Color Plates I:15-8 and 15-10, I:338
Sural artery flap, for foot reconstruction, VI:1435-1436, 1439f
Sural flap, for lower extremity reconstruction, VI:1377-1378, 1378f
Sural nerve, neuroma of, VII:945
Sural neurocutaneous flap, for foot reconstruction, VI:1419, 1422f
Surgeon. *See also* Ethics; Professionalism.
    contacts with, I:134-136
    peer review of, I:133-134
    summary suspension of, I:134
    termination of, I:135
Surveys, I:40-41, 40f, 41t, 47
Sushruta, I:27
Suspensory ligament, penile, VI:390
    release of, VI:391-393, 391f-393f
Sutter implant, for osteoarthritis, VII:714, 717
Sutures, I:760-761. *See also* at specific procedures.
    absorbable, I:761, 761t
    antibiotic-coated, I:763
    colon cancer recurrence and, I:1059, 1059f
    nonabsorable, I:761, 762t
Swallowing, III:923
    after esophageal reconstruction, III:1018
    cleft palate and, IV:254-255
Swan-neck deformity, VII:413-414, 663, 664f
    ORL reconstruction in, VII:414, 414f
    pathomechanics of, VII:403, 405f
    treatment of, VIII:548t, 550-551
Swanson implant, for osteoarthritis, VII:713-717, 714f-716f, 718t

Sweat glands, I:294f
  in skin grafts, I:312
  occlusion of, after laser resurfacing,
      II:370
  tumors of, V:258-261, 259f, 260f, 298,
      298f, VII:960, 961f, 964-965
Sweating, I:857
  in complex regional pain
      syndrome/reflex sympathetic
      dystrophy, VII:846
Symblepharon conformers, III:745
Symbrachydactyly, VIII:82t, 110-131, 353-
      355, 353f, 354f
  classification of, VIII:111, 111t, 112f,
      113f
  clinical presentation of, VIII:114-116,
      115f, 117f-119f
  etiology of, VIII:111, 114
  in Poland syndrome, VIII:110-111
  incidence of, VIII:111
  treatment of, VIII:116-131, 116t, 117f-
      120f
    fifth digit in, VIII:126
    hypoplastic digits in, VIII:121-125,
        122f-124f
    hypoplastic nubbins in, VIII:121
    in adactylic hand, VIII:126
    in monodactylic hand, VIII:126
    nonvascularized toe transfer in,
        VIII:121-125, 122f-124f
    prosthesis for, VIII:130f, 131
    tendon transfers in, VIII:126
    thumb in, VIII:125
    toe transplantation in, VIII:126-129,
        129f, 131
  vs. constriction ring syndrome, VIII:196
Sympathectomy
  in complex regional pain
      syndrome/reflex sympathetic
      dystrophy, VII:851-852
  in hand frostbite, VII:652
  in vasospastic disease, VII:817-818,
      817f-819f
  Leriche, in vasospastic disease, VII:817
  periarterial, in vasospastic disease,
      VII:817-818, 818f, 819f
Sympathetic block, in complex regional
      pain syndrome/reflex sympathetic
      dystrophy, VII:853-855
Sympatholytics
  in complex regional pain
      syndrome/reflex sympathetic
      dystrophy, VII:855-857
  preoperative, I:171
Symphalangism, VIII:265-269, 266f
  clinical presentation of, VIII:265-267,
      266f
  genetics of, VIII:265
  nonhereditary, VIII:265
  outcomes of, VIII:268-269
  treatment of, VIII:267-268, 268f
Syndactyly, VIII:139-180
  anatomy of, Color Plate VIII:204-1,
      VIII:139-141, 140f, 148-149
  bone configurations in, VIII:149
  classification of, VIII:139-141, 140f
  complex, VIII:139-140, 140f
  digital nerves in, VIII:149
  etiology of, VIII:141
  fascial interconnections of, VIII:148-149

Syndactyly (Continued)
  in Apert syndrome, IV:99, VIII:144-146,
      144f, 145f, 146f, 170-175, 171t,
      172t, 173f-176f, 363-365, 363f
  in Freeman-Sheldon syndrome,
      VIII:147, 148f
  in Poland syndrome, VI:488, VIII:141-
      144, 142f, 143f, 144t, 175, 177,
      177f
  incidence of, VIII:39, 40t, 41t, 141
  recurrent, VIII:169-170, 170f
  simple, VIII:139, 140f
  skeletal anatomy of, VIII:139-140,
      140f
  soft tissue anatomy of, VIII:139, 140f
  thumb-index, VIII:140-141, 168-169
    mild, VIII:159, 160f
    moderate, VIII:159-160
    severe, VIII:160-161, 161f, 162f
  treatment of, VIII:149-180
    fingernails in, VIII:168
    fingertips in, VIII:168
    historical perspective on, VIII:150-
        159, 152f-158f
    in Apert syndrome, VIII:170-175,
        171t, 172t, 173f-176f
    in Poland syndrome, VIII:175, 177,
        177f
    in two- and three-digit hand,
        VIII:168, 169f
    interdigital release in, VIII:161-167,
        163f-167f, 169-170, 170f
      anesthesia for, VIII:161
      dissection for, VIII:162-163, 166f,
          167f
      dressing for, VIII:166-167
      flap inset for, VIII:166
      marking for, VIII:161-162, 164f
      nail folds in, VIII:162-163, 166f,
          167f, 168
      outcomes of, VIII:169-170, 170f
      skeletal correction for, VIII:166
      skin grafts for, VIII:166, 168
    outcomes of, VIII:168-170, 170f
    principles of, VIII:159, 159t
    skin graft in, VIII:166, 168
    thumb-index web release in,
        VIII:159-161, 160f-162f, 168-169
    timing of, VIII:149-150, 150f, 151f
    web creep after, VIII:169-170, 170f
Syndrome, definition of, IV:94
Synechiae
  with laser resurfacing, II:375, 375f
  with nasal fracture, III:208
Synkinesis, in facial paralysis, III:890
Synovectomy, arthroscopic, at wrist,
      VII:131
Synovial sarcoma
  in children, V:14
  of head and neck, V:119
  of upper extremity, VII:70, 75f, 972-
      973
Synovial sheaths, of hand, VII:29, 32, 47
Synovitis, silicone, vs. hand infection,
      VII:769
Synpolydactyly, Color Plates VIII:201-2
      and 201-3, VIII:20-21, 21t, 235, 236f,
      237f, 240f, 241f. See also Polydactyly;
      Syndactyly.
Syringoma, V:258

Syrinx, vs. nerve entrapment syndromes,
      VII:881
Systemic lupus erythematosus, IV:555-556,
      566f-567f. See also Hemifacial
      atrophy.
  wound healing in, I:937

T
T-cell lymphoma, cutaneous, V:300, 300f
T tubules, I:606, 606f
Tacrolimus, I:275t, 276-277
Tagliacozzi, Gaspare, I:27, 28f
Tamoxifen, in breast cancer, VI:671
Tantalum implants, I:752
Tar burns, I:831
Tarsal strip lateral canthoplasty, II:843t,
      846-847, 846f, 847f
Tarsal tunnel, VII:917
Tarsal tunnel release, in diabetes mellitus,
      VI:1448, 1448f
Tarsal tunnel syndrome, VII:876t, 917-
      922
  diagnosis of, VII:917-918
  incision for, VII:919-920, 920f
  management of, VII:918-920, 918f, 919f,
      922t
  pain in, VII:920, 921f
Tarsals, VI:1410, 1413f
Tarsorrhaphy
  in lagophthalmos, III:895
  in secondary lower lid canthopexy,
      II:821, 821f
Tattoo, traumatic, III:12-13, 12f
Tattooing, in areola reconstruction, Color
      Plate VI:139-1, VI:814, 814f-816f
Tazartoene, II:395
Tear film, evaluation of, II:93-94, 93f
Tear trough, II:92-93, 92f
Tear trough deformity, II:97
  implant for, II:97, 97f
  postblepharoplasty, II:805-807, 806f,
      807f
Tearing, with facial paralysis, III:883-884
Teeth. See Tooth (teeth).
Telangiectasias, VIII:378, 380, 380f
Tele-home care, I:1142
Tele-prison care, I:1142
Telemedicine, I:837-838, 1137-1145
  applications of, I:1142-1143
  barriers to, I:1143-1145
  benefits of, I:1137, 1138t
  cost-effectiveness of, I:1144
  definition of, I:1137
  emergency, I:1142
  for surgery, I:1157, 1158f
  historical perspective on, I:1137-1138
  insurance payments and, I:1144
  Internet in, I:1140-1142
  legal issues of, I:1144
  methods of, I:1139-1140, 1139t
  rural, I:1142
  staff resistance to, I:1145
  technophobia and, I:1144
  transfer modalities in, I:1138-1139,
      1139t
  video conferencing systems in, I:1139-
      1140, 1139t, 1142-1143, 1143f
  wireless, I:1140
Telepsychiatry, I:1142
Teleradiology, I:1142

Temperature
 body
  anesthetic effects on, I:186-187
  core, I:858
  regulation of, I:186-187, 856-857
 digital, VII:798
  in vasospastic disease, VII:816
 environmental, cold injury and, VII:648
Temple-zygoma junction, II:216-217, 217f
Temporal bone, IV:71
Temporal brow lift, II:62-63, 63f
Temporal fascia, II:82-83, 216-217, 217f,
  III:608, 608f
Temporal frontal scalp flap, for lip
  reconstruction, III:823, 827f
Temporal hollowing, porous polyethylene
  implant for, III:561, 561f
Temporal line, brow anatomy and, II:53,
  54f
Temporalis, III:608-609
Temporalis flap, for head and neck
  reconstruction, I:421, V:223-225
Temporalis transplantation
 in facial paralysis, III:906, 910, 910f
 in lagophthalmos, III:894, 895f
Temporo-occipital scalp flap, III:620
Temporomandibular joint. See also
  Temporomandibular joint
  dysfunction.
 anatomy of, III:535-537, 536f, 537f
 ankylosis of, III:182, 414f, 418, 543
 imaging of, III:542
 internal derangement of, III:537-539,
  538f, 538t, 539f
 palpation of, III:542
 range of motion of, III:542
 reconstruction of, III:543, 544f
Temporomandibular joint dysfunction,
  III:537-544
 ankylosis in, III:543
 arthroscopy in, III:542-543
 avascular necrosis in, III:543-544
 condylar abnormalities in, III:539
 condylar dislocation in, III:544
 condylar fracture in, III:539-541, 540f
 condylar reconstruction in, III:544
 congenital abnormalities in, III:539
 coronoid enlargement in, III:539
 imaging in, III:542
 inflammatory, III:537
 internal derangement in, III:537-539,
  538f, 538t, 539f
 medical management of, III:542
 myofascial, III:537
 open arthrotomy in, III:543
 oral examination in, III:542
 osteoarthritis in, III:541
 osteoarthrosis in, III:539, 540f
 patient history in, III:541
 physical examination in, III:541
 rheumatoid arthritis in, III:541, 541f
 surgical management of, III:542-544
Temporoparietal fascia, II:53, 55f, III:607,
  608, 608f, VII:336f
Temporoparietal flap
 calvarial, I:688-691, 690f, 691f
 fascial, I:585, 587-588
  for facial reconstruction, V:223
  for scalp reconstruction, III:617-618,
   618f

Temporoparietal flap (Continued)
  for upper extremity reconstruction,
   VII:333, 335, 336f-341f
 for forehead reconstruction, I:371, 372f
Tenascin, in nerve regeneration, VII:480
Tendinitis
 elbow, VII:904, VIII:558, 559f
 hand, VII:54, VIII:559-561, 559f-561f
 in musician, VII:702
 wrist, VIII:560-561
Tendon(s), I:591-601. See also specific
  tendons.
 anatomy of, I:591-592, 592f
 blood supply of, I:591-592
 collagen of, I:592, 593f
 débridement of, I:875-876, 875f-880f
 extrinsic healing of, I:594
 healing of, I:594-595
 histology of, I:592-594, 593f, 594f
 injury to, I:595-600. See also at Extensor
  tendon(s); Flexor tendon(s).
 intrinsic healing of, I:594
 light microscopy of, I:594, 595f
 moment arm of, VII:28, 28f
 nutrition for, I:594
 of hand, VII:29-32, 30f, 31f. See also
  Extensor tendon(s); Flexor
  tendon(s).
 repair of, I:595-600
  allograft in, I:599-600
  blood supply in, I:595-596
  early motion in, I:596
  flexor sheath in, I:596, 596f
  guidelines for, I:595
  suture technique in, I:596-597, 597f-
   598f
  synthetic grafts in, I:600
  tendon grafting in, I:598-599, 599f
  tenolysis in, I:597-598
  tensile stress in, I:596-597, 597f-598f
  timing of, I:595
 transfer of, VIII:453-486. See also Hand
  reconstruction, tendon transfer in.
Tendon graft, I:598-599, 599f
 for flexor tendon reconstruction,
  VII:384-386, 385f. See also Flexor
  tendon reconstruction.
 for index finger abduction, VIII:479
 for upper extremity injury, VII:322
Tendon sheath, I:591, 593f
 fibroma of, VII:953, 953f
 giant cell tumor of, VII:955-956, 955f
Tendon transfer, VIII:453-486. See also
  Hand reconstruction, tendon transfer
  in.
Tennis elbow, VII:904, VIII:558, 559f
Tennison cheiloplasty, IV:204-205, 341-
  342, 342f
Tenoarthrolysis, in Dupuytren disease,
  VII:752
Tenolysis, I:597-598
Tenosynovitis, VII:675-688
 extensor tendon, VII:675-684, 676f. See
  also De Quervain syndrome.
  anatomy in, VII:675-676, 676f
  fifth dorsal compartment, VII:676f,
   683
  first dorsal compartment, VII:676-
   680, 676f. See also De Quervain
   syndrome.

Tenosynovitis (Continued)
  fourth dorsal compartment, VII:676f,
   682-683
  second dorsal compartment, VII:676f,
   680-681, 681f
  sixth dorsal compartment, VII:676f,
   683-684
  third dorsal compartment, VII:676f,
   681-682, 682f
 flexor tendon, VII:46-47, 684-686, 684f,
  686f
  pyogenic, VII:773, 773f, 774f, 780-
   781, 781f
  stenosing, VIII:560, 561f
Tenotomy, I:608
Tensor fascia lata flap, I:584-588
 for abdominal wall reconstruction,
  I:380-381, 380f-381f, 447, 447t,
  449f, 585, 586f, 985, 987f, VI:1188-
  1191, 1188f-1190f
 for groin and perineal reconstruction,
  I:451
 for lower extremity reconstruction,
  VI:1370-1371, 1371f
 for pressure sore treatment, I:465,
  VI:1338, 1340f-1342f, 1345, 1345f
 harvesting of, I:585, 587f
 historical perspective on, I:584
 indications for, I:585
 outcomes of, I:585, 586-587, 587f
 use of, I:585, 586f
Tensor veli palatini
 anatomy of, IV:58t, 59f, 60t, 61-62, 62f,
  72, 73f-75f, 312f
 magnetic resonance imaging of, IV:65,
  67f
Teratogens, IV:11-12
 in craniofacial microsomia, IV:113-114,
  114f
Teratoma, V:5-6
 nasal, V:112-113
 nasopharyngeal, III:766, 766f
 pericardial, fetal, I:1126
 sacrococcygeal, I:1127-1128
Tessier, Paul, I:32
Testis (testes)
 autotransplantation of, VI:1245-1246,
  1245f
 blood supply of, VI:1201-1204, 1201f-
  1205f
 cancer of
  gynecomastia and, VI:528-529
  polythelia and, VI:510
 embryology of, VI:1261, 1262f
 lymphedema of, VI:1255-1256
 protective withdrawal of, VI:1198-1199
 reattachment of, VI:1230-1232, 1233f
 tunica vaginalis of, VI:1201
Tetanus, prophylaxis for, VII:424, 424t
Tetracaine, I:190t
 for facial anesthesia, III:7-8, 7t
Tetraplegia, upper extremity function
  restoration in, VIII:507-540
 active grasp for, VIII:518, 520, 520f
 elbow extension in, VIII:512-518, 513f-
  515f, 517f, 519f, 540
  biceps to triceps transfer for,
   VIII:517-518, 519f
  deltoid to triceps transfer for,
   VIII:512-517, 513f-515f, 517f

Tetraplegia, upper extremity function restoration in (Continued)
functional evaluation before, VIII:511, 511f
functional neuromuscular stimulation for, VIII:536, 538, 539f
grasp and refined pinch for, VIII:535, 538f
grasp and release for, VIII:529-535
extensor phase of, VIII:530
flexor phase of, VIII:530-532, 532f-534f
House intrinsic tenodesis for, VIII:531-532, 533f-534f
in IC group 3, VIII:531-532, 532f-534f
in IC group 4 and 5, VIII:532-535, 536f-538f
in stable CMC joint, VIII:535, 536f-538f
in unstable CMC joint, VIII:534-535
intrinsic stabilization for, VIII:530-531
Zancolli lasso procedure for, VIII:531, 532f
guidelines for, VIII:512
historical perspective on, VIII:507-509, 508f
in IC groups 0, 1, and 2, VIII:518, 520-529, 520f-523f, 525f-529f
in IC groups 3, 4, and 5, VIII:529-535, 532f-534f, 536f-538f
in IC groups 6, 7, and 8, VIII:535, 538f
International Classification for, VIII:509-510, 509t
key pinch for, VIII:521-527, 522f, 540
brachioradialis to FPL transfer for, VIII:527-529, 528f, 529f
Brand-Moberg pollicis longus tenodesis for, VIII:508-509, 508f, 522, 524-527, 525f-527f
flexor pollicis longus tenodesis for, VIII:522, 524-527, 525f-527f
in IC group 1 and 2, VIII:521-522, 522f, 523f, 524-527, 525f-527f
in IC group 2 and 3, VIII:527-529, 528f, 529f
split FPL to EPL interphalangeal stabilization for, VIII:522, 523f
motor examination for, VIII:511, 511f
patient evaluation for, VIII:510-512, 511f
results of, VIII:538, 540
team for, VIII:510
timing of, VIII:510
winch procedure for, VIII:518, 520, 520f
wrist-driven flexor hinge splint in, VIII:508, 508f
wrist extension for, VIII:520-521, 521f
TGIF gene, IV:3
Thalidomide, III:638, VIII:61
Thenar flap
for fingertip reconstruction, VII:162-163, 163f, 164f
reverse-flow, for finger reconstruction, VII:228, 229f, 230f-231f
Thenar muscles, VII:32
Theophylline, in obstructive sleep apnea, III:776

Thermal injury. See Burns; Facial burns; Hand burns.
Thermography
in complex regional pain syndrome/reflex sympathetic dystrophy, VII:846
in hand frostbite, VII:649, 650f
Thermometry, in flap monitoring, I:497
Thermoplastics, I:756-758, 756f, 758f, 759f
Thermoset implants, I:760
Thigh, liposuction for, VI:231-232, 232f-234f, 250-251, 250f, 276f, 282-288, 284f, 285f, 286f, 287f
Thigh flap
anterior, for pressure sores, VI:1347, 1349, 1349f, 1350f
for penile reconstruction, VI:1226-1227, 1229f
gluteal, for pressure sores, VI:1323f, 1324t, 1325, 1327, 1331f, 1332f, 1338, 1343f
lateral
for esophageal reconstruction, III:1012-1013
for lower extremity reconstruction, VI:1377, 1377f
for neck reconstruction, III:1045, 1046f
for oral cavity reconstruction, III:941-942, 944-948, 948f, 949f
transverse, for breast reconstruction, VI:1055f, 1056f-1057f, 1057-1058, 1058f, 1063
medial, for lower extremity reconstruction, VI:1376-1377, 1377f
Thigh lift, VI:257-271
complications of, VI:269-271
consultation for, VI:257-258, 258t
contraindications to, VI:259
indications for, VI:259
lateral tension abdominoplasty for, VI:260
medial, VI:265-268, 267f, 268f
patient selection for, VI:259
photography for, VI:258
physical examination for, VI:258
transverse, Color Plate VI:125-4, VI:262-265, 265f, 266f
Thiopental, I:172, 172t
Thoracic dystrophy, asphyxiating, VI:484-485, 484f, 485f
Thoracic ectopia cordis, VI:482-483, 483f
Thoracic outlet syndrome, VII:876t, 906-909, 908f
diagnosis of, VII:880-881, 907-908
in musician, VII:702
management of, VII:908, 909f
pathophysiology of, VII:907
scapular winging in, VII:908
vascular, VII:810-813, 813f
Thoracoabdominal intercostal nerves, VI:1178
Thoracodorsal nerve, in latissimus dorsi flap, VI:830-831
Thoracoepigastric flap
for chest reconstruction, I:990
for complex post-mastectomy defect, VI:773, 776, 776t, 777f-780f

Thorax
anatomy of, VI:411-413, 412f
congenital anomalies of, VI:457-509, 458t. See also at Rib(s); Sternum.
embryology of, VI:457
expansion of, in Jeune syndrome, VI:485, 485f
fetal, I:1122-1125, 1123f
heart outside of, VI:482-483
muscles of, congenital disorders of, VI:485-509. See also Poland syndrome.
neuroma of, VII:943-944
Three-flap technique
for forehead reconstruction, III:716, 717f
for scalp reconstruction, III:613, 616f
Thromboangiitis obliterans, VI:1475, VII:814-815, 814f
Thrombocytopenia, kaposiform hemangioendothelioma and, V:36
Thrombocytopenia-absent radius syndrome, VIII:62, 326
Thromboembolism, VI:175-178, 177t, 178f
abdominoplasty and, VI:362, 378
Thrombolysis, in upper extremity ischemia, VII:802, 804
Thrombophlebitis
after breast augmentation, VI:30
septic, in burns, I:829
Thrombosis
arterial, VII:808-813, 810f-812f
flap, I:486-488, 487f
Thromboxane A_2, I:488, VII:797
Thumb(s). See also Finger(s); Hand(s).
absent. See Thumb(s), hypoplastic.
amputation of, VII:253-258, 254t. See also Thumb reconstruction.
burn-related, VII:627-630, 629f
in constriction ring syndrome, VIII:203, 205, 355-360, 356f-359f. See also Constriction ring syndrome.
intrauterine, VIII:185
level of, VII:254-256, 256f, 257f, 306
physical examination in, VII:256
prostheses for, VIII:592, 595f-597f
radiography in, VII:256
vascular anatomy in, VII:256, 258
anatomy of, VII:22-24, 23f, 254, 255f, VIII:327f
Apert, VIII:298, 298f, 363-365, 363f
aplasia of, VIII:331-332, 333f, 338-339. See also Thumb(s), hypoplastic.
arterial supply of, VII:795, 795f
carpometacarpal joint of
dislocation of, VII:433-434
fracture-dislocation of, VII:434-436, 435f
clasped, VIII:280, 282-286, 283f-286f, 564
commissural ligaments of, VII:732, 732f
constriction ring of, VIII:355-360, 356f-359f. See also Constriction ring syndrome.
cylinder grasp of, VII:254, 255f
deviation of, VIII:294-298, 295f, 298f. See also Clinodactyly.

Thumb(s) (Continued)
  duplication of, VIII:215-229. See also
    Polydactyly, radial (thumb).
  extension of, tendon transfer for,
    VIII:483, 484f
  extensor tendon injury of
    zone II, VII:415
    zone III, VII:415-417
    zone IV, VII:417
    zone V, VII:417-418
  extrinsic extensor muscles of, VII:25
  fascia of, VII:732, 732f
  flexion-adduction of, tendon transfer
    for, VIII:478-479
  flexion of, tendon transfer for, VIII:483,
    485f
  floating, VIII:324f, 327f, 330-331, 333f,
    338
  fracture-dislocation of
    at carpometacarpal joint, VII:434-
      436, 435f
    at metacarpophalangeal joint,
      VII:440-441, 441f
  fracture of, metacarpal, VII:425-426,
    426f
  hypoplastic, VIII:323-366
    classification of, VIII:323-324, 324f
    clinical presentation of, VIII:326-335
    etiology of, VIII:324, 325t
    in Apert syndrome, VIII:298, 298f,
      363-365, 363f
    in Fanconi anemia, VIII:325
    in Holt-Oram syndrome, VIII:326
    in Pfeiffer syndrome, VIII:363-365,
      363f
    in thrombocytopenia-absent radius
      syndrome, VIII:326
    in VACTERL, VIII:325
    incidence of, VIII:324
    malformation associations with,
      VIII:324, 325t
    treatment of, VIII:332, 334-338
      first web space deficiency in,
        VIII:339-340
      IP joint motion in, VIII:343
      MP joint instability in, VIII:340-
        341, 341f
      palmar abduction in, VIII:342-344,
        342f
      pollicization in, VIII:343-350
      principles of, VIII:332
      timing of, VIII:334, 334f
    type I (mild), VIII:324f, 326, 327f,
      328f
      treatment of, VIII:334-335, 335f
    type II (moderate), VIII:324f, 326,
      327f, 328, 329f, 330f
      treatment of, VIII:335-336
    type III (severe), VIII:324f, 327f, 328-
      330, 331f, 332f
      metacarpophalangeal joint
        instability in, VIII:340-341,
        341f
      treatment of, VIII:336-338, 337f,
        338f
    type IV (floating thumb), VIII:324f,
      327f, 330-331, 333f
      treatment of, VIII:338
    type V (aplasia), VIII:331-332, 333f
      treatment of, VIII:338-339

Thumb(s) (Continued)
    type VI (central deficiency), VIII:350-
      355, 351, 352f. See also Cleft
      hand; Symbrachydactyly.
    type VII (constriction ring
      syndrome), VIII:355-360, 356f-
      359f. See also Constriction ring
      syndrome.
    type VIII (five-fingered hand),
      VIII:360, 361f, 362f
    type IX (radial polydactyly),
      VIII:360-362. See also
      Polydactyly, radial (thumb).
    type X (syndromic), VIII:363-365,
      363f, 364f
  in cleft hand, VIII:350-353, 351f, 352f
  in mirror hand, VIII:253, 254f
  in motor nerve palsy, VII:34
  intrinsic muscles of, VII:34
  key pinch of, VII:254, 255f, VIII:521,
    522f. See also Key pinch.
  ligaments of, VII:23-24
  loss of, VII:253-258, 254t
    level of, VII:254-256, 256f, 257f
    physical examination in, VII:256
    radiography in, VII:256
    vascular anatomy in, VII:256, 258
  metacarpophalangeal joint of
    dislocation of, VII:437-438, 437f-439f
    fracture-dislocation of, VII:440-441,
      441f
    instability of, in thumb
      reconstruction, VIII:340-342,
      341f
    osteoarthritis of, VII:724, 725f
  motion of, VII:23, 24, 34
  opposition of, VII:254, 255f. See also Key
    pinch.
    abductor digiti quinti minimi transfer
      for, VIII:342, 342f
    after reconstruction, VII:276f
    flexor digitorum superficialis transfer
      for, VIII:342-343
  ossification centers of, VIII:323
  osteoarthritis of, VII:724, 724f, 725f
  prosthetic, I:786-787, VII:284-285
  reconstruction of, VII:281-292, 295-315,
    304t. See also Thumb
    reconstruction.
  replantation of. See also Finger
    replantation.
    flap coverage for, VII:329f
    indications for, VII:566
    outcome of, VII:581
  rope avulsion injury to, VII:581
  symbrachydactyly, VIII:353-355, 353f,
    354f
  synovial sheath of, VII:29
  three-point pinch of, VII:254, 255f
  trigger, VII:686-688, 686f, VIII:280-282,
    281f, 282f
  triphalangeal, VIII:229-232, 231f, 254-
    261
    associated anomalies with, VIII:254
    classification of, VIII:254-255
    clinical presentation of, VIII:255, 255f
    incidence of, VIII:254
    treatment of, VIII:255-261, 256f, 256t,
      257f-261f
    type I, VIII:255, 255f, 256t

Thumb(s) (Continued)
    type II, VIII:255f, 256t, 257f
    type III, VIII:255, 255f, 256t, 257,
      258f
    type IV, VIII:255f, 256t, 257, 259, 259f
    type V, VIII:256t, 259, 260f, 261f
    type VI, VIII:256t, 259
  web space of
    burn scar contracture of, VII:621-623,
      622f
    deficiency of, VIII:339-340
    in cleft hand, VIII:97-98, 97f
    release of, VIII:159-161, 160f-162f,
      335f, 339-340
      in Apert syndrome, VIII:172
    Z-plasty for, I:252f, VII:621-623, 622f
Thumb-in-palm deformity, VIII:548t, 549-
  550, 564
Thumb reconstruction, VII:281-292, 295-
  315, 304t
  acute, VII:283-284
  age and, VII:282
  associated diseases and, VII:282
  contraindications to, VII:283t
  digital transposition for. See Thumb
    reconstruction, pollicization for.
  distraction lengthening for, VII:291-292,
    628-629
  function after, VII:306
  goals of, VII:282, 282t
  gracilis muscle transfer for, VIII:500-
    501, 501f
  historical perspective on, VII:295-302,
    296f-299f, 300, 301f-304f, 302
  indications for, VII:283t, 306, 315
  injury-related factors and, VII:282
  interphalangeal joint in, VIII:343
  lateral arm flap for, VII:330f, 331f, 332f-
    333f
  lengthening technique in, VII:291-292
  Loda technique of, VII:285, 286f-287f
  occupation and, VII:282
  osteoplastic, VII:289-291, 290f-291f,
    295-296, 296f, 297f, 306, 307f, 630
  phalangealization for, VII:295, 296, 298f,
    299f
    in burn injury, VII:628
  pollicization for, VII:285-289, 286f-289f,
    300, 301f-304f, 302, 304t, 306, 308f-
    314f, VIII:343-350
    age at, VIII:348
    care after, VIII:347-348
    closure in, VIII:346f, 347
    complications of, VIII:348
    dissection for, VIII:344
    in burn injury, VII:628, 629f
    incisions for, VIII:343-344, 347f-348f
    index digit in, VII:303f-304f, 308f,
      309f, 311f-314f
    index finger inadequacy and,
      VIII:348-350, 349f
    muscle rebalancing in, VIII:346f, 347
    of intact finger, VII:285, 286f-289f
    of mutilated finger, VII:285-289,
      289f-290f
    outcomes of, VIII:348
    ring digit in, VII:307f, 310f
    scar contracture with, VII:288
    skeletal shortening for, VIII:346f, 347
    web construction in, VIII:346f, 348

Thumb reconstruction *(Continued)*
  preparation for, VII:258
  radial forearm flap for, VII:290, 290f-291f
  rein technique of, VII:285, 286f-287f
  second-toe transfer for, VII:271-272, 273f, 296-297, 298f
  secondary, VII:284-292. *See also* Thumb reconstruction, osteoplastic; Thumb reconstruction, pollicization for.
  sensibility and, VII:281-282
  toe transfer for, VII:258-269, 338, 344f-345f, 345, 346f, 348, 630
    anesthesia for, VII:258
    appearance outcomes in, VII:277-278, 277f
    closure for, VII:268, 268f
    complications of, VII:275, 275t
    contralateral thumb size in, VII:258, 259f
    donor site outcomes in, VII:276-277
    donor site repair in, VII:267-268, 269f
    functional recovery after, VII:276
    hand dissection in, VII:259-261, 260f, 261f
    historical perspective on, VII:296-297, 299f
    incision markings for, VII:259, 260f
    osteotomy in, VII:264, 265f, 266f
    outcomes of, VII:275-278
    partial, VII:272-273, 273t, 274f
    plantar dissection in, VII:264
    postoperative management in, VII:273-275
    radiography in, VII:258, 259f
    rehabilitation after, VII:275
    sensory recovery after, VII:275-276
    subjective results in, VII:277-278
    toe dissection in, VII:261-265, 261f-263f, 265f
    transfer technique in, VII:265-268, 266f, 266t, 267f, 268f
    trimmed toe technique in, VII:270-271, 271f, 272f, 277f
    wraparound flap technique in, VII:268, 270, 270f, 277f
  vs. amputation, VII:282
  vs. no reconstruction, VII:284-285
Thyroglossal duct cyst, III:767, 1029, 1029f, 1030f
Thyroglossal remnants, V:4
Thyroid cartilage reduction, in male-to-female transformation, VI:1315
Thyroid gland
  arterial supply of, I:344
  cancer of, in children, V:16
  lingual, III:767
Thyroid-stimulating hormone, in temperature regulation, I:856
Tiagabine, in complex regional pain syndrome/reflex sympathetic dystrophy, VII:858
Tibia
  distal, fracture of, I:1008, 1010, 1011f-1014f
  for bone graft, I:673t, 680, 681f
Tibial artery, Color Plates I:15-8 and 15-9, I:338
Tibial recurrent artery, Color Plate I:15-8, I:338

Tibialis anterior flap, I:389f
Tight lip, after cleft lip repair, IV:350
Tinel sign
  after peripheral nerve repair, VII:506
  in brachial plexus injury, VII:525
Tissue engineering, I:765, 1081-1103
  bioreactor in, I:1085-1086, 1086f
  cell-polymer constructs in, I:1081-1082, 1082f
    construction of, I:1085-1086, 1086f
  cells in, I:1083-1085, 1084f
    seeding of, I:1085-1086, 1086f
  hydrogels in, I:1083, 1093-1095, 1095f, 1095t
  myoblasts in, I:1096-1097, 1097f
  of blood vessels, Color Plate I:37-2, I:1089-1091, 1090f, 1092f
  of bone, I:1100-1101, 1102t, 1103f
  of cartilage, Color Plate I:37-3, I:1097-1099, 1098f, 1099t
  of dermis, I:1087-1089, 1087t, 1088f
  of fat tissue, I:1095-1096
  of keratinocytes, I:1087-1088, 1087t
  of organoids, I:1096-1097
  of peripheral nerves, I:1091-1093, 1093t, 1094f
  of skeletal muscle, I:1096-1097, 1097f
  of soft tissue, I:1093-1096, 1095f, 1095t
  polymer scaffolds in, Color Plate I:37-1, I:1082-1083, 1083t
  stem cells in, I:1084-1085, 1085f
  Web sites on, I:1086
Tissue expansion, I:361, 380-384, 380f-386f, 539-556
  biology of, I:540-543, 540f-545f
  bone response in, I:541
  complications of, I:565-566, 920-921
  cytoskeleton in, I:542, 544f
  dermis response to, I:541
  epidermis response to, I:540-541
  expanders for, I:543-544, 544f, 546
  failure of, I:384, 920-921
  filling ports with, I:546
  flap compromise with, I:566
  flap planning for, I:545
  for full-thickness skin graft, I:547
  for myocutaneous flaps, I:547
  growth factors in, I:542, 544f
  historical perspective on, I:539-540
  implant exposure after, I:566
  implant failure with, I:566
  implant inflation for, I:546
  implant overinflation for, I:546
  implant with, I:543-544, 545
  in breast reconstruction, I:557-561, 559f, 560f. *See also* Expander-implant breast reconstruction.
  in burn reconstruction, I:546, 555f
  in cheek reconstruction, III:833, 841f-842f
  in children, I:546-547
  in ear reconstruction, I:557
  in extremities, I:563-565
  in forehead reconstruction, I:551
  in head and neck reconstruction, I:547-548, III:1034-1035, 1035f-1036f
  in hypoplastic breast, I:561-563
  in irradiated chest wall, I:561
  in lateral face and neck reconstruction, I:551, 553, 554f, 555f

Tissue expansion *(Continued)*
  in male pattern baldness, I:551, III:629-630
  in nose reconstruction, I:553, 556f
  in periorbital reconstruction, I:556-557
  in Poland syndrome, I:563, 564f
  in scalp reconstruction, I:548-551, 549f-551f, III:618-619, 619f
  in trunk and abdomen, I:563, 565f
  infection with, I:565-566
  mitosis in, I:543
  molecular basis for, I:542-543, 544f, 545f
  muscle response to, I:541, 541f
  principles of, I:544-546
  protein kinase C in, I:542
  safety of, I:384
  ultrastructure of, I:542
  vascular response to, I:541-542, 542f, 543f
Tissue plasminogen activator, in frostbite, VII:652
Titanium implants, I:752, 752t
  for facial defects, Color Plate I:27-2, I:773-774, 773f, 774f
Tobacco. *See also* Cigarette smoking.
  head and neck cancer and, V:159
  oral cavity cancer and, III:918
Toe(s), VI:1410, 1413f
  pressures of, VI:1412
Toe fillet flap, for foot reconstruction, VI:1424, 1425f
Toe flaps
  fillet, for foot reconstruction, VI:1424, 1425f
  for finger reconstruction, VII:237, 239t, 240-244, 240f-243f
  lateral first-toe, for finger reconstruction, VII:237, 241f, 242
  neurovascular island, for foot reconstruction, VI:1424-1425, 1426-1427, 1426f, 1430f
  second-toe, for finger reconstruction, VII:237, 240f, 242-244, 243f
Toe transfer
  for constriction ring syndrome, VIII:179, 179f, 357f, 359-360, 359f
  for finger reconstruction, VII:216, 217f, 244-247, 244f-247f, 338, 344f-345f, 345, 346f, 348
  for metacarpal hypoplasia, VIII:59-60, 60f
  for symbrachydactyly, VIII:126-129, 129f, 131
  for thumb reconstruction, VII:258-269. *See also* Thumb reconstruction, toe transfer for.
  multiple, for finger reconstruction, VII:244-247, 244f-247f
Tolerance, immunologic, I:278-279, 285
Tomography, of hand and wrist, VII:65, 66f
Tongue. *See also* Oral cavity.
  advancement of, in obstructive sleep apnea, III:789-791, 790f, 791f
  anatomy of, III:920-922, 921f, V:163f, 164, 164f
  arterial supply of, Color Plate I:15-13, I:343, 343f, 343t
  base of, V:165, 165f
  dysfunction of, V:166

Tongue (Continued)
  reconstruction of, III:924-925, 927-928, 929f, 941, 942f-944f. See also Oral cavity reconstruction.
    rectus abdominis flap for, III:941, 942f-944f
    skin graft for, III:927-928, 929f
  trauma to, III:37
  tumors of, V:166-167, 166f
Tongue flap, for lower lip reconstruction, V:383, 385, 385f
Tongue-lip adhesion procedure, in Robin sequence, IV:514-515, 516f
Tonic-clonic movements, ketamine-related, I:175
Tonsillar pillars, V:165, 165f
Tonsilloadenoidectomy, in craniofacial clefts, IV:422
Tonsils, V:165, 165f
Tooth (teeth). See also Orthodontics; Orthognathic surgery.
  aesthetic analysis of, II:4t, 13, 13f-15f, 23-24, 25f
  anatomy of, III:920, 921f
  cephalometric analysis of, II:23-24, 25f
  cracks in, with laser resurfacing, II:375-376
  examination of
    in craniosynostoses, IV:497
    in temporomandibular joint dysfunction, III:542
    preoperative, I:168
  fracture of, in children, III:407, 409
  fracture-related fixation of, III:118, 120-128, 155
    acrylic splints in, III:127, 129f
    anatomy for, III:118, 120-122, 120f-122f
    arch bar method wiring in, III:123-126, 124f-127f
    Eyelet method wiring in, III:122-123, 123f
    Gilmer method wiring in, III:122, 122f
    intermaxillary fixation screw in, III:128, 130f
    monomaxillary vs. bimaxillary, III:128
    orthodontic bands in, III:127, 128f
    wiring techniques in, III:122-128, 122f-127f
  implantation of
    after mandibular reconstruction, III:985-986, 986f, 987f
    osseointegrated, I:524, 524f
    recombinant bone morphogenetic proteins with, I:662-663
  injury to
    in children, III:405-409, 406f-408f
    with orthognathic surgery, II:684
  malocclusion of
    class I, II:649, 650f
    class II, II:649, 650f
    class III, II:649, 650f
    in condylar process fracture, III:515
    in mandibular fracture, III:185-186, 187f
    in maxillary fracture, III:239, 240f, 252-253, 252f
    in panfacial fracture, III:257, 257f

Tooth (teeth) (Continued)
    in pediatric facial fracture, III:411-412
    in zygoma fracture, III:213
    transverse dimension of, II:649, 650f
    vertical dimension of, II:649, 650f
    with condylar process fracture, III:515
  overbite of, II:13, 15f
  overjet of, II:13, 15f
  reimplantation of
    in children, III:406f, 409
    in mandibular fracture treatment, III:155
  roots of, in mandibular fracture treatment, III:187
Torsoplasty, circumferential, VI:171-172, 172f, 173f
Torticollis, III:398, 1032-1033, 1033f, IV:98-99
Torus mandibularis, V:11
Torus palatinus, V:11
Total anterior tenoarthrolysis, in Dupuytren disease, VII:752
Total body surface area, in burn assessment, I:813-814, 814f, 815f
Tourniquet, for hand surgery, VII:115-118, 116f
Toxic epidermal necrolysis, I:793-799
  ABCs in, I:797
  classification of, I:793-794, 794t
  clinical presentation of, I:795-796, 796f
  corticosteroid therapy in, I:798
  cyclosporine in, I:799
  definition of, I:793-794
  differential diagnosis of, I:796-797
  drugs in, I:794-795, 798
  epidemiology of, I:794-795
  infection in, I:795-796, 799
  intravenous immune globulin in, I:799
  nutrition in, I:798-799
  ocular care in, I:799
  ocular sequelae of, I:796
  oral hygiene in, I:798
  pathogenesis of, I:795
  plasmapheresis in, I:799
  prognosis for, I:799
  sequelae of, I:796
  treatment of, I:797-799, 798f
  wound care in, I:797-798, 798f
Toxic shock syndrome, VII:762
  after laser resurfacing, II:372
TP53 gene, VII:988
Trace metal deficiency, wound healing and, I:221
Trachea
  arterial supply of, Color Plate I:15-13, I:343-344, 343t
  embryology of, III:1026-1027
  endoscopic clip for, in fetal diaphragmatic hernia, I:1124
  ligation of, in fetal diaphragmatic hernia, I:1123-1124
  occlusion of, in fetal diaphragmatic hernia, I:1123-1124
  stenosis of, in pediatric facial trauma, III:398
Tracheal intubation, I:176-177
  in children, III:395, 397-398, 397f
Tracheoesophageal fistula, congenital, III:1026-1027

Tracheostomy
  in burn treatment, I:829
  in craniofacial microsomia, IV:523
  in micrognathia, III:777
  in obstructive sleep apnea, III:786, 791-794, 793f, 794f
  in pediatric facial trauma, III:397
  scar after, revision of, I:255, 257f, 258, 258f
Tragus deformity, after face lift, II:732-734, 733f, 734f
TRAM flap. See Transverse rectus abdominis myocutaneous (TRAM) flap.
Tramadol, in complex regional pain syndrome/reflex sympathetic dystrophy, VII:860
Transblepharoplasty, II:63-64
Transconjunctival blepharoplasty, II:122-124, 124f
Transcutaneous electrical nerve stimulation
  in complex regional pain syndrome/reflex sympathetic dystrophy, VII:855
  in hand therapy, VIII:572
Transcutaneous oxygen tension, in foot, VI:1414-1415
TransCyte
  in burn treatment, I:824t, 825
  in wound healing, I:1018
Transference, I:70-71
Transforming growth factor-β
  exogenous, I:664-665
  in bone repair, I:656t, 663-665
  in fetal wound healing, I:218
  in wound healing, I:212t, 215-216, 1018
  osteogenic protein 1 with, I:663
Transforming growth factor-β3, in palatal fusion, IV:8
Transoral resection, in oral cavity cancer, V:177, 177f, 178f
Transplantation, I:269-285
  antibody screening for, I:274
  basal cell carcinoma and, V:396
  crossmatching for, I:274
  historical perspective on, I:269-270
  immunologic screening for, I:273-274
  immunologic tolerance in, I:278-279, 285
    anergy and, I:279
    clonal deletion and, I:278-279
    suppression and, I:279
  immunology of, I:270-279
    B lymphocytes in, I:271-272
    blood group antigens in, I:271
    complement in, I:272
    dendritic cells in, I:272
    granulocytes in, I:271
    immunoglobulins in, I:272
    macrophages in, I:271
    major histocompatibility complex in, I:270-271
    minor histocompatibility antigens in, I:271
    natural killer cells in, I:271
    rejection cascade in, I:271-273
    skin-specific antigens in, I:271
    T lymphocytes in, I:272-273

Transplantation *(Continued)*
immunosuppression for, I:274-278,
274t, 275t, 285
anti-interleukin-2 in, I:277-278
antilymphocyte globulin in, I:277
azathioprine in, I:275t, 276
corticosteroids in, I:275-276, 275t
cyclosporine in, I:275t, 276
mycophenolate mofetil in, I:275t, 276
OKT3 in, I:277
rapamycin in, I:275t, 277
tacrolimus in, I:275t, 276-277
major histocompatibility complex in,
I:273-274
nomenclature for, I:270
of bone, I:280-281, 692. *See also* Bone
graft.
of cartilage, I:281. *See also* Cartilage
graft.
of composite tissues, I:282. *See also*
Microvascular surgery.
of hair, III:628-629, 628f
of limb, I:283-285, 283t
of muscle. *See* Flap(s).
of nerve, I:281-282, 735, VII:500-503,
501f, 502f. *See also* Nerve graft.
of skin, I:279-280. *See also* Skin graft.
rejection of, I:271-273
acute, I:273
chronic, I:273
skin cancer and, V:396, 397
squamous cell carcinoma and, V:397
Transversalis fascia, VI:91, 1176, 1176f
Transverse carpal ligament, VII:29, 30f
Transverse flank-thigh-buttock lift, Color
Plate VI:125-4, VI:262-265, 265f, 266f
Transverse flap, for back reconstruction,
VI:442, 446f
Transverse lines, postblepharoplasty
recurrence of, II:814
Transverse pedicle flap, for nasal
reconstruction, V:349, 359f-360f
Transverse rectus abdominis myocutaneous
(TRAM) flap, I:433, 436f-440f, 440,
VI:712-761, 712f, 714f-719f
advantages of, I:433
complications of, I:440, VI:713, 717f,
751, 751t, 843, 847, 865, 872, 993-
995
contraindications to, I:433, VI:713,
731t
delayed (free), VI:1001-1020
breast support after, VI:1015
care after, VI:1014-1015
contraindications to, VI:1024
dissection for, VI:1006-1012, 1009f-
1012f
donor site closure for, VI:1012-1013,
1013f
fascia-sparing flap for, VI:1002, 1005f
flap elevation for, VI:1006, 1008,
1008f-1010f
flap inset for, VI:1013-1014, 1013f-
1015f
flap transfer for, VI:1011-1012
liposuction after, VI:1015
mound reduction after, VI:1017,
1018f-1019f
muscle-sparing flap for, VI:1002,
1003f

Transverse rectus abdominis myocutaneous
(TRAM) flap *(Continued)*
nipple reconstruction with, VI:1019-
1020
opposite breast surgery with, VI:1017,
1019
pain control after, VI:1014
pedicled, VI:1001, 1002f, 1002t
planning for, VI:1004, 1006-1007,
1007f
pocket dissection for, VI:1006
rationale for, VI:1001-1002, 1002t
recipient vessels for, VI:1004, 1006,
1006f
result of, VI:1002, 1003f, 1019f
revisions of, VI:1015-1017, 1016f-
1019f
V to Y island flap after, VI:1015-1017,
1016f-1017f
delayed (pedicled), VI:714f-716f, 973-
997
abdominal examination for, VI:979
abdominal wall strength after, VI:994-
995
anatomic considerations in, VI:976
anesthesia for, VI:980
bilateral, VI:721f, 987, 989f, 990f
bipedicled, VI:721f, 733-736, 733f-
735f, 740f, 761f, 983, 983t, 987,
987f-990f
blood donation in, VI:730
body habitus in, VI:977-978, 978f
chest dimensions and, VI:978
chest marking in, VI:725
collagen vascular disease and, VI:979
complications of, VI:713, 717t, 993-
995
contraindications to, VI:979
contralateral unipedicled, VI:981-983,
982f, 984f
decision for, VI:997
donor site closure for, VI:983, 993
expander-implant procedure with,
VI:952, 955f-959f, 956
expander in, VI:977
fat necrosis after, VI:994
flap folding in, VI:992
flap orientation in, VI:991-993, 992f
flap shaping in, VI:991, 993
hernia after, VI:994-995
historical perspective on, VI:974
implant in, VI:738, 742f-743f, 952,
955f-959f, 956
indications for, VI:973-974, 974t
ipsilateral unipedicled, VI:981-983,
981f, 985f, 986f
marking for, VI:720, 721f, 722-723f
mastectomy scar in, VI:977, 977f,
978f, 990-991, 991f
muscle-sparing flap for, VI:982-983,
982f
nerve supply in, VI:976
nipple reconstruction with, VI:985f,
986f, 993
obesity and, VI:977-978, 978f, 995
oblique flap orientation in, VI:991f,
992
partial flap loss after, VI:995
patient positioning for, VI:980-981
patient satisfaction after, VI:996-997

Transverse rectus abdominis myocutaneous
(TRAM) flap *(Continued)*
patient selection for, VI:979, 979f,
980f
pregnancy after, VI:996
preoperative preparation for, VI:979-
980
radiation therapy and, VI:978, 978f,
979f, 994, 996
results of, VI:714f-716f, 719f, 721f-
724f, 752f
secondary shaping in, VI:993
skin necrosis after, VI:994
skin-sparing mastectomy and,
VI:976-977
smoking and, VI:995-996
strategic delay in, VI:717, 718f-719f
transverse flap orientation in, VI:991-
992, 992f
unipedicled, VI:981-983, 981f, 982f,
984f-986f
vascular patterns of, VI:974-976, 974t,
975t, 976t
volume assessment in, VI:987, 990
weight loss and, VI:730
historical perspective on, VI:686, 689f
immediate (free), VI:849-872
abdominal wall repair after, VI:859,
862, 865
alternatives to, VI:1053-1065, 1054f
anesthesia for, VI:853
care after, VI:862, 863f-864f
complications of, VI:865, 872
contraindications to, VI:850
deep venous thrombosis after,
VI:872
disadvantages of, VI:850
dissection for, VI:853-854, 855f-858f
fat necrosis after, VI:865
flap design for, VI:851, 852f
flap insetting for, VI:858-859, 861f
flap loss after, VI:865
flap shaping for, VI:858-859, 861f
flap thrombosis after, VI:872
hematoma after, VI:872
hernia after, VI:872
indications for, VI:850
infection after, VI:872
inframammary fold sutures for,
VI:853, 854f
marking for, VI:852-853, 853f
mastopexy with, VI:859
nipple reconstruction in, VI:862,
864f, 865
patient assessment for, VI:850-851
patient positioning for, VI:853
pulmonary embolism after, VI:872
rationale for, VI:849-850, 850f
recipient site for, VI:851-852, 852f
results of, VI:866f-871f
second stage of, VI:862, 865
vascular anastomosis for, VI:854, 858,
859f, 860f
immediate (pedicled), VI:676f, 712f,
835-847
abdominal closure for, VI:840-841,
842f
abdominal wall complications of,
VI:843, 847
anatomy for, VI:836-838, 836f, 837f

Transverse rectus abdominis myocutaneous (TRAM) flap *(Continued)*
bipedicled, VI:720, 731t, 738, 741f, 842-843, 844f
donor site closure in, VI:747, 747f, 748f
inset of, VI:751, 758, 759f, 760f
blood donation in, VI:730
complications of, VI:713, 843, 847
dissection for, VI:839-840, 839f-842f
goals of, VI:838
historical perspective on, VI:835
indications for, VI:713, 731t, 835-836
markings for, VI:720, 725, 838-839, 839f
placement of, VI:751, 753f, 841-842
planning for, VI:838-839, 839f
results of, VI:753f-754f, 844f-846f
types of, VI:836, 838
unipedicled, VI:730-731, 731t
immediate-delayed, VI:977, 978
indications for, I:433, VI:713, 731t
radiation therapy and, VI:670, 670t, 978, 978f, 979f, 994, 996
results of, VI:959-960, 960f, 960t
technique of, VI:730-758. *See also* Transverse rectus abdominis myocutaneous (TRAM) flap, delayed; Transverse rectus abdominis myocutaneous (TRAM) flap, immediate.
abdominal marking for, VI:720, 721f, 725, 725f
anesthesia in, VI:731
arc of rotation in, VI:738
bipedicled, VI:733-736, 733f-735f, 738, 740f, 741f
closure for, VI:747-749, 747f, 748f
flap inset for, VI:751, 758, 759f-761f
chest preparation in, VI:722f, 725, 736-738, 736f-737f
contralateral symmetry procedures in, VI:724f, 725
donor site closure in, VI:738, 744f-745f, 746-751, 746f-752f
flap elevation in, VI:725f-730f, 731-736, 732f-735f
flap inset in, VI:751, 753f-758f, 758, 759f-761f
flap transposition in, VI:736-738, 736f-737f, 739f-743f
implant in, VI:738, 742f-743f
inferior margin and, VI:725
perforator vessels in, VI:732, 732f
postoperative management in, VI:758, 761
preoperative markings in, VI:720, 721f-722f, 725, 725f
selection of, VI:720
skin island in, VI:713, 717-720, 717f, 718f
strategic delay in, I:371, VI:717, 718f-719f
supercharging and, VI:720
umbilical inset in, VI:749-751, 750f, 751f
vascular anatomy in, VI:717-718, 720, 729f-730f
Transversus abdominis, VI:91, 1176-1177

Trapeziotrapezoid ligament, VII:456f
Trapezius flap, I:423
for back reconstruction, VI:441, 443f
for chest reconstruction, I:990
for facial reconstruction, I:423, 428f-430f, III:833, 846f
for head and neck reconstruction, I:423, 428f-430f, III:1055-1062, 1055f-1061f, V:222-223, 223f, 226t
for mandible reconstruction, III:961, 962
for scalp reconstruction, III:620
Trapezius transfer, for obstetric brachial plexus palsy, VII:557, 559f
Trastuzumab, VI:671
Traumatic tattoo, III:12-13, 12f
Treacher Collins syndrome, III:778, IV:30, 31f, 33-35, 34f-35f, 100-101
airway in, IV:507
cheek region in, IV:506, 506f
choanal atresia in, IV:422, 422f
colobomas in, IV:427, 427f, 428f, 506, 506f
dysmorphology of, IV:504-507, 505f, 506f
ear in, IV:506-507
embryology of, IV:11
evaluation of, IV:507
eyelid deformities in, IV:426-427, 427f, 428f, 506, 506f
full-thickness transposition flap for, IV:427, 428f
musculocutaneous flap for, IV:426, 428f
Z-plasty for, IV:426, 427f
facies of, IV:504, 505f
genetics of, IV:413-414
mandibular defects in, IV:505-506, 506f
maxillary defects in, IV:505, 505f
nasopharyngeal intubation in, IV:416, 422
nose in, IV:507
orbital defects in, IV:505, 505f
pharynx in, IV:507
reconstruction for, IV:418t, 504-511
centrofacial flattening procedure in, IV:509, 509f
cheek procedures in, IV:511, 512f
ear procedures in, IV:509-510
eyelid procedures in, IV:510, 511f, 512f
integral procedure in, IV:509, 510f
mandibular distraction osteogenesis in, IV:509
nasal procedures in, IV:510-511
orbital bone grafting in, IV:431-432, 432f, 433f, 508-509, 508f
pericranial flaps in, IV:511, 512f
results of, IV:446, 453f, 454, 454f
timing of, IV:507
vascularized vs. nonvascularized bone graft in, IV:507-508, 508f
temporal region in, IV:506, 506f
zygomatic defects in, IV:30, 31f, 504-505, 505f
Trench foot, I:858-859
Tretinoin, II:395, V:405
Triamcinolone, after lower lid blepharoplasty, II:818

Triangular fibrocartilage complex, VII:21
tears of
arthroscopic débridement of, VII:129-130, 129f, 130f
arthroscopic repair of, VII:130-131, 131f-134f
radial, VII:131, 133f, 134f
ulnar, VII:130-131, 131f, 132f
ulnar plus variance and, VII:133, 135f
Triazine, teratogenicity of, IV:113, 114f
Tricalcium phosphate implants, I:693t, 697, 755
Triceps reconstruction, VIII:502
Trichiasis, II:91
Trichion, II:3f, 3t
Trichloroacetic acid injury, to hand, VII:654
Trichoepithelioma, V:260, 260f
Trichorhinophalangeal syndrome, VIII:21t
Tricyclic antidepressants, in complex regional pain syndrome/reflex sympathetic dystrophy, VII:858-859
Trigeminal nerve, IV:81-82
anatomy of, II:85-86, 86f
in facial trauma, III:4, 4f, 5
injury to, with orthognathic surgery, II:684
neuroma of, VII:944
Trigeminal nerve block, I:191-192, 192f
Trigger finger, VII:684-686, 684f, 686f, 702, VIII:560, 561f
Trigger points, in complex regional pain syndrome/reflex sympathetic dystrophy, VII:833-835
Trigger thumb, VII:686-688, 686f, VIII:280-282, 281f, 282f
Trigonocephaly, IV:137t, 154-158, 156f-160f, 472-474, 475f, 476f
Triphalangeal thumb, VIII:229-232, 231f, 254-261. *See also* Thumb(s), triphalangeal.
Triquetrocapitate ligament, VII:456f
Triquetrohamate ligament, VII:456f
Triquetrolunate ligament, dissociation of, VII:468
Triquetrum, VII:19
evaluation of, VII:54
fracture of, VII:466-467
in children, VIII:424
Reagan-Linscheid test of, VII:54
Trochanter
for bone graft, I:673t, 684-685
pressure sores of, I:999t, 1000, VI:1338, 1340-1346, 1340f-1346f
Trochlea, II:80
Tropocollagen, in wound healing, I:213
Trumpet nail, VII:202f, 203-204, 203f
Trumpet sign, VII:549
Trunk
liposuction for, VI:273-282, 280f, 281f, 283f
care after, VI:289-290
complications of, VI:274-275, 275t
fat assessment for, VI:274
gender-related variations in, VI:277-278, 278f-279f
infiltration for, VI:277
patient selection for, VI:273-275, 274f, 274t
physical examination for, VI:273, 274f

Trunk (Continued)
    pinch test in, VI:289
    planning for, VI:275
    power-assisted, VI:275
    principles of, VI:288-289
    ultrasound-assisted, VI:275
    wetting solution for, VI:276-277, 277t
    tissue expansion in, I:563, 565f
Trunk lift, VI:257-271
    complications of, VI:269-271
    consultation for, VI:257-258, 258t
    contraindications to, VI:259
    indications for, VI:259
    lateral tension abdominoplasty for,
      VI:260
    patient selection for, VI:259
    photography for, VI:258
    physical examination for, VI:258
    transverse, Color Plate VI:125-4,
      VI:262-265, 265f, 266f
Truth telling, I:123-124
Tuberculosis, in children, V:2
Tuberous breasts, I:562-563, VI:513-522
Tufted angioma, V:36-37
Tumors. See Cancer and specific sites and
    cancers.
Tunnel procedure, in auricular
    reconstruction, III:686-687, 688f-692f
Tuohy needle repair, for triangular
    fibrocartilage tears, VII:130-131,
    132f
Turbinate flap, for unilateral cheiloplasty,
    IV:184, 184f, 185f, 189f, 190f
Turbinate hypertrophy, III:765
Turbinectomy, II:524
Turner syndrome
    pterygium colli in, III:1027, 1027f-1028f
    venous malformation in, V:47
Turribrachycephaly, IV:477, 495, 496f. See
    also Craniosynostosis
    (craniosynostoses), syndromic.
Twin studies, of craniofacial microsomia,
    IV:115
Twin-twin transfusion syndrome, I:1129-
    1130
TWIST gene, IV:92, 93t
Two-flap technique, of palatoplasty,
    IV:259, 260f

U

UBE3A gene, I:53
Ulcer(s)
    diabetic, I:942-943, 943f, 981, 982f
    digital, in Raynaud disease, I:905-906,
      906f
    foot, I:866, 868f, 943, 943f, 981, 982f
    gastrointestinal, with burns, I:829
    hemangioma and, V:28, 28f
    lower extremity
      arterial, wound healing and, I:903-
        904, 904f, 963, 965f-966f
      carcinoma and, I:916, 916f
      diabetic, I:942-943, 943f, 981, 982f
      ischemic, I:903-904, 904f
      venous, wound healing and, I:906-
        907, 906f, 907f, 964
    Marjolin, I:916, 917f, III:612, V:275,
      276f, 437-439, 437f, 437t, VI:446-
      447, 447f, VII:614
    of pyoderma gangrenosum, I:940, 940f

Ulcer(s) (Continued)
    pressure, I:942, 942f, 999-1000, 999t,
      1001f-1004f, VI:1317-1352. See also
      Pressure sores.
    radiation-induced, I:850-852, 851f
Ulna
    fracture of, in children, VIII:420-423,
      422f
    lengthening of, VIII:74f, 75, 77f
    radius fusion to. See Radioulnar
      synostosis.
    shortening of, in lunotriquetral
      instability, VII:135
    straightening of, VIII:75
    vascular territories of, I:335-336
Ulnar abutment syndrome, VII:133, 135f
Ulnar artery, Color Plates I:15-4 and 15-5,
    I:335
    anatomy of, VII:34-35, 792
    aneurysm of, VII:813-814
    dominance of, VII:796-797
    in scleroderma, VII:84f
    post-traumatic aneurysm of, VII:894
    pseudoaneurysm of, VII:83f
    thrombosis of, VII:808-810, 810f-812f
Ulnar deficiency, VIII:101-110
    at elbow, VIII:103, 107, 110
    at forearm, VIII:103, 105f, 106f, 107,
      110, 110f
    at hand, VIII:103, 104f, 107, 109f
    at shoulder, VIII:105f, 106f, 107
    at wrist, VIII:103, 107, 110
    classification of, VIII:101, 102f
    clinical presentation of, VIII:103-107,
      104f-106f
    etiology of, VIII:101-102
    incidence of, VIII:40t, 101
    treatment of, VIII:107, 109f
Ulnar dimelia. See Mirror hand.
Ulnar forearm flap
    for esophageal reconstruction, III:1013
    for penile reconstruction, VI:1235-1237,
      1236f, 1238f, 1240f
Ulnar impaction syndrome, VII:19, 19f
Ulnar nerve
    anatomy of, VII:38-39, 40f, 41, 472
    entrapment of, VII:893-902
    evaluation of, VII:50, 51f, 52f
    fascicular pattern of, VII:475
    injury to, VII:34. See also Ulnar nerve
      palsy.
      nerve transfer for, VII:503-504, 504f
      neuroma-in-continuity with, VII:494,
        495f
      outcomes of, VII:508-509
    laceration of, VII:39, 41
    repair of, I:736
      nerve transfer for, VII:503-504, 504f
      outcomes of, VII:508-509
    tourniquet-related injury to, VII:117
Ulnar nerve block
    at elbow, VII:103-104, 104f
    at wrist, VII:105, 105f
Ulnar nerve graft, in brachial plexus injury,
    VII:530, 531f
Ulnar nerve palsy
    high
      high radial nerve palsy with, tendon
        transfer for, VIII:482
      tendon transfer for, VIII:479, 481

Ulnar nerve palsy (Continued)
    low
      low median nerve palsy with, tendon
        transfer for, VIII:481-482
      tendon transfer for, VIII:471-472,
        472f, 475-476, 476f
Ulnar parametacarpal flap, for finger
    reconstruction, VII:231, 237, 238f
Ulnar recurrent artery, Color Plates I:15-4
    and 15-5, I:335
Ulnar variance, VII:19, 19f
Ulnocapitate ligament, VII:454, 454f
Ulnocarpal ligament plication, in
    lunotriquetral instability, VII:135
Ulnolunate ligament, VII:454, 454f
Ulnotriquetral ligament, VII:454, 454f
Ultrasonography
    in arteriovenous malformation, VIII:398
    in breast cancer, VI:633-635, 634t, 639
    in flap monitoring, I:497t, 498-499
    in hemangioma, V:26-27, VIII:371, 373
    in ischemia, VII:798, 800
    in lymphatic malformation, VIII:392
    in salivary gland tumors, V:74
    in venous malformation, V:49, VIII:383
    of breast implants, VI:637
    prenatal, Color Plates I:36-1 to 36-6,
      I:1067-1072
      ethical issues in, I:1071
      fetal outcome and, I:1071-1072
      four-dimensional, Color Plate I:36-4,
        I:1069
      in congenital hydronephrosis, I:1126,
        1127
      in surgery, I:1118, 1120
      indications for, I:1067, 1068f
      limitations of, I:1069-1070, 1070t
      measurements on, I:1067-1068
      three-dimensional, Color Plates I:36-
        1 to 36-7
      two-dimensional, I:1069, 1070t
      types of, I:1069
Ultrasound-assisted liposuction, VI:196-
    197, 196f, 197f, 387
    for lower extremity, VI:275
    for trunk, VI:275
    large-volume, VI:248-251, 249f, 249t,
      250f, 251f
Ultrasound therapy
    in hand healing, VIII:571-572
    in tendon healing, I:595
Ultraviolet radiation
    actinic keratosis and, VII:960
    skin cancer and, V:274, 274t, 275, 290-
      291, 393
    skin exposure to, II:386-388, 387f, 388f-
      390f
Umbilicoplasty, VI:105-108, 106f-108f,
    149-152, 150f, 172-174
    secondary, VI:188-189, 189f
Umbilicus, VI:89
    in abdominoplasty, VI:126, 126f, 136f,
      137f, 139, 172-174, 377-378, 378f
    in Baroudi abdominoplasty, VI:147,
      147f
    ischemia of, after abdominoplasty,
      VI:377, 379
    malposition of, after abdominoplasty,
      VI:378-379
    pathology of, VI:93

Unicoronal synostosis, IV:469, 471-472, 473f, 474f

Uniparental disomy, I:53

Unna boot, I:964

Upper extremity. *See also* Arm(s); Elbow; Finger(s); Hand(s); Shoulder; Thumb(s); Wrist.
  body contouring of, VI:291-313, 292f, 292t, 293f
  brachioplasty for, VI:300, 306f, 307f, 308, 309f, 310f-311f. *See also* Upper extremity, liposuction for.
  embryology of, VIII:3-22, 6f-10f, 11t, 12f, 277-280
    anterior-posterior axis in, VIII:17, 19, 19f
    arterial, VIII:13, 14f
    dorsal-ventral axis in, VIII:19
    HOX genes in, VIII:19-20, 20f
    molecular, VIII:16-20, 18f-20f
    muscle, VIII:15-16, 15f-17f
    neural, VIII:13, 15
    progress zone model of, VIII:17, 18f
    proximal-distal axis in, VIII:19-20, 20f
    skeletal, VIII:11-13, 13f
    stages of, VIII:11, 11t, 12f
  gunshot injury to, I:1008, 1009f
  laser resurfacing of, II:367
  liposuction for, VI:291-313, 292f, 292t, 293f
    complications of, VI:292t, 312
    in group 1 patients, VI:296-300, 296f-303f
    in group 2 patients, VI:300-308, 304f-308f
    in groups 3 and 4 patients, VI:308-312, 309f-313f
    in lymphedematous arm, VI:292, 312
    measurements for, VI:294, 294f
    muscle tone and, VI:294
    patient evaluation for, VI:293-296, 293t, 294f, 294t
    patient's weight and, VI:295
    photography for, VI:295-296, 295f
    pinch test for, VI:294, 296, 296f
    skin tone and, VI:294
    superwet solution for, VI:297, 297t
  lymphangioma of, I:983, 984f
  lymphedema of, VII:995-1004. *See also* Lymphedema, upper extremity.
  muscle transfers in, I:390, 400f-402f, 405, VIII:489-506. *See also* Arm(s), muscle transfer in.
  prostheses for, I:781-788, VIII:573-580. *See also* Prostheses, upper extremity.
  reconstruction of. *See* Upper extremity reconstruction.
  tendon transfer in, VIII:453-486. *See also* Hand reconstruction, tendon transfer in.
  tissue expansion in, I:563-565
  tumors of, VII:949-974. *See also specific tumors.*
    benign, VII:950, 952-960
      evaluation of, VII:949-950, 950t
      fibrous, VII:952-956, 952f-955f
      treatment of, VII:950

Upper extremity *(Continued)*
  bone, VII:979-991
    benign, VII:983-991, 984f-987f
    biopsy of, VII:980-981
    evaluation of, VII:979-981, 980f
    malignant, VII:988-991, 989f, 990f
    reconstruction after, VII:982-983
    resection of, VII:981-982, 982t
    staging of, VII:981, 981f
  evaluation of, VII:949-952, 950t, 951f
  malignant, VII:950-952, 951t, 960-973, 960t
    evaluation of, VII:949-952, 951t, 952f
    melanoma, V:326-327, 330f-332f
    pigmented, VII:959-960
    sweat gland, VII:960, 961f
    vascular, VII:956-958, 957f, VIII:370-378, 372f-375f, 377f-379f
  vascular anomalies of, VIII:369-413, 370t. *See also* Capillary malformations; Hemangioma; Vascular malformations; Venous malformations.
  vascular system of
    anatomy of, VII:792-796, 793f-795f
    variations in, VII:795
    embryology of, VII:792
    territories of, Color Plates I:15-4 to 15-7, I:334-337
  wound healing in, I:1008, 1009f, 1010f

Upper extremity reconstruction, VII:317-348. *See also* Arm(s), mangling injury to; Finger reconstruction; Hand reconstruction; Thumb reconstruction.
  anesthesia for, VII:87-106. *See also* Anesthesia, upper extremity.
  arterial anastomoses for, VII:323-324
  bone grafting in, VII:321
  care after, VII:323
  débridement and, VII:320
  delayed, VII:319
  double-toe transfers for, VII:348
  early, VII:319-320
  fibula transfer for, VII:335, 342f
  flaps for, VII:322-323. *See also at specific flaps.*
    fascial and fasciocutaneous, VII:326-335, 329f-341f
    muscle, VII:323, 324-326, 325f-328f
  fracture fixation in, VII:321
  free tissue transfer for, VII:323-324
  functional, VII:335, 338, 342-348, 342f-347f, VIII:489-506. *See also* Arm(s), muscle transfer in.
  in tetraplegia. *See* Tetraplegia.
  joint reconstruction in, VII:338, 345
  lateral arm free flap for, VII:328, 330, 330f-333f
  musculotendinous, VII:322
  nerve grafting in, VII:322
  patient evaluation for, VII:318
  planning for, VII:318-319
  provisional revascularization and, VII:320-321
  ribbon sign in, VII:322
  skeletal stabilization and, VII:321
  soft tissue, VII:322-324
  tendon transfer in, VIII:453-486. *See also* Hand reconstruction, tendon transfer in.

Upper extremity reconstruction *(Continued)*
  thumb reconstruction in, VII:345, 348. *See also* Thumb reconstruction.
  timing of, VII:319-320
  toe transfer for, VII:338, 344f-347f, 345, 348. *See also at* Thumb reconstruction.
  vascular, VII:321-322

Urethra, male. *See also* Hypospadias.
  anatomy of, VI:1261
  embryology of, VI:1261, 1263f
  lymphatic supply of, VI:1206
  reconstruction of, VI:1239, 1242f
    genital flaps for, VI:1223, 1225f-1226f, 1226-1227
    in epispadias, VI:1207-1208
    in hypospadias, VI:1259-1277. *See also* Hypospadias.
    meshed split-thickness graft in, VI:1246, 1246t, 1247f-1249f

Urethral valves, posterior, I:1126

Urinary retention
  epidural block and, I:194-195
  spinal block and, I:194-195

Urinary tract obstruction, in fetus, I:1126-1127, 1126t

Urine, fetal, I:1126-1127, 1126t

Urogenital tract abnormalities, microtia and, III:638-639

Urokinase, in upper extremity ischemia, VII:802, 804

Utilitarianism, I:98, 98t

Utilities, in medical decision-making, I:42, 42f, 43f

Uvula, IV:60t, 72
  anatomy of, IV:58f, 59f, 60t, 62, 63f, 312f
  magnetic resonance imaging of, IV:65, 66f

Uvulopalatopharyngoplasty, in obstructive sleep apnea, III:787-789, 788f

V

V-Y flap, I:367, 369f
  for fingertip reconstruction, VII:159-161, 159f, 160f
  for foot reconstruction, VI:1425, 1427, 1427f, 1428f, 1431f
  for penile reconstruction, VI:391-393, 391f, 392f, 398-399
  for pressure sore treatment, VI:1324t, 1334, 1337f-1339f, 1338, 1341f, 1342f, 1345, 1345f

VACTERL association
  hypoplastic thumb in, VIII:325
  radial defects in, VIII:62, 80, 81f

Vacuum-assisted closure, I:886-888, 887f-889f, 950-952, 951f-953f, 954t

Vagina. *See also* Vaginal reconstruction.
  anatomy of, VI:1296, 1296f

Vaginal reconstruction
  acquired defects, I:404f, VI:1295-1304
    anatomy for, VI:1296, 1296f
    complications of, VI:1303-1304
    consultations for, VI:1297
    defect assessment in, VI:1295-1296, 1296f
    delayed healing after, VI:1303
    flap loss after, VI:1303

Vaginal reconstruction (Continued)
for type IA defects, VI:1296f, 1297, 1298f, 1299f
for type IB defects, VI:1296f, 1297-1299, 1298f, 1300f
for type IIA defects, VI:1296f, 1298f, 1299, 1301, 1301f
for type IIB defects, VI:1296f, 1298f, 1301, 1302f, 1303f
goals of, VI:1297, 1297t
gracilis flap for, VI:1301, 1302f, 1303f
rectus myocutaneous flap for, VI:1299, 1301, 1301f, 1303
sexual function after, VI:1303-1304
Singapore flap for, VI:1297, 1298f, 1299f
congenital defects, VI:1281-1289
Abbe-McIndoe procedure in, VI:1282-1285, 1282f-1285f
full-thickness skin grafts in, VI:1285
gracilis flap for, VI:1285-1286, 1286f, 1287f
historical perspective on, VI:1281-1282
intestinal flaps for, VI:1289
rectus abdominis flap for, VI:1286-1289, 1287f, 1288f
Vaginectomy, in female-to-male transformation, VI:1311-1312
Vaginoplasty, in male-to-female transformation, Color Plates VI:156-3 to 156-7, VI:1312-1314, 1313f, 1314f
Valerian, VI:176t
Validity, of questionnaire, I:40-41, 40f
Valproic acid, in complex regional pain syndrome/reflex sympathetic dystrophy, VII:858
Valvular heart disease, preoperative evaluation of, I:168, 169t
Van der Woude syndrome, IV:102-103
Vascular anatomy, I:317-361. See also Vascular territories.
angiosome concept in, Color Plate I:15-2, I:332-344, 336f
clinical implications of, I:333-334
arterial territories of, I:322-324, 325f
basic research on, I:321-332
cadaver for, I:322, 322f
radiographs for, I:322, 323f-325f
comparative, I:330-332, 332f-335f
cutaneous perforators of, Color Plate I:15-1, I:322
course of, I:322-324, 325f
direct, Color Plate I:15-1, I:323
indirect, I:323
source arteries of, Color Plate I:15-2, I:322
historical perspective on, I:13-18, 15f-18f, 21f-23f, 317-321, 318f, 320f, 321f
nerves and, I:326-327, 328f
of dog, I:331, 333f, 334f, 335f
of duck, I:331, 333f
of muscles, I:325-330, 327f, 328f
of pig, I:331, 332f, 334f, 335f
of rabbit, I:331, 333f, 334f, 335f
venosomes of, Color Plate I:15-3, I:332
venous drainage of, I:324-326, 326f, 327f

Vascular anomalies, V:19-61, VIII:369-413, 370t. See also Capillary malformations; Hemangioma; Vascular malformations; Venous malformations.
nomenclature for, V:19-20
Vascular arcades, I:348-350, 348f-353f
Vascular endothelial growth factor
in bone repair, I:655, 657t, 658
in fetal wound healing, I:218
in wound healing, I:212t, 216
microvascular surgery and, I:521
Vascular endothelial growth factor, in hemangioma, V:20
Vascular graft, tissue-engineered, Color Plate I:37-2, I:1089-1091, 1090f, 1092f
Vascular malformations, V:6-8, 8f, 37-61, VIII:378-413. See also specific malformations.
capillary, V:37-41. See also Capillary malformations.
combined (eponymous), VIII:407-413, 409f-412f, 413t
head and neck, III:774-775
macrodactyly and, VIII:309-310, 311f, 312f, 316-317
pathogenesis of, VIII:378
venous, V:47-51. See also Venous malformations.
vs. hemangioma, V:19-20, 25, 26f
Vascular prosthesis, infection of, I:919-922, 921f, 996-999, 998f-999f
Vascular territories, I:334-344
angiosomes of, I:332-334
arterial, Color Plates I:1-1 and 15-1, I:323-324, 325f
arterial arcades in, I:348, 348f, 349f
arterial radiation in, I:345, 346f
clinical applications of, I:355-361
for composite flaps, I:359-361, 360f
for fasciocutaneous flaps, I:358-359
for liposuction, I:361
for musculocutaneous flaps, I:359, 360f
for perforator mapping, I:355
for skin flap dimensions, I:356-358, 357f, 358f
for skin flap selection, I:355-356, 356f
for tissue expansion, I:361
comparative anatomy of, I:330-332, 332f, 333f
connective tissue framework and, I:344-345
directional veins in, I:350
forearm, I:334-337
clinical implications of, I:336-337
donor site morbidity and, I:336-337
free flap donor sites and, I:337
of bones, I:335-336
of muscles, Color Plates I:15-5 to 15-7, I:335
of skin, Color Plate I:15-4, I:334
Volkmann ischemic contracture and, I:337
growth effects on, I:347-348, 347f
head and neck, Color Plate I:1-1, I:339-344
of anterior neck muscles, Color Plate I:15-13, I:343-344, 343t
of internal nose, Color Plate I:15-13, I:343

Vascular territories (Continued)
of lateral muscles, Color Plate I:15-13, I:342-343
of muscles, I:341-343, 342t, 343t
of muscles of facial expression, Color Plate I:15-12, I:340f, 341-342
of muscles of mastication, Color Plate I:15-12, I:342
of ocular muscles, I:342
of palate, I:343-344
of posterior neck muscles, Color Plate I:15-13, I:342
of salivary glands, I:344
of skin, Color Plate I:15-12, I:340-341, 340f, 341f
of superficial musculoaponeurotic system, Color Plate I:15-12, I:340-341, 340f, 341f
of thyroid gland, I:344
of tongue, I:343, 343f
historical perspective on, I:317-321, 318f-321f
in dog, I:330-332, 333f
in duck, I:330-332, 333f
in pig, I:330-332, 332f
in rabbit, I:330-332, 333f
law of equilibrium in, I:350
lower leg, I:337-339
clinical implications of, I:339
compartment syndromes and, I:339
flap donor sites and, I:339
knee-related anastomoses and, I:339
of muscles, Color Plates I:15-9 to 5-11, I:338, 338t
of skin, Color Plate I:15-8, I:337-338, 339
nerves and, Color Plate I:15-15, I:327-330, 345-347, 346f, 355
oscillating avalvular veins in, I:351, 354f
supply constancy in, I:350
tissue mobility and, I:345
venous, I:324-327, 326f, 327f
venous arcades in, I:348-350, 351f-353f
venous convergence in, I:345
venous flow in, Color Plate I:15-14, I:350-351, 354-355, 354f
Vascular tumors, VII:956-958, 957f
Vascularized bone flap, I:380t, 387, 390, 390f, 391f-399f
fasciocutaneous flap with, I:390
fibula for, I:390, 390t, 393f-395f
iliac crest for, I:390, 390t, 395f-396f
radius for, I:390, 390t
rib for, I:390, 391f, 392f
scapula for, I:390, 390t, 397f-399f
Vasculitis
hypersensitivity, I:939
lower extremity, VI:1476, 1478f
wound healing and, I:938-939, 938t
Vasoconstriction, cold injury and, I:857, VII:647, 648
Vasodilation, cold injury and, I:857
Vasospasm, in microvascular surgery, I:515-516, 516f
Vasospastic disease, VII:815-819
diagnosis of, VII:816
secondary, VII:816-817
sympathectomy in, VII:817-818, 818f, 819f

Vastus lateralis flap, for pressure sore treatment, VI:1345-1347, 1346f

Veau-Wardill-Kilner (pushback) technique, of palatoplasty, IV:258-259, 259f

Vecuronium, I:180, 180t

Vein(s). *See also* Vascular anatomy; Vascular territories.
arcades of, I:348-350, 351f-353f
avalvular, oscillating, I:351, 354f
connective tissue relation of, I:344-345
convergence of, I:345
cutaneous, Color Plate I:15-14, I:324-327, 326f, 355
directional, I:350
muscular, I:326, 327f, 354

Vein graft
for arterial reconstruction, VII:806
for upper extremity injury, VII:321-322

Velocardiofacial syndrome, IV:102

Velopharyngeal apparatus, IV:311-335
anatomy of, IV:72-76, 73f-75f, 311, 312f, 313f
assessment of, IV:313-317, 314f-317f
dysfunction of
cinefluoroscopy in, IV:317, 317f
in submucous cleft palate, IV:317-318
nasopharyngeal endoscopy in, IV:315-317, 317f
perceptual speech evaluation in, IV:313
pressure-flow measurement in, IV:314-315, 314f-316f
terminology for, IV:311
treatment of, IV:318-335
comparative outcomes of, IV:333-334
palatal lengthening procedures in, IV:332
posterior pharyngeal flap in, IV:318-324, 320f-323f, 333-334
posterior pharyngeal wall augmentation in, IV:332
prosthetic management in, IV:332-333
selection of, IV:334-335
sphincter pharyngoplasty in, IV:325-332, 326f-329f, 333-334

Velopharyngeal insufficiency, cleft palate and, III:777

Veloplasty, intravelar, IV:261, 262f

Venae communicantes, I:349-350, 352f, 353f

Venography, in venous malformations, V:49

Venosomes, Color Plates I:15-2 and 15-3, I:332

Venous conduit, for nerve repair, VII:499-500

Venous flap, I:412, 413f

Venous insufficiency, VI:1464-1473. *See also* Lower extremity, chronic venous insufficiency of.

Venous malformations, V:6, 8f, 47-51, VIII:381-389, 382f-390f
angiography in, VIII:383-384, 387f
cerebral, V:47
clinical presentation of, V:47-49, 49f, VIII:381-383, 382f, 383f

Venous malformations *(Continued)*
coagulopathy and, V:49
cutaneous-mucosal, V:47
familial, V:47
genetic factors in, V:47
in Klippel-Trenaunay syndrome, V:56-60, 59f
in Maffucci syndrome, V:55-56, 57f
laser therapy in, V:50
macrodactyly in, VIII:310, 313f
magnetic resonance imaging in, V:49, 49f, VIII:383, 384f
management of, V:49-51, 50f
of extremities, V:48, 49f
of gastrointestinal tract, V:47, 48, 48f, 50-51
of head and neck, V:48, 49f
operative management of, V:50-51, 50f
pathogenesis of, V:47
phlebography in, VIII:383
phleboliths in, V:49, 49f
radiologic features of, V:49, 49f
sclerotherapy in, V:50, 50f, VIII:384-385, 386f
surgery in, VIII:385-389, 386t, 387f-390f
ultrasonography in, VIII:383

Ventilation, mechanical
in burn treatment, I:829
in toxic epidermal necrolysis, I:797

Ventricular fibrillation, in hypothermia, I:858

Ventriculomegaly, fetal intervention for, I:1128-1129

Ventriculoradial dysplasia syndrome, radial defects in, VIII:62

Veratrum californicum, teratogenicity of, IV:12

Vermilion. *See also* Lip(s).
deficiency of
after cleft lip repair, IV:343-346, 344f-348f
after unilateral cheiloplasty, IV:208, 209f
in cleft lip, IV:172f, 173
malalignment of, after cleft lip repair, IV:342-343, 342f-344f
reconstruction of, III:801, 805, 805f, 806f

Vermilion triangular flap, IV:189-190, 190f-192f

Verruca vulgaris, Color Plate V:112-1, V:252, 253f, VII:194

Verrucous carcinoma, V:162, 294, 294f

Verrucous nevus, V:257, 257f

Vertex, II:3f, 3t

Vertical subsigmoid ramus osteotomy, IV:443-444, 444f

Vesalius, Andreas, I:14-15, 14f, 15f

Vesicant agents, hand injury from, VII:653t, 654

Veto cell, I:279

Video stroboscopy, in head and neck cancer, V:227

Videotaping, of musicians' hand, VII:696

Vincristine, in kaposiform hemangioendothelioma, V:36

Vincula, VII:29, 31f

Violent behavior, I:86-87

Violinist, hand disorders in, VII:694, 700f

Viral infection. *See also* Human immunodeficiency virus (HIV) infection.
cutaneous, Color Plate V:112-1, V:252-254, 253f
hemangioma and, V:21
laser resurfacing and, II:342, 345, 346f, 372
of hand, VII:768, 784-785
of perionychium, VII:194, 196f

Virtue, I:100-101. *See also* Ethics.

Viscerocranium, IV:9, 10f, 11

Vision
in fibrous dysplasia, V:101, 101f
in frontobasilar region fracture, III:335-338
in orbital fracture, III:273, 326-327

Visual acuity, assessment of, II:90-91

Visual fields, assessment of, II:90

Vitamin A, VI:175, 177t
deficiency of, wound healing and, I:220
teratogenicity of, IV:12

Vitamin B$_1$, deficiency of, wound healing and, I:220

Vitamin B$_2$, deficiency of, wound healing and, I:220-221

Vitamin B$_6$, deficiency of, wound healing and, I:220

Vitamin C
deficiency of, wound healing and, I:220
for skin rejuvenation, II:400-401, 401

Vitamin E, VI:175, 177t
in breast pain, VI:355
in Dupuytren disease, VII:740

VM-plasty, canthal web treatment with, III:60, 61f-62f

Vocal cords
cancer of, V:241-246, 241f, 244f-247f, 244t, 245t
in gastroesophageal reflux disease, III:771
paralysis of, III:769

Voice alteration, in male-to-female transformation, VI:1316

Volar V-Y flap, for fingertip reconstruction, VII:160-161, 160f

Volkmann ischemic contracture, I:337
vs. reflex sympathetic dystrophy/chronic regional pain syndrome, VII:848-849, 849f

Voltage, VII:598

Volume-outcome analysis, in evidence-based decision-making, I:43-44, 43t, 48

Vomer, IV:70, 70f

Vomer flaps, with palatoplasty, IV:261-262

Vomiting, postoperative, I:201-202
prevention of, I:184, 185t

Von Langenbeck technique, of palatoplasty, IV:258, 258f

Vulvobulbocavernosus flap, for vaginal reconstruction, VI:1285

W

Waist-to-hip ratio, VI:119, 120f, 126

Wallerian degeneration, VII:929-930, 932f

Wart, Color Plate V:112-1, V:252, 253f, VII:194
senile, V:253-254, 254f

Wartenberg sign, VIII:478

Wartenberg syndrome, VII:902-904, 903f, 905f

Warthin tumor, V:77, 81f

Watson scaphoid shift test, VII:54, 458, 459f

Webbing
after blepharoplasty, II:106
digital. *See* Syndactyly.

Weber-Fergusson incision, in paranasal sinus cancer, V:248, 248f

Wedge osteotomy, in Dupuytren disease, VII:751

Weight gain, abdominoplasty and, VI:376

Weight loss
abdominoplasty after, VI:167-172. *See also* Gastric bypass surgery, abdominoplasty after.
liposuction for. *See* Liposuction, large-volume.

Werner syndrome, V:401

White blood cells, in wound healing, I:210-211, 210f, 211f, 212t

White phosphorus injury, to hand, VII:654

Whitnall, superior transverse ligament of, II:133

Wick lymphangioplasty, VII:1002, 1002f

Wide lip, after cleft lip repair, IV:350-351, 351f

Winch procedure, in tetraplegic patient, VIII:518, 520, 520f

WireFoam splint, for finger contracture, VII:667-668, 667f

Wise-pattern marking, for breast reduction, VI:558-559, 560f

Witch's chin deformity, III:833, 854f-857f

Wood's lamp, in corneal evaluation, II:93

World War I, I:28-29

World War II, I:31-32

Worthen flap, for forehead reconstruction, III:708, 709f

Wound(s), I:223-226. *See also* Wound healing.
acute, I:299, 949
assessment of, I:864-866
blood flow to, assessment of, I:865, 866f, 867f
cellulitis of, assessment of, I:864, 865f
chronic, I:223, 299-300, 949-950
skin cancer and, V:275, 276f
closed, care for, I:222-223
complex, I:901
depth of, I:864-865, 866f
Doppler evaluation of, I:865, 866f
erythema of, I:864
exudate of, laser resurfacing and, II:368-369
factitial, I:944
fetal, Color Plate I:11-1, I:217-218, 217f
in epidermolysis bullosa, I:804
in toxic epidermal necrolysis, I:797-798, 798f
infection of, I:220, 911-918, 912-913t, 914f, 915f, 916t
culture for, I:882
débridement and, I:881-882, 881f
hydrogen peroxide for, I:882, 882f
spread of, I:879-880
management of, I:863-897. *See also* Wound(s), problem.

Wound(s) *(Continued)*
antibiotics in, I:224-225, 883-884, 884t, 950, 954-955
cleansing in, I:871, 872f
collagenases in, I:225-226
débridement in, I:300, 863-883, 955-958, 956f
for acute wound, I:880-881
for bone, I:876, 878-879, 879f
for chronic wound, I:882-883
for fascia, I:875
for infected wound, I:881-882, 881f, 882f
for skin, I:873-875, 874f
for subcutaneous tissue, I:875
for tendon, I:875-876, 875f-878f
gauze dressing for, I:873
infection assessment and, I:879-880
nonsurgical tools for, I:873
techniques of, I:866-868, 870f
tools for, I:870-872, 870f-872f
wound assessment for, I:864-866, 865f-868f
dressings in, Color Plate I:32-1, I:224, 225t, 873, 883-886, 885t
gene therapy in, I:226
growth factors in, I:226
hyperbaric oxygen in, I:893, 895-897, 952-954, 954f
irrigation in, I:950, 951f
skin replacement in, I:224, 225t, 890, 892-893, 894f, 896f
systemic antibiotics in, I:954-955
topical treatment in, I:223-225, 883-884, 884t, 950
vacuum-assisted closure in, I:886-888, 887f-892f, 950-952, 951f-953f, 954t
nerve assessment of, I:865-866, 867f, 868f
problem, I:219-221, 901-1020
abdominal wall surgery and, I:983, 985, 986f-989f
Achilles tendon rupture and, I:1010, 1012, 1015f
acne keloidalis nuchae and, I:944
animal bites and, I:926-928, 928t
aplasia cutis congenita and, I:944
arterial insufficiency and, I:219, 902-906, 904f, 963-964, 965f-966f
arteriovenous malformation and, I:945, 946f
atherosclerosis and, I:903-904, 905f
bites and, I:926-928, 927t, 928t
bowel resection and, I:993f-994f, 993
branchial cleft cyst and, I:945
burns and, I:930-931, 930f, 931f, 1000, 1004-1006, 1005f-1006f
cavity persistence and, I:919, 919t, 920f, 921f, 983, 985-992, 986f-992f
cellular impairment and, I:981
chemotherapy and, I:221, 911, 937
chest wall defects and, I:985, 990, 991f
collagen disorders and, I:902-903, 938, 938f, 939f
congenital abnormalities and, I:944-948
connective tissue diseases and, I:937-938
copper deficiency and, I:919
corticosteroids and, I:221

Wound(s) *(Continued)*
definition of, I:901
diabetes mellitus and, I:942-943, 943f
drug abuse and, I:914
drug effects and, I:905
endothelial cell disorders and, I:910
envenomation and, I:931-932, 933f-935f, 1016-1017
extravasation and, I:932, 935f, 936, 936f, 1012, 1016, 1016f
extrinsic factors in, I:903t, 924-937, 925t, 926f, 927t, 928t, 929t, 930f-936f, 999-1017, 999t, 1001f-1016f
fibroblast disorders and, I:910
fistula and, I:922-924, 922t, 923f, 924f, 967, 970f-971f
fracture and, I:1008-1010, 1009f-1012f
gastrointestinal tract defects and, I:993-995, 994f
gastroschisis and, I:945, 948, 948f
gout and, I:943
gunshot injury and, I:926, 926f, 1006-1008, 1007f-1009f
hemangioma and, I:945
heparin and, I:936
hidradenitis suppurativa and, I:940, 941f
human bites and, I:926-928, 927t
human immunodeficiency virus infection and, I:940-941, 941f
immune deficiency and, I:940-942, 941f
immunosuppressants and, I:221, 941-942
impaired cellular function and, I:908, 910-911, 910f
in diabetes mellitus, I:219-220, 981, 982f
in legs, I:219-220
in perineum, I:967, 974f
in Raynaud disease, I:905-906, 906f
infection and, I:220, 911-918, 912-913t, 914f, 915f, 916t, 974, 976-981, 987f-980f
intrinsic factors in, I:901-919, 902t, 903t, 904t
ischemia and, I:903-904
keratinocyte disorders and, I:910
leukemia and, I:916, 918
lymphatic insufficiency and, I:907-908, 908f, 909f, 964
lymphatic malformation and, I:945
macrophage deficiency and, I:908
malignant disease and, I:916-918, 916f-918f, 981, 983, 984f
malingering and, I:944
malnutrition and, I:220-221
management of, I:948-1020
antibiotic-impregnated beads in, I:955, 956f
clinical assessment for, I:948-949
débridement in, I:955-958, 957f, 958t, 959f-962f
electrical stimulation in, I:1019-1020, 1019t
flaps in, I:962-963, 962f, 963f
hyperbaric oxygen in, I:952-954, 954f
irrigating systems in, I:950, 951f
nonoperative, I:950-955, 951f-954f

Wound(s) (Continued)
    reconstructive planning in, I:958, 962-963, 962f, 963f
    skin substitutes in, I:1018-1019
    stem cell therapy in, I:1019
    systemic antibiotics in, I:954-955
    timing of, I:949-950
    tissue expansion in, I:962-963, 962f, 963f
    topical antimicrobial agents in, I:950
    topical growth factors in, I:1017-1018
    vacuum-assisted closure in, I:950-952, 951f-953f
  mechanical factors in, I:919-924, 919t, 920f-924f, 983, 985-999, 986f-989f, 991f-999f
  medications and, I:936-937
  metabolic diseases and, I:942-943, 943f
  neurologic disorders and, I:942, 942f
  neutrophils and, I:908
  nicotine and, I:905
  nutritional disorders and, I:918-919, 918f, 981
  obesity and, I:221, 943
  omphalocele and, I:945, 947f
  organ system failure and, I:943-944
  osteomyelitis and, I:914-915, 915f
  perineal defects and, I:990, 992f, 993
  platelet disorders and, I:910
  postsurgical, I:928-929, 929f
  pressure disorders and, I:219, 942, 942f, 999-1000, 999t, 1001f-1004f
  prosthesis exposure and, I:919-922, 921f, 922f, 995-999, 995f-999f
  protein levels and, I:918
  pyoderma gangrenosum and, I:940, 940f
  pyogenic granuloma and, I:945
  radiation therapy and, I:220, 904-905, 910-911, 911f, 967, 968f-969f, 972f-976f, 974
  rheumatoid arthritis and, I:937-938
  scleroderma and, I:937
  sepsis and, I:911
  sinus tracks and, I:945
  soft tissue infection and, I:911, 914, 914f
  spina bifida and, I:945
  sternal infection and, I:915-916, 915f, 916t
  steroids and, I:936-937, 941-942
  systemic lupus erythematosus and, I:937
  temperature extremes and, I:930-931, 930f-932f, 1000, 1004-1006, 1005f-1006f
  thromboxane A_2 and, I:905
  tissue pressure and, I:929-930, 929t, 930f
  tobacco use and, I:905
  trauma and, I:902-903, 925-928, 926f, 927t, 928t, 1006-1012, 1007f-1015f
  vascular anomalies and, I:945
  vascular insufficiency and, I:219-220, 901-906, 904f-907f, 963-964, 965f-966f
  vasculitis and, I:938-939, 938t
  vasoconstriction and, I:905-906, 906f

Wound(s) (Continued)
  venous insufficiency and, I:906-907, 906f, 907f, 964
  vitamin A deficiency and, I:918
  vitamin B_1 deficiency and, I:918
  vitamin B_2 deficiency and, I:918-919
  vitamin B_6 deficiency and, I:918
  vitamin C deficiency and, I:918, 918f
  warfarin and, I:936
  zinc deficiency and, I:919
  Semmes-Weinstein monofilament testing of, I:865-866, 867f
  simple, I:901
  stable, I:949-950
  transition, I:217
  unstable, I:901, 949-950
Wound healing, I:209-230, 883-897. See also Scar(s).
  adult, I:209-217, 210f
    contraction in, I:213-214, 213f
    epithelialization in, I:214
    extracellular matrix in, I:216-217
    fibroblast growth factors in, I:212t, 216
    fibroplasia in, I:211-213, 211f
    granulation in, I:213
    growth factors in, I:212t, 215-216
    inflammatory phase of, I:209-211, 210f, 211f, 212t
    insulin-like growth factor in, I:216
    platelet-derived growth factor in, I:212t, 215
    proliferation phase of, I:211-214, 211f, 213f
    regulation of, I:215-217
    remodeling phase of, I:214-215, 214f, 215f
    transforming growth factor-β in, I:212t, 215-216
    vascular endothelial growth factor in, I:212t, 216
    vs. fetal, I:217-218
  copper in, I:919, 919t
  endothelial cells in, I:910
  excessive, I:221-222, 226-230, 227t
    prevention of, I:227, 228t, 230
    treatment of, I:227-230, 228t, 229f
  extracellular matrix in, I:214
  failure of. See Wound(s), problem.
  fetal, I:217-218, 217f
    fibroblasts in, I:217-218
    growth factors in, I:218
    hyaluronic acid in, I:218
    inflammation in, I:218
  fibroblasts in, I:910
  fluid administration and, I:903
  growth factors in, I:888-890
  impairment of. See Wound(s), problem.
  in animals, I:213
  in irradiated tissue, I:841
  keratinocytes in, I:910
  macrophages in, I:908, 910f
  neutrophils in, I:908
  of closed wounds, I:222-223
  of open wounds, I:223-226
  platelets in, I:910
  radiation effects on, I:844-845
  scarless, Color Plate I:11-1, I:217-218, 217f
  tensile strength with, I:215, 215f

Wound healing (Continued)
  tissue oxygenation and, I:902, 904f, 944
  vitamins in, I:918-919, 919t
  zinc in, I:919, 919t
Wrinkles (rhytids). See also Face lift.
  botulinum toxin injections for, II:69-70, 69f, 281, 343t
  chemical peels for, II:258-259, 343-344, 343t, 379-380, 379t, 380f
  collagen injections for, II:258
  dermabrasion in, II:281
  fat injections for, II:258
  forehead, II:48-50, 49f, 67-68, 68t
  laser resurfacing for, II:339-380. See also Facial resurfacing.
  nonsurgical treatment of, II:257-259
  peels for, II:258-259
  perioral, II:280-281, 281f
  periorbicular, II:242, 243f
  phenol-croton oil peel for, II:280-281, 281f
Wrist. See also Hand(s).
  anatomy of, VII:19-21, 19f, 20f, 29-32, 30f, 31f, 453-456, 454f-457f
  angiography of, VII:80, 82, 83f, 84f, 649
  arthroscopy of, VII:125-137
    anatomy for, VII:126-128, 127f
    diagnostic, VII:125-126, 128-129
    in abrasion chondroplasty, VII:134
    in carpal instability, VII:134-135
    in distal radius fracture, VII:136
    in ganglionectomy, VII:136
    in loose body removal, VII:131, 133
    in lunotriquetral instability, VII:135-136
    in proximal row carpectomy, VII:133
    in radial triangular fibrocartilage complex tear, VII:131, 133f, 134f
    in radioscaphoid impingement, VII:133
    in scaphoid fracture, VII:136-137
    in synovectomy, VII:131
    in triangular fibrocartilage complex débridement, VII:129-130, 129f, 130f
    in triangular fibrocartilage complex repair, VII:130-131, 131f-134f
    in ulnar shortening, VII:133, 135f
    in ulnar triangular fibrocartilage complex tear, VII:130-131f, 131f, 132f
    indications for, VII:125-126, 126t
    portals for, VII:126-128, 127f, 127t
    staging, VII:126
    surgical, VII:126, 128-129
    technique of, VII:128-129
  ballottement tests for, VII:54
  biomechanics of, VII:456-458, 457f, 458f
  chondromalacia, VII:134
  congenital amputation at, VIII:56-60
  degrees of freedom of, VII:22
  dorsal compartments of, VII:456, 457f
  evaluation of, VII:458-459, 459f
  extension of, in tetraplegic patient, VIII:520-521, 521f
  extrinsic ligaments of, VII:454-455, 454f
  flexion deformity of, VIII:548-549, 548t
  flexion of, VII:403, 405f
  fracture of, VII:460-467
    arterial injury with, VII:804

Wrist (*Continued*)
carpal, VII:464-467, 465f, 466f
distal radioulnar, VII:463-464, 463f
distal radius, VII:136, 460-463, 461f, 462f, VIII:562
evaluation of, VII:458-459, 459f
internal fixation for, VII:139-150, 140t. *See also* Finger(s), fracture of, internal fixation for.
scaphoid, VII:68, 136-137, 464-465, 464f, 465f
ganglion of, VII:136
in musicians' hands, VII:702
giant cell tumor of, VII:70, 71f, 74f
greater arc of, VII:19, 20f
hemorrhage in, VII:68, 69t
imaging of, VII:55-84
angiography in, VII:80, 82, 83f, 84f
computed tomography in, VII:66, 68, 68f
magnetic resonance angiography in, VII:79-80, 80f, 81f
magnetic resonance imaging in, VII:69-79, 69t, 70t, 71f-78f, 79t
plain film radiography in, VII:55-65, 56f-65f. *See also* Wrist, plain film radiography of.
radionuclide imaging in, VII:65-66, 67f
tomography in, VII:65, 66f
ultrasonography in, VII:68-69
in burned hand treatment, VII:616
in mirror hand, VIII:251, 253
in obstetric brachial plexus palsy, VII:557, 561f, 562
injury to, VII:459-468
computed tomography in, VII:458
fracture. *See* Wrist, fracture of.
magnetic resonance imaging in, VII:458-459
patient history in, VII:458
physical examination in, VII:458, 459f
sprain, VII:459-460
intrinsic ligaments of, VII:20, 21, 455-457, 456f
joints of, VII:453-454
Kleinman-Reagan shear test of, VII:458
ligaments of, VII:20-21, 454-456, 454f-456f
dissociation of, VII:467-468, 467f, 468f
loose bodies of, VII:131, 133
lymphangioma of, VII:80, 81f
midcarpal clunk test of, VII:458
motion of, VII:20, 41
neuroma of, VII:940-941, 943f
ossification centers of, VIII:423, 423f
osteoarthritis of, VII:707-725. *See also* Hand(s), osteoarthritis of.
osteochondroma of, VII:985, 986f
osteomyelitis of, VII:78, 78f
plain film radiography of, VII:57-65, 58f-61f, 458, 460f
capitolunate angle on, VII:58, 61f
carpal arcs on, VII:58, 60f
carpal height on, VII:57, 58f
carpal tunnel view for, VII:61, 63, 63f
palmar tilt on, VII:58, 59f
radiolunate angle on, VII:58, 61f

Wrist (*Continued*)
radioulnar inclination on, VII:57-58, 59f
rheumatoid arthritis on, VII:63, 63f
scapholunate angle on, VII:58, 61f
specialized views for, VII:61-63, 62f, 65
ulnar deviation for, VII:61, 62f
ulnar variance on, VII:58, 59f
reconstruction of, after tumor resection, VII:983
retinacular system of, VII:29-32, 30f, 31f
extensor tendon injury under, VII:418-420, 419f, 456
rheumatoid arthritis of, VII:63, 63f
sprains of, VII:459-460
tendinitis of, VIII:560-561
tendons of, VII:456
ulnar deficiency of, VIII:103
Watson scaphoid shift test of, VII:458, 459f

X

X chromosome disorders, I:52, 53f
Xeroderma pigmentosum, Color Plate V:113-3, III:612, V:279-280, 399, 400f

Y

Y chromosome disorders, I:52
Yeast infection, after laser resurfacing, II:371, 371f
Young face-old forehead deformity, II:749-751, 750f
Young face-old mouth deformity, II:751
YV-plasty, in scar revision, I:255-258, 255f-258f

Z

Z-plasty
for axillary contracture, VII:632
for burn-related thumb contracture, VII:621-623, 622f
for constriction ring syndrome, VIII:198, 199f, 200f
for facial scar, I:248, 249f-250f
for neck scar, I:251, 254f
for penoscrotal web, VI:400f, 401-402
for scar revision, I:244, 245f, 248-254, 248t, 249f-254f, 251t, 257f, 258f
for tuberous breasts, VI:517, 518f
four-flap, I:251, 252f
in palatoplasty, IV:259-261, 261f
in Treacher Collins syndrome, IV:426, 427f
multiple, I:251, 252f-254f
planimetric, I:248, 252f
skew, I:251
Zancolli lasso, VIII:473-475, 474f, 531, 532f
Zenker diverticulum, III:994, 995f
ZEUS Robotic Surgical System, I:1155
ZIC2 gene, IV:3
Zone of fixation, brow anatomy and, II:53, 54f
Zygoma. *See also* Zygomatic arch.
anatomy of, III:208-212, 209f-212f
fracture of, III:580
bleeding in, III:227
blow-in, III:214
butterfly rim fragment in, III:214

Zygoma (*Continued*)
classification of, III:212-213, 212t
complications of, III:227-229, 228f
computed tomography in, III:214, 215f
diagnosis of, III:213-214, 215f
diplopia in, III:210-212, 211f, 213, 227-228, 228f
ecchymosis in, III:213
edema in, III:213
globe in, III:210-212, 211f, 213, 227-228, 228f
hematoma in, III:209, 210f, 214
in children, III:397f, 424-432, 425f-426f
infraorbital nerve in, III:212, 212f, 213, 229
malocclusion in, III:213
mechanisms of, III:208-209, 213
oral-antral fistula in, III:227, 229
palpation in, III:213-214
radiography in, III:214
scarring with, III:227, 228f
treatment of, III:214, 216-226
anterior approach for, III:216-218, 217f, 218f
buttress articulations in, III:216
Carroll-Girard screw in, III:217, 217f
complications of, III:227-229, 228f
coronal incision for, III:218
delayed, III:224, 226
Dingman approach for, III:218-219
endoscopically assisted, III:219
fixation for, III:219-224, 221f-223f
in compound comminuted fracture, III:224
in high-energy fracture, III:224, 225f-227f
intraoral approach for, III:219
K-wire fixation for, III:220
malposition after, III:228-229
maxillary sinus approach for, III:219
pin fixation for, III:220
plate and screw fixation for, III:220-224, 221f-222f, 229
scarring after, III:227, 228f
zygomaticofrontal suture diastasis and, III:217-218, 218f
in craniofacial microsomia, IV:120
Zygomatic arch. *See also* Zygoma.
fracture of, III:209-210, 210f, 211f, 580
endoscopic management of, III:491-492, 494f-503f
contraindications to, III:491-492
indications for, III:491-492
results of, III:492
technique of, III:492, 494f-503f, 504f
in panfacial fracture, III:258-259, 259f
treatment of, III:221, 223f, 224, 227f, 580
Zygomatic-cutaneous ligament, II:217, 219f
Zygomatic ligaments, II:169, 170f, 172, 173f
Zygomaticofrontal suture, diastasis of, III:217-218, 218f
Zygomaticomaxillary suture, in maxillary fracture, III:239
Zygomaticotemporal nerve, II:57, 58f
Zygomaticus major, III:888-889, 888t